CONTENTS

CONTENTS IN BRIEF

SECTION 1

SECTION 2

SECTION 3

NURSING
PI

HOS
The
Seco

Edited by

Margaret F. Alexander CBE FRCN BSc PhD RN RM RNT
Visiting Professor, Department of Nursing and Community Health,
Glasgow Caledonian University, Glasgow

Josephine N. Fawcett BSc (Hons) RN MSc RNT
Lecturer, Department of Nursing Studies,
University of Edinburgh, Edinburgh

Phyllis J. Runciman BSc MSc MPhil RN RM RHV RNT
Senior Lecturer — Research, Department of Health and Nursing,
Queen Margaret University College, Edinburgh

CHURCHILL
LIVINGSTONE

EDINBURGH LONDON NEW YORK PHILADELPHIA ST LOUIS SYDNEY TORONTO 2000

CHURCHILL LIVINGSTONE An imprint of Harcourt Publishers Limited

First published 1994
Second edition 2000
Reprinted 2001 (twice)

ISBN 0 443 06013 4

British Library Cataloguing in Publication Data
A catalogue record for this book is available from the British Library

Library of Congress Cataloging in Publication Data
A catalog record for this book is available from the Library of Congress

Note
Medical knowledge is constantly changing. As new information becomes available, changes in treatment, procedures, equipment and the use of drugs become necessary. The editors, the contributors and the publishers have taken care to ensure that the information given in this text is accurate and up to date. However, readers are strongly advised to confirm that the information, especially with regard to drug usage, complies with the latest legislation and standards of practice.

The publisher's policy is to use **paper manufactured from sustainable forests**

Printed in Spain

CONTRIBUTORS

Erica S. Alabaster MSc DipN(Lond) RN RNT DANS RCNT WNBCert ITEC MIFA
Lecturer, School of Nursing and Midwifery Studies, University of Wales College of Medicine, Cardiff
32 The chronically ill person

Douglas Allan MN BEd RNT RN RMN
Lecturer, Department of Nursing and Community Health, Glasgow Caledonian University, Glasgow
9 The nervous system

Dorothy Armstrong MN BSc RN CritCareCert
Nurse Teacher, Critical Care Course, Royal Infirmary of Edinburgh, Lothian University Hospitals NHS Trust, Edinburgh
18 Shock

John Atkinson BA PhD RN NDNCert DipEd DNT
Senior Lecturer, Adult Nursing, Department of Nursing, Midwifery and Healthcare, University of Paisley, Ayr
37 The person with HIV/AIDS

Sue Bale BA RN NDN RHV DipN
Nursing Director, Wound Healing Research Unit, University of Wales College of Medicine, Cardiff; Senior Lecturer, School of Care Sciences, University of Glamorgan, Pontypridd
23 Wound healing

Joyce M. Brown BSc RN DN ONC DipNurs
Service Manager, Orthopaedic Supported Discharge Service, Western Infirmary, North Glasgow University Hospitals NHS Trust, Glasgow
10 The musculoskeletal system

Karen L. Burnet MSc BSc RN
Nurse Practitioner in Breast Care, Oncology Centre, Addenbrook's Hospital, Cambridge
7 Part 2 The breast

Bernadette M. Byrne BSc OncCert RN
Clinical Nurse Specialist, Imperial Cancer Research Fund, Oncology Department, Western General Hospital, Lothian University Hospitals NHS Trust, Edinburgh
31 The patient with cancer

Roseanne Cetnarskyj BSc SPQ (Genetic Nursing) RN
Clinical Nurse Specialist, S. E. Scotland Genetic Department, Western General Hospital, Lothian University Hospitals NHS Trust, Edinburgh
6 Genetics Section on 'Huntingdon's disease'

Charmaine Childs MPhil PhD BNurs RN
Medical Research Council Trauma Group, North Western Injury Research Centre, Manchester; Honorary Research Fellow, Department of Child Health, University of Manchester, Manchester
22 Temperature control

S. Jose Closs BSc(Hons) MPhil PhD RN
Director of Nursing Research, School of Healthcare Studies, University of Leeds, Leeds
25 Sleep

Margaret M. Colquhoun MA MN RN RM
Nurse Lecturer in Palliative Care, St Columba's Hospice, Edinburgh; Honorary Lecturer, Queen Margaret University College, Edinburgh
33 The patient who needs palliative care

David B. Cooper RMN FETC
Freelance consultant /lecturer/author on substance use issues and mental health
36 People who use and abuse substances

Aileen E. Crosbie BA HVD OHNC RN
Formerly Senior Clinical Nurse Specialist in Genetics, Department of Clinical Genetics, Western General Hospital, Lothian University Hospitals NHS Trust, Edinburgh
6 Genetic disorders

Claire Dibbs RN
Formerly Research Nurse, Molecular Endocrinology Department, Medical Research Council, Imperial College School of Medicine, Hammersmith Hospital, London
5 Part 1: Endocrine and metabolic disorders

Frances M. Davidson RSCN RN RCNT RNT
Lecturer, Faculty of Health Studies, Napier University - Livingston Campus, St John's Hospital, Livingston
30 The patient with burns

Christine Docherty BN RN RSCN DipN
Senior Charge Nurse, Dermatology Unit, Ninewells Hospital, Tayside University Hospitals NHS Trust, Dundee
12 Skin disorders

Helen A. S. Dougan BEd DipCNE RN RCNT RNT
Senior Nurse Lecturer in Palliative Care, St Columba's Hospice, Edinburgh; Honorary Lecturer, Queen Margaret University College, Edinburgh
33 The patient who needs palliative care

Fiona M. Duke BSc MSc DipEd RN RMN RNT RCNT ENB237
Nurse Lecturer, Napier University, Livingston Campus, St John's Hospital, West Lothian Healthcare NHS Trust, Livingston
11 Blood disorders

Sue Duke BSc(Hons) MSc RN RNT PGDE
Lecturer Practitioner, Oxford Radcliffe Hospitals NHS Trust and School of Health Care, Oxford Brookes University, Oxford
19 Pain

Cynthia B. Edmond BA MSc GradDipEd RN RNT RM(Aust.) Cert.Admin(Aust.) MCN(NSW) FRCNA
PhD student, Glasgow Caledonian University, Glasgow
Formerly Freelance Lecturer and Clinical Nurse, Edinburgh; Lecturer, Department of Health Occupations, University of Newcastle, New South Wales, Australia
3 The respiratory system

Elizabeth S. Farmer PhD RN SCM DN
Senior Lecturer, Department of Nursing and Midwifery, University of Stirling, Highland Campus, Inverness
35 The older person

Catriona Fulton BSc MSc RN
Staff Nurse, Intensive Care Unit, Royal Infirmary of Edinburgh, Lothian University Hospitals NHS Trust, Edinburgh
29 The critically ill patient

Ruth F. M. Gardner RN OND OStJ
Advanced Ophthalmic Nurse Practitioner, Eye Department, St John's Hospital at Howden, West Lothian Healthcare NHS Trust, Livingston
13 Disorders of the eye

Mary Gobbi DipN DipN(Ed) MA(Ed) PhD RN ENB100
Lecturer in Nursing and Head of Critical Care Nursing Department, School of Nursing and Midwifery, University of Southampton, Southampton
20 Fluid and electrolyte balance
21 Nutrition

Margaret Harris MSc RN DipN(Lond) DipSS CertEd RNT RCNT
Formerly Nurse Teacher, Continuing Education, University of Wales College of Medicine, Cardiff
35 The patient in need of rehabilitation

Rhoda Hodgson RN CertCouns
Nurse Photo-therapist and Senior Charge Nurse, Photobiology and Dermatology Unit, Ninewells Hospital, Tayside University Hospitals NHS Trust, Dundee
12 Skin disorders

Evelyn Howie RN SCM
Ward Sister, Royal Infirmary of Edinburgh, Lothian University Hospitals NHS Trust, Edinburgh
4 The gastrointestinal system, liver and biliary tract

Liz Jamieson BSc(Hons) RN ONC RNT DipProfStud
Lecturer/Programme Organiser, Department of Nursing and Community Health, Glasgow Caledonian University, Glasgow
10 The musculoskeletal system

Rosemary Kelly RN SCM
Sister, Canniesburn Plastic Surgery Unit, North Glasgow University Hospitals NHS Trust, Glasgow
15 Disorders of the mouth

Vivian Leefarr BA(Hons) DipCouns BAC RegIndCouns United Kingdom Register of Counsellors (UKRC)
Nurse and Health Visitor, Counsellor in General Practice, Inverness; Sister, Child Development Unit, Raigmore Hospital NHS Trust, Inverness
17 Stress

Kathleen Liddle RN CritCareCert DipAdvNurs
Cystic fibrosis liaison sister, Western General Hospital, Lothian University Hospitals NHS Trust, Edinburgh
6 Genetics Section on 'Cystic fibrosis'

Cath M. McFarlane MBA RN ONC SCM
Directorate Manager, Medicine for Elderly, Glasgow Royal Infirmary, North Glasgow University Hospitals NHS Trust, Glasgow
10 The musculoskeletal system

Rosemary McIntyre DipM(Lond) MN PhD RN NDN(CERT) RNT
Head of Studies (Scotland), Marie Curie Cancer Care, Edinburgh
5 Endocrine and metabolic disorders Part 2: Diabetes mellitus

Anne C. H. McQueen BA MSc MPhil RN SCM DipCNE RCNT RNT
Lecturer, Department of Nursing Studies, University of Edinburgh, Edinburgh
7 Part 1: The reproductive systems

Margot E. A. Miller RN RCNT
Clinical Nurse Practitioner, Centre for Liver and Digestive Disorders, Royal Infirmary of Edinburgh, Lothian University Hospitals NHS Trust, Edinburgh
4 The gastrointestinal system, liver and biliary tract

Mary B. Murchie RN SCM
Formerly Ward Sister, Hepato-biliary Unit, Royal Infirmary of Edinburgh, Lothian University Hospitals NHS Trust, Edinburgh
4 The gastrointestinal system, liver and biliary tract

Marie-Noelle Orzel MSc PGDE RN RSCN
Assistant Director of Nursing, Oxford Radcliffe Hospitals NHS Trust, Oxford
27 The patient who experiences trauma

Lesley Pemberton MEd RN RCNT DipN(Cert) FETC Teacher's Cert ENBN17
Formerly Senior Lecturer, Acute and Critical Care Nursing, University of Central Lancashire, Preston
28 The unconscious patient

Muriel E. Reffin EN RN
Ward Sister, Gartnavel General Hospital, North Glasgow University Hospitals NHS Trust, Glasgow
14 Disorders of the ear, nose and throat

Billie Reynolds
Formerly, Haemophilia Unit, Royal Infirmary of Edinburgh, Lothian University Hospitals NHS Trust, Edinburgh
6 Genetics Section on 'Haemophilia'

Sheila E. Rodgers MSc BSc(Hons) RN
Lecturer, Department of Nursing Studies, University of Edinburgh, Edinburgh
27 The patient facing surgery

Lesley Selfe BSc(Hons) RN
Senior Lecturer, School of Nursing Practice Development and Midwifery, University of Northumbria at Newcastle, Newcastle upon Tyne
8 The urinary system

Anna M. Serra MSc RN RNT
Senior Lecturer, Education Department, Marie Curie Centre Edenhall, London
14 Disorders of the ear, nose and throat

Marion C. Stewart BA MSc RN SCM
Nursing Officer, Control of Infection, Highland Acute Hospitals NHS Trust, Raigmore Hospital, Inverness
16 The immune system and infectious disease

Kathy Strachan BA MEd DipEd RN RNT RCT
Senior Lecturer and Programme Organiser for DipHE(Nursing), Glasgow Caledonian University, Glasgow
5 Endocrine and metabolic disorders Part 2: Diabetes mellitus

Margaret A. Studley BSc(Hons) CertEd RN OND RNT RCNT
Lecturer, Adult Branch, Faculty of Health Studies, Napier University, Edinburgh
13 Disorders of the eye

Jean Swaffield BSc(Hons) MSc RN RSCN DN DNT PWT FETC
Formerly Senior Lecturer, School of Nursing and Midwifery, University of Glasgow, Glasgow
24 Continence

David R. Thompson BSc MA PhD RN FRCN FESC
Professor of Nursing, Department of Health Studies, University of York, York
2 The cardiovascular system

Colin Torrance DipLScN BSc PhD RSCN RN
Professor of Advanced Nursing Practice, La Trobe University Clinical School of Advanced Nursing Practice, Melbourne, Australia
21 Nutrition

Rosemary A. Webster BSc RN
Clinical Nurse Specialist, Coronary Care Unit, Leicester General Hospital, Leicester
2 The cardiovascular system

ACKNOWLEDGEMENTS

The editors would like to extend particular thanks to the advisors listed here, who gave assistance with specific chapters.

For assistance with *Section 1 Care of Patients with Common Disorders*:

Allan MacDonald BSc PhD
Reader, School of Biological Sciences and Biomedical Sciences, Glasgow Caledonian University, Glasgow

David Scott BSc(Pharm) MSc PhD MRPharms MIBiol CBiol
Lecturer, School of Biological Sciences and Biomedical Sciences, Glasgow Caledonian University, Glasgow

Iain C. Wilkie BSc PhD
Senior Lecturer in Physiology, School of Biological Sciences and Biomedical Sciences, Glasgow Caledonian University, Glasgow

The editors would also like to thank all who kindly granted permission to borrow material such as illustrations and tables from existing publications, with particular thanks to Kathleen J. W. Wilson for the many illustrations taken from Wilson K J W and Waugh A 1996 Ross & Wilson: Anatomy and physiology in health and illness, 8th edn. Churchill Livingstone, Edinburgh.

The editors wish to record their thanks to those authors who contributed to the original chapters in the first edition and whose work has provided the foundation for the current volume. These are:

Shirley Alexander
Pat Ashworth
Teresa Barr
Kathryn Carver
Elizabeth Craig
Catherine Crosby
The late Margaret Cutler
Eleanor Hayes
Margaret Kindlen
Anne Lowie
Carol Mackinnon
Janice McCall
Moira Mennie
Ruth Miller
Maureen Morrison
Anne E. Murdoch
Joanna Parker
Carmen Rose
Kate Seers
The late Anne Shackleton
Theyaga Shandran
Frances Smithers
Roger Watson

PREFACE

While no single text can encompass the wealth of knowledge that underpins the practice of nursing, we believe that the second edition of this text will be valuable not only for student nurses, but also for the established practitioner, the nurse returning to practice and nurse educators, all of whom face the challenge of new knowledge.

The structure of the book

As in the first edition, the book is divided into three sections which are progressive in nature, encouraging the reader to move from the broad approach of Section 1 to a more in-depth appreciation of specific nursing issues in Sections 2 and 3. There is sufficient cross-referencing to encourage readers to make links and pursue lines of enquiry.

Section 1 — Care of patients with common disorders

The decision to adopt the systems approach for this section was not taken lightly, given that nursing is moving away from the medical model. Our reasoning is that nurses must come to terms with medical terminology and classifications, and have a thorough grounding in disease pathology, in order to work effectively in the health care team and give sensitive and appropriate nursing care.

All the chapters in this section contain information on the following:

- anatomy and physiology
- pathophysiology
- medical management
- nursing priorities and management.

Only essential anatomy and physiology have been presented, as an aid to rational decision-making. There are recommendations for further reading where more detail is desired. We have been selective about the disorders chosen, concentrating on those that illustrate common presenting features and related principles of care. The nursing priorities and management section is the most important. The wording of the heading reminds the student of the need to set priorities depending on the individual's unique needs and circumstances.

Section 2 — Common patient problems and related nursing care

This section presents another way of examining nursing and builds on the foundations laid in Section 1. The focus is on common patient problems, which are not merely physiological in origin, but also arise from the subtle, complex interplay of social, psychological and economic factors. Some of these problems have a high profile, such as stress and pain. Others, such as nutrition and sleep, are often relatively neglected but are nevertheless very much the concern of nurses. These problems are not confined to, or only evident in, hospital care. They are part of life and may be experienced in many settings and at any time. Throughout the section, both the nurse's and the patient's perspectives have been considered and the focus is on research-based problem-solving.

Section 3 — Nursing patients with special needs

Some of the most challenging areas of nursing are explored in this section. By addressing special needs, the broad spectrum and contrasts of adult nursing are revealed. Such needs, some long-term in nature, often make the greatest demands on the nurse's clinical and interpersonal skills. Section 3 challenges stereotypes and examines values and beliefs, raising awareness of the moral decision-making which underlies so much of day-to-day nursing practice.

Key features

In harmony with our commitment to exploring the different ways of knowing about nursing, certain features have been retained throughout the book. These include interactive material; illustrations, tables and care plans, the latter written in such a way as to be useful both as an educational and as a practice tool; boxes, which include, for example, accounts of personal 'lived experience' and research abstracts; references, further reading and useful addresses.

The contributors and advisors

More than 70 nurse authors have contributed to the significant updating of this text. They are from all areas of nursing: hospital and community practice, education and research. We pay sincere tribute here to their knowledge, experience and skills and thank them for their key contributions to this text.

We owe a sincere debt of gratitude to the advisors who read and commented on the manuscript during its revision. Their names are listed in the Acknowledgements section. We also greatly appreciated the informal advice we received from academic and clinical colleagues, and as editors we have been delighted by the value placed on this book by readers, particularly the students, who are our future.

Whether you read this book, therefore, as a novice nurse, an expert practitioner, a preceptor or a teacher, it will provide a wealth of knowledge, derived from many sources: from professional nursing practice, from research and from the experiences of countless patients and clients.

Edinburgh 2000

Margaret F. Alexander
Josephine N. (Tonks) Fawcett
Phyllis J. Runciman

ABOUT THE BOOK

The key features shown on the sample pages below make the text easy to read, quick to refer to and useful for revision.

Main text

This has been broken up as follows:

- colour headings—used to identify main headings and to highlight the 'Nursing priorities and management'
- different style of type—information on 'Anatomy and physiology' and 'Medical management' in Section 1
- bullet-point lists
- Reference and Further Reading lists—at ends of chapters
- Useful Address lists—at ends of selected chapters.

Displayed material

Case History

Self-assessment Question

Answer at end of book

Further reading

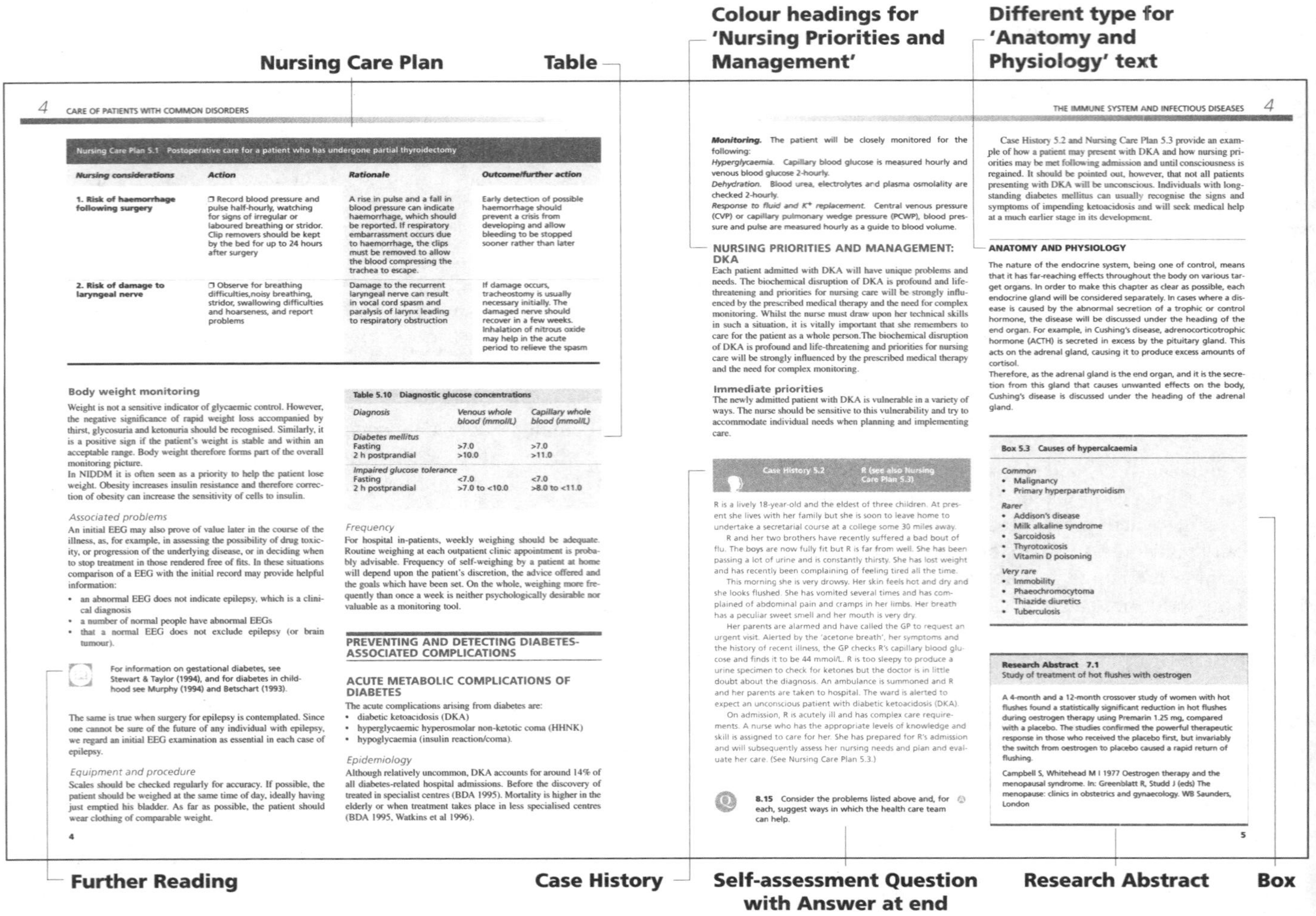

4 CARE OF PATIENTS WITH COMMON DISORDERS

Nursing Care Plan 5.1 Postoperative care for a patient who has undergone partial thyroidectomy

Nursing considerations	*Action*	*Rationale*	*Outcome/further action*
1. Risk of haemorrhage following surgery	❐ Record blood pressure and pulse half-hourly, watching for signs of irregular or laboured breathing or stridor. Clip removers should be kept by the bed for up to 24 hours after surgery	A rise in pulse and a fall in blood pressure can indicate haemorrhage, which should be reported. If respiratory embarrassment occurs due to haemorrhage, the clips must be removed to allow the blood compressing the trachea to escape.	Early detection of possible haemorrhage should prevent a crisis from developing and allow bleeding to be stopped sooner rather than later
2. Risk of damage to laryngeal nerve	❐ Observe for breathing difficulties,noisy breathing, stridor, swallowing difficulties and hoarseness, and report problems	Damage to the recurrent laryngeal nerve can result in vocal cord spasm and paralysis of larynx leading to respiratory obstruction	If damage occurs, tracheostomy is usually necessary initially. The damaged nerve should recover in a few weeks. Inhalation of nitrous oxide may help in the acute period to relieve the spasm

Body weight monitoring

Weight is not a sensitive indicator of glycaemic control. However, the negative significance of rapid weight loss accompanied by thirst, glycosuria and ketonuria should be recognised. Similarly, it is a positive sign if the patient's weight is stable and within an acceptable range. Body weight therefore forms part of the overall monitoring picture.

In NIDDM it is often seen as a priority to help the patient lose weight. Obesity increases insulin resistance and therefore correction of obesity can increase the sensitivity of cells to insulin.

Associated problems

An initial EEG may also prove of value later in the course of the illness, as, for example, in assessing the possibility of drug toxicity, or progression of the underlying disease, or in deciding when to stop treatment in those rendered free of fits. In these situations comparison of a EEG with the initial record may provide helpful information:

- an abnormal EEG does not indicate epilepsy, which is a clinical diagnosis
- a number of normal people have abnormal EEGs
- that a normal EEG does not exclude epilepsy (or brain tumour).

For information on gestational diabetes, see Stewart & Taylor (1994), and for diabetes in childhood see Murphy (1994) and Betschart (1993).

The same is true when surgery for epilepsy is contemplated. Since one cannot be sure of the future of any individual with epilepsy, we regard an initial EEG examination as essential in each case of epilepsy.

Equipment and procedure

Scales should be checked regularly for accuracy. If possible, the patient should be weighed at the same time of day, ideally having just emptied his bladder. As far as possible, the patient should wear clothing of comparable weight.

Table 5.10 Diagnostic glucose concentrations

Diagnosis	*Venous whole blood (mmol/L)*	*Capillary whole blood (mmol/L)*
Diabetes mellitus		
Fasting	>7.0	>7.0
2 h postprandial	>10.0	>11.0
Impaired glucose tolerance		
Fasting	<7.0	<7.0
2 h postprandial	>7.0 to <10.0	>8.0 to <11.0

Frequency

For hospital in-patients, weekly weighing should be adequate. Routine weighing at each outpatient clinic appointment is probably advisable. Frequency of self-weighing by a patient at home will depend upon the patient's discretion, the advice offered and the goals which have been set. On the whole, weighing more frequently than once a week is neither psychologically desirable nor valuable as a monitoring tool.

PREVENTING AND DETECTING DIABETES-ASSOCIATED COMPLICATIONS

ACUTE METABOLIC COMPLICATIONS OF DIABETES

The acute complications arising from diabetes are:

- diabetic ketoacidosis (DKA)
- hyperglycaemic hyperosmolar non-ketotic coma (HHNK)
- hypoglycaemia (insulin reaction/coma).

Epidemiology

Although relatively uncommon, DKA accounts for around 14% of all diabetes-related hospital admissions. Before the discovery of treated in specialist centres (BDA 1995). Mortality is higher in the elderly or when treatment takes place in less specialised centres (BDA 1995, Watkins et al 1996).

4

THE IMMUNE SYSTEM AND INFECTIOUS DISEASES 4

Monitoring. The patient will be closely monitored for the following:

Hyperglycaemia. Capillary blood glucose is measured hourly and venous blood glucose 2-hourly.

Dehydration. Blood urea, electrolytes and plasma osmolality are checked 2-hourly.

Response to fluid and K^+ replacement. Central venous pressure (CVP) or capillary pulmonary wedge pressure (PCWP), blood pressure and pulse are measured hourly as a guide to blood volume.

NURSING PRIORITIES AND MANAGEMENT: DKA

Each patient admitted with DKA will have unique problems and needs. The biochemical disruption of DKA is profound and life-threatening and priorities for nursing care will be strongly influenced by the prescribed medical therapy and the need for complex monitoring. Whilst the nurse must draw upon her technical skills in such a situation, it is vitally important that she remembers to care for the patient as a whole person.The biochemical disruption of DKA is profound and life-threatening and priorities for nursing care will be strongly influenced by the prescribed medical therapy and the need for complex monitoring.

Immediate priorities

The newly admitted patient with DKA is vulnerable in a variety of ways. The nurse should be sensitive to this vulnerability and try to accommodate individual needs when planning and implementing care.

Case History 5.2 R (see also Nursing Care Plan 5.3)

R is a lively 18-year-old and the eldest of three children. At present she lives with her family but she is soon to leave home to undertake a secretarial course at a college some 30 miles away.

R and her two brothers have recently suffered a bad bout of flu. The boys are now fully fit but R is far from well. She has been passing a lot of urine and is constantly thirsty. She has lost weight and has recently been complaining of feeling tired all the time.

This morning she is very drowsy. Her skin feels hot and dry and she looks flushed. She has vomited several times and has complained of abdominal pain and cramps in her limbs. Her breath has a peculiar sweet smell and her mouth is very dry.

Her parents are alarmed and have called the GP to request an urgent visit. Alerted by the 'acetone breath', her symptoms and the history of recent illness, the GP checks R's capillary blood glucose and finds it to be 44 mmol/L. R is too sleepy to produce a urine specimen to check for ketones but the doctor is in little doubt about the diagnosis. An ambulance is summoned and R and her parents are taken to hospital. The ward is alerted to expect an unconscious patient with diabetic ketoacidosis (DKA).

On admission, R is acutely ill and has complex care requirements. A nurse who has the appropriate levels of knowledge and skill is assigned to care for her. She has prepared for R's admission and will subsequently assess her nursing needs and plan and evaluate her care. (See Nursing Care Plan 5.3.)

8.15 Consider the problems listed above and, for each, suggest ways in which the health care team can help.

Case History 5.2 and Nursing Care Plan 5.3 provide an example of how a patient may present with DKA and how nursing priorities may be met following admission and until consciousness is regained. It should be pointed out, however, that not all patients presenting with DKA will be unconscious. Individuals with long-standing diabetes mellitus can usually recognise the signs and symptoms of impending ketoacidosis and will seek medical help at a much earlier stage in its development.

ANATOMY AND PHYSIOLOGY

The nature of the endocrine system, being one of control, means that it has far-reaching effects throughout the body on various target organs. In order to make this chapter as clear as possible, each endocrine gland will be considered separately. In cases where a disease is caused by the abnormal secretion of a trophic or control hormone, the disease will be discussed under the heading of the end organ. For example, in Cushing's disease, adrenocorticotrophic hormone (ACTH) is secreted in excess by the pituitary gland. This acts on the adrenal gland, causing it to produce excess amounts of cortisol.

Therefore, as the adrenal gland is the end organ, and it is the secretion from this gland that causes unwanted effects on the body, Cushing's disease is discussed under the heading of the adrenal gland.

Box 5.3 Causes of hypercalcaemia

Common
- Malignancy
- Primary hyperparathyroidism

Rarer
- Addison's disease
- Milk alkaline syndrome
- Sarcoidosis
- Thyrotoxicosis
- Vitamin D poisoning

Very rare
- Immobility
- Phaeochromocytoma
- Thiazide diuretics
- Tuberculosis

Research Abstract 7.1
Study of treatment of hot flushes with oestrogen

A 4-month and a 12-month crossover study of women with hot flushes found a statistically significant reduction in hot flushes during oestrogen therapy using Premarin 1.25 mg, compared with a placebo. The studies confirmed the powerful therapeutic response in those who received the placebo first, but invariably the switch from oestrogen to placebo caused a rapid return of flushing.

Campbell S, Whitehead M I 1977 Oestrogen therapy and the menopausal syndrome. In: Greenblatt R, Studd J (eds) The menopause: clinics in obstetrics and gynaecology. WB Saunders, London

5

NURSING PRACTICE: AN INTRODUCTION

1

Margaret F. Alexander
Josephine N. Fawcett
Phyllis J. Runciman

CHAPTER CONTENTS

Unless we are making progress in our nursing every year, every month, every week, take my word for it we are going back (Florence Nightingale in 1914, cited in Skeet 1980, p. 100).

The main purpose of this book is to explore ways of knowing about nursing. It is about developing ways of thinking, learning and exploring critically and creatively the nurse's role in helping individuals to maintain good health, to recover from episodes of ill-health, to cope day by day with chronic illness and to experience dignity and comfort at life's end.

As editors, we had certain goals:

- to reflect the changing context and dynamic nature of nursing and health care
- to present the knowledge and skills required for competent, evidence-based practice in a variety of settings, in hospital and at home
- to demonstrate the essential contribution of research in practice
- to demonstrate nursing as an integral part of multidisciplinary care
- to value the individual 'lived experience' of health and illness, and the importance of listening carefully to the patient's voice
- to encourage constructive reflection on practice.

The fundamental principles of nursing care in the community and in hospital are given. These lay the essential foundation for competent practice as a nurse, for continuing professional education and for advanced and specialist nursing skills, in whatever context.

The changing context of nursing

The focus of this book is on health care in the UK and on the context in which nursing takes place — the society which it serves, its values and mores.

Changes which are significant include:

- demographic shifts, with more and more people living to a greater age
- altered patterns of health and disease
- major technological and medical advances in a climate of cost-containment
- greater emphasis on the community context of care
- increasing demands from patients/clients and carers for a greater understanding of their health and the health care experience
- acknowledgement of the individual's role in promoting and maintaining his or her own health.

As in all professions, nurses must be proactive in recognising change and, indeed, in bringing about and influencing change, since it is only by understanding and reacting creatively and intelligently that a profession can remain dynamic and healthy.

Partnerships

In the UK, many of the major changes in health care delivery have been the result of new government initiatives and legislation. One of the UK government's main aims in recent years, and indeed an aim of the World Health Organization (WHO 1998), has been to encourage partnerships between health care professionals. Partnership is fundamental to initiatives such as clinical governance and managed clinical networks (SODoH 1998) and nurses need to examine and understand these concepts. With the increasing emphasis on quality assurance and the resulting growth in the number of clinical guidelines, nurses must be aware of the potential tensions between using such guidelines or protocols and the exercise of clinical freedom and professional judgement. The emphasis on partnership means that nurses in hospital and in the community are having to find new ways of working with colleagues in the NHS, in social services and in the independent and voluntary sectors. Nurses therefore have to address questions such as:

- Is there proper assessment of need?
- Are the right services being developed to ease the transition between hospital and home?
- Is priority being given to providing practical support for carers?

- Are the different sectors clear about their responsibilities and is there good coordination of services?
- Is there a potential conflict between value for money and the caring ethic?

At the direct care-giving level, Christensen's (1993) research into nurse–patient partnership as a model for practice draws our attention to the quality of individual interactions between nurse and patient. Her keen and informed observations of nursing illuminate what she terms as a 'passage' or 'shared journey' as nurse and patient, from their different perspectives, work their way together through a health-related experience.

At global level, the World Health Organization has repeatedly stressed the importance of the contribution of nurses, who are at the forefront of change in improving health and caring for those who are ill, and the need for all health care professionals to work in partnership. Empowerment of individuals and communities is imperative if the targets of 'HEALTH21' (WHO 1998), the health policy for the WHO European Region for the 21st century, are to be achieved.

Health and illness

As more becomes known about disease processes, there is a growing appreciation of the extent to which some diseases can be prevented by adopting a healthy lifestyle. Nurses, in particular those working in the community, have always been concerned to convey health messages to their patients. Now health promotion has become a part of what it means to be a nurse in any setting. From having been 'add-on extras', especially for nurses working in acute care, health promotion and education have assumed a central place in all nursing activities. Promoting health is a complex process (Kelly 1990). As our understanding of health grows, some fascinating questions emerge: why does disease develop in some healthy individuals and not in others, and how is it possible that people manage to be healthy in the face of so much disease? (Kelly & Charlton 1992). At a more fundamental level, why do such stark inequalities of health status persist between people and communities? Health and ill-health are now known to be influenced by a wide range of factors in people's life circumstances — economic, social, cultural, educational, psychological and genetic (DoH 1999, SODoH 1999). Nurses, then, have two related functions in health promotion: to be aware of the broader concepts of health currently being debated, and at the same time to be ready to respond in a very practical, everyday way to patients' growing desire for more health-related information. Nurses have an increasingly important role in advising 'well' individuals about health, and nurse-led initiatives, such as asthma clinics and preoperative assessment clinics, are now commonplace.

The settings: hospital and home

Although the majority of nurses in the UK work primarily in hospital, the demarcation between hospital and community interventions is increasingly blurred, and all nursing students in the UK are being prepared to work in both settings. This necessarily means thinking in new ways about the individual, the family and the community and about the lives of people as they come into and move within the nursing and health care systems.

For example, a major factor is early discharge from hospital. Patients are now staying in hospital wards for much shorter periods for a number of reasons, both practical and political. The trend towards the use of minimally invasive techniques and new advances in treatment have shortened recovery times for many patients. There is also an increasing adherence to the belief that, wherever possible, people should be cared for in their own homes, where they can retain maximum independence and be closer to their loved ones. New technologies have migrated from hospital to the patient's own home and this is one of the major challenges for nurses, patients and carers. For most people, therefore, a hospital stay may be a very brief life episode. For others, periodic visits to hospital will become a regular, almost routine, part of life, and for some individuals hospital itself may become a home. This blurring of the boundary between 'hospital' and 'home' has made it essential for nurses to interpret their knowledge and skills for use in a range of settings.

The patient's experience

The shift toward community care has far-reaching implications for many traditional views of health and illness and for the way in which the patient's role is conceptualised. The image of the helpless person in a hospital bed — a passive recipient of paternalistic beneficence from the medical and nursing professions — has lost its validity.

Patients are becoming empowered within the health care system, many exploiting information technology. As knowledgeable 'consumers' of health care, they present a new challenge to both doctors and nurses. They have high expectations of what that system can offer them, and demand a high level of professionalism and accountability from all practitioners. More than ever before, patients and their carers are recognising their own need for information about health, illness, treatment options and support systems. They are becoming more involved in decision-making regarding care and expect to be given the opportunity to make informed choices. For patients with chronic disease, there is an increased emphasis on maintaining independence in the activities of living for as long as possible. These changes have placed new demands upon patients and their carers, requiring them to adopt a more participatory role and to take greater responsibility in matters related to health and health care. At the same time, the need for nurses to be well-informed, to provide up-to-date patient education and to promote healthy lifestyles has become particularly urgent. However, the notion of empowerment and the participatory role has to be thought of carefully in the context of increasing social inequalities and the impact of these on people's health and access to information and to care (Macintyre 1997).

Constructive reflection

Some of the most sensitive insights of experienced nurses come from their careful, thoughtful analysis of daily work — its highs and its lows, its achievements and its frustrations. Much can be learned from the telling of nursing stories and the recounting of 'critical incidents'. These processes bring the practice of nursing alive and raise important questions about giving and receiving nursing and health care. What is it like to live with a particular disability? What are the challenges and priorities in caring for someone with such a problem? Could situations such as these be prevented? How can an acceptable quality of life be achieved for such patients?

Throughout this text we have incorporated stories — vignettes — which illustrate richly, often in people's own words, the lived experience of health and illness at home and in hospital. Working so closely with people in health and illness can be immensely satisfying, but also profoundly distressing; telling the stories of the day to those who have had similar work experiences and who share the same code of patient confidentiality can be immensely therapeutic.

It is vital to the progress of our profession that we learn to reflect upon our experience. The nurturing of the ability to reflect constructively upon practice is fundamental to the development of sound professional judgement, decision-making, risk management and the selection of priorities for care. One of the hallmarks of a 'profession' is its ability to draw together a body of knowledge and experience, a kind of accumulated wisdom in which all its members may share.

In conclusion...

In all our care-giving, to speak of the wholeness of nursing intervention is not to minimise the importance of individual aspects of care. Every nursing action is vital to achieving excellence in care. The poet William Blake (1757–1827) wrote that 'art and science cannot exist but in minutely organised particulars'. This book strives to illuminate many of the particulars of nursing, but in the context of the whole. It responds to the challenges of the new millennium, and the need to find a meeting point between our professional skills and expertise and the patient's lived experience.

Nursing must never be seen as 'a given', but as always evolving. Practice must never be viewed complacently; its rationale must always be sought. The ways of thinking and learning, implicit in the whole approach of this book, are ways intended to encourage in the reader a love of learning, of questioning, of searching for 'the best available knowledge' which will inform nursing practice.

Nursing is a profession that must change and develop to meet the health care needs of the society it seeks to serve. The knowledge needed for nursing, therefore, can never be static but will also change and develop, and those who pursue such knowledge will undertake a journey which has no ending: a journey of discovery and challenge. As editors, we hope this book opens up further vistas and gives pointers towards the goal of ever better standards and quality of care.

To all our readers, never lose the gift of curiosity!

REFERENCES

Christensen J 1993 Nursing partnership: a model for nursing practice. Churchill Livingstone, Edinburgh

Department of Health (DoH) 1999 Saving lives: our healthier nation. Cm 4386. The Stationery Office, London

Kelly M 1990 The World Health Organization's definition of health promotion: three problems. Health Bulletin (Edinburgh) 48: 176–180

Kelly M, Charlton B G 1992 Health promotion: time for a new philosophy. The British Journal of General Practice 42(359): 223–224

Macintyre S 1997 The Black Report and beyond: what are the issues? Social Science Medicine 44(6): 723–745

Scottish Office Department of Health (SODoH) 1998 Acute Services Review report. The Stationery Office, Edinburgh

Scottish Office Department of Health (SODoH) 1999 Towards a healthier Scotland. Cm 4269. The Stationery Office, Edinburgh

Skeet M 1980 Notes on nursing: the science and the art. Churchill Livingstone, Edinburgh

World Health Organization 1998 HEALTH21 — health for all in the 21st century. European Health for All series, no. 6. World Health Organization, Copenhagen

CARE OF PATIENTS WITH COMMON DISORDERS

SECTION 1

SECTION CONTENTS

THE CARDIOVASCULAR SYSTEM

2

David R. Thompson   Rosemary A. Webster

INTRODUCTION

The cardiovascular system consists of the heart and blood vessels. It is a closed circuit and is responsible for ensuring that blood flows throughout the body.

Heart and circulatory disease, termed cardiovascular disease (CVD), includes all the diseases of the heart and blood vessels. The two main diseases in this category are coronary heart disease (CHD) and stroke, but CVD also includes congenital heart disease and a range of other diseases of the heart and blood vessels.

Diseases of the heart and circulatory system are the main cause of death in the UK, accounting for some 300 000 deaths per year, approximately half of all deaths. Coronary heart disease alone is the most common cause of death in the UK, accounting for 1 in 4 deaths in men and 1 in 5 deaths in women (British Heart Foundation 1998).

Because cardiovascular disease is so prevalent in Western industrial societies, it is likely to be encountered by all nurses, whether hospital- or community-based. This is particularly true now that an increasing percentage of the population is over 60 years old, an age group in which cardiovascular disease is very common. But it also affects the younger population, being the main cause of premature death and handicap in the UK. There are marked regional variations in death rates. East Anglia, the south-east and the south-west of England have the fewest deaths from heart disease; Northern Ireland, the north of England and Scotland have the most. There is also a clear difference between socio-economic groups in the prevalence of cardiovascular disease, with the lowest incidence among the professional groups and the highest among the unskilled manual group.

The burden imposed by cardiovascular disease on the National Health Service (NHS) is substantial. The annual cost of health service resources for treating coronary heart disease is at least £1600 million (Maniadakis 1997). Hospital care accounts for just over half these costs and other financial costs include the economic effect of premature deaths, sickness and retirement from work. It is estimated that the working days lost to CHD cost British industry £3 billion per annum in lost production (British Heart Foundation 1998). CVD also has an immense impact on society in human terms. Bereavement, disability, changing roles within the family and society, and fear are some examples of its consequences.

Many cardiovascular diseases take the form of progressive debilitating illness, often becoming chronic with acute episodes. Individuals are faced with the prospect of a lifelong problem. In contrast, a heart attack (myocardial infarction, MI) is often sudden and unexpected, arousing acute distress in the individual and family as they confront a life-threatening crisis. Nurses, as one of the largest groups of health professionals, must inevitably bear some responsibility for helping to reduce the mortality, morbidity and personal suffering caused by cardiovascular disease. Ashworth (1992) identifies ways in which nurses can intervene to contribute to such a reduction:

- facilitating lifestyle adjustment to enable people to attain and maintain a level of health compatible with their personal goals
- assisting people to modify the demands of the activities of living, to balance with their capacity to meet them
- modifying the environment to achieve for each person the optimum possible environment within available resources
- providing physical treatment and monitoring for pathophysiological conditions
- reassuring, supporting and comforting patients and their families.

This chapter is based upon a nursing framework of activities of living. This framework reflects Roper et al's (1996) activities of daily living model of nursing, which is used by many UK nurses caring for people with cardiovascular disorders. Roy's (1984) adaptation model and Orem's (1991) self-care model have also been used. Whilst the activity of living based models have been criticised for being too simplistic and not placing enough emphasis on psychosocial aspects of care, they continue to be a helpful basis for nursing assessment and care planning.

Cardiovascular nursing in many areas is evolving as nurses move on from practising the skills of advanced life support, cannulation and phlebotomy to taking responsibility for decisions which influence patient care management. The specialised nature of much cardiovascular nursing with established post-basic education opportunities, coupled with lower nurse–patient ratios, may in some part explain the ongoing development of nursing roles in these areas. Primary nursing lends itself to the environment that is often found on cardiovascular units. Here, there is potential for therapeutic nurse–patient relationships to develop which can be used effectively in health promotion and psychological support (Broomfield 1996a). Increasingly, experienced nurses are managing admission and discharge of patients from specialist units through triage and fast-tracking; others are prescribing thrombolytic therapy for acute MI patients (Caunt 1996) and coordinating outpatient clinics and rehabilitation programmes.

There is an increased focus on examining the patient's experience, from onset of symptoms at home to discharge and follow-up, from a multiprofessional perspective, in an attempt to provide seamless high-quality evidenced-based care — 'process management' and 'managed care' are terms which refer to this method of coordinating care. The pivotal tool for these approaches is the 'critical pathway' or 'integrated care pathway', which is used by medical, nursing and other professionals to standardise treatment plans, record progress against these standards, monitor deviations from this standard and document care (Kegel 1996). Despite concerns that this will limit individualised care, reduce nursing to a series of tick boxes and limit effective communication, many areas are replacing traditional nursing care plans with care pathways. For an example of a critical pathway for a patient with an acute MI, see Figure 2.10 (p. 26).

For more information on critical pathways see Walsh (1998).

The chronic nature of a large proportion of cardiovascular disease means that health professionals within the hospital see only episodes within the total spectrum of care. Much is carried out in the community by the primary health care team, who will focus upon health education and promoting lifestyle adaptation and coping. It is therefore important that when people with cardiovascular problems are admitted to hospital, emphasis is placed on a holistic multidisciplinary assessment so that staff have an understanding of their home, family and work circumstances. Preparing for return to their own environment with an optimum level of independence together with any necessary support requires good liaison between the hospital and community health care teams.

ANATOMY AND PHYSIOLOGY OF THE HEART

The heart is a muscular pump that generates pressure changes resulting in the propulsion of blood around the vascular system. The right side of the heart pumps blood around the pulmonary system where gaseous exchange takes place and then on to the left side of the heart. The left side of the heart operates under much greater pressure to enable it to pump blood around the systemic circulation. The various chambers of the heart are illustrated in Figure 2.1.

The heart is composed of three layers:

- *Pericardium* — a thick fibrous outer layer that protects the heart from injury and infection.
- *Myocardium* — a muscular layer that varies in thickness throughout the heart. The atria, which act as filling chambers, have a thin layer of myocardium as they do not, in the fit individual, have to generate high pressures. In the ventricles, the muscular layer is

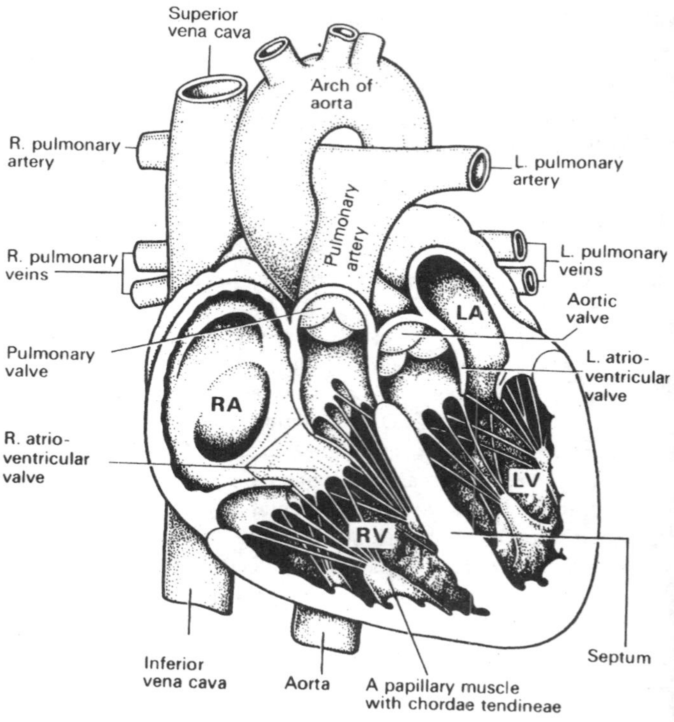

Fig. 2.1 The internal anatomy of the heart. (Reproduced with kind permission from Wilson 1996.)

better developed, particularly on the left side, which is larger and thicker than in the right side, as a more forceful contraction is required to pump blood through the systemic circulation.

- *Endocardium* — a thin layer of endothelium and connective tissue lines the inner chambers of the heart and coats the valves, which open and close to ensure a forward flow of blood at all times.

Coronary blood supply

Like all major organs, the heart requires blood flow to maintain cellular activity. The myocardium cannot derive oxygen and nutrients from the blood within the chambers. It receives its blood supply from the right and left coronary arteries which arise from the aorta just beyond the aortic valve (see Fig. 2.2).

The left coronary artery runs towards the left side of the heart and divides into two major branches: the left anterior interventricular branch or left anterior descending artery (LAD) and the circumflex artery (CX). The LAD follows the anterior ventricular sulcus and supplies blood to the interventricular septum and the anterior walls of both ventricles. The CX follows the coronary sulcus and supplies blood to the lateral and posterior regions of the left atrium and left ventricle. The right coronary artery (RCA) runs to the right side of the heart and divides into two branches: the posterior interventricular artery and the marginal artery. The more important posterior interventricular artery follows the posterior interventricular sulcus to the apex of the heart and supplies blood to the posterior ventricular walls. It is near the apex of the heart that the posterior and anterior interventricular arteries merge. The marginal artery follows the coronary sulcus and supplies the right ventricle. It is the RCA that normally supplies the sinoatrial and atrioventricular nodes (see Fig. 2.3, p. 10).

After passing through the capillary bed, the blood drains into the cardiac veins. These join to form the coronary sinus on the posterior surface of the heart from where venous blood drains into the right atrium.

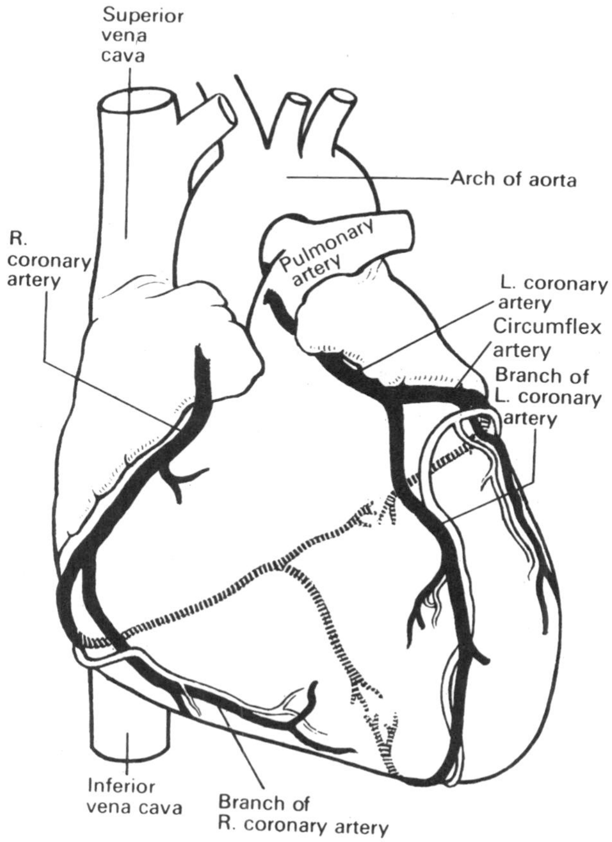

Fig. 2.2 The coronary circulation. (Reproduced with kind permission from Wilson 1998.)

Structure and function of cardiac valves

The atrioventricular valves, i.e. the tricuspid and the mitral, function in a similar manner. During ventricular diastole (relaxation), they act as a funnel to promote rapid filling of the ventricles. Most of ventricular filling is passive. During ventricular systole (contraction), intraventricular pressure rises, pushing the cusps, which are restrained by the chordae tendineae, back and up towards the atria, thus preventing back-flow of blood during systole. These valves can withstand high pressure, since their surface area is much greater than the orifice itself.

The semilunar valves, i.e. the pulmonary and the aortic, have three cusps each. They are closed during ventricular diastole. Once ventricular contraction begins, the intraventricular pressure rises, and when it exceeds that in the aorta and the pulmonary artery, the semilunar valves are forced open and blood is ejected. After ventricular systole, the pressures in the aorta and pulmonary artery exceed those in the left and right ventricles, respectively. Retrograde blood flow therefore occurs due to the difference in pressure, which fills the valve cusps and snaps them home.

Pathological processes may result in valves becoming stenotic or incompetent. The term 'stenotic' means that the valve orifice has been narrowed, impeding blood flow; 'incompetent' or 'insufficient' refers to the fact that the cusps no longer prevent back-flow of the blood to the lower pressure areas. The haemodynamic consequences of stenosis and incompetence depend upon which valve is affected.

The conducting system of the heart

It is important that the contraction of the atria and ventricles is organised to ensure that filling and emptying of the chambers is coordinated and controlled.

Cardiac cells contract and relax as a result of a stimulus response system. The heart consists of two major types of cardiac cells: unspecialised myocardial cells, which are designed for contraction, and automatic cells, which specialise in impulse formation.

The main bulk of the atria and ventricles consists of unspecialised myocardial cells. Adjacent myocardial cells are held together by a complex system of projections known as intercalated discs with relatively low electrical resistance. These permit the movement of ions (electrically charged particles), which facilitates the propagation of action potentials from one myocardial cell to another. The main ions involved in the generation of a cardiac action potential are sodium (Na^+), potassium (K^+) and calcium (Ca^{2+}). In the normal resting state, the myocardial cell is said to be polarised, and due to the distribution of ions across its cell membrane, it is negatively charged on the inside (intracellular) and positively charged on the outside (extracellular). When electrical activation of the cell occurs, changes in the cell membrane permeability result in the movement of ions, with a resulting change in electrical polarity. The membrane is now said to be depolarised and has an intracellular positive charge and an extracellular negative charge. Return to the resting state for each cell is called repolarisation and involves active pumping of ions against concentration gradients.

For further details of the cardiac action potential, consult Jowett & Thompson (1995).

As the myocardial cells are knitted closely together, the electrical stimulation of any one single cell causes the action potential to be propagated through all adjacent cells, eventually reaching the entire lattice work of the myocardium.

The automatic cells regulate the contraction of the myocardial cells by providing the initial electrical stimulation. They do not contribute significantly to the cardiac contraction itself. These cells possess three specific properties:

- automaticity — the ability to generate action potentials, spontaneously and regularly
- excitability — the ability to respond to electrical stimulation by generating an action potential
- conductivity — the ability to propagate action potentials.

The electrical charge on the surface of an automatic cell leaks away until a certain threshold is reached, when spontaneous complete depolarisation occurs over the whole cell surface and spreads to adjacent cells, both automatic and unspecialised. The automatic cell with the most rapid leak of charge becomes the principal pacemaking cell. Normally this is located within the sinoatrial node.

The automatic cells are found in the cardiac conducting system (see Fig. 2.3), which consists of:

- sinoatrial (SA) or sinus node
- atrioventricular (AV) junction (the AV node and bundle)
- ventricular conducting tissue (the right and left bundle branches).

Sequence of excitation

Depolarisation begins at the SA node and spreads through both atria. The activating impulse travels at a rate of about 1 m/s and reaches the most distant portion of the atria in about 0.08 s. The atria and ventricles remain electrically separate except via the AV junction, which allows the action potential to be conducted from the atrial to the ventricular conducting system. When the impulse reaches the AV node, there is a delay of about 0.04 s to allow blood flow from the atria to the ventricles. After emerging from the AV node, the impulse enters the rapidly conducting tissue of the bundle of His and the right and left bundle branches. The rapid spread of the impulse throughout the ventricles means that the entire ventricular mass is depolarised almost simultaneously, which is necessary for efficient contraction and pumping.

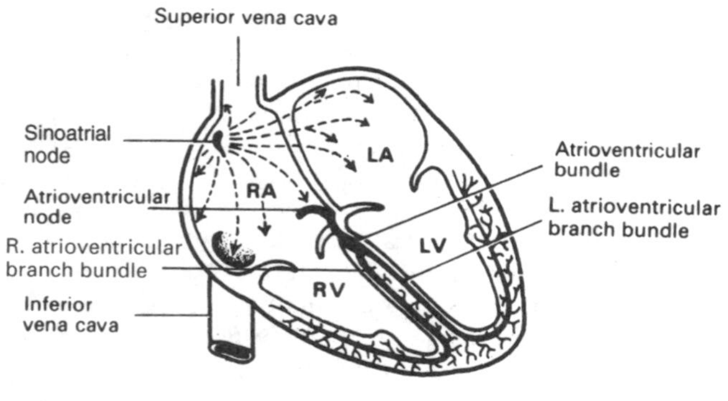

Fig. 2.3 The conducting tissues of the heart. (Reproduced with kind permission from Wilson 1996.)

Electrocardiography

Electrocardiography is the graphic recording from the body surface of potential differences resulting from electrical currents generated in the heart. This recording may be displayed on special graph paper or on an oscilloscope (monitor) and is known as an electrocardiogram (ECG). An ECG is a graphic record of electrical changes at the skin surface plotted against time. The main value of the ECG is in the detection and interpretation of cardiac arrhythmias, diagnosis of coronary heart disease and assessment of ventricular enlargement (hypertrophy).

The sequence of electrical events produced at each heartbeat has arbitrarily been labelled P, Q, R, S and T (see Fig. 2.4).

The P wave is associated with atrial activation. The width of the P wave represents the time necessary for the atrial activation process. Following atrial depolarisation, an absence of electrical activity is noted on the ECG for a brief period, representing the passage of the impulse through the AV node. The PR interval (measured from the beginning of the P wave to the beginning of the QRS complex) is the time taken for the action potential to spread from the SA node, through the atrial muscle and the AV node, down the bundle of His and into the ventricular muscle mass.

The Q, R and S waves are associated with ventricular activation. The first downward deflection after the P wave is always labelled the Q wave and the R wave is the first upward deflection. If a negative deflection follows an R wave, it is labelled an S wave. The width of the QRS complex shows how long the action potential takes to spread through the ventricles.

The ST segment, a flat line between the S wave and the T wave, represents the early phase of ventricular muscle repolarisation, or recovery.

The T wave represents the actual recovery of the ventricular muscle. Occasionally, a U wave can be observed following the T wave. The origin of this wave is not well understood, but it is considered significant in a state of hypokalaemia.

For more details on the ECG, see Erickson (1996a).

Excitation–contraction coupling

Excitation–contraction coupling is the term used to describe the link between the electrical events and the contraction of the myocardial

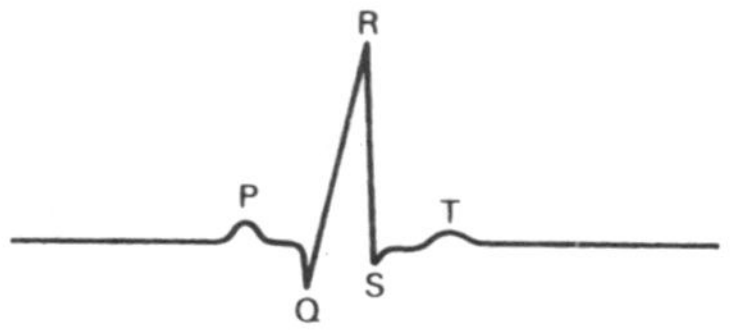

Fig. 2.4 ECG of one cardiac cycle. (Reproduced with kind permission from Boore et al 1987.)

muscle. When an action potential passes over the cardiac muscle cell membrane, it is able to pass into the interior of each muscle cell down a series of fine branching tubules until it reaches the cell's contractile elements and stimulates the release of calcium ions. Calcium ions act as a catalyst for the chemical reaction that activates the sliding of thin muscle filaments (myofilaments) over each other to produce contraction. The strength of myocardial contraction is thus partly dependent on the intracellular concentration of free calcium ions.

Cardiac cycle

The cardiac cycle is the cyclical contraction (systole) and relaxation (diastole) of the two atria and the two ventricles. Each cycle is initiated by the spontaneous generation of an action potential in the sinoatrial node.

During diastole, each chamber fills with blood. Diastole usually lasts about 0.4 s, and during this time blood enters the relaxed atria and flows passively into the ventricles. During ventricular diastole, the mitral and tricuspid valves are open and the aortic and pulmonary valves are closed.

Blood is expelled from the chambers during systole. The atria contract fractionally before the ventricles and complete ventricular filling. The ventricles then begin to contract. Increasing pressure in the ventricles closes the mitral and tricuspid valves so that all four valves are closed. This is known as the isometric phase of ventricular contraction because the volume of blood in the ventricles remains constant. Ventricular pressure continues to rise until eventually the pulmonary and aortic valves are forced open and blood is ejected into the pulmonary artery and aorta. When the ventricles stop contracting, the pressure within them falls below that in the major blood vessels, the aortic and pulmonary valves close and the cycle begins again with diastole (see Fig. 2.5).

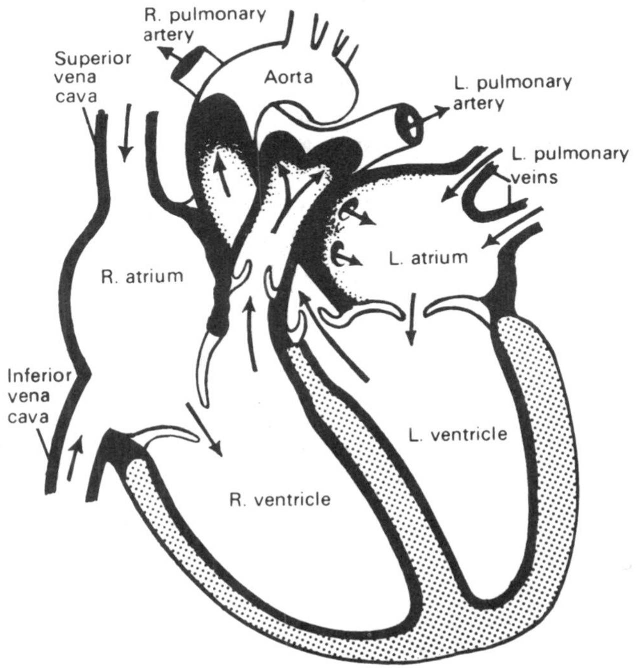

Fig. 2.5 Blood flow through the heart. (Reproduced with kind permission from Wilson 1996.)

The normal heart rate is about 70 beats/min in the resting adult, with each cardiac cycle lasting about 0.8 s. With each ventricular contraction, 65–75% of the blood in the ventricle at the end of diastole is ejected. This is usually a volume of 70–80 mL of blood and is known as the stroke volume.

Cardiac output is the volume of blood ejected from one ventricle in 1 min. Although cardiac output is a traditional measure of cardiac function, it differs markedly with body size. Thus, a more informative measure is the cardiac index, which is the cardiac output per minute per m^2 of body surface area. Usually it is about 3.2 L/m^2.

The primary factors which determine cardiac output are:

- preload — the amount of tension on the ventricular muscle fibres before they contract, determined primarily by the end-diastolic volume (EDV)
- afterload — the resistance against which the heart must pump. Major components of afterload are:
  —blood pressure in the aorta
  —resistance in the peripheral vessels
  —the size of the aortic valve opening
  —left ventricular size
- contractility of the heart
- heart rate.

Within physiological limits, the volume of blood pumped out by a ventricle is the same as that entering the atrium on the same side of the heart, i.e. cardiac output matches venous return. This principle is often referred to as the Frank–Starling law of the heart. This means that the heart is able to adapt to changing loads of inflowing blood from the systemic and pulmonary circulations. Within certain limits, cardiac muscle fibres contract more forcibly the more they are stretched at the start of contraction. Once the venous return increases beyond a certain limit, the myocardium begins to fail. This regulation of the heart in response to the amount of blood to be pumped is known as intrinsic regulation.

Q **2.1** What are the main factors that determine cardiac output?

Regulation of cardiac function by the autonomic nervous system

The autonomic nervous system alters the rate of impulse generation by the SA node, the speed of impulse conduction and the strength of cardiac contraction. It regulates the heart through both sympathetic and parasympathetic nerve fibres. The sympathetic fibres supply all areas of the atria and ventricles, and effects on the heart include increased heart rate, increased conduction speed through the AV node and increased force of contraction. Parasympathetic impulses are conducted to the heart via the vagus nerve and affect primarily the SA node, the AV node and the atrial muscle mass. Parasympathetic stimulation produces decreased heart rate, decreased conduction rate through the AV node and decreased force of atrial contraction.

Sympathetic and parasympathetic control of the heart occurs by reflexes coordinated in the medulla oblongata of the brain. The group of neurones in the brain that affect heart activity and the blood vessels is known as the cardiovascular centre. This centre receives information from various sensory receptors. Baroreceptors alter their rate of impulse generation in response to changes in blood pressure and chemoreceptors respond to changes in the chemical composition of the blood.

For further reading, see Herbert & Alison (1996).

ANATOMY AND PHYSIOLOGY OF THE BLOOD VESSELS

Systemic circulation

The systemic circulation is a high-pressure system that supplies all the tissues of the body with blood. It consists of the arteries, arterioles, capillaries, venules and veins. Blood flows through the system because of a downward pressure gradient from the aorta to the superior and inferior venae cavae. Arteries distribute oxygenated blood from the left side of the heart to the tissues, and veins convey deoxygenated blood from the tissues to the right side of the heart. Adequate perfusion resulting in oxygenation and nutrition of body tissues is dependent in part upon patent and responsive blood vessels and adequate blood flow.

Arteries and arterioles

Arteries are thick-walled structures that carry blood from the heart to the tissues. The major arteries leading from the heart branch to form smaller ones, which eventually give rise to arterioles. The walls of the arteries and arterioles are divided into three layers:

- the inner layer provides a smooth surface in contact with the flowing blood
- the middle layer, the thickest, consists of elastic fibres and muscle fibres. The elasticity of the arterial wall enables it to recoil during ventricular relaxation and maintain blood flow
- the outer layer of connective tissue anchors the vessel to its surrounding structures.

There is much less elastic tissue in the arterioles than in the arteries. The middle layer of the arteriole wall consists primarily of smooth muscle which, by contraction and relaxation, controls the vessel's diameter. Arterioles regulate the pressure in the arterial system and the blood flow to the capillaries. The arterioles respond to local conditions such as a decrease in oxygen concentration or an increase in the concentration of carbon dioxide or other waste products. This ensures that a tissue that needs extra oxygen receives extra blood flow.

Arterioles will sometimes respond to changes in blood pressure. A local increase in blood pressure will cause the arterioles to constrict, in order to protect the smaller vessels in the tissue from increased pressure. If pressure in the arterioles suddenly decreases, the arterioles will dilate to ensure that the tissue receives sufficient blood flow for nutrition. This local regulatory mechanism is sometimes referred to as autoregulation and is an important factor in determining relatively constant blood flow despite alterations in arterial pressure. The sympathetic nervous system will also influence the diameter of the arterioles. Increased sympathetic stimulation to blood vessels usually produces constriction, whereas decreased sympathetic stimulation results in vasodilatation.

Capillaries

The velocity of the blood is at its slowest in the capillaries, thus allowing sufficient time for exchange of materials between the blood and the interstitial space. Capillary walls lack muscle. They consist of a single layer of cells and have a large total surface area. Their thin walls allow efficient transport of nutrients to the cells and the removal of metabolic wastes. The density of capillary networks varies in different tissues.

Veins and venules

Capillaries join together to form larger vessels called venules, which in turn join to form veins. The walls of the veins are thinner and a lot less muscular than the arteries. This allows the veins to distend more, which permits storage of large volumes of blood in the veins under low pressure. Approximately 75% of total blood volume is contained in the veins. Some veins are equipped with valves to prevent the reflux of blood as it is propelled towards the heart. The sympathetic nervous system can stimulate venoconstriction, thereby reducing venous volume and increasing the general circulating blood volume. This adjustment of the total volume of the circulatory system to the amount of blood available to fill it contributes to the regulation of blood pressure.

Blood pressure

Blood pressure refers to the hydrostatic pressure exerted by the blood on the blood vessel walls and is a function of blood flow and vascular resistance. As most of the resistance to blood flow is due to the peripheral vessels, especially the arterioles, it is often described as the total peripheral resistance, as in the equation:

$$\text{mean arterial pressure} = \text{cardiac output} \times \text{total peripheral resistance}$$

Blood pressure varies in different blood vessels. However, clinically the term 'blood pressure' refers to systemic arterial blood pressure.

Arterial blood pressure

Arterial blood pressure fluctuates throughout the cardiac cycle. The maximum pressure occurs after ventricular systole and is known as the systolic pressure. Systolic pressure is dependent on the stroke volume, the force of contraction and the stiffness of the arterial walls. The level to which arterial pressure falls before the next ventricular contraction is the minimum pressure, known as the diastolic pressure. Diastolic pressure varies according to the degree of vasoconstriction and is dependent on the level of the systolic pressure, the elasticity of the arteries and the viscosity of the blood. Alterations in heart rate will also affect diastolic pressure. A slower heart rate produces a lower diastolic pressure as there is more time for the blood to flow out of the arteries. The difference between the systolic and diastolic blood pressures is known as the 'pulse pressure'. The average pressure attempting to push the blood through the circulatory system is known as the 'mean arterial pressure'.

Blood pressure values

There is no such value as a 'normal' blood pressure, as it varies both from person to person and in individuals from moment to moment, under different circumstances. Normal blood pressure is said to range from 100/60 mmHg to 150/90 mmHg. Factors such as age, sex and race influence blood pressure values. Pressure also varies with exercise, emotional reactions, sleep, digestion and time of day.

The predominant mechanisms that control arterial pressure within the 'normal' range are the autonomic nervous system and the renin–angiotensin–aldosterone system.

Baroreceptors in the aortic arch and the carotid sinus respond to changes in arterial pressure and relay impulses to the cardiovascular centre in the medulla oblongata of the brain. When the arterial pressure is increased, baroreceptor endings are stretched and relay impulses that inhibit the sympathetic outflow. This results in a decreased heart rate and arteriolar dilatation and the arterial pressure returning to its former level. If the blood pressure remains chronically high, the baroreceptors are reset at a higher level and respond as though the new level were normal.

When blood flow to the kidneys decreases, with a fall in blood pressure, renin is released. Renin is an enzyme which acts on a blood protein angiotensinogen, which is converted to angiotensin I and then, by another enzyme, to angiotensin II. Angiotensin II produces an elevation in blood pressure by direct constriction of arterioles. Angiotensin II also directly stimulates the release of the hormone aldosterone from the adrenal cortex which leads to renal retention of sodium and water. This increases extracellular volume, which in turn increases the venous return to the heart, thereby raising stroke volume, cardiac output and arterial blood pressure. The kidneys respond to an increase in arterial pressure by excreting a greater volume of fluid. This decreases the extracellular fluid, resulting in a lower venous return and reduced cardiac output until arterial pressure is returned towards normal.

Further details of blood pressure regulation can be found in Herbert & Alison (1996).

DISORDERS OF THE CARDIOVASCULAR SYSTEM

Atherosclerosis

Atherosclerosis is a complex, chronic disease of the arteries characterised by endothelial injury, the accumulation of lipids and fibrous tissue in the form of atheromatous plaques, and the thickening and hardening of the vessel walls with resultant loss of elasticity (see Figs 2.6 and 2.7). The aetiology of atherosclerosis remains unclear, and although several theories have been put forward to explain its pathogenesis, it is not fully understood.

Further details of the pathogenesis of atherosclerosis can be found in Jowett & Thompson (1995).

2.2 How early in life has evidence of atheromatous change in the blood vessels been found?

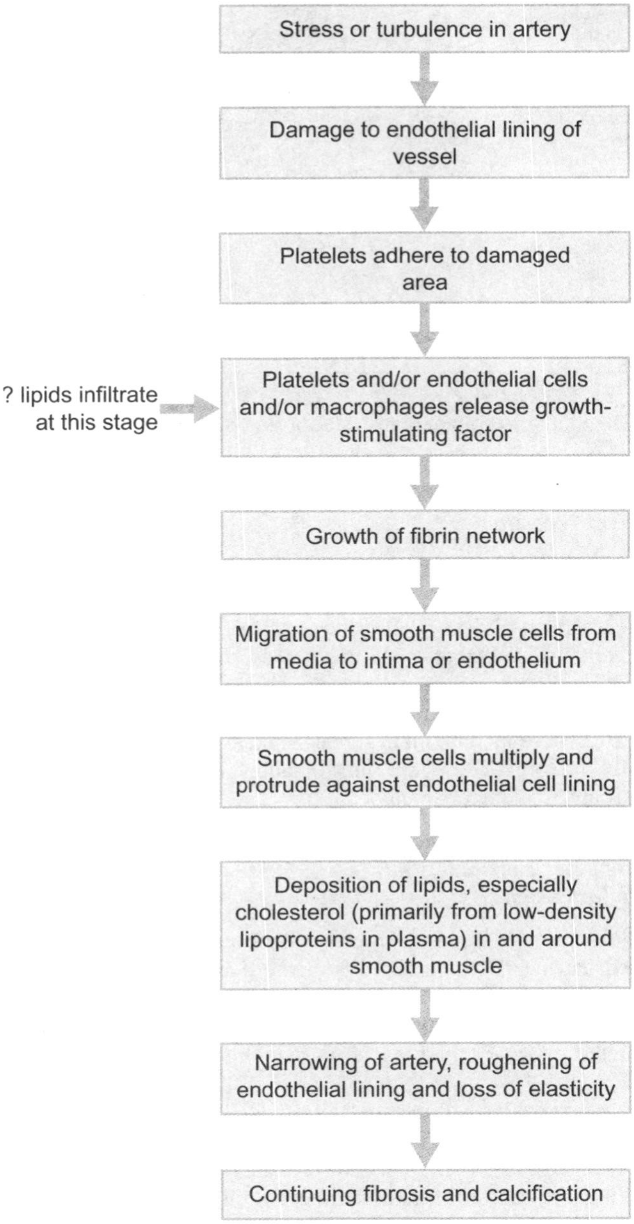

Fig. 2.6 Probable course of events in the development of atheroma. (Reproduced with kind permission from Boore et al 1987.)

Atherosclerosis is responsible for most coronary artery and ischaemic heart disease and much peripheral and cerebrovascular disease. Emboli may arise as a result of pieces of dead tissue from the damaged arterial wall breaking off. With progression of the process, the lining of the vessel wall may become eaten away and, especially if the blood pressure is elevated, the vessel may become permanently dilated and weakened in the form of an aneurysm. Vessels may become blocked or stenosed or, as a result of endothelial damage and platelet adhesion, an ulcer-like site can develop, leading to thrombus formation. Thrombosis may cause complete obstruction or undergo spontaneous thrombolysis. This dynamic process occurs over a period of hours to days, preceding an acute coronary event or spontaneous resolution.

Myocardial ischaemia

Traditionally, myocardial ischaemia is defined as a condition of the heart in which there is an imbalance between oxygen supply and demand. However, such a definition excludes the removal of metabolites, particularly heat and carbon monoxide, which are an important function of myocardial blood flow.

Oxygen demand depends mainly upon heart rate, myocardial contractility and tension in the myocardial wall. Oxygen supply to the myocardium varies with coronary blood flow. The heart extracts the maximum amount of oxygen from its blood supply and is dependent upon an increased volume of blood in times of increased demand. Myocardial blood supply may be compromised by abnormalities of the vessel wall, in blood flow or in the blood itself.

Localised myocardial ischaemia may be intermittent and have reversible effects, but it causes decreased myocardial function. Ischaemia results in acidosis and the rapid accumulation of potassium in the extracellular space. Pain is usually experienced after about a minute of myocardial ischaemia.

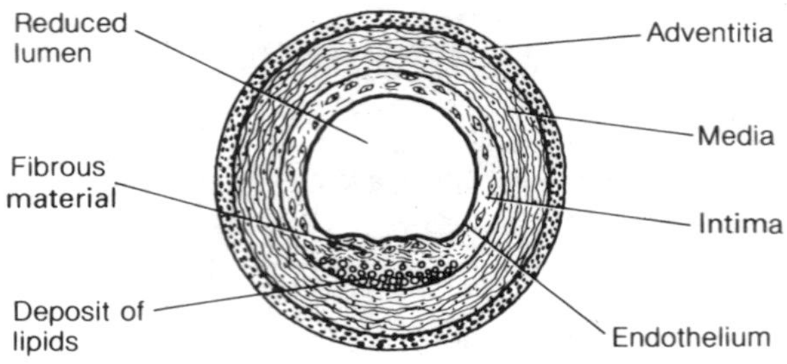

Fig. 2.7 Cross-section of an artery. (Reproduced with kind permission from Boore et al 1987.)

There are three main manifestations of ischaemic heart disease:

- angina pectoris
- acute myocardial infarction
- sudden death.

Risk factors

Epidemiological studies have sought to find associations between coronary heart disease (CHD) and physical, biochemical and environmental characteristics of a population or individuals. As a result, predictive variables, termed risk factors, have been defined, which have been shown to be associated with the development of disease. These include male gender, increasing age and a positive family history. These are unavoidable risk factors; however, modifiable risk factors include:

- hypercholesterolaemia
- cigarette smoking
- hypertension.

Such risk factors are extremely common in the UK. It is estimated that nearly three-quarters of the population have a raised serum cholesterol level (greater than 5.2 mmol/L). The average diet in the UK is unhealthy. In particular, fat intake, especially of saturated fat, is too high and fruit and vegetable consumption is too low.

Almost a quarter of the deaths from CHD in men are attributable to smoking (British Heart Foundation 1999) and there is a marked social class difference in smoking habits.

Almost a quarter of adults in the UK either have raised blood pressure (more than 160/95 mmHg) or are being treated for raised blood pressure. For each 5 mmHg reduction in blood pressure, the risk of CHD is reduced by about 16% (British Heart Foundation 1999).

Other main risk factors are:

- obesity
- lack of physical exercise
- stress
- diabetes mellitus.

Major geographical variations in the incidence of CHD are apparent. Mortality rates from CHD have been falling in the UK since the late 1970s; however, the rates in the UK are very close to the top of the international league table. Scotland, Northern Ireland and the north of England have the highest mortality rates, and the south-east has the lowest. Mortality from CHD differs significantly between ethnic groups. It is highest in men and women born in the Indian subcontinent and is also raised in Irish- and Polish-born immigrants. Risk factors need to be viewed in conjunction with each other, as their effect is cumulative. Although, by definition, each risk factor associates positively with increased risk of CHD, it does not follow that risk factors are causal. It is also important to remember that a significant number of patients presenting with CHD do not have identifiable risk factors and that standard risk factors explain less than half the disease (Box 2.1).

Box 2.1 Risk factors associated with coronary heart disease

Genetic
- Race
- Gender
- Family history

Medical
- Diabetes mellitus
- Hypertension
- Hyperlipidaemia
- Hypercholesterolaemia
- Hypothyroidism
- Gout

Social
- Geographical location
- Living conditions
- Occupation
- Stress

Personal
- Age
- Smoking
- Diet:
  - —obesity
  - —fat intake
  - —salt intake
  - —fibre intake
  - —alcohol intake
- Lack of exercise
- Lack of relaxation
- Oral contraception

2.3 Health promotion may be defined as efforts to enhance positive health and prevent ill-health, through the three overlapping spheres of:
- health education
- prevention
- health protection.

The health promotion movement stresses the importance of 'empowerment', of enabling people to make choices and to determine their own lives.

Discuss the three spheres in relation to the promotion of cardiovascular health.

2.4 'Empowering' people is neither simple nor easy. What might hinder people from taking greater control over their health and what might encourage them to do so?

For more information on health promotion in hospital, see McBride (1995), and in the community see Kelly (1992). The use of health education materials is discussed in Buxton (1999).

Angina pectoris

Angina pectoris is a discomfort or pain resulting from a transient, reversible episode of inadequate coronary circulation occurring as a result of an imbalance between oxygen supply and demand. It is a symptom rather than a disease and it is estimated that 2 million people in the UK suffer from it (British Heart Foundation 1999).

PATHOPHYSIOLOGY

Inadequate supply of oxygen is usually the result of coronary artery obstruction caused by atherosclerosis, although spasm or thrombus may also contribute to the obstruction. Severe anaemia and hypoxia can also produce a decreased myocardial oxygen supply. Increased demand for myocardial oxygen may be the result of a variety of clinical conditions, including tachycardia, hypertension, valvular stenosis, left ventricular hypertrophy and hyperthyroidism.

Anginal pain at rest or during minimal exertion is known as unstable, crescendo or pre-infarction angina. Despite the last term, not all patients with this syndrome subsequently sustain a myocardial infarction, but its occurrence does highlight a group of patients at increased risk.

Common presenting symptoms. The presentation and history vary and may mislead the practitioner initially if a thorough examination is not undertaken. History is usually of increasing discomfort over a period of time, often related to specific events. The presenting features indicate a deficiency in the oxygen supply, such as:

- Episodic pain or discomfort occurring centrally in the chest, often described as 'dull', 'aching' or a 'tight band'. This may radiate to the arms, particularly the left arm, jaw or neck. It is often induced by exercise or emotion and relieved by rest. The pain takes many forms (see Table 2.1). Typically, the duration of an anginal attack is 2–5 min.
- Breathlessness on exertion, e.g. walking uphill, or in cold weather.
- Discomfort in the epigastric region after a heavy meal.

Table 2.1 Classification of angina pectoris

Classification	*Characteristics*
Stable angina	Condition in which the frequency and severity of angina remains well controlled and unchanged over several months
Unstable angina	Condition in which the pain is increasing in frequency, severity and duration. Occurs with less activity or at rest
Crescendo angina	Form of angina where chance of AMI occurring within a few days is high
Angina decubitus	Pain occurring when lying down
Atypical angina (Prinzmetal's angina)	Unusual form where pain occurs at rest or long after activity has ceased. Accompanied by transient ST segment elevation. Coronary artery spasm without underlying disease is often the cause
Intractable angina	Continued pain with increasing frequency, despite treatment

MEDICAL MANAGEMENT

Investigations are as follows:

Electrocardiogram. The recording is invariably normal between attacks of angina, but during an episode of pain, the segment between the end of the QRS complex and the beginning of the T wave may be depressed (ST depression). The T wave may also be flattened or inverted.

Exercise tolerance test. This is a means of assessing the heart's response to increased demand. The test is based on the theory that patients with ischaemic heart disease will produce marked ST-segment depression on the ECG when exercising. The test is considered negative if there are no significant ECG abnormalities and the patient experiences no significant symptoms. Three common methods of exercise testing include:

- climbing stairs
- pedalling a stationary bicycle
- walking a treadmill.

These methods are familiar to the general public as recommended ways of promoting cardiovascular fitness. Aerobic exercise is now a common leisure pursuit. In the exercise tolerance test, the ECG, heart rate and blood pressure are recorded while the patient engages in some form of exercise (physiological stress). The principle is that coronary arteries that may be occluded will be unable to meet the heart's increased oxygen demand during exercise, resulting in chest pain, fatigue, dyspnoea, excessive heart rate (tachycardia), a fall in blood pressure or the development of arrhythmias. The test is stopped if any of these occur, or before, at the patient's request. The patient needs to have the procedure explained in detail before the test. The term 'stress' test is best avoided as it may sound ominous and increase patient anxiety. The patient should be advised to avoid a heavy meal prior to the test and to wear loose-fitting clothes. The procedure takes about 30 min.

Holter monitoring. Continuous monitoring of the ST segments of the ECG can be used to detect transient changes compatible with ischaemia.

Coronary angiography. This involves the injection of contrast medium into the heart during cardiac catheterisation. The procedure shows the shape and size of the heart chambers and will pinpoint any stenosis or occlusion in the coronary arteries. This test is described in Box 2.2.

Diagnosis. Angina is diagnosed by the characteristic chest pain, which is induced by exercise and relieved by rest. Exercise testing only confirms angina if it produces pain or ECG changes during the test. Angiography in the absence of clinical symptoms confirms the presence of myocardial ischaemia, not of angina. The differential diagnosis is very important at this stage.

The pain of angina may be confused with the pain of oesophagitis or the pain of peptic ulceration. Patients, fearing a 'heart attack', may choose to interpret the pain as 'a little indigestion'.

Treatment. Stable angina may be managed by the GP. Unstable angina (see Table 2.1) requires admission to a specialised unit to avert myocardial infarction and any sequelae.

The aim of treatment is:

- to restore and maintain cardiac output necessary for normal living activities
- to reduce the workload of the heart
- to bring back into balance oxygen supply and demand.

Box 2.2 Cardiac catheterisation

Purpose
Cardiac catheterisation involves the insertion, usually under screening, of a fine, flexible, radio-opaque catheter into one or more of the heart chambers. The catheter is inserted via a peripheral vein or artery under sterile conditions in a cardiac catheterisation laboratory. The right and left side of the heart may be investigated separately or together. The procedure is performed to:

- visualise the heart chambers and vessels by means of a radio-opaque substance under X-ray control (angiography)
- measure pressure and record waveforms from the cavity of the heart
- obtain blood samples from the heart.

Cardiac catheterisation will always be performed on a prospective candidate for coronary artery bypass graft surgery and it is also used to evaluate the effect of thrombolytic agents. Angiography involves injecting contrast medium into the heart during cardiac catheterisation in order to pinpoint any stenosis or occlusion. It is recommended for patients with significant angina.

Procedure
Cardiac catheterisation is usually carried out under local anaesthesia, but the patient is usually asked to fast for 4–6 h to prevent aspiration, should cardiac arrest occur. The groin area will be shaved. The procedure is performed by a cardiologist and takes about 90 min. The patient will be asked to wear a gown and should be prepared to lie flat on her back on a hard table during the procedure. She needs to be warned to expect a sudden burning sensation as the dye is injected into the heart. Angina may occur as a result of the catheter blocking the artery.

Following the procedure the patient may require analgesics and should be allowed to rest. A pressure dressing will be applied to the wound site, which needs to be observed for excessive bleeding. The limb needs to be kept straight for 1–2 h to prevent turbulence of blood flow at the incision site. If the catheter is inserted via the femoral artery, the patient is advised to rest in bed for 6–8 h to prevent flexing the hip and possible artery occlusion. The patient is usually discharged the following day.

Possible complications
Complications are uncommon but can include:

- transient cardiac arrhythmias
- perforation of the heart
- syncope
- emboli.

A reaction to the dye may produce symptoms ranging from a rash to anaphylaxis.

Treatment is achieved by:

- medication to optimise cardiac function by relieving the pain of angina and improving myocardial perfusion (Table 2.2)
- reduction in activity
- reducing risk factors
- surgical intervention — percutaneous transluminal coronary angioplasty (PTCA) or coronary artery bypass graft (CABG) surgery (see pp. 19 and 20).

Patients who persist with ST depression despite full anti-anginal therapy should be considered for urgent coronary angiography and possible angioplasty or CABG. Elective referral for angiography is warranted for those with a positive exercise test and on maximum drug therapy.

Q **2.5** (a) Read Case History 2.1(A). What is the significance of this result?
(b) What other tests might be requested?
(c) What are Mr B's risk factors for ischaemic heart disease?
(d) How would you discuss the results of this test with Mr B?

NURSING PRIORITIES AND MANAGEMENT: ANGINA

The major goals for the patient are to:

- prevent or minimise chest pain
- cope with the anginal pain and any other symptoms
- reduce anxiety
- be aware of the underlying nature of the disorder
- understand the prescribed care and be able to make informed decisions about future lifestyle.

Nursing input will vary according to the type of contact a person has with health care services. Practice nurses and occupational health staff may be the main source of professional information and support for those in the community. Admission to hospital is likely to occur only if the angina is uncontrolled or further investigation is warranted.

Nursing assessment should pay particular attention to those activities that have been found to precede and precipitate attacks of angina pain and associated symptoms, so that a logical programme of prevention can be worked out with the patient, who needs to feel in control of her condition and to regain a realistic outlook for the future.

Maintaining a safe environment

The effect of angina on the person and on those around her needs to be considered. The patient needs to know both how to prevent attacks and how to manage them when they occur. As the nurse will not witness many of the attacks, it should be impressed upon the patient that their management lies with her and her family. As much of the nursing management involves advice about potential adaptations in lifestyle, the family members require the same information and support as the patient.

The individual needs to be advised to plan her daily activity around adequate rest periods. If she cannot avoid activities liable to precipitate an attack, then she should rest before and after the activity. For example, a large family gathering such as a wedding can be very stressful, with socialising, a large meal to eat and a lot of preparation. As much time as possible should be spent quietly, with rest periods after dressing, after the meal, etc. Explaining to other members of the family the reason for this is better than suffering an attack during the proceedings.

Taking glyceryl trinitrate (GTN) prophylactically is often the best way of managing this. Further manipulation of the individual's environment can take place; for example, if climbing stairs induces angina and the bathroom is downstairs and the bedroom upstairs, it may help to dress in a downstairs room, as climbing stairs after a hot bath is very likely to induce an attack. Advice on the practical aspects of daily routine can be given during history-taking.

Table 2.2 Drugs used in angina

Drug group	*Role in angina*	*Physiological action*	*Comments*
Nitrates			
Glyceryl trinitrate (GTN) (spray or tablets)	Used for relief of angina Administered as spray form or tablet under tongue to ensure rapid release into the bloodstream GTN can be given i.v., maintenance dose 6–10 mg/h	Venodilatation with consequent reduction in preload Also causes systemic arteriolar vasodilatation with decrease in afterload	Tablets need to be stored correctly Tablets lose potency over time and if exposed to light They should not be kept for more than 2 months, should be stored in an airtight container and not exposed to light
Suscard buccal	Slow-release form of nitrate placed in the buccal cavity	As above Used for effect for 4–5 h	
Isosorbide mononitrate (oral or i.v.)	Used for prevention of angina Oral administration	As above Used as longer-term control	Patient can develop tolerance
Beta-blockers (e.g. atenolol 50–100 mg)	Used in preventing angina Administered once or twice daily Dose lower than for hypertensive patients	Block sympathetic stimulation, so slowing heart rate and reducing oxygen demand	Need to be used with caution in patients with chronic obstructive airways disease
Calcium antagonists	Used in preventing angina	Interfere with calcium transfer across the cell membrane, causing relaxation of arteriolar smooth muscle, thus reducing afterload. Affects rate of action potential and reduces oxygen demand	
Anticoagulant therapy			
Aspirin	Small dose taken daily to protect against MI	Aspirin prolongs the prothrombin time as well as decreasing platelet viscosity	Small dose should not affect stomach lining
Intravenous or subcutaneous low molecular weight heparin	Started early in unstable angina to inhibit thrombus formation		

Case History 2.1(A) Mr B

Mr B is a 55-year-old factory foreman who regards himself as being fit and well for his age. He plays badminton at the local sports club two or three times a week and enjoys taking his dog on regular rambles. He does not smoke and, being aware of factors leading to heart disease, has tried to reduce the fat intake in his diet over the past few years. His father died of a heart attack at the age of 73. Mr B's company offer regular medical checks to screen for health problems and on his last visit he underwent an exercise test. After 5 min of the test he felt short of breath. He was noted to have ST-segment depression.

A change of occupation is sometimes necessary following a diagnosis of angina; it could, for example, be unsafe to drive public transport vehicles. This double blow can be very difficult for the person to accept. The occupational health nurse can help, as he will be aware of other areas to which the individual can be relocated. If retraining is required social worker and retraining counsellors should be involved as early as possible.

Mobility

Exercise is the most common cause of an attack, and patients need to be advised to stop and rest rather than attempting to work through the pain. The patient should understand how to use GTN both to prevent and to treat an attack. If the patient takes GTN prior to an activity likely to cause angina, she may prevent an attack and still complete the activity. However, the patient needs to appreciate that she should not use GTN to over-exercise, but to maintain a reasonable quality of life and to achieve some feeling of control over the condition. She should be encouraged to keep records of the activities that induce angina. These can be reviewed with her practitioner to provide a reliable assessment of angina and of the effectiveness of therapy. Knowledge of her limitations gives the patient some feeling of control over her own life and she can then attempt to extend them by altering her daily routine.

Many of the heavier household tasks induce angina, e.g. shopping, ironing and vacuuming, and often make patients feel threatened. A basket with wheels can be used to transport shopping, and other such simple measures are easily adapted into people's lifestyles. Help from other family members or domestic help in the home may be another solution.

Breathing

In some individuals, angina presents as, or is accompanied by, difficulty in breathing. This is often worse in cold or windy weather. Such individuals need to be advised against walking great distances in these conditions. Smokers need to be clear about the association between ischaemic heart disease and cigarette smoking, so that they can make informed decisions about stopping.

Cigarette smokers have a 2–3 times greater risk of death from ischaemic heart disease than non-smokers. The risk is greater in young adults and in those who smoke more than 20 cigarettes a day. Nicotine stimulation results in an increase in heart rate, cardiac output, blood pressure and coronary blood flow. Carbon monoxide attaches itself to the haemoglobin molecule and therefore reduces its ability to transport oxygen.

The nursing history should include information as to whether the patient has tried to give up smoking before, and if so, how she planned to stop, how long she was able to stop, what support she received and why she started smoking again. Any perceived benefits of smoking, e.g. stress reduction, need to be discussed and plans for stopping based on experience gained in conjunction with new information and advice given.

Q **2.6** Many strategies for giving up smoking exist. Not all will suit every would-be non-smoker. What strategies can you identify? The following articles describe approaches used by a health visitor and by coronary care nurses, respectively: Gallop (1993) and Clark et al (1994).

Diet and nutrition

Obese people develop cardiovascular disease more frequently than do others. Obesity also denotes an increased likelihood of hypertension, hyperlipidaemia and diabetes mellitus. Total blood cholesterol levels have been shown to be associated with ischaemic heart disease mortality and morbidity (Box 2.3). However, there is a negative association between one category of lipoproteins, high-density lipoproteins (HDLs), and coronary heart disease: the risk of the disease is lower when the concentration of HDLs is raised. Early conclusions that cholesterol and saturated fat in the diet raise cholesterol and fat levels in the blood and therefore promote atherosclerosis are now the topic of much controversy. It has been recommended that consumption of saturated fatty acids and total fat be reduced to 11 and 35%, respectively, of food energy. Dietary advice needs to take into account personal preferences and domestic, socioeconomic and cultural factors. Alterations to general eating habits are preferable to restrictive diets. Sensible dietary advice includes:

- losing excess weight
- reducing fat, particularly saturated fat intake
- reducing salt intake
- increasing fibre intake.

Eating more fish, poultry, vegetables, grains, cereals and fruit should be encouraged. Keeping within an ideal body weight range and taking suitable physical exercise are logical recommendations (see Ch. 21).

Large meals may trigger an attack of angina, so small, frequent meals are preferable. It can be difficult to motivate people to change their diet. Involving the family is very important, particularly the person primarily responsible for buying food and preparing meals.

The patient who presents to the medical services with epigastric pain may have angina, particularly if the history is vague. Diagnosis requires history-taking skills and spending time with the patient.

Alcohol intake should be discussed with the individual. In small quantities, alcohol has a vasodilatory effect which is beneficial in CHD, so a small nightcap will help to relax the patient and aid sleep. However, heavy drinkers are at risk of hepatic dysfunction.

The patient should know whether her medication should be taken before or after meals and its effect with alcohol.

Work and recreation

The person with angina has to come to terms with the progressive nature of the disease. People with limited energy reserves may

Box 2.3 Understanding cholesterol

Definition: a steroid found in animal fats and most body tissues, especially nervous tissue.

Cholesterol has received rather bad publicity in recent years because of the role it has been found to play in the formation of atheromatous plaques, but it must be remembered that, although it is not used as an energy fuel, cholesterol is an important dietary lipid, essential in maintaining homeostatic mechanisms in the body. It is a vital constituent of cell membranes and forms the structural basis of many steroid hormones and bile salts.

The recommended daily intake of cholesterol for adults is approximately 250 mg or less. However, cholesterol is not only obtained from the diet but is synthesised in the liver, the intestinal mucosa and, to a lesser degree, other body cells. It is excreted from the body in bile salts.

Cholesterol, like fatty acids and glycerol, is insoluble in water and therefore cannot circulate freely in the bloodstream. It is transported, bound to small lipid proteins (lipoproteins), which are essentially of high-density or low-density compositions. Low-density lipoproteins (LDLs) are responsible for transporting cholesterol to the peripheral tissue so that it is available for membrane synthesis, hormone synthesis and storage, for later use. Excessive cholesterol leads to 'dumping' of the excess in the lining of the blood vessels, e.g. the coronary arteries. High-density lipoproteins (HDLs) have a different function in that they transport cholesterol from the peripheral tissue to the liver to be broken down. HDLs have been described as scavenging excess cholesterol for disposal.

High levels of total serum cholesterol have been repeatedly shown to be associated with the development of coronary artery disease and myocardial infarction. However, it is not enough merely to measure cholesterol, but rather the form in which it is being transported. HDLs can be thought of as beneficial because they promote the degradation and removal of cholesterol. On the other hand, LDLs, when excessive, can lead to a potentially serious deposition of cholesterol in the artery walls.

Although it is now regarded as important to limit our dietary cholesterol, severe restriction does not lead to a correspondingly dramatic drop in plasma cholesterol. This is because, although cholesterol production is to some extent adjusted by a feedback mechanism such that a high dietary intake will inhibit hepatic synthesis, the liver will always produce a certain amount irrespective of the diet.

It would seem that the factor that has the most significant effect on plasma cholesterol is the amount of saturated and unsaturated fat in the diet. Saturated fats, found essentially in animal produce, stimulate the hepatic synthesis of cholesterol whilst inhibiting its removal. In contrast, unsaturated fats, found in vegetable oils, enhance the excretion of cholesterol in the bile salts, thereby reducing cholesterol levels.

Other factors also appear to affect plasma cholesterol levels. Stress, coffee and smoking are thought to be implicated in increased levels of LDLs. Regular aerobic exercise has been associated with the lowering of LDLs and raising of HDLs.

If research continues to support the above findings, there are clear implications for the role of the nurse in promoting nutritional health and well-being.

Further reading: Pharaoh & Hollingworth (1996).

put all their effort into work and find they have little left for leisure pursuits. The nurse's role is to assist the individual to assess her lifestyle and make decisions about priorities and possible changes. Those with sedentary lifestyles should be advised to take regular exercise, such as walking to work, climbing the stairs, swimming and cycling. Some apparently sedentary jobs may be mentally exhausting, which can put severe strain on the compromised myocardium and lead to an anginal attack. Planning the day is important, to allow for quiet periods, particularly before and after long meetings or heavy business lunches. For certain personality types, therapy such as relaxation techniques or yoga may help.

If a change of occupation or early retirement is proposed as the only solution, the person may resist, particularly if she is the family breadwinner.

Rest and sleep

Taking frequent naps throughout the day is often better than a longer sleep at night. The bedroom should be well ventilated but not cold or draughty (see Ch. 25).

Expressing sexuality

In some people with angina, sexual intercourse can trigger an attack. This can be stressful for both the sufferer and her partner. Prophylactic use of GTN and some planning may help. The couple may have to adapt their usual position or the partner may have to take on a more dominant role. Touching and caressing may replace full intercourse while satisfying both.

This subject needs delicate handling but must be addressed, as the individual's perceived view on this aspect of daily living can affect all other aspects. A man receiving beta-blocker therapy may suffer from impotence and the reason for this should be explained.

An important related aspect of sexuality is role reversal, e.g. if a housewife has to hand over some of her tasks and feels threatened, or where the family breadwinner is forced to give up work. This may greatly affect self-esteem.

The fear of dying

People who have angina may have difficulty coming to terms with the fact that they have a progressive disease affecting their heart and most probably other parts of their body as well. Angina can progress to myocardial infarction, which can cause death. This has to be discussed with the person to keep the situation in perspective. If she feels in control over some aspects of the condition to help prolong life, e.g. stopping smoking or altering her diet, she will possibly cope better than the person with a strong family history over which she has no control. Encouraging the patient to discuss her fears may help her to cope with them or alert the nurse to the fact that expert counselling is required.

Communication

Getting to know the person as an individual is important if appropriate support is to be given. She needs to be guided towards pinpointing aspects of lifestyle that will be affected by angina and then learning through discussion and counselling how to minimise their effect. If the person can communicate what causes pain, what relieves it, etc., management is often simplified. Anxiety will reduce the ability to communicate, particularly when in an unfamiliar environment, such as the occupational health department or hospital. The use of a scoring table or a continuum for assessing and comparing attacks of angina may prove beneficial for monitoring the effect of therapy.

Personal hygiene and dressing

Here again, the key is living within the constraints of the condition. The person should be advised against locking the bathroom door whilst in the bath so that help can reach her if necessary. Other family members must remember this and respect privacy. Spacing activities throughout the day rather than rushing to do everything first thing in the morning may minimise the occurrence of symptoms.

Constrictive clothing may induce breathlessness and chest tightness, and so should be avoided; however, the person should be advised to wrap up warmly in cold weather to limit increased workload on the heart for thermoregulation.

Elimination

Diuretic therapy may be indicated if there is a degree of cardiac failure present (p. 39). The timing of ingestion of these drugs can be controlled by the angina sufferer so that the ensuing diuresis does not disrupt daily routine.

Straining at stool should be avoided. A healthy diet will help, but the judicious use of a mild aperient may be indicated.

Q

2.7 Read Case History 2.1(B).
(a) What pre-procedure preparation is required?
(b) How would you describe the procedure to the patient and his family?
(c) What complications should you aim to prevent post-procedure?

Case History 2.1(B) Mr B — invasive treatment for angina

Mr B has now had the following investigations, all of which are normal: chest X-ray, ECG, cardiac enzymes (p. 24) and weight. His serum lipids are high, so, having had dietary advice, he has begun drug therapy to reduce these levels.

Cardiac catheterisation revealed that he had an 85% reduction of the lumen of the left coronary artery main stem. Mr B is advised that he should undergo percutaneous transluminal coronary angioplasty (PTCA). This is planned for the next day.

Cardiac catheterisation

The patient should be fully informed about the procedure (see Box 2.2, p. 16), its findings and their implications. Nurses need to be aware of the possible complications and place particular importance on pain relief.

See De Jong & Morton (1997) for a research-based protocol for post-catheterisation nursing care.

Percutaneous transluminal coronary angioplasty (PTCA) (Box 2.4)

The patient will need to have the procedure explained so that she is fully aware of both the benefits and drawbacks. The importance of reporting any pain or discomfort during or following PTCA should be stressed. Pain is most likely to be experienced when the balloon is inflated over the narrowed area and the patient should be warned of this. Nitrate therapy is used for pain relief.

The patient may require assistance with various activities of living whilst mobility is temporarily limited. She is likely to be

Box 2.4 Percutaneous transluminal coronary angioplasty (PTCA)

Purpose
PTCA is a technique involving the introduction of a balloon catheter into the coronary artery up to the site of a coronary stenosis, where it is inflated. This process produces compression and redistribution of the lesion and a substantial increase in the size of the lumen. PTCA may be performed to relieve the symptoms of angina if medication is ineffective, or it may be performed soon after successful thrombolysis (see p. 25) to restore perfusion to the ischaemic zone.

Procedure
PTCA is carried out under local anaesthetic in a cardiac catheterisation laboratory. If the procedure is planned, the patient will be admitted to hospital the day before and asked to starve for 6–8 h prior to the procedure. This is in case of complications necessitating bypass surgery.

Usually, two arterial catheters are used: a guiding catheter and a dilating catheter. The guiding catheter is inserted, usually in the leg, and advanced to the coronary artery to be dilated. The dilating catheter is then inserted and manipulated into the stenotic area of the artery. Angiography is performed and heparin administered to avoid clot formation at the catheter site. When the dilatation catheter is placed over the stenosis, it is inflated for 5–6 s and then deflated. Blood flow around the balloon is assessed by angiography. Once it has been decided that maximum dilatation has been obtained, the catheters are removed.

Following this procedure, the patient is usually routinely attached to a cardiac monitor for 24 h. Peripheral pulses are frequently checked for occlusive thrombus at the insertion site. The patient is advised to rest for 4–6 h, lying as flat as is comfortably possible, to keep the leg used for catheter insertion straight in order to minimise the risk of thrombus formation at the insertion site. The introducer sheath is often left in situ for 2–3 h, until the effects of heparin have been reduced.

The patient should be encouraged to drink extra fluid to help eliminate contrast medium.

Because of the risk of thrombosis and coronary artery spasm after angioplasty, patients are often prescribed calcium antagonists and antiplatelet agents.

Re-stenosis occurs in 15–30% of patients, more frequently within the first few months. Repeat angioplasty may be appropriate for some patients.

Possible complications
Complications tend to be sudden and include:

- myocardial infarction
- chest pain
- vagal reaction
- intimal injury
- bleeding at the puncture site
- occlusive thrombus at the puncture site
- coronary artery spasm
- coronary artery dissection.

fully mobile the day after the procedure and to be discharged home after 2 days. Discharge planning should include teaching about medication, risk factor modification and follow-up assessment (Jensen et al 1993). An exercise test may be performed prior to discharge, and a thallium scan, which detects myocardial perfusion, can give further information as to the patency of the vessel.

If re-stenosis does occur, the procedure can be repeated.

Coronary artery stents

Laser angioplasty and coronary artery stents are increasingly being used as an alternative to conventional angioplasty. There are two main types of stent — coil and mesh — which are inserted into the widened coronary artery during cardiac catheterisation. Intravascular ultrasound is useful for accurate placement of the stent.

Patient management is similar to angioplasty, although more time may have to be spent in hospital in order for the patient to be stabilised on warfarin. De Feyter et al (1996) provide an overview of coronary artery stenting.

Coronary artery bypass grafting (CABG)

This is now a routine operation performed on patients whose angina is severely limiting their lifestyles but whose left ventricle is functioning reasonably. It may also be carried out in an emergency on patients who have uncontrolled angina after an AMI or who have experienced complications after angioplasty. The procedure is described in Box 2.5.

Bypass surgery is a potentially traumatic event, and prior to the procedure the nurse must address any worries or concerns that the patient may have. Pre-admission education programmes have been found to be beneficial in reducing anxiety in some patients (Nelson 1996); a visit to the operating theatre and the ITU may also help. Male patients need to know that their chest will be shaved prior to the operation. Patients also need to know that they may be asked to take a bath using antibacterial soap. An aperient may be required to reduce the likelihood of postoperative abdominal discomfort. Patients will be asked to fast prior to surgery and may benefit from a sedative to help them relax the night before.

The nurse should prepare the patient for what to expect on regaining consciousness, i.e. an endotracheal tube, chest drains, intravenous infusions, arterial lines, urinary catheter, cardiac monitoring, and possibly a nasogastric tube. The patient should be taught breathing, coughing and leg exercises.

After the operation, nursing objectives include:

- pain relief (see Hancock 1996a,b)
- fluid management — patients can quickly become dehydrated
- assistance with activities of living
- psychological support — patients may become disoriented and confused and need help coming to terms with the effect of the operation (Laitinen 1996)
- preparation for discharge home.

Patients should be told to expect pain from the sternotomy for several weeks, leg swelling, and discomfort on coughing or lifting the hands above the head. Short-term anxiety and depression may occur if the person feels that recovery is slower than anticipated. The spouse and other family members will also need information and support.

Minimally invasive cardiac surgery. Some centres in the UK are now performing keyhole surgery on patients with coronary artery disease. This has the advantage of reducing patient problems associated with sternotomy, including less pain, increased mobility and a reduced hospital stay. The left internal mammary artery is grafted through an incision between the fourth and fifth intercostal spaces. Pre- and postoperative care is similar to that in conventional cardiac surgery.

Revascularisation without cardiopulmonary bypass. This procedure involves a median sternotomy and limited thoracotomy and is a new alternative to the conventional approach (Campanella 1997). Potential advantages include decreased transfusion requirements, reduced incidence of low cardiac output syndrome, shorter hospital stay and lower costs.

Box 2.5 Coronary artery bypass graft surgery (CABG)

Purpose

Coronary artery bypass graft surgery is a technique in which an occluded or stenosed section of a coronary artery is bypassed using part of a vein or artery from elsewhere in the body. Most commonly the long saphenous vein is used, although increasingly the internal mammary artery is being considered. The objectives of CABG are:

- restoration of perfusion and increased oxygenation to the ischaemic myocardium in the peri-infarction patient
- relief of angina pectoris
- improvement of functional status and quality of life
- prolongation of life.

Surgery is only feasible if the risk of the operation is less than continuing with medical therapy. The procedure tends to be offered to those who have:

- symptoms despite maximum therapy
- triple vessel disease or left main stem coronary artery stenosis
- unstable angina.

Procedure

During surgery, the heart is exposed by median sternotomy, the aorta clamped off and cardiopulmonary bypass maintained via cannulae in the descending aorta. The body temperature may be reduced to 32°C and cardiac arrest induced with potassium.

Revascularisation with arterial grafts is becoming more common, as they last longer (10–15 vs. 5–10 years for veins). The internal mammary artery is biologically superior for grafting compared with the saphenous vein.

The artery or vein being used is harvested whilst the chest is being opened. The distal end of the bypass graft is sutured to as many vessels as required. The aorta is then unclamped, the patient rewarmed (if cooling has been used) and normal cardiac rhythm re-established by internal defibrillation. The proximal ends of the grafts are sutured to the ascending aorta and cardiopulmonary bypass is then stopped, the cannulae removed and the chest closed. The whole operation takes up to 4 h.

The patient is normally cared for in an intensive care unit after the procedure and will be ventilated until she is haemodynamically stable. An arterial line and pulmonary artery flotation catheter will be used to monitor cardiac pressures for 24 h.

The patient will usually be able to eat a solid diet on the first or second day. Activity is increased as tolerated over the first 2 days and early mobilisation is encouraged. Patients are often fit for discharge home after about a week.

Possible complications

Complications include:

- leakage at the incision site, producing discomfort and shock
- hypertension as a result of increased sympathetic activity
- hypotension as a result of reduced cardiac output following hypothermia
- pain at both the graft and incision sites
- post-pump cardiotomy syndrome (up to 3 months)
  —problems with coordination
  —loss of memory
  —loss of sense of taste
  —disturbance of vision
- shortness of breath due to heart failure or chest infection.

Fast-tracking. Patients are increasingly being 'fast-tracked' after cardiac surgery (Howard 1996). This focuses on early extubation and a move away from elective overnight ventilation post-surgery. The recovery of low-risk patients can therefore be managed without overnight admission to the ITU.

Q

2.8 In a group, discuss whether someone with persistent angina who continues to smoke warrants CABG.

2.9 Find out the relative costs of PTCA and CABG. What are the advantages and disadvantages of each procedure?

2.10 Read Case History 2.1(C).

(a) What information will Mr B require before discharge on the following:
- cardiac catheterisation site
- reasons for failure of angioplasty and what this implies
- imminent surgery.

(b) What other health professionals might you contact to provide him with information and support?

Case History 2.1(C) Mr B

Mr B's angioplasty is unsuccessful, as it has not been possible to enter the left coronary artery (LCA) and pass the balloon over the occlusion. The patient is returned to the ward after 2 h in the cardiac catheterisation room. He is told that he can go home that evening and is asked to return in 2 weeks for cardiac surgery.

The procedures outlined above unfortunately do not stop the process of atherosclerosis; they only delay it and aim to provide the sufferer with a good quality of life for a while. All procedures can be repeated, but ultimately the blood supply may become insufficient to sustain the ventricle so that cardiac failure ensues.

ACUTE MYOCARDIAL INFARCTION (AMI)

Myocardial infarction, also known as a heart attack or a coronary, refers to the death or necrosis of a portion of myocardium as a result of reduction, interruption or cessation in blood flow. Nearly all the deaths from CHD are the result of an AMI. In the UK, some 300 000 people suffer an AMI each year, of which about 50% are fatal. In 25–30% of cases, the patient with AMI dies before reaching hospital (British Heart Foundation 1998).

PATHOPHYSIOLOGY

Myocardial cells require a constant supply of oxygen and nutrients in order to generate the high-energy phosphate compounds required for contraction. Generally, myocardial cells are irreversibly injured by 30–40 min of total ischaemia. It is now clear that AMI almost always results from total occlusion of a coronary artery by a thrombus, usually at the site of a recently cracked or fissured atheromatous plaque. If the lumen of an artery is blocked for about 20 min, and blood supply by the small vessels of the surrounding collateral circulation is inadequate, MI may develop. Surrounding the area of necrotic tissue there is usually a zone of injury. This

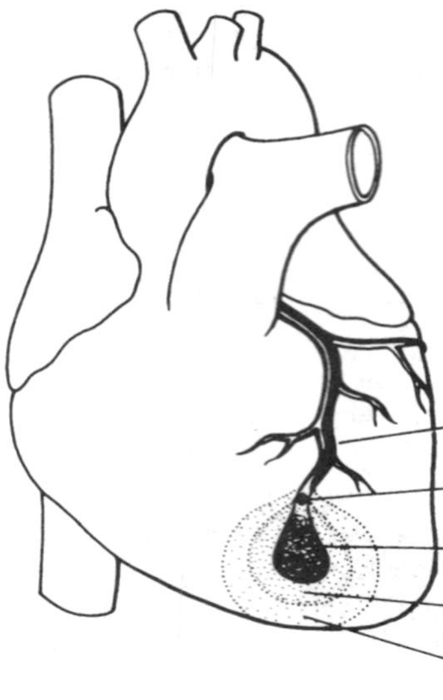

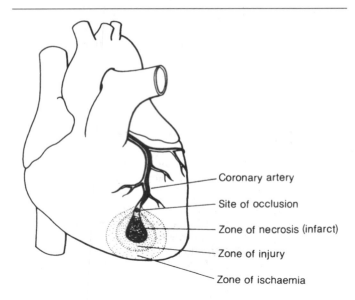

Fig. 2.8 Zones of necrosis, injury and ischaemia. (Reproduced with kind permission from Boore et al 1987.)

tissue cannot contract but may be salvaged if an adequate blood supply can be quickly established and is sometimes known as 'hibernating' myocardium. The ischaemic zone separates the zone of injury from undamaged tissue. This tissue can usually be salvaged if treatment is prompt (see Fig. 2.8).

During the first 6 h after the onset of symptoms, the affected myocardium becomes oedematous and swells. There is a shift in the distribution of sodium and potassium ions and an increased risk of arrhythmias. A summary of events following an AMI is given in Table 2.3. The infarcted area is replaced by fibrous scar tissue over the course of 3–6 weeks.

The site of infarction depends on the coronary artery which has become occluded. The extent of infarction, and therefore the amount of muscle involved, depends on the artery involved, the previous rate of progression of the disease and the effectiveness of the surrounding collateral circulation. In over 50% of fatal MIs, death occurs in the first hour after the attack, usually as a result of a cardiac arrhythmia.

Common presenting symptoms. Myocardial infarction can occur both in people who are known to have angina and in those who are not. Pain is usually experienced about 60 s after the onset of ischaemia and occurs in the majority of people suffering an AMI, but is less likely to be experienced in the elderly or in those with diabetes. Pain typical of MI often:

- occurs at rest
- awakens the individual from sleep
- is unrelieved by rest or nitrates
- lasts longer than 20 min
- is described as crushing, vice-like, tight or constricting in nature
- may radiate to the arms and neck.

Other signs and symptoms may include:

- shortness of breath at rest, on exertion or when lying flat
- hyperventilation as a result of anxiety
- change in cardiac rhythm or rate
- change in blood pressure
- change in level of consciousness
- increased anxiety or restlessness
- pallor
- sweaty or clammy skin
- nausea and vomiting
- cyanosis.

Table 2.3 Events following AMI. (Adapted, with kind permission, from Boore et al 1987)

Length of time following AMI	*Event*
0–6 h	Cellular breakdown No electrical impulses conducted Necrosis occurs
24 h	Phagocytosis occurs in the infarcted area
5 days	Area infiltrated by fibroblasts, capillaries and collagen tissue Reperfusion of capillaries
2–3 weeks	Fibrosis occurs
2–3 months	Ventricular scarring

MEDICAL MANAGEMENT

Diagnosis of AMI may be difficult in the early stages. The ECG may be non-diagnostic and the pain difficult to quantify. Biochemical markers (cardiac enzymes) may also be non-specific. Therefore, high-risk patients with atypical presentations need to be observed closely.

The modern management of AMI has been divided into three overlapping stages:

- treatment of the acute attack through:
  —relief of symptoms by analgesics (opiates) plus antiemetic; oxygen and nitrates
  —monitoring for and treating life-threatening complications
  —modification of the infarct process by means of improved blood supply, thrombolysis, aspirin or PTCA
  —reduction of oxygen demand by rest and beta-blockade and alteration of early physiological changes by angiotensin-converting enzyme inhibition (ACE inhibitors)
- risk stratification (1–6 weeks)
- secondary prevention (1 week onwards).

Patients should ideally be managed on a coronary care unit (CCU) and preferably be admitted there directly. In hospitals where suspected AMI patients are admitted to A&E departments, nurses have a role in identifying patients experiencing an acute cardiac event so that they can then be moved quickly to the CCU, a process known as 'fast-tracking'. Fast-tracking has implications for training and resources for paramedic personnel and staff in A&E departments and admission wards.

History and examination. The history provides subjective information about the presenting symptoms, previous patterns of health and illness, and the activities of living. A family history of ischaemic heart disease together with risk factor identification and social and psychological background adds to the picture.

It may be inappropriate to obtain a full history if the patient is in pain or acutely ill. An initial assessment can be enough to set early priorities, without a full physical examination or diagnostic tests.

Clinical examination includes:

- observation of general appearance, build, body posture and facial expression

- assessment of the location, nature and severity of the pain, any relieving or aggravating factors, and attempted methods of pain relief
- observation of other signs of reduced cardiac output
- vital signs — arrhythmias are common; blood pressure may be low with reduced cardiac output or high due to pain and anxiety
- temperature — slight pyrexia is a common response to muscle damage
- auscultation — usually performed by medical staff, this involves using a stethoscope to listen to the sounds the heart makes throughout the cardiac cycle, to identify heart murmurs produced by changes in the force and direction of blood flow
- palpation — usually performed by medical staff and involving a systematic examination of the chest to feel for abnormal vibrations or pulsations.

Investigations. These are as follows:
Electrocardiogram may show characteristic changes, pinpointing the area of ventricle affected. The ECG is an imperfect diagnostic tool and, as early ECGs may appear normal, a series is necessary. The classic infarct change is ST elevation (see Fig. 2.9).
Blood tests

- *Cardiac enzymes.* Myocardial necrosis results in the release of certain intracellular enzymes into the circulating blood. The rate and pattern of release are important (see Table 2.4). The traditional role of biochemical testing has been to provide retrospective confirmation of the presence or absence of AMI through sequential measurement of cardiac enzymes on consecutive days. Modern analytical equipment now allows for conventional enzymes to be measured in minutes. Bedside analysis is possible, with rapid diagnosis having implications for patient triage and shortening length of hospital stay. Increasingly, measurement of cardiac troponins is allowing cardiac damage to be diagnosed with high sensitivity and specificity. Measurement of cardiac troponin T and cardiac troponin I also allows prognostic risk stratification of patients with unstable angina.
- *White cell count.* This is usually elevated for the first few days following AMI.
- *Erythrocyte sedimentation rate (ESR).* This usually rises after the first few days and may remain elevated for several weeks.
- *Glucose.* Stress-related hyperglycaemia is common in the acute phase following infarction. Previously undetected diabetes is found in about 5% of coronary patients admitted to hospital.
- *Electrolytes.* It is important to know the serum sodium and potassium levels, as these electrolytes can have a major effect on cell excitability.
- *Lipids.* The important lipids in ischaemic heart disease are plasma cholesterol and triglycerides. Total cholesterol should be measured within the first 24 h and a full lipid profile done at 6–8 weeks.

Chest X-ray may show evidence of pulmonary oedema or hypertrophy.
Prevention of complications. AMI is a very serious condition in the early stages, although the risks diminish rapidly after the first 48 h. AMIs affect different areas of the heart and therefore put the patient at risk of various complications. Careful observation of the patient will help in the prevention, or at least early treatment, of these complications to prevent them becoming life-threatening.

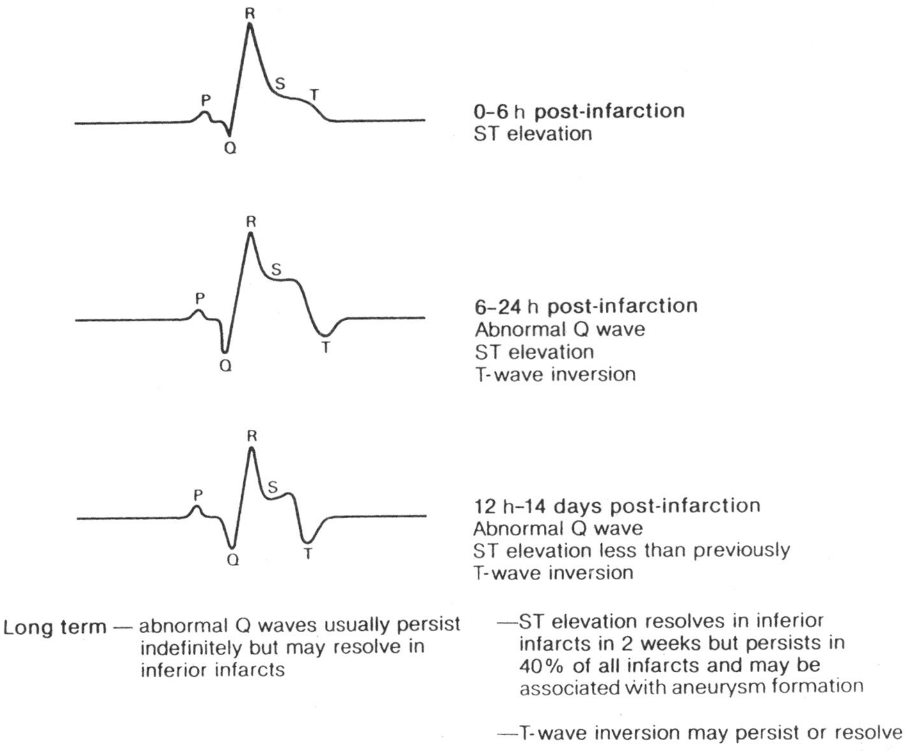

Fig. 2.9 ECG changes in myocardial infarction. (Reproduced with kind permission from Boore et al 1987.)

Table 2.4 Changes in enzyme levels following AMI

	Released into circulation		
Enzyme	*Initially*	*Peaks*	*Range (normal)*
Creatinine phosphokinase (CPK)	6 h	18–36 h	200–1000 u/mL (100 u/mL)
Serum aspartate transferase — formerly glutamic oxaloacetic transaminase (SGOT)	12–24 h	36–48 h	>100 u/ml (50 u/mL)
Lactic dehydrogenase (LDH)	2–3 days	7 days	

NURSING PRIORITIES AND MANAGEMENT: THROMBOLYTIC THERAPY

The nurse needs to be aware of patient selection criteria and be able to assist in identifying patients who are candidates for therapy (Box 2.6). An awareness of contraindications for therapy and of the importance of initiating therapy as soon as possible after the onset of chest pain is also necessary. Mortality in patients given thrombolytic drugs sufficiently early is one-third less than in those left untreated. Nurses in some CCUs are taking on the responsibility of prescribing thrombolytic therapy in accordance with agreed protocols (Quinn 1995, Rhodes 1998). The nurse should explain to the patient the benefits and potential problems of this therapy. It is important that the nurse is aware of possible complications so that he can monitor and observe appropriately.

On discharge, people who have been thrombolysed receive a card, indicating what drug they received and when. It may be inappropriate for them to have a second treatment with certain thrombolytics. Thrombolysis does not have any effect on the underlying cause of thrombus formation and re-occlusion remains a problem. Heparin, warfarin and aspirin have been used to reduce re-thrombosis and there is increased interest in drugs that act directly on the thrombus. Patients may require subsequent mechanical recanalisation with either PTCA (rescue angioplasty) or surgery.

Primary angioplasty

Angioplasty used instead of thrombolytic therapy in acute infarction results in better patency and causes fewer strokes. Patients most likely to gain from this procedure are those with cardiogenic shock, anterior infarcts and the elderly. However, primary angioplasty is unlikely to become widely available because most patients with MI are admitted directly to hospitals without intervention facilities (De Belder & Thomas 1997).

For further information on the use of thrombolytic therapy, see Kynman (1997).

NURSING PRIORITIES AND MANAGEMENT: AMI

Most patients admitted to hospital are likely to benefit from admission to a CCU for monitoring and thrombolytic therapy. These units were first established in the 1960s in order to provide surveillance from skilled personnel with electrocardiographic and resuscitation facilities in a specialised setting.

Possible patient problems include:

- pain and discomfort
- fear and anxiety
- decreased activity levels
- lack of knowledge and understanding
- misconceptions
- altered activities of living
- loss of control
- ineffective or inappropriate coping responses.

Immediate priorities

The priorities on admission to hospital include:

- cardiac monitoring (see Table 2.5); ECG
- establishment of intravenous access
- relief of pain and anxiety
- thrombolytic therapy
- decrease in the workload of the heart.

Nursing management reflects the above and is also aimed at:

- observation for signs of complications
- rehabilitation and recovery.

For a critical care pathway illustrating the management of AMI, see Figure 2.10.

Maintaining a safe environment

The nurse is responsible for the patient's safety. This involves being aware of possible complications and how they are likely to present. The temptation to respond to monitor tracings without concurrently assessing the patient should be avoided.

Pain control. The patient must be kept free from pain. It is a sign of ongoing myocardial ischaemia and should be controlled. Patients should be told of the importance of reporting pain.

Accurate pain assessment is essential to ensure that appropriate analgesics are given. Assessment scales, where patients rate their pain numerically, can be useful. Pain can be difficult to assess and nurses have been shown to be unreliable in assessing cardiac pain (O'Connor 1995), although this can be improved with appropriate education (Thompson et al 1994). Ischaemic pain can easily be confused with pain from other sources, particularly pericarditic or pleuritic pain (see Table 2.6). Opiates are the first-line analgesics for ischaemic pain, and diamorphine i.v. is the drug of choice. It is likely to produce beneficial effects through:

- decreasing anxiety through action on the central nervous system
- vasodilatation of the peripheral circulation
- central nervous system sedation and primary analgesia through stimulation of opiate receptors.

Intravenous diamorphine reaches its peak effect within 20 min of administration. Undesirable effects include:

- nausea and vomiting, due to reduced gut motility, so it should be given with an antiemetic
- depressant effects on the central nervous system, so the antidote naloxone should be available
- hypotension, if vasodilatation occurs alongside hypovolaemia
- dry mouth and slow heart rate as a result of decreased sympathetic activity.

Q **2.11** In a group, discuss how the management of cardiac ischaemic pain might differ between the person cared for on a CCU and someone cared for on a general medical ward.

Box 2.6 Thrombolytic therapy

Purpose

The primary aim in limiting infarct size is the rapid recanalisation of the occluded coronary artery. Occlusion is most often caused by a thrombus at the site of a ruptured atheromatous plaque. The aim of thrombolysis is to induce dissolution of the thrombus through the administration of an intravenous drug in order to establish recanalisation and provide subsequent reperfusion to the ischaemic zone. Thrombolysis is the single most important advance in coronary care since defibrillation, resulting in increased survival and quality of life.

Action

Optimal benefit results when the thrombolytic drug is given promptly after the onset of chest pain, although it is considered worthwhile administering the treatment up to 12 h later. The main thrombolytic drugs currently available are:

- *Streptokinase* — to date, the most widely tested and used, and also the cheapest. It is a bacterial protein whose administration results in a systemic lytic state, with reduced levels of circulating fibrinogen and clotting factors V and VIII. Once given, a patient cannot receive this drug again for at least 4 years.
- *Recombinant tissue-type plasminogen activator (tPA)* — a naturally occurring human protease that is fibrin-specific and thus works predominantly on the clot, with less risk of systemic bleeding.
- *Reteplase* — a new generation thrombolytic which appears to be as effective as streptokinase. It has the advantage that it can be given as a bolus and is non-antigenic.

Patient selection

Patients considered to be having an acute myocardial infarction, with the onset of symptoms within the previous 12 h. Contraindications include:

- active or recent bleed
- major surgery or trauma within the previous month
- cerebrovascular accident within the previous 3 months
- severe systemic hypertension.

Reperfusion

Signs and symptoms of reperfusion may include:

- abrupt cessation of chest pain
- reperfusion arrhythmias or conduction disturbances
- rapid return of the ST segment to normal
- improved left ventricular function
- an early peak in cardiac enzymes as a result of enzymes being washed out of the infarct area by the reperfused artery.

Complications

These include:

- bleeding episodes (including rarely cerebral bleeds)
- reperfusion arrhythmias
- allergic reactions
- hypotension.

Table 2.5 Observing the cardiac monitor[a]

Parameter	*Aspect to note*
Rate	Is it fast/slow/normal?
Rhythm	Is it irregular/regular?
P waves	Are they present/absent?
QRST complex	Is each complex preceded by a P wave? Is each complex the same?
PR interval	Is it normal/prolonged?
Ectopics (extras)	Are there any extra P waves or extra QRST complexes?

[a]While observing, note whether the patient is experiencing any symptoms, such as pain, shortness of breath or light-headedness.

Patients need to know that they may experience episodes of angina pain after discharge. They should be aware of the importance of reducing activity if pain occurs and feel confident to use glyceryl trinitrate (GTN). They should also know how to distinguish between angina and another heart attack. GTN, available in tablet or spray form, should be taken for angina pain and patients need to appreciate that it is not addictive and will not mask the symptoms of a heart attack. GTN can also be taken before doing something known to produce pain. It should be taken sublingually and the person should sit down before taking it, to minimise the risk of fainting. Any pain should be resolved 5–10 min after taking the drug; if not, a further dose should be taken. Once the pain has gone, any remaining tablet should be spat out or swallowed.

GTN can produce unpleasant side-effects such as flushing and headache due to generalised vasodilatation. Paracetamol can be taken to ease a headache. Medical help should be obtained if pain is still present after 20 min. An ambulance is usually quicker than the general practitioner and patients should not hesitate to call 999. For effective use, GTN in tablet form needs to be:

- stored in a cool glass container without cotton wool
- stored at a temperature not exceeding 25°C
- replaced after 8 weeks of opening the bottle.

Observation of all vital signs is aimed at early detection of complications.

Pulse. The ECG will be continuously monitored on a screen. Knowledge of the normal rhythm is vital and diagnosis of arrhythmias is part of the CCU nurse's role.

Deviations from the normal must be noted and the patient's concurrent condition assessed. Someone who is in pain or who is anxious may be tachycardic (heart rate >100 beats/min) and the heart rate is likely to fall once analgesics have been given.

Blood pressure. Recording the patient's blood pressure is a means of assessing how effectively blood is being pumped from the left ventricle. Frequency of recordings needs to be balanced against the patient's need for undisturbed rest. A fall in blood pressure may indicate that further damage or complications are occurring and that there is a reduced supply to the vital organs. Cardiac output can also be assessed by examining perfusion in the peripheries.

Temperature. Pyrexia as a response to muscle damage is normal in the first 48 h, following which it should settle. Continued pyrexia may indicate pericarditis.

Respiration. The patient with AMI is given oxygen therapy in conjunction with analgesics on admission, to ensure oxygen uptake in the lungs is optimised. Dyspnoea may indicate hypoxia or the onset of pulmonary oedema, which is a serious complication. It can also be induced by anxiety. Raised anxiety levels in coronary

Care categories	Admission Day 1	Day 2	Day 3	Day 4/5	Day 5/6
Hospital location	CCU	Ward	→	→	Home
Personnel	Appropriate specialists	Cardiac rehabilitation Dietician Social services if necessary Physiotherapy/OT	→	→	→
Tests	12-lead ECG Chest X-ray, O_2 sat Cardiac enzymes × 2 FBC, U&Es Cholesterol	12-lead ECG Cardiac enzymes × 1 U&Es Echocardiogram	12-lead ECG	12-lead ECG	Risk stratification via exercise, stress testing and thallium imaging Cardiac catheterisation if necessary
Activities	Bed rest and commode privileges	Sit in chair Self-care in bed/chair	Sit in chair ad lib Walk in bed area	Self-care as tolerated Walk to bathroom then walk in ward Supervised activity	Shower with supervision Walk in ward Climb stairs with supervision
Assessments	Pain assessment Vital signs/weight	→ Cardiac monitoring Intake/output	→	→	→
i.v. fluids and other medications	Oxygen Aspirin ? Thrombolytic s.c. Heparin Anxiolytic Diamorphine ß-blocker	Oxygen prn Aspirin s.c. Heparin Anxiolytic GTN prn s/l ß-blocker Stool softener	Oxygen prn Aspirin Anxiolytic GTN prn s/l ß-blocker ? ACE inhibitor ? Stool softener	Aspirin Anxiolytic GTN prn s/l ß-blocker ? ACE inhibitor ? Stool softener	Aspirin GTN prn s/l ß-blocker ? ACE inhibitor Anxiolytic prn ? Lipid lowering drug
Diet	As tolerated (may feel nauseous)	→	→	→	→
Discharge planning	Evaluate social support and living conditions for after discharge	→	Evaluate need and initiate necessary home care (nursing, social services)	Determine discharge date Discuss with family	Arrange transport Check outpatient appointment Check cardiac rehabilitation follow-up
Teaching	Explain nature of illness and CCU environment	Explain causes of MI Explain reasons for and expected outcomes of therapy	Begin medication, diet and activity teaching	Risk factor analysis and modification Recovery over next few weeks How to manage any post-discharge symptoms	Reinforce discharge teaching to accommodate transition home Provide resource options for continued support and education after discharge
Psychosocial support	Encourage patient and family to express concerns Provide appropriate information Develop therapeutic relationship	→	→	→	→

Fig. 2.10 Critical care pathway for myocardial infarction.

Table 2.6 Characteristics of chest pain

Description	*Location*	*Medical diagnosis*
Tight, like a band around the central chest Precipitated by cold, exercise, large meals, emotion Usually relieved by rest and GTN	Central chest Radiating to jaw, shoulders and arms usually on left side	Angina pectoris
As above, but not relieved by GTN or other measures. Lasts longer and is more severe	As above	Myocardial infarction
Stabbing or burning pain Worse on deep inspiration, often relieved by bending forwards	Substernal and often affecting the trapezius muscle and upper abdominal area	Pericarditis
Sudden sharp pain, worsened by inspiration Dyspnoea, cough, cyanosis and possible haemoptysis	Lateral, very often	Pulmonary embolus
Excruciating pain 'burning' towards the spine	Intrascapular region	Dissecting aneurysm

patients admitted to hospital have been well documented, with serial measurements generally showing that anxiety is highest on admission to the CCU (Thompson 1990). To exclude anxiety from masking more serious complications, the patient may benefit from the use of anxiolytics for a short period, particularly at night. Pain must also be controlled.

Ongoing care

The majority of life-threatening problems develop within the first 36 h, and after this time the patient will be transferred to the ward. The move is likely to induce anxiety and the patient will be aware that the nurse–patient ratio has been reduced. Explaining that the immediate danger period is over and that she is now beginning to recover will help to convey optimism to the patient and family. Ideally, the transfer can be planned well in advance and the nursing staff on the ward should take time to discuss natural fears and vulnerability (Jenkins & Rogers 1995).

These same feelings are likely to resurface as the time of discharge from hospital approaches and again nursing staff must prepare both the patient and the family to resume their life as an integral unit.

Both in the CCU and on the ward the patient should have within reach articles she is likely to need, e.g. a glass of water, a book or an oxygen mask. This minimises danger and inconvenience when trying to reach these articles.

Any restrictions, such as not smoking and limiting activity, should be fully explained. Although certain activities should ideally be avoided, the patient may feel less stress if permitted a low level of involvement; for example, the businessperson who requires to continue working may rest more easily if she has some contact with her secretary.

Communicating

Someone who has suffered an AMI is likely to be worried about the eventual outcome. Some people are able to express their feelings openly, but others find this difficult. The nurse should try to probe beneath outward signs such as hostility, withdrawal and denial to ensure they are not masking fear. He should keep the patient informed of her progress and how it will affect her stay in hospital. Communication skills are important to CCU nurses and answers to questions should be honest and supportive. The hospital chaplain or the patient's own spiritual adviser may be of help in this area.

Communication must also extend to the family members. They experience shock and anxiety on seeing their loved one in such an environment and will fear for her survival. Involving family members, particularly the partner, in information-giving and support can significantly reduce distress at this time (Thompson 1990). Spending time with the relatives, both when they are visiting and when they are alone, may allow fears and worries to be expressed. Frequent and adequate information about the equipment and the patient's progress is vital. The family member whose trust is gained can be a source of information to the nurse and an ally in helping to reduce anxiety in the patient. Unrestricted visiting for designated close family members is also useful in reducing anxiety.

Appropriate advice for the patient and family in hospital may include (see Research Abstract 2.1):

- explaining the structure and function of the heart as a pump, where it lies in the body and how it works
- explaining how a heart attack occurs, narrowing of the coronary arteries, obstruction and heart muscle damage
- describing symptoms and explaining terminology
- outlining the reasons for admission and treatment
- explaining possible angina and shortness of breath that may be experienced after discharge
- explaining the healing process, muscle damage, swelling, scar formation and the healing period
- discussing the outlook for the future and the need to accept the illness
- describing the likely mobility level
- explaining the reasons for stopping smoking
- explaining how to recognise possible limiting factors in physical activity
- giving advice on diet, social activities and sexual life
- giving advice on resuming work
- being prepared for changes in mood, e.g. anxiety and depression (see Bennett & Mayfield 1998)
- preparation of the partner and family.

Preparation for discharge

Patients and their families need to be prepared for rehabilitation and recovery. Patients' needs for information and support should be assessed individually as people cope differently. For example, women have been found to have different concerns from men (Radley et al 1998).

Issues to be addressed include:

- concerns about resumption of activities, including return to work and sexual activity
- overprotectiveness by the family
- use of medication, including GTN

Research Abstract 2.1
Patient education after myocardial infarction

How do you decide the content of a patient education programme? What do you teach? Do patients feel that they need or want to know the information you provide? What do patients actually learn? When is the best time to learn?

In a study of 30 post-MI patients, Chan (1990) explored the views of patients pre- and post-discharge regarding how important and how realistic it was to learn the material presented.

It was found that most content areas, e.g. anatomy and physiology, diet, medication, physical activity, psychological factors and risk factors, were viewed as important for learning pre-discharge. However, all content areas were not of equal value. Some items such as 'how the heart works' and 'what the heart looks like' were given low ratings. This might have been related to different basic levels of insight and understanding of the body and disease processes. It may not always be wise, therefore, to introduce basic concepts of normal heart function before discussing myocardial infarction. What the nurse thinks is important may not be what the patient most wants to know.

It was also found that it was more realistic for patients to learn about illness and its management during early convalescence than before discharge. Readiness to learn and timing of teaching are therefore as important as content of teaching. Pre-discharge, patients may be physically debilitated and psychologically stressed and therefore less able to attend to teaching and learning. Follow-up education to reinforce and extend hospital-based education is important. Patient education pre- and post-discharge should be carefully planned and evaluated.

Chan V 1990 Content areas for cardiac teaching: patients' perceptions of the importance of teaching content after myocardial infarction. Journal of Advanced Nursing 15(10): 1139–1145.

- lifestyle changes
- uncertainty about informing the insurance company and Department of Social Security
- the need for definite guidelines about the amount of weight to lose and how to stop smoking.

Both community and hospital nurses have a role in tackling many of the above issues, so that the sufferer and family are equipped to cope with recovery and future lifestyle (Duddy & Parahoo 1992). Conflicting information needs to be avoided. There is an increasing number of coronary rehabilitation nurses who visit both in hospital and at home. The first 2 or 3 weeks at home can be the most stressful for the person and the family, particularly the partner, as they attempt to come to terms with a frightening and often unexpected event (Thompson et al 1995). Coronary rehabilitation programmes that offer individualised packages of information and support on both a one-to-one and group-session basis, in addition to a graduated programme of exercises, have the potential to restore the individual to an optimum level of recovery (physical, emotional, economic and vocational) and to minimise the risk of the underlying disease progressing. It is now recommended that every major district hospital treating people with heart disease should provide such a cardiac rehabilitation service (Thompson et al 1996). Home-based programmes involving cassette tapes and a manual have been shown to be effective for those not able to access a group programme (Lewin et al 1992, Linden 1995). Nurses working in primary care are also potential sources of support, particularly in the area of secondary prevention (Fullard 1998).

For further information on cardiac rehabilitation, see Thompson et al (1997).

2.12 Find out about cardiac rehabilitation services offered locally. What do you think are the benefits of such a programme? See Pell (1997) for a review of the effectiveness of cardiac rehabilitation.

Mobility

In hospital. While experiencing symptoms such as pain and dyspnoea, the patient should remain in bed and receive analgesics and oxygen therapy. The reasons for limiting activity (and that it is only for a short period) should be explained. As symptoms resolve, activity levels can increase.

In recent years, the trend has been towards early resumption of activity. This allows the patient to carry out activities such as washing, using the commode and carrying out passive and active limb exercises. Periods of gentle activity should be followed by frequent rest periods and all activity should be stopped if the patient experiences pain, dyspnoea or palpitations. The ability to increase activity gradually is a positive reinforcement for recovery and the patient's family will also experience relief at seeing the patient regain independence.

By the time of discharge, usually after 5 or 6 days, the person should be fully independent in the activities of daily living.

Some centres have programmes in which the patient can chart her progress towards specific goals (see Box 2.7). In other centres, activity is increased on a much less formal basis and the nurse can point out to the patient that she is making progress. Realistic aims, both pre- and post-discharge, are important.

The patient should be prepared to have good and bad days and be aware of symptoms that suggest she is doing too much, such as pain, palpitations, dyspnoea, fatigue and dizziness.

At home. Graduated physical activity should permit a return to previous daily activities over a 4–12 week period and, if applicable, return to work after 6–8 weeks. The ultimate aim should be to take some exercise at least three times a week. Recommended exercise, after 6–8 weeks, includes walking, swimming, and cycling, for 15–20 min at a time.

The activity plan for convalescence should be based on a knowledge of the person's functional capacity, interests, previous lifestyle, needs for the future and home environment. Any inhibiting factors such as arthritis also need to be acknowledged. Many hospitals now offer formal structured exercise programmes as part of a coronary rehabilitation programme. However, such programmes might not begin for 3–6 weeks after discharge and the patient needs specific advice to prepare for the first few weeks at home. For example, most patients will be able to walk 2 miles a day at the end of 4 weeks. Patients can resume driving 4 weeks after an uncomplicated MI, although HGV drivers have to show evidence of a negative exercise test. Return to work provides increased self-satisfaction, restored self-respect and relief from financial worries, although early retirement may be a more realistic option for some. Occupational health and community nurses can support the patient and family throughout convalescence.

For further information on the effects of exercise on CHD, see Davies (1997). See Allaker (1995) for information on the effects of exercise motivation and adherence in cardiac rehabilitation, and Jolliffe & Taylor (1998) for a review of the relationship between physical activity and cardiac rehabilitation.

The aim for all patients is that they will be able to resume their daily lifestyle without physical symptoms, but this depends on their residual left ventricular function. An important part of the rehabilitation process is teaching the person and family how to live with these new limitations. If there is residual ischaemic tissue and angina, drug therapy will help to control this (see p. 17).

Breathing
Oxygen therapy should be given alongside analgesics, to ensure maximal relief of pain. A semi-upright position also eases breathing. Smoking is not permitted if oxygen therapy is being given and the patient should be encouraged to give up this habit. Anxious people often hyperventilate and, here, deep breathing exercises may help.

Sleeping
The importance of punctuating exercise with rest periods is vital and people should be encouraged to have catnaps at home. In hospitals, night sedation may help the patient to settle in a strange environment where noise levels are often high. Interventions need to be coordinated to allow the patient undisturbed periods of rest. A patient who is unable to sleep at night often becomes worried and anxious. An observant nurse can talk to the patient and help to put these fears into perspective.

Fear of dying
This is a very real fear for someone who has had an AMI (Thompson et al 1995). Once the initial fear has subsided, the patient has to come to terms with the cause of the AMI and the consequences of atherosclerosis. Complications with a high mortality rate occur at two stages:

- in the first 48 h, when cardiogenic shock and arrhythmias cause death
- 7–10 days later, due to myocardial rupture and ventricular septal defect.

Family fears of death must also be discussed. If not put into perspective, relatives can become overprotective once the person returns home.

Diet and nutrition
In the early stages of AMI, the patient may have little appetite and opiates may induce nausea. Antiemetics should always be given in conjunction with opiates. Dietary advice needs to be tailored to the individual and will be similar to that given to those with angina pectoris.

Diabetic patients are likely to have raised blood glucose levels following a heart attack. There is evidence that rigorous control of plasma glucose by insulin infusion followed by subcutaneous insulin can have a significant effect on long-term prognosis, and therefore patients' blood glucose levels need to be monitored closely and insulin therapy altered accordingly (see Yudkin 1998).

Eliminating
Fluid balance is a vital means of assessing renal function, as 25% of cardiac output goes to the kidneys. If left ventricular function is compromised, fluid intake may be restricted to prevent the onset of cardiac failure and pulmonary oedema (p. 37). Electrolyte balance must also be maintained within normal limits and any deviations from normal acted upon.

Potassium regulation is important in the cardiac patient, as both low and high levels of serum potassium lead to life-threatening arrhythmias. Hypokalaemia causes ECG changes and increases the susceptibility to digoxin therapy and therefore toxicity. It can result from acidosis and diuretic therapy with insufficient potassium replacement. Hyperkalaemia in the cardiac patient also results in bradycardia and heart block, and leads to other

Box 2.7 A typical exercise programme for a patient following acute myocardial infarction

Phase 1 (in the coronary care unit)

Step 1
- Rest in bed. Out to chair for short periods
- 2-hourly passive range of motion exercises
- Twice-daily breathing exercises
- Independent with personal cleansing at bedside, i.e. wash hands and face
- Use bedside commode

Step 2
- Up to sit unlimited by bedside
- Walk around bed area

Phase 2 (in the ward area)

Step 3
- Walk to bathroom/toilet
- Personal cleansing in bathroom on chair

Step 4
- Unrestricted walking in ward area
- Sit in day room if desired
- Shower/bath unaided

Step 5
- Climb one flight of stairs
- Increase exercises, e.g. use of exercise bike

Phase 3 (early days at home)

Step 6 (first week at home)
- Stay within own home/garden
- Use the stairs 2–3 times daily
- Undertake any activity that involves standing for short periods, e.g. washing up, dusting, shaving
- Keep as active as possible and walk around little and often

Step 7 (second week)
- Walk approximately 100 yards on flat ground, increasing by approximately 10 yards daily, e.g. walk to the corner shop
- Use stairs 4–5 times daily

Step 8 (third week)
- Walk 250–300 yards, two or three times a day
- Use stairs as normal
- Begin to do light shopping, gardening or housework
- Take a bus

Step 9 (fourth week onwards)
- Begin to resume a normal way of life; participate in most normal daily activities, avoiding heavy gardening, moving heavy furniture, etc.
- Begin to take regular exercise, e.g. swimming and walking, progressing gradually
- Start driving again

ventricular arrhythmias. Causes include renal failure and tissue breakdown, which leads to large amounts of intracellular potassium being released into the circulation.

Sodium levels also require to be kept within normal limits. Assessment for obvious signs of fluid overload, such as oedema in the ankles and other dependent parts, and a daily weight check are also part of fluid-balance monitoring.

An increased workload is placed on the heart if there is straining at stool to aid defaecation. Aperients may be used to soften stools and attention should be paid to diet. A commode is usually easier to use than a bedpan and even someone confined to bed is likely to expend less energy using a commode than balancing on a bedpan.

Personal hygiene

Initially the patient with AMI will be dependent on nursing staff, but this is one of the first areas where independence can quickly be regained. It is possible even in bed to wash the face and upper body and by discharge to be fully independent. It is safer not to lock the bathroom door, in case of emergency, and the family should discuss how to maintain the person's privacy while using the bathroom.

Expressing sexuality

Although discussion of this intimate aspect of life is often difficult, sexual counselling should be an integral part of cardiac rehabilitation (Thompson & Webster 1992). The severity of the infarction and resulting cardiac decompensation are much less important causes of sexual debility than the person's psychological state. Reasons for not resuming previous levels of activity include:

- fear of chest pain or another heart attack
- feelings of depression
- partner concern about symptoms
- lack of, or poor, sexual advice from health professionals.

The energy levels and demands placed on the heart during sexual intercourse are comparable to walking briskly or climbing two flights of stairs. It is very rare for sexual intercourse to trigger off another heart attack and as a general guide sex can usually be resumed about 2 weeks after discharge, although touching and caressing may be comfortable for some earlier than this.

The subject of sex is best approached as a routine part of the rehabilitation of all coronary patients and their partners. The patient needs to feel at ease and the nurse needs to be well informed and prepared for questions. Written information may be useful as a starting point for discussion (Albarran & Bridger 1997). The aim of sexual advice is to restore the couple as nearly as possible to pre-infarction levels of sexual activity (Jones 1992).

Complications of AMI

There are a considerable number of complications of AMI, listed in Box 2.8. It is not possible to look at each one in detail, but the nurse should be able to recognise and report the following major problems and carry out the appropriate nursing intervention.

Cardiac arrest

Cardiac arrest may be defined as failure of the heart to pump sufficient blood to keep the brain alive. The three main mechanisms of cardiac arrest are:

- ventricular fibrillation (VF)
- ventricular asystole
- electromechanical dissociation (EMD).

Box 2.8 Complications of acute myocardial infarction

- Sudden death
- Arrhythmias
- Cardiac failure
- Hypoxia
- Hypotension
- Cardiogenic shock
- Papillary muscle insufficiency
- Ventricular septal defect
- Ventricular aneurysm
- Myocardial rupture
- Pulmonary embolus
- Pericarditis
- Deep vein thrombosis
- Post-MI syndrome
- Emotional difficulty

Brain death usually occurs because of the failure of oxygenation of brain cells associated with either failure in ventilation or failure of the heart to pump oxygenated blood to the brain. The brain can tolerate only 4–6 min of anoxia. The signs of cardiac arrest are:

- abrupt loss of consciousness
- absent carotid and femoral pulses
- absent respirations.

A rapidly developing pallor often associated with cyanosis follows. Apnoea, gasping and gagging may occur.

The risk of sudden death in AMI patients is great. In 25% of cases, this occurs within minutes of the onset of pain, before the patient has reached hospital. The nurse must be familiar with resuscitation procedures within the hospital but should also know how to perform basic cardiopulmonary resuscitation (CPR) without hospital technology. If he can administer CPR in the community setting, someone's life may be saved. Training programmes in basic CPR for lay people are aimed at reducing this very high early mortality rate, as are the development of trained paramedical staff in ambulances, mobile coronary care units and defibrillators in public places.

Nurses working in cardiac wards are increasingly expanding their roles to incorporate advanced life support skills. To be effective, regular training update is necessary (ideally 6-monthly), particularly for those who do not use these skills frequently (Broomfield 1996b, Inwood 1996).

The risk of sudden death remains high for the first 24 h, following which it rapidly diminishes. In the CCU, cardiac arrest may be anticipated; in the ward it is often diagnosed by the nurse, who finds the patient unconscious and pulseless. This is an emergency and every nurse is responsible for:

- recognising that cardiac arrest has occurred
- knowing the procedure for summoning help within the hospital
- commencing effective resuscitation.

The priorities of CPR are:

- airway
- breathing
- circulation.

The nurse is also responsible for maintaining the person's comfort and dignity, anticipating events and procedures, and giving care and support to the patient and relatives after the event.

Restoration of an oxygenated blood supply to the brain involves artificial ventilation and external cardiac massage.

Medical help should be summoned once it has been established that the patient is not breathing. Presence of breathing is assessed by looking for a rise and fall in the chest wall, listening for any breath sounds and feeling for any expelled air.

Artificial ventilation involves:

- maintaining a clear airway through the removal of loose-fitting dentures, food, sputum, vomit or other debris
- performing the head tilt/chin lift (or the head tilt/jaw thrust if suspected spinal injury) method to allow maximum air entry with the patient in a supine position
- inserting an oesophageal airway, laryngeal mask or endotracheal tube if available
- ventilating the patient mouth to mouth, mouth to mask or with a self-expanding bag and valve mask and pure oxygen if available
- observing for a rise and fall in the patient's chest wall.

The patient should be given two effective rescue breaths (determined by a rise and fall in the patient's chest wall) before assessing for signs of circulation. Each rescue breath should last about 2 s, with a pause of 2–4 s before the next breath.

Circulation is assessed by feeling for a carotid pulse for up to 10 s. If there is no pulse then external cardiac massage needs to be commenced.

External cardiac massage can only provide limited cardiac output. If the arrest is witnessed, an initial blow to the chest (precordial thump) may be attempted, as this may restore the heart rhythm and takes only seconds to perform. Blood flow during cardiac massage is thought to occur due to increased intrathoracic pressure rather than direct heart compression. External cardiac massage involves:

- placing the patient supine on a firm surface
- placing the heel of one hand on the lower half of the patient's sternum, and the other hand on top of the first
- keeping the rescuer's arms straight and elbows locked
- kneeling level with the patient and applying firm downward pressure, depressing the sternum approximately 4–5 cm
- compressing the sternum at a rate of about 100/min.

The European Resuscitation Council (1998) recommends a cycle of two inflations followed by 15 compressions for one rescuer and one ventilation to five compressions for two rescuers (Fig. 2.11).

Drug therapy. Ideally, all drugs used during CPR are best administered through a central line to ensure swift distribution, as circulation time is greatly reduced. CPR should continue for 3 min to allow circulation of the drug.

Defibrillation involves the delivery of a direct current (DC) shock to the heart through the chest wall. This causes depolarisation of all the myocardial cells that are able to respond to a stimulus, thereby terminating the fibrillation and allowing the normal conducting pathways to regain control of the heart. Monophasic defibrillation, with the current going one way through the heart muscle, is increasingly being replaced with equipment that delivers a shock in two directions (biphasic). This means that lower energy levels are required and damage to myocardial muscle is reduced. The current can be delivered through hand-held paddles placed over gel pads or via pads stuck to the patient's chest. One pad should be placed below the right clavicle and the other over the apex of the heart in the fifth intercostal space. Ideally, the first shock should be administered within 90 s of the cardiac arrest. Precautions should be taken to ensure that floor surfaces are dry and all personnel warned that the shock is about to be delivered. Defibrillators that interpret the patient's heart rhythm and advise about defibrillation are increasingly available in areas where health professionals are less experienced in advanced life support and also in public places such as shopping centres and airports.

After-care. After successful resuscitation, the patient will require skilled nursing care. Full recovery can only be said to have occurred when the patient is fully conscious, with full cardiac, cerebral and renal function. The chances of achieving this are greatly enhanced if the patient is in a CCU where the arrest is witnessed and treatment initiated promptly. Success is less likely in the street where resources are limited.

Several body systems need assessment post-arrest, including the cardiovascular, renal, respiratory and central nervous systems. The patient may have been incontinent, have a sore chest and feel exhausted and somewhat embarrassed by her current state. An assessment of her level of orientation, recall, anxiety and general feelings should be made. The psychological support needed will vary. Relatives and witnesses to the arrest and the resuscitation attempt will also need support.

Ethical considerations. Unsuccessful resuscitation attempts do not enhance the dignity that is hoped for when we die. The appropriateness of merely prolonging the process of dying is often the subject of heated debate. The decision not to resuscitate should involve the patient and the family and be documented to avoid confusion. Policy also needs to be reviewed on at least a 24-h basis.

The joint statement of the British Medical Association and the Royal College of Nursing (1993) on CPR points out that 'do not resuscitate' (DNR) orders may be a potent source of misunderstanding and dissent amongst doctors, nurses and others involved in the care of patients. Issues surrounding this dilemma include whether resuscitation is appropriate, involvement of the patient and family in the decision-making process and communication difficulties between doctors and nurses once the decision is made (Mason 1996). Increasingly, living wills are being made by patients, and nurses need to be aware of the significance of these when making decisions about resuscitation.

2.13 Read the guidelines for decision-making in the joint statement. What are your local policies on CPR? How are decisions made in individual situations?

2.14 Should relatives be permitted to witness resuscitation attempts? See Connors (1996).

For further information on resuscitation, see Baskett & Strunin (1997).

Cardiogenic shock

This is a serious degree of heart failure, precipitated by extensive left ventricular damage in which the cardiac output is not sufficient to give an adequate blood pressure to maintain perfusion. The patient develops clinical shock with low urine output, cold clammy skin and hypoxia. Lactic acid is produced in the skeletal muscle beds as the metabolism changes, giving rise to a metabolic acidosis. This process is cyclical with the heart continually trying to pump harder for an ever falling stroke volume (see Ch. 18).

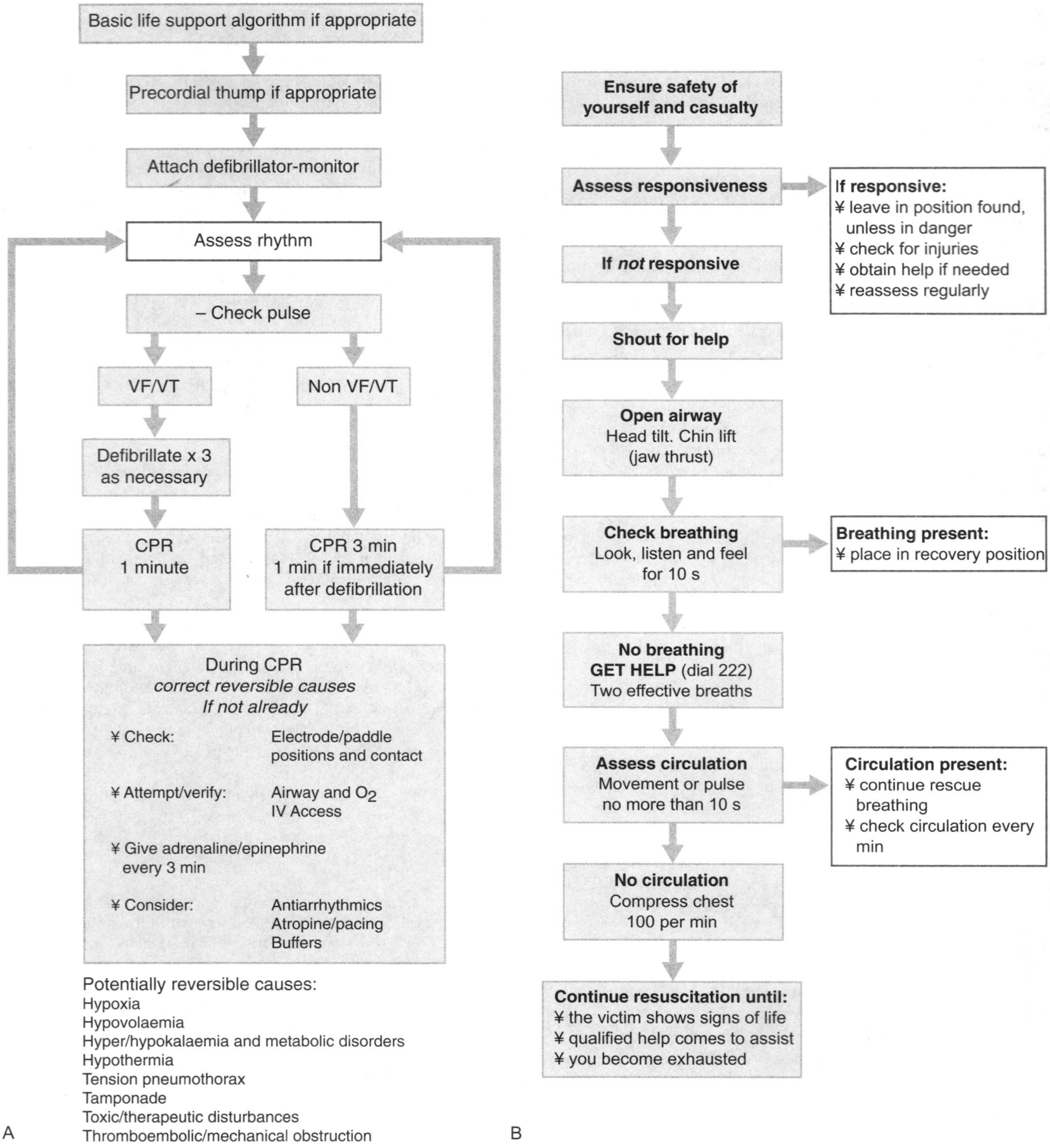

Fig. 2.11 Algorithm for the management of cardiac arrest in adults. (A) Basic life support. (B) Advanced life support. (Reproduced with kind permission from the European Resuscitation Council 1998.)

PATHOPHYSIOLOGY

Clinical features. In the early stages, the patient may be restless and agitated, followed by mental confusion and lethargy as cerebral hypoxia increases. The skin becomes cold and clammy to touch.
Examination. There will be signs of central cyanosis. Vital recordings will reveal a rapid, thready pulse, hypotension, tachypnoea and hypothermia. Urinary output will be reduced.

MEDICAL MANAGEMENT

The priorities are to:

- enhance cardiac output
- restore tissue perfusion
- effect a diuresis through increased renal flow.

The last of these is achieved by drug therapy, often requiring manipulation of multiple drugs to obtain the best effect for the patient. The aim is to improve cardiac output using inotropic drugs such as adrenaline, dopamine and dobutamine. These drugs, often given via a central line, improve cardiac output by increasing contractility and often heart rate, which increase the demand on the myocardium for oxygen. Cardiac output can also be improved by using vasodilators to reduce afterload. The use of nitrates will have the additional benefit of dilating coronary arteries, so increasing the supply of oxygen to the myocardium. Diuretics are widely used in cardiac shock to induce a diuresis and maintain glomerular filtration. The patient will require urinary catheterisation to assess hourly urine output and may be haemodynamically monitored using a pulmonary artery flotation (Swan–Ganz) catheter (see Ch. 18). If pharmacological intervention is ineffective in treating cardiogenic shock then more invasive therapy such as the intra-aortic balloon pump (IABP) or ventricular assist device may be required. Some patients may be appropriate for PTCA.

The outlook for patients developing cardiogenic shock is poor and mortality is high, as the process is very difficult to reverse.

NURSING PRIORITIES AND MANAGEMENT: CARDIOGENIC SHOCK

The priority in caring for these patients is prevention or early recognition of the signs that shock is developing (O'Neal 1994).
Observation. Recording and assessment of all vital signs are important. The pulse will initially be rapid and thready as a compensatory response to the falling cardiac output; in the late stages, bradycardia develops.

Initially, systolic and later diastolic pressure will fall. A fall in pulse pressure of more than 30 mmHg may be an indication that shock is developing in the hypertensive patient. The initial response to hypoxia is tachypnoea, which later becomes shallow and irregular. Some patients may benefit from oxygen therapy. Urine output falls as a result of the falling cardiac output.

Nursing management of these patients requires careful observation and recording of response to drug therapy. Patients are likely to become increasingly drowsy, confused, immobile and dependent on nursing care. They may also be lethargic or semi-conscious. Anxiety and fear need to be recognised and addressed (Williams 1992).

Small doses of opiates may promote comfort and rest. The relatives need time spent with them to explain the condition of their loved one and how they can best help. The hospital chaplain may provide comfort for the patient and family at this time.

Medical complications of AMI

This group of complications results in reduced cardiac output because there is specific failure of one area of myocardium.
Myocardial rupture. This very rare complication results in instantaneous death. It usually occurs 8–10 days after an extensive infarction in a heart with poor collateral blood flow. Necrosis occurs before fibrosis of the myocardium is complete, causing muscle rupture and the pumping of blood into the pericardium.
Ventricular septal defect. This occurs more frequently than rupture but in some cases is amenable to treatment. The pathophysiology is the same as that for myocardial rupture, with a hole developing in the septum separating the right and left ventricles. The right ventricle has to cope with increased pressures and blood volumes while the left ventricle suffers a fall in cardiac output. Rapid onset of cardiogenic shock may be the result. Operative repair can be undertaken but the mortality rate is high. If the patient can be supported for 2–4 weeks by aggressive medical management until the septum has become fibrosed, then the surgical results are slightly better.
Papillary muscle rupture. Loss of blood supply to the muscle supporting the mitral valve leads to prolapse and malfunctioning of the valve. If acute rupture occurs then sudden death may result. Surgical repair can be attempted, but again survival rates are low.
Ventricular aneurysm. This occurs when the infarction involves the full thickness of the myocardium. As the necrotic tissue is replaced by fibrous tissue, it is subject to the high pressures in the left ventricle. This fibrous tissue balloons out to form a blood pouch, which does not contract. Blood stagnation in this pouch leads to the development of thrombi, which may embolise. If a large area of myocardium is affected then it can lead to cardiac failure; if the aneurysm is near the papillary muscle or mitral valve then incompetence will result. Surgical resection can be undertaken successfully with some of the smaller aneurysms.
Pericarditis. This is thought to be due to an autoimmune reaction in which antigens from the damaged myocardium cause inflammation of the pericardium. The patient presents with pain at any time from 24 h to 1 week after the AMI. On examination, a 'friction rub' caused by friction between the pericardium and myocardium is often heard and is often accompanied by an unresolving post-infarction pyrexia. Medical treatment and nursing care involve treating the pain with analgesics and anti-inflammatory drugs such as aspirin and indomethacin. Reassurance that the pain is not an extension of the AMI is important.
Emboli. Embolism of a pulmonary or systemic vessel can occur after AMI. Emboli arise from clots forming in the healing myocardium or from circulatory stasis causing clot formation in the lower limbs. Nursing care involves maintaining passive exercises on the patient, whose mobility is restricted. The use of anti-embolism stockings should be considered. It is now becoming common practice for all post-AMI patients and those with known CHD to be given aspirin, which, taken daily, is thought to be effective in reducing clot formation. In most patients this may be sufficient, but in people with pulmonary emboli or who are known to have mural thrombi, a more aggressive approach to anticoagulation is required.

ARRHYTHMIAS

The term arrhythmia is used to imply an abnormality in either electrical impulse formation or electrical impulse conduction within the heart. An arrhythmia may cause an effect by any one of the following changes:

- change in heart rate
- increase in myocardial oxygen requirement
- decrease in myocardial blood flow
- loss of synchronicity of ventricular contraction.

PATHOPHYSIOLOGY

Clinical features. The clinical manifestation of an arrhythmia depends on the ventricular rate, the conduction of the myocardium and the psychological response of the patient. Patient problems include:

- palpitations
- dizziness
- faintness
- shortness of breath
- chest pain
- headache
- reduced activity tolerance
- anxiety.

Nursing assessment includes the apparent effect of the arrhythmia on the patient, a history of any past experiences of the problem, a knowledge of any relevant medications or other treatments and identification of any possible precipitating factors.

In cardiac disease, the normal sinus mechanism can be altered if the disease affects the heart's specialised conduction tissue. Various conditions result in specific conduction disturbances, and while this chapter cannot deal with them all, it will concentrate on a few of the more common ones with which the nurse should be familiar. In interpreting heart rhythms, the method used must be systematic and consider all components of the ECG complex.

Normal sinus rhythm should be recognisable to all nurses, as patients attached to cardiac monitors are increasingly nursed on general wards. The nurse's priorities are to:

- recognise and immediately report anything abnormal
- assess quickly the effect of the abnormality on the patient and take the appropriate action.

The normal electrocardiogram and the basic rules for observing cardiac monitors discussed earlier in the chapter apply here.

Sinus arrhythmias

The sinoatrial node is under autonomic control, primarily vagal, but is influenced by sympathetic stimulation, temperature, oxygen saturation and other metabolic changes. Sinus arrhythmias are often secondary to these influences.

Sinus arrhythmias are characterised by a constant PR interval but progressive beat-to-beat change in R–R intervals. During expiration, the reflex discharge of the vagal nerve slows the sinus mechanism; during inspiration this influence is diminished, allowing a speeding up of the sinus rhythm.

Sinus bradycardia

This meets the requirements for sinus rhythm but the rate is less than 60 beats/min. It may result from increased vagal tone but also results from hypothermia, certain medications, e.g. beta-blockers, raised intracranial pressure and inferior MI. Some individuals may experience sinus bradycardia when sleeping. It may be the norm in athletes.

Sinus tachycardia

This also fits the criteria for sinus rhythm, but this time the rate is greater than 100 beats/min. It is a direct result of decreased vagal tone and often a response to sympathetic stimulation.

NURSING PRIORITIES AND MANAGEMENT: SINUS ARRHYTHMIAS

Sinus arrhythmias tend to be observed and not treated directly. They are not life-threatening and resolution of the primary cause resolves the arrhythmia. Atropine i.v. is given for symptomatic sinus bradycardia.

Atrial arrhythmias

Atrial flutter

This is characterised by rapid and regular atrial excitation at a level above 200 beats/min. The AV node is not capable of conducting atrial rates above this level. The atrial waves form a sawtooth pattern. Ventricular deflections usually occur regularly within the atrial pattern and the block is described as a ratio, e.g. 4:1, which means 4 P waves per QRS complex.

Almost always associated with organic disease, it is not a stable rhythm and progresses to atrial fibrillation.

Atrial fibrillation

When individual muscle fibres of the atria or ventricles contract independently, they are said to be 'fibrillating'. There is rapid disorganised atrial depolarisation because the atrial tissues have lost synchrony with each other. The atrial waves can occur up to 600 times per minute. Ventricular depolarisation is also irregular as a result of the variable response at the AV node, but the QRS complex is normal. It occurs in congestive cardiac failure and mitral valve disease, and often presents with ischaemic changes in old age.

MEDICAL MANAGEMENT

Atrial fibrillation can severely compromise cardiac output, as the loss of the effect of atrial systole can reduce stroke volume by up to 25%. With chronic atrial fibrillation, the danger of thrombi forming in the atria and then embolising is high.

Treatment is aimed at reducing the rapid ventricular rate through chemical or DC cardioversion (Box 2.9) to revert to sinus rhythm. Cardioversion after digoxin therapy may precipitate ventricular fibrillation if large doses of digoxin have been used. Anticoagulation in the form of heparin or warfarin may be prescribed to reduce the risk of thrombi.

NURSING PRIORITIES AND MANAGEMENT: DC CARDIOVERSION

The procedure should be fully explained to the patient so that she is aware of what to expect. The thought of an anaesthetic and an electric current being put across the heart may be frightening. Care should be taken to ensure that the area is dry and that all personnel are warned that the shock is about to be delivered. The patient is likely to want to know the outcome of the procedure and this should be explained. Topical creams may help to ease any chest soreness.

Q **2.15** Clarify the differences between emergency defibrillation and elective cardioversion.

Box 2.9 Cardioversion

Purpose
The term 'cardioversion' is used to mean the delivery of a specific and predetermined amount of energy to the heart, timed (synchronised) in such a way that the shock is delivered well away from the vulnerable period of the T wave on the ECG. It is usually performed electively, with the patient lightly anaesthetised. This differs from defibrillation, which usually involves the delivery of a larger amount of electricity to a patient in ventricular fibrillation without anaesthetic, as the patient is usually unconscious. Elective cardioversion is used to treat supraventricular and ventricular arrhythmias.

Electrical treatment has the advantage that it is free from pharmacological side-effects.

Procedure
Cardioversion usually takes place at the patient's bedside. The patient is asked to remove any dentures or restrictive clothing. An ECG will be performed before and after the procedure, and the patient attached to a cardiac monitor throughout. Oxygen is given both before and after the procedure. A light anaesthetic is usually given and the patient asked to fast for 4–6 h. Resuscitation equipment needs to be on hand. The defibrillator is set to the required output and the paddles are placed in position on gel pads, usually with one below the right clavicle and the other over the apex of the heart in order to depolarise an optimum mass of myocardial cells. The patient is usually awake and talking 5–10 min after the procedure, although nausea and vomiting are not uncommon, as are a sore throat from the endotracheal tube and chest wall soreness due to the cardioversion. Cardioversion is often performed on a day-case basis.

AV junctional arrhythmias

The AV node, unlike the SA node, normally has no pacemaking role. Impulses must travel in both directions to stimulate atrial and ventricular contractions, so the position of the P wave varies. The QRS complex is of normal configuration and duration since the normal conduction pathway is followed below the AV node.

Junctional (nodal) tachycardia is similar to sinus tachycardia. Nodal tachycardia can occur in paroxysms or sustained rates. The rate is usually around 120–200 beats/min. The significance of the arrhythmia depends on its haemodynamic effect.

Supraventricular tachycardia. This applies to rapid arrhythmias that originate above the His bundle. Because of their rapid rate, P waves are difficult to see and often coincide with the previous T wave. The QRS is of normal configuration.

Medical management of supraventricular tachycardia aims to reduce the rapid ventricular rate using carotid sinus pressure or antiarrhythmic drugs, e.g. amiodarone, adenosine or digoxin. If these measures are unsuccessful then cardioversion may be indicated.

Ventricular arrhythmias

In these rhythms the ectopic focus arises below the AV node.

Ventricular tachycardia. The QRS complex looks wide and bizarre. The rate is regular at around 140–200 beats/min. It is generally caused by an irritable or ischaemic myocardium. Treatment, if the patient is symptomatic, is with immediate synchronised cardioversion and/or intravenous lignocaine. Other medication includes amiodarone and mexiletine. Persistent episodes of ventricular tachycardia may be treated with override pacing or ablation therapy (where the ectopic focus or source of the arrhythmia is identified and removed).

Ventricular fibrillation. In this rhythm, there are no distinguishable complexes on the screen and only an erratic baseline trace is evident. Treatment is by immediate initiation of resuscitation procedures and defibrillation.

Cardiac electrophysiology studies and ablation processes

Electrophysiology studies involve the introduction of an intravenous or intra-arterial catheter with multiple electrodes positioned at various intracardiac sites for the purpose of recording or initiating electrical activity from specific areas of the atria or ventricles. These studies are performed on patients with arrhythmias which are resistant to drug therapy, in order to identify the nature of the rhythm disturbance — also known as cardiac mapping.

Ablation therapy requires the delivery of a high-energy electric shock through a catheter in order to produce localised tissue damage in the unstable area identified as producing the arrhythmia.

For more details of these procedures see Lane (1997).

Implantable cardioverter defibrillators

The implantable cardioverter defibrillator is an electronic device used to detect and terminate potentially lethal arrhythmias through the delivery of an electric shock. Current models weigh less than 200 g and are implanted without open chest procedures. They are particularly suitable for patients who have survived one episode of cardiac arrest not thought to be the result of MI and for those with recurrent episodes of ventricular tachycardia unresponsive to optimal drug therapy. Appropriate patients are likely to need individualised information and support to enable them to cope with the concept of being dependent on the device.

For more information, see Stephenson & Combs (1996).

Heart block

This arrhythmia results when there is a delay or interruption of impulse conduction from the atria to the ventricles at the AV node. It is described as:

- first-degree heart block
- second-degree heart block
- complete heart block.

Heart block is usually a complication of myocardial infarction.

First-degree block appears as a prolonged PR interval with a mild bradycardia. It is asymptomatic and seldom requires treatment.

Second-degree block appears as occasional blocking; for example, there may be alternate conducted and non-conducted atrial beats, giving twice as many P waves as QRS complexes. The patient may have no symptoms and require no treatment. If a fall in blood pressure or other signs of reduced cardiac output develop, the heart block is treated pharmacologically with isoprenaline or by the insertion of a pacemaker (see Box 2.10).

Complete heart block exists when atrial and ventricular activity are uncoordinated. The atria and ventricles are electrically dissociated and desynchronised, with a subsidiary pacemaker developing in the ventricles. Cardiac output is reduced and the patient is haemodynamically compromised. The ventricles often contract at

Box 2.10 Pacemaker insertion

Purpose
Pacemakers are used to gain control over the electrical activity of the heart. They have two basic components:

- a pulse generator containing a power source and electrical circuitry
- one or two pacing leads, each with an electrode on its tip.

Pacemakers may be either temporary or permanent, depending on whether the pulse generator is located externally or implanted. If pacing is planned for a short duration, an external source is used to deliver electricity to the heart via the skin. When long-term control of the heart is required, a permanent pacemaker is implanted. The two most common modes of pacing are:

- demand (ventricular inhibited) — senses intrinsic cardiac rhythm and stimulates myocardial depolarisation and contraction as necessary
- fixed rate — fires at a predetermined rate, irrespective of intrinsic cardiac activity.

Temporary pacing
This is used to maintain cardiac output during episodes of extreme bradycardia, heart block and asystole. It may also be used for the suppression of tachyarrhythmias, which are resistant to drug therapy. It is usual for a special room to be set aside for temporary cardiac pacing, with ECG monitoring, fluoroscopy and resuscitation equipment being readily available.

Most commonly, a bipolar catheter is inserted into the subclavian vein, external jugular vein or antecubital fossa under local anaesthesia. The catheter is then passed into the right atrium and thence through the tricuspid valve and into the apex of the right ventricle, where the tip of the catheter is lodged against the ventricular wall. The external end of the catheter is stitched into place at the skin surface. The bipolar catheter is stimulated by the pacemaker's external pulse generator. Verification of pacing is judged from the appearance of a pacing spike preceding the QRS complex of the ECG. Pacing 'threshold' is obtained by determining the lowest voltage needed to elicit a paced beat, ideally less than 0.5 V. The threshold needs to be checked at least every 12 h, as it may increase over time.

Possible complications
These include arrhythmias, failure of the electrode to sense the heart's own electrical activity, failure of the electrode to generate a contraction, abdominal muscle twitching, pneumothorax and infection.

Permanent pacing
The decision to implant a permanent pacemaker is made after careful patient assessment. It is usually offered to patients with symptomatic bradycardias and heart block. The modern pacemaker is a small metal unit weighing between 30 and 130 g. It is powered by a lithium battery with a life of up to 15 years. Two types of pulse generator currently available are:

- single chamber with an electrode placed in either the atrium or the ventricle
- dual chamber with electrodes situated in both chambers.

The pacemaker is usually implanted under local anaesthesia in a cardiac catheterisation laboratory. The pulse generator is implanted in a subcutaneous pocket, usually under the clavicle, axilla or abdominal wall. The procedure is usually performed on a day-case basis.

a rate of less than 40 beats/min and a pacemaker requires to be inserted immediately to restore cardiac output. The nurse's role is one of observation, reporting and patient support.

For further details of cardiac arrhythmias and the appropriate medication, see Erickson (1996b) and Stanley (1996), respectively.

NURSING PRIORITIES AND MANAGEMENT: HEART BLOCK

The nursing management involves anticipating and resolving patient problems, monitoring the patient, including her response to treatment, and providing information and support.

Pacemakers

Nursing considerations include assessing pacemaker function, ensuring patient comfort and safety, preventing and dealing with complications, and teaching the patient about her condition and its management. The patient needs to be prepared for the procedure, even if it is done as an emergency (see Box 2.10).

Following pacemaker insertion, the patient should be attached to a cardiac monitor to assess whether the pacemaker is functioning properly. Cardiac output needs to be assessed frequently by recording the patient's blood pressure and asking her to report any symptoms of faintness, dizziness, chest pain or shortness of breath.

Limited mobility may make the patient more dependent on nursing care for a while. She should be aware of how long the temporary pacing is likely to continue and appreciate what is likely to happen next.

Removal of the temporary pacemaker is performed at the patient's bedside under aseptic conditions.

Permanent pacing

Initially, the nursing considerations are similar to those for temporary pacing. Some patients will be helped by a visit from a person who already has a permanent pacemaker, and also by being given an opportunity to handle a pacemaker. The patient needs to be reassured that the pacemaker will not be damaged by day-to-day activities. She should be taught to take her own pulse and be aware of the signs of reduced cardiac output. Signs of infection, such as redness or increased soreness at the implantation site, should also be reported. The importance of follow-up appointments should be explained. It is also useful to warn people that the pacemaker may trigger off alarms at airports.

HEART FAILURE

The term 'heart failure' is used to describe a clinical syndrome which results from an inability of the heart to provide an adequate cardiac output for the body's metabolic requirements.

The diagnosis of heart failure is not difficult to make, but discovering the underlying cause can be. Heart failure can result from primary heart disease or from non-cardiac causes (see Box 2.11). Many of these conditions are very common, particularly in the elderly. They are often found in combination, making their individual contribution to the heart failure difficult to assess. Non-cardiac causes include chronic obstructive airways disease (COAD), hyperthyroidism and chronic anaemia (see Chs 3, 5 and 11).

PATHOPHYSIOLOGY

Heart failure can involve either ventricle independently or both together. Pure left or right ventricular failure may not exist for long

Box 2.11 Primary cardiac conditions causing heart failure

Right heart failure
- Pulmonary hypertension secondary to left heart failure
- Congenital heart defect
- Thromboembolism
- Cor pulmonale
- Atrial septal defect
- Pulmonary venous stenosis

Left heart failure

Ventricular origin
- Coronary artery disease
- Aortic or mitral valve disease
- Congenital heart defect
- Hypertension
- Ventricular septal defect

Atrial origin
- Atrial myxoma
- Mitral stenosis

because of their dependence on each other to maintain adequate blood flow. It is useful to look at the heart as two pumps. The left ventricle can cope better with alterations in pressure and the right with alterations in volume. Failure of the left side of the heart causes accumulation of blood in the left ventricle and left atrium with subsequent congestion of the lungs. Right-sided failure, where the right ventricle cannot effectively transfer deoxygenated blood to the pulmonary circulation, subsequently causes congestion of the circulation in the rest of the body (systemic circulation).

Cardiac reserve. The function of the heart is to pump blood to the body at sufficient volume and pressure to perfuse the tissues with oxygen. The requirements of many tissues are fairly constant, but the needs of the skeletal musculature vary with the level of physical activity. An increase in activity leads to an increase in cardiac output, this capacity to increase being the 'cardiac reserve'. The increase results mainly from increased heart rate and contractile force as a direct result of sympathetic nervous system (SNS) stimulation. In the patient with heart failure, the cardiac reserve is used to maintain baseline cardiac function and so the ability to respond to increased activity is limited. When the baroreceptors at various points in the body sense a fall in pressure and therefore a fall in cardiac output, the principal response is to increase stimulation of the SNS, followed up by a longer-term response.

Myocardial dilatation. Increased stretching of the myocardial cells, which occurs immediately after a sudden reduction in the ability to expel the stroke volume, increases their force of contraction and increases the cardiac output correspondingly. This compensatory mechanism becomes limited as myocardial oxygen demand increases.

Renal response. Reduced cardiac output has a depressant effect on the kidneys, which will not improve until the cardiac output returns to normal. The fall in blood pressure and sympathetic constriction of renal arterioles reduce the glomerular filtration rate (GFR). Reduced blood flow through the kidneys leads to increased angiotensin production, increased secretion of aldosterone and therefore increased sodium and water reabsorption. The fluid retention in itself does not interfere with the pumping ability of the heart, but it does increase venous return. The rise in extracellular fluid and blood volume increases systemic filling pressures, so more of the cardiac reserve has to be used to maintain perfusion, further reducing the heart's ability to respond to increased physical activity.

Congestive cardiac failure (CCF). This term describes a state in which there is both right and left ventricular failure with a corresponding combination of systemic and pulmonary symptoms.

Myocardial hypertrophy. In response to the increased workload, the individual myocardial cells enlarge, thus increasing the total amount of contractile tissue. This compensation is usually of a temporary nature, and at this stage the prognosis is poor.

Oedema. In order to understand oedema, the nurse must first understand the normal tissue fluid exchange that occurs between the capillaries and the cells to ensure that nutrients, O_2 and H_2O are delivered to the cell and waste products are removed.

Oedema may result when anything increases the flow of fluid from the bloodstream and impairs its return. One of the commonest causes is CCF, where the failure of the pump to move the blood volume forward results in back pressure, which raises the hydrostatic pressure such that it exceeds the colloidal pressure created by plasma proteins. As a result, the excess tissue fluid formed accumulates and cannot be drained away completely by the lymphatic system.

In the early stages of heart failure, patients may complain of 'puffy ankles', being unable to fit comfortably into their shoes. There will also be sacral oedema.

Pulmonary oedema. As systemic arterial pressure (and therefore afterload) increases, so does pressure in the left heart. Increased left ventricular end-diastolic pressure (LVEDP) results in increased pulmonary pressure and an accumulation of blood in the lungs. If the pulmonary pressure rises above 28 mmHg, there is movement of fluid from the capillaries into the alveoli and interstitial spaces. This causes pulmonary oedema. If this occurs as an acute event, it can lead to death in 30 min. In the congestive failure situation, it is a chronic progressive state where the reduced lung compliance and high pulmonary pressure lead to increased right heart pressures and blood congestion on this side. This further raises pressure in the systemic circulation, making the whole process one of cyclical deterioration. As the systemic pressure rises, there is movement of fluid into the tissues giving rise to peripheral oedema. This is initially gravitational, but as the condition progresses the oedema becomes more widespread (see Fig. 2.12).

Common presenting symptoms. The presentation and history will depend on which side of the heart is failing. It may present gradually, as occurs in the ageing process, or suddenly, manifesting as acute pulmonary oedema:

- Fatigue on exertion, dyspnoea with mild exercise and paroxysmal nocturnal dyspnoea are common early signs of failure of the left ventricle.
- Fatigue, awareness of fullness in the neck and abdomen, and ankle swelling are early signs of failure of the right ventricle.

Features appearing in systemic examination are listed in Table 2.7.

Q **2.16** How do the features of nursing assessment relate to and complement the doctor's examination?

MEDICAL MANAGEMENT

Investigations. The main concern is to identify the primary cause of failure and to ensure that correctable lesions are treated and contributing factors eliminated if possible.

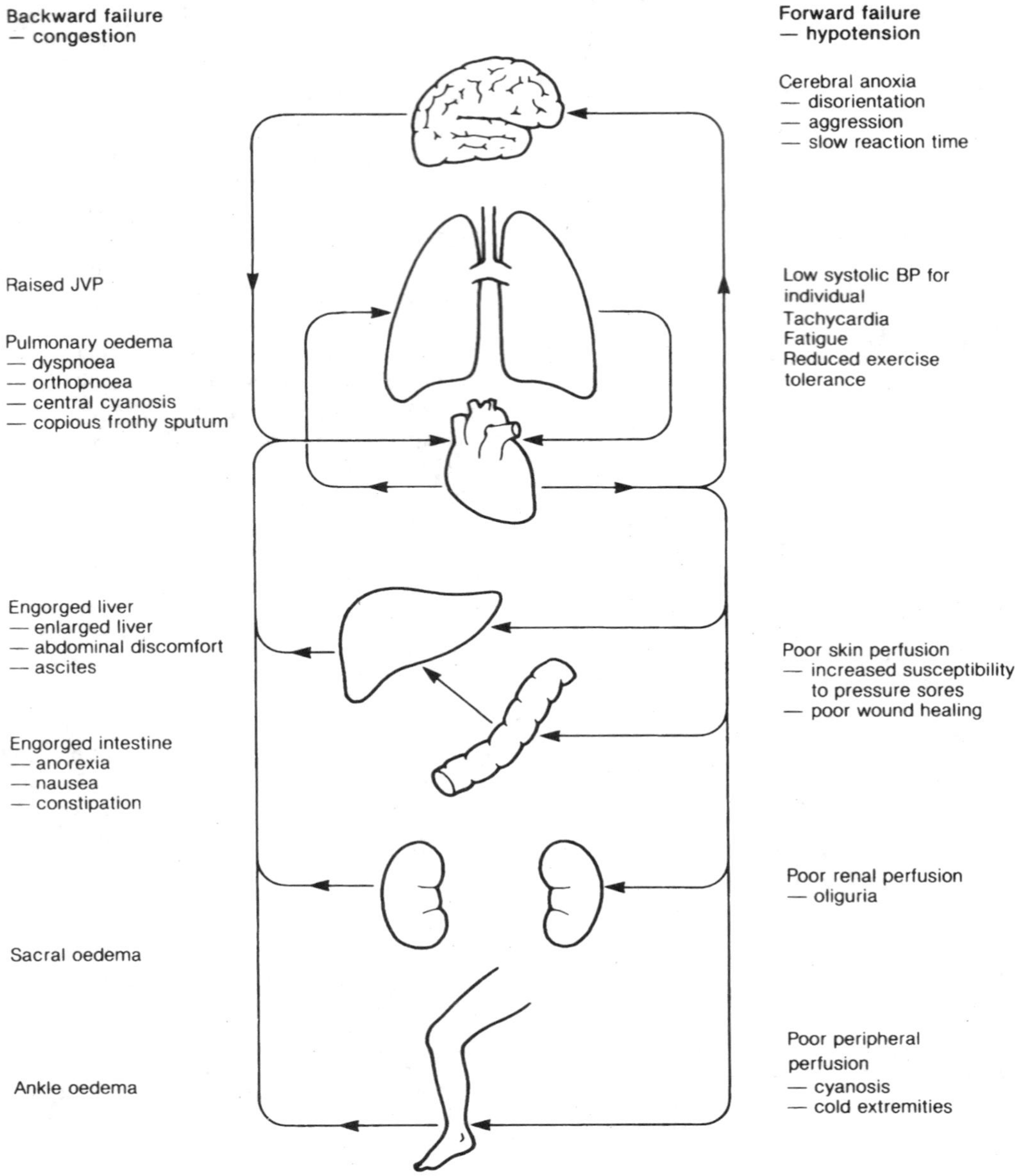

Fig. 2.12 Clinical effects of decompensatory phase of ventricular failure. (Reproduced with kind permission from Boore et al 1987.)

ECG. There may be no specific abnormalities, but indications of ventricular hypertrophy, heart block and acute MI may help to pinpoint the aetiology of the heart failure.

Other investigations include chest X-ray, auscultation and palpation.

Treatment. The main treatment approaches are:

- oxygenation to improve myocardial contractility
- rest to reduce cardiac rate and work
- digoxin to increase myocardial contractile force and efficiency
- diuresis of excess fluid in conjunction with restricted salt intake
- correction of arrhythmias.

A combination of digitalis and diuretic therapy has been the standard management of heart failure. Digoxin helps to increase the strength of myocardial contraction and slows the heart rate by increasing vagal activity. Diuretics help by increasing water loss. More recently, the use of ACE inhibitors has increased life expectancy.

For the pharmacological aspects of management of heart failure, see Stanley (1996).

NURSING PRIORITIES AND MANAGEMENT: HEART FAILURE

Nurse-led multidisciplinary intervention in chronic heart failure is likely to yield substantial benefits for patients and family members, including reduced hospital admission rates, improved quality of life and cost savings (McMurray & Stewart 1998).

Table 2.7 Systemic examination in heart failure

System	*Points to note*	*Rationale*
CVS	Chest X-ray	Evaluation of chamber enlargement Indication of primary cardiac abnormality
	Auscultation	Arrhythmia (especially AF) common
	Vital signs	Venous hypertension common Observe jugular venous pressure
	Presence of oedema	Visible oedema in dependent parts (e.g. ankles, hands and sacrum) in bed-bound patients is a sign of inability to excrete sufficient water
Respiratory	Wheeze, bronchospasm	Possible increased pulmonary fluid
	Paroxysmal nocturnal dyspnoea	Evidence of poor LV compensation
	Amount and consistency of sputum	Evidence of pulmonary oedema
	Pleural effusion on right side	Often found in patients with CCF
	Chest X-ray	Recognition of oedema
GIS	Diet	Sodium control is an important part of controlling fluid retention
	Palpation of abdomen	Signs of hepatic and splenic engorgement Presence of ascites
GUS	Micturition	Frequency and amount of urine passed; vital to assess effect of diuretic therapy
MS	Physical activity levels	Often severely limited by reduced cardiac reserve
CNS	Mental status	Signs of cerebral hypoxia
Skin	Skin integrity	Risk of pressure sores and delayed healing

Ongoing concerns

Patients with heart failure have a chronic condition that is likely to deteriorate. It is estimated that the average life expectancy of a patient with heart failure is 4–5 years. Patients and their families will need information and support to help them retain their independence for as long as possible. Patients with heart failure are not routinely offered cardiac rehabilitation and there is a need to evaluate the impact of such a service for this group of patients (Bowman et al 1998).

For a review of the information and support needs of this group of patients, see Hagenoff et al (1994).

Maintaining a safe environment

The prime concern is to restore haemodynamic stability, using a combination of drugs to optimise cardiac function and control fluid loss through the kidneys. The effects of this therapy should be regularly assessed and practice nurses may be involved in monitoring the patient's weight, heart rate and rhythm. People living with heart failure should be taught how to monitor their pulse and to check their ankles for signs of oedema.

In the patient admitted to hospital with an acute exacerbation of heart failure, the manipulation of medication will form a major part of therapy. Sensitive day-to-day nursing care will depend on having a sound understanding of medication and its effects.

Breathing

The patient will often describe breathlessness, especially on exertion, as the main symptom. Control of fluid balance and reducing energy demands may help to minimise the symptoms, and the patient should be encouraged to stop smoking.

Acute left ventricular failure leading to pulmonary oedema results in marked respiratory distress, agitation and production of copious frothy sputum. The priority is to reduce both the psychological and respiratory distress, using i.v. morphine, diuretics and oxygen therapy. Being with the patient and explaining what is being done in a reassuring way can allay anxiety and help the person through the alarming experience.

In hospital, the nurse is responsible for:

- ensuring that respiration is recorded regularly
- assessing the patient's subjective feelings about her breathing
- reporting acute episodes of dyspnoea
- administering oxygen therapy to help reduce anoxia (cautiously, in the patient with COAD)
- assessing the nature and amount of sputum
- working in partnership with the physiotherapist to apply chest physiotherapy and nasopharyngeal suctioning to help with sputum clearance.

Sleeping

Respiratory distress is often worse at night when the patient lies flat, and paroxysmal nocturnal dyspnoea is a very frightening experience. Sleeping supported with extra pillows helps. Patients with congestive failure may not sleep for long periods. Many doze for periods during the day. Some people stay in a chair at night, instead of going to bed, because of their respiratory distress. These factors should be remembered when patients are taken to hospital. A restless patient awake in bed at 02.00 h may get more rest if she follows her normal pattern and is not constricted by hospital policy.

Elimination

Accurate estimation of fluid losses in conjunction with daily weights provides information on the effectiveness of diuretics; output should be in excess of 30 mL/h. Input of fluid and sodium should be restricted. Restricting sodium intake also often reduces the patient's thirst, which is very important if fluid intake is to be restricted to around 1 L/day. The knowledge that fluid is being restricted is almost guaranteed to make someone want to drink more. The use of loop diuretic therapy, such as frusemide, will cause loss of potassium. Potassium supplements are given and serum levels of potassium closely monitored to ensure they remain within normal limits, 3.5–5.5 mmol/L (see Ch. 20). To assist in the accurate assessment of haemodynamic status, a central venous catheter or pulmonary artery pressure catheter may be inserted.

Constipation should be avoided.

Oedema

Daily assessment of the extent of oedema will indicate the effectiveness of therapeutic intervention. All dependent areas should be assessed, including the spine and sacrum, if the patient is bedbound. Patients at home should be taught how to monitor weight and the signs of oedema.

Diet and nutrition

The patient should be encouraged not to use salt at the table and to reduce the amount used in cooking. Herbs or salt substitutes can be used to add taste instead. In hospital, a low-salt diet may be rigidly enforced if the oedema is severe. Obese patients should also be on a reduced-calorie diet, to prevent further strain on the heart. Iron intake may need to be assessed if the person is anaemic.

Mobility

Rest is important for patients with congestive heart failure, in order to reduce the cardiac workload and oxygen demand. In the acute phase complete bed rest is advocated until pulmonary oedema is controlled. Activity is gradually increased until tolerated without signs of physical difficulty. A patient confined to bed or chair rest requires pillows for support, to keep her breathing comfortable. With cardiac beds, both foot and head ends can be altered, helping to relieve respiratory distress, while aiding the peripheral drainage of fluid. Ankle swelling can be significantly reduced by walking and elevating the feet when sitting down.

Work and leisure

People with heart failure may require help to live within their activity limits and to come to terms with the fact that they have a progressive disease for which there is no cure. Many people consider they are doomed to, and a few adopt, the role of invalid and dependant. The response to gradually increased activity is assessed to calculate the patient's functional capacity (see also the section on mobility for people with AMI, p. 28).

Personal hygiene

A patient with congestive failure can usually retain independence in this area by taking certain precautions. Showers demand less energy expenditure than a bath, and a seat in the shower is helpful. A common difficulty is in drying the lower half of the body, because bending affects respiration, but by sitting, all parts of the body can be reached.

Someone with oedema will have very fragile, papery skin in the affected areas and great care must be taken not to break the skin by too much rubbing. Soap also has a drying effect on the skin; emulsifying oils may be better.

Communication

The importance of information being exchanged between the patient, family and health professionals cannot be overemphasised. It should be remembered that heart failure is a progressive disease which affects many old people. The restrictions on mobility may confine these people to their home, further isolating them. Community nurses, health visitors and practice nurses are increasingly involved in health assessment and screening of old people at home. Their assessment needs to take careful account of the social and psychological consequences, as well as the physical consequences, of disease processes and disability. It may be possible to arrange for attendance at a day hospital for those who wish it, or for a charity group such as Age Concern or the WRVS to provide transport to social events or day centres.

Expressing sexuality

The patient's role within the family may have to alter as the disease increasingly restricts activities. Women may have to give up some household tasks to partners or to a home help. This can further demoralise them and requires tactful support from family and health professionals. Sexual activity may need to be modified if the individual's activity levels decrease or shortness of breath becomes a problem. The nurse needs to be equipped to offer realistic, non-judgmental advice (Jaarsma et al 1996).

For further information on the management of heart failure see Dahlen & Roberts (1995a,b).

VALVULAR DISORDERS

Most adult valvular disease is either congenital or acquired. The effects of congenital problems largely manifest themselves in childhood and so are excluded from discussion here.

The major causes of valve pathology are rheumatic heart disease (RHD), subacute bacterial endocarditis (SBE) and, to a lesser extent today, syphilis. Major disruption can also result from papillary muscle dysfunction following AMI or penetrating chest wounds, when onset of symptoms can be sudden and severe.

Rheumatic heart disease

Rheumatic fever (RF) is usually a childhood ailment. It is closely associated with streptococcal pharyngitis and so shows seasonal variation with a peak in colder months. It may take up to 10 years before the signs of heart disease appear, but 25% of those affected may have died by then. Most of the rest go on to develop RHD and within two decades most will have died from heart failure, cerebral embolisation and respiratory failure.

PATHOPHYSIOLOGY

The connective tissue of heart, joints and skin respond to infection by a proliferative and exudative inflammatory response with oedema and fragmentation of collagen fibres. The arthritic pain flits from joint to joint. Fever is low grade. All layers of the heart can be affected. Endocarditis is most common, usually affecting the left side and involving the mitral valve, although any valve is at risk. The valve leaflets become oedematous with small, firmly attached vegetations. In the acute stages, this results in incompetence of the valve. Subsequent fibrosis deforms and thickens the leaflets and shortens the chordae tendineae, leading to stenosis with or without incompetence (Majeed 1989).

MEDICAL MANAGEMENT

Prophylactic antibiotic cover is instituted following the first occurrence of RF, and if this prevents recurrence then most of those who develop endocarditis will have normal hearts in the long term. Outbreaks are now more common in developing countries than they are in the West, especially within communities that are becoming progressively urbanised. Poor housing and socioeconomic conditions exacerbate the problem. Prevention would have to take these factors into account to be effective.

Infective endocarditis

The majority (75%) of cases are streptococcal or staphylococcal infections, although an increasing number of infective agents are being isolated, due to increasingly invasive medical techniques, such as in dental treatment or urinary investigation. Intravenous drug users also introduce bacteria into their systems through contaminated needles.

PATHOPHYSIOLOGY

As well as being a cause of valvular disorder, those who have pre-existing valve disease or congenital lesions are more at risk of developing bacterial endocarditis, as the underlying structures are already damaged and the blood flow is more turbulent. Certain sites are more favoured than others for bacterial proliferation. When blood flows from a high-pressure to a low-pressure system via a narrow orifice, the organisms tend to gather on the low-pressure side. If a high-pressure jet or regurgitant stream is created due to, for example, valve dysfunction, then satellite colonies will be seeded in the endothelial wall where the jet hits. In aortic regurgitation, for example, blood flows back from the high-pressure aorta via the supposedly closed aortic valve to the low-pressure left ventricle. Colonisation by bacteria would most likely occur on the ventricular surface of the aortic valve. Similar patterns can be elicited for other areas of dysfunction.

The vegetations of infective endocarditis, in contrast to those in RHD, are large and friable and can aggregate to form up to 6 cm masses. This poses a double threat to the patient in that they:

- are more likely to embolise
- may cause ventricular insufficiency themselves by prolapsing into the valve orifice and obstructing flow.

Common presenting symptoms. Presentation may be slow and insidious, with general malaise, weight loss, lethargy, intermittent, often low-grade pyrexia, profuse sweating and joint pain. Microembolisation may manifest as splinter haemorrhages of the nail beds. If the infection has eroded tissue close to the valves where the conduction system lies, there may be evidence of rhythm and conduction disturbances. Evidence of embolisation may be seen in renal, cerebral, pulmonary and gastrointestinal systems. Myocardial infarction may also result from septic embolisation of the coronary arteries. Heart failure secondary to valve failure varies in its severity, depending on the valve affected and the acuteness of onset, and may give rise to shortness of breath and ankle oedema.

MEDICAL MANAGEMENT

Investigations should include ECG, chest X-ray and echocardiography. Cardiac catheterisation is also necessary in those who will be referred for surgery to assess valve function, ventricular function and the patency of coronary arteries. Intravenous routes are usually used for long-term administration of antibiotic therapy. Patients need to be advised about the importance of regular dental hygiene and prophylaxis when undergoing surgical procedures.

For more information on infective endocarditis, see Thompson & Webster (1992).

MEDICAL MANAGEMENT OF VALVULAR DISORDERS

The aim is to improve the haemodynamics by improving any aberrant rhythm, e.g. atrial fibrillation (AF), by digitalisation or cardioversion. This reduces the heart rate, allowing more time for filling the coronary arteries in the longer diastolic period. Atrial contribution to cardiac output is regained. Congestive failure is relieved by diuretics and physical demands by reduced activity. Oxygen therapy may be of use to those with pulmonary congestion. Fever should be investigated and treated appropriately. Anticoagulation may be commenced on those with evidence of previous embolisation, those in AF and those in low output states with left and right failure. The latter may require inotropic support to increase cardiac output and renal perfusion. Sudden onset with pulmonary oedema, e.g. with papillary muscle rupture post-AMI, requires artificial ventilation, full monitoring, afterload reduction and the possible aid of an intra-aortic balloon pump (IABP) as in cardiogenic shock (see Ch. 18) to gain time prior to urgent surgery.

Those with chronic disease processes may be maintained on medication. Increasing interest is being shown in the technique of balloon valvuloplasty for stenotic valves where a catheter is introduced across the valve, the balloon is inflated and the calcified stenosis cracked and opened up.

In the mitral position, the approach is across the septum, while with the aortic valve the catheter is introduced retrogradely. Problems include:

- bradycardias
- profound hypotension when the balloon is inflated
- embolisation
- tamponade
- possible myocardial rupture.

The aim, to increase the functional area of the valve and therefore cardiac output, has met with some success. It may find application in the treatment of elderly people with aortic stenosis, for whom a full operation would hold too many risks but whose life expectancy would be short without it. It has the advantage of a short hospital stay and the prompt resumption of normal life, compared with an operation. An alternative would be prosthetic valve replacement (Kolvekar & Forsyth 1991).

NURSING PRIORITIES AND MANAGEMENT: VALVULAR DISEASE

Breathing

Shortness of breath, often initially on exertion, is the hallmark of progressive heart failure. In some patients, sudden valvular failure may result in an alarming onset of breathlessness. In others, it is a slow progressive problem which starts with breathlessness on exertion and eventually also breathlessness at rest. Orthopnoea (breathlessness in the supine position) may also occur and the increasing number of pillows people require is an indicator of the progression of their disease. Diuretic therapy is used to reduce fluid in the pulmonary interstitium. Sudden valve failure can be very alarming and these patients may require an urgent operation. They should be within sight of the nursing staff and have means of summoning help. An upright position, well supported by pillows, helps chest expansion. Observations should include:

- the depth, rate and pattern of respirations
- the colour of the person's mucous membranes and peripheries
- the quantity of sputum produced and its nature
- any evidence of infection.

The white frothing sputum of pulmonary oedema is characteristic of heart failure. Oxygen therapy may improve symptoms. Some people find the masks very claustrophobic and may benefit from nasal cannulae if low-flow oxygen is all they require.

Breathlessness may be precipitated by alterations in heart rate, especially the irregularity of atrial fibrillation. Pulse oximeters are often used to monitor heart rate and oxygen saturation by the use of non-invasive skin probes. Their accuracy depends, in part, on the adequacy of the circulation through the skin and so they are less suitable for those who have poor peripheral circulation. When the circulation is poor, the probes should be moved from finger to finger regularly to avoid skin damage.

Diet and nutrition

General fatigue may be the major limiting factor in maintaining adequate nutrition. Small, frequent meals may be more easily digested. They should be high in protein and carbohydrate, especially if the metabolism is raised by fever. Long-term mitral insufficiency does not allow sufficient forward flow of oxygenated blood to nourish the peripheries. The nutritional state of people with valvular disorders should be optimised prior to surgery. Liver failure may already be a problem due to right-sided heart failure, which is secondary to primary left-sided failure. Altered function affects the liver's ability to metabolise and synthesise basic substrates of cellular construction and function.

The advice of the dietician may be valuable. High-protein, commercially available drinks can be given to supplement the diet; however, fluid restriction might also be necessary to prevent pulmonary oedema. Fluid restriction and oxygen therapy often leave the mouth dry, and sucking ice or frozen fruit juice helps to keep the mouth as fresh as possible, while minimising fluid intake.

Personal hygiene

The ability to look after personal hygiene may be limited by fatigue and breathlessness. The district nursing team can help at home with bathing and can arrange, through the occupational therapist, to provide aids that make getting in and out of baths easier. Helping patients in this way allows nurses to assess perfusion of the peripheries. Those with fever or who experience sweating associated with aortic insufficiency may need more frequent attention to personal freshness.

Sleeping

It can be difficult to sleep due to shortness of breath, even when sitting upright. Each person may have to amend daily activities to allow for periods of rest. Nursing care should be similarly planned.

Mobility

Movement may be limited by the symptoms of the individual. If restricted to bed rest, deep breathing and leg exercises should be encouraged. People whose activities are limited at home might benefit from a home help or may be eligible for mobility allowance. Advice can be sought from the social services department.

Local authorities issue car stickers for the disabled, to allow greater access to public amenities in prohibited zones.

Wheelchair use. Access to public buildings is slowly improving; public planning incorporates wheelchair access, and many older buildings have been adapted to cater for the less mobile. Lists of places that are suitable for access are available. Wheelchairs can also be provided to enable people to tour exhibitions or to travel more easily between trains and aircraft, and most large travel organisations provide this service. Holiday brochures often specify which hotels are easily accessible. The Red Cross also hires out wheelchairs and aids for limited periods.

For patients who have had surgery, mobility is regained gradually. Each person should set herself the daily goal of walking a little further. Strenuous exercise should be avoided until the sternum heals; for example, any sport involving swinging movements of the arms, such as golf, could prevent the bone edges from knitting together. Some surgeons restrict strenuous exercise for longer, since they feel too great a gradient can be developed across the prosthetic valve.

Work and recreation

Some lines of work may prove too strenuous, necessitating a change of job. After cardiac valve surgery, the patient will be unable to return to work for at least 3 months. Returning part-time is desirable, as people often tire easily at first. This can gradually be increased back to full-time. Very physical work is to be avoided for about 6 months. The employer might be able to find a lighter task for these people to do initially but still involve them in the working environment. Some work is forbidden after cardiac surgery, e.g. an HGV licence cannot be held. Advice from the social worker about claiming social security allowance and information about retraining schemes can be given, if appropriate. Worry about loss of income can add to the stress of undergoing major surgery.

Maintaining a safe environment

Once a prosthetic valve is in situ, the recipient should be aware of how to avoid putting the valve and herself at risk. Anticoagulation is routine for life in those with metal valves, and for a shorter time for those with tissue valves. The person should understand the action of the drugs and their potential risks. She should also be aware of the risk of infection and should inform other health professionals, e.g. dentists, that she has a prosthetic valve and is taking warfarin. Antibiotic cover is given for dental treatment and any other invasive investigation.

For further details on the use of anticoagulants, see Stanley (1996).

Driving is to be avoided until the sternum heals, as sudden movement, e.g. to avoid an accident, could disrupt sternal wire sutures, as could sudden impact to the chest. A small pillow between the seat belt and the chest can reduce friction on the wound, but does not necessarily absorb impact. Eyesight, especially of those who wear glasses, and concentration span are both affected for some weeks after cardiopulmonary bypass.

Expressing sexuality

In relation to sexual activity, avoiding strain on the sternal suture line is the most important limitation until the bone heals, but after that, resumption of relationships should not be excluded. Intimacy between couples can be maintained without full intercourse prior to this. Fear that the valve will fail under exertion should be allayed. Some surgeons do not recommend that young women with prosthetic valves become pregnant, because of the increase in circulating volume and cardiac workload. However, successful pregnancies have been completed and obviously this should be as planned an event as possible. Women of child-bearing age are given tissue valves, as this allows the period of anticoagulation to be relatively short. Warfarin is teratogenic, especially during the first trimester of pregnancy. Oral contraceptives also inhibit the effects of warfarin. Some may find the prospect of sharing a bed with a partner who 'ticks' off-putting, especially as increases in heart rate can be clearly heard, which can increase fears that catastrophic events will take place during intercourse.

These people can be reassured that the metallic noise becomes softened with time. As a last resort, tissue valves might be considered, although they have a shorter life span and would require replacement within a few years.

Valve stenosis and incompetence

Aortic stenosis

PATHOPHYSIOLOGY

The left ventricle becomes progressively hypertrophied, working at a higher pressure to eject blood past the stenosed valve. The chamber size of the ventricle is reduced by the increased muscle mass, which may itself contribute to outflow obstruction. This state is asymptomatic until the orifice is reduced to 0.5–0.7 cm^2 (normal 2.6–3.5 cm^2) when the patient may experience angina as oxygen supply does not meet demand.

The other major effect is syncope, as cardiac output fails to rise in response to exercise. Hypertrophy may progress to decompensation and heart failure with rising LVEDP and pulmonary oedema. Aortic stenosis is also associated with occult gastrointestinal bleeding. The reason for this is still unclear, however the problem subsides with valve replacement (Tuchek 1991).

Mitral stenosis

PATHOPHYSIOLOGY

In this condition, the left atrium has to eject through a resistant valve. Left atrial pressure rises, and the atrium distends and eventually decompensates, with fibrous tissue interspersed between cardiac muscle. Conduction becomes aberrant and atrial fibrillation results. This decreases cardiac output as there is no atrial contribution to ventricular filling. If sinus rhythm persists, evidence of atrial hypertrophy can be seen on the ECG. Since conduction takes longer to spread across the enlarged left atria, the P wave becomes broadened and bifid. Left atrial pressure rises further with the stasis of blood within the chamber. This pressure increase is transmitted to the pulmonary vasculature, where vascular resistance rises with resultant greater right-sided afterload and possible failure. Acute elevations of pressure with exercise, for example, will precipitate pulmonary oedema. Stasis of blood allows the formation of mural thrombus within the atria. The obvious danger is that this may be dislodged and carried forward into the systemic circulation with profound ischaemic consequences for the area supplied by the vessel embolised (see Case History 2.2).

Q

2.17 The continuing care of people with valvular disorders is essentially carried out in the community. The desired outcome for someone like K, in Case History 2.2, is that:

- she enjoys a full and happy life within the limitations imposed by her disorder
- she can cope with the medications and dietary restriction
- she maintains medical and nursing advice and support.

Which members of the primary health care team will support K? What would their priorities be in caring for K at home?

Aortic incompetence

PATHOPHYSIOLOGY

Left ventricular end-diastolic pressure (LVEDP) is approximately one-eighth of the concomitant aortic pressure, and therefore any breach of the valve would allow large amounts of blood to flow back into the ventricle. The ventricle dilates to accommodate this volume, LVEDP rises, stroke volume increases and so does systolic pressure. Diastolic pressure within the aorta is low because of regurgitation, and therefore there is a wide pulse pressure, often about 190/50 mmHg. Chronic gradual aortic incompetence (AI) is well tolerated, but if there is an acute onset, left ventricular failure (LVF) quickly develops. AI also occurs when the valve annulus becomes dilated so that the cusps cannot coapt, e.g. in connective tissue disorders, syphilis and aortic dissection.

Mitral incompetence

PATHOPHYSIOLOGY

This allows back-flow of blood to the left atrium in systole, where regurgitated blood and the normal atrial volume mix and return to the ventricle during atrial systole. In order to cope with this increased load, the ventricle hypertrophies and then dilates. Forward flow diminishes, with progressive failure of the ventricle and with back-flow into the atria at systole. Weight loss and

Case History 2.2 — K — living with mitral stenosis

K is an infant-school teacher in her early 30s. When she was 12 she developed rheumatic fever, thought to have resulted from a streptococcal throat infection, although it was not a common disorder and no-one else in her family had ever suffered from it. At that time she was in hospital for several weeks and left with inflammation of her mitral valve (valvulitis) which caused a progressive narrowing (stenosis) of her mitral valve over the years. On auscultation, K's mitral stenosis was identified by the characteristic diastolic murmur.

Until the age of 25, K felt quite healthy and often wondered just why she had to have regular medical checks and be prescribed antibiotics so quickly when some minor infection occurred. However, in her late 20s she began to experience breathlessness after various activities with the children at school. She often had to sit down, feeling light-headed, and developed a persistent, irritating cough. At first she dismissed it, but eventually she contacted her GP. Investigations showed that K's stenosis of the mitral valve was becoming worse and that she was developing the early signs of heart failure.

As a result of K's mitral stenosis, the pressure in the left atrium, pulmonary veins and capillaries increases. The left atrium dilates, fluid may accumulate in the alveoli, the pulmonary artery pressure rises, and the right ventricle hypertrophies. Systemic effects become apparent in the form of peripheral oedema, ascites and hepatic engorgement. Atrial fibrillation can occur which may potentiate pulmonary oedema and systemic emboli.

Managing such symptoms will include the use of digoxin to control atrial fibrillation, diuretics, a low-sodium diet and anticoagulant therapy. K will have to adjust her lifestyle to accommodate her valvular disorder but she will be at home.

lethargy are marked as the heart can no longer provide the nutrition the blood usually carries. The left atrium dilates, and changes in conduction and rhythm occur.

Tricuspid stenosis and incompetence

PATHOPHYSIOLOGY

These both result in increased right-sided pressure, with evidence of stasis and engorgement of the portal and peripheral circulations, e.g. ascites, liver dysfunction and peripheral oedema. If the right atrium becomes hypertrophied due to tricuspid stenosis, the P wave on the ECG will become peaked. The majority of right-sided failure is usually secondary to failure on the left; however, there is an increase in bacterial endocarditis of the right heart, with the increasing use, or abuse, of intravenous drugs.

HYPERTENSION

Hypertension is difficult to define and there is controversy as to what level of pressure, systolic or diastolic, constitutes hypertension (Fahey & Peters 1996). The technique of measuring blood pressure can also vary, resulting in differences, principally in diastolic definition. The scope of the problem may well be underestimated since the majority of people are without symptoms until target organs are affected. They then present with major consequences such as renal failure, ischaemic heart disease, cerebral emboli or infarction.

Being aware of associated predisposing factors may enable health workers to target screening towards at-risk groups, as they will be largely unaware of the problem.

Associated factors

Several factors associated with hypertension have been identified:

- obesity
- sodium intake
- alcohol
- genetic factors
- smoking
- stress.

Obesity

The interaction between obesity and hypertension is not fully understood. Overweight adolescents are at significant risk of later hypertension. Those involved in health education and school nursing may play an important part in educating children about diet and exercise in general. An increased intake of sodium is consumed in general overeating and it is thought that the sodium pump may become impaired in this group. However, this is a reversible situation and blood pressure decreases with weight loss (Richards et al 1996).

Sodium intake

The link between sodium and hypertension may result from increased sodium and water retention by the kidneys in response to an increased sodium load. Sodium accumulates within the arterial walls of hypertensive people. These vessels then become more responsive to substances that cause vasoconstriction. People who reduce their sodium intake also reduce their blood pressure. High sodium intake is a feature of Western lifestyle and more isolated peoples with a lower intake have a lower incidence of hypertension; once they adopt a Western diet the incidence rises. Compliance with low-sodium diets is poor, as they are so unpalatable. Emphasis is now laid on not adding salt after cooking and salt substitutes are widely available. There is a generally increased awareness of the contents of packaged foodstuffs; clear product labelling helps people at risk to identify substances that contain sodium.

An increase in potassium intake through consumption of fruits, vegetables and beans is reported to be beneficial in lowering blood pressure (Lydakis et al 1997).

Alcohol

The contribution of alcohol is difficult to assess, as there is a tendency to underreport alcohol consumption due to social pressures. However, blood pressure rises with increasing intake and a reduction in intake reverses this.

Genetic factors

A family history of hypertension predisposes individuals to the same condition. Certain ethnic groups are more susceptible to the condition: the black population in the USA has a 50% greater prevalence than their white counterparts. It appears that the mean resting renal blood flow of normotensive individuals with hypertensive parents is greater than those with normotensive parents. The kidneys' ability to handle sodium is also thought to be genetically influenced.

Smoking

Nicotine promotes catecholamine release and so increases heart rate and blood pressure.

Stress

This is presumed to relate to increased sympathetic outflow (see Ch. 17). Certain occupations are associated with a higher risk of developing hypertension, e.g. crane drivers and air traffic controllers. People who work in noisy overstimulating environments also run a higher risk of occupational stress, especially if the tasks are repetitive and monotonous.

PATHOPHYSIOLOGY

Although difficult to define in terms of elevated blood pressure, hypertension is commonly classified according to cause:

- Primary or essential hypertension refers to a raised blood pressure where no cause can be found.
- Secondary hypertension is a result of the underlying conditions, most commonly:
  —renal disease (see Ch. 8)
  —an adrenaline-secreting tumour, e.g. phaeochromocytoma in the adrenal medulla
  —diseases of the pituitary or adrenal cortex, where there is an elevation of glucocorticoids (see Ch. 5)
  —coarctation (narrowing) of the aorta
  —hyperthyroidism (see Ch. 5).

  Hypertension can also be classified according to severity:

- *mild* — when elevation of blood pressure is only moderate and occurs over a long period of time
- *malignant* — when there is a sudden and severe blood pressure elevation.

The malignancy does not refer to cellular changes but to the fact that this is a life-threatening condition. Whatever form of hypertension is diagnosed, the concern is always the effect of this high blood pressure:

- on the heart, where the increased demand on its pumping capacity can lead to ventricular hypertrophy
- on the brain, where any elevation of blood pressure could precipitate a cerebral catastrophe (see Ch. 9).

Other organs that give rise to concern are the kidneys, where the delicate function of the nephrons can be impaired by constant high pressure, and the eyes, where fine retinal vessels may rupture and significantly impair vision.

Common presenting symptoms. People who are aware that they have a condition that predisposes them to hypertension will have been alerted to this potential problem and the symptoms may be more readily appreciated. However, many may be completely unaware of their hypertensive state, either having no symptoms at all or dismissing complaints such as headaches, vertigo, nosebleeds and fatigue.

MEDICAL MANAGEMENT

Examination. The elevated blood pressure may only be noticed at some routine examination for another reason, such as insurance cover. A single elevated reading does not justify a diagnosis of hypertension since anxiety about the examination itself may be the temporary cause; however, the person should be reassessed at a later date. Examiners should also be aware of the possible contribution their own technique and instrument calibration may make to errors in estimation, e.g. using inappropriately sized cuffs.

Generally, hypertension is defined by grading, with arbitrary cut-off points according to diastolic pressure, as follows:

- mild: 95–104 mmHg
- moderate: 105–120 mmHg
- severe: >120 mmHg.

The higher the diastolic pressure, the greater the risk of CVA, renal failure, coronary artery disease and heart failure.

Treatment of hypertension has been shown to reduce the relative risks of cardiovascular mortality and morbidity by 30% (Collins & Peto 1994). The management of the patient with hypertension is generally the responsibility of the primary health care team and hospitalisation is not usually required.

Investigations include:

- blood pressure monitoring
- chest X-ray and ECG to determine the degree of left ventricular hypertrophy and heart failure
- full blood count, electrolytes, urea or nitrogen and creatine, to exclude secondary causes and renal effects of the disease process
- urinalysis with microscopy, 24-h collections for creatinine clearance and vanillylmandelic acid (VMA)
- intravenous pyelogram (IVP) to assess renal perfusion.

Treatment depends largely on how elevated the blood pressure is. Guidelines produced as a result of clinical drug trials tend to produce conflicting recommendations (Jackson & Sackett 1996). The emphasis is on targeting treatment at those people who have absolute risk of cardiovascular disease (Fahey & Peters 1996).

Mild elevation. Advice focuses on modifying lifestyle to minimise the individual's risk factors. Regular 6-monthly follow-ups to reinforce the information and check the blood pressure may be all that is required. Practice nurses may find a developing role as counsellors as GP practice moves more towards preventive medicine.

The benefit of drug treatment for diastolic pressures under 100 mmHg is still uncertain. Over that level it is accepted for men between 45 and 65 years of age.

Moderate elevation is treated largely with thiazide diuretics or cardioselective beta-blockade along with general advice on risk reduction. If the desired level of pressure is not achieved with these agents alone, then they can be tried in combination. Long-acting preparations allow a once-daily dose, which the patient might prefer. Failing this, a third-line drug is introduced. This is often a calcium channel blocker, which promotes vasodilatation of the coronary bed and peripheries.

Angiotensin-converting enzyme (ACE) inhibitors block the conversion of angiotensin I to angiotensin II. Thus vasoconstriction is reduced and the blood pressure becomes normal.

If these measures fail to control pressure, or if there is severely raised diastolic pressure, the patient will be referred to specialised clinicians. Investigation for secondary causes of hypertension should ensue promptly. Tests should include assays for evidence of renal disease, primary aldosteronism, hypothyroidism and phaeochromocytoma, while urgent assessment and control of blood pressure take place. It may be that this is a side-effect of other treatment, e.g. oral contraception. Only 4–5% of women taking 'the pill' develop overt hypertension due to oestrogen ingestion, but it may take several months for it to settle. Other forms of contraception should be advised. Hypertension is also one of the signs of pre-eclampsia of pregnancy.

Overzealous treatment to achieve good blood pressure figures, rather than a good effect for the individual, should be avoided. Many people with hypertension have coexisting CHD, even if asymptomatic, and since the extraction of oxygen within the coronary circulation is close to maximum at rest, lowering the blood pressure may further compromise the coronary circulation, causing myocardial ischaemia.

Malignant elevation. At any point in primary hypertension, sudden acute elevation of pressure can occur. This malignant hypertension can rapidly become life-threatening. Death can ensue from CVA or from the cerebral oedema of hypertensive encephalopathy. Hypertension generally promotes the progression of atherosclerosis. Sudden increased pressure in vessels already compromised may lead to rupture or embolisation of existing thrombus. The importance of this depends on where the emboli occlude. Renal function is usually already impaired by renal artery sclerosis and the effects of chronic hypertension. Further occlusion of the afferent arterioles exacerbates the situation by stimulating increased renin release, which in turn contributes to the hypertensive state. Increased pressure may result in internal haemorrhage and infarction of the kidneys.

The progress of the increasing pressure is mirrored in changes to the vessels of the optic fundi, termed hypertensive retinopathy. Once papilloedema occurs, intracranial pressure has increased and the individual may complain of blurring of vision. Prognosis at this point is poor.

Management of hypertensive crisis

The aim of medical and nursing management of this life-threatening condition is a controlled reduction in blood pressure, with monitoring of other systems in order to minimise further damage or to prevent it from occurring (O'Donnell 1990, Uber & Uber 1993). Cerebral function should be assessed continuously. Blood pressure should be monitored, preferably by direct arterial cannulation, at least every 15 min to assess the efficacy of drug therapy. Cardiac demand should be reduced as much as possible by bed rest and sedation. Straining at stool should be avoided. The patient should have urinary catheterisation and frequent observation of urine output. Twenty-four hour urine collection should be commenced for excretory products of catecholamines, such as VMA, levels being twice that of normal in the presence of adrenal tumours, such as phaeochromocytoma. The nurse should also be alert for haematuria or any other sign of blood loss. Complaints of ischaemic chest pain should be investigated and treated as already described.

Anxiolytic drugs may benefit people whose condition is exacerbated by anxiety.

NURSING PRIORITIES AND MANAGEMENT: HYPERTENSION

Where hypertension is secondary to an underlying condition, nursing priorities will reflect the needs of the primary problem. Hypertension will affect lifestyle and sense of well-being in many ways.

Since people with hypertension present in various ways, it is difficult to generalise about their management plans.

The experience of pain

Pain control is appropriate in those experiencing headaches or anginal pain, with or without palpitations. Oral analgesics can be prescribed to combat the headaches although the prescription may have to be tailored to the individual, to find an effective agent. This symptom may only lessen once the level of hypertension is controlled and this may motivate the patient to comply with other treatments. Angina will be approached as previously discussed and will also be helped by other treatments aimed at lowering blood pressure, e.g. beta-blockade.

Diet and nutrition

Dietary changes are aimed at the reduction of obesity, the control of any underlying problem such as diabetes, and the reduction of the salt content. A diet rich in fruits, vegetables and low-fat dairy food with reduced saturated total fat can substantially lower blood pressure (Cutler et al 1997). It is best to involve the whole family, as it is less socially disruptive if everyone can continue to sit down to the same meals together. Also, the hereditary aspect of hypertension would indicate that it is in the whole family's interest to prevent the problem developing. No salt added at table, or salt substitutes, are advised (see p. 44). The nurse may be able to assist patients in interpreting labels on food products.

Moderating alcohol intake is advised. This may be difficult for some, where entertaining forms a great part of their work; however, low-alcohol wines and beers are increasingly available.

Elimination

Diuretic drugs can result in the need to pass urine at socially inconvenient times. This can often be avoided if the drugs are taken first thing in the morning, so that their effect is largely over by the time the person leaves home. Discussing the person's daily routine and flexibility in the timing of treatment to adapt to the person's lifestyle can result in greater compliance with treatment. It is often difficult for an asymptomatic individual to realise the importance of continuing with medication, especially if there are undesirable side-effects. It is often best to broach the subject of side-effects before they occur and to point out that other drugs can be tried if one medication does not suit.

Diuretics, apart from potassium-sparing varieties, promote the excretion of potassium in the urine. Low levels of K can result in muscle weakness and fatigue and cardiac arrhythmias. It is therefore important that potassium supplementation is also adhered to by those taking diuretics. Many products combine both diuretic and potassium. A list of foods rich in potassium, e.g. bananas, can be supplied.

Sleeping

Relaxation and rest are important. Daily routines should be examined in order to find appropriate periods for rest. Night sedation may be necessary to ensure adequate sleep, although the patient should be encouraged to maintain her own relaxation habits, e.g. soaking in a warm bath. Referral to agencies that practise relaxation and stress management techniques may be of benefit to some (see Ch. 17).

Work and leisure

Some working environments may add to the stress that individuals experience. Work routines should be re-examined to see if more opportunity exists for delegation of work and for rest. Smoking may be a habit engendered by stress and reinforced by working with a group of people in similar positions. Finding interests other than work may help the 'workaholic'. Sporting hobbies should be encouraged, as exercise will increase cardiac fitness as long as strenuous exercise is not embarked on without advice.

Breathing

Every effort should be made to stop smoking. Various approaches exist, from cigarette substitutes to hypnosis, acupuncture and sheer will power. People should be encouraged to find their own way and, as in changing eating habits, the whole family can also be involved here.

Beta-blockade, using the non-cardioselective varieties, may result in bronchospasm. This side-effect could be extremely alarming if the patient is not aware of the possibility.

Expressing sexuality

Anxiety and tension between couples may lead to sexual dysfunction. Openness on the part of health professionals may help couples to feel they can discuss their fears with these professionals and with each other. Beta-blockade may also cause impotence.

Q **2.18** Health education leaflets related to cardiovascular disease are widely available. Where do these leaflets come from? Who uses them? Do health professionals and the public find them useful? Explore these questions during your placements in community and hospital.

See Buxton (1999), pp. 47–50.

AORTIC ANEURYSMS

PATHOPHYSIOLOGY

The aorta is divided into three segments:

- the ascending aorta
- the arch
- the descending aorta, which consists of abdominal and thoracic portions.

Aneurysms are also classified by shape, as being:

- fusiform — involving a complete circumferential section
- saccular — describes an outpouching from one weakened area.

Saccular aneurysms can be tied off surgically at the neck of the sack, while fusiform types require excision and replacement with a tubular graft. If the graft is required close to the aortic valve, a composite prosthetic valve and tube graft may be employed, with reimplantation of the coronary arteries if necessary.

There are several causes of aneurysm formation:

- *Atherosclerotic disease*. This is the major cause of aneurysms, especially of the descending portion, 75% of the aorta being below the level of the diaphragm. Plaque formation reduces the nutritional supply to the aortic wall by hampering diffusion of nutrients from blood in the lumen.
- *Turbulence around bifurcations*.
- *Hypertension and medial degeneration*. The medial layer of the vessel wall undergoes degenerative changes associated with ageing. Since this is the layer that, due to its elasticity, withstands the most pressure, degeneration allows the wall to dilate. This often occurs without symptoms and may be found on routine examination. The patient is often hypertensive. Increased blood pressure, especially diastolic pressure, reduces the blood flow to the medial layer, which becomes ischaemic and weakened.
- Cystic medial degeneration also occurs as a consequence of connective tissue diseases, e.g. Marfan's and Ehlers–Danlos syndromes. These affect the ascending aorta and may cause the annulus of the aortic valve to dilate. This may result in an incompetent valve, as the cusps cannot completely cover the larger area. First presentation may be as a consequence of valvular failure.
- *Infection*. Aneurysms due to syphilis and other infectious causes are less prevalent today; they largely affect the ascending aorta.

Abdominal aortic aneurysms (AAAs)

PATHOPHYSIOLOGY

Common presenting symptoms. The majority of AAAs are without symptoms, but a pulsating abdominal mass may be felt when lying in bed. Pain relates to compression of neighbouring organs. It is severe, unrelated to movement and radiates through to the low back, and possibly down into the thighs and buttocks. Presentation may be as ischaemia of end organs whose arterial supply originates within the aneurysmal section. Ischaemia may also be the result of embolisation of thrombus that gathers in the dilated portion due to sluggish blood flow and turbulence around atherosclerotic plaques. Half of the dilatations greater than 6 cm will rupture within a year, so prompt surgical management is called for. Surgical repair involves performing a laparotomy and exposing the whole aneurysm, clamping above and below the swelling and removing the thrombus. A graft is laid within the aneurysmal sac and sutured in place. The sac is trimmed and sewn over the graft. Elderly or cardiorespiratory-compromised individuals may be unsuitable for surgical repair. Endovascular repair involving stent insertion into the affected lumen may be more appropriate for these patients (Ransome 1996). The risk of spontaneous dissection is that severe blood loss, hypotension and death will supervene. Emboli may enter the inferior vena cava and result in pulmonary infarction. Mortality in ruptured aneurysms is high. Emergency management aims to stabilise blood pressure by large volume infusion of colloid or other volume expanders, the use of military anti-shock trousers (MAST) and pharmacological support with inotropic drugs. Surgical repair should not be delayed.

MEDICAL MANAGEMENT

Investigations prior to planned surgery include X-ray, which will highlight any vessel calcification, echocardiography, ultrasound and CT scanning, all of which are non-invasive. Some centres also perform angiography; however, this may precipitate embolisation. Full cardiac investigation is required since atherosclerosis is a diffuse disease. Correction of any coronary insufficiency is recommended prior to surgical non-emergency aneurysm repair, since postoperative mortality is largely due to myocardial infarction.

Thoracic aneurysms

The aetiology is similar to aneurysms in the abdomen. False thoracic aneurysms can be secondary to blunt or penetrating injury to the chest in road traffic accidents, although they are more often associated with true rupture of the aorta, from which mortality is high. Some thoracic aneurysms are stabilised by surrounding tissue which can allow time for the patient to present at cardiothoracic services.

PATHOPHYSIOLOGY

Atherosclerosis affects the arch and descending thoracic aorta, while cystic medial degeneration and infections are found as causative agents in the ascending portion.

Common presenting symptoms depend on the site of occurrence. Chest X-ray shows a widened mediastinum. Dilatation causes pressure on other structures: bronchospasm may result from deviation of the trachea; secretion retention and alveolar collapse from obstruction; shortness of breath, and even haemoptysis, if erosion occurs into the left main bronchus. Obstruction of the oesophagus may present as dysphagia, while fainting may be the result of reduced cardiac output due to obstruction of the superior vena cava.

Dissecting aortic aneurysms

PATHOPHYSIOLOGY

Tears in the intima due to the forces of hypertension and the degenerative changes already discussed allow a column of blood to enter and disrupt the media, creating a false lumen. Classification is by site of the tear. In addition to previously discussed predisposing diseases, there is a higher, but as yet unexplained, incidence of dissection among pregnant women.

Common presenting symptoms depend upon the site and severity of the rupture. Severe anterior chest pain can be mistaken for AMI, but it is often described as tearing in nature. Pain may migrate as the dissection progresses. Alterations of neurological function may reflect involvement of the vessels originating from the arch of the aorta. As the dissection progresses, loss of peripheral pulses and palpable blood pressure will track its course. Renal artery dissection or occlusion will result in acute renal failure, exacerbated by the effects of profound hypotension. Alterations in rhythm or degrees of heart block may result from septal disruption as a consequence of aortic valve regurgitation. Leakage into the pericardium or pleural space manifests as compression known as tamponade. The signs of cardiac tamponade are:

- hypotension
- tachycardia
- raised CVP/JVP
- oliguria
- peripheral vascular constriction
- fall in peripheral temperature.

MEDICAL MANAGEMENT

Investigations are identical to those used in AAAs.

Treatment. Operative correction is urgently required. If hypertension persists, this should be controlled by the use of arterial vasodilators, intensively and invasively monitored. If hypotension and collapse has supervened then intervention is as for AAAs.

NURSING PRIORITIES AND MANAGEMENT: AORTIC ANEURYSMS

Preoperative care

Although this type of aneurysm is the most life-threatening, any vessel may become aneurysmal.

Pain control

The pain is often described as ripping or tearing in nature. Its location varies according to the section of artery affected and may progress as the dissection progresses. Intravenous opiate is the appropriate measure, but the patient may be so shocked that immediate operative procedure is of greater priority.

Anxiety and fear of dying

The prospect of surgery is extremely frightening, whether emergency or elective, and this should be acknowledged by carers. Operations carry high risks, but there is often no alternative intervention. Those going for elective procedures may wish access to legal advisors. The need for spiritual care should also be recognised. There may be times when a dignified, peaceful death is more appropriate than surgery.

Maintaining a safe environment

Rupture of an aneurysmal vessel is a potentially catastrophic and largely unpredictable event. Those with known aneurysms that do not yet merit surgery should be aware of signs that indicate a progression of their disease. Control of hypertension by medication is indicated and should be adhered to (see p. 45).

Breathing

Shortness of breath may be experienced by those with aneurysms of the thoracic aorta as the vessel impinges on the trachea. This may also result in bronchospasm. Rupture of the vessel can create a fistula into the bronchus, with resulting haemoptysis. Changing the person's position to allow maximal lung expansion may help. Oxygen therapy will often be required. Bronchodilators may be of limited use, as the problem is mechanical rather than irritant. Chest infection due to atelectasis as the lung is collapsed under the weight of the expanding aorta is to be expected. Since maintaining the airway is a potential problem, an airway, suction equipment, an Ambu-bag and other resuscitation equipment should be available.

Mobility and rest

Anxiety may prevent the patient from sleeping, so sedation may be helpful if the blood pressure is not adversely affected. The patient's condition can be so unstable that performing routine care can exhaust her. Plan care so that people are left in peace for periods. Nurses sometimes have to accept that their patient's condition will not allow care that would otherwise be thought essential, e.g. pressure area care. Consider the use of aids such as air-fluidised beds to dissipate pressure on what is often already poorly perfused skin.

Elimination

Since approximately 25% of cardiac output perfuses the kidneys, urine output is a useful and important reflection of cardiac function. Accurate observation and recording of fluid balance are essential.

Hygiene

Because of poor status and poor tissue perfusion, this is an area where the patient becomes dependent on a nurse to maintain standards of personal hygiene.

Expressing sexuality

People attending electively for resection of abdominal aneurysms may be offered counselling before surgery. There is a possibility of impotence and paraplegia postoperatively if the arterial supply to the spinal cord is interrupted. It is possible to arrange storage in sperm banks against this eventuality. These issues need to be handled with sensitivity by the nurse.

Surgical intensive care

If the patient's condition has deteriorated and surgery is necessary, she is completely dependent on hospital staff for circulatory support. Accurate haemodynamic assessment is essential. Careful observation and documentation of the response to drug therapy and large-volume colloid infusion are essential. This may require invasive monitoring and the specialist nursing skills of the intensive therapy unit, and the patient should be moved to such a unit as soon as is feasible. This can mean journeys of several hours by road or air, a daunting prospect for patient and escorting staff alike. It often necessitates the separation of the patient from her family at a time of great stress, so every effort should be made to ensure effective communication. The management of cardiogenic shock is described in Chapter 18. Postoperative care is similar to that following cardiac surgery (see Nursing Care Plan 2.1).

PERIPHERAL VASCULAR DISEASE

Arterial and venous peripheral disease can occur alone or together and it is important to be able to differentiate between the two (Bright & Georgi 1992).

Revise the vascular anatomy of the lower limbs (Wilson & Waugh 1996). See Gibson & Kenrick (1998) for patients' experiences of living with peripheral vascular disease

ARTERIAL DISEASE

Arterial occlusions

Like the rest of the cardiovascular system, the lower limbs may also be affected by atherosclerosis. Symptoms of impaired blood supply may be slow to appear if collateral circulation has had time to develop.

Arteriosclerosis obliterans

PATHOPHYSIOLOGY

This is the state of chronic occlusive atheroma of the arteries supplying the extremities. Peripheral artery occlusive disease affects approximately 12% of the population. Turbulence at bifurcations, as occurs in larger vessels, predisposes to intimal changes. There is also a degenerative element in its development. The same process is found in the cerebral and visceral arteries. The factors influencing its development have been discussed in the section on CHD and hypertension. It is typically a disease of middle-aged to elderly men, who may be hypertensive, diabetic, have a diet high in lipids and who smoke, resulting in greater risk of atherosclerosis.

Nursing Care Plan 2.1 B is a 54-year-old unemployed welder who had an abdominal aortic aneurysm repair 36 hours previously. This was an elective operation and involved the insertion of a synthetic graft. Since the operation B has been cared for in an intensive care unit. He had artificial respiratory support on a ventilator up until 12 hours ago. A urinary catheter, nasogastric tube and central venous pressure line were inserted in theatre. B's wife and family are very concerned about his condition and his wife is spending most of the day at his bedside

Nursing considerations	*Action*	*Rationale*	*Expected outcome*
1. Potential problem of hypovolaemic shock	❒ Continue to monitor vital signs, noting for: • fall in blood pressure • increase in heart rate ❒ Observe for fall in hourly urine output ❒ Observe for changes in mental state: restlessness, confusion ❒ Note and report significant changes in temperature ❒ Observe for signs of peripheral oedema and cold, pale peripheries ❒ Observe wound site for excessive leakage ❒ Give intravenous fluids as prescribed ❒ Continue with central venous pressure recordings, noting and reporting trends	Hypovolaemic shock may arise due to excessive blood loss/ inadequate fluid replacement	Stable vital signs Urine output >30 mL/h Stable neurological function
2. Possibility of developing hypertension	❒ Regular measurement of blood pressure ❒ Monitor effects of any hypertensive drug therapy ❒ Ensure that B knows to report any pain/discomfort. Assess and plan intervention, and evaluate pain relief measures ❒ Observe wound site regularly for any sign of suture line being under stress due to increased blood pressure ❒ Attempt to limit anxiety by providing information and support, and creating a calm, relaxed atmosphere for B and his family	May have been hypertensive prior to operation Systemic vascular response may increase as a result of: • decreased circulatory volume • increased sympathetic tone as a stress response To control/relieve pain and anxiety	Vital signs within normal limits Is pain-free, comfortable and relaxed
3. Risk of infection	❒ Monitor temperature recordings at regular intervals ❒ Give prophylactic antibiotics ❒ Observe sites of intravenous and arterial access for redness/ inflammation ❒ Observe colour and consistency of urine	Risk of infection due to: • surgical procedure • immobility • urinary catheterisation • venous and arterial convolution	Remains apyrexial and free from infection
4. Possibility of gastrointestinal disturbance	❒ Note nature of stools, especially diarrhoea and bloody stools ❒ Observe for increase in abdominal girth ❒ Maintain position and patency of nasogastric tube, gradually introducing fluids orally ❒ Ensure that B knows to report abdominal pain ❒ Ensure B is aware of the planned timescale for resuming eating and drinking	May develop as a result of handling the colon during surgery with resultant oedema May develop as a result of antibiotics	Remains free from gastrointestinal disturbance

(cont'd)

Nursing Care Plan 2.1 *(cont'd)*

Nursing considerations	*Action*	*Rationale*	*Expected outcome*
5. Possibility of difficulty in breathing	❒ Ensure B knows to report any difficulty breathing ❒ Observe respiratory rate and chest expansion ❒ Offer oxygen therapy ❒ Encourage turning 2-hourly to promote postural drainage ❒ Encourage deep breathing and coughing ❒ Liaise with physiotherapist regarding chest physiotherapy	Wound may limit deep breathing Abdominal distention may raise the diaphragm, reducing breathing capacity Signs of heart failure may suggest a rupture into the vena cava	Is comfortable when breathing Displays no evidence of cyanosis or heart failure
6. Potential problem of pain/discomfort	❒ Ensure B knows to report any pain/discomfort ❒ Give prescribed analgesics on a regular basis for abdominal pain at incision site ❒ ECG if B experiences chest pain ❒ Observe for signs associated with ischaemic pain: shortness of breath, nausea and vomiting	May experience abdominal pain at wound site May experience ischaemic chest pain as a result of decreased coronary artery blood flow	Is pain-free and comfortable
7. Potential problem of renal impairment	❒ Maintain record of fluid input and output ❒ Record weight at the same time daily ❒ Give intravenous fluids at the rate prescribed ❒ Note trends in urine output in relation to blood pressure and rates of drug infusion	May develop renal impairment as a result of embolisation; fall in blood pressure; trauma to the renal artery during surgery; or preoperative renal ischaemia due to renal artery involvement in development of aneurysm	Urine output >30 mL/h
8. Reduced mobility	❒ Assist to maintain desired activities of living: hygiene, personal grooming, mouth care, etc. ❒ Place objects within reach. Offer access to radio, papers, books as requested ❒ Liaise with physiotherapist ❒ Formulate plan for gradually increasing mobility, beginning with sitting out of bed for short periods ❒ Involve family members in care, if acceptable to them ❒ Encourage frequent changes in position whilst in bed ❒ Advise how to support wound when moving about	Mobility is reduced as a result of monitoring equipment, intravenous lines, urinary catheter, abdominal discomfort and uncertainty as to permitted safe level of movement	Effects of limited mobility will be minimised Mobility levels will be gradually increased
9. Anxiety and lack of information	❒ Explain all treatment and expected course of hospital stay to B and his family ❒ Encourage B's family to visit when they can promoting a welcoming and open atmosphere ❒ Develop one-to-one relationship between nurse and B to foster open communication and individualised support and information giving ❒ Provide realistic outlook for future and recovery	B and his family are likely to be anxious about the outcome of the operation and the future The ITU environment may exacerbate these feelings	B and his family will appear to be coping effectively with the operation and recovery B and his family will express that they feel able to cope and state that they understand the operation, treatment and plans for recovery

The result of increasing occlusion of the vessels, with medial calcification and loss of elastic fibres, is the slowing of blood flow. The blood becomes hypercoagulable. Thrombosis of the deep veins may occur, secondary to sudden arterial thrombosis. The ischaemia of surrounding tissue is evidenced by skin and muscle atrophy, loss of subcutaneous fat deposits and ischaemic neuropathy. Severe occlusion will result in gangrene, usually first seen at the toes, then extending into the foot and leg. At the boundary between viable and necrotic tissue, an area of inflammation is often seen. The extent of the ischaemia will depend on how quickly occlusion developed and how extensive collateral circulation has become. Gangrene occurs when insufficient oxygen is conveyed to the tissue to sustain its life. This can be exacerbated by any other superimposed demand, e.g. infection, when oxygen demand rises but cannot be sustained by an impaired blood flow. Diabetic patients are more prone to infected ulceration in association with gangrene (see Ch. 5). Vasoconstriction should be avoided if at all possible.

Common presenting symptoms may occur gradually or with sudden acute thrombosis, which may be the first indication of a process that has been silently progressing for some time (see Table 2.8).

Pain: intermittent claudication. This is exercise-induced pain in muscle groups distal to the occluded vessel. Its nature varies from a numb cramp to severe pain. It is a manifestation of increased oxygen demand with exercise and the subsequent accumulation of metabolic wastes. This is relieved by rest. The calf muscles are the most commonly affected, but thigh and buttock muscles can also be involved, depending on the site of occlusion. The distance the individual can walk on the flat before onset of symptoms (claudication distance) is an indication of the progress of the disease. Pain may eventually occur at rest, most often in the toes and foot and particularly at night when it interferes with sleep. Pain may become severe and difficult to contain when gangrene intervenes. However, a degree of neuropathy reduces sensation and may make the person unaware of the progressive gangrenous changes. Any exercise that can be tolerated should be encouraged.

MEDICAL MANAGEMENT

Investigations

Pulses should be assessed at rest in a warm room. They may remain intact until two-thirds of the lumen is occluded. Posterior tibial, popliteal and femoral pulses should be included in the examination (dorsalis pedis pulses are not consistently present in all people). The volume of the pulses should be compared, as well as simple absence or presence. Many people find it difficult to differentiate between their own pulses and the patient's, and increasing the examiner's rate by exercising can help in this situation. Bruits may also be heard over areas of turbulence in arteries that are still pulsating.

Colour and temperature. As occlusion develops, the feet, and especially the toes, may be red in colour. This can later develop into bluish mottled areas or areas of pallor. With sudden occlusion, pallor may be marked. Elevation of legs with severe occlusion results in deathly pallor. Once legs return to the dependent position, colour normally returns. Superficial veins normally refill within 15 s, but in these cases it may take a minute or more. In severe cases, the limbs may become a cyanotic red colour (rubor). Temperature changes accompany reduced blood flow with cool pale extremities.

Chest X-rays will show calcification of the vessel wall.

Doppler ultrasound. When low-intensity sound is directed through the tissue towards a blood vessel, sound waves strike moving blood cells and are transmitted back. The frequency of the sound waves that are reflected changes in proportion to the velocity of the blood. Sound waves diminish in arterial occlusion and stenosis.

Arteriograms are usually performed in order to assess the occlusion prior to surgery.

Table 2.8 Presenting features of arterial and venous peripheral vascular disease. (Adapted from Bright and Georgi 1992.)

Assess	*Arterial disease*	*Venous disease*
Pain	Acute: sudden, severe pain, peaks rapidly Chronic: intermittent claudication; rest pain	Acute: little or no pain; tenderness along course of inflamed vein Chronic: heaviness, fullness
Impotence	May be present with aortoiliac femoral disease	Not associated
Hair	Hair loss distal to occlusion	No hair loss
Nails	Thick, brittle	Normal
Skeletal muscle	Atrophy may be present; may have restricted limb movement	Normal
Sensation	Possible paraesthesia	Normal
Skin colour	Pallor or reactive hyperaemia (pallor when limb elevated; rubor [red] when limb dependent)	Brawny (reddish-brown); cyanotic if dependent
Skin texture	Thin, shiny, dry	Stasis dermatitis; veins may be visible; skin mottling
Skin temperature	Cool	Warm
Skin breakdown (ulcers)	Severely painful; usually on or between toes or on upper surface of foot over metatarsal heads or other bony prominences	Mildly painful, with pain relieved by leg elevation; usually in ankle area
Oedema	None or mild; usually unilateral	Typically present, usually foot to calf; may be unilateral or bilateral
Pulses	Diminished, weak, absent	Normal
Blood flow	Bruit may be present; pressure readings lower below stenosis	Normal

Other examinations include ECG, a full blood count, urea, electrolytes and blood sugar estimation.

Treatment. Underlying disease states, e.g. diabetes and infection, should be as well controlled as possible. Advice aimed at minimising symptoms and the risk of extending atherosclerosis should be given, as follows:

- Modify the diet to reduce lipid intake.
- Avoid:
  —cigarette smoking
  —tight clothing
  —cold temperature
  All of these lead to vasoconstriction.
- Avoid direct use of heat because of the risk of burns in a limb with decreased sensation.
- Promote increased blood supply by a generally warm environment and elevation of the head of the bed.
- Avoid maintaining a completely dependent position since the resultant oedema will further reduce circulation.
- Encourage exercise up to the limit of pain, partly to maintain joint and muscle function and to promote collateral circulation. By walking three to four times a day, ischaemic time will decrease and pain control can also be improved by increasing blood flow; however, ischaemic pain is notoriously difficult to manage and may require opiate analgesics and night sedation.
- Avoid trauma to the impaired limb.
- Avoid ill-fitting shoes; referral to a chiropodist may be required.

Following assessment, sympathectomy may be considered to increase blood flow by obliterating neural control of vasoconstriction.

Percutaneous transluminal balloon angioplasty (PTBA) is a minimally invasive treatment for patients with atherosclerotic peripheral vascular disease. This surgical technique involves placing an intra-arterial balloon within an obstructing arterial lesion and forcibly dilating the balloon under fluoroscopy. In selected patients, the use of an intravascular stent may be an alternative to traditional bypass.

If the occlusion is sudden and acute and the viability of the limb is in question, then surgical intervention will be required to bypass the occlusion using either saphenous vein or prosthetic material, e.g. a femoropopliteal bypass. Endarterectomy of the vessel may be performed first to core out the atheroma of the vessel.

Prior to surgery the patient may undergo arteriography and should be rehydrated and have blood coagulation status assessed. There is a strong association with CHD, so full cardiac assessment is required prior to operation. If the lesion is localised and accessible, embolectomy under local anaesthesia may be sufficient to reperfuse the limb. In this procedure, a catheter is inserted into the artery up to the level of the occlusion when the balloon at the end is inflated, aiming to fracture the plaque. Inflammation and re-endothelialisation occur secondary to this. Fibrinolytic drugs can be infused at the site of the occlusion. The advantage of embolectomy is that general anaesthesia can be avoided; however, reocclusion occurs more frequently than with bypass grafting.

For more information on symptom distress, mood and discharge information needs after peripheral arterial bypass see Galloway et al (1995).

Pain may become so severe and gangrene so advanced that the limb is no longer viable and amputation may become unavoidable. Bypass grafting may minimise the extent of amputation by restoring circulation, e.g. to a foot, but losing some of the toes. Amputation of a limb is traumatic for anyone but may be accepted as a relief from intolerable pain. It may, however, require skilled counselling before this fact can be faced by the patient and the full support of rehabilitation and limb-fitting services postoperatively (see Ch. 10).

Q **2.19** Find out about the rehabilitative care for any patient who has had amputation of a lower limb and is adapting to the use of a prosthesis.

For more information on the care of a patient faced with the prospect of amputation, see Donohue (1997a–d).

Thromboangiitis obliterans or Buerger's disease

This occlusive inflammatory disease has no known cause. It manifests in a younger population than atherosclerosis, is predominant in men and is strongly associated with smoking. It is postulated that carbon monoxide has a toxic effect on the arterial wall and nicotine has vasoconstrictive effects. In contrast to atherosclerosis, it affects small and medium vessels of the extremities. It is not a diffuse disease since only segments of arteries develop lesions. Thrombosis is a secondary feature. The lumen may become occluded and the intima thickened but the medial wall structure remains intact, in contrast to atherosclerotic disease. The diagnosis can often be made on the basis of a careful history and physical examination. Occasionally, arteriography is warranted to confirm the diagnosis. The patient is strongly advised to stop smoking. Besides the general treatment approaches used in ischaemic diseases of the limbs — antibiotics, antirheumatics and corticosteroids — some specific surgical procedures may be considered.

Raynaud's disease

This is a vasospastic condition, usually occurring in young women and more prevalent in cool, damp climates. A distinction should be made between Raynaud's phenomenon, which results in no permanent damage, and Raynaud's disease, the more advanced condition associated with permanent damage. Constriction of the arterioles associated with cold and emotional stress results in colour changes, usually in the hands. The fingers become pale and cold, but pulses are intact. Cyanosis may also be a feature. Pain is not always present, but function may be lost. Similar episodes of vasospasm can be found secondary to scleroderma, some neurological conditions and in some occupational groups, e.g. those that use pneumatic vibrating tools. Treatment includes avoiding the situation that triggers the problem. This may mean a change in occupation, giving up smoking and keeping warm. Vasodilating drugs, including calcium channel blockers (e.g. nifedipine), and sympathectomy have been tried as means of improving the circulation. The nurse's primary role is patient education so that the onset of symptoms associated with this disease can be identified and minimised.

For a discussion of the nurses' role in patient education in this disease, see Kaufman (1996).

NURSING PRIORITIES AND MANAGEMENT: ARTERIAL DISEASE

Almost all the activities of life are affected by the distress of arterial disease.

Case History 2.3 Mrs C

Mrs C is 75, living alone in a large apartment. She has extensive arterial disease and is awaiting admission for femoropopliteal artery bypass surgery. The community nurse and occupational therapist carry out a personal and environmental assessment pre-surgery. During their home visit, they note many environmental hazards that could cause accidents and lower limb damage.

Maintaining a safe environment

Possible loss of sensation increases the risk of trauma to tissue that has reduced ability to combat infection and to heal. The person's home and work circumstances can be considered, and hazards minimised (see Case History 2.3). Useful advice includes the following points:

- Toenails may be best cut by the chiropodist in case soft tissue injury is inflicted, especially as some people with atherosclerotic disease, with or without diabetes, may also have poor sight.
- Caution should be exercised with electric blankets, hot water bottles, open fires and hot baths, as burns may not be felt.
- Cold can also be damaging.
- Constrictive clothing, e.g. tight underwear, is best avoided.
- Sitting cross-legged causes constriction of lower limb circulation.
- Remaining in one position for any length of time puts pressure on one area of tissue, allowing ischaemic changes to occur.
- Bed cradles can be used to support bedclothes without causing constriction.

2.20 Drawing on your experience of visiting old people at home, identify the range of possible hazards.

Think of your own home and work environment. How aware are you of actual and potential damage to your lower limbs from knocks, friction, pressure and cuts?

Health professionals try to act in the best interests of their patients but may fail to assess the situation adequately. For example, the community nurse slipped on Mrs C's rug (Case History 2.3), which was lying in the centre of the highly polished hallway floor. She promptly rolled up the rug and put it away in a cupboard.

2.21 How might Mrs C feel in that situation?

In fact, Mrs C quickly returned the rug to the hallway floor, saying: 'Don't worry, that lovely rug was my mother's. I never set foot on it. I just walk round the edge. I'll be quite safe, but you be careful.'

Pain control

The pain of claudication is relieved by rest; however, exercise to the limit of pain is to be encouraged in the hope of developing increased perfusion and collateral circulation. Controlling ischaemic pain is essential and will often require the use of opiate analgesics, which may cause drowsiness as a side-effect. Keeping warm, especially for people affected by vessel spasm, and positioning the affected limb in a dependent position from time to time are also advised. Anti-inflammatory drugs are used in diseases with an inflammatory response. Distraction techniques can also be helpful (see Ch. 19).

Eating and drinking

Excessive weight increases circulatory demand, and people with diabetes need to be particularly careful about what they eat. Dehydration contributes to the process of clot formation because of increased blood concentration, so taking plenty of liquids is recommended. A balanced diet, including the vitamins and trace elements that aid tissue healing and integrity, can help to prevent aggravation of symptoms (see Ch. 23). People with hyperlipidaemia could be encouraged to follow the diet suggested for those with coronary heart disease (CHD) and may also be prescribed drugs to reduce their lipid levels.

Sleep

This is often impaired by pain. Elevating the bed head is suggested to increase flow (see also Ch. 25).

Breathing

Smoking reduces the amount of oxygen the haemoglobin can carry and nicotine results in venous spasm. Encouraging the patient to give up smoking may therefore produce benefits.

See Parry et al (1998) for a discussion of the impact of smoking on an individual with arterial disease.

Mobility

Maintaining as great a degree of mobility as possible can help to prevent general stiffness of all joints, which can develop if they are underutilised. Muscle wasting and weakness are associated problems; the patient can be encouraged to carry out a wide range of joint exercises.

Hygiene

Careful attention to hygiene helps to prevent infection, especially if the person is diabetic. After bathing, the skin should be thoroughly dried, especially between the toes. This gives the opportunity to assess the skin for any signs of ischaemia. Points to note are as follows:

- bath water should be neither too hot nor too cold
- tight socks with elastic tops cause constriction
- clean clothing, daily, is preferred
- plastic shoes encourage sweating and maceration of the skin as water cannot evaporate.

Work

Consideration should be given as to the physical demands and environmental hazards at the person's work. Strong analgesics may also impair work performance and safety.

Discharge planning

After successful surgery, it is important to consider how vascular improvement can be maintained to ensure a reasonable quality of life and prevent further hospital admissions.

VENOUS DISEASE

Venous insufficiency

Venous disease results from:

- obstruction, by thrombus or thrombophlebitis
- incompetence of valves in the veins.

2.22 Read Case History 2.4 and consider the following questions:
(a) What is meant by the term gangrene?
(b) Mr L was suffering from the pain of ischaemia prior to surgery. What was meant by phantom limb pain and how do you think such pain could be alleviated?
(c) Can you explain, in physiological terms, why his aching legs were relieved by rest?
(d) Describe the tests Mr L might have undergone to assess his arterial insufficiency?
(e) How does smoking affect feet?
(f) What vasodilatory medication might have been prescribed?
(g) What was the surgery Mr L underwent?
(h) It was clear that Mr L found it almost impossible to change his lifestyle. What role do you think hospital and community nurses can play in helping someone like Mr L?
(i) Outline a plan of care for Mr L for the immediate postoperative period after an above-knee amputation of his right leg.

2.23 What kind of discharge planning would be appropriate for Mrs C (see Case History 2.3) following femoropopliteal bypass grafting?

Some diseases, such as varicose veins, may seem trivial but can contribute to day-to-day discomfort and absence from work. Other venous diseases are associated with chronic health problems, such as venous ulcers, or a sudden medical emergency, such as pulmonary embolus following deep vein thrombosis.

Deep vein thrombosis (DVT)

Clot formation is more likely to occur when flow is reduced within the veins. This can occur due to obstruction and stasis but is also associated with increased blood viscosity, slower flow and damage to the endothelial wall of the vessel. Hypercoagulability may be a feature of dehydration or malignant disease. It seems that there is also an imbalance between fibrinolysis and coagulation in the postoperative patient, which predisposes them to DVT. Trauma may be mechanical or chemical. The increasing use of vascular cannulae predisposes the patient in hospital to the irritant effects of pharmacological preparations, the plastic of the cannula itself and the possibility of intimal trauma at insertion.

Stasis allows clotting factors that normally would be cleared from the circulation to remain active for longer. The effects of the muscle pumps of the leg and negative intrathoracic pressure during inspiration normally promote venous return. Any situation that obliterates their action predisposes to stasis of the venous circulation. Immobility and the recumbent position are frequently features of the postoperative patient and the elderly. Muscle relaxant drugs used during surgery abolish the muscle pump, and breathing is under positive pressure when ventilated mechanically. Stasis is more common in the dilated portions of varicosities. Mechanical obstruction to flow can be seen in pregnancy and abdominal tumours.

For further information on assessing patients at risk of DVT, see Autar (1998).

Case History 2.4 — Peripheral vascular disease: Mr L's memories

Mr L lay back on his hospital pillow, wishing he was at home. The powerful analgesic was at last easing the pain in his gangrenous foot. Tomorrow he would have surgery that would rid him of the limb, but losing a limb had been difficult to come to terms with — and what was this phantom pain he had heard so much about?

Thirty years ago Mr L had been strong and fit, fond of long country walks and watching football. His first complaint had been aching legs after his long walks, but it hadn't lasted long and was easily relieved by sitting down. However, the aching became a great deal worse and his walks became shorter and shorter. Fond of his food, he had gained weight and spent more of his leisure time smoking.

His GP had described his symptoms as intermittent claudication or limping. He had said it was due to impairment of the blood supply to his lower limbs and had organised several tests to confirm this. At first the treatment had seemed quite easy. Mr L had to cut down on his smoking, alter his diet to avoid rich and fatty food that could 'clog up' his arteries and avoid extremes of temperature, which would make the symptoms worse.

It had been hard to stick to his diet and give up smoking and, seeing no visible evidence of it working, he had soon abandoned this. The ache in his legs eventually became worse, developing into excruciating pain. At night he had to sit up in bed and hang his legs down to cool them and ease the pain. The GP had given him tablets to help dilate the blood vessels but they hadn't helped and not long afterwards he had found himself facing an operation to improve the blood supply.

Mr L hadn't minded the operation too much. One of his veins had been used to bypass the occlusion in the artery of his thigh. He had thought this rather clever at the time and he had quickly felt the benefits. After the operation he had felt much more enthusiastic about changing his lifestyle. The surgeon had stressed that the success of the operation in the long term would depend on his ability to stop smoking, and he had, for a while. Friends and family had said he looked so much better but somehow it didn't last. He had lost weight but just couldn't stop smoking. He had known the pain was coming back. His toes were looking discoloured and often felt either very sensitive or numb. The skin on his right leg, particularly, was thin and dry and there had seemed to be less muscle. Once again, he had found himself in hospital, the circulation to his lower limbs being thoroughly assessed.

The night before his operation he was unable to sleep and feared both the immediate and long-term future.

MEDICAL MANAGEMENT

The affected area will be tender, swollen and hot. D-dimer, a fibrin degradation product, is used as a diagnostic aid. Once diagnosed, treatment includes pain relief and anticoagulation, first with heparin and later with warfarin; bed rest with leg elevation will be necessary until swelling and pain subside. Bed rest may prevent the thrombus dislodging, resulting in embolisation, usually of the lungs.

Early ambulation, especially of the elderly postoperative patient, helps prevent stasis. Sized-to-fit, knee-length graded compression stockings should be worn (see Cowan 1997) and prophylactic subcutaneous heparin is almost a routine postoperative prescription. Avoidance of dehydration, external pressure, immobility in those at risk, and careful observation are all part of the preventive management.

Chronic venous insufficiency

Of those suffering from chronic venous insufficiency, most will have had episodes of DVT previously. Pressure within the venous system remains high, resulting in increased capillary pressure and allowing chronic oedema to develop. The valves and elastic fibres of the vein wall are also destroyed by thrombophlebitis, aggravating the situation. Accumulation of interstitial fluid increases pressure locally. Eczema may occur secondary to this, possibly with pruritus. Owing to stasis, red blood cells may be trapped and haemolysed. This manifests as areas of brown pigmentation (haemosiderin). Melanin may also be deposited. Prolonged oedema reduces the nutrition available to subcutaneous tissue, which then fibroses. This induration further prevents drainage of any oedema.

Venous ulcers. Ulceration may follow trauma or dermatitis of such an area. Ulcers are commonly seen around the internal malleolus and tend to recur in the same place, as the scar tissue is atrophic.

See Hollingworth (1998) for information on the aetiology of leg ulcers.

Infection of ulcers is common. Venous ulceration is a major problem, particularly in the elderly population, with district nurses spending up to 50% of their time treating venous leg ulcers (Peters 1998). Compression therapy is considered to be the most appropriate non-invasive treatment of leg ulcers (Gould et al 1998), although appropriate patients may benefit from surgery.

MEDICAL MANAGEMENT

Prompt and correct treatment of thrombophlebitis goes a long way to prevent chronic venous insufficiency. Pain is worse in the dependent position, so elevation of the limb when seated and regular walking should be advised. Prolonged standing should be avoided.

Oedema is treated by elevation during bed rest. Once it is reduced, support stockings should be fitted. Any infection should be isolated and treated with appropriate medication. If varicose veins contribute to ulceration, they may be dealt with surgically. Chronic ulcers may have to be skin-grafted.

Further details of the nursing care of individuals who live with chronic arterial and venous ulcers are given in Chapter 23.

Varicose veins

Varicosities are long and tortuously dilated veins. They are partly due to the effects of gravity. Dilatation causes the valves to become incompetent and retrograde flow is no longer prevented. It has a genetic component: about half the sufferers will have a family history of varicosities. The hormonal changes in pregnancy also reduce venous tone, while the obstruction to venous return by the gravid uterus combines to increase pregnant women's susceptibility. Simple obesity has a similar obstructive effect. Standing for prolonged periods maximises the force of gravity. Thrombophlebitis of the deep veins increases venous pressure, while inflammation destroys valve tissue. This increase in pressure is transmitted to the superficial veins which, being relatively less supported by surrounding structures, dilate. Most people complain of dull aching in their legs. Trauma may result in significant blood loss and should be guarded against. Ulcers are rare. Some individuals are concerned by appearance. Elevation and support stockings may help the aching and reduce oedema.

MEDICAL MANAGEMENT

If symptoms persist, the most common management is the surgical stripping and ligation of the varicose vein. For some, the injection of a sclerosing agent would be considered. Treatment is increasingly being carried out on a day surgery basis and this has an impact on nursing care priorities both in hospital and at home. There is potentially less time for providing accurate information to patients about the disease process, treatment options and interventions for its prevention. (For further information on surgical intervention see Ch. 26.)

For a review of the treatment and prevention of varicose veins, see Johnson (1997).

NURSING PRIORITIES AND MANAGEMENT: VENOUS INSUFFICIENCY

Mobility

Mobility should be maintained as much as possible. Patients should be advised to elevate the legs when sitting, in order to increase venous return and reduce oedema, and to avoid standing for long periods. After an operation for ligation of varicosities, measures to prevent DVT should be considered. The patient will be advised to:

- walk a prescribed distance of perhaps 2 miles daily
- avoid standing for long periods
- always elevate the feet when sitting.

(See Nursing Care Plan 2.2.)

Eating and drinking

Adequate hydration and balanced nutrition assist flow and maintain vessel integrity. Some supplementation of vitamins, trace elements and iron may have to be considered in the elderly.

Maintaining a safe environment

Avoidance of trauma and infection is important, as in arterial disease. Blood loss can be severe, even from venous circulation.

Working

Occupations that involve standing for long periods, e.g. shop assistants, may present a problem. Prophylactic use of support hose by at-risk groups may be something the occupational health nurse could advise.

Pain control

Bed rest or limb elevation reduces the throbbing pain of venous insufficiency. Walking rather than standing is advisable. Supportive anti-embolism stockings, by aiding venous return, reduce the feeling of pressure in the legs. However, they can be hot and uncomfortable. Once any oedema has reduced, the patient should be measured again, to ensure that the stockings fit properly and are still therapeutic. Similarly, swollen legs should not be squeezed into elastic stockings that have become too small. Anti-inflammatory drugs may be prescribed to settle the inflammatory process of thromboembolism.

Nursing Care Plan 2.2 J is a 68-year-old lady admitted to hospital 2 days previously for surgical stripping and ligation of varicose veins in her left leg. J lives alone and is concerned about how she will cope after discharge

Nursing considerations	*Action*	*Rationale*	*Expected outcome*
1. Pain/discomfort	❒ Explain normal pains/sensations likely to be felt over forthcoming days/weeks ❒ Ensure support stockings are fitted correctly ❒ Give analgesics to promote pain-free movement of affected extremities ❒ Inspect bandages regularly for bleeding	It is normal for the leg to feel painful and be very bruised. This may be a problem in the groin, particularly if the support stocking ends over a bruise Complaints of patchy numbness are to be expected, but these disappear over a year Sensation of pins and needles or hypersensitivity to touch in the involved extremity may indicate a temporary or permanent nerve njury as a result of surgery; the saphenous vein and saphenous nerve are in close proximity	Ultimately, is pain-free and comfortable Feels informed about the pains/sensations to expect Wears support stockings correctly
2. Leg needs to be supported	❒ Elevate leg 30° to provide adequate support for whole leg ❒ Leg to be encased in pressure bandage from toe to groin for about a week, followed by knee level stockings for 3–4 weeks after surgery ❒ Ensure J has adequate supply of stockings	Long-term elastic support after discharge will promote circulation and limit likelihood of recurrence	Is aware of the importance of supporting the leg
3. Fear/difficulty in walking	❒ Encourage J to walk with normal gait, offering support if necessary ❒ Encourage short frequent walks to regain confidence and promote circulation ❒ Give analgesics to ease movement of affected extremity ❒ Advise to continue leg exercises after discharge	Early ambulation needs to be encouraged to promote circulation	Feels confident about walking and is able to walk without discomfort
4. Potential for recurrence of varicosities	❒ Advise J to continue to avoid activities that cause venous stress by obstructing blood flow: • avoid wearing tight socks or tight girdle • avoid sitting or standing for long periods of time • avoid dangling legs (causes stasis of blood in lower leg) • avoid crossing legs at the knee for long periods whilst sitting (decreases circulation by 15%) ❒ Elevate foot of bed 15–20° at night ❒ Avoid excessive weight gain ❒ Wear elastic support tights ❒ Attend outpatient follow-up visits every 6 months ❒ Avoid knocking/damaging leg	It is possible that varicosities may recur, therefore conservative measures learned perioperatively need to be continued	Recurrence of varicosities will be avoided Will feel confident about practising preventive measures
5. Coping after discharge	❒ Ensure that she knows what to expect after discharge ❒ Discuss availability of support from family and neighbours after discharge; assist in coordinating these resources ❒ Discuss feelings about wearing support bandages; arrange to talk to someone who has previously had this operation to talk through feelings ❒ Arrange for district nurse to visit after 12–14 days to remove sutures ❒ Advise about keeping bandage dry when washing ❒ Ensure she is aware of outpatient follow-up	May feel isolated after support of hospital May feel embarrassed about having to wear support stockings May have difficulty coping with activities of living at home Sutures are removed after 2 weeks	Feels more confident about coping after discharge home

Lifestyle issues

Women taking oral contraception run a slightly increased risk of DVT, especially if there is a family history of thrombosis. If a DVT was to develop then oral contraception would have to be discontinued and another form adopted. Pregnant women are also more prone to DVT and varicose vein formation. The cosmetic effect of these problems can prove very upsetting, as wearing thick white stockings is far from attractive. Trousers and opaque-coloured tights may make them more acceptable. The perfect compression stocking, which would be easy to put on, comfortable to wear, give adequate graduated compression and look fashionably sheer, has not yet been invented!

REFERENCES

Albarran J A W, Bridger S 1997 Problems with providing education on resuming sexual activity after myocardial infarction: developing written information for patients. Intensive and Critical Care Nursing 13: 2–11

Ashworth P 1992 Cardiovascular problems and nursing. In: Ashworth P M, Clarke C (eds) Cardiovascular intensive care nursing. Churchill Livingstone, Edinburgh, pp 1–19

Bennett P, Mayfield T 1998 Mood and behaviour following first myocardial infarction. Coronary Health Care 2(4): 210–214

Boore J R P, Champion R, Ferguson M C (eds) 1987 Nursing the physically ill adult: a textbook of medical-surgical nursing. Churchill Livingstone, Edinburgh

Bowman G S, Thompson D R, Lewin R J P 1998 Why are patients with heart failure not routinely offered cardiac rehabilitation? Coronary Health Care 2: 187–192

Bright L D, Georgi S 1992 Peripheral vascular disease: is it arterial or venous? American Journal of Nursing 92(9): 34–47

British Heart Foundation 1998 Coronary heart disease statistics. British Heart Foundation, London

British Heart Foundation 1999 Statistics database. British Heart Foundation, London

British Medical Association and Royal College of Nursing 1993 Cardiopulmonary resuscitation: a statement. BMA/RCN, London

Broomfield R 1996a The named nurse in the coronary care setting. Professional Nurse 11(4): 256–258

Broomfield R 1996b A quasi-experimental research to investigate the retention of basic cardiopulmonary resuscitation skills and knowledge by qualified nurses following a course in professional development. Journal of Advanced Nursing 23: 1016–1023

Campanella C 1997 Port access coronary artery surgery and mitral valve surgery. Cardiology News 10: 9–12

Caunt J 1996 The advanced nurse practitioner in CCU. Care of the Critically Ill 12: 136–139

Collins R, Peto R 1994 Antihypertensive drug therapy: effects on stroke and coronary heart disease. In: Swales J D (ed) Textbook of hypertension. Blackwell Scientific Publications, Oxford, pp 1156–1163

Connors P 1996 Should relatives be allowed in the resuscitation room? Nursing Standard 10(44): 42–44

Cowan T 1997 Compression hosiery. Professional Nurse 12(12): 881–886

Cutler T M, Windhausser M M, Lin P H, Jaranja N 1997 A clinical trial of the effects of dietary patterns on blood pressure. DASH Collaborative Research Group. New England Journal of Medicine 336: 1117–1124

De Belder A J, Thomas M R 1997 Primary angioplasty for the acute myocardial infarction. British Journal of Hospital Medicine 58: 35–38

De Feyter P, Ruygrok P N, Mills P 1996 Some thoughts on the present and future of coronary artery stenting. Heart 75: 356–358

Duddy I, Parahoo K 1992 The evaluation of a community coronary specialist nursing service in Northern Ireland. Journal of Advanced Nursing 17(3): 288–293

European Resuscitation Council: Basic Life Support Working Group 1998 The 1998 European Resuscitation Council guidelines for adult single rescuer basic life support. British Medical Journal 316: 1870–1876

Fahey T P, Peters T J 1996 What constitutes hypertension? Patient based comparison of hypertension guidelines. British Medical Journal 313: 93–96

Fullard E M 1998 Organisation of secondary prevention of coronary heart disease in primary care. The nurses' perspective. Coronary Health Care 2(4): 177–236

Gould D J, Campbell S, Newton H, Duffelen P, Harding E F 1998 Setopress vs Elastocrepe in chronic venous ulceration. British Journal of Nursing 7(2): 66–70, 72–73

Hancock H 1996a The complexity of pain assessment in the first 24 hours after cardiac surgery: implications for nurses. Part 1. Intensive and Critical Care Nursing 12: 295–302

Hancock H 1996b The complexity of pain assessment and management in the first 24 hours after cardiac surgery: implications for nurses. Part 2. Intensive and Critical Care Nursing 12: 346–353

Howard C 1996 Fast-track care after cardiac surgery. British Journal of Nursing 4: 1112–1117

Inwood H 1996 Knowledge of resuscitation. Intensive and Critical Care Nursing 12: 33–39

Jaarsma T, Dracup K, Walden J, Stevenson W 1996 Sexual function in patients with advanced heart failure. Heart and Lung 25: 262–270

Jackson R T, Sackett D L 1996 Guidelines for raised blood pressure. Evidence based or evidence burdened? British Medical Journal 313: 64–65

Jenkins D A, Rogers H 1995 Transfer anxiety in patients with myocardial infarction. British Journal of Nursing 4: 1248–1252

Jensen K, Banwart L, Venhaus R, Popkess-Vawter S 1993 Advanced rehabilitation nursing care of coronary angioplasty patients using self-efficacy theory. Journal of Advanced Nursing 18: 926–931

Jones C 1992 Sexual activity after myocardial infarction. Nursing Standard 6(48): 25–28

Kegel L S 1996 Case management, critical pathways and myocardial infarction. Critical Care Nurse 16: 97–104

Kolvekar S, Forysth A 1991 Valvular surgery. Nursing Standard 5(32): 48–49

Laitinen H 1996 Patients' experience of confusion in the intensive care unit following cardiac surgery. Intensive and Critical Care Nursing 12: 79–83

Lewin B, Robertson I M, Cay E L, Irving J B, Cambell M 1992 A self help post MI rehabilitation package. The heart manual: effects on psychological adjustment, hospitalisation and GP consultation. Lancet 339: 1036–1040

Linden B 1995 Evaluation of a home based rehabilitation programme for patients recovering from acute myocardial infarction. Intensive and Critical Care Nursing 11: 10–19

Lydakis C, Lip G Y H, Beevers M, Beevers D G 1997 Diet, lifestyle and blood pressure. Coronary Health Care 1: 130–137

McMurray J J V, Stewart S 1998 Nurse-led multidisciplinary intervention in chronic heart failure. Editorial. Heart 80: 430–431

Majeed H A 1989 Acute rheumatic fever. Medicine International 70: 2910

Maniadakas N 1997 Coronary heart disease statistics: economic costs supplement. British Heart Foundation, London

Mason S 1996 The ethical dilemma of the do not resuscitate order. British Journal of Nursing 6: 646–649

Nelson S 1996 Pre-admission education for patients undergoing cardiac surgery. British Journal of Nursing 5: 335–340

O'Connor L 1995 Pain assessment by patients and nurses, and nurses' notes on it, in early acute myocardial infarction. Intensive and Critical Care Nursing 11: 183–191

O'Donnell M E 1990 Assessment of the patient with malignant hypertension. Dimensions of Critical Care Nursing 9(5): 280–286

O'Neal P V 1994 How to spot early signs of cardiogenic shock. American Journal of Nursing 94(5): 36–41

Orem D 1991 Nursing, concepts of practice, 2nd edn. McGraw-Hill, New York

Peters J 1998 A review of the factors influencing nonrecurrence of venous leg ulcers. Journal of Clinical Nursing 7(1): 3–9

Quinn T 1995 Can nurses safely assess suitability for thrombolytic therapy? A pilot study. Intensive and Critical Care Nursing 11: 126–129

Radley A, Grove A, Wright S, Thurston H 1998 Problems of women compared to those of men following first myocardial infarction. Coronary Health Care 2(4): 202–209

Ransome P 1996 Transluminal aortic stenting. Nursing Standard 23(11): 52–53

Rhodes M A 1998 What is the evidence to support nurse-led thrombolysis? Clinical Effectiveness in Nursing 2(2): 29-77

Richards R J, Thakur V, Reison E 1996 Obesity related hypertension: its physiological basis and pharmacological approaches to its treatment. Journal of Human Hypertension 10(suppl. 3): 559–564

Roper N, Logan W W, Tierney A J 1996 The elements of nursing, 4th edn. Churchill Livingstone, Edinburgh

Roy C 1984 Introduction to nursing: an adaptation model. Prentice Hall, New Jersey

Thompson D R 1990 Counselling the coronary patient and partner. Scutari, London

Thompson D R, Bowman G S, Kitson A L, de Bono D P, Hopkins A 1996 Cardiac rehabilitation in the United Kingdom: guidelines and audit standards. Heart 75: 89–93

Thompson D R, Ersser S J, Webster R A 1995 The experiences of patients and their partners one month after a heart attack. Journal of Advanced Nursing 22: 707–714

Thompson D R, Webster R A 1992 Caring for the coronary patient. Butterworth-Heinemann, Oxford

Thompson D R, Webster R A, Sutton T W 1994 Coronary care unit patients' and nurses' ratings of intensity of ischaemic chest pain. Intensive and Critical Care Nursing 10: 81–88

Tuchek M F 1991 Valvular heart disease in the older adult: a case study presentation. Nursing 4(1): 58–68

Uber L A, Uber W E 1993 Hypertensive crisis in the 1990s. Critical Care Nursing Quarterly 16(2): 27-34

Williams K (ed) 1992 The community prevention of coronary heart disease. HMSO, London

Wilson K J W 1996 Ross & Wilson anatomy and physiology in health and illness, 8th edn. Churchill Livingstone, Edinburgh

Yudkin J S 1998 Managing the diabetic patient with acute myocardial infarction. Diabetic Medicine 15: 276-281

FURTHER READING

Allaker D 1995 Enhancing exercise motivation and adherence in cardiac rehabilitation. In: Coates A, McGee H, Stokes H, Thompson D R (eds) BACR guidelines for cardiac rehabilitation. Blackwell Science, Oxford, pp 92–101

Autar R 1998 Calculating patients' risk of deep vein thrombosis. British Journal of Nursing 7(1): 7–12

Baskett P J, Strunin L (eds) 1997 Resuscitation. (BJA in association with Resuscitation Council (UK)). British Journal of Anaesthesia 79: 2

Bennett P 1996 Counselling for heart disease. British Psychological Society, Leicester

Berne R M, Levy M N 1997 Cardiovascular physiology, 7th edn. Mosby, St Louis

Brown L (ed) 1998 Cardiac intensive care. WB Saunders, Philadelphia

Buxton T 1999 Effective ways to improve health education materials. Journal of Health Education 30: 47–50

Clark J M, Rowe K, Jones K 1994 Evaluating the effectiveness of coronary care nurses' role in smoking cessation. Journal of Clinical Nursing 2: 313–322

Dahlen R, Roberts S 1995a Nursing management of congestive heart failure. Part 1. Intensive and Critical Care Nursing 11: 272–279

Dahlen R, Roberts S 1995b Nursing management of congestive heart failure. Part 2. Intensive and Critical Care Nursing 11: 322–328

Davies B 1997 The effects of exercise on primary and secondary coronary heart disease. Coronary Health Care 1: 60–78

De Jong M J, Morton P G 1997 Research analysis: control of vascular complications after cardiac catheterisation. A research-based protocol. Dimensions of Critical Care Nursing 16: 170–181

Donohue S J 1997a Lower limb amputation 1. indications and treatment. British Journal of Nursing 6(17): 970–972, 974–977

Donohue S J 1997b Lower limb amputation 2. Once the decision to amputate has been made. British Journal of Nursing 6(18): 1048–1052

Donohue S J 1997c Lower limb amputation 3. The role of the nurse. British Journal of Nursing 6(21): 1171–1174, 1187–1191

Donohue S J 1997d Lower limb amputation 4. Some ethical considerations. British Journal of Nursing 6(22): 1311–1314

Erickson B A 1996a Introduction to electrocardiography. In: Kinney M R, Packa D (eds) Andreolis' comprehensive cardiac care, 8th edn. CV Mosby, St Louis, pp 58–85

Erickson B A 1996b Disrhythmias. In: Kinney M R, Packa D (eds) Andreolis' comprehensive cardiac care, 8th edn. CV Mosby, St Louis, pp 86– 220

Gallop M 1993 Kissing the weed goodbye. Health Visitor 66(3): 97–98

Galloway S, Bubela N, McKibbon A, Rebeyka D, Saxe-Braithwaite M 1995 Symptom distress, anxiety, depression and discharge information needs after peripheral arterial bypass. Journal of Vascular Nursing 13(2): 35–40

Gibson J M, Kenrick M 1998 Pain and powerlessness: the experience of living with peripheral vascular disease. Journal of Advanced Nursing 27: 737–745

Hagenoff B D, Feutz C, Conn V S, Sagehorn K K, Moranviulle-Hunziker M 1994 Patient education needs as reported by congestive heart failure patients and their nurses. Journal of Advanced Nursing 19: 685–690

Herbert R, Alison J 1996 Cardiovascular function. In: Hinchliff S M, Montague S E, Watson R (eds) Physiology for nursing practice. Baillière Tindall, London, pp 375–451

Hinchliff S M, Montague S E, Watson R (eds) 1996 Physiology for nursing practice, 2nd edn. Baillière Tindall, London

Hollingworth H 1998 Venous leg ulcers. Part 1. Aetiology. Professional Nurse 13(8): 553–558

Johnson M T 1997 Treatment and prevention of varicose veins. Journal of Vascular Nursing 15(3): 97–103

Jolliffe J, Taylor R 1998 Physical activity and cardiac rehabilitation: a critical review of the literature. Coronary Health Care 2(4): 179–186

Jowett N, Thompson D R 1995 Comprehensive coronary care, 2nd edn. Scutari Press, London

Kaufman M W 1996 Raynaud's disease: patient education as a primary nursing intervention. Journal of Vascular Nursing 14: 34–39

Kelly M P 1992 Health promotion in primary care: taking account of the patient's point of view. Journal of Advanced Nursing 17(11): 1291–1296

Kinney M R, Packa D (eds) 1996 Andreolis' comprehensive cardiac care, 8th edn. CV Mosby, St Louis

Kynman G 1997 Thrombolysis: the development of unit guidelines. Intensive and Critical Care Nursing 13: 30–41

Lane P 1997 Cardiac electrophysiology studies and ablation procedures: a literature review. Intensive and Critical Care Nursing 13: 224–229

McBride A 1995 Health promotion in hospitals: the attitudes, beliefs and practices of hospital nurses. Journal of Advanced Nursing 20: 92–100

Parry O, Kenicer M, Haw S, Richmond C, Isles C 1998 A 56 year old arteriopath who is unable to stop smoking. Coronary Health Care 2(4): 215–220

Pell J 1997 Cardiac rehabilitation: a review of its effectiveness. Coronary Health Care 1: 8–17

Pharoah P B, Hollingworth W 1996 Cost effectiveness of lowering cholesterol. British Medical Journal 312: 1443–1448

Stanley R 1996 Cardiovascular drugs. In: Kinney M R, Packa D (eds) Andreolis' comprehensive cardiac care, 8th edn. CV Mosby, St Louis, pp 415–469

Stephenson N, Combs W J 1996 Artificial pacemakers and implantable cardioverter defibrillators. In: Kinney M R, Packa D (eds) Andreolis' comprehensive cardiac care, 8th edn. CV Mosby, St Louis, pp 220–255

Thompson D R 1994 Death and dying in critical care. In: Millar B, Burnard P (eds) Critical care nursing. Baillière Tindall, London, pp 234–249

Thompson D R, Bowman G S, DeBono D P, Hopkins A 1997 Cardiac rehabilitation: guidelines and audit standards. Royal College of Physicians, London

Thompson D R, Webster R A 1992 Infective endocarditis. In: Ashworth P M, Clarke C (eds) Cardiovascular intensive care nursing. Churchill Livingstone, Edinburgh

Viney C 1996 Nursing the critically ill. Baillière Tindall, London

Walsh M 1998 Models and critical pathways in clinical nursing – conceptual frameworks for care planning. Baillière Tindall, London

Wilson K J W, Waugh A 1996 Ross and Wilson anatomy and physiology in health and illness, 8th edn. Churchill Livingstone, Edinburgh

THE RESPIRATORY SYSTEM

3

Cynthia B. Edmond

INTRODUCTION

The respiratory system is one of the most vital systems in the human body. In health, it functions automatically and usually without our awareness. There are, however, few disease processes that do not have some disruptive effect on the respiratory system. There are also many respiratory disorders relating to environmental pollution, trauma, infection, genetic susceptibility and primary disease, as well as conditions secondary to other diseases. Although causative agents differ, the aetiology of each condition follows certain common patterns. To know the anatomy and physiology of the respiratory system is to understand how respiratory disorders inevitably relate to breakdown in ventilation, gaseous exchange or pulmonary perfusion. Symptoms differ only in degree and effect, and the treatment of symptoms will always have certain basic aims.

The effects of respiratory disorders range from the minor discomforts of the common cold to the distressing and life-threatening symptoms associated with respiratory failure. All are disabling to some extent to the individual and his family. As respiratory conditions and diseases cover such a broad spectrum and are common in both community and hospital settings, it is essential that nurses have a broad knowledge base relating to the basic concepts of normal respiration and an understanding of the factors that can lead to respiratory dysfunction.

Research indicates that some of the more serious respiratory disorders are related to lifestyle and are actually preventable. This chapter will therefore emphasise and outline various approaches to health promotion and disease prevention and the nurse's expanding role, opportunities and challenges in this field. It will also explore some of the more common disorders and, in discussing them, draw out the basic principles of management for all respiratory disorders. Although the emphasis is on nursing management, implicit in all discussions is the assumption that nurses work in close collaboration with other health care professionals and, in many instances, are responsible for coordinating the work of the whole team.

As you read this, you are probably unaware that you are breathing quietly and effortlessly; once you become attentive to the process of breathing, however, you can voluntarily vary the depth and pace of your respirations. You can sigh, cough or hold your breath for a time, and you can force air out through your vocal chords and sing or shout. When you go to sleep tonight, you can be reasonably confident that you will continue to breathe automatically and wake up in the morning feeling refreshed and well. However, if for any reason your respiratory system were to break down, this whole picture would change. Case History 3.1(A) gives some insight into a patient's perspective on an acute episode of respiratory distress.(See p. 73)

The essential elements of life support are the essential elements of respiration. Airway, breathing (ventilation) and circulation are the ABC of life support. If any one of the three is cut off or becomes dysfunctional, the others are of no use and an emergency situation exists which requires instant action if irreparable brain damage and death are to be prevented. An airway must be established and the individual's breathing and circulation restored in order to get oxygen to the vital organs and tissues.

3.1 What is the critical response time in cardiopulmonary resuscitation (CPR) if you are to prevent irreparable brain damage? Refer to your first aid manual and, with the guidance of your teacher, be sure to practise CPR regularly throughout your nursing career: it is an essential procedure.

3.2 As well as following up suggested reading and activities, you may find it useful to compile an information folder on essential procedures relating to respiratory care as you work your way through this chapter. It is also very important when you are in the clinical area to observe the patients who are undergoing these procedures, to note their reactions and the effects of the procedures on them, and to talk to them about how they feel. Analyse the context. Reflect on your experiences and make notes of critical incidents. Include these in your folder too. Discuss them with your preceptor or teacher.

ANATOMY AND PHYSIOLOGY

The reader is advised to review the anatomy and physiology of the respiratory system as a whole and to use a model of the thoracic cage to establish the relationship between all the structures illustrated in Figure 3.1. This section is intended as an overview of the most relevant points relating to normal respiratory function. Two texts that can be consulted in conjunction with the present discussion are suggested below.

For further information, see Rutishauser (1994) and Wilson & Waugh (1996).

Physiology of respiration

A continuous supply of O_2 and the elimination of CO_2 are necessary for the survival and functioning of body cells. The respiratory system in conjunction with the red blood cells (RBCs) of the circulatory system is responsible for this vital exchange. The process of respiration involves both external and internal respiration. External respiration involves oxygenation of the pulmonary capillary blood supply and elimination of CO_2 by diffusion across the alveolar and capillary membranes. Internal respiration involves the exchange of O_2 and CO_2 at the cellular level and the use of O_2 and production of CO_2 in the tissues (see Fig. 3.2).

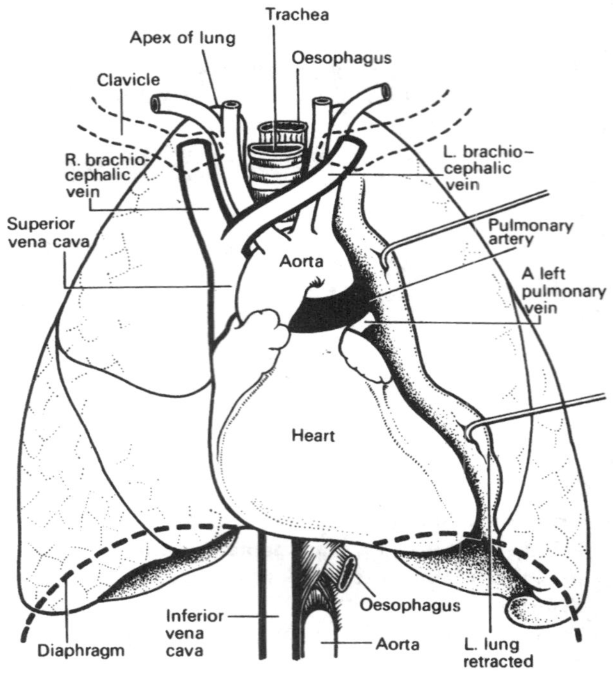

Fig. 3.1 Organs associated with the lungs. (Reproduced with permission from Wilson 1990.)

External respiration

External respiration involves ventilation, gaseous exchange and perfusion of the lungs with blood.

Ventilation is the process which moves air in and out of the lungs via the airways. This process is powered by the respiratory muscles — mainly the diaphragm and the intercostal muscles — which work together to increase and decrease the size of the thoracic cavity. They are responsive to both voluntary and involuntary central nervous system (CNS) control. The thoracic cavity is lined with parietal pleura and the lung surfaces have a covering of visceral pleura. The negative pressure and serous lubricant between the parietal and visceral pleura have the effect of 'sticking' the lungs to the thoracic wall so that they expand and contract with these ventilatory movements. In health there is only a potential space between the pleural layers.

Central control. Most of the time the involuntary system maintains the regular automatic breathing cycle and is controlled by respiratory centres in the brain (see Fig. 3.3). These centres receive information from sensory receptors throughout the respiratory system and from chemoreceptors located in the carotid arteries, aorta and medulla.

The sensory receptors in the respiratory system itself monitor local irritants and lung expansion. A cough, for example, is a reflex response to airway irritants and a natural defence mechanism to clear the airways. The chemoreceptors monitor the levels of CO_2, O_2 and H^+ in the blood and of H^+ in the CSF, and alter ventilation of the lungs to restore a normal balance of gases (see Table 3.1).

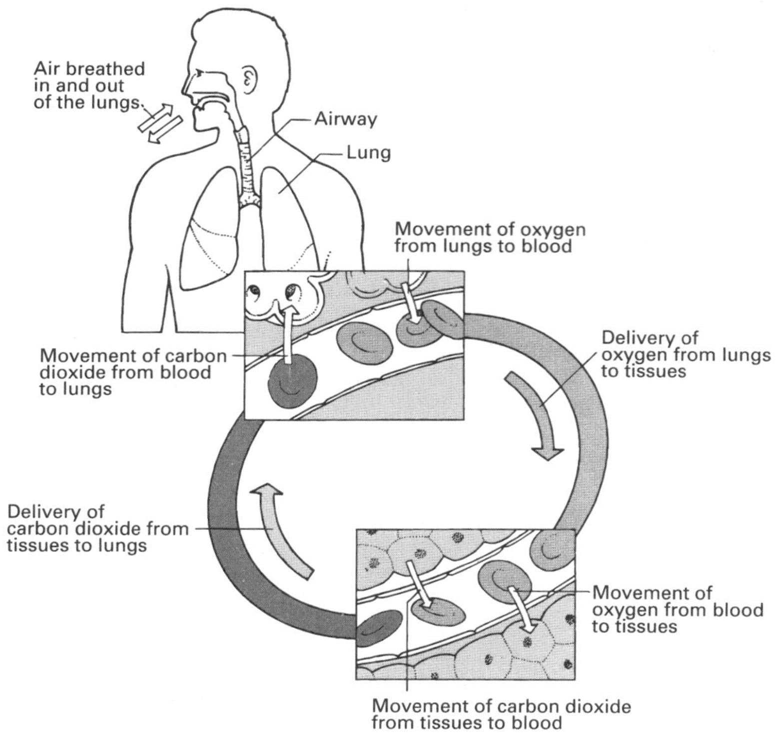

Fig. 3.2 Transport of oxygen and carbon dioxide between the lungs and the tissues. (Reproduced with permission from Rutishauser 1994.)

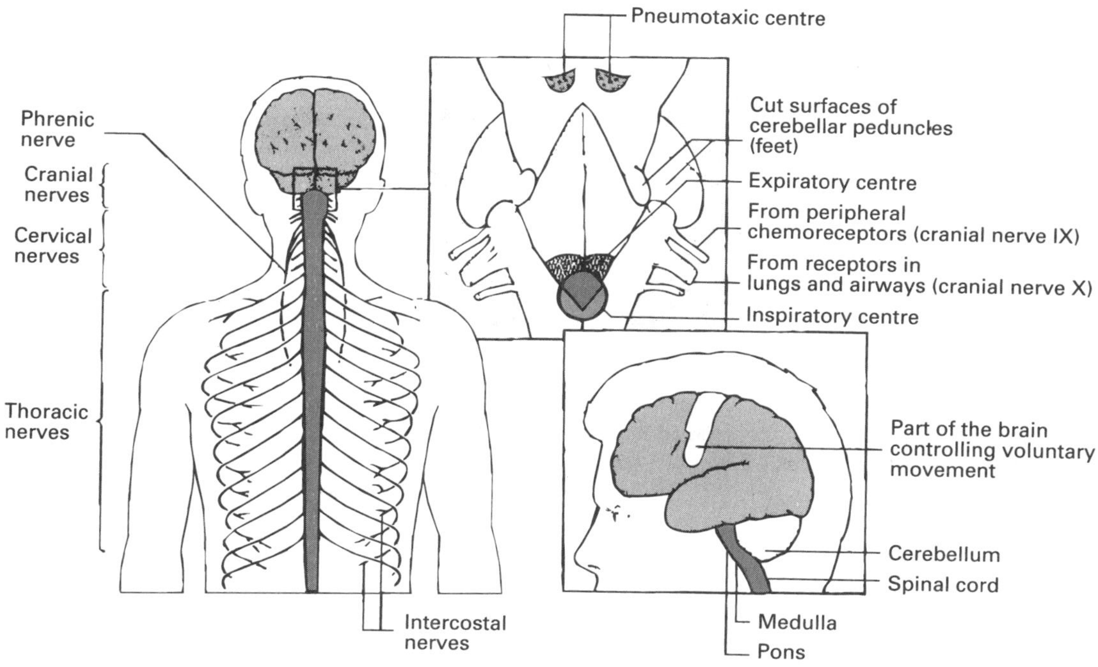

Fig. 3.3 Parts of the nervous system involved in controlling breathing: brain, brain stem, spinal cord and nerves. The enlarged inset shows the position of the respiratory centres in the medulla and pons of the brain stem as viewed from behind (the cerebellum, which sits on top of this, is not shown). (Reproduced with permission from Rutishauser 1994.)

Table 3.1 Sensory receptors involved in the control of breathing. (Reproduced with permission from Rutishauser 1994)

Type	*Location*	*Stimulus*	*Effect on breathing*
Within the respiratory system			
Irritant receptor	Airway epithelium — Nose	Inhaled particles and vapours	Sneeze
	Airway epithelium — Trachea		Cough
	Airway epithelium — Bronchioles		Increased rate and depth
Stretch receptors	Airway smooth muscle	Inflation	Slowed down
J receptors	Alveolar wall	Interstitial oedema Pulmonary emboli	Rapid and shallow
Muscle spindles	Respiratory muscles	Elongation of the muscles	Made smoother and more efficient
Elsewhere			
Chemoreceptors	Carotid artery Aorta	↑ CO_2, ↓ O_2, ↑ H^+ in blood	Increased rate and depth
	Brain (medulla)	↑ H^+ in CSF	Increased rate and depth

Lung volume capacity and compliance. It is important to bear in mind the basic principles relating to lung volume capacity and compliance and to recognise the significance of their measurement. They are important factors in ventilation and are often affected by respiratory disorders.

The volume of air breathed in and out and the number of breaths per minute vary from one individual to another according to age, size and activity. Normal, quiet breathing gives about 15 complete cycles per minute in the adult. Lung volume can be assessed in the following terms (see also Fig. 3.4 and Box 3.1):

- *Tidal volume (TV).* This is the amount of air that passes in and out of the lungs during each cycle of quiet breathing (approximately 500 mL in the adult). Exchange of gases takes place only in the alveolar ducts and sacs. The rest of the air passages are known as 'dead space' and contain about 150 mL of air.
- *Inspiratory capacity.* This is the amount of air that can be inspired with maximum effort. This consists of tidal volume plus the inspiratory reserve volume (IRV).
- *Functional residual capacity (FRC).* This is the amount of air remaining in the air passages and alveoli at the end of quiet respiration; it is composed of expiratory reserve volume (ERV) and residual volume (RV). The RV prevents collapse of the alveoli and makes continuous gaseous exchange possible as the alveolar gas mix remains constant.
- *Vital capacity (VC).* This is the TV plus the IRV and ERV.
- *Total lung capacity (TLC).* With maximum effort the adult lungs can hold 4–6 L of air. Most of this can be forcibly expelled, leaving a RV of about 1 L.

Lung expansion and recoil. Elastic fibres in lung tissue and the surface tension of the fluid lining the alveoli give the lungs their natural recoil tendency. Ease of expansion and recoil depends on normal compliance and elasticity and on the presence of surfactant in the fluid lining the alveoli. Compliance can be reduced by the stiffening of normally soft alveolar tissue due to pulmonary oedema or to the ageing process. Conversely compliance can be increased by extreme softening due to loss of lung tissue, as in emphysema.

Surfactant is a mixture of substances, mainly lipoproteins, secreted by cells of the alveolar epithelium, which lowers the surface tension of the alveolar fluid, making it easier for the alveoli to expand. Lack of surfactant in premature infants results in alveoli that remain collapsed (atelectasis) and leads to a ventilatory problem known as infant respiratory distress syndrome. A surfactant deficiency can also occur in adults as a response to severe shock, trauma or massive blood transfusion. This leads to increasing ventilatory difficulty, with rapid, shallow breathing and ineffectual respiration — a critical condition known as adult respiratory distress syndrome (ARDS) which may require artificial ventilatory support.

Ventilation, then, depends on CNS control, functioning respiratory muscles and adequate volume capacity of the lungs. Conditions which affect ventilation include some neurological diseases, diaphragmatic compression from constricting dressings or appliances, injuries to the chest wall, lungs or diaphragm, obstructive airways diseases such as asthma, space-occupying lesions, thoracic deformities and severe pain. In addition, certain narcotic drugs, such as morphine, are known to depress the central respiratory centre.

Gaseous exchange is the second vital component in the respiratory process. By a process of diffusion, O_2 passes from the alveoli into the bloodstream and CO_2 passes from the bloodstream into the alveoli. This exchange is dependent on adequate perfusion by the pulmonary blood supply.

Perfusion, i.e. the volume of blood passing through the lungs, determines the amount of O_2 taken into the body and the amount of CO_2 eliminated. In health, regulatory mechanisms ensure a balance between ventilation and perfusion such that well-ventilated parts of the lung receive an adequate blood supply and blood does not pass through the pulmonary circulation without being oxygenated (termed 'shunting'). Shunting occurs where there is an area of consolidation, as in pneumonia; although there is adequate perfusion there is no ventilation.

Q **3.3** Revise the properties of gases.

Gaseous exchange and lung perfusion. Each microscopic, grape-like alveolus is surrounded by an intimate structural network of capillaries which together provide the lungs with an enormous

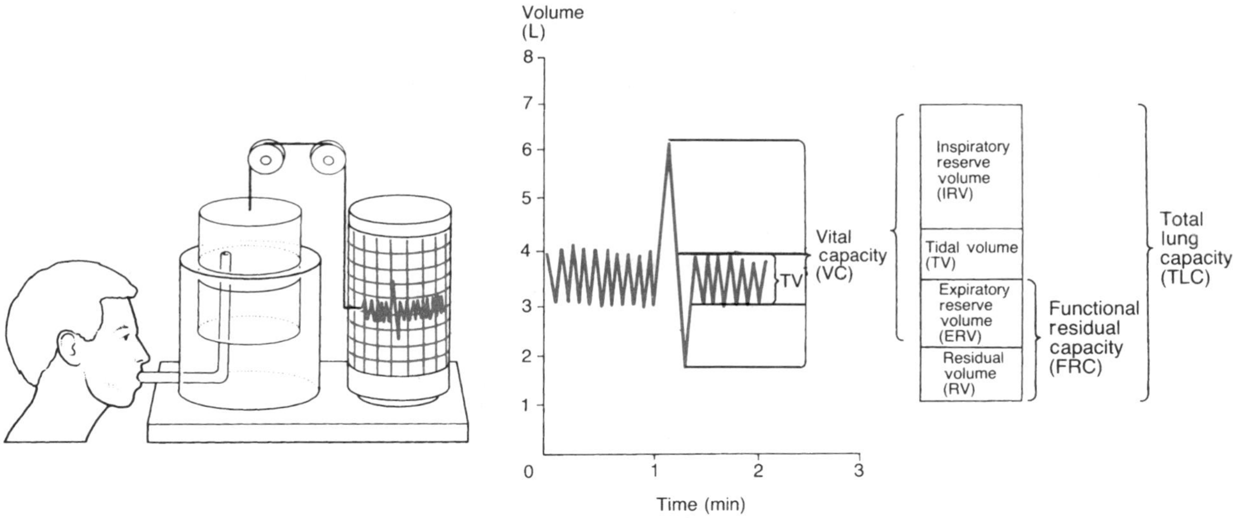

Fig. 3.4 Measurement of lung volumes by spirometry. The spirometer consists of a cylinder filled with air which is inverted into a container of water. As air is breathed in and out, the cylinder rises and falls. This movement is inscribed on the chart fixed to a slowly revolving drum. Note: the valves in the system and the CO_2 absorbant within the spirometer are not shown. (Reproduced with permission from Rutishauser 1994.)

Box 3.1 Assessment of air flow

Vital capacity
This is the sum of inspiratory reserve volume, tidal volume and expiratory reserve volume, about 4800 mL.

Peak expiratory flow rate (PEFR), or peak flow
This is an expression of the maximum rate of air flow when the individual is breathing out as hard and fast as possible, starting with full lungs. The normal range is 400–600 L/min. PEFR is measured with a simple instrument called a peak flow meter. Patients with diseases such as asthma are taught to record their own peak flow at regular intervals. A fall in PEFR provides a warning of bronchospasm before breathlessness occurs and therefore alerts patients to use prescribed bronchodilator drugs or to seek medical advice before the condition worsens. PEFR measures are also recorded before and after administration of bronchodilatory drugs to assess their effectiveness.

Forced expiratory volume (FEV)
This is the proportion of vital capacity that can be forcibly expelled from the lungs as measured at 1 and 3 s: FEV_1 and FEV_3, respectively. Normal FEV_1 is approximately 80% of the vital capacity and FEV_3 is about 100%. Where the airways are narrowed, as in asthma or in the presence of tumours, the FEV values will be lower.

capacity for gaseous exchange. This exchange is smooth and uninterrupted because the composition of the alveolar air remains constant due to the tidal ebb and flow of inspired air and the residual volume (RV) which is warmed and saturated with water vapour. As indicated in Figure 3.5, the gases in the blood leaving the lungs are in equilibrium with the air in the alveoli.

See Rutishauser (1994), Chapter 7, for a detailed explanation of gaseous exchange.

The total pressure exerted in the walls of the alveoli by the mixture of gases in air is the same as atmospheric pressure (100 kPa). Each gas in the mixture exerts a part of that total pressure proportional to its concentration; this is known as its partial pressure (*P*).

Arterial blood gas (ABG) levels. As a nurse you may be involved in interpreting blood gas results, administering oxygen and monitoring respirators. A working knowledge of the properties of gases, of partial pressure and of gaseous exchange is essential (see Table 3.2).

Internal (cellular) respiration

Cellular respiration is an essential part of the whole process of respiration.

The haemoglobin of the red blood cells (RBCs) carries O_2 to the tissues where, by the process of diffusion, gaseous exchange takes place between the arterial end of the capillaries and the tissue fluid. CO_2, which is one of the waste products of carbohydrate and fat metabolism in the cells, transfers to the venous capillary blood, where it is carried to the lungs in three ways, i.e.:

- dissolved in the blood plasma
- combined with haemoglobin
- in combination with sodium as sodium bicarbonate.

These processes are described more fully in Rutishauser (1994, pp. 154–155) where a clear description of both the oxygen–haemoglobin dissociation curve and the carbon dioxide dissociation curve is given.

PRINCIPLES OF NURSING MANAGEMENT IN THE PREVENTION AND TREATMENT OF RESPIRATORY DISORDERS

There are two main areas of nursing concern:

- health promotion and disease prevention
- developing clinical skills in order to ensure competent care.

The first concern will be addressed in relation to preventing serious respiratory diseases caused by environmental pollution and cigarette smoking; the second concern will be addressed in relation to specific respiratory disorders later in the chapter.

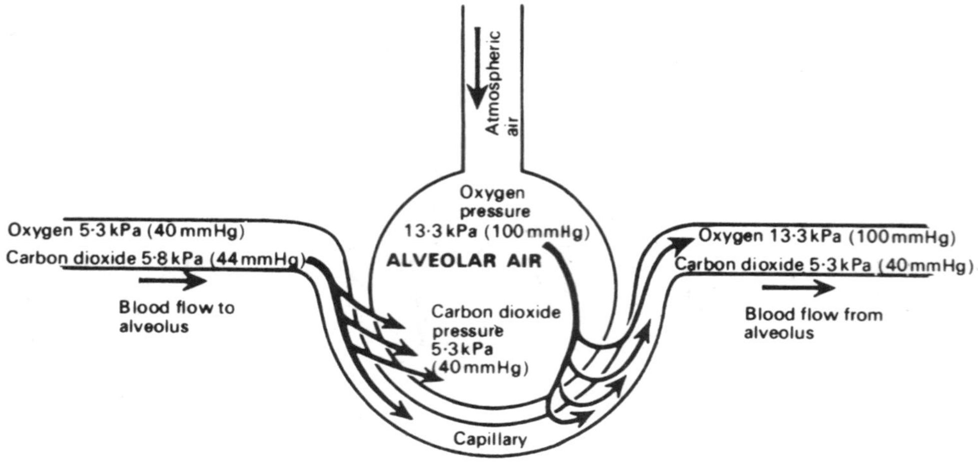

Fig. 3.5 Diagram of the interchange of gases between air in the alveoli and the blood capillaries. (Reproduced with permission from Wilson 1990.)

Table 3.2 Composition of air. (Reproduced with permission from Rutishauser 1994)

	Dry atmosphere		*Alveolar air (37°C)*	
	%	kPa[a]	%	kPa[a]
Oxygen	21	21	13.2	13.2
Carbon dioxide	0.04	0.04	5.3	5.3
Nitrogen[b]	79	79	75.2	75.2
Water vapour	?[c]	?[c]	6.3	6.3

[a] Assuming barometric pressure is 100 kPa.
[b] Includes <1% rare gases (argon, helium, etc.).
[c] Amount of moisture in atmosphere depends on humidity and temperature. If moisture is present, percentage of other constituents will then be correspondingly decreased.

Conceptual framework

It is assumed that in all care planning for patients with respiratory disorders, whether in the hospital or in the community, an appropriate driving philosophy and model of nursing care will be adopted. It is suggested, for example, that a modified version of Orem's (1971) classic philosophy of promoting independence and balancing self-care deficit with nursing compensatory intervention could be appropriate in the care of an asthma patient (see Table 3.3). For example, on admission during an acute attack of asthma (Case History 3.1(A)), C is unable to meet his self-care needs and requires major compensatory intervention by both medical and nursing staff. As he recovers, the deficit is reduced and nursing intervention (always in collaboration with other members of the health care team) moves through partly compensatory to supportive-educative as he is prepared for discharge home and is more able to control his asthma and maintain a higher degree of independence (see Case History 3.1(B), p. 76, and Collaborative Care Plan 3.1, p. 77).

The nurse's role in health promotion and disease prevention

Promoting health and preventing disease are vital to the social and economic well-being of our society and their importance is being reflected in government legislation and the development of large-scale screening and health education programmes. With the cost of health care soaring, it makes good sense to prevent disease where possible rather than treating the consequences. This is particularly true of some respiratory diseases and nurses are well placed in their many roles in the hospital and community to plan an active and expanding role in the area of primary health care (Buck 1997).

Downie et al (1996) describe three basic orientations for health education: disease orientation, risk factor orientation and health orientation (see Box 3.2). The evidence suggests that while each of these models has a valid place, a comprehensive and collaborative approach is necessary to tackle the complexities of most health-related issues. Government initiatives are aimed at preventing specific diseases and eliminating risk factors while health-oriented programmes initiated by the health professionals reinforce government policies by offering a more positive focus and satisfying outcome for the individual. Information should be presented in an innovative and effective way, which means that nurses must make sure they have accurate information, good teaching skills and adequate resources.

In modern industrial society, environmental pollutants and cigarette smoking are two of the major risk factor areas which can affect the health of the respiratory system. What happens when the lungs are continually exposed to such irritants? Firstly there is an increase in mucus secretion. The cilia, which normally clear the air passages of mucus, become coated and dysfunctional and eventually die. The presence of irritants and excess mucus causes inflammation and narrowing of the airways and disrupts gas diffusion. Cigarette smoke also contains carbon monoxide (CO), which binds easily to haemoglobin and displaces oxygen. Other chemicals in tobacco smoke cause vasoconstriction and constriction of the airways. Constant inflammation with formation of fibrous tissue and permanent narrowing of the airways lead to chronic bronchitis. Alveolar tissue is destroyed, reducing lung area and resulting in emphysema (see p. 70). These destructive changes are irreversible, although further destruction can be avoided by eliminating the cause: a concept simple in theory but difficult to put into practice.

Table 3.3 Orem's basic nursing system. (Orem 1971)

Nurse action		*Some characteristics of patient*		*Patient action*
Nurse action intense	→	Patient unable to meet own self-care needs —state of coma —inability to make decisions Wholly compensatory system		Patient action limited
Nurse action shared	→	Patient has limited ability to meet self-care needs —limited knowledge —limited ability to ambulate and to perform manipulative skills Partly compensatory system	←	Patient action shared
Nurse action supported	→	Patient can accomplish self-care —has learned new self-care activities —needs limited help in decision-making Supportive-educative system	←	Patient action intensive

Box 3.2 Orientations for health education

Downie et al (1996) describe the following orientations for health education:

1. *Disease-oriented education.* This approach aims to prevent specific diseases. The emphasis is on measuring success in terms of progress towards target rates for morbidity and mortality.
2. *Risk factor-oriented education.* Efforts are aimed at eliminating particular risk factors to prevent associated diseases.
3. *Health-oriented education.* The aim is to enhance positive health as well as to prevent ill-health. This orientation recognises the physical, mental and social facets of both positive and negative health and acknowledges that:
   - Provision of information is not enough. The educational process needs to be participatory, to help people clarify their values (e.g. how they see themselves and their health) and acquire and develop life skills (e.g. decision-making and assertiveness). The educator seeks to understand people's perspectives and opinions, to respect them rather than correct them or blame them for their behaviour
   - There are major constraints to freedom of choice in health-related behaviour (e.g. sociopolitical factors).

Environmental pollution and health

Exhaust fumes from motor vehicles are a major source of air pollution in cities in the UK and other heavily populated countries in the world. Government intervention is needed to control this and other environmental pollutants such as dust, smoke, chemical fumes, agricultural pollutants and cigarette smoke. Nurses can actively and usefully support such intervention through early detection of risk factors, innovative local intervention and health education in the hospital, the workplace, the school and the home.

Many industrial workplaces expose employees to pollutants such as dust, chemicals and toxic fumes. Miners of nickel, coal, cobalt and radium are exposed to fluorocarbons, which have been shown to be related to an increased incidence of serious lung disease, including carcinoma (Kidd 1989). Agricultural workers are exposed to biohazards such as grain dust, bacteria and their metabolites (endotoxins), fungi and their metabolites (glucans) and storage mites; they are also exposed to airborne insecticides, fungicides and pesticides and to animal parasites and debris. Epidemiological and clinical studies have identified strong associations between agricultural exposure and chronic bronchitis, asthma, hypersensitivity pneumonitis and organic dust toxic syndrome (Zejda & Dosman 1993).

Occupational health and community nurses have a responsibility to educate workers and managers about environmental hazards and to press for the use of appropriate protective clothing and respiratory masks and for improved working conditions and leisure facilities.

The home also can be full of respiratory risk factors. Use of aerosol hair and body sprays and household cleaning products together with sidestream cigarette smoke can be a constant source of respiratory irritation for the whole family. Again, it is the community nurse who can advise and educate families.

Cigarette smoking and health

There is increasing evidence that smoking relates directly to the high incidence of lung cancer, which kills about 300 people a day in the UK alone (Pollock 1993, Buck 1997). The sidestream smoke inhaled in passive smoking has a higher concentration of some toxic and carcinogenic substances than has mainstream smoke, which is significant for families and workmates of smokers. The evidence is that both active and passive smoking by pregnant women have detrimental effects on the unborn child and are clearly associated with low birth weight and perinatal morbidity and mortality (Jones & MacLeod-Clark 1993). Maternal smoking has been linked to sudden infant death syndrome (SIDS) and passive smoking to a high incidence of childhood asthma (Azizi 1993). Passive smoking can also be linked to a high incidence of coronary heart disease in adults (Kawachi et al 1997: see Research Abstract 3.1).

Q **3.4** Scan current journals for articles relating to smoking and health.

In spite of an observed long-term decline in overall UK smoking rates because of voluntary agreements on tobacco advertising restrictions and health promotion initiatives, there is still an increase in numbers of young teenage smokers and a more recent trend towards an increase in the smoking rates of graduates and young professionals (Buck 1997, National Asthma Campaign 1997). Although the government is pledged to ban overt cigarette advertising and tobacco company sponsorship of sporting events, there are no restrictions on how smoking can be portrayed in

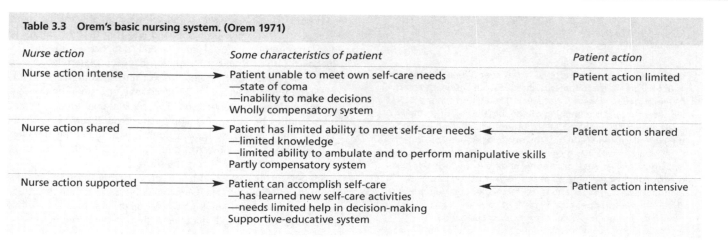

Research Abstract 3.1
Passive smoking doubles the risk of heart disease

Cardiovascular and respiratory diseases are often associated with the same causative agents and this would appear to be the case in cigarette smoking. A study of 32 000 nurses in the USA indicates that passive smoking can double the risk of coronary heart disease through regular exposure to sidestream smoke in the workplace and the home. The nurses aged between 36 and 61 were asked whether they had been exposed to passive smoking either at work or at home and how regularly this had occurred and were followed over a 10-year period with biannual questionnaires about risk factors for heart disease. During this 10-year period, 152 cases of coronary heart disease occurred, resulting in 25 deaths. Previous research has established that women who smoke are four or five times more at risk of coronary heart disease than those who have never smoked, but previous studies on passive smoking have been less conclusive.

Kawachi I, Colditz G A, Speizer F E et al 1997 A prospective study of passive smoking and coronary heart disease. Circulation 95(10): 2374–2379.

popular magazines through association with fashion, music and media personalities. This kind of covert advertising is thought to be very powerful with women and the two groups identified above.

Evidence points to the *contextual* determinants of the addictive habit of cigarette smoking. It is not enough to inform people of the devastating consequences of smoking. Most people are well aware of these. Rather a comprehensive and concerted attempt must be made to define the factors that initiate a smoking habit and the contexts that sustain it and to change these. Accordingly, the government, in its White Paper *The Health of the Nation* (Department of Health 1992, see also Graham 1993), put forward policies for the reduction of morbidity and mortality from cigarette smoking. The key target is for a 40% reduction in the overall consumption of cigarettes from 98 billion in 1990 to 59 billion by the year 2000.

In order to achieve this target, the government set up an interdepartmental workforce to coordinate the policies of the ministries involved. These ministries include education (relating to the National Curriculum), employment (workplace and personnel smoking policies), the treasury (tax increases), environment (smoking in public places) and trade and industry (affecting exports and jobs). Many of these policies have been put into effect and, in addition, the government is to legislate against tobacco advertising and tobacco firms supporting sporting events. Research in countries such as New Zealand, Australia, Canada, Finland and Norway supports the assumption that advertising bans do produce significant reductions in smoking rates. In the USA, leading tobacco companies have reached agreement with 40 states to acknowledge the health risks, pay millions of dollars in compensation, drastically alter their marketing programmes and submit to the regulatory heel of the Food and Drug Administration (Smolowe 1997).

Nursing intervention. As indicated above, in addition to government initiatives, nursing involvement should aim for the positive benefits of the 'health orientated education model' to define individual and group needs and work out appropriate participatory action (Downie et al 1996). Midwives have a unique opportunity to be closely involved with the family in both the antenatal and postnatal periods to promote the health of the mother and the newborn. Early screening and advice are essential and time spent defining specific social problems and ensuring that the family is given appropriate referral and social support is invaluable. Blackburn (1993) found a correlation between material stressors and a high incidence of smoking in working class mothers, where a cigarette represented a well deserved treat or a small luxury that countered a sense of deprivation. These social conditions demand understanding and innovative approaches from health professionals, who must appreciate how difficult it is to break the smoking habit as nicotine is a powerful and addictive stimulant and does have a stress-relieving effect in the short term.

School nurses can begin health education early in the child's life and involve the parents. Unfortunately, research into the effectiveness of school anti-smoking education programmes shows disappointing results and indicates that more comprehensive interventions will be needed to curb teenage smoking (Nutbeam et al 1993, Buck 1997). Conveying information to young people demands a creative approach and may involve promoting sporting and other leisure time activities for both parent and child. Community nurses can be active in defining social needs, lobbying local councils to provide recreational and child care facilities and giving time to individuals to lessen their sense of isolation.

Q **3.5** Design a health education programme for early teenage children. What activities would you include? What teaching aids would you use? Access current websites that cover health promotion initiatives and look for local advertisements regarding one-to-one helplines.

The nurse's role in developing clinical skills

In order to ensure that patients receive skilled nursing care, it is necessary for nurses to have a working knowledge of the disease processes involved in respiratory health breakdown. They also need to be able to work cooperatively with doctors and other health team personnel through an understanding of medical management and to be able to deliver a holistic nursing assessment and management plan as part of a collaborative team approach. These issues are addressed below with the emphasis on nursing management.

COMMON RESPIRATORY DISORDERS

Respiratory disorders involve a breakdown in the integrity of the alveolar walls. They either cause or are caused by oedema, the presence of exudate, or by inflammation, resulting in scarring and alteration in the process of gaseous exchange. Causes of respiratory inflammation are varied and range from common diseases such as 'the flu' and colds to bronchitis, pneumonia, tuberculosis, cystic fibrosis and the opportunistic infections of AIDS and other immunosuppressive conditions. While causative factors, organisms or irritants differ, the aetiologies of respiratory disorders are similar and they are, in varying degrees, similar in their clinical manifestations. Assessment of respiratory function is central to all clinical care (see Box 3.3).

The incidence of emphysema and malignancy due to environmental pollutants and cigarette smoking appears to have increased significantly in recent years (Pollock 1993, Buck 1997). Additionally, the lungs are often involved in terminal or critical illness where pulmonary oedema, bronchitis, pneumonia or atelectasis (collapse of alveoli) may develop.

Box 3.3 Respiratory assessment: a clinical skill central to all patient care

- Visual observation
- Respiratory rate, rhythm and depth
- Breath sounds
- Use of ancillary muscles
- Sputum and secretions
- Causes of variation from normal, e.g. pain, anxiety, disease
- Respiratory history
- Arterial blood gases
- Pulse oximetry
- Chest X-ray
- Pulmonary lung function tests
- Bronchoscopy
- Imaging, e.g. CT scan, MRI

Common clinical manifestations of all of these disorders include varying degrees of breathlessness, cough and sputum production, dyspnoea (difficulty in breathing), tachypnoea (increased respiratory rate), cyanosis (blue discoloration of the skin), hypoxia (low O_2 concentration in the tissues) and hypercapnia (high concentration of CO_2 in arterial blood).

For a detailed account of respiratory assessment, see Field (1997).

Wherever there is disruption of the respiratory process, there is the probability that oxygen therapy will be necessary to relieve breathlessness and improve tissue perfusion (Allan 1989) (see Box 3.4).

Each of the processes involved in external respiration — ventilation, gaseous exchange and circulatory perfusion — is a critical component in maintaining the life and function of body cells. Disruption in any of these processes results in respiratory disorders of varying severity.

INFECTIONS OF THE RESPIRATORY SYSTEM

Infections of the upper respiratory tract are dealt with in Chapter 14. This chapter will focus on bronchitis, pneumonia and tuberculosis.

Acute bronchitis and tracheobronchitis

Acute bronchitis is the inflammation of the mucous membranes of the bronchial tree. Tracheobronchitis, as the name implies, affects the trachea as well as the bronchi. Both conditions are associated with infections of the upper respiratory tract (see Ch. 14) but may also occur as a result of atmospheric pollutants, cigarette smoking or when some other chronic respiratory disorder already exists. They can affect people of all ages and are usually only of real concern in the very young, the very old and the debilitated. A normally healthy person will usually recover quite quickly. The concern in terms of health promotion is to ensure that acute bronchitis does not develop into bronchopneumonia and that acute attacks do not become so frequent that the condition becomes chronic (see p. 70).

PATHOPHYSIOLOGY

Common presenting symptoms. The individual feels generally unwell with, initially, a dry painful cough and a moderate pyrexia.

Box 3.4 Oxygen (O_2) therapy

The need for O_2 therapy arises when oxygen transport to the tissues is insufficient due to breakdown in either the respiratory or the circulatory systems. Clinical signs and blood gas levels are the main indicators of degree of hypoxia. Profound hypoxaemia will cause death in minutes, whereas death from carbon dioxide (CO_2) narcosis is a more lengthy process (see Box 3.5).

The aim of O_2 therapy is to administer sufficient oxygen to maintain tissue oxygenation at a functional level and eliminate detrimental compensatory responses to hypoxaemia, and to prevent serious or irreparable damage to vital organs and tissues.

The percentage of oxygen that is to be delivered is carefully determined, either by circumstances (as in life-threatening emergencies, where 100% pure oxygen may be given initially) or by carrying out arterial blood gas (ABG) measurement or percutaneous oximetry and prescribing oxygen accordingly. An oximeter is a small, non-invasive device which can register arterial oxygen saturation through the skin using a clip-on sensor (see Cowan 1997).

For therapeutic purposes, the range of prescription is usually between 24 and 60% of O_2. Hyperbaric oxygen (oxygen given at greater than 1 atmosphere absolute) may be used to improve oxygen perfusion of the tissues by increasing the dissolved oxygen in the blood, as in treatment of CO poisoning or deep-sea divers' 'bends'.

In certain conditions, the amount of oxygen given is determined by prior knowledge of adverse effects. For example, in patients with known COAD (see p. 69) it is dangerous to give too much oxygen, and in premature babies high oxygen saturation is known to cause blindness.

Means of giving oxygen include nasal cannulae, oxygen masks, oxygen tents, non-invasive positive pressure ventilation (NIPPV), mechanical ventilators and hyperbaric oxygen chambers. Each of these devices can deliver controlled amounts of oxygen and is selected according to overall patient requirements and tolerance.

Humidification chambers attached to the oxygen equipment ensure that the oxygen is humidified before being inhaled. In mechanical ventilators it is also warmed and therefore enters the respiratory tract as vapour, fully saturated and at body temperature.

Oxygen toxicity

The lungs may be damaged if high concentrations of oxygen are given over several days. This is thought to increase alveolar permeability so that capillary walls break down and fluid and blood accumulate. Severe cases may progress to pneumonia, fibrosis, pulmonary hypertension and right-sided heart failure.

The cough becomes increasingly productive as the inflamed mucosal cells pour out mucus and the sputum produced becomes increasingly mucopurulent. Bronchospasm can occur, causing wheezing and a degree of dyspnoea.

MEDICAL MANAGEMENT

Investigations. For otherwise healthy individuals, investigations are usually unnecessary. However, if marked mucopurulent sputum is produced, a sputum culture will be taken to identify the causative organism. A chest X-ray may also be required.

Treatment. The treatment is aimed at relieving the symptoms. Bed rest is advocated until the pyrexia has resolved. Moist inhalations can relieve the bronchial symptoms and a high fluid intake is encouraged. Expectorants will also help to relieve the congestion, and antibiotic therapy will be prescribed and taken as appropriate.

NURSING PRIORITIES AND MANAGEMENT: ACUTE BRONCHITIS AND TRACHEOBRONCHITIS

The nurse's priority will be for those vulnerable individuals for whom acute bronchitis could prove serious. Overexertion must be avoided and such patients may need support with expectoration and maintaining respiratory hygiene. Optimal nutritional and fluid intake will aid recovery and help to prevent further infection.

When the individual is well enough, advice should be given as to how further attacks can be avoided. The avoidance of cigarette smoke, dusty, ill-ventilated, cold or crowded environments is encouraged but is not always easy to achieve. The advice given and the outcomes aimed for must be realistic and tailored to the lifestyle and socioeconomic circumstances of the individual. An influenza vaccination may prove an effective preventive measure in particularly vulnerable individuals.

Pneumonia

Pneumonia is an infection of lung tissue and is most usefully classified according to the causative organism, which may be bacterial or viral. However, it can be further defined according to the area of lung that is involved, i.e. bronchopneumonia or lobar pneumonia.

Bronchopneumonia

PATHOPHYSIOLOGY

Bronchopneumonia is characterised mainly by patchy areas of consolidated lung tissues. Causative organisms are bacterial and fungal and include staphylococci, pneumococci, streptococci, *Haemophilus influenzae* and *Candida*. It usually occurs in individuals weakened by other conditions and often in the very old, the very young, the unconscious, and as a result of a pre-existing disease, such as chronic bronchitis, atelectasis or carcinoma in adults, or infectious diseases in infants.

Clinical features. These vary in severity depending on the overall condition of the patient but include varying degrees of pyrexia, cough with copious purulent sputum, exhalatory râles, dyspnoea and tachypnoea. Consolidation of the lower lobes is found on auscultation.

MEDICAL MANAGEMENT

The causative organism is isolated by sputum culture and sensitivity and appropriate antibiotic therapies are commenced. The patient's general condition is improved by attention to nutrition, hydration and physiotherapy.

NURSING PRIORITIES AND MANAGEMENT: BRONCHOPNEUMONIA

The patient with bronchopneumonia will be very ill and he and his family will need a great deal of comfort and reassurance. Attention to personal hygiene and physical comfort is important. The patient should be turned or encouraged to move regularly. A sitting position, where possible, will make breathing easier and, if oxygen is prescribed, this therapy should be monitored carefully. Aids to prevent pressure sores developing should be selected judiciously (see Ch. 23).

Bronchopneumonia can be prevented in many hospitalised high-risk patients by thorough nursing assessment and meticulous nursing care.

Lobar pneumonia

PATHOPHYSIOLOGY

This is an acute bacterial infection which sometimes involves a whole lobe. It occurs mainly in young adults (usually males) but its full-blown effects are uncommon now because of the early and effective use of antibiotics. However, if left untreated lobar pneumonia can progress to further areas of consolidation as well as to pleurisy, pericarditis, bacteraemia and possibly death.

Viral pneumonia: primary atypical pneumonia (PAP)

PATHOPHYSIOLOGY

In viral pneumonia, the inflammatory reaction is localised within the septal walls of the alveoli and there is no exudate. This is its point of difference from other types of pneumonia and the reason why it is known as 'atypical'. There are many known and highly contagious viruses which can begin as a 'common cold' and progress to more severe respiratory tract infections — which may include PAP in susceptible individuals. These viral agents include *Mycoplasma pneumoniae*, influenza types A and B, respiratory syncytial virus (RSV), rubella and varicella, *Rickettsia* and echoviruses. PAP was responsible for the highly fatal influenza pandemics of the early and middle 1900s.

Clinical features. Symptoms include pyrexia, muscular pains, headaches and a dry, hacking cough. Treatment is symptomatic with attention given to general nutrition, hydration and antibiotic treatment of any intercurrent bacterial infections. The disease runs its course and, except in the weaker individual, resolution is expected. However, the patient may be left feeling weak and exhausted for some time afterwards.

NURSING PRIORITIES AND MANAGEMENT: PAP

Susceptible individuals — the aged, the debilitated and health workers at high risk of infection — should be encouraged to attend the practice nurse clinic for a course of 'flu' vaccinations in preparation for the winter months or where epidemics are forecast.

Most individuals with PAP can be treated at home. Some may need nursing advice or assistance to carry out the activities of daily living and to ensure they are properly nourished and hydrated. Individuals nursed at home can be referred back to their GP if medical treatment becomes necessary.

Tuberculosis (pulmonary)

Tuberculosis (TB) is a chronic infectious disease mainly of the lungs (pulmonary tuberculosis) but can infect other parts of the body (miliary tuberculosis). In the early part of the 20th century, it was common in developed as well as developing countries. With the advent of compulsory chest X-ray, bacille Calmette–Guérin (BCG) vaccination and effective drug treatment, the incidence in developed countries became almost negligible. However, since the discontinuation of compulsory screening and treatment of the adult population and increased immigration from developing countries, there has been a significant increase in incidence. The disease is rife in developing countries and, in many, is complicated by the susceptibility of AIDS victims to respiratory infections (Cayla et al 1993).

PATHOPHYSIOLOGY

Tuberculosis is a notifiable disease caused mainly by *Mycobacterium tuberculosis*, although *Mycobacteria avium* and *bovis* can also cause the respiratory form. The disease is characterised by two types of lesions: exudative and productive.

The exudative lesion arises from the inflammatory process in which the bacterial organism is surrounded by fluid containing polymorphonuclear leucocytes and monocytes. If the lesion fails to heal, it may become necrosed and develop into a productive lesion (tubercle).

A tubercle consists of a fibrous or a soft outer cover with a core of giant cells, lymphocytes, monocytes, fibroblasts and epithelioid cells. The mycobacterium can live in the centre of this tubercle for years. The soft tubercle can rupture and spread its contents into surrounding tissue. Spread of infection is by direct contact with the infected tissue, by the bloodstream or by the lymphatics. Spread to others is by droplet infection from coughing or saliva.

Clinical features vary in severity, depending on the virulence of the organism and the susceptibility of the individual. Manifestations include a productive cough, sometimes with bloodstained sputum; fatigue; weight loss; low-grade evening fever; night sweats and pleuritic pain. Advanced cases will manifest wheezing and râles, deviation of the trachea, pulmonary consolidation and haemoptysis (frank bleeding from the lungs).

MEDICAL MANAGEMENT

Investigations. A Mantoux skin test may be performed (see below). Specimens of sputum, gastric washings or a lymph node biopsy may be sent for bacteriology. Chest X-ray will indicate the condition of the lungs.

Treatment. The patient is isolated until there is complete compliance with the drug therapy (usually 2–4 weeks). Drugs used include isoniazid, rifampicin, streptomycin, ethambutol and pyrazinamide. Until the specific sensitivity is determined, the patient is usually on a rotating regimen of several of these drugs because of the high probability of bacterial resistance to some combinations. Therapy will then continue with long-term treatment with at least two of the drugs. Regular clinic attendance and supervision of treatment are mandatory. Contacts are traced and tested and treated if necessary.

NURSING PRIORITIES AND MANAGEMENT: PULMONARY TUBERCULOSIS

Prevention

Prevention is based upon public health education and on screening and vaccination to protect those at risk. Nurses are actively involved in these programmes in clinics and schools.

Schoolchildren, health care workers and contacts of people identified as having TB are screened by the Mantoux skin test. This test uses a single intradermal injection of purified protein derivative (PPD). The result is read within 24–72 h. If the area of induration is 10 mm or more, the test is positive, which indicates either that a past subacute infection stimulated present immunity or that present infection exists which needs treatment. In the case of past infection, the result signifies that there is good immunity and vaccination is not necessary. An area of 5 mm in a person recently exposed to tuberculosis indicates that a course of prophylactic treatment should be given. A negative Mantoux test (i.e. no reaction) indicates that there is no natural immunity and the BCG vaccination is necessary.

Management of a newly diagnosed patient

This patient will be isolated for 2–4 weeks and barrier-nursed (see Ch. 16, p. 592). He will need reassurance that treatment will be effective, as well as rest, diversionary therapy, good nourishment and administration of prescribed drugs. He should be encouraged to retain his independence in activities of daily living. When he is discharged home, he will need minimal community nurse support and advice but must attend the chest clinic for check-ups regularly. All sputum must continue to be disposed of as advised by the chest clinic and the patient must use tissues and cover his mouth when coughing.

OBSTRUCTIVE DISORDERS OF THE AIRWAYS

'Chronic obstructive airways disease' (COAD) is a term used to describe a group of disorders which cause obstruction to air flow. Included in this group are chronic bronchitis, emphysema, asthma and bronchiectasis. In chronic bronchitis the inflammation and constant productive cough obstructs air flow; in emphysema the overdistended alveoli with reduced permeability results in impaired gaseous exchange; in asthma there is both inflammatory reaction and bronchospasm; and in bronchiectasis there are chronic copious secretions filling the lungs. Bronchiectasis is usually a separate condition, but the others often coexist and complicate each other in presenting as a set of symptoms commonly termed COAD or COPD (chronic obstructive pulmonary disease) (British Thoracic Society 1997).

Chronic bronchitis

The definition of chronic bronchitis is the presence of a persistent productive cough for at least 2 months over 2 consecutive years. It can occur in any age group but is common in middle-aged men and amongst cigarette smokers and people exposed to high levels of environmental pollution.

PATHOPHYSIOLOGY

Chronic irritation causes hypertrophy and hyperplasia of the mucous glands of the tracheobronchial tree, which results in excessive mucus production and impaired ciliary action. The bronchi and bronchioles are usually the most severely affected and may become blocked with purulent mucus. This, together with the resultant oedema and congestion, can affect respiratory defence mechanisms and predispose to recurrent bacterial and viral infections.

Clinical features. A chronic productive cough with mucopurulent sputum may persist for years, accompanied by gradual and increasing airway resistance and functional impairment. Untreated, this will lead to increasing dyspnoea, hypoxia and hypercapnia.

MEDICAL MANAGEMENT

Management is to advise the patient to avoid the causal irritant, if this is possible, and to treat the symptoms. This may involve prescribing physiotherapy, bronchodilatory drugs, antibiotics and oxygen therapy.

NURSING PRIORITIES AND MANAGEMENT: CHRONIC BRONCHITIS

Prevention of deterioration

The patient is advised and supported in avoiding causative agents.

When identifying patient problems and nursing priorities, it is useful to consider chronic bronchitis and emphysema together, as the two conditions often coexist (Jess 1992).

Pulmonary emphysema

Pulmonary emphysema is a chronic destructive disease of the respiratory bronchioles, alveolar ducts and alveoli. It is most common in those aged over 40 and is often associated with other chronic lung disorders. There are two main types of pulmonary emphysema, which may coexist and which are exacerbated by persistent and severe coughing: alveolar emphysema and centrilobar emphysema.

Alveolar emphysema

PATHOPHYSIOLOGY

In this form of emphysema, the walls between adjacent alveoli break down, the alveolar ducts dilate and there is loss of interstitial elastic tissue. This results in distension of the lungs and loss of normal elastic recoil and therefore trapping and stagnation of alveolar air. As alveoli merge, there is loss of surface area for gaseous exchange, and this is further reduced by loss of permeability of the stretched and damaged alveolar walls. Predisposing factors include cigarette smoking, genetic deficiency of α_1-antitrypsin (making the individual more susceptible to environmental pollutants), acute lower respiratory inflammatory conditions and chronic coughing (which puts pressure on the already stretched tissues).

Q **3.6** Maintaining a clear airway by regular aspiration of tracheal secretions is a common nursing procedure. As a rule of thumb, the procedure should not be carried out for more than 10–15 s at a time, with adequate periods of rest in between. What is the reason for this? (Refer back to residual volume and the composition of alveolar air.) A full description of tracheal suctioning can be found in Jamieson et al (1999).

Centrilobar emphysema

PATHOPHYSIOLOGY

This type of emphysema involves irreversible dilatation of the bronchioles in the centre of the lobules, which affects airway pressure and ventilation efficiency. Predisposing conditions include recurrent bronchiolitis, pneumoconiosis and chronic bronchitis.

Clinical features. Emphysema becomes symptomatic when about one-third of the lung parenchyma is affected. The patient is dyspnoeic, and in advanced cases the slightest physical activity can cause severe respiratory distress and cyanosis. Ventilation is forced and exhalation is particularly lengthy and difficult. The patient learns to push the air out through pursed lips, which automatically brings the upper abdominal muscles into play and helps maintain positive pressure in the airways. The hyperinflation of the lungs makes the chest barrel-shaped and rigid and exerts pressure on thoracic structures so that neck and facial veins are distended. There is a chronic, productive cough and wheezing. Abnormal ventilation:perfusion ratios result in chronic hypoxia (low O_2 in tissues), hypercapnia (high CO_2) and polycythaemia. The clinical picture representing this is of peripheral cyanosis (due to low O_2) and facial flushing (because CO_2 is a vasodilator). Respiratory acidosis may occur in acute exacerbations of the disease, although the body may adapt its buffer system to some extent given the chronic nature of the condition.

The patient is weakened by constant respiratory effort and unable to tolerate normal basic activities of daily living. Laughing and coughing may stimulate life-threatening attacks, and respiratory failure is always a possibility.

MEDICAL MANAGEMENT

Investigations. History, symptoms and clinical examination are diagnostic. Pulmonary function tests (spirometry) indicate the type and extent of restricted function: reduction in all parameters indicates obstructive disease because of the prolonged exhalation time, and reduced FEV_1 (forced expiratory volume in 1 s) and FVC (forced vital capacity) indicate restrictive disease. Blood gas analysis and chest X-ray will confirm the stage and effect of the disease and influence treatment.

Treatment. Oxygen is prescribed according to individual need and blood gas results (see Box 3.4). It is given in strictly controlled percentages because of the importance of the 'hypoxic drive' in COAD patients and the fact that too much oxygen can knock out this drive, resulting in carbon dioxide narcosis and respiratory arrest (see Box 3.5). Oxygen may be required constantly both in hospital and at home.

Bronchodilator drugs and antibiotics may be prescribed, and physiotherapy is essential.

Q **3.7** How would you explain the concept of hypoxic drive and its importance for self-treatment to a patient with COAD who is about to be sent home on O_2 therapy?

NURSING PRIORITIES AND MANAGEMENT: EMPHYSEMA AND CHRONIC BRONCHITIS

Major considerations

Reassurance and support

In advanced cases of emphysema, the patient will be constantly striving for breath and will need maximum reassurance and calm support. His lifestyle will be drastically curtailed and every effort should be made to make a realistic assessment of his capabilities and need for assistance in designing his care plan. His limitations may be extreme and affect even minor activities such as eating, drinking, combing hair, brushing teeth and moving about the room. Time should be spent helping, observing and listening.

Oxygen therapy

Procedures such as non-invasive positive pressure ventilation (NIPPV) have been found to have significant beneficial effects for patients with acute exacerbations of COAD and other respiratory disorders where the patient has intact swallowing, cough and gag reflexes. NIPPV is a method of administering oxygen under positive pressure via a nasal mask and, because it does not require the patient to be intubated, is increasingly carried out on general medical wards (Place 1997) (see Research Abstract 3.2 and Fig. 3.6).

Box 3.5 Carbon dioxide narcosis. (Reproduced with permission from Rutishauser 1994)

In healthy people, when CO_2 levels rise, the respiratory rate increases. This increase allows excess CO_2 to be blown off by the lungs. However, in chronic obstructive airways disease (COAD), where chronic ventilatory problems result in constantly high levels of arterial CO_2, this mechanism becomes blunted and eventually Pco_2 has no effect on the respiratory centre in the brain.

With severe CO_2 retention, the respiratory drive is created by the low Po_2 stimulating the carotid and aortic bodies. This is known as the 'hypoxic drive'. A high concentration of O_2 will suppress this hypoxic drive, and if Po_2 is raised even to normal, breathing becomes shallow and more and more CO_2 is retained, further depressing the respiratory centre, and a condition known as carbon dioxide narcosis develops. This is characterised by increasing drowsiness and eventual death.

The hypoxic drive must always be considered when O_2 is prescribed for patients with COAD. Usually this is not more than 24% of O_2 — slightly more than the 21% in room air — which is enough to improve oxygenation without eliminating the hypoxic drive. Prior to and during O_2 therapy, it is essential to determine arterial blood gas levels and to prescribe O_2 accordingly. The correct percentage is ensured by using controlled-flow O_2 masks and other appliances.

Research Abstract 3.2
Positive benefits of non-invasive positive pressure ventilation (NIPPV)

(a) A prospective randomised controlled trial using NIPPV was carried out in a group of 60 patients with chronic obstructive airways disease. Those who received NIPPV showed a reduction in Pco_2 and breathlessness, a significant rise in pH and a reduced mortality.

Bott J, Carrol M P, Conway J H et al 1993 Randomised controlled trial of nasal ventilation in acute ventilatory failure due to chronic obstructive airways disease. The Lancet 341 (8860): 1555–1557.

(b) A prospective randomised controlled trial in 41 patients with COAD found that the use of NIPPV reduced the incidence of endotracheal intubation and the mortality rate.

Wysocki M, Tric I, Wolff M A et al 1995 Non-invasive pressure support ventilation in patients with acute respiratory failure. Chest 107: 761–768.

For further information, see Place (1997).

Oxygen should always be administered strictly according to the prescribed amount, because of the danger of switching off this patient's hypoxic drive. It is vital that the nurse understands this and can explain it in simple terms to the patient, especially if he is to use and control his own oxygen supply at home. The patient and his family will need both verbal and written information and plenty of opportunity for discussion (see Box 3.6). A controlled percentage face mask (Ventimask) is usually used for this purpose.

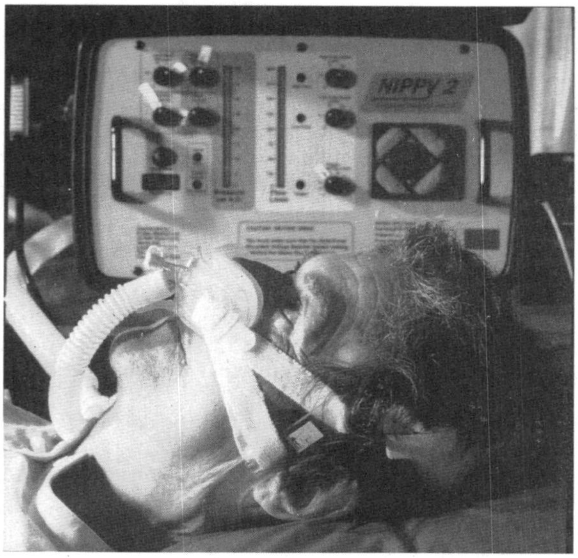

Fig. 3.6 Non-invasive positive pressure ventilation (NIPPV). *Establishing NIPPV:* **(1)** The first few hours of treatment are the most important. Get this right and the effectiveness of the treatment will be significantly enhanced. **(2)** Sit by the side of the patient and watch the respiratory pattern. Adjust the machine to mimic the patient's inspiratory and expiratory phases and his respiratory rate. **(3)** Choose a mask that best suits the patient. Masks can either be full-face or just cover the nose. An additional variant comes in the form of nasal plugs, where the mask fits snugly into the nostrils. **(4)** Allow the patient to hold the mask firmly to his face until his confidence rises. **(5)** Give the patient a thorough explanation of the procedure to help relieve his anxiety and try to ensure he is as comfortable as possible. (Reproduced with kind permission of the author and *Nursing Times*, from Place 1997.) *Photograph: Ben Edwards.*

Arterial blood gas analysis

Arterial blood gas (ABG) analysis is the most reliable way to monitor blood gas levels and the nurse should be prepared to follow the required procedure for obtaining the blood sample (see Box 3.7). A basic understanding of normal levels is also assumed.

The nurse must be aware that cyanosis may be a late sign of hypoxia and should not be relied upon as an early indicator. As a rule of thumb, cyanosis is usually noticeable when the concentration of deoxygenated haemoglobin in blood exceeds 50 g/L. The distinction between central and peripheral cyanosis is an important one. Central cyanosis is due to low oxygen content of the arterial blood (hypoxic hypoxia) and can be determined by inspecting the tongue and mucous membranes of the eye in addition to the skin. Peripheral cyanosis is due to a sluggish circulation (stagnant hypoxia) where release of oxygen from the blood is slowed down even though the arterial oxygen content may be normal, as for example in cardiac failure and shock.

For further information see Margereson & Esmond (1997a,b,c): NT Learning Curve, Unit 43, Parts 1–3.

Positioning and breathing

The patient will be more comfortable sitting up and well supported by pillows. He may find breathing easier if he leans forward on an overbed table with his elbows extended to the side.

Box 3.6 Patient teaching in O_2 therapy. (Reproduced with permission from Rutishauser 1994)

Increasingly, patients go home on O_2 therapy and will need information on how to get a supply of medical O_2 and how to set it up at home. The following instructions, which should accompany the patient, should be discussed fully and reinforced on every contact.

Instructions for home use of oxygen

- Oxygen is highly combustible. Do not use it near a fire or open flame. Post a 'no smoking' sign on the cylinder and explain to relatives and friends the reason for so doing. Electrical appliances and kinetic toys that may produce a spark are also a source of danger.
- Adjust the flow meter to the flow rate the doctor prescribes and do not change it without her consent.
- Keep water in the humidifier to the correct level and change it daily.
- NOTIFY DOCTOR if any of the following occur:
  —you have increased difficulty breathing
  —you feel unusually restless or upset
  —your breathing becomes irregular
  —you feel abnormally drowsy
  —your lips or fingernails look blue
  —you have trouble concentrating or you become confused.

Do not assume that you will feel better if you take more oxygen. This may not be the case and you should consult your doctor or go to the nearest casualty department immediately.

Box 3.7 Monitoring arterial blood gas levels (ABGs)

In the clinical situation, ABG levels can be monitored by laboratory blood gas analysis.

Blood is drawn from the radial or femoral artery, or from an established arterial line, using a heparinised syringe. Care is taken not to draw air into the syringe, which is capped and sent for immediate analysis.

Following the procedure, firm pressure must be applied to the puncture site for at least 5 min, as the artery may spurt significantly.

If the patient is on oxygen therapy, it is important to make sure that he has been having the prescribed amount for at least 15 min before the sample is drawn and to maintain that amount during the procedure. If he has been on a mechanical ventilator for a session of intermittent positive pressure breathing (IPPB), the nurse should wait at least 20 min before taking a sample and 20 min after commencing ventilation or post-tracheal suctioning. The prescribed amount of oxygen or the IPPB should be noted on the laboratory request form.

Emphysematous patients tend to take short, shallow breaths and should be taught diaphragmatic breathing to improve and slow down ventilation. Pursed-lip exhalation is helpful because it improves positive airway pressure and brings the abdominal muscles into play.

Chest physiotherapy

The physiotherapist will teach the patient deep breathing and coughing exercises and postural drainage techniques. Frappage (patterns of clapping the chest wall) may be necessary to loosen tenacious secretions. These exercises should be reinforced by nursing staff and the patient should be taught to perform them independently so that he can continue them after discharge home.

Patient education

The patient should understand the disease process and the aims of treatment. If the disease is in the early stages, removal of predisposing factors such as cigarette smoking will help to prevent further deterioration. If the condition is advanced, the patient may need help to adapt to a severely compromised lifestyle and to preserve what pulmonary function he has. Ensuring that the patient obtains optimal relief from his symptoms and is given adequate psychological support will present a considerable challenge for the nurse. The whole health care team will often be involved in providing support, advice and practical help to the whole family.

Asthma

Asthma is a common chronic inflammatory condition of the airways which is characterised by bronchospasm, severe dyspnoea, wheezing, chest tightness and expiratory exertion. As a result of inflammation, the airways are hyperresponsive and narrow easily in response to a wide range of provoking stimuli. Although much is known about asthma, it is a complex condition about which much remains to be understood.

Broadly speaking, there are two types of bronchial asthma: extrinsic and intrinsic. The extrinsic form occurs in children and young adults who are hypersensitive to foreign proteins such as dust mites, pollens, animal dander and feathers. Familial allergic tendencies can often be traced. Intrinsic or chronic asthma occurs later in life and is often associated with chronic respiratory inflammatory disease. Although there is no history of childhood asthma, there may be a family history of asthma and allergic tendencies. In many cases the role of allergens is still suspected. A large group of asthma sufferers are found to be vulnerable to stimuli of both extrinsic and intrinsic origin. There is increasing evidence that the psychosomatic element is negligible and can no longer be regarded as a major causative factor in most cases (Barnes 1993).

Recent research suggests that there is a critical trigger time early in the development of asthma when, if steroid therapy is introduced, the process can not only be controlled but 'turned off' so that the condition does not progress or recur. However, there continues to be some resistance to steroid therapy from the general public, especially in relation to treating children. This is because of the misconceived fear of side-effects, which in fact are minimal with inhaled steroids (Barnes 1993).

The National Asthma Audit 1996 (National Asthma Campaign 1997) states that over 3 million people in the UK have asthma; 1.5 million of these are children. The annual cost to the National Health Service of treating asthma is now in excess of £1000 million and morbidity is extensive, with an estimated 200 000 sufferers disabled by it. Despite the increasing incidence of asthma in the UK (especially in children and occupational asthma), there has been a significant decrease in mortality in all age groups except the elderly. Mortality was estimated at 1665 in 1994 (214 fewer than in 1993) and this downward trend continues. It is attributed to increased awareness of the disease, early use

Case History 3.1(A) C

C was brought into the A & E Department one night by his wife, and this is the account of his first severe asthma attack:

'I just couldn't get my breath .. I was panicking and really scared. My chest felt it was in a steel vice ... I was wheezing and gasping for air and just couldn't move it in or out. The nurse took one look and got action straight away. The room was swirling ... I thought I was a gonner ... and I passed out.

'When I came to, they'd put some powerful medication through a drip in my arm and an oxygen tube in my nose. I began to feel the panic again but then realised that the breathing was getting easier, and that calmed me down. That was my first bad attack of asthma and I never want to go through that again. I ended up in the Intensive Care and my family were worried sick.

'Two years before this we'd been through a rough time ... I was made redundant from my regular job ... been unemployed then got this other job which I'm not happy with ... there's a lot of dust and fumes around. I'd started to wheeze and cough a fair bit and the GP said it was asthma ... which was a bit of a shock at my age – 40 years old! It must run in the family, though. Dad has asthma but I thought I'd got away with it. Anyway, the doctor had given me some pills and a puffer, which helped at times but I must admit I wasn't really good at taking them. The severe attack, though, made me want to know more about it so that it doesn't happen again.'

of preventive medication and emphasis on rapidly establishing control of symptoms and then 'stepping down' treatment to the lowest dose to maintain adequate control. As yet there is no cure for asthma, although in the majority of cases where there is well-informed medical and nursing management and effective patient education and compliance, the disease can be well controlled.

PATHOPHYSIOLOGY

The immunoglobulin IgE is present in small amounts in normal sera but in increased amounts in asthma sufferers. In allergic extrinsic asthma, the disease process involves inhalation of antigens (allergens) which are absorbed by the bronchial mucosa and trigger production of IgE antibodies. These antibodies bind to mast cells and basophils around the bronchial blood vessels. When the allergen is encountered again, the antigen–antibody reaction releases histamines and bradykinin, resulting in bronchial muscle spasm, oedema and excessive secretion of thick mucus. In many cases, the severity of attacks lessens with age and good treatment unless other factors are involved.

There are various theories of the pathogenesis of intrinsic asthma. Allergens may be implicated. Whatever the cause, the bronchi and bronchioles are chronically inflamed, oedematous, full of mucus and subject to bronchospasm. Air is trapped in the alveoli and expiration is difficult. The disease can be progressive and impaired ventilation can result in hypoxia, hypertension and right-sided heart failure.

Clinical features. Asthma attacks can last for minutes, hours or days (status asthmaticus). They manifest as paroxysms of severe ventilatory difficulty with rapid, laboured breathing accompanied by wheezing. Expiration is forced and prolonged due to bronchospasm, hyperinflated lungs and trapped alveolar air. This may be accompanied by a dry or moist cough. There may be extreme anxiety, sweating, dyspnoea, orthopnoea and peripheral cyanosis with hypoxia and hypercapnia. Tachycardia is common because of anxiety and hypoxia and may be increased by bronchodilatory drugs such as salbutamol (Walker 1997). If there is no response to treatment, exhaustion will occur rapidly and may be followed by respiratory failure.

MEDICAL MANAGEMENT

Investigations. Diagnosis is by typical clinical presentation and past history. After an attack has subsided, lung function tests such as FEV_1 will be helpful in establishing the degree of impairment and in monitoring response to treatment. Prolonged FEV_1 indicates loss of elasticity of lung tissue. Chest X-rays will indicate clarity of lung fields and size of the heart. Skin sensitivity tests and history of exposure to specific allergens may help in isolating and avoiding triggering factors.

Treatment. Because of the complexity of asthma and concern about the continuing high incidence of mortality, a group of experts from the British Thoracic Society, the Research Unit of the Royal College of Physicians of London, the King's Fund Centre and the National Asthma Campaign drew up a comprehensive set of guidelines for the treatment of adult asthma. Their main concerns were that there was underuse of inhaled and oral corticosteroid treatment, underuse of objective measures of severity of asthma and inadequate supervision. These guidelines are available to all GPs, A&E departments and respiratory units.

For further information, see British Thoracic Society (1997).

3.8 Obtain the British Thoracic Society (BTS) guidelines for the management of asthma and study them carefully. Add the BTS guideline charts to your information folder.

The best treatment for asthma is avoidance of the cause, if this is known. In the event of an attack, initial treatment is usually with a bronchodilatory drug such as salbutamol and possibly a corticosteroid drug such as beclomethasone (an anti-inflammatory) given via a nebuliser or metered dose inhaler. First aid and home treatment can include steam inhalation to relax muscle spasm and loosen secretions. Severe cases may be treated in the A&E department, where oxygen therapy may be given in addition to nebulised or i.v. drugs. Oxygen is usually given at 4–6 L/min and by intranasal catheter because of the claustrophobic effect of oxygen face masks. ABGs will be analysed and oxygen prescribed accordingly. If the patient falls within the diagnostic category of COAD, care must be taken not to overprescribe because of possible compromise of hypoxic respiratory drive (see Box 3.5).

The majority of patients are treated by their GP and can administer their own treatment at home and avoid asthma attacks (see Box 3.8). Severe cases are referred to specialist respiratory units. Once diagnosed, if the patient does not respond to the usual prescribed

Box 3.8 Self-management of asthma. (Reproduced with kind permission from the British Thoracic Society 1997)

1. As far as possible, patients should be trained to manage their own treatment rather than be required to consult the doctor before making changes.
2. The patient should have a relevant understanding of the nature of asthma and its treatment. This would include:
   - training in the proper use of inhaled treatment and the use of a peak flow meter
   - knowledge of the difference between relieving and anti-inflammatory therapies
   - instruction to ensure recognition of signs that asthma is worsening, especially the significance of night-time symptoms and of changes in peak expiratory flow (PEF).
3. Patients should be given adequate opportunity to express their expectations of treatment and to hear how far those expectations can be met. They should have a balanced view of the possible side-effects of the treatments.
4. Education and training of the patient are the responsibility of the doctor but can profitably be shared with specially trained health care professionals. Advice should be consistent, and repeated. It should be supported by written or audiovisual material. The patient should be acquainted with the resources of the National Asthma Campaign.
5. Patients who have required, or who are likely to require, a course of systemic corticosteroid treatment should be trained to initiate or increase inhaled and oral corticosteroid treatment themselves under specified pre-arranged circumstances as outlined in a self-management plan.
6. The three elements of a self-management plan are:
   - symptom, peak flow and drug usage monitoring leading to
   - the patient taking pre-arranged action according to
   - written guidance.

   Such self-management plans should be carefully discussed with the patient and written down individually or by using a National Asthma Campaign Adult Asthma Card. The plans should include information about how and where to obtain urgent medical attention.
7. Patients should regard the plan of management as subject to a process of continuing but orderly review in which they play an active part. Review of a patient's progress at a pre-arranged visit to the doctor should include review of:
   - symptoms, especially nocturnal
   - interference with normal activities (e.g. work loss)
   - the patient's own record of treatment changes
   - peak flow recordings
   - understanding of asthma
   - understanding of management
   - inhalation skills
   - the action to be taken by the patient if pre-arranged signs of deterioration develop.
8. Requests for help from a patient with asthma should be accorded the highest priority by doctors. Other health care workers should be aware that medical help may be required promptly in the event of worsening asthma.
9. Patients with brittle asthma (sudden severe attacks) should be under active specialist care, always carry an emergency kit, have a written action plan and wear a Medic-Alert disc.

treatment and notices a significant drop in his peak flow reading or experiences increasing difficulty, he may present and self-admit to the respiratory unit where he is known or to the nearest A&E department (see Fig. 3.7).

NURSING PRIORITIES AND MANAGEMENT: ASTHMA

Major considerations

The first priority of nursing intervention is to ensure that the individual experiencing an asthma attack is seen by a doctor as soon as possible. The condition can deteriorate rapidly.

Giving psychological support

An attack of asthma is extremely frightening. The patient will be fighting for breath and is often panic-stricken. It is vital for the nurse to maintain a calm and reassuring manner. The nurse with a sound knowledge base will be able to anticipate the course of the attack and the patient's reactions to it, and thus will be better equipped to help him to remain calm. The nurse should stay with the patient at all times.

Positioning and monitoring

The patient should sit up well supported by pillows or lean forward on an overbed table. Vital signs, oxygen therapy and ABGs should be monitored constantly and interpreted intelligently. The nurse should be on the alert for any sign of deterioration.

Assisting with inhalation technique

The nurse should make sure that the patient is using his nebuliser or inhaler correctly (see Box 3.9 and Figs 3.8 and 3.9). There are different kinds of inhalation delivery systems and it is essential to follow the manufacturer's instructions specific to each type. A common cause of failed home treatment is that the patient does not use his inhaler correctly and therefore does not get his full dose of the drug (Newman et al 1991). There is some debate about which kind of metered dose inhaler is best, but the weight of opinion gives preference to the breath-actuated pressurised aerosol for patients with poor inhaler technique. Between 40 and 50% of patients have poor technique which can be improved by changing from the conventional metered dose inhalers to the breath-actuated pressure inhaler and being given proper instruction in its use (Crompton 1991). Large-volume 'spacer devices' (Fig. 3.9) are being used more frequently with metered dose inhalers. They are recommended for patients who have difficulty coordinating their inhaler technique or who have hand disabilities. The technique allows the propellant time to evaporate before the medication is inhaled and therefore reduces the systemic effects of steroids but delivers a higher dose of medication. The chlorofluorocarbon (CFC) carrier substance for inhaled drugs is currently being replaced by a non-CFC propellant (British Thoracic Society 1997).

Practice nurses, community nurses and hospital nurses are in a good position to make a realistic assessment of patient capabilities and inhaler technique and to give advice accordingly. The effectiveness of received medication can be determined by measuring lung function (peak flow) before and after inhalation. Patients can be taught to do this themselves and to record the results. A multidisciplinary care plan and critical pathway based on the latest British Thoracic Society's Asthma Guidelines should be developed to ensure research-based practice, consistency of care and cost-effectiveness (see Case History 3.1(B) and Collaborative Care Plan 3.1).

Thorax 1997;52 (Suppl 1) S15

Chart 5

Asthma in accident and emergency departments

ASTHMA CAN KILL

Immediately measure peak expiratory flow

>75% predicted mild

50–75% moderate

33–50% severe

<33% life threatening

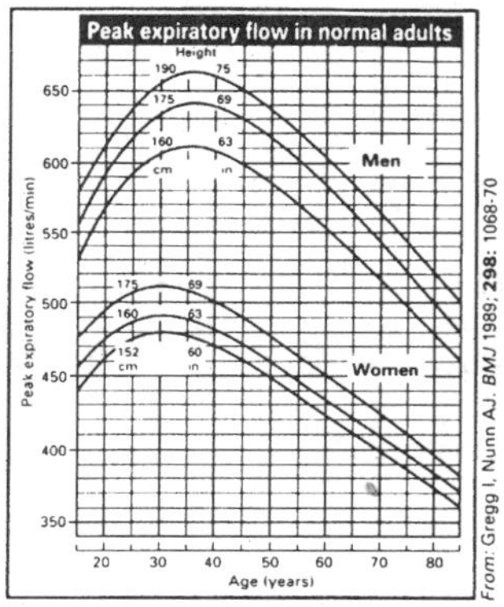

POSSIBLE DISCHARGE

ADMIT

USUAL INHALED BRONCHODILATOR

NURSE TO GIVE NEBULISED SALBUTAMOL 5 mg OR TERBUTALINE 10 mg WITH OXYGEN AS DRIVING GAS

Any severe or life threatening features

Features of severe asthma
- Cannot complete sentence in one breath
- Respirations ≥25/min
- Pulse ≥110 beats/min

Life threatening features
- Silent chest, cyanosis, feeble respiratory effort
- Bradycardia or hypotension
- Exhaustion, confusion, or coma

Keep under observation 60 min.

If patient stable and PEF >75%

Wait 30 minutes

If PEF 50–75% repeat nebulised β agonist. Give prednisolone tablets 40 mg. Wait 30 minutes

If worse or PEF ≤50%

Caution:
Patient with severe or life threatening attacks may not be distressed and may not have all these abnormalities. The presence of any should alert the doctor

If stable or improving and PEF >75%

If PEF 50–75% wait 60 min

If patient stable or improving and PEF >60%

If worse or PEF ≤60%

ARTERIAL BLOOD GAS MARKERS OF SEVERITY
- Normal (5–6 kPa, 36–45 mm Hg) or high $Paco_2$
- Severe hypoxia (Pao_2 <8 kPa, 60 mm Hg) irrespective of oxygen treatment
- Low pH (or high H^+)

No other investigations are needed for immediate management

DISCHARGE

Mild
- Ensure patient has usual treatment supply and inhaler technique is correct, advise full compliance, instruct relatives if appropriate
- Give note for GP, advise early consultation, recommend PEF charting, advise registration with GP
- Tell patient to return immediately if asthma worsens and be admitted

Moderate
- As for mild, plus:
- Prednisolone tablets 30–40 mg, regular inhaled corticosteroid, and β agonist as necessary.
- Consider referral to chest clinic

MANAGEMENT

Immediate:
- Oxygen 40–60% in all cases
- Salbutamol 5 mg or terbutaline 10 mg via oxygen driven nebuliser
- Prednisolone tablets 30–60 mg or intravenous hydrocortisone 200 mg, or both

If life threatening features present:
- Add ipratropium 0.5 mg to nebulised β agonist
- Give intravenous aminophylline 250 mg over 20 minutes or salbutamol or terbutaline 250 μg over 10 minutes. Caution when giving bolus aminophylline if patient is already taking theophyllines
- Chest radiography to exclude pneumothorax

ADMIT

DISCHARGED PATIENTS NEED EXTRA CARE AS MORTALITY IS HIGH IN THIS GROUP

PATIENTS SHOULD BE ACCOMPANIED BY A NURSE OR DOCTOR AT ALL TIMES

NATIONAL ASTHMA CAMPAIGN

Working for Healthier Lungs

This chart is appropriate for patients from puberty onwards

in association with the General Practitioner in Asthma Group, the British Association of Accident and Emergency Medicine, the British Paediatric Respiratory Society and the Royal College of Paediatrics and Child Health

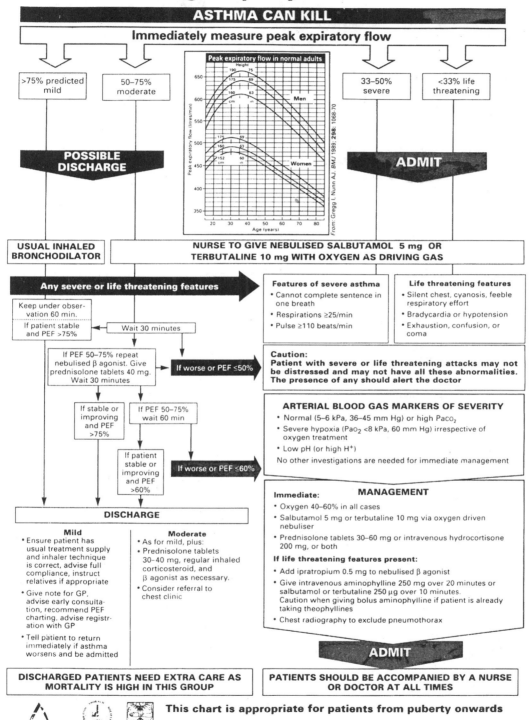

Fig. 3.7 Management of asthma in accident and emergency departments. (Reproduced with kind permission from BMJ Publishing Group.)

Box 3.9 Assisting a patient to use a nebuliser

A nebuliser attached to a flow of oxygen or air converts a liquid into an aerosol mist. The medication is prescribed by the doctor along with 2–3 mL of normal saline. The procedure may be coordinated with chest physiotherapy, and peak flow of tidal volume may be measured and recorded before and after the treatment. The equipment is assembled according to the procedure illustrated in Figure 3.8.

The medication is checked and drawn up into a syringe and diluted with the prescribed 2–3 mL of normal saline. If two medications are prescribed, they should not be mixed together. Separate nebulisers should be used and the bronchodilator drug given first.

- The equipment and purpose of the medication is explained to the patient. The medication is put into the nebuliser, which is assembled and attached to the oxygen or air supply. If oxygen is used, a 'no smoking' sign is displayed and the reason explained. Air is used instead of oxygen if the patient has chronic obstructive airways disease (COAD) because of the danger of disrupting his hypoxic drive (see Box 3.5).
- Peak flow is measured if required and the best of three attempts is charted.
- The patient sits up in a comfortable position.
- The oxygen flow meter is adjusted to 5 L to ensure vaporisation of the medication.
- The nurse observes to ensure that there is a fine vapour coming from the nebuliser and encourages the patient to breathe it in through the mouthpiece if possible. If this is too difficult, he may use an oxygen mask instead. The patient is instructed to breathe normally, taking an occasional deep breath. If the patient is on a respirator, a nebuliser can be introduced into the ventilator circuit.
- The nurse should stay with the patient until all the medication is nebulised and observe his respirations. She should ask him how he feels and encourage him to cough and expectorate if he has mucus in his lungs. A clean sputum container should be ready to hand.
- Half an hour after the treatment, peak flow readings are taken again and the best of three is charted.
- The procedure is documented and the equipment washed and dried and stored in the patient's locker until needed again.

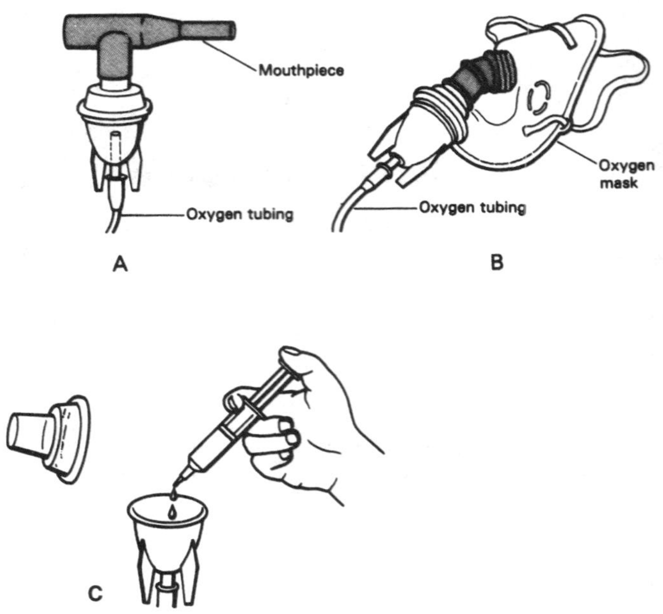

Fig. 3.8 Nebulisers. A: Nebuliser attached to a mouthpiece. B: Nebuliser attached to an oxygen mask. C: Nebuliser taken apart to introduce a prepared medication. (Reproduced with permission from Jamieson et al 1999.)

Case History 3.1(B) C's story *(cont'd)*

At the team conference just before C was discharged from hospital, he made the following comments:

'I just did not realise how important it was to know about asthma — and in particular to know about how it affects me and how the medications work. I hadn't given it much thought really before this severe attack and usually just had a few more puffs with the inhaler when I thought I needed them.

'When I first came to this ward I remember how surprised I was that the other patients seemed to know so much and take such an active part in their own treatment. I thought you came into hospital to have things done to you, not to learn how to do it yourself, but I see now. They treated the unit a bit like a "club". Mostly they'd been in before and their good-natured "advice" was a great help, especially when I got depressed about being stuck with asthma. I realised it wasn't the end of the world.

'Knowing about asthma makes me feel more in control; and now I've learnt how to use the inhaler properly and the peak flow meter, and you've explained what my safe limits are, I shall know what to do in future. Having it all written down, too, is somehow reassuring. I certainly don't want another episode like this last one, so it's worth taking a bit more time to understand things and look after myself. I don't intend to let asthma rule my life, though, but I will change my job and try to look after my general health more.'

Health education

The adequacy of asthma patients' knowledge of their disease and its treatment and of their compliance with drug therapy has been called into question by Tettersell (1993). In particular, her research indicates that instructions given by nurses are poorly understood (see Research Abstract 3.3).

A telephone information line was set up in 1990 by the National Asthma Campaign to answer questions about the disease and its treatment. This line continues to be inundated with calls for information relating to the disease and its treatment, medication, delivery systems, peak flow readings, asthma in schools and many other related topics. The calls have been from asthma sufferers themselves, from mothers of children with asthma, from relatives and from health professionals (Crone et al 1993, National Asthma Campaign 1997).

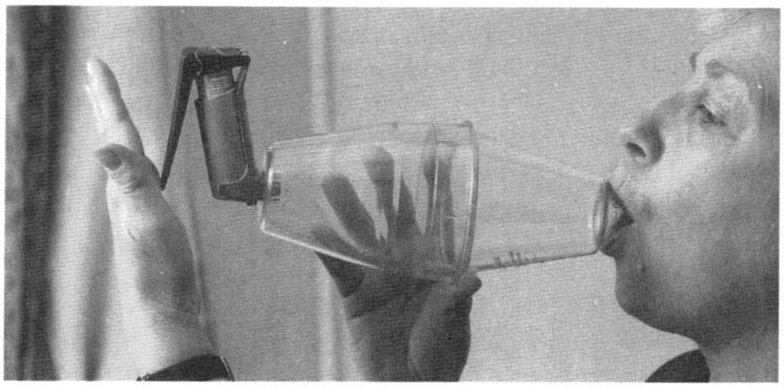

Fig. 3.9 Spacer device. (Reproduced with kind permission from MacDonald 1997 and *Nursing Times*.) *Photograph: Laurence Bulaitis*

Using your spacer: *Advice to patients:*
(1) Make sure your inhaler fits your spacer device.
(2) Shake inhaler before attaching it to spacer.
(3) Attach inhaler to spacer and place mouth over spacer mouthpiece.
(4) Squirt inhaler once and medication enters spacer.
(5) Optimal breathing patterns:
(a) take in one big breath to inhale medication; or
(b) within a count of 5, take in a breath and hold it for a count of 10; or
(c) if short of breath, just breathe normally and squirt inhaler once when comfortable to do so.

Care of spacer device: Wash and rinse once each week and dry in air. Do not wipe dry as this increases electrostatic charging of spacer wall and reduces drug delivery. Spacers should be replaced every 6–12 months (British Thoracic Society 1997).

Multidisciplinary Collaborative Care Plan 3.1 C: acute asthma. (BTS critical pathway will be developed using BTS guidelines.)

Problem focus	***Medical***	***Nursing***	***Patient***	***Physiotherapy***	***Social work***
Transfer from ICU for stabilisation and establishment of self-care treatment regimen following an acute severe asthma attack	• Priority if called to review patient's condition	Coordinate team care • educative-suppportive role • priority to any signs of deteriorating condition. Action STATIM • monitor vital signs and respiratory status		• Ensure clear airways — deep breathing, coughing exercises, use of ancillary muscles	• Problem with work environment
Patient involvement and understanding essential regarding: • disease process • symptoms • management • interpretation of symptoms and PEF • specific drug actions and side-effects • written self-care plan and action to be taken when pre-arranged signs of deterioration are evident	• Select and prescribe treatment and drugs • Discuss with patient and care team: —asthma disease process —treatment and action of drugs —taking and monitoring peak expiratory flow (PEF) — significance —nebuliser technique • Monitor ABGs • Establish individual acceptable range PEF • Establish written self-care plan for patient and action to be taken	• Reassurance • Reinforce and repeat doctor's explanations in lay terms • Teach use of peak flow meter. Repeat significance of PEF readings • Teach use of nebuliser and inhaler • Coordinate physio and medication times • Assist with ABGs • Medications as prescribed • Monitor effects • Assist C to work out role in care team and express questions and concerns • Contact Asthma Campaign • Assist with written self-care plan	• Cooperate with health care team to learn more about: —asthma —treatment —management —using nebuliser/ inhaler —recording PEF and what readings signify Work out action to take at set points • Ask questions — discuss results • Practise use of equipment • Talk to social worker and get advice on work and family problems • Help to work out written self-care plan • Aim to control asthma and avoid further severe attacks	• Coordinate physiotherapy with inhalation regimen. Assist with nebuliser technique • Discuss general fitness • Teach C respiratory mechanics and exercises	• Advise on family benefits • Funding for peak flow meter • Advise on job change

Research Abstract 3.3
Asthma patients' knowledge in relation to compliance (Tettersell 1993)

Patient knowledge about asthma and its treatment and treatment compliance levels were assessed among 100 moderate to severe asthmatics recruited from general practice. Postal questionnaires were used. Non-compliance was found to be high, with 39% of patients omitting to take their asthma treatment as prescribed. Reasons given were 'believing the drugs not to be necessary' and 'forgetting'. Almost half the cohort admitted a reluctance to use their inhalers in public and a third stated a preference for tablets. The highest compliers were respondents who reported never receiving an explanation about the condition. The level of patient knowledge had no significant effect on compliance with drug therapy, although it did correlate with ability to manage asthma attacks. The majority of patients believed they would know how to manage an attack, but when 'scored' on actual ability only 34.4% were deemed to be safe. Less than half the patients who had had asthma explained to them reported to have understood the initial explanation. Explanations made by nurses were particularly poorly understood. Health professionals need to look both to their teaching techniques and to methods other than education in isolation as a means of improving patient compliance. Since the GP contract was introduced in April 1990, nurses working in general practice have become increasingly involved with health education as part of health promotion and chronic disease management clinics. This study highlights the need for a more comprehensive approach to patient education and more research into contextual factors involved in non-compliance.

Tettersell M J 1993 Asthma patients' knowledge in relation to compliance with drug therapy. Journal of Advanced Nursing 18(1): 103–113.

Box 3.10 Audit of asthma care

Audit has shown that specialist care of adults admitted with asthma is associated with improved outcomes (British Thoracic Society 1997).

In hospital, audit should be of the process of care. The British Thoracic Society (BTS) audit tool allows assessment of eight criteria:
- Peak expiratory flow (PEF) recorded on admission
- Arterial blood gases measured in patients with S_aO_2 <92%
- Systemic steroids administered within 1 h of admission
- PEF serially recorded so that variability can be calculated
- Inhaled steroids prescribed on discharge
- Oral steroids prescribed on discharge
- Follow-up appointment planned
- Self-management plan given

In general practice, audit will include:
- An asthma register
- An ability to determine the frequency of attendance with asthma
- Information on the prescribing of both preventive and relieving medication
- Information on outpatient referral rates and admission to hospital
- Agreed strategies for coping with patients at risk of developing severe attacks or showing features which have recognised associations with asthma deaths

Specialist training

Audit has shown that specialist care of adult patients admitted with asthma is associated with improved outcome. The British Thoracic Society (BTS) recommends that health care personnel such as ambulance officers, A&E staff, practice nurses and school nurses should have specific training in asthma care and be enabled to follow the guidelines that they recommend (British Thoracic Society 1997) (see Box 3.10).

BRONCHOGENIC CARCINOMA

Bronchogenic carcinoma can be of primary origin, as discussed above, or can occur as secondary metastatic spread from other primary sources.

PATHOPHYSIOLOGY

Bronchogenic carcinomas are classified according to their basic cell type, i.e. squamous cell adenocarcinoma (the most common), undifferentiated carcinoma, and large- and small-cell carcinoma. The tumour presents as a cauliflower-shaped mass which slowly infiltrates the lung parenchyma. Because this form of cancer is difficult to detect in the early stages, it has a high potential for metastatic spread before being discovered.

Common presenting symptoms. The patient presents with a persistent cough of several months' duration which may be accompanied by haemoptysis (bloodstained sputum), chest pain, hoarseness and breathlessness. There may also be weight loss, anaemia, pleural effusion and bone pain. The patient will look generally unwell (see Case History 3.2).

MEDICAL MANAGEMENT

Investigations. Diagnosis is confirmed by auscultation (listening to the chest with a stethoscope), chest X-ray or CT scan and sputum cytology. A bronchoscopy (direct visualisation of the trachea and bronchi using a bronchoscope, i.e. a flexible tube with a light source) may be performed. A small piece of lung tissue (biopsy) may be taken via the bronchoscope and sent for pathology.

Treatment. A full explanation of the diagnosis and prognosis will be given to the patient and his family, who will be involved in decision-making regarding treatment. About 15% of primary lung tumours can be treated successfully by surgical removal. This will involve either lobectomy (removal of the affected lobe) or pneumonectomy (removal of the whole lung) followed by cytotoxic chemotherapy. Where there is invasive and metastatic spread, the treatment is usually conservative, involving chemotherapy, deep X-ray, intervention to alleviate symptoms, and pain control (see Chs 19 and 31).

Q

3.9 Discuss the social problems contributing to M's heavy smoking habit (Case History 3.2). What additional problems were created by her early death and what impact could it have on her children? What kind of interventions are called for, and by whom? Consider the ethical dilemmas that a community nurse could be faced with in offering support and advice, remembering the fine balance between beneficence and patient autonomy and the fact that most of this life drama was played out in M's own home.

Case History 3.2 Mrs M

M was 40 years old, mother of an 18-year-old son and two daughters aged 17 and 15. Her son was unemployed and had been involved in one or two minor skirmishes between his local gang and the police. The girls were still at school. M's husband walked out on her 8 years ago and she had supported her family as best she could on social benefits and the occasional odd job.

They lived in a high-rise housing estate in the inner city area. She seldom went out except to get bare necessities and to window shop during the daytime. It wasn't safe for a woman at night in that part of town. She spent a lot of time in front of the television. She had smoked heavily for the past 10 years, saying it was her only luxury and that when she tried to cut down she got 'stressed out of her mind'.

Recently she had lost a lot of weight and had been breathless after climbing the stairs to the flat. She had had a 'smoker's' cough for years and been prone to 'chest colds', but when she started to find breathing painful she visited her GP asking for antibiotics for her 'chest infection'.

A series of tests (chest X-ray, sputum culture and lung scan) showed that she had advanced bronchogenic carcinoma. She was immediately referred to the oncology department at the local hospital, where further tests showed that she had bony metastases (secondary cancer in the bones). Having discussed a range of options for treatment, which included chemotherapy and irradiation therapy and their side-effects, she elected not to have any treatment except pain relief when the symptoms got worse.

M's symptoms and breathing difficulties quickly did get worse and her few activities were severely curtailed. She insisted on staying at home until a week before her death and she died 6 months after she had been diagnosed. Apart from her three children and an elderly mother in a nursing home, there were no other relatives to call upon.

NURSING PRIORITIES AND MANAGEMENT: CARE OF THE PATIENT FOLLOWING LOBECTOMY

General perioperative care is as described in Chapter 26. The reader should also review the position and function of the structures illustrated in Figure 3.1.

Specific considerations

The following points are of particular importance in postoperative management following lobectomy:

- The physiotherapist will manage the pre- and postoperative chest physiotherapy; however, the role of nursing staff in giving assistance and ensuring continuity is extremely important.
- Chest surgery can be very frightening and the patient and his family will need careful explanations and constant reassurance.
- In order to allow full expansion of the operated lung, the patient must be nursed in a semi-upright position, well supported with pillows, following a lower lobectomy. Following an upper lobectomy, the patient must be nursed in the position requested by the surgeon.
- If oxygen therapy is required it will be prescribed by the doctor. The nurse will need to monitor the equipment, the amount given and the effect of the therapy on the patient.
- There are usually two chest drains in situ, one anterior to the apex and one posterior to the base. These are attached to underwater seal drainage and pleural suction (see Fig. 3.10). Their purpose is to allow air to escape from the lobectomy space and to allow drainage of haemoserous fluid caused by the surgical procedure. Management of underwater seal drainage is discussed in detail in Box 3.11 (p. 82).
- The patient can sit out of bed and walk short distances while the drains are in place, but care must be taken not to put traction on the tubes and to keep the drainage system below the level of the chest. Two pairs of chest drain clamps should accompany the patient at all times.

For further information, see Campbell (1993).

NURSING PRIORITIES AND MANAGEMENT: CARE OF THE PATIENT FOLLOWING PNEUMONECTOMY

Specific considerations

Postoperative positioning

It is vital to find out whether the pericardium has been opened during the operation or not. If it has been opened the patient must not be allowed to lie on the operated side because of the danger of herniation of the heart through the pericardium and a mediastinal shift (i.e. a shifting of the heart and greater vessels into the pleural space, causing kinking of the vessels and acute circulatory failure).

Unless otherwise indicated by the surgeon, the best practice is to nurse the patient upright, well supported by pillows.

Chest drains

Usually there are no drainage tubes in position, the main aim being for the space to fill with haemoserous fluid. This will slowly become organised into fibrous tissue and, together with contraction of the intercostal and diaphragmatic muscles and gradual slight shift of the mediastinum, will eventually fill the residual space.

However, if chest drains are in position, they will be attached to an underwater seal drainage system and double-clamped. There may be a request that the clamps be released for brief periods at given times to allow escape of excess fluid and air. If this is the case, the nurse must stay with the patient during the unclamped period and be prepared to clamp the tubings immediately if the patient is about to cough. Because a cough is a full inspiration followed by forced expiration, it will force air from the lung space out through the drainage tube, allowing a sudden mediastinal shift, which could be fatal.

Other considerations

The knowledge that he has lost an entire lung can cause a patient to panic and to be extremely agitated. It is vital for the nurse to remain with the patient as much as possible and to maintain a calm and reassuring manner. She may need to explain that the lung space will be allowed to fill slowly with blood and serum which, over the following few weeks, will undergo fibrosis.

There may be a degree of post-anaesthetic atelectasis (collapse of the alveoli) in the remaining lung, causing breathlessness. Oxygen will be given as prescribed.

Pain can be severe following this pneumonectomy and prescribed pain relief should be given promptly. It should be borne in mind that effective pain control will help to promote calm, relaxed breathing and is therefore important to the patient's recovery (see Ch. 19).

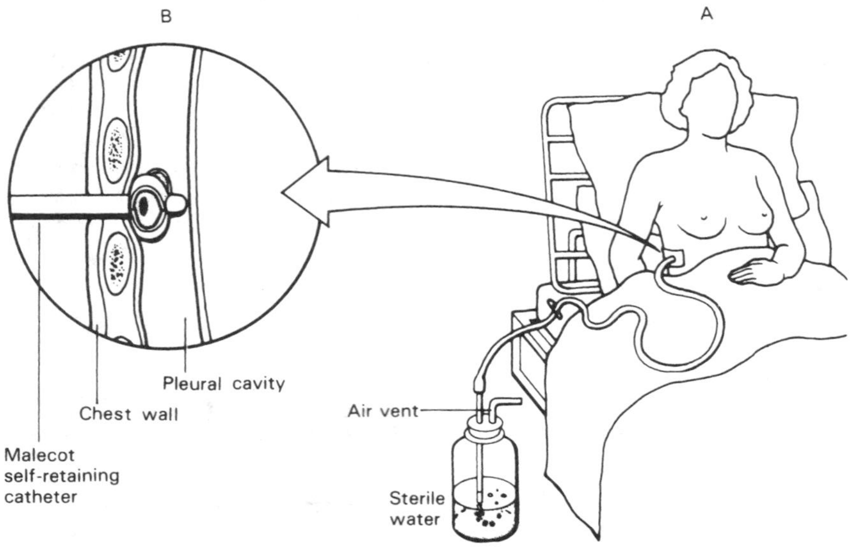

Fig. 3.10 Underwater seal chest drainage. A: Drainage system in position. B: Detail of the position of the catheter. (Reproduced with permission from Jamieson et al 1999.)

RESPIRATORY EMERGENCIES

This section begins with a brief consideration of chest injuries, pulmonary oedema and respiratory failure. An introduction to endotracheal intubation and mechanical ventilation is also given. Pulmonary embolism, a fairly common and potentially lethal complication of surgery and trauma, is discussed in Chapter 26.

CHEST INJURIES

Fractured ribs and flail chest

PATHOPHYSIOLOGY

Any injury to the thoracic cavity has the potential to compromise respiratory function. Penetrating injuries caused by knives, bullets, fractured ribs or sharp objects can disrupt ventilatory mechanisms or pierce vital structures, resulting in collapse of the lung or abnormal collections of blood or air in the pleural cavity. Non-penetrating injuries caused by blunt trauma or crushing can also disrupt ventilatory mechanisms, especially if the diaphragm or other structures are ruptured or contused. Both types of injury will involve dysfunctional pain, and both will restrict surface area and gaseous exchange.

Clinical features. Signs and symptoms shared by all chest injuries include varying degrees of dyspnoea, chest pain, cyanosis, hypoxia, tachycardia and possibly haemoptysis.

MEDICAL MANAGEMENT

Investigations. Diagnosis is confirmed by chest X-ray and the degree of hypoxia is determined by blood gas analysis.

Treatment. Simple fractured ribs are usually stable and heal without intervention. Compound fractured ribs may cause a pneumothorax (see below).

When several successive ribs are fractured and become dissociated completely from the rest of the rib cage, the condition is known as flail chest and is characterised by paradoxical breathing (see Fig. 3.11).

NURSING PRIORITIES AND MANAGEMENT: FRACTURED RIBS AND FLAIL CHEST

Providing there are no complications or other serious injury, the patient with fractured ribs can be nursed at home. Flail chest, however, is often associated with more serious chest trauma requiring hospital care.

The main aim of nursing care is to promote rest and control pain until the intercostal muscles have had a chance to stabilise the fractured ribs. In the case of flail chest, the patient will need bed rest and probably narcotic pain relief by i.m. injection. In some cases, patient-controlled analgesia (PCA) may be appropriate.

The patient should be advised to avoid heavy lifting or exertion until the fractures are healed.

Pneumothorax and haemopneumothorax

PATHOPHYSIOLOGY

The term 'pneumothorax' refers to the presence of air in the pleural space, and 'haemopneumothorax' refers to the presence of blood and air in the pleural space. Both conditions cause partial or complete collapse of the lung on the affected side.

In 'tension pneumothorax', the opening into the pleural space from either the lung or the outside chest wall acts as a one-way valve and sucks air into that space during inhalation but does not allow it to escape during exhalation. Gradually there is a build-up of air in the affected side and a mediastinal shift occurs with resultant cardiopulmonary compromise.

Clinical features. An open pneumothorax is characterised by the presence of an open wound and a sucking sound as air is drawn into the pleural cavity. In a closed pneumothorax, air enters the space from torn lung tissue and there is little or no movement on the affected side.

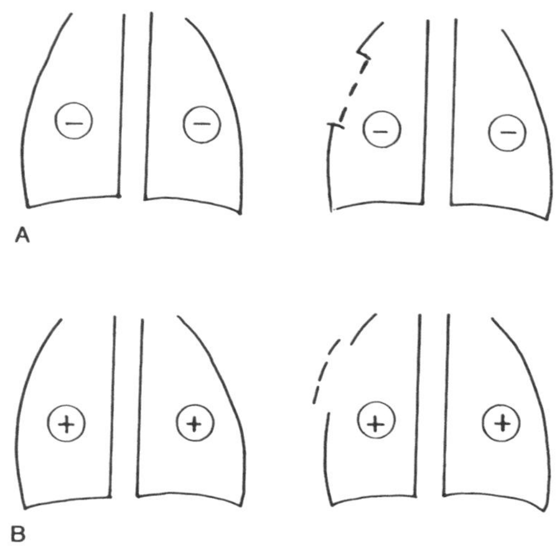

Fig. 3.11 Paradoxical breathing. A: On inhalation, the rib cage expands to create a negative pressure in the lungs and thus sucks in air. This negative pressure also draws in the dissociated ribs. B: On exhalation, the rib cage contracts to expel air from the lungs, but the resultant positive pressure also forces out the dissociated ribs. (Reproduced with permission from Game et al 1989.)

MEDICAL MANAGEMENT

First aid. The patient is kept in an upright position or lying on the affected side. Penetrating foreign bodies are not removed until intensive care facilities are available, in case their removal causes massive haemorrhage or mediastinal shift. Open wounds can be covered by a clean occlusive dressing; this must be released at intervals to avoid a tension pneumothorax developing.

On admission to the A&E department, the patient will have a chest X-ray. An apical intercostal chest drain will be inserted and connected to an underwater drainage system. If there is a haemopneumothorax, the patient will require a second chest drain in the basal chest wall. Narcotic analgesia will usually be necessary to manage the patient's pain and anxiety.

NURSING PRIORITIES AND MANAGEMENT: PNEUMOTHORAX AND HAEMOPNEUMOTHORAX

Specific considerations

General principles of care for the initial period will be as described in Chapter 27. Specific considerations are as follows.

Observation and monitoring

Constant vigilance must be maintained in observing for any change in respiratory status. These injuries are potentially life-threatening and the patient should never be left unattended. Changes in respiratory patterns, symptoms and vital signs should be monitored frequently and action taken accordingly.

Assisting with insertion of a chest drain

The patient will usually be given a narcotic analgesic to relax him and relieve the pain. This will also result in slower, deeper and more effective breathing. The nurse assisting should offer simple explanations and reassurance. If possible, the patient should be sat up so that he can lean his arms forward on an overbed table. This will help to expand the thoracic cavity and provide good support for the patient. The pressure needed to pierce the chest wall is unpleasant but should not be painful. The nurse assembles all the equipment. Often a complete, sterile chest drain set is kept prepackaged in the A&E department. Before the chest drain is inserted, the drainage system should be opened, connected and the drainage jar filled with sterile water to the requisite level. The whole system should be carefully checked to ensure that it is airtight. A local anaesthetic is then given at the chosen site, a small incision made, and the chest drain inserted into the pleural cavity, connected to the underwater drainage system and sutured in place (see Box 3.11 and Fig. 3.10). A chest X-ray is carried out to confirm the correct position.

Assisting with removal of a chest drain

This procedure must be carried out by two people, usually a doctor and an experienced nurse. A careful explanation of the procedure should be given to the patient and he should be shown how to practise the Valsalva manoeuvre (forcible exhalation against a closed glottis). Alternatively, he can be asked to take in a deep breath and hold it, as this prevents a rush of air into the puncture site and is more easily controlled than the Valsalva manoeuvre. An occlusive dressing and airtight tape must be ready to be applied to the insertion site. The purse-string suture is located and the retaining suture removed. The drain is steadied, and as the patient performs the Valsalva manoeuvre the drain is quickly removed and the purse-string suture tied to close the insertion hole. The dressing and airtight tape are then applied firmly. The patient should be observed carefully following the procedure. A check X-ray may be performed.

PULMONARY OEDEMA

Pulmonary oedema (excess fluid in lung tissue) is associated with many conditions, including inflammatory response to infections, shock, cardiac failure, nephrotic syndrome and severe allergic reactions.

PATHOPHYSIOLOGY

The lungs are susceptible to oedema because of the minimal tissue resistance offered by the thin alveolar cells and the capillary walls. The condition is akin to drowning in that the lungs are full of water, blood and mucus. Pulmonary oedema is usually acute and life-threatening, as it disrupts gaseous exchange.

Clinical features. The patient presents with a moist cough that produces copious, frothy, pink sputum. He is dyspnoeic, tachycardic and extremely distressed.

MEDICAL MANAGEMENT

Diagnosis is made on presenting signs and symptoms, auscultation, chest X-ray and medical history. The main principles of treatment are to remove the water from the lungs and to assist the respiratory process. Treatment consists of sitting the patient upright, giving oropharyngeal suction, diuretic therapy, narcotic analgesics, bronchodilator drugs and oxygen. In severe cases, it may be necessary to intubate and mechanically ventilate the patient.

NURSING PRIORITIES AND MANAGEMENT: PULMONARY OEDEMA

As pulmonary oedema is usually associated with cardiovascular disease, specifically left ventricular failure, the principles of nursing management are discussed in Chapter 2.

Box 3.11 Care of underwater seal drainage

Basic principles

The drainage system is sterile throughout. It is completely assembled prior to the chest drain being inserted. Connections are airtight and sealed with transparent tape to allow inspection. Water level in the drainage bottle or device is determined by hospital policy but should be at least enough to submerge the drainage tube by 2.5 cm. In the case of prepacked drainage units, the manufacturer's instructions should be followed. The water acts as a valve and prevents air re-entering the pleural space. The outlet tube allows expelled air to escape. Drainage may be by gravity and respiratory movements or may be assisted by attaching a vacuum pump to the outlet tube. Single-, two- and three-bottle systems are available.

The chest drain is sutured in place and has an additional purse-string suture around the skin entry site. A sterile dressing surrounds the entry site.

Nursing management

- Give a full explanation and reassurance to the patient to allay his anxiety and gain his cooperation.
- Administer pain relief as required.
- Keep the patient sitting up, well supported by pillows whilst he is in bed, and encourage deep breathing and coughing exercises as discussed with the physiotherapist.
- Ensure that two pairs of chest drain clamps accompany the patient at all times in case of accidental disconnection. If the system becomes disconnected, air will be drawn into the interpleural space, extending the pneumothorax.
- When clamping is necessary, the clamps must not be left on for long periods as a tension pneumothorax may develop (see p. 80). The patient must never be left unattended while the tubing is clamped.
- Ensure that the drainage system is always kept below the level of the chest to prevent back-flow into the interpleural space.
- Check regularly to ensure that the system is airtight and the water level is correct.
- Note the presence of bubbling. If the tube is bubbling, air is being evacuated from the pleural space. If there are no bubbles, there should be a swinging movement of fluid in the down-tube which reflects the pressure changes in the pleural cavity with respiration. The amount of fluid swing should lessen as the lung re-expands. If there are no bubbles and there is no fluid swing, this means either that the drainage tube is blocked or that the lung is fully expanded. Chest X-ray will confirm.
- Prevent accidental disconnection by:
  - —supporting the chest drain with adhesive tape on the chest wall, taking care to loop and not bend it
  - —securing the tubing to the bedclothes or the patient's clothes with tape and pins, taking care not to pierce the tubing
  - —stabilising the drainage jar by housing it in a special cradle on the floor.
- Maintain patency by gently lifting sections of the tubing at regular intervals to facilitate the gravitational drainage of blood and viscous fluid.
- Maintain sterility when changing the down-tube and drainage bottle.
- Measure and record the amount and consistency of drainage.

RESPIRATORY FAILURE

If impending respiratory failure is recognised early then the actual state can be avoided; nurses should be alert for the following clinical signs:

- the patient appears restless and confused
- there is an increase in respiratory rate with laboured ventilatory effort and use of auxiliary respiratory muscles (sternomastoid and abdominal muscles)
- forced and abnormal movement of the diaphragm
- flaring nostrils with each breath
- pale or cyanosed and clammy skin.

Where impending respiratory failure is suspected, sedation must be withheld as it will further depress respiratory function. Arterial blood gas levels (ABGs) will confirm the diagnosis.

Respiratory failure is indicated where there is respiratory acidosis with a falling pH, Po_2 below normal and raised Pco_2. Untreated, the condition will worsen steadily, and increasingly difficult ventilatory effort will leave the patient exhausted and hypoxic, and he will eventually become comatosed and die. However, patients with impending respiratory failure are normally intubated and mechanically ventilated and are nursed in ITU. Only then can sedation be given with safety.

In order to cut down on dead space and improve respiratory efficiency, a tracheostomy (opening into the trachea) is usually performed. Refer to Chapter 14 for indications for a tracheostomy and nursing management of a patient with a tracheostomy.

EMERGENCY AIRWAY MANAGEMENT, ENDOTRACHEAL INTUBATION AND MECHANICAL VENTILATION

Nursing priorities and management

The nurse must be prepared at all times to perform emergency airway procedures and to assist in endotracheal intubation and mechanical ventilation. These procedures are reviewed in Boxes 3.12 and 3.13 (see also Fig. 3.12).

For further information, see McGarvey (1990), Armstrong & Salmon (1997) and Inwood & Cull (1998).

3.10 When a patient is mechanically ventilated, and in certain other instances, it is necessary to flood the lungs with pure oxygen both before and after carrying out aspiration. What is the reason for this? (See Ch. 29.).

GENETIC DISORDERS OF THE RESPIRATORY SYSTEM

There is considerable evidence of genetic predisposition and susceptibility to some of the more common respiratory diseases such as asthma. Of the classic genetic disorders, cystic fibrosis has the most dramatic and distressing impact on the respiratory system. This is a disease which disturbs the mucus-producing glands throughout the body, particularly those of the respiratory tract. For a full description of the disease process and its nursing management, see Chapter 6.

3.11 To complete your essential procedures folder, scan current nursing and medical journals and identify recent trends in nursing involvement and the delivery of health care. Can you relate these to the management of respiratory disorders?

Box 3.12 Endotracheal intubation and mechanical ventilation

Endotracheal intubation and mechanical ventilation are both specialist procedures and will be performed and monitored by doctors and nurses specially trained in this area. However, it is necessary for the generalist nurse to be familiar with the relevant procedures and equipment in order to be prepared to assist in emergency situations and to better understand the needs of the patient who has been intubated and ventilated during general anaesthesia.

Endotracheal intubation

Maintenance of equipment

Equipment on resuscitation trolleys and in the anaesthetic room must be checked regularly to ensure that it is complete and functional. Equipment must include a full range of sizes of both nasal and oral endotracheal (ET) tubes, at least two laryngoscopes with a supply of new batteries, universal connectors, catheter mounts, 20 mL syringes, artery forceps, Magill intubating forceps, introducers, masks, oral airways, laryngeal spray, suction, lubricant and scissors.

Assisting the anaesthetist

During induction of general anaesthesia, the anaesthetist will select the appropriate tube for the patient and will test and lubricate it. The nurse will ensure that suction is available and hold the prepared tube ready to hand for the anaesthetist. The patient is given a full explanation and should be continually reassured until the i.v. anaesthetic, muscle relaxant and anaesthetic gas have taken effect. The anaesthetist will visualise the vocal chords with the laryngoscope, introduce the ET tube, inflate the cuff and connect the ET tube to the anaesthetic machine. The nurse may be requested to apply cricoid pressure during induction of the anaesthetic in order to prevent regurgitation of stomach contents, especially in emergency cases. Pressure is applied using the thumb and forefinger and continued until the patient is asleep and the cuff of the ET tube has been inflated.

Extubation

Following extubation, the nurse must be alert for complaints of sore throat due to damage to the tracheal mucosa, or oedema of the larynx leading to tracheal obstruction. The nurse should raise the head of the bed unless this is contraindicated and report the symptoms to the surgical team.

Mechanical ventilation

There are many reasons why a patient may need mechanical help with respiration. Extrapulmonary causes which affect the respiratory process include:

- those which affect the respiratory control centres in the brain, e.g. CNS disease, brain contusion or haemorrhage, drug overdose or anaesthesia
- those of neuromuscular origin which cause respiratory paralysis, e.g. Guillain–Barré syndrome, myasthenia gravis, poliomyelitis, organic phosphate poisoning and cervical spine injury
- those which restrict expansion of the thoracic cavity, e.g. musculoskeletal injuries such as extensive flail chest and ruptured diaphragm.

In addition, disorders which affect gaseous exchange can result in severe hypoxia. These include adult respiratory distress syndrome (ARDS), cardiac disease resulting in pulmonary oedema, smoke inhalation and respiratory infection in a patient with chronic obstructive airways disease (COAD).

When a patient needs help to breathe, he may be intubated and attached to a mechanical ventilator. The ventilator will simulate the bellows action normally provided by his diaphragm and thoracic cage and will deliver oxygen-enriched air to his lungs. The type of ventilator used will depend on the specific needs of the individual and will be prescribed by the respiratory specialist. The patient will be nursed in the intensive therapy unit (ITU) and will need specialist nursing care, the principles of which are described in Chapter 29.

Box 3.13 Emergency airway management

Emergency airway management is an essential clinical procedure. The nurse must be familiar with the assembly and use of the hand-held resuscitator known as the AMBU bag and should always be aware of its location in her work area. In cases of respiratory arrest, the AMBU bag will ensure more effective ventilation. The procedure for its use is as follows:

- First, clear the airway of any obstruction, mucus or vomitus. Position the patient to open the airway and insert an oral pharyngeal airway (Brook or Guedel).
- Position the face mask to seal the mouth and nose and compress the AMBU bag with the other hand every 5 s. This will deliver approximately 1 L of air with each compression. A smaller bag is used for a child. Oxygen may be attached to the AMBU bag if available.
- Should you need to aspirate mucus from the patient's airway, do so via the oropharyngeal airway. Avoid nasotracheal suctioning where possible because this can stimulate the sensory receptors of the vagus nerve, causing disordered heart rate and rhythm — usually bradycardia (slowing).

CONTINUITY OF CARE: HOSPITAL AND COMMUNITY

Communication between hospital and community health care teams is vital for continuity and ultimate effectiveness of care, and issues relating to discharge planning, accountability and ethical implications are outlined in Box 3.14.

Q

3.12 During your community placement, ask your community nursing team leader to discuss her practice profile with you.

Select two respiratory care patients from the profile and then collect as much relevant

Q

3.12 (*Cont'd*)

information about the type of statutory and voluntary services available for these particular patients as you can and add this to your resource folder.

Compare your findings with those of your colleagues who may have had placements where the emphasis and case load were different.

Suggested resource people: Local Council of Social Services Directory of Statutory and Voluntary Services, GP surgeries, local libraries, health education libraries, day hospitals, community nursing services.

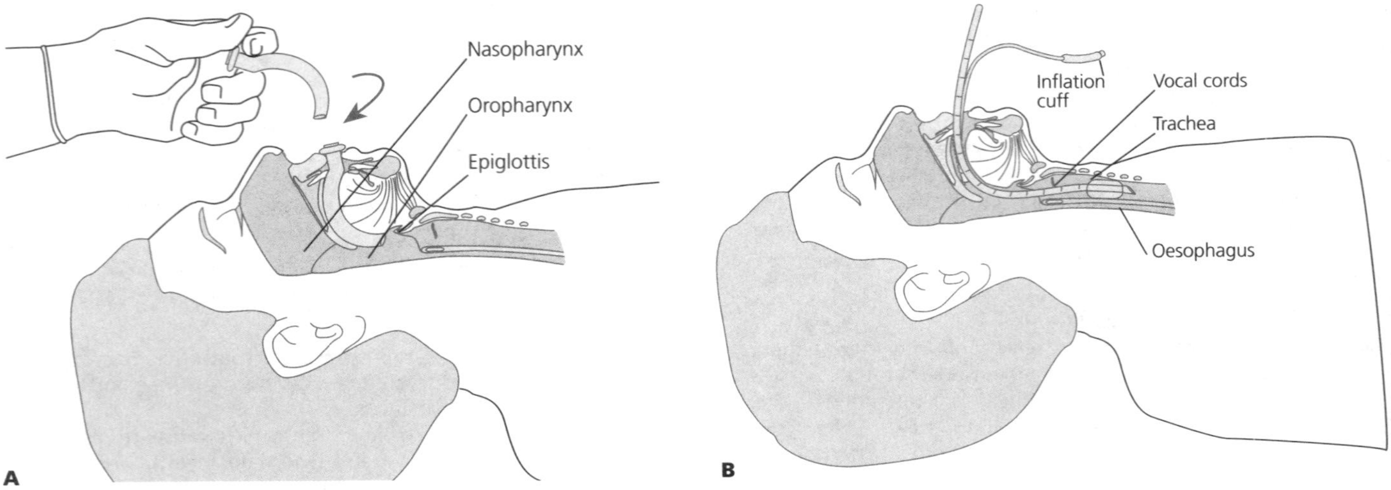

Fig. 3.12 Maintaining an airway. (Reproduced with permission from Inwood & Cull 1998). Illustrator: Peter Gardiner

Box 3.14 Principles of nursing management: dimensions of community respiratory care

Recent trends have highlighted certain basic issues involved in management of respiratory disorders in the community. These trends include early discharge home from hospital, a higher incidence of severe and chronic respiratory disorders being cared for in the home, and respiratory consultants visiting patients in the community and working alongside GPs, practice nurses and clinical nurse specialists (King's Health Care 1993).

The discharge process

Patient education

Teaching self-care and teaching relatives to assist with care should be commenced early during hospitalisation so that an acceptable level of proficiency is achieved before discharge and problems are identified and addressed.

Liaison between hospital and home

When a patient is discharged home following acute hospital care, it is vital that there is close liaison between the hospital and the community health care teams. Ideally, the community nurse or another member of the multidisciplinary community care team is allocated time to visit the patient while he is still in hospital and to participate in planning for his discharge. At the very least, the community nurse should have direct patient and family contact before the patient is discharged home. She may already know them and therefore be able to provide valuable input into discharge planning. The earlier this is done, the better, so that arrangements can be made to have the necessary equipment and services in place.

In addition to basic aids to daily living, special equipment such as that required for oxygen therapy, inhalation and nebulisation therapy, airway suctioning or mechanical ventilation can be installed before the patient is discharged, and the patient and carers taught to manage it efficiently.

Linking

Knowing and utilising all the statutory and voluntary support bodies that are available and appropriate to the patient and his family are crucial in ensuring effective community care.

Practice profile

A descriptive and statistical record, the practice profile is compiled by each community nurse and is a vital tool in overviewing case type, frequency and workload, and in planning maximum and effective use of resources and skill mix.

Documentation

Respiratory disorders and their management in the home can carry a fair degree of risk and hazard.

Documentation is important in all areas of nursing as a basis for accountability and quality assurance, but for the community nurse, detailed and accurate records are even more essential as she often practices alone and is especially vulnerable to the complex legal and ethical dimensions involved in entering a person's home and administering treatment and advice. Great care must be taken to ensure that entry and treatment are with that person's consent and cannot be construed as intrusion or assault or, conversely, that the care given cannot be described as negligent.

CONCLUSION

In health we are seldom aware of the functioning of our respiratory system, but disorders and diseases that affect respiration have the potential to affect every aspect of daily living. Airway, breathing and pulmonary circulation are the ABC — the essential elements — of survival.

This chapter has emphasised the importance of a thorough understanding of the anatomy and physiology of the respiratory system — particularly its physiology, for to understand the function of the system is to understand the profoundly disrupting effects that respiratory disorders can have for the individual's health and well-being. A sound knowledge base in respiratory care must inform nursing interventions in every field of practice. Whether working with children or adults, in general practice or a hospital ward, in educational programmes or in an industrial setting, the nurse must be prepared to recognise and to act upon any compromise, whether chronic or acute, in respiratory function. The potential for nursing intervention will range from resuscitative procedures in an emergency to giving day-to-day advice on the prevention or management of respiratory disease.

The nursing role today encompasses both community-based primary health care and the specialised 'high-tech' skills required in acute care. Nurses are developing new interdependent and independent roles every day to meet the demands of new approaches to health care delivery. Increasingly, they are being employed in community and specialist clinics to screen, advise, immunise and treat patients and to promote disease prevention and health education. At the same time, technological and medical advances are demanding a higher level of clinical nursing skills.

This chapter has illustrated two of the major principles in nursing management of respiratory disorders: disease prevention and health promotion, and the active, reflective acquisition of a sound knowledge base and clinical skills. Although the emphasis has been on nursing management, the implicit assumption is always that nurses work in close collaboration with other health care professionals and, in many instances, will be responsible for coordinating the work of the whole team.

REFERENCES

Allan D 1989 Making sense of oxygen delivery. Nursing Times 85(18): 40–42

Azizi B H O 1993 The effects of passive smoking on children's health: the evidence. Paper given 27th Congress of Medicine (Aug), Kuala Lumpur

Barnes P 1993 Asthma prevention. Paper given at 27th Congress of Medicine (Aug), Kuala Lumpur

Blackburn C 1993 Gender, class and smoking cessation work. Health Visitor 66(3): 83–85

Bott J, Carrol M P, Conway J H et al 1993 Randomised controlled trial of nasal ventilation in acute ventilatory failure due to chronic obstructive airways disease. The Lancet 341(8860): 1555–1557

British Thoracic Society 1997 The British guidelines on asthma management. Thorax 52(suppl. 1)

Buck D 1997 The cost-effectiveness of smoking cessation interventions: what do we know? International Journal of Health Education 35(2): 44–51

Campbell M J, Cogman G R, Holgate S T, Johnston S I 1997 Age specific trends in asthma mortality in England and Wales 1983–1995: results of an observational study. British Medical Journal 314(7092): 1439–1441

Cayla J A, Jansa J M, Artazcoz L, Plasencia A 1993 Predictors of AIDS in cohort of HIV-infected patients with pulmonary or pleural tuberculosis. Tubercle and Lung Disease 74(2): 113–119

Cowan T 1997 Pulse oximeters. Professional Nurse 12(10): 744–750

Crompton G 1991 Turbuhaler: the essential issues. Paper given at International Symposium of Medicine (June), Sydney

Crone S, Partridge M, McLean F 1993 Launching a national helpline. Health Visitor 66(3): 94–96

Department of Health 1992 The health of the nation. HMSO, London

Downie R S, Tannahill C, Tannahill A 1996 Health promotion, models and values, 2nd edn. Oxford University Press, Oxford

Game C, Anderson R E, Kidd J R 1989 Medical-surgical nursing: a core text. Churchill Livingstone, Edinburgh

Graham H 1993 Women's smoking: government targets and social trends. Health Visitor 66(3): 80–82

Jamieson E M, McCall J M, Blythe R, Whyte L A 1999 Guidelines for clinical nursing practices related to a nursing model, 3rd edn. Churchill Livingstone, Edinburgh

Jess L W 1992 Chronic bronchitis and emphysema: airing the differences. Nursing 92, 22(3): 34–41

Jones K, MacLeod-Clark J 1993 Smoking and pregnancy: the role of health professionals. Health Visitor 66(3): 88–90

Kawachi I, Colditz G A, Speizer F E et al 1997 A prospective study of passive smoking and coronary heart disease. Circulation 95(10): 2374–2379

Kidd J R 1989 Chronic disorders of the lung. Ch. 39. In: Game C, Anderson R E, Kidd J R (eds) Medical-surgical nursing: a core text. Churchill Livingstone, Melbourne

King's Health Care 1993 Chest disease: a consultant at work in the community. In: A review of quality initiatives. King's College Hospital, London

MacDonald P 1997 Asthma in older people. Nursing Times 93(19): 42–43

McGarvey H 1990 Making sense of endotracheal intubation. Nursing Times 86(42): 35–37

National Asthma Campaign 1997 Factsheet: National Asthma Audit 1996. Providence House, London

Newman S P, Weise A W B, Talace N, Clarke S W 1991 Improvement of drug delivery with a breath actuated pressurised aerosol for patients with poor inhaler technique. Paper for 3M Health Care, Department of Thoracic Medicine, Royal Free Hospital and School of Medicine, London

Nutbeam D, Macaskill P, Smith C, Simpson J, Catford J 1993 Effectiveness of school smoking education programmes. Health Visitor 66(3) (Recent papers)

Orem D E 1971 Nursing: concepts of practice. McGraw-Hill, New York

Place B 1997 The skill behind the mask. Nursing Times 93(26): 31–32

Pollock D 1993 Curbing the death merchants. Health Visitor 66(3): 86–87

Rutishauser S 1994 Physiology and anatomy: a basis for nursing and health care. Churchill Livingstone, Edinburgh

Smolowe J 1997 Sorry, pardner. Time 149(26): 29–30

Tettersell M J 1993 Asthma patients' knowledge in relation to compliance with drug therapy. Journal of Advanced Nursing 18(1): 103–113

Walker J 1997 ABPI data sheet compendium. Datapharm, London

Wilson K J 1990 Ross and Wilson anatomy and physiology in health and illness, 7th edn. Churchill Livingstone, Edinburgh

Wysocki M, Tric I, Wolff M A et al 1995 Non-invasive pressure support ventilation in patients with acute respiratory failure. Chest 107: 761–768

Zejda J E, Dosman J A 1993 Respiratory disorders in agriculture. Tubercle and Lung Disease 74(2): 74–83

FURTHER READING

Armstrong R F, Salmon J B (eds) 1997 Critical care cases. Oxford University Press, Oxford

Amos A 1993 Youth and style magazines: hooked on smoking. Health Visitor 66(3): 91–93

Badnall P, Haslop A 1987 Chronic respiratory disease: educating patients at home. Professional Nurse 2(9): 293–296

British Thoracic Society 1997 The British guidelines on asthma management. Thorax 52(suppl. 1)

Brunner L S, Suddarth D S 1991 The Lippincott manual of medical-surgical nursing, 2nd edn. Harper & Row, London

Campbell J 1993 Making sense of underwater sealed drainage. Nursing Times 89(9): 34–36

Field D 1997 Every breath you take. Nursing Times 93(26): 28–30

Game C, Anderson R E, Kidd J R (eds) 1989 Medical-surgical nursing: A core text. Churchill Livingstone, Melbourne

Inwood H, Cull G 1998 Advanced airway management. Professional Nurse 13(8): 509–513

Jamieson E M, McCall J M, Blythe R, Whyte L A 1999 Guidelines for clinical nursing practices related to a nursing model, 3rd edn. Churchill Livingstone, Edinburgh

Kendrick A H 1992 Simple measurements of lung function. Professional Nurse 6: 395–404

Lee R N F, Graydon J E, Ross E 1991 Effects of psychological well-being, physical status and social support on oxygen dependent COPE patients' level of functioning. Research in Nursing and Health 14: 323–328

McDermott J 1993 Setting up a no smoking support group. Health Visitor 66(3): 99–100
McGarvey H 1990 Making sense of endotracheal intubation. Nursing Times 86(42): 35–37
Margereson C, Esmond G 1997a Professional development 'learning curve' 1(3), Unit 43: 5–8. Chronic obstructive pulmonary disease: Part 1. Knowledge for practice. Nursing Times 93(19)(suppl.)
Margereson C, Esmond G 1997b Professional development 'learning curve', Unit 43. Chronic obstructive pulmonary disease: Part 2. The role of the nurse. Nursing Times 93(20): 67–70
Margereson C, Esmond G 1997c Professional development 'learning curve', Unit 43. Chronic obstructive pulmonary disease: Part 3. Professional issues. Nursing Times 93(21): 57–62
Place B 1997 The skill behind the mask. Nursing Times 93(26): 31–32
Place B, Cornock M 1997 Critical timing. Nursing Times 93(26): 28–30
Price J 1993 Joint account. Nursing Times 89(13): 44–46
Rutishauser S 1994 Physiology and anatomy: a basis for nursing and health care. Churchill Livingstone, Edinburgh
Stevenson G 1992 Infection risks in respiratory therapy. Nursing Standard 6(18): 32–34
Yeaw E M J 1992 Good lung down. American Journal of Nursing 92(3): 27–29
Williams S J 1989 Chronic respiratory illness and disability: a critical review of the psychological literature. Social Science and Medicine 28: 791–803
Wilson K J, Waugh A 1996 Ross and Wilson anatomy and physiology in health and illness, 8th edn. Churchill Livingstone, Edinburgh

USEFUL ADDRESSES

National Asthma Campaign Helpline
National Asthma Campaign
Providence House
Providence Place
London N1 0NT

Local Council of Social Services
Dept of Statutory and Voluntary Services
Your Town

THE GASTROINTESTINAL SYSTEM, LIVER AND BILIARY TRACT

4

Evelyn Howie Margot E. A. Miller Mary B. Murchie

INTRODUCTION

The study of the gastrointestinal (GI) system is essential to nursing practice, as the digestive processes are the means by which foods and liquids are digested and absorbed and then transported by the blood for cellular metabolism. Nutrition and dietary factors are integral to the care of individuals receiving treatment for diseases affecting either the digestive system itself or other systems of the body.

Because the GI system comprises a large number of organs with a range of interrelated functions, disorders can produce diverse and often distressing symptoms, some of which may cause people considerable embarrassment, leading them to restrict their social lives. Symptoms include pain, dysphagia, anorexia, loss of weight, heartburn, vomiting, constipation and diarrhoea.

Disorders of the GI system may be acute, presenting as life-threatening emergencies, or chronic, requiring long-term management and sometimes admission to hospital for more intensive treatment and/or surgical intervention. The specific needs of patients with GI disorders will vary, although in GI surgery there are general principles of perioperative care which can be followed. Although many advances in pharmacological treatment have been made over the years, surgery is still the treatment of choice for some conditions, allowing many patients to make a complete and rapid recovery. For those patients whose condition is such that palliative surgery is the only option, skilled nursing care will be required both in the hospital and in the community.

Essential to human health and well-being is the ability to maintain a regular intake of a balanced diet, and the nurse working in a community or hospital setting is in a key position to advise individuals on the constituents of such a diet and how it may be achieved. The nurse is also in a good position to provide explanations of any investigations, treatments, diagnoses and prognoses, and to follow up any information given by medical colleagues. The principles of holistic care should be adhered to and a process of continuous assessment, planning, intervention and evaluation followed. This process should be flexible, allowing priorities to be changed as the patient's condition and circumstances evolve.

This chapter begins with a review of the basic anatomy and physiology of the GI tract and its related structures, describing the basic functions of that system and how the specialised organs and tissues which it comprises contribute to its effective functioning. The disorders of the GI system, liver and biliary tract that will most commonly be encountered by nurses in hospital or community settings are then described. A separate chapter has been devoted to disorders of the mouth and its related structures (Ch. 15) and it is vital that nurses caring for patients undergoing surgery, the terminally ill or those with GI and related disorders should appreciate the importance of giving careful attention to mouth care.

ANATOMY AND PHYSIOLOGY

The gastrointestinal or digestive tract runs from the mouth to the anal canal and includes the oesophagus, the stomach, the duodenum and the small and large intestines. The ancillary organs of digestion which are connected to, but do not form part of, the digestive tract include the liver, the pancreas and the gall bladder. In this chapter, the spleen will also be considered alongside the GI system.

The digestive tract is responsible for taking in food and fluids at the mouth (ingestion), breaking up the food into pieces of a manageable size, extracting the nutritional content of the food and expelling residues and waste products from the rectum via the anus (defaecation). This section will briefly describe the structure and function of the different components of the digestive tract in order to help the reader understand the adverse effects of diseases of this organ system.

The mouth

The mouth carries out three functions in the process of digestion (see Ch. 15): mechanically breaking down food (chewing or mastication); initiating the chemical breakdown of food (salivation); and swallowing food (deglutition) to allow it to proceed on its journey through the digestive tract.

Movement of food within the mouth is achieved mainly by the tongue, which is largely composed of skeletal muscle. The tongue is also a sensory organ, allowing the taste, texture and temperature of food and fluids to be perceived. The sensation of taste is enabled by the fungiform papillae, or taste buds, which house the relevant sensory nerve endings. The filiform papillae give the tongue a roughness which allows it to be used for manipulating semi-solid food (see Ch. 15).

Saliva is released from three pairs of glands located around the lower jaw. These are, moving anteriorly, the parotid, the submandibular and the sublingual glands. A constant stream of saliva is released into the mouth, of which the submandibular glands contribute about 70% in the absence of a food stimulus. However, the sight, smell or presence of food in the mouth will stimulate the parotid glands to make the major contribution.

Saliva is a mildly alkaline and slightly viscous fluid which serves to keep the mouth moist and clean. It is mildly antibacterial. In digestion, it helps to lubricate food prior to swallowing and, since it contains the enzyme amylase, it also initiates the digestion of starch.

The final process in which the mouth participates is that of swallowing, whereby food is passed into the oesophagus. After food has been sufficiently chewed, which is partly a subjective decision and partly determined by the texture of the food ingested, it is formed into a ball (bolus) between the palate and the tongue and pushed to the back of the mouth by the tongue. The swallowing reflex is initiated by the bolus touching the oropharynx and involves the following steps: the temporary cessation of breathing; the soft palate shuts off the nasal passage; the raising of the larynx and the lowering of the epiglottis to protect the trachea; and the opening of the upper oesophageal sphincter to receive the bolus of food.

The oesophagus

The oesophagus is a hollow, muscular tube connecting the pharynx to the stomach. It exists solely to enable the passage of food between these two areas and performs no digestive or absorptive roles. The oesophagus is composed of three layers of tissue: an inner mucosal layer with an underlying submucosal layer; a middle muscular layer; and an outer connective tissue layer. The mucosal layer contains glands which secrete mucus for the lubrication of food as it passes down the oesophagus. The submucosal layer provides a nerve and blood supply. The muscles of the middle layer are arranged both circularly and longitudinally. The composition of this layer changes throughout the length of the oesophagus in such a way that there is more striated, or voluntary, muscle at the pharyngeal end. Towards the stomach end, the muscle becomes predominantly and then entirely smooth, or involuntary.

The propulsion of food towards the stomach is achieved by peristalsis, which can be described as follows:

1. A descending wave of contraction of circular muscle narrows the lumen of the oesophagus, thereby compressing the bolus of food
2. This is preceded by contraction of the longitudinal muscles to widen the lumen in order to receive the bolus.

Peristalsis is entirely under involuntary control. Relaxation of the lower oesophageal sphincter allows food to enter the stomach (see Fig. 4.1).

The stomach

Digestion continues in the stomach when the bolus of food enters through the lower oesophageal sphincter. The basic structure of the stomach is illustrated in Wilson & Waugh (1996). On the inner surface of the stomach, a mucosal, secretory, layer of tissue is supplied with blood vessels and lymph glands by an underlying submucosal layer. Between the mucosal layer and the outermost, peritoneal layer lies a muscular layer, which is itself composed of three layers: an inner layer of oblique fibres, a middle layer of circular fibres and an outer layer of longitudinal fibres. These layers of muscle allow increasingly stronger waves of contraction in three directions to mix the food in the stomach and allow maximum contact with gastric juice. Innervation of the stomach is from a branch of the Xth cranial (i.e. vagus) nerve, which provides parasympathetic nerve endings that stimulate the secretory cells of the stomach. The internal surface area of the stomach is increased by the arrangement of folds (rugae) in the lining.

Cells in the mucosa of the stomach produce mucus, hydrochloric acid and pepsinogen. This mixture is referred to as 'gastric juice' and, when combined with food in the stomach, as 'chyme'. Hydrochloric acid helps to maintain the acidity of the stomach at a

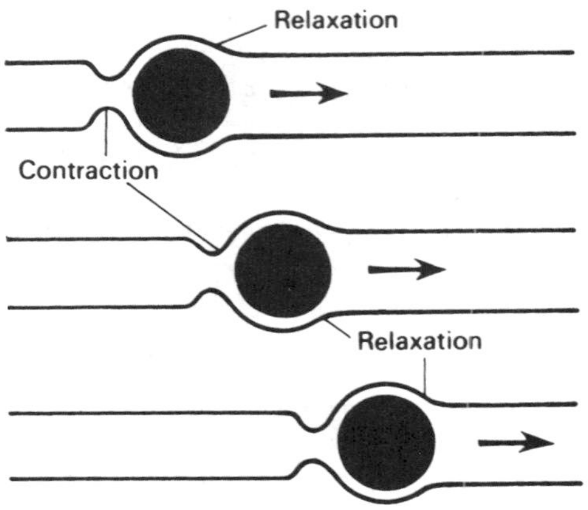

Fig. 4.1 Illustration of the movement of the bolus through the oesophagus by peristalsis. (Reproduced with kind permission from Wilson & Waugh 1996.)

pH of about 2. At this level of acidity, the pepsinogen, an inactive precursor, is converted to pepsin, a protein-digesting enzyme which works optimally at this pH. The stomach, therefore, is mainly responsible for initiating protein digestion, although some carbohydrate digestion can continue inside a bolus of food by the action of any salivary amylase which has not yet become inactivated by the acidity of the stomach.

Release of gastric juice by the stomach mucosa is stimulated by the sight, smell and thought of food. This is known as the cephalic phase of digestion. The gastric phase of digestion begins when food reaches the stomach and continues until chyme enters the duodenum, where the intestinal phase of gastric digestion begins. The length of time taken to empty the stomach is variable and depends on the composition of the meal eaten. An average time for emptying of the stomach after a meal is about 4 h. Emptying takes place through the pyloris. The pyloric region holds about 30 mL of chyme; with each wave of contraction in the stomach about 3 mL of chyme is released into the duodenum. This process is regulated by the pyloric sphincter.

Digestion in the stomach is controlled by several factors. The presence of food in the stomach stretches the stomach wall, activating stretch receptors and stimulating the release of gastric juice. A hormone called gastrin is released by the stomach walls; this also stimulates the release of gastric juice. The presence of food substances such as protein and caffeine also stimulates gastrin release. Waves of contraction in the stomach are also increased by stretching of the stomach wall and by the presence of protein. On the other hand, low pH inhibits gastrin release. Both the cephalic and gastric phases of digestion can be inhibited by emotional factors. The stomach is not involved in the main process of absorption, although some water, alcohol and certain drugs, such as aspirin, are absorbed in the gastric phase.

The intestinal phase of digestion begins when chyme enters the duodenum. The main effect on gastric digestion of the entry of food into the duodenum is inhibitory. The enterogastric reflex, which is mediated via the medulla, leads to the inhibition of gastric secretion. In addition, the presence of food in the duodenum stimulates the release of three hormones — secretin, cholecystokinin and gastric inhibitory peptide — all of which inhibit gastric juice secretion and reduce gastric motility (see Fig. 4.2).

The small intestine

Extending from the pyloric sphincter to the ileocaecal valve, the small intestine is responsible for the completion of digestion, the absorption of nutrients and the reabsorption of most of the water which enters the digestive tract. The duodenum, which takes up the first 25 cm or so of the small intestine, plays a key role in the process of digestion. It collects chyme from the stomach and is the site where the secretions of the gall bladder and the pancreas are mixed with chyme. These secretions enter the duodenum through the ampulla of Vater (the joining of the common bile duct and the pancreatic duct), which meets the duodenum at the duodenal papilla. The emptying of the gall bladder is regulated by the sphincter of Oddi at the duodenal papilla.

In common with the remainder of the small intestine, the duodenum has a mucosal layer, a submucosal layer, a muscular layer and a peritoneal layer. Unlike the remainder of the small intestine, however, the duodenum is relatively immobile. Its regulatory role is fulfilled when the stimulus of chyme entering the duodenum triggers the enterogastric reflex as well as stimulating the release of gastrin, secretin, cholecystokinin and gastric inhibitory peptide. The effects of cholecystokinin and secretin on the functioning of the stomach have been mentioned (p. 88). Secretin also stimulates the cells of the liver to secrete bile, and cholecystokinin stimulates the release of digestive enzymes by the small intestine.

Chyme is very acidic because of its high concentration of hydrochloric acid. When it enters the duodenum, it is brought to a neutral pH by the effect of alkaline bicarbonate released by the pancreas. The effect of bile is to emulsify fats in the chyme,

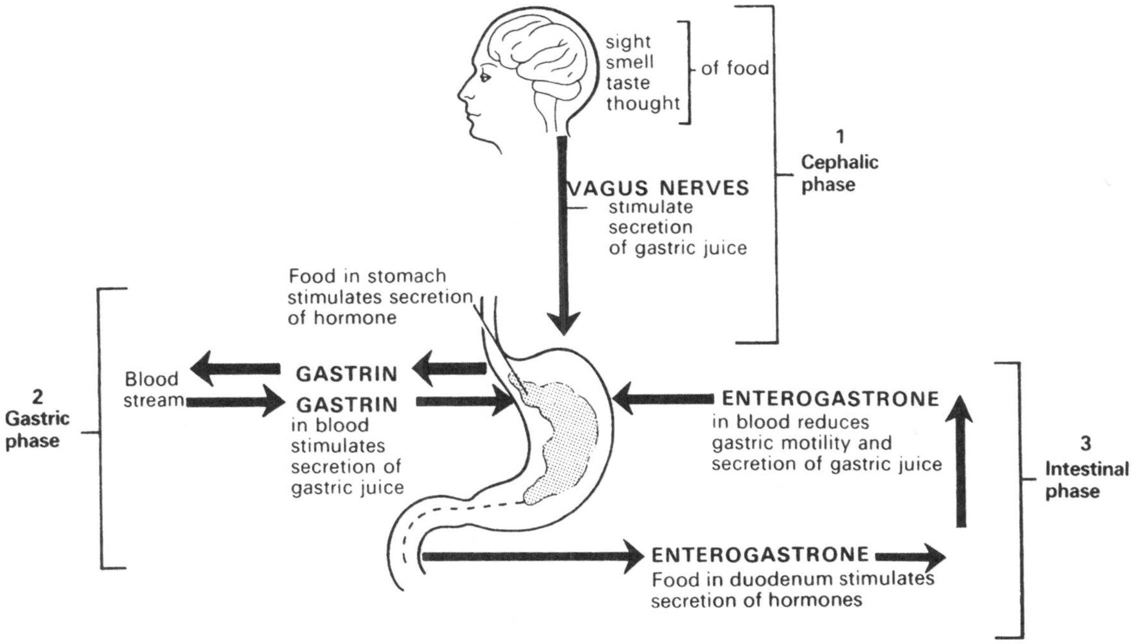

Fig. 4.2 The phases of secretion of gastric juices. (Reproduced with kind permission from Wilson & Waugh 1996.)

i.e. to break up fat globules into smaller particles more amenable to the effects of fat-digesting enzymes. The enzymes of pancreatic juice can then begin to digest their respective food substances in the duodenum; this action is continued as the chyme is passed down the small intestine.

The first two-fifths of the small intestine following the duodenum is called the jejunum and the remaining three-fifths the ileum. Two types of movement, segmentation and peristalsis, take place in the small intestine; these, respectively, mix and move the food along the tract.

Secretory cells of the mucosa of the small intestine release a slightly alkaline juice containing mainly water and mucus. The remaining enzymes of digestion in the GI tract are located on the microvilli, which are microscopic finger-like projections of the cell membrane. The enzymes of the small intestine complete the digestion of all components of the diet, including protein, fat, carbohydrate and nucleic acids.

Absorption takes place along the full length of the small intestine, and 90% of all the products of digestion are absorbed here. The products of digestion are amino acids and peptides from protein; fatty acids and monoglycerides from fats; hexose sugars from carbohydrates; and pentose sugars and nitrogen-containing bases from nucleic acids. About 7.5 L of water are secreted into the small intestine daily and 1.5 L ingested. As only about 1 L enters the large intestine, the major portion of the water is reabsorbed in the small intestine. Absorption takes place at the villi, which greatly increase the digestive and absorptive area of the small intestine. Each villus contains an arteriole and a venule connected by a capillary network, and a central lacteal, which is a projection of the lymphatic system. Short-chain fatty acids, amino acids and carbohydrates are absorbed directly into the bloodstream. Triglycerides, which form structures called chylomicrons, are absorbed into the lacteals and then enter the bloodstream where the thoracic lymphatic duct empties into the left subclavian vein (see Fig. 4.3).

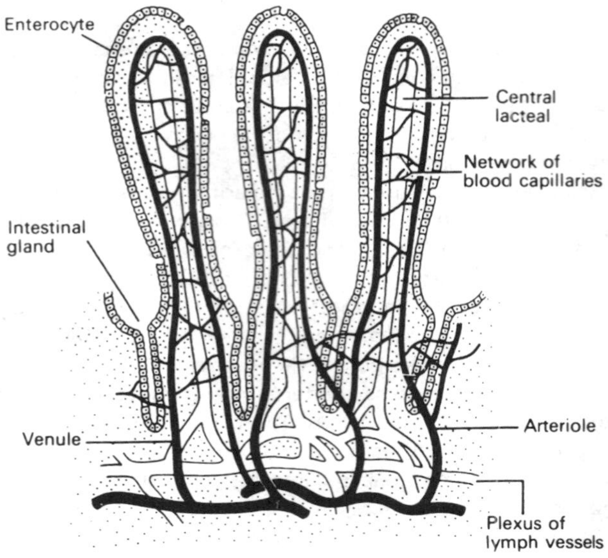

Fig. 4.3 A highly magnified view of the villi in the small intestine. (Reproduced with kind permission from Wilson & Waugh 1996.)

The large intestine

With most of the nutrients removed, the indigestible residue of food from the small intestine passes through the ileocaecal valve and enters the large intestine. The mesentery attaches both the small and large intestines to the rear wall of the abdomen and provides both with their blood supply.

The large intestine can be divided into four portions: the ascending, the transverse, the descending and the pelvic (or sigmoid) colon. The curves joining the ascending with the transverse colon and the transverse with the descending colon are referred to as the right and left colic flexures, respectively. Near the ileocaecal valve, two features can be identified: the caecum, which is a pouch below the ileocaecal valve; and the appendix, which is a finger-like projection of the caecum. The descending colon leads to the sigmoid colon, which terminates in the rectum. Three muscular bands called the taeniae coli run the length of the large intestine. These maintain a slight longitudinal tension in the large intestine and give it its characteristic segmented appearance (haustration). The rectum stores food residue as faeces before expulsion via the anus. The anal canal, which opens externally at the anus, controls evacuation and has an internal anal sphincter of smooth muscle and an external anal sphincter of skeletal muscle.

In common with the small intestine, the large intestine has mucosal, submucosal, muscular and peritoneal layers, but it differs in appearance from the small intestine in that there are no villi. The large intestine is designed mainly for the absorption of water and the lubrication of food residue as it is passed, by the mass action of food entering at the ileocaecal valve, to the rectum. Any nutrients which do enter the large intestine are broken down by commensal bacteria, causing the gases methane, hydrogen, carbon dioxide and sulphur dioxide to be produced. Food can take up to 24 h to pass through the large intestine.

When faeces reaches the rectum, a reflex is initiated whereby stretch receptors in the wall of the rectum send signals to the brain informing it of the presence of faeces. However, the desire to expel faeces (defaecation) can be suppressed until the time and place are appropriate. When it is appropriate to defaecate, the internal anal sphincter automatically relaxes and the external anal sphincter, under voluntary control, is relaxed. Intra-abdominal pressure is increased as the individual breathes in and holds the breath against a closed glottis (Valsalva's manoeuvre), and faeces are expelled from the rectum via the anal canal (see Fig. 4.4).

The hepatobiliary system, pancreas and spleen

The liver

With the exception of the skin, the liver is the largest single organ in the body. It is located mainly in the upper right quadrant of the abdomen, just below the diaphragm, and weighs about 1.5 kg. It is a compact lobular organ with large right and left lobes and two smaller caudate and quadrate lobes. Blood is supplied to the liver by the hepatic artery (oxygenated), as well as by the hepatic portal vein, which carries blood containing the products of digestion from the small intestine directly to the liver. The hepatic portal system also collects blood from the lower oesophagus, the stomach, the spleen and the large intestine.

Each lobe of the liver is subdivided into functional units called lobules. In these lobules, branches of the hepatic artery, the hepatic portal vein and a bile duct run concurrently in a structure known as the portal triad. All of the blood entering the liver mixes in spaces called sinusoids and is then drained into a central vein. Bile is manufactured by liver cells and secreted into transport channels (canaliculi), which then empty into the bile ducts.

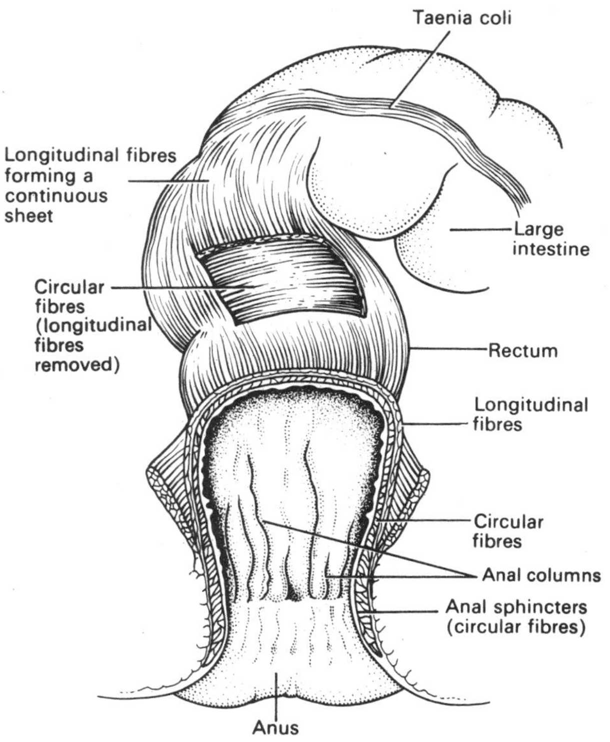

Fig. 4.4 The arrangement of muscle fibres in the colon, rectum and anus (sections have been removed to show layers). (Reproduced with kind permission from Wilson & Waugh 1996.)

A major metabolic role with respect to carbohydrates, fats and proteins is played by the liver. The liver stores some glycogen and also forms part of the monophage/macrophage system which scavenges old erythrocytes, leucocytes and bacteria.

The gall bladder

Lying underneath the liver, the gall bladder has the function of storing and concentrating bile, which is composed principally of bilirubin (derived from the breakdown of haemoglobin from erythrocytes) and bile salts (formed from excess steroid hormones). The gall bladder is a pear-shaped sac about 10 cm long. It lacks a submucosal layer but, in common with other parts of the digestive system, has a middle muscular layer comprising smooth muscle under vagal and hormonal control. Vagal stimulation causes the gall bladder to contract. The mucosal surface area of the gall bladder is increased by the presence of rugae; this promotes the reabsorption of water and a 10-fold concentration of the bile which enters from the cystic duct. The liver secretes bile at a rate of about 1 L per 24 h, but the capacity of the gall bladder is only 30 mL. Bile ducts in the right and left lobes of the liver empty their contents into the right and left hepatic ducts, respectively, which join to form the common hepatic duct. Bile is taken by the cystic duct from the common hepatic duct to the gall bladder, where it is stored and water is reabsorbed. When the gall bladder is stimulated, it contracts and the bile travels to the duodenum down the common bile duct. The release of bile is stimulated by cholecystokinin and secretin.

The pancreas

The pancreas, which lies below and behind the stomach, manufactures and releases pancreatic juice containing enzymes (including enzymes which digest protein, carbohydrate, fat and nucleic acids) and bicarbonate. These constituents of pancreatic juice are produced in the acinar cells of the pancreas.

The exocrine function of the pancreas is discrete from its endocrine function whereby insulin and glucagon are secreted into the bloodstream in response to fluctuating blood glucose levels. The exocrine secretory functions of the pancreas are under vagal and hormonal control. The initial stimulus for the release of pancreatic juice is food entering the duodenum and stimulating the release of cholecystokinin and secretin. Cholecystokinin is responsible for stimulating the release of the pancreatic enzyme portion of pancreatic juice and secretin is responsible for the release of bicarbonate. The pancreatic duct (which delivers pancreatic juice to the duodenum) and the common bile duct join at the ampulla of Vater. Release of bile and pancreatic juice into the duodenum is controlled by the sphincter of Oddi. This sphincter, a ring of smooth muscle, is relaxed by cholecystokinin.

The spleen

The spleen is composed of lymphatic tissue and lies in the upper left quadrant of the abdomen, between the stomach and the diaphragm. It is richly supplied with blood via the splenic artery. Blood flow through the spleen is slowed down by the fact that it must pass through sinuses in which the monophage/macrophage system scavenges old erythrocytes and pathogenic particles and passes the breakdown products on to the liver via the hepatic portal system.

DISORDERS OF THE GASTROINTESTINAL TRACT

DISORDERS OF THE MOUTH

The mouth and tongue are often examined by the physician during clinical examination, as local abnormalities or indications of disease elsewhere can often be detected in this manner. For example, a dry, furred tongue can indicate the presence of a digestive problem or dehydration.

Patients with gastrointestinal and liver disease require meticulous attention to oral hygiene as the mouth can be affected both directly (as in Crohn's disease) and indirectly (as in vitamin and iron deficiency in malabsorption and GI haemorrhage). Patients on steroid and immunosuppressive therapy are also prone to infections of the mouth and oesophagus.

The principles of mouth care and the treatment of a range of disorders affecting the mouth and related structures are described in detail in Chapter 15.

For further reading on oral care, see Turner (1996).

DISORDERS OF THE OESOPHAGUS

Because the oesophagus has a relatively narrow lumen, any obstruction rapidly affects the passage of food. The two most common symptoms which are experienced by patients with diseases of the oesophagus are dysphagia and pain. The term dysphagia refers to difficulty in swallowing. This can present in varying degrees, ranging from slight and intermittent difficulty in swallowing solid food to total occlusion of the oesophagus, preventing the patient even from swallowing saliva. Oesophageal pain can be extremely severe and should not be underestimated. There are three main presentations:

- A burning pain (known as 'heartburn') felt high in the epigastrium and behind the sternum. This is usually due to the reflux of gastric contents and sometimes radiates to the neck and to one or both arms.
- A deep, boring, gripping pain across the front of the chest which may radiate to the back, neck or arms. This is usually due to spasm of the oesophageal muscle and is similar in nature to the pain of angina pectoris.
- Pain behind the sternum on swallowing, especially hot liquids. This is usually due to oesophagitis.

Oesophageal moniliasis

This condition is caused by the yeast-like fungus *Candida* (*Monilia*) *albicans*. Those who may be vulnerable to this condition are:

- patients with chronic oesophageal obstruction — oesophageal dysfunction causes stasis of saliva and food particles, which predisposes to infection
- patients with immunosuppressive disorders, e.g. diabetes mellitus, leukaemia, lymphoma, AIDS
- patients taking immunosuppressive therapy, e.g. chemotherapy or corticosteroids
- debilitated patients receiving long-term antibiotic therapy.

PATHOPHYSIOLOGY

Common presenting symptoms. These will vary according to the severity of the infection, but may include dysphagia, heartburn and retrosternal pain. *Candida* affecting the mouth will show as white patches on the mucosa. A mild fever may be present.

MEDICAL MANAGEMENT

Diagnosis will be made using endoscopy, when biopsies will be taken. Treatment is with antifungal oral antibiotics such as nystatin suspension, amphotericin lozenges or parenteral fluconazole.

NURSING PRIORITIES AND MANAGEMENT: OESOPHAGEAL MONILIASIS

The priority of nursing care is to minimise the dysphagia and pain experienced on eating and drinking. The patient should be given a soft diet tailored to her likes and dislikes. Supplemental drinks should also be given to ensure weight loss does not occur. Oral hygiene is, of course, extremely important. Patients who prefer to wear their dentures at all times may have to be persuaded of the benefits of removing them at night, as the constant pressure and friction from the presence of dentures could exacerbate the problem.

Hiatus hernia and gastro-oesophageal reflux

A hernia is the protrusion of an organ through the wall of the cavity which contains it. It may apply to any part of the body but is most commonly thought of in terms of abdominal hernias, which are discussed later in this chapter (see p. 110).

A hiatus hernia results from herniation of a portion of the stomach through the oesophageal hiatus in the diaphragm. The opening of the diaphragm normally encircles the oesophagus tightly, and therefore the stomach lies within the abdominal cavity. When the opening through which the oesophagus passes becomes enlarged, part of the stomach protrudes into the thoracic cavity.

PATHOPHYSIOLOGY

Hiatus hernias occur most frequently from middle age onwards. They are four times more common in women than in men and are often found in association with obesity. Burkitt et al (1996) suggest that the pressure of intra-abdominal fat is a contributory factor. Such hernias can also result from a congenital abnormality presenting in early infancy. Hiatus hernias can be described as 'sliding' or 'rolling', the former being by the far the most common. In sliding hernias, the oesophageal sphincter mechanism is defective, causing reflux of acid-peptic stomach contents.

Clinical features. Although many individuals with a hiatus hernia are symptomless, the most common and significant symptom is heartburn as a result of the reflux oesophagitis. It occurs after eating and can be initiated by bending over and lying down. Waterbrash (pyrosis) and a feeling of fullness are common, but dysphagia is a relatively uncommon symptom. Bleeding may also be a feature, involving a chronic, small loss leading to anaemia. This may occur particularly in the elderly patient with reflux oesophagitis.

MEDICAL MANAGEMENT

Investigations. Diagnosis is by medical history, barium swallow and meal or endoscopy.

Treatment. In mild cases, it may be sufficient simply to advise the individual to make certain lifestyle adjustments, e.g. losing weight if appropriate, taking small meals at more frequent intervals, wearing loose clothing and avoiding bending over from the waist. Sleeping well supported by pillows is also helpful. It is essential for the individual not to smoke. Drug therapy may include antacids and/or acid-inhibiting drugs.

Failure of medical treatment still remains a significant indication for surgery to reduce the hernia and re-form the angle between the oesophagus and stomach. The procedure is fundoplication (Griffiths & Raimes 1997), commonly performed by laparoscopic technique. During the operation, a cuff of stomach is wrapped around the lower end of the oesophagus to tighten up the junction between the oesophagus and the stomach, thereby reducing the risk of reflux.

NURSING PRIORITIES AND MANAGEMENT: GASTRO-OESOPHAGEAL REFLUX

In many individuals, reflux occurs, without associated hiatus hernia, due to obesity, pregnancy or the use of drugs that may relax the gastro-oesophageal sphincter, e.g. anticholinergic drugs. Reflux can be most distressing and is often mistaken for angina. Most people are able to manage their symptoms by conservative means. For example, raising the head of the bed may be all that is needed to relieve symptoms at night. However, if reflux is chronic or severe, the inflammation of the oesophagus can lead to fibrosis and narrowing of the oesophagus, the development of dysphagia and a predisposition to malignant change (see p. 94).

Preoperative preparation

Preparation for surgery will be as for elective abdominal surgery on the GI tract (see p. 806 and Nursing Care Plan 26.1, p. 811).

Postoperative management

This is the same as that for patients undergoing laparoscopic surgery.

Adequate analgesia using opiate analgesics by patient-controlled analgesia (PCA) or i.m. administration must be given to ensure that the patient is pain-free and hence able to cooperate in deep breathing and coughing exercises. Causes of postoperative pain are described in Table 26.7 (p. 823). Analgesics commonly used in postoperative pain control are listed in Table 26.6 (p. 822).

The i.v. infusion must be monitored to ensure adequate hydration. Oral fluids may be withheld for 24 h. As bowel sounds return, sips of water can be given, increasing to 30 mL of water hourly and then greater amounts as they are tolerated. The nasogastric tube, if used, is removed at the discretion of medical staff, usually as the volume of gastric aspirate decreases.

Following this operation, patients will often have some difficulty in swallowing solid foods, but these symptoms usually settle within approximately 1 month of surgery. Approximately 5% of patients will have persistent problems with the expelling of wind orally following surgery. This is termed 'gas bloat' and can be significantly reduced by encouraging the patient not to swallow air while eating or drinking and to reduce the intake of carbonated drinks. Prior to discharge the patient should be advised to take small, regular meals and to avoid heavy lifting. Return to normal activities will be possible as soon as the discomfort from the abdominal wounds has settled, normally 5–10 days following laparoscopic surgery and 2–6 weeks following conventional surgery.

Achalasia

PATHOPHYSIOLOGY

This is a relatively rare motility disorder of the oesophagus (incidence = 1:100 000) (Heading & Tibaldi 1998). The cause is unknown but the essential pathophysiology is a loss of inhibitory innervation of the oesophageal body and the lower oesophageal sphincter (LOS). This impairment results in a loss of oesophageal peristalsis and failure of the LOS to relax. Unopposed cholinergic innervation can then compound the increased LOS pressure.

The condition can be complicated by respiratory pneumonitis and, very rarely, by oesophageal carcinoma.

Clinical features are as follows:

- dysphagia for solids and often liquids
- intermittent retrosternal chest pain
- regurgitation of oesophageal contents (especially at night)
- aspiration of oesophageal contents
- weight loss.

MEDICAL MANAGEMENT

Treatment. There is no cure for achalasia and medical treatment is aimed at reinstating acceptable swallowing for the patient.

The principal treatment at present is pneumatic dilatation of the LOS and this seems to be effective in 60% of patients (Heading & Tibaldi 1998). Oesophageal perforation is a serious, but rare, complication of this procedure. Where dilatation is unsuccessful, a Heller's myotomy may be performed.

Smooth muscle relaxants such as nitrates or nifedipine can be used in the short term to provide some relief from dysphagia whilst awaiting treatment.

Recent studies have shown that endoscopic injection of botulinum toxin is a safe and effective treatment for achalasia (Annesse et al 1996, Cuilliere et al 1997). This treatment inhibits the cholinergic effect on the LOS.

NURSING PRIORITIES AND MANAGEMENT: ACHALASIA

Nursing input is aimed at helping the patient come to terms with, and cope with, an imperfect swallow, although to many patients, the fact that they can swallow at all is a significant improvement on their pre-treatment condition.

The patient should be encouraged to eat slowly and wash food down with fluids. Dietetic referral may be necessary for patients with extreme weight loss prior to treatment and who require dietary supplementation.

For further reading on disorders of oesophageal motility, see Heading (1999).

Carcinoma of the oesophagus

The majority of carcinomas of the oesophagus occur in the elderly. Men are affected more frequently than women. This form of cancer is extremely unpleasant and distressing. The patient will rapidly becoming emaciated due to difficulty in eating and drinking, and skilled nursing care is essential to comfort and support the patient as she copes with these and other effects of the illness. Several predisposing factors for oesophageal cancer have been identified:

- smoking — this form of cancer is more prevalent among individuals who smoke (Kjaerheim et al 1998)
- alcohol consumption — individuals who have had a high intake of alcohol are more likely to develop a malignant tumour; in England, a high incidence of oesophageal cancer among publicans and brewers has been noted
- achalasia of the cardia, gastro-oesophageal reflux, Paterson–Kelly (Plummer–Vinson) syndrome and previous trauma — these are all associated with an increased risk of oesophageal cancer.

PATHOPHYSIOLOGY

Squamous cell carcinoma and adenocarcinoma form the majority of malignant oesophageal tumours, squamous cell carcinoma being the most common (Gore 1997). In squamous cell carcinoma, 10% occur in the upper oesophagus, 45% in the mid-oesophagus, and 45% in the lower end. Most adenocarcinomas occur in the lower third of the oesophagus and at the gastro-oesophageal junction and can account for approximately 34% of all oesophageal cancers (Gore 1997). The primary tumour can spread locally up or down the oesophagus and through its wall to the trachea, bronchi, pleura, aorta and lymph vessels. Distant metastases may occur in the liver and lungs.

Common presenting symptoms. The most prominent presenting feature is dysphagia. In the initial stages, this symptom will occur only occasionally and the individual will probably not seek medical help. As the disease progresses and the tumour enlarges, dysphagia will increase and become a constant feature. There will be regurgitation of food, and vomiting and pain will become intense, indicating a spread of the cancer to surrounding tissues. Because of the dysphagia the patient will be anorexic and lose weight rapidly. Many patients develop a cough due to pressure on the bronchus and a chest infection due to aspiration of oesophageal contents. Haematemesis and melaena occasionally occur as a result of an ulcerated tumour.

Box 4.1 Endoscopy in GI medicine

Endoscopy refers to the visualisation of the interior of the body cavities and hollow organs by means of a flexible fibre-optic instrument (endoscope). The use of this technique has contributed greatly to diagnosis and therapy in many areas of medical practice. For use in the gastrointestinal tract, the endoscope is variously designed to view the oesophagus, the stomach, the duodenum, the colon and the rectum. It is also possible, by a modification of the gastroduodenoscope, to visualise the pancreatic and common bile duct; this is called endoscopic retrograde cholangiopancreatography (ERCP). Although most endoscopes are flexible, a rigid instrument may be used for a sigmoidoscopy. For further information, see Forrest et al (1995).

MEDICAL MANAGEMENT

Investigations. Diagnosis is confirmed by oesophagoscopy (see Box 4.1), during which biopsies will be taken. Computed tomography (CT) scan may be used to help identify local and metastatic spread to surrounding tissues. Bronchoscopy may be performed if the tumour is in the upper zone. This will identify whether the bronchus has been invaded and will have a bearing on treatment and care.

Endoscopic ultrasonography is becoming a recognised diagnostic tool for the staging of oesophageal and gastric carcinomas.

Treatment. As the prognosis is poor, treatment is directed mainly towards the relief of symptoms. Each patient is carefully assessed as to the extent of the disease before a treatment plan is chosen and commenced. Time is also spent on improving the general nutritional state of the patient by either nasogastric or parenteral feeds.

Surgical intervention will be attempted if the tumour is resectable and if there is no local spread or metastases (see Fig. 4.5).

Radiotherapy may be used if the tumour is radiosensitive, i.e. a squamous cell carcinoma. This treatment is usually used for tumours of the upper third of the oesophagus, but is also sometimes used for the relief of pain.

Malignant dysphagia may be relieved by oesophageal dilatation, endoscopic or open insertion of a stent, or tumour ablation with laser, heat, diathermy or injection of cytotoxic substances (Griffin & Raimes 1997).

NURSING PRIORITIES AND MANAGEMENT: CARCINOMA OF THE OESOPHAGUS

The 'typical' patient with this distressing form of cancer will be miserable and emaciated, her life dominated by the symptoms of the disease and by the thought that there is no cure. However, by adopting a caring and sensitive approach, the nurse can do much to alleviate the patient's physical and emotional suffering (Lindars & Sergeant 1994).

Q **4.1** Mr J is a 65-year-old, newly retired accountant, with a wife and two married sons. He has recently been diagnosed as having oesophageal cancer with metastases in the bronchus and lungs. What would you consider to be the main priorities of his nursing care?

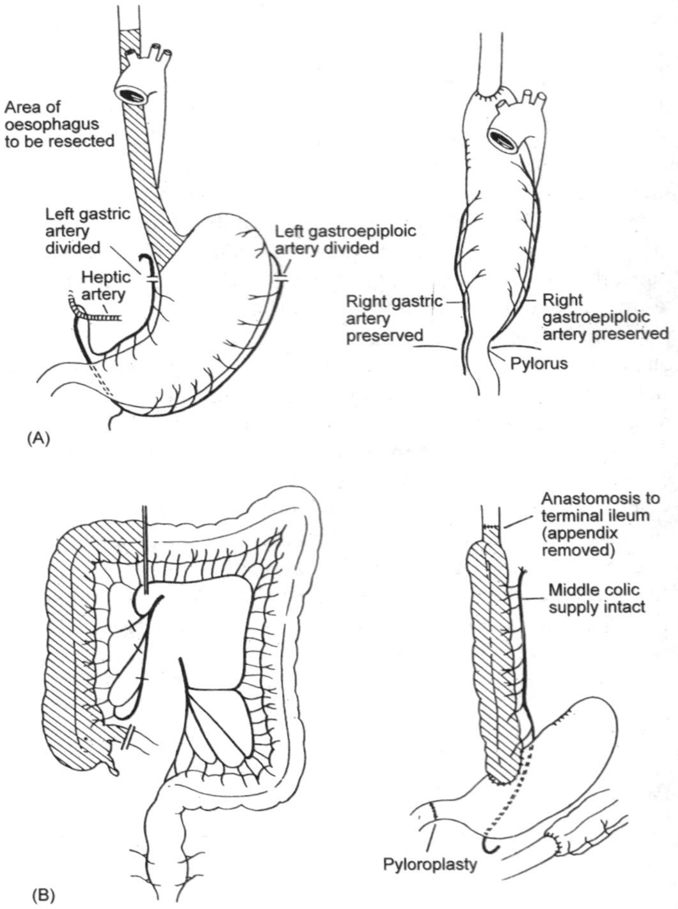

Fig. 4.5 Oesophagectomy and methods of reconstruction. A: Replacement by stomach. B: Replacement by colon. (Reproduced with kind permission from Forrest et al 1991.)

Major patient problems

Dysphagia

The first step in nursing care is to assess the extent of the dysphagia and whether the patient's nutritional intake is adequate. The patient's weight should be recorded and noted in relation to her pre-illness weight. An accurate account of daily dietary intake should be taken (the dietician may help with this) and a description made of the consistency of the food she is able to swallow. If she can manage semi-solids, she will be able to take an adequate diet if careful thought is put into its components; for example, large chunks of meat, 'stringy' foods such as oranges, and 'stodgy' foods such as scones should be avoided. The patient should be encouraged to take fluids with meals and to chew foods twice as long as normal. It may be necessary to provide a liquidised diet. If the patient cannot afford to purchase a liquidiser, one can be borrowed from the Macmillan Nursing Service. The patient should be weighed weekly.

At a later stage, the patient will only be able to swallow liquids and should be supplied with a variety of nutritionally supplemented liquids. Unfortunately, most of these drinks (e.g. Enlive, Ensure) are quite sweet and the patient may soon tire of them. However, Build Up is now also available in savoury flavours and tonic water can be added to supplements to give a fresher taste.

Eventually, total dysphagia will occur. It cannot be overemphasised what a miserable condition this is. Nursing management is discussed on page 94.

In the case of a bolus obstruction, it may be necessary to perform an endoscopy to relieve the obstruction. The insertion of a stent is often used to relieve dysphagic symptoms. The oesophagus is dilated at endoscopy and the tube inserted. Following this procedure, the patient will lose the action of the gastro-oesophageal sphincter and will therefore suffer from reflux. The head of the bed should be elevated at all times. She will be prescribed an H_2 blocking agent (e.g. cimetidine) to help prevent reflux oesophagitis; this should be given in syrup form. She should be encouraged to eat a semi-solid diet and to chew food well. The patient should take carbonated drinks with every meal as this helps keep the stent clear.

Immediately after the insertion of a stent, the patient may suffer quite severe discomfort and it may be necessary to give an analgesic injection, e.g. i.m. pethidine. A chest X-ray will be performed and the patient should not be allowed any food or fluid until this has been done in case of perforation of the oesophagus.

For further information, see Donahue (1990).

Pain

In the earlier stages, if pain is present, mild analgesics such as paracetamol given in dispersible form may be all that is necessary. As the disease advances, opiates may be required. Initially, the patient may be able to swallow a morphine suspension, but if total occlusion of the oesophagus occurs, it may be necessary to give the morphine by injection. The most effective and convenient way of administering this is by the s.c. route via, for example, a Graseby syringe driver. This delivers a constant level of opioid and readily allows for a 'booster' dose to be given as necessary, to avoid the distress of breakthrough pain. The patient will be able to be at home, if circumstances allow, with a community nurse visiting daily to change the syringe. If necessary, an antiemetic can also be added to the syringe driver.

Psychological distress

Time must be set aside to allow these patients to express their thoughts, fears and anger, which may be directed towards either the distressing nature of their symptoms or the poor prognosis of the disease, or perhaps both. In the final stages of the disease, every effort should be made to allow the patient to die in the environment of her own choosing. If she wishes to be at home, a Macmillan or Marie Curie nurse can provide the support and medical and nursing care required.

For further information, see Fletcher & Freeling (1988) and Savage (1992).

Traumatic conditions of the oesophagus

Foreign bodies

Most cases of foreign bodies being lodged in the oesophagus involve children who have swallowed small items such as buttons or safety pins. Adults also occasionally swallow such items, but more frequently present with a blockage caused by an unchewed bolus of food (usually meat).

MEDICAL MANAGEMENT

History and examination. The patient's description of what occurred and the symptoms that followed are very important in diagnosis. Symptoms may range from mild discomfort to severe pain, dysphagia and haemorrhage. Diagnosis may be made by a plain X-ray, but in the case of a bolus of food, barium examination may be required.

Treatment. Once haemodynamic stability is ensured, the foreign body can be removed using endoscopic technique, taking care not to cause further damage (especially if the object is sharp). If a food bolus proves to be the problem, gas-producing pellets may be swallowed which can push the bolus on into the stomach.

NURSING PRIORITIES AND MANAGEMENT: FOREIGN BODIES

The patient may be very distressed and extremely anxious for the offending object to move either up or down. She may be in considerable pain, and analgesics such as i.m. pethidine may be required. The nurse should observe for signs of shock, denoting perforation.

Corrosive agents

Strong acids or alkalis may be swallowed accidentally or deliberately. Accidental cases usually involve children who have drunk cleaning fluids left within reach. Deliberate ingestion by an adult may indicate a serious psychological disturbance requiring professional intervention and probably psychiatric referral after the initial treatment.

MEDICAL MANAGEMENT

First aid measures include ensuring a clear airway and allowing nothing to be taken orally. It is vital that the patient is not made to vomit, as this would only exacerbate the corrosive damage. Immediate referral to the emergency services is essential. On admission to hospital, the antidote specific to the chemical will be administered, but gastric lavage should be avoided.

Longer-term treatment will probably involve dilatation of the oesophagus to relieve fibrosis and stricture. Occasionally a gastrostomy tube must be inserted for feeding purposes until the oesophageal tissue has healed.

NURSING PRIORITIES AND MANAGEMENT: CORROSIVE AGENTS

The key components of care will be:

- maintenance of a clear airway
- observation for shock
- analgesics (i.m. or i.v.)
- nil orally
- antibiotic therapy for infection.

Observations of pulse and blood pressure should be made half-hourly until the patient's condition is stable. A raised temperature may indicate severe inflammatory changes, infection or abscess formation.

Anxiety and fear will be a major feature; the support, reassurance and understanding shown by nursing and medical staff will help to allay these feelings.

Oesophageal perforation

PATHOPHYSIOLOGY

Instrumental perforation may occur during endoscopy, especially if the oesophagus is friable due to disease. There is an increased risk of perforation with oesophageal dilatation and the insertion of an oesophageal tube in the palliative management of patients with oesophageal carcinoma.

Spontaneous perforation may occur following a sudden increase in oesophageal pressure caused by vomiting, straining, convulsions or blunt abdominal pressure, e.g. steering wheel pressure in a car accident.

Clinical features. The individual will experience severe pain, which may be accompanied by dyspnoea, cyanosis, dysphagia and fever due to leakage into the mediastinum.

MEDICAL MANAGEMENT

Treatment will be centred on managing potential shock, providing analgesics and prescribing antibiotic therapy. If perforation is severe, surgery may well be required. Such a patient may be acutely ill and require intensive nursing support (see Ch. 29).

Conservative management includes the administration of broad-spectrum antibiotics and preventing the patient from taking anything orally. These patients are fed either parenterally or by a feeding jejunostomy.

DISORDERS OF THE STOMACH AND DUODENUM

Disorders of the stomach and duodenum are the most common organic disorders of the GI tract. They are considered together here because disorders of one organ commonly affect the other. The overall incidence of acute upper gastrointestinal haemorrhage in the UK is 103/100 000 adults per year. The incidence rises with age and the overall mortality is 14% (Rockall et al 1995).

Gastritis

PATHOPHYSIOLOGY

Gastritis is an inflammatory condition of the stomach which may be acute or chronic. Acute gastritis is commonly caused by the ingestion of an irritant substance such as aspirin or an anti-inflammatory drug, or by the excessive intake of alcohol. Chronic gastritis develops over many years and is found in patients with pernicious anaemia, autoimmune disorders, chronic alcohol abuse, peptic ulceration and gastric cancer, and following gastric surgery.

Clinical features. The outstanding presenting symptom in gastritis is abdominal pain, accompanied by a feeling of distension, nausea, vomiting and anorexia. However, in chronic gastritis, the patient is often asymptomatic. Where symptoms are present, these are the same as those found with acute gastritis, pain being associated with eating and often being described as 'indigestion'.

MEDICAL MANAGEMENT

Investigations. Diagnosis is made endoscopically by gastric biopsy. *Helicobacter pylori* is found in the biopsy of many patients with chronic gastritis, and if confirmed, antibiotic therapy will be prescribed.

Treatment. An antacid may be prescribed to relieve discomfort and an H_2 blocker such as cimetidine prescribed to prevent histamine from stimulating the gastric parietal cells to secrete hydrochloric acid. Most important is dietary advice, as the patient should avoid causative agents such as alcohol and highly spiced foods.

NURSING PRIORITIES AND MANAGEMENT: GASTRITIS

In the very acute stage, when vomiting is present, an antiemetic will be given and i.v. fluid replacement therapy may be necessary for a short time. Frequent mouthwashes are given and an appropriate diet gradually reintroduced. The opportunity should be taken to explore the patient's dietary habits and to promote a healthy eating pattern. This is particularly important where the problem of alcohol abuse has been identified.

Peptic ulcer

A peptic ulcer occurs in those parts of the digestive tract which are exposed to gastric secretions, namely the stomach and duodenum.

Until recently, peptic ulcer disease was thought to be a chronic relapsing condition that required long-term acid suppression therapy and often major surgical intervention. There was also an associated mortality due to major gastrointestinal haemorrhage and development of gastric cancer.

The identification of the *Helicobacter pylori* bacterium (Marshall & Warren 1984) and its association with peptic ulcer disease has radically altered the management of this condition in the 1990s, especially with the shift in focus in the NHS from secondary to primary care.

PATHOPHYSIOLOGY

Peptic ulcer formation requires both the presence of gastric acid and damage to the mucosal defence barrier. *H. pylori* is known to be a major factor in causing this damage and is present in 95–100% of all duodenal ulcers and 75–80% of gastric ulcers (Tytgat et al 1993). Gastric irritant drugs like aspirin and non-steroidal anti-inflammatories (NSAIDs) are also known to cause mucosal damage. Cigarette smoking is considered to have a causative influence in the development of peptic ulcers and there is growing evidence that it prevents the healing of gastric and duodenal ulcers (Haslett et al 1999). The exact mechanisms by which this occurs are not clear, but it is known that long-term smoking increases gastric secretion and interferes with the actions of H_2-receptor antagonists.

The gastric mucosa is, in part, protected by being buffered by food, and erratic dietary habits may contribute to ulcer formation. There is also some conflicting evidence as to whether emotional factors such as stress and anxiety are also causative factors (see Box 4.2).

In *H. pylori* infection, the bacteria burrow beneath the mucosal layer and release a toxin that results in a local inflammatory and systemic immune response. Consequently there is inhibition of the release of somatostatin, a gastric hormone that inhibits gastric acid formation, and oversecretion results. The *H. pylori* survives in this acid climate by enzymatically creating an alkaline microenvironment.

It was once believed that ulcers could not develop in the absence of gastric acid (achlorhydria) found in some conditions such as pernicious anaemia and gastric mucosal atrophy (Schwarz's dictum: 'no acid, no ulcer'). Research has shown that while this dictum holds for duodenal ulcers, gastric ulcers can be found in non-acid states (Bynum 1991).

Box 4.2 Stress ulceration

Unlike other forms of peptic ulceration, stress ulcers are superficial in nature and are often referred to as erosions, since they do not penetrate muscle layers. Although their cause is still not clear, it is believed that an emotional or physical stressor can give rise to ischaemia and vasospasm of the gastric microcirculation. This impairs the natural mucosal resistance such that acid pepsin is able to diffuse into the epithelial cells of the gastric lining. Within a clinical setting, these ulcers tend to occur after major surgery, trauma, burns or severe illness and commonly present with bleeding (which may be dramatic). The recognition of such a life-threatening occurrence will be less likely if the patient has been receiving prophylactic i.v. H_2 antagonist medication. See Kalder (1985) for further information.

Chronic peptic ulcers penetrate through the mucosa to the muscle layers. They can damage blood vessels and cause bleeding. In the duodenum, they are found immediately beyond the pylorus and in 10–15% of cases are multiple. The resulting fibrosis can lead to pyloric stenosis, which in turn can lead to gastric outlet obstruction. Gastric ulcers are found on the lesser curvature of the stomach in 90% of cases.

Common presenting symptoms. The individual with a chronic peptic ulcer will describe a pattern of episodic pain and dyspepsia. Pain is a classic symptom and is described as a burning or boring pain in the epigastrium; often the patient points directly to where the pain is felt. The pain is sometimes more diffuse or radiates through to the back.

While studies show the relationship to food and mealtimes to be variable, the person with a duodenal ulcer is more likely to feel pain and 'hunger feelings' about 2–3 h after a meal, whereas with a gastric ulcer, pain is felt about 30–60 min after a meal and is not relieved by more food. Sometimes patients admit to inducing vomiting in an attempt to relieve the pain. Persistent non-induced vomiting of large amounts indicates an obstruction to the pylorus: pyloric stenosis.

Other common features are belching and regurgitation which causes heartburn.

MEDICAL MANAGEMENT

Investigations. A full medical history will be taken. An accurate diagnosis is made by endoscopy and/or barium meal.

Diagnosis of *H. pylori* infection can be made by blood or serum tests for antibodies, and at endoscopy by taking a biopsy from the stomach lining and subjecting it to the rapid urease test, which detects the enzyme that *H. pylori* produces (also known as the CLO test).

'Breath test'. This is a non-invasive test that detects isotopic carbon dioxide after ingestion of radiocarbon-labelled urea. The *H. pylori* enzyme splits the carbon from the urea. It is then carried as carbon dioxide via the blood to the lungs, where it can be detected in exhaled breath. These tests are specific, as no other bacterium is known to produce the urease enzyme.

A full blood count is taken for haemoglobin estimation.

Treatment. This is dependent on the cause and severity of the ulcer. Removal of the causative factor followed by healing of the ulcer is the main aim of treatment, e.g. eradication therapy in *H. pylori* or discontinuation of NSAIDs or aspirin followed by acid-suppressing medication.

Advice should also be given on avoiding known aggravating factors, such as smoking and erratic dietary patterns. Patient compliance with drug therapies is crucial to the success of *H. pylori* eradication and ulcer healing, and therefore patient education is essential. In some cases, surgical intervention may be necessary.

Drug therapy may include:

- Antacids for the relief of dyspepsia. Many preparations are based on magnesium and may result in a degree of diarrhoea.
- H_2-receptor antagonists, e.g. cimetidine and ranitidine. These assist in ulcer healing by preventing histamine from stimulating the gastric parietal cells to secrete hydrochloric acid.
- A proton pump inhibitor (i.e. omeprazole) to inhibit the release of hydrochloric acid from the parietal cells.
- Eradication therapy is now the standard treatment for *H. pylori*.

First-line treatment lasts for 1 week and consists of:

- proton pump inhibitor (lanzoprazole/omeprazole) twice daily
- amoxycillin 500 mg three times daily
- metronidazole 400 mg three times daily.

In patients with penicillin allergy, it is common practice to substitute clarithromycin 500 mg twice daily for amoxycillin. Note that long-term acid-lowering therapy may be required if there are complicating factors, e.g. NSAID therapy.

Repeat endoscopy is essential to confirm that healing has occurred.

For further information, see University of York (1995), Cottrill (1996) and MacConnachie (1997).

Surgical intervention. Indications for surgery for peptic ulcer are as follows:

- failure of response to medical therapy
- recurrence
- development of complications, i.e. perforation, haemorrhage, pyloric stenosis.

The aim of surgical intervention is to reduce acid and pepsin secretion. This is achieved by interrupting the vagus nerve or by resection of the gastric acid-producing section of the stomach. The options for surgical intervention in peptic ulceration are summarised in Table 4.1.

NURSING PRIORITIES AND MANAGEMENT: PEPTIC ULCER

Preoperative preparation (see Case History 4.1)

The patient who is to undergo an elective procedure is normally admitted 1 day prior to surgery. This allows time for final medical examinations to be made regarding the individual's fitness for the operation and for receiving a general anaesthetic. Blood is taken for grouping and cross-matching.

A full nursing assessment is made and a care plan is formulated to meet the specific needs identified as well as to fulfil standard preoperative nursing requirements (see Ch. 26). Explanations are given of the timescale for the preparation which will take place. If the patient is a smoker and has still not stopped, the importance of doing so now is explained.

Preparation of the GI tract will include nil orally for at least 4–6 h preoperatively (see Ch. 26, p. 808). On the morning of the operation, the patient is prepared for theatre. A nasogastric tube is passed perioperatively.

Table 4.1 Surgical procedures used in the treatment of peptic ulceration. (After Whitehead 1988 and Forrest et al 1995)

Site	*Elective*	*Emergency*
Gastric	Partial gastrectomy, or truncal vagotomy and pyloroplasty, or gastrojejunostomy	Partial gastrectomy Excision of gastric ulcer with truncal vagotomy and pyloroplasty or gastrojejunostomy Simple closure
Duodenal	Highly selective vagotomy Truncal vagotomy and pyloroplasty, or gastrojejunostomy Partial gastrectomy	Simple closure with truncal vagotomy and pyloroplasty, or gastrojejunostomy

Case History 4.1 — Mr R

Mr R has been diagnosed as having a duodenal ulcer with pyloric stenosis. He is 54 years old. He has lost a lot of weight over the last few months as a result of vomiting and does not eat much now. He is very thin and is also very anxious. He admits that he smokes 30–40 cigarettes a day and has difficulty sleeping. He has difficulty in hearing but does not use a hearing aid. His particular identified care needs are:

- relief of pain
- relief of anxiety caused by difficulty in hearing the doctor's explanations
- breathing exercises pre- and postoperatively, especially in view of his smoking
- pressure area care due to weight loss
- optimal maintenance of nutritional status
- getting adequate sleep.

Prior to emergency surgery, regular observations are made of blood pressure and pulse in order to detect any deterioration in the patient's condition. Analgesics are given for pain relief, and clear, concise explanations are given to the patient and her relatives regarding treatment.

4.2 In the light of Mr R's identified needs in Case History 4.1, create a plan for this patient's preoperative care in hospital.

Postoperative management

On the patient's return to the ward, the nurse will monitor and/or observe the following:

- airway, blood pressure and pulse
- the nasogastric aspirate
- bleeding and drainage from the wound
- skin colour
- the i.v. infusion and site
- urinary output.

During the first 24–48 h, these observations are maintained, decreasing in frequency as haemodynamic stability is regained.

The nasogastric tube is usually left on free drainage between aspirations to allow air to escape. The aspirate should be observed for colour and amount. Normally the aspirate diminishes and bowel sounds are heard within 24–48 h. Should large amounts of aspirate continue to be obtained, this would indicate that absorption from the stomach is not occurring; it may also indicate the onset of paralytic ileus (see Ch. 26, p. 824).

Fluids are withheld for at least 24 h, after which period, if bowel sounds have returned, sips of water may be given. Water may then be given at hourly intervals, beginning with 30 mL and gradually increasing the amount until free fluids are well tolerated. Light, easily digested food is gradually introduced and the patient is encouraged to eat, but is told to avoid drinking fluids for at least half an hour after meals (see 'dumping syndrome' below).

Care should be taken that the nasogastric tube is positioned comfortably and well supported. Nasal care is given as required. Oral hygiene is also very important and the mouth should be kept clean and moist using mouthwashes or by brushing the teeth if the patient can tolerate this.

The i.v. infusion must be maintained as prescribed to preserve fluid and electrolyte balance and prevent dehydration while oral fluids are not being taken.

4.3 What observations could the nurse make of the patient that would indicate whether adequate fluid intake is being maintained? (See Ch. 20.)

Following surgery, patients should be encouraged to sit up, get out of bed and take a few steps as soon as possible. They should also be encouraged to breathe deeply and cough to clear the lungs of anaesthetic gases and excess mucus. These measures will help to prevent chest infection. Gentle activity also helps to prevent the development of deep vein thrombosis. Adequate analgesia and holding the wound firmly when the patient moves or coughs will encourage the patient to cooperate with postoperative therapy.

Dumping syndrome

Dumping syndrome is a postoperative complication of gastric surgery which occurs following eating. Symptoms are varied and may consist of a feeling of epigastric fullness and discomfort, sweating, an increase in peristalsis, a feeling of faintness and sometimes diarrhoea.

These symptoms occur within 10–15 min of eating and usually settle within 30–60 min. Patients frequently have to lie down until symptoms subside. The symptoms are caused by the sudden emptying of hyperosmolar solutions into the small bowel, resulting in rapid distension of the jejunal loop anastomosed to the stomach and a withdrawal of water from the circulating blood volume into the jejunum to dilute the high concentration of electrolytes and sugars.

The symptoms of dumping may be alleviated by eating smaller portions of food more frequently, reducing carbohydrate intake and avoiding fluids during meals. If symptoms persist, changes in dietary intake and further surgery may eventually be indicated.

Discharge planning

Patients who have undergone surgery for peptic ulceration are generally fit to be discharged 5–7 days after the operation. However, elderly patients and those with intercurrent disease may need a longer period in hospital. Therefore, it is important for the nurse to be fully aware of the patient's social circumstances from the time of admission so that adequate preparation for discharge can be made and potential problems anticipated, e.g. will the patient need transport home; is a home help required; does the patient have young children? Again, communication with the patient's relatives or friends can be extremely helpful in planning for discharge.

Q **4.4** In view of the patient profile given in Case History 4.1, what advice should be given to Mr R prior to his discharge?

An outpatient follow-up appointment may be arranged so that the success of the surgery can be assessed and the patient's rehabilitation monitored. The general practitioner is always advised of the patient's surgery and discharge and of any special after-care that may be required. If continuing care of the wound is required, it will be arranged with the community nursing team or practice nurse.

Complications of peptic ulcer

The three major complications of peptic ulcer are:

- haemorrhage
- perforation
- pyloric stenosis.

Haemorrhage

Severe abdominal bleeding is a life-threatening emergency. Immediate measures must be taken to replace blood loss and arrest the bleeding (see Ch. 18, p. 638).

MEDICAL MANAGEMENT

Careful assessment of the extent of the bleeding is made, and fibre-optic endoscopy may be used to identify the exact site. In the first instance, an i.v. infusion is commenced and blood transfusion given if the patient is shocked. Intravenous ranitidine is commenced to reduce gastric secretion. Hourly drinks and a light diet are commenced when bleeding has stopped. Surgery is undertaken as an emergency if the bleeding does not cease. Elective surgery at a later date may be advised for patients who do not respond to conservative treatment.

NURSING PRIORITIES AND MANAGEMENT: ABDOMINAL HAEMORRHAGE

Major nursing considerations

Nursing and medical staff must promptly implement resuscitative techniques as necessary. Oxygen therapy should be commenced and maintained at the prescribed rate. Blood pressure, pulse and respirations should be checked and recorded frequently to assess the patient's general condition and to observe for continuing haemorrhage. Central venous pressure monitoring may also be instituted.

Any vomit should be observed for amount and for the presence of fresh blood or a 'coffee ground' appearance. If the bleeding is severe and vomiting is continuous, a nasogastric tube will be passed to determine blood loss and to prevent further vomiting. Stools should be observed for melaena.

Pain is usually severe, requiring opiate analgesic relief. The patient should be monitored for response to analgesics (see Ch. 19, p. 665).

Urinary output must be monitored, as hypotension can affect renal function, diminishing filtration. A urinary catheter should be passed to assist in monitoring output.

Intravenous plasma protein substitutes or whole blood and plasma should be given promptly to restore circulating blood volume. Continuous monitoring must be maintained.

Efforts should be made to allay the patient's anxiety. Ongoing explanations will help to reassure her and her relatives that appropriate treatment is available and that everything possible is being done to arrest the bleeding.

When the patient's condition has stabilised, preparation for surgery can be finalised. Alternatively, if conservative treatment has been successful, surgery may be avoided.

Perforation

PATHOPHYSIOLOGY

A perforated ulcer allows the duodenal and gastric secretions to leak into the peritoneal cavity, resulting in peritonitis.

Perforation of a duodenal ulcer is 2–3 times more common than perforation of a gastric ulcer (Burkitt et al 1996).

Common presenting symptoms. Haemorrhage is not a constant feature and the patient may have had very few symptoms. The major presentation is the onset of severe epigastric pain, which becomes generalised abdominal pain and tenderness made worse by any movement. Therefore, the patient typically stays remarkably still, as a result of which the abdomen develops a 'board-like' rigidity — a classic sign.

MEDICAL MANAGEMENT

Diagnosis is usually confirmed by plain erect X-ray of the upper abdomen. In a positive diagnosis, this will show air collected under the diaphragm. If the diagnosis is uncertain, barium examination may be undertaken; gastroscopy, which requires inflation of the stomach, is contraindicated. Emergency surgery is the usual course of action, either to repair the perforation or to make a more extensive intervention.

NURSING PRIORITIES AND MANAGEMENT: PERFORATION

Nursing care will include the following:

- giving resuscitative therapy as necessary
- giving oxygen therapy
- monitoring blood pressure and pulse for shock
- giving i.v. fluids to correct electrolyte imbalance
- providing analgesics
- passing a nasogastric tube and performing aspiration to empty the stomach and prevent further peritoneal contamination
- commencing antibiotic therapy as prescribed
- preparing the patient for surgery
- giving careful explanations and calm reassurance.

Pyloric stenosis

PATHOPHYSIOLOGY

This complication of peptic ulceration is less common than haemorrhage or perforation, and most people associate the disorder with the congenital hypertrophy of the pylorus that sometimes occurs in male babies. The stenosis occurs in the first part of the duodenum and in adults is due to repeated healing and breakdown of a chronic peptic ulcer. The build-up of fibrous tissues causes the stenosis, which results in partial or complete obstruction to the gastric outlet.

Common presenting symptoms include a feeling of fullness after meals, anorexia and occasional vomiting, which progresses to an overdistended stomach full of partly digested food, and projectile vomiting.

MEDICAL MANAGEMENT

Investigations. Diagnosis is by clinical examination and a barium meal.

Treatment. Dehydration and electrolyte imbalance, which may be severe due to the vomiting, are corrected by i.v. fluids. A nasogastric tube is inserted to alleviate vomiting. Once the patient is stable, surgical intervention may be necessary to prevent further ulceration and ensure gastric drainage. The most common procedures are vagotomy and pyloroplasty or vagotomy and gastrojejunostomy (Forrest et al 1995, Burkitt et al 1996).

Q **4.5** What would you consider to be the nursing priorities for a patient with pyloric stenosis in the time before surgical intervention is undertaken?

Carcinoma of the stomach

Gastric carcinomas are more common in men than in women and are usually found in 55- to 70-year-olds. The highest incidence is in Japan. A diet high in carbohydrates and low in fat, fresh fruit and vegetables is thought to predispose to gastric cancer. An increased risk is associated with pernicious anaemia, chronic gastritis and following gastric surgery. The incidence is greater in individuals with blood group A (Forrest et al 1995).

PATHOPHYSIOLOGY

Gastric carcinomas are almost always adenocarcinomas derived from the mucus-secreting cells of the gastric glands; 60% occur at the pylorus or in the antrum, 20–30% in the body and 5–20% in the cardia. The tumour spreads along the gastric wall to the duodenum and oesophagus and through the wall to the peritoneum. Adjacent organs become infiltrated. Metastatic spread may occur locally to neighbouring organs, within the peritoneal cavity, or via the lymphatic or blood vessels to the liver, lungs and bones. In most countries, the overall cure rate for gastric cancer remains around 10%. However, the results from Japan present a more encouraging picture, with an overall 5-year survival rate of over 50% (Griffin & Raimes 1997).

Common presenting symptoms. The most common symptoms are anorexia, loss of weight and epigastric pain. Often such symptoms are either rationalised as trivial or tolerated despite the distress they cause; consequently, there may be considerable delay before the patient seeks medical help. By this time, the disease may be well advanced and may have spread to adjacent organs. Dysphagia indicates that the cardia of the stomach is involved. Vomiting suggests obstruction by a tumour at the gastric outlet.

MEDICAL MANAGEMENT

Investigations. Diagnosis can be made by medical history, clinical examination and a barium meal, usually confirmed by CT scanning. Fibreoptic gastroscopy allows direct inspection and a biopsy to be taken.

Treatment. The prognosis is poor. A partial or total gastrectomy — which is either palliative or so-called curative, depending on the extent of the tumour — may be undertaken. Details of surgery are given in Figure 4.6 (see also Griffin & Raimes 1997). Sadly, for some patients the carcinoma is so advanced that surgical intervention is inappropriate.

NURSING PRIORITIES AND MANAGEMENT: CARCINOMA OF THE STOMACH

See Chapter 26 for details of perioperative nursing priorities in abdominal surgery.

Long-term care after palliative surgery

Major patient problems

After the patient has been discharged home, it is very likely that the symptoms of the cancer will gradually increase. Skilful and sensitive nursing care will be required to help the patient to remain as comfortable and free from anxiety as possible.

Pain from the tumour, metastases and ascites can be relieved initially by oral morphine sulphate (MST) Continus, progressing,

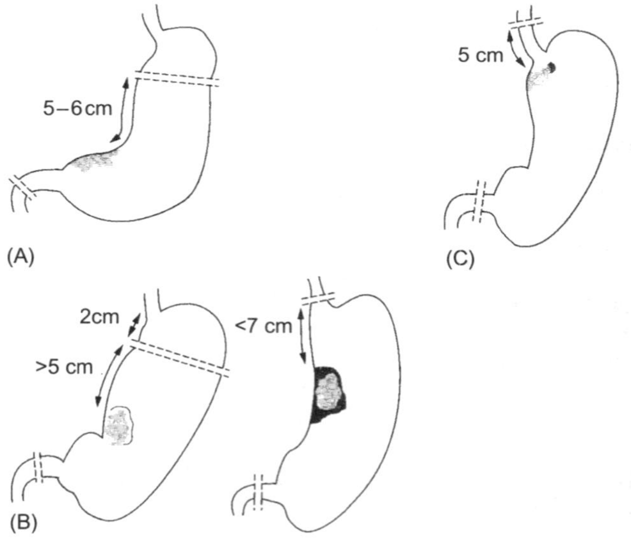

Fig. 4.6 Surgical resection for carcinoma of the stomach. A: Antral carcinoma — subtotal gastrectomy and resection of the first part of the duodenum. B: Carcinoma of the middle third — subtotal or total gastrectomy depending on the proximal margin of resection. C: Carcinoma of cardia — total gastrectomy and resection of lower oesophagus. (Reproduced with kind permission from Griffin & Raimes 1997.)

as the need arises, to the judicious use of analgesics (usually diamorphine). This is usually given subcutaneously via a syringe driver. Such delivery gives a consistent level of analgesia and is often the key factor in enabling the patient to be pain-free and to remain at home.

Dietary intake may prove a problem. Persistent nausea and vomiting may develop and be difficult to control. Regular and pre-emptive antiemetic medication can be most beneficial. Meals should be small and attractively served at times when the effect of antiemetics is at its optimal level. Nutritious drinks such as Ensure and Enlive can help to supplement nutrition without extra effort on the part of the patient.

Diarrhoea and constipation can both occur. A common side-effect of opiate analgesics is constipation, for which an oral laxative should be prescribed. Orally or rectally administered medications can help to control these symptoms, as can dietary care.

Mouth infection. As in all malignant disease, candidiasis is very common. Nystatin lozenges or suspensions may be given after meals and oral hygiene and dental/denture care must be meticulously maintained (see Ch. 15, p. 559).

Ascites. For some patients, there may be the added distress of ascites, which is an accumulation of serous fluid within the peritoneal cavity which can cause pressure on other abdominal organs and the respiratory system. Abdominal paracentesis, whereby the ascitic fluid can be drained off, may be preferred to relieve the symptoms. Diuretics may also be used.

Psychological distress. The support of the community nursing team and perhaps the Macmillan or Marie Curie nursing services can prove indispensable in giving the patient the confidence to remain at home rather than in hospital. The daily visits of such a nurse, as well as ensuring that the practical aspects of care are achieved, give the patient and her family the opportunity to talk about their fears and worries. The visiting nurse is in an ideal position to monitor the well-being of both parties and to recognise when plans of care should be renewed. Chapters 31 and 33 explore many ways in which a sensitive continuity of care can be achieved, whether in hospital, at home or in a hospice.

DISORDERS OF THE SMALL AND LARGE INTESTINES

Unlike disorders of the upper GI tract, in which the major problem is that of ingestion of nutrients, disorders of the small and large intestines result in problems of absorption of nutrients or the transit and elimination of bowel contents. People suffering from such problems complain of varying degrees of abdominal pain and discomfort, diarrhoea and/or constipation. Often the symptoms are insidious and/or embarrassing, such that they are ignored or tolerated and not mentioned even to close relatives. Health education strategies must strive to overcome this and encourage the early reporting of symptoms before serious and perhaps irreversible changes have occurred. Examples of this are continuing efforts to promote the early detection of colorectal cancer. Mant et al (1992), for example, describe a trial to predict patient compliance with faecal occult blood screening.

Malabsorption syndrome

PATHOPHYSIOLOGY

Malabsorption syndrome may result from any of the following causes:

- Incomplete digestive processes, which may be due to:
  - —damage or dysfunction of the pancreas
  - —reduction or absence of bile salts to emulsify fats for absorption; this can occur in biliary obstruction, liver disease or extensive resection of the small bowel
  - —excessive transit time, impairing optimal absorption; this can occur in disorders of metabolic rate, inflammatory bowel disease and even prolonged and excessive stress
- Faulty absorption of nutrients due to:
  - —damage to the absorptive surfaces, as in inflammatory bowel disease and coeliac disease
  - —impaired enzyme activity, e.g. in lactose intolerance
  - —resection of the absorptive surfaces, e.g. in inflammatory bowel disease.

Common presenting symptoms. Malabsorption may not be immediately or directly observable, but indicative features would include loss of weight together with abdominal distension, oedema and fatty diarrhoea (steatorrhoea). There is general malaise and lack of energy, which may be easiest to detect in children. In children, growth failure may also be obvious and anaemia and vitamin deficiency will be apparent.

The symptoms that tend to prompt the individual to seek medical advice are the distressing diarrhoea and general malaise. Parents will very quickly seek advice if their child fails to thrive.

MEDICAL MANAGEMENT

Investigations. When a careful history and clinical examination suggest malabsorption, the following diagnostic tests will be carried out to determine the cause:

- faecal fat estimation
- glucose and lactose tolerance tests
- haematological studies
- radiological and barium studies
- endoscopic examination and biopsy.

Treatment. The form of treatment offered will clearly depend upon the cause of the malabsorption. In coeliac disease, where there is a sensitivity to gluten, or in lactose intolerance, the advice seems simple: avoid foods containing the offending element. However, for the person, such advice is not always easy to follow and her condition can potentially cause disruption and stress in everyday life, undermining her sense of well-being.

Where malabsorption is part of, or has resulted from, some other disorder, nutritional supplementation may be required on a temporary or permanent basis.

NURSING PRIORITIES AND MANAGEMENT: MALABSORPTION SYNDROME

Major considerations

The assessment and planning of care will necessarily focus on the problems of nutritional impairment, diarrhoea and any associated feeling of embarrassment, anger or despair. For some, pain will be a distinctive feature, in which case providing analgesics must be a priority.

A full nutritional assessment should be made (see Ch. 21) with the assistance of the dietician. While assessing eliminatory function, efforts should be made to minimise the physical misery and embarrassment caused by diarrhoea. Attention to hygiene and the provision of soothing creams for any excoriation can make all the difference. General malaise can be helped by ensuring rest and relaxation; this is not always easy, as the investigations may be many and frequent. Supporting the patient through such tests and ensuring her full understanding will help her to cope and to maintain a positive attitude.

Counselling and teaching will be a priority once the problem and treatment have been determined. This is especially important as discharge approaches and the patient begins to take responsibility for dietary modification. Support in the community can be given by the community nurse, GP and self-help groups, but probably the best support can be gained from the people closest to the patient. The involvement of family and significant friends in any teaching and health promotion programme should be encouraged.

Inflammatory bowel disease: Crohn's disease and ulcerative colitis

Inflammatory bowel disease is the term used to describe the two chronic and debilitating conditions, Crohn's disease (CD) and ulcerative colitis (UC). Both disorders are relatively common in developed countries and commonly affect people in young adulthood. The prevalence of both conditions, especially CD, appears to have risen in the last 40 years. In Western populations, the incidence of CD is 1/1500 and of UC 1/1000 (Kamm 1996). As yet no definitive cause has been found. Genetic factors, autoimmunity, diet, bacteria, allergens and stress have all been implicated and probably all play a part. It would seem that UC and CD are different manifestations of the same disease; UC, however, affects primarily the descending colon and rectum, whereas CD can affect any part of the GI tract from the mouth to the anus.

PATHOPHYSIOLOGY

In UC, inflammatory changes occur in the mucosa and submucosa. These changes are diffuse, with widespread superficial ulceration. In CD, the inflammatory changes seem to affect isolated segments of all layers of the intestinal tract. The damaged mucosa develops granulomata, which give the bowel a cobblestoned appearance. Fibrosis and narrowing of the tract can occur and the transmural damage can lead to fistula formation whereby abnormal passageways develop between loops of the bowel.

In UC, the rectum is almost always involved (proctitis) and a variable amount of the rest of the colon (the full colon can be affected). The inflammatory process affects primarily the mucosa and is continuous. Initially, there is reddening and oedema of the mucosa with bleeding points. This is followed by ulceration, which is usually superficial. In very acute disease, especially of the transverse colon, there may be gross dilatation (toxic dilatation) causing the bowel wall to become thin and rupture. In chronic disease, the colon becomes shortened and narrowed. It should be noted that when Crohn's disease affects the colon or rectum, the presentation, treatment and prognosis are very similar to that of UC.

Common presenting symptoms. Whether the diagnosis is UC or CD, the presenting symptoms are very similar. Diarrhoea is pronounced, especially in UC where it is often combined with rectal bleeding. Abdominal pain is also present and is often the dominant feature in CD, where a persistent low-grade 'grumbling' pain can be quite debilitating. Tenesmus, the painful and ineffectual straining to empty the bowel, may be a feature. However, the problems that often take the patient to the doctor are general malaise, low-grade fever and weight loss. In addition, there may be extraintestinal symptoms such as joint pain, skin breakdown and inflammation of the eyes which, when combined with the GI symptoms, become too much to bear and affect the individual's ability to work and to enjoy social activities. (It is the presence of the extraintestinal symptoms which suggests that inflammatory bowel disease may be an autoimmune disorder.)

Sometimes the disease is in quite an advanced state before help is sought. In such situations, the symptoms may reflect the more serious complications of rectal abscesses, fissures, fistulae or even obstruction and perforation, which will constitute an abdominal emergency.

MEDICAL MANAGEMENT

Investigations. History and examination suggesting inflammatory bowel disease prompt hospital admission for diagnostic tests. Haematological studies will reveal a raised WBC, a raised ESR, a raised platelet count and lowered Hb, B_{12} and zinc. There is often hypoproteinaemia.

Q **4.6** Can you explain these abnormalities in the blood picture?

Other investigations will include:

- examination of the diarrhoea for blood, fat and infective agents
- radiological and barium examination to reveal characteristic features of inflammatory bowel disease
- endoscopic examination — proctoscopy, sigmoidoscopy and colonoscopy, often combined with radionuclide imaging (great care must be taken with such examinations, which are in fact contraindicated in fulminating disease due to the risk of perforation of the bowel)
- ultrasound and CT scanning to determine abscess formation.

Treatment. As there is no real cure for inflammatory bowel disease, the aim of medical intervention is to bring about remission of active disease and maintain this for as long as possible. This may involve the initial correction of fluid and electrolyte imbalance (see Ch. 20), malnutrition and anaemia. Close observation will be made for signs of obstruction or perforation.

Treatment strategies will have the following aims:

- Relieving abdominal pain by the judicious use of analgesics.
- Controlling the inflammation by the use of steroid therapy and 5-amino-salicylic-acid (5ASA) drugs like mesalazine and sulphasalazine. Anti-inflammatory treatment can be given orally or rectally. The aim is to bring the inflammation under control with steroids and then to maintain remission with 5ASAs, thus avoiding long-term steroid usage. The immunosuppressant drug azathioprine is used in severe cases and when the patient cannot tolerate steroids.
- Preventing thrombosis in the acute stage due to thrombocytosis — s.c. heparin 5000 U twice daily.
- Restoring nutritional and fluid and electrolyte status. In fulminating disease, enteral nutrition may not be possible and parenteral nutrition will be required (see Ch. 21, p. 713). If enteral nutrition is possible, an elemental diet free of residue may be necessary for a short while before a low-residue diet can be reintroduced. As the inflammation settles, dietary restrictions can be reduced. During any quiescent phase, a 'normal' healthy diet is recommended. Such a diet should have sufficient kilocalories to

restore and maintain weight, as well as being high in protein and carbohydrate and low in fat. Supplements of vitamins, iron, folic acid, zinc and potassium will usually be required.

Surgical intervention. Surgery is required in 20–30% of patients with inflammatory bowel disease, but it is always preferred that any surgery be postponed for as long as possible. As a result, living with this condition can mean living with the constant anxiety that symptoms will become severe and complications arise. Surgery becomes unavoidable when:

- acute episodes fail to respond to medical treatment and there is a deterioration, leading to generalised debility, malnutrition, fluid and electrolyte disturbance and anaemia
- obstruction is acute and/or fails to resolve by conservative means
- perforation occurs
- toxic megacolon occurs — the colon hypertrophies and dilates and could rupture
- fistulae develop — these may be internal or enterocutaneous
- abscesses fail to respond to intensive treatment
- malignant changes are considered to be a risk.

The choice of operation will depend on the extent and severity of the disease. It is now generally accepted that the emergency operation of choice is colectomy with terminal ileostomy and preservation of the rectum. This leaves open for the future the option of proctectomy, ileorectal anastomosis or ileoanal anastomosis. Elective surgery may include total proctocolectomy with permanent ileostomy, colectomy with ileorectal anastomosis or restorative proctocolectomy with ileoanal reservoir.

Great strides have been made in recent years to develop sphincter-preserving operations which avoid a stoma (Salter 1990, Moreno et al 1996) (see Box 4.3). Salter (1990) discusses the possible alternatives to conventional stoma formation, recognising the undoubted impact stoma formation can have on the patient's self-concept and body image (Price 1990).

In CD, the patient may undergo more than one operation over many years, as surgery may initially be limited to resection of the affected segments of the bowel. However, because the disease affects the total GI tract, alternatives to stoma formation are not so easily achieved (Salter 1990).

Box 4.3 Ileal pouch–anal anastomosis (Moreno et al 1996)

The surgical management of chronic ulcerative colitis and familial adenomatous polyposis was revolutionised in 1978 by the introduction of the ileal pouch–anal anastomosis, following proctocolectomy and avoiding the necessity of a permanent stoma. Factors such as age, concurrent medical conditions and, most importantly, anal sphincter function are to be considered. Patient selection is of paramount importance to achieve good results. The use of a temporary ileostomy is recommended in most patients to prevent pelvic sepsis. Small bowel obstruction, pelvic sepsis, fistula formation and pouchitis are the most common complications. Sexual dysfunction represents a major concern for younger patients in need of this kind of surgical treatment. The primary advantages of this technique are that the disease is removed completely, adequate reservoir is restored and transanal defaecation and faecal continence are re-established, avoiding the necessity of a permanent stoma.

This procedure is not used in Crohn's disease because of the risk of disease recurrence in the pouch.

NURSING PRIORITIES AND MANAGEMENT: INFLAMMATORY BOWEL DISEASE

General considerations

The nursing care of patients with inflammatory bowel disease is essentially symptomatic and must be individualised. Assessment will focus on nutritional status, pain and discomfort, eliminatory patterns, how much the person knows about the condition and how she has been coping with it. It will also be important to get to know the patient and her lifestyle, likes and dislikes, and to identify any sources of stress in her daily life. For some patients, developing a treatment plan will be much easier if a trusting relationship is developed with the nurse. Having a 'named nurse' can be a great comfort and support in coping with the stress of being hospitalised and undergoing a range of often exhausting investigations for which fasting and bowel preparation is required (see Case History 26.4, p. 803).

Confirmation of diagnosis can be a great source of relief in some patients, many of whom may have thought they had a much more serious illness. However, they will now have to accept the reality of a condition that is with them for life. Time must be spent on a regular basis helping the patient to adjust and to plan positively for the future. The National Association for Colitis and Crohn's Disease (NACC) can offer a great deal of support to both patients and their families (see 'Useful addresses').

In addition, nursing priorities must include assessing and relieving pain; providing comfort measures that will promote rest; ensuring a high standard of personal hygiene; and providing emotional support to both the patient and her family.

It is essential that privacy and ease of access to a toilet or commode is ensured, as the patient will be embarrassed and sensitive about the frequent bowel movements. The patient should be encouraged to maintain an adequate nutritional intake. Small snacks between meals will help to increase calorie intake. The provision of regular oral hygiene and antiseptic mouthwashes is essential to prevent moniliasis. The use of an oil-based barrier cream will help to prevent excoriation around the anal area. Fatigue will be a constant feature. A tactful approach when disturbing an exhausted patient in order to carry out essential care is helpful in gaining her cooperation, although she may appear unappreciative of the nursing care being carried out.

Nursing care in acute episodes

During fulminating episodes, the patient may be acutely ill. Abdominal pain can be severe and diarrhoea unremitting, and the presence of fissures, fistulae and rectal abscesses may make the symptoms worse. Dehydration and electrolyte imbalance must be corrected and nutritional status maintained by the parenteral route. The patient will be prone to infection, and the nurse should be alert for signs of pyrexia and tachycardia which may indicate the presence of infection. Toxic megacolon, when the colon becomes grossly dilated, is a life-threatening medical emergency which can result in perforation, haemorrhage and septicaemia. A sudden reduction in bowel motions or bowel sounds in the acutely ill patient should alert the nurse to the possible onset of this grave complication. Pain and abdominal distension are not always present. This complication will require immediate surgical intervention.

Monitoring

Specific monitoring of the patient's physical condition would include:

- recording of vital signs, particularly any elevation in temperature or pulse rate or signs of impending shock

- recording fluid intake and output. This would include all fluid replacement, whether i.v. or oral, and all losses: urine, liquid diarrhoea and fistula loss. A drop in urine output may indicate fluid depletion. However, if parenteral nutrition is necessary, signs of fluid overload could occur (see Ch. 20, p. 683)
- recording frequency and nature of diarrhoea on a stool chart.

Perioperative care

The essential principles of perioperative care are discussed in Chapter 26. In inflammatory bowel disease there are additional concerns of which the nurse must be aware. Many patients are physically debilitated and, should they present as an abdominal emergency, it may not be possible to improve this state prior to surgery (see Case History 26.2, p. 801). The psychological preparation for surgery that may involve stoma formation is essential even if time is limited. If optimal time is available, such preparation, in which the stoma therapist plays a key role (see Box 4.4), has been shown to have a very beneficial effect in helping the patient come to terms with and manage the stoma.

For further information, see Price (1990) and Myers (1996).

Stoma care

Postoperatively, the nurse must maintain close observation of the stoma to ensure that it is viable and has a good blood supply. The stoma should be pink; if it darkens in colour this indicates that the blood supply is threatened. Initially the stoma will be oedematous, but should reduce over a few days. A clear drainage stoma bag will be in position to allow good observation of the stoma. If an ileostomy has been formed, digestive enzymes will be present and fluid faeces will become copious, and therefore care must be taken that the skin is protected by the correct application of the stoma bags. The stoma is formed so that it is approximately 3.5 cm long, thus protecting the surrounding skin. However, care is still necessary to protect the skin and position the appliance. No pressure should be put on the stoma during care.

The patient should be reassured that the output from the stoma will reduce and will become more 'paste-like' in consistency as the small intestine recovers and adjusts. The stoma nurse can demonstrate the various appliances available so that the patient has a supply of the most suitable ones prior to discharge. Initial care of the stoma is given by the nursing staff, with the patient gradually taking over under supervision and then performing care independently before going home. Continuity of care is given in the community by the primary health care team and the stoma therapist. Advice is also available from the ward staff as required.

Dietary advice should be given by the dietician before discharge, and the patient and her family should be advised of the long recovery and adjustment time that will be required before a return to good health and a full lifestyle can be achieved.

For further information, see Kelly & Henry (1992).

4.7 Arrange to accompany a stoma nurse specialist on a follow-up visit if possible.

4.8 Ensure you are aware of the different stoma appliances which are available to ostomists. What are the arrangements for the supply and disposal of the appliances?

Box 4.4 The role of the stoma nurse

Psychological preparation for ileostomy and colostomy is essential. The need for information, for emotional support and to develop new skills is vital for the total well-being of the patient (Price 1990).

The stoma therapist is a nurse who specialises in the care of patients who undergo stoma surgery. In the case of elective surgery, she will visit the patient and her family prior to the operation to give information and support. It is essential that the patient is fully informed of the surgical options available to her so that she can give her informed consent to treatment. Clear explanations can help to ensure that the patient understands the changes in body function that will take place and help her to adjust to the accompanying alteration of body image and self-concept. The individual should be given the opportunity to voice her feelings and concerns. The individual's spouse or partner should be included in these discussions, and topics such as sexuality and fertility should be covered. Referral for specialist counselling may be made as required. Part of the stoma nurse's function is to liaise with other members of the health care team in hospital and in the community, in order to ensure that optimal care and support are given during the patient's treatment and rehabilitation.

The stoma nurse is usually involved in helping to choose the stoma site; this decision should be made after observing the patient standing, walking and sitting, rather than just lying in bed (Nichols 1996). The chosen stoma site should be marked before the patient is transferred to theatre. The various appliances which are available should be demonstrated before the operation, and, if it seems appropriate, it may be helpful for an individual who has a stoma to visit the patient to talk about what it is like to cope with a stoma in day-to-day living and to reinforce the fact that general health will improve after the surgery.

Research has shown that adequate counselling and education prior to surgery have a positive effect upon the individual's ability to cope following the procedure.

4.9 As part of your community studies, find out the allowances and benefits to which a person with Crohn's disease may be entitled.

Diverticular disease

Diverticular disease presents as small hernias or outpouchings of the mucosa through the muscular wall of the bowel. These occur predominantly in the sigmoid and descending colon. The presence of uncomplicated diverticulae with minimal or no symptoms is known as diverticulosis. If inflammation occurs, causing severe symptoms, the condition is referred to as diverticulitis and, if persistent, will be considered a chronic inflammatory disease. However, it is often impossible to distinguish one condition from the other on radiological examination, and hence it is useful to include both active and asymptomatic disease in the term 'diverticular disease'.

It is thought that a diet low in fibre is a major factor in the development of the disease. Research has shown that people with diverticular disease have diets low in fresh fruit and vegetables, brown bread and potatoes, and high in meat and milk products. It is also thought that chronic constipation and the excessive use of purgatives may cause diverticular disease by raising intraluminal pressure. Women are affected more often than men.

PATHOPHYSIOLOGY

It is thought that a low volume of colonic content leads to a reduction in the diameter of the colon. Increased luminal pressure during segmentation causes herniation of the mucosa through the muscle wall. Faeces may collect in the hernia, causing inflammation, perforation and abscess formation, the formation of fistulae into the small intestine, bladder or vagina, and peritonitis. Repeated attacks can eventually lead to obstruction.

Common presenting symptoms include the presence of intermittent grumbling, spasmodic pain in the left iliac fossa or suprapubic region, and a mass may be palpable on abdominal or rectal examination. Constipation, intermittent constipation or intermittent diarrhoea are usual. The majority of patients with diverticular disease are asymptomatic, but Figure 4.7 shows the range of clinical presentations that can occur.

MEDICAL MANAGEMENT

Investigations. Diagnosis is made by barium enema. Sigmoidoscopy is undertaken to exclude cancer. Colonoscopy is indicated when there is rectal bleeding or where a carcinoma is suspected. Most individuals are treated in the community by their GP.

Treatment. The main treatment is dietary. The individual should increase her intake of fibre, including unprocessed bran, wholemeal bread, fruit and vegetables, and should drink plenty of water. Antispasmodics such as propantheline bromide can be used. It must be emphasised that stimulant laxatives should not be used as they increase the pressure in the muscular wall of the colon and can cause more herniation of the mucosa.

In severe exacerbations, admission to hospital may be necessary if there is marked abdominal pain and pyrexia. Treatment will include broad-spectrum antibiotics, i.v. infusion and nasogastric aspiration until the inflammation settles. Although many people who live with diverticular disease feel able to cope and have no difficulty in adhering to dietary advice, for about 25% of sufferers complications do occur and surgical intervention will be required. Those complications that may necessitate surgery are shown in Figure 4.7(C)–(H). Depending on the nature and severity of the problem, resection and temporary or permanent stoma formation may be necessary.

Q

4.10 Possible surgical procedures for diverticular disease might include:

(a) colectomy
(b) 'Hartmann's' procedure (see Ch. 26)
(c) transverse loop colostomy.

An anxious elderly patient cannot remember what the surgeon actually said in describing these operations. How would you explain the nature and purpose of these procedures to the patient?

Irritable bowel syndrome

PATHOPHYSIOLOGY

Irritable bowel syndrome (IBS) is the commonest disease diagnosed by gastroenterologists and is an interaction of three major mechanisms: psychosocial factors, altered gut motility and altered sensory gut function (Camilleri & Choi 1997). Organic bowel disease is excluded when making the diagnosis. The syndrome is thought to affect about 1 in 4 of the population (Jones & Lydeard 1992), although not all consult a doctor. In IBS, the disorders of gut

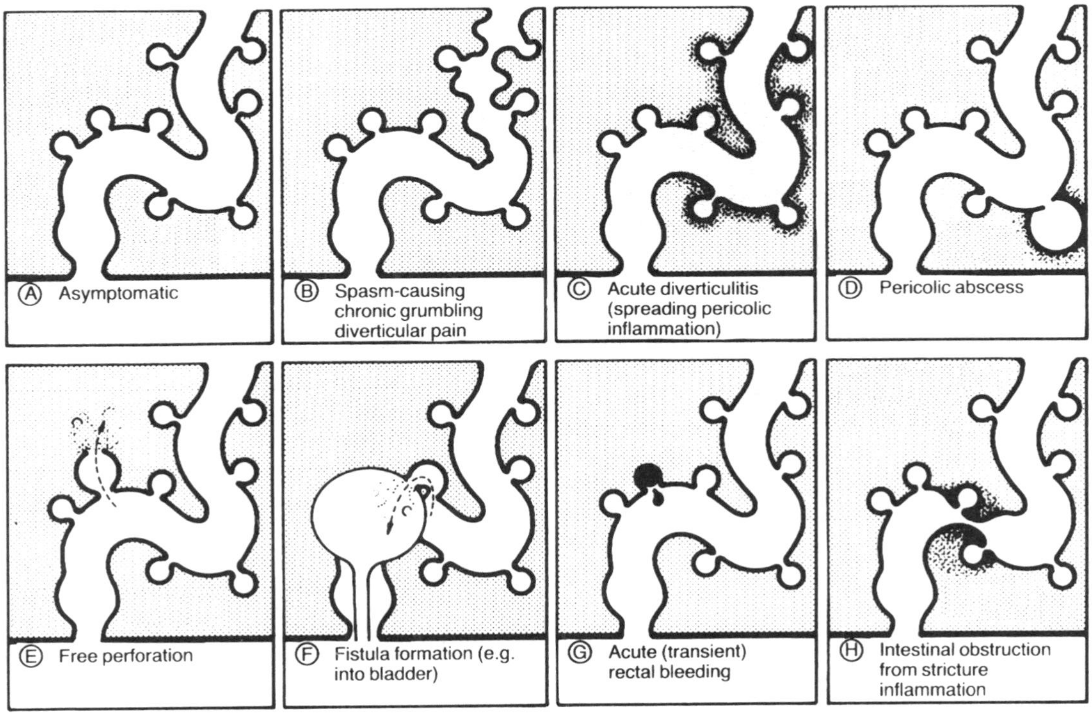

Fig. 4.7 Clinical presentations in diverticular disease. (Reproduced with permission from Burkitt et al 1996.)

motility and sensation are mediated by psychological stress factors such as anxiety and depression, although other gut irritants, some food types and alcohol can exacerbate symptoms.

Common presenting symptoms are:

- diarrhoea and/or constipation
- abdominal pain (often relieved by defaecation)
- abdominal distension
- sensation of incomplete evacuation.

MEDICAL AND NURSING MANAGEMENT

Investigations include a careful history, noting details of the individual's physical symptoms, life stressors and reactions to these, and general personality. Sigmoidoscopy is always performed, and if the patient is over 40 years old with a relatively short onset of symptoms, a barium meal and follow-through and a barium enema are performed to exclude any other cause, e.g. a tumour.

Once the diagnosis is confirmed, time is spent discussing the symptoms and findings and reassuring the patient that there is no underlying pathology.

Treatment is aimed at control of the predominant symptoms. If this can be achieved by avoiding known aggravating factors such as certain foodstuffs or psychological stressors, then the need for pharmaceutical intervention can be avoided. However, if no particular factor can be identified then antidiarrhoeal agents, bulking agents and antispasmodics can be employed.

Use of alternative therapies such as hypnotherapy have been shown to have significant value in symptom control in IBS (Houghton et al 1996). However, nurses must remember to be realistic when discussing coping strategies with patients, as alternative therapies are not readily available on the NHS and can be very expensive.

Appendicitis

The appendix develops from the dependent pole of the caecum as a blind-ended tube. It has a large amount of lymphoid tissue in its walls and is covered by the peritoneum. The appendix is described as vestigial in that it constitutes the remnant of a structure whose function is no longer required.

Inflammation of the appendix is the most common cause of abdominal sepsis in developed countries. The concern is always that the inflamed appendix might rupture, causing peritonitis. Appendicitis is a life-threatening condition and constitutes a surgical emergency.

Although in many people the appendix has virtually disappeared by their middle years, appendicitis can occur at any age. It is rare in infancy and less common in later life, but in the UK can affect 12–15% of those aged 8–15 years. Its prevalence is thought to be closely related to refined Western diets where faecolith residues are retained in and obstruct the lumen of the blind-ended appendix. The incidence of appendicitis does appear to have fallen significantly over the past 10 years, perhaps reflecting the promotion of a healthier diet that is high in fibre. Less commonly, viral infections, contaminated food and intestinal (tape) worms can precipitate appendicitis.

PATHOPHYSIOLOGY

When the lumen of the appendix becomes obstructed, bacteria proliferate and cause an acute inflammatory response. The local end arteries become thrombosed and gangrene sets in. This in turn leads to perforation and localised peritonitis. If left untreated, this becomes generalised peritonitis (see Box 4.5 and Fig. 4.8).

Common presenting symptoms. Appendicitis can occur 'out of the blue'. Many an anecdote tells of individuals who at 21.00 h were happily enjoying an evening at the theatre or a restaurant and at 03.00 h found themselves in a hospital bed minus their appendix.

For others, symptoms of colic and fever may 'grumble' on for some time before an acute episode occurs. In such cases, the obstruction has perhaps been partial and the inflammation transitory. These recurrent episodes can result in adhesions forming which can cause further problems (see Box 4.6).

The classic and cardinal features are usually seen in the young person and readily 'diagnosed' even by family and friends (see Case History 4.2).

Box 4.5 Peritonitis (inflammation of the peritoneum)

Acute peritonitis

Acute peritonitis is commonly caused by irritating substances, often bacterial in nature, entering the abdominal cavity due to:

- perforation of an organ by either trauma or disease, e.g. a penetrating injury, a perforated appendix, duodenal ulcer, or ruptured fallopian tube as a result of an ectopic pregnancy
- gangrene of an organ such as might occur in a strangulated hernia
- septicaemia, which may have originated in another part of the body.

The peritoneum becomes inflamed, inciting a dramatic increase in the production of serous fluid. This rapidly becomes infected and purulent in the presence of bacteria, (typically *Escherichia coli* and *Bacteroides*). Toxins are absorbed from the inflamed and oedematous peritoneum and large amounts of fluid are lost into the peritoneal cavity, leading to paralytic ileus, abdominal distension, hypovolaemia, fluid and electrolyte imbalance and loss of protein.

Immediate and intense pain are felt at the site, followed by vomiting, pyrexia, extreme weakness and shock. Diagnosis is essentially clinical, supported by X-ray examination to detect the presence of free air, fluid levels, abdominal masses and perforations.

Treatment is by a combination of surgery, i.v. antibiotic therapy and specific intervention for the underlying cause. The peritoneal cavity may need to be opened to remove the toxic material and allow drainage of the peritoneal cavity. Supportive therapy includes i.v. fluids to maintain fluid and electrolyte balance, nasogastric aspiration to relieve distension, oxygen therapy and analgesics. If the patient continues to remain pyrexial, tachycardic and in pain, an abdominal abscess should be suspected as a complication.

Chronic peritonitis

This is far less common than acute peritonitis but may occur in association with tuberculosis (see Ch. 3) or as a complication of some long-standing irritant such as peritoneal dialysis or a foreign body. Symptoms are less severe and include low-grade fever, vague pain and malaise. Treatment will essentially depend on the cause.

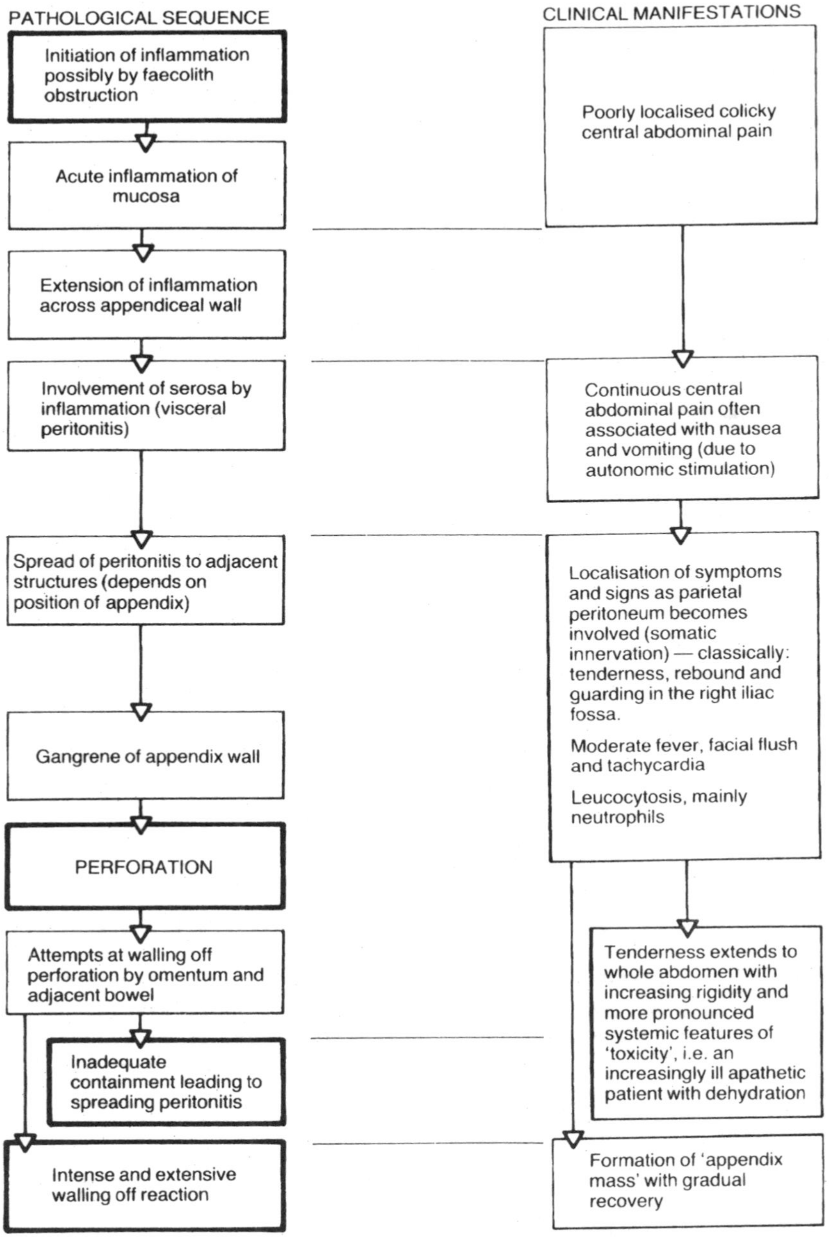

Fig. 4.8 The pathophysiology and clinical manifestations of acute appendicitis. (Reproduced with permission from Burkitt et al 1996.)

4.11 After reading Case History 4.2, try to answer the following questions:

(a) How do you account for the discomfort affecting P's right leg?
(b) Why would any delay in admitting P to hospital have been unwise?
(c) Why might P have experienced postoperative urinary retention? (See Ch. 26, p. 824.)

MEDICAL MANAGEMENT

Investigations. Diagnosis is essentially clinical; following a careful history and examination, only essential investigation will be carried out to confirm diagnosis. If this is in doubt, ultrasound or laparoscopic techniques may be employed.

Surgical intervention. Appendicectomy is the treatment of choice. To remove the offending appendix, a small incision is made, the appendix 'delivered' and the stump sutured. The cavity will be irrigated and a drainage tube inserted if any infected material is evident.

Box 4.6 Adhesions

An adhesion is the union of two surfaces that are normally separate. In the abdomen they are commonly the result of abdominal surgery, injury or inflammation. As healing occurs, fibrous scar tissue develops which may adhere to adjoining tissue, e.g. loops of bowel. These adhesions can distort tissue and, by so doing, impair function, e.g. the transit of intestinal contents. Adhesions may be asymptomatic, but they occasionally cause obstruction and require surgical division.

Such fibrous bands can also occur around pelvic organs, in the pleura, the pericardium and in damaged joints.

NURSING PRIORITIES AND MANAGEMENT: APPENDICITIS

As appendicitis so often presents as an emergency, the patient may have to be prepared quickly. Every detail of safe physical preparation must be attended to, but psychological support must not be considered 'a luxury we can't afford'. The skilled nurse will blend clinical and interpersonal skills to support the patient and her family during this crisis.

In the majority of cases, postoperative recovery will be uneventful and rapid. Pain relief should be ensured and vital signs monitored at frequent intervals until stability is restored (see Ch. 26, p. 816).

Complications

Should perforation and peritonitis occur (see Box 4.5), the patient may become seriously ill. Intestinal peristalsis will be halted and the risks of dehydration, electrolyte imbalance and septicaemic shock are very real. Treatment will involve the removal of the appendix and toxic material, drainage of any abscess and the administration of systemic antibiotics. Oxygen therapy will be necessary and vascular volume will be restored and maintained intravenously. Opiate analgesics will be given to ensure pain is not allowed to exacerbate an already serious situation. Fortunately, with effective and prompt intervention, the mortality rate of such complications is low.

Abdominal hernia

In the discussion on hiatus hernia (see p. 92), a hernia was defined as the protrusion of an organ through the structures that normally contain it. Abdominal hernias occur where there is an acquired or congenital weakness in the muscle wall of the abdomen, allowing an outpouching of peritoneum to form a sac (see Fig. 4.9). Acquired weakness can occur in any condition that may result in chronically raised intra-abdominal pressure (e.g. chronic cough, constipation or heavy lifting) or where abdominal muscle weakness has developed (e.g. obesity, old age, illness or pregnancy). An untreated hernia may progress to contain peritoneal contents, typically the small or large bowel. The major concern is that, due to twisting and/or constriction at the neck of the sac, the blood supply becomes impaired at that site. Unless this is immediately resolved, all of the symptoms of intestinal obstruction will occur (see Box 4.7).

Q **4.12** How would paralytic ileus be managed?

Case History 4.2 P

P, an active 13-year-old boy, complained of having pains in his stomach and of feeling sick. He refused his breakfast and was reluctant to go to school. Kept at home 'just in case', he was listless and vomited the soup he tried at lunchtime. His friends came round after school; for a while he seemed to 'pick up' and laughter was heard from his room. However, by 20.00 h he could localise the pain to his right side. He curled up on the sofa and complained particularly when he tried to straighten out his right leg.

His mother, suspecting appendicitis, called the doctor. By the time the GP arrived, P was flushed, vomiting and in considerable pain, especially when the GP tried to examine his abdomen. He was immediately admitted to hospital, where he went directly to theatre. His designated nurse ensured that both he and his mother understood what was to happen. P's mother was relieved to know that an analgesic could now be given but understood that P's description of the pain had been important in aiding diagnosis. The reader may wish to refer to Attard et al (1992) and Jones (1992) for further debate on this issue. P was not given any bowel preparation, as it would only aggravate the condition. He had not eaten since lunchtime but, because he had vomited and on examination appeared dehydrated, an i.v. infusion was started to correct any fluid and electrolyte imbalance (see Ch. 20). Intravenous antibiotics were administered in the perioperative period.

P appeared to cope well but was clearly comforted by his mother's presence; she helped him into his theatre gown and promised to safeguard his precious watch. Once prepared, P was taken to theatre, returning to the ward in the early hours of the next day. P's mother decided to go home, having reassured P that she would be back in the morning.

P recovered rapidly and there had been no evidence of perforation or peritonitis (see Box 4.5). He required little analgesic relief but the nurse remained observant lest he was just putting on a brave face. The fluid balance record was maintained while the i.v. infusion continued, but this was discontinued after 24 h. By the next day, P was out of bed and taking a light diet and wanting to go home. His only problem had been an initial inability to pass urine which he found unpleasant and embarrassing. However, standing out of bed made things easier. The nurse running water from the tap, however, didn't impress him at all.

P was discharged on the third postoperative day. His sutures were dissolvable and would therefore not need to be removed. The discharge advice for this normally active boy was to ensure that he was not overly active too soon and his nurse took time to explain again that healing would not be fully complete for about 4–6 weeks.

PATHOPHYSIOLOGY

The most commonly occurring types of abdominal hernia may be described as follows.

Inguinal hernia. This type of hernia may be indirect or direct, the former being the more common. In indirect inguinal hernia, congenital abdominal weakness causes the hernial sac to protrude through the inguinal ring and follow the round ligament or spermatic cord. A direct inguinal hernia protrudes directly through the posterior ring. Inguinal hernias are far more common in men

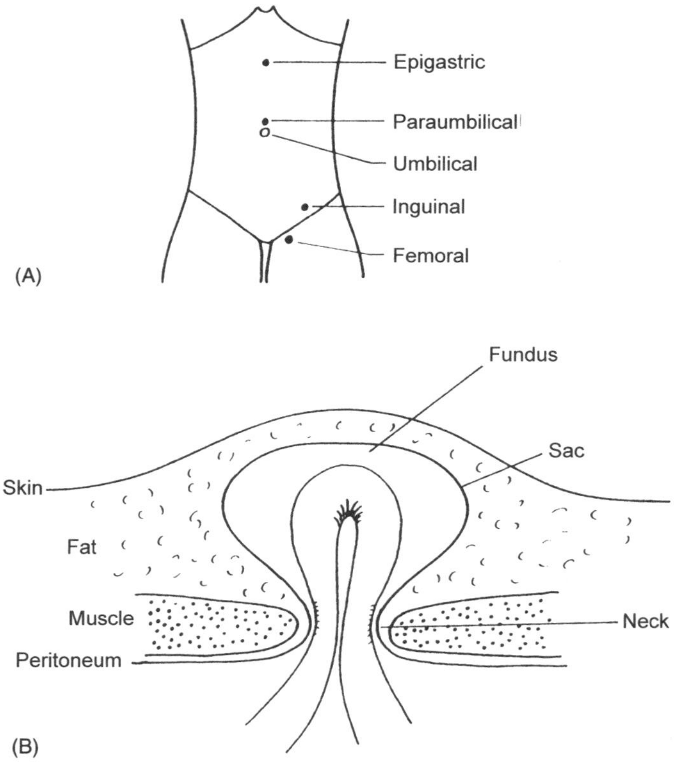

Fig. 4.9 A: Common abdominal wall hernias. B: The principles of the anatomy are the same in each case, although there are obviously individual differences. There is a protrusion of the peritoneum through a natural gap or weakness in the muscle wall of the abdomen. This gap narrows the sac of peritoneum into a neck before it opens out into the fundus. The sac may or may not contain some of the contents of the peritoneal cavity, e.g. omentum, small bowel. (From Whitehead 1988, reproduced with kind permission from Edward Arnold.)

than in women. Burkitt et al (1996) noted that about 7% of surgical outpatient consultation and 12% of UK operating time are accounted for by the repair of inguinal hernias.

Femoral hernia. This type of hernia is considered to be acquired, resulting from herniation through the femoral canal. This canal is wider in women, making such herniation more commonly a female complaint. Femoral hernias also have a greater risk of complications.

Umbilical hernia. Many infants are born with an umbilical hernia. This normally disappears in the first year of life without surgical repair. Acquired umbilical hernias can develop in overweight individuals or in those with abdominal ascites (see p. 119).

Incisional hernia. Following abdominal surgery, the incision site is a point of potential weakness. This becomes a problem if the patient experiences postoperative problems such as impaired healing (especially if drainage of the wound has been required), abdominal distension or generalised debility.

4.13 It is often difficult to picture the anatomical features of inguinal or femoral hernias. Review again normal abdominal anatomy with the help of your physiology textbook and take time to understand for yourself how hernias develop.

Box 4.7 Intestinal obstruction

Intestinal obstruction occurs when the normal transit of intestinal contents is impeded due to mechanical obstruction, vascular occlusion or impaired innervation. Obstruction may be partial or complete.

Mechanical obstruction

Intraluminal causes
- Neoplasms
- Strictures
- Foreign bodies
- Faeces
- Intussusception: a telescoping of one part of the bowel into another part.

Extramural causes
- Adhesions
- Strangulated hernia
- Volvulus: twisting of the bowel (see Roberts 1992)
- Neoplasms outwith the intestinal tract.

When the obstruction occurs, the affected intestine becomes distended with GI secretions (as much as 8 L is formed each day). As the fluid accumulates, the pressure rises and the bowel responds by attempting to propel the contents forward. This serves only to increase secretions; eventually, the increase in pressure increases capillary permeability and fluid is forced out into the peritoneal cavity. The distension may cause respiratory embarrassment. Severe abdominal colic is experienced. If the obstruction is in the small bowel, vomiting occurs. Obstruction in the large bowel results in distension with air and faeces, and the eventual increase in pressure results in necrosis and the threat of perforation. The outcome of unresolved obstruction will be electrolyte imbalance, hypovolaemia and possibly peritonitis.

Vascular occlusion

Obstruction may occur if there is vascular occlusion of the major mesenteric blood supply by a thrombus or embolus. It is the resulting ischaemia that leads to obstruction. Although there is pain, there is no distension. As the condition deteriorates, the pain may actually decrease. If undiagnosed, gangrene and bacteraemia develop as toxins from the lumen invade the peritoneum and are absorbed into the bloodstream. If surgical intervention is not prompt, death may result. It should also be noted that any mechanical obstruction, such as strangulation, that impairs blood supply carries with it a significant mortality risk.

Impaired innervation: paralytic ileus

Paralytic ileus will occur when trauma, inflammation or pain in the thoracolumbar region interferes with the normal innervation of the bowel. It can therefore be a complication of such conditions as back and chest injury, renal pathology and peritonitis. Temporary (paralytic) ileus that follows the necessary handling of the bowel in certain abdominal surgical procedures usually resolves in 12–48 h (see Ch. 26, p. 824). Paralytic ileus will result in marked distension, causing discomfort and respiratory embarrassment.

Treatment

Treatment will essentially involve the correction of fluid and electrolyte imbalance, the relief of the distension and pain, and surgical intervention to address the cause.

Reducible and irreducible hernias. In the early stages, a hernia may often be reducible, i.e. with manual palpation or a change to standing posture the sac will return to the abdominal cavity. However, as the hernia becomes larger and adhesions form, this becomes impossible and the hernia is described as irreducible or incarcerated. If the blood flow is then impaired and obstruction occurs, the hernia is described as strangulated.

Common presenting symptoms. The term hernia is usually familiar to the public and the diagnosis, therefore, is often of no surprise. However, familiarity with the term must not be confused with full understanding of the condition. Many may live with the condition for some time, not appreciating the related problems that could occur. Often it is only when symptoms of local pain and tenderness occur that medical advice is sought. By that time the hernia will probably have become irreducible.

MEDICAL MANAGEMENT

The traditional treatment of choice is surgical repair, herniorrhaphy being the usual procedure. The abdominal contents are returned, the sac excised (herniotomy) and the abdominal wall repaired and strengthened with sutures. Laparoscopic technique is the more recent approach to hernia repair. The minimally invasive nature of such surgery is proving increasingly beneficial to the patient.

If surgery is contraindicated, a supporting truss may be worn to keep the hernia reduced and the patient free of symptoms. However, this option is not ideal. Surgery under epidural or local anaesthetic for those patients with chronic respiratory or cardiac problems has greatly improved patient outcome and obviated the need for many people to wear a truss.

Strangulation of a hernia. This life-threatening complication presents with all of the symptoms of intestinal obstruction, i.e. vomiting, severe abdominal pain, distension and absolute constipation. The patient rapidly becomes shocked, dehydrated and pyrexial. Diagnosis is made by history and clinical examination. A plain X-ray may identify the location and the associated distended loops of bowel. Rapid preparation for surgery will be necessary and definitive therapy will include oxygen, opiate analgesics, i.v. correction of fluid and electrolyte balance, nasogastric aspiration and antibiotic administration. Surgery may well necessitate resection of the affected bowel and intensive nursing care will probably be required in the early postoperative period.

When such an occurrence is unexpected, relatives will find it especially hard to cope and will need regular contact with nursing staff for information, explanation and support. The patient is often too ill to appreciate more than simple, gentle communications.

NURSING PRIORITIES AND MANAGEMENT: ABDOMINAL HERNIA

Perioperative care

Ideally, the surgery will be elective and the patient fit. Care must be taken to ensure the patient is not suffering from a chest complaint, allergy or severe smoker's cough. In such situations, surgery should be postponed, as postoperative coughing could threaten the integrity of the repair. Smoking is always discouraged, even if for only the perioperative period, and the physiotherapist and nurse should teach the patient how to support the wound and flex the hip on the affected side should coughing or sneezing occur. Postoperative recovery is usually uneventful and the patient up and walking the next day. Potential problems that must be recognised are urinary retention, infection of the wound and pain (particularly scrotal pain when inguinal herniorrhaphy has been performed). A scrotal support used in conjunction with analgesics usually eases the pain.

Q **4.14** What specific nursing care is required if the patient has had her hernia repaired under epidural anaesthetic?

Hernia repair should never be considered lightly. Often surgery is more complicated than anticipated and the patient may experience considerable postoperative pain and temporary loss of peristalsis. If this is the case, postoperative recovery will necessarily take a little longer (see Ch. 26).

Discharge advice

Time must be taken to ensure that the patient and her family understand the precautions that must be taken to ensure optimal recovery and well-being. Although activity is encouraged, lifting or straining must be avoided. Elderly men may be troubled by an enlarged prostate gland and may strain to pass urine (one operation may well lead to another). Equally, coughs, colds, known allergens and constipation — i.e. anything that might raise intra-abdominal pressure during the weeks of healing — should be avoided if at all possible. The time allocated to give advice and support prior to discharge presents an ideal opportunity for general health promotion (e.g. on smoking, diet and alcohol) and, in the vulnerable patient, for a sensitive reappraisal of home circumstances and community support.

Colorectal cancer

Neoplasms, both benign and malignant, can occur in the large bowel. The concern with benign neoplasms such as polyps is that, if they are extensive, large and of prolonged duration, there is a propensity for malignant change to occur. As a result, if polyps are diagnosed, they are usually removed surgically. Malignant tumour of the large bowel — colorectal cancer — is second only to cancer of the lung in causing death from malignant disease in Western society. It is the second most common cause of cancer-related deaths in Scotland (SIGN 1997). Although it affects all age groups, it is uncommon under the age of 40.

Cancer can affect any part of the large bowel but is most common in the rectum and sigmoid colon (Forrest et al 1995). It affects men and women equally, but rectal carcinoma is more common in men and colonic carcinoma is more common in women.

The exact cause of colorectal cancer is unclear. As it is virtually unknown in rural communities in the developing world, its association with the Western diet is increasingly accepted. The early work of Burkitt (1971), relating low-fibre diets to disease, has proved very influential. Certainly, a low-residue diet prolongs transit time in the intestine, thus allowing any potential carcinogen increased contact with the intestinal mucosa. Colorectal cancer is also associated with other disorders of the bowel, e.g. ulcerative colitis, adenomatous polyps and, significantly, the hereditary disorder known as familial polyposis (see Ch. 6).

PATHOPHYSIOLOGY

The tumours arise from the epithelial cells of glandular tissue — adenocarcinomas. As they grow, they progressively obstruct the bowel by extending into the lumen or spreading circumferentially to form a ring-like stricture (see Box 4.7). Metastatic spread is by direct infiltration of local tissues and organs, lymphatically or via the portal circulation.

Common presenting symptoms. Unfortunately, patients tend not to present until the disease is at an advanced stage. The symptoms are subtle, gradual and easily ignored or explained away. Symptoms will vary somewhat according to the site of the tumour but will essentially involve an alteration in bowel habit. Constipation alternating with diarrhoea is the common concern, combined with rectal bleeding and excess mucus in the stool. Pain is not a common feature and, perhaps due to this, medical advice is often not sought until either the patient is very anaemic and debilitated or the symptoms associated with obstruction are marked.

MEDICAL MANAGEMENT

Investigations. Many patients will present with a palpable mass that can be detected on abdominal or rectal examination. Specific investigations to confirm diagnosis will include barium studies, sigmoidoscopy, colonoscopy and biopsies. CT scan, chest X-ray and ultrasound scan will be necessary to seek metastases, particularly in the lung and liver. For the latter, liver function tests will also be carried out.

Staging. The staging of the carcinoma is based on histological examination of a resected specimen (see Ch. 31). For colorectal cancer, Dukes' staging is the most widely used (Forrest et al 1995). At its simplest, it describes four stages:

- A — the tumour is confined to the bowel mucosa and submucosa
- B — the tumour has invaded the bowel wall to serosa but there is no lymph node involvement
- C — spread to involve lymph nodes
- D — distant metastases or severe local or nodal spread makes surgical 'cure' impossible.

Treatment. Surgical removal of the tumour is the only effective management. The type and extent of surgery will depend on the site of the tumour. It may be possible for resection and end-to-end anastomosis to be performed (e.g. see Fig. 4.10), but often stoma formation is necessary on a temporary or permanent basis.

See also Forrest et al (1995), pp. 430–435, for further detail.

4.15 Turn to Chapter 26 and read Case History 26.2 (p. 801). Mrs B represents a common clinical reality. She had felt unwilling to talk about her symptoms, hoping they were just haemorrhoids. Ultimately she required emergency intervention and a stoma formation for which she was totally unprepared. Can you think (or discuss as a group) how such a situation might have been prevented?

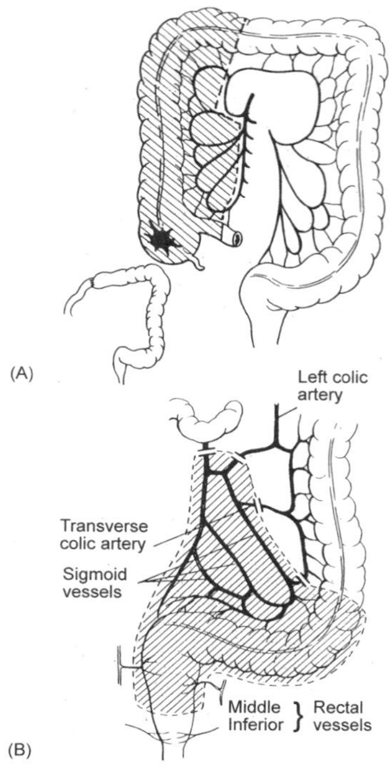

Fig. 4.10 A: Right hemicolectomy for carcinoma of the caecum. B: Anterior resection of rectum for carcinoma of the middle third of the rectum. (Reproduced with kind permission from Forrest et al 1995.)

NURSING PRIORITIES AND MANAGEMENT: COLORECTAL CANCER

Major considerations

Giving psychological support

The realisation that seemingly minor ailments are actually symptoms of cancer is most stressful for any individual. From the moment a patient is referred, as an outpatient or in-patient, a sensitive and tactful approach is of paramount importance. This is not easy: Wilkinson (1992) suggests that many nurses still feel ill-equipped in terms of their ability to communicate effectively with cancer patients. Psychological care needs to include the family and significant others in order to develop a trusting relationship. The beneficial effect of spending time to allow fears to be expressed and explanations and support to be given cannot be overstated.

Perioperative care

The principles of perioperative nursing care are given in Chapter 26. If surgery is to include stoma formation, this will present a further source of stress. A cooperative team approach by the diverse health care professionals involved will greatly assist the patient's physical and psychological recovery and adjustment to what may prove to be major and perhaps only palliative surgery. For the specific input of the stoma therapist, see Box 4.4.

Discharge planning

For those patients for whom cure is not a possibility, planning for discharge and home care should aim to maximise their independence and quality of life for as long as possible. This requires the coordination and integration of hospital and community services, and a respect for the wishes of both the patient and her family. The reader is referred to Case History 31.4 (p. 934) for a more detailed examination of this issue.

Health promotion

Great efforts are being made to detect colorectal cancer early, when its prognosis is so much more favourable. Factors that are being addressed include fostering awareness of early warning signs and counselling those people who might be especially at risk. Preventive measures also include providing advice concerning diet and health screening.

ANORECTAL DISORDERS

Anorectal conditions such as haemorrhoids, abscesses, fissures, fistulae and sinuses are relatively common and always distressing, but are often tolerated for many months or even years before professional help and advice are sought.

Haemorrhoids

PATHOPHYSIOLOGY

Haemorrhoids, commonly called 'piles', are generally considered to be varices of the superior haemorrhoidal veins as a result of congestion of the venous plexus. It would seem that, yet again, a lack of dietary fibre is the most important predisposing factor (see Box 4.8). The resulting chronic constipation and straining during bowel movements raises intra-abdominal pressure, leading to venous plexus engorgement. The bulging mucosa is dragged down and, as the condition worsens, the haemorrhoids prolapse into the anal canal. Other conditions that can lead to or aggravate the congestion are pregnancy (where the development of haemorrhoids is often neglected), tumours and cardiac failure.

Haemorrhoids may be internal or external. Internal haemorrhoids are classified according to the degree to which they prolapse into the anal canal. External haemorrhoids occur outside the anal canal and are less common.

Common presenting symptoms. Commonly the patient complains of 'fresh' blood in her bowel movements, which at first may be thought to be due simply to the passing of constipated motions. The experience of prolapse, at first transient, becomes increasingly

Box 4.8 Constipation

Constipation may be defined as difficult and infrequent defaecation. The following factors can contribute to its development.

Diet
A diet which is low in fibre and bulk predisposes to small faecal bulk. A low fluid intake also contributes to small bulk. Small bulk predisposes the GI tract to reduced peristaltic action and slow passage of contents along the colon. Epidemiological studies indicate that low-fibre diets contribute to many of the GI diseases found in the Western world, such as diverticulosis, appendicitis and haemorrhoids.

Exercise
Lack of exercise contributes to reduced peristalsis, due to reduced muscle tone of the bowel and abdominal muscles. Individuals who take less exercise include the elderly and those who are ill or have a physical disability. Hospital patients are, in general, restricted in their mobility, given their environment and their medical condition, and investigations and treatment often predispose patients to constipation.

Elimination habits
Neglecting to empty the rectum when the stimulation caused by faeces therein (the 'call to stool') is ignored results in constipation; if this occurs repeatedly, faecal impaction can result. Watery diarrhoea, caused by the breakdown of faecal material proximal to the hard impacted mass, can bypass the mass. Impacted faeces can press on the urethra and cause retention of urine (see also Ch. 24).

Socioeconomic factors
Nutritional and dietary intake is determined by eating patterns formed in childhood and influenced by familial and social norms and income levels. A low income can result in the exclusion of fresh fruit and vegetables, which can be relatively expensive, from the diet. Low-income families and elderly people living alone may have to make difficult choices in spending their limited resources on food, heating and clothing. Lack of transport or reduced mobility can also limit shopping expeditions and therefore the choice of foods. The elderly person living alone may be less likely to cook nutritious meals for a number of reasons, e.g. lack of motivation, poor appetite and limited mobility.

Medication
Many drugs have side-effects which cause constipation; these include ganglion-blocking drugs, psychotropic drugs, muscle relaxants, and morphine and its derivatives.

Dentition
Poor dentition makes chewing difficult, especially where there has been dental clearance and dentures do not fit well or comfortably. This can result in the avoidance of fresh fruit and vegetables, and an emphasis on soft, easily chewed foods which do not add fibre to the diet.

Motility of colon
A reduction of muscle tone can result in the faecal mass not being propelled along the colon. Peristalsis and propulsion of faeces are increased after meals, but only in those individuals who are physically active (Holdstock et al 1970).

The bowel may become obstructed by a growth, a hernia or by adhesions following surgery. In addition, spasticity can occur in inflammatory conditions such as appendicitis or diverticulitis.

Rectal conditions
Local conditions such as haemorrhoids or anal fissure which cause pain on defaecation can result in avoidance of defaecation with eventual constipation.

Prevention and treatment

Dietary advice is important in the prevention of constipation. Wholemeal bread, fresh fruit and vegetables, and cereals such as porridge oats and All Bran are important. Unprocessed bran can also be added to soups or stews. The individual should be advised to drink plenty of fluid throughout the day. Elderly persons who have urinary incontinence tend to take inadequate fluid in an attempt to avoid being incontinent of urine.

The importance of emptying the bowel regularly and of not ignoring the call to stool should be emphasised. The individual should be encouraged to take as much physical exercise as possible.

The initial treatment of constipation can include the use of laxatives. Bulk-forming preparations such as Fybogel and stimulant laxatives such as bisacodyl by mouth or by rectum may be used initially. Where there is a faecal mass, rectally administered faecal softeners such as arachis oil may be necessary.

Any condition, such as haemorrhoids, anal fissure or diverticulosis, which is predisposing the individual to constipation should be treated.

frequent and is associated with pain, the discharge of mucus and pruritus. Often such symptoms have been managed by over-the-counter (OTC) remedies such as creams to reduce the itching and pain, but it is not common for the patient to be aware of the significance of changing her diet (Hope 1993). Should the haemorrhoidal vessels thrombose, pain is always severe and it may only be at this stage that the patient seeks help.

MEDICAL MANAGEMENT

Investigations. History and examination will be carefully carried out to exclude other pathologies, particularly a carcinoma. Rectal examination, proctoscopy and sigmoidoscopy will confirm the diagnosis.

Treatment. If the haemorrhoids are identified in their early stages, management requires no more than attention to the patient's diet and perhaps a bulk laxative. If the constipation is corrected, the problem will usually resolve but the patient must understand this and feel confident in her ability to alter her diet. The practice nurse can play an important part in patient education and in arranging a follow-up visit to monitor the patient's well-being.

Surgical intervention. The following surgical treatments may be used to resolve haemorrhoids that do not respond to conservative management:

- *Injection*. For haemorrhoids in the early stages, injection of the haemorrhoidal veins with an irritant solution provokes fibrosis and atrophy with minimal discomfort.
- *Band ligation*. Bands are applied to the mucosa-covered haemorrhoidal pedicle, constricting the vessels, which then eventually shrink.
- *Infrared coagulation*. Infrared radiation is applied in pulses to the haemorrhoid by means of a fibreoptic probe. This causes coagulation and shrinkage.
- *Haemorrhoidectomy*. The above interventions are the most commonly used and can be carried out on an outpatient basis. If, however, the haemorrhoids are not amenable to such therapies, haemorrhoidectomy to ligate and excise the haemorrhoids may be required. If thrombosis has occurred, this procedure will be required immediately.

NURSING PRIORITIES AND MANAGEMENT: HAEMORRHOIDS

General considerations

Whether it is the cause or the effect, it is most important that difficulty with defaecation is effectively corrected. Measures to achieve this include:

- increasing dietary fibre
- maintaining a high fluid intake (2–3 L/day)
- prescribing a stool softener to facilitate water and fat absorption into the faeces
- ensuring sufficient exercise and activity.

In addition, nursing priorities must include measures to alleviate pain and itching, to ensure good personal hygiene, to provide appropriate privacy in a hospital setting and to prevent infection.

Preoperative preparation (see Box 4.9)

If surgery is required, the aim of nursing care in the preoperative period is to control the patient's acute symptoms and to ensure that she feels comfortable and free from any distress when defaecating. One of the major postoperative fears in any form of anorectal surgery is the pain that might be experienced upon the first bowel movement. Time is well spent explaining postoperative care and how any pain and discomfort will be relieved or minimised. The patient is very often comforted merely by the fact that the nurse understands her fears and has the knowledge and skill to help her to manage the problem.

Postoperative care (see Box 4.9)

Care priorities in the postoperative period include:

- the relief of pain and promotion of comfort
- the prevention of postoperative haemorrhage
- the prevention of postoperative urinary retention
- the prevention of infection
- the promotion of optimal faecal elimination
- patient education prior to discharge vis-à-vis lifestyle and diet.

Q

4.16 Anaesthesia and pain may inhibit urination in the early postoperative period. What support and interventions might be considered?

4.17 What would be the key points in any pre-discharge advice and support given to a patient following anorectal surgery?

Other common anorectal disorders

Fissure in ano

PATHOPHYSIOLOGY

This is a tear in the lining of the lower anal canal. Pain is experienced only on defaecation. The cause of a primary fissure is uncertain, but it often follows an episode of constipation and the forceful passage of a hard stool. It is a common complication of Crohn's disease.

Common presenting symptoms. The main symptom is extreme pain on defaecation which persists for some hours. Rectal bleeding may be seen on defaecation.

MEDICAL MANAGEMENT

Anal fissures can heal spontaneously with the local application of creams or suppositories. Constipation is treated and then avoided by a high-fibre diet. Surgical treatment is a lateral internal sphincterectomy.

Fistula-in-ano

PATHOPHYSIOLOGY

A fistula is an opening between two epithelial surfaces. The cause is uncertain, but it may be associated with an infection which produces an abscess which then tracks. Fistulae are associated with Crohn's disease, ulcerative colitis and HIV infections.

Common presenting symptoms. Commonly an abscess is present, as well as pain, rectal discharge and excoriation of skin, and prorates.

MEDICAL MANAGEMENT

The fistula is laid open and heals gradually by granulation over some weeks.

Pilonidal sinus

PATHOPHYSIOLOGY

This is a sinus which contains hair and occurs in the natal cleft. The hair curls and penetrates the skin, causing irritation. Secondary infection is common, which can lead to a pilonidal abscess.

Common presenting symptoms. The individual will experience localised pain which is throbbing in nature. The site will be tender to the touch if an abscess is present. A discharge is often the first sign that a sinus is present.

MEDICAL MANAGEMENT

Antibiotic therapy is given prior to surgery if an infection is present, followed by excision of the sinus when the infection has cleared.

DISORDERS OF THE HEPATOBILIARY SYSTEM

DISORDERS OF THE LIVER

The liver can be affected by a large number of diseases, some of which are more commonly encountered than others. Because of the large number of functions which the liver performs, there are infinite combinations of manifestations, both specific and non-specific. The onset illness may be acute, as in an acute attack of viral hepatitis, or chronic, where disease processes have been progressing for many years before symptoms become evident. A patient with advanced chronic liver disease but who has little or no symptoms is said to be 'compensated'. When the liver begins to fail and symptoms appear, the patient is then said to be 'decompensating'.

Manifestations of liver disease

Non-specific symptoms such as anorexia, nausea, lethargy, malaise and vomiting are common. Weight loss also occurs in chronic liver disease, notably in malignant disease.

Specific features include enlargement of the liver, portal hypertension with associated ascites and splenomegaly, oesophageal varices and hepatic encephalopathy.

ACUTE LIVER DISEASE

Acute hepatitis

PATHOPHYSIOLOGY

Hepatitis denotes inflammation of the liver which may be acute or chronic. Globally, viruses are the most common cause of acute hepatitis, but the disease may also be a response to certain drugs (see Box 4.10) and alcohol. All types of hepatitis will cause similar symptoms, which can range from being absent or negligible to severe and possibly life-threatening, as in fulminant hepatic failure which, fortunately, is very rare. Many patients with acute hepatitis will not require hospitalisation and some will not even contact a doctor. For patients who do have symptoms, they are generalised, as follows:

- *Prodromal illness*. Flu-like symptoms lasting 2–7 days in hepatitis A virus (HAV), and slightly longer in hepatitis B virus (HBV). Symptoms include headache, low-grade fever (37.5–38.5°C), nasal congestion, sore throat, anorexia, lethargy, mild upper abdominal pain or discomfort (right hypochondrium), arthralgia and arthritis. As the liver has no sensory innervation, pain is caused by stretching of the liver capsule. In inflammatory conditions like hepatitis, it is usually perceived as a dull ache in the right upper quadrant. However, in malignancy it can be very severe.

Box 4.9 Principles of nursing care for patients undergoing perianal surgery

Preoperative preparation
- Ensure the patient's privacy to reduce embarrassment
- Give analgesics for the acute pain which is often present
- Provide bowel preparation. This may include the administration of suppositories or an enema to clear the rectum. Some surgeons prefer not to give any bowel preparation prior to haemorrhoidectomy so that evacuation of the bowel after surgery can occur more quickly

Postoperative care
- Observe for haemorrhage during the first 24 h by monitoring vital signs and checking the anal area
- Give analgesics as this area can be very painful after surgery
- On the first postoperative day, the patient is encouraged to bathe
- Assess the patient for urinary retention
- Assess for return of bowel movement
- Administer a bulk-forming aperient to facilitate easier bowel evacuation. Analgesics may be required prior to the first bowel movement
- Give the patient a bath after the bowels have opened to keep the area clean and to relieve discomfort
- Advise the patient on avoiding constipation

Box 4.10 Drug-induced hepatitis

Hepatitis may be caused by any drug, but the more common culprits include analgesics such as paracetamol taken in excess, psychotropic drugs such as the phenothiazines, antibiotics such as erythromycin, and anaesthetics such as halothane. Any patient with hepatitis should be questioned regarding drugs taken recently, including those taken without medical advice, and including herbal remedies.

In most incidences of any drug-induced hepatitis, the biopsy shows changes as for viral hepatitis. However, some drugs will also cause fatty changes in the liver cells.

- *The icteric phase*. Prodromal symptoms usually disappear. Jaundice, of varying intensity, occurs but rarely causes plasma bilirubin to be above 200 mmol/L. Jaundice is a yellowing of the skin and mucous membranes and occurs when the bilirubin level in the blood exceeds 50 mmol/L. There are three distinct types:
  —haemolytic jaundice: caused by excessive red cell destruction
  —hepatocellular jaundice: hepatocyte destruction renders the liver unable to transport bilirubin
  —cholestatic jaundice: caused by obstruction to the flow of bile through the liver ducts due to cirrhosis or malignancy. Obstruction of the larger extrahepatic ducts may be caused by gallstones or cancer of the head of pancreas.
- *The convalescent phase*. Occurs approximately 2 weeks after onset of jaundice. Jaundice lessens and eventually disappears. Other symptoms resolve.

Postviral syndrome. It is recognised that hepatitis is a common cause of a postviral syndrome in which, despite liver function tests returning to normal, lethargy persists for some months. Patients need to be reassured firmly, as many feel that they have developed chronic liver disease.

MEDICAL AND NURSING MANAGEMENT

There is no specific treatment for acute hepatitis, but advice can be given to help the patient cope with her illness. Drugs thought to have caused the hepatitis should be stopped, and no other drugs should be taken without medical advice. Whilst strict bed rest is not necessary, it is advisable for the patient to rest as much as possible and to avoid strenuous exercise. The patient may have an intolerance to fatty foods. A well-balanced, high-calorie diet should be encouraged. Alcohol should be totally avoided, as it can slow recovery and exacerbate symptoms. If required, referral can be made to the 'alcohol liaison sisters', who provide counselling and support for patients with alcohol dependency problems. The patient should be given education on the transmission routes of the hepatitis viruses in order that hygiene precautions may be taken (see section on hepatitis viruses. Restrictions on certain professional and sexual activities may also be required.

Fulminant hepatic failure

PATHOPHYSIOLOGY

This is a rare condition which results in sudden massive necrosis of liver cells and severe impairment of hepatic function. The most common causes are drug-induced hepatitis and viral hepatitis; all other causes are extremely rare.

Clinical features. The patient develops encephalopathy, in which confusion leads to stupor and progresses rapidly to coma. Jaundice and fetor hepaticus are present and ascites may develop later. Abnormal neurological signs, cerebral oedema, hypoglycaemia, circulatory and renal failure and coagulation defects develop.

MEDICAL MANAGEMENT

The medical management of fulminant hepatic failure is supportive care and management of complications such as infection. Liver transplant should be considered if early improvement does not occur, so that patients can be transferred to a transplant centre before severe coma occurs.

The prognosis is extremely poor, with the survival rate being approximately 10% once deep coma has occurred. However, patients who do survive recover normal hepatic structure and function. Liver transplantation allows 48–71% of patients to survive (Williams & Wendon 1994).

The nursing care of these patients is highly specialised and is of paramount importance to the patient's recovery. For this reason, patients with fulminant hepatic failure must be nursed in a specialist liver or intensive therapy unit.

Future management: the bioartificial liver. As many patients die before a suitable liver transplant can be found, research is ongoing to find a treatment to support the patient until either a donor is found or the liver repairs itself enough to support life. The most likely treatment will be the bioartificial liver (Plevris et al 1998).

The bioartificial liver will work on similar principles to renal dialysis. However, as there is no known artificial filter that can imitate the many functions of the hepatocyte, real hepatocytes (most likely porcine) will be used.

These will be loaded into a haemofiltration device known as a bioreactor and, using a delivery system similar to renal dialysis, blood will be pumped through the bioreactor and back into the patient.

This project is still very much in the early research stages, with many practical problems to be solved before human trials can begin.

VIRUSES THAT CAUSE HEPATITIS

All the hepatic viruses can cause a similar initial illness. The differences between them would appear to be their modes of transmission and progression of disease:

- *Common viruses*
  - —hepatitis A
  - —hepatitis B
  - —hepatitis C
  - —hepatitis D (delta)
- *Uncommon viruses*
  - —hepatitis E
  - —hepatitis F
  - —Epstein–Barr (EB) virus
  - —cytomegalovirus (CMV)
  - —measles.

Hepatitis A

PATHOPHYSIOLOGY

Hepatitis A is an acute condition of which a chronic form does not occur. It is usually a mild illness, often occurring in epidemics in communities such as schools, prisons, army camps and psychiatric institutions. It is transmitted by the faecal–oral route. The incubation period is 2–7 weeks, with faeces being the most important infective material. The person becomes infectious 2–3 weeks prior to the onset of the clinical illness and remains so for 2 weeks thereafter. Blood and urine are rarely infectious. Male homosexuals are at risk of hepatitis A due to oral–anal contact. Patients with hepatitis A are usually only mildly unwell and are rarely admitted to hospital.

MEDICAL MANAGEMENT

Investigations. The diagnosis of hepatitis A virus (HAV) depends on the presence of antibodies to HAV in the patient's blood. The presence of anti-HAV IgM denotes recent or current infection. It is present from 1 week before onset of the clinical illness and disappears after approximately 3 months. The presence of anti-HAV IgG denotes previous infection and remains positive for life.

Precautions. If hospitalisation is required, the patient is usually independent and therefore the risk of infection is low. However, if a patient has diarrhoea and requires nursing assistance, the following precautions should be taken:

- plastic gloves and aprons to be used for all procedures
- linen and disposable wipes to be disposed of as per local policy
- thorough handwashing after patient contact.

Immune serum globulin i.m. can prevent hepatitis A if given within a few days of exposure. A vaccine has now been developed which will give protection for 5–10 years and is recommended for food handlers, travellers in high-risk areas and homosexual men.

Hepatitis B

PATHOPHYSIOLOGY

Hepatitis B can cause acute or chronic infection. According to the British Liver Trust, approximately 10% of infected adults will become chronic carriers, of which there are an estimated 350 million worldwide and 1 in 1000 of the population of the UK. The virus is transmitted by the parenteral route. Patients receiving blood or blood products and i.v. drug abusers who share needles are greatly at risk. Tattooing can also spread the virus. The virus is present in body fluids such as saliva, urine and semen and therefore the disease can be spread by close personal contact, e.g. sexual intercourse (especially homosexual), and in areas of overcrowding, poverty and poor sanitation. The disease can also be transmitted from mother to baby either at birth or soon afterwards. Faeces will not transmit infection provided they are free of blood. The incubation period is approximately 2–6 months.

MEDICAL MANAGEMENT

Investigations. The most important test in the diagnosis of hepatitis B virus (HBV) is for the hepatitis B surface antigen (HBsAg) in the blood. This appears from one to several weeks before the onset of the clinical illness and disappears 1–12 weeks later. However, this may not be present in patients who either clear the virus from the blood quickly or present late. It is therefore also necessary to look for antibodies to the hepatitis core antigen (anti-HBc). The presence of anti-HBc IgM denotes acute HBV; anti-HBc IgG denotes chronic HBV.
Precautions. There is great risk to medical and nursing staff when dealing with blood, blood products, body fluids and open wounds, e.g. venepuncture sites, skin lesions, and ulcers on injection sites of i.v. drug abusers. Care should also be taken in areas where the patient's identity is unknown, e.g. casualty departments. All precautions should be taken as per individual hospital policies, and hospital staff should be vaccinated against HBV infection.

Hepatitis B immune globulin i.m. can prevent hepatitis B if given within a few days of a high-risk exposure (e.g. a 'sharps' injury). Vaccination provides good long-term immunity but booster doses are needed every 3–5 years.
Treatment. At present, interferon is the only treatment for HBV and this will be considered in more detail in the HCV section below.

4.18 A staff member sustains a 'sharps' injury. What procedure should be followed and how can the individual be prevented from developing hepatitis?

Hepatitis C

The hepatitis C virus (HCV) was identified in 1989 and is now known to be responsible for 90% of what was known as non-A, non-B hepatitis (Blair & Hayes 1997).

PATHOPHYSIOLOGY

Like HBV, HCV is transmitted parenterally and the highest incidences are in i.v. drug users (IVDUs) and people who received blood products before 1991 when screening became available. Other risk factors include body piercing, tattooing, needlestick injuries and previous immunisation. Unlike HBV, sexual transmission appears to be low in HCV.

Acute infection occurs in about 10% of patients, but about 80% will go on to develop chronic infection. Of these, approximately 20% will develop cirrhosis after 20 years of infection. There is also an increased risk of hepatocellular cancer associated with chronic HCV infection (Chen et al 1997).

MEDICAL MANAGEMENT

Investigations. Diagnosis is made serologically by the presence of antibodies to HCV. A positive anti-HCV test will then be confirmed by a technique which amplifies nucleic acids, known as the polymerase chain reaction (PCR) test. However, a negative PCR test does not necessarily indicate absence of the disease (Haydon et al 1998). Liver biopsy can be useful for staging the extent of any liver damage.
Treatment is aimed at interrupting viral replication and/or increasing the immune response to HCV. The only licensed drugs for this purpose at present are alpha-interferon and ribavirin. Many different trials have been held using various regimens. One example is a 6-month course of 3 mega-units of interferon s.c. three times per week plus ribavirin 1000 mg—1200 mg twice daily. Trials are in progress using combinations of interferon with other antiviral agents such as amantadine. It is believed that combination therapies may improve the response rate (Blair & Hayes 1997).

Nursing support is vital for patients undergoing interferon therapy. There are many associated side-effects and the patient will require regular haematological monitoring and help and advice on coping with physical side-effects. The common side-effects are:

- flu-like symptoms and poor appetite — these can be reduced by taking paracetamol
- fatigue
- reduction of the white cell and platelet count
- mood lowering and depression
- thyroid dysfunction.

All side-effects are reversible on stopping treatment.

The patient will require education on self-injection techniques and the safe disposal of equipment. Advice on diet and lifestyle may be necessary and the patient should be encouraged to avoid alcohol and drugs.

Hepatitis D (delta) virus

The delta virus occurs either simultaneously with an acute hepatitis B infection or as an added infection in a chronic hepatitis B carrier. It never occurs when the B virus is not present. It is diagnosed by the presence of anti-delta (anti-HD) in the blood.

Further information on the less common hepatitis viruses can be found in Shearman et al (1997).

CHRONIC LIVER DISEASE

Chronic hepatitis

Hepatitis is referred to as chronic when the patient still has clinical symptoms or abnormal liver function tests 6 months after the onset of the illness. The main causes of chronic hepatitis are:

- the B, C and D viruses as already described.
- autoimmune hepatitis
- drug-related hepatitis
- cryptogenic hepatitis.

Autoimmune hepatitis

PATHOPHYSIOLOGY

The cause of this disease is unknown. It is a chronic condition but may present as an 'acute' illness similar to acute viral hepatitis. This 'acute' onset is probably an exacerbation of long-standing but asymptomatic disease. It is identified by detecting non-organ-specific antibodies to nuclei, smooth muscle and occasionally liver-kidney microsomes. About 80% of those affected are women and about 20% have other autoimmune disorders, e.g. rheumatoid arthritis and ulcerative colitis.

Prognosis is dependent on the severity of the inflammatory activity. Patients with severe multilobular necrosis on biopsy generally develop cirrhosis within 5 years.

Clinical features. Patients who present with an 'acute' illness will show the signs and symptoms similar to those of an acute hepatitis (p. 115); however, other features such as ascites and hypoalbuminaemia may be present and indicate the chronic nature of the disease.

MEDICAL MANAGEMENT

Steroids and immunosuppressive drugs (prednisolone and azathioprine) are used to achieve remission. The doses are gradually reduced until a maintenance dose is achieved. If cirrhosis is present, treatment will include symptomatic relief of the manifestations of chronic liver disease.

NURSING PRIORITIES AND MANAGEMENT: AUTOIMMUNE HEPATITIS

Nursing intervention is dependent on the severity of the illness. Initially the patient may require full nursing care and nutritional support. Occasionally a high-dependency setting may be appropriate.

As the patient improves, education regarding the condition is important to help her to understand the symptoms and the need for long-term steroid therapy. Alcohol should be avoided, especially if there is cirrhosis.

Alcoholic hepatitis

PATHOPHYSIOLOGY

Clinical features. This condition usually follows years of alcohol abuse and often a recent prolonged bout of heavy drinking. The patient will complain of anorexia, vomiting, lethargy, diarrhoea and upper abdominal pain. A fever will be present and the patient will appear generally unwell and malnourished. Signs of chronic liver disease may be present, i.e. ascites and oedema, encephalopathy, jaundice and spider telangiectasis. GI bleeding may occur from erosions or peptic ulceration, and also as a result of bleeding tendencies due to the liver's inability to synthesise adequate clotting factors.

The diagnosis is made from an accurate picture of the patient's alcohol intake (often obtained from relatives and friends), liver function tests and liver biopsy if the patient's clotting time allows.

Cirrhosis of the liver

Cirrhosis or scarring of the liver is an irreversible condition caused by many hepatic diseases. There are many clinical manifestations, which vary with the severity and duration of the disease. Alcohol is the commonest cause, with the other major players being viral hepatitis, primary biliary cirrhosis, autoimmune hepatitis and haemochromatosis.

PATHOPHYSIOLOGY

Prolonged low-grade inflammation causes progressive scarring and destruction of the liver cells. The remaining liver cells proliferate to form nodules; this results in the liver becoming irregular and distorted in shape. The blood vessels are also destroyed. The resistance to the flow of blood increases, which in turn leads to portal hypertension (see p. 120). The major complications of cirrhosis result from the hepatocellular failure, portal hypertension and portal systemic shunting. These are ascites, GI bleeding, hepatic encephalopathy, renal dysfunction and hepatocellular carcinoma.

Common presenting features. As the disease progresses, the patient feels increasingly fatigued and lethargic. Anorexia, nausea and weight loss are common. Jaundice, bruising, spider telangiectasis and finger clubbing are also seen. Pruritus is a common symptom of cirrhosis (see Nursing Care Plan 4.1) and is probably caused by bile salt deposition in the skin. It is a feature of cholestasis but is not always accompanied by jaundice. It is especially troublesome in primary biliary cirrhosis. Endocrine abnormalities such as gynaecomastia and impotence in males and amenorrhoea and infertility in females can also develop.

MEDICAL MANAGEMENT

The aim of treatment is the removal of any identifiable cause such as alcohol abuse and the management of the major symptoms and complications. Liver transplantation is considered when earlier treatment fails. Considerable counselling and support may be required to eliminate an alcohol problem and improve nutrition. The medical and nursing management of the major complications of cirrhosis of the liver are considered in more detail below.

Ascites

Ascites is the abnormal accumulation of serous fluid within the peritoneal cavity and is a serious prognostic development (Jalan & Hayes 1997). It results from a combination of the following factors:

- raised portal pressure
- increased lymphatic pressure in the liver
- low plasma protein — albumin
- sodium retention.

Box 4.11 gives further details on pathophysiology.

MEDICAL MANAGEMENT

The main components of treatment are restriction of sodium intake, restriction of fluid intake, administration of diuretics and abdominal paracentesis (in refractory ascites — see Box 4.12).

NURSING PRIORITIES AND MANAGEMENT: ASCITES

Major considerations

The main aims of nursing care are as follows:

- To promote bed rest in the position most comfortable for the patient. The legs should be elevated to help reduce peripheral oedema. The semi-prone position improves kidney perfusion and also the venous return to the heart, which in turn promotes a diuresis.
- To provide pressure area care. This is vital because of the oedema and the patient's likely reluctance and difficulty in moving.
- To obtain baseline observations before commencing treatment. This should include the patient's weight and a record of the extent of ascites and oedema.
- To encourage the patient to eat a diet very low in salt. Daily sodium intake must be restricted to 60 mmol, and to 40 mmol in severe ascites.
- To ensure that the patient manages the restriction in fluid intake and understands why it is necessary. It is important to help the patient to 'pace' the fluid intake throughout the day. NB — it is also important that the patient's family and friends are made aware of diet and fluid restrictions.

Nursing Care Plan 4.1 Care plan for an elderly man with liver failure due to alcoholic cirrhosis

Problem (actual/potential)	***Reason***	***Nursing action***
1. Anxiety, anger and fear	Due to: lack of knowledge, fear of the unknown and perhaps denial of the reality of his condition	❒ Encourage fears to be expressed and questions to be asked. Explain all procedures and maintain a non-judgemental approach. Confidence will be restored and he will feel better able to cope
2. Loss of self-concept: **• body image** **• role performance** **• self-identity** **• self-esteem (McClane 1987)**	Due to: physical alteration resulting from jaundice, ascites and weight loss. Loss of libido, impotence and gynaecomastia due to retention of oestrogens normally broken down in the liver	❒ Restore optimal liver function ❒ Provide a trusting relationship ❒ Refer to a specialist counsellor as appropriate
3. Pain and discomfort	Due to: • the enlarged liver that stretches the liver capsule (the liver itself has no sensory nerve innervation) • biliary obstruction secondary to the cirrhosis gastritis due to alcohol abuse • oedema, ascites, bowel disturbance, dyspepsia and itching	❒ Relieve pain and discomfort via: • comfort measures such as positioning, gentle movement and distraction techniques • medication for pruritus —sodium bicarbonate baths —calamine lotion —cholestyramine which binds the bile —salts in the intestines —antihistamines • analgesics, used with caution to avoid hepatotoxic effects
4. Insomnia	Due to: pain, anxiety, dyspnoea induced by ascites, itching and the strange environment	❒ Relieve pain, anxiety, dyspnoea and itching (see above) ❒ Provide optimal peace and quiet when appropriate
5. Nutritional impairment: anorexia, anaemia and weight loss	Due to: the inability of the liver to perform its metabolic functions and the reduction in production of bile. Iron, vitamin B_{12} and red blood cells are reduced. Fetor hepaticus (a bad taste in the mouth and bad breath)	❒ A diet high in calories • protein* to restore plasma proteins • glucose, thought to aid liver cell recovery ❒ Supplements, e.g. vitamins and iron ❒ Low salt to reduce oedema ❒ Controlled fat intake according to degree of jaundice ❒ Small tempting meals ❒ Oral hygiene ❒ Monitoring of weight *If ammonia levels rise and features of encephalopathy present, protein reduced to 20 g per day If anaemia becomes severe a blood transfusion and oxygen therapy may be required
6. Fluid and electrolyte imbalance and impaired tissue perfusion	Due to: • reduced arterial flow, portal hypertension, ascites • salt retention due to loss of detoxification of aldosterone and the triggering of the renin–angiotension mechanism	❒ Reduce salt intake to no added salt (NAS) or less as necessary ❒ Fluid restriction (1–1.5 L/day) if hyponatraemia develops ❒ Gentle use of diuretics ❒ Paracentesis if necessary
7. Infection	Due to: loss of Kupffer cell function and lymphocyte production and exacerbated by nutritional, circulatory and respiratory impairment	❒ Hygiene maintained at a high standard. Strict asepsis with any invasive techniques. Regular monitoring of vital signs ❒ Chest physiotherapy as appropriate ❒ Infection screening as appropriate ❒ Antibiotics if necessary but used with caution
8. Impaired skin integrity	Due to: oedema, loss of protein, jaundice, weight loss and bleeding tendency (see problem 11)	❒ Regular relief of pressure ❒ Sensitive care of the skin, nails and when shaving ❒ Use of emollients ❒ Optimal positioning and repositioning
9. Immobility	Due to: malaise, weakness, ascites, dyspnoea and perhaps confusion	❒ Ensure optimal activity and rest. Provide companionship ❒ Relieve symptoms as described

Nursing Care Plan 4.1 *(cont'd)*

Problem (actual/potential)	*Reason*	*Nursing action*
10. Impaired detoxification of natural and medicinal substances	Due to: liver cell damage	❐ Careful and tactful enforcement of abstinence from alcohol ❐ Vigilance with all medications
11. Tendency to bleed that might be insidious or dramatic leading to hypovolaemic shock	Due to: • portal hypertension and development of oesophageal varices • gastritis • loss of clotting factors • inadequate absorption of vitamin K • reduced reserves of blood in the liver	❐ Regular monitoring of vital signs ❐ Monitoring of any vomit for blood, fresh or digested ❐ Skin and mucous membranes observed for bruises or bleeding ❐ Give vitamin K as necessary ❐ Manage hypovolaemic shock (see p. 638) should severe bleeding occur
12. Encephalopathy • **lethargy** • **flapping tremor (asterixis)** • **irrational behaviour** • **aggression** • **loss of ability to perform daily duties**	Due to: inability of the liver to convert ammonia to urea. Ammonia levels rise to such a level that cerebral cell damage occurs due to nitrogenous neurotoxins Note: 1 A GI bleed constitutes a 'high protein meal' and will exacerbate encephalopathy 2 Infection will exacerbate encephalopathy by inducing a catabolic state 3 Hypoxia will exacerbate encephalopathy	❐ Careful monitoring of behaviour and ability to communicate effectively ❐ Observe for precipitating factors, e.g. 1, 2 or 3 ❐ Manage encephalopathy: • reduce protein intake • give rectal and colonic washouts, if necessary, to remove blood from bowel • give oral lactulose, an osmotic laxative, to reduce ammonia by acidification of bowel environment and to help evacuate bowel contents, *and/or* . . . • give oral neomycin (poorly absorbed from the gut) to reduce intestinal flora • monitor level of consciousness (LOC) • ensure safety and comfort

Box 4.11 Ascites

The term ascites refers to a marked increase in the volume of fluid in the peritoneal cavity. This is usually due to an underlying disease in which the total body fluid is increased, such as cardiac failure, cirrhosis or nephrotic syndrome, or to a local disease in the peritoneum, such as malignancy, or an infection such as tuberculosis.

In health, serous fluid is continually produced in the peritoneal cavity and is sufficient to provide lubrication only, but ascites occurs when fluid enters the peritoneal cavity more quickly than it can be returned to the circulation by the capillaries and lymphatics. Fluid normally leaves a capillary at its arteriolar end and returns at its venous end but, in cirrhosis, portal hypertension and hypoalbuminaemia combine to reduce the re-entry of peritoneal fluid at the venous end. The presence of ascites in liver disease is a poor prognostic sign as it implies poor liver function and portal hypertension.

Severe ascites can cause great discomfort: dyspnoea, anorexia and the ability to eat only small meals, inhibited mobility and discomfort when lying in bed or sitting upright in a chair. If pain occurs, it is often felt in the back. Many of the symptoms correspond to the discomfort of full-term pregnancy! Increased intra-abdominal pressure also leads to hernias, especially at the umbilicus.

Ascitic fluid in cirrhosis is usually straw-coloured; blood-stained ascites indicates malignant disease; bile staining indicates a communication with the biliary system; and cloudy fluid denotes infection. Chylous ascites, which has a milky appearance, is caused by lymphatic obstruction.

Box 4.12 Abdominal paracentesis

In intractable ascites, i.e. when sodium restrictions and diuretic therapy have little effect, it is possible to drain the fluid from the peritoneal cavity by means of a catheter inserted through the abdominal wall. This procedure is known as abdominal paracentesis. Such patients are already hypoproteinaemic and the sudden loss of fluid and protein by paracentesis is likely to lead to a shift of both from the rest of the body into the abdominal cavity, sometimes with consequent hypovolaemia, shock and even death. The protein is therefore replaced at the time of paracentesis by an infusion of salt-poor albumin. The patient's blood pressure should be monitored closely and the fluid drained no more quickly than at a rate of approximately 2 L/h. Strict aseptic technique should be used when inserting the catheter to avoid introducing infection which can lead to bacterial peritonitis. This procedure requires cooperation from the patient to lie relatively still in bed while the catheter is in situ over several hours. She will require help from the nursing staff to remain comfortable over this period. Any leakage on removal of the catheter can be collected in a drainable bag, e.g. a stoma bag, until the puncture site heals (usually within 48h).

- To administer diuretics as prescribed. Spironolactone is the drug of choice because of its potassium-sparing properties. Fluid loss is measured by weighing the patient at the same time each day in similar clothes.
- Pain may be mild and responsive to non-opioid analgesics. However, in malignant disease it can be severe and difficult to control. Strong analgesics and small doses of prednisolone are used to control this severe pain.

Gastrointestinal bleeding

GI bleeding is a direct result of portal hypertension. It may be slow and insidious, as in portal hypertensive gastropathy, or sudden and catastrophic, as in major oesophageal or gastric variceal rupture.

PATHOPHYSIOLOGY

Portal hypertension occurs when there is an obstruction in the intrahepatic or extrahepatic circulation. Hepatic cirrhosis accounts for over 90% of cases of intrahepatic hypertension in this country. Extrahepatic portal hypertension is less common. In adults it is usually due to thrombosis (as occurs in polycythaemia rubra vera), local inflammation or sepsis (as in pancreatitis), or invasion by malignant tumours.

Common clinical features. The cardinal signs of portal hypertension are splenomegaly (enlargement of the spleen), hypersplenism (splenomegaly and a deficiency in one or more types of blood cells) and a portosystemic collateral circulation. The collateral vessels open up to decompress the portal system and are present throughout the abdomen. They are, however, most problematic at the gastro-oesophageal junction where they can rupture and cause massive haemorrhage.

MEDICAL MANAGEMENT

Investigations. Portal hypertension is diagnosed by medical history, palpation of the abdomen, and ultrasound when splenomegaly is demonstrated. Angiography of the portal venous system will determine the cause and site of the obstruction. Endoscopy will demonstrate gastro-oesophageal varices. Hypersplenism will cause thrombocytopenia and leucopenia. Anaemia may also be present.

Treatment. The presenting symptoms are treated. Bleeding from oesophageal varices is treated by blood transfusion and by variceal eradication. This can be done endoscopically by either injection sclerotherapy or band ligation. Balloon tamponade and drugs such as vasopressin are used only to stop active bleeding until eradication treatment is commenced. Patients who do not respond to endoscopic management of their varices will be treated with a transjugular intrahepatic portosystemic stent (TIPSS).

Sclerotherapy is a treatment for oesophageal varices involving the injection of an irritant solution. This causes thrombosis and obliteration of the varicosed veins.

Banding has been introduced recently for the long-term treatment of varices as it has fewer complications than sclerotherapy.

Splenectomy is particularly valuable where there is a regional portal hypertension due to obstruction in the splenic vein.

Transluminal intrahepatic portasystemic stent shunt (TIPSS). This is a radiological intervention whereby a metal stent is deployed in the liver and connects the portal and systemic veins. It is effective in lowering the portal pressure and thus controlling variceal bleeding and re-bleeding. It is associated with a low complication and mortality rate (Redhead et al 1993).

For further information, see Miller (1996).

NURSING PRIORITIES AND MANAGEMENT: OESOPHAGEAL VARICES

If the patient is vomiting profusely from bleeding oesophageal varices, a high-flow suction catheter should be available for intermittent suction and maintenance of a clear airway.

Blood pressure and pulse should be observed quarter-hourly and the nurse should be alert for signs of hypovolaemic shock (see Ch. 18). Intravenous fluids and a blood transfusion should be maintained and an accurate record of all fluid intake and output kept. A urinary catheter is passed and urine output measured hourly during the acute phase, as underperfusion of the kidneys due to shock can cause renal impairment.

The patient is fasted prior to transfer to theatre for endoscopic eradication of varices. Standard preparation is followed and on return to the ward, a clear airway and nil by mouth must be maintained until sensation and the ability to swallow have returned. The nurse will observe closely for recurrence of bleeding.

Because of the experience of either vomiting blood or passing melaena, the patient will be extremely anxious. A calm approach and clear explanations of treatment and care will be essential in order to help relieve the natural fears that extensive bleeding causes.

Should the bleeding not be arrested endoscopically, a gastric or oesophageal tamponade is used to stop the bleeding by balloon tamponade, i.e. compression. A Sengstaken or Minnesota tube is passed well into the stomach and the gastric balloon inflated to approximately 300 mL of air. Gentle but firm traction is applied to maintain the balloon at the oesophagogastric junction. The oesophageal balloon is inflated only if bleeding persists, as it carries a risk of oesophageal perforation. Great care is required when inflating the oesophageal balloon (no more than 30 mL of air) and it must be deflated for 30 min every 4 h. The nurse will monitor the inflation pressures and times and move the tube from side to side in the mouth every hour to prevent pressure sores from forming.

The tube should be in situ no more than 12 h and immediate therapy is required on removal, i.e. endoscopic eradication or TIPSS.

Anxiety and agitation can be relieved by small i.v. doses of a benzodiazepine sedative such as midazolam. As patients with liver disease are very sensitive to sedatives, the benzodiazepine antagonist flumazenil should be immediately available. Antiemetics such as metoclopramide should be given if the patient is nauseated and retching, as this increases the pressure in the varices and could cause further haemorrhage.

For further information, see Dewar (1985) and Stanley & Hayes (1997).

Hepatic encephalopathy

PATHOPHYSIOLOGY

Hepatic encephalopathy (HE) is a neuropsychiatric syndrome that occurs only in significant liver disease. It may be overt or subclinical and is potentially fully reversible (Jalan & Hayes 1997). The subclinical form can be difficult to diagnose but the overt form can lead to bizarre and even violent behaviour. The exact cause is unclear, but one popular theory is that gut-derived neurotoxins that the failing liver has been unable to neutralise somehow cross the blood–brain barrier and cause changes in cerebral neurotransmission (Jalan & Hayes 1997). This gives rise to a range of behaviour patterns that are graded 1–4 in order of severity, as follows:

1. lack of awareness, euphoria, short attention span and impaired ability for simple arithmetic

2. lethargy, apathy, disorientation in time and place, personality change and inappropriate behaviour
3. semi-stupor, somnolence, confusion and gross disorientation
4. coma.

MEDICAL MANAGEMENT

Medical treatment is aimed at reversing the commonly known precipitating factors of HE, which are:

- protein loading
- GI bleeding
- sepsis
- dehydration
- blood chemistry imbalances
- use of sedatives
- constipation.

NURSING PRIORITIES AND MANAGEMENT: HEPATIC ENCEPHALOPATHY (HE)

Detection, avoidance and management of the above factors can be largely nurse-led. The better the nurse knows his patient, the easier it will be for him to detect subtle changes in the patient's personality and to reverse the encephalopathic process before coma develops. It is useful to involve family and friends in the monitoring process.

Good dietary advice is essential, not only to avoid protein excess but also to maintain a high calorie intake to avoid tissue catabolism. Constipation should be avoided and lactulose can be used to promote one to two bowel movements per day. Lactulose is especially beneficial following GI bleeding, as it alters bowel pH which alters colonic bacterial metabolism so that less ammonia is produced. A GI bleed represents a large protein load in the bowel.

Close monitoring of fluid balance and daily weight is important to avoid dehydration, especially in patients on diuretic therapy or undergoing abdominal paracentesis.

Strict aseptic technique should be used for all invasive procedures and any focus of infection promptly reported and treated. A safe environment must be maintained for the patient at all times as she may be confused and unsteady on her feet.

For further information on HE, see Shearman et al (1997).

Cancer of the liver

Tumours of the liver can be either primary or secondary growths. The liver is the most common site for metastatic spread and patients often present with symptoms from the secondary rather than the primary lesion.

Primary tumours

Hepatocellular carcinoma is the principal primary tumour. It is one of the major cancers of the world but the incidence varies greatly between countries. The highest risk populations are in sub-Saharan Africa and eastern Asia and males are more commonly affected than females (Chen et al 1997). Chronic hepatitis B and C virus infections are the main causes of the cancers in high-incidence areas. Hepatocellular carcinomas also occur in haemochromatosis and alcoholic cirrhosis of the liver.

PATHOPHYSIOLOGY

The tumour is highly vascular and occurs most frequently in the right lobe. It invades the hepatic and portal vein. The obstruction to these vessels results in portal hypertension. There may be local spread to the peritoneum or metastatic spread to the lungs or lymphatic system.

MEDICAL MANAGEMENT

Investigations. A very high serum alpha-fetoprotein (AFP >200 ku; normal: 2–6 ku) is diagnostic. Ultrasound with fine-needle aspiration or biopsy at laparoscopy is performed to obtain cells for histological examination. Ultrasound, CT scan and angiography are needed to define the extent of liver involvement and venous invasion prior to a decision being taken on treatment.

Treatment. The first objective is to see whether the tumour is localised sufficiently in the liver to be resected surgically (see Box 4.13). Unfortunately, surgery is usually impossible, either because liver involvement is too extensive or because metastasis to other organs has occurred. Some patients may benefit from chemo-embolisation of the vessels supplying the tumour, but as this treatment can have unpleasant side-effects, it is often reserved for patients with hepatic symptoms (see Box 4.14). Medical therapy also aims to relieve symptoms such as pain or ascites.

Secondary tumours

These are the most common malignant liver tumours and can originate from a primary growth in any part of the body.

PATHOPHYSIOLOGY

Multiple deposits are usually found and may be sited anywhere in the liver. The histology of the cells may indicate the primary site; however, the cancer cells may be anaplastic, giving no indication of their origin.

Box 4.13 Surgical resection of liver tumours

Resection of liver tumours constitutes major surgery. In some cases, complete removal of the tumour may be possible, depending on the site and size of the tumour and on liver function. Resection is contraindicated in patients with extensive liver cirrhosis.

Because the liver has a good capacity to regenerate, following small hepatic lobectomy the prognosis is relatively good if all of the tumour has been resected. More extensive resections carry a higher mortality rate.

The nursing management of a patient following major liver surgery is intensive and should be carried out in a specialist unit.

Box 4.14 Hepatic artery ligation and tumour embolisation

Hepatic artery ligation may give worthwhile palliation in patients with hepatocellular carcinoma. Following ligation, tumour necrosis occurs. This treatment is contraindicated in patients with portal vein obstruction and cirrhosis because of the ensuing massive hepatic necrosis.

Tumour embolisation may also provide worthwhile palliation. During hepatic angiography, a gelatin sponge is injected into the branches of the hepatic artery, causing tumour infarction.

Chemotherapy may also be used; if so, the drug is delivered directly into the tumour to avoid systemic side-effects.

Clinical features are as for primary malignant tumours, with signs of associated cirrhosis. Pain is often the most common symptom for which the patient seeks medical help. The abdomen will become distended due to the enlarged liver, peritoneal invasion and ascites. The patient will have difficulty in bending and is usually anorexic. Jaundice may be present. Weight loss is usually marked.

MEDICAL MANAGEMENT

Diagnosis is by fine-needle aspiration under ultrasound imaging to obtain cells for histology. If the primary site is unknown and causing no symptoms, but there are metastatic deposits in the liver, the patient is not subjected to investigations to locate the primary tumour, as outcome is determined by the spread to the liver.

Treatment must generally be restricted to symptom control, although occasionally a localised metastasis from the colon can be resected.

NURSING PRIORITIES AND MANAGEMENT: CANCER OF THE LIVER

Major patient problems

Nursing management is aimed at symptom control as well as providing the emotional support patients require when facing a terminal illness. Time should be spent with the patient so that she has the opportunity to express her thoughts, fears and anger. As the prognosis of this form of cancer is so poor, this patient may be left with a very short time to put her affairs in order and to prepare herself and her loved ones for her impending death. Her family and friends will also need support from nursing and medical staff.

Initially, the patient may be able to attend to her own needs, and may also be able to return home. However, repeated admission may be necessary for abdominal paracentesis (see Box 4.12). As the disease advances, she will become progressively more dependent on nurses and/or relatives for care. Due to extreme weight loss, much attention is required in maintaining intact pressure areas, and oral hygiene should be given regularly in the hope of preventing moniliasis. At this point, the patient and her family may appreciate the privacy of a single room, but this should not be undertaken without prior discussion with them.

DISORDERS OF THE BILIARY SYSTEM

Q **4.19** With the help of your physiology textbook, review the structure and function of the biliary system.

Cholelithiasis

Cholelithiasis (the presence of gallstones) is the commonest disorder of the biliary tree. It is more prevalent among women than men and its incidence appears to be increasing. In developed countries, at least 20% of women over 40 will develop gallstones. Until about 20 years ago, the most likely person to develop gallstones was an obese woman in her 40s with fair skin ('fair, fat, female and 40'). This categorisation is now considered outdated as, for unknown reasons, gallstones are affecting people at a much younger age.

PATHOPHYSIOLOGY

Gallstones are formed from the constituents of bile salts. There are three main types:

- mixed stones (mainly cholesterol): 80%
- pure cholesterol stones (a 'solitaire' that fills the gall bladder): 10%
- pigmented stones ('jack stones', black and shiny): 2–3%.

Stones vary in size and shape, and may be solitary or multiple. Their colour can vary from yellow to dark brown.

Biliary colic

Gallstones can be asymptomatic but more often they cause biliary colic or an acute or chronic cholecystitis. Cholecystitis can also, less commonly, be caused by trauma and, even more rarely, by tumours.

PATHOPHYSIOLOGY

Biliary colic is caused by a transient obstruction of the gall bladder from an impacted stone.

Common presenting symptoms. The patient complains of a sudden onset of severe gripping pain in the right hypochondrium which often radiates to the back. It can be associated with nausea and vomiting. The pain may vary in intensity and can last for several hours. The pain will ease when the stone either passes into the common bile duct or falls back into the gall bladder.

MEDICAL MANAGEMENT

The patient will recover quickly, but repeated bouts of colic are common. Following investigations a cholecystectomy may be performed.

Acute cholecystitis

PATHOPHYSIOLOGY

It is thought that, in this condition, gallstones irritate the mucous membrane of the gall bladder, which then becomes inflamed.

Common presenting symptoms. The patient presents with an acute illness which is severe in nature. She may be in shock due to pain and vomiting.

A mass may be felt and Murphy's sign (a catching of the breath at the height of inspiration when the gall bladder is palpated) is usually positive. The pain will be severe in the right hypochondrium and may radiate to the right shoulder tip.

Tenderness and guarding of the whole abdomen may be present and the patient may not tolerate examination. Sweating and pallor may be present.

Pyrexia and tachycardia will be present due to infection. Jaundice may be present if there is obstruction of the common bile duct; in this case the patient will have a history of pale stools and dark urine. A history of fatty intolerance may also be given; the pain often starts following a fatty meal.

MEDICAL MANAGEMENT

Investigations. Tests that may be used to establish a diagnosis are as follows:

- blood tests — liver function tests, serum amylase and white blood count
- ultrasound
- CT scanning
- endoscopic retrograde cholangiopancreatography (ERCP)
- intravenous cholangiogram (used occasionally)
- oral cholecystogram (less common).

Ultrasound is now the main investigative procedure for patients with suspected gallstones. It is non-invasive, causes minimal discomfort to the patient and can be used on both jaundiced and non-jaundiced patients. It can identify stones in the gall bladder, thickening of the gall bladder wall and intra- and extrahepatic duct dilatation. It can be done quickly and is relatively inexpensive.

Treatment. Cholecystectomy is indicated in patients with biliary colic or acute cholecystitis and may be undertaken early in the acute admission or as an elective procedure. Antibiotic cover is always given. Moreover, with an 'early' cholecystectomy, the patient is not at risk of further attacks of acute cholecystitis while waiting for elective surgery. Removal of gallstones can also be performed by ERCP and sphincterotomy. In more specialised centres, surgeons are now performing laparoscopic cholecystectomy.

Laparoscopic cholecystectomy. The advantages to the patient of this procedure are:

- reduced stay in hospital
- early mobilisation with lower risk of complications
- minor nature of surgical wounds
- reduced need for opioid analgesics
- speedy return to normal life.

The procedure is performed with the patient under general anaesthetic. The surgeon passes a laparoscope into the abdomen at the umbilicus. The abdomen is then insufflated with CO_2 to allow clear visualisation of the gall bladder.

Three more incisions are made in the region of the right hypochondrium to allow instruments to be manipulated. The cystic artery is identified and ligated. The cystic duct is identified, at which stage an intraoperative cholangiogram can be done to check for stones in the common bile duct. If stones are present, these can be removed.

By careful dissection, the gall bladder is then removed from the liver bed. It is brought to the undersurface of the umbilicus, where the stones are extracted and the gall bladder removed.

All stab wounds are then closed with a subcutaneous suture. On return from theatre, immediate nursing care is as for any routine general anaesthetic.

Free fluids can be given when the patient has fully recovered from the general anaesthetic. Normal diet is commenced the following day. Most patients are discharged on the first or second postoperative day.

For further information, see Johnson (1993).

NURSING PRIORITIES AND MANAGEMENT: ACUTE CHOLECYSTITIS

Immediate concerns

Patients experiencing an acute episode of cholecystitis will be severely ill and will be referred to hospital as quickly as possible after being seen by their GP. The priorities of care while the attack is being managed before surgical intervention include the following:

- administration of an i.m. opiate analgesic at frequent intervals
- hourly recording of vital signs until the patient's condition stabilises
- fasting the patient and commencing i.v. fluids
- careful monitoring of fluid and electrolyte balance
- i.v. administration of a broad-spectrum antibiotic
- if vomiting is persistent a nasogastric tube may be passed and an antiemetic given.

Major patient problems

The patient will be restless due to the pain and will be unable to make herself comfortable. She should be nursed in bed in the most comfortable position for her and given regular analgesics. Fear of pain and of the unknown increases pain (see Ch. 19). It is therefore vital to explain what is happening and to assure the patient that her condition can be treated. When the condition is stable, she should be introduced to her surroundings and given information about the ward.

Once the acute phase has passed, fluids can be given and foods gradually reintroduced. The i.v. infusion may be discontinued when the patient can manage an adequate oral intake. Intravenous antibiotics are usually given for 5 days and then discontinued.

Sweating can be a problem and frequent washes and changes of bedclothes may be necessary to keep the patient comfortable. Oral hygiene should be maintained as necessary.

While the patient is in bed she should be encouraged to change her position at frequent intervals to alleviate pressure. She should be taught gentle leg exercises to prevent deep venous thrombosis. If she can tolerate taking deep breaths to avoid pulmonary complications, she should be encouraged to do so. Smoking should be discouraged.

Perioperative care

Cholecystectomy is carried out on patients with acute cholecystitis to relieve symptoms and prevent complications. Exploration of the common bile duct may be undertaken if there is evidence of stones in the common bile ducts. Open cholecystectomy used to be one of the most common surgical operations, however since the advent of laparoscopic cholecystectomy in 1978, the use of this operation has fallen sharply (Forrest et al 1995).

Nursing care following an open cholecystectomy

In this procedure, the surgeon approaches the gall bladder through a subcostal paramedian or midline incision. An intraoperative cholangiogram is performed to identify any stones in the common bile duct. If stones are present, the surgeon will explore the duct, remove the stones, insert a T-tube and bring the long leg of the tube out through a stab wound in the abdominal wall and then connect it to a drainage bag. It is vital that this tube is not removed accidentally (see Box 4.15). A T-tube cholangiogram is done 8–10 days postoperatively to ensure patency of the duct prior to removal. If the ducts are stone-free, the tube will be removed following instructions from the surgeon (see Fig. 4.11).

Immediate postoperative care is as for any major abdominal surgery requiring general anaesthesia. Adequate analgesia is vital so that the patient can perform deep breathing and coughing exercises to prevent atelectasis and pneumonia. In most cases, the anaesthetist will perform an intercostal nerve block and top it up at regular intervals so that the patient is pain-free. This can be supplemented with i.m. or i.v. analgesia given regularly over the first 24–48 h. The nurse should check at regular intervals that the incision site and surrounding area are numb to ensure the intercostal nerve block is working effectively. The patient should be raised to an upright position and encouraged to do her breathing exercises to prevent pulmonary complications.

There is usually a wound drain inserted into the gall bladder bed. Careful observation of the colour and amount of blood draining

Box 4.15 Management of a T-tube

A T-tube is inserted into the common bile duct following exploration. This tube is necessary as a 'safety valve' because following surgery the duct will become inflamed and oedematous, blocking the flow of bile into the duodenum. Approximately 300–500 mL of bile should drain in the first 24 h. This amount will gradually decrease over the next 8–10 days as the patency of the duct returns. An accurate recording of the amount of bile drainage must be made. The presence of insufficient or excessive bile must be reported. When there is a sudden cessation of bile drainage, a kinked or compressed tube must be suspected.

It is also important to support the bile drainage bag at all times to prevent traction on the tube and accidental removal. An aseptic technique must be used when emptying or changing the bag. Daily cleaning of the skin at the drain site is necessary and the nurse should check for bile leakage from around the tube, inflammation, or excoriation of the skin. Any excess tubing should be coiled and taped to the abdomen. Prior to removal, a T-tube cholangiogram will be done to check the patency of the bile duct and the flow of bile into the duodenum. If the duct is patent, the tube is removed. If there are residual stones in the duct, the T-tube is left in situ. These residual stones may pass spontaneously into the duodenum; otherwise it will be necessary to remove them under X-ray vision.

Prior to performing a T-tube cholangiogram some surgeons ask for the T-tube to be clamped for 24 h. This procedure is, however, becoming less common. If there is any complaint of abdominal pain whilst the tube is clamped, it must be respected and the clamp removed immediately.

The patient will require an analgesic 30 min before the tube is removed. The skin suture is removed and a firm steady pressure applied to the tube. The nurse should observe the amount of bile leakage following removal and apply a sterile dressing. Observation of the patient for any signs of biliary peritonitis should be made for 24 h.

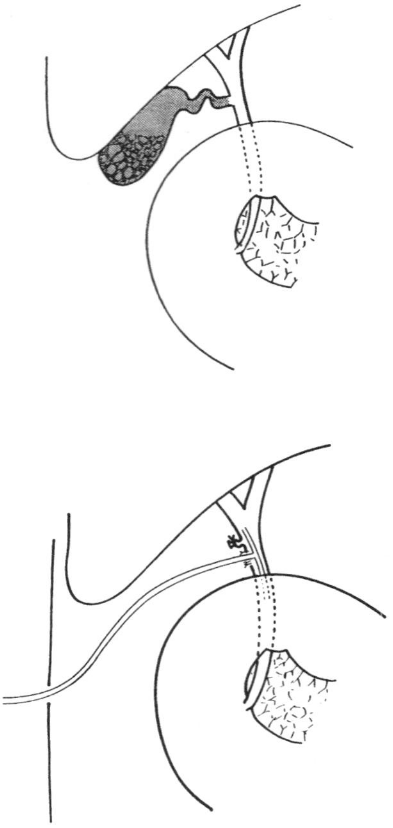

Fig. 4.11 The T-tube in the common bile duct. (Reproduced with kind permission from Forrest et al 1995.)

postoperatively is vital. Excessive drainage of bright red blood must be reported immediately to the surgeon. This drain is usually removed 24–48 h postoperatively.

Other considerations. The patient may be commenced on fluids gradually after the first 24 h (30–60 mL/h). If this is tolerated, free fluids may be commenced. Diet is gradually increased over the next 3 days. A nasogastric tube is not used unless the patient shows signs of paralytic ileus. In this case the patient should be fasted, a nasogastric tube passed and the stomach kept empty.

Sutures are removed 7–10 days postoperatively unless, as has become more common, a subcutaneous suture is used, in which case there will be no need to remove it. If the wound is dry and clean, the dressing can be removed 24–48 h postoperatively and the wound left exposed.

Depending on the patient's fitness and age, she can usually be discharged within 6–10 days. Discharge plans will need to be discussed with relatives or carers. The patient must be instructed to do no heavy lifting for 4–6 weeks to avoid wound herniation. Normal diet is allowed. In an uncomplicated recovery, the patient should be fit to return to work 4–6 weeks later. A detailed discharge summary will be sent to the GP, who will then certify when the patient is fit for work. A follow-up appointment will be given for 4 weeks after discharge so that the surgeon can make sure that the outcome is satisfactory (see Case History 4.3).

Chronic cholecystitis

PATHOPHYSIOLOGY

Chronic cholecystitis is caused by the presence of stones in the gall bladder. In this condition the gall bladder wall becomes thickened and fibrosed.

Common presenting symptoms. The patient may present with biliary colic but more often complains of pain in the right upper quadrant of the abdomen, often following a big meal. There will be a history of fat intolerance, flatulence and heartburn. Abdominal distension may also be a problem following meals.

The pain is less severe than in acute cholecystitis and patients often put up with their symptoms for years before seeking medical advice. In chronic cholecystitis, the patient's general condition must be taken into account, particularly if she is elderly or suffering from other medical conditions which may increase the risks of surgery.

MEDICAL MANAGEMENT

Investigations. Tests and investigations are as for acute cholecystitis.

Treatment. Usually the diseased gall bladder is removed, either by an open cholecystectomy or, more commonly now, by a laparoscopic cholecystectomy.

Case History 4.3 Mrs G

Mrs G had suffered from episodes of cholecystitis and biliary colic for many months before she finally went to her GP. She was a busy mother of three and, as she recounted at a later date, 'There really was no time to be going to the doctor. Besides, the pain always went eventually, especially if my husband rubbed my back up between the shoulder blades.'

Eventually, when she felt so ill that she was forced to stay in bed, she 'gave in'.

The investigations and surgery passed uneventfully in surgical terms, as she had been quite well and free from symptoms at the time of admission. Unlike her sister in London, she had had an open cholecystectomy. It was the first time she had had an operation and, although she thought the nurses were wonderful and had explained everything, she later remarked: 'No one ever tells you just how awful the first day after the operation really is.'

Within 10 days, Mrs G was at home once more, delighted that at least her sutures were dissolvable ones. She knew that she must not do too much lifting and that although she should have a normal diet, she should avoid fatty foods as they might make her feel 'squeamish'. 'It's like only having weak washing-up liquid to deal with greasy dishes instead of good concentrated liquid,' she explained to a friend.

Three weeks after discharge, she visited the doctor. She was quite distressed and reported the following problems: 'I keep having episodes of diarrhoea and I'm so tired. No one said who was going to do the hoovering or put the shopping away in those high cupboards. The family think I'm back to normal because the wound is healed but I am so tired still. Everything is an effort.'

For further information, see Smith (1992).

Choledocholithiasis

Stones in the bile duct occur in about 10–15% of patients with gallstones.

PATHOPHYSIOLOGY

Common presenting symptoms. Colicky pain occurs if the stones impede the flow of bile through the sphincter of Oddi. Impaction of a stone at the sphincter will cause jaundice. The patient will have pale, fatty stools and dark urine. Some stones will clear spontaneously following passage into the small intestine.

If the stone becomes impacted, the bile duct will become dilated. Infection can cause cholangitis with rigors, severe pain and jaundice. Acute pancreatitis may develop due to obstruction of the sphincter of Oddi and reflux of bile salts into the pancreatic ducts (see p. 126).

MEDICAL MANAGEMENT

Investigations are as for acute and chronic cholecystitis.

Treatment. Removal of the stones via ERCP and sphincterotomy to allow the stones to pass freely into the small intestine will be carried out either prior to surgery or in cases where surgery is contraindicated.

For further information, see Garden (1997).

Tumours of the biliary tract

Cancer of the gall bladder

PATHOPHYSIOLOGY

This is a rare cancer and is nearly always related to gallstones. It is more common in females than in males. Signs and symptoms are consistent with those for gallstones and a history of persistent obstructive jaundice may be present. A mass may be palpable. In most cases, surgery is not a chosen treatment and survival rates are poor. Eighty per cent of gall bladder tumours are adenocarcinomas. As with other tumours, the involvement of lymph nodes and the presence of metastases will determine the patient's prognosis.

Cancer of the bile duct (cholangiocarcinoma)

PATHOPHYSIOLOGY

The cause of bile duct cancer is unknown. It is more common in the elderly, and men are affected more than women. It is a rare cancer but its incidence appears to be increasing. Tumours can arise from the intra- or extrahepatic biliary tree. Direct spread and metastases are present in at least half of the patients who go for surgery.

MEDICAL MANAGEMENT

Treatment. As cancer of the bile ducts carries a poor prognosis, treatment is usually in the form of palliative therapy. Jaundice is a very distressing symptom and if this is not treated the patient may die from liver failure.

For some patients, palliation can be achieved by the insertion of a stent, either by ERCP or by percutaneous transhepatic techniques (PTC). In a few cases where the tumour is at the lower end of the common bile duct, a radical resection in the form of a Whipple resection may be possible (see Fig. 4.12). This is major surgery and should be considered only if the tumour is localised and if the patient is fit for surgery.

Tumours of the upper biliary tract are resectable in only 10% of cases. Following resection of the tumour, a Roux loop of jejunum is anastomosed to the biliary tract or, in some cases, the left hepatic duct. A hepaticojejunostomy then restores the continuity of

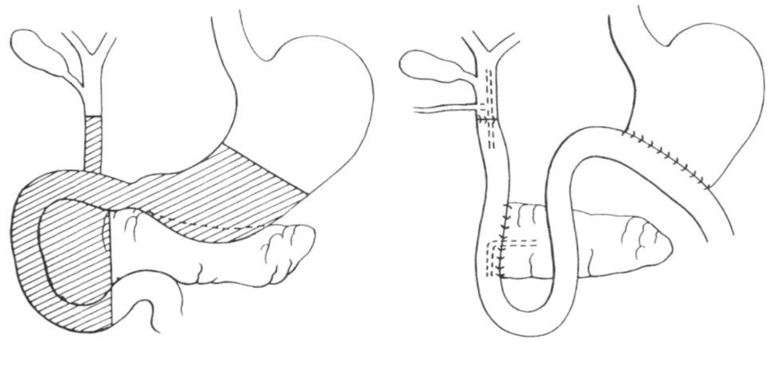

Fig. 4.12 Whipple's procedure. This extensive procedure involves resection of the head of the pancreas, the duodenum and the antrum of the stomach, as well as removal of the gall bladder. Reconstruction is carried out with choledochojejunostomy, pancreatojejunostomy and gastrojejunostomy. This is a major operation which carries a relatively high mortality rate. Leakage from the anastomosis, abscess formation and fistula are the main complications. (Reproduced with kind permission from Forrest et al 1995.)

the small intestine. A hepaticojejunostomy can also be performed to bypass the tumour and achieve palliation. Radiotherapy and chemotherapy have not been shown to improve survival.

NURSING PRIORITIES AND MANAGEMENT: CHOLANGIOCARCINOMA

The patient with a diagnosis of cholangiocarcinoma will require specialised nursing care. Only a few of these patients will be considered for major resection, following which they should be cared for in a high-dependency ward or an intensive care unit. In some cases the patient is prepared for major resection but at the time of surgery it is discovered that only a bypass of the tumour may be carried out safely. These patients are usually devastated by this turn of events and require a great deal of support. Following palliation, jaundice will subside and the patient's appetite will improve. For a few months the patient may feel so well that she becomes unrealistic about the prognosis. Few patients survive more than a year following palliation. Following resection, the outlook is better. Good family support is necessary. It is important to take an honest approach and to give explanations to the patient and her family as they request it. It will be necessary to spend time with the patient and her relatives to answer their questions and offer support. Close communication with the GP is also important so that community care can be provided when necessary.

DISORDERS OF THE PANCREAS

Pancreatitis

Inflammation of the pancreatic gland may be acute or chronic. Acute pancreatitis can range from mild oedema to severe necrosis and haemorrhage. Following an attack, the gland returns to normal. Chronic pancreatitis is associated with permanent anatomical and functional abnormality. The patient usually suffers from relapsing attacks with relative good health between episodes.

Acute pancreatitis

Acute pancreatitis can be life-threatening, with approximately 1 in 4 presenting with severe disease; of these, 1 in 4 will die (Forrest et al 1995). It can affect all adult groups. In the UK its two main causes are gallstones and excessive alcohol consumption. Other causes are infection, trauma, drugs (e.g. steroids), hyperparathyroidism, hyperlipidaemia, pancreatic cancer and investigation procedures. ERCP is now the third defined cause of pancreatitis in modern practice (Garden 1997).

PATHOPHYSIOLOGY

The pancreatic enzymes trypsin and lipase, which are normally activated in the duodenum, are prematurely activated within the pancreas, causing autodigestion of the gland. This autodigestion leads to varying degrees of oedema, haemorrhage, necrosis, abscess and cyst formation in and around the pancreas. Spasm of the sphincter of Oddi with reflux of duodenal contents into the pancreatic duct is thought to be an important factor in this enzyme activation. Gallstones and alcohol are two contributing factors to spasm. Passage of stones down the common bile duct may also promote reflux of infected bile along the pancreatic duct when these ducts form a common channel to the ampulla of Vater.

Activated enzymes such as trypsinogen and chymotrypsinogen, phospholipase, elastase and catalase are responsible for increased capillary permeability. This permits large volumes of fluid to escape into the peritoneal and retroperitoneal cavity, causing damage to the surrounding tissue. This severe loss of circulating fluid leads to hypovolaemic shock and predisposes the individual to acute renal failure, which may result from local intravascular coagulation in the renal vascular bed. Development of pulmonary oedema with left-sided pleural effusion may result from release of toxins. The release of lipase causes fat necrosis in the omentum and areas adjacent to the pancreas. Calcium soaps become sequestered in areas of fatty necrosis, which may result in the development of hypocalcaemia.

MEDICAL MANAGEMENT

History and examination. The patient usually presents with epigastric pain of acute onset radiating to the back, associated with nausea and vomiting. She may have a history of biliary tract disease or alcohol abuse.

Acute pancreatitis is often associated with severe shock. There may be signs of dehydration with rapid pulse and respiration, hypotension and pyrexia. Marked abdominal tenderness is usually present in the upper abdomen, which may appear distended. Bruising around the umbilicus (Cullen's sign) and in the loin region (Grey Turner's sign) are rare late manifestations of acute pancreatitis. ***Investigations*** include blood analysis, urinalysis, X-ray ultrasound and CT scan, as follows:

- Serum lipase is one of the most reliable markers of acute pancreatitis.
- A serum amylase of above 1000 IU/L in the past 48 h is strongly suggestive of acute pancreatitis. Normal levels are 100–300 IU/L. Urinary amylase can remain elevated for 10–14 days.
- Plain X-ray films of the abdomen can reveal distended loops of small bowel with paralytic ileus. Chest X-ray may reveal left-sided pleural effusion.
- Urea and electrolyte levels are important indicators of the state of hydration and are necessary for the correct management of the patient.
- A raised white blood cell count ($9–20 \times 10^9$/L) reveals an active inflammatory process.
- Hyperglycaemia and glycosuria are often present but are transient.
- Arterial blood gases may reveal severe hypoxia.
- Abdominal ultrasound and CT scan are used to detect the presence of peripancreatic collections and pancreatic necrosis.

Treatment

Conservative management. Acute pancreatitis is usually managed conservatively; for mild attacks, treatment is generally symptomatic. The principles of management are as follows:

- *Pain relief.* This is usually provided in the form of opiate analgesics. Morphine and pethidine can cause some spasm at the sphincter of Oddi, but they are frequently prescribed and are effective (Forrest et al 1991).
- *Correction of shock.* If haemorrhagic pancreatitis is diagnosed, shock is treated by the administration of large volumes of crystalloids, plasma, dextran or blood in order to maintain circulatory blood volume and adequate urine output. Oxygen therapy is essential to correct the associated hypoxia. Po_2 saturation levels should be monitored. Hypoxaemia may develop insidiously such that respiratory failure (ARDS) can develop. Arterial blood gases are closely monitored in case ventilatory support is required (see Chs 2, 18 and 29).
- *Suppression of pancreatic function.* The patient is fasted to decrease stimulation of pancreatic enzymes and a nasogastric tube is passed if the patient is vomiting persistently.

- *Controlling infection.* When there is evidence of infection, a broad-spectrum antibiotic is prescribed. For the majority of patients this supportive treatment will settle the acute attack and surgical treatment will not be necessary. If there is any doubt about the diagnosis, a laparotomy may need to be performed to exclude other causes of peritonitis, such as perforated peptic ulcer and mesenteric ischaemia.
- *Monitoring blood glucose levels.* This must be performed as secondary diabetes can sometimes develop, requiring insulin therapy.
- *Monitoring cardiac status.* This will be required if electrolyte derangement is such as to cause potentially lethal dysrhythmias.

Surgical intervention. At an early stage in management, gallstones as a cause of the acute attack are excluded by ultrasound scanning. Cholecystectomy during the course of the patient's admission is now advocated to avoid recurrent problems following discharge. Patients with gallstone pancreatitis can usually be identified by their slow clinical progress and by the use of various clinical and biochemical prognosis factors.

Early ERCP may demonstrate the presence of stones in the common bile duct, which can be extracted by a small balloon catheter or basket following sphincterotomy. The complication of peripancreatic necrosis or abscess can be detected by radiological imaging (see Appendix 1). Most patients will require necrosectomy (i.e. the removal of necrotic tissues) and drainage at laparotomy. It may be wise to put in place a gastrostomy and jejunostomy tube at this time, as recovery is slow and the patient may require prolonged nutritional support (see Ch. 21).

NURSING PRIORITIES AND MANAGEMENT: ACUTE PANCREATITIS

Major considerations (see Case History 4.4)

The care of patients with acute pancreatitis will vary according to the severity of the attack. Some individuals present with vague abdominal pain which resolves quickly. More often, patients present with severe epigastric pain, often radiating to the back, and with vomiting and shock. It should be borne in mind that the severity of the attack is not always easily judged by an initial assessment and that these patients therefore require close observation.

Priorities of nursing care are:

- to relieve pain and promote comfort (See Nursing Care Plan 4.2)
- to monitor vital functions
- to restore and maintain haemodynamic status, i.e. to restore volume deficit, correct electrolyte imbalance and correct impaired gaseous exchange
- to restore and maintain adequate nutrition
- to prevent or minimise potential complications (see Box 4.16)
- to prevent the development of pressure sores
- to maintain the nasogastric tube (if present) and provide frequent mouthwashes and oral hygiene
- to monitor blood sugar level in order to detect secondary diabetes
- to support the patient in maintaining personal hygiene
- to help the patient to be up and about as early as possible.

As the patient's general condition improves, clear oral fluids can be introduced, gradually progressing to a light diet.

An episode of pancreatitis can be a very traumatic time for both the patient and her family, who may have been unaware of the important functions that the pancreas performs. It is important to explain the rationale of all procedures and investigations carefully to alleviate anxiety. Showing the patient diagrams can be very helpful. The patient may be very worried about her work, family and financial situation, and a visit from the social worker may be of value. Patients with alcohol-associated acute pancreatitis may, with their consent, be referred for counselling to address their dependency problem (see Ch. 36).

It is important to reduce the noise level on the hospital ward to a minimum to allow patients to get adequate sleep (see Ch. 25). It may be advisable to give some form of night sedation. Restricting visits by family and friends to short periods during the day will reduce the strain on the patient during visiting hours. Communication with the family is of course vital. On the patient's admission to the ward, the nurse should introduce himself to the relatives and give a full explanation of what has occurred. Medical staff should be available to give regular updates on the patient's condition.

Case History 4.4 — Mr N (see also Nursing Care Plan 4.2)

Mr N, aged 36, is admitted with a history of sudden, central abdominal pain which is only partially relieved by sitting forward and hugging his knees. He describes the pain as 'boring through his back'. His skin is pale and clammy and his respirations rapid and shallow, his pulse is rapid and there is marked hypotension. Mr N is clearly in an advancing state of shock. In addition, he is nauseated and repeated vomiting has led to increasing dehydration, exacerbating his shocked state.

Further considerations

When the acute episode has resolved, and if gallstones are present, an early elective cholecystectomy with possible exploration of the common bile duct will be undertaken.

If the attack has been due to alcohol, the patient must be advised prior to discharge to abstain totally or risk a life-threatening recurrence. Advice regarding return to work is important. The patient often feels tired and it is often advisable for her not to return to work for perhaps 4–6 weeks. The patient will be reviewed in the outpatient clinic initially at 3–4 weeks. A detailed account of her management will be sent to the GP so that continuity of care can be maintained.

For further information, see Garden (1997).

Chronic pancreatitis

Chronic pancreatitis is a relatively rare condition in the UK but its incidence is increasing due to the increase in alcohol consumption.

However, the mechanism by which alcohol damages the pancreas is poorly understood.

PATHOPHYSIOLOGY

Chronic pancreatitis leads to permanent damage of the gland with replacement by fibrotic tissue and calcification. The ducts become narrowed and the flow of pancreatic juice is obstructed. The cells slowly stop secreting pancreatic juice. The obstructed ducts can give rise to recurrent attacks of pancreatitis lasting a few days.

Nursing Care Plan 4.2 Care of a patient with acute pancreatitis. (See Case History 4.4): The management of pain

Nursing consideration	*Action*	*Rationale*	*Desired outcome*
1. *Pain* Mr N has severe and potentially excruciating pain due to autodigestion of the pancreas, the 'chemical burn' of pancreatic exudate, inflammation, and distension caused by an adynamic bowel	❐ Rapidly assess and then monitor verbal and non-verbal evidence of pain, noting factors that either aggravate or ease the pain	To assist in achieving effective pain relief	Mr N's pain is relieved, as evidenced by the verbal communication, body relaxation and corresponding changes in vital signs
	❐ Give the prescribed analgesic	All opiates may cause some spasm of the sphincter of Oddi, but they are very effective (Forrest et al 1995). As analgesia is achieved, smaller and less frequent doses may be given	
	❐ Give other adjuvant medication, e.g. antibiotic therapy, sedative agents, H_2 antagonists, antiemetics	Such agents may be used to help control the acute attack and associated symptoms, particularly pain	
	❐ Pass an NG tube and aspirate stomach contents	This will relieve the pain associated with distension and minimise pancreatic stimulation	
	❐ Position Mr N as comfortably as possible, minimising any unnecessary activity	Pain will be minimised, as will Mr N's metabolic rate and pancreatic activity	

Common presenting symptoms. The patient usually presents with a history of severe epigastric pain, often radiating to the back. The pain is often eased by bending forward. Nausea and vomiting may also be present. A history of recent alcohol abuse may be given.

Q **4.20** Why might bending forward ease the pain in chronic pancreatitis?

Weight loss is common and may be due to the pain or to malnutrition associated with alcohol. Malabsorption is also present as a result of pancreatic insufficiency. The stool may be pale and offensive and difficult to flush away. This type of bowel movement is known as steatorrhoea and is due to a high undigested fat content. It is often a distressing feature for the patient.

Diabetes mellitus develops in approximately one-third of these patients and may require treatment. Transient jaundice may be present due to inflammation of the head of the pancreas, which obstructs the common bile duct. The presence of jaundice may be upsetting for some people, who feel 'dirty' or 'old' due to the discoloration of the skin and the marked yellowness of the sclera.

MEDICAL MANAGEMENT

Investigations. Clinical assessment is as follows:

- plain abdominal X-ray may show speckled calcification of the pancreas
- ultrasound scan and CT scan may show an enlarged, swollen gland
- ERCP is performed to outline the pancreatic duct if surgery is contemplated
- faecal fat estimation may reveal malabsorption
- fasting blood sugars are assessed and a glucose tolerance test may be necessary.

Treatment. Management of chronic pancreatitis is mainly symptomatic. The patient should be advised to stop drinking alcohol and may need professional counselling to this end. Replacement of pancreatic enzymes with a commercial preparation may help to alleviate the steatorrhoea and reduce pain. Good control of diabetes will be necessary.

Pain control can be difficult, since some of these patients are addicted to opiates. Help from a pain control specialist is valuable. In a small number of patients in whom severe pain persists, surgery will be indicated. It may be necessary to resect the head of the gland (Whipple's procedure; see Fig. 4.12) or the body and tail (distal pancreatectomy). Adequate drainage of the duct (pancreatojejunostomy) may be undertaken where ERCP shows the pancreatic duct to be dilated. A total pancreatectomy is rarely undertaken due to the consequent permanent diabetes and exocrine insufficiency.

NURSING PRIORITIES AND MANAGEMENT: CHRONIC PANCREATITIS

Nursing management of an acute attack in relapsing pancreatitis is similar to that for acute pancreatitis.

Major patient problems

Pain

Pain is often constant in nature, radiating through to the back. It is often described as being like a sharp knife twisting in the gut and presents a major challenge to pain control. Assisting the patient into a comfortable position often helps. The patient may find that bending forward while leaning on a bed table helps. The use of a heat pad to the back may give some relief, and NSAIDs such as diclofenac sodium (Voltarol) in suppository form can be of value. It is often necessary to use opioid drugs to alleviate pain or it may be necessary to seek advice from a pain specialist. Many hospitals now have pain teams that can advise on all aspects of pain management.

Box 4.16 Complications of acute pancreatitis

Pancreatic pseudocyst
This condition develops in about 10% of patients following acute pancreatitis or an exacerbation of chronic pancreatitis. A pseudocyst is a sac containing pancreatic juice, debris and blood within a lining of inflammatory tissue, directly connecting with a pancreatic duct. Small pseudocysts are often asymptomatic, but large cysts can compress surrounding structures, often causing pain, nausea, vomiting and, occasionally, obstructive jaundice. A raised serum amylase will be present. Ultrasound scan can be used in diagnosis and monitoring. Surgery is necessary if the cyst is symptomatic, since there is a danger that it may rupture or precipitate haemorrhage. Surgery consists of drainage of the pseudocyst into the stomach (cyst gastrostomy) or duodenum (cyst duodenostomy).

Pancreatic abscess
This is a more serious complication of acute pancreatitis. The patient is usually very ill, with pyrexia, a raised white blood cell count and tachycardia. Early diagnosis by CT scanning and the use of aggressive surgical intervention have improved mortality rates. Surgery consists of extensive drainage and debridement of infected tissues. Multiple large drains are used to drain the abscess cavity. Peritoneal lavage with normal saline 0.9% warmed to body temperature can be used to irrigate the cavity. Adequate nutrition following surgery is vital. Most surgeons establish a feeding jejunostomy and gastrostomy tube during surgery.

Pancreatic necrosis
This complication is a major cause of death in acute pancreatitis. Early diagnosis is essential. The patient often fails to improve with conservative management. A persistent pyrexia, raised white blood cell count, tachycardia, hypotension and poor respiratory function are ominous signs. At laparotomy, necrotic tissue is removed, peritoneal lavage is carried out and the pancreatic bed adequately drained. A feeding jejunostomy and gastrostomy tube are inserted.

In some cases, the surgeon may opt to leave the wound open to allow for packing of the wound and to minimise the need for repeated laparotomies to deal with recurrent intra-abdominal sepsis.

Duodenal ileus
Due to persistent pancreatic inflammation, duodenal ileus may persist. Nutritional status will need to be maintained either by parenteral means or by jejunostomy feeding. A gastroenterostomy may need to be performed.

Haemorrhage
Severe bleeding may occur from gastric or duodenal ulceration. Prophylactic i.v. cimetidine is given to patients with acute pancreatitis. On rare occasions, haemorrhage may occur into a pseudocyst or by erosion of a blood vessel by the inflammatory process.

Alcohol dependency

Alcohol abuse is the most common cause of chronic pancreatitis. Total abstinence will help to resolve the pain. If the patient has had a recent 'binge', sudden withdrawal may precipitate delirium tremens. Mild sedation is frequently used to prevent this. Expert help may be necessary to assist the patient to overcome her alcohol problem.

Patient education is vital in view of the progressive destruction of the gland by this disease. Family life is usually already disrupted by the patient's alcohol abuse, and help from a social worker will be useful in assisting the patient and her family to cope with the situation. Good liaison with the GP is important so that support can be continued in the community. Caring for these patients can present a professional and personal challenge to members of the multidisciplinary team, who may feel inclined to blame the patient for her illness (see Ch. 36).

The patient's nutritional intake must be assessed. The patient is weighed and a well-balanced diet low in fat is given once the acute attack has resolved. Pancreatic enzyme supplements can be prescribed and taken prior to meals to aid absorption of nutrients. This should also alleviate the steatorrhoea. Concurrent administration of an H_2-receptor antagonist may improve the efficacy of these supplements.

Cancer of the pancreas

Tumours of the pancreas can arise from exocrine or endocrine tissue. Benign tumours are very rare. Insulinoma arises from the islet cells and results in oversecretion of insulin, causing hypoglycaemia. Gastrinomas also arise from the islet of Langerhans cells, secreting gastrin and giving rise to Zollinger–Ellison syndrome. Adenocarcinoma is by far the most common malignant tumour of the exocrine pancreas.

The cause of pancreatic cancer is unknown, but smoking and a high-fat, high-protein diet are thought to increase the risk. It is twice as common in men as in women and its incidence is increasing; over 6000 people die from pancreatic cancer in the UK each year (Garden 1997). It is the fourth most common cause of cancer deaths in men in the UK and the sixth most common in women. It mainly affects individuals aged 50–70 years.

PATHOPHYSIOLOGY

Adenocarcinoma of the pancreas arises from the ductal tissue and is more commonly located in the head of the gland. Lesions frequently obstruct the pancreatic duct, causing chronic pancreatitis. The carcinoma can also obstruct the bile duct, giving rise to obstructive jaundice. Cancer of the pancreas carries a poor prognosis because the disease has often spread to nearby organs by the time a diagnosis is made. Surgical resection has not been shown to improve the rate of survival. However, cancer of the duodenum, lower bile duct and periampullary regions often present earlier with obstructive jaundice, and surgical resection offers a much better prognosis.

Common presenting symptoms. Jaundice is often the symptom with which the patient first presents to her GP. The urine is dark in colour, the stool pale and fatty, and the skin and sclera have a yellowish tinge. Severe itch can be a very distressing symptom.

Severe weight loss and anorexia are associated with vague epigastric pain, often radiating to the back. Initially pain is intermittent, but gradually it becomes constant and severe.

MEDICAL MANAGEMENT

Investigations are as follows:

- blood is taken for liver function tests and to check for the presence of a coagulation defect
- an ultrasound scan will detect a dilated biliary tree and exclude the presence of gallstones
- a CT scan may demonstrate a pancreatic mass, local invasion by tumour, or metastases

- pancreatic tissue may be obtained for cytology by using CT scan or ultrasound-guided fine-needle aspiration
- ERCP can be used to define the site of obstruction and obtain biopsies.

Treatment. Relief of obstructive jaundice and pain control are all that can be offered to the majority of patients with pancreatic cancer. ERCP with stenting of the biliary tree can relieve obstructive jaundice and may reduce the necessity for surgical intervention. Chemotherapy has been used but appears to have little effect. Surgery is usually palliative but jaundice may be relieved by cholecystojejunostomy or choledochojejunostomy.

In a minority of cases, pancreatoduodenal resection (Whipple's procedure) may be worthwhile, if the tumour is less than 2 cm in diameter and confined to the head of the pancreas (see Fig. 4.12).

NURSING PRIORITIES AND MANAGEMENT: CANCER OF THE PANCREAS

Investigative procedures are extensive and surgery in the majority of cases only offers palliation. The nurse has a very important role in helping the patient and her family to cope during this very difficult time.

Major patient problems

Anxiety

Patients with pancreatic cancer are usually very anxious. They may have no previous history of illness and often deny the diagnosis. They are often the breadwinner in the family and may even be approaching retirement. They may have difficulty coming to terms with the diagnosis and are often angry and withdrawn, especially with close family members. Relatives often feel shut out and helpless. The nurse can help by offering support and advice to both the patient and the family members, who should be encouraged to discuss the illness and its implications.

Extensive discussion with the patient and her relatives prior to surgery is necessary. Some patients are prepared for a Whipple's procedure but then at surgery it is found that the disease is more extensive than expected and a bypass is all that can be safely attempted. This is devastating for the patient and her family, who will have built up hopes for recovery.

Pain

Pain is often persistent, particularly when the disease is at an advanced stage. Oral opioids may be given and titrated to the patient's specific needs. Progression to s.c. diamorphine may be necessary as the disease advances and an oral laxative will also be given to prevent the side-effect of constipation.

As the disease advances, pain may become more difficult to control. A coeliac plexus nerve block may also be of benefit.

Close monitoring of the effectiveness of pain control is essential to ensure that the best possible quality of life can be maintained for the patient (see Ch. 19). If the patient is discharged home, liaison with the primary health care team is essential to ensure that full continuity of care is achieved. As the condition of the patient deteriorates, a decision will be taken as to the best care option available (see Ch. 33).

Jaundice

Jaundice (see p. 114) is usually persistent and accompanied by severe pruritus. The itching is usually all over the body and the patient often scratches until the skin bleeds. She may be so distressed by it that she thinks it will drive her mad. Every effort should be made to relieve itching which is believed to be caused by a deposition of bile salts in the skin. Antihistamines are used but they can cause sedation. A twice-daily bath with added sodium bicarbonate is very effective. Calamine lotion or Eurax cream applied locally may help. Night sedation is important as itching is often worse at night.

Following ERCP and stenting, the jaundice and itch will subside over 7–10 days. The patient will feel much better as soon as the itch disappears and as the jaundice fades.

Anorexia and weight loss

Poor appetite and subsequent weight loss are further distressing aspects of the disease. Meals should be small and attractively presented. Liaison with the dietician is necessary. High-protein drinks between meals may be tolerated well. If weight loss is severe, special care should be taken to prevent the development of pressure sores. Malaise associated with anorexia and weight loss will increase the patient's dependency; nurses and other carers will need to offer more and more assistance with many aspects of daily life (see Box 4.17).

For further reading on cancer care, see David (1995).

DISORDERS OF THE SPLEEN

Trauma

The spleen is highly vascular and is one of the organs most frequently damaged by abdominal trauma. In 20% of patients who present with splenic injury, associated rib fractures are found on X-ray examination. The spleen is particularly susceptible to injury when pathologically enlarged.

PATHOPHYSIOLOGY

Injury to the spleen can result in rupture, evulsion from its pedicle or tearing beneath the capsule, with possible formation of a subcapsular haematoma.

Delayed rupture of the spleen occurs in about 5% of patients and is thought to be caused by haematoma bursting through the capsule wall. This usually occurs within 2 weeks of injury, but in a few cases can be delayed for months or even years.

Box 4.17 Reversal of cancer cachexia in pancreatic cancer

Cancer cachexia is characterised by numerous metabolic abnormalities which would appear to be driven by cytokines such as interleukin-6 and also, perhaps, specific tumour-derived factors (McNamara et al 1992). The resulting alterations in energy balance and loss of lean tissue very much impair the individual's quality of life and shorten survival.

Conventional nutritional supplements for cachexia have failed to demonstrate any significant benefit in terms of nutritional status. While previous studies have shown that the administration of oral eicosapentaenoic acid (EPA) will stabilise weight in patients with advanced cancer, a recent pilot study undertaken by Barber et al (1999) combining EPA with a conventional nutritional supplement has demonstrated that this combination may indeed reverse cachexia in advanced pancreatic cancer.

Common presenting symptoms. Rupture and evulsion of the spleen cause immediate intraperitoneal bleeding. As blood spreads throughout the peritoneal cavity, signs of haemorrhage and hypovolaemic shock may develop. Patients generally present as an acute abdominal emergency.

The patient experiences abdominal pain with particular tenderness in the left upper quadrant. Referred pain is often felt in the left shoulder tip. Bruising to the abdomen may or may not be evident.

MEDICAL MANAGEMENT

Treatment. Injury to the spleen is an indication for splenectomy, provided the organ cannot be conserved. The tendency now is to conserve splenic tissue if at all possible by suturing capsular tears or by performing a partial splenectomy. This is because of the risk of systemic infection following splenectomy (Forrest et al 1995). Another method used following injury is to wrap the spleen in an absorbable haemostatic mesh.

NURSING PRIORITIES AND MANAGEMENT: TRAUMA

General considerations

The patient may be in a distressed and anxious state and reassurance should be given by the nurse. Holding the patient's hand and offering encouragement may help to relieve some of the anxiety, whilst measures should be taken by medical and nursing staff to establish and administer i.v. fluids along with blood and blood products as required. Oxygen therapy is commenced to raise the circulating levels and a urinary catheter is inserted to assess renal function. Blood pressure, pulse, respirations and Po_2 saturations should be closely monitored and any changes reported quickly. A nasogastric tube may be passed to empty the stomach contents and prevent aspiration. Analgesics to relieve pain should be given and their effect monitored.

Relatives should be kept informed of what is happening and comfort and support given during this stressful and worrying time.

Perioperative care

Any clotting defect which may be present is rectified and, once the patient's condition has stabilised, she is prepared for surgery. Close observation of the patient is required throughout this period. If at all possible, it is helpful to allow close relatives to see the patient before surgery as this may relieve a little of both their and the patient's anxiety. Postoperative care is as for abdominal surgery requiring general anaesthesia and the patient will usually be nursed in a high-dependency area (see Nursing Care Plans 26.2, p. 816, and 26.4, p. 820).

Non-acute presentation

Not all patients present with splenic injury in such a dramatic way. If a diagnosis is difficult to establish and splenic injury is suspected, vigilant and careful observation of the patient is vital. The patient will be admitted to hospital for close observation, which includes frequent monitoring of blood pressure, pulse, respiration and Po_2 saturations. Any pain experienced by the patient should be monitored, noting its site, type and duration. Whether the pain is increasing or decreasing may be relevant. Analgesics may initially be withheld, as they may mask the true situation. The patient will be fasted during this period of observation and should be given frequent oral hygiene.

Any change in the patient's condition should be reported immediately as, following rupture, temporary improvement in the patient's condition may precede sudden deterioration.

Hypersplenism

Hypersplenism is a syndrome consisting of splenomegaly and pancytopenia. The bone marrow is normal and no autoimmune disease is present.

PATHOPHYSIOLOGY

Primary hypersplenism is due to hypertrophy of the spleen as a response to the need to destroy abnormal blood cells. Secondary hypersplenism occurs when inappropriate cell destruction is secondary to splenic enlargement; this condition may complicate inflammatory disorders such as rheumatic fever and malaria.

In portal hypertension, splenic congestion frequently leads to splenomegaly and hypersplenism. Other conditions causing splenic enlargement are haemolytic anaemias, idiopathic thrombocytopenic purpura, myelofibrosis and lymphomas. Tumours, cysts and splenic abscesses are rarely found.

Clinical features. The effects of hypersplenism include expansion of the blood volume to fill the increased vascular spaces. There is increased pooling of blood in the cells with excessive destruction, possibly induced by metabolic damage as the cells are packed tightly together in the enlarged spleen. Increased amounts of urobilinogen are present in the urine. Blood analysis will show anaemia, leucopenia and thrombocytopenia, and marrow turnover will be increased.

MEDICAL MANAGEMENT

Splenectomy may be undertaken in many of these conditions, although removal of a grossly enlarged spleen carries an appreciable risk. Close liaison is necessary between the haematologist and the surgeon.

NURSING PRIORITIES AND MANAGEMENT: HYPERSPLENISM

Perioperative care

In preparation for elective splenectomy, a full assessment of the patient's blood count and coagulation status must be made. In the presence of any bleeding tendency, a transfusion of blood or platelets may be administered. In patients with thrombocytopenia, platelets should be made available for use to cover the intra- and postoperative phase.

An anti-pneumococcal vaccine is given to prevent or minimise chest infection postoperatively. The H. Influenza Type B vaccine is also given prophylactically.

Preparation for surgery is as for abdominal surgery requiring general anaesthesia. A nasogastric tube is passed because of handling of the stomach during surgery and the subsequent risk of aspiration of stomach contents.

In the postoperative period, the physiotherapist plays an important role in the care of these patients because of the increased risk of collapse of the left lower lobe of the lung. The nurse must encourage the patient to perform deep breathing exercises and aid expectoration between physiotherapy sessions. Some doctors advise the administration of low-dose heparin in all patients undergoing splenectomy as there will be a transient increase in platelet and leucocyte levels. The nurse must therefore be aware of the importance of passive exercises whilst the patient is on bed rest and encourage movement and early ambulation. Another complication which can follow splenectomy is pancreatitis caused by the handling and bruising of the tail of the pancreas during surgery. Therefore the nurse must be alert to any change in the patient's condition, especially any increase or change in the nature of the pain experienced.

Due to the loss of lymphoid tissue, there is an increased risk of infection. As most infections occur within 3 years of splenectomy, some surgeons advise the use of prophylactic penicillin for this period, or even longer. This cover is mandatory when the patient is a child.

REFERENCES

Annesse V, Basciani M, Perri F et al 1996 Controlled trial of botulinum toxin versus placebo and pneumatic dilatation in achalasia. Gastroenterology 111: 1418–1424

Attard A R, Corlett M J, Kidner N J, Leslie A P, Fraser I A 1992 Safety of early pain relief for acute abdominal pain. British Medical Journal 305(6853): 554–556

Barber M D, Ross J A, Voss A C, Tisdale M J, Fearon K C H 1999 The effect of an oral nutritional supplement enriched with fish oil on weight loss in patients with pancreatic cancer. British Journal of Cancer 81(1): 80–86

Blair C, Hayes P 1997 Hepatitis C. Current concepts. Proceedings of the Royal College of Physicians of Edinburgh 27: 300–310

Burkitt D P 1971 Epidemiology of cancer of the colon and rectum. Cancer 28: 3–13

Burkitt H G, Quick C R G, Gatt D 1996 Essential surgery: problems, diagnosis and management, 2nd edn. Churchill Livingstone, Edinburgh

Bynum T E 1991 Non acid mechanisms of gastric and duodenal ulcer formation. (Review). Journal of Clinical Gastroenterology 13(suppl. 2): S56–64

Camilleri M, Choi M 1997 Review article: irritable bowel syndrome. Alimentary Pharmacology and Therapeutics 11: 3–15

Chen C, Yu M, Liaw Y 1997 Epidemiological characteristics and risk factors of hepatocellular carcinoma. Journal of Gastroenterology and Hepatology 12(9–10): S294–308

Cuilliere C, Ducrotte F, Metman E et al 1997 Achalasia: outcome of patients treated with intersphincteric injection of botulinum toxin. Gut 41: 87–92

David J 1995 Cancer care. Chapman and Hall, London

Forrest A P M, Carter D C, McLeod I B 1991 Principles and practice of surgery, 2nd edn. Churchill Livingstone, Edinburgh

Forrest A P M, Carter D C, McLeod I B 1995 Principles and practice of surgery, 3rd edn. Churchill Livingstone, Edinburgh

Garden O J 1997 (ed) Hepatobiliary and pancreatic surgery. WB Saunders, London

Griffin S M, Raimes S A 1997 Upper gastrointestinal surgery. WB Saunders, London

Gore R M 1997 Oesophageal cancer. Clinical and pathologic features (review). Radiologic Clinics of North America 35(2): 243–263

Haslett C, Chilvers E R, Hunter J A A, Boon N A 1999 Davidson's principles and practice of medicine, 18th edn. Churchill Livingstone, Edinburgh

Haydon G, Jarvis L, Blair C, Simmonds P, Harrison D, Simpson K, Hayes P 1998 Clinical significance of intra-hepatic hepatitis C virus levels in patients with chronic HCV infection. Gut 42: 570–575

Heading R, Tibaldi M 1998 Oesophageal symptoms and motility disorders. Medicine 26(7): 1–6

Holdstock D J, Misciewicz J J, Smith T, Rowlands E N 1970 Propulsion (mass movements) in the human colon and its relationship to meals and somatic activity. Gut 11: 91–99

Hope J 1993 The counter revolution. BBC Good Health (March): 36–38

Houghton L A, Heyman D, Whorwell P 1996 Symptomatology, quality of life and economic features of irritable bowel syndrome – the effect of hypnotherapy. Alimentary Pharmacology and Therapeutics 10: 991–995

Jalan R, Hayes P 1997 Hepatic encephalopathy and ascites. The Lancet 350(1): 1309–1315

Jones P F 1992 Early analgesia for acute abdominal pain. British Medical Journal 305(6860): 1020–1021

Jones R, Lydeard S 1992 IBS in the general population. British Medical Journal 304: 87–90

Kamm M A 1996 Inflammatory bowel disease Martin Dunitz, London

Kelly M P, Henry T 1992 A thirst for practical knowledge: stoma patients' opinions of the services they receive. Professional Nurse 7(6): 350–356

Kjaerheim K, Gaard M, Andersen A 1998 The role of alcohol, tobacco and dietary factors in upper aerogastric tract cancers: a prospective study of 10,900 Norwegian men. Cancer Causes and Control 9(1): 99–108

Lindars J, Sergeant T 1994 Quality of life in patients with oesophageal carcinoma. Nursing Times 90(43): 31–32

McClane A M (ed) 1987 Classification of nursing diagnoses: proceedings of the seventh conference. Mosby, St Louis

McNamara M J, Alexander H R, Norton J A 1992 Cytokines and their role in the pathophysiology of cancer cachexia. Journal of Parenteral and Enteral Nutrition 16: 505–555

Mant D, Fuller A, Northover J, Astropp P 1992 Patient compliance with colorectal cancer screening in general practice. British Journal of General Practice 42: 18–20

Marshall B J, Warren J R 1984 Unidentified curved bacilli in the stomachs of patients with gastritis and peptic ulceration. Lancet 1: 1311–1315

Moreno E F, Dominguez J M, Sagar P M, Pemberton J H 1996 Update on ileal pouch-anal anastomosis. Revista de Gastroenterologia de Mexico 61(4): 387–393

Nichols R J 1996 Surgical procedures. In: Myers C (ed) Stoma care nursing: a patient-centred approach. Arnold, London

Plevris J, Schina M, Hayes P 1998 Review article: the management of acute liver failure. Alimentary Pharmacology and Therapeutics 12: 405–418

Redhead D N, Chalmers N, Simpson K, Hayes P 1993 Transjugular portasystemic stent shunting (TIPSS). A review. Journal of Interventional Radiology 8: 37–41

Roberts M K 1992 Assessing and treating volvulus. Nursing 92 22(2): 56–57

Rockall T, Logan R, Devlin H, Northfield T 1995 Incidence and mortality from acute upper gastrointestinal haemorrhage in the United Kingdom. British Medical Journal 311(6999): 222–226

Salter M 1990 Current trends in stoma care. Nursing Standard 4(22): 22–24

Scottish Intercollegiate Guidelines Network 1997 Colorectal cancer. SIGN, Edinburgh

Tytgat G, Lee A, Graham D 1993 The role of infectious agents in peptic ulcer disease. Gastroenterology International 6: 76–89

Whitehead S 1988 Illustrated operation notes. Edward Arnold, London

Wilkinson S 1992 Confessions and challenges. Nursing Times 88(35): 24–28

Williams R, Wendon J 1994 Indications for orthotopic liver transplantation in fulminant hepatic failure. Hepatology 20: 55–105

Wilson K J W, Waugh A 1996 Ross & Wilson anatomy and physiology in health and illness, 8th edn. Churchill Livingstone, Edinburgh

FURTHER READING

Burkitt D P 1982 Don't forget the fibre in your diet. Dunitz, London

Cottrill M R B 1996 Helicobacter pylori. Professional Nurse 12(1): 46–48

Dewar B J 1985 Management of oesophageal varices. Nursing Times 81(22): 32–35

Donahue P A 1990 When it's hard to swallow: feeding techniques for dysphagia management. Journal of Gerontological Nursing 16(4): 6–9, 41–42

Fletcher C, Freeling P 1988 Talking and listening to patients: a modern approach. Nuffield Provincial Trust, London

Forrest A P M, Carter D C, MacLeod I B 3rd (eds) 1995 Principles and practice of surgery. Churchill Livingstone, Edinburgh

Garden O J (ed) 1997 Hepatobiliary and pancreatic surgery. WB Saunders, London

Hayward J C 1975 Information: a prescription against pain. Royal College of Nursing, London
Heading R C 1999 Disorders of oesophageal motility. In: Bianchi Porro G, Isselbacher K J (eds) Gastroenterology and hepatology. Clinical medicine series. McGraw-Hill, Milan
Health Education Authority 1989 Can you avoid cancer: a guide to reducing your risks. HEA, London
Howard V 1989 Making sense of endoscopic retrograde cholangiopancreatography. Nursing Times 85(9): 49–51
Johnson P 1993 Laparoscopic cholecystectomy. Nursing Standard 7(22): 26–29
Kalder P K 1985 Stress ulcers. Critical Care Nursing Currents 3(3): 13
Kelly M P, Henry T 1992 A thirst for practical knowledge: stoma patients' opinions of the services they receive. Professional Nurse 3: 350–356
MacConnachie A M 1997 Eradication therapy in peptic ulcer disease. Intensive and Critical Care Nursing 13: 121–122
Miller F 1996 Using a stent to treat patients with portal hypertension. Nursing Standard 10(26): 42–45
Moorhouse P J, Geissler A C, Doenges M E 1988 Acute pancreatitis. Journal of Emergency Nursing 14(6): 387–391
Myers C 1996 Stoma care nursing. Arnold, London
Norris H T (ed) 1991 Pathology of the colon, small intestine and anus, 2nd edn. Churchill Livingstone, Edinburgh
Savage J 1992 Advice to take home. Nursing Times 88(38): 24–27
Price B 1990 Body image: nursing concepts and care. Prentice Hall, UK
Shearman D J C, Finlayson N, Camilleri M 1997 Diseases of the gastrointestinal tract and liver, 3rd edn. Churchill Livingstone, Edinburgh
Smith S 1992 Tiresome healing. Nursing Times 88(36): 24–28
Spross J A, Manolatos A, Thorpe M 1988 Pancreatic cancer: nursing challenges. Seminars in Oncology Nursing 4(4): 274–284
Stanley A, Hayes P 1997 Portal hypertension and variceal haemorrhage. Lancet 350: 1235–1239
Thomas S 1992 A new development in radiology: TIPS. Nursing Standard 7(2): 25–28
Turner G 1996 Oral care. Nursing Standard 10(28): 51–54
University of York, NHS Centre for Reviews and Dissemination 1995 Helicobacter pylori and peptic ulcer. Effectiveness Matters 1(2)

USEFUL ADDRESSES

British Colostomy Association
15 Station Road
Reading RG11 1LG

Ileostomy Association (IA Ileostomy and Internal Pouch Support Group)
Amblehurst House
Blackscotch Lane
Mansfield, Notts
NG18 4PF

National Association for Colitis and Crohn's Disease (NACC)
98A London Road
St Alban's
Hertfordshire AL1 1NY

IBS Network
Northern General Hospital
Sheffield S5 7AU

The Coeliac Society
PO Box 220
High Wycombe
Bucks AL1 1NX

British Liver Trust
Ransomes Europark
Ipswich IP3 9QG

ENDOCRINE AND METABOLIC DISORDERS

5

Claire Dibbs
(Part 1 Endocrine and metabolic disorders)
Rosemary McIntyre, Kathy Strachan
(Part 2 Diabetes mellitus)

PART 1
ENDOCRINE AND METABOLIC DISORDERS

INTRODUCTION

Endocrinology is the study of hormones (or chemical messengers) secreted by endocrine cells and neurones. These hormones maintain homeostasis by acting on and coordinating activity within target organs or tissues.

Endocrinology is a relatively new and rapidly growing field. Considerable progress is being made, with important implications for other areas of medicine, e.g. neuroendocrinology, which in turn has important applications within psychiatry. Advances are constantly being made in this field and current research into the genetic causes of many endocrine conditions is moving forward. Indeed, the site of the mutation in the gene that causes one of the syndromes of multiple endocrine neoplasia (MEN) has been discovered. Identifying carriers of the mutation will allow biochemical screening of individuals before they are symptomatic, therefore providing an opportunity for earlier treatment (Bassett et al 1998). This topic is not discussed in this chapter, as it is not within its scope. However, this is certainly an area from which future treatments of endocrine disease will come. There are other areas of endocrinology that are not covered in this chapter, mostly rare conditions. They have been omitted simply to make the chapter manageable. A list of further reading at the end of the chapter will give the enthusiastic reader plenty of scope for further study.

A new area to be considered is the effect on the endocrine system of exposure to the human immunodeficiency virus (HIV) and subsequent development of the acquired immune deficiency syndrome (AIDS). This may involve any part of the endocrine system and, because endocrine disease may not be easy to identify in the severely ill patient, it may be overlooked. Treatment of the underlying disease may help to improve the quality of the patient's life. The adrenal gland is found to be infected with cytomegalovirus at postmortem in 37–88% of patients. Medication used in concurrent fungal infection (e.g. ketaconazole) may inhibit cortisol synthesis, resulting in adrenal insufficiency. Indeed, adrenal insufficiency is seen in up to 5% of patients (Grinspoon & Bilezikian 1992).

Apart from diabetes mellitus and thyroid disorders, endocrine problems are not common. Many endocrine disorders are rarely seen and may be difficult to diagnose. As a result, patients may be referred by their general practitioner or local hospital to specialist centres for the often complicated and exhaustive tests necessary for diagnosis. For the patient, this has the advantage of offering highly specialised care, although conversely it also means that relatively few nurses have the opportunity to treat and care for people with these disorders.

However, given the wide-ranging effects of endocrine dysfunction, it is important that all nurses have a general understanding of endocrinology. Endocrine diseases can affect every system of the body, causing disfigurement and a change in body image or even posing a threat to life. These disorders can seriously affect the patient's psychological outlook, either as a direct result of the illness or by virtue of the individual's reaction to it.

It is well documented that individuals react differently to being ill. Some view their situation as a challenge, while others see it as a punishment, react with anger or try to apportion blame. Anger may be directed at family members or at nursing and medical staff (Sinclair & Fawcett 1991). This situation may be exacerbated by an unstable mental state, mood swings, depression or frank psychosis, which may, in fact, be sequelae of the disorder. The nurse must be aware of this possibility and react accordingly, offering support and understanding to the patient and his relatives. Explanations that the underlying illness may be influencing the patient's mood may help him and his relatives to cope.

As the tests and investigations required to diagnose some of the rarer endocrine conditions are often long and exhausting, clear explanations are essential so that the patient understands the need for them and the procedures that will be followed. This will help to reduce anxiety and increase the patient's confidence in the health care team. The psychological support that the nurse can offer this group of patients cannot be overemphasised. From experience, these patients are often young and probably otherwise in good health, and therefore the impact of endocrine disease on the body image and/or self-esteem should not be underestimated. For example, patients experiencing sexual dysfunction may feel embarrassed to talk to and seek support from family members and friends — in such cases, support from the health care professional is crucial.

ANATOMY AND PHYSIOLOGY

The nature of the endocrine system, being one of control, means that it has far-reaching effects throughout the body on various target organs. In order to make this chapter as clear as possible, each endocrine gland will be considered separately. In cases where a disease is caused by the abnormal secretion of a trophic or control hormone, the disease will be discussed under the heading of the end organ. For example, in Cushing's disease, adrenocorticotrophic hormone (ACTH) is secreted in excess by the pituitary gland. This acts on the adrenal gland, causing it to produce excess amounts of cortisol. Therefore, as the adrenal gland is the end organ, and it is the secretion from this gland that causes unwanted effects on the body, Cushing's disease is discussed under the heading of the adrenal gland.

Hormones

The endocrine system is one of the two major control systems of the body, the other being the nervous system. The nervous system mediates its activity by means of nerves directly supplying the organs and structures to which it relates. The endocrine system operates by a system of hormones, which are secreted into the bloodstream for transport to their respective target organs.

The endocrine glands and their anatomical position are shown in Figure 5.1.

Action

Although the hormones are carried to every cell in the body, they affect only those cells or organs upon which they have an excitatory or inhibitory action. This system allows individuals to respond to changes in their environment and is important in controlling growth and development, sexual maturation and homeostasis.

Many hormones are bound to proteins within the circulation. It is generally thought that only unbound or free hormones are biologically active, and that binding serves as a buffer against very rapid changes in plasma levels of a hormone. This principle is important in the interpretation of many tests of endocrine function.

Control

Most hormone systems are controlled by a feedback system which ensures that hormone levels, whilst fluctuating, remain within a mean (see Table 5.1). Figure 5.2 illustrates how negative feedback operates in the hypothalamic–pituitary–thyroid axis.

Pattern of secretion

Hormone secretion is either continuous or intermittent. An example of the former is the secretion of thyroxine by the thyroid gland,

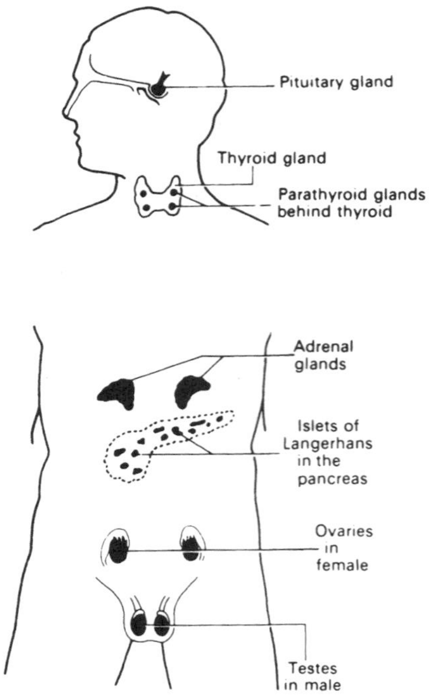

Fig. 5.1 The endocrine glands and their location in the body. (Reproduced with kind permission from Wilson & Waugh 1996.)

Table 5.1 List of normal ranges (these may vary for different laboratories). (Reproduced with kind permission from Besser & Trainer 1995)

Hormone			*SI units*
Aldosterone (normal diet)	Pose	Upright (4 h) Supine (30 min)	330–830 pmol/L 135–400 pmol/L
Cortisol	Time	09.00 h 18.00 h 00.00 h (asleep)	200–700 nmol/L 100–300 nmol/L <50 nmol/L
11-deoxycortisol	Time	09.00 h	26–46 nmol/L
Dehydroepiandodterone (DHEA)	Time	09.00 h	7–31 nmol/L
DHEA sulphate	Population	Women Men Prepubertal	3–12 μmol/L 2-10 μmol/L <0.5 μmol/L
Androstenedione	Population	Adults Prepubertal	3–8 nmol/L <1 nmol/L
Oestradiol	Population	Prepubertal Women Postmenopausal Follicular Mid-cycle Luteal Men	<20 pmol/L <100 pmol/L 200–400 pmol/L 400–1200 pmol/L 400–1000 pmol/L <180 pmol/L
Progesterone	Population	Women Follicular Luteal Men	 <10 nmol/L >30 nmol/L <6 nmol/L
Testosterone	Population	Prepubertal Men Women	<0.8 nmol/L 9–35 nmol/L 0.5–30 nmol/L
ACTH	Time	09.00 h	<18 pmol/L
FSH	Population	Prepubertal Women Postmenopausal Follicular Mid-cycle Luteal Men	<5 U/L >30 U/L 2.5–10 U/L 25–70 U/L >0.3–2.1 U/L 1–7 U/L
GH	Fasting between pulses		<1 mU/L
LH	Population	Prepubertal Women Postmenopausal Follicular Mid-cycle Luteal Men	<5 U/L >30 U/L 2.5–10 U/L 25–70 U/L <1–13 U/L 1–10 U/L
Prolactin			<360 mU/L
TSH			0.4–5 mU/L
Thyroxine (free)			10–20 pmol/L
Tri-iodothyronine (free)			5–10 pmol/L
Catecholamines	Taken with patient cannulated and lying for 30 min prior	Adrenaline Noradrenaline	0.03–1.31 nmol/L 0.47–4.14 nmol/L

in which hormone levels over a day, month or year show very little variation. Intermittent secretion is seen in three forms: circadian, menstrual and pulsatile.

Other factors which affect hormone secretion include stress, disease, trauma, surgery or emotional upset. As in any complex regulatory system, it is likely that disequilibrium in endocrine function will have important consequences. Disorders of the endocrine system may be categorised most simply as those involving overproduction (hypersecretion) and those involving underproduction (hyposecretion).

See Hinchliff et al (1996), Section 2.6. pp. 203–244

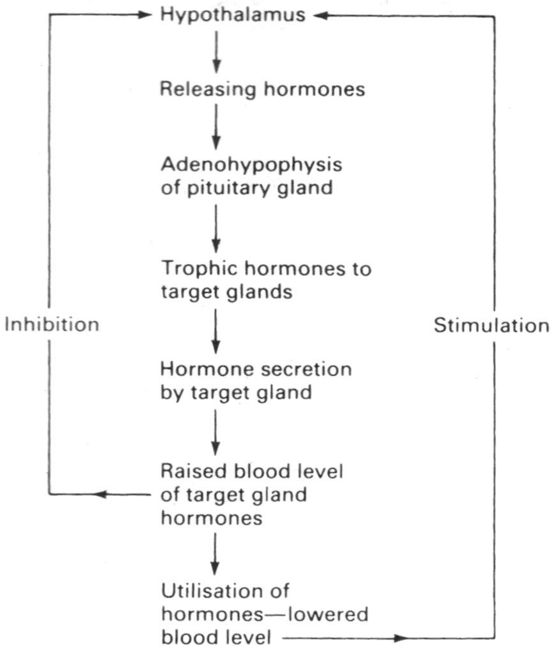

Fig. 5.2 Negative feedback regulation of the secretion of anterior pituitary hormones. (Reproduced with kind permission from Wilson & Waugh 1996.)

DISORDERS OF THE PITUITARY GLAND AND HYPOTHALAMUS

As stated above, disorders of the endocrine system result in either an oversecretion or an undersecretion of a hormone. Therefore, in principle, treatment should be straightforward, either replacing the missing hormone or removing, or suppressing the source of, the oversecretion. Recent advances have made the treatment of the wide range of endocrine disorders more successful, and the outlook for those suffering from them is becoming ever more hopeful.

Hypersecretion of a hormone usually arises from a so-called 'functioning' pituitary adenoma. As this adenoma grows, it is likely to 'crowd out' the normal function of other areas of the pituitary, and as a result progressive hypopituitarism occurs. This failure of the pituitary hormones occurs in a characteristic sequence (Besser & Thorner 1995). Usually secretion of gonadotrophins is lost first, followed by thyroid-stimulating hormone (TSH) and then ACTH. Prolactin deficiency is rare (except as seen postpartum in Sheehan's syndrome). The stage at which GH secretion is lost is difficult to ascertain as, except in the growing child, symptoms of GH deficiency rarely manifest themselves in a way that is obvious to the patient.

ANATOMY AND PHYSIOLOGY

The existence of the pituitary gland has been known of for at least 2000 years. It lies immediately below the hypothalamus in the pituitary fossa. It is connected to the hypothalamus by the pituitary stalk and consists of two lobes — anterior and posterior — which function independently of each other (see Fig. 5.3). In the developing fetus the anterior lobe is formed from Rathke's pouch, which grows upwards and becomes separated from the oropharynx

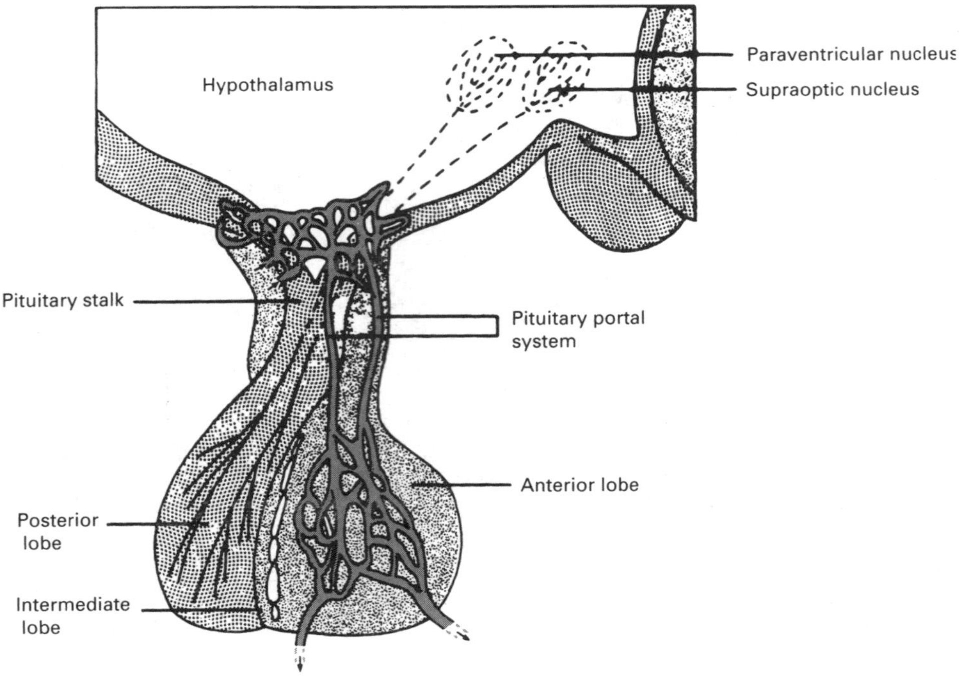

Fig. 5.3 Position of the pituitary and its associated structures. (Reproduced with kind permission from Wilson & Waugh 1996.)

to become the adenohypophysis. The posterior lobe is a downgrowth from the forebrain, which becomes the neurohypophysis. The posterior pituitary contains nerve fibres which grow into it from the hypothalamus via the pituitary stalk. The hormones secreted by the pituitary gland, together with their action, are listed in Table 5.2.

The hypothalamus is part of the floor of the third ventricle of the brain. It is an area of specialised cells or nuclei which produce hormones. These hormones regulate pituitary function and act as releasing factors for the anterior pituitary hormones (see Fig. 5.4). The hypothalamus also controls many centres for functions such as appetite, thirst, temperature regulation, sexual activity, sleeping and waking.

The pituitary stalk carries blood to both lobes of the pituitary in a portal system by which the hypothalamic releasing or inhibitory hormones are carried to the anterior pituitary. The trophic hormones produced in the anterior pituitary stimulate the peripheral endocrine glands. The posterior pituitary acts as a reservoir for antidiuretic hormone (ADH) vasopressin and oxytocin.

The optic chiasma sits just above the pituitary fossa. Therefore, an expanding lesion from the pituitary or the hypothalamus may result in a defect in the visual fields because of pressure on the optic nerve or optic chiasma.

Hypersecretion or hyposecretion of hormones or local effects of a tumour will disturb the balance of the system.

HYPERSECRETION OF THE ANTERIOR PITUITARY HORMONES

Hypersecretion of adrenocorticotrophic hormone: Cushing's disease

Cushing's disease is found when an excess of glucocorticoid secretions is stimulated by an ACTH-producing adenoma of the pituitary. As the clinical features are similar to those of Cushing's syndrome, this disease will be discussed under 'Disorders of the adrenal cortex' (p. 150).

Hypersecretion of growth hormone: acromegaly and gigantism

Aetiology

Hypersecretion of growth hormone (GH) causes gigantism and acromegaly. If excessive secretion occurs before fusion of the bony epiphyses, this is termed gigantism. It is extremely rare. Acromegaly caused by excess secretion of GH after fusion of the epiphyses is seen in about 40 per million of the population. Gigantism probably constitutes only 1% of this number. A distinction must be made between those who are constitutionally tall, i.e. individuals who have two tall parents, and those suffering from gigantism. Individuals with pituitary disease can easily grow to a height in excess of 2 m, and some to over 2.4 m.

PATHOPHYSIOLOGY

Clinical features. Acromegaly can remain undetected for years, as its onset is insidious. It causes enlargement of all systems and structures of the body except the nervous system. The effects of the disorder include:

- enlargement of bones and soft tissues, seen especially as an overgrowth of the supraorbital ridge, a broadening of the nose, prognathism and interdental separation
- enlargement of the hands and feet, resulting in the need for larger gloves, rings and shoes
- osteoarthritis (commonly)
- weight gain
- cardiomegaly
- hypertension
- excessive sweating
- hyperprolactinaemia with menstrual disturbances and amenorrhoea in women
- loss of libido

Table 5.2 Hormones of the pituitary gland and their action

Hormone	*Action*
Anterior lobe	
Growth hormone (GH)	Pulsatile release. Does not have a single target gland but acts on a variety of tissues, e.g. bone, viscera and soft tissues. It is particularly important in children to stimulate growth. Action in adults recently thought to involve maintenance of cardiovascular activity, fat deposition and muscle development
Prolactin (PRL)	Main action is to stimulate lactation in females, also stimulates corpus luteum to secrete progesterone
Adrenocorticotrophic hormone (ACTH)	Secreted under circadian rhythm. Stimulates the adrenal cortex to secrete corticosteroids
Luteinising hormone (LH)	Promotes ovulation; stimulates formation of the corpus luteum
Follicle-stimulating hormone (FSH)	Stimulates the production of sex hormones and contributes to regulation of the menstrual cycle in women. In women, stimulates the production of ovarian follicles and secretion of oestrogen; in men, promotes the production of spermatozoa
Thyroid-stimulating hormone (TSH)	Stimulates the thyroid to release thyroxine
Posterior lobe	
Vasopressin — also called antidiuretic hormone (ADH)	Controls water homeostasis in the body by regulating water reabsorption from the renal tissues
Oxytocin	Induces uterine contraction during labour and ejection of milk from breasts postpartum

- diabetes mellitus (in 25% of patients due to insulin resistance as a result of high GH levels)
- enlarged pituitary fossa.

Common presenting symptoms. The patient will present with a number of symptoms. Most commonly, the enlargement of the hands and feet and changed appearance will have been noticed and commented on by relatives and friends. Other conditions for which the patient will initially seek help may be related to osteoarthritis or cardiovascular problems. In women, amenorrhoea may prompt a visit to the GP. Changes in the field of vision may have been noticed. Often old photographs of the individual can be useful to the doctor in reaching a provisional diagnosis.

MEDICAL MANAGEMENT

Investigations. Diagnosis can be confirmed following clinical examination and tests of pituitary function. On clinical examination, all or some of the features listed above will be evident. Skull X-rays and magnetic resonance imaging (MRI) may show an enlarged pituitary fossa. Measurement of GH levels will show uniformly elevated levels throughout the day, which are not suppressed to undetectable levels following glucose administration (as in normal individuals). Further tests of pituitary function may be carried out in specialist centres to confirm the diagnosis and establish whether the normal pituitary is compromised.

See Bouloux & Rees (1994).

Treatment. In untreated acromegaly, mortality is nearly doubled in comparison with the normal population. Therefore, early treatment is recommended. The aim of treatment is to relieve symptoms and resolve the associated metabolic abnormalities, e.g. diabetes mellitus.

Treatment may take the form of surgery, radiotherapy or drug therapy. Hypophysectomy via the trans-sphenoidal route, which has a low morbidity and mortality, is the surgical procedure most commonly used. Drug therapy using oral bromocriptine has been shown to reduce tumour size as well as lowering GH levels. Octreotide, a relatively new drug, is a synthetic compound which mimics the hypothalamic growth hormone release-inhibiting hormone (GHRIH). Octreotide has to be given by regular subcutaneous (s.c.) injection or continuous s.c. infusion and various studies have shown that GH levels decrease within 2 h of s.c. injection (Ho et al 1990, Newman et al 1995).

Usually, surgery and radiotherapy are used in conjunction, as tumour regrowth often occurs following surgery alone. Drug therapy is then used to control residual excess GH secretion, as radiotherapy only lowers GH levels gradually. Hypopituitarism may occur as a result of either treatment. In patients unfit for surgery, drug therapy alone may be used.

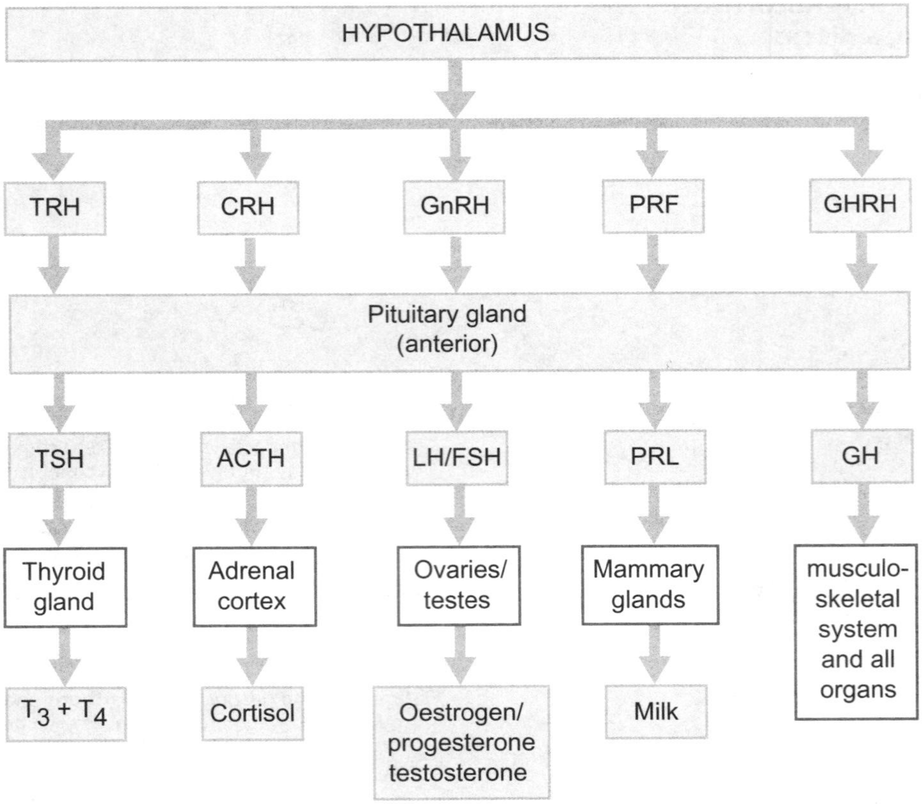

Fig. 5.4 Schematic diagram showing the relationship between the hypothalamus, the pituitary gland and their target organs. TRH, thyrotrophin-releasing hormone; CRH, corticotrophin-releasing hormone; GnRH, gonadotrophin-releasing hormone; PRF, prolactin-releasing factor; GHRH, growth hormone releasing hormone; TSH, thyroid-stimulating hormone; ACTH, adrenocorticotrophin-releasing hormone; LH/FSH, luteinising hormone/follicle-stimulating hormone; PRL, prolactin; GH, growth hormone.

NURSING PRIORITIES AND MANAGEMENT: ACROMEGALY

Major considerations

Giving psychological support

Change in body image is an important feature of this disorder. Most probably the individual will have considerable difficulty in coming to terms with his changed appearance and will be anxious about the investigations he must undergo and the treatment that may be required.

It is important to create a relaxed environment and to reduce anxiety by spending time with the patient and his family, explaining the reasons for his changed appearance, the effect of therapy and the expected treatment outcome. They will be reassured to hear that biochemical cure may result in a return to a more normal appearance, although the degree will depend on the stage of the disease at the beginning of treatment. Some symptoms, such as sweating, may be cured almost immediately, while others (especially bony changes) may take years to resolve.

Some patients benefit from meeting others who have been treated successfully and nursing staff should try to arrange this. The personal experience of one former female patient — whose shoe size was reduced by two sizes in 6 months — is the kind of success story which might boost the morale of a newly diagnosed patient.

Perioperative care

The reader is referred to Chapter 26 for principles of preoperative preparation and postoperative care, and to Chapter 23 for information on wound healing. Specific postoperative observations include neurological monitoring, with special care being taken to observe for leakage of cerebrospinal fluid from the nose (Baxter 1994). The patient is nursed well supported on pillows to ensure that an upright position is maintained.

Recovery is usually rapid and the patient is discharged home on the fourth or fifth postoperative day.

5.1 Miss W, aged 45 years, has been diagnosed as having acromegaly. She has undergone trans-sphenoidal hypophysectomy for the removal of a GH-producing adenoma.

Identify the specific or potential problems and devise a plan to meet her care needs. What long-term treatment and care will she require? (See Nursing Care Plan 5.1, p. 147.)

Prolactin hypersecretion

Aetiology

It is now known that prolactin is the commonest hormone to be secreted by pituitary tumours and that tiny prolactinomas, which may be as small as 2–3 mm in diameter, occur frequently (Haslett et al 1999). However, a wide variety of drugs and diseases can cause high prolactin levels. Before carrying out extensive investigations for pituitary disease, it is important to exclude physiological causes such as hypothyroidism and to take a detailed drug history. Drugs that block the dopamine receptor, such as chlorpromazine and metoclopramide, elevate prolactin levels.

PATHOPHYSIOLOGY

Hyperprolactinaemia in women causes galactorrhoea and amenorrhoea; lack of ovulation due to prolactin interfering with LH and FSH acting on the ovary results in infertility (Haslett et al 1999). In men, the galactorrhoea is not so pronounced, but there is a decreased sperm count and infertility.

Common presenting symptoms include, in women, amenorrhoea, infertility, hirsutism and acne, and in men, impotence, infertility and gynaecomastia.

MEDICAL MANAGEMENT

Investigations. When other causes of the presenting symptoms have been excluded, prolactin levels should be measured in the unstressed patient. Because venepuncture is stressful, an intravenous cannula is placed in the patient's arm and the patient allowed to rest for 30 minutes prior to the blood sample being taken. The patient should not smoke or drink tea or coffee in this period. If the prolactin levels are raised, a lateral skull X-ray should be taken. If this shows a large pituitary fossa, tests of other pituitary functions should be carried out to see if other pituitary hormones are affected (see Cushing's disease, p. 152). Visual field tests may also be carried out to exclude pressure on the optic chiasma. High-resolution CT scanning and MRI will usually show even a small tumour. Prolactinomas are almost always benign.

Treatment. The aim is to lower the excessive levels of prolactin, to reduce the tumour size and to restore to normal levels those deficiencies that may have resulted from the presence of the tumour. Reduction of tumour size and lowering of hormone levels may be achieved by drug therapy alone. Prolactinomas respond well to bromocriptine. Surgery is usually not performed until the tumour has been reduced in size, and is carried out via the trans-sphenoidal route.

NURSING PRIORITIES AND MANAGEMENT: PROLACTIN HYPERSECRETION

Specific nursing care is aimed at ensuring that the medication regimens are followed correctly in order to avoid side-effects. Blood pressure is observed, bearing in mind that a postural drop may occur. Bromocriptine can be poorly tolerated in many people. There should be a slow increase in dosage, the first doses being given whilst eating and on retiring to prevent the common symptoms of postural hypotension and gastric irritation. The dosage can then be built up gradually to 2.5 mg three times a day.

See Besser & Thorner (1995).

HYPOSECRETION OF THE ANTERIOR PITUITARY HORMONES

Hypopituitarism

The term hypopituitarism refers to partial or total deficiency of anterior pituitary hormone secretion. It may be associated with pathological processes that destroy the pituitary itself or with disturbance of the hypothalamic control of the pituitary. Total failure of all hormone production is termed panhypopituitarism.

Aetiology

As already stated, hypopituitarism is most commonly caused by the presence of a pituitary tumour. These are frequently benign. Pituitary carcinoma is very rare indeed. Benign microadenomas having no clinical effects are surprisingly common and are found in up to 23% of people at postmortem (Bouloux & Rees 1994).

PATHOPHYSIOLOGY

Pituitary tumours can vary greatly in size and may extend outside the pituitary fossa to compress surrounding structures. They are generally classified as functioning or non-functioning, depending on whether they produce a hormone, e.g. GH or prolactin.

Common presenting symptoms. Symptoms caused by local compression may arise (see Ch. 9, p. 362), but the individual usually presents with signs associated with pituitary hormone deficiency. The precise symptoms will vary in accordance with the particular hormone that is deficient (see Table 5.3).

MEDICAL MANAGEMENT

Investigations. Diagnostic investigations include field of vision testing and biochemical investigation to determine the severity and degree of pituitary failure and to distinguish between isolated hormone failure and complete anterior failure. Skull X-rays, CT scanning and MRI are also carried out.

Treatment. The choice of treatment will depend on the diagnosis of the cause of the pituitary failure and will aim to relieve the clinical effects and symptoms experienced by the patient. Treatment may involve surgery, radiotherapy to reduce the tumour and drug therapy to replace the deficient hormones (see Table 5.4).

Table 5.3 Symptoms associated with anterior pituitary hormone hyposecretion

Deficiency	*Symptoms*
LHFSH	*Men* Poor libido and impotence Infertility Small soft testicles Loss of secondary sexual hair *Women* Amenorrhoea Infertility Dyspareunia Breast atrophy Loss of secondary sexual hair
TSH	*Children* Growth retardation *Adults* Decreased energy Constipation Sensitivity to cold Dry skin Weight gain
ACTH	*All* Weakness Tiredness Dizziness on standing Pallor Hypoglycaemia
GH	*Children* Growth retardation Short stature *Adults* Cardiovascular activity Muscle development Fat distribution General sense of well-being

NURSING PRIORITIES AND MANAGEMENT: HYPOPITUITARISM

Major considerations

Giving information

Effective nursing intervention depends upon the establishment of a good nurse–patient relationship in a friendly environment. As the effects of hypopituitarism can be widespread, causing diverse physical and psychological changes which can be difficult to comprehend, it is important to ensure that all of the patient's questions are answered in a way that is understood. Open and frank discussion about changes in body image and sexuality is essential to the individual concerned. The nurse should be aware that short stature is not always caused by a simple deficiency in the production of GH. Other factors may come into play, requiring different investigations and treatment approaches (see Box 5.1 and Table 5.5).

Clear, ongoing explanations of the extensive and possibly uncomfortable investigations will help to relieve the patient's anxiety. The presence of a nurse familiar to the patient during these investigations can be reassuring.

Table 5.4 Hormone replacement therapy. (Reproduced with kind permission from Besser & Cudworth 1990)

Deficient hormone	*Replacement*	*Check*
Anterior pituitary Women LH FSH	Ethinyloestradiol Medroxyprogesterone	*Libido and symptoms of deficiency
Men LH FSH	Testosterone	*Libido and potency
Children ACTH TSH	GH Hydrocortisone Thyroxine	Growth chart Cortisol levels throughout the day T_3 and T_4 levels
Posterior pituitary ADH	Desmopressin	Plasma and urine osmolality

*For men and women, the only treatment of associated infertility entails regular injections of the deficient pituitary hormones (mainly FSH in the form of Pergonal or Metrodin) or, if the defect is hypothalamic, hourly parenteral injection of a gonadotrophin-releasing hormone via an implanted pump.

Box 5.1 Growth hormone deficiency and short stature

Normal growth results from a number of interacting factors; therefore short stature cannot be attributed simply to underproduction of GH from the pituitary.

From childhood into adulthood, growth relies on both extrinsic and intrinsic factors such as the height of the individual's parents, dietary intake and absorption, emotional or psychological problems, endocrine conditions such as hypothyroidism, and skeletal disorders or other congenital abnormalities (see Table 5.5).

All children should be measured before commencing school in pre-school clinics and during school attendance in order to determine their pattern of growth. Most children fall within a statistically derived height–distance curve: those thought to be shorter than average should have their height measured at regular intervals so that their growth velocity can be calculated. In those children who are failing to grow, a diagnosis will need to be made in order to commence the appropriate therapy.

Table 5.5 Types of short stature: features, diagnosis and management

Type	*Description*	*Investigations*	*Management*
Disproportionate short stature	Short limbs and backs, e.g. hypochondroplasia	Full skeletal survey with interpretation by a specialist	In the past, little could be done for the classic 'dwarf', but recently experimentation in bone lengthening has been successful in increasing height by up to 15 cm
Systemic causes of growth delay normal	In systemic disease, there is often delayed skeletal maturation, e.g. Crohn's disease, asthma, dietary deficiency	These causes should all be eliminated by routine investigation, including jejunal biopsy if Crohn's is suspected	Once treated, the short child with systemic disease should catch up and reach his normal growth
Psychological and emotional deprivation	This is commonly recognised in infancy. Behavioural abnormalities may be displayed. Short stature and delay in maturity may result	Detailed investigations may not be necessary if emotional disturbance can be identified	Support for the family including counselling for the parents may be necessary and could require cooperation from the child's school, etc. In the ward environment, an observant nurse may well identify interaction difficulties and should always be aware of the child who has been non-accidentally injured, whose parents may be seeking help from outside agencies
Hormone deficiency	Important hormones required for growth are thyroid hormone, growth hormone (GH) and sex hormones. The child may display characteristic features of deficiency	Investigations include skeletal X-ray (to determine bone age) and testing of the hypothalamopituitary axis to check GH secretion	Replacement of the deficient hormone may be required to promote growth. GH is given by injection three times a week
Laron dwarfism	This occurs when GH is produced, but due to receptor failure the child cannot respond to it	On testing, GH levels are normal, even high, but the child appears very small	The child does not respond to GH. Both the child and family require sensitive handling and emotional support as the child will remain small while moving into adulthood. Intellect will usually be normal
Pseudo-hypoparathyroidism	The child has a short stature and round face, is obese, has short metacarpals and is below normal intelligence	X-rays show subcutaneous calcification. It is caused by the patient having resistance to the action of parathyroid hormone. PTH levels will be high and calcium levels low	High doses of vitamin D treat the condition
Cushing's syndrome	Typical Cushing's appearance	This is extremely rare. Investigations as for Cushing's syndrome in adults will be undertaken (see Table 5.7)	The treatment is the same as for adults
Constitutional growth delay	The child appears small and in proportion with no unusual features	Hand and wrist X-ray shows retarded bone development. GH levels and hypothalamopituitary tests are normal	Once the child reaches puberty and experiences the associated growth spurt that accompanies it, the eventual height will be within the normal range

As the prospect of neurosurgery or radiotherapy is frightening for most people, careful preoperative preparation must include an explanation of procedures, the nature of immediate postoperative care and the expected long-term outcome. Reminding the patient that his symptoms will be relieved by surgery, radiotherapy and hormone replacement therapy will be of considerable psychological benefit.

Supporting the patient in ongoing replacement therapy

Gonadotrophins. Replacement of gonadotrophins is reasonably straightforward, requiring a once daily tablet or a monthly injection.
Growth hormone. GH is generally only given to children prior to fusion of the epiphyses. Synthetic GH is administered by injection. The child and his parents will be taught how to carry this out at home, where supervision and support will be given by the community health team. There is some argument as to the value of GH replacement in the adult. In 1962, Raben described increased activity, vigour and a sense of well-being in a hypopituitary female aged 35 years. Until 1988 it was claimed that low levels of GH had little or no effect in adults, but studies have shown that replacement GH therapy in growth hormone-deficient individuals has profound effects. It is now apparent that GH deficiency is associated with changes in body composition, bone density, lipid metabolism, physical performance and cardiovascular function (Grinspoon & Bilezikian 1992), and recombinant hGH treatment has become more widely available and used (Bengtsson et al 1993). However, the enormous expense of GH treatment makes its widespread use in the adult unlikely.
Cortisol. Hydrocortisone is given to those who have ACTH deficiency. The dose can be variable and cortisol levels should be checked frequently. The omission of even one dose may have serious consequences. Such patients should be advised to carry a steroid card and to wear a Medic-Alert bracelet at all times.
Thyroid hormones. Thyroid replacement is given as an oral medication. As the half-life of thyroxine is very long, the occasional missed dose is not critical.

Replacement of deficient hormones should alleviate symptoms, allowing the patient to lead a normal life within the community. It is essential that the individual feels free to contact the appropriate doctor or specialist unit at any time to discuss his condition or any related anxieties. As pituitary disease is a lifelong condition that will require ongoing monitoring, hospital attendance may be frequent. It helps if visits and tests are coordinated so that they can be kept to a minimum; at the same time, advice and support must be given promptly when required so that the patient can lead as normal a life as possible.

DISORDERS OF THE POSTERIOR PITUITARY: ANTIDIURETIC HORMONE (ADH) VASOPRESSIN SECRETION

All the conditions caused by disorders of antidiuretic hormone (ADH) secretion or activity are uncommon. These disorders include:

- deficiency of hypothalamic secretion of ADH (central diabetes insipidus)
- nephrogenic diabetes insipidus — a condition in which the renal tubules are insensitive to the action of ADH
- inappropriate/excessive secretion.

Causes include pituitary tumours, infection, surgery, trauma, renal disease and some drugs.

Diabetes insipidus

PATHOPHYSIOLOGY

Clinical features. Deficiency of antidiuretic hormone (ADH) leads to polyuria, nocturia and a compensatory polydipsia. Urine output may reach 10–15 L or more per day, leading to severe dehydration if the individual's fluid intake is restricted in any way.

MEDICAL MANAGEMENT

Investigations. Diagnosis may be made by single paired urine and plasma osmolality, obviating the need for the more stressful and prolonged water depletion test. Plasma osmolality will show high concentration and urine will be dilute.
Treatment is by the administration of synthetic vasopressin (desmopressin or DDAVP) 10–20 μg one to three times daily by the intranasal route. Initially, it is best given at night. It can also be given i.m. or s.c. at one-tenth of the dose.

Syndrome of inappropriate antidiuretic hormone (SIADH)

The causes of SIADH are many, but include oat cell carcinomas, pneumonia, TB, meningitis, head injury, porphyria and some chemotherapeutic agents such as vincristine.

PATHOPHYSIOLOGY

Clinical features. SIADH usually presents with vagueness, confusion, nausea and irritability and if not corrected leads to epileptiform attacks and coma. It is caused by an excess of ADH, leading to hyponatraemia as a result of dilution. Biochemical investigation will reveal low plasma sodium, low plasma osmolality and high urine osmolality. Blood pressure, serum potassium levels, kidney function and adrenal function will be normal.

MEDICAL MANAGEMENT

Medical intervention may include:

- fluid restriction to 500–1000 mL/day
- treatment of the underlying cause
- administration of demeclocycline to inhibit the action of ADH on the renal tubules
- administration of hypertonic saline infusions (in severe cases).

NURSING PRIORITIES AND MANAGEMENT: VASOPRESSIN SECRETION

Major considerations

The nurse's interventions will include accurate recording of fluid intake and output with the full cooperation and participation of the patient. It is essential for the patient to have easy access to toilet facilities. Samples of urine will be required for osmolality assessment.

The nurse will also be involved in medication administration and education of the patient with regard to self-administration of medicines, continued measurement of fluid balance, and regular weight recording. Most patients thereby rapidly become aware if the therapy is no longer working and will contact their GP or the specialist physician supervising their care.

DISORDERS OF THE THYROID GLAND

ANATOMY AND PHYSIOLOGY

The thyroid gland produces the hormones tri-iodothyronine (T_3) and thyroxine (T_4). As these control metabolism, overactivity or underactivity will have significant effects.

The thyroid sits anteriorly to the larynx and is attached to the thyroid cartilages and the trachea. It consists of two lobes connected by an isthmus (see Fig. 5.5). Structures which lie in close proximity include the oesophagus, the parathyroid glands, the recurrent laryngeal nerves and the carotid artery. These may all be affected by enlargement of the gland.

The thyroid receives a rich blood supply from the superior thyroid arteries, which branch from the external carotid arteries, and from the inferior thyroid arteries, which branch from the subclavian arteries. Each lobe is filled with hollow vesicles called follicles, which produce and store the thyroid hormones as thyroglobulin. Between the follicles is parafollicular material, which secretes the hormone calcitonin; this together with parathormone from the parathyroid glands is involved in the metabolism of calcium.

The thyroid hormones are synthesised from within the gland. This synthesis is dependent on the availability of iodine in the diet. Dietary iodine is absorbed from the small intestine, changed to iodide and transported in the blood to the thyroid gland, where it is taken up by the thyroid cells.

More T_4 than T_3 is produced, but T_4 is converted in some tissues to the more biologically active T_3. Over 99% of all thyroid hormone is bound to plasma proteins by thyroid-binding globulins. Only the free hormone is available for use by the tissues.

Q **5.2** Describe how the thyroid hormones T_3 and T_4 are controlled.

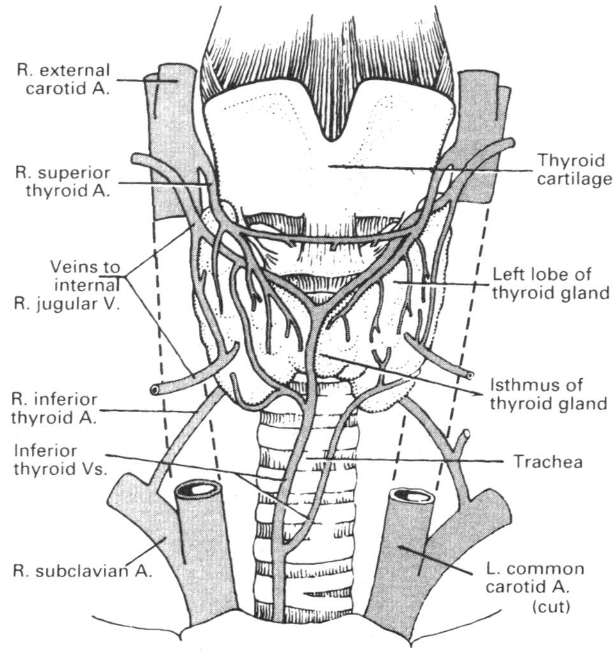

Fig. 5.5 The thyroid gland and associated structures. (Reproduced with kind permission from Wilson & Waugh 1996.)

HYPERSECRETION OF THE THYROID HORMONES

Hyperthyroidism (or thyrotoxicosis) and diabetes mellitus are the most prevalent of the endocrine diseases. (Diabetes mellitus is discussed in detail in Part 2 of this chapter.) The most common cause of hyperthyroidism is intrinsic thyroid disease; pituitary causes are extremely rare. Hyperthyroidism is a condition in which there are high levels of circulating thyroid hormones. It predominantly affects females aged between 30 and 50 years, but can occur at any age in either sex.

Graves' disease

Graves' disease is the most common form of hyperthyroidism. It is an autoimmune disorder, associated with a diffuse enlargement (or goitre) of the gland, in which antibodies behave like TSH, stimulating thyroid hormone production. Graves' disease tends to run in families and may be associated with ophthalmic features, e.g. retro-orbital inflammation leading to periorbital oedema.

Toxic multinodular goitre

This type of goitre is characterised by an asymmetrical nodular thyroid enlargement. It tends to occur in an older age group than those with Graves' disease.

Toxic adenoma (solitary nodule)

This type of tumour constitutes about 5% of thyroid disease. In these cases, a thyroid nodule may act autonomously and produce excess levels of thyroid hormone, leading to suppression of the normal thyroid.

PATHOPHYSIOLOGY

In hyperthyroidism, high levels of circulating thyroid hormones stimulate cell metabolism, resulting in a high metabolic rate. TSH secretion is suppressed. The cardiovascular system is affected, and tachycardia and atrial fibrillation are common. Patients will complain of general fatigue, although they may become more active and find that they are unable to rest for long. They may become exophthalmic due to periorbital oedema, causing lid retraction and limited upward gaze. If the eyelids are unable to close, corneal ulceration can occur.

Common presenting symptoms. Patients will have noticed a variety of symptoms, notably increased irritability, inability to relax and sleep, heat intolerance with excessive sweating, weight loss despite an increased appetite, and perhaps a feeling of shakiness and a fine tremor of the hands. Eye changes may be present. An enlargement of the gland may have been noticed. If it is pressing on the trachea, there may be some breathlessness.

MEDICAL MANAGEMENT

Investigations. Clinical examination will confirm the tachycardia and fibrillation, enlarged thyroid and ophthalmic signs. The skin will be hot and moist and a fine tremor of the outstretched hands may be discernible. Diagnosis is confirmed by elevated serum T_4.

Treatment. The three approaches to treatment in hyperthyroidism are:

- antithyroid drug therapy
- surgery
- radioactive iodine therapy.

Drug therapy. Antithyroid drugs (carbimazole 30–40 mg daily or propylthiouracil 300–600 mg daily) are prescribed to inhibit the synthesis of thyroid hormones. The patient will continue to take the drug until a euthyroid state (i.e. normal thyroid function) is achieved, after which the serum T_4 and the drug dose are monitored to ensure that the patient remains euthyroid and to avoid over- or under-medication. Treatment usually continues for some months, with monitoring by the patient's GP and regular outpatient visits. The patient is warned to report unexplained fever or a sore throat, as the major side-effect of antithyroid drugs is agranulocytosis, which occurs in roughly 1 in 1000 patients (see Ch. 11, p. 463).

Symptomatic control of tachycardia is obtained by administration of beta-blockers such as propranolol until thyroid hormone levels are normal.

Surgical intervention. Partial thyroidectomy is performed only after drug therapy has produced a euthyroid state. In some centres, the patient is given potassium iodide for 1–2 weeks before surgery, which will inhibit thyroid hormone release, reduce the size and vascularity of the gland and reduce the risk of postoperative haemorrhage.

About 75% of patients are cured by surgery. Partial thyroidectomy is also a useful treatment for patients with large or unsightly goitres — complications of this procedure include postoperative haemorrhage, recurrent laryngeal nerve palsy, hypocalcaemia and hypothyroidism.

Radioactive iodine therapy. Iodine-131 (^{131}I) acts by destroying functioning cells or by inhibiting their ability to replicate. It is usually administered as a single capsule on an outpatient basis. Patients are advised to avoid eating for 3–4 h after administration to allow adequate absorption of the iodine; they are also advised to drink at least 2 L of fluid over the next 24 h and to pass urine frequently in order to excrete free circulating radioactive iodine as rapidly as possible.

Patients present a radiation hazard for approximately 1 week following this treatment. In some centres, anything more than a minimal dose requires that patients are admitted for a few days until they are no longer significantly radioactive. This type of therapy is used when surgery is not appropriate, but it is not usually offered to women of child-bearing age.

NURSING PRIORITIES AND MANAGEMENT: HYPERTHYROIDISM

Major nursing considerations

Preoperative preparation (see also Ch. 26)

Patients are admitted to hospital 1–2 days prior to surgery. Although euthyroid, they may well be over-anxious about surgery, and a quiet area of the ward should be reserved for them.

Blood pressure and pulse are monitored to ensure that patients are euthyroid, and deep breathing exercises should be taught and practised. The nurse should also demonstrate the postoperative positioning and support of the head and neck to prevent strain on the sutures.

Postoperative care (see also Ch. 26)

Features of postoperative nursing care specific to patients who have undergone partial thyroidectomy are described in Nursing Care Plan 5.1.

CARCINOMA OF THE THYROID GLAND

Carcinoma of the thyroid gland is rare, comprising around 1% of all cancers (Haslett et al 1999). In the UK, it causes approximately 400 deaths per annum, compared with 35 000 from carcinoma of the lung. It is three times more common in females than males and, apart from anaplastic carcinoma, tends to occur in a much younger age group (20–40 years) than most other malignancies.

The five common types of thyroid carcinoma are:

- papillary
- follicular
- anaplastic
- lymphomatous
- medullary cell.

PATHOPHYSIOLOGY

Papillary or follicular carcinomas usually present with a rapidly growing lump which can cause hoarseness or difficulty in swallowing. Papillary carcinoma may prove fatal due to lymphatic spread to the trachea. Metastases commonly involve the brain, liver, lungs and bones and are more common with follicular carcinomas.

Common presenting symptoms. Often the patient will have noticed a small nodule or swelling in the neck. He may be euthyroid or he may have symptoms associated with either hyper- or hypothyroidism.

MEDICAL MANAGEMENT

Investigations. Tests of thyroid function (T_3, T_4, and TSH levels) are carried out and are followed by radiological examination of the neck. Needle biopsy and aspiration may be used to give a firm diagnosis and differentiate between the types. Isotope scanning will generally appear as 'cold' on scanning, but only 10% of such cold nodules are malignant. Many are cysts, and operative exploration may be avoided if aspiration cytology is normal.

Treatment. The treatment of choice is near-total thyroidectomy. This is usually followed by a large dose of ^{131}I to isolate any thyroid remnant. Any tissue showing radioiodine uptake subsequently must be assumed to be recurrent disease, and further ^{131}I may be therapeutically taken up by the tumour tissue. The thyroidectomy is performed first on the principle that only when normal thyroid tissue has been removed will malignant tissue take up the ^{131}I in a concentration high enough to cause destruction.

Follow-up is important and will usually be carried out at 6-monthly intervals initially. During this time, replacement of thyroid hormone will be with T_3 (this has a shorter half-life than T_4 and allows scanning to be repeated with ^{131}I). Any local recurrence will be treated with a further dose of ^{131}I and scanning repeated.

With early treatment, thyroid carcinoma has a relatively good prognosis.

NURSING PRIORITIES AND MANAGEMENT: CARCINOMA OF THE THYROID GLAND

Major considerations

Caring for the patient receiving ^{131}I therapy

The patient and his family should be given clear explanations regarding the effect of ^{131}I, the reasons for being nursed alone with restricted access for staff and visitors, and procedures to follow in the handling of body fluids. It should be explained to the patient that he cannot be discharged until his radiation level is safe.

Nursing Care Plan 5.1 Postoperative care for a patient who has undergone partial thyroidectomy

Nursing considerations	*Action*	*Rationale*	*Outcome/further action*
1. Compromise of airway as a result of anaesthesia and surgery to the neck area	❒ Sit the patient in an upright position with plenty of support for the neck. Oxygen may be ordered for 1–2 h after surgery	Support of the head will reduce strain on the suture line and improve the comfort of the patient, who may be very anxious about moving the neck	The airway will remain clear and strain on the suture line will be minimal
2. Risk of haemorrhage following surgery	❒ Record blood pressure and pulse half-hourly, watching for signs of irregular or laboured breathing or stridor. Clip removers should be kept by the bed for up to 24 hours after surgery	A rise in pulse and a fall in blood pressure can indicate haemorrhage, which should be reported. If respiratory embarrassment occurs due to haemorrhage, the clips must be removed to allow the blood compressing the trachea to escape. The wound should be covered with saline-soaked gauze and the patient returned to theatre immediately	Early detection of possible haemorrhage should prevent a crisis from developing and allow bleeding to be stopped sooner rather than later
3. Risk of tetany due to accidental removal of the parathyroid glands	❒ Observe closely for tetany, including tingling of fingers and toes, a positive Chvostek's sign (facial asymmetry on tapping of the cheek) or Trousseau's sign (inflation of blood pressure cuff causes spasm of hand) (See Box 5.4)	Sudden drop in calcium levels can lead to tetany, resulting in airway obstruction and, if left untreated, fitting and death	Early indications of lowered calcium levels should be reported, allowing treatment in the form of i.v. calcium gluconate to be given
4. Risk of thyroid crisis (This is now rare due to improved postoperative preparation of the patient about to undergo thyroid surgery. It is a life-threatening situation)	❒ Measure pulse, blood pressure, temperature and respiratory rate half-hourly, reducing as recovery allows	As a result of trauma to the , thyroid enormous amounts of the thyroid hormones are released into the bloodstream, causing tachycardia, a rise in blood pressure and hyperpyrexia (up to 41°C). The patient appears very restless and irritable. Death may result from heart failure	Once thyroid crisis has been diagnosed, treatment must be commenced immediately with i.v. beta-blockers (propranolol in high doses), carbimazole, steroid therapy (i.m. hydrocortisone 100 mg)
5. Risk of damage to laryngeal nerve	❒ Observe for breathing difficulties,noisy breathing, stridor, swallowing difficulties and hoarseness, and report problems	Damage to the recurrent laryngeal nerve can result in vocal cord spasm and paralysis of larynx leading to respiratory obstruction	If damage occurs, tracheostomy is usually necessary initially. The damaged nerve should recover in a few weeks. Inhalation of nitrous oxide may help in the acute period to relieve the spasm

Immediately prior to administration of the dose, TSH may be given, which will increase the uptake. Measures should be taken to prevent constipation, as this inhibits the subsequent excretion of radioactive material. A high fluid intake should be encouraged to promote a good urinary output. Commodes and bedpans should be designated for the patient's exclusive use. All body fluids will be highly radioactive following ^{131}I administration and the patient should be encouraged to bath or shower regularly to remove contaminated perspiration.

The patient should be nursed in a single room with a minimum of equipment in it. Film badges should be worn at all times by staff members to indicate radiation exposure. Duties should be coordinated so that each staff member spends a minimum amount of time with the patient.

As with all endocrine disease, prompt treatment should result in complete alleviation of all signs and symptoms; the patient should be reassured to this end whilst undergoing treatment. Follow-up after treatment is essential. Nursing staff should encourage the patient to attend outpatient or GP clinics as advised. The patient should be reassured that, particularly with localised disease from a papillary carcinoma, the probability of 'cure' is extremely high (Mallett & Bailey 1996).

J Schafer, My Story, Thyroid Papillary Carcinoma — http://oncolink.upenn.edu/disease/thyroid/index.html.

SIMPLE GOITRE

A goitre is an enlargement of the thyroid gland. It can occur without over- or underactivity of the gland. If the goitre is large, it may exert pressure on surrounding structures, causing respiratory distress or dysphagia.

HYPOSECRETION OF THE THYROID HORMONES

Underactivity of the thyroid gland may be primary, resulting from disease of the thyroid, or secondary, due to pituitary failure.

Aetiology

Primary hypothyroidism as a result of autoimmune disease is the commonest cause of thyroid underactivity. It is often termed 'Hashimoto's thyroiditis' and is often associated with other autoimmune disease. It is six times more common in women than in men.

Hypothyroidism (myxoedema) may also be caused by previous treatment for thyrotoxicosis by means of surgery or radioactive iodine.

Iodine deficiency is another cause of hypothyroidism and is due to insufficient dietary intake of iodine. This leads to reduced thyroid hormone production. Goitre is a common feature of this condition. Endemic hypothyroidism is occasionally seen in areas where iodine levels in the water supply are low (usually inland areas far from the sea). This was once a problem in Derbyshire. It is still seen in some areas such as the Andes, the alpine areas of Europe, the Himalayas and some parts of central Africa.

Congenital hypothyroidism occurs in approximately 1 in 4000 live births and usually results from congenital absence of the thyroid gland; it can also be caused by certain genetic enzyme defects. Some drugs may also induce hypothyroidism — for example, lithium carbonate (used in bipolar disorders), because of its high iodine content, can result in goitrous hypothyroidism (Haslett et al 1999).

PATHOPHYSIOLOGY

Congenital hypothyroidism results in cretinism; if it is not detected and treated early, the child will not develop fully, either mentally or physically. Most centres now screen for hypothyroidism in neonates.

In primary hypothyroidism (myxoedema), serum T_4 is low and levels of TSH are high. The effect on the cardiovascular system results in low blood pressure, bradycardia and cardiomegaly. The metabolic rate is low, resulting in lethargy, weight gain and sensitivity to cold.

Common presenting symptoms. The onset of myxoedema is slow and insidious. Because the affected individual is often elderly, it may be accepted as a normal part of ageing and it may be some time before a medical opinion is sought. The patient may report sensitivity to cold, weight gain, a general slowing down of body functions, lethargy, depression and an inability to 'think quickly'. His face will be puffy in appearance and his hair sparse, coarse and brittle. He may also notice an unattractive thickening of the skin.

In severe hypothyroidism, the patient may be admitted in a coma and perhaps be thought to be suffering from hypothermia. This represents a medical emergency in which intensive treatment and care are essential.

Diagnosis of hypothyroidism is confirmed by low plasma levels of T_4 and raised TSH levels.

MEDICAL MANAGEMENT

Treatment. Hypothyroidism is treated with replacement doses of thyroid hormone (thyroxine) commencing with a low dose and increasing to 150 mg daily. To ensure that the patient is euthyroid, both T_4 and TSH levels should be checked.

NURSING PRIORITIES AND MANAGEMENT: HYPOTHYROIDISM

It is usual to treat patients on an ongoing basis in the community. The community nursing team should follow up medical treatment and explanations and ensure that patients understand the reasons for the thyroxine replacement therapy and the importance of attending for regular checks to ensure that a euthyroid state is achieved and maintained.

DISORDERS OF THE PARATHYROID GLANDS

ANATOMY AND PHYSIOLOGY

The parathyroid glands are situated on the posterior lobes of the thyroid gland. They are usually four in number; however, more than four glands occur in up to 6% of normal individuals. This has been attributed to division of the glands during development. The blood supply is from the inferior and superior thyroid arteries.

The glands secrete parathormone (PTH), which is the most important hormone involved in calcium metabolism. Parathormone maintains plasma calcium levels within normal limits. It acts predominantly on the kidney tubules to increase reabsorption of calcium but also increases gut absorption of calcium and mobilises it from bone. Calcium levels of plasma will therefore rise, and this in turn suppresses PTH secretion; conversely, a fall in plasma calcium will stimulate the secretion of the hormone. In most instances, raised levels of calcium in the plasma are caused by hyperparathyroidism and malignancy.

Vitamin D and calcitonin are also involved in calcium metabolism (see Box 5.2).

HYPERSECRETION OF THE PARATHYROID GLANDS

Hypercalcaemia

PATHOPHYSIOLOGY

In most instances, raised levels of calcium in the plasma are caused by hyperparathyroidism or are secondary to malignancy (see Box 5.3). Mild hypercalcaemia, which is often symptomless, occurs in about 1 in 1000 of the population (Kumar & Clark 1998).

Even mild symptoms can lead to an early diagnosis, thanks to advanced chemical analysis techniques; this means that it is now extremely rare to see the severe renal and bone problems associated with hypercalcaemia that occurred in the past.

Common presenting symptoms. Patients may present with symptoms of malignancy or of hypercalcaemia, including:

- constipation
- depression
- drowsiness, coma
- excessive calcium intake
- malaise
- nausea, vomiting

Box 5.2 Vitamin D and calcitonin in calcium metabolism

Vitamin D is found in two forms: cholecalciferol (vitamin D_3), which is formed predominantly in the skin by the action of sunlight, and ergocalciferol (vitamin D_2), which is synthetic and added to food. It is the skin-synthesised form which is of greatest importance and is perhaps best considered as a hormone.

Vitamin D is biologically inactive; only when it is metabolised by the liver (to form mildly active 25-hydroxy-cholecalciferol) and the kidney (to form very active 1,25-dihydroxycholecalciferol) does it have any action on calcium metabolism. The active metabolite increases calcium absorption from the gut and is essential for bone formation.

If 1,25-dihydroxycholecalciferol is present in excess, it causes increased resorption of calcium from bone, leading to hypercalcaemia. The kidney is able to detect rising levels and ceases production of the active form, producing an inactive form until the levels drop.

Bone is constantly being re-formed by deposition and resorption of calcium. Calcitonin reduces the resorption of calcium from bone. Local stress, such as weight-bearing, is important in this process. Prolonged inactivity or immobility can result in calcium being lost from bone, while exercise increases bone formation and remodelling.

Box 5.3 Causes of hypercalcaemia

Common
- Malignancy
- Primary hyperparathyroidism

Rarer
- Addison's disease
- Milk alkaline syndrome
- Sarcoidosis
- Thyrotoxicosis
- Vitamin D poisoning

Very rare
- Immobility
- Phaeochromocytoma
- Thiazide diuretics
- Tuberculosis

- nocturia
- polydipsia, polyuria
- psychosis
- weakness.

MEDICAL MANAGEMENT

Investigations. Diagnosis is based on medical history, clinical examination and tests to ascertain the cause.

Treatment. Hypercalcaemia caused by malignancy is usually seen only in advanced carcinoma when bony metastases have occurred. If possible, it should be treated, as this may improve the quality of the patient's life. Adequate hydration is of great importance and, in itself, is often enough to relieve the symptoms of the hypercalcaemia. Other treatments include oral phosphate and steroid therapy. However, recent studies have established that the biphosphonate drugs (pamidronate, etidronate) are highly effective in lowering malignant hypercalcaemia, although the best routes of administration are still under investigation.

Primary hyperparathyroidism

This condition is caused by the overproduction of PTH by the parathyroid glands. It affects three times more women than men and its incidence increases with age. It is usually idiopathic (Haslett et al 1999).

MEDICAL MANAGEMENT

Treatment. Surgery is indicated for the management of hypercalcaemia due to excessive PTH secretion, as no long-term drug therapy is available. However, asymptomatic hypercalcaemia is treated conservatively and monitored in the GP surgery or outpatient department.

Following parathyroidectomy, hypocalcaemia of either a transient or permanent nature may ensue. This should be treated promptly to prevent tetany occurring. If severe hypocalcaemia occurs, i.v. calcium gluconate (10 mL of 10%) should be given immediately. Vitamin D and oral calcium supplements will be required. Calcium levels should be monitored closely until they have stabilised.

NURSING PRIORITIES AND MANAGEMENT: PRIMARY HYPERPARATHYROIDISM

Major considerations

The investigations required to make a diagnosis of hypercalcaemia may sometimes require hospital admission, particularly if the hypercalcaemia is severe and/or is thought to be secondary to malignancy. The patient will probably have been unwell for some time and will be feeling very tired and weak on admission.

Careful explanations of the investigations and treatment are required. It is particularly important for the accuracy of the urine tests that the urine collections are completed properly, and it is therefore essential that this is explained clearly and fully understood by the patient.

If surgery is undertaken, the perioperative care is the same as for thyroidectomy. In addition, regular assessment for impending hypocalcaemia is made (see Box 5.4).

Box 5.4 Detecting increased neuromuscular irritability (tetany) due to hypocalcaemia

Positive Chvostek's sign
The nurse can test for this sign by tapping the person's facial nerve about 2 cm anterior to the ear lobe. If hypocalcaemia (or hypomagnesaemia) is present, unilateral twitching of facial muscles, especially around the mouth, may be observed.

Positive Trousseau's sign
This may be observed when taking the blood pressure of a person with a low calcium level which, as yet, is not producing observable effects. The sphygmomanometer cuff is inflated around the person's arm and pressure is increased to above systolic pressure for 2–3 minutes. The constrictive effect of the inflated blood pressure cuff exacerbates the hypocalcaemia in the limb distal to the cuff. During blood pressure recording or shortly afterwards, muscular contraction or twitching will be noticed in the limb concerned.

Secondary and tertiary hyperparathyroidism

Secondary hyperparathyroidism occurs due to disease causing hypocalcaemia, e.g. in vitamin D deficiency or in renal disease. The parathyroid glands strive to keep the calcium levels up, while calcium remains normal or is frankly low. Rarely, this leads to permanent hypercalcaemia, termed tertiary hyperparathyroidism. This is often seen in patients with renal failure.

HYPOSECRETION OF THE PARATHYROID GLANDS

Hypocalcaemia

This is a rarer biochemical abnormality than hypercalcaemia. It is most commonly caused by renal failure but also occurs transiently, following surgery to the neck. As an idiopathic condition, it is often associated with other autoimmune features. It may be related to disorders elsewhere and not those associated with the parathyroid glands. It may also be due to severe vitamin D deficiency, an inability to convert dietary vitamin D into the active form (see Box 5.2).

Rickets and osteomalacia

These are diseases of calcium and phosphorus metabolism resulting from a deficiency in vitamin D intake and synthesis. It may be questionable to discuss these under the heading of endocrinology, but as they are usually seen and treated by endocrinologists, as opposed to other physicians, it is worth considering them in this chapter.

Vitamin D deficiency during growth produces rickets in the growing skeleton. In childhood, rickets produces soft, painful bones which are readily bent; this is seen especially in the weight-bearing bones and may give rise to gross deformities. In the adult, osteomalacia is the result; symptoms are generally diffuse bone pain and myopathy.

Rickets does not now occur commonly in the endogenous population of the UK due to better nutrition and, possibly, to a reduction in industrial pollution which allows more sunlight through. It is, however, sometimes seen in the Asian community in the UK, particularly in individuals with an increased vitamin D requirement, e.g. babies, children and pregnant women. The exact explanation for its prevalence is not clear, but it may be associated with an inability to synthesise vitamin D, as it occurs predominantly in people who eat a strict vegetarian diet.

Treatment is by vitamin D replacement, and prophylaxis is the aim in known vulnerable groups.

DISORDERS OF THE ADRENAL GLANDS

ANATOMY AND PHYSIOLOGY

The adrenal glands are situated on the upper part of the kidneys. They are highly vascular and derive their blood supply from the renal arteries, the inferior phrenic arteries and directly from the aorta; they are drained by the suprarenal veins (see Fig. 5.6). The adrenal glands have a composite origin. The cortex (the outer part) has the same embryonic site of origin as the gonads. The medulla (the inner part) is derived from neural crest cells which have migrated from the developing neural tube and have become enclosed within the cortex. The secretions, and therefore the actions of the two separate parts of the glands, are quite different and will be discussed separately.

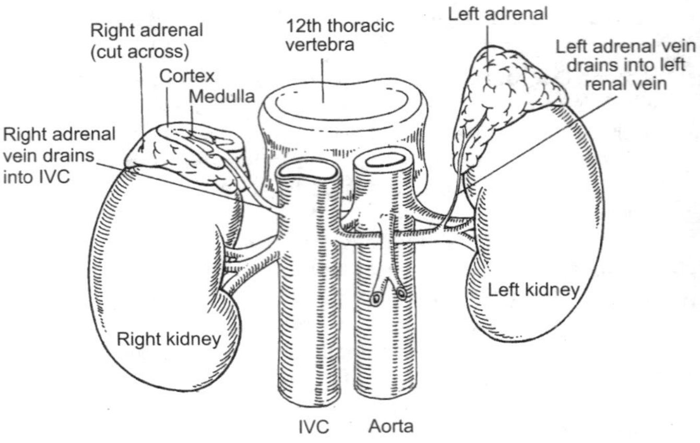

Fig. 5.6 The adrenal gland and associated structures. IVC, inferior vena cava. (Reproduced with kind permission from Jeffcoate 1993.)

The adrenal cortex

The adrenal cortex produces three types of hormone, collectively termed corticosteroids:

- mineralocorticoids
- glucocorticoids
- gonadotrophins (sex hormones).

Mineralocorticoids. The most important of the mineralocorticoids is aldosterone, which is the most potent regulator of sodium and potassium and hence of the acid–base balance of the body. Aldosterone acts on the distal convoluted tubules of the kidney and stimulates the cells to reabsorb and thus conserve sodium.

Glucocorticoids such as cortisol (the principal glucocorticoid), cortisone and hydrocortisone have varied and wide-ranging actions, many of which are not yet fully understood. They are essential to life and, in their absence, blood sugar falls, blood pressure and blood volume falls, sodium excretion increases and muscle contractility decreases. Death ensues due to low blood volume and myocardial weakness and shock. If present in excessive amounts, an opposite set of changes occurs. Blood volume expands, blood pressure rises, potassium falls, glycogen storage is increased, blood sugar levels rise, connective tissue is reduced in quality and strength, and immunity is impaired. Wound healing and the process of inflammation are also inhibited.

It appears that glucocorticoid effects are concerned with intermediary metabolism, inflammation, immunity and connective tissue healing (see Fig. 5.7).

Gonadotrophins. The adrenal glands, in addition to the gonads, produce male sex hormones. The effects are typical in the male, but in the female excessive production may have a virilising effect.

The adrenal medulla

Adrenaline, noradrenaline and dopamine (the catecholamines) are secreted by the adrenal medulla. Eighty per cent of adrenomedullary secretion is adrenaline, most noradrenaline and dopamine being secreted by neurones and functioning as neurotransmitters.

In normal secretion, adrenaline probably has some effect on mean blood pressure as, although it increases systolic pressure, it

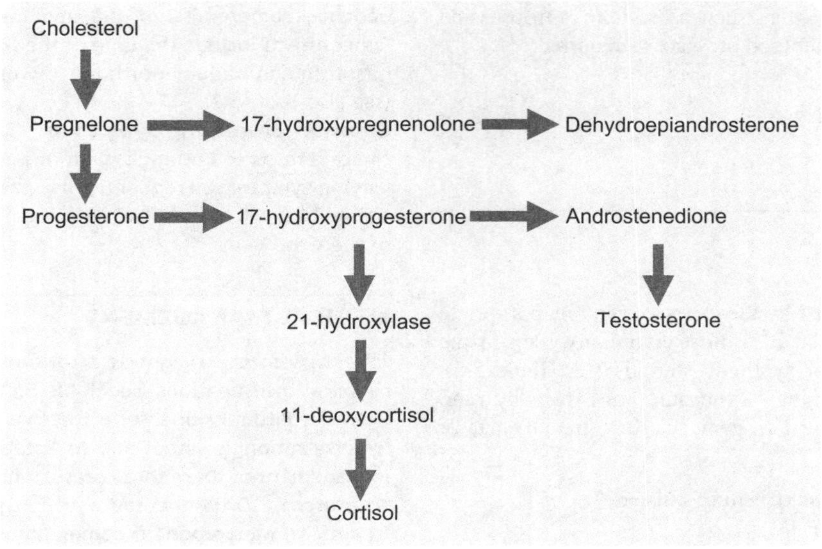

Fig. 5.7 Simplified schematisation of cortisol synthesis. (Adapted from O'Riordan et al 1982.)

decreases diastolic pressure. When secreted under the control of the sympathetic nervous system (see Ch. 9, p. 360) it causes tachycardia, decreased gut motility and the closure of sphincters in the gut, pupil dilation, bronchodilation and piloerection.

Noradrenaline raises both diastolic and systolic blood pressure but has less effect on gut motility and does not produce bronchodilation.

The difference between the effects of adrenaline and noradrenaline is partly explained by the presence of receptors on the surface of effector cells (i.e. those cells on which adrenaline and noradrenaline have their effect). These are termed α- and β-adrenoreceptors. Noradrenaline is most active at α-adrenergic receptors and adrenaline at β-adrenergic receptors. In addition, most cardiac receptors are termed B_1, to distinguish them from bronchodilator B_2 adrenoreceptors.

HYPERSECRETION OF THE ADRENAL GLANDS

The adrenal medulla

The main effect of the catecholamines (adrenaline, noradrenaline and dopamine) which are secreted by the adrenal medulla is on the cardiovascular system and the central nervous system, and on carbohydrate and lipid metabolism. Together, adrenaline and noradrenaline prepare the body for the 'fight or flight' response.

Phaeochromocytoma

Phaeochromocytoma is a very rare condition which causes about 1 in 1000 cases of hypertension (Kumar & Clark 1998). In this condition, a tumour of the adrenal medulla produces excessive adrenaline and noradrenaline. The tumour is small, with about 10% being multiple tumours and 10% being malignant.

PATHOPHYSIOLOGY

Clinical features. The tumour produces the clinical effects of excessive catecholamine secretion. Hypertension and hypertensive retinopathy are common.

Common presenting symptoms. Patients may present with anxiety, palpitations and panic attacks. Throbbing headaches, sweating and pallor are also common. There may be a history of high blood pressure. Patients may present as an acute emergency (Spencer et al 1993).

MEDICAL MANAGEMENT

Investigations. A careful history and clinical examination may lead the physician to suspect a phaeochromocytoma. Investigations include 24-h urine collections for catecholamines or their major metabolite, vanillylmandelic acid (VMA). Normal levels of catecholamine secretion virtually exclude a diagnosis of phaeochromocytoma. Abdominal X-rays and a CT scan may show a tumour of the medulla.

Treatment includes surgical removal of the tumour or administration of β-adrenoreceptor blocking drugs (e.g. propanolol).

NURSING PRIORITIES AND MANAGEMENT: PHAEOCHROMOCYTOMA

Major considerations

The first priority of care is to limit anxiety as much as possible and to nurse the patient in a quiet, non-stressful environment. Clear, concise explanations of the reasons for the symptoms will help to relieve the anxiety.

Observations of blood pressure and pulse should be recorded 4-hourly, and any sweating or flushing noted. Antihypertensive drug therapy must be maintained as the risk of postoperative hypotensive collapse is reduced by adequate preparation with adrenoreceptor blocking drugs.

A care plan should be devised such that the patient can be as independent as possible in self-care tasks. Preoperative preparation is as for general abdominal surgery (see Ch. 26). Specific postoperative care includes $\frac{1}{2}$-hourly recording of blood pressure to observe for immediate postoperative hypotensive collapse brought on by the reduced blood volume characteristic of chronic vasoconstriction. Specialist drugs such as sodium nitroprusside should be available to control blood pressure as required.

See Spencer et al (1993).

The adrenal cortex

Cushing's syndrome

Cushing's syndrome is caused by the excessive and inappropriate circulation of glucocorticoids. It is most commonly seen in the therapeutic administration of synthetic steroids (see Table 5.6). Spontaneous causes of Cushing's syndrome are extremely rare. The major causes, excluding iatrogenic causes, are (Kumar & Clark 1998):

- pituitary-dependent disease (Cushing's disease)
- ectopic ACTH production
- adrenal adenoma
- adrenal carcinoma
- alcohol-induced.

PATHOPHYSIOLOGY

Clinical features. Increased plasma cortisol levels have wide-ranging clinical effects on most systems of the body, i.e. altered fat and carbohydrate metabolism, diabetes mellitus and obesity, wasting of muscles, retention of sodium leading to hypertension, oedema, compromise of the immune system and osteoporosis. Other effects include thinning of the skin with bruising or purpura, hirsutism and oligomenorrhoea in women and impotence in men (see also Table 5.7).

Common presenting symptoms. Because of the wide-ranging clinical effects of Cushing's syndrome, the patient can present with varying symptoms. Frequently, the patient will complain of infections which will not resolve, weight gain, bruising and discoloration of the skin.

MEDICAL MANAGEMENT

Investigations. Diagnosis is confirmed by radiological and biochemical investigations (see Table 5.8). The differential diagnosis between pituitary disease, ectopic ACTH production and adrenal hypersecretion is important to establish as the treatment and management of these three causes will vary considerably.

Treatment. Drug therapy and surgery are the main forms of treatment. Metyrapone is commonly used to lower cortisol levels. An alternative approach is to remove completely intrinsic cortisol and supplement levels with an oral steroid.

Trans-sphenoidal surgery is the treatment of choice for removal of an ACTH-producing tumour of the pituitary. The antifungal drug ketaconazole is now widely used due to its activity in inhibiting steroidogenesis in the steroid synthesis pathway (see Fig. 5.7). Surgery for removal of a benign adenoma offers a good chance of cure, but adrenal carcinoma carries a poor prognosis. The drug mitotane (o'p'DDD) is adrenolytic.

Table 5.6 Unwanted effects of steroids on the systems of the body[a]

System	*Pathological effect*	*Comments*
Endocrine	Suppression of endogenous steroid production Diabetes Weight gain Amenorrhoea	Therapy should always be withdrawn gradually to enable the hypothalamic–pituitary–adrenal axis to recover
Cardiovascular	Elevation of blood pressure	Due to sodium retention
Gastrointestinal	Peptic ulceration/GI bleeding	
Renal	Polyuria Glycosuria	
Central nervous	Mood change Change in sleep pattern Appetite stimulation	May manifest itself as euphoria, depression and even so-called steroid psychosis
Musculoskeletal	Muscle wasting Osteoporosis Pathological fracture	Muscle wasting can be seen in proximal muscle; often severely affected patients cannot rise from a squatting position
Skin	Bruising Striae Thinning Poor wound healing 'Moonface' and acne	Skin becomes friable and may tear easily
Immune	Suppression	May mask signs of infection

[a]The use of steroids in medicine has proved to be beneficial in a wide variety of diseases, from asthma to bowel disease, and as an adjunct to other treatment in cancer therapy. They can provide effective pain relief in chronic musculoskeletal conditions. However, their use should be judicious and all patients having steroid therapy in the long term should be monitored and supervised. Short-term treatment (such as therapy used in the relief of an acute asthma attack) does not require such long-term follow-up. In the long term, use of steroid therapy (natural or synthetic) will mimic Cushing's syndrome, so-called iatrogenic disease.

All patients on steroid therapy should wear a 'Medic-Alert' bracelet, and told to inform other doctors or dentists that they are on steroid therapy. Surgery or intercurrent illness will require dose increases to mimic the body's normal response to stress.

Table 5.7 Signs and symptoms of Cushing's syndrome

Symptoms or sign	*Aetiology*
Muscle wasting which can be demonstrated by the patient being unable to stand from a squatting position	Catabolic effect of the steroids
Osteoporosis which can be so severe as to result in spontaneous fracture of vertebrae or ribs	Protein loss from the skeletal matrix
Skin thinning and purple striae, plethora, easy bruising and purpura	Atrophy of the elastic lamina allows disruption of the dermis so capillaries can be seen below the surface. Weakening of the capillaries leads to easy bruising (often without trauma)
Oedema	Weakening of the capillaries
Poor wound healing, immunocompromisation	The lymphocytes are destroyed, lowering the ability to fight infection. Signs of infection, e.g. swelling and redness, are masked
Obesity and 'buffalo hump' (pad of fat across shoulders)	Altered metabolism of fat. Fat is laid down over the trunk. Lipid levels may be raised
Hypertension	Sodium-retaining properties of glucocorticoids
Diabetes mellitus	Alteration in the normal metabolism of carbohydrate and the increased conversion of protein to carbohydrate
Depression, euphoria and frank psychosis	Unknown
Change in libido, impotence, oligomenorrhoea and infertility Excess hair growth, hair loss (particularly of the male pattern type in women)	Due to the general hormone imbalance that is occurring. This is seen in Cushing's but is not solely due to cortisol overproduction

Table 5.8 Radiological and biochemical tests for differential diagnosis of Cushing's syndrome

Test	*Findings indicative of Cushing's syndrome*
Radiological Adrenal CT scan	Adrenal adenomas and carcinomas are usually large and detectable on a CT scan
Skull X-ray	It is difficult to detect these often small pituitary tumours; 90% of X-rays are normal
CT scan of head and pituitary fossa, MRI scan	High-resolution scanning and increasingly sophisticated techniques often allow an enlarged pituitary to be detected
Chest X-ray	May show a bronchial carcinoma which may be a source of ectopic ACTH production
Venous catheterisation	This technique may be of value in confirming by blood sampling a pituitary origin of ACTH production as well as locating an ectopic source
Biochemical Dexamethasone suppression test	Under the principle that as a result of the feedback system high levels of steroids will switch off ACTH production and therefore steroid production, failure of suppression indicates Cushing's syndrome and at a higher dose may indicate pituitary disease. Ectopic ACTH production is not suppressed with a low or a high dose
Circadian rhythms	Patients with Cushing's syndrome may lose the normal variation in levels of cortisol. These should be measured at 09.00 h and at 24.00 h when the patient is sleeping and not warned. The patient should have been in hospital for at least 48 h before commencement of this test
Insulin tolerance test	This test, in which a dose of i.v. insulin is given, demonstrates that the normal rise in cortisol levels to hypoglycaemia is absent and will differentiate between true Cushing's, depression and alcohol-induced pseudo-Cushing's. It is performed mainly in specialist centres as a high level of supervision is required, and certain baseline measurements of pituitary function and confirmation of a normal ECG are recommended to ensure the patient's safety
Glucose tolerance test	This test will indicate that glucose metabolism is impaired; indeed, most people with Cushing's syndrome show a diabetic tendency
Urine collection	24-h urinary collections are performed and should show an elevation in excreted steroids. Accuracy in this test is difficult to achieve as it relies on the patient managing a complete, uncontaminated 24-h collection

Following adrenalectomy, patients will require lifelong hydrocortisone and mineralocorticoid replacement therapy. They must always wear a Medic-Alert bracelet and carry a steroid card, and they should be informed of the dangers of hypocortisolaemia, which is a life-threatening condition.

Management of ectopic ACTH syndrome. This condition most often occurs in patients with an oat cell carcinoma of the lung. The neoplastic cells themselves produce ACTH and give rise to Cushing's syndrome. Care is as for malignant disease (see Ch. 31), taking into account the additional complications of Cushing's syndrome.

There is another subgroup of patients with ectopic ACTH production from less malignant tumours (the so-called carcinoid tumours) who present with a more classical Cushing's syndrome and who may survive for many years with appropriate chemotherapy.

NURSING PRIORITIES AND MANAGEMENT: CUSHING'S SYNDROME

Major considerations

The main aim of nursing care is to relieve the symptoms of the disease. On admission, a full nursing history is taken and the patient's needs thoroughly assessed to provide a basis for a care plan. A major consideration will be the psychological impact of the illness, e.g. as related to a change in body image. Providing clear ongoing explanations of the hormonal changes that the patient is experiencing and of the investigations and subsequent treatment that he will undergo will go a long way toward providing psychological support.

Ongoing follow-up after discharge from hospital is essential. Initially, 3-monthly tests will be carried out, gradually reducing to an annual check. If adrenalectomy or pituitary surgery has been performed, precautions will need to be taken regarding hydrocortisone replacement; this must be explained in detail. An information leaflet can be useful as a reference for the patient when at home. This should tell the patient when to increase the therapy, e.g. during illness, and when to seek medical advice.

Q

5.3 Recall the physical symptoms that commonly occur in Cushing's syndrome. Identify the potential care needs that the patient will have and formulate a care plan responsive to those needs (see Case History 5.1 and Nursing Care Plan 5.2).

HYPOSECRETION OF THE ADRENAL HORMONES

Addison's disease

Addison's disease is a rare condition in which there is total destruction of the adrenal cortex resulting in failure of cortisol secretion. It may occur at any age and is more common in females. Autoimmune adrenalitis is the most common cause in the developed world. Adrenal destruction by adrenalytic drugs such as mitotane (o'p'DDD), malignant disease or malignancy are rare causes.

PATHOPHYSIOLOGY

Clinical features. High levels of ACTH result in pigmentation of the skin and mucous membranes. Glucocorticoid, sex steroid and mineralocorticoid production is reduced. Plasma levels of proteins are low, and plasma levels of potassium are high, with serum urea being elevated due to volume depletion.

Common presenting symptoms. The onset of the disease is usually insidious, often starting with a feeling of general malaise and weakness. The discolouring of the skin will have been noticed, especially in the palmar creases and on the inside of the lips and cheeks. Some patients present as medical emergencies with Addisonian crisis, in which there is hypotensive collapse, abdominal pain and fever (O'Donnell 1997).

MEDICAL MANAGEMENT

Investigations. Diagnosis is by clinical examination and blood tests to confirm high levels of ACTH and low levels of cortisol.

In the short Synacthen test, a dose of 250 mg of tetracosactrin (synthetic ACTH) is given i.v. or i.m.; blood samples for plasma cortisol taken at 30 and 60 min after its administration will show a failure of the adrenal glands to respond to the stimulus of the parenteral ACTH.

Treatment is by long-term replacement doses of mineralocorticoid and glucocorticoid. This should lead to an improvement in the patient's well-being. Levels of hydrocortisone should be checked regularly to ensure the dose is correct. Mineralocorticoid replacement with fludrocortisone should be checked by regular blood pressure readings (which should show no postural hypotension) and by measurement of plasma renin.

Addisonian crisis. Adrenal crisis is a life-threatening event. It occurs in such situations as injury infections, anaesthesia and surgical procedures where, unlike in the healthy individual, the stress response does not occur. The absence of the cortisol surge to a major stressor results in a severely shocked patient. Addisonian crisis requires immediate intervention. Treatment aims to restore steroid, sodium and glucose levels to within normal range by i.v. administration of 100 mg hydrocortisone, and i.v. infusion of normal saline given quickly with dextrose if glucose levels are low. Hydrocortisone is then given i.v. or i.m. 6-hourly until the patient is stable, following which the steroid replacements can be given orally and mineralocorticoid introduced.

NURSING PRIORITIES AND MANAGEMENT: ADDISON'S DISEASE

Major considerations

Careful observation of temperature, pulse, and standing and lying blood pressure should be made. A raised temperature will indicate signs of infection which the patient may not be able to fight effectively. Any postural drop in blood pressure should be reported immediately.

The steroid replacement therapy should be administered with the patient's involvement so that he will have a full knowledge of drug dosage and timing and techniques for self-administration before discharge. The patient should be issued with a steroid card and advised to carry this and to wear a Medic-Alert bracelet on his wrist or ankle at all times.

An ampoule of hydrocortisone 100 mg should be kept at home in case of serious illness or trauma, and the GP or community nurse called to administer it. It may also be of value to teach a member of the family how to do this.

It is vital that the patient has a thorough understanding of his condition and the signs associated with complications. This will help to restore confidence and enable him to return to a full and active life.

Case History 5.1 J

J was a 20-year-old woman admitted to the unit following transfer from her local hospital with a history of weight gain, hirsutism, acne on her back and face, pain and increasing weakness in her limbs, amenorrhoea and depression.

She was transferred in a wheelchair, being unable to walk at this point. Her parents and her fiancé accompanied her.

Once J was settled into the unit, clinical examination showed her to have centripetal obesity, severe acne, marked facial hair and some loss of occipital hair. She had severe pitting oedema of her ankles and had been amenorrhoeal for 6 months. Purple striae were present on her abdomen and thighs, and bruising was noticeable on her shins. She was unable to stand from the squatting position, indicating marked proximal myopathy. She was tearful and anxious and complained of a poor sleep pattern and waking at about 04.00 h. Observations showed her to be hypertensive at 170/110 mmHg; pulse and temperature were normal. J had some photographs of herself taken at her engagement party some 4 months before, showing a pretty, very slim, smiling young woman.

She was helped to settle into the unit and her nurse sat with her and explained the investigations that were to be performed. As many of these involved multiple venepunctures, she was reassured that a local anaesthetic cream would be applied. (It is inadvisable to leave cannulae in situ as the risk of infection in someone who is immunocompromised is great.)

On the first day blood tests showed that J's baseline cortisol levels were well above the normal range. Her haemoglobin, liver function, urea and electrolytes were measured, as well as her sex hormone levels and thyroid function. A measurement of ACTH was made and found to be extremely high. Skull and chest X-rays were performed.

An insulin tolerance test showed elevated cortisol levels throughout with no response to hypoglycaemia. A glucose tolerance test showed elevated glucose levels throughout; glycosuria was present 1 h post-glucose load. This had not resolved at 2 h, indicating a diabetic tendency.

On the third and fourth days, blood was taken at 09.00 h, 18.00 h and 24.00 h and repeated the next night, the midnight samples being taken when J was asleep. This was to establish her circadian rhythm; the results showed that the levels of ACTH and cortisol did not fall at night and remained high throughout the day.

The finding that both the ACTH levels and the cortisol levels were high indicated that the high cortisol levels were being driven by ACTH. The source of the ACTH had to be established.

During this time J was seen by a psychiatrist, who established that she was depressed but not suicidal. Medical staff kept her informed about the results of her tests and their implications; further explanations were given by her nurse. A CT scan the following day showed an enlarged pituitary gland.

Based on this it was decided that petrosal sinus sampling would be performed and samples taken for ACTH and cortisol after a catheter had been inserted into the right groin. The procedure was explained to J and her consent obtained. Her right groin was shaved and she was fasted overnight. Samples were taken at various points, including the petrosal sinuses (the point nearest the pituitary gland on both the left and right sides). No sedation is permitted prior to this test as it interferes with the results and so extremely detailed explanation of the procedure was required to gain J's confidence and understanding. She was accompanied by her nurse, who remained with her throughout the procedure. When assayed, the results showed a higher level of ACTH on the left side of the pituitary.

Once a source had been found for the excess ACTH, J could be started on drug therapy to control her symptoms. She was started on metyrapone 500 mg t.d.s. and her cortisol levels were checked daily to ensure she did not become hypocortisolaemic.

After review of her results and X-rays, it was suggested that to try to remove the pituitary tumour would be the best treatment option. After discussion with J, her consent for the operation was obtained. It was explained to her and her fiancé that there was a possibility that she may become deficient in all pituitary hormones following the surgery, including those which would affect her fertility. In this eventuality hormone replacement could be given.

A small adenoma was removed from the left side of her pituitary gland. On return from theatre J was nursed on the neurosurgical ward initially. Hydrocortisone injections were given (100 mg every 6 h for 48 h) to ensure that if the tumour had been removed, J's cortisol levels would not fall too rapidly and predispose her to an Addisonian crisis. J returned to the endocrine unit looking rather bruised around the eyes and wearing a nasal bolster but otherwise well. Nursing staff continued to monitor her lying and standing blood pressures. Temperature and pulse were checked 4-hourly and nasal discharge was observed and tested for signs of CSF leak.

Three days postoperatively J's hydrocortisone was withdrawn. A measurement of her 09.00 h cortisol and ACTH was taken the next day. Her cortisol level was very low and correspondingly J felt weak and light-headed. Her blood pressure showed a postural drop. The next morning the exercise was repeated and the results were the same. J was losing weight around her face and her ankle oedema was reduced. She said she felt very positive for the first time in months and was sleeping well. On the afternoon of the fourth postoperative day, she became weak and dizzy and felt nauseated. Her blood pressure was measured and found to be low. She was laid down and the doctor informed. It was felt that an Addisonian crisis was impending and so a blood sample was taken for cortisol measurement and J was commenced on oral prednisolone. Some days later all of J's hormone levels were checked and, as she felt well on her replacement therapy, she was discharged home to the care of her family. It was arranged for her to return to the ward in 12 weeks' time.

By the time J returned for this visit, she had lost a considerable amount of weight, was walking unaided, had lost most of her facial hair and had started menstruating. Her steroid therapy was stopped and close observation maintained to observe for impending adrenal crisis. A blood test 48 h later indicated that her cortisol levels were in the normal range. It was decided to repeat all the pituitary function tests done prior to the surgery. These showed all hormones to be in the normal range and responses to hypoglycaemia, as demonstrated by the insulin tolerance test, to be intact. This showed that the pituitary had recovered its normal function. J was discharged home with a regular follow-up in-patient appointment every 12 weeks to ensure that all was well.

Some months after, the nurses received an invitation to J's wedding and 1 year later J was the very proud mother of a baby daughter.

Nursing Care Plan 5.2 Care of a patient with Cushing's syndrome

Nursing considerations	*Action*	*Rationale*	*Expected outcome*
1. Pain from fractured vertebrae or ribs as a result of osteoporosis	❒ Provide immediate pain relief. Administer as prescribed, noting the efficacy ❒ Handle and position the patient carefully	Pain will cause the patient discomfort and will increase anxiety. Pain relief will reduce this. Fractured ribs will cause shallow breathing and will increase chances of chest infection. Gentle handling will reduce distress and prevent further fractures	The patient should be pain-free and comfortable and his anxiety reduced
2. Infection as a result of immunocompromisation	❒ Make 4-hourly recordings of temperature, pulse and blood pressure. Report any variation from the normal range immediately	Death from overwhelming infection can occur. Signs of infection will be masked, so infection may be advanced before signs are seen	Any infection will be identified early and correct treatment commenced
3. Damage to skin as a result of skin thinning and oedema or poor wound healing	❒ If the patient is immobile, care of pressure areas will be required to prevent tissue damage. Legs will need to be elevated to relieve the oedema and any wounds will require scrupulous aseptic technique when dressed	Tissue will be rapidly broken down and slow to heal, so preventive measures are essential. Susceptibility to infection requires precautions to prevent introduction of infection	Further tissue damage will be prevented and any present source of infection healed as rapidly as possible
4. Hypertension	❒ Record blood pressure readings 4-hourly after 10 min lying flat and 1 min standing. Report levels beyond the normal range or postural deficit	Increasing blood pressure may lead to stroke or heart failure and if persistently high will need to be treated with drugs. Postural deficit will indicate a problem with sodium excretion or retention	Blood pressure levels will remain within acceptable limits
5. Diabetes mellitus as a result of abnormal carbohydrate metabolism	❒ Record pre- and postprandial blood sugar levels and perform daily urinalysis	Persistently high blood sugars will lead to the complications of diabetes mellitus and may need to be treated with insulin	Blood sugar levels will remain within the normal range
6. Psychosis and mental disorder	❒ Ascertain the patient's psychological status early on. A psychiatric opinion should be obtained. Mood swings and bizarre behaviour should be reported. The patient may be so disturbed as to require 24 h psychiatric nurse observation	The patient's psychological state may change rapidly and close observation for this is necessary. Some patients can become suicidal	The patient will not be a danger to himself or others and his safety is maintained at all times

Q

5.4 With a colleague, undertake a role-play exercise by acting out the education of the patient regarding steroid therapy. Formulate an information sheet which could be given to patients prior to discharge.
5.5 Check within the local hospital context what advice is available for patients with Addison's disease. Where do patients obtain the Medic-Alert bracelet from? Are these patients exempt from prescription charges?

CONGENITAL ADRENAL HYPERPLASIA (CAH)

This is a condition caused by a deficiency in one of the enzymes involved in cortisol synthesis. It is an inherited disorder and is thought to occur in about 1 in 5000 of the population in Europe.

PATHOPHYSIOLOGY

To understand CAH it is necessary to understand the biosynthesis of steroids. If, as can be inferred from Figure 5.7, the enzyme 21-hydroxylase is absent (to take the most common deficiency as an example), cortisol will not be produced in sufficient quantity. By means of the negative feedback system, ACTH production will be increased to stimulate the production of cortisol. This in turn will lead to hypertrophy of the adrenal cortex and elevated levels of 17-hydroxyprogesterone, androstenedione and testosterone — the hormones occurring before the enzyme block. This will result ultimately in virilisation.

Common presenting symptoms. If severe, CAH presents at birth with sexual ambiguity. In the female, the high level of androgens present cause clitoral hypertrophy and fusion of the labial folds. The syndrome may not be recognised in the male. Internal genitalia may develop normally. If a diagnosis is not made at birth, a genotypical female may be labelled male. Furthermore, the individual may go into adrenal crisis and die if not treated with corticosteroids.

Other problems which may occur because of the excessive circulating sex hormones are primary amenorrhoea in girls, precocious puberty and short stature due to premature fusion of the bony epiphyses.

MEDICAL MANAGEMENT

Investigations include blood tests to confirm high levels of ACTH and 17-hydroxyprogesterone. Replacement of the glucocorticoid is usually given in the form of prednisolone to suppress the ACTH production and thereby reduce the overstimulation of the adrenals. Other corticosteroids may be used.

NURSING PRIORITIES AND MANAGEMENT: CONGENITAL ADRENAL HYPERPLASIA (CAH)

General considerations

Information should be given to the individual regarding steroid replacement therapy (details of which can be read under 'Hypopituitarism', p. 141). Nursing care should concentrate on the psychological support which will be required, especially if the diagnosis is made late.

The psychosocial implications of CAH are considerable, and formal counselling and psychotherapy should be made available. In female patients, some of the effects of virilisation are not reversible with drug therapy; plastic surgical repair may therefore be necessary. This is particularly important as the patient approaches adulthood, as sexual intercourse may be rendered difficult, painful or impossible.

DISORDERS OF THE GONADS

ANATOMY AND PHYSIOLOGY

The gonads — ovaries in the female and testes in the male — are described in Chapters 7 and 8.

DISORDERS OF SEXUAL DIFFERENTIATION

In normal development, gonadal and phenotypic sex follow an orderly process of development determined by chromosomal sex at the moment of conception (see Ch. 6).

During the early stages of fetal life the gonad has the potential to develop female or male characteristics. In the presence of another X chromosome (i.e. 46, XX) or the absence of another chromosome (i.e. 45, XO), development will follow the female pattern. The presence of two X chromosomes is, however, necessary for normal ovarian function.

By the second month of fetal development the genital organs are undifferentiated duct systems termed the Müllerian and Wolffian ducts. In the normal female, as development progresses, the Wolffian system regresses and the Müllerian system develops to form the fallopian tubes, the uterus and the upper vagina. The external genitalia undergo little change.

In the male, the Müllerian system regresses and the Wolffian system develops to form the testes, vas deferens, prostate and seminiferous tubules. The genital tubercle present in both systems forms the clitoris in the female and the penis in the male.

There is evidence to suggest that the normal development of a male child is hormone-dependent. It appears that testosterone inhibits the regression of the Wolffian duct and stimulates its development into the male sexual structures. In contrast to this, the ovary is not affected by hormones in utero.

Abnormalities of sexual differentiation may present with abnormal genitalia at birth, growth disturbance in childhood or abnormal secondary sexual development.

Abnormalities of gonadal development

True hermaphroditism (i.e. the presence of both male and female sexual characteristics in the same individual) is extremely rare. It occurs when both the Müllerian and Wolffian systems continue to develop. Ovotestes may exist or an ovary on one side and a testis on the other.

Chromosomal abnormalities

Chromosomal abnormalities affecting sexual differentiation may briefly be described as follows:

Klinefelter's syndrome. A condition in which phenotypical males have two X and one Y chromosomes.

Turner's syndrome. A condition in which the individual is phenotypically female, but has the genotype XO. Affected individuals are of short stature with a 'web neck' and may have widely spaced nipples and peripheral oedema. The ovaries are atrophic and serum LH and FSH levels are elevated.

Kallman's syndrome. There is a normal karyotype but a deficiency of gonadotrophins. This condition is sometimes termed hypogonadotrophic hypogonadism. Typically, the individual has a partial defect in the sense of smell. Normal function can be resumed with replacement of LH and FSH. Fertility is possible.

Testicular feminisation. This is a syndrome of androgen resistance. The karyotype is male and testes are present, but because of tissue resistance to circulating androgens at puberty, breast tissue develops although pubic hair does not. Due to tissue insensitivity the regression of the Müllerian system occurs but the Wolffian system does not develop and a blind-ended vagina results. The gonads may become malignant and are usually removed at the onset of adult life.

NURSING PRIORITIES AND MANAGEMENT: DISORDERS OF SEXUAL DIFFERENTIATION

Whilst disorders of the gonads rarely are life-threatening or require admission to hospital, the psychological implications for individuals and their families cannot be overemphasised.

The role of the nurse in the investigation and treatment of these conditions is to offer psychological support to the individuals concerned in an environment which is both relaxed and supportive.

Counselling on an informal and formal basis is essential during investigations, when complete privacy must be ensured. Feelings of inadequacy regarding sexuality and low self-esteem are common. An approach which demonstrates empathy with the individual helps to create a positive image during the initial examinations and investigations and subsequent treatment.

EATING DISORDERS

The discussion of eating disorders in this chapter may seem controversial as endocrine disorder is often a manifestation of an eating disorder (e.g. amenorrhoea in the patient with anorexia).

However, the interface between the two is complicated and as many patients may be seen in endocrine units, eating disorders are worth considering here.

Recent studies into the role of the hypothalamus have highlighted the influence it has on appetite control. It is now almost certain that the hypothalamus has a function in some eating disorders. Recent hypotheses include the identification of a negative feedback system involving specific proteins known as leptins that may be malfunctioning in the obese patient (Glick 1995).

ANOREXIA NERVOSA

Anorexia nervosa is an eating disorder characterised by self-inflicted starvation and a relentless pursuit of thinness (Bruch 1973).

Epidemiology

Anorexia nervosa is seen in all social classes and in both sexes. However, only 5–10% of cases occur in males and there is a higher prevalence in social classes 1 and 2 (Edwards et al 1995). Bruch (1973) indicated that anorexic individuals tend to be young girls who come from highly successful families in which the parents have high expectations of their children.

Aetiology

Contributory factors in the development of anorexia nervosa include:

- Family background, parental pressure, sibling disability, parental overprotection and negative changes within family relationships (Horesh et al 1996)
- The onset of puberty and psychosexual development in which there is denial and avoidance of sexuality marked by the development of the breasts and change of shape of hips and thighs
- Sociocultural expectations — there is an enormous emphasis on thinness in society's image of female beauty.

Recent studies also suggest that there is a genetic risk factor for anorexia. Studies of twins in the USA suggest that about half the risk of developing this eating disorder is inherited (Berretini & Kaye 1998).

PATHOPHYSIOLOGY

There is a complex relationship between nutritional, endocrine and psychological factors in this condition. Disorders in nutritional status result from prolonged insufficient intake of carbohydrates, fats and other nutrients. Metabolic disturbances (e.g. hypokalaemia) can occur following self-induced vomiting or the continual use of laxatives.

Clinical features. Endocrine dysfunction appears to relate to weight loss and affects the hypothalamopituitary–gonadal axis. Blood tests reveal low circulating levels of LH, FSH and oestradiol. Injections of gonadotrophin hormone stimulate a rise in these, indicating that hypothalamic function is affected and the pituitary response is intact. Amenorrhoea occurs as a result of this disturbance, secondary to the loss of body fat. The individual's metabolic rate slows down, resulting in hypotension, bradycardia, reduced core body temperature and cold extremities.

Individuals with anorexia nervosa often have underlying depression. It would seem that their psychological symptoms are aggravated by the undernutrition, and some professionals argue that patients are more receptive to psychological help when they are better nourished. The characteristic mental state involves a denial of the illness, a failure to recognise the need for treatment and a need to exercise control over eating behaviour. The individual will have a distorted body image and insist that her cachectic body appears obese.

Common presenting symptoms. Most frequently, the anorexia will have been present for some months before individuals can be persuaded to see their GP. A determination to lose weight coupled with the desire to change the shape of the body is typical, as is the denial of any problem or illness. Sufferers will claim to 'feel fat' even when they are obviously underweight or emaciated. In women, amenorrhoea, typically beginning 3–6 months from the start of weight loss, will be found.

MEDICAL MANAGEMENT

History and investigation. Diagnosis is reached after investigations have proved that there is no underlying cause for the weight loss. Objective criteria have been developed to aid diagnosis. These include:

- a determination to diet and lose weight and maintain the weight loss
- a change of body shape to one of extreme thinness
- distorted body image
- avoidance of sexuality
- amenorrhoea in female patients.

Treatment. Depending on the severity of the weight loss and its effect on general health, the patient is managed as an outpatient or in-patient in a specialist mental health unit.

It is commonly accepted that an eclectic approach to treatment is useful. This may involve cognitive–behavioural approaches, social reality and individual and family therapy. Restoring body weight and nutritional status will be at the centre of whatever approach is used. If the weight loss has led to physiologically life-threatening conditions such as hypokalaemia or renal failure, it may be necessary to correct fluid and electrolyte imbalance by i.v. fluids and to improve nutritional status by parenteral or nasogastric feeding for as short a time as possible. (Given the invasive nature of these procedures, they can be psychologically damaging for the individual.)

A multidisciplinary team approach in which dieticians, occupational therapists, medical staff and nurses work together with the anorexic individual in an agreed and consistent framework is essential. Current therapy combines the use of psychotherapy and the use of antidepressants in the serotonin uptake inhibitor group. This is thought to be proving successful as serotonin is known to be a modulator of eating behaviour (Bardin et al 1997). Other studies have looked at the maintenance of weight using drugs that act on serotonin uptake (O'Dwyer et al 1996).

NURSING PRIORITIES AND MANAGEMENT: ANOREXIA NERVOSA

Major considerations

The main aims of nursing care for individuals with anorexia nervosa are:

- to establish a good relationship with the patient
- to restore body weight and nutritional status
- to establish a good eating pattern and the enjoyment of mealtimes
- to eliminate self-induced vomiting and the use of laxatives
- to help the individual to acquire a positive self-image.

Because of their condition, patients will often present strong arguments as to why they cannot eat and will resort to devious methods to avoid taking in calories. Visits to the toilet after eating (to vomit or to dispose of food not eaten) should be observed for and prevented. It is important that mealtimes are handled in a relaxed manner; and realistic goals should be set and agreed to by each patient, with regard to foods eaten and weight gain. A written contract can help to create a climate of trust and help to prevent manipulation of staff and parents.

As goals are met and maintained, short stays with the family can be arranged. If these visits are successful, plans can be made for discharge home. Continued support and monitoring of nutritional and weight status is essential, as relapse is common among anorexics.

BULIMIA NERVOSA

Bulimia nervosa is an eating disorder characterised by episodes of binge eating, self-induced vomiting and the use of laxatives. While in both anorexia and bulimia there is an exaggerated concern with weight and body shape, these are separate conditions. Further reading on both subjects is suggested at the end of the chapter.

ACKNOWLEDGEMENTS

The author would like to thank the Molecular Endocrinology team at the Medical Research Council, Hammersmith Hospital, London, for their advice and assistance.

REFERENCES

Bassett J H D, Forbes S A, Pannett A A J et al 1998 Characterization of mutations in patients with multiple endocrine neoplasia type I. American Journal of Human Genetics 62: 232–244
Baxter M A 1994 Acromegaly and hypophysectomy: a case report. Association of American Nurse Anaesthetists 62(2): 182–185
Bengtsson B A, Eden S, Lon L et al 1993 Treatment of adults with growth hormone deficiency with recombinant hGH. Journal of Clinical Endocrinology and Metabolism 76: 309–317
Berretini W, Kaye W 1997 Directions in Psychiatry (Winter issue). http://www.cmch.com./articles/eatdis2
Besser G M, Cudworth A G 1990 Clinical endocrinology. Lippincott, Philadelphia
Besser G M, Thorner M O 1995 Clinical endocrinology. Gower, Aldershot
Besser G M, Trainer P J 1995 The Barts endocrine protocols. Churchill Livingstone, Edinburgh
Bouloux P M G, Rees L M 1994 Diagnostic tests in endocrinology and metabolism. Chapman and Hall, London
Bruch H 1973 Eating disorders. Basic Books, New York
Glick M E 1995 Fat, body weight regulated by a newly discovered hormone. http://www.rockefeller.edu/pubinfo/ob/rel.htlm
Grinspoon S K, Bilezikian J P 1992 HIV disease and the endocrine system. New England Journal of Medicine 327: 1360–1365
Haslett C, Chilvers C R, Hunter J A, Boon N A 1999 Davidson's principles and practice of medicine. 18th edn. Churchill Livingstone, Edinburgh
Ho K Y, Weissberger A J, Marbach P, Lazarus M B 1990 Therapeutic efficacy of the somatostatin analog SMS 201–995 (octreotide) in acromegaly. Annals of Internal Medicine 112: 173–181
Horesh N, Apter A, Ishai J et al 1996 Abnormal psychosocial situations and eating disorders in adolescence. Journal of the American Academy of Child and Adolescent Psychiatry 35(7): 921–927
Jeffcoate W 1993 Lecture notes on endocrinology, 5th edn. Blackwell Scientific Publications, Oxford
Kumar P, Clark M 1998 Clinical medicine, 4th edn. WB Saunders, Edinburgh
Li J, Li L Y, Son C, Banks P, Brodie A 1992 4- pregnene-3-one 20 beta-carboxaldehyde:a potent inhibitor of 17-alpha-hydroylase/C17,20 lyase and of 5-alpha reductase. Journal of Steroid Biochemistry and Molecular Biology 42: 313–320
Mallet J, Bailey C (eds) 1996 Manual of clinical nursing procedures, 4th edn. Blackwell Science, Oxford
Newman C B, Melmed S, Snyder P J et al 1995 Safety and efficacy of long term octreotide therapy in acromegaly: results of a multicentre trial in 103 patients. Journal of Clinical Endocrinology and Metabolism 80: 2768–2775
O'Donnell M 1997 Emergency! Addisonian crisis. American Journal of Nursing 97(3): 41
O'Dwyer A M, Lucie J V, Russell G F 1996 Serotonin activity in anorexia nervosa after long term weight restoration: response to D-fenfluramine challenge. Psychological Medicine 26(2): 353–359
O'Riordan J L H, Malan P G, Gould R P 1982 Essentials of endocrinology. Blackwell Scientific, Oxford
Sinclair H C, Fawcett J N 1991 Altschul's psychology for nurses, 7th edn. Baillière Tindall, London
Spencer E, Pycock C, Lyttle J 1993 Pheochromocytoma presenting as acute circulatory collapse and abdominal pain. Intensive Care Medicine 19(6): 356–357
Bardin C et al 1997 Current therapy in endocrinology and metabolism, 6th edn. Mosby, St Louis
Wilson K J W, Waugh A (eds) 1996 Ross & Wilson: anatomy and physiology in health and illness, 7th edn. Churchill Livingstone, Edinburgh

FURTHER READING

Agana-Defensor R, Proch M 1992 Pheochromocytoma: a clinical review. Clinical Issues in Critical Care Nursing 3(2): 309–318
Bayliss R I S, Tunbridge W M G 1991 Thyroid disease: the facts, 2nd edn. Oxford University Press, Oxford
Behi R 1989 Treatment and care of thyroid problems. Nursing (Oxford) 3(41): 4–6
Besser G M, Thorner M O 1995 Clinical endocrinology. Gower, Aldershot
Bouloux P M G, Rees L M 1994 Diagnostic tests in endocrinology and metabolism. Chapman and Hall, London
Bryant S O, Kopeski L M 1986 Psychiatric nursing assessment of the eating disorder client. Topics in Clinical Nursing 8(1): 57–66
Chambers J K 1987 Metabolic bone disorders: imbalances of calcium and phosphorus. Nursing Clinics of North America 22(4): 861–872
Costin C 1996 The eating disorder source book: a comprehensive guide to the causes, treatments and prevention of eating disorders. Lowell House, Harvard
Counsell C M, Gilbert M, Snively C 1996 Management of a patient with a pituitary tumour resection. Dimensions of Critical Care Nursing 15(2): 75–81
Crowther J H 1992 The etiology of bulimia nervosa. Hemisphere, London
DeRubertis F R 1985 Hypocalcemia: etiology and management. Hospital Medicine 21(3): 88–90, 95–97, 100

Edwards C R, Lincoln D W 1992 Recent advances in endocrinology and metabolism. Churchill Livingstone, Edinburgh
Epstein C D 1991 Fluid volume deficit for the adrenal crisis patient. Dimensions of Critical Care Nursing 10(4): 210–217
Francis B 1990 Hypothyroidism. Advancing Clinical Care 5(2): 29–30
Goldberger J, Goldberger S 1989 Iatrogenic thyroid dysfunction: a case study. Hospital Practice 24(9): 30, 35
Graves L 1990 Disorders of calcium, phosphorus and magnesium. Critical Care Nursing Quarterly 13(3): 3–13
Grinspoon S 1999 Advances in recombinant human growth hormone replacement therapy in adults. http://neurosurgery.mgh.harvard.edu/e-f-944.htm
Grinspoon S K, Bilezikian J P 1992 HIV disease and the endocrine system. New England Journal of Medicine 327: 1360–1365
Hall R, Besser M (eds) 1989 Fundamentals of clinical endocrinology, 4th edn. Churchill Livingstone, Edinburgh
Halloran T H 1990 Nursing responsibilities in endocrine emergencies. Critical Care Nursing Quarterly 13(3): 74–81
Hardcastle W 1989 Management of Addison's disease. Nursing (Oxford) 3(41): 7–9
Hinchliff S M, Montague S E, Watson R 1996 Physiology for nursing practice, 2nd edn. WB Saunders, Philadelphia
Kessler C A 1992 An overview of endocrine function and dysfunction. Clinical Issues in Critical Care Nursing 3(2): 289–299
Kessler C M 1988 Protecting the adrenalectomy patient. Nursing 18(12): 64L
Kiecolt-Glaser J, Dixon K 1984 Postadolescent onset male anorexia. Journal of Psychosocial Nursing and Mental Health Services 22(1): 10–13, 17–20
Moroney J 1991 Living with anorexia and bulimia. Manchester University Press, Manchester
Nalbach D A, Carson M A 1991 Prolactinoma: a review and case study. Critical Care Nurse 11(9): 48–49, 52–57
Nusbaum J G, Drever E 1990 Inpatient survey of nursing care measures for treatment of patients with anorexia nervosa. Issues in Mental Health Nursing 11(2): 175–184
Reasner C A 1990 Adrenal disorders. Critical Care Nursing Quarterly 13(3): 67–73
Rice V 1991 Hypercalcaemia. Canadian Intravenous Nurses Association Journal 7(1): 6–8
Schafer J 1997 My story, thyroid papillary carcinoma. http://oncolink.upenn.edu/disease/thyroid/index.html
Sheppard M C, Franklyn J A (eds) 1988 Clinical endocrinology and diabetes. Churchill Livingstone, Edinburgh
Smith J E 1990 Pregnancy complicated by thyroid disease. Journal of Nurse-Midwifery 35(3): 143–149
Smith-Rooker J L, Garrett A, Hodges L C 1993 Case management of the patient with a pituitary tumour. Medsurg Nursing 2(4): 265–274
Spencer E, Pycock C, Lyttle J 1993 Pheochromocytoma presenting as acute circulatory collapse and abdominal pain. Intensive Care Medicine 19(6): 356–357
Szmukler G I 1985 The epidemiology of anorexia nervosa and bulimia. Journal of Psychiatric Research 19:143–153
Walker M 1990 Women in therapy and counselling: out of the shadows. Eating disorders; women, food and the world. Open University Press, Milton Keynes, ch 7
Walpert N 1990 An orderly look at calcium metabolism disorders. Nursing 20(7): 60–64
Walworth J 1990 Parathyroidectomy: maintaining calcium homeostasis. Todays O R Nurse 12(4): 20–24, 31–33
Yeomans A C 1990 Assessment and management of hypothyroidism. Nurse Practitioner 15(11): 8, 11–12
Yucha C, Blakeman N 1991 Pheochromocytoma: the great mimic. Cancer Nursing 14(3): 136–140

USEFUL ADDRESSES

Medic Alert Foundation
9 Hanover Street
London
W1R 9HF

The Pituitary Foundation
PO Box 1944
Bristol
BS99 2UB

UK Child Growth Foundation
2 Marfield Avenue
Chiswick
W4 1PW
Tel: 0181 995 0257

PART 2
DIABETES MELLITUS

INTRODUCTION

The British Diabetic Association (BDA) describes diabetes mellitus as a condition in which the amount of glucose in the blood is abnormally high because the body is no longer able to adequately use it as fuel (BDA 1995). This elevated blood glucose (hyperglycaemia) and other biochemical abnormalities which occur are a consequence of the deficient production or action of insulin, a hormone that controls glucose, fat and amino acid metabolism. The BDA estimates that, within the UK, there are 1.38 million adults with known diabetes (BDA 1995).

Diabetes classification

Various classifications exist for diabetes mellitus, none of which is entirely satisfactory. In the past, the patient's age at diagnosis was the main classification criterion. Accordingly, diabetes was described as being either of 'juvenile onset' or 'maturity onset'. Specific diagnostic and treatment characteristics were ascribed to each type. This classification is now obsolete and has been replaced by the WHO classification (WHO 1985) which recognises the main types of diabetes as follows:

- insulin-dependent (type 1)
- non-insulin-dependent (type 2)
- malnutrition-related
- impaired glucose tolerance
- gestational
- secondary to other diseases and conditions.

For information on gestational diabetes, see Stewart & Taylor (1994), and for diabetes in childhood see Murphy (1994) and Betschart (1993).

ANATOMY AND PHYSIOLOGY

For a detailed study of normal anatomy and physiology, the reader is referred to Tortora & Grabowski (1996).

The pancreas

The pancreas combines both exocrine and endocrine functions. Exocrine tissue is responsible for the secretion of enzymes which are transported in ducts to the duodenum where they play a vital role in the digestion of food (see p. 91). The endocrine function of the pancreas is concerned with the secretion of hormones. Clusters of endocrine tissue, the islets of Langerhans, are found scattered throughout the pancreas. There are two principal types of cells contained within the islets: beta cells (β cells), which secrete insulin, and alpha cells (α cells), which secrete glucagon. Each has a role in the regulation of blood glucose.

Blood glucose regulation

Within a 24-h period, the healthy human being will alternate between the 'fed state' and the 'fasting state' several times. In the 2 h following a meal the blood glucose will tend to rise as absorption of nutrients takes place. This is termed the postprandial or fed state. Once absorption has peaked, blood glucose levels will tend to fall and will not rise again until the next meal is taken. This is termed the preprandial or fasting state. In health these fluctuations are very slight.

Insulin and glucagon are principally (but not exclusively) responsible for blood glucose regulation.

Insulin

Insulin, which could be described as an anabolic hormone, is secreted in response to a rising blood glucose level. Its functions are (Table 5.9):

- to facilitate glucose uptake by the cells
- to promote glycogenesis, i.e. the conversion of glucose to glycogen for storage in the liver and skeletal muscle
- to promote protein synthesis
- to promote conversion of glucose to triglycerides for ultimate storage as body fat.

All of these functions have the effect of preventing an abnormal rise in blood glucose (hyperglycaemia) during the postprandial period (see Fig. 5.8). Insulin secretion is highest in the fed state and lowest in the fasting state.

Glucagon

Glucagon could be described as a catabolic hormone. It is secreted in response to a falling blood glucose level and has the following functions:

- to promote the conversion of stored glycogen to glucose (glycogenolysis) and its release from the liver
- to promote fat and protein breakdown in order to provide an alternative source of glucose (lipolysis and gluconeogenesis)
- to influence the generation of ketone bodies (ketogenesis). In total or near-total insulin lack, these weak acids are produced as a result of the chemical processes involved in fat breakdown.

The actions of glucagon and the other stress (counter-regulatory) hormones are all geared towards preventing an abnormal fall in blood glucose (hypoglycaemia). Glucagon secretion is highest in the 'fasting state' and lowest in the 'fed state'.

Q **5.6** Imagine that 1 h ago you finished a three-course meal. What hormonal response would you expect from the islet cells in the pancreas right now?

Other influences on blood glucose regulation

The anterior pituitary secretes two hormones of significance to blood glucose regulation, as follows:

- *Somatotrophin (growth hormone)*. This hormone tends to raise blood glucose and is therefore described as diabetogenic in action and anti-insulin in effect. It influences blood glucose in two main ways:
  —by promoting glycogen-to-glucose conversion (glycogenolysis)
  —by inhibiting muscle glycogen storage.
- *Adrenocorticotrophic hormone (ACTH)*. This hormone stimulates the adrenal cortex to release cortisol (see below). A negative feedback mechanism operates in response to the circulating levels of cortisol in the blood.

The adrenal cortex secretes a group of hormones known as glucocorticoids, the most significant of which is cortisol. Cortisol is released in a diurnal rhythm such that secretion is higher in the mornings and lower in the evenings (see p. 150).

Like glucagon, cortisol is a catabolic hormone. Secretion is increased during periods of physical or psychological stress, when its effect is to raise the blood glucose level in an effort to meet the additional metabolic demands posed by the stressed state. Cortisol causes stored glycogen to be converted to glucose and promotes the breakdown of fat (lipolysis) and protein (gluconeogenesis), thus providing an alternative source of glucose to meet the energy needs of the cells.

The adrenal medulla secretes adrenaline and noradrenaline, which together are known as catecholamines. These 'fight or flight' hormones are catabolic in their action. In response to stress they

Table 5.9 The physiological effects of insulin. (Reproduced with kind permission from Watkins et al 1996)

Process	*Action*	*Tissue*
Effects on carbohydrate metabolism		
Glucose transport	↑	Adipose, muscle
Glycolysis	↑	Adipose, muscle
Glycogen synthesis	↑	Adipose, muscle, liver
Glucose oxidation via pentose phosphate pathway	↑	Liver, adipose
Glycogen breakdown	↓	Muscle, liver
Glycogenolysis, gluconeogenesis	↓	Liver
Effects on lipid metabolism		
Lipolysis	↓	Adipose
Fatty acid synthesis	↑	Adipose, liver
Low-density lipoprotein synthesis	↑	Liver
Lipoprotein lipase	↑	Adipose
Cholesterol synthesis	↑	Liver
Effects on protein metabolism		
Amino acid transport	↑	Muscle, adipose, liver, others
Protein synthesis	↑	Muscle, adipose, liver, others
Protein degradation	↓	Muscle
Urea formation	↓	

↑, increase; ↓, decrease.

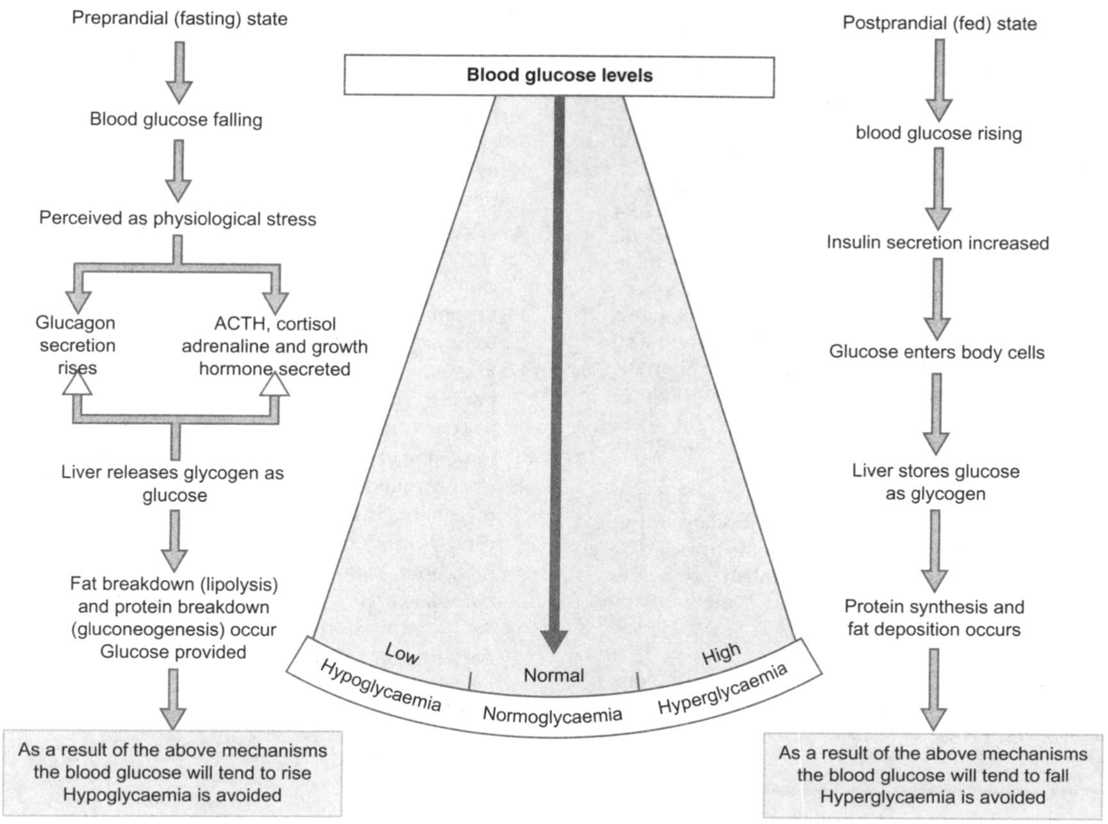
Preprandial (fasting) state
Blood glucose falling
Perceived as physiological stress
Glucagon secretion rises
ACTH, cortisol adrenaline and growth hormone secreted
Liver releases glycogen as glucose
Fat breakdown (lipolysis) and protein breakdown (gluconeogenesis) occur Glucose provided
As a result of the above mechanisms the blood glucose will tend to rise Hypoglycaemia is avoided
Blood glucose levels
Low
Normal
High
Hypoglycaemia
Normoglycaemia
Hyperglycaemia
Postprandial (fed) state
blood glucose rising
Insulin secretion increased
Glucose enters body cells
Liver stores glucose as glycogen
Protein synthesis and fat deposition occurs
As a result of the above mechanisms the blood glucose will tend to fall Hyperglycaemia is avoided

Fig. 5.8 The regulation of blood glucose in health.

place the body and brain in a state of 'high alert', causing blood glucose to rise as glycogen stores are released and fat/protein breakdown occurs. This increases the amount of available glucose and helps to prepare the body to meet increased energy demands (see p. 617).

The liver and skeletal muscle. About 60% of absorbed nutrients are laid down as reserves in order to meet energy demands during fasting. Under the influence of insulin, the liver and, to a lesser extent, skeletal muscle can store glucose in the form of glycogen. The liver is also involved in protein and fat synthesis for subsequent storage.

During fasting, or in response to stress, glucagon (and other stress hormones) will promote the release of liver and muscle glycogen in the form of glucose. The liver also contributes to the chemical processes of gluconeogenesis by which body stores of fat and protein are converted to glucose (see Fig. 5.8).

INSULIN-DEPENDENT DIABETES MELLITUS (IDDM)

Aetiology

The pathogenesis of insulin-dependent diabetes mellitus is complex and has been the subject of extensive study. It is currently thought that a genetic predisposition to the disease, possibly combined with environmental triggers, activates mechanisms which lead to progressive loss of pancreatic β cells (see Box 5.5). In IDDM, insulin secretion is totally (or almost totally) absent, and as a result lifelong treatment with insulin is required.

The precise cause of damage to the pancreatic β cells remains uncertain. Interest has been shown in viral factors, e.g. Coxsackie and mumps viruses, and in toxic chemicals. There have been reported seasonal differences in the incidence of IDDM in the UK, with the peak in the autumn and winter months. Whilst the exact reason for this is unclear it has been suggested that 'it might represent the unmasking of a latent diabetes by non-specific virus infection' (Watkins et al 1996). Indeed, the peak incidence of enterovirus occurs in late summer and early autumn (Haverkos 1997).

PATHOPHYSIOLOGY

Whatever the underlying trigger in IDDM, the cause remains unknown. Islet cell destruction, however, is the problem. This may be a gradual process in which there may be several years between the onset of the β cell destruction and the appearance of clinical symptoms. However, individuals often present with initial symptoms when the demand for insulin has been increased, e.g. in response to a physical or psychological stress such as illness, trauma, surgery, pregnancy or bereavement. In such cases, the additional metabolic demands posed by the stressed state can no longer be met by the failing pancreas and symptoms of diabetes become evident for the first time.

Once insulin has been started and good control achieved, the remaining β cell mass can temporarily provide sufficient insulin to meet the body's demands. In this case the external insulin can be

Box 5.5 Insulin-dependent diabetes mellitus: the genetic link

An increased risk of developing IDDM is likely if a first-degree relative such as a parent or sibling also has the disease, and approximately 15% of those with IDDM in the UK have a positive family history (Watkins et al 1996). A genetic susceptibility has been traced to the DR3 and DR4 genes in the human leucocyte antigen (HLA) located on chromosome 6 (Green 1996). Studies have revealed that in identical twins identified as HLA-DR3 'types' and in whom one suffers from IDDM there is a high incidence of diabetes mellitus affecting the second twin. The HLA-DR3 group also show persistent islet cell antibodies, indicating that genetic and immunological (possibly autoimmune) susceptibilities probably coexist. Within the general population it has been found that autoimmune disorders occur more frequently in people identified as HLA-DR3 types (see Ch. 16).

Twins identified as HLA-DR4 types have fewer autoimmune symptoms and rarely show islet cell antibodies. In this group it is less common for the second twin to be affected by IDDM. Given the identical genetic endowment shared by the twins, this suggests that the genetic tendency is mediated by environmental influences (Bodansky 1994, Green 1996; see also Ch. 6).

The HLA tissue-typing system referred to above is the one used to match potential organ donors with recipients. This helps to minimise the risk of rejection by the recipient's immune system.

reduced or stopped on occasions. Unfortunately this 'honeymoon period' is short-lived and as the β cell mass continues to wane, the symptoms will reappear, necessitating lifelong treatment with insulin (Watkins et al 1996).

The effects of lack of insulin. The signs, symptoms and clinical features of IDDM can best be explained in terms of the effects of insulin lack, as described in the following (clinical features are given in italic):

1. In the face of insulin lack, body cells are unable to obtain glucose for metabolism.
2. Glucose which is unable to enter cells accumulates in the blood, causing an abnormally high blood glucose level — *hyperglycaemia*.
3. Increased amounts of glucose are filtered at the glomeruli. The capacity of the kidneys to reabsorb glucose (the renal threshold for glucose) is exceeded and glucose appears in the urine — *glycosuria*.
4. Glucose is highly osmotic, i.e. it attracts and holds water to itself. As glucose is lost in the urine, large volumes of water are lost with it — *polyuria*.
5. As fluid loss continues, the patient will begin to experience symptoms of dehydration, the most common of which is copious drinking in response to severe thirst — *polydipsia*.
6. The cells' requirements for glucose are not being met. The counter-regulatory response is an increased secretion of glucagon and other stress hormones.
7. Under the influence of these hormones specific mechanisms come into play:
   - glycogen is converted to glucose and is released by the liver (*glycogenolysis*)
   - glucose is produced from the breakdown of body fat and protein (*gluconeogenesis*)
   - the patient's appetite may increase (*polyphagia*).
8. These efforts to meet the demands of the cells for glucose have the combined effect of raising the blood glucose even higher.
9. *Weight loss* occurs due to the depletion of body fat and protein stores. This, together with cell deprivation of glucose and fluid–electrolyte imbalance, causes *muscle weakness* and *exhaustion*.
10. In the absence of insulin, fat breakdown results in the production and accumulation of ketone bodies (β-hydroxybutyric acid, acetoacetic acid and acetone). This leads to *ketonaemia* and *ketonuria*. Additionally, acetone excreted by the lungs gives a characteristic sweet, *'pear drop' odour* to the breath.
11. Ketone bodies are weak acids which release free hydrogen ions to cause the serious condition of *metabolic acidosis* to develop.
12. Excess acidity of the blood causes a respiratory response. The patient *hyperventilates*, i.e. respirations become faster and deeper (Kussmaul's respirations), which is a very useful way of removing H^+ from the blood.
13. Uncontrolled lipolysis, gluconeogenesis, ketogenesis and glycogenolysis combine to raise the blood glucose level still further, increase osmotic diuresis, and exacerbate dehydration and metabolic acidosis. This is a life-threatening situation known as *diabetic ketoacidosis* (DKA; see p. 173).
14. As a result of these profound biochemical disturbances, the patient may experience *nausea and vomiting* and *colicky abdominal pain*.
15. Unless a diagnosis is reached and urgent medical treatment is established, the patient will progress to *coma* and then ultimately to death.

Onset and progress of the disease. Although the onset of IDDM (type 1 diabetes mellitus) may appear abrupt, the patient may have had undetected clinical signs, such as glycosuria, in the absence of actual symptoms over a period of months or years. Once symptoms do appear, the disease will usually have a rapid progression. However, there will be variations in severity, some patients being much more acutely ill than others at the time of diagnosis.

The patient with IDDM may visit his general practitioner (GP) complaining of thirst, an increase in the amount of urine passed and weight loss. He may also complain of feeling exhausted. The GP is likely to have the patient's urine tested for glucose and ketones. Blood glucose will also be measured. The presence of ketonuria and hyperglycaemia combined with symptoms of polyuria and thirst will usually be sufficient evidence upon which to refer the patient to a diabetes consultant. In hospital, following a full assessment, treatment can be commenced and the patient's response to therapy closely monitored (see p. 172 for diagnostic and monitoring tests). Although most patients are referred to hospital, admission is not automatic. Some newly diagnosed patients with IDDM are managed as outpatients under the care of community staff.

Recently, diabetic care has been focused on the nurse-led diabetic centres and patients less often require admission to hospital, unless particularly unwell (Craddock 1996). The members of the diabetes care team in the hospital and community will have specialist knowledge about diabetes management. The central objective of care will be to help the patient acquire the knowledge and skills needed to resume an independent lifestyle. The patient will usually be asked to attend the diabetic outpatient clinic at specified intervals or, if unable to do so, may be visited at home by the diabetes nurse specialist. A shared care approach between community and diabetes specialist centres is essential for the ongoing care, treatment supervision and evaluation of progress.

Many patients with IDDM are acutely ill at the time of diagnosis. This may be because initially the symptoms are not recognised or because the patient has an underlying sepsis. Onset can be so rapid that the patient may have progressed to full-blown DKA and may be drowsy or unconscious when the GP is first contacted. This extremely serious situation will require urgent hospital admission to stabilise and control the acidosis.

NON-INSULIN-DEPENDENT DIABETES MELLITUS (NIDDM)

Aetiology

The aetiology of NIDDM (type 2 diabetes mellitus) is also unclear but it seems likely that several factors combine to cause susceptibility to the disease. Although these factors are not fully understood, they differ from those thought to cause IDDM.

Genetic factors leading to susceptibility. Despite the fact that no HLA markers have been found for NIDDM, there is undoubtedly a genetic component in its aetiology (WHO 1994, Watkins et al 1996). An abnormality on the insulin gene found on chromosome 11 has been suggested as a cause, but whatever the exact mechanism it seems that genetic factors are more important in NIDDM than in IDDM. In one of the largest studies on diabetes in identical twins, Barnett et al (1981) found 55% discordance one twin affected in IDDM, whilst in NIDDM almost complete concordance both twins affected was found, suggesting that in NIDDM genetic factors are the chief determinants of the disease.

There is one unusual form of type 2 diabetes which has a clearly established autosomal dominant form of inheritance. It is non-insulin-dependent, commonly develops in those under 25, and is given the rather anomalous title of 'maturity onset diabetes of the young' (MODY) (see Watkins et al 1996, BDA 1997).

Age. The prevalence of NIDDM rises significantly with increasing age and can be as high as 1 in 10 in the over-70s (BDA 1996). Glucose metabolism is known to become less efficient from the third or fourth decade of life onwards and this deterioration accelerates in people over 60 years of age. Whilst this alteration in glucose tolerance may not in itself be pathological, when compounded by other factors (see below) it can contribute to the onset of symptoms of diabetes.

Insulin resistance. In NIDDM, tissue sensitivity to insulin may decline. The result is that hyperglycaemia can occur even when the circulating levels of insulin are normal or raised. Several reasons have been suggested for the development of insulin resistance; these include resistance in peripheral tissues in obesity, the effects of ageing and the presence of anti-insulin antibodies in the blood. Whatever the cause, the result is the inefficient use of available insulin.

β cell deficiency. Up to 70% of patients with NIDDM show β cell deficit. The effect of this deficit is often that the initial postprandial surge in insulin is lost (Jones 1987).

Obesity. Obesity is known to induce insulin resistance in body cells. However, only a minority of obese people develop NIDDM and only around 60% of people with the disorder are obese. Glucose tolerance decreases as weight increases and can be reversed as weight loss occurs. Fat distribution would appear to be significant in that there is a relationship between central obesity and diabetes and those who are 'apple-shaped' with a waist:hip ratio of 0.9 are more prone to NIDDM (Watkins et al 1996).

Ethnic and environmental factors. There are wide geographical variations in the incidence of type 2 diabetes. In western Europe and in the USA, 1–2% of the population develop NIDDM, but in certain circumscribed societies incidences of up to 40% have been reported, e.g. among the Pima Indians of North America and the Nauru Islanders of the Pacific, where gross obesity is also very common. These remarkably high prevalences are probably due to the exposure of genetically isolated, diabetes-predisposed populations to influences such as a 'Westernised' diet and reduced physical activity. In many developing and newly industrialised nations, NIDDM is thought to be epidemic (Griggs 1998). In the UK, people of Asian origin have two to four times the risk of developing NIDDM (BDA 1995).

PATHOPHYSIOLOGY

NIDDM usually presents in those over the age of 40 and most commonly in people over 60. Typically the patient is overweight.

The signs, symptoms and clinical features of NIDDM, although still marked, are less severe than those of IDDM and are due to the more gradual onset and the effects of hyperglycaemia arising from a relative deficiency of insulin. In NIDDM there is still some insulin being secreted; as a result, ketogenesis is inhibited and, as the hyperglycaemia is less severe, dehydration is also much less common.

The effects of a relative lack of insulin are as follows:

1. Hyperglycaemia-related symptoms. Nocturia, polyuria and thirst may develop gradually. The patient, who is often obese, may initially be gratified to note that weight loss is occurring.
2. Genital or oral fungal infections. Candidal infections are common and result in the distressing symptoms of pruritus vulvae in the female and balanitis in the male. The sugar-rich urine around the genitalia appears to provide the yeast with favourable conditions in which to multiply.
3. Staphylococcal skin infections, commonly resulting in boils and abscesses, may provide the initial stimulus for the patient to visit the GP.
4. Non-specific symptoms such as tiredness and lethargy are also frequently reported. The cause is uncertain, but altered fluid and electrolyte balance may be responsible. Visual disturbance may occasionally be reported, as hyperglycaemia may cause opacity of the optic lens and accommodation may be affected by dehydration of the lens fluid (Craddock 1996).

Symptom-related complications. At the time the patient first seeks medical attention, evidence of vascular and neurological complications such as proteinuria, sexual dysfunction, retinopathy and peripheral neuropathy may already have developed. Such patients have probably had asymptomatic diabetes with persistent hyperglycaemia for several years prior to diagnosis.

Onset and progress of the disease. NIDDM may present in several ways. A diagnosis will usually be made on the evidence of glycosuria and a fasting or random blood glucose of more than 8 mmol/L and 11 mmol/L, respectively, in laboratory tests. The presence of symptoms and an elevated blood glucose of >11 mmol/L together are diagnostic of diabetes (Watkins et al 1996). These criteria, however, are currently under review (BDA 1997).

Ketonuria is not a feature, as in NIDDM ketogenesis is inhibited by the presence of even small amounts of insulin.

Asymptomatic glycosuria may be discovered as an incidental finding, e.g. during a routine medical examination. Such a finding would normally prompt capillary or venous blood glucose analysis. Only if the results were equivocal would an oral glucose tolerance test be necessary to confirm the diagnosis.

MALNUTRITION-RELATED DIABETES MELLITUS (MRDM)

This name is given to a collection of clinical features that affect young people who live in developing tropical countries. The sufferer is typically below 30 years of age, has a body mass index of less than 20, has moderate to severe hyperglycaemia, is not prone to ketosis in the absence of precipitating factors, requires a large dose of insulin for metabolic control and often has a history of malnutrition in infancy (WHO 1994). MRDM has been subdivided into two types: fibrocalculous pancreatic diabetes and protein-deficient pancreatic diabetes. For further information, see Tripathy & Samal (1997).

IMPAIRED GLUCOSE TOLERANCE (IGT)

It is not clear why some people may have blood glucose results at or just above the upper limit of 'normal'. Inconclusive results in the absence of symptoms may not necessarily be judged abnormal. For example, since glucose tolerance is known to decline with age and obesity, such factors would be considered in the overall assessment. To help determine to which category the patient should be assigned, an oral glucose tolerance test may be carried out (see Table 5.10).

It is known that some people with IGT will go on to develop diabetes mellitus and that they may have a greater risk of developing atherosclerosis.

Onset and progress of the disease. Although it is clearly desirable that people should be spared the negative consequences of being inappropriately labelled as 'diabetic', they should nonetheless have access to regular medical screening and should be offered information about the prevention of atherosclerosis and its consequences (see Ch. 2, p. 13). These health promotion functions will normally be carried out by the practice nurse or the GP and community nursing staff, although in some areas the patient may also be asked to attend a diabetic clinic periodically. An annual review may be carried out at the diabetic centre.

IGT has implications for women who are planning to conceive. Current evidence suggests that it is important to correct hyperglycaemia and ensure tight control of blood glucose prior to conception to reduce the risk of fetal abnormality (Parker 1996). Pre-conception advice should be made available and the patient's blood glucose brought within normal limits before conception and closely monitored throughout her pregnancy. Care of this kind may be provided at a combined 'diabetic-obstetric' clinic.

Table 5.10 Diagnostic glucose concentrations

Diagnosis	*Venous whole blood (mmol/L)*	*Capillary whole blood (mmol/L)*
Diabetes mellitus		
Fasting	>7.0	>7.0
2 h postprandial	>10.0	>11.0
Impaired glucose tolerance		
Fasting	<7.0	<7.0
2 h postprandial	>7.0 to <10.0	>8.0 to <11.0

In the absence of diabetic symptoms, abnormality in both 2 h postprandial and fasting blood sugar is required to establish the diagnosis of diabetes mellitus.

DIABETES MELLITUS SECONDARY TO OTHER DISEASES AND CONDITIONS

PATHOPHYSIOLOGY

In IDDM the fault is to be found in the islets of Langerhans where β cell output of insulin is either absent or insufficient to meet the needs of the cells. In NIDDM the islet cells may still produce insulin, but in insufficient amounts, or its function may be hindered in some way. In contrast, hyperglycaemia in secondary diabetes may be iatrogenic, i.e. occurring as a side-effect of certain drugs, or be secondary to other disease. Some drugs, notably steroids, have a diabetogenic effect. The thiazide group of diuretics have been known to worsen established diabetes and in some elderly patients may actually hasten the onset of the disease. Excess secretion or administration of glucocorticoids, aldosterone, catecholamines or growth hormone will have a diabetogenic effect and can result in hyperglycaemia. Diabetes may therefore be a feature of Cushing's syndrome, Cushing's disease, phaeochromocytoma, primary aldosteronism and acromegaly (see Ch. 5, part 1).

Pancreatitis and carcinoma of the pancreas may greatly reduce the number of functioning β cells and result in impaired insulin secretion. Chronic hepatic disease will have considerable consequences for carbohydrate, protein and fat metabolism. Glycogenesis and glycogenolysis may both be impaired and consequently hyperglycaemia and hypoglycaemia frequently feature in chronic disorders of the liver (see Ch. 4). Chronic renal failure can cause impaired glucose tolerance and insulin resistance, although the underlying mechanism by which this occurs is unclear.

Finally, there are a few rare genetic disorders which give rise to secondary diabetes. Friedreich's ataxia, an inherited disorder of balance and movement, is one example. Another is a condition with an autosomal character which is referred to by the acronym DIDMOAD as it incorporates diabetes insipidus, diabetes mellitus, optic atrophy and deafness.

Onset and progress of the disease. This is characterised by hyperglycaemia with glycosuria. Associated features such as thirst and polyuria may be experienced, and in hepatic disease the patient may also experience hypoglycaemic episodes, with symptoms such as trembling, sweating and clouding of consciousness. The underlying disease process will influence the nature and severity of the symptoms. Urinalysis and blood glucose will be monitored and dietary adjustment may be prescribed; this may be combined with oral hypoglycaemic medication or insulin therapy.

MANAGEMENT STRATEGIES IN DIABETES MELLITUS

Diabetes care in Europe and in the UK has been largely influenced by the St Vincent declaration (see Box 5.6). Such was the concern over the duration and quality of life of people with diabetes that the countries concerned pledged to deploy resources for its resolution and to intensify research into prevention and cure of diabetes and its complications.

Diabetes management requires a multidisciplinary approach. For those patients who are not acutely ill at the time of diagnosis, management may be provided entirely within the community setting. However, many patients are more acutely ill at the time of onset and require hospital care to allow close monitoring of the effects of early treatment.

Box 5.6 The St Vincent Declaration (Krans et al 1992)

In 1989, representatives of government health departments were among the signatories of the St Vincent declaration. This document was prepared under the aegis of the WHO and the International Diabetes Federation. It stated that:

> Diabetes mellitus is a major and growing European health problem...at all ages and in all countries. It causes prolonged ill health and early death. It threatens at least 10 million European citizens. ...a major reduction in this heavy burden of disease and death can be achieved. Countries should give formal recognition to the diabetes problem and deploy resources for its solution. Plans for the prevention, identification and treatment of diabetes and particularly its complications – blindness, renal failure, gangrene and amputation, aggravated coronary heart disease and stroke – should be formulated at local, national and European regional levels.

General goals for people with diabetes mellitus

- Sustained improvement of health experience and a life approaching normal expectation in quality and quantity
- Prevention and cure of diabetes and of its complications by intensifying research effort.

The signing of this declaration has led to an increased awareness of the problems associated with diabetes and research into the best way to achieve the published goals.

The professionals in the diabetes care team will share common goals for care, each contributing expertise in accordance with the patient's individual needs. It is worth remembering, however, that the patient is the most important member of the diabetes care team, and full participation by the patient is necessary to achieve the following aims:

- Attainment and maintenance of normoglycaemia
- Monitoring of response to therapy
- Prevention and detection of diabetes-associated complications
- Facilitation of self-care through education
- Promotion of social and psychological adjustment.

ATTAINING AND MAINTAINING NORMOGLYCAEMIA

There are three main therapeutic approaches to this management:

- dietary therapy
- oral hypoglycaemic therapy
- insulin therapy.

DIETARY THERAPY

Dietary modification is an important management strategy, whether used alone or combined with other therapies. Once the diagnosis of diabetes mellitus has been confirmed, the patient is usually referred to a dietician, who is often a diabetes specialist. The dietician will assess the patient's calorific and nutritional needs, taking into account such factors as age, gender, lifestyle, religious or ethnic influences and current dietary habits. Recommendations for a healthy diet are centred around:

- foods containing complex carbohydrates, e.g. bread, cereal, potatoes, pulses
- free foods, e.g. some fruits and vegetables
- foods to avoid, e.g. simple sugars found in confectionery, alcohol and biscuits.

Establishing and maintaining links with the dietician will help to promote a well-informed, positive and flexible approach to diabetes management.

The patient should be helped to understand how diet can influence current and future well-being. For some obese patients with NIDDM, dietary therapy alone may bring the disorder under control. An individually formulated reduced-calorie diet which is low in fat and refined carbohydrate and high in fibre will usually be recommended. Such a diet should have the effect of slowing down the rate of glucose absorption and reducing obesity. As a result, the demand for insulin should be reduced and cell sensitivity to insulin improved.

Soluble fibre as found in peas, beans and lentils appears to have a beneficial effect on both blood glucose and blood cholesterol. The insoluble fibre found in cereals, wholegrain bread and fresh fruit and vegetables provides energy, helps to avoid constipation and, especially if combined with a diet low in salt and saturated fat, helps to reduce diabetes-associated cardiovascular risk (Abraham & Levy 1992).

Diet combined with medication

When dietary modification is combined with oral hypoglycaemic or insulin therapy, the patient will need additional education so that carbohydrate intake can be distributed fairly evenly throughout the day and is consistent from day to day. It is particularly important that the patient knows that food must be taken following insulin or oral hypoglycaemic drugs to avoid a dangerous fall in blood glucose (hypoglycaemia).

The glycaemic index of food

This may be considered in formulating dietary allowances. It is known that different carbohydrate-rich foods affect the blood glucose in different ways. Glucose has been given a glycaemic index of 100 and other carbohydrate foods are measured against this to reveal their relative potential to raise blood glucose. Pulses and bran have a low glycaemic index and are therefore recommended, whilst refined sugars have a very high glycaemic index and are therefore not advised except when a sharp rise in blood glucose is desired, e.g. to treat hypoglycaemia (Fuller 1990, Frost 1997). For this reason the use of 10 g carbohydrate exchanges is no longer advocated. What is important, especially for those on insulin therapy, is that the intake of carbohydrate is consistent from day to day and that it is taken regularly.

Team approach to dietary therapy

Although the dietician is the key professional in dietary management, it often falls to the hospital or community nurse to offer advice. Although standardised diet sheets have given way to a more individualised approach, some patients find it useful to have some form of checklist to guide them in their decisions. The BDA provides useful guidelines relating to diet in diabetes (see Aitken 1997 and 'Useful addresses', p. 193).

'Diabetic' foods can be rather expensive and are not actually necessary. Indeed, it may be worth bearing in mind that the type of diet recommended for people with diabetes could equally be commended to the general population. Such a diet is nutritious, promotes health and well-being and helps to prevent obesity, high blood pressure and heart disease (see Box 5.7).

Box 5.7 Recommendations for people with diabetes (Nutrition Sub-Committee of the BDA's Professional Advisory Committee 1990)

BDA recommendations on diet: summary
- Include more complex carbohydrates in diet
- Reduce total fat intake
- Include less fat from animal sources in diet
- Balance the distribution and timing of carbohydrates with medication
- Follow a high-fibre/low-fat diet to assist weight loss
- Reduce sodium intake
- Consume alcohol only in modest amounts
- Avoid specialist diabetic products — they are unnecessary and can be misused
- Obtain individualised dietary advice

The best carbohydrates for a diabetic diet
- Wholegrain or fibre-enriched breakfast cereals
- Wholemeal flour and bread
- Wholewheat pasta
- Brown rice
- Dried/baked beans and pulses
- Fruit
- Vegetables
- Biscuits and snack bars made with fibre-rich ingredients

ORAL HYPOGLYCAEMIC THERAPY

Oral hypoglycaemic medication can be effective only if β cells are capable of secreting some insulin. This form of therapy is therefore used exclusively for patients with NIDDM. In IDDM the underlying problem is total (or near-total) insulin lack, and insulin replacement therapy is the only suitable treatment.

Day (1991) recommends that in the absence of persistent symptoms, dietary treatment should continue for at least 3 months before drug therapy is commenced. Oral hypoglycaemic therapy would then be reserved for patients with NIDDM who have persistent hyperglycaemia despite a period of dietary adjustment.

Four main groups of oral agents are available for use in the UK (see Table 5.11).

The sulphonylureas

This is the most common group.

Mode of action. These drugs stimulate the β cells of the pancreas to secrete more insulin in response to blood glucose levels. It has been suggested that this group of drugs may increase the sensitivity of muscle, liver and fat cells to insulin and reduce the hepatic metabolism of insulin (Paterson 1990, Cantrill 1994).

Side-effects. The most common side-effect is hypoglycaemia. This can be minimised by starting the patient on the lowest dose possible and gradually increasing the amount over a period of weeks. As sulphonylureas lower blood glucose it is important that the patient and his carers are aware of the risks of hypoglycaemia. The medication should be taken with or just before food. The relationship between exercise, medication and diet will form an important part of the patient teaching programme (see p. 186).

Other side-effects are uncommon but include weight gain, gastrointestinal disturbance and skin rash. Facial flushing following alcohol ingestion can occur with chlorpropamide. It should be noted that the effect of sulphonylureas is potentiated by other protein-bound drugs, e.g. warfarin. This interaction increases the amount of available sulphonylurea and may therefore cause hypoglycaemia (Paterson 1990).

The biguanides

These are less popular than the sulphonylureas as they are more liable to cause side-effects. Only one, metformin, is in regular use in the UK.

Mode of action. The way in which the biguanides work is unclear but it is thought to involve reduced glucose absorption in the gut and inhibition of gluconeogenesis in the liver. Some improvement in cell sensitivity to insulin has also been suggested (Paterson 1990). Metformin tends to be used to treat obese patients who show persistent hyperglycaemia despite treatment with diet alone or with diet combined with one of the sulphonylureas.

Table 5.11 Oral hypoglycaemic agents. (Reproduced with kind permission from Watkins et al 1996)

Drug	*Dose range (mg/day)*	*Special points*
Sulphonylureas		
Glipizide	2.5–40	Hepatic metabolism; short half-life; useful for the elderly and in renal failure
Gliclazide	40–320	
Tolbutamide	500–2000	
Chlorpropamide	100–500	Not in common use, very long half-life; flushing with alcohol
Glibenclamide	2.5–15	Long half-life; renal excretion; unsuitable in the elderly or those with renal failure
Tolazamide	100–750	Not in common use
Gliquidone	15–180	
Glibornuride	12.5–75	
Glymidine	500–2000	
Biguanides		
Metformin	1000–2000	Used in obesity; not used in renal or cardiac failure
Glucosidase inhibitors		
Acerbose	150–300	
Guar gum		
Guarem	15 000	Not in common use
Guarina	15 000	

Side-effects. Medication-induced hypoglycaemia is very uncommon with biguanide therapy but vitamin B_{12} malabsorption and gastrointestinal upsets such as anorexia, dyspepsia, nausea and diarrhoea are common. Lactic acidosis is a rare but very serious side-effect (Cantrill 1994).

Aplha-glucosidase inhibitor

Acerbose is the most recent addition to the pharmacological management of NIDDM. It is used when there is inadequate control of blood glucose with diet alone or using diet in combination with other oral hypoglycaemics.

Mode of action. Acerbose acts by delaying the breakdown of starch and sucrose into monosaccharides which can be absorbed in the small intestine. In the diabetic patient, the effect is to reduce the postprandial peak in blood glucose.

Side-effects. The most common side-effect is flatulence.

Guar gum

Guar gum acts by reducing the absorption of carbohydrate and thereby may reduce hyperglycaemia. The clinical effectiveness is very limited and the role of guar gum in diabetes is minor. The flatulence caused by ingestion of the quantity of guar gum required often makes its use intolerable (Watkins et al 1996).

INSULIN THERAPY

Insulin therapy is essential to maintain life, and will be required throughout life, for all patients with IDDM. Insulin cannot be given orally as its protein structure would be inactivated by digestive enzymes. Parenteral administration will therefore be necessary and normally takes the form of subcutaneous (s.c.) injection.

Patients with NIDDM may become 'insulin requiring' during periods of stress or illness or when other therapeutic approaches cease to control their symptoms. This does not change the classification of their disorder, despite the (often temporary) requirement for insulin.

The objectives of insulin therapy are:

- to maintain blood glucose within normal limits
- to relieve hyperglycaemia-associated symptoms
- to correct metabolic/biochemical disturbances
- to prevent diabetes-associated complications.

Types of insulin

In the past all insulin preparations were derived from animal sources, mainly beef and pork. Genetic engineering and other advanced techniques have resulted in the production of biosynthetic human insulin and purified or highly purified pork and beef insulin. This has been a welcome development and has significantly reduced the adverse effects experienced by some patients on insulin therapy.

Throughout western Europe it is mostly human insulins which are used. Although patients may still develop insulin antibodies whilst taking human insulin, the titres are much lower and no significant side-effects are noted. Insulins are manufactured in various forms: soluble, isophane, insulin zinc suspension, and ready-mixed in combination. All are cloudy except soluble insulin which is clear in appearance.

Duration of action

There are many insulin preparations on the market. These may be categorised as short-acting, intermediate-acting or long-acting (see Fig. 5.9).

Short-acting insulins (soluble) are clear solutions. They have a rapid onset of action and when injected subcutaneously their maximal effect occurs in 3–4 h but can last up to 8 h.

Short-acting insulin may be prescribed in the following ways:

- once daily — given in the morning in combination with a long-acting insulin
- twice daily — given in the morning and evening in combination with an intermediate-acting insulin
- by multiple injection regimen — three or four injections of short-acting insulin given about 30 min prior to each meal; this is usually combined with a single daily dose of long-acting insulin given at bedtime for overnight release
- by continuous s.c. infusion using an insulin pump (for selected patients judged likely to benefit from this form of therapy)
- intravenously — during acute metabolic emergencies when immediate insulin effect is required, e.g. in diabetic ketoacidosis (DKA).

Intermediate and long-acting insulins are cloudy. Their onset of effect is delayed for 1–2 h. The intermediate-acting insulins achieve maximum effect in 4–6 h and have a duration of action of 12–20 h. Long-acting insulins have their maximum effect in 8–12 h and a duration of action of up to 36 h.

Intermediate-acting insulins come in three main forms:

- Isophane insulin comes as a suspension of insulin with protamine. This is a useful type of insulin to use in combination with short-acting insulin. It provides a stable solution in which each insulin retains its own pharmacological properties even when mixed and stored in the same syringe.
- Lente insulins are complexed with zinc in two forms: amorphous 30% and crystalline 70%. The zinc binds the insulin, and as a result onset of action is delayed and the duration extended.
- Ready-mixed insulins include a combination of soluble and intermediate-/long-acting insulins in varying amounts. Many are now available in 'pen' form and for some patients may be easier to administer.

Long-acting insulin suspensions have a greatly extended period of action and can therefore be given once daily. However, tight control may be more difficult and this method of administration may be more suitable for the elderly or some NIDDM patients who can no longer achieve control with diet and/or oral hypoglycaemic therapy (Watkins et al 1996).

Q **5.7** Using the *British National Formulary* (BNF) or a current pharmacology text (e.g. Trounce 1997) draw up a table which illustrates examples from rapid-, medium- and long-acting insulins and indicate the species (source), onset and duration of action.

Administering insulin

The aim in administering insulin therapy is to achieve the best possible control of blood glucose without causing distressing hypoglycaemia. Ideally, the treatment should mimic the physiological response to normal variations in blood glucose.

In the healthy person, 30–40 IU of insulin is secreted by the pancreas each day. During the fasting state there is a continual but low secretion of insulin. Following meals a surge in blood glucose results in increased insulin secretion.

Frequency

To mimic normal blood glucose fluctuations, a single injection of insulin with a 24-h period of action, such as Human Ultratard (insulin zinc suspension crystalline), could be given once daily

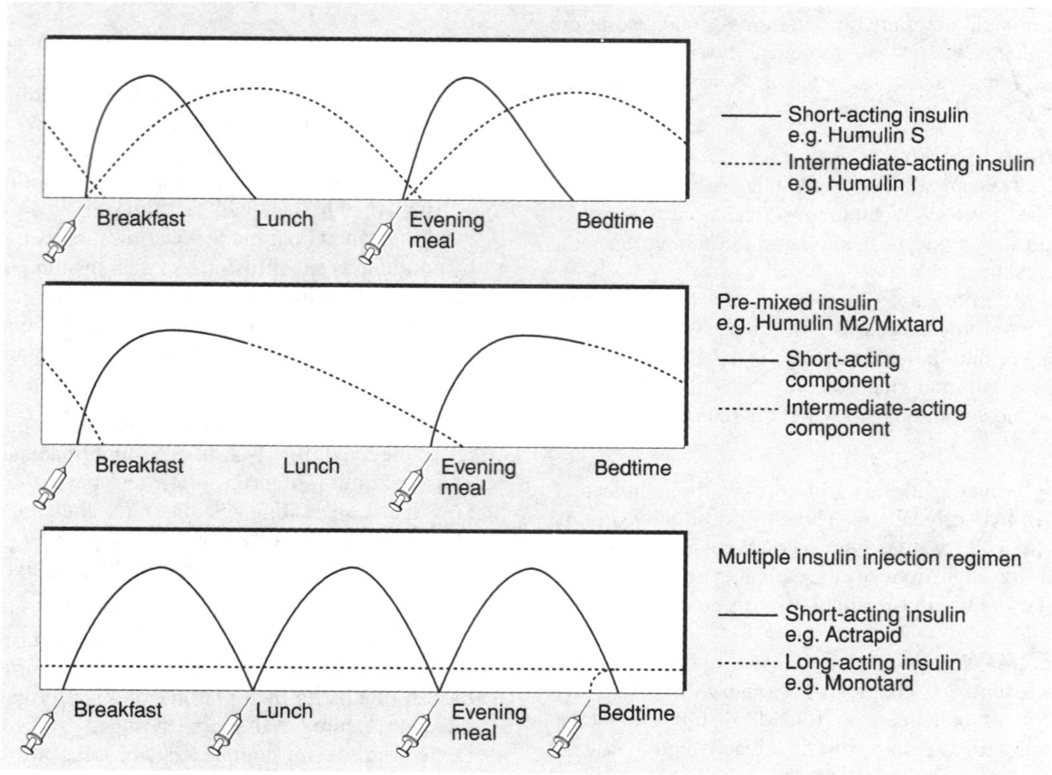

Fig. 5.9 Duration of action for short-, intermediate- and long-acting insulins.

in combination with quick-acting insulin with a short (2–4 h) duration of action, such as Human Actrapid (neutral insulin injection), before each meal. This multi-injection system has considerable advantages, not least of which are patient autonomy and flexibility of mealtimes. Patients using this system usually carry a precharged pen-type injection device such as the NovoPen or the B-D Pen. This allows administration of insulin to be discreet and adaptable to the day-to-day changes in the patient's activity levels, eating pattern and lifestyle. This system is most effective with patients who are able to monitor blood glucose closely and to adjust diet and insulin accordingly and does not, therefore, suit everyone. For many patients, twice-daily injections remain the favoured regimen, whereas some, especially elderly patients, who have perhaps been required to progress to insulin from diet and/or oral therapy, will be more willing to accept once-daily injections.

Mixing insulin

It is not advisable to mix zinc-based insulins and soluble insulins in a syringe for later use, as free zinc in the suspension can bind to the soluble insulin, extending the onset and duration of action. The injection should be given just after preparation. This problem does not arise with isophane insulins as they do not contain zinc (see Fig. 5.10).

Q **5.8** What effect might such contamination have on the onset, effect and duration of action of the clear insulin and on the patient's blood glucose level?

Pre-mixed insulin. Various fixed ratios of short to intermediate-acting insulins are available. Pre-mixed solutions are available for use with either syringe or pen injection devices. Such preparations are popular but it is still common practice for insulin mixtures to be prepared by the patient or carer where fine adjustment of the dosage of each type of insulin is required.

Dosage will be carefully worked out and adjusted on an individual basis, taking account of blood glucose levels, ketonuria, lifestyle, and growth and development needs. The very real risk of hypoglycaemia needs to be addressed. Insulin must be followed by food within 15–30 minutes of administration if a serious fall in blood glucose is to be avoided. The patient and his carers will need information about how they can achieve a balance of food, exercise and insulin to avoid detrimental swings in blood glucose.

Injection sites

Insulin is given by s.c. injection. The most common sites for injection are the upper arms, the upper thighs, the abdominal wall and the buttocks. Overuse of one site can lead to fat hypertrophy, loss of sensitivity and impaired/erratic absorption of insulin. For this reason 'site rotation' is advised (see Fig. 5.11). Insulin is more rapidly absorbed from the abdomen and arm, and therefore the thigh and buttock are more useful for evening injections.

Injection technique

Cleansing the skin with alcohol is not considered advisable as this hardens it. Moreover, whilst this may be a local infection control policy in some areas, especially for in-patients, there is evidence

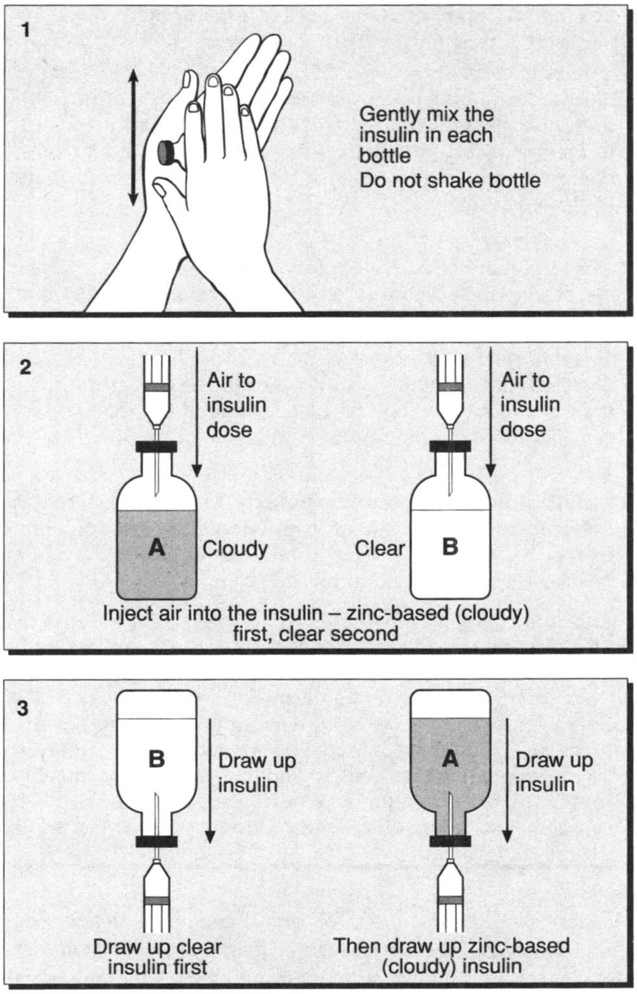

Fig. 5.10 Mixing clear and zinc-based (cloudy) insulin. This technique avoids 'contaminating' the clear (rapid-acting) insulin with zinc-based (cloudy) insulin and thus extending the onset and duration of action.

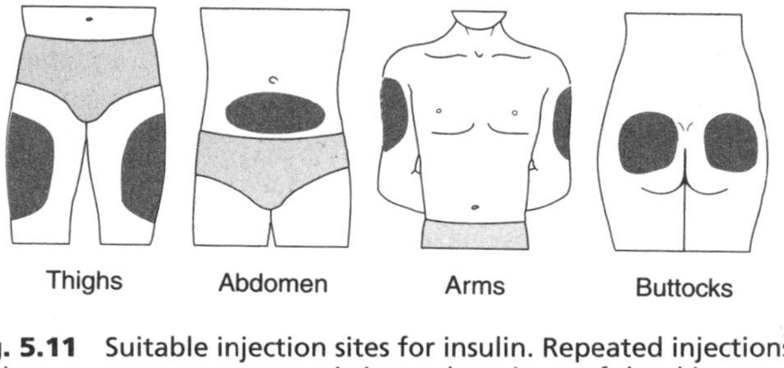

Fig. 5.11 Suitable injection sites for insulin. Repeated injections in the same area may cause pitting or lumpiness of the skin.

that this practice does not significantly alter the minimal risk of infection (Borders et al 1984). To reduce discomfort, some patients find it helps to stretch or, alternatively, gently pinch up a mound of skin before injection. The latter is preferred in that it is more likely to ensure s.c. administration. The syringe should be held like a dart and the needle inserted straight into the subcutaneous tissue. Insulin syringes currently in use in the UK have short, fine needles attached, thus avoiding the penetration of muscle. The insulin should be injected steadily over 3–5 s and the needle withdrawn smoothly. If slight leakage or bleeding occurs, gentle pressure can be applied using a clean cotton wool ball. Teaching the newly diagnosed insulin-dependent patient how to self-administer insulin is a significant part of diabetes education (see p. 186). For some patients, learning this skill is the most difficult part of adjusting to the diagnosis.

The care setting. The insulin-dependent patient may be managed in the primary care setting provided adequate supervision and support can be given to both patient and family during the early stages of treatment. It is still common for initial stabilisation on insulin to take place within the hospital setting and for outpatient attendance to be advised to allow for regular screening for diabetes-related complications. If ketoacidosis or dehydration is present, management in hospital will be essential.

MONITORING RESPONSE TO THERAPY

METHODS

The methods used for monitoring glycaemic control include:

- urinalysis
- blood glucose monitoring
- glycosylated protein estimation
- body weight monitoring.

Urinalysis

Urine tests are performed to detect the presence of glucose and ketones. (In order to screen for possible renal complications of diabetes mellitus, urine may also be tested for protein.) Urine testing is simple, inexpensive, non-invasive, easy to teach and generally acceptable to patients. It requires a degree of manual dexterity, adequate vision (including colour vision) and urinary continence. It also requires the ability to interpret and act upon results. Its usefulness is limited by variations in the renal threshold but it is still regarded as a fairly useful monitoring device for those patients for whom strict glycaemic control is not critical (Higgins 1994).

Equipment

Chemically impregnated dipsticks (e.g. Diastix) are the usual means of testing for glucose and, where necessary, for ketones. It should be noted that dipsticks for testing urine glucose levels may be rendered insensitive by the presence of heavy ketonuria. As a result some centres still prefer urine glucose to be checked using Clinitest tablets, believing them to be more accurate. The manufacturer's instructions for use and storage of urine testing materials must be followed precisely in order for reliable results to be obtained.

Interpretation

The absence of glycosuria merely indicates a blood glucose level below the renal threshold for glucose, which in most people is around 10 mmol/L. Urinalysis cannot therefore detect hypoglycaemia. For this reason some physicians and diabetes nurse specialists recommend that elderly patients on oral hypoglycaemic therapy show occasional slight traces of glycosuria — but no more than 0.25%. This reassures the patient and the staff that an overdosage of oral hypoglycaemic medication is not being given.

Recording
Urinalysis results should be accurately recorded on the appropriate chart. The patient should also keep a record of results, as this can prove useful for analysis and discussion at the diabetic clinic or surgery.

Blood glucose monitoring
The value of blood glucose monitoring is reflected in the rapid increase in its practice by patients, doctors and nurses over the past 10 years.

Advantages
Blood glucose monitoring offers increased patient involvement in diabetes management and helps to improve day-to-day glycaemic control. The patient can enjoy greater flexibility at mealtimes and can participate safely in strenuous exercise. Blood glucose monitoring can also give warning of impending metabolic crisis and guide subsequent intervention.

Disadvantages
Blood glucose monitoring requires a fair degree of manual dexterity, visual acuity, cognitive ability and motivation. It is invasive and some patients find it uncomfortable and unacceptable. It is also more expensive than urinalysis and can potentially provide inaccurate information due to errors in technique (see Box 5.8). In the current climate of concern over blood-borne infections such as hepatitis B and C, HIV and AIDS, protective gloves must be worn by staff performing this procedure.

Equipment
This includes:

- finger-pricking devices for obtaining a capillary blood sample
- reagent strips impregnated with chemicals that change colour according to the glucose content in the blood
- meters that employ microtechnology to provide an accurate reading and visual display of the capillary blood glucose.

Reagent strips and lancets are available on prescription, but battery-operated glucose meters must be purchased by the patient and can be expensive. Some clinics lend meters to patients to provide added security during periods when particularly close monitoring is needed. This may be following diagnosis, during illness or periods of instability, or when the type or dosage of insulin is being changed.

Frequency
In most situations, preprandial and bedtime tests are sufficient if combined with occasional postprandial tests. Once glycaemic control is established, the frequency of monitoring should be reviewed. During periods of metabolic crisis, blood glucose monitoring may be carried out hourly.

Method
The patient should wash his hands with warm soapy water before the test is carried out. A drop of blood of sufficient size should be obtained and the procedure detailed in the manufacturer's directions followed precisely (Craddock 1996). If a nurse is conducting the test, she should wear gloves.

Blood glucose monitoring provides a simple and, if performed correctly, reliable method of monitoring glycaemic control. A suitable system of recording results must be devised. Some meters can store results in the memory but for the most part a written record should be kept for analysis. The nurse or patient carrying out the procedure should know the levels above and below which specific actions should be taken. Although primarily a tool to monitor diabetic control, blood glucose monitoring enables the individual to learn how blood glucose levels fluctuate in different situations (Craddock 1996). For further information on blood glucose measuring systems, see Batki et al (1998).

Box 5.8 Accuracy of blood glucose monitoring

Studies (cited by Rayman 1989) revealed that 50% of blood glucose tests performed by hospital nurses differed from laboratory findings by more than 20%. As the meters used were found to be accurate the errors were attributed to poor operator technique. The main causes of inaccuracy were identified as follows:

Sticky fingers
Finger contamination with foodstuffs can lead to falsely elevated blood glucose results. It is therefore essential that the patient washes his hands before the test.

Smeared test strips
Blood should be allowed to drop onto the test strip rather than being smeared on. Patchy coverage of the reagent pad can lead to inaccurate results.

Incorrect calibration
Manufacturers of meters compensate for slight differences between batches of reagent strips by using calibration numbers or bar codes. The meter should be recalibrated when a new batch of strips is begun.

Incorrect timing
Precise timing is essential for accuracy. The manufacturer's instructions should be followed exactly.

As treatment may be based on the reported results it is clearly important that all those involved in carrying out this procedure should be adequately instructed and observed by an experienced supervisor who can correct any faults in technique. Only then should a nurse (or patient) be deemed competent to carry out and record blood glucose results.

Glycosylated protein estimation
Glucose in solution binds to protein by a process of glycosylation. The rate at which proteins bind glucose is directly related to the current glucose concentration in the blood. The blood proteins in which glycosylation is most readily measured are haemoglobin, albumin and fructosamine. The normal ranges vary according to the laboratory technique and reference ranges should therefore be provided by the laboratory undertaking the test.

Advantages
Measurement of glycosylated proteins provides an independent check of other measures of glycaemic control. It gives an indication of control over a period of time and not merely a one-off recording as in plasma glucose estimation (Higgins 1994). Additionally, it provides a tool to assess the effects of interventions such as diet, drugs or education.

Disadvantages
Anything which interferes with normal haemoglobin levels (such as haemorrhage or anaemia) could potentially distort glycosylated haemoglobin results. Similarly, conditions which influence serum albumin levels, such as renal or hepatic disease, may result in problems in interpreting glycated albumin results.

Body weight monitoring

Weight is not a sensitive indicator of glycaemic control. However, the negative significance of rapid weight loss accompanied by thirst, glycosuria and ketonuria should be recognised. Similarly, it is a positive sign if the patient's weight is stable and within an acceptable range. Body weight therefore forms part of the overall monitoring picture.

In NIDDM it is often seen as a priority to help the patient lose weight. Obesity increases insulin resistance and therefore correction of obesity can increase the sensitivity of cells to insulin. Weight reduction alone may bring the blood glucose down within normal limits.

Associated problems

Social attitudes can lead to overweight people feeling stigmatised. As a result, guilt or low self-esteem may affect the patient's response to dietary advice. It is important that nurses involved in monitoring the patient's weight in the home, clinic or hospital adopt a sensitive approach. Public weighing and castigation of patients for lack of 'success' have no place in diabetes care. Punitive attitudes and inflexible advice only confirm guilt feelings in the patient, further lowering self-esteem (Thomas 1994).

Equipment and procedure

Scales should be checked regularly for accuracy. If possible, the patient should be weighed at the same time of day, ideally having just emptied his bladder. As far as possible, the patient should wear clothing of comparable weight.

Frequency

For hospital in-patients, weekly weighing should be adequate. Routine weighing at each outpatient clinic appointment is probably advisable. Frequency of self-weighing by a patient at home will depend upon the patient's discretion, the advice offered and the goals which have been set. On the whole, weighing more frequently than once a week is neither psychologically desirable nor valuable as a monitoring tool.

PREVENTING AND DETECTING DIABETES-ASSOCIATED COMPLICATIONS

ACUTE METABOLIC COMPLICATIONS OF DIABETES

The acute complications arising from diabetes are:

- diabetic ketoacidosis (DKA)
- hyperglycaemic hyperosmolar non-ketotic coma (HHNK)
- hypoglycaemia (insulin reaction/coma).

Diabetic ketoacidosis (DKA)

This condition can be defined as uncontrolled hyperglycaemia accompanied by dehydration and acidosis.

Epidemiology

Although relatively uncommon, DKA accounts for around 14% of all diabetes-related hospital admissions. Before the discovery of insulin, DKA was invariably fatal. Even today it carries a significant threat to life, with a mortality rate of approximately 7% when treated in specialist centres (BDA 1995). Mortality is higher in the elderly or when treatment takes place in less specialised centres (BDA 1995, Watkins et al 1996).

Aetiology

Around 25% of patients admitted with DKA have previously undiagnosed diabetes (Watkins et al 1996). In patients with established diabetes, DKA can be precipitated by infection, myocardial infarction, stroke or physical or emotional trauma, as these increase stress hormone secretion. Stress hormones raise the blood glucose and increase insulin requirements. DKA may therefore be caused by an inadequate dosage of insulin being taken during periods of illness or other major stress, or by insulin being omitted altogether.

In 10–15% of admissions with DKA, the underlying cause of the crisis remains undiscovered. Fluctuations in diabetes control are common during adolescence and this is reflected in the number of young people admitted to hospital with DKA. DKA is the most common cause of death in children and adolescents with IDDM (Betschart 1993).

Q **5.9** Consider why diabetes may be unstable during adolescence.

PATHOPHYSIOLOGY

The symptoms of DKA are a consequence of the combined effect of insulin lack and increased secretion of catabolic hormones. As a result, two major biochemical derangements occur simultaneously:

- Accelerated gluconeogenesis and glycogenolysis cause hyperglycaemia, which in turn results in osmotic diuresis, electrolyte disruption and dehydration.
- Increased fat breakdown (lipolysis) results in the formation of ketone bodies which are weak acids and cause metabolic acidosis (see Box 5.9).

Q **5.10** Explain the pathophysiological basis for the signs, symptoms and clinical features of diabetic ketoacidosis (see Peragallo-Dikko 1995).

MEDICAL MANAGEMENT

Reversing the hyperglycaemia. Rapid-acting insulin is administered to lower blood glucose. Initially, approximately 6 IU/h is given via i.v. infusion pump (0.1 IU/kg per hour). The insulin dose will later be varied in accordance with the blood glucose level. If blood glucose does not fall within 2 h and true insulin resistance is present, the insulin dose may be increased to 12 IU/h. Capillary blood glucose should be checked hourly. Venous blood glucose and plasma potassium (K^+) is measured 2-hourly.

Rehydrating. Sodium chloride (NaCl) 0.9% is given by rapid i.v. infusion, e.g. 1–2 L may be given over the first hour, and then 1 L hourly for 2–5 h. The rate is then adjusted according to the patient's state of hydration. When blood glucose falls below 15 mmol/L, the sodium chloride is replaced by i.v. dextrose 5–10%.

Replacing potassium. Derangements in plasma potassium can vary. Hyperkalaemia may be evident in the very early stages due to severe acidosis, but once rehydration is underway, hypokalaemia is usual and may be severe. Intravenous potassium chloride (KCl) is prescribed in accordance with the blood biochemistry. Initially 10–30 mmol/h may be administered within the i.v. fluids. Ideally this should be by a regulated infusion delivery system.

Monitoring. The patient will be closely monitored for the following:

Box 5.9 The development of diabetic ketoacidosis (DKA)

The key precipitating factors are inadequate supply of insulin and increased demand for insulin, often in combination. These are often triggered by:
- infection (especially respiratory, urinary or abscesses)
- trauma or surgery
- severe illness, e.g. myocardial infarction or cerebrovascular accident
- failure to take sufficient insulin.

As a result of *reduced insulin* and *increased stress hormone levels*, cells will be unable to utilise glucose, glycogen will be converted to glucose, protein will be broken down to provide glucose (gluconeogenesis) and fat will be broken down (lipolysis) releasing ketone bodies. The combined effects of these events are:
- hyperglycaemia and hyperketonaemia
- osmotic diuresis
- fluid and electrolyte disruption
- catabolism/wasting
- acidosis.

As a result the patient will exhibit the following symptoms, signs and clinical features:

Symptoms	Signs and clinical features
• Polyuria	• Hyperglycaemia and glycosuria
• Polydipsia	• Polyuria progressing to oliguria
• Lethargy/weakness	• Ketonuria
• Nausea/vomiting	• Ketone breath (sweet fruity odour)
• Abdominal colic	• Weight loss
• Muscle cramps	• Hypokalaemia
	• Hypotension and tachycardia
	• Acidaemia
	• Rapid, deep (Kussmaul's) respirations
	• Evidence of intercurrent infection/illness
	• Skin flushed and warm
	• Hypothermia may develop
	• Drowsiness progressing to coma

Hyperglycaemia. Capillary blood glucose is measured hourly and venous blood glucose 2-hourly.
Dehydration. Blood urea, electrolytes and plasma osmolality are checked 2-hourly.
Response to fluid and K^+ replacement. Central venous pressure (CVP) or capillary pulmonary wedge pressure (PCWP), blood pressure and pulse are measured hourly as a guide to blood volume. A 12-lead ECG is performed and continuous cardiac monitoring commenced to detect cardiac arrhythmias associated with serum potassium lack or excess (see p. 684).
Acidosis. Arterial or venous blood gases and hydrogen ion (H^+) concentration are checked 1–2-hourly.
Underlying infection. A chest X-ray is performed. Blood cultures, urine and sputum specimens and a throat swab are sent to microbiology. Temperature, pulse and respiration are recorded hourly.
Ketosis and renal function. Urine is tested for glucose, ketones, protein, urea and electrolytes. In addition, urine volumes may be measured hourly.
Additional therapy which can be used in the treatment of DKA includes:
Sodium bicarbonate. This is not routinely used as it may exacerbate tissue hypoxia and hypokalaemia. As overcorrection may result in alkalosis, sodium bicarbonate is usually reserved for the treatment of very severe acidosis where the pH is below 7.0 and hydrogen ion concentration exceeds 100 mmol/L (Marshall 1993; see also Ch. 20, p. 687).
Broad-spectrum antibiotics. These may be given if infection is suspected and as a prophylaxis against supervening infection.
Anticoagulants. Low-dose heparin 5000 IU s.c. twice daily may be given (especially if the patient is elderly or deeply comatose) to reduce the risks of circulatory complications of dehydration and immobility.
Oxygen therapy. This will be administered in accordance with blood gas results.
Nasogastric aspiration will be performed to protect the airway if the patient is vomiting, drowsy or unconscious.
Urinary catheterisation. Urine volume is measured hourly as severe dehydration carries a risk of acute renal failure.
Space blanket. This may be used if the patient is hypothermic due to the vasodilatory response to acidosis.
Subsequent medical management of DKA will address the following concerns:
Insulin. When blood glucose is below 15 mmol/L, it is common to change the i.v. prescription to a regimen which combines glucose, potassium and insulin (GKI 'cocktail'). A typical cocktail would consist of 500 mL dextrose 10% plus 20 units of soluble insulin plus 20 mmol of potassium chloride (KCl) given via regulated infusion 4-hourly.
Fluid and electrolytes. If the patient is still dehydrated, or severely hyponatraemic, further i.v. sodium chloride 0.9% can be given in combination with the GKI cocktail. Plasma electrolytes, osmolality and glucose levels will be checked 4- to 6-hourly. Capillary blood glucose is monitored (visually or by meter) 2-hourly. The GKI cocktail and infusion rate will be adjusted in accordance with blood glucose and other biochemical results. When the patient is deemed to be clinically and biochemically stable, s.c. insulin and an oral diet are resumed. The i.v. GKI therapy is discontinued 1 h after the first s.c. injection of insulin.
Prevention. Once the patient is stable, every effort is made to discover the cause of DKA and, if possible, to prevent recurrences. For many patients, however, the experience of DKA is what first makes them aware that they have diabetes mellitus.

NURSING PRIORITIES AND MANAGEMENT: DKA

Each patient admitted with DKA will have unique problems and needs. The biochemical disruption of DKA is profound and life-threatening and priorities for nursing care will be strongly influenced by the prescribed medical therapy and the need for complex monitoring. Whilst the nurse must draw upon her technical skills in such a situation, it is vitally important that she remembers to care for the patient as a whole person.

Immediate priorities

The newly admitted patient with DKA is vulnerable in a variety of ways. The nurse should be sensitive to this vulnerability and try to accommodate individual needs when planning and implementing care.

Case History 5.2 and Nursing Care Plan 5.3 provide an example of how a patient may present with DKA and how nursing priorities may be met following admission and until consciousness is regained. It should be pointed out, however, that not all patients presenting with DKA will be unconscious. Individuals with long-standing diabetes mellitus can usually recognise the signs and symptoms of impending ketoacidosis and will seek medical help at a much earlier stage in its development.

Further considerations

When the patient is alert and able to respond, the focus of care will change. The nurse will work with the patient, the dietician and the medical staff to stabilise blood glucose and to monitor the effects of therapy.

The subsequent care of the patient in hyperglycaemic crisis, whether due to DKA or HHNK, will be similar in many respects and is described on page 176.

Hyperglycaemic hyperosmolar non-ketotic coma (HHNK)

This term refers to uncontrolled hyperglycaemia and dehydration in the absence of ketonaemia.

Epidemiology

HHNK is less common than DKA. It most commonly occurs in people with undiagnosed NIDDM (O'Hanlon-Nichols 1996) and as such tends to affect an older age group. Mortality rates as high as 70% have been reported (Peragillo-Dittko 1995).

Aetiology

Severe physical or psychological stress such as cerebrovascular accident (CVA), myocardial infarction, trauma or bereavement can precipitate HHNK (as in DKA). Thiazide diuretic therapy has also been found to precipitate HHNK in some people.

Case History 5.2 **R (see also Nursing Care Plan 5.3)**

R is a lively 18-year-old and the eldest of three children. At present she lives with her family but she is soon to leave home to undertake a secretarial course at a college some 30 miles away.

R and her two brothers have recently suffered a bad bout of flu. The boys are now fully fit but R is far from well. She has been passing a lot of urine and is constantly thirsty. She has lost weight and has recently been complaining of feeling tired all the time.

This morning she is very drowsy. Her skin feels hot and dry and she looks flushed. She has vomited several times and has complained of abdominal pain and cramps in her limbs. Her breath has a peculiar sweet smell and her mouth is very dry.

Her parents are alarmed and have called the GP to request an urgent visit. Alerted by the 'acetone breath', her symptoms and the history of recent illness, the GP checks R's capillary blood glucose and finds it to be 44 mmol/L. R is too sleepy to produce a urine specimen to check for ketones but the doctor is in little doubt about the diagnosis. An ambulance is summoned and R and her parents are taken to hospital. The ward is alerted to expect an unconscious patient with diabetic ketoacidosis (DKA).

On admission, R is acutely ill and has complex care requirements. A nurse who has the appropriate levels of knowledge and skill is assigned to care for her. She has prepared for R's admission and will subsequently assess her nursing needs and plan and evaluate her care. (See Nursing Care Plan 5.3.)

Dietary indiscretion such as a marked increase in refined carbohydrate intake (perhaps over Christmas or a holiday period) may account for the onset of HHNK. Some patients give a history of drinking large volumes of sugar-containing drinks in an effort to quench an ever-increasing thirst.

In 50% of patients the cause of this metabolic disturbance will remain unknown.

PATHOPHYSIOLOGY

HHNK may develop gradually over a period of hours or days (O'Hanlon-Nichols 1996). This is similar to DKA, in which the symptoms of uncontrolled diabetes appear over a period of days, although the course of the illness occasionally, and especially in the young, can develop over a few hours (Watkins et al 1996). Whilst there is no clear-cut distinction between DKA and HHNK, the variation is in the extent of the biochemical abnormalities (Marshall 1993, O'Hanlon-Nichols 1996).

The gradual onset in HHNK is probably due to the patient being less obviously 'ill' in the absence of ketosis. The signs and symptoms are similar to those found in DKA, with the following notable exceptions:

- ketonuria is absent or slight
- severe weight loss is unusual
- in the absence of the serious symptoms of ketosis, the blood glucose may be even higher than in DKA before the patient feels ill and seeks medical attention; indeed blood glucose is commonly over 60 mmol/L (Watkins et al 1996)
- physiological response to dehydration can be more marked due to the degree of hyperglycaemia and to age-associated intolerance to fluid and electrolyte disruption
- symptoms associated with ketonaemia/acidosis will not be in evidence.

Q **5.11** Given the above differences, draw up a list of signs, symptoms and clinical features of HHNK. Compare this with the list given for DKA and discuss the reasons for the differences.

The features of HHNK may be further described as follows:

Hyperglycaemia can be severe but develops gradually. Although some insulin is still being secreted, there is a relative insulin deficiency and the blood glucose continues to rise. The severe hyperglycaemia in HHNK is due to the combined effects of cellular resistance to insulin and the generation of glucose by stress hormone-driven glycogenolysis and gluconeogenesis.

Hyperosmolality. Normal plasma osmolality is around 285–295 mmol/kg. This is calculated using a formula which takes account of the sodium, potassium, urea and glucose levels in the blood. Hyperglycaemia accounts for much of the hyperosmolar state in HHNK. The high blood glucose will exert an osmotic pull and as a result fluid is drawn out of the cells into the circulation. Initially this will cause an increase in the glomerular filtration rate and large volumes of fluid will be lost by osmotic diuresis. As a result, the patient will develop polyuria, thirst, dehydration and hypovolaemia.

Hypernatraemia. The normal range for plasma sodium (Na^+) is 135–145 mmol/L. In HHNK, Na^+ may be raised above this level. Hypernatraemia can develop in response to a reduction in circulatory volume — in order to conserve a falling blood volume, aldosterone is secreted by the adrenal cortex, causing the kidney to retain sodium and excrete potassium (see p. 316).

Nursing Care Plan 5.3 Nursing care for R, a patient with DKA, during the first 24 h after admission (see Case History 5.2)

Nursing considerations	*Action*	*Rationale*	*Evaluation*
Impaired consciousness	❒ Position and support R in semi-prone or lateral position ❒ Keep artificial airway in position until voluntarily expelled ❒ Perform oropharyngeal suction if secretions are audible ❒ Provide nasogastric (NG) aspiration ❒ Continuously monitor colour and breathing ❒ Administer oxygen as prescribed, ensuring that fire safety rules are observed ❒ Monitor neurological status hourly. Record/report findings	To prevent asphyxia and prevent aspiration of secretion/vomitus Due to unconscious state and recent vomiting To correct hypoxia and prevent O_2 combustion To detect improvement/deterioration in conscious level	Skin colour and respirations are normal Risk factors eliminated Blood gases improving R is progressively more responsive
Hyperglycaemia and ketonaemia	❒ Administer prescribed rapid-acting insulin i.v. by infusion pump ❒ Monitor capillary blood glucose hourly; record/report findings	To correct hyperglycaemia and ketonaemia To evaluate response to insulin therapy and prevent hypoglycaemia	Trends indicate blood glucose returning to within the normal range
Fluid deficit/replacement	❒ Administer i.v. fluids as prescribed. Observe venepuncture site for redness, swelling or extravasation. Record all fluids in fluid balance chart ❒ Monitor CVP, BP, breathing, temperature; observe neck veins, skin colour and urine volumes ❒ Catheterisation usually prescribed if unconsciousness persists and if patient is oliguric ❒ Test urine hourly for ketones; record results	To correct hypovolaemia To monitor effects of fluid replacement To monitor renal function and detect renal insufficiency (urine <30 mL/h)	No discomfort or swelling of venepuncture site Vital signs are returning to within their normal ranges Urine volume >30 mL/h Ketonuria diminishing
Electrolyte imbalance/ replacement	❒ Observe effects of potassium replacement; provide continuous cardiac monitoring ❒ Report tall peaked T wave (indicates hyperkalaemia) ❒ Report flattened or inverted T wave (indicates hypokalaemia) ❒ REPORT ECG CHANGES PROMPTLY (see Ch. 2, p. 33)	Overzealous K^+ replacement can cause ventricular fibrillation, leading to cardiac arrest Persistent hypokalaemia due to inadequate K^+ replacement can result in heart block, which may lead to cardiac arrest	K^+ should be 3.5–5 mmol/L Cardiac monitor should display normal tracing
Probable current infection/ potential risk of infection	❒ Collect throat swab, catheter specimen of urine and, when consciousness returns, a specimen of sputum. Monitor TPR. Doctor will collect a specimen for blood culture ❒ Administer prescribed antibiotics and note/report side-effects ❒ Reduce risks of infection by high standards of nursing care (e.g. personal and catheter hygiene)	To detect/monitor current infection To safely administer therapy To prevent hospital-acquired infection	Specimen analysis Blood culture results and TPR normal Patient infection-free

By the time the patient comes to medical attention, the period of osmotic diuresis has usually passed and dehydration has developed. As a result the glomerular filtration rate falls, oliguria develops and blood urea rises. The combined effect of fluid loss, raised sodium levels, high blood glucose and raised plasma urea is that the blood becomes highly 'concentrated', i.e. hyperosmolar (hyperosmotic).

Non-ketosis. The production of ketones (ketogenesis) will be inhibited by the presence of insulin. Insulin also enables the small amount of ketones which result from lipolysis to be metabolised, thus preventing their accumulation in the blood.

Impaired level of consciousness. This occurs due to the effects of dehydration (hyperosmolality) on brain cells, impairing cerebral function and leading ultimately to coma.

Nursing Care Plan 5.3 *(cont'd)*

Nursing considerations	*Action*	*Rationale*	*Evaluation*
Inability to meet or communicate comfort needs	❐ Ensure bed is smooth, cool and crease-free. Provide regular position change and use of pressure-relieving aids to protect skin. Ensure careful positioning of limbs	To promote general comfort	Skin unblemished and free from discomfort
	❐ Wash, rinse and dry skin; observe for signs of pressure	To protect skin from damage	
	❐ Clean oral cavity 2-hourly. Lubricate lips. Clean nostrils and apply lubricant	To prevent oral and nasal discomfort and drying due to O_2 and the effects of dehydration and nasogastric tube	Oral/nasal mucosa intact
	❐ Keep hair groomed in preferred style. Use R's own nightwear. Maintain privacy throughout	To maintain R's individuality/ dignity	Patient feels/looks comfortable
Fear and shock as consciousness returns and diagnosis becomes apparent	❐ Display calm, empathic manner. Provide brief, clear explanations of reason for hospital admission and current care and treatment ❐ Provide access to parents and family	To convey positive attitudes To provide relevant information	R appears less acutely distressed
	❐ Encourage patient to verbalise concerns and express emotions ❐ Avoid bombarding R with information at this stage ❐ Show sensitivity to the emotional needs of this vulnerable young patient	To recognise R's rights as an individual	R is able to express her needs
R's parents are anxious and shocked due to their daughter's hospitalisation and diagnosis	❐ Provide a comfortable, private waiting area for parents ❐ Explain (briefly at this stage) what has happened to their daughter ❐ Encourage/accept verbalisation of fears and expression of emotions	To provide essential information to answer immediate concerns	Parents are reassured and able to meet with and support their daughter
	❐ Provide access to R and to medical staff ❐ Supply information about the ward/hospital (booklets etc.) ❐ When parents feel able to cooperate, complete admission documentation and patient profile ❐ Assure parents of access to nursing staff to answer their questions as they occur ❐ Arrange a visit from the diabetes nurse specialist at a mutually suitable time	To establish a trusting relationship, facilitate early educational interventions and offer support to the family	Parents' immediate needs have been met; they appear to feel supported

MEDICAL MANAGEMENT OF HHNK

This follows a similar approach to that of DKA, with some important differences, and centres on the following concerns.

Rehydration. The fluid deficit is vast and can be as much as 8–12 L. Replacement must, however, be approached with a degree of caution, given the risks associated with over-vigorous fluid replacement to which elderly patients are especially vulnerable:

- Sodium chloride 0.9% (normal saline) is given if plasma Na^+ levels are either not yet known or lower than 145 mmol/L.
- If plasma sodium is higher than 145 mmol/L then half-strength normal saline (0.45% NaCl) may be given. This approach is controversial in view of the risks it carries. Rapid reduction in plasma osmolality can result in fluid moving from the vascular compartment into the cells. This may result in hypovolaemia and cerebral oedema (Marshall 1993).

Replacement of potassium. As potassium levels are so variable and unpredictable in HHNK, extreme care is required during replacement to monitor cardiac effects. Continuous cardiac monitoring is strongly recommended.

Insulin therapy. As in DKA, a dose of 6 IU/h of soluble insulin is given until the blood glucose falls below 15 mmol/L, after which a GKI 'cocktail' is given (see p. 174).

Anticoagulant therapy. A major cause of death in HHNK is thrombosis (often pulmonary or cerebral), which is presumed to result from dehydration and hyperosmolality. Patients who are comatose or who have serum osmolality in excess of 360 mOsm/L should receive full-dose heparinisation. Heparin 5000 IU s.c. may be given 8-hourly to patients with lesser degrees of hyperosmolality as a means of preventing intravascular coagulation (Marshall 1993).

Other therapy and monitoring is as for ketoacidosis.

NURSING PRIORITIES AND MANAGEMENT: HYPERGLYCAEMIC HYPEROSMOLAR NON-KETOTIC (HHNK) COMA

Aspects of medical management which have implications for the planning of nursing care include:

- i.v. infusion (fluid replacement)
- i.v. insulin (by infusion pump)
- heparin (s.c. or by i.v. infusion pump)
- central venous pressure (CVP) monitoring
- cardiac monitoring
- urinary catheterisation
- oxygen therapy
- nasogastric aspiration (if patient is unconscious).

Immediate priorities

These interventions will need appropriate attention to ensure the safety and comfort of the patient. In addition, the patient is likely to be vulnerable due to an impaired level of consciousness, dehydration, electrolyte imbalance, the hazards of immobility and diabetes-associated risk factors. Nursing interventions will therefore include the following.

Monitoring consciousness level

In patients with HHNK the level of consciousness is of particular importance as there is a risk of cerebral thrombosis due to the combined effects of immobility, dehydration and diabetes-associated atherosclerosis (see Chs 9 and 29).

Another reason for vigilance is that the patient may be prescribed an i.v. infusion of half-strength normal saline aimed at reducing hyperosmolality. As explained above, if the fall in plasma osmolality is too rapid, cerebral oedema can develop, raising intracranial pressure. The nurse should therefore promptly report any evidence of deterioration in the patient's neurological function (see p. 856).

Monitoring dehydration and electrolyte balance

The nurse should observe for the following warning signs:

Evidence of persistent hypovolaemia. Hourly monitoring is usual. The nurse should report hypotension, a rapid thready pulse, a CVP reading lower than 5 cmH_2O and a urine volume of less than 30 mL/h. Measures to raise blood volume and blood pressure will probably be prescribed. This can include rapid infusion of i.v. fluids or plasma. Such treatment will require close monitoring in order to detect circulatory overload (see below).

Evidence of fluid overload. The nurse should promptly report a rising CVP, especially if this is accompanied by breathlessness, moist breath sounds, distended neck veins and a full pulse. These may indicate that fluid replacement has been too vigorous, causing overexpansion of the circulatory volume and placing strain on the left ventricle (see p. 683).

Evidence of electrolyte disruption. Changes in pulse rate and rhythm should be reported promptly, along with ECG changes associated with hypokalaemia and hyperkalaemia (see Nursing Care Plan 5.1), in order to allow adjustment to therapy and to prevent development of life-threatening cardiac dysrhythmias.

Monitoring response to insulin

Capillary blood glucose should be measured hourly to assess the response to i.v. insulin and to prevent overcorrection leading to hypoglycaemia. Accurate measurement and recording of blood glucose will provide the basis for adjusting insulin dosage.

Preventing complications

Many patients with HHNK are elderly and are especially vulnerable to the effects of hospitalisation and the complications of immobility. Maintenance of comfort and hygiene, including oral care, is of great importance.

Diabetes can cause impairment in circulation and sensation, placing the skin at particular risk. Avoidance of skin damage is therefore a priority. The patient's position should be frequently altered, suitable pressure-relieving devices should be used and the skin, clothing and bedding should be kept cool, clean and dry.

Care is required when lifting, moving or positioning the patient to avoid damage to skin, muscles or joints. Particular attention should be paid to avoiding damage to the heels. Due to vascular and neurological changes, the feet of people with diabetes require particular attention to avoid serious complications (see p. 184).

Atherosclerosis is common in patients with diabetes, thus placing them at particular risk of vascular complications. Passive limb exercises whilst the patient is unconscious, and active limb movements when he is able to cooperate, will help to prevent venous stasis, which may result in deep vein thrombosis and pulmonary embolism. The nurse and the physiotherapist will both be involved in encouraging limb exercises.

Breathing exercises are also important as elderly bedfast patients are at considerable risk of developing chest infections. Moreover, elderly people, and in particular those with diabetes, are less able to resist infection and tend to recover less quickly than younger non-diabetic people.

Monitoring the patient for pyrexia or other evidence of infection will allow prompt intervention. It is also important to ensure that the care environment and the standards of nursing care provided are such that infection risks are minimised.

Providing psychological support

The experience of a hyperglycaemic crisis can cause great distress not only to the patient but also to his family and close friends. Adopting a warm, empathic approach and accepting the fears of the patient and his family is important if trust and rapport are to be established. The nurse should provide essential information using brief, clear explanations. Access to medical staff and information about the ward or hospital should be provided.

Further considerations in DKA and HHNK

When the patient is deemed to be clinically and biochemically stable on the basis of observation, bedside monitoring and laboratory tests, ongoing care is planned to address changing needs. If urine volumes are satisfactory, the urinary catheter is removed. The nasogastric tube is removed and oral fluids are offered. Diet is introduced under the guidance of the dietician. When oral intake is adequate and blood urea and electrolyte levels are within normal limits, the i.v. fluids will usually be discontinued.

Subcutaneous insulin
This will replace the i.v. insulin when the patient is well enough to eat. Prescribing insulin is the responsibility of the physician but the nurse will be closely involved in monitoring patient response by frequent estimation of blood glucose. The nurse may also be required to adjust the insulin dosage within guidelines laid down in the written prescription.

Oral hypoglycaemic therapy
If possible, the patient is re-established on oral hypoglycaemic therapy. However, some patients may need to continue insulin therapy for some time before changing back to oral medication. Others may need to make a permanent change to insulin therapy in order to achieve better control of blood glucose levels.

Restoration of self-care
The physician, diabetes nurse specialist, dietician and ward nurses will initiate the process of preparing the patient to assume responsibility for self-care, but the major contribution will be made by the GP and the community nursing staff once the patient returns home.

Patient education
The newly diagnosed patient will require information about how a balance between activity, food and medication can be achieved with the help of frequent blood glucose monitoring. This is especially important for patients with IDDM.

Once the crisis has passed, perhaps the most important aspect of care is to prevent further episodes of DKA or HHNK. This involves identifying the events which led up to the crisis and analysing, together with the patient, where action might have been taken to avert the crisis or obtain help at an earlier stage. Glycosylated protein estimation can provide useful information about glycaemic control over the preceding weeks, as can the patient's record book containing blood glucose and urinalysis results.

It is all too easy to be wise in retrospect. It is therefore not helpful to blame the patient for any episode of DKA or HHNK. To do so would be to lose the benefits of a potentially valuable teaching situation.

Emotional support
If severe underlying emotional distress or disturbance has precipitated the metabolic crisis then the patient's difficulties may need to be sensitively explored. In accordance with the patient's wishes, appropriate counselling facilities may be provided. The newly diagnosed patient will require emotional support as he prepares to meet the immediate practical demands imposed by his disorder.

Hypoglycaemia (insulin reaction/coma)
Hypoglycaemia is a condition in which blood glucose is lower than the normal fasting range of 3.5 mmol/L. In reality, symptoms of hypoglycaemia rarely occur until the blood glucose falls below 3 mmol/L.

Epidemiology
Hypoglycaemia is the most common complication of insulin therapy and is a rare but serious complication of oral sulphonylurea therapy. It can also feature in diabetes secondary to other disorders, e.g. in patients with certain liver diseases. More than 90% of people with IDDM suffer episodes of symptomatic hypoglycaemia but it can also affect people with NIDDM who are treated with insulin or oral hypoglycaemics (Macheca 1993).

Aetiology
There are three main causes of hypoglycaemia (see Box 5.10):

- excess insulin
- insufficient food
- unusual exercise/activity.

PATHOPHYSIOLOGY

People tend to respond idiosyncratically to falling blood glucose. Symptoms will often be absent until the blood glucose is lower than 3 mmol/L. In long-standing diabetes mellitus the sensitivity of response to hypoglycaemia can become blunted, and the patient may remain asymptomatic even when the blood glucose falls below 2 mmol/L (although at this level some signs may be obvious to others).

Onset and progression. Symptoms may develop over a very short period of time, usually 5–15 min. This can be contrasted with DKA and HHNK, both of which have a more insidious onset.

Endocrine/autonomic response. Glucagon and other stress hormones (including adrenaline) are secreted in response to falling blood sugar. These hormones potentiate the effects of the sympathetic nervous system to cause the following symptoms:

- full, bounding pulse
- palpitations
- sweating and trembling
- 'butterflies' in the stomach
- hunger pangs (sometimes).

Central nervous system response. As brain cells are unable to use alternatives to glucose for metabolism, a fall below the normal blood sugar will cause symptoms of cerebral dysfunction (neuroglycopenic symptoms) such as:

- headache
- lack of concentration
- dizziness
- unsteady gait
- slurred speech
- tingling around the lips.

Box 5.10 Hypoglycaemia: classification and causes

Classification
- *Asymptomatic*: biochemical hypoglycaemia without symptoms
- *Mild*: easily recognised and corrected by the patient
- *Severe*: patient conscious but requiring help from others
- *Comatose*: cerebral function severely affected by glucose lack

Causes
- Too much insulin
- Wrong type of insulin
- Inappropriate combination of insulins
- Excess dosage of oral sulphonylureas
- Delayed or missed meal
- More than usual amount of exercise
- Alcohol ingestion, especially when hungry
- Stress, such as hypothermia

In addition, observers may notice abnormalities such as:

- irrational behaviour
- muscle twitching/seizures
- automatism
- extreme drowsiness or coma.

Some of these symptoms and signs could, with disastrous consequences, be mistakenly attributed by others to excess intake of alcohol.

Loss of sensitivity to symptoms. Recently diagnosed patients tend to rely on endocrine/autonomic symptoms such as sweating, tremor and palpitations to alert them to a fall in blood glucose. However, after some years, patients may become less sensitive to these responses and come to rely on central nervous system (neuroglycopenic) signs such as visual blurring and dizziness to alert them to impending hypoglycaemia. Symptoms can also be masked by:

- *Neuropathic changes*. As the patient's ability to perceive the neurological early warning symptoms of hypoglycaemia may be impaired by diabetic neuropathies, progression to irrational behaviour, automatism and coma can occur.
- *Alcohol*. If the patient is known to have drunk alcohol or his breath smells of alcohol, this can mask the symptoms of hypoglycaemia and lead others to mistake hypoglycaemia for intoxication.
- *Ageing*. In older people hypoglycaemia can develop rather more insidiously and the symptoms can be mistaken for failing mental function.
- *Time of day*. Nocturnal hypoglycaemia most often occurs between 03.00 and 05.00 h and may pass unnoticed, although symptoms such as night sweats, restlessness, stertorous breathing and headaches on waking may give the patient an indication of its occurrence.

Other forms of hypoglycaemia can be attributed to:

- *Nocturnal hypoglycaemia*, which may be characterised by night sweats and morning headache, accompanied by a high glucose level. This causes rebound hyperglycaemia and is attributed to an increase in the release of counter-regulatory hormones during the night to correct the hypoglycaemia. This is known as the Somogyi phenomenon (Macheca 1993, Appleton & Jerreat 1995).
- *Sulphonylurea hypoglycaemia* — chlorpropamide and glibenclamide, even at normal therapeutic doses, have been implicated in severe, prolonged hypoglycaemic coma. This risk is increased in elderly people and in those with poor renal function. This can lead to prolonged hypoglycaemia and even death (Appleton & Jerreat 1995).

MEDICAL MANAGEMENT

Treatment of hypoglycaemia is simple and the effects are dramatic and gratifying. Nevertheless, the risks posed by hypoglycaemic coma and the importance of early detection and intervention must be stressed.

Hypoglycaemia can be treated with oral carbohydrate, s.c. or i.m. glucagon, or i.v. glucose — depending on the stage and severity.

The conscious patient should be given rapidly absorbed glucose together with a more gradually absorbed form of carbohydrate, e.g. Dextrosol tablets followed by a glass of milk or fruit juice and a biscuit or sandwich. If a meal has been missed this should be taken at the earliest opportunity.

The confused or drowsy patient. If he is too drowsy to eat or drink safely, the patient can be given glucagon 1 mg by s.c. injection. This will have the effect of raising the blood glucose. Relatives can be taught how to administer glucagon.

The unconscious patient. Medical help should always be sought for the unconscious patient, although if hypoglycaemia is known to be the problem, glucagon should be given whilst the doctor is awaited and the patient should be placed in the recovery position until consciousness returns. Nothing should be given orally whilst the patient is unconscious.

If glucagon is unavailable, or fails to bring a response within 10–15 min, 30–50 mL of glucose 50% may be injected i.v. by the doctor. This treatment will usually raise the blood glucose enough for the patient to regain consciousness. When unconsciousness persists, hospital admission will be necessary.

The hospitalised patient with hypoglycaemic coma. A specimen of blood will be taken for estimation of blood glucose. Continuous i.v. infusion of dextrose 10–20% will be commenced and the patient's response monitored by frequent measurement of capillary blood glucose.

Unfortunately, 1–2% of hospitalised patients fail to respond promptly to therapy. For these patients, other causes of coma such as alcohol or drug overdose, hypothermia or cerebral haemorrhage should be excluded. As cerebral oedema can accompany prolonged hypoglycaemia and as persistent attacks of hypoglycaemia may result in cognitive impairment, an i.v. infusion of mannitol (a hyperosmotic fluid) may be given (Richmond 1996).

NURSING PRIORITIES AND MANAGEMENT: HYPOGLYCAEMIA

In hypoglycaemic coma the period of extreme vulnerability tends to be short. Nevertheless, the nurse must take the patient's vulnerabilities into account in nursing interventions by:

- ensuring the patient's safety and comfort
- monitoring the patient's consciousness level
- administering prescribed therapy
- monitoring capillary blood glucose
- investigating the cause of the hypoglycaemic coma
- providing information and encouragement for the patient to help improve diabetes control.

Metabolic complications of diabetes vary in cause, severity and outcome. All indicate a lack of stability of diabetes control which requires investigation and possibly subsequent modification of treatment or lifestyle.

For a detailed account of the causes, symptoms, treatment and management of hypoglycaemia, see Macheca (1993) and Appleton & Jerreat (1995).

CHRONIC COMPLICATIONS OF DIABETES MELLITUS

This section will consider chronic complications of diabetes mellitus which result in pathological changes in large blood vessels (macroangiopathies), small blood vessels (microangiopathies) and nerves (neuropathies). Although the exact mechanism underlying pathological changes is unknown, poor glycaemic control is thought to be responsible for the metabolic, neurological and vascular changes that occur (Watkins et al 1996).

The recently reported Diabetes Control and Complications Trial (Diabetes Control and Complications Research Group 1993) demonstrated that tight control of blood glucose prevented or delayed the onset of complications in IDDM, particularly retinopathy, neuropathy and nephropathy. However, the risk of severe hypoglycaemic attacks increased threefold.

In September 1998, the United Kingdom Prospective Diabetes Study Group (UKPDS) reported their findings in relation to the reduction of long-term complications in patients with type 2 diabetes. It was found that, through tight control of blood glucose and maintenance of blood pressure within normal limits, the risk of deaths related to diabetes could be reduced. Additionally, the long-term complications of diabetes such as heart disease and stroke and the loss of sight and kidney damage could also be reduced (see Turner et al 1998, UKPDS 1998).

Q

5.12 Discuss the potential risks of poor diabetes control.

Detailed management of specific diabetes-related complications will not be provided in this chapter. All are dealt with fully elsewhere in this book. The reader is therefore urged to consult the relevant chapters for detailed coverage of these disorders.

Atherosclerosis

Epidemiology

Although atherosclerosis is not peculiar to diabetes, it is known that myocardial infarction, cerebrovascular accident (CVA) and gangrene are relatively frequent complications and are major causes of death in people with diabetes. Atherosclerosis develops at a much younger age in people with diabetes than in non-diabetic individuals; this is most noticeable in females.

Both types of diabetes carry increased risk, but those with NIDDM show the strongest tendency to develop atheroma. This is probably due to age-related factors and perhaps also to the effects of long-standing asymptomatic hyperglycaemia prior to diagnosis. In IDDM, microvascular disease such as retinopathy usually precedes evidence of atherosclerosis.

Aetiology

In diabetes, blood lipids and clotting factors may be elevated (Donnelly 1992). The ability to break down fibrin can also be impaired. Blood platelets tend to be stickier and platelet aggregation is often increased. Factors such as smoking, obesity and hypertension further increase the risk. A diabetic smoker, for example, is 10 times more likely to have a major vascular event than a diabetic non-smoker (Abraham & Levy 1992).

Onset and progress of the disease

The development and vascular distribution of atherosclerosis in diabetes are similar to what is found in non-diabetic people, the exception being the more severe peripheral arterial involvement which may affect the lower limbs of some people with diabetes.

Cardiovascular disease

When compared with the general population, diabetes in men is associated with a two to threefold risk of developing coronary heart disease. In premenopausal women this is increased to four to five times the risk if the woman has diabetes (BDA 1995). In a recent study coordinated by the WHO, it was found that of a group of 497 people aged 35–54 with diabetes at 8-year follow-up, the prevalence of cardiovascular disease was 45%; 43% had coronary heart disease, 4.5% cerebrovascular disease and 4.2% had peripheral vascular disease (BDA 1995). Atherosclerosis of the coronary vessels can impair oxygen delivery to the myocardium, resulting in angina pectoris or myocardial infarction. Due to the effects of autonomic neuropathy the patient may develop a cardiac arrhythmia and may have a 'silent' (painless) myocardial infarction. Indeed, mortality after myocardial infarction is twice as high in the diabetic than in the non-diabetic person (Department of Health/BDA 1995).

Cerebrovascular disease

Strokes are about twice as common in people with diabetes when compared with the general population. Hypertension is probably the most important causative factor; those factors which contribute to the development of atherosclerosis are also important.

Retinopathy

Diabetic retinopathy occurs in 12% of people with IDDM and in 5% of those with NIDDM, after 30 years of having diabetes (MacCuish 1992). It is the most common cause of blindness among those who are registered blind between the ages of 20 and 65 years (Perry & Tullo 1995). Retinopathy results from changes in the small blood vessels of the retina (retinal microangiopathy) and can be classified as:

- background (non-proliferative) retinopathy
- maculopathy
- proliferative retinopathy.

Background retinopathy

Background retinopathy rarely causes a major threat to vision unless the macula is affected. In the early stages of retinopathy, the capillaries of the retina become more permeable. This can cause fluid exudation (hard exudates) into the vitreous humour. Retinal veins may swell at localised spots, giving the appearance of 'beading'. Microaneurysms can develop; these can rupture, causing small bleeds. Arteriolar occlusions may appear as 'cotton wool spots' on the retina. More spots occur in rapidly developing retinopathy or where there is coexisting hypertension. Evidence of venous bleeding and 'cotton wool' spots suggests progression to preproliferative retinopathy.

Maculopathy

Maculopathy can cause significant visual loss. In this condition, oedema, haemorrhages and exudates are concentrated on the macular area of the retina.

Proliferative retinopathy

Microvascular disease of the retina can result in areas of hypoxia. This will give rise to the compensatory development of new blood vessels (neovascularisation) which grow forward from the retina to invade the vitreous body. These new vessels are fragile and poorly supported; consequently, haemorrhages into the vitreous body are common. Progressive traction on the retina can result in retinal detachment. Proliferative retinopathy and retinal detachment will seriously threaten vision.

MEDICAL MANAGEMENT

The main priorities in the treatment of diabetic retinopathy are to reduce the risk of haemorrhage and to limit new vessel growth into the vitreous body. Photocoagulation by means of laser technology can be used to treat all forms of retinopathy. Treatment should be considered in all patients with visual potential (Hamilton & Ubig 1991, Phillips 1994; see also Ch. 13, see p 520).

Screening. Phillips (1994) reported that the majority of cases of blindness as a consequence of diabetic retinopathy could have been prevented or delayed by timely and appropriate management. Annual ophthalmoscopic examination is therefore strongly advised. Where glycaemic control is poor, more frequent eye examinations may be recommended.

Retinal photography can be carried out annually and it is now possible to do this using non-mydriatic retinal cameras which allow the retina to be photographed without prior dilatation of the pupil. The BDA has already sponsored 10 mobile units to carry out photographic screening for retinopathy (Lovelock 1990).

Prevention. The patient should be aware of the established link between poor blood glucose control and retinopathy and of the importance of promptly reporting changes in vision. A full eye examination is recommended at least once yearly, either by an ophthalmologist or an optician. As eye tests for patients with diabetes are free of charge, the optician should be made aware that the patient has diabetes. The risks of retinopathy increase if the patient is hypertensive. The benefits of following medical advice and treatment with regard to blood pressure regulation should therefore be explained.

Other eye disorders

Although retinopathy poses the main threat to vision in diabetes there is also an increased risk of cataracts and glaucoma. The reasons why this should be so are not entirely clear. It is possible that glycosylation of protein in the optic lens can cause the opacities of cataract (Hamilton & Ubig 1991). The management of cataracts and glaucoma are described in full in Chapter 13.

Sadly, many patients with diabetes do ultimately suffer partial or total blindness. Maintaining independence in relation to diabetes management and general self-care will present quite a challenge. Davis (1989) describes various devices which can enable the blind or partially sighted patient to draw up and administer insulin and to monitor blood glucose. These include 'click-count' syringes, the dial-a-dose NovoPen and B-D Pen, insulin cartridges and even a 'talking' blood glucose meter. Although audible blood glucose meters are available, the challenge is in teaching a patient to accurately place a blood sample on a reagent strip (Hall & Waterman 1997).

The nurse caring for the blind diabetic patient should work with him to seek out ways of reducing his dependence on others. The BDA and the Royal National Institute for the Blind (RNIB) can provide invaluable up-to-date information about the help currently available for blind diabetic patients.

Diabetic nephropathy

Diabetic nephropathy accounts for 25% of all patients who require renal support therapy. Whilst IDDM is responsible for most cases of renal failure in those under 50 years of age, there is an increasing number of NIDDM patients who are prone to this complication. Recently the number of patients with IDDM who develop nephropathy has declined, and with good control and good quality care this number could be reduced to as low as 10% (Watkins et al 1996).

AETIOLOGY AND PATHOPHYSIOLOGY

The kidneys of people with diabetes are vulnerable with respect to the following:

- *Microvascular changes.* Damage to the capillaries in the glomeruli can occur. The basement membrane initially thickens and in the later stages nodules of glycoprotein are deposited in the glomerular capsule. As a result the filtering capacity of the glomeruli is reduced.
- *Macrovascular changes.* Atheromatous changes in renal vessels can lead to poor renal perfusion which will ultimately impair renal function.
- *Hypertension.* A common feature in diabetes, hypertension can contribute to kidney damage and, conversely, can also result from kidney damage.
- *Urinary tract infection.* This can occur for several reasons:
  —diabetes-associated predisposition to infection
  —damaged renal tissue vulnerable to infection
  —the need for catheterisation during metabolic crisis
  —atonic bladder associated with autonomic neuropathy, causing urinary stasis and ascending urinary tract infection.

Screening

Proteinuria. This is the clinical hallmark of diabetic renal disease. Urine testing for albumin should be undertaken at each clinic visit and at least once a year for all patients with diabetes. A positive dipstick test for albuminuria suggests the need for more detailed biochemical analysis to provide quantitative information about the extent of protein loss from the kidney. Many centres still collect, or ask the patient to collect, urine over a 24-h period to measure total protein excretion.

Microalbuminuria. For several years before albuminuria becomes detectable, microalbuminuria may be present, indicating early pathological changes within the kidneys. Testing kits are available to detect microalbuminuria in the clinic or GP surgery. If a positive result is obtained, laboratory methods which quantify microalbuminuria are then used (Doyle 1991, Marshall 1991; see Eccles 1995 for a review of tests).

Blood/urine biochemistry. Estimation of plasma and urine urea, creatinine, electrolytes and osmolality can be undertaken. Serum albumin will also usually be measured if either albuminuria or oedema is present.

Blood pressure. All patients with proteinuria should have their blood pressure measured at every clinic or surgery visit. Many patients with evidence of proteinuria are in their 30s or 40s. The Scottish Intercollegiate Guidelines Network (SIGN 1997) recommend that, in the presence of microalbuminuria, blood pressure should be treated when greater than 120/70 mmHg in IDDM patients and 140/90 mmHg in NIDDM patients.

MEDICAL MANAGEMENT

Diabetic renal disease is treated in the same way as renal disease in the non-diabetic population. The reader is referred to Chapter 8 for detailed coverage of early, advanced and end-stage renal failure. Only diabetes-related points will be mentioned in the short sections which follow.

Treatment choices for the patient in end-stage renal failure include haemodialysis, continuous ambulatory peritoneal dialysis (CAPD) or renal transplant using live or cadaver donors.

Renal transplantation using a live donor offers the best treatment for suitable patients. Careful selection of patients is important, given that other major diabetes-related complications usually coexist with the renal disease. Virtually all diabetic patients with end-stage renal failure have retinopathy, and 20–30% are blind. Retinopathy alone would not militate against active treatment by dialysis or renal transplantation but the presence of carcinomatosis, advanced dementia or severe cerebrovascular disease would do so. The prognosis in, for example, severe cardiovascular disease is also poor (Watkins et al 1996).

Blood glucose control in people with Diabetic Nephropathy

Insulin requirements. These can be difficult to predict. To enable insulin dosage adjustments to be made, frequent blood glucose monitoring will be required. Multiple injections using a pen injection device or continuous s.c. infusion may be advised to enable adjustments to be made more readily.

Oral hypoglycaemics. Due to the danger of lactic acidosis, metformin (a biguanide) should not be used for patients with renal impairment. Chlorpropamide (a sulphonylurea) should also be avoided as it is mainly excreted by the kidneys and in renal failure can accumulate in the blood, causing serious hypoglycaemia. It may be necessary for some patients in renal failure whose diabetes was previously controlled by oral medication to be changed to insulin therapy.

NURSING PRIORITIES AND MANAGEMENT: DIABETIC NEPHROPATHY

When renal function is impaired, diabetes control should be closely monitored by regular blood glucose measurement and urinalysis. Measurement and recording of fluid intake and output and body weight may be required to monitor renal function. Dietary and fluid restrictions may be imposed due to renal impairment. Patients and their families should be made aware of the vital importance of these measures.

Specific aspects of nursing care in renal failure can be found in Roberto (1990), Trusler (1992) and King (1997).

Prevention of renal failure

By identifying early renal impairment by screening for microalbuminuria, making efforts to improve diabetes control and detecting and treating hypertension, it is possible to prevent or delay the progression of renal disease (Diabetes Control and Complications Research Group 1993).

Medical and nursing staff should exercise extreme caution in the introduction and subsequent care of urinary catheters in order to prevent infection. Prompt treatment of any established urinary tract infection will normally be required to minimise damage.

5.13 Suggest three treatment approaches which may be used in end-stage renal failure in a diabetic person and discuss the potential lifestyle implications of each form of treatment.

For further information on renal disease in diabetes mellitus, see Hoops (1990), Roberto (1990), Trusler (1992), Coates (1996) and Warmington (1996).

Diabetic neuropathy

Aetiology

Although the cause of diabetic neuropathy is uncertain, it is known that nerve function in the diabetic patient deteriorates in response to pressure, metabolic changes and ischaemia (Watkins et al 1996). The incidence of diabetic neuropathy is known to rise in line with the duration of diabetes and with increasing age. A popular theory is that nerve damage occurs as a result of the accumulation of metabolites of glucose (such as sorbitol), causing osmotic swelling and subsequent damage to the nerve cell. Ischaemia as a cause of diabetic neuropathy, however, remains controversial but must be considered a contributory factor (Watkins et al 1996).

PATHOPHYSIOLOGY

Structural damage occurs which affects the Schwann cells and causes segmental areas of demyelination to appear, thus impairing conduction of the nerve impulses (Porth 1994). The types of neuropathy which may occur are as follows:

Peripheral neuropathies. These principally affect the lower extremities and play a major part in the aetiology of diabetic foot problems. They can affect either sensory or motor nerves and the patient's symptoms will reflect this.

Polyneuropathy This term refers to widespread neuropathic changes affecting many nerves. Again, the lower extremities are often affected (peripheral polyneuropathy).

Mononeuropathies. It is possible for a single nerve to display evidence of damage. An example of mononeuropathy is the ptosis (drooping eyelid) and diplopia which can occur as a result of third cranial nerve damage (see Table 5.12).

Autonomic neuropathies. Damage can also develop within the autonomic nervous system, causing a wide range of symptoms in many different sites. Sexual impotence, atonic bladder and silent myocardial infarction are examples of conditions associated with autonomic neuropathy (see Table 5.12).

Prevention

Whether or not diabetic neuropathy can be prevented is a contentious issue. Most experts agree that neuropathies seem to be more prevalent and more severe in poorly controlled diabetes. This may suggest that if the blood sugar is kept within the normal range and other sensible measures such as avoiding smoking are employed then the risk of neuropathy developing may be reduced. However, once neuropathies have developed, the damage cannot be reversed and means must be sought to help the patient deal with the particular problems which the neuropathy presents.

MEDICAL MANAGEMENT

Diabetic neuropathy can affect virtually any part of the body. Management, which is essentially symptomatic, may involve the interdisciplinary efforts of the diabetes care team. A variety of treatment approaches may be adopted, including medication, surgery and physiotherapy.

NURSING PRIORITIES AND MANAGEMENT: DIABETIC NEUROPATHY

Devising ways to meet the particular comfort needs of the patient will be a central focus for nursing care. Reducing the risk of accidental tissue damage arising from severe sensory impairment will also be a priority.

Neuropathies can seriously interfere with lifestyle and with emotional well-being. An example of this is neuropathic impotence which develops gradually over a period of months or years and which, once established, is permanent and irreversible (Watkins et al 1996). This can be devastating for both the patient and his partner. Nurses in particular can strive to improve their sensitivity to the verbal and non-verbal cues which may indicate the patient's concerns in this area. Management includes professional sexual counselling and a range of treatment options that include suction devices, penile

Table 5.12 Diabetic neuropathy

Type of neuropathy	*Body system/part affected*	*Symptoms/signs*	*Special points*
Peripheral neuropathies Polyneuropathies: • Sensory	The lower extremities are the most frequently affected area	Reduced sensation: numbness, heaviness, insensitivity to heat, cold, and pressure Increased sensation: tingling, burning, pain (worse at night)	Serious risk of tissue damage as a result of heat, cold or pressure
• Motor —Amyotrophy —Muscle wasting	Muscles of the pelvic girdle Muscles of the hands and feet	Severe muscle wasting and pain Loss of strength in hand grip Changes in walking pattern Pressure points altered Painless foot ulcers can develop	Physiotherapy Aids to assist hand grip Chiropody Adapted footwear Care of the feet
Neuropathic arthropathy	Joints in the feet; 'Charcot's joints'	See 'The diabetic foot'	
Mononeuropathies: • Sensory	Femoral, sciatic, radial or ulnar nerve 3rd cranial nerve	Acute pain with sudden onset Weakness and paralysis Ptosis: drooping of the upper eyelid	Provide pain relief Improve diabetes control Refer to an ophthalmologist
• Motor	3rd, 4th and 6th cranial nerves	Squint: diplopia	
Autonomic neuropathies	*Cardiovascular system* • Heart and blood vessels • Vasomotor centre	Postural hypotension Tachycardia at rest Painless myocardial infarction Reduced perspiration in lower extremities Increased perspiration in upper extremities	Symptoms such as syncope, dizziness and sweating; can be confused with hypoglycaemia
	Gastrointestinal system • Stomach	Diabetic gastroparesis (delayed emptying) Nausea, anorexia Feeling of fullness	Altered absorption rate of nutrients can affect diabetes control
	• Bowel	Constipation Nocturnal diarrhoea	Adjust diet
	Urinary system • Bladder	Loss of sensation Incomplete emptying Retention of urine Atonic bladder Sphincter incompetence	Urinary stasis creates risk of infection which may lead to renal damage
	Reproductive system • Male genitalia	Sexual impotence Retrograde ejaculation Infertility	Neuropathic, vascular and psychological factors usually coexist

injections or implants (Tiley 1997). Recently, pharmacological preparations, e.g. Sildenafil (Viagra), have been added to the treatment options and have improved sexual function in 50–60 %of men with diabetes. However, it is expected that those men who have not responded to other therapies and who have severe vascular disease will not respond to Sildenafil either (BDA 1998a).

The diabetic foot (see Table 5.13)

Disorders of the foot in diabetes can occur as a result of neuropathic and vascular changes. Generally, these two complications coexist, namely neuropathic ulcers and neuropathic arthropathy.

Neuropathic ulcers

Painless neuropathic ulcers can develop from chemical, thermal or mechanical injury. Forces applied to the foot can result in callus formation. As a result of sensory impairment, the patient is usually unaware of the developing callosity. Mechanical forces continue to be applied to the damaged area, resulting in inflammation, abscess formation and, eventually, ulceration.

MEDICAL MANAGEMENT OF NEUROPATHIC ULCERS

An infected ulcer in the foot requires urgent medical attention. Bedrest or the use of non-weight-bearing crutches is usually prescribed. A wound swab will be taken to identify infective microorganisms and to allow appropriate antibiotic therapy to be commenced. It may be necessary to undertake surgical debridement and drainage of pus. A serious complication of neuropathic ulcer is necrotising anaerobic infection and gangrene.

Once the acute situation has resolved it will be necessary to ensure redistribution of the weight-bearing forces on the vulnerable foot by the use of specially constructed shoes or moulded

Table 5.13 Clinical signs in the diabetic foot. (Reproduced with kind permission from Kinson & Nattrass 1984)

	Ischaemia	*Neuropathy*
Pain	Considerable	Relatively free
Deformity	Nil	May be present
Skin	Thin Rubor on dependency Blanches on elevation	Often callus formation Normal colour
Temperature	Feels cold	Feels normal
Subcutaneous tissues	Atrophic	Normal
Peripheral pulses	Absent	Present

insoles. If recurrence of neuropathic ulceration is to be avoided, regular follow-up by a chiropodist will be required. The patient will also need supplementary information and advice on foot care.

Neuropathic arthropathy (Charcot's joint)

A trivial injury such as that caused by tripping or bumping into something can lead to the development of a hot, red and swollen (yet usually painless) joint in the foot. Gradually the joint structure is destroyed and major deformities of the foot result. The metatarsal and tarsal joints are the most commonly affected. The extent of the joint destruction can be discovered by the use of X-rays and bone scans.

MEDICAL MANAGEMENT OF CHARCOT'S JOINT

Rest, antibiotics and non-steroidal anti-inflammatory drugs (NSAIDs) such as indomethacin may be prescribed. Adapted footwear will usually be prescribed once ambulation is possible. Prevention of further joint damage will be attempted by education and by arranging supervision by a chiropodist.

Ischaemia

The ischaemic foot results from atherosclerotic changes in the distal vessels of the legs. Poor delivery of oxygen leads first to pain in the calf and foot during walking (claudication); later, when blood flow is further impaired, pain will be experienced during rest. Localised pressure can result in ulceration; this can be complicated by secondary infection and gangrene. The foot feels cold and foot pulses may be absent. Colour changes occur in the skin and pain can be severe and unremitting.

MEDICAL MANAGEMENT OF THE ISCHAEMIC FOOT

This can include reducing oxygen demand of the tissues by rest and by cooling the area. Antibiotics to treat infection and analgesics for pain will be prescribed. Vascular reconstructive surgery may be attempted (see Ch. 2). In severe cases, where the pain is intolerable or where sepsis is life-threatening, amputation may need to be considered.

Prevention of foot problems

The diabetic foot is vulnerable on several counts. Sensory impairment can result in accidental injury remaining undetected until catastrophic damage has occurred. Vascular insufficiency deprives distal cells of their metabolic requirements, causing devitalisation of the tissue. Finally, healing of established injury may be delayed and the tendency to infection is increased. These factors can result in major complications such as gangrene developing from relatively minor injuries. The key to preventing serious diabetes-related complications in the lower limbs lies in providing education for professionals, patients and their families/carers. Patients may benefit from the advice given in Box 5.11.

Infection

Infection can be viewed as a precipitating or a complicating factor in diabetes mellitus. In established diabetes it can precipitate a metabolic crisis; in undiagnosed diabetes, it can herald the onset of symptoms.

Stress hormones such as ACTH, cortisol and catecholamines will be released in response to severe infection. These hormones will raise the blood glucose by the processes of glycogenolysis and gluconeogenesis. The resulting increase in insulin demand will present a challenge to an already malfunctioning pancreas, and as a result metabolic crisis may ensue.

Infection as a complicating factor

Evidence on whether diabetic people are more prone to developing infection than non-diabetic people is somewhat conflicting. It has

Box 5.11 Measures to protect the feet in diabetes

General measures
- Do not smoke
- Take a healthy diet with lots of fibre and not too much fat
- Try to keep body weight within normal limits
- Exercise. Try to keep active. This will help the circulation
- Get blood pressure and blood fats checked regularly

Footwear
- Try to get shoes which don't pinch anywhere and which allow all toes to move freely. Break in new shoes very gradually
- Ensure that socks or stockings fit comfortably. Change them daily
- Change footwear as soon as possible if wet
- Avoid walking barefoot; wear slippers and beach shoes to prevent injury

Foot care
- Bathe feet daily using lukewarm (not hot) water and soap
- Pat feet dry gently; pay special attention to the area between the toes
- Apply a lanolin-based moisturising cream daily to avoid dryness and keep the skin supple
- Avoid exposing feet to excess heat or cold
- Avoid sunburn to the feet and legs
- Cut nails straight across while they are still soft from bathing
- Inspect feet daily for blisters, corns, calluses, cracks or redness (a mirror can help in seeing the underside of the foot)
- If a minor cut or abrasion does occur, wash thoroughly and cover with a clean dressing. See your doctor if the cut has not healed in 48 h
- Your chiropodist should be consulted for treatment of ingrown toenails, corns, calluses or verrucae (no home remedies, please)
- A doctor or nurse should be consulted if foot problems such as tingling, numbness, swelling, pain or loss of feeling develop
- Remember: most people with diabetes never have any trouble with their feet. Take reasonable care of your feet and they will reward you by lasting a lifetime!

been suggested that people with diabetes have normal immune systems but have an impairment in their 'first-line' defences against infection, i.e. bactericidal activity linked to the inflammatory response and phagocytosis. The action of leucocytes is impaired in the presence of an abnormally high blood glucose (Robertson 1995). High blood glucose also presents a favourable environment for bacteria by influencing the growth of microorganisms and increasing the severity of the infection (Porth 1994). Poor blood glucose control does seem to be linked to increased infection rates. In addition, host defences against infection may be further compromised by microvascular and neuropathic changes associated with diabetes. A good example of this is the diabetic foot.

Q

5.14 Why would microvascular and/or neuropathic changes cause an increased susceptibility to infection?
5.15 Identify the most common infections which affect people with diabetes. Discuss why this should be so.
5.16 Explain the way in which infection can have an impact on diabetic control and consider the role of the nurse in minimising the effect of intercurrent infections (see Wood 1997).

Summary

Chronic complications of diabetes can have important implications for the planning of nursing care. Whether the patient is at home or in hospital, the nurse should carefully assess his nursing needs, giving special consideration to risks associated with impaired circulation and sensation, increased risk of infection and delayed healing (see Ch. 23). Recognition of these risk factors will enable care to accommodate the patient's particular vulnerabilities and will help to ensure that suitable educational support is provided.

FACILITATING SELF-CARE THROUGH EDUCATION

In some hospital and community settings the overall coordination of patient teaching is undertaken by the diabetic nurse specialist working closely with the specialist dietician and the patient's physician. In many cases, however, the care of diabetic patients will be undertaken by community and hospital nurses who are not specialists as such in diabetes care. All such nurses may be required to undertake a teaching role and must therefore ensure that their own knowledge base is adequate.

Assessment

Before embarking on a teaching programme, the nurse must determine the needs of the patient and his family for information, and plan teaching strategies that will make the learning experience pleasant and effective (Ley 1997). By establishing a rapport with the patient and family, the nurse will be better able to assess the patient's needs in relation to:

- current level of knowledge about diabetes
- understanding about the reasons for prescribed treatment
- knowledge and skills required for self-care
- emotional response to the diagnosis
- social support from family and friends
- barriers to learning, e.g. sensory loss, mobility and manipulation problems, language difficulties, reading and writing difficulties and intellectual impairment.

Planning a teaching programme

Personnel

Any member of the diabetes care team may be involved in teaching the patient and his family about diabetes. However, it is likely that the main responsibility for patient teaching will rest with the nursing staff, and in particular with the diabetes nurse specialist. It is essential that the nurse and patient work in partnership, the aim of which is to empower the patient to play a leading part in his own management (Shillitoe 1994). Developing knowledge and skills in the management of diabetes is therefore a prerequisite for the patient.

Materials and methods

An impressive array of informative and attractive booklets is available, mainly sponsored by manufacturers and written by diabetes health care professionals. These provide visual back-up for teaching and discussion sessions. Video programmes can sometimes be provided for patients to view individually or in groups. The BDA is a good source of educational materials (see 'Useful addresses', p. 193).

Teaching sessions

Sessions should be short and information presented in small, easily assimilated and integrated sections with teaching points categorised into lists. Ordering presentation so that the most important point is always raised first can help the patient to prioritise information. Being direct and specific will aid retention, as will using simple words and brief sentences. Before going on to a new topic, the instructor can use sensitive questioning to check the patient's recall and understanding of the material already covered (Ley 1997).

Staff members should be consistent in the information which they provide. Adopting a friendly manner and taking time to talk about non-medical matters can relax the patient and set the scene for a more productive teaching session. It is important to consider the age group for which teaching materials have been designed in order to avoid giving offence.

The programme

The teaching programme should be tailored to suit the patient's individual needs but is likely to include some of the following topics:

- defining diabetes mellitus
- medication in diabetes mellitus
  - —oral hypoglycaemics
  - —insulin therapy
    - why insulin?
    - types of insulin
    - storage and administration of insulin
- the diet–insulin–exercise balance (see Box 5.12)
- monitoring blood glucose and urinary glucose
- recognising hypoglycaemia and hyperglycaemia
- avoiding complications
- health screening.

Q

5.17 J is 15 years old and has insulin-dependent diabetes. He plays football for the school team, enjoys partying and goes swimming once a week. Discuss with your colleagues how a short teaching session might be prepared to help J understand the significance of exercise to overall diabetes control, personal well-being and the prevention of chronic complications (see Britt 1998 and 'Additional resources', p. 193, for educational material).

Box 5.12 Exercise in diabetes

A clear understanding of the role of exercise in blood glucose control is essential for every diabetic patient. The nurse must find a way of explaining this role that is appropriate to the learning needs of individual patients. The analogy of 'fuel intake' (food) and 'energy output' (activity/exercise) is often useful for the purposes of illustration.

What happens during exercise?
When energy output is low, the demand for fuel in the form of glucose is also low. However, during bursts of activity the demand for glucose will rise. The rate at which glucose is taken up by the cells is influenced by medication (insulin or tablets). If available supplies of glucose are depleted and are not replaced, the patient's blood glucose will fall (hypoglycaemia).

Avoiding exercise-induced hypoglycaemia
The person on insulin therapy should be advised to monitor blood glucose before and after strenuous exercise and to take in extra carbohydrate to avoid hypoglycaemia caused by exercise or unusual activity. A quickly absorbable form of glucose such as Dextrosol tablets (or a chocolate bar) may be used to augment diet and prevent an abrupt fall in blood glucose. Another less commonly employed strategy to avoid exercise-induced hypoglycaemia is for insulin dosage to be slightly reduced prior to planned and prolonged strenuous activity. Blood glucose should then be monitored to gauge the effects of the insulin reduction.

Patients on oral sulphonylurea therapy may, less frequently, also experience exercise-induced hypoglycaemia and consequently may need to adjust their carbohydrate intake to meet the additional energy demands imposed by the exercise (see Hillson 1992, Kenwright 1997).

PROMOTING PSYCHOLOGICAL AND SOCIAL ADJUSTMENT

The emotional impact of diabetes mellitus

When diabetes is first diagnosed, the patient and his family are presented with a challenge on two distinct but equally important levels.

First, they are faced with the practicalities of learning a whole new 'science', for that is how some patients describe grappling with terminology and treatment. The significance of 'hypos', 'hypers', ketones, carbohydrates, insulin injections, urine testing and blood glucose monitoring all need to be understood and new and complex skills must be mastered.

Secondly, the patient has to absorb the emotional impact of being diagnosed with a chronic illness that will not go away. The patient may experience a variety of emotions. Self-image can be affected as the patient absorbs the new 'diabetic self'. One patient described this as feeling 'vulnerable and mortal', summing up her initial response to the diagnosis in this way: 'Since I was given the result it seemed as if my whole personality had changed. I wasn't the same as everyone else. I was a diabetic!' (Bow 1989).

Guilt reactions are not unusual. Patients may blame themselves (unjustifiably) for bringing on the disease. This may be compounded by the fact that some patients believe that health professionals also blame the individual for poor control (Richmond 1996). The newly diagnosed patient with diabetes can experience a sense of loss akin to grief. Feelings of numbness, denial, anger and depression are common. A previously untrammelled lifestyle may have to be replaced by a life of enforced order. Kelsall (1990) described the depression which she experienced after being diagnosed and suggested that to tell a patient who is depressed about her diabetes to 'pull herself together' is as unreasonable as telling her to make her own insulin. Cox (1990), Shillitoe (1995) and Maffeo (1997) give detailed accounts of how the diagnosis of diabetes mellitus can affect patients and their families.

However, it should be noted that not all patients react in a wholly negative way to their diagnosis. Maclean & Orem (1988) cited several examples of patients who have enjoyed an enhanced self-image and who appear to have experienced personal growth as they successfully rose to the challenges presented by diabetes.

How an individual will cope with a diagnosis of diabetes will be influenced by a variety of personal and social factors but perhaps most importantly by how he perceives and evaluates problems (see Ch. 17). This in turn will be influenced by his attitudes and beliefs with regard to illness. We may consider these attitudes with reference to the following concepts:

- locus of control
- the health belief model.

Locus of control

Many people believe that they exert a good degree of control over what happens to them and that by their own actions they can influence events. Those who take this view might be said to have an 'internal' locus of control and tend to be highly self-directing and self-motivated (Niven & Robinson 1994). This can have implications for treatment compliance and self-care. Such people will tend to seek out information and will strive to master difficult tasks; they are often quick to achieve and maintain stability of blood glucose control in the early post-diagnostic period.

In contrast, patients with an 'external' locus of control believe that events happen due to circumstances which are beyond their control (Niven & Robinson 1994). They view themselves as passive victims rather than active agents. Such patients may experience problems in achieving good control of blood glucose in the early stabilisation period and, accordingly, require relatively frequent hospital admissions.

Some studies suggest that, in the long term, patients with an external locus of control can maintain good diabetes control, as they will be inclined to adhere rigidly to instructions. In contrast, patients with an internal locus of control, having achieved control of their diabetes, are more likely to experiment with and manipulate their treatment independently, knowing and accepting the risks to stability which this degree of self-direction may bring (Kelleher 1988, Shillitoe 1995).

Health beliefs and compliance

The long established health belief model (see Fig. 5.12) provides one means of examining the issue of patient compliance with medical therapy in diabetes mellitus (Becker et al 1979). Kelleher (1988) reported non-compliance rates in diabetes treatment ranging between 30 and 60% and linked these rates to health beliefs. Those who regard their diabetes as 'serious' are more likely to comply with a treatment regimen, whereas non-compliance is more often found in people who do not regard their diabetes as serious or who, having weighed up the personal cost, view the loss of lifestyle choices as too high a price to pay for good control of blood glucose.

It is well known that behaviour in the present is relatively insensitive to the threat of long-term consequences. Additionally, one cannot be certain that by providing information health care professionals will ensure treatment compliance. Cognitive dissonance (Festinger 1957) is an accepted phenomenon. Few users of alcohol or tobacco, for example, would deny knowledge of the risks involved, but many consciously elect to exercise their freedom of choice with regard to actual behaviour. Similarly, patients with diabetes, even if well informed, may consciously decide not to comply with diabetes treatment.

By contrast, some people with diabetes become engaged in a battle for perfection in blood glucose control and come to regard any evidence of imbalance as a personal failure. Such individuals may find that guilt plays an increasingly significant role in their lives. Maclean & Lo (1998) have reported that attitude to health professionals was a common factor in both success and failure of compliance.

Q

5.18 What may lead you to decide whether a patient has an external or an internal locus of control or what his 'health beliefs' are? What relevance may such judgements have for the ways in which you provide care and information for the patient? (Read from the following authors: Oberle (1991), Woolridge et al (1992), Niven & Robinson (1994) and Smith & Draper (1994).)

Relationships

Family relationships

If the family unit was previously stable, diabetes is unlikely to have an adverse effect on family relationships. Indeed, patients who enjoy good social support from their families show enhanced stability and are more likely to comply with health maintenance behaviours (Maclean & Lo 1998).

However, the very nature of diabetes, with its attendant rules and restrictions, may allow the disorder to be used by family members or the patient as a means of manipulation or self-assertion. This rather unhealthy state of affairs is more likely to occur where family relationships were difficult prior to the diagnosis of diabetes.

Sexual relationships

Although embarking on a sexual relationship is anxiety-provoking for many people, it raises particular concerns for people with diabetes. Uncertainty may be felt about when, and if, to tell the other person about the diabetes. Practical issues such as what to do if a 'hypo' develops when out on a date (or, even worse, during lovemaking) may cause real worry. Having to explain such things as set eating and injection times or dietary restrictions may cause embarrassment and may be seen as interfering with the spontaneity of a budding relationship. Waterson (1995) gives a frank account of the impact of diabetes on lifestyle.

A comprehensive overview of research into diabetes-related sexual problems and an account of various management strategies is provided by Bancroft (1989).

Family planning

People with diabetes can have healthy, happy families just like anyone else. Prospective parents may worry about passing on their diabetes to the baby. Genetic counselling may be offered to enable the couple to make an informed decision (see Ch. 6). A discussion of genetic and other pregnancy-associated risks is provided by Parker (1996).

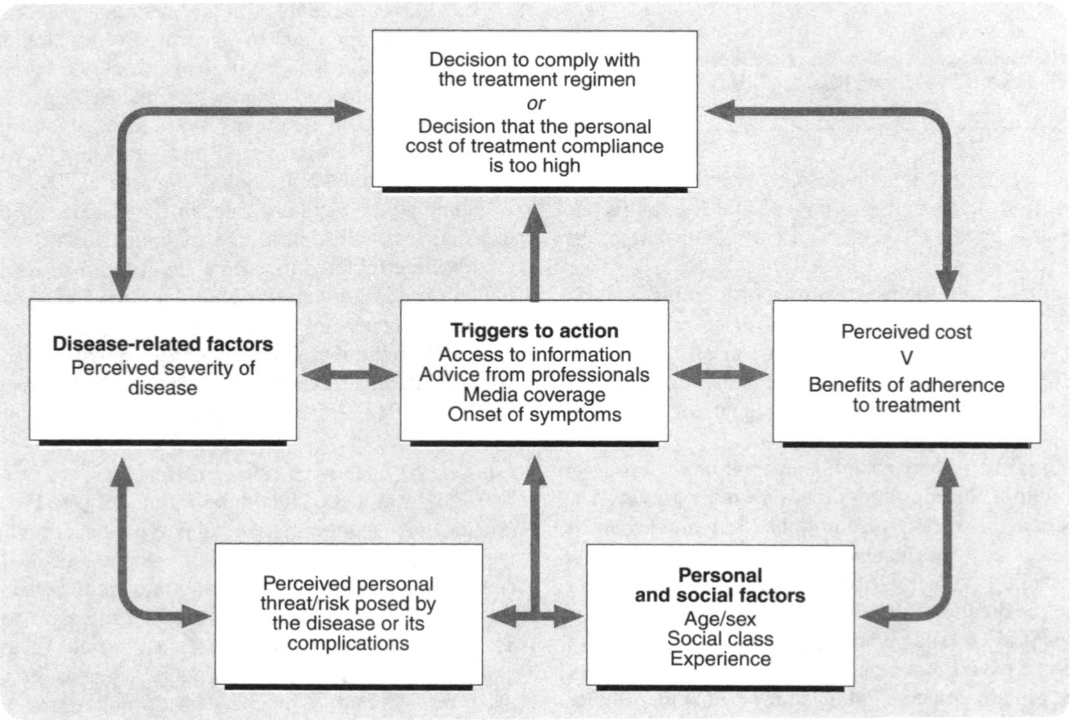

Fig. 5.12 The health belief model, summarised.

Pre-conception. Ideally the couple should attend a pre-conception clinic to reduce the risks to mother and baby. Strict control of blood glucose before conception greatly helps towards improving the outcome of the pregnancy (Parker 1996). When pregnant, the woman should be cared for by a specialist team, e.g. specialist diabetes midwives, diabetologists and obstetricians.

For further information on pre-pregnancy monitoring in diabetes, see Parker (1996) and for a discussion of gestational diabetes see Stewart & Taylor (1994). The SIGN guidelines (1996) on the management of diabetes in pregnancy details the management of both.

Contraception. General advice may be offered by nurses and doctors in both community and hospital settings. The family planning clinic may also offer advice. If oral contraceptives are used it is important to monitor blood and urine glucose more frequently than usual, as some of these drugs alter glycaemic control. Risks to the vascular system associated with oral contraception should be discussed; some centres do not prescribe the combined contraceptive pill because of this.

Social relationships

Patients with diabetes quite naturally resist being singled out and labelled. This can create real difficulties. On the one hand, coping with diabetes means that the individual may have to rely on others should a crisis occur. On the other hand, the person with diabetes may resent being treated differently from others. The patient's adjustment within his social milieu will involve a complex interplay of personal and social factors; the degree of success will vary considerably from person to person.

Access to counselling should be provided for those people who are experiencing relationship difficulties arising from their diabetes.

5.19 What do you understand by the term 'labelling'? Why do you think people with diabetes may be concerned about being labelled?

See Stockwell (1972), World Health Organization (1985), pp. 73–76, Bruhn (1991), Niven & Robinson (1994) and Waterson (1995).

Lifestyle implications

Employment

In view of the risk of hypoglycaemia, people with insulin-dependent diabetes are barred from vocational driving, airline piloting and deep sea diving, and from working on offshore oil rigs, at heights or near dangerous moving machinery. Diabetes would also exclude an applicant from joining the UK armed forces or the police. For further information see Shaw (1997).

Driving

The driver vehicle licensing authority in Swansea (DVLA) must, by law, be informed when a driver is diagnosed as having diabetes mellitus. Diabetic people whose disease is controlled by insulin are not permitted to hold a full licence but will be issued with a licence for a period of 1–3 years to allow periodic review by the DVLA. A medical practitioner may be required to advise on the stability of the driver's diabetes control prior to relicensing.

Box 5.13 The British Diabetic Association (BDA)

The BDA is a charitable organisation which raises money for diabetes research and provides information and advice for people with diabetes and professionals involved in their care. As well as being a national organisation, it has local branches throughout the UK. Different sections cater for particular groups, e.g. teenagers. The BDA offers help and advice on a wide variety of topics such as monitoring and treatment approaches, insurance, holidays and travelling abroad.

Full members of the BDA receive the bi-monthly journal *Balance* free of charge. This is an excellent publication which provides a forum for diabetic people and their families to exchange ideas and keep up-to-date with current progress in diabetes management. *Balance* is also produced on audiotape for visually impaired subscribers.

Since 1990, patients who have diet-controlled diabetes have been entitled to hold an unrestricted car driving licence but must notify the DVLA if they develop relevant disabilities (Sheppard 1998).

Insurance

The BDA have their own insurance broker who can advise on any insurance-related matter (see Box 5.13).

Travel

Altered mealtimes, travelling across different time zones, and dietary and climatic changes may all have an effect on diabetes stability. Blood glucose monitoring is an excellent way of monitoring diabetes control. All the requirements for medication and monitoring should be carried in hand luggage as suitcases may get lost in transit and the baggage hold is too cold for transporting insulin (Kelleher 1995). For further information on travel see *Useful Holiday Tips* published by the BDA (1998b).

Eating out

Flexible insulin therapy and home blood glucose monitoring (HBGM) has simplified eating out for diabetic people. Most restaurant menus offer enough variety and choice to allow customers with diabetes to enjoy, without worry, the social benefits of having a meal with friends.

Smoking

People with diabetes are at greater risk than others of developing vascular and neuropathic disorders. Smoking compounds these risks. The health care team should try to discourage smoking and should discuss the availability of resources to provide support whilst the patient is trying to give up smoking. However, it must be accepted that the patient has freedom of choice and may decide to continue to smoke against advice.

Identification

Patients should be encouraged to carry a card or wear a Medic-Alert pendant to identify themselves and to give details of the type of diabetes they have and its management.

CONCLUSION

Research in diabetes care is at an exciting stage. Pancreatic transplantation has been carried out successfully on thousands of diabetic patients and has become accepted therapy for certain types of patients (American Diabetic Association 1998). Pancreatic transplant can greatly improve the quality of life for IDDM patients. Whilst transplant can remove the threat of acute complications, there is little evidence that transplant will delay or prevent the long-term complications experienced by IDDM patients. Pancreatic transplant should be considered for those patients with end-stage renal failure who have had or who plan to have a renal transplant, since pancreas-only transplant would require lifelong immunosuppression to prevent rejection and recurrence of β cell destruction. Work is progressing in the field of islet cell transplantation, and although this has been done successfully on humans the work is still largely experimental (Jaremko & Rorstad 1998). Drawbacks include the large number of β cells required, shortage of donors and problems with immune rejection.

Research on the artificial pancreas has almost reached reality. For an artificial pancreas to be successful it would require a glucose sensor, an implantable insulin pump and a control system. To date, a practical and reliable glucose sensor has not been perfected. Research in molecular genetic engineering is being directed towards the production of surrogate β cells with insulin-producing and glucose-sensing functions, and also towards a polymer matrix, able to release insulin in direct response to glucose concentrations (see Jaremko & Rorstad 1998).

As a result of the Diabetes Control Complications Trial (DCCT) there is now greater awareness of the impact of tight glucose control on the chronic complications of diabetes. The Diabetes Mellitus, Insulin Glucose Infusion in Acute Myocardial Infarction Study Group (DIGAMI) recently reported a reduction in mortality of 11% in patients treated by insulin-glucose infusion followed by subcutaneous insulin after acute myocardial infarction (Malmberg 1997).

Insulin analogues have now been introduced (e.g. Humalog). These substances are quicker in onset and shorter in action than conventional insulins and are thought to reduce the incidence of hypoglycaemic attacks.

For further information on insulin analogues see Gale (1998).

Feasibility studies into the use of nasal insulin, inhaled and oral insulins have produced interesting preliminary findings – inhaled insulin for meal coverage with short-acting insulin appears to have the best outlook (Saudek 1997).

The ultimate hope is that diabetes will at some future date be preventable. Researchers continue to seek definitive answers to the questions surrounding aetiological factors with a view to finding ways of manipulating these factors to prevent the disease developing.

Recent trends in health care provision

The political and economic climate in the UK over the last decade has given rise to significant changes in the structure and function of the primary care team and has shifted the focus of health care toward the community setting. These changes are reflected in trends in diabetes care (Powell 1991a,b) and a significant innovation has been the developing role of the diabetes nurse specialist who 'can transform the standard of diabetic care, achieving liaison between hospital, general practitioner and patients at home and offering a wide range of clinical and educational expertise' (Watkins et al 1996).

The growth in the number of practice nurses has made it possible for some GPs to run their own clinics for diabetic patients. In some areas, community dieticians and chiropodists are available for consultation in the health centres where clinics are run.

Community nurses and health visitors may find themselves, to an increasing extent, taking high-quality diabetes care directly into the patient's home. Effective hospital–community liaison will become especially important to ensure continuity for the patient in 'shared care'.

Whatever the care setting, it is important that the patient has access to facilities for estimation of glycated haemoglobin and microalbuminuria and for screening for retinopathy and foot-threatening neuropathic or vascular disease. It seems likely that integrated hospital and community care will offer the best use of resources for diabetes screening. However, dealing with a severe metabolic crisis such as DKA will remain the province of the hospital.

Continuing education for all members of the diabetes care team must be a priority. Diabetes specialist nurses can make a significant contribution in the education of their colleagues. Nursing care in diabetes should have a firm research base. Nurses require a clear understanding of the scientific aspects of the disorder and its management if safe care is to be provided. Diabetes care is, however, more than science. Providing the support which will enable the patient to move away from the despondency and fear which frequently accompany diagnosis towards independence and autonomy is surely the art of nursing care in diabetes mellitus.

REFERENCES

Abraham R, Levy D 1992 Cardiovascular disease in diabetes – a practical approach. Diabetes Care 1(4): 8–10
Aitken G 1997 Nutrition and diabetes: putting guidelines into practice. British Journal of Nursing 6(18): 1035–1040
American Diabetes Association 1998 Pancreas transplantation for patients with diabetes mellitus. Diabetes Care 21(suppl 1): 79
Appleton M, Jerreat L 1995 Hypoglycaemia. Nursing Standard 10(5): 36–40
Bancroft J 1989 Human sexuality and its problems. Churchill Livingstone, Edinburgh, ch 11, pp 552–562
Barnett A H, Eff C, Leslie R D, Pyke D A 1981 Diabetes in identical twins. Diabetologia 20(2): 87–93
Batki A, Garvey K, Thomason H et al 1998 Blood glucose measuring systems. Professional Nurse 13(12): 865–873
Becker M H, Maiman L A, Kirscht J P et al 1979 Patients' perceptions and compliance. In: Shillitoe R W 1988 (ed) Psychology and diabetes. Chapman & Hall, London, p 197
Betschart J 1993 Children and adolescents with diabetes. Nursing Clinics of North America 28(1): 35–44
Bodansky J 1994 Diabetes, 2nd edn. Wolfe, London
Borders L M, Bingham P R, Riddle M C 1984 Traditional insulin use practices and the incidence of bacterial contamination. Diabetes Care 7(2): 121–127
Bow M 1989 One drop = 12.5. Balance 113: 52–53
British Diabetic Association 1995 Diabetes in the United Kingdom – 1996. BDA, London
British Diabetic Association 1996 Counting the cost – the real impact of non insulin dependent diabetes. BDA/Kings Fund, London
British Diabetic Association 1997 Two more diabetes genes identified. Diabetes Update Spring: 1–3
British Diabetic Association 1998a Sildenafil (Viagra) – guidelines for use (online – http://www.diabetes.org.uk/whats_new/4/viagra.htm) (accessed 1.2.99)
British Diabetic Association 1998b Useful holiday tips. BDA, London
Britt P 1998 Group education sessions better than one-to-one? Diabetic Nursing 27: 12–13
Bruhn J G 1991 Nouns that cut: the negative effects of labelling by allied health professionals. Journal of Allied Health 20(4): 229–231

Cantrill J 1994 Perfecting the match – choosing the right tablets. Diabetes Care 3(2): 8–9
Coates V 1996 Diabetic renal failure. Practice Nurse 12(4): 263–267
Cox S 1990 How I coped emotionally with diabetes in my family. Diabetic Nursing 1(4): 7–8
Craddock S 1996 Diabetes mellitus at diagnosis. Nursing Standard 10(30): 41–48
Davis R 1989 Equipment guide for administering insulin. Professional Nurse 5(2): 91–92, 94
Day J 1991 Improving self management (symposium). The Practitioner 235: 775–779
Department of Health/British Diabetic Association 1995 St Vincent Joint Task Force for Diabetes: the report. DoH/BDA, London
Diabetes Control and Complications Research Group 1993 The effect of diabetes on the development and progression of long term complications in insulin dependent diabetes. New England Journal of Medicine 329: 977–986
Donnelly D 1992 Insulin resistance and blood pressure. British Journal of Hospital Medicine 47(1): 9–11
Doyle A 1991 Microalbuminuria in diabetic patients. Nursing Times 87(28): 43
Eccles L 1995 Assessment of screening tests for microalbuminuria – a nurse's view. Diabetic Nursing 19: 4–6
Festinger L 1957 A theory of cognitive dissonance. Stanford University Press, Stanford, CA
Frost G 1997 A new look at the glycaemic index. Diabetic Nursing 24: 2–4
Fuller N 1990 The glycaemic index – how dietary carbohydrates raise the blood glucose. Diabetic Nursing 1(5): 3–5
Gale E 1998 Insulin inspro: the first insulin analogue to reach the market. Practical Diabetes International 13(4): 122–124
Green A 1996 Prevention of IDDM: the genetic epidemiologic perspective. Diabetes Research and Clinical Practice 34(suppl): S101–106
Griggs K 1998 Global contender. Nursing Times 94(22): 65–66
Hall B, Waterman H 1997 The psychosocial aspects of visual impairment in diabetes. Nursing Standard 11(39): 40–43
Hamilton H, Ubig M 1991 The eye in diabetes. The Practitioner (Symposium) 235: 780–782
Haverkos H W 1997 Could the aetiology of IDDM be multifactorial? Diabetologia 40(10): 1235–1240
Higgins C 1994 Blood and urine tests for diagnosis and monitoring of diabetes. British Journal of Nursing 3(17): 886–892
Hillson R 1992 Diabetes, sport and exercise. Diabetes Care 1(4): 4–5
Hoops S 1990 Renal and retinal complications in insulin-dependent diabetes mellitus; the art of changing the outcome. Diabetes Educator 16(3): 221–233
Jaremko J, Rorstad O 1998 Advances toward the implantable artificial pancreas for treatment of diabetes. Diabetes Care 21(3): 444–449
Jones D B 1987 Aetiology of diabetes. Update 35(10): 1012–1014
Kelleher A 1995 Planning for trouble-free travel. Diabetes Care Team 4(2): 6–7
Kelleher D 1988 Diabetes. The experience of illness series. Routledge, London, chs 2, 4, 5
Kelsall L 1990 Understanding anxiety. Balance 114: 28–29
Kenwright D 1997 The value of exercise. A personal experience. Diabetic Nursing 26: 14–15
King B 1997 Preserving renal function. Registered Nurse 60(8): 34–39
Kinson J, Nattrass M 1984 Caring for the diabetic patient. Churchill Livingstone, Edinburgh
Krans H M J, Porta N, Keen H (eds) 1992 Diabetes care and research in Europe. The St. Vincent Declaration action programme. World Health Organization Regional Office for Europe, Copenhagen
Ley P 1997 Communicating with patients: improving communication, satisfaction and compliance. Croom Helm, London, ch 2
Lovelock L 1990 A day in the life of: mobile eye screening technician. Balance 116: 26–27
MacCuish 1992 Early detection and screening for diabetic retinopathy. Eye 7: 254–259
Macheca M K K 1993 Diabetic hypoglycaemia: how to keep the threat at bay. American Journal of Nursing 21(2): 34–39
Maclean D, Lo R 1998 The non-insulin-dependent diabetic: success and failure in compliance. Australian Journal of Advanced Nursing 15(4): 33–42
Maclean H, Orem B 1988 Living with diabetes: personal stories and strategies. University of Toronto Press, Toronto, ch 3
Maffeo R 1997 Helping families cope with type 1 diabetes. American Journal of Nursing 97(6): 36–39
Malmberg K 1997 Prospective randomised study of intensive insulin treatment on long term survival after acute myocardial infarction in patients with diabetes mellitus. British Medical Journal 314: 1512–1515
Marshall S 1991 Microalbuminuria. Diabetes Nursing 2(3): 13–14
Marshall S 1993 Hyperglycaemic emergencies. Care of the Critically Ill 9(5): 220–223
Niven N, Robinson J 1994 The psychology of nursing care. BPS/ MacMillan Press, London, pp 171–173
Nutrition Sub-committee of the BDA's Professional Advisory Committee 1990 Dietary recommendations for people with diabetes: an update for the 1990s. BDA, London
O'Hanlon-Nichols T 1996 Hyperglycaemic hyperosmolar non-ketotic syndrome. American Journal of Nursing 96(3): 38–39
Oberle K 1991 A decade of research in locus of control: what have we learned? Journal of Advanced Nursing 16(7): 800–806
Parker C 1996 Pre-pregnancy monitoring for women with diabetes. Professional Care of Mother & Child 6(5): 135–138
Paterson K R 1990 Non-insulin-dependent diabetes in the nineties. Practical Diabetes 7(5): 200–202
Peragallo-Dittko V 1995 Diabetes 2000. Acute complications. Registered Nurse 58(8): 36–40
Perry J P, Tullo A B 1995 Care of the ophthalmic patient, 2nd edn. Chapman and Hall, London
Phillips W B 1994 Ocular manifestations of diabetes mellitus. Journal of Ophthalmic Nursing & Technology 13(6): 255–261
Porth L 1994 Pathophysiology, concepts of altered health status. JB Lippincott, Philadelphia, ch 46
Powell J 1991a Mini clinics in general practice. The Practitioner 235: 766–772
Powell J 1991b Shared care. The Practitioner 235: 761–762
Rayman G 1989 Hospital inpatient monitoring of diabetes. Practical Diabetes 6(2): 62–64
Richmond J 1996 Effects of hypoglycaemia: patients' perceptions and experiences. British Journal of Nursing 5(17): 1054–1059
Roberto P L 1990 Diabetic nephropathy: causes, complications and considerations. Nursing Clinics of North America 2(1): 89–95
Robertson C 1995 Diabetes 2000 – chronic complications. Registered Nurse 58(9): 34–40
Saudek C D 1997 Novel forms of insulin delivery. Endocrinology and Metabolism Clinics of North America 26(3): 599–610
Scottish Intercollegiate Guidelines Network 1997 Management of diabetic renal disease, no. 11. SIGN, Edinburgh
Shaw H 1997 Employment and diabetes. Diabetic Nursing 25: 2–4
Sheppard D 1998 Diabetic drivers: get up to date with the new regulations. Journal of Diabetes Nursing 2(1): 9–11
Shillitoe R 1994 Counselling people with diabetes. BPS, Leicester
Shillitoe R 1995 Diabetes mellitus. In: Broome A, Llewelyn S (eds) Health psychology, processes and applications, 2nd edn. Chapman and Hall, Glasgow, ch 11, pp 197–200
Smith R, Draper P 1994 Who is in control? An investigation of nurse and patient beliefs relating to control of their health. Journal of Advanced Nursing 19(5): 884–892
Thomas D 1994 Dietary care – negotiation or prescription? Diabetes Care 3(3): 8–9
Tiley S 1997 Impotence: what is it? Diabetic Nursing 25: 5–7
Trounce J 1997 Clinical pharmacology for nurses, 15th edn. Churchill Livingstone, Edinburgh
Trusler L A 1992 Management of the patient receiving simultaneous kidney-pancreas transplantation. Critical Care Nursing Clinics of North America 4(1): 89–95
United Kingdom Prospective Diabetes Study Group 1998 Intensive blood glucose control with sulphonylureas or insulin compared with conventional treatment and risk of complications in patients with type 2 diabetes (UKPDS 33). Lancet 352(9131): 837–853
Warmington V 1996 Renal patients in the community. Practice Nurse 11(9): 620–622, 623
Waterson J 1995 Funny you don't look like a diabetic. Ashgrove Press, Bath
Watkins P J, Drury P L, Howell S L 1996 Diabetes and its management, 5th edn. Blackwell Science, Oxford
Woolridge K L, Wallston K A, Graber A L, Brown A W, Davidson P 1992 The relationship between health beliefs, adherence and metabolic control of diabetes. Diabetes Educator 118(6): 495–500
World Health Organization 1985 Diabetes mellitus: technical report series 727. WHO, Geneva
World Health Organization 1994 Prevention of diabetes mellitus: technical report series 844. WHO, Geneva

FURTHER READING

Diabetes — causes and management

Appleton M, Jerreat L 1995 Hypoglycaemia. Nursing Standard 10(5): 36–40

Andreani D, Di Mario U, Pozzilli P 1991 Prediction, prevention and early intervention in insulin-dependent diabetes. Diabetes/Metabolism Reviews 7(1): 61–77

Betchart J 1993 Children and adolescents with diabetes. Nursing Clinics of North America 28(1): 35–44

British Diabetic Association 1997 Two more diabetes genes identified. Diabetes Update Spring: 1–3

Craddock S 1996 Diabetes mellitus at diagnosis. Nursing Standard 10(30): 41–48

Gadsby R 1994 Primary care holds the key to DCCT improvements. Diabetes Care (3): 4–5

Gale E 1998 Insulin inspro: the first insulin analogue to reach the market. Practical Diabetes International 13(4): 122–124

Haverkos H W 1997 Could the aetiology of IDDM be multifactorial? Diabetologia 40(10): 1235–1240

Hayden S 1996 Gene discoveries unlock door to prevention. Diabetes Care Team 5(2): 4–5

Jaremko J, Rorstad O 1998 Advances toward the implantable artificial pancreas for treatment of diabetes. Diabetes Care 21(3): 444–449

Macheca M K K 1993 Diabetic hypoglycaemia: how to keep the threat at bay. American Journal of Nursing 93(4): 46–50

Murphy H 1994 Diabetes in childhood. British Journal of Nursing 3(17): 892–896

Oberle K 1991 A decade of research in locus of control: what have we learned? Journal of Advanced Nursing 16(7): 800–806

Parker C 1996 Pre-pregnancy monitoring for women with diabetes. Professional Care of Mother & Child 6(5): 135–138

Richmond J 1998 The effects of hypoglycaemia. A study of four case histories. Diabetic Nursing 28: 12–13

Scottish Intercollegiate Guidelines Network 1997 Management of diabetic renal disease, no. 11. SIGN, Edinburgh

Sonksen P, Fox C, Judd S 1991 The comprehensive diabetes reference book for the 1990s. Class Publishing, London

Stewart M, Taylor R 1994 Gestational diabetes mellitus. Professional Care of the Mother and Child 4(5): 136–138

Thomas L 1993 An overview of current reasearch into diabetes. Professional Nurse 9(1): 15–19

Tortora G T, Grabowski S R 1996 Principles of anatomy and physiology, 8th edn. Harper Collins, New York

Tripathy B, Samal K 1997 Overview and consensus statement on diabetes in tropical areas. Diabetes/Metabolism Reviews 13(1): 63–76

Foot care

Bradshaw T W 1998 Aetiopathogenesis of the Charcot foot: and overview. Practical Diabetes International 15(1): 22–24

Foster A 1997 Psychological aspects of treating the diabetic foot. Practical Diabetes International 14(2): 56–58

Hamer S 1998 Choosing the right foot ulcer dressing. Diabetic Nursing 28: 7–9

Jones R B, Gregory R, Murry K J et al 1995 A simple rule to identify people with diabetes at risk of foot ulceration. Practical Diabetes International 12(6): 256–258

Knowles A 1995 Foot problems: prevention is better than cure. Diabetes Care Team 4(1): 4–5

Monitoring/education

Batki A, Garvey K, Thomason H et al 1998 Blood glucose measuring systems. Professional Nurse 13(12): 865–873

Day J L 1996 All this education: is it worthwhile? Practical Diabetes International 13(4): 125–127

Higgins C 1994 Blood and urine tests for diagnosis and monitoring of diabetes. British Journal of Nursing 3(17): 886–892

Thompson A 1993 Setting standards in diabetes education. Nursing Standard 7(43): 25–28

Infection

Wood J 1997 Coping with intercurrent infection. Diabetic Nursing Issue 26: 11–13

Health belief model

Niven N, Robinson J 1994 The psychology of nursing care. BPS/ Macmillan Press, London

Rosenstock I M, Strecher V J, Becker M H 1988 Social learning theory and the health belief model. Health Education Quarterly 15(2): 175–183

Lifestyle implications

Aitken G 1997 Nutrition and diabetes: putting guidelines into practice. British Journal of Nursing 6(18): 1035–1040

British Diabetic Association 1998 Diabetes and travel. Diabetic Nursing 28

Hillson R 1992 Diabetes, sport and exercise. Diabetes Care 1(4): 4–5

Kenwright D 1997 The value of exercise. Diabetic Nursing 26: 14–15

Shaw H 1997 Employment and diabetes. Diabetic Nursing 25: 2–4

Labelling

Bruhn J G 1991 Nouns that cut: the negative effects of labelling by allied health professionals. Journal of Allied Health 20(4): 229–231

Maclean H, Orem B 1988 Living with diabetes: personal stories and strategies. University of Toronto Press, Toronto, ch 4

Stockwell F 1972 The unpopular patient. Royal College of Nurses/DHSS, London

World Health Organization 1985 Diabetes mellitus. Technical Report Series 727. WHO, Geneva, pp 73–76

Surgery

Marshall S 1996 The peri-operative management of diabetes. Care of the Critically Ill 12(2): 64–68

Metcalf L 1993 Operations manager. Nursing Times 89(5): 40, 42, 44

Saltiel-Berzin R 1992 Managing a surgical patient who has diabetes. Nursing 92 22(4): 34–42

Wound healing

Norris S O, Provo B, Stotts N A 1990 Physiology of wound healing and risk factors that impede the healing process. Clinical Issues in Critical Care Nursing 1(3): 545–552

Rosenberg C S 1990 Wound healing in the patient with diabetes mellitus. Nursing Clinics of North America 25(1): 247–261

Silhi N 1998 Diabetes and wound healing. Journal of Wound Care 7(1): 47–51

Renal failure

Coates V 1996 Diabetic renal failure. Practice Nurse 12(4): 263–267

Hoops S 1990 Renal and retinal complications in insulin-dependent diabetes mellitus: the art of changing the outcome. Diabetes Educator 16(3): 221–233

King B 1997 Preserving renal function. Registered Nurse 60(8): 34–39

Parsons B 1995 Microalbuminuria – the case for screening. Diabetes Care Team 4(1): 3

Roberto P L 1990 Diabetic nephropathy: causes, complications and considerations. Nursing Clinics of North America 2(1): 55–66

Robertson C 1995 Diabetes 2000 – chronic complications. Registered Nurse 58(9): 34–40

Trusler L A 1992 Management of the patient receiving simultaneous kidney-pancreas transplantation. Critical Care Nursing Clinics of North America 4(1): 89–95

Warmington V 1996 Renal patients in the community. Practice Nurse 11(9): 620–622, 623

Waterston J 1995 Funny you don't look like a diabetic. Ashgrove Press, Bath

Psycho-social aspects

Munday H 1996 Psychosocial aspects of diabetes care. Diabetic Nursing 23: 13–15

Shillitoe R 1995 Diabetes mellitus. In: Broome A, Llewelyn S (eds) Health psychology: processes and application, 2nd edn. Chapman and Hall, Glasgow, ch 11

ADDITIONAL RESOURCES AND USEFUL ADDRESSES

Sources of information
General Practitioner Information Pack
Directory of Diabetes Specialist Nurses
Both available free of charge to health care professionals from:
British Diabetic Association
10 Queen Anne Street
London W1M 0BD

Diabetes in General Practice — clinical series
Royal College of General Practitioners
14 Princes Gate
Hyde Park, London SW7

The Diabetes Handbook
Non-insulin Dependent Diabetes
Insulin Dependent Diabetes
Both by Dr John L Day, available from the BDA

Magazines & journals
Practical Diabetes International
PMH Publications Ltd
PO Box 100
Chichester
West Sussex

Diabetes Update
Published twice a year by the BDA and mailed free on request

Diabetes Care Team
Colwood House
Medical Publications (UK)
The Mitfords
Basingstoke Road
Three Mile Cross
Reading
Berks RG7 1AT

Balance
Published by the BDA (bi-monthly)
Mailed free of charge to members of the BDA

Diabetic Nursing — The Journal for all Nurses involved in Diabetes Care
PMH Publications Ltd
PO Box 100
Chichester
West Sussex
(Sponsored by MediSense)

Sources of educational material, etc.
General information on diet, living with diabetes etc.
The British Diabetic Association
10 Queen Anne Street
London W1M 0BD

Measurement of insulin and injection technique
Diabetes Care Division
Becton Dickinson (UK) Ltd
21 Between Towns Road
Cowley
Oxford OX4 3LY

Insulin and mode of action
Eli Lilly & Co Ltd
Dextra Court
Chapel Hill
Basingstoke, Hants

Novo Nordisk Pharmaceuticals Ltd
Novo-Nordisk House
Broadfield Park
Brighton Road
Pease Pottage
Crawley
West Sussex RH11 9RT

Blood & urine glucose monitoring
Bayer plc
Diagnostics Division
Bayer House
Strawberry Hill
Newbury
Berkshire RG14 1JA

Roche Diagnostics Ltd
Bell Lane
Lewes
East Sussex BN7 1LG

Oral hypoglycaemics
Servier Laboratories Ltd
Fulmer Hall
Windmill Road
Fulmer
Slough SL3 6HH

Foot care
Customer Services Department
Scholl (UK) Ltd
475 Capability Green
Luton
Beds LU1 3LU

GENETIC DISORDERS

6

Aileen Crosbie

Roseanne Cetnarskyj (Section on 'Huntington's disease')
Kathleen Liddle (Section on 'Cystic fibrosis')
Billie Reynolds (Section on 'Haemophilia')

INTRODUCTION

Genetics is the study of genes and their relationship to hereditary characteristics. Genes are units of deoxyribonucleic acid (DNA) found in the chromosomes within the nuclei of living cells. They carry coded information which influences physical and psychological characteristics such as eye colour and temperament and also susceptibility to many major life-threatening diseases.

The aims of this chapter are:

- to provide a basic outline of the mechanics of genetic inheritance
- to raise awareness of the genetic aspects of common diseases
- to describe a small number of classic but rare genetic disorders
- to introduce the principles of cancer genetics
- to outline nursing roles in health promotion and genetic counselling
- to discuss the future potential of gene therapy, genetic engineering and the ethical issues involved therein.

A Working Party for the British Medical Association (BMA 1992) reported that genetic and genetically influenced disease affected 1 in 20 people by age 25 and possibly 2 in 3 people in their lifetime. It also predicted that recent and rapidly evolving advances in genetic science will make possible an era of genetically informed health care, disease modification and genetic engineering that will have major implications for medical management and nursing involvement.

Because of the wide range of genetic influences in health and disease, nurses in most areas of practice will have occasion to apply their understanding of genetics. In the community, nurses are involved in screening for and recognising inherited traits and in providing counselling to promote optimum levels of health. Inheritance of a predisposition to common diseases such as heart disease, cancer, diabetes and asthma is more complex than that of classic genetic disorders and has a much higher incidence. Environmental and other triggering factors will determine whether a predisposition manifests in actual disease. Nurses must promote awareness and modification of these environmental factors to help the public avert some of the consequences of their genetic make-up.

Nurses in the fields of learning difficulty, psychiatry, community and health visiting may be involved with families in which there is an existing classic genetic disorder. Nurses in hospital wards, in particular midwives and those working in gynaecology units, may be involved with patients who have miscarried or terminated a pregnancy with a genetic abnormality or who have infertility problems. Nurses in acute and long-term care may be involved with the management of the more distressing classic genetic diseases.

Within the specialised field of genetics, there is the more focused role of the specialist nurse, who is involved in non-directive counselling, diagnosis and support of individuals and families with genetic disorders.

THE MECHANICS OF GENETIC INHERITANCE

Chromosomes

Each human cell contains 46 chromosomes within its nucleus, with the exception of the gametes (sex cells), which contain 23. Of the 46 chromosomes, 23 come from one parent and 23 from the other. These chromosomes are paired, giving 22 pairs called autosomes 1–22 and one pair of sex chromosomes, either XX for females or XY for males.

By staining, photographing and arranging according to size, the chromosomes extracted from a cell can be organised into a karyotype. A normal female karyotype would be reported as 46, XX and a normal male karyotype as 46, XY (see Fig. 6.1). Chromosomal abnormalities can be identified by this method.

Cell division

To understand the mechanisms of genetic inheritance, it is necessary to be familiar with the basic processes of cell division, i.e. mitosis and meiosis.

Mitosis is the normal process of cell division for growth and replacement whereby two replica daughter cells, each with 46 chromosomes carrying identical hereditary information, are derived from a parent cell.

Meiosis is the process of cell division which results in the production of gametes (ova or spermatozoa), each having one copy of each chromosome found in somatic cells, i.e. 23. New pairings are established when gametes come together at fertilisation. Reshuffling of chromosomal material results in the individual differences seen in offspring, whilst familial genetic patterns are still maintained. If meiosis is not successful, one gamete may end up with an abnormal number of chromosomes or with malformed chromosomes. The results of this are seen in the classic chromosome disorders.

Chromosomal abnormalities often lead to miscarriage, usually early in pregnancy. Some result in various manifestations of genetic abnormality. An example is Down's syndrome, or trisomy 21, where the infant has 47 chromosomes, with three copies of chromosome 21.

DNA and RNA

In 1944, chromosomal nucleic acid was shown to be the carrier of genetic information. Two types are recognised: DNA (deoxyribonucleic acid) and RNA (ribonucleic acid).

A molecule of DNA is composed of two nucleotide chains spiralled round one another to form a double helix. Genes are carried in this DNA. In humans, the total length of DNA in a set of 46 chromosomes is 3000 million base pairs. If stretched out, this would be 1.74 m in length. The average gene contains perhaps 2000 base pairs. If the total length of DNA were stretched out from Glasgow to London, a distance of 400 miles, then each gene would take up approximately 12 inches.

Genes

Genes are units of DNA which carry coded hereditary information and are carried on the chromosomes. As chromosomes are paired, each pair carries two copies of each gene (with the exception of the genes on sex chromosomes in males). Each gene is located at a specific point on a chromosome known as its locus. Chromosomes can, for identification purposes, be divided into numbered chromosome regions and bands so that, if known, the position of genes can be charted (see Fig. 6.2). Genes at the same locus on chromosomes are called alleles. If the two alleles at a locus are identical, the individual is said to be homozygous at that locus and if they are non-identical, the individual is said to be heterozygous.

With the exception of identical twins, each individual carries unique sequences, or patterns, of minisatellite DNA. These genetic patterns can be recorded by a technique known as DNA fingerprinting and can identify individuals, as for example in forensic medicine or paternity testing (see Box 6.1).

There are at least two kinds of genes: structural genes which specify protein synthesis; and genes that act as 'switches' to activate or deactivate structural genes and maintain homeostasis.

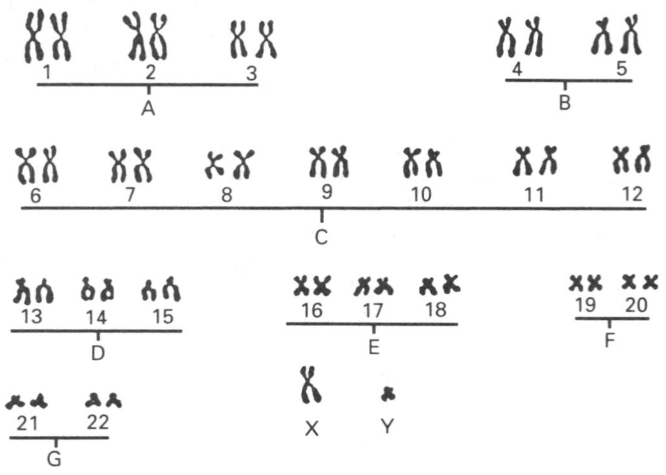

Fig. 6.1 Karyotype of a normal male.

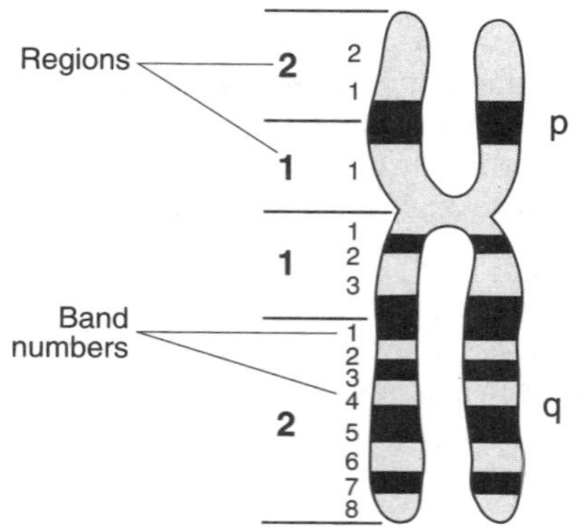

Fig. 6.2 The X chromosome: regions and bands. Each chromosome has a narrow waist called the centromere and a long and a short arm. The short arm is labelled p (from the French *petit*) and the long arm is labelled q. The tip of each arm is called a telomere. Chromosomes can be divided for reporting purposes into numbered chromosome regions, with region 1 closest to the centromere. Each region is further divided into bands.

Box 6.1 DNA fingerprinting

Paternity testing has been revolutionised by the technique known as DNA fingerprinting. Throughout the human genome, there are repeats of short sequences (tandem repeats) called minisatellite DNA. They have no known function but are valuable tools for genetic analysis. After DNA digestion with a restriction enzyme and electrophoresis, a DNA minisatellite probe will identify multiple DNA fragments from many chromosomal regions. The number and size of these fragments are unique to each individual, except for identical twins. In other words, one can generate a unique genetic fingerprint specific only to that individual. Each band is inherited from one parent and therefore a putative father can be either excluded or positively identified. DNA can be extracted from dried bloodstains or semen; for this reason this technique has had important implications for forensic medicine.

The coded information carried by the structural genes is translated with the help of RNA into specific proteins. The RNA becomes a mobile copy of the corresponding encoded blueprint in the DNA (messenger RNA, or mRNA). Some of these proteins are enzymes that catalyse specific chemical reactions. Others form part of the structure of body cells and tissues. Together they determine appearance and behaviour. Molecular biology has been able to describe the process of enzyme movement and matching of chemical bases along the coding strand of the DNA double helix which is involved in translating genetic codes into mRNA for protein synthesis.

With the progress in recent years, the positions of more human genes have been located, but only a relatively small number of the 6000 recognised genetic disorders have been traced to particular malfunctioning genes. The Human Genome Project (HGP), a worldwide effort of coordinated research based in the USA, aims to map all genes on the human chromosomes and determine the DNA sequence of around 3 billion base pairs.

For information on the Human Genome Project, see Peters & Hadley (1997).

GENETIC MODIFICATION AND GENE THERAPY

Techniques have been perfected for targeting and cutting out fragments of DNA containing one or more genes from one organism and joining them artificially to another. This results in what is known as recombinant DNA (rDNA). By modifying genes, it is possible to alter the proteins they produce and alter the structure or chemical function of the organism.

The importance of genetic coding for specific proteins is illustrated in a condition called phenylketonuria (PKU), where the absence of gene coding for the enzyme that converts the amino acid phenylalanine to tyrosine results in an accumulation of phenylalanine in the blood of newborn babies with this recessive gene condition. This affects the brain, causing severe learning difficulties. Babies can be tested routinely on the fifth day of life for high levels of phenylalanine in the blood and, when detected early, the effects of PKU can be prevented with a phenylalanine-free diet.

Applications of genetic modification

For many years, innocuous bacteria and viruses have been used as the workhorses of molecular biology to ferry genetic material from one species to another or to grow genetically determined proteins. The hormone insulin used in the treatment of diabetes and once extracted from the pancreases of pigs and cows is now manufactured by growing bacteria into which a human insulin gene has been inserted. Interferons used to treat some forms of cancer and the human luteinising hormone used to treat infertility are other examples of the use of genetic modification in pharmaceuticals. Gene modification also has applications in agriculture, where it can be used to improve strains of livestock and plants, introducing characteristics such as resilience against disease.

Genetic biotechnology also has the potential to do great harm, if we consider the destructive potential of genetically engineered microbes and biological aberrations that can be produced in large numbers and released accidentally or intentionally with devastating effect in biological warfare. Recently, there has also been controversy over the use of genetically engineered seeds for crops and vegetables and over genetically modified food ingredients.

Human gene therapy

There are a number of ways in which human gene therapy could potentially be used (Greener 1993). Theoretically, defective genes could be deleted from somatic cells, genetic defects corrected or missing genes introduced. This would affect only the individual being treated and has been judged by controlling committees as acceptable practice in most cases. A missing gene could be transferred to a recipient from a healthy donor's cell, as demonstrated by a breakthrough in gene therapy when the missing ADA (adenosine deaminase) gene was transferred using an innocuous virus as the vector.

In germ-line therapy, which would involve genetic modification of the embryo, there is the potential for aberrations to be created which would become part of every nucleated cell and be passed on to future generations. This has been declared unacceptable because of the unforeseeable long-term consequences, the ethical implications of research on human embryos and the prohibition on human cloning (Pennisi & Williams 1997).

Eugenics, the science of attempting to improve the human race either by encouraging individuals deemed to be superior to reproduce or by attempting to prevent individuals with characteristics considered to be undesirable from reproducing, is the subject of perennial controversy. This ideal influenced sociopolitical movements of the 20th century, most notably Nazism, with tragic effect. As genetic science rapidly advances, its potential applications within eugenic thinking must continue to be scrutinised.

Ethical considerations

Genetic modification and gene therapy are subject to strict guidelines and controls by governmental and scientific bodies. The principles of regulating new technologies are established in the international forum by the United Nations and by international scientific bodies. The European Community has issued a number of directives to be translated into national legislation for the control of biotechnology. The UK has a medical ethics committee — the Clothier Committee — to monitor the ethical implications of the application of genetic technology in specific cases.

A British Medical Association investigating committee (BMA 1992) recommended that 'the regulation of genetic modification should be conducted in an open, democratically accountable and representative fashion' in order to ensure that the public are fully informed and as an additional safeguard to community interest. It also stipulated that genetic screening should always be accompanied by non-directive counselling.

CATEGORIES OF GENETIC DISORDERS

The three main categories of genetic disorders are:

- chromosomal anomalies
- single gene or Mendelian disorders
- multifactorial or polygenic disorders.

Chromosomal anomalies

Autosomal variations

Numerical autosomal chromosome variations. Abnormalities can arise if, during meiosis, non-disjunction takes place and both of one pair of chromosomes pass to one gamete and the other gamete does not get a copy of that chromosome. If fertilisation takes place, the zygote will then have either three copies of the chromosome (trisomy) or only one copy (monosomy). One example of a trisomy is Down's syndrome (an extra copy of chromosome 21) with its characteristic appearance, a degree of mental handicap, and sometimes cardiac and intestinal abnormalities.

Autosomal chromosomal deletions and translocations. Structural variations arise if a piece of a chromosome breaks off and attaches itself to another chromosome. This will result in the gamete either having part of a chromosome missing (a deletion) or having a rearrangement (a translocation).

A balanced translocation causes no abnormality because no chromosomal material is gained or lost. However, there will be a higher risk that when the individual has a child an unbalanced chromosome form will arise, causing spontaneous abortion or a syndrome with both physical and mental handicap.

Chromosomal abnormalities are often found in spontaneously aborted fetuses. The risk of a couple having a second affected child with a chromosomal abnormality is usually regarded as low, but if one of the parents is found to carry a balanced translocation, that risk is greatly increased. However, this occurs in only 5% of chromosomal abnormalities. The risk to other family members of having an affected child is even lower, unless there is a familial history of translocation. In this situation, all relatives should have their chromosomes checked for the abnormality if they so wish.

Sex chromosome variations

Although the psychological implications of the diagnosis of a sex chromosome anomaly are profound, the problems caused by these abnormalities tend to be less severe than those resulting from autosomal abnormalities. Consequently, a significant number of people may have a sex chromosome anomaly without being aware of it. We now know that numerical abnormalities of the sex chromosomes are not as uncommon as was once believed.

A diagnosis can be made during routine antenatal screening, but as some chromosome disorders cause infertility they may be detected for the first time at infertility clinics.

Some result in a degree of retarded or excessive growth, in which case diagnosis may be made at a paediatric growth or endocrine clinic. It is rare for sex chromosome abnormalities to recur in a family, even in the offspring of affected fertile individuals.

Serious cognitive impairment has not been found and long-term information on prognosis and achievements is becoming available. A slightly lower mean IQ has been demonstrated, as has an increase in learning difficulties. The latter can usually be helped with remedial support at school. However, should more than one extra sex chromosome be present, learning difficulties and/or physical abnormality are more likely.

An example of a sex chromosomal anomaly is Klinefelter's syndrome (an extra copy of the X chromosome in a male) with normal appearance and usually a normal level of intelligence. The personality may be more reticent. After puberty the testes are small, facial hair is scant and sometimes there can be a degree of breast enlargement. Most of those with Klinefelter's syndrome are infertile, but it is important to note that sexual performance is not impaired.

Mosaicism occurs when an individual has two different cell lines resulting in a certain percentage of abnormal cells, the remainder of the cells being normal. This may result from somatic mutation.

Single gene or Mendelian disorders

These disorders are caused by a defect in one of our 60 000–100 000 genes. The risk of offspring being affected is usually high and can be calculated if the mode of inheritance and a detailed family history (including a family tree or pedigree) are known. A risk factor can also be given for other members of the family.

The inheritance of single-gene disorders can be:

- autosomal dominant
- autosomal recessive
- X-linked.

Autosomal dominant inheritance

Autosomal dominant conditions are caused by a defect in a dominant gene on one of the 44 autosomes. One gene on a pair of autosomes will be normal while the corresponding gene on the other of the autosome pair will be defective. If the defective gene is dominant, it will overrule the normal gene. As a result, the individual will usually both carry the condition and suffer from it.

Those who have the defective dominant gene will have a 1 in 2 chance of passing it on to their offspring. This is because during meiosis only one of each pair of chromosomes will pass to each ovum or sperm. Whether the disease is transmitted from the parent will depend on whether the ovum or sperm contains the chromosome with the normal gene or the chromosome with the defective gene.

It is important to note that this amounts to a 50% probability in each pregnancy. If there are two children, it is not inevitable that one will be affected and the other will not. It could be that both have the disorder, both are free of it, or one will have it and one will not.

As the defect is on an autosome rather than a sex chromosome, the sex of the individual is of no consequence to inheritance. A child of either sex can inherit the disorder; if he or she does, then once again, the chance of passing it on to a child of either sex will be 50%.

If an individual is proved beyond doubt not to have the disorder, and therefore not to have the defective gene, he or she cannot pass on the disease. Dominant gene faults cannot skip a generation and reappear again. In some instances, this may appear to happen, because with some conditions it is possible for an individual with an affected parent to show no detectable signs of the disease and yet pass it on to the next generation. In this case, the gene fault must have been present in all three generations but has not resulted in causing the disease in each. This is known as 'reduced penetrance' or 'non-penetrance'. Defective genes may sometimes show a variation in expression of the disease from very severe to barely detectable. This is known as 'variable expressivity'. Non-penetrance and variable expressivity are complicating features in diseases inherited as autosomal dominants.

In some conditions, the nature of the gene defect allows it to become enlarged as it passes down the generations. This is termed 'anticipation' and tends to result in a more severe form of the resulting disease.

If the gene mutation responsible for causing a condition has been located and identified, it becomes possible to perform direct gene testing on a blood sample to confirm a diagnosis. This eliminates the element of doubt present when diagnosis relies on the detection of varying signs and symptoms. The number of genes responsible for classic genetic disorders which have been located is still small but is steadily increasing.

The age of onset of dominantly inherited conditions can also be variable. With some conditions, symptoms may not appear until young adulthood or middle age. Examples of these are myotonic dystrophy and Huntington's disease.

A defective gene can be caused by a new mutation, i.e. the genetic anomaly causing the defect has occurred for the first time in an individual rather than being passed down by a parent.

Autosomal recessive inheritance

Autosomal recessive conditions are caused by a defect in a recessive gene on an autosome. An individual can have a copy of a defective gene on one of a pair of autosomes and a corresponding normal gene on the other of the pair. As the defective gene in this case is recessive, the normal gene will overrule the defective gene. As a result, the individual will carry the disorder but will not suffer from it. It is unlikely that he or she will be aware of this situation.

A problem may arise if two parents who carry the same recessive gene defect have children, because it is possible for both parents to pass the defective recessive gene on to the child. The child will then have two copies of the defective gene with no normal gene to compensate and will suffer from the condition.

When both parents carry the same defective recessive gene, there is a 1 in 4 risk in each pregnancy that a child will suffer from the disorder. Again, chance has no memory. There is unlikely to be a family history of the condition and often the parents will become aware that they are carriers only after the birth of a child affected with the recessive genetic disorder.

Consanguinity, including interfamily marriage, such as between cousins, increases the risk of a recessive disorder because both parents could have inherited the defective gene from a common ancestor. The overall increase in risk to offspring of parents who are first cousins is moderately low, i.e. 3% above the risk to the general population.

Some recessive defects are more common in certain ethnic groups, e.g. thalassaemia, sickle cell disease and Tay–Sachs disease.

Many recessive disorders are severe, including complex malformation syndromes and recognised inborn errors of metabolism.

X-linked recessive inheritance

X-linked recessive disorders are caused by a defect in a recessive gene on the X chromosome. If a female has a recessive gene defect on an X chromosome, she will have a corresponding normal gene on her other X chromosome. This will overrule the defective gene such that she will be a carrier of the disease but is unlikely to suffer from it. Manifesting carriers have occasionally been reported but they are not common.

In order to be male, a fetus must get a Y chromosome from its father. If a carrier female passes on her X chromosome with the defective gene to a son, his Y chromosome will have no corresponding gene to compensate for it and consequently he will suffer from the disease associated with the gene defect. If, however, she passes on her X chromosome with the normal gene to her son, there will be no defect and no disease.

To be female, a fetus must get an X chromosome from its father. If a carrier female passes on her X chromosome with the defective gene to a daughter, the X chromosome from her father with the normal gene will overrule the defective gene, but she will still be a carrier like her mother. If, however, the mother passes on her X chromosome with the normal gene to her daughter, there will be no defect to be transmitted to the next generation. The risk to the offspring of a female carrier of an X-linked recessive condition is therefore 50% of having an affected male child and 50% of having a carrier female child. Thus the woman has an overall risk of 1 in 4 of having an affected child.

In the case of an affected male with an X-linked condition, all of his daughters will be carriers but none of his sons will either be affected by or carry the disease, except in the unlikely event of the mother being a carrier of the same disease.

If the defect occurs for the first time in the affected boy and is not found in his mother's blood sample, it will have been caused either by a new mutation or by a mutation which has arisen in the cells of his mother's ovaries. The latter is termed gonadal mosaicism. There will be no risk to the wider family but the possibility of gonadal mosaicism means that one can rarely rule out the mother having another affected son or carrier daughter.

If the mother of an affected boy is known to be a carrier, it is possible that her female relatives may also be carriers with similar risks of passing on the defective gene.

X-linked dominant disorders and Y-linked disorders have been described but are rare.

Multifactorial or polygenic disorders

In many disorders, genetic and environmental factors combine to give rise to disease. Risks of recurrence of these disorders within a family are generally regarded as being moderately low, the greatest risk being to first- and second-degree relatives (approximately 1%). Empirical risks may be used when estimating recurrence. It is rare for third-degree relatives to have a recurrence risk of over 1%.

When environmental factors are known (e.g. diet, smoking and exercise in coronary heart disease), these can be modified with beneficial effect. However, this approach is not possible for the majority of multifactorial disorders.

Factors which increase the risk of multifactorial disorders in relatives are (Harper 1993):

- the genetic component of the disease
- the closeness of the relationship to the affected person
- the presence of the disorder in more than one family member
- the severity of the condition in the affected person
- the presence of the disorder in a person not of the sex usually affected.

Common disorders which are considered to be multifactorial in origin include:

- asthma
- coronary artery disease
- congenital heart disease
- diabetes
- essential hypertension
- schizophrenia
- cleft lip and palate
- neural tube defects.

TESTING FOR GENETIC DISORDERS

Testing for genetic disorders can be divided into four main categories:

Antenatal testing (also referred to as prenatal testing) is used to predict whether a fetus is affected by a genetic disorder or is carrying a defective gene which will cause it to become affected by a genetic disorder (see Case History 6.1). A woman's chance of having a baby with an abnormality recognisable at birth is 1 in 40. This risk excludes those genetic disorders not recognisable at birth, e.g. familial adenomatous polyposis, Huntington's disease and familial hypercholesterolaemia. The aim of prenatal diagnosis is prevention by early detection and intervention.

Diagnostic testing is used to find out whether or not an individual has a particular genetic disorder and often relies on the presence or absence of signs and symptoms. The type of testing necessary will be determined by the kind of defect likely to be found. Relatives of those affected by genetic conditions often have to be assessed in this way to ascertain whether they have the same condition in a different form and are at risk of passing it on. Diagnostic testing in the form of direct gene testing is now available for a small but increasing number of conditions, e.g. Huntington's disease and myotonic dystrophy.

Pre-symptomatic or predictive testing is used to predict whether or not an individual at risk of inheriting a genetic disorder has inherited the defective gene before there are any signs or symptoms of the disorder itself. The benefits of pre-symptomatic testing are clear where treatment is available to prevent the occurrence of the disease. However, when no treatment can be prescribed to prevent, cure or alleviate the disease, much thought has to be given to the advisability of having a test and the recommended test protocol must be adhered to. Some of those at risk of progressive debilitating genetic disease prefer to know what lies in store for them, so that they can make appropriate decisions regarding careers, pregnancy and housing, while others prefer not to know.

Carrier testing is used to find out whether an individual carries a particular defective autosomal recessive or X-linked recessive gene defect. It has mainly been used for conditions known to be a high risk within certain ethnic groups. However, it can also be used for close relatives of couples who have an affected child, providing there is a test available which will detect that particular gene fault. As more genes become isolated and testing becomes simpler and more routine, carrier testing for the more common conditions such as cystic fibrosis may become widely available.

Case History 6.1 S and P

S is 30 years old. She and her husband have been trying to conceive a child for the past 5 years of an 8-year marriage. After undergoing infertility investigations, S conceives. She is booked to have her baby at her local maternity hospital. At the booking clinic, she receives a package of leaflets explaining various screening tests available to her during her pregnancy. S opts for shared antenatal care between her GP and obstetrician. An ultrasound scan is offered as part of routine antenatal care to check that the baby is healthy. Unfortunately this reveals that the fetus has anencephaly.

S and P are seen immediately by the obstetrician, who gently but frankly explains the results of the scan and the options open to them. They understand that they have a choice of terminating the pregnancy or allowing nature to take its course, knowing that the infant cannot survive. The obstetrician leaves them to discuss this with one another in private. A midwife who specialises in the care of couples undergoing prenatal diagnosis and who is a trained counsellor is close at hand to offer practical comfort and information on how a termination would be carried out, how long it would take, and the intensity of discomfort that would be experienced. The hospital's methods of inducing labour and procedures for delivery are discussed.

Although there are no legal requirements to cremate or bury a baby born dead before 28 weeks, it is explained to the couple that they could, if they wish, have a funeral and/or a burial service. The hospital chaplain is available to discuss any aspects of religious or personal beliefs S and P have and the arrangements that could be made. S and P find that knowing the plan of care for their infant from beginning to end helps them to come to a decision with regard to continuing or ending the pregnancy.

S and P decide that terminating their long-awaited and much-wanted pregnancy is for them the only acceptable option.

Techniques for genetic testing

There is no broad-based test which can be used to screen for all genetic disorders at once. Indeed, for many disorders there is at present no test available. Where testing is feasible, it is a specific test for a specific disorder and, in some cases, will indicate a greatly increased or decreased likelihood of inheriting or carrying a disorder rather than confirming or eliminating its presence.

The main techniques used in testing for genetic disorders are:

- chromosomal analysis or karyotyping (see Fig. 6.1)
- family-based DNA linkage studies (see Box 6.2)
- direct gene testing
- clinical examination
- biochemical tests
- radiography
- ultrasonography.

Table 6.1 lists the commonly used sources of tissue for chromosomal analysis.

Box 6.2 Predictive testing using DNA technology

Small blood samples (20 ml) are obtained from the at-risk individuals being tested and as many close relatives as possible. At a minimum, the affected and unaffected parents and one affected sibling, or the affected parent and an 'escapee' sibling, would be needed, although this would rarely be enough to work on. In the absence of these individuals, other relatives might be sufficient for establishing the linkage. The more close relatives available, the higher the probability that the test will be informative. Leucocytes are isolated from the blood and the DNA is then cut into fragments using several restriction enzymes. The resulting fragments are placed in a solution containing a specific fragment of DNA (the 'probe' or 'marker'), which binds to its complement on the fragments. The probe or marker is radioactively labelled, and so allows the pattern of cleavage of the DNA to be visualised using X-ray film. There are a finite number of cleavage patterns, six being that most frequently found. The pattern which links the altered gene differs among families. Based on pedigree analysis, we can often determine which pattern is inherited along with the altered gene.

Table 6.1 Commonly used sources of tissue in human chromosome studies

Source	*Cell*	*Application*
Blood	T lymphocytes	Routine analysis
Skin	Fibroblasts	Suspected mosaicism
Bone marrow	White cells etc.	Leukaemia
Amniotic fluid	Shed epithelial cells	16–20 week fetus
Chorionic villi	Trophoblast	8–12 week fetus
Buccal smear	Shed epithelial cells	Sex chromatin

Techniques for antenatal diagnosis

Diagnostic ultrasound

Various abnormalities can be detected using high-resolution ultrasound imaging. Congenital abnormalities can, in some instances only, be detected by ultrasound scans from around 14 weeks' gestation.

Conditions detectable by ultrasound scanning include:

- skeletal abnormalities, e.g. severe short-limbed dwarfism, osteogenesis imperfecta
- neural tube defects, e.g. spina bifida
- major organ malformations, e.g. severe congenital heart disease, renal agenesis
- polyhydramnios (excess amniotic fluid)
- oligohydramnios (decreased amniotic fluid)
- hydrops (abnormal accumulation of serous fluid in a body cavity or tissues).

Amniocentesis

During pregnancy, fetal cells slough off into the amniotic fluid. It is possible to withdraw a sample of amniotic fluid between 16 and 20 weeks' gestation and to culture and test the fetal cells for chromosomal abnormalities. Alpha-fetoprotein (AFP) levels can be measured to detect neural tube defects such as spina bifida. Amniocentesis has the potential to diagnose around 200 genetic disorders. The risk of spontaneous abortion after the procedure is estimated to be less than 1%.

Conditions detectable by amniocentesis include:

- chromosomal disorders, using karyotyping
- inherited diseases, using biochemical and DNA studies
- open neural tube defects: indicated by amniotic fluid AFP.

Chorionic villus sampling (CVS)

This is carried out between 10 and 12 weeks of pregnancy and is thus termed first-trimester prenatal diagnosis. Essentially, this test provides the same diagnostic information as amniocentesis but gives a quicker result as the cells grow faster; however, it is not suitable for diagnosing all genetic disorders, e.g. neural tube defects.

Under ultrasound guidance, a catheter is inserted through the abdomen or the cervical os to the placental insertion site. Villi are aspirated and the cells are analysed. Conditions detectable by CVS are chromosomal disorders (using karyotyping) and inherited diseases (using DNA studies).

Transabdominal CVS can be done at any stage of pregnancy, providing the placenta is in an accessible position. Some pregnancies are more suitable for transcervical sampling and others for transabdominal sampling. Depending upon the type of analysis, results may be available within days. The risk of spontaneous abortion after CVS is estimated to be 2–4%.

Fetal blood sampling

This is occasionally used for diagnosis of disorders when DNA diagnosis is not possible. Under ultrasound guidance a special sampling needle is passed transabdominally. A fetal vessel near the umbilical cord insertion is punctured and fetal blood is withdrawn. This is carried out at 18 weeks' gestation. (See Proud (1995)).

GENETIC COUNSELLING

Referrals for genetic counselling may be made by family doctors, specialist consultants (e.g. paediatricians, obstetricians, cardiologists), other genetic centres, and also as self-referrals.

Nurses in the community, midwifery, learning disability and psychiatric nursing, and in hospital settings are in a strategic position to detect disease patterns and risk factors. In their interactions with patients and their families, nurses may have occasion to suspect the possibility of the occurrence of classic genetic disease within a family. The following indications should alert the nurse that referral for genetic counselling may be appropriate:

- family history of classic genetic disease
- newly diagnosed genetic disorder
- older women seeking advice on pregnancy and fetal abnormalities
- cousin relationships
- ethnic groups with a high incidence of a particular disorder
- presence of dysmorphic features
- unexplained mental retardation
- unexplained stillbirth
- recurrent miscarriages
- family history of structural chromosomal abnormality.

Once a need for specialist genetic counselling has been identified, appropriate referral should be organised in consultation with other members of the health care team. Where family members express concern or the need for more information, it may be helpful to refer them as well.

General practitioners and specialist consultants are concerned mainly with diagnosis and illness management. Ideally, the doctor actively treating the patient will introduce the idea of a genetic aspect to the condition, but it will be members of the specialist genetic unit who will allocate the length of time necessary for this aspect to be dealt with adequately and who will follow up other family members who may be at risk of contracting the illness or passing it on.

The patient for whom a genetic counselling referral has been suggested may not understand what this means and why it is necessary. An initial response may be concern that a directive will be given as to the pattern of any future reproduction. An important part of the genetic nurse's role is to allay this fear.

Q

6.1 A family history reveals a high incidence of heart disease in a particular client's family. Although he has no signs of heart disease at this point in time, it is possible that he may have inherited a genetic predisposition. He also has several relevant environmental risk factors: he is overweight, smokes heavily and takes little exercise. What might you predict his chances to be of developing serious heart disease? What specific action could you as a nurse take to promote his health and prevent serious disease developing?

Box 6.3 Drawing up a family tree

- Always take details from both sides of the family.
- Go back at least three generations.
- Record dates of birth rather than ages if possible.
- Record those who have died, plus cause and age of death.
- Ask specifically about infant deaths, stillbirths and miscarriages.
- Ask directly about consanguinity (marriage between relatives, e.g. cousins).
- Record maiden name of women.
- Check that the father of an individual is the person you would expect him to be. Assume nothing. Mistaken paternity causes inaccurate information to be given.

The clinical genetic team

Most genetic units provide a regional service which covers a wide range of disorders and serves a large geographical area. Staff include:

- clinical medical geneticists
- specialist nurses
- genetic associates without a nursing or medical background who have undergone specific training in genetic counselling at MSc level
- scientists
- data managers
- laboratory staff
- administrative staff.

The main aspects of the team's work are:

- making or confirming diagnoses
- estimating risks of either contracting the condition or passing it on
- giving information about the condition
- giving information about testing
- giving information about screening
- exploring options
- giving support.

The medical staff will be more involved in the accurate diagnosis of a condition and will estimate the risk to the patient or relatives of contracting the disease and/or passing it on to their children. Specialist nurses may be in a better position to explain why tests are necessary or what they will involve and thus allay unnecessary anxiety.

The role of the specialist practitioner nurse in genetics

Information-gathering

An essential part of the counselling process is obtaining a full family history, including the presence of risk factors in the individual's environment. This is often collected by specialist nurse practitioners working in genetic units. A family tree giving a diagrammatic representation of familial relationships over several generations is useful in demonstrating a pattern of inheritance of family traits and recurrent diseases. Points to remember when drawing up a family tree are listed in Box 6.3. Symbols used to indicate key information in family trees are shown in Figure 6.3.

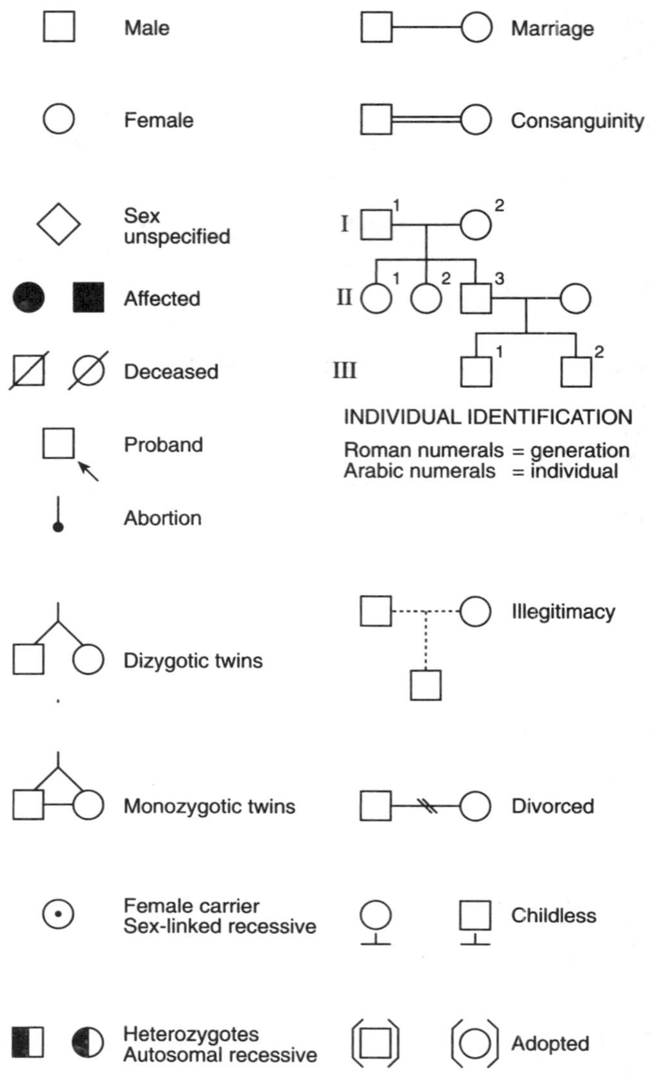

Fig. 6.3 Symbols used in family trees for genetic assessment.

Education

The specialist nurse practitioner may be asked to speak about genetic issues to students, qualified nurses and other professionals in a formal setting, or on a one-to-one basis with a colleague involved with a patient with a genetic condition who asks for specific information. He may also be requested to set up training courses and study days, as well as to research and pass on information about rare genetic conditions to colleagues and students. He will have access to textbooks, journals and to individual experts in given fields not always available to others. The specialist nurse practitioner will have an important role in giving the patient information about the nature of her disorder and the mechanics of genetic transmission. During a routine procedure, such as taking a blood sample, patients may ask questions or refer to worries and concerns, providing the nurse with an opportunity to give information and reassurance and to clarify issues that may be creating anxiety.

Counselling individuals and families

The giving of information by way of genetic counselling is mainly the role of the medical geneticist. However, in some centres, genetic counselling may be the responsibility of experienced genetic nurses in cases where the genetic situation is estimated to be straightforward, e.g. genetic counselling for hereditary cancers. Nurse practitioners also have an important role to play in decision-making and pre-symptomatic testing. Genetic counselling aims to be non-directive. Families are presented with information in a way they understand and are encouraged to explore in detail all the paths open to them (Clarke 1991). There is little done in the way of physical care by the staff in genetic departments. Options that may be relevant to individuals or family members include:

- delaying a decision until more facts are available
- pre-symptomatic testing
- ascertainment of carrier status
- planning a screening programme
- antenatal diagnosis
- termination of affected pregnancies
- planning a pregnancy without any form of testing
- limitation of size of family by contraception or sterilisation (male or female)
- artificial insemination
- ovum donation and in vitro fertilisation.

It should be borne in mind that a risk that seems overwhelmingly high to some couples may be acceptable to others in a similar situation.

When a difficult decision has to be made, such as whether to terminate an established pregnancy, it is helpful to the individuals concerned if the nurse makes it clear that he will support them whatever their decision. Often in these circumstances, couples are inundated with advice from others who, for various reasons, are seeking to influence their decision. It may come as a relief that the only decision the genetic nurse is interested in is that of the couple.

Record-keeping

Accurate record-keeping is important. In genetic units, records are kept literally for generations. The specialist genetic nurse will also be involved in maintaining genetic registers of inherited diseases. Increasingly, statistics are asked for, such as the uptake of testing for specific conditions, the estimated number of individuals at high risk of a particular condition or the workload engendered by a new scientific breakthrough.

Policy-making

As a practitioner in a rapidly developing field, the specialist nurse may also become involved in policy-making at a local and national level, particularly now that there is greater awareness of genetic implications among both professionals and the general public. The Association of Genetic Nurses and Counsellors (AGNC) has a membership of over 100 nursing and non-nursing genetic counsellors who work in this speciality. The AGNC is part of the larger organisation, The Human Genetics Association, and is presently addressing the issue of the lack of formal training in genetic nursing.

Special components of genetic counselling

The work of the genetic counselling team has many interrelated aspects which require a high level of clinical expertise, excellent communication skills and scrupulous professionalism in the handling of confidential information. Some special components of genetic counselling may be outlined as follows:

- Maintaining a detailed specialist knowledge of genetic conditions and keeping abreast of advances in research. Worldwide cooperation in the study of these rare conditions has contributed greatly to the advancement of knowledge. Research findings can lead to changes in the understanding of a disease and its inheritance patterns which may alter risk calculation.
- Recognising disease patterns within a family illustrating a particular mode of inheritance which may point to health implications for the wider family, e.g. a risk of polyposis coli or hypercholesterolaemia.
- Calculating risks to family members. Not only is the presenting patient given genetic counselling, but consideration is given to each member of the wider family, e.g. siblings, parents' siblings and offspring of these individuals. This is most important in conditions such as Huntington's disease, where healthy relatives may be at risk of becoming affected by the same disease process.
- Allocating sufficient time to consider all implications of a disease or disease risk.
- Linking family pedigrees. Identifying those at risk of a disorder in a family and linking different branches of the same kinship are, now that more direct gene tests are available, less important components of the work with some conditions. However, it is of great importance when working with familial cancers (see pp. 215–217). Confidentiality regarding individuals' diagnoses, genetic status or attendance at clinics must be strictly maintained.
- Storing family information throughout generations. Strict control is maintained over access to genetic disease registers. Maintenance of these registers allows all individuals on a register to be contacted if new tests or treatments become available and enables family members to be offered genetic counselling at an appropriate age via their parents.

The role of the nurse in clinical genetics was first discussed by Farnish (1988) and recently by Skirton et al (1997).

Genetic counselling has been defined as (Harper 1993):

> the process by which patients and relatives at risk of a disorder that may be hereditary are advised of the consequences of the disorder, the probability of developing the disorder and of the ways in which this can be prevented or ameliorated.

The genetic counselling procedure

When families or individuals are referred for genetic counselling, information from them must be obtained in order to be able to give accurate information about the condition, the recurrence risks to future children, and the availability and accuracy of genetic tests.

The genetic counselling procedure can be divided into three phases:

- obtaining the family history
- the counselling appointment
- family follow-up.

Family history

Information about family members can be obtained in a variety of ways:

- at a home visit
- at a clinic appointment
- by telephone
- by the patient filling in a postal questionnaire.

Home visits are preferred by both patients and nurse practitioners, but because of the amount of professional time and travelling involved, priority may have to be given to those who have suffered recent bereavements, who are handicapped or ill, or who are from lower socioeconomic groups. In the home environment, a more sensitive appraisal can be made of the family's level of knowledge, their educational, socioeconomic and cultural background, and their religious beliefs, all of which have a direct bearing on the counselling approach.

A family history clinic appointment is the next best alternative. Patients are seen face to face in unthreatening surroundings and time can be given to explore the emotional issues surrounding the family situation. It is essential that the purpose of the appointment is given in the appointment letter and the information which is required by the genetic unit is clearly listed. In order to confirm the diagnosis and to assess the mode of inheritance of the condition, it is necessary to obtain details about other family members who may be similarly affected (see Box 6.3 and Fig. 6.3). Information about one relative should never be given to another relative without the knowledge and consent of the former.

It is of benefit to ask what has already been explained to the patient or family about the condition. This will confirm their level of understanding of the basic facts.

Family information can also be collected by telephone or by sending out forms to be completed. The lack of individual contact and the associated communication problems make these methods of obtaining information less satisfactory.

The counselling appointment

If possible, the nurse who obtained the family history should be present during the consultation in case there is difficulty in comprehension due to problems with intellect, anxiety, accompanying children or a language barrier. The clinical geneticist will re-check the family history with the patient, making amendments or additions as necessary. On completion of the data-gathering process, questions of an open-ended style can be used to ascertain the clients' experience and understanding of the disorder.

If the diagnosis is clear at this stage, the information-giving aspects of genetic counselling can begin. The clinician explains how the diagnosis was determined and what the implications are for the individual or couple, their children and other family members. All aspects are carefully explored and reassurance is given that further opportunities to reiterate and explore the information will be made available.

If the diagnosis is unclear, physical examinations may be necessary to confirm or negate it. Laboratory tests or other diagnostic procedures may be requested and consultation with medical specialists in other fields may be necessary to obtain sufficient information for accurate diagnosis and estimation of risks. In a substantial number of cases, a definite diagnosis cannot be made, making it impossible to give a definite estimation of risk of recurrence.

Letters are sent to the individual or couple, the referring doctor and the general practitioner after the consultation, summarising the information given.

Family follow-up

Short-term follow-up by the genetic nurse may be considered necessary in certain situations, where there is difficulty in comprehension, unresolved grief, where problems are evident in coming to terms with the situation, or a couple have a difference of opinion regarding which option to follow.

Future contact may be necessary when further pregnancies are embarked upon, especially in high-risk disorders. It may be that antenatal testing is offered and found to be acceptable. At times like this the couple may find it beneficial to talk the situation through with a specialist nurse already known to them (see Case History 6.2).

Family contact may result when an individual has been asked to inform relatives who may be at risk or from whom blood samples are needed for DNA-based family studies. Confusion can arise following requests for blood samples. Those samples needed for DNA linkage tests do not get 'tested' themselves. There will be no individual diagnostic results. The blood samples are used only for family linkage, as a kind of comparison between those known to be affected by the disease and those known not to be affected. However, it can be very difficult for the individuals concerned to grasp why they will not get a result from their own blood sample.

Long-term follow-up for family support by a genetic nurse specialist may be indicated in some circumstances.

Case History 6.2 — B and R

B studied hard at university to become a dentist. She specialised in maxillofacial surgery and then entered private practice. She met and married R when she was 37 years old. Despite having a busy career and an active social life, B was keen to have a baby. Because of her age, she thought she would first consult her doctor. B's GP assured her that there was no reason why she should not have a healthy pregnancy, but there was one problem: at B's age she had an increased risk of having a baby with a chromosome abnormality such as Down's syndrome. 'I think,' said her GP, 'you would be better advised of the risks and the various options open to you and R by our clinical geneticist.'

B and R met the clinical geneticist 3 weeks later and listened carefully to her explanation of the potential problem of a pregnancy resulting in a chromosome abnormality at B's age. The geneticist then explained that they could consider prenatal testing to check the baby's chromosomes, and described the procedures and timing for chorionic villus sampling (CVS) and amniocentesis.

B and R discussed the possibility of prenatal testing, should B become pregnant. Indeed, B was successful in becoming pregnant, and at 9 weeks of pregnancy she underwent CVS. The tissue sample was sent to the genetics laboratory for analysis. Two weeks later, B and R met the obstetrician to discuss the results of the karyotype. 'The chromosomes all look normal,' she said. 'Would you like to know if the baby is a girl or a boy?' B looked at R, and they both shook their heads. They had already decided to continue the rest of the pregnancy in as normal a way as possible.

The psychological impact of diagnosis

When individuals are given a diagnosis of genetic disease, their lives are changed radically. For the person shown to have a particular disorder, the expectation of a reasonably long and healthy life may be replaced by the terrifying prospect of progressive disability and premature death. For a parent, the anticipation of a child's day-to-day struggle to remain active or even simply to survive may seem too much to bear. For a young couple whose hopes for parenthood have been dashed, the future may suddenly seem empty. Any genetic illness will affect each member of a family in a different way; for many, the diagnosis will require that extremely difficult and painful decisions concerning family planning are made. Each person's reaction will be unique, even though the person's situation may not be new to the professional. It is essential for the nurse to allow time for feelings of disbelief, anger, grief or even hopelessness to be expressed.

Examples of feelings and worries that may be experienced by individuals who have received a diagnosis related to a genetic disease are listed below, but while such reactions may be anticipated, they must not be presumed. The specialist nurse must ensure that each person's priorities and concerns have been understood and are sensitively and honestly addressed.

- *Being diagnosed as having a progressive illness*
  'How bad will I get?'
  'Will I be able to keep working?'
  'Will I live to see my children grow up?'
  'Will my children have it too?'
- *Being told that one is a carrier of a defective gene or a balanced chromosome translocation*
  'It is my fault.'
  'I feel I have caused my child to be like this.'
- *Being told one's parent has a tragic illness such as Huntington's disease or cerebellar ataxia*
  'Will I end up exactly the same?'
  'Are my children going to get this disease too?'
- *A stillbirth or neonatal death.* The hopes and aspirations of the future lie buried with the child. Friends and relatives do not know what to say to the couple and find it difficult to cope with the situation.
- *The diagnosis of a mentally and/or physically handicapped child*
  'Will nothing make her the child we hoped for?'
  'Will she ever go to normal school or even walk, talk and dress herself?'
  'What if another child is affected too?'
- *An elective mid-trimester termination of pregnancy for fetal abnormality.* The pregnancy which has been terminated was a wanted baby and the so-called mini-labour endured is little different from normal labour, except there is no baby at the end of it to make up for all the suffering. It may help if the fetus is given a name and there is the comforting ritual of a funeral.

The psychological implications of termination of pregnancy

The last circumstance listed above is the one faced by the couple described in Case History 6.1 (p. 200). We might consider a little more closely the emotional and psychological needs of a couple in this situation to illustrate how the nurse, as an impartial professional, can provide invaluable support.

Every couple faces their own unique situation. Professionals become familiar with these situations, but for the couple it is a lonely and sad episode with an inevitably unhappy end. A couple's particular circumstances determine their own special needs. Furthermore, a couple is composed of two individuals whose reactions and needs may vary. Most have the following basic needs:

- to be able to trust in those caring for them
- to have time to reflect upon their loss
- to be supported in coming to terms with feelings of guilt
- to be allowed to remember
- to assimilate the events.

Trust. A couple will be more reassured if they feel they can trust those professionals caring for them and their unborn child. Facts should always be given frankly and honestly. Empathy is a comfort: the nurse should not be afraid to show his feelings. He should ask the couple what they feel are their own special needs at each stage of the episode and work with them to devise a care plan which meets their physical, emotional and spiritual needs, and those of their unborn child.

Reflection upon loss. Couples need to reflect upon what the loss of their baby means to them individually and as a couple. Couples will work through their loss in their own way: by tears, silence, anger and perhaps hostility. Some may prefer to be alone with their grief, but many have a profound need to talk through their experience and to explore what this baby meant to them. Was this a long-awaited pregnancy? Was it unplanned? Did they know beforehand there was a risk to their infant? Have they arrived at this juncture unaware and shocked? What were their plans and aspirations for this child?

Feelings of guilt. The couple should be encouraged to re-examine any mistaken ideas they may have about their infant's disorder. If the fetal disorder was due to teratogenic effects (e.g. drugs or viral infection), the parents should be allowed to examine the circumstances of how this occurred. They should be helped to find out what kind of social support network is available to them. Is there someone who can give emotional support at home? Is there a local self-help group which gives ongoing support to those who have experienced termination of pregnancy as a result of fetal abnormality?

A licence to remember. Creating memories is now recognised as making a therapeutic contribution to the grieving process. The couple can be encouraged to accept tangible evidence of their experience, e.g. sonograms or fetal monitor strips. Some may decline the offer initially, only to request the same later.

If a couple lose a baby late in pregnancy, they should be asked if they wish to see and hold their baby. The midwife can hold the baby first, allowing the parents to adapt to the situation. Some couples may wish to see the abnormality and others not. The couple should always be asked what they feel their special needs are.

Assimilation of the events. Putting the events into order is a normal and very necessary process for any couple in coming to terms with their grief. Every story needs a beginning, a middle and an end. Talking through the sequence of events is an enormously therapeutic exercise for many, and those undertaking the support of couples in the days and months after termination of pregnancy need to recognise and positively encourage this healing process. Years afterwards, the story will continue to be retold. If we give couples the right support at the right time, it can be remembered and related by two individuals who are emotionally healed (White-van Mourik et al 1992).

CLASSIC GENETIC DISORDERS AND THEIR MANAGEMENT

Although there are over 6000 described classic genetic disorders, even the more common ones are comparatively rare. Nevertheless, their occurrence, or fear of their occurrence, can have devastating effects on the individuals concerned and their families. The aim of the following sections is to illustrate the principles of nursing management in this complex and specialised area of care by focusing on five disorders, namely:

- cystic fibrosis
- haemophilia A
- myotonic dystrophy
- Huntington's disease.
- the familial cancers.

CYSTIC FIBROSIS

Cystic fibrosis (CF) is a single-gene, autosomal recessive disorder which disturbs the mucus-producing glands throughout the body, leading to respiratory problems, incomplete digestion and abnormal sweating. In the UK, it affects 1 in 2500 newborns and about 1 in 25 individuals carry a CF gene.

There is no complete cure for CF and, if untreated, a child may die at a young age from severe lung infection. A small number of patients are not diagnosed until their adult years. Over the past several decades, CF treatment has steadily improved, and today, life expectancy in the UK is 30 years. Despite this, affected individuals continue to have numerous medical problems requiring exhaustive and expensive therapy.

PATHOPHYSIOLOGY

In CF there is a defect in the passage of sodium and chloride ions in and out of the epithelial cells of a number of organs which affects fluid secretion in various glands.

Common presenting symptoms. The majority present in early life with recurring respiratory problems, frequent bulky offensive-smelling stools and failure to gain weight satisfactorily. A small number are not diagnosed until adulthood (Dodge et al 1993).

Clinical features. The air passages of people with CF secrete large amounts of thick, sticky mucus which plugs up the small airways and creates an ideal environment for bacterial infection in the respiratory tract. In the intestine, thick, abnormal mucus is also produced which clogs the ducts leading from the pancreas to the intestine. Food is incompletely digested; weight loss occurs despite a good appetite, and fatty, bulky, foul-smelling stools are passed. The pancreas regresses and may be completely destroyed; however, 10–20% of patients retain at least partial pancreatic function. The incidence of CF-related diabetes mellitus rises with life expectancy, with up to 50% of those surviving into their third decade displaying abnormal glucose tolerance. Five per cent of patients develop hepatic cirrhosis; some of these go on to develop portal hypertension and splenomegaly. Oesophageal varices may develop in these patients, which can be fatal. The sweat glands also malfunction, secreting too much chloride and sodium in the sweat.

Most males with CF are infertile, as a result of an abnormality of the epididymis and vas deferens which end in blind channels instead of leading through to the urethra. In the female, fertility can be impaired because thick cervical mucus impedes the passage of spermatozoa. Delayed secondary sexual development is an almost universal finding in adolescents.

The gene responsible for cystic fibrosis is on chromosome 7 and has been labelled the 'cystic fibrosis transmembrane regulator' gene (CFTR).

The clinical consequences of CF are outlined in Figure 6.4.

Prognosis. Increasing numbers of affected individuals with CF are surviving into their 30s and 40s, but some still die as young children. The psychological burden of living with a debilitating disease which needs constant drug therapy and physiotherapy is great for both

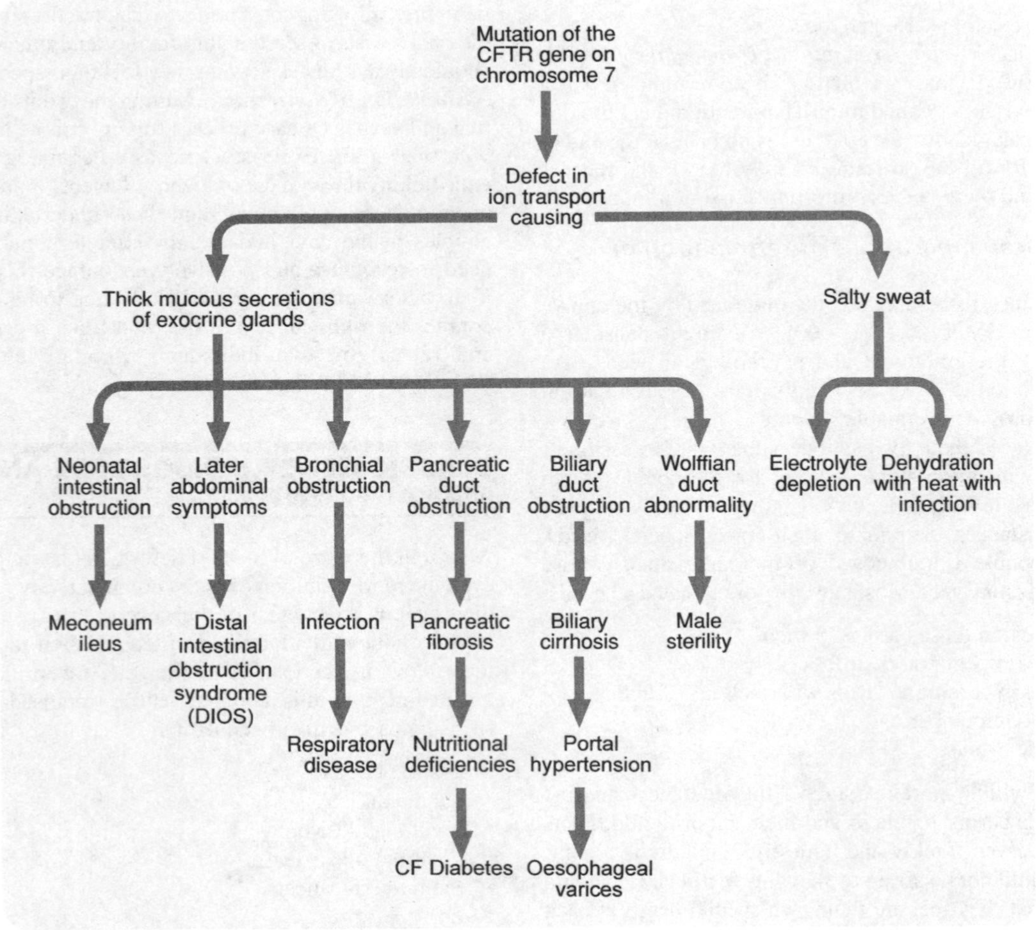

Fig. 6.4 Clinical consequences of cystic fibrosis.

those affected and their families, particularly during adolescence. However, there is great camaraderie among the adult members of the associations for CF adults. Fifty per cent of adults are reported as being employed, 18% unemployed, only 3.6% unable to work through illness and the remainder are students or housewives (Harris & Super 1991).

MEDICAL MANAGEMENT

Investigations. Until the CFTR gene was identified, testing to determine levels of salt and chloride in the sweat was the single most important method for diagnosing CF. A sweat salt abnormality is present from birth in almost all affected individuals and persists throughout life.

In CF the potential difference between interstitial fluid and the respiratory surface epithelium is abnormally large. This can be measured in the nasal epithelium and may aid diagnosis.

Other supporting evidence is based on X-ray examination and sputum cultures. There may also be pancreatic insufficiency or recurrent respiratory infection. In some cases there may be a family history of CF.

Genetic diagnosis. At least 600 different mutations within the CFTR gene have been found. One common mutation, called Delta 508, is found in 75% of the affected UK population. This mutation, along with a number of others, allows us to detect most affected individuals by analysing their DNA. At present, most suspected CF cases are diagnosed by a combination of sweat test and genetic testing.

Surgical intervention. Heart–lung transplant has brought renewed hope for CF sufferers, but it may also cause new problems as a direct result of the surgery or from tissue rejection. Moreover, there are psychosocial problems which can be difficult to foresee. The idea of a heart–lung transplant should be introduced very sensitively, as consenting to this procedure is a very grave decision. Who should make it? Patients, relatives and professionals may have differing viewpoints and conflicting emotions (see Case History 6.3). The overwhelming shortage of cadaveric donor organs has resulted in the use of living donor transplants, which creates further ethical dilemmas. About 80% of those who have a transplant survive and for the families of those who do not there is the comfort of knowing that everything possible has been tried.

Aims of treatment. The overall aim of management is to help affected individuals reach adulthood, leading as normal a life as possible with minimal dependency. The ultimate aim is self-advocacy, and from the time of diagnosis this concept should be instilled in the parents and, in turn, in the child and adolescent. These aims are attained by a multidisciplinary team whose skills, along with close cooperation between the parents, patient and family, are put into action from the time of diagnosis. Regional cystic fibrosis treatment centres lead the way in management.

The treatment programme. At a regular clinic visit the patient is weighed, lung function tests are carried out and sputum is sent for culture and sensitivity. At regular intervals, exercise testing and chest X-rays are carried out and blood is taken for biochemistry and haematology. A standard form is used to record findings, including details of physical examination. Aspects of dietary regimens and physiotherapy techniques are checked and specific problems requiring detailed involvement of particular team members identified.

Improved survival is largely due to effective antibiotic treatment against staphylococcal and pseudomonal infections. Centres vary in their policies for antibiotic therapy, some believing in continuous treatment and others using large doses of antibiotics only when infection occurs. Once *Pseudomonas* colonises the lungs, it is almost impossible to eradicate and causes deterioration of lung function. Many CF centres practise segregation of patients in hospital and at clinics to reduce the incidence of cross-infection.

Case History 6.3 — Individuals with CF: J, A and S

J thought about a heart–lung transplant for over a year but elected not to attend for assessment at the transplant centre. She eventually chose to discontinue active treatment because she wished to avoid coping with a protracted terminal illness. J died in relative peace and dignity in her local hospital within a short time.

A was keen to find out if he was a suitable candidate for transplant and was very pleased to be accepted and placed on the waiting list. Everything in the family centred around waiting for the moment when the buzzer to call him to the transplant unit would burst into sound. 'I won't let you down, Mum. I'll keep alive until they find a donor,' he promised solemnly. Alas, A ran out of time and was unable to keep his promise.

S was one of the lucky few. He underwent a heart–lung transplant and experienced the added bonus of giving his own heart to save someone else. S can do all sorts of things now, just like his schoolmates. But for how long? Will signs of rejection show up when next he attends for follow-up, or in a few years, or never? His parents alternate between happiness and despair, but never have complete relief.

To reduce the length of stay in hospital, parents and older children are taught to administer their own antibiotic drugs intravenously so that treatment initiated in hospital can be completed at home. This allows patients to feel more in control of the situation and less dependent on hospital staff. An implantable venous reservoir has greatly improved home intravenous treatment and compliance. Nebulised antibiotics have been shown to be effective, but require a special compressor and nebuliser system.

Pancreatic enzyme supplements are taken at regular intervals throughout each meal. The amount of capsules required varies greatly between individuals. Small snacks between meals require a lower dose of capsules.

Genetic screening. To have cystic fibrosis, an individual must inherit one copy of the mutated gene from each parent (see Fig. 6.5). It is a recessive disease where both parents are carriers or heterozygotes and have a CF gene on one chromosome 7 and a normal gene on the other chromosome 7. Carriers have no symptoms of the disease, as the normal gene compensates fully for the CF gene (see p. 199).

Using DNA from a mouthwash sample, it is possible to detect 85% of those who carry a CF gene by testing for the most common CF mutations. (It is not practicable to test routinely for all 600.) If both partners are found to be carriers, they are given the option of prenatal diagnosis. Pilot screening programmes designed to test individuals in the general population have been carried out in the UK in two ways. The first screened pregnant women in an antenatal booking clinic. The partners of women identified as carriers were then offered screening. This can also be done as 'couple screening' where a couple are screened together and their combined risk of having an affected child is given (Livingston et al 1994). The second approach offered screening through GP practices to men and women of child-bearing age with the advantage of screening prior to pregnancy (Harris & Super 1991). The psychological aspects are being carefully monitored (Mennie et al 1993).

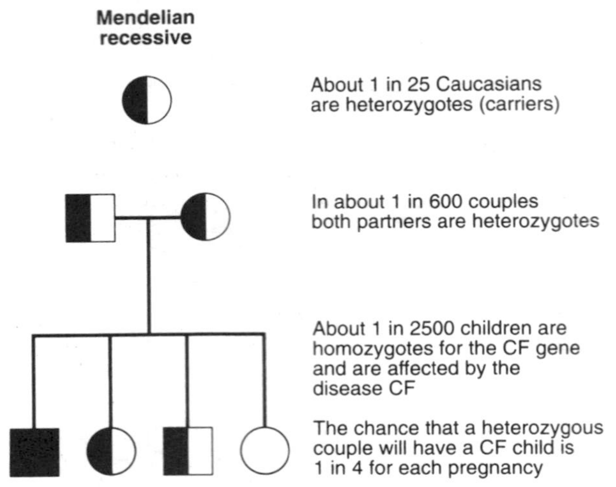

Mendelian recessive
About 1 in 25 Caucasians are heterozygotes (carriers)
In about 1 in 600 couples both partners are heterozygotes
About 1 in 2500 children are homozygotes for the CF gene and are affected by the disease CF
The chance that a heterozygous couple will have a CF child is 1 in 4 for each pregnancy

Fig. 6.5 Genetic inheritance of cystic fibrosis.

NURSING PRIORITIES AND MANAGEMENT: CYSTIC FIBROSIS

Life-threatening concerns

Cystic fibrosis is a long-term, life-threatening multisystem disorder and there are a number of essential areas of management.

Respiratory infection

Persistent recurrent lower respiratory tract infections result in lung damage and impaired function.

Physiotherapy is an essential part of respiratory tract management and should be carried out at least twice daily at home to keep the airways clear of mucus and allow maximum entry of air. Postural drainage, in which the patient is placed in a variety of positions and treated by percussion, allows gravity to assist in the clearance of each lung segment (see Fig. 6.6). The patient assumes each position for a minimum of 10–15 min. In each treatment session, only one area (right and left) should be cleared, i.e. both bases or both mid-zones. Subsequent sessions should cover the remaining areas so that all lung areas are covered in a day. Breathing exercises incorporating a cycle of deep breathing, relaxed breathing and the forced expiratory technique (FET) are fundamental to these sessions. Children from the age of 3 years are taught how to carry out this exercise (see Box 6.4). Much time is spent with parents and children educating them in physiotherapy techniques, as this is a key element of the treatment programme.

Exercise. It has been shown that regular exercise not only increases the efficiency of the lungs, heart and circulation but also improves the general physique and self-esteem. Activities must complement, not replace, physiotherapy and it is helpful to remember that it is when the patient is well that physiotherapy and muscle training are important (Harris & Super 1991).

Nutritional management. It has been shown that CF patients require 25–50% more than the normal daily food allowance because a significant amount of nutritional intake is lost in frequent, bulky, greasy stools. Individuals with CF have a higher resting energy requirement, and extra energy is also needed to combat chest infections. Pancreatic enzyme preparations are now so effective that fat absorption can reach 80–90% of normal. Three daily

Box 6.4 The forced expiration technique (FET)

1. Patient takes a medium inspiration (not a deep one)
2. Patient gives a forced and slightly prolonged expiration (called a huff)
3. Patient coughs, and can expel more sputum than coughing alone allows
4. Patient should alternate this with gentle diaphragmatic breathing

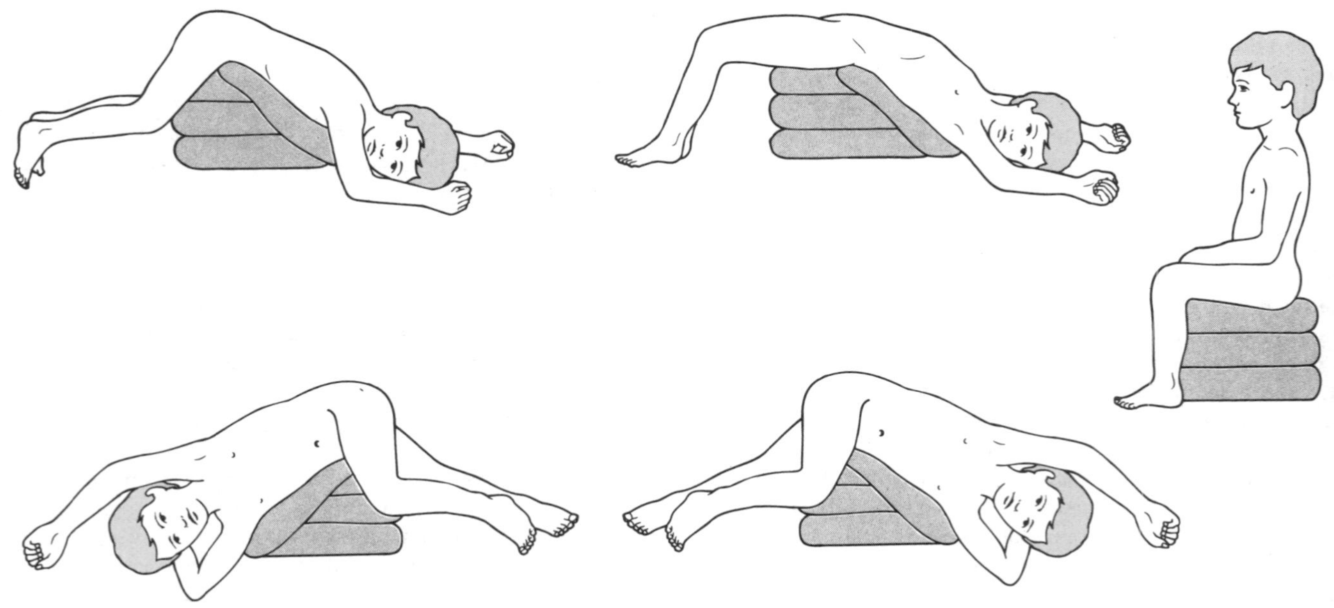

Fig. 6.6 Postural drainage techniques used in the treatment of cystic fibrosis.

meals and supplemental snacks are usually required to bring the energy level up to that desired. Fat-soluble vitamin supplements are given to compensate for loss in the stools. Salt depletion can occur in hot weather and as a result of strenuous exercise, and salt supplements are recommended where appropriate.

Enteral feeding is encouraged in children who fail to gain weight over a 6-month period and in adults who are chronically underweight (body mass index <19), either by the nasogastric route or through a gastrostomy tube. Good nutrition correlates positively with fewer respiratory exacerbations.

Control of diabetes

An annual oral glucose tolerance test is recommended for patients over 10 years of age. If a modest glucose intolerance is demonstrated, no action is taken other than the monitoring of blood glucose levels twice weekly. If patients progress to develop diabetes, insulin is the treatment of choice and the dose is adjusted to control blood glucose levels rather than restriction of diet as with conventional diabetes mellitus. Secondary diabetic complications are rare (Koch & Lang 1995).

Liver disease

Significant disease may already have occurred by the time the liver function tests (LFTs) become abnormal. Ursodeoxycholic acid may improve the LFTs but long-term effects are unclear. Sclerosis can be performed to halt variceal bleeding. Surgical portosystemic shunting may be considered for those with portal hypertension. Liver transplant is an option in end-stage disease and has been found to be associated with an improvement in lung function post-surgery (Westaby 1995).

Psychosocial considerations

Patients, parents and siblings are profoundly affected by the psychosocial and emotional stresses of living with CF. The CF nurse is in an ideal position to recognise that problems exist, and to plan and implement measures to help. Case History 6.4 describes some of the difficulties that might be faced by a teenage boy with CF, and how the sensitive intervention of a specialist nurse might help.

Young female adults with CF have similar problems to those described in Case History 6.4. They develop later than their peers and although they can reproduce, unlike their male counterparts, a pregnancy in a CF woman will often cause deterioration in health and is a time for close cooperation between the CF multidisciplinary team and the obstetrician, as the increased cardiac output and changes in pulmonary function associated with normal pregnancy can cause problems. The mechanical reduction in lung volume as the growing uterus encroaches on the thorax further reduces pulmonary function. Moreover, the woman with CF must also

Case History 6.4 G

G is a small, thin, red-haired 16-year-old in his fourth year at high school. He is judged to be academically average by his headmaster. G is a particularly keen cyclist and is a member of the school cycling team. He was diagnosed as having CF when he was 3 years old. Since that time, his care has been shared by his GP, the local hospital and the regional cystic fibrosis centre. G attends the centre every 3 months. At these visits he is due a chest X-ray. Then lung function tests are carried out and blood is taken for analysis. The physiotherapist checks G's breathing exercises, postural drainage and FET technique. He then sees the dietician, who checks his height and weight and discusses his diet and pancreatic enzyme and vitamin supplements. The chest physician in charge of the centre also examines G, who has been admitted four times in the past 2 years for intensive i.v. antibiotic therapy for *Pseudomonas* respiratory infection. On these occasions G was successfully treated with the antibiotic ciprofloxacin.

Today, G is going to talk to the specialist nurse, who is going to suggest that she introduce G to a careers guidance officer. She knows G well and has already submitted a report to the careers office. G has had periods of absence from school when his condition necessitated hospital admission. Some teaching was given while he was in hospital and he has had extra tuition at home. His father helps him with his physiotherapy and has a close relationship with his son.

The specialist nurse knows from discussions with G's parents that G is quite sensitive about his illness. Firstly, he is smaller and thinner than his schoolmates. He weighs 50 kg and is currently 5′ 4″ tall. His friends have entered puberty at the normal time, but G has no sign of secondary sex characteristics. Naturally, he is self-conscious about this, particularly when using the communal shower and changing rooms at school. Reassurance from the consultant and his parents that he will catch up with his peers, probably continuing to grow after they have stopped, is small consolation.

For a time G had shown signs of depression and had entered a period of non-compliance in his physiotherapy, diet and pancreatic enzyme supplements. It was then that G's parents had contacted the centre and asked the specialist nurse to visit. She was in the process of setting up a group for CF teenagers from within her own and a neighbouring region. The object of the group was to meet socially and discuss any issues which the group or a particular teenager or young adult wanted to discuss. Reluctantly, G went along to the first meeting. He met several people he had seen before at the CF centre but there were some unfamiliar faces. The meeting opened with one young man volunteering to describe an average day in his life:

> The moment I get up, I start my treatment. I start with nebulised Ventolin so that I can do my physio without wheezing and feeling my chest tight. Then comes the physio followed by the nebuliser with my antibiotics. After that I have breakfast and swallow my pancreatin capsules. I take the capsules to school with me to take with my lunch and any snacks. I stay on 2 nights a week after school for games. Most of the time I can manage, although periodically I have to give up because of wheezing. I hope to sit my Standard Grades this year, and I am having extra tuition because I got behind last year with my studies due to numerous hospital admissions for i.v. therapy. The moment I arrive home it is a repeat of the morning's treatment routine. Sometimes I feel very despondent and wonder if it is all worthwhile. My best friend at school wants us to go along to the local disco, but I don't suppose any girl will look twice at me. I am smaller than all the other lads my age and I feel very self-conscious.

This was exactly how G felt about having CF and he felt greatly comforted by hearing this young man put into words his own frustrations at this stage in his life.

consider the impact of her shortened life expectancy upon her children, as progression of the disease may prevent her from carrying out day-to-day care of her child. Those who become pregnant require increased supervision, as more physiotherapy is needed and antibiotic therapy must be carefully selected.

Adult males with CF are now in a position to seek help at assisted reproduction clinics where techniques such as artificial insemination by donor (AID) and microscopic epididymal sperm aspiration (MESA) with intracytoplasmic sperm injection (ICSI) are allowing fatherhood to become a reality. These techniques are expensive, not always easily available and raise further ethical dilemmas.

Outlook for the future

Identification of the CFTR gene is already leading to a clearer understanding of the variability of clinical manifestations. In time we should gain a clearer understanding of the role of the CFTR gene in the control of ion transport. Chemical therapies aimed at improving the impaired ion transport, e.g. nebulised amiloride and uredinetriphosphate (UTP), are new drugs being used in trials. The ultimate aim, however, is treatment. Research on the introduction of normal CFTR genes by aerosol inhalation into the stem cells of the lungs of CF patients is in progress. Whatever the future, the identification of the CF gene gives hope for a greater understanding of the disease and more effective treatment.

For further reading on CF, see Harris & Super (1991).

HAEMOPHILIA

Haemophilia is a name given to a group of genetic disorders of blood coagulation. The most common types are haemophilia A (see Fig 6.7), haemophilia B and von Willebrand's disease. The mode of inheritance of haemophilia A and haemophilia B is X-linked, which explains why males are predominantly affected, although it is possible for female carriers to have mild symptoms.

von Willebrand's disease is caused by mutations of the von Willebrand factor gene on chromosome 12. Different families may show autosomal dominant or autosomal recessive inheritance patterns, depending on the type of mutation. Although rarer, the recessive forms which result from homozygous mutations tend to result in a severe form of the disease.

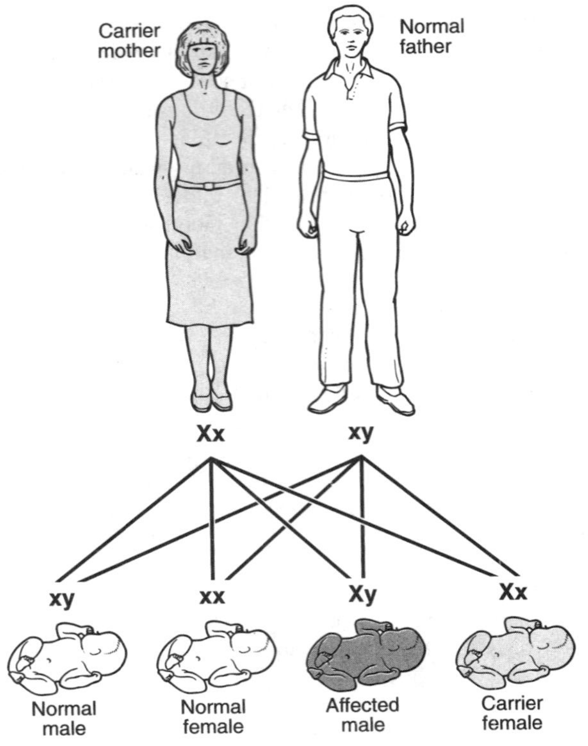

Fig. 6.7 Genetic inheritance of haemophilia A.

PATHOPHYSIOLOGY

Haemophilia A is characterised by a low or absent level of clotting factor VIII (FVIII) and by a prolonged activated thromboplastin time (APTT). The less common haemophilia B is clinically identical to haemophilia A, with the missing or deficient clotting factor being Christmas factor, factor IX (FIX). The severity of the disease can differ, with severe haemophiliacs having a FVIII level of less than 2%, those with moderate haemophilia a FVIII level of 2–5%, and those with mild haemophilia having FVIII levels above 5%.

Common presenting symptoms. In haemophilia, although factor VIII levels are reduced at birth, babies rarely present with bleeding from the umbilical cord. In infancy, unexplained bruising or prolonged bleeding from cuts or abrasions may be early indications and there may be a family history of bruising and bleeding. Severely affected children will bleed spontaneously and may present with haematomas or bleeding into the joints — haemarthrosis. Although the severity of the disease is variable, it is constant within a family. Individuals with severe haemophilia can suffer a bleeding episode at any time and those over school age tend to be aware of this happening even before physical signs appear. Some experience a tingling sensation at the onset of a spontaneous bleed and feel pain as blood begins to fill the joint cavity. As the bleeding progresses, the pain increases, the joint may feel hot or warm to touch and may begin to swell and restrict movement.

Patients with von Willebrand's disease suffer mainly from prolonged mucosal bleeding such as epistaxis, bleeding gums, gastrointestinal bleeding, haematuria or menorrhagia, while joint and muscle bleeds are more rare.

Prognosis. The life expectancy of those with haemophilia should not differ from that of the average person, and most haemophiliac males now reach adult life with only a moderate degree of disability. This contrasts greatly with the past when it was a debilitating condition which resulted in a shortened lifespan (Harper 1993).

MEDICAL MANAGEMENT

Diagnosis. Any individual with prolonged or unexplained bleeding should be tested for haemophilia. Specific factor assays are carried out in haematology laboratories. It is important to note that females with normal FVIII/FIX levels can still be carriers.

Treatment of a joint bleeding episode. If a joint bleeding episode is severe enough to warrant admission, FVIII/FIX levels and full blood count should always be monitored before and after treatment is administered. Intravenous treatment with the appropriate factor concentrates should be given for bleeding into a joint, any bleeding into muscles or injuries to the head, eye, mouth, tongue or neck. Should open surgery be required, this treatment will be needed until the wound has healed. It is imperative that pain is controlled and activity reduced by resting the affected joint, supporting it with pillows and applying cold packs or crushed ice.

The use of aspirin must be avoided and intramuscular injections should never be given as they will cause a haematoma. Any weight or pressure on the joint must be avoided and, after the acute phase has passed, referral made to the physiotherapist. Some haemophiliac patients develop inhibitors to FVIII and therefore require careful monitoring.

Complications of joint bleeds. When a bleed occurs within a joint, the ligaments become stretched due to swelling, the patient stops using the joint because of severe pain and the ligaments become slack and wasted. The joint, being no longer supported adequately, becomes susceptible to injuries which cause further bleeding. Blood enters the joint space causing damage to the articular cartilage, the synovium and the joint surface. The joint space becomes smaller, leading to permanently restricted movement, and cysts can develop. Repetitive bleeding episodes result in arthritis, particularly if not adequately treated.

Complications of muscle bleeds. Untreated muscle bleeds can cause contractures, leading to loss of use of the affected limb, e.g. 'foot drop' from a bleed into the calf muscle, or 'claw hand' from a bleed into the forearm. Bleeding into muscles can weaken them, rendering them unable to support joints and causing risk of joint damage. Muscle bleeding can also cause compression, leading on to nerve damage and permanent palsy. If blood is lost into a large muscle it can cause a drop in haemoglobin level, and if blood loss is rapid, hypovolaemic shock can occur. Pressure on surrounding tissues during a bleeding episode may lead to formation of a fibrous capsule around the lesion and cause a muscle cyst.

NURSING PRIORITIES AND MANAGEMENT: HAEMOPHILIA

The haemophilia centre

There is a network of haemophilia centres throughout the UK that aim to provide the best possible care and management of haemophilia patients. The support given by specialist staff alleviates the fears of families with new diagnoses, and the reassurance provided as an ongoing service for long-term patients is greatly valued. At the reference centre, potential patients are tested for haemophilia by using specific factor assays, new patients are registered and special medical cards issued. Some of the initial investigations include specialised laboratory tests which cannot be carried out in smaller centres. These reference centres provide a 24-h emergency service by a multidisciplinary team of consultant haematologist, specialist nurse, social worker, physiotherapist, dentist and orthopaedic surgeon. Patients are reviewed on a regular basis and lasting relationships are formed with the nursing staff, as this service is likely to be continued throughout the patients' entire lives (see Box 6.5).

Box 6.5 Aims of the haemophilia centre

- To provide a 24-h clinical service
- To coordinate services
- To act as a resource/reference centre for patients and families, family doctors, employers, schools, dentists and community services
- To advise on problems and to undertake specialised or general surgery
- To provide additional services, e.g. carrier detection and prenatal diagnosis
- To maintain links with schools, employment agencies, social and voluntary services

Home treatment

Many parents and adult patients are selected for home treatment after being taught and carefully supervised until becoming proficient in all aspects of care including performing venepuncture. This allows immediate treatment of bleeding episodes and consequently the need for less factor concentrate. Pain is minimised and hospitalisation often avoided. Self-management of treatment allows a degree of control over the disorder, raises self-confidence and increases independence. However, prompt attendance at the haemophilia centre is advised for more serious bleeding episodes, particularly of the head, neck, tongue, throat and eyes.

Genetic screening

Haemophilia is a sex-linked recessive disorder, the gene responsible being on the X chromosome. As males have only one X chromosome, affected males will pass the faulty gene to each of their daughters. All daughters will be carriers and are termed obligate carriers. These daughters have a 1 in 4 chance of producing a son with haemophilia and a 1 in 4 risk of having a carrier daughter. All sons of a man with haemophilia will be unaffected, as they inherit his Y chromosome which does not carry an affected gene. Fifty per cent of affected males carry a detectable alteration (an inversion in the DNA) in the haemophilia gene. Prenatal diagnosis is possible for carrier women by chorionic villus sampling at 10 weeks or amniocentesis at 14 weeks, to obtain material for genetic analysis by looking for a particular gene inversion in the DNA of the fetus. In families where there is no gene inversion, linked markers can be used in DNA-based family linkage analysis if there is a suitable family structure. Carrier testing is also available for other female relatives. These tests are offered by specialised genetic units (Bonthron et al 1997).

Outlook for the future

The problem of blood-borne viruses

In the past, freeze-dried factor concentrates were made from large donor pools with the disadvantage that if there was an infective agent present it would contaminate the whole batch. As a result, many patients receiving factor concentrates were exposed to hepatitis viruses, which caused some to be at risk of progressive liver disease. All who receive, or are likely to receive, factor concentrates are now immunised against hepatitis A and B.

The impressive advances in treatment were for a time overshadowed by the situation between 1979 and 1984 when large numbers of haemophiliacs were infected with the AIDS virus from the use of contaminated blood and blood products; many lives were lost. This radically altered the attitude of affected families and the community at large to haemophilia (Harper 1993). The stigmatisation which resulted should no longer now exist, as continuing research has enabled the artificial production of recombinant factor concentrates. These have all the advantages of plasma-derived factor concentrates but lack the disadvantages. At present, although costly, they are available. This is a positive step that gives hope that all patients with haemophilia will receive only safe recombinant factor concentrates in the future.

MYOTONIC DYSTROPHY

Myotonic dystrophy is a progressive neuromuscular disease. Myotonia is the name given to a particular type of muscular stiffness in which the muscle contracts normally but is unable to relax normally. Dystrophy is a weakening and wasting of the muscles. It is caused by an enlargement of a section of DNA within the myotonic dystrophy gene.

The muscles particularly involved are:

- the facial muscles
- the sternomastoid muscles
- the distal limb muscles.

Involvement of other body systems is common. Associated problems may include:

- cataracts
- hormonal problems
- cardiac problems
- gastrointestinal tract involvement
- learning difficulties (in children with the congenital form)
- sleep disturbance
- anaesthesia risks
- auditory involvement.

The age of onset is variable but the majority of those who have the myotonic dystrophy gene show some symptoms by the time they reach adult life. It is important to be aware that it can occur in neonates and young children as the severe congenital form (Harper 1989). These cases are usually the offspring of an affected mother because the altered gene is more unstable in females.

There is great variation in severity: some people with the myotonic dystrophy gene can be so mildly affected that they are unaware of it, while others can have major problems. As inheritance is autosomal dominant, an affected individual of either sex has a 50% risk of passing the gene on to a child of either sex (see p. 198).

Other forms of progressive muscular dystrophies include:

- Duchenne muscular dystrophy — the severe, childhood, X-linked recessive form
- Becker muscular dystrophy — the less severe, adult, X-linked recessive form
- fascioscapulohumeral dystrophy — a less severe autosomal dominant form.

Prevalence

Myotonic dystrophy is no longer thought to be a rare disorder and is regarded as the most frequently occurring muscular dystrophy of adult life. Precise figures are not easy to find and are likely to be underestimations because of the variation of expression: 1 in 8000 has been suggested (Harper 1989).

New mutations are thought to be rare and it should be assumed that all cases have been transmitted unless there is positive evidence to the contrary.

PATHOPHYSIOLOGY

Characteristic changes in the muscle tissue of those with myotonic dystrophy can be seen on microscopic examination. It is likely that a defect in the muscle cell membrane is responsible for both the muscle wasting and the myotonia.

Electrical studies show a specific disturbance leading to failure of muscle relaxation. This seems also to point to the muscle cell membrane as the site of the problem (Harper 1989).

MEDICAL MANAGEMENT

Tests and investigations used to diagnose myotonic dystrophy are as follows:

Direct gene testing. The gene responsible for myotonic dystrophy has been identified. It lies on the long arm of chromosome 19 and has an interesting feature, a sequence of three bases, CTG, that is repeated a variable number of times in different individuals. Normal people may have between five and 37 copies of the repeat. Patients with myotonic dystrophy have between 50 and several thousand copies. This resembles the abnormal gene found in Huntington's disease, but in myotonic dystrophy the number of repeats is much greater. There is a rough correlation between the number of copies and the severity of the disorder, and several thousands of repeats are found in infants with the congenital form.

Physical examination will demonstrate the presence of muscle weakness. Patients are asked to grip an object firmly and then let go. If myotonia is present, there will be a delay of several seconds in relaxation of the muscle. Percussion of the tongue may show a persistent furrow.

Slit lamp examination is an important aid in the differentiation of atypical cases of myotonic dystrophy and in its detection in asymptomatic patients. The lens opacities have a characteristic refractile, multicoloured appearance when viewed through a slit lamp (Harper 1989).

Electroretinography is a sensitive method of detecting retinal changes when cataract obscures an ophthalmoscopic view.

Electrocardiography will detect cardiac abnormalities such as arrhythmias, conduction defects and varying degrees of heart block.

NURSING PRIORITIES AND MANAGEMENT: MYOTONIC DYSTROPHY

Major considerations

Management of complications

It is important that medical problems are diagnosed early and treated appropriately to prevent exacerbation and to avoid complications. This should be stressed both to those at risk and to those already affected. The severe degree of apathy characteristic of myotonic dystrophy can be a major obstacle to overcome and can be responsible for low attendance rates and lack of compliance with treatment.

Myotonic dystrophy affects a number of body systems and thus requires careful management both in day-to-day living and when particular medical problems arise. The nurse should be aware of the following points:

- Breathing exercises may help to combat the tendency to hypoventilation found in many patients with myotonic dystrophy. Postural drainage (see Fig. 6.6) will reduce the effect of bronchial aspiration of food and secretions.
- Below-knee calipers and toestrings or plastic moulded splints may help to control foot drop.
- Beta-adrenergic blockers and and calcium channel blockers, e.g. verapamil, have been used to control cardiac arrhythmia. The use of selected beta-adrenergic stimulants in the form of bronchodilator agents should be avoided because of the risk of arrhythmias.
- Cardiac pacemakers are inserted when there is evidence of conduction defects.
- Cataract surgery is necessary for many of those with myotonic dystrophy.
- Problems with anaesthesia usually arise because the surgeons and anaesthetists are unaware that the patient has a neuromuscular disorder. The wearing of a bracelet to alert people in case of accidents requiring surgery may save lives.
- Special obstetric care is necessary during pregnancy and delivery.

- A high-fibre diet will help to alleviate constipation. Laxatives may be necessary but liquid paraffin should be avoided because of the risk of bronchial aspiration.
- Sternomastoid weakness makes the use of headrests in cars imperative.

Psychological support

The diagnosis of a hereditary, slowly progressive muscle disorder of varying severity with associated abnormalities of other body systems can have a profound psychological effect upon a family.

Living with myotonic dystrophy is not easy either for those affected, who have little energy, little motivation, and can find daily living an overwhelming effort, or for their partners or offspring. To live with someone who has an expressionless face, a monotonous voice, a marked lack of enthusiasm and who keeps falling asleep may put a great strain on a relationship. The sympathy and understanding necessary for both partners may be in short supply.

Patient education

It is likely that several members of a family will be shown to have the myotonic dystrophy gene. Explanations will be sought for variations in the severity of the condition and for the apparently unrelated associated medical problems encountered. Although medical staff will relate the initial information to family members, many will ask the nurse for further explanation, advice and reassurance.

When giving information to family members, care must be taken to avoid causing excessive anxiety by giving the impression that everyone with the myotonic dystrophy gene will experience every complication seen in textbooks or information leaflets. As the cardiac muscle can be impaired, sudden death from myocardial infarction is a possibility but is by no means inevitable. Only a few of those affected will require wheelchairs, and removal of cataracts to restore sight is now a routine procedure with a high success rate.

In some areas, the Muscular Dystrophy Group, a charitable organisation, supplies a family care officer to advise families with muscular dystrophy who may have a wealth of knowledge about muscle conditions, including myotonic dystrophy, to pass on.

See Van Haastregt et al (1994).

HUNTINGTON'S DISEASE

Huntington's disease (HD), previously known as Huntington's chorea, is a progressive neurodegenerative disorder first described by George Huntington, an American physician, in 1872. Affected individuals in the later stages have severe involuntary movements, speech and swallowing difficulties, as well as emotional and psychiatric disturbances and dementia. It is an autosomal dominant condition caused by a gene abnormality on chromosome 4 and tends to progress slowly over 15–20 years. A common cause of death is aspiration pneumonia. The incidence in the UK varies beween 5 and 10 per 100 000 (Harper 1996).

PATHOPHYSIOLOGY

Cell death occurs in the region of the putamen and the caudate nuclei of the brain. Atrophy of the caudate nuclei can be demonstrated using computed tomography (CT scan) 5 or more years after symptoms have been present (Furtado & Suchowerski 1995).

Common presenting symptoms. Affected individuals present with physical, cognitive or emotional symptoms, or a combination of these. Those in the early stages of the disease may have symptoms so mild that they are unaware of them, such as restlessness, small involuntary movements of limbs or face, slight forgetfulness or mild depression. Those who do not seek help until the later stages may by then have striking involuntary movements. These very high amplitude movements are termed choreic, meaning dance, and are sudden, quick, unintended movements of almost any part of the body which become more marked if the patient is under additional stress. Voluntary movements become clumsy and slow, response time is delayed and the ability to perform fine hand movements accurately is lost. Gait becomes impaired with slow, short, widely based steps performed irregularly. There may be marked depressive illness, decreased cognitive speed, personality changes and inability to make reasonable judgements, all of which cause problems for those in employment. It may be only when looking back after a diagnosis that relatives recall changes which occurred some years previously but were not viewed as significant. It is common for those with obvious signs, or those who have been diagnosed, to deny symptoms (see Box 6.6).

MEDICAL MANAGEMENT

Noticeable symptoms of Huntington's disease usually appear from 40 to 50 years of age (Tibben et al 1993). It is possible for onset to be earlier or later and there is also a rare childhood form. Most studies show a mean age of onset of between 35 and 44 years, but the concept of a 'zone of onset' which spans several years rather than a definitive point of onset is useful (Harper 1996).

Due to its insidious nature, affected individuals may be several years into the disease before HD is thought of, especially if there is no prior knowledge of family history of the disease. It is difficult to confirm the diagnosis on signs and symptoms, because many of these can be due to other causes and are not obvious on neurological examination. Research has shown that early symptoms can be detected by specific neuropsychometric evaluation and this can be a helpful assessment for those having relationship difficulties at work or home. Previously, a diagnosis of HD was considered only with a definite family history of the illness in addition to signs and

Box 6.6 Common symptoms of Huntington's disease

Physical
- Involuntary movements of arms and legs
- Slurring of speech
- Unsteady gait
- Swallowing difficulties
- Difficulty with coordination

Cognitive
- Short-term memory loss
- Difficulty in carrying out two tasks at once
- Loss of drive and initiative
- Loss of self-awareness

Emotional
- Depression
- Irritability
- Apathy
- Personality change
- Lack of inhibition

symptoms, but could be confirmed only by postmortem examination of the brain. Since the discovery of the HD gene in 1993, a diagnosis can be made with a blood test. A diagnosis of HD has an impact on every member of a family. Affected individuals have to cope with a prolonged debilitating illness, partners may become long-term carers, all children have a 50% chance of developing the illness themselves and grandchildren are at 25% risk.

Integrated care pathways, i.e. structured patient records designed to promote standardisation of diagnosis, screening and management of specific conditions, are being used for a number of illnesses in some UK hospitals. These are being developed in Scotland for certain genetic diseases (Campbell et al 1998). The HD care pathway recommends referral to a multidisciplinary team, with speech therapist, physiotherapist, dietician, social worker and psychologist, who will support the HD family through the progression of the disease. A full range of supportive nursing and social care can improve the patient's situation dramatically (Skirton & Glendinning 1997).

Investigations. Since 1993, direct gene testing has been available at genetic centres throughout the UK. The mutated HD gene is expanded because it contains an excess number of trinucleotide repeats, making it unstable and causing it to malfunction. Previously, DNA-based family linkage analysis was used, but with this technique testing was not possible for all families. Three categories of testing can now be offered: diagnostic, pre-symptomatic and prenatal testing.

Diagnostic testing for HD. This is carried out by a direct gene test to confirm whether an individual who appears to be showing symptoms of HD has the enlarged HD gene. The test should only be carried out with informed consent, with the patient's relatives having been informed of the implications to other family members should the test confirm the diagnosis of HD.

Pre-symptomatic testing. This test is available to all asymptomatic individuals over 18 years of age at high risk of having inherited the HD gene and is only carried out in clinical genetic units. Those who elect to have a pre-symptomatic test (PST) must follow a strict test protocol produced from a set of guidelines which recommend several interviews with genetic staff to discuss the advantages and disadvantages of testing before a blood sample is taken. From start to finish, the test programme normally takes a minimum of 3 months, which ensures that decisions about testing and the implications of an unfavourable result are not taken lightly (see Case History 6.5). A significant number of test candidates decide not to continue with testing, although the majority proceed and get a result (Tibben et al 1993). Follow-up support is offered by the genetic team. The knowledge gained from HD testing experience has been used as a model for methods of dealing with other adult onset diseases.

Antenatal testing. A gene-positive parent can have an antenatal direct gene test performed via CVS or amniocentesis on a fetus. It must be understood that if a gene-positive pregnancy were to be allowed to continue to full term, a pre-symptomatic test would have been carried out without the permission of that baby. An antenatal exclusion test is available for those at 50% risk who wish to have a baby who does not carry the HD gene, but who do not want to know their own HD status. DNA samples are needed from both parents and from both grandparents on the HD side of the family. Family linkage analysis is used to determine the source of the gene which the fetus has inherited from its 'at risk' parent. If the fetus has inherited a gene from the grandparent who does not come from an HD family, it is free of risk and the pregnancy is continued. If it inherits a gene from the grandparent with HD, it is at 50% risk, like its 'at risk' parent (we do not identify whether it is the grandparent's HD gene or the normal gene), and the pregnancy can be terminated. The timing of this test is crucial and should be discussed with a geneticist prior to pregnancy or soon after confirmation.

Case History 6.5 J

J is 33 years old. Her father suffers from HD and is cared for in a hospital for the chronically ill. Her younger sister, P, has minimal signs of the disease and the diagnosis has been confirmed by direct gene testing which shows that she is carrying the HD gene. J has asked her general practitioner if she can be referred for genetic counselling. J is seen at the genetic department and is given information on the HD pre-symptomatic test protocol. She decides to go ahead with the test programme and understands that it involves four counselling sessions with staff in the genetic unit, including one with a specialist psychiatrist who will assess her coping mechanisms. Three months later, at the end of the programme, she is still sure that she wants a test because, for her, the uncertainty of being at risk of HD is even worse than knowing for certain that she has inherited the altered gene and therefore will definitely develop HD at some time in the future.

Treatment. There is no medication which can halt or cure HD, but scientists are hopeful that research into what causes the brain cells to die will be the next step in the search to find a cure. It is possible to treat symptoms such as depression, psychosis or emotional problems. The movement disorder is more difficult to manage using drugs because of side-effects. The Scottish Huntington's Association (SHA) and the Huntington's Disease Association (HDA) produce information booklets giving advice on pharmacological and non-pharmacological interventions. There are no known medications which treat the cognitive deterioration caused by the effects of brain cell death.

NURSING PRIORITIES AND MANAGEMENT: HUNTINGTON'S DISEASE

Major considerations

General care and personal hygiene

To ensure the best quality of life, use should be made of the multidisciplinary team. Nurses with skills in both adult and mental health nursing can play a major role in the care of the HD patient and will complement each other's skills. In the latter stages, help is needed with skin care and oral hygiene, with trimming of finger and toenails, grooming and styling of hair, applying make-up, choosing and taking care of clothes, dressing and toileting. Many patients lose their ability to self-assess and make judgements about personal appearance. Efforts can be made to find out what they were like when well and to encourage them to look attractive, enjoy life and to feel good about themselves.

Many HD patients smoke, but because of their involuntary movements they have difficulty using ashtrays and may drop lighted cigarettes. Smoking aids will help prevent burning accidents, attractive clothes protectors worn at mealtimes keep clothing clean for longer, and easily laundered clothing is less of a problem for carers if frequent changes are necessary. Help is needed with cleaning teeth and regular dental checks will ensure that loose teeth are dealt with promptly, particularly if there is difficulty in swallowing.

Incontinence tends to be the result of the inability to reach the toilet in time and the difficulty in adjusting clothing or undoing buttons and zips rather than loss of control. However, other causes, such as infection, should be considered. Protective underwear is available and an incontinence advisor should be consulted wherever possible.

If professional carers view HD patients as valued individuals whose dignity and autonomy must be respected and who still have basic rights and responsibilities with interpersonal relationships, relatives observing them caring for their loved one and seeing proactive methods of care being used may be helped to look upon the situation more positively (Chiu 1991). Children of affected individuals not only have the responsibility of caring, but also carry the additional stress of knowing that there is a high risk of them suffering the same fate. If professionals can promote care of HD patients as a challenging but rewarding experience, relatives at risk may feel more secure knowing that sensitive care and management are possible. The SHA and the HDA have a network of advisors, many with a nursing background, who offer support, advice, education and information.

Communication

Speech becomes slurred in the later stages, causing difficulty in communication which is extremely distressing for both patients and carers (France 1993). Speech and language therapists should be involved from early on in the disease process to show affected individuals and carers exercises which help to maintain intelligible speech. Speech deterioration can be monitored and the suggestion of a communication aid made. No single communication aid has been shown to be helpful for all HD patients, and therefore a variety should be tried. It is important to ask them to repeat words slowly and to listen carefully with no distractions. Speech is more difficult to understand if patients are anxious, in a new environment or meeting new people, and although they may not initiate a conversation, they enjoy being included. As time must be given for them first to absorb information and then to answer, only one question should be asked at a time.

Swallowing

Many in the middle to late stages of the disease experience difficulty with swallowing which is alarming for both carer and patient. A speech and language therapist can carry out a swallowing assessment and a video fluoroscopy in order to advise patients and carers about the consistency of food and to minimise swallowing problems. Advice can be given on positioning for eating and on the need for thickeners and how to use them.

Diet

Many lose weight in the early stages of the disease and require extra calories despite eating a well balanced diet. Some have an insatiable appetite and yet continue to lose weight. Dieticians can offer samples for tasting and advise family doctors about prescribing dietary supplements which enable large amounts of calories to be consumed in small volumes. This is particularly helpful if swallowing is a problem. Dieticians can show carers how to produce an appealing meal which is safe to eat. When patients are no longer able to feed themselves, the issue of help with feeding needs to be discussed sensitively and assistance given. However, some degree of independence can be maintained by allowing patients to feed themselves with finger-buffet-type snacks.

Mobility

A physiotherapist should be involved to encourage mobility and promote confidence about moving around. Wide spaces are needed to accommodate the ataxic gait and to prevent patients from constantly bumping into walls and furniture. Nurses can learn a basic mobility programme to use in the ward.

The occupational therapist can provide aids for daily living such as smoking aids, toilet seating, bath seating and non-slip matting, and in addition will have a vital role in the seating assessment of HD patients whose constant movements do not allow them to sit still. There are many excellent chairs on the market which cater for different needs, however it is essential to have a chair for a trial period before making a definite order. Seating assessment should also include provision of a safe eating position, and patients with swallowing difficulties should never be allowed to lie down for at least 20 minutes after eating or drinking.

Social and family support

Social work input at an early stage should ensure that families are receiving all services and financial benefits available. The NHS and Community Care Act of 1990 was designed to allow more ill and disabled patients to live at home. It is possible for care packages to be put together which provide help for patients and carers and allow home life to be extended. The cognitive impairment seen is similar to many early-onset dementias and includes lack of concentration, difficulties with memory, temper outburst, difficulty in initiating action, poor road sense and inability to carry out more than one task at a time. However, the ability to recognise friends and family is never lost, which is of great comfort to relatives. If long-term care is being considered, professional support during decision-making is helpful and financial assistance may be needed from the social work department.

CANCER GENETICS

The majority of human cancers have both sporadic and genetic components. The latter may be due to inherited changes in the genes directly involved in normal cellular growth and proliferation or to genetic changes resulting in the increased possibility of a mutation in the genes related to cell growth. The formation of a human cancer is a multistep process and is the result of a series of mutations in a single cell (see Ch. 31). Genes with a positive effect on growth and proliferation of cells are known as oncogenes, and those with a negative effect on growth and proliferation of cells are known as tumour suppressor genes or anti-oncogenes. Activation of oncogenes and inactivation of tumour suppressor genes are both important in the formation of the malignant cell (Hodgson & Maher 1993).

The aims of cancer genetics are:

- the identification of a subgroup of the population who are at significantly increased risk of developing cancer
- reduction of mortality from the common cancers (breast, ovarian, colorectal) by appropriate screening or surgery for those at high risk
- reassurance and discharge from screening for those not at increased risk compared with the general population.

Factors which suggest a predisposition to cancer are:

- a family history with an autosomal dominant pattern of inheritance on one side of the family of the same cancers or cancers with a known association, e.g. breast and ovarian (familial clustering is not conclusive as it can result from a shared environment)
- onset of cancer at a young age (under 50 years)
- the presence of multiple primary tumours or bilateral tumours
- two or more rare cancers in the same family
- the detection of an identifiable gene fault in a tumour of an affected family member.

Familial breast cancer

It is believed that dominantly inherited genes are responsible for about 5–10% of breast cancers and up to 25% of those diagnosed at under 30 years (Claus et al 1991). The BRCA1 gene was cloned in 1994 (Futreal et al 1994) and is thought to account for 2% of all breast cancers and to be present in most breast and/or ovarian cancer families. Over 100 different mutations have been identified so far. The overall risk of breast cancer for those with a BRCA1 mutation is thought to be 85% by 70 years, and of ovarian cancer to be 63% by 70 years. There is also an increased risk of colon and prostate cancer. The BRCA2 gene has also been identified and more genes are being searched for. It is thought that BRCA2 is present in families who have a male member with breast cancer.

Screening for early detection

Annual mammography can be offered to women over 35 and under 50 years whose family history fits the criteria which suggest they are at increased risk. However, the younger the woman is, the more difficult it is to detect a tumour at an early stage and no form of screening is ever 100% effective. The National Screening Programme starts at 50 years for all women (See Ch. 7).

Criteria for referral to a familial breast cancer clinic for screening and advice are:

- one first-degree relative who developed breast cancer at under 40 years
- two first- or second-degree relatives on the same side of the family who developed breast cancer at under 60 years or with ovarian cancer
- three first- or second-degree relatives on the same side of the family with breast or ovarian cancer at any age
- one first-degree relative with breast cancer in both breasts
- one first-degree male relative with breast cancer.

The alternative choice — prophylactic surgery

Women who have, or are likely to have, gene mutations may elect for prophylactic mastectomies. This may seem a drastic course of action, but it is acceptable to some women who have seen a number of their relatives suffer from breast cancer.

Some personal experiences are described in Marteau & Richards (1996).

It must be remembered that it is not possible to remove every single cell of breast tissue, and therefore a slight residual risk of cancer will remain.

Aspects for discussion regarding this are (Eeles 1996):

- which surgical technique should be used — subcutaneous or total mastectomy
- whether surgery can remove enough breast tissue to prevent development of invasive breast cancer
- how psychological complications can be minimised.

Familial ovarian cancer

Screening

This can be offered to women over 25 years of age whose family history fits the criteria which suggest they are at increased risk. It takes the form of annual gynaecological examinations, ultrasound scans of the ovaries and measurements of the blood level of an enzyme called CA125. Screening has not yet been proven to be effective and should be carried out as a research programme which evaluates the results.

Criteria for referral to a familial ovarian cancer clinic for screening and advice are:

- two first-degree relatives with ovarian cancer on the same side of the family
- one first-degree relative with ovarian cancer and one first-degree relative who developed breast cancer under the age of 50
- one first-degree relative with ovarian cancer and two first- or second-degree relatives who developed breast cancer under the age of 60
- members of a family where a recognised breast/ovarian cancer gene fault has been identified.

Surgical intervention for ovarian cancer

Prophylactic oophorectomy is considered by proven gene carriers and by some at high risk who have completed their family. Gynaecologists may be reluctant to operate on women under 35 years. Hormone replacement therapy (HRT) is recommended for premenopausal women to reduce side-effects and mortality and morbidity from cardiovascular disease, but opinions differ as to the best regimen (see Ch. 7). There have been a few reports of ovarian-type cancers in women who have had prophylactic oophorectomy, and therefore a small residual risk remains after this procedure (Eeles 1996).

Hereditary non-polyposis cancer of the colon (HNPCC)

Approximately 10–15% of colorectal cancer is due to HNPCC. The younger the individual is when the bowel cancer develops, the more likely it is to be HNPCC. At under 30 years of age, it will almost definitely be HNPCC, and at under 40 there is a good chance it could be HNPCC. The risk also increases with the number of close relatives with bowel cancer. There is a known association with endometrial and ovarian cancer. There are at least four different genes implicated in HNPCC. Individuals with an HNPCC mutation are believed to have a high risk of bowel cancer, with a greater risk in men. For women with HNPCC mutations, the risk of uterine cancer has been shown to be greater than that of bowel cancer (Dunlop et al 1997). Two-yearly colonoscopic examination, with removal of polyps or early surgery as soon as cancer is detected, has been shown to be effective in reducing mortality and morbidity (see Ch. 4).

Criteria for referral to a family history clinic for screening and advice on HNPCC are:

- one relative with colon cancer diagnosed under 45 years
- two first-degree relatives on the same side of the family with bowel cancer.

Screening for those at high risk or proven HNPCC gene carriers

Colonoscopic screening has been shown to be very effective and should start at 25 years and be repeated 2- to 5-yearly. Endometrial screening by annual endometrial biopsy and ultrasound scanning is also advised for women who have the HNPCC gene.

Familial adenomatous polyposis coli (FAPC)

This is a rarer autosomal dominant condition, characterised by the presence of hundreds or thousands of polyps, some of which will eventually become cancerous, which can usually be detected at under 20 years. Annual colonoscopy and eventually prophylactic colectomy are indicated. It can also present in the upper gastrointestinal tract. Direct gene testing is now possible in many families.

Direct gene testing for breast, ovarian or colorectal cancer

This is, at present, scientifically feasible for only a very few large families who have been involved in research, but availability and demand will grow. Testing for cancer susceptibility may on the surface seem an attractive option but requires a great deal of thought. Knowledge of greatly increased risk of cancer may cause great anxiety for certain personalities. People want a test to reassure them that all is well and are not necessarily prepared for an adverse result. There should always be several counselling sessions before a test is performed, and the disadvantages of screening procedures, such as the risk of perforation of the bowel, should be explained (Biesecker 1997).

For further information on cancer genetics, see Williams (1997).

CONCLUSION

The use of scientific knowledge raises ethical and moral problems, particularly in the field of human genetics, where every advance has an enormous potential for good and evil. Recognition of the destructive potential of genetic engineering has prompted the imposition of strict controls on biotechnology and genetic research. This chapter has presented an outline of current developments in genetics and molecular biology and has outlined nursing involvement in genetic counselling and care of patients with genetic disorders. Although progress is rapid, there is much work to be done before the aims of The Human Genome Project can be achieved. It is essential that nurses keep themselves informed. As public awareness grows and families look for informed discussion, nurses involved in every branch of health care will need to develop an awareness of genetic influences in health and disease and of achievements in genetic science (Box 6.7).

Box 6.7 A brief overview of some of the achievements in genetic science

- Production of drugs and chemicals for treatment of disease
- Research leading to a better understanding of common diseases and their genetic component and of rare classic genetic disorders
- Prenatal diagnosis of carriers of genetic disorders
- Methods of antenatal testing so that parents have the choice of termination or acceptance of pregnancy
- Genetic screening to detect correctable genetic deficiencies, e.g. phenylketonuria
- DNA fingerprinting
- Testing for adult-onset genetic disorders
- Gene therapy to modify cells to either correct or prevent genetic disease
- Genetically engineered microbes and biological aberrations that can be used in mass environmental or human destruction

Discussion of a few classic genetic disorders has emphasised the importance of nursing intervention, ranging from non-directive counselling and support from specialist nurses to input from nurses in every branch, who will be involved in recognition, treatment, referral and support to promote optimal levels of health.

6.2 Refer to the list of achievements in genetic science in Box 6.7 and decide which involve major ethical issues. Discuss these with your colleagues.

REFERENCES

Biesecker B B 1997 Genetic testing for cancer predispositions. Cancer Nursing 20(4): 285–296

Bonthron D, Fitzpatrick D, Porteous M, Trainer A 1997 Clinical genetics – a case-based approach. WB Saunders, Philadelphia

British Medical Association 1992 Our genetic future: the science and ethics of genetic technology. Oxford University Press, Oxford

Campbell H, Hotchkiss R, Bradshaw N, Porteous M 1998 Integrated care pathways. British Medical Journal 316(7125): 133–137

Chiu E 1991 Caring for persons with Huntington's disease. Huntington's Disease Society of America, New York

Clarke A 1991 Is non-directive counselling possible? The Lancet 338(8773): 998–1001

Claus E B, Risch N, Thompson W D 1991 Genetic analysis of breast cancer in the cancer and steroid hormone study. American Journal of Human Genetics 48(2): 232–241

Dodge J A, Brock D J H, Widdicombe J H 1993 Cystic fibrosis – current topics. John Wiley, Chichester

Dunlop M D, Farrington S M, Carothers A D et al 1997 Cancer risk associated with germline DNA mismatch repair gene mutations. Human Molecular Genetics 6(1): 105–110

Eeles R (ed) 1996 Genetic predisposition to cancer. Chapman and Hall, London

Farnish S 1988 A developing role in genetic counselling. Journal of Medical Genetics 25: 392–395

France J K 1993 Huntington's disease: helping the patient retain function. American Journal of Nursing 93(8): 62–64

Furtado S, Suchowerski O 1995 Huntington's disease: recent advances in diagnosis and management. Canadian Journal of Neurological Sciences 22: 5–12

Futreal P A et al 1994 BRCA1 mutations in primary breast and ovarian carcinomas. Science 266(5183): 120–122

Greener M 1993 Gene therapy: the dawn of a revolution. Professional Nurse 8(12): 784–787

Harper P 1989 Myotonic dystrophy. WB Saunders, London

Harper P 1993 Practical genetic counselling, 4th edn. Butterworth-Heinemann, Oxford

Harper P 1996 Huntington's disease, 2nd edn. Harcourt Brace, London

Harris A, Super M 1991 Cystic fibrosis – the facts. Oxford University Press, Oxford

Hodgson S, Maher E 1993 A practical guide to human cancer genetics. Cambridge University Press, Cambridge

Koch C, Lang S 1995 Other organ systems. In: Hodson M, Geddes D (eds) Cystic fibrosis. Chapman and Hall, London

Livingston J, Axton R A, Gilfillan A et al 1994 Antenatal screening for cystic fibrosis; a trial of the couple model. British Medical Journal 308: 1459–1462

Mennie M, Compton M, Gilfillan A et al 1993 Prenatal screening for cystic fibrosis: psychological effects on carriers and their partners. Journal of Medical Genetics 30: 543–548

Pennisi E, Williams N 1997 Will Dolly send in the clones? Science 275(5305): 1415–1416

Skirton H, Barnes C, Curtis G, Walford-Moore J 1997 The role and practice of the genetic nurse: report of the AGNC Working Party. Journal of Medical Genetics 34(12): 141–147

Skirton H, Glendinning N 1997 Using research to develop care for patients with Huntington's disease. British Journal of Nursing 6(2): 83–90

Tibben A, Frets P G, van de Kamp J J et al 1993 Presymptomatic DNA testing for Huntington's disease: pre-test attitudes and expectations of applicants and their partners in the Dutch programme. American Journal of Medical Genetics 48(1): 10–16

Westaby D 1995 Liver and biliary disease. In: Hodson M, Geddes D (eds) Cystic fibrosis. Chapman and Hall, London

White-van Mourik M, Connor J M, Ferguson-Smith M A 1992 The psychosocial sequellae of a second-trimester termination of pregnancy for foetal abnormality. Prenatal Diagnosis 12: 189–204

FURTHER READING

Beischer N A 1997 Obstetrics and the newborn, 2nd edn. WB Saunders, London

Clarke A 1994 Genetic counselling – practice and principles. Routledge, London

Connor S 1993 Gene found for Huntington's chorea. British Medical Journal 306(6882): 878

Crauford D, Tyler A 1992 Predictive testing for Huntington's disease: protocol of The Huntington's Disease Prediction Consortium. Journal of Medical Genetics 29: 915–918

Emery A 1994 Muscular dystrophy – the facts. Oxford University Press, Oxford

Guilbert P, Cheater F 1990 Health visitors awareness and perception of clinical genetic services. Journal of Medical Genetics 27(8): 508–511

Harper P, Clarke A 1997 Genetics, society and clinical practice. Bios Scientific Publications

Harris H, Scotcher D, Hartley N, Wallace A, Crawford D, Harris R 1993 Cystic fibrosis carrier testing in early pregnancy by general practitioners. British Medical Journal 306(6892): 1580–1583

Harris A, Super M 1991 Cystic fibrosis – the facts. Oxford University Press, Oxford

Kingston H 1994 ABC of clinical genetics. British Medical Journal, London

Korf B 1996 Human genetics – a problem-based approach. Blackwell Science, Oxford

Marteau T, Drake H, Bobrow M 1994 Counselling following diagnosis of fetal abnormality: the differing approaches of obstetricians, clinical geneticists and genetic nurses. Journal of Medical Genetics 31: 864–867

Marteau T, Richards M (eds) 1996 The new genetics: a users' guide. Cambridge University Press, Cambridge

Morris J 1995 Cost effectiveness of antenatal screening for cystic fibrosis. British Medical Journal 311: 1460–1464

Muscular Dystrophy Group 1994 Fact sheet CMY1 Mar.94 1/5. Muscular Dystrophy Group, London

Peters K F, Hadley D 1997 The Human Genome Project. Cancer Nursing 20(1): 62–75

Proud J 1995 Ethics and obstetric ultrasound. British Journal of Midwifery 3(2): 79–82

Van Haastregt J C, de Whitte L P, Terpstra S J et al 1994 Membership of a patient organisation and well-being. Patient Education and Counselling 24: 135–148

Williams J K 1997 Principles of genetics and cancer. Seminars in Oncology Nursing 13(2): 68–73

USEFUL ADDRESSES

Association of Cystic Fibrosis Adults (UK)
Alexandra House
5 Blyth Road
Bromley
Kent
BR1 3RS

Contact a Family
The CaF Directory of Specific Conditions and Rare Syndromes in Children with their Family Support Networks
170 Tottenham Court Road
London
W1P 0HA

Down's Syndrome Association
153–155 Mitcham Road
London
SW17 9BG

Haemophilia Society
123 Westminster Bridge Road
London
SE1 7HR

Huntington's Disease Association
108 Battersea High Street
London
SW11 3HP

Scottish Huntington's Disease Association
Thistle House
61 Main Road
Elderslie
PA5 9BA

Muscular Dystrophy Group of Great Britain and Northern Ireland
35 Macaulay Road
London
SW4 0QP

The Muscular Dystrophy Group
7–11 Prescott Place
London
SW4 6BS

Association of Genetic Nurses and Counsellors
Ruth Cole
Clinical Genetics Unit
Birmingham Woman's Hospital
Edgbaston
Birmingham
B15 2TG

THE REPRODUCTIVE SYSTEMS AND THE BREAST

7

Anne C. H. McQueen
(Part 1 The reproductive systems)
Karen L. Burnet
(Part 2 The breast)

PART 1
THE REPRODUCTIVE SYSTEMS

INTRODUCTION

Any threat to an individual's reproductive capacity affects that person's body image, self-esteem and gender identity. Since they are influenced by personal attitudes, social customs and cultural background, different people respond differently to such a threat.

Reproduction of the human species involves a complex series of events affected by physical and psychological capacities and the state of health. One's attitude towards sexual reproduction, underlying beliefs held and feelings experienced are influenced by cultural norms, current social values, religious background, lifestyle and parental and peer pressure.

A raised awareness of the human immunodeficiency virus (HIV) and increased incidence of acquired immune deficiency syndrome (AIDS) have stimulated greater discussion about sexual practices and ways of decreasing the incidence of sexually transmitted diseases (STDs). Although human sexual behaviour is now more openly debated in the media, there is still a hesitancy to discuss the subject on a personal level, even within health care settings (Thurlow 1992).

For some people, having their own children and raising a family are perceived as important and enjoyable parts of their role in life. For others, these things are undesirable or inconsequential. For yet others, they may be desirable but unobtainable, giving rise to much sadness and regret.

While some couples desperately want children, others try to prevent pregnancy and childbirth. Thus the demands of society can help to shape medical science, but this is also influenced by the economic situation, available technology and political ideology of the time (Allan & Jolley 1982, Stacey 1988).

The ethos of disease prevention is favoured in health care. Screening for early detection and treatment is advisable where feasible, but in some cases disease is far advanced before diagnosis. While scientific advances are made and more sophisticated technology becomes available, there are real economic constraints on practical therapeutics, and choices must be made when resources are not available for general clinical application. In addition, the accelerated progress of science and technology creates ethical issues that society has not had time to debate and fully explore as a basis for action and future directions in health care. The Joint Report of the Council of Scientific Affairs and the Council on Medical Service (1992) recognises that the proliferation of health care technology, accompanied by the need for cost containment, calls for thorough evaluation of new technologies in terms of safety and effectiveness for clinical use.

Advances, however, have allowed patients a shorter stay in hospital, and to be treated as day patients or outpatients. This inevitably has implications for nursing and patient care following hospital treatment. Nurses are continually called upon to adapt to the dynamic nature of nursing in a society of flux.

This chapter presents an overview of the anatomy and physiology of the female reproductive system and addresses common disorders of the reproductive organs.

NB The anatomy and physiology of the male reproductive system appear in Chapter 8.

ANATOMY AND PHYSIOLOGY OF THE FEMALE REPRODUCTIVE SYSTEM

The primary function of the reproductive system is the propagation or continuation of the human species. Sexual drive and anticipated pleasure help to meet the reproductive need. The female reproductive system is structured to produce gametes (ova or eggs), to receive the male penis during sexual intercourse and to facilitate the passage of sperm. It accommodates and promotes the growth of the embryo before birth and feeds the newborn infant.

These complex functions are maintained by the following structures (see Figs 7.1 and 7.2):

- the internal organs
  —the ovaries
  —the uterus
  —the uterine (fallopian) tubes (or oviducts)
  —the vagina.

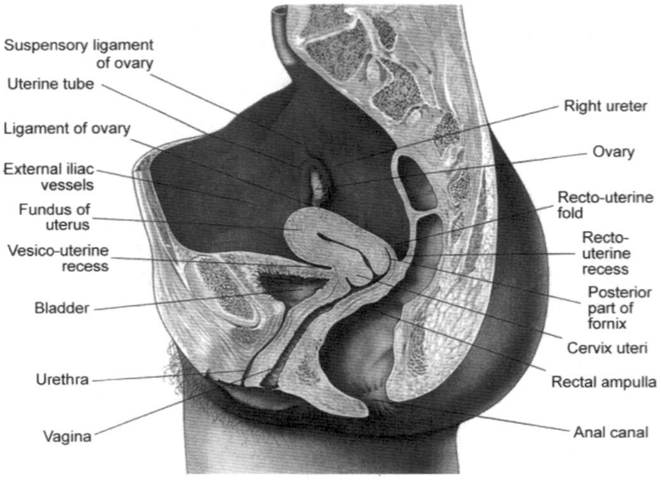

Fig. 7.1 The relationships of the female reproductive organs: sagittal section. (Reproduced with kind permission from Wilson & Waugh 1996.)

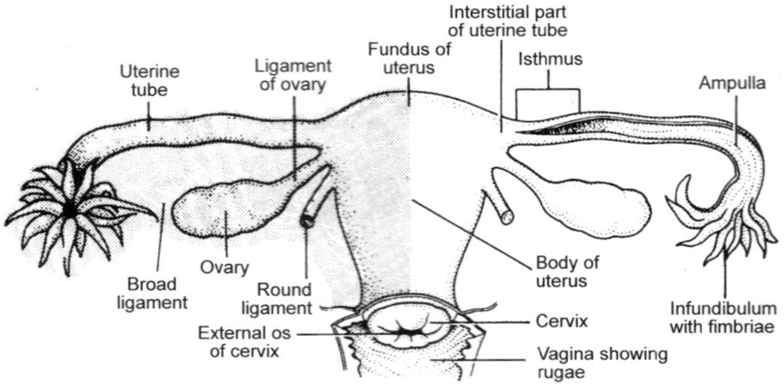

Fig. 7.2 The organs of the female reproductive system and attachments. (Reproduced with kind permission from Wilson & Waugh 1996.)

- the external organs
  —the vulva
  —the mammary glands or breasts.

The ovaries

Women have two ovaries, which are the size and shape of large almonds, one on either side of the uterus.

The surface of the ovary consists of a single layer of germinal epithelium surrounding connective tissue that forms the stroma of the ovarian cortex and medulla. The ovarian follicles develop in the cortex. A woman is born with approximately 100 000 follicles, although the number of follicles may fall to approximately 30 000 by adolescence. Each follicle contains an immature ovum known as an oocyte. The medulla, in the centre of the ovary, consists of fibrous connective tissue, blood vessels and nerves.

The production of ova and hormones

The ovary has two functions:

- ovum production
- internal secretion of hormones.

Ovum production. The ovarian cycle begins at around 12–13 years of age. Follicles begin to mature under the influence of the follicle-stimulating hormone (FSH) and luteinising hormone (LH), released by the anterior pituitary gland. During the cycle, follicles can pass through five stages (see Fig. 7.3):

- *primary follicle* — each oocyte is surrounded by a thin layer of epithelial cells
- *developing follicle* — the follicular epithelium proliferates, the oocyte moves to a side position, and a fluid-filled cavity develops within the epithelium
- *mature (Graafian) follicle* — the follicle reaches its maximum size
- *corpus luteum* — a yellow mass which forms in the ovarian follicle after ovulation
- *corpus albicans* — scar tissue on the surface of the ovary when the degenerated corpus luteum atrophies.

The maturing follicle is surrounded by a layer of ovarian tissue, known as the theca. Several follicles may develop together but only one will mature fully, while the others regress. The mature follicle

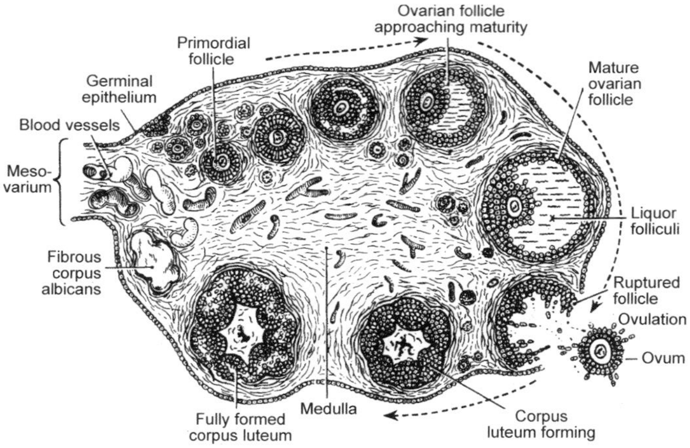

Fig. 7.3 Sequence of development of the ovarian cycle. (Reproduced with kind permission from Wilson & Waugh 1996.)

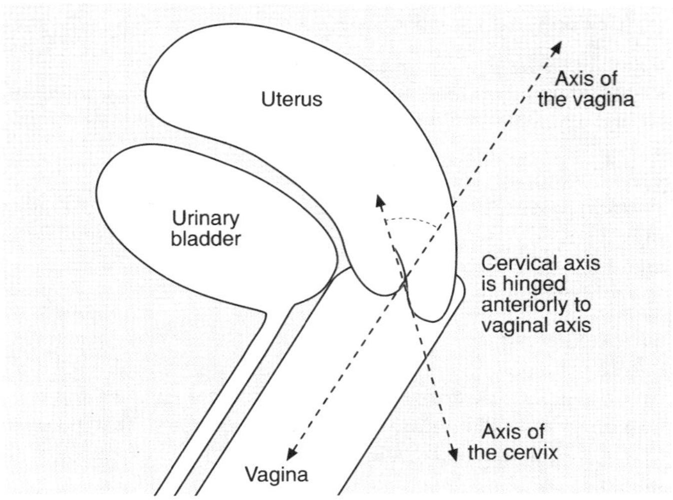

Fig. 7.4 The anteverted position of the uterus.

(Graafian follicle) ruptures at the surface of the ovary and discharges the ovum and fluid into the peritoneal cavity. This process is called 'ovulation'.

Wafting movements of the finger-like ends of the uterine tubes assist the transfer of the ovum into the tube (oviduct). It is thought that fertilisation of the ovum usually occurs in the ampulla of the uterine tube.

The ruptured follicle contracts around leaked blood after discharging the ovum. The epithelial cells (granulosa) multiply and the corpus luteum is formed under the influence of LH, secreted by the anterior pituitary gland. The corpus luteum synthesises steroid sex hormones for at least 8–10 days. If the ovum is not fertilised, the corpus luteum degenerates, stops its hormone production and forms scar tissue called the 'corpus albicans' near the surface of the ovary. If the ovum is fertilised, the corpus luteum continues to develop, increasing its size and hormone production for about 2 months.

Secretion of hormones. The production of sex hormones is influenced by the hypothalamus of the brain. The hypothalamus produces gonadotrophin-releasing hormone, which stimulates the anterior pituitary gland to release FSH and LH. FSH stimulates the initial development of ovarian follicles and their secretion of oestrogen. LH stimulates further development of the ovarian follicles, initiates ovulation and incites production of ovarian hormones. FSH and LH control the secretion of two types of ovarian steroid hormones: oestrogens and progestogens.

The oestrogens. Oestrogens have three main functions:

- development and maintenance of female reproductive structures
- control of fluid and electrolyte balance
- increase of protein anabolism.

The compound secreted by the theca interna cells of the developing follicle is oestradiol, and its metabolite or waste product is oestriol. Many other oestrogens may be identified in the urine. Oestradiol is also produced by theca interna cells that invade the corpus luteum.

The progestogens. The main compound of this group is progesterone. It is produced by the luteinised granulosa cells of the corpus luteum. The metabolite of progesterone is pregnanediol, which is also excreted in the urine.

The uterus (see Figs 7.1 and 7.2)

The uterus is a pear-shaped organ approximately 7.5 cm long. It has three main parts:

- the fundus
- the body
- the cervix.

The uterine tubes enter the uterus at its upper outer angles or cornua. The body of the uterus narrows towards the cervix and this area is known as the isthmus. The cavity of the uterus connects with the cervical canal at the internal os. The cervical canal opens into the vagina via the external os. The cervix occupies the lower third of the uterus and half of the cervix projects into the vagina. The uterus normally lies in an antiverted position, almost at right angles to the vagina (see Figs 7.1 and 7.4).

Structure

The uterus has three coats:

- endometrium — mucous lining
- myometrium — smooth muscle
- parietal peritoneum — serous coat.

Endometrium. This is the tissue lining the uterus. This mucosa is continuous with the vagina and the uterine tubes. There are three layers of endometrial tissues:

- the compact surface layer — partially ciliated, simple columnar epithelium (stratum compactum)
- the spongy middle layer — composed of loose connective tissue and glands (stratum spongiosum)
- the dense, inner layer — responsible for the regeneration of the endometrium after menstruation (stratum basale).

During menstruation the compact and spongy layers slough away from the inner layer. The thickness of the endometrium varies from 0.5 mm just after menstrual flow to about 5 mm near the end of the endometrial cycle.

Myometrium. The myometrium is formed from three layers of muscle fibres that extend in all directions:

- the outer layer of longitudinal fibres
- the intermediate layer, in which fibres run irregularly, transversely and obliquely
- the inner layer of circular fibres.

Parietal peritoneum. Peritoneum forms the external coat of the uterus but does not cover the lower anterior quarter of the uterus and the cervix.

Blood supply

The blood supply to the uterus is from the uterine artery, a branch of the internal iliac artery. Veins accompany the arteries and drain into the internal iliac veins. Tortuous arterial vessels enter the layers of the uterine wall and divide into capillaries between endometrial glands.

Nerve supply

The nerves supplying the uterus and the uterine tubes are formed from parasympathetic fibres from the sacral outflow and sympathetic fibres from the lumbar outflow.

Supporting structures

The uterus is maintained in position in the pelvis by fascia and muscle structures (see Fig. 7.5). The uterine ligaments are:

- *the broad ligament* — a fold of peritoneum and fibromuscular tissue extending from the uterus to the pelvic side wall
- *the cardinal ligaments* — these are formed by dense fascia at the base of the broad ligaments, from the cervix to the pelvic side wall
- *the round ligaments* — these extend from the anterior cornua of the uterus forwards and down through the inguinal canal to the subcutaneous fat of the labia majora

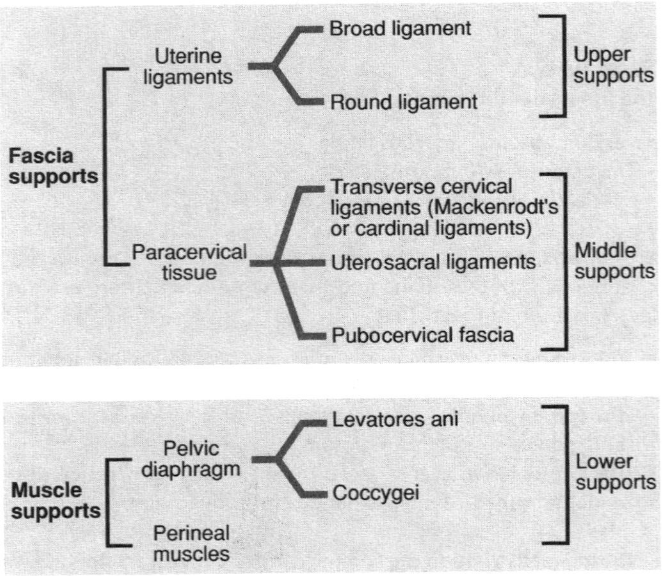

Fig. 7.5 The supports of the uterus.

- *the uterosacral ligament* — this passes from the cervix and cardinal ligaments backwards to the sacrum, dividing to pass around the rectum
- *the pubocervical ligament* — this passes from the anterior cervix forwards to the pubic bone, dividing to pass around the urethra.

These ligaments support the position of the uterus within the pelvis. Paracervical tissue, fatty and connective tissue form a supportive sling allowing the uterus to pivot either backwards or forwards. This gives the uterus mobility anteriorly and posteriorly. Lateral and downward movements are limited by the muscles of the pelvic floor.

The axis of the vagina is considered to be a straight line that is related to the axis of the cervix. When the cervical axis is hinged anterior to the vaginal axis, the uterus is 'anteverted' (see Fig. 7.4), which is its normal position. When the cervical axis is hinged backwards to lie posterior to the vaginal axis, the uterus is 'retroverted'. This can be a normal position for the uterus to occupy provided that the retroversion is mobile and not fixed.

Functions

The functions of the uterus are:

- menstruation — sloughing off of compact and spongy layers of endometrium attended by bleeding from torn vessels
- maintenance of pregnancy — an embryo implants itself in the endometrium and takes all its nourishment throughout fetal life
- initiation of labour — it develops powerful, rhythmic contractions of the muscular wall for the birth of the infant.

The uterine tubes (fallopian tubes or oviducts)

(see Fig. 7.2)

The uterine tubes (10–14 cm long) turn posteriorly as they extend laterally from the cornua (or horns) of the uterus towards the lateral pelvic wall. The ends open as funnel-shaped structures with finger-like projections (fimbriae). The broad ligament of peritoneum forms the outer serous layer of the tubes. The middle coat, of muscular tissue, is arranged in two layers; an outer longitudinal layer and an inner circular layer. The lining of mucous membrane, comprised mainly of ciliated columnar epithelium and secretory cells, lies in folds. The lumen of the tube is narrow. The ends of the tubes are mobile and at ovulation the fimbriae enfold the adjacent ovary to take up the released ova.

Functions

The functions of the uterine tubes are to convey ova from the ovary to the uterus and to allow the sperm and ova to meet for fertilisation within the tube. Passage of the ova along the tube is facilitated by the action of cilia and peristalsis.

The vagina

The vagina is a fibromuscular channel extending downwards and forwards from the cervix to the labia, thereby connecting the internal and external reproductive organs. The cervix of the uterus is inserted into the upper end of the vagina, known as the vault. This creates anterior, posterior and lateral fornices (see Fig. 7.1). The anterior wall of the vagina is approximately 7.5 cm and the posterior wall about 9 cm in length. The vagina is composed mainly of smooth muscle with a lining of mucous membrane arranged in folds or rugae. In the virginal state a fold of mucous membrane, the hymen, forms a border around the external opening of the vagina, partially closing the outlet. Normally the anterior and posterior walls lie in apposition but the vagina is capable of considerable distension during childbirth.

The vagina is kept moist during the reproductive years by mucus from the cervix and transudation of fluid through the vaginal wall. Glycogen produced in the vagina is fermented by the Doderlein bacilli (normally inhabiting the vagina) to produce lactic acid. This maintains a slightly acid environment in the vagina, inhibiting the growth of other microorganisms.

Functions

The vagina:

- receives semen from the male, deposited in the posterior fornix during sexual intercourse
- provides an outlet for the fetus and other products of conception
- provides an outlet for menstrual flow
- provides a barrier to infection.

The vulva

The vulva comprises the female external genital organs, consisting of:

- the mons pubis
- the labia majora
- the labia minora
- the clitoris
- the fourchette
- the urinary orifice
- the vaginal orifice
- Bartholin's glands.

The pelvic floor

The pelvic floor is formed by tissues which fill the pelvic outlet and support the pelvic organs.

The levator ani muscles form a broad muscular sheet extending from the pubic bone to the sacrum and coccyx and laterally to the pelvic walls. The urethra, vagina and rectum perforate this muscular sheet.

The superficial perineal muscles lie under the levator ani muscles. They pass from the pelvic side walls, the pubis and the sacrum to unite centrally between the vagina and the rectum, where they form the superficial part of the perineal body.

The perineal body consists of wedge-shaped muscle and fibrous tissue lying between the lower vagina and lower rectum.

The endometrial cycle

The ovarian cycle (see 'Ovarian functions', p. 220) and the endometrial cycle together constitute the menstrual cycle. The endometrial cycle is driven by the hormonal events of the ovarian cycle and can be divided into four phases:

- the menstrual phase
- the proliferative phase (follicular or pre-ovulatory)
- the secretory phase (luteal or post-ovulatory)
- the ischaemic phase.

The menstrual phase

Menstruation is believed to be caused by low levels of progesterone and oestrogens causing vasospasm of arteries to the endometrium. The menstrual phase lasts for 3–6 days and is characterised by bleeding from the uterus. Fifty to sixty millilitres of blood are lost at each menstrual period. Necrotic parts of the compact and spongy layers of endometrium slough away leaving a thin, bleeding area of tissue. By the third day of menstruation new epithelial cell growth has begun to cover the disorganised basal layer of endometrium. By the fifth day, epithelium covers the whole surface.

The proliferative phase

The proliferative phase begins while bleeding is still continuing. It is a time of regrowth of endometrium under the control of oestradiol from the maturing follicle. The growth of epithelium, glands, blood vessels and connective tissue produces thickening of the endometrium. This phase extends to the 14th or 15th day of the cycle, when the peak of proliferation is reached.

The secretory phase

Soon after ovulation, glycoprotein secretory granules appear in the endometrium and can be seen with an electron microscope as large, clear vacuoles developing under the nuclei. Progesterone produced by the corpus luteum promotes the secretory phase. The endometrial glands become enlarged, the arteries coil, connective tissue hypertrophies, and tissues rich in glycogen become oedematous. Seven to 8 days following ovulation, the endometrium is 5–6 mm in depth and is in a state of readiness to implant a fertilised ovum. If implantation occurs, the corpus luteum continues to produce progesterone and maintains the pregnancy (see Fig. 7.6.)

The ischaemic phase

In the absence of implantation, the corpus luteum degenerates and the production of oestrogen and progesterone declines. A leucocytic infiltration of the endometrium takes place, the stroma starts to disintegrate, oedema disappears and the endometrium shrinks. Vasoconstriction occurs. There is lack of nourishment to the

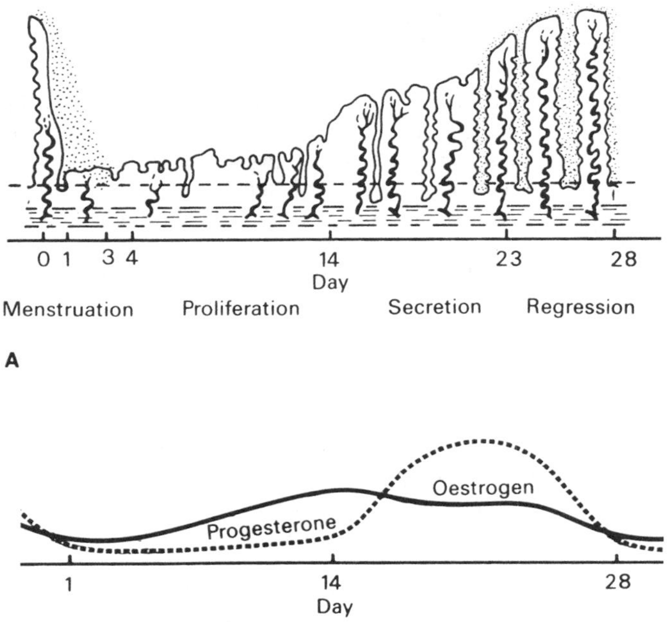

Fig. 7.6 The hormonal control of the menstrual cycle. (Reproduced with kind permission from Wilson & Waugh 1996.)

endometrium and it begins to slough and separate and menstruation begins again 14 (±1) days after ovulation. This time relationship is constant. Fluctuations in the length of the cycle occur in the preovulatory phase, as follicles may not mature at the same rate each month. Thus there may be variation in the time of onset of menstruation. Most women establish an average pattern that is normal for each, although many young women have irregular patterns.

The menarche

In Western cultures, girls first menstruate, or reach the menarche, within the age range of 9–16 years. Nutrition and body weight influence menstruation and sexual development. This has cultural ramifications in that amenorrhoea and infrequent menstruation are more common in developing countries, especially in the rural areas (Helman 1997). The onset of menstruation may be delayed by intensive physical activity.

Some oestrogen synthesis stimulates early physical sexual changes to occur some time before the first menstruation. There may be follicular growth and some oestrogen withdrawal bleeding to give the early periods of the first few months. These periods are anovular, ovulation having not yet occurred. Such periods are painless. More discomfort may be experienced with the menstruation that follows ovulation. A rise in basal temperature may be a guide to whether ovulation has occurred.

Variation in menstrual cycle length occurs in response to significant life events. Excitement, stress, anxiety or change of environment can delay the maturing of a follicle, ovulation and menstruation. Excessive exercise, as in athletes, can result in irregular periods, anovulatory cycles and amenorrhoea.

The climacteric and menopause

The word climacteric comes from the Greek word *klimacter*, meaning a step or rung of a ladder. This signifies a step or phase in life from the child-bearing years to a period of infertility associated with age-related changes. The process of the climacteric is usually gradual and may extend over several years. Most women experience the climacteric or perimenopause over a period of 2–3 years, but it may extend over 10 years. During this time the body adjusts to lower levels of oestrogen.

The ageing process of the ovaries results in ripening of fewer follicles and a decreased stimulation by the pituitary hormones. The ovaries atrophy and less oestrogen is released into the circulation. Initially this reduced oestrogen level in the blood results in excessive production of follicle-stimulating hormone (FSH) from the anterior pituitary gland, and this feedback mechanism can continue for several years. The withdrawal of oestrogen and the increase in pituitary hormone contribute to the changes associated with the climacteric.

The menopause is sometimes confused with the climacteric. However, the menopause is defined as the cessation of menstruation and is marked specifically by the date of the last menstrual period. It follows, then, that the time of the menopause or last menstrual period can only be identified in retrospect some months after the event. The menopause is only one effect of the climacteric. 'Postmenopausal' is a term applied to events occurring after menstruation has stopped for at least a year.

The menopause (last menstrual period) signifies the end of a woman's reproductive capacity. This normally occurs between 45 and 55 years of age, with the mean age for cessation of periods being 51 years. This has remained constant for many years (Abernethy 1997).

A premature menopause is one which occurs before the age of 40 years. This can occur naturally or may be induced iatrogenically. The age of menarche, socioeconomic factors, race, use of oral contraceptives and number of pregnancies appear to have no affect on whether a woman has an early or late menopause (Abernethy 1997).

Endocrine changes influencing the climacteric

Endocrine changes occur prior to changes in a woman's menstrual pattern when there is an alteration in the ratio of the pituitary gonadotrophins (FSH and LH). FSH levels begin to rise between the ages of 35 and 40 years, affecting the oestrogen feedback mechanisms and resulting in altered ovarian function. As a consequence, some anovular menstruation occurs and there is a reduction in progesterone produced by the theca-lutein cells. During this period the amount of oestrogen produced shows considerable fluctuation.

Although ovarian cycles may become anovular many years before the menopause occurs, women between the ages of 40 and 45 can still become pregnant as regular ovulation may continue.

Eventually there is further deterioration in ovarian response to the pituitary gonadotrophins and disturbance to the feedback between the hypothalamus–pituitary and the ovaries. There is then a further alteration to the FSH:LH ratio, with an elevation in LH and a steep rise in FSH. However, fewer follicles are stimulated so oestrogen secretion is reduced. The fluctuations in oestrogen production, while following a gradual decline, alter the menstrual pattern in many women, showing considerable variation amongst women until the menopause.

After the menopause there is continued secretion of oestradiol and oestrone, although in varying and declining amounts. Oestrone becomes the predominant oestrogen. Small amounts of oestrogen can be found in the blood and urine of postmenopausal women. Some of this oestrogen may be derived from adrenal activity and the conversion of some androgens into oestrogen. Some oestrogen may be produced by residual ovarian stroma.

Uterine bleeding patterns

The climacteric is characterised by irregular menstruation. Periods may become scanty, or bleeding may be heavy. The menstrual cycle shortens, associated with a decrease in oestradiol secretion. As this continues, LH levels rise and then menstrual cycles lengthen. Anovulatory cycles result in oestrogen-withdrawal bleeding patterns, irregular cycles with intermittent and prolonged spotting (low oestrogen profile) or prolonged amenorrhoea followed by sudden, profuse bleeding (high oestrogen profile).

Somatic changes associated with the climacteric

The somatic changes associated with the climacteric occur as a consequence of a decrease in circulating oestrogen and an increase in gonadotrophins. Since the diurnal secretion of oestrogen varies from woman to woman, the changes experienced vary in severity but are progressive.

The ovaries atrophy and follicles disappear or fail to respond to gonadotrophins. Uterine atrophy is accompanied by a transformation of the muscle fibres to fibrous tissue. The endometrium becomes thinner. The cervix tends to remain dilated and the external os more lax. The fallopian tubes become smaller and the fimbriated ends retract from the ovaries. Atrophy of the vaginal epithelium results in thinning of the vaginal wall, a loss of folds, elasticity and lubrication and an increase in pH. Vaginal dryness can result in pruritus and dyspareunia. Loss of acidity within the vagina allows organisms to multiply more easily. There is an increase in connective tissue beneath the mucosa, causing narrowing and shortening of the vagina. The vagina is more prone to ulceration and bleeds easily to touch. Senile vaginitis may occur in elderly women. The labia become thin and lose their sexual responsiveness. Skin over the vulva loses support due to a decrease in subcutaneous tissue and lack of tone of the underlying tissues. Hair growth in this area decreases with advancing years. The muscles and connective tissue of the pelvic floor lose tone and elasticity, and consequently become less effective in supporting the pelvic contents. The urethral mucosa may also show atrophic changes, resulting in symptoms of urethritis and cystitis, although no bacteria are isolated in the urine. In the breasts, subcutaneous fat is reabsorbed and glandular tissue atrophies.

Some of these physiological changes, resulting in lack of lubrication, loss of libido and dyspareunia, can contribute to sexual problems for the woman. Hormone replacement therapy may be a possible treatment option or psychosexual counselling may be of benefit. Many factors contribute to a satisfying sex life; satisfaction in a relationship, psychological well-being and emotional security can all make a significant contribution, illustrating the need for a holistic approach.

Vasomotor disturbances

Vasomotor disturbances commonly accompany the climacteric changes. Hot flushes (or hot flashes) are the most common but perspiration, headache, fainting and palpitation may also be experienced. Hot flushes can start with a sensation of extreme warmth in the chest, quickly followed by flushing of the face and neck. The feeling of heat may become generalised. This is caused by dilatation of the blood vessels to the skin and an increased blood flow. The flush may be accompanied by sweating and palpitations. Dizziness and nausea may also be experienced. Shivering is often reported after the flush, probably due to compensatory constriction of the blood vessels. Hot flushes and sweats are embarrassing and uncontrollable and are experienced by 75% of women, many of whom receive no special treatment. If untreated, vasomotor symptoms will eventually subside with no long-term effects (see Box 7.1).

Box 7.1 Hot flush changes

A technique has been standardised for the continuous recording of skin temperature and conductance. Meldrum et al (1979) showed that the first change was an increase in perspiration (conductance), followed by a rise in finger temperature and then a decrease in the central core (ear drum) temperature. The mean temperature increase during the flush was 2.7°C and lasted an average 3.1 min. The subjective 'flash' was usually noted a minute before and ended a minute after the temperature rise, and lasted an average 2.6 min. Consistently correlated with patients' subjective feelings was change in:

- conductance (98%)
- skin (82%)
- core temperature (81%).

There was a marked increase in the blood flow of the hand, with the onset of symptoms. This was sustained for 3–4 min, with return to control level 6 min after symptoms abated. The blood pressure was unaltered during the flush. It was suggested that the flush occurred because of a downward setting of the hypothalamic temperature-regulating centre. The reason for change was unknown.

Research Abstract 7.1
Study of treatment of hot flushes with oestrogen

A 4-month and a 12-month crossover study of women with hot flushes found a statistically significant reduction in hot flushes during oestrogen therapy using Premarin 1.25 mg, compared with a placebo. The studies confirmed the powerful therapeutic response in those who received the placebo first, but invariably the switch from oestrogen to placebo caused a rapid return of flushing.

Campbell S, Whitehead M I 1977 Oestrogen therapy and the menopausal syndrome. In: Greenblatt R, Studd J (eds) The menopause: clinics in obstetrics and gynaecology. WB Saunders, London

Although research into the possible relationship between low levels of oestrogens and hot flushes has been inconclusive, oestrogen therapy can improve symptoms. For example, in blind crossover studies, symptoms recurred when patients were given placebos (Notelovitz 1986) (see Research Abstract 7.1). In addition to oestrogen therapy, other treatments, such as vitamin E and/or B_6, clonidine, plant oestrogens, propanolol and oil of evening primrose, have been used.

Emotional changes

Some women complain of irritability, anxiety, difficulty in concentration, dizziness, a bloated feeling and depressive feelings after the menopause. In addition to hormonal changes occurring at the perimenopause, women may also be facing other psychological or social changes which can affect their emotional state. It is difficult to establish a causal relationship between oestrogen deficiency and the emotional behaviour of women, but the metabolic products of oestrogen, the catecholestrogens, may have a secondary regulatory role in neurotransmitter activities that influence mood and feelings of well-being (Notelovitz 1986).

When talking to someone about the climacteric, the normality of the stage of development should be emphasised. The need to maintain a positive outlook and to continue with activities should be encouraged. Some women regret their loss of fertility and perceive changes as the beginning of old age.

Nurses can give information, reassurance and support to women at this time by:

- establishing the patient's concerns and problems
- using a counselling approach to respond to the patient's expression of feelings
- providing information about self-help in overcoming hot flushes and sweating, e.g.:
  —wearing cotton, rather than nylon, loose clothing, and short sleeves rather than long
  —wearing light layers of outer clothing that can be removed as required
  —avoiding wearing a bra or pantie-girdle
  —using light bedclothes rather than a duvet so that covers can be shed if necessary, or using a duvet with a low tog rating if preferred
  —sleeping with a bedroom window open
  —keeping living and working areas at lower air temperatures
  —taking cool showers twice a day rather than a hot bath

—minimising alcohol intake, hot curries and foods containing ginger
—using self-relaxation techniques.

The long-term effects of oestrogen withdrawal are considered as disorders of the menopause.

CONDITIONS AFFECTING MENSTRUATION

The term 'gynaecology' means the study of woman. It includes evaluating normal and abnormal functions and the treatment of disorders.

Amenorrhoea

Secondary sexual development is usually complete in girls by the age of 16 years and menstruation is the last sign to appear. Amenorrhoea means the absence of menstruation and is a symptom, not a disease. It is described as primary or secondary.

Primary amenorrhoea is defined as non-appearance of menstruation in a female by the age of 16 years. A delay in the onset of menstruation may be a cause of concern. There may be an anatomical fault or some disturbance in hormonal secretions. Delayed puberty may be familial or constitutional. Secondary amenorrhoea is the absence of menstruation for a period of time which is twice the length of the normal menstrual cycle for a woman who has previously menstruated. Thus, if two or more menstrual periods are missed then secondary amenorrhoea may be said to exist. This often means that the woman may wait until menstruation has been absent for a year before seeking investigation.

Physiological amenorrhoea

Amenorrhoea is physiological before puberty, during pregnancy and lactation, and after the menopause. Inheritance, race, climate and general nutrition influence when menstruation begins. The potential for maturation of ovarian tissue is in place before birth. After puberty, full regulation of ovarian activities by the hypothalamus and pituitary gland is achieved and menstrual cycles are established, but the exact time for this is unpredictable.

A parent may take a teenage girl to see her GP because of concern over delay in the onset of menstruation. The daughter may compare her own late development with that of a sister or her peers at school and may feel abnormal. The doctor may undertake a general physical examination to be able to reassure the patient that other secondary sex characteristics are already present and that the onset of menstruation will follow in due course. Advice can be given about reducing anxiety, which may delay the onset of menstruation. If secondary sex characteristics or menstruation fail to develop, the doctor will refer the young woman to a consultant gynaecologist and endocrinologist for a programme of investigations.

During pregnancy

After ovulation has occurred, the lining cells of the ovarian follicle are stimulated by LH to develop the corpus luteum which produces progesterone. This hormone in turn stimulates the endometrium and its secretory glands into a state of readiness to receive the fertilised ovum from the uterine tube. When the fertilised ovum becomes embedded in the wall of the uterus, it produces the hormone human chorionic gonadotrophin (HCG). This hormone enables the corpus luteum to continue its production of progesterone for 3–4 months until the placenta grows and produces its own progesterone and oestrogen. The presence of the growing fetus and the continued production of progesterone prevent the loss of endometrium and the menstrual flow.

Amenorrhoea is frequently one of the first symptoms that lead a woman to suspect that she is pregnant. Levels of HCG in the urine provide a positive diagnosis when a test for pregnancy is completed in the clinic or laboratory. The doctor usually confirms the pregnancy by abdominal palpation and a vaginal examination, when the uterus is found to be increased in size.

During lactation

Mothers who totally breast feed their baby may not ovulate or menstruate during the first 6 months after the birth or until they start to wean the baby. Breast feeding therefore exerts a measure of birth control, but it cannot be recommended as 100% effective as a contraceptive. Total nipple stimulation is important for suppression of ovarian function. The suckling stimulus to the nipple leads to a neurohormonal reflex production of prolactin by the anterior pituitary gland and the consequent maintenance of high circulating levels of prolactin inhibits gonadotrophin hormone release, preventing ovulation and menstruation. However, Hartmann (1991) states that fertility may return as early as 2 weeks after birth in some women who are fully breast feeding their infants. Farrer (1990) indicates that most women will ovulate before their first menstruation following childbirth.

Suppression of the ovaries declines where supplements comprise more than 50% of the diet of the baby who is breast feeding. The incidence of ovulation and the risk of pregnancy then rise rapidly.

A poor state of nutrition in the mother is also known to inhibit ovulation, particularly in developing countries (Lunn et al 1980, 1981, Lunn 1992). To ensure contraception during the period of lactation, the mother may be advised to use a barrier method. The progestogen-only pill is considered safe during lactation since it does not affect the milk supply and only insignificant quantities enter the milk. The combined oral contraceptive pill, however, inhibits lactation and small quantities enter the milk (Everett 1997).

After the menopause

The menopause, or date of the final menstrual period, may not be fully acknowledged until a year without periods has passed. Many women pass this milestone without regrets and without unpleasant physical symptoms. Medical intervention may be sought if physical discomfort such as hot flushes, headaches or sweating is experienced.

Information and support from the nurse, outlined earlier in this chapter (p. 225), can be helpful.

Pathological amenorrhoea

Uterine lesions, congenital abnormalities

PATHOPHYSIOLOGY

Congenital absence of uterus and vagina may occur, although ovaries and secondary sex characteristics have developed. ***Primary deficiency of endometrium.*** A diagnostic test can be performed by giving ethinyl oestradiol 0.05 mg by mouth, twice a day for 21 days. If withdrawal bleeding occurs within 7–10 days then there is not a failure of endometrium but probably failure of stimulation by the ovaries. If there is no bleeding, an endometrial problem exists. The endometrium may be absent, deficient or unable to be stimulated by oestrogen. In this case, the amenorrhoea is entirely of uterine origin.

Ovarian lesions

Failure of normal development is a rare condition of the ovary. Chromosomal abnormalities such as Turner's syndrome may occur.

PATHOPHYSIOLOGY

Turner's syndrome is a condition that results from the absence of one female chromosome. The chromosome complement is written as 45XO. The woman is reported to be 'chromatin-negative'. The condition shows infantile development of the genitalia, absence of breasts, short stature and a webbed neck. Congenital cardiac lesions may be associated with it (see Ch. 5).

MEDICAL MANAGEMENT

Treatment is to induce sexual maturation by administering oestrogen. Ethinyl oestradiol 0.01 mg twice daily, in 3-week cycles, is given for several months, and then norethisterone is added for the last 10 days of each cycle.

Arrhenoblastoma

PATHOPHYSIOLOGY

Arrhenoblastoma is a masculinising tumour of the ovary, which may cause amenorrhoea because of the high production of androgenic hormones. Most ovarian tumours, even if they are bilateral, do not usually destroy all active ovarian tissue and so would not usually cause amenorrhoea.

MEDICAL MANAGEMENT

Surgical removal of the ovary is generally the treatment for this condition, although Tita et al (1996) reported a case of neoplasm removal and subsequent therapy.

Surgical removal of both ovaries (bilateral oophorectomy), which may be associated with the removal of the uterus and fallopian tubes (hysterectomy with bilateral salpingo-oophorectomy), will result in amenorrhoea.

Effects of irradiation. Direct irradiation of the ovaries, for the treatment of tumour, or indirect irradiation from treatment of other pelvic organs, bladder or rectum may cause amenorrhoea. Accidental irradiation may occur in women whose work exposes them to radiation sources.

Pituitary disorders (see also Ch. 5)

Deficiency of gonadotrophin secretion may occur without deficiencies of other trophic hormones. No cause may be found but it is often associated with emotional responses.

Infantilism may result from congenital failure of the pituitary gland, causing dwarfism, lack of sexual development and amenorrhoea. Follicle-stimulating hormone (FSH) is absent or low. Oestrogens may be undetectable in the urine.

Fröhlich's syndrome is a disturbance of the hypothalamus, resulting in underdevelopment of genital tissues, amenorrhoea, obesity, hirsutism and retardation of mental responses.

Ischaemic necrosis of pituitary tissue may result from thrombosis of pituitary vessels following profound shock and anaemia, often due to severe postpartum haemorrhage. The production of trophic hormones ceases or is reduced. The condition is characterised by lethargy, weight gain, reduced metabolic rate, hypotension and amenorrhoea. Hormone therapy gives some psychological benefit only, by withdrawal bleeding effects.

New growths of the pituitary cause acromegaly and amenorrhoea, with signs of Cushing's syndrome due to effects on the suprarenal glands.

Other endocrine disorders

Adrenogenital syndrome results from overactivity of the adrenal cortex due to the presence of a tumour or hyperplasia. Excessive production of androgens occurs, giving signs of virilism — a deepening voice, hirsuteness, an enlarged clitoris and the development of acne and amenorrhoea.

Cushing's disease is caused by hyperplasia of the adrenal cortex, which leads to an excess of glucocorticoids, stimulating the conversion of protein into carbohydrate. Obesity, glycosuria, hypertension, increased androgen activity and amenorrhoea from regressive changes in the genital organs are the main features of the condition.

The following endocrine disorders may also be accompanied by amenorrhoea:

- Addison's disease
- myxoedema
- thyrotoxicosis
- diabetes mellitus.

Emotional stress

PATHOPHYSIOLOGY

Emotional disturbance is likely to affect menstrual function through the hypothalamic–pituitary axis since the hypothalamus controls the output of gonadotrophins from the pituitary gland. Emotional distress caused by some traumatic event, such as receiving bad news or being involved in a major disaster, may contribute to amenorrhoea. If a woman has sexual intercourse without contraception, the fear of becoming pregnant may itself cause temporary amenorrhoea.

MEDICAL MANAGEMENT

Following discussion with the doctor, it is expected that the patient will understand and be reassured about the effects of stress on menstruation. When she makes a positive adjustment to the critical event that has preceded the problem, physical and mental relaxation will promote a spontaneous return of menstruation.

Anorexia nervosa (see also Ch. 5)

PATHOPHYSIOLOGY

Anorexia nervosa is a psychiatric illness characterised by extreme weight loss and dislike for foods, particularly carbohydrates. It occurs most commonly in adolescent girls and is associated with dieting routines and distortion of body image. There is failure in hypothalamic stimulation of LH release and amenorrhoea occurs.

MEDICAL MANAGEMENT

Patient management may initially be carried out by a physician who has been investigating the patient's weight loss, but when a diagnosis is made care is usually maintained by a psychiatrist. A behavioural therapy programme is negotiated with the patient to ensure an improvement in food intake, while a cognitive therapist may assist her to think more rationally and improve her feelings of self-esteem and her body image. Positive physical and psychological changes can promote a return to menstruation.

Psychotic illness

PATHOPHYSIOLOGY

Psychotic illness may be a cause of amenorrhoea. The person with a schizophrenic reaction may not menstruate for many months or years. A life crisis can contribute to disturbances in the activity of neurotransmitter catecholamines in the brain. The chemistry of the hypothalamic–pituitary axis may be disrupted, resulting in amenorrhoea.

MEDICAL MANAGEMENT

The psychiatrist would check that a pregnancy has not developed in the patient with a psychotic reaction. A reliable source of information will be needed, whether the patient herself or her partner. A laboratory pregnancy test may be necessary. The acute symptoms of the patient's illness may be treated by neuroleptic drugs or psychotherapeutic intervention. A return of the normal menstruation pattern would be expected when the body chemistry becomes more stable.

Severe general illness

PATHOPHYSIOLOGY

The stress of severe illness may induce ineffective functioning in multiple body organs and may temporarily suppress menstrual function. Stress, as experienced by prisoners of war or refugees, associated with malnutrition, minimal protein and vitamin intake, leads to amenorrhoea.

MEDICAL MANAGEMENT

The amenorrhoea is secondary to the general illness. Thus the particular illness condition must be treated before the amenorrhoea can be relieved. The influences of emotional and physical stress are complex, and sometimes assisting the patient to relax and lower anxiety levels may promote menstruation before the general illness is fully relieved.

NURSING PRIORITIES AND MANAGEMENT: AMENORRHOEA

The nurse caring for a patient with amenorrhoea may do so in any of the hospital specialities or in the community — the nursing management will be similar in all of these locations.

Assessment

As part of routine assessment of the patient, the nurse should enquire about the date of the last menstrual period and whether there are any problems with menstruation. The nurse should ascertain whether the patient has any knowledge of the reason for the absence of menstruation. As the patient shares information, the nurse should be able to establish how the patient feels about the amenorrhoea that is described. The patient may not regard amenorrhoea as a problem or, conversely, it may be a source of some distress. Assessment should take account of her lifestyle, including nutrition, eating pattern, body weight, level of exercise and any stressful life events.

Care planning

In negotiation with the patient, the nurse should plan time to give her information about the absence of menstruation. This can perhaps be associated with potential worries about the condition. The patient's level of anxiety should be documented in the plan. The nurse may wish to emphasise the need for self-relaxation and may teach a simple relaxation exercise. Relaxation audiotapes may be available from the physiotherapy department, occupational therapy or the department of clinical psychology.

If, following a medical assessment, puberty is deemed to be delayed, reassurance and counselling are part of nursing care. Nurses can encourage optimism, provide general information about diet, exercise and lifestyle, and offer support, but in some cases skilled counselling may also be of value.

Evaluation of care

The patient's long-term goal of 'a return of the menstrual period' may not be achievable within the early weeks of care and should be modified to include a short-term realistic target. This may include an evaluation of the level of anxiety experienced by the patient. Nurse and patient should negotiate a goal statement suited to the individual patient. This goal should be evaluated daily, to check on the response to self-relaxation activity during the first 2 days of care. The patient may need more help from the nurse and new target times for evaluation of goal achievement will then need to be set.

The patient should be asked to report menstruation. Achievement of such a long-term goal may occur as a result of medical treatment, particularly if hormonal or anxiolytic sedative drugs have been prescribed.

Cryptomenorrhoea

This is a condition of concealed menstruation and it is important to differentiate it from amenorrhoea. Menstrual blood is unable to pass through the vagina due to an obstruction. This may be due to an imperforate hymen, a transverse vaginal membrane, complete or partial vaginal atresia. Incomplete canalisation of the lower end of the Müllerian cords will result in atresia of the upper vagina. There may be a complete absence of the vagina or cervical stenosis after cautery to the cervix or amputation of the cervix.

PATHOPHYSIOLOGY

In this condition, the uterus, ovaries and the pituitary gland are functioning normally, but the menstrual outflow is obstructed. Conditions such as an imperforate hymen or a transverse vaginal septum will result in an accumulation of blood in the vagina (haematocolpos). In addition to vaginal distension, retrograde flow to the fallopian tubes (haemosalpinx) and accumulation of blood may cause pelvic congestion and displacement of structures. Symptoms are cyclical pain and lower abdominal swelling.

MEDICAL MANAGEMENT

The condition is relieved by surgical drainage. There is a risk that the fallopian tubes may be damaged due to retrograde flow and consequent distension.

NURSING PRIORITIES AND MANAGEMENT: CRYPTOMENORRHOEA

Assessment

The patient will be admitted as an emergency for early transfer to the operating theatre. The nurse assessing the patient on admission will encounter the following symptoms:

- pelvic pain
- potential retention of urine from pressure on the urethra
- anxiety about the condition, the strange environment and unknown procedures.

Care planning

If time allows before transfer to the operating theatre, the relief of the patient's pain will be a priority, according to medical prescription.

A comforting, positive attitude of open regard shown by the nurse may help to reduce the patient's anxiety. Giving information will prepare the patient for the procedures to be expected before surgery and in the first 24 h after the operation (see Ch. 26).

A urethral catheter may be introduced unless there is an obstruction of the urethra. This may be undertaken once the patient is anaesthetised. An empty bladder facilitates the work of the surgeon and reduces risk of injury to the bladder.

Postoperative care

This will ensure the patient's safe recovery from anaesthesia and that pain is fully relieved. The patient's vaginal blood loss will be observed and documented. The patient should quickly recover, without any complications of anaesthesia or surgery.

Full information should be given about what the surgery entailed and expected future progress.

Evaluation of care

The patient should quickly achieve the following outcomes:

- freedom from pain
- minimal blood loss, reducing daily
- no nausea or vomiting
- return to self-care activities within 24 h
- no hospital-acquired infection
- able to explain, before discharge, the action to be taken if the condition recurs
- discharge within 4 days or less, with an outpatient clinic appointment for 1 month's time.

If these outcomes are not achieved then discharge will be delayed while care is modified, until the patient's condition improves. Surgical treatment should result in subsequent menstrual blood flow per vagina.

Dysmenorrhoea

Dysmenorrhoea is pain associated with menstruation. Many women experience minor discomfort associated with menstruation, but dysmenorrhoea is more disabling. Before the start of the period, the breasts may feel larger and ache; there may also be feelings of abdominal distension, constipation may be a problem, and the woman may feel unwell. The symptoms may persist for 1–2 days and are relieved or replaced by the symptoms of backache, frequency of passing urine and loose bowel action, with the onset of menstruation.

For some women, the first hours or the first day are the most painful. Dragging sensations from the umbilical area down to the groins and thighs may be experienced, or the pain may be severe, colicky or spasmodic in nature across the abdomen and back. The pain may be so distracting as to interfere with the woman's usual daily activities. Dysmenorrhoea is a major contributing factor to absenteeism among schoolgirls and working women.

Two types of dysmenorrhoea are described:

- primary dysmenorrhoea (spasmodic) is due to physiological activities of the menstruation, with muscle contraction
- secondary dysmenorrhoea (congestive) is associated with organic pelvic disease.

Research Abstract 7.2
Knowledge and attitudes about female health among girls

Questionnaires were completed by 74 girls between the ages of 11 and 17 years regarding their knowledge of personal health and attitudes towards issues of contraception and sexually transmitted diseases. Before the study, 47 girls had begun menstruating. The average age of menarche was 12 years. Negative feelings towards menstruation were expressed by the majority of girls who had not yet started their periods. These feelings stemmed from lack of knowledge, anxiety about peer group attitudes, and fear of the 'pains' that were expected as an inevitable part of menstruation. Similar negative feelings were also expressed by the girls who had started their periods. They also mentioned 'loss of freedom' during periods and the 'messiness' of menstruation. Nine positive responses towards menstruation were recorded and associated with growing up. Knowledge about the menstrual cycle and the hormones involved varied but in a number of cases appeared limited. There was evidence that myths about menstruation still exist; they were told 'not to run about a lot, or do sport'. The research findings do not support the belief that the menarche is a positive event and that adolescents perceive menstruation as normal. The negative views of those who had begun menstruating focused mainly on pain and inconvenience. It is questioned whether negative attitudes result from the experience of pain or whether pain is a result of women's negative attitudes. Nurses should be aware of the perceptions, anxieties and special health education requirements of teenage girls.

Smithson A 1992 Girls will be women. Nursing Times 88(6): 46–48

Primary dysmenorrhoea

This is seen in young women in their late teens and early 20s. At first they may have anovulatory, pain-free menstruation. Later, when ovulation becomes established, they experience pain 24 h before the flow begins. The pain is of the severe colic type over the lower abdomen, often radiating to the thighs and back, and lasts for at least 12 h. Nausea, fainting and diarrhoea may accompany the acute phase and the girl looks pale and drawn with a tense facial expression.

PATHOPHYSIOLOGY

Misconceptions about the physical changes of menstruation and the way they should be managed may underlie painful periods (Brown & Woods 1984, Smithson 1992; see also Research Abstract 7.2). Therefore, problems associated with environment, parental pressures and the patient's attitude towards and beliefs about menstruation and sexual matters should be explored.

In the days prior to menstruation, there is a build-up of progesterone and a raised level of prostaglandins in the endometrium. As menstruation begins, the progesterone level is lowered and arterioles in the uterus go into spasm. Muscle ischaemia results and can produce uterine pain similar to that of angina. Circulation of blood to the endometrium decreases during uterine contractions; a correlation had been found between minimal endometrial blood flow and maximal pain, supporting the view that hypercontractility, resulting in ischaemia, is the cause of primary dysmenorrhoea

(Lundstrom 1981, Lumsden 1985). It is now generally agreed that this hypercontractility in primary dysmenorrhoea is associated with excessive prostaglandin production (Rees 1988).

Primary dysmenorrhoea is due to excess prostaglandin (F_2); the circulating prostaglandin may also cause nausea, vomiting, diarrhoea or faintness.

Muscular incoordination may be the result of improper functioning of the autonomic nervous system. This may cause spasm of muscles of the uterine isthmus and of the internal os.

Rarely, dysmenorrhoea may be due to an obstruction to the flow of blood as a result of a clot being lodged in the cervix. Other possible causes include pelvic inflammatory disease, endometriosis and congenital abnormalities.

MEDICAL MANAGEMENT

Detailed interviews are needed with the girl and her mother, separately and together. In this way, shared and different attitudes to the subject can be identified and problems defined. Vaginal or rectal examinations will be carried out.

Efforts are made to educate the girl and her mother, as necessary, about normal menstrual function. It is important to test their understanding by giving them opportunities for feedback about attitudes and old wives' tales. A period of rest and the application of warmth to the abdomen or back may be helpful. The need to rest should not be used as an excuse for avoiding school or work. Regular exercise, the avoidance of constipation and the prevention of anxiety and tension are emphasised. Exercise encourages the release of endogenous endorphins which have natural analgesic properties. A series of exercises to stretch the ligaments that support the uterus in the pelvis may relieve menstrual pain. Attention should be paid to maintaining good posture.

Treatment. Non-habit-forming analgesics can be of value, particularly aspirin, which reduces prostaglandin synthesis. An anti-prostaglandin synthetase inhibitor such as mefenamic acid or naproxin may be prescribed to reduce the pain. Mephanemic acid can be taken three times per day, the analgesic effect persisting for longer than that of asprin (Trounce 1997). Antispasmodic drugs such as hyoscine butylbromide may help with colicky pain. In cases of severe pain, the combined oral contraceptive pill may be taken for 6 months to suppress ovulation and reduce blood loss. This relieves pain for that period, and when normal cycles return, the pain should be less severe. Progesterone alone may be given to the young girl whose skeletal growth is incomplete. Progesterone from day 5 to day 25 will relax the arteriole spasm in the myometrium without inhibiting ovulation. It is thus also useful for those with pain who wish to become pregnant.

Dilatation and curettage may be performed to relieve cervical spasm or obstruction but is not advised as a routine intervention in dysmenorrhoea, due to the risk of incompetence of the cervix. In severe cases, hysteroscopy may be necessary to exclude uterine pathology. A laparoscopy may be required to exclude endometriosis (found to occur 3–4 years after the onset of menstruation; Hoshiai et al 1993). A pregnancy and vaginal delivery may improve or cure primary dysmenorrhoea.

NURSING PRIORITIES AND MANAGEMENT: PRIMARY DYSMENORRHOEA

Assessment

An assessment should be made of the general health of the patient. The nurse should enquire about any difficulties with menstrual periods and document the date of the last menstrual period. The patient's own description of the nature of her painful periods should be recorded along with any observations she makes about her physical and emotional symptoms on particular days of the cycle. Any medication used for pain relief or contraception, and its effectiveness, should be noted. Dietary habits and usual exercise activities are also relevant. By sensitively questioning the patient as to whether she has any special worries or has recently experienced any stressful events, useful information may be obtained for inclusion in planning care. Tension affects the perception of pain and when this is alleviated, by talking freely with an empathetic listener, the patient may experience some relief.

Asking the patient to suggest possible reasons for her pain should give the nurse insight into the patient's need for information about normal functioning and alternative ways of coping with pain.

Care planning

The care plan should be designed in collaboration with the patient. The degree of pain experienced will influence the care required. It may be necessary to help the woman recognise signs of impending menstruation so that analgesia can be taken in time to prevent pain. The nurse and patient should discuss strategies other than pharmacological interventions to relieve pain and how these can be incorporated in the care plan.

The stress of hospital admission or the illness condition may induce menstruation at an earlier date than expected and when the patient is more highly dependent. The nurse may then have to write up appropriate interventions to ensure the patient is 'pain-free' or 'pain is reduced to a tolerable level'. The patient's preferred methods of pain relief should guide the nursing actions planned.

The patient's need for health education should feature in the care plan and an outline teaching plan should be completed in preparation for the patient's discharge. Important issues for inclusion are as follows:

- Give a simple explanation of the functioning of hormones in the menstrual cycle and the effects of excessive prostaglandins; perhaps use diagrams.
- Discuss the beneficial effects of a diet adequate in fibre, vitamins and polyunsaturated fats, and low in sodium chloride.
- Compare the patient's present level of physical exercise with that of a more beneficial programme. Explain the effects of exercise and good posture in stimulating the function of all organs and the release of pain-relieving endorphins (see Ch. 19).
- Teach a simple relaxation exercise. Ask the patient to practise the exercise regularly. Explain the effects of muscular relaxation in counteracting anxiety or tension and muscle spasm. Refer to massage and local heat application.
- Discuss the use of drugs that reduce the development of prostaglandins, particularly any drug prescribed for the patient.
- Ask the patient to explain, in her own words, some of the changes she would like to make in future. Reinforce her understanding and resolve, and check whether she needs further explanation.

Evaluation of care

A pain verbal rating scale, such as the visual analogue scale (VAS, 0–10), from 'no pain' to 'intolerable pain' could be used by the patient to evaluate her experience of pain and the goal of reduced pain (see Ch. 19). If the goal is not achieved it may be necessary for the doctor to change the analgesic prescribed. Relaxation exercises should be used while the effects of analgesics are awaited. The pain the patient is experiencing whilst menstruating in hospital may be aggravated by the illness causing admission. There may be many factors in the care plan that are interdependent and need to be reviewed when setting further goals.

The achievement of the patient's goals will be her first step in a change of lifestyle. Further support and encouragement may be given by her mother, friend, partner, a school or practice nurse or the GP.

Secondary dysmenorrhoea

PATHOPHYSIOLOGY

Secondary dysmenorrhoea is experienced in later menstrual life by women in their mid-20s after previous years of painless menstruation. Woman usually complain of a dragging pain in the lower abdomen, pelvic area and breasts, accompanied by headache. The pain occurs some days before the menstrual flow and may continue throughout the period.

The condition is usually associated with some pelvic pathology, although anxiety or depression can be aggravating factors.

Adenomyosis. A state of increased tension in the uterine muscles, due to accumulating blood in the cystic spaces.

Fixed retroversion of the uterus can cause severe pain, especially if associated with a low-grade pelvic infection.

Partial stenosis of the cervix, following cautery or cone biopsy.

Endometriosis interferes with normal rhythmic contractions of the uterus.

Pelvic congestion, due to increased blood supply to the uterus, and menorrhagia.

Pelvic inflammation, particularly salpingitis, might contribute to pain.

Fibromyomata and polyps interfere with normal rhythmic contractions of the uterus and cause muscular spasms as the uterus attempts to empty itself of the abnormal tissue.

MEDICAL MANAGEMENT

History and examination. A detailed history of the problem is recorded and a full physical examination is completed. An accurate history of the pain is important, noting the age of onset, and the site, radiation, duration, character and time of onset in the menstrual cycle. The doctor seeks information about any related symptoms, possible abnormal uterine bleeding, pain on sexual intercourse (dyspareunia), pruritus and premenstrual tension.

Treatment. Medical treatment may involve examination under anaesthetic, dilatation of the cervix and curettage of endometrium. A laparoscopy may be performed when endometriosis is suspected. The presence of fibroids or polyps will be treated appropriately (see p. 248). Pelvic inflammation can be treated by antibiotics. An analgesic drug can be prescribed that is suitable for inhibiting prostaglandin synthesis, e.g. mefenamic acid.

NURSING PRIORITIES AND MANAGEMENT: SECONDARY DYSMENORRHOEA

On assessment, actual or potential pain episodes will be identified as a problem. Goals and interventions will be similar to those described for primary dysmenorrhoea, particularly education for the maintenance of personal health. Additional problems will be identified and appropriate nursing interventions planned depending on the specific underlying pathology and the treatment interventions recommended.

Social and psychological issues to be addressed in nursing vary with women's individual circumstances and needs. For example, a woman in her mid-20s may be anxious about a young family at home and worried about whether her partner will be able to cope with his work, the children and the chores, as well as visiting the hospital. The nurse may need to spend time with both the woman and her partner, together and separately, to establish whether any community support is needed until the woman is able to continue with her responsibilities at home. The nurse must be alert to the potential needs of the patient's children and may need to contact the health visitor about the family. Immigrant families may rely more heavily on support of their extended family so the burden of care is shared and there may be less need for support services.

Preoperative and postoperative care planning will be needed if surgical procedures are planned. Communicating information about examinations and any surgical procedures is part of the nurse's role. The nurse needs to be able to promote trust and develop a warm relationship with the patient, so that she can counteract the patient's fears and communicate effectively. The patient should be encouraged to express her feelings and thoughts and the nurse should be alert to the need for the patientto gain new knowledge to cope better with her physical sexual needs.

Opportunities for counselling and teaching should feature in the care plan. At the time of discharge the patient's future prospects for an improved pattern of menstrual cycles should appear much improved.

ABNORMAL UTERINE BLEEDING

Abnormal uterine bleeding is described according to the rhythm or pattern of the blood loss episodes:

- *Menorrhagia* refers to heavy or profuse menstrual bleeding. The flow of blood occurs at normal intervals but is increased in amount or duration.
- *Polymenorrhoea* describes menstrual periods that occur with a frequency of less than 21 days.
- *Polymenorrhagia* refers to periods that are both heavy and frequent.
- *Metrorrhagia* describes irregular or unusual bleeding from the uterus between periods.
- *Dysfunctional uterine* bleeding is the descriptive diagnosis used when no organic cause for the abnormal bleeding can be identified.

When abnormal uterine bleeding occurs, the passing of blood clots from the uterus is significant. The menstrual flow is greater than normal if the usual anti-clotting agents released by the endometrium are not able to control the volume or rate of flow of the blood.

Menorrhagia

PATHOPHYSIOLOGY

There is hormonal imbalance from any variation in the pattern of oestrogen and progesterone secretion; it is usually of endocrine origin with oversecretion of gonadotrophins. Emotional stress may result in excesses of these hormones being produced.

Ovarian lesions are of two types:

- *Polycystic growths* — may disturb the normal production of ovarian hormones and excessive endometrial growth occurs.
- *Immature follicles* — may fail to result in ovulation. The corpus luteum fails to form, so progesterone cannot be produced.

Oestrogen levels continue to rise and there is a proliferation of the endometrium.

Uterine lesions consist of the following types:

- *Fibroids* — increase the surface area of the endometrium that bleeds with greater flow. They may prolong the flow by restricting or disturbing contractions.
- *Polyps* — increase the surface area of endometrium.
- *Adenomyosis* — interferes with contractions by infiltrating the myometrium with endometrial cells.
- *Multiparity* — may result in loss of tone in the uterine muscle fibres. These may be replaced by fibrous tissue which will interfere in the normal contractions.
- *Developmental disorders*, e.g. a bicornuate, septate or duplicated uterus — may impede contractions.
- *Endometriosis* — this is a condition in which ectopic endometrium deposits may be found in the muscle wall or in scattered areas of the pelvic cavity; it is accompanied by increased blood supply to the uterus.
- *Tumour formation* — increases blood supply and bleeding.
- *Intrauterine contraceptive devices* — cause some irritation of the endometrium. Excessive bleeding may be problematic during the first 3 months after insertion.
- *Fallopian tubal ligation* — involves some alteration in the course of blood vessels that increases uterine blood supply. Following the operation, menstruation is usually heavier and may lead to the need for hysterectomy in some women.

MEDICAL MANAGEMENT

Medical examination seeks evidence of stress, worry or tension in the patient and will try to establish whether bleeding is a problem of quantity or rhythm, or both. Pelvic examination may reveal tenderness, masses or irregularities. If no pelvic abnormality is found, then a provisional diagnosis of dysfunctional uterine bleeding is made.

Investigations. Special investigation is made of haemoglobin level and full blood count to assess any anaemia present. An examination is carried out under anaesthetic (EUA) and a diagnostic curettage is performed to show the endometrial response to hormones and to exclude carcinoma. The curettage may identify uterine polyps. An estimation of urinary gonadotrophins, oestrogens and progestogens as indicators of hormonal activity may be completed.

Treatment. Depending upon the amount of blood lost, it may be necessary to nurse the patient in bed and to administer an anxiolytic sedative drug as prescribed to encourage relaxation and reduce stress responses. Any anaemia identified should be corrected as appropriate. The dilatation and curettage investigation may in itself relieve the problem, especially in cases of an endometrial polyp.

Hormone therapy may be given. Progesterone may be prescribed to provide a balance with oestrogens and reduce excessive endometrial growth. One of the combined contraceptive pills may be given to suppress hormone production, e.g. norethisterone 10–20 mg daily for 10 days, from the 15th day of the cycle. Progestogen administration will modify flow in heavy, but regular, cycles and acts as a haemostatic in dysfunctional uterine haemorrhage.

Endometrial ablation is a more recent treatment option for menorrhagia. This is also known as hysteroresection or transcervical resection of the endometrium (TCRE). Having been assessed as suitable for this treatment, the woman may be prescribed danazol 4–6 weeks in advance of the procedure to reduce endometrial thickening. The minimally invasive surgery involves the use of a hysteroscope and other instruments to remove the endometrial lining. This is monitored on a video screen. Following the procedure slight vaginal bleeding can be expected for a few days. Menstrual periods will become lighter or may cease, but dysmenorrhoea and premenstrual symptoms may continue. This procedure may require to be repeated at a later stage or a hysterectomy may eventually be necessary. Disadvantages of this procedure include the possibility of severe haemorrhage or uterine perforation which would necessitate hysterectomy at the time of TCRE. Women should therefore be aware of this before consenting to the procedure.

When a hysterectomy is deemed necessary it may be possible to undertake this without major surgery. This is achieved by means of laparoscopic surgery. There are several variations of laparoscopic hysterectomy which may involve the whole procedure being completed laparoscopically or a varying number of stages being completed vaginally. This requires insertion of a number of small trochars through the abdominal wall, providing entry sites for instruments. The viewing laparoscope is inserted below the umbilicus, two other insertion sites will be positioned just above the pubic hair line and accessory insertion sites will be used for electrosurgical techniques, a stapling device or to insert sutures via the abdominal cavity. The procedure is performed using video monitoring. The woman can be discharged from hospital within 2 days.

If large fibroids or endometriosis exist, an abdominal hysterectomy is required. Alternatively, in the case of fibroids, a myomectomy may be appropriate. Here the fibroids are shelled out of the myometrium. This conserves the uterus for child-bearing in younger women.

Metrorrhagia

PATHOPHYSIOLOGY

Lowered oestrogen level may occur just prior to the formation of the corpus luteum, resulting in vaginal blood spotting at the time of ovulation.

Changes in the cervix, e.g. inflammation, erosion, polyps or carcinoma, may cause slight bleeding, especially after intercourse or vaginal examination.

Changes in the vagina, e.g. inflammation, ulceration and atrophy, may cause bleeding.

New growth. Endometrial carcinoma is a major cause of irregular bleeding.

Complications of an early pregnancy. As an ovum settles into the endometrium, slight bleeding may occur. This loss may be repeated during several months of the pregnancy. Haemorrhage might also occur due to an abnormal positioning of the placenta, known as 'placenta praevia' (see Farrer 1990).

MEDICAL MANAGEMENT

Investigations. A visual examination of the vagina and cervix with a lighted vaginal speculum is usually an early investigation. A more detailed examination is possible with binocular magnifying microscopy, using the colposcope apparatus and completing the colposcopy examination. Magnification of the cervix allows for early diagnosis of cervical neoplasia through observation of the epithelial vascular pattern, surface contour and colour, which change with the neoplastic process. In 95% of patients, premalignant intraepithelial neoplasia is visible only through the colposcope.

Punch biopsies are taken for histological examination. The cytology laboratory examination of tissue complements the colposcopy observations. The Papanicolaou (Pap) smear test is a routine investigation to evaluate changes in cells shed or scraped from the cervix. A high vaginal swab of secretions will allow the identification of bacterial infection, fungal or parasitic infestations.

The dilatation and curettage operation will provide evidence to support any further investigations that may be necessary.

Treatment. Infections of the reproductive tract will be treated with the broad-spectrum antibiotic to which the organism is sensitive. Infestation with vaginal thrush (candidiasis) is relieved by nystatin pessaries. *Trichomonas vaginalis* is treated with metronidazole (Flagyl).

In ovulation spotting, small quantities of oestrogen may be given for 6–7 days, 3 days before ovulation.

Any malignant changes that are identified are usually treated by surgical excision, following which radiotherapy or cytotoxic drug treatment may be advised.

PREMENSTRUAL SYNDROME

Premenstrual syndrome (PMS) refers to a group of symptoms occurring in the latter half of the cycle, 2–12 days prior to menstruation, and subsiding soon after the menstrual flow begins. As luteal phase symptoms, they are not present for longer than 16 days. There is a symptom-free week following menstruation. The symptoms are diverse and vary from one woman to another, but also show variability from cycle to cycle in individual women with respect to severity, timing and duration. Definitions and diagnostic criteria show wide variation, causing problems with respect to establishing the true prevalence. Reported prevalence varies from 5 to 97%.

In establishing a diagnosis, Reid (1991) stresses the importance of the severity of symptoms experienced by women, since many experience premenstrual symptoms which are relatively mild and do not cause a notable problem. True PMS is said to affect 40% of women, approximately 5–10% being severely incapacitated during this phase of their cycle (Reid & Yen 1981). Symptoms of PMS frequently start after discontinuing the oral contraceptive pill or after a pregnancy, and become progressively worse with age.

Abraham (1987) subdivides symptoms as follows:

- nervous tension, mood swings, irritability and anxiety
- weight gain, swelling of extremities, breast tenderness, abdominal bloating and pelvic pain
- headache, craving for sweets, increased appetite, heart pounding, fatigue and dizziness or fainting
- depression, forgetfulness, confusion, crying and insomnia.

Symptoms can cause serious social disturbance within the family, at school or at work. Leather et al (1993) found that symptoms of PMS had greatest effect in the home, with 82% of women reporting relationships with their partners to be seriously affected and 61% reporting relationships with their children to be severely affected.

There may also be disturbed body image and low self-esteem. The woman may have been seeking help from her GP for recurring symptoms for at least six previous menstrual cycles before the diagnosis is made.

PATHOPHYSIOLOGY

Numerous theories have been suggested to explain PMS, but despite extensive research the precise cause remains unknown. PMS is concluded to be a multifactorial psychoneuroendocrine disorder.

The range of theories of PMS refer to imbalances, excesses or deficiency states and resulting physical changes (see Box 7.2).

Box 7.2 Theories related to premenstrual syndrome

Imbalance
- Oestrogen/progesterone
- Prostaglandins

Excess
- Aldosterone
- Angiotensin II
- Oestrogen
- Androgen
- Antidiuretic hormone
- Endorphin
- Prolactin

Deficiency
- Progesterone
- Androgen
- Essential fatty acid
- Blood glucose
- Magnesium
- Endorphin
- Zinc
- Vitamin B6

Physical changes
- Sodium and water retention
- Abnormal water distribution
- Leakage of albumin/tissue fluid
- Allergy related to progesterone
- Dietary abnormality
- Serotonin or aspartine neurotransmitter disturbance

Prostaglandins are produced in response to changing levels of oestrogen and progesterone. They exert sedative effects on the central nervous system and affect both aldosterone and ADH activity. If premenstrual changes are influenced by prostaglandins, it may be the balance between the prostaglandins that is of greatest importance.

Fluid retention or redistribution. Since the 1930s it has been suggested that PMS might be related to hormones responsible for fluid retention, but research studies can only suggest that there may be a redistribution of body fluids in intracellular and extracellular compartments. They have failed to demonstrate a pattern of fluid retention in most women who suffer from PMS.

Hypoglycaemia. Research studies have shown abnormalities of glucose metabolism in the luteal phase of the menstrual cycle and concluded that exaggerated glucose swings during the luteal phase might account for premenstrual hypoglycaemic symptoms. However, it has been concluded that there is not a causal relationship with PMS, but perhaps some concurrence between it and glucose metabolism (Reid et al 1986).

Vitamin B_6 (pyridoxine) deficiency. Vitamin B_6 is involved in the production of brain biogenic amines. It increases inhibitory amines such as dopamine and serotonin, and also acts as a coenzyme in converting excitatory amino acids to corresponding inhibitory amino acids, with sedative effects. Several PMS behavioural symptoms represent an excitatory state of the central nervous system and vitamin B_6 can reduce the excitatory biogenic amines. However, there is little scientific data to support the theoretical assumption that vitamin B_6 relieves PMS symptoms.

Research suggests a central neurotransmitter abnormality, causing a reduced platelet uptake of serotonin and reduced peripheral

Research Abstract 7.3
Beta-endorphins in premenstrual syndrome

In a study by Chuong et al (1985), 20 symptomatic and 20 control patients were studied for levels of several peptides, including beta-endorphin, on days 7 and 25 of the menstrual cycle. There were no significant differences between the two groups in the follicular phase of the study. In the control patients, beta-endorphins were higher in the luteal or premenstrual phase than in the follicular phase, but in the symptomatic PMS patients, the beta-endorphin levels fell in the luteal phase.

The difference between PMS patients and controls during the luteal phase was significant.

Chuong C J, Coulam C B, Kao P C, Bergstahl E J, Go V L W 1985 Neuropeptide levels in premenstrual syndrome. Fertility and Sterility 44(6): 760–765

blood serotonin levels found in the luteal phase of the cycle in women with PMS (Menkes et al 1992, Sundblad et al 1992).

Progesterone withdrawal. Although many researchers have suggested that PMS is the result of unopposed oestrogen effects, due to deficiency of progesterone production, many PMS patients have been shown to have adequate corpus luteum functioning. This suggests that it may be the rate of fall of progesterone level during the late luteal phase that is causative in PMS rather than a deficiency state.

Endorphin withdrawal. Endorphins are a group of substances which are endogenous opioid peptides. They appear to be important in the physiology of pain and mood change. Studies have shown that there is a change in endorphin levels in women who experience PMS, endorphins declining as the cycle progresses or in the week preceding menstruation (Giannini et al 1984, Facchinetti et al 1987). The endorphin theory is said to be one of the most credible for PMS (see Research Abstract 7.3).

O'Brien (1987) suggested that PMS is probably related to ovarian function, which in turn is linked to gonadotrophins, which may well be dependent on endorphin function. The current state of knowledge suggests that the primary causal factor lies somewhere in the hypothalamo–pituitary–ovarian mechanism or in the higher centres which influence it. While researchers have been keen to find one reason for PMS, it is possible that there is a combination of physical, psychological and social factors at play.

MEDICAL MANAGEMENT

Current treatment recommended focuses on identifying and controlling individual symptom clusters. Drug treatments are used cautiously. Many research studies have shown marked placebo effects of 40–60% in PMS sufferers. The patient–doctor relationship is thought to be an important influence on some women, who may be relieved that their condition is being taken seriously. Knowing that many other women also suffer is helpful and anticipation that some symptoms may improve, may relieve some tension.

Investigations. A thorough examination is required to accurately diagnose PMS and exclude or identify any underlying pathology. The patient may be treated by her GP or be referred to a PMS clinic. Other medical, psychiatric and gynaecological conditions must be excluded or be identified as coexisting with PMS.

A general physical examination of the patient is completed. Breast cancer must be excluded, as hormone-dependent cancers may be stimulated by therapy. A patient with pelvic pain may have an inflammatory condition, or endometriosis, that needs further investigation. Some patients may have a depressive illness, as well as PMS. This may be referred to as secondary PMS; the depressive symptoms persist through what is expected to be a symptom-free week in the cycle.

Estimations of oestrogen, progesterone, prolactin, gonadotrophin or electrolytes are not usually helpful in making a diagnosis of PMS. However, if there is research taking place in the PMS clinic, patients may be asked to give blood specimens as part of a series of investigations and treatments. Although research results are inconclusive about hormonal factors in PMS, hormonal treatments are still used and patients expect to receive hormone therapy.

Treatment. An integrated treatment programme can be adopted whereby patients are asked to record in a diary, on a daily basis, personal experiences in mood, behaviour, thinking patterns and physical discomforts, for at least 3 months. Symptom clusters and symptom-free times can be thus easily identified.

In addition, women should be advised to:

- take regular exercise
- avoid coffee, tea and chocolate
- take a diet that is low in sugars and high in lean proteins
- take vitamin supplements B_6 and E_1 and the mineral magnesium
- restrict salt intake
- limit fluid intake
- chart their weight daily
- avoid alcohol and smoking
- avoid stress.

These general measures contribute to good health and can maximise physical and psychological well-being.

While some women have found evening primrose oil to relieve symptoms of PMS (Campbell et al 1997), the beneficial effects have not been substantiated in research (Khoo et al 1990, Robinson & Garfinkel 1990, Budeiri et al 1996). Robinson & Garfinkel (1990) included factors such as diet, exercise and stress control in their recommendations for effective management of PMS.

Women may recognise factors that aggravate or trigger their symptoms. They learn to cope and live with their condition and may not report back to the clinic or need further treatment. Knowing that professional help remains available to them gives confidence.

Some women find aromatherapy helpful for specific PMS symptoms, such as headache or fluid retention. A few drops can be added to bathwater or mixed in a massage oil. Clary sage, rosemary or peppermint can be used to relieve headache; fennel, juniper or geranium to reduce fluid retention; bergamot, jasmine and clary sage to elevate mood; and lavender and rose to help balance hormone production (Rich 1996). Essential oils should not be used directly on the skin without diluting in water or carrier oil, and instructions on the bottle should be followed to reduce the risk of any skin sensitivity.

Drug treatments used in PMS depend partly on the preference of the doctor providing care and the particular cluster of symptoms experienced by the patient. Many women who have already tried over-the-counter remedies expect or request hormonal treatment. The patient needs to know that the doctor may not find the right medication at first.

Hormonal treatment of PMS is as follows:

- Some doctors continue to use progesterone or progestogen for all PMS symptoms. The drug may be given orally, by injection, by suppository, in the combined contraceptive pill or by means of an implant.

- The drug danazol, which inhibits pituitary gonadotrophin secretion, is prescribed selectively for some patients, particularly those with severe mastalgia and other PMS symptoms (Halbreich et al 1991). Danazol completely suppresses the menstrual cycle and reduces breast tenderness, but varying degrees of improvement in other symptoms have been documented. Patients are advised to use alternative, non-hormonal contraceptive methods. The major disadvantage of danazol is that high doses cause masculinisation. Treatments at low dosage, not greater than 400 mg daily, can reduce symptoms in some women (Deeny et al 1991) without the masculinisation effects. Other minor side-effects such as nausea, dizziness and rashes are troublesome to certain patients, who need to discontinue treatment.
- Analogues of gonadotrophin-releasing hormone (GnRH), such as buserelin, if given continuously and in high doses, will inhibit the release of gonadotrophins and so suppress follicular development, ovulation and the endocrine changes of the cycle.
- GnRH analogue may be administered by nasal inhalation or as a depot preparation. Muse et al (1984) treated eight patients with clear-cut PMS symptoms. Controlled suppression of the cycle was achieved and nearly all symptoms were greatly reduced. A temporary, reversible 'medical oophorectomy' is produced by this treatment. The treatment is expensive. GnRH analogue can only be used as a short-term therapy, otherwise postmenopausal symptoms will develop.
- Oestrogen therapy, in the form of transdermal patches or subcutaneous implants, can be used to suppress menstruation. Natural oestrogen administered by this route avoids the liver and so prevents problems with clotting factors and lipid metabolism. For women with a uterus, the use of this percutaneous oestrogen therapy requires to be complemented by the use of cyclical progestogen, to prevent endometrial hyperplasia. Unfortunately some women experience mild PMS-like symptoms during this phase of the treatment.
- Bromocryptine is a stimulant of dopamine receptors in the brain and also inhibits the release of prolactin by the pituitary. The role of prolactin in PMS is poorly understood, but bromocryptine has been shown to be effective in the treatment of breast symptoms. Sondheimer et al (1988) suggest that some patients are helped simply by reassurance that the breast symptoms are not cancer but normal fluctuations in breast activity.

Diuretic treatment. In women who have a measured weight increase the diuretic spironolactone may be prescribed. This drug has an adrenocortical and anti-androgen action. Some investigators have found it to be useful for symptoms of depressed mood.

Analgesic treatment. Where pain is a primary symptom, the anti-inflammatory analgesic and prostaglandin inhibitor mefenamic acid may be helpful, but research as to how many PMS symptoms this drug will relieve is contradictory. There is agreement that the drug is of benefit for some PMS symptoms.

Psychological support. Supportive psychotherapy and techniques that improve coping skills and stress management should be part of the care programme. Patients have found self-help groups of benefit. Relaxation exercises undertaken together and assertiveness training may be part of the total programme. People who experience secondary PMS, whereby their unhappy mood and agitated behaviours persist throughout their cycles, may need the clinical help of a psychiatrist. Rational emotive therapy and antidepressant medication may be necessary to relieve symptoms.

Surgery. In cases of severe PMS or those compounded by other gynaecological problems, hysterectomy with bilateral salpingo-oophorectomy followed by hormone replacement therapy may be considered. Oophorectomy must be included to prevent the ovarian cycle, otherwise the cyclical problems will persist.

NURSING PRIORITIES AND MANAGEMENT: PMS

Assessment

The nurse may encounter many women who experience PMS symptoms which they have not discussed with their doctors. Nurses have opportunities to provide such women with information that may enable them to modify their lifestyles. Suggesting daily recording of physical changes, discomforts, emotional feelings and behaviour can help with personal assessment.

Care planning

A supportive–educative approach should be used. This combines the giving of information and advice, but also allows the woman to suggest how best the aims can be achieved in her particular circumstances. The nurse should discuss options with particular care to avoid causing any financial embarrassment to the woman who may have little money to spare from her family budget for vitamin supplements or evening primrose oil, which are available without a prescription.

Useful advice includes the following:

- Undertake physical exercise as a stimulant to the circulatory system, improving functioning of all bodily organs and relieving congestion. As a result concentration and sleep should improve, and feelings of well-being may increase.
- Reduce fat, sugar, salt, coffee and tea consumption.
- Aim to eat five servings of fresh fruit and vegetables per day (Williams 1995).
- Reduce smoking and alcohol intake.
- Avoid stressful situations to reduce tension and feelings of frustration, particularly at trigger times in the cycle.
- Incorporate relaxation exercises.
- Obtain massage, carried out by a partner, nurse or therapist.

A counselling approach by the nurse can encourage the woman to verbalise her preferred choices appropriate to her individual programme. Information should be given to the patient about the nature of any drugs prescribed, their action and possible side-effects. Referral to a health visitor may be necessary if the patient requires continuing support at home. The availability and possible value of self-help groups can also be discussed with the woman, but the value of family support, emphasised in some cultures, should not be undermined.

Evaluation of care

The patient should be guided into self-evaluation of progress during the week when she is usually symptom-free. Any measures taken will be recalled and any physical or emotional changes that the patient has recorded in the daily diary will be noted. These can be related, where possible, to the actions the patient has taken, and conclusions drawn. Some symptoms may have greatly improved, but there may be no feeling of improvement in other areas. The patient must be congratulated on her personal achievements, as appropriate, and encouraged to sustain any changes in lifestyle that are thought to have had a beneficial effect.

Where unresolved problems remain, the exposure to each planned action should be reviewed and the action modified for a further interval. Evidence of a sustained unhappy mood or other severe symptoms should be referred to the GP or PMS clinic doctor. The patient may need the added interventions of a psychiatrist or psychotherapist. With support, and medication if necessary, most women are able to achieve some measure of improvement.

DISORDERS OF THE MENOPAUSE

Physiological, psychological and social changes associated with the menopause have been described earlier. The long-term effects of oestrogen withdrawal on women's health will now be addressed.

Decreased oestrogen formation is associated with the development of osteoporosis and cardiovascular disease, resulting in an increased risk of bone fractures, myocardial infarction, angina and stroke. The literature suggests that there is some cultural variation in the experience of postmenopausal symptoms and in the incidence of disorders related to the withdrawal of oestrogen (Lock 1994, Robinson 1996, Chow et al 1997). Gasperino (1996) proposes that there is ethnic variation as well, suggesting, for example, that the greater bone and muscle mass and lower fat, as a percentage of body weight, in black women is relevant to the lower incidence of osteoporosis and cardiovascular disease in this ethnic group.

Factors contributing to an increased risk of osteoporosis and cardiovascular disease include:

- inherited factors
- sedentary lifestyle
- low calcium intake
- low body weight
- early menopause
- cigarette smoking
- excessive salt intake
- excessive stress
- high protein
- alcohol
- caffeine
- pre-existing disorders of the kidney or thyroid, rheumatoid arthritis and diabetes.

Osteoporosis

Osteoporosis is a disease characterised by a decrease in bone density per unit volume predisposing to fracture with minimal trauma. The demineralisation and consequent weakening of bone are more marked in trabecular bone. The most common sites for fractures are the wrist, spine and hip, causing pain, deformity and hospitalisation. The report of a World Health Organization (WHO) Scientific Group (1996) noted that the prevalence of osteoporosis and hip fracture varies by country and by population group within countries, osteoporosis being rare in Africa, frequent in India and most common in Europe and North America. Whitehead & Godfree (1992) indicated that 40–50% of British women will suffer an osteoporotic fracture before 75 years of age.

Oestrogens play an important part in achieving a strong bone structure. They determine the sensitivity of bone to parathyroid hormone, limit resorption of bone and increase calcium absorption from the gut. In early adult life, the rate of bone formation exceeds that of resorption to build up strong bone. When oestrogen levels decline prior to the menopause, bone resorption increases and bone loss accelerates after the menopause. This is most marked in the first years after the menopause when there is a significant decline in oestrogen. During the first 5–10 years after the menopause, bone density decreases significantly. Thereafter the rate of bone loss gradually decreases. Lower oestrogen levels are a major factor contributing to osteoporotic fractures in women (Rosenberg et al 1995). Failure to achieve maximum skeletal mass in early adulthood will be aggravated by oestrogen deprivation after the menopause.

Cardiovascular disease

Before the age of 50, deaths from breast cancer outnumber deaths from ischaemic heart disease and stroke in women, but in postmenopausal women the mortality rate for arterial disease greatly exceeds that of breast cancer. Jacobs & Loeffler (1992) suggested that 60% of deaths in women over the age of 65 are due to cardiovascular causes.

Withdrawal of oestrogen at the menopause causes changes in lipid and lipoprotein metabolism, resulting in a low HDL/LDL ratio. Such metabolic disturbances contribute to the incidence of cardiovascular disease in this group (Stevenson 1996). Oestrogen replacement therapy in postmenopausal women has been shown to improve serum lipid profiles. It is therefore suggested that hormone replacement therapy can have a favourable effect on cardiovascular health (Rosano et al 1996, Stevenson 1996).

MEDICAL MANAGEMENT: LONG-TERM EFFECTS OF THE MENOPAUSE

Although the long-term effects of oestrogen withdrawal occur years after the menopause, they have potentially serious implications for health, quality of life and mortality.

Hormone replacement therapy. Once bone loss has occurred it cannot be replaced. There is evidence that oestrogen prevents bone loss in early menopausal women (Stevenson et al 1990) by decreasing the rate of bone resorption. Prophylactic hormone replacement therapy (HRT) has therefore been recommended. Whilst this can be commenced at any time after the menopause, it is most effective if started at the time of the menopause or shortly after, as this is when bone loss occurs most rapidly.

Other therapies which reduce the rate of bone resorption are calcitonin and bisphosphonates. Calcitonin can prevent postmenopausal trabecular bone loss (MacIntyre et al 1988, Overgaard et al 1989) by decreasing osteoclast activity. Bisphosphonates also inhibit osteoclast activity and can be used as a preventive measure or as treatment in established osteoporosis (Reginster et al 1989).

Epidemiological studies have suggested that oestrogen replacement can decrease the risk of cardiovascular disease after the menopause (Hunt et al 1990, Stampfer & Colditz 1991). Finucane et al's (1993) results from a national cohort suggest a decreased risk of stroke in postmenopausal women on hormone therapy. Nabulsi et al (1993) suggested that taking oestrogen postmenopausally can reduce the risk of coronary artery disease by 42%, and if progestin is included the benefits may be even greater. The main beneficial effects on the cardiovascular system appear to be on vessel walls, blood flow and lipid metabolism (Whitehead & Godfree 1992).

Oestrogens used in HRT are natural oestrogens which mimic 17-beta oestradiol, oestradiol and oestrone, the main oestrogens produced by the ovary. Oestrogen therapy is administered continuously.

Progestogens are given for 12–14 days per month on a cyclical basis to women with a uterus, for endometrial protection, reducing the risk of erratic bleeding, endometrial hyperplasia and endometrial cancer (Whitehead et al 1990). This results in a withdrawal bleed. Livial (Tibilone) is a synthetic steroid with properties of oestrogen, progestogen and androgen; if taken continuously, it should not cause a withdrawal bleed.

Oestrogens are available orally, as a subcutaneous implant, a transdermal patch, a vaginal cream and a percutaneous gel. A nasal spray has been subject to trial (Gangar & Penny 1995). Oral oestrogen passes through the liver before entering the general circulation. Other routes avoid the liver and potentially reduce the risk of disturbed liver functioning.

Progestogens are available as tablets or a transdermal patch in association with oestrogen. An intrauterine device containing levonorgestrel in the stem, released through the membrane, may provide a useful source of progestogens for women on HRT (Gangar & Penny 1995). By introducing progestogen directly into the uterus, the systemic side-effects can be eliminated.

Short-term hormone therapy may be prescribed for specific menopause symptoms such as hot flushes and atrophic vaginitis, for as long as treatment is required.

Long-term HRT is required in women under 40 years who have had a premature menopause, occurring naturally, as a result of surgery or iatrogenically. In addition, it is increasingly being considered prophylactically to reduce the risk of osteoporosis and cardiovascular problems following the menopause.

While HRT confers benefits for both short-term and longer-term effects of the menopause (see Research Abstracts 7.1 and 7.4), it can also have side-effects, and risks are associated particularly with long-term use. In addition, there are some contraindications to be considered regarding the use of HRT.

Research Abstract 7.4
Transdermal administration of oestrogen/progestogen hormone replacement therapy

Sixteen symptomatic, postmenopausal patients (median age 54.1 years) applied the oestradiol transdermal therapeutic system (TTS) 50 mg/day for 14 days via patches to the buttocks. They were then given two combined norethisterone acetate–oestradiol patches (approximately 50 mg of oestradiol and 0.2–0.3 mg of norethisterone) daily for a further 14 days. The treatment was repeated for five cycles. All but one of the patients had regular withdrawal bleeding. Fourteen patients had endometrial biopsy samples taken during the fifth treatment cycle. No sample showed proliferative or hyperplastic features. The patients also underwent metabolic studies. The effects of transdermal norethisterone acetate on postmenopausal symptoms of hot flushes, night sweats and vaginal dryness, and on lipid metabolism and psychological status were determined by comparing effects in the oestrogen-only phase and in the combined phase. The effects were very mild. Three patients experienced skin irritation. The findings show that transdermal progestogen, at a lower dosage, can be successfully administered in hormone replacement therapy to prevent endometrial proliferation while minimising the adverse effects that may be seen with oral administration.

A small number of patients participated in this preliminary study. Caution is therefore needed in drawing broad conclusions.

Whitehead M I, Fraser D, Schenkel L, Crook J, Stevenson J C 1990 Transdermal administration of oestrogen/progestogen hormone replacement therapy. Lancet 335: 310–312

Although there are many preparations of HRT available for long-term benefits, the reported compliance rate is poor, with a significant number of women discontinuing therapy. Hall & Spector (1992) claim that only 26% of women prescribed HRT take the treatment beyond 1 year and a National Opinion Poll (1992) survey indicated that 50% of women discontinue HRT within 6 months. Treatment is abandoned because of the side-effects experienced or because of fear of risks associated with the treatment. Possible side-effects include:

- breast pain/tenderness
- leg cramps
- vaginal discharge
- vaginal bleeding
- fluid retention/bloating
- mood changes
- increased appetite.

Such side-effects might be reduced or eliminated by changing to a different preparation. However, women are encouraged to persist with one form of therapy for at least 3 months as some of the early side-effects can be temporary.

While it is acknowledged that unopposed oestrogen increases the risk of endometrial cancer, if progestogens are administered for 12–14 days of the cycle, this risk is eliminated (Whitehead et al 1990) (see Research Abstract 7.4). The link between HRT and breast cancer is more controversial. The general view, on the basis of current research, is that there appears to be no increased risk with short-term therapy (up to 10 years) but that there may be a slightly increased risk if taken for more than 10 years (Harris et al 1992, Yang et al 1992, Colditz et al 1995).

Contraindications to HRT are usually described as absolute or relative. Absolute contraindications generally include:

- pregnancy
- undiagnosed endometrial bleeding
- endometrial cancer
- breast cancer
- severe active liver disease
- porphyria.

While HRT is not recommended for women with these problems, individual women may still wish to take HRT for severe acute symptoms or for protective effects. Such women are referred to a specialist centre to be fully informed and closely monitored if they decide to embark on the therapy. Possible contraindications are identified to highlight the likelihood of complications, to ensure that underlying disorders are treated or monitored, and to monitor the appropriate therapy, which may differ from uncomplicated cases, if the woman and her doctor decide on HRT. Caution is therefore required in prescribing HRT in association with the following:

- endometrial hyperplasia, endometriosis or fibroids
- hypertension — treat prior to HRT
- clotting problems — refer to a haematologist (Whitehead & Godfree 1992)
- diabetes — monitor glucose levels to identify any change required in insulin
- gallstones — may be aggravated, rather than develop as a new disease (Whitehead & Godfree 1992); if treated, they are not of concern
- otosclerosis — Whitehead & Godfree (1992) recommend referral to an ENT specialist since they have anecdotal experience of increasing deafness in such patients.

Some GPs prescribe hormone replacement therapy directly, while others refer women to menopause clinics, which have become established in many hospitals throughout the UK.

Menopause clinics. Many hospitals now provide menopause clinics that are staffed by a gynaecologist with a special interest in the management of problems associated with the menopause. Specially trained nurses and paramedic personnel contribute to the overall assessment and care of those attending the clinics and attempts are made to provide a cost-effective service. Treatments can be more easily controlled and supervised within such a clinic, protocols are established, dietetic and diagnostic facilities are more available, and screening, general health and patient education programmes can be introduced.

NURSING PRIORITIES AND MANAGEMENT: THE POSTMENOPAUSAL WOMAN

Women should be encouraged to make an informed choice about HRT. The role of the nurse involves the development of trust within the nurse–patient relationship and the giving of information to enable women to come to an informed decision. The educative and supportive aspects of the self-care nursing model (Orem 1991) are useful. Whilst not recommending HRT for all postmenopausal women, it is not justifiable to withhold treatment from a fully informed patient who requests it. However, HRT will only be fully evaluated after a further two decades of use (Purdie 1990).

Since women worry about the risks of HRT, the nurse should raise these, both to allow a discussion of personal feelings and to clarify any misunderstandings. It is important to warn about the early side-effects of the sudden rise in oestrogen levels at the start of HRT. Women should understand that there are a range of medications, doses and types of HRT, so that if one is found to be unacceptable, another regimen may be tried.

The following is a guide for nurses interviewing women facing the menopause:

- Provide information and advice according to the problems and concerns of individual women and any ongoing postmenopausal symptoms.
- Encourage a healthy lifestyle and continuing health awareness.
- Give dietary information to encourage selecting low-fat, calcium-rich foods; explain physiological links to vascular conditions and the maintenance of bone mineral content.
- Check the patient's usual physical exercise pattern; reinforce the need for regular exercise, stressing the importance of the pull of muscle on bone for bone formation and health; discuss a weight-bearing exercise programme.
- Discuss the benefits and possible side-effects of HRT.
- Explain the need for self-examination of breasts and teach the technique.
- Provide opportunities for questions.
- Check the patient's understanding of the information given by encouraging feedback.
- Give the patient a copy of free booklets prepared by the HEA (HEB in Scotland), relating to the menopause and a healthy lifestyle (such as *The Time of Your Life, Well Woman, Eat to your Heart's Content, Look after Yourself*).
- Give the patient the name and telephone number of a person to contact in the event of any problem occurring.

DISORDERS OF THE FEMALE REPRODUCTIVE SYSTEM

GYNAECOLOGICAL CANCER

Cancer is a state of overgrowth of tissue resulting from disorganised cell division (see Ch. 31). Normal mechanisms limit tissue cell reproduction so that the number of cells produced is relative to the number of cells that die. In some circumstances, the restraining mechanism of a cell may be faulty. The cell is then able to multiply without restriction or concern for balancing body requirements.

The organs of the female reproductive system are susceptible to benign or malignant overgrowth of tissues. Cancerous or malignant tumours are generally differentiated from benign tumours by the following properties:

- they are not encapsulated and invade tissues in which they arise
- they show disorderly reproduction
- they tend to show loss of structural differentiation
- they can produce metastases.

The cervix, body of the uterus, ovary and vulva are potential sites for primary cancerous growth.

Carcinoma of the cervix

The cervical tissue is at particular risk of carcinomatous change. Each year there are approximately 2000 deaths in England and Wales from carcinoma of the cervix, and approximately 4500 new cases are registered. The incidence of invasive cervical cancer appears to be falling but there is a notable increase in the incidence of pre-invasive cancer (Blake et al 1998).

Cancer of the cervix occurs most often in women between 30 and 50 years of age. It is preceded by a pre-invasive condition that can be simply and effectively treated if identified by cervical cytological screening. Although there is difficulty in providing a high-quality smear and programmes can still be improved in terms of accessibility and education for all women, cervical cytology remains the most effective screening test in medical oncology, contributing to a reduction in the morbidity and mortality rates of cervical cancer (Masood 1997).

Pre-invasive cancer of the cervix

PATHOPHYSIOLOGY

The endocervical canal is lined with columner epithelium one cell thick. Deep branching glands, called compound racemose glands, exist within these cells and secrete alkaline mucus. Adenocarcinoma, which is relatively rare, arises within these cells (5–12% of cervical cancers). This type of cancer is not normally diagnosed from a cervical smear.

The area where the columnar cells of the endocervix join with the squamous cells of the ectocervix is called the squamocolumnar junction (SCJ). A natural physiological process exists whereby the columnar cells migrate down to the ectocervix, moving the SCJ to a new position and causing a red area of columnar epithelium around the cervical os (Hopwood 1990). The migrated columnar cells then start to break down in the acid environment of the vagina and the squamous cells beneath grow to replace them. This area where the normal replacement of the columnar cells with squamous cells takes place is called the transformation or transitional zone and is most commonly where pre-cancerous changes occur. Cervical smears must therefore be taken from this area using specially shaped instruments.

A specific segment of DNA (the fundamental genetic material of all cells), known as an 'oncogene', has been identified as giving a cell its cancer potential. Adolescence, the time of menstruation, the first pregnancy and the prenatal period are times of maximum cellular activity in the cervix, when the tissues are more sensitive to a carcinogen that has been sexually transmitted and more prone to genetic mutation.

The relationship between cervical squamous pre-cancer and sexual intercourse appears to be conclusive since the condition is virtually unknown in celibate women. Epidemiological observations indicate that the age of onset of intercourse and the number of sexual partners influence the development of cervical pre-cancer and cancer (Lewis & Chamberlain 1995). The condition is also more common in lower socioeconomic groups. The more sexual partners the woman has had, the more likely she is to be exposed to the unknown carcinogen(s). Two viruses have been proposed as possible carcinogens:

- the human papilloma virus (HPV) (Eluf-Neto et al 1994)
- the herpes simplex virus type 2 (Hildesheim et al 1991, Jones 1995).

The specific high-risk viruses thought to be linked with cervical cancer — HPV16, 18, 31 and 33 — cannot be identified from a cervical smear test alone. The DNA needs to be examined.

Studies of the role of the male sexual partner suggest the possible transmission of viruses but also refer to the possible carcinogenic effect of human sperm. It is suggested that the basic proteins of histone and protamine fraction of the sperm heads may act as carcinogens. Some men may be high-risk sexual partners (French et al 1982). Barrier methods of contraception can be advised to offer protection.

There is a possible increased risk of cervical cancer associated with cigarette smoking although there may be several coexisting factors contributing to the risk (Phillips & Smith 1994, Szarewski et al 1996). Factors currently considered to be important are listed in Box 7.3. These factors may change as research continues.

Carcinoma of the cervix is now classified as a preventable disease if certain examinations are undertaken regularly by women. Cervical cancer that is identified in the pre-invasive stage is curable.

Common presenting symptoms. The earliest knowledge that a woman may have of a malignant change in the cervix may be from a report on a cervical smear test. A clear vaginal discharge may occur in the early stages, whereas later the discharge may be bloodstained or have a bad odour. Irregular vaginal bleeding may be associated with prolonged menstruation, occur between periods, follow sexual intercourse, or be postmenopausal. Pain may be experienced when metastases are present or if there is nerve involvement.

Where there is advanced disease, venous or lymphatic obstruction may lead to extensive oedema within the pelvis. Blocked ureters may result in renal failure, and the spread of growth may lead to fistula formation between the vagina and rectum, or the vagina and the urinary bladder, in which case incontinence will be unavoidable. Massive haemorrhage may occur and death may be related to kidney failure or intestinal complications.

Box 7.3 Risk factors and possible causes of carcinoma of the cervix. (Reproduced with kind permission from Shingleton & Orr 1987)

Risk factors
- Early intercourse (before 17 years of age)
- Multiple sexual partners
- Early pregnancy
- Living in an urban environment
- Low socioeconomic status
- Smoking
- Immunosuppression
- Use of oral contraception
- Previous abnormal smear
- Failure to participate in screening
- Nutritional deficits — vitamins A, C, folic acid
- High-risk male partner
- In utero diethylstilboestrol exposure

Possible causes
- Human papilloma virus
- Herpes simplex virus
- Sperm from high-risk tissue-type male
- Smoking
- In utero exposure to diethylstilboestrol
- Immune deficiency

MEDICAL MANAGEMENT

Investigations. The following procedures may be completed:

- Papanicolaou smear test
- colposcopy and biopsy
- Schiller test
- histological examination of smears and tissue specimens.

Papanicolaou (Pap) smear test. Papanicolaou and Traut showed the value of smears in detecting cervical cancer as early as 1941, but it was not until 1964 that cervical screening was introduced in the UK. During the 1980s a number of initiatives were introduced in the UK to improve the organisation of cervical screening services and reduce mortality from cervical cancer. In 1985, district health authorities in England and Wales and health boards in Scotland were awarded responsibility for setting up computer-managed systems for the call-up and recall of women for cervical screening (DHSS 1985). Women are generally recalled on a 3- or 5-yearly basis depending on the health authority or health board. In 1988 the government instructed district health authorities and health boards to offer cervical screening to women aged 25–64 years (20–60 years in Scotland) by 31 March 1993 (DHSS 1988). The 1990 contract for general practice (Health Departments of Great Britain 1989) reiterates this recommendation, with target payments being awarded to GPs on the basis of the percentage of women on their lists being adequately screened within a certain time.

On the basis of research, Day (1989), Cancer Research Campaign (1994) and Ibbotson & Wyke (1995) recommend that women between 20 and 64 years old should have a smear test every 3 years. This takes account of cost-effectiveness of the service and benefits to women. However, for maximum personal benefit women may wish to have a Pap test every 1–2 years from the time they are sexually active until the age of 70. Women who are not or have never been sexually active are excluded. A woman who has had a total hysterectomy for benign reasons will not require subsequent smear tests, but if a hysterectomy has been performed for pre-cancer or cancer, subsequent vault smears should be taken. Women who have had a subtotal hysterectomy will still require to have cervical smear tests.

All those who take smears must be adequately trained in the procedure and many courses are available for nurses in the UK. The

Box 7.4 Papanicolaou smear test results in graded classes

Class 1	Cells are normal in appearance
Class 2	Abnormal cells are present but are not malignant; the patient may have suffered from vaginal inflammation
Class 3	Abnormal cells are present and are suggestive of malignancy
Class 4	Abnormal cells are present and appear to be malignant
Class 5	Abnormal cells are present and definitely malignant

Box 7.5 Histology of cervical intraepithelial neoplasia (CIN)

Current terminology for cervical intraepithelial neoplasia describes three grades of change as part of a continuum of pre-invasive disease:

- CIN1 corresponds to mild dysplasia
- CIN2 corresponds to moderate dysplasia
- CIN3 corresponds to severe dysplasia and carcinoma in situ

Royal College of Nursing (1994) acknowledges that this requires a knowledgeable practitioner who can understand and interpret results, communicate results to women, make appropriate follow-up arrangements and implement fail-safe recommendations.

The cells identified from the cervical smears are classified as shown in Box 7.4. This information is supplemented as appropriate with the histological grade of pre-invasive disease, i.e. CIN1, CIN2 or CIN3 (see Box 7.5).

Women may be asked to have a smear test repeated. This may occur in cases where there is an inconclusive diagnosis or if minor cytological abnormalities are detected. In cases of moderate dysplasia or worse, the woman should immediately be referred for colposcopy, for more detailed examination.

Schiller test. Iodine 3.5% is used to stain normal cells of the cervix. Abnormal cells will not pick up the colour because they do not contain glycogen. A section of tissue is taken for histology.

Colposcopy and biopsy. Every woman who has an abnormal smear test result should be examined with the colposcope, but the high incidence of cervical cell abnormalities makes this an unrealistic expectation. Colposcopy is recommended immediately for all women with a smear that suggests CIN2 or CIN3.

Colposcopy is examination of the vagina and cervix using magnification and illumination, to identify and assess pre-invasive changes. Saline may be applied to the cervix to identify blood vessel patterns there. Acetic acid is applied to the transformation zone, mucus is removed with a cotton wool ball or a swab and the area is carefully examined for abnormal epithelium. Iodine can be used to outline abnormalities. Several biopsies are taken from abnormal areas. Histological examination of the biopsies will confirm the diagnosis of pre-invasive disease. If the transformation zone cannot be completely visualised because it extends too high in the cervical canal, a cone biopsy is performed for diagnosis.

A diagnostic biopsy method may be that of punch biopsy or low-voltage diathermy loop excision biopsy. The punch biopsy tends to crush the sampled tissue and may not include stroma which can lead to missing invasive disease. The diathermy loop excision method can provide tissue samples of better size and allows better control of bleeding.

Treatment options

Conservative treatment. Pre-invasive cancer of the cervix that can be fully visualised within the transformation zone can be treated by destruction of the entire transformation zone down to a depth of 6 mm. This depth will ensure the destruction of diseased crypts and glands without destroying normal tissue. Accurate assessment of depth is difficult. Conservative treatment is important to the woman who has not yet started a family and who needs to avoid developing an incompetent cervix to prevent loss of a future pregnancy.

The following destructive treatment methods may be used:

Cryotherapy. Cryonecrosis is produced by crystallisation of intracellular water using nitrous oxide or carbon dioxide. Freeze–thaw–freeze techniques produce the best results. Little or no analgesia is required. There is, however, some concern about the adequacy of the technique; reported cure rates are between 27 and 96% (Charles & Savage 1980). Patients can expect a copious watery vaginal discharge after this procedure.

Electrocoagulation diathermy. Temperatures of over 700°C are used to induce tissue destruction to a depth of at least 7 mm. As the procedure is painful, it is carried out under general anaesthesia. Bleeding and discharge can be expected in the postoperative period. A high success rate is achieved: 88–97% (Woodman et al 1985).

Cold coagulation. A thermasound heated to 120°C is applied for 20 seconds to five areas of the surface of the cervix. The procedure is completed under local anaesthetic and has a reported cure rate of 94% (Gordon & Duncan 1991).

Laser vaporisation. The carbon dioxide laser may be applied to the cervix to ablate the pre-invasive cancer by causing intracellular water to boil, create steam and explode cells. The laser power may be pulsed or be continuous in use. The depth of tissue destruction can be controlled. The procedure can be performed under local anaesthetic. Postoperatively, primary or secondary haemorrhage may occur. A 94% success rate has been reported (Baggish et al 1989).

Excision of the transformational zone. This procedure can be performed using laser or a diathermy loop. The latter method is easier to perform and more economical in terms of time. Large loop excision of the transformation zone (LLETZ) may be achieved under colposcopic guidance by low-voltage diathermy. It may be an alternative to cone biopsy. The wire loop is introduced into the cervix and taken slowly across it, enveloping the transformation zone, which may be removed in one or several pieces. The procedure is performed under local anaesthetic. A bloodstained vaginal discharge usually follows for 1–2 weeks. Severe secondary haemorrhage may occasionally occur.

Cone biopsy. When a transformation zone is not fully visible for colposcopy then an excisional method of treating the pre-invasive cancer has to be used. A cone or cylinder of tissue is removed, either by laser or by a scalpel after the application of Lugol's iodine to the tissues. The entire transformation zone is excised, which provides a large specimen for histological examination and allows confirmation that all diseased tissue has been removed or that the disease was more extensive than originally diagnosed. The procedure, performed under a general anaesthetic, may be complicated by secondary haemorrhage, infection, cervical stenosis or incompetence. Care is required to prevent uterine perforation and pelvic abscess.

NURSING PRIORITIES AND MANAGEMENT: PRE-INVASIVE CARCINOMA OF THE CERVIX

The person with pre-invasive cancer is treated as an outpatient or may be admitted and discharged within 1 day. Diagnosis, treatment and follow-up are completed in separate visits to a colposcopy clinic. Information about appointments and details of cervical smears, colposcopy procedure and possible treatment of the condition is usually sent to the patient in advance of attendance at the clinic. An appointment for colposcopy is given to correspond with the middle of the menstrual cycle, which is a favourable time for the procedure. The nurse will need to reinforce the information given when the patient attends the clinic, to ensure that the patient understands the procedures planned and the expected outcome.

Opportunities need to be provided for patients to express any concerns. Anxiety levels amongst women presenting for colposcopy have been found to be higher than those of women going for surgery, concerns about the procedure being as great as those about the illness condition (Marteau et al 1990). The nurse can seek to reduce the patient's anxiety to an acceptable level. Sensitive approaches are required to help the patient to express her feelings and think rationally about the future after treatment.

When the patient feels more calm, other information can be given, as it is more likely to be retained. The nurse should tell the person to expect vaginal discharge and some bleeding after the treatment, and explain what to do if bleeding becomes suddenly very heavy or if she suspects she has an infection. The opportunity for health promotion regarding possible smoking can be taken.

Arrangements for a follow-up cervical smear test are discussed as part of the pre-discharge routine, as well as the need for future annual check-ups.

Invasive carcinoma of the cervix

PATHOPHYSIOLOGY

Commonly, carcinoma develops from the vaginal surface of the cervix, and less often from the cervical canal. It may form an ulcer on the cervix or become a fungating cauliflower-type growth and is of the squamous cell type. Tissues become eroded and infected, forming an unpleasant vaginal discharge.

The carcinoma spreads by direct infiltration of surrounding tissues and via lymphatic vessels. Blood-borne metastases in more distant organs occur less often. The prognosis for cervical cancer relates to the extent of the growth at the time of diagnosis rather than to the histological type of the cancer. The international classification of carcinoma of the cervix is shown in Box 7.6 (see also Ch. 31).

Box 7.6 International classification of carcinoma of the cervix

Stage 0	Pre-invasive carcinoma, also known as carcinoma in situ (CIN3)
Stage IA	Microinvasive carcinoma; less than 5 mm in depth
Stage IB	Neoplasm confined to the cervix
Stage IIA	Neoplasm has infiltrated adjacent parametric tissue or upper vagina; if the carcinoma is endocervical then it has extended up into the uterus in this stage
Stage IIB	Tumour extending to the parametrium but not to the pelvic wall
Stage IIIA	Lower third of the vagina is involved or the parametrium
Stage IIIB	Involves lymph nodes as far as the pelvic wall or there are isolated metastases in the pelvis, often obstructing a ureter
Stage IVA	Spread of growth to adjacent organs
Stage IVB	Spread to distant organs

Common presenting symptoms. A woman may have no particular symptoms at the time a cervical smear result confirms that cancer of the cervix exists. On the other hand, she may visit the doctor because of irregular vaginal bleeding, perhaps associated with sexual intercourse, micturition or defaecation. An ulcerated area or an overgrowth of tissue on the cervix may be directly visible to the doctor on examination using a vaginal speculum.

A vaginal discharge becomes more continuous, a thin blood-stained loss may change to a thicker, brown, offensive discharge or heavier bleeding episodes. Lower abdominal pain develops as the growth increases in size, spreads and exerts pressure on surrounding structures. Very severe lower back and sciatic pain may occur and lymphatic nodes adhere to the sacral plexus. Pressure on the pudendal nerve and blood vessels causes obstruction to the venous return and oedema of the legs.

Incontinence of urine and faeces may occur as the bladder and rectum are inflated with growth or react to radiation side-effects. Ureters may become blocked and renal failure may ensue.

MEDICAL MANAGEMENT

Investigations. A number of investigations are required before any treatment is planned to establish the spread or otherwise of the disease. A chest X-ray and intravenous pyelogram are completed to gain information of obstruction of the flow of urine from the kidneys, which indicates involvement of the parametrium. A cystoscopy may be performed. A lymphangiogram and a CT scan will assist with identification of disease spread to lymph nodes.

The patient with carcinoma of the cervix requires a general physical examination and a thorough pelvic examination. Haematological and blood chemistry and nutritional studies will be completed. An examination under anaesthetic (EUA) is carried out at the time of cone biopsy or the insertion of radioisotopes. The EUA increases the accuracy of identifying the stage of development of the growth. It allows better examination of the upper vagina and improved palpation of the abdomen, pelvis and enlarged pelvic, inguinal and para-aortic lymph nodes. Fine-needle aspiration of nodes under sonar or CT guidance may be performed to delineate the spread of the cancer. The information gained is used to confirm, modify or extend treatment plans.

Serum markers. Tumour-derived and tumour-associated markers in the plasma of patients with carcinoma of the cervix continue to be studied and reported on in the medical literature (Ngan et al 1996, Sliutz et al 1997). Individual marker levels may be used at the assessment stage, in the planning of treatment, when monitoring the response to treatment and in the follow-up years of care. Marker measurement values tend to increase with the stage of disease and decrease with effective treatment. Initial levels before treatment may be an aid to prognosis. The following are examples of serum markers that may be studied:

Carcinoembryonic antigen (CEA). Squamous cell carcinoma and adenocarcinoma have significantly different capacities for CEA release (Kjorstad & Orjasaester 1984).

Plasma histaminase falls during radiotherapy with a value that is inversely proportional to the radiation response (Birdi et al 1984).

Tumour-associated antigen (TA-4) provides a means for monitoring squamous cell tumours (Maruo et al 1985).

Immunosuppressive acid protein (IPA). It has been reported that patients with recurrent cervical cancer showed elevated IPA, whilst 83% of patients previously treated but without evidence of recurrence did not have elevated levels (Sawada et al 1984).

***Treatment* options:**

Surgery. When the carcinoma is confined to the cervix, resection of the malignant tissue is necessary. This may be achieved by laser beam therapy, cone biopsy of the endocervical tissue or amputation of the cervix. Where there is extension of the growth up into the uterus, hysterectomy and removal of pelvic lymph nodes will be necessary.

Radical surgery may be planned for some patients who are at earlier stages of the disease and are more generally fit. This surgery may be combined with radiotherapy as tumours of the cervix are particularly radiosensitive. Care is jointly planned by the surgeon and radiotherapist. The Wertheim–Bonney–Meigs operation involves removal of the uterus, cervix, the upper third of the vagina, pelvic cellular tissue lateral to the uterus and vagina, and the uterosacral and cardinal ligaments. The lymphatic glands in the obturator fossae and along the external and internal iliac vessels are removed. The ovaries are preserved in premenopausal women.

To facilitate the excision of the cervix, vagina and supporting ligaments, the ureters are dissected free during the operation. Postoperatively there may be a breakdown of the ureteric anastomosis, leading to a urinary fistula. The autonomic nerve supply to the bladder may be disturbed resulting in incomplete bladder emptying as a complication.

Pelvic exenteration. Where there is extensive recurrent disease, an anterior pelvic exenteration may be performed, involving removal of all the reproductive organs and the urinary bladder. The ureters are implanted into an artificial bladder fashioned from a loop of ileum. If the rectum is also removed, a terminal colostomy is formed. This extremely radical surgery may be combined with cytotoxic drug therapy using cisplatin and other chemotherapeutic agents.

Radiotherapy. Stages III and IV of carcinoma of the cervix are usually inoperable. Palliative irradiation therapy is then indicated. Radiotherapy is initially to reduce the size of tumour, inhibit its growth and reduce its blood supply before surgical removal by hysterectomy. Caesium-137 rods may be inserted under general anaesthetic into the uterine cavity and vaginal vault to provide a radiation dose to the whole pelvis. The treatment will reduce the blood supply to the growth and exert a lethal effect on the cancer cells. Hysterectomy may be performed after local irradiation by caesium or standard supervoltage techniques. Cytotoxic drug treatments are also used as necessary, in combination with other therapies. The surgeon may fashion a ureteric transplant or a colostomy that will provide more physical comfort for the patient in the later phase of the illness.

Radiation may also be administered via sophisticated machinery such as the Cathetron, which can pass high-intensity radiocobalt radiation from a protected store along ducts to applicators already positioned in the uterus and vagina. The patient is treated in a protected room, reducing radiation risks to others.

The dose of radiation necessary to kill the tumour cells may leave a very low level of protection for healthy tissue cells. Short- or long-term radiation reactions may be induced by therapy. The bladder and rectal tissue may become swollen, inflamed, friable or fibrosed and there is a risk of the development of a fistula. The patient may become distressed by urinary problems or diarrhoea. Symptoms are relieved as they occur. Minor surgical repair operations may be necessary. The patient's general comfort is of prime importance.

NURSING PRIORITIES AND MANAGEMENT: HYSTERECTOMY

Preoperative care

Assessment

The patient who is to have a hysterectomy for carcinoma of the cervix will be admitted to the ward with enough time to allow for necessary medical investigative procedures to be carried out before the operation. She is likely to be physically fairly independent of the nurse for her personal care but will need to be introduced to the new surroundings of the ward.

The assessment process will identify the patient's individual problems and needs for nursing assistance and support. She will be invited to share details of her menstrual history, the date of her last menstrual period, the events leading up to admission and the current degree of vaginal blood loss or discharge. The patient who has previously been prescribed an oral contraceptive drug will have been advised to discontinue the contraceptive pill and use an alternative barrier method for 6 weeks prior to the operation to reduce the risk of thrombus formation during surgery or in the postoperative period. The nurse should check that this advice has been followed.

The ward may provide useful guidelines for the nurse to follow in assessing a patient's gynaecological details.

Identification of actual and potential problems

The summary of patient problems at the end of the assessment will reflect the stage of the cervical carcinoma. Problems of distressing pain in the back or abdomen, poor appetite and weight loss, as described in the medical history section earlier in this chapter, are associated with later stages of the disease. The patient may identify few actual problems herself but may agree with the nurse that she has some special needs at this time that will be part of her care plan.

Anxiety. In anticipating hysterectomy, the woman may experience considerable anxiety related to surviving the operation and the illness condition. A change in body image may occur, a sense of loss and some alteration in sexuality and sexual identity may be feared. The woman's loving relationship with her partner may appear to be threatened by the surgery, particularly if her child-bearing potential is lost. Anxiety may also be focused on the family members who remain at home: how will the children and her partner cope whilst she is in hospital? She may be worried that her illness will affect her ability to work and support the family in future. A gentle approach by the nurse may help the patient to speak about her main concerns. Being able to do this at the time of assessment may be the first step towards making a positive adjustment and thereby reducing anxiety. The nurse will be able to plan to utilise opportunities to help the patient manage her anxiety during the hospital period.

The need for information. In preparation for surgery, the patient will need information about the events to be expected during both the lead-up to the operation and the recovery period. The benefits of planned information-giving preoperatively, based on nursing research findings, are described in Chapter 26. Opportunity must be given for the patient to ask questions and express fears.

She will need to know about pain relief, e.g. by her own patient-controlled analgesia system (PCA) or epidural analgesia. Time should be taken to explain that sexual relations with her partner will still be possible after hysterectomy and refashioning of the vagina. An information booklet explaining the operation and its resultant internal changes and answering many questions about the future should be provided for the patient to read at her leisure. This provides a permanent reminder of what she may have been told and reinforces her understanding.

The surgeon will advise when sexual intercourse may be resumed. Normally this will be several weeks after the operation, to allow internal healing and to reduce the incidence of infection. The patient will benefit from knowing that a sexual climax will again be achievable even though the uterus has been removed. The nurse can explain that the pleasurable sexual experience is achieved from the stimulation of the external clitoris within the vulva and the psychological experience associated with stimulation of the penis in the vagina. The patient may already be aware of this, but will be pleased to know that the experience should not change. It is helpful if the patient's partner can be included in the information-giving session. The patient may then approach surgery more calmly and confidently, and recover with minimal physical or emotional problems (see also Research Abstract 7.5).

The need for exercise and mobilising skills. Patients will have limited mobility in the first 48 h after a hysterectomy. There will be a risk of venous stasis and pressure sore development. Patients should be encouraged to practise foot and leg exercises before the operation, so that they understand how to carry out the exercises while resting in bed after surgery. If appropriate, use of the contraceptive pill, with its potential risk of deep vein thrombosis, will already have been discontinued and a short course of subcutaneous heparin may be prescribed prophylactically. Patients will also benefit from experiencing how it feels to be moved and lifted by nurses and a mechanical hoist, and from knowing what they can do to assist the process. This should help to reduce apprehension about being moved at a time when dependent and in some pain. A visit by the physiotherapist will prepare the patient for moving, deep-breathing and coughing exercises to be used after the operation. Smokers will be asked to stop.

Protection from hazards. The person preparing for and undergoing hysterectomy needs to be safeguarded from misidentification and wrong operation. The patient must wear an identification bracelet at all times and this must be strictly checked at strategic times in the immediate preoperative period. The nurse responsible for planning care writes specific instructions for maintaining patient safety. Many hospitals and NHS Trusts use a preoperative checklist or protocol for every patient preparing for surgery. Such protocols have been agreed by ward nurses, anaesthetic and theatre staff and reflect the quality standard of patient safety to be achieved. A record of safety checks is retained in the patient's care plan.

The doctor is responsible for fully informing the patient about the planned operation and is required to obtain the patient's informed consent in writing. The nurse preparing the patient checks that the consent form has been signed before completing the other major surgery preoperative procedures (described in detail in Ch. 26). The patient will wear anti-embolism stockings to counteract venous stasis during the operation period. A premedication is given as prescribed. The patient relaxes in bed until she leaves the ward escorted by her nurse who completes a safe transfer to the operating theatre staff.

Postoperative care

The patient's individual needs and actual problems will transfer from a preoperative care plan to a postoperative care plan, but a major new focus will be that of maintaining a safe internal and external environment for the patient. There are a number of potential problems that will feature in the care plan and will have been explained to the patient preoperatively. The general care of a patient following major abdominal surgery is described in Chapter 26 and in Nursing Care Plan 7.1.

Research Abstract 7.5
A study of self-concept and social support after hysterectomy

Webb & Wilson-Barnett (1983) studied depression, self-concept and sexual life in 128 women during recovery from hysterectomy as part of a nursing study. At the time of operation, 103 were premenopausal and 102 were sexually active. The women were interviewed 1 week and 4 months after the hysterectomy. The results showed that women felt physically and emotionally much better, were less tired and irritable, had gone back to work and had resumed leisure and social activities. Responses showed that:

- 94% were happy to have no more periods
- 84% were glad they could no longer become pregnant
- 90% of those who were sexually active said their sex life was now as good as, or even better than, previously
- 92% were glad they had the operation.

The small numbers who gave 'negative' replies to these questions were still not completely recovered and gave this as the reason for their answers. They referred to physical complications of wound, urinary or vaginal infections which delayed recuperation rather than the psychological problems suggested in medical studies.

In studying the social support of these women results showed:

- 70% had been told 'old wives' tales' of pessimistic outcomes; 11% felt there was some truth in them after their own experiences
- 23% of partners (n = 103) had been given no extra help in the home.

The greatest area of dissatisfaction was in the lack of information from doctors and nurses. Women would have liked guidance on what they could do, how they might feel as they progressed and what symptoms or complications could occur.

The Roy adaptation nursing model was used in the care of a patient following hysterectomy (Webb 1988).

Webb C, Wilson-Barnett J 1983 Self concept, social support and hysterectomy. International Journal of Nursing Studies 20(2): 97–107

Carcinoma of the body of the uterus

Carcinoma of the body of the uterus is more common with advancing age, most cases occurring in the sixth and seventh decades (Blake et al 1998). The condition is associated with infertility, diabetes mellitus, oestrogen replacement therapy, obesity and hypertension. An excess of oestrogen is common to all the risk factors. As women are living longer, the present rate is expected to increase.

PATHOPHYSIOLOGY

The columnar epithelium that covers the surface of the endometrium and forms the lining of the glands gives origin to the carcinoma of the body of the uterus. The growth is usually an adenocarcinoma. In a small number of cases of adenocarcinoma, there may be a squamous metaplasia. This squamous element may be benign or malignant.

Nursing Care Plan 7.1 Care of a patient following a hysterectomy

Potential problems	*Expected patient outcomes*	*Nursing care*	*Rationale*
1. Irregularity in vital signs	❒ Pulse and BP measurements are within acceptable limits for the patient ❒ Blood loss through wound or drainage tubes is minimal in any 24 h	Record BP and pulse: ______ Inspect wound/drains Observe for any pv loss Record temperature: ______	Haemorrhage due to loss of haemostasis at operation site would result in hypovolaemia, requiring blood transfusion. Fine drainage tube is in position in wound. Pyrexia may occur due to infection in chest, urinary tract, wound or veins
2. Body fluid imbalance	❒ No sign of dehydration or fluid overload ❒ Patient is adequately hydrated ❒ Signs of fluid overload are detected from fluid balance record	Maintain intravenous therapy as prescribed Observe i.v. puncture site for signs of infection or fluid being given extravenously Record fluid intake and output Dress cannula site with: _____ Change giving set: ______	Major surgery depletes body potassium, sodium and water levels Fluid and electrolyte replacement is needed by the intravenous route
3. Patient to have nil by mouth	❒ Peristalsis returns within 48 h	Patient to be given no fluid or food by the oral route until prescribed by doctor Record any bowel activity	Peristaltic movement of the intestines stops when the abdomen is opened and the gut is handled. Food and fluid, if taken, could not be digested. Bowel sounds are heard when peristalsis returns. Patient passes gas
4. Urinary bladder is drained by a self-retaining catheter (suprapubic or transurethral) **Risk of bladder dysfunction after catheter removal** **Risk of urinary tract infection**	❒ Urine drains freely to minimise pressure on operation sites ❒ Urine is clear and has low bacterial count	Observe and record urinary output Obtain catheter specimen of urine: __________ for laboratory culture and sensitivity Complete catheter toilet: ___ Remove catheter on: ______	During the radical hysterectomy the ureter is either partially dissected to allow resection of the medial portion of the cardinal ligament, or more extensively dissected to sever the cardinal ligament at the pelvic side wall. There may be oedema and bruising of posterior urethral wall. Diminished bladder sensation, reduced bladder compliance and stress incontinence may occur. Urinary tract infection is a risk with a catheter in the urinary bladder
5. Possibility of patient becoming distressed or uncomfortable due to postoperative pain	❒ Patient expresses verbally or by body language that pain has decreased to an acceptable level on a pain scale of 1 = 'low' to 5 = 'high'	Remind the patient of the availability of analgesia Reposition the patient as necessary for comfort Give analgesia as prescribed or supervise the patient-controlled analgesia system (PCA) Ask patient if analgesia is adequate using pain scale 1 = 'low' to 5 = 'high'	Patients have different pain tolerance levels. It may not be possible to keep the patient pain-free at all times. A degree of pain control that is acceptable to the patient should be planned
6. Limited mobility with risk of: **• venous stasis** **• pressure sores**	❒ No limb tenderness, pain, swelling or redness during hospital stay ❒ Moves safely within limits allowed ❒ Pressure areas remain intact	Supervise limb exercises whilst patient in bed, to be performed __ -hourly Move patient to relieve pressure over bony prominences: 2-hourly Anti-embolism stockings to be worn until _______ Mobilisation programme: ______________________ ______________________	The patient who is immobilised by major surgery and confinement to bed may experience reduced muscular stimulation to the venous system. The blood flow in the veins of the limbs is slowed down, increasing the potential for blood clot formation, inflammation of the vein and surrounding tissues (phlebitis and cellulitis) with accompanying

Nursing Care Plan 7.1 *(cont'd)*

Potential problems	***Expected patient outcomes***	***Nursing care***	***Rationale***
			swelling and pain and possible embolism. Body pressure exerted over pressure areas for more than 2 h will result in compromising the blood supply to the tissues and the development of pressure sores. Exercising of limb muscles and the wearing of anti-embolism stockings are preventive measures that reduce risk. Measures to relieve pressure over pressure areas are effective in preserving skin and other tissue integrity
7. Needs information or new skills in readiness for discharge	❐ With information/ instruction/practice will be able to function independently in:_____ _____ _____ by discharge on:_____	Patient preparation: _____ _____ _____ _____	Depending upon progress during the hospital stay, the patient will need an individualised pre-discharge programme. Advice and counselling in areas of the activities of living may be needed. Personal care, including wound management, the importance of exercise and restricting of lifting activity, should be related to the surgical removal of ligaments and supporting structures in the pelvis and the slow healing of abdominal muscle and other tissues The patient may be discharged with a suprapubic catheter in situ. Practice will be needed in the management of the closed drainage system. The patient may have the support of a community nurse when at home to complement self-care. The patient will need to know what to do if problems occur, and who to contact: GP or hospital. The patient should be encouraged to ask questions and talk about any concerns. Information about a local group of the Hysterectomy Association should be provided should the patient feel in need of support and social contact. Medical staff will need to give specific instructions about when sexual intercourse may be resumed and what follow-up surveillance will be maintained in the observation for recurrence of disease; 20-year follow-up may be achieved

Box 7.7 International classification of endometrial cancer

Stage 0	Carcinoma with no stromal invasion
Stage I	Carcinoma confined to the body of the uterus; the cancer is also graded according to histological type, as follows: *Grade 1* — well-differentiated adenocarcinoma *Grade 2* — moderately differentiated adenocarcinoma with partly solid areas *Grade 3* — predominantly solid or entirely undifferentiated carcinoma
Stage II	The carcinoma involves the cervix as well as the corpus
Stage III	The carcinoma has extended outside the uterus, but not outside the pelvis
Stage IV	The carcinoma has involved the bladder or the rectum or has been extended outside the pelvis.

Endometrial carcinoma develops in an atrophic senile uterus. The lesion penetrates the endometrium, spreads laterally and grows slowly. With time it penetrates the myometrium deeply, reaching the peritoneal covering, and the lymphatic glands become involved. Secondary deposits may affect pelvic and aortic lymph nodes and the ovary. Metastases to the lung, bone, liver or brain may be late, blood-borne complications (see Box 7.7).

Common presenting symptoms. From the age of 45 years, a woman expects changes in the menstrual cycle related to the menopause. The early signs of carcinoma of the uterus may be difficult to distinguish from the changes of the climacteric. Unexpected or irregular vaginal bleeding is a significant sign. Bleeding that is too heavy, occurs too often or happens after cessation of periods at the menopause needs to be investigated. Low abdominal pain may be a late experience for the woman with uterine carcinoma. The vaginal discharge may be clear or brown with an offensive odour.

MEDICAL MANAGEMENT

Investigations. In some cases a routine cervical smear test may yield the first evidence of malignant endometrial cells. Initial investigations include a transvaginal scan (TVS) and endometrial biopsy. If the endometrial biopsy is insufficient for histological identification of malignant cells or if there is thickening of the endometrium shown on the TVS (indicative of pathology), the diagnosis can be concluded by a hysteroscopy followed by dilatation and curettage of the endometrium.

Total hysterectomy. Cancer of the uterus is usually treated by total hysterectomy and bilateral salpingo-oophorectomy, i.e. surgical removal of the uterus, cervix, fallopian tubes and ovaries. The abdominal or vaginal surgical approach may be used. A vaginal hysterectomy is suitable if the uterus is small and not distended with bulky tumour.

Extended hysterectomy. An extended hysterectomy also includes removal of pelvic lymph nodes. Surgical treatment may be combined with radiotherapy to the pelvic wall. Alternatively, the uterine tumour may be irradiated to shrink it and deplete its blood supply before surgery. Postoperative radiotherapy may be given either as external beam only or in combination with vault caesium.

Cytotoxic and hormonal drug treatments. Cytotoxic drugs may be used as early as possible following surgery to counteract metastatic seeding. Carcinoma of the endometrium is often sensitive to hormone therapy. High doses of medroxyprogesterone acetate (Depo-Provera) or hydroxyprogesterone caproate (Delalutin) may suppress the progress of the disease in advanced cases and limit metastatic activity. The 5-year survival rates in women treated for early cancer of the uterus are 60–70%.

NURSING PRIORITIES AND MANAGEMENT: CARCINOMA OF THE UTERUS

The nursing care of the patient with cancer of the uterus involves pre- and postoperative care for hysterectomy. Care will be individualised but will be similar to that for the patient with carcinoma of the cervix (see p. 241).

Total or extended hysterectomy does not involve dissection of the ureters, as in radical hysterectomy. The patient should therefore have less difficulty with recovery of bladder function postoperatively, as there will be no disturbance of the nerve supply or any bladder wound. A self-retaining urethral catheter may be used in the first few days, to avoid distending the urinary bladder and exerting pressure on the posterior urethral wall, which may be swollen and bruised.

A haematoma in the vault of the vagina is a potential complication of vaginal hysterectomy. This will result in prolonged abdominal discomfort, raised body temperature and a sustained feeling of being unwell, until the haematoma is diagnosed and drained.

The patient will need information about her progress at regular intervals in the postoperative period. Of particular concern may be the need to have cytotoxic drug therapy at an early, vulnerable stage after major surgery. The patient may feel greatly debilitated by the side-effects of nausea and vomiting. Psychological support from the nurse should help the patient to view the chemotherapy as the final safety net in the treatment process. Positive improvements should be seen within 3 months of treatment being completed. Medical follow-up will be essential to monitor progress and identify early signs of recurrent disease.

Malignant disease of the ovary

Ovarian cancer is more common in developed than in developing countries (Lambert et al 1992). A relationship is said to exist between multiple ovulation in women in well-nourished communities and the incidence of ovarian cancer, the disease being more common in the better-nourished and upper social groups. Pregnancy and the oral contraceptive pill have a protective effect. The condition is more common in infertile and nulliparous women and in women who have not taken a sexual partner. A previous problem of endometriosis of the ovary is linked to malignant change. The peak incidence is between 50 and 70 years of age (Blake et al 1998).

To date there is no effective sceening procedure for early detection of this disease in the population. The tumour is widespread before symptoms appear. As a result, late detection of the condition prohibits effective treatment and the mortality rate is higher than for other genital malignancies.

PATHOPHYSIOLOGY

Ovarian tumours comprise tissues of the normal ovary, most commonly arising from the epithelial lining. The tumour may occur unilaterally or bilaterally. Carcinoma developing in other organs can metastasise to the ovary. Carcinoma of the body of the uterus may spread directly to the ovary, although this is less common with carcinoma of the cervix or vagina. The pylorus, sigmoid colon, rectum, gall

Box 7.8 International classification of ovarian cancer

Stage I	Disease limited to one or both ovaries
Stage II	Growth extending beyond the ovaries but confined within the pelvis
Stage III	Growth with widespread intraperitoneal metastases
Stage IV	Cases with other distant metastases and/or parenchymal liver involvement

bladder, breast and kidney are very possible sites of primary growth. The lymphatic channels and blood vessels facilitate the spread of ovarian cancer. Box 7.8 gives the classification of ovarian cancer.

Ovarian cancer is histologically classified according to the type of cell from which it originates, the most common source being surface epithelium, which is formed from embryonic mesothelium. Three types of tumour may develop:

- serous (tubal)
- endometrioid (endometrial)
- mucinous (endocervical).

Serous papilliferous carcinoma. The malignant serous tumour is the commonest type of primary ovarian cancer and often affects both ovaries. The growth penetrates the capsule of the ovary and projects on the outside surface. Tumour cells are disseminated into the peritoneal cavity to form multiple seedling metastases. In most cases there is rapid spread in the peritoneal cavity. The peritoneum secretes excessive amounts of fluid into the abdominal cavity.

Serous papilliferous cystadenoma. The cysts of this serous new growth contain many papillary processes and are lined with a single layer of cubical epithelium on a vascular connective tissue base. The epithelium resembles that of the fallopian tube, the cells being ciliated.

Mucinous cystadenoma. Mucinous tumours are formed from columnar epithelium, similar tissue to that of the endocervix. The tumours are described as multilocular because they consist of several cysts clustered together and separated from each other by a septum. The cysts have mainly fibrous tissue walls and contain viscid mucin, a glycoprotein. This tumour can grow to a very large size.

Mucinous cystadenomas may rupture spontaneously or be damaged during surgery, spilling epithelial cells into the peritoneum where seeding and further growth takes place with secretion of mucin that may form a jelly-like mass in the abdominal cavity.

Mucinous carcinoma. Approximately 10% of ovarian cancer is classified as mucinous and 5% of mucinous cysts are found to be malignant (Lewis & Chamberlain 1995). Many of these tumours tend to be identified at an early stage of growth, which gives a better prognosis for the patient.

Endometrioid carcinoma. In the ovary, this type of cancer histologically resembles adenocarcinoma of the endometrium of the uterus. The tumour consists of tubular gland cells as found in the endometrium. It may be secondary to uterine disease or it may be a primary ovarian growth that coexists with cancer in the body of the uterus.

Germ cell tumours. Similar tumours may arise in the germ cells of either sex and may be benign or malignant. Benign conditions are very common, while malignancy is rare. The commonest type of germ cell tumour is the dermoid cyst or cystic teratoma. Dermoid cysts, which are discussed in more detail later in the chapter, usually occur in the ovary but are very rare in the testis. The malignant teratoma is more common in the testis.

Amongst the malignant germ cell tumours, the highest incidence is of the dysgerminoma which histologically resembles a seminoma of the testis. It shows large round cells separated by fibrous septa and is highly malignant, perforating its capsule and spreading cells into the blood and lymphatics.

MEDICAL MANAGEMENT

Ovarian cancer is insidious in its growth and the woman may be quite free from discomfort or suspicion of disease until it has reached an advanced stage. Approximately 70% of women have the disease diagnosed when it has spread beyond the ovaries (Blake et al 1998). The late symptoms that appear are related to increased pressure in the abdominal-venous channels, causing oedema in the legs and pain from pressure on nerves to the legs. Metastatic growth in the peritoneum will contribute to extensive ascites, abdominal pain, frequency of micturition, nausea, vomiting, emaciation and breathlessness. A thrombosis may form in an iliac vein or in the inferior vena cava. If growth has spread to other organs then other symptoms may occur, such as obstruction of the small bowel or the colon.

Investigations. A full pelvic examination is necessary, with palpation of the ovaries. Ultrasonic scanning and laparoscopy are useful diagnostic procedures. A Pap smear may show ovarian malignant cells in a specimen taken from the posterior fornix of the vagina. X-rays of the pelvis and vertebrae may show bony metastases. An intravenous pyelogram may be performed to assess the degree of involvement of the urinary system. A ureter may become obstructed and hydronephrosis may occur. A full blood count and serum biochemistry are included in investigations and tumour markers have a place in diagnosis. Ovarian tumours are always surgically removed. It is important that the ovary and peritoneal cavity should be fully assessed to define the spread of the disease.

Treatment. When malignant disease of the ovary is diagnosed, both ovaries need to be removed and total hysterectomy completed. The tumour may involve the peritoneum or other organs, and as much malignant tissue as possible will be removed. The infracolic omentum should be removed since it is a common site for microscopic disease (Blake et al 1998). Adjuvant chemotherapy is normally given except in early stages of the disease. Radiation is generally confined to palliation. In advanced states, palliative treatment only may be possible. Abdominal paracentesis may be performed to relieve the pain and respiratory distress caused by ascites. Hospital admissions are arranged as needed to make patients more comfortable. They may be cared for in a hospice or live their last months with their families at home.

NURSING PRIORITIES AND MANAGEMENT: OVARIAN CANCER

In addition to physical care, the patient with ovarian cancer will need much psychological support from the nurse. The anxieties associated with investigations, diagnosis and the effects of hysterectomy and cytotoxic drug therapy will need to be anticipated and managed in all aspects, as described earlier in the chapter. The patient may make a full recovery quite quickly or, if secondary disease remains, may be debilitated for longer. She may or may not be aware of the seriousness of the cancer condition, as full details of the illness may have been withheld in her best interests. However, openness is generally found to be more helpful for both the patient and her carers (Glaser & Strauss 1965, Hinton 1980, Knight & Field 1981, McQueen 1997).

The nurse will work towards helping the patient make physical and emotional adjustments. Attention will be given to the relief of pain, nausea and vomiting after surgery and chemotherapy. As physical problems are relieved, the patient may cope better emotionally, but in terminal cases, time is needed to adjust to the sad news. If a warm, trusting relationship has been developed with the nurse at the acute stage of treatment, it will sustain the patient who needs to return to the ward to continue with cytotoxic drug therapy or for palliative paracentesis. This can be emotionally demanding for the nurse but can also provide immense satisfaction, and patients appreciate the time and individualised attention given to their emotional needs (McQueen 1995). The terminal patient may choose to spend her last days at home with her family and with the support of the community nursing service; alternatively, she may wish to stay in the familiar surroundings of the ward with staff who are known to her and able to cope with her needs. In caring for terminally ill patients, the nurse's empathetic feelings extend to the patient's family, and part of holistic patient care incorporates the giving of information and support to the relatives (McQueen 1997).

BENIGN TUMOURS OF THE UTERUS

Endometrial polyps

Polyps are benign neoplasms of the endometrium of the uterus. They may develop from an overgrowth of endometrial glands and stroma. The polyp may produce a stalk and may descend towards the vulva. Single or multiple polyps may occur, commonly in women of any age group. Vaginal bleeding may be slight but occurs between menstrual periods or following coitus. The patient can be anaesthetised and the polyp removed from the uterus by twisting it off at its stalk or by curettage of the endometrium. Recurrent multiple polyps may undergo malignant change. Histological examination of all polyps is routine.

Fibromyomata

Myomata or fibroid tumours of the muscle of the uterus can occur in women between 35 years of age and the onset of the menopause. The growth of fibroids is stimulated by ovarian hormones, particularly oestrogens. Women who have not had children are more liable to develop such tumours.

PATHOPHYSIOLOGY

The fibroid is spherical in shape and firm in consistency. Some fibroids are small, while others may grow large enough to fill the abdominal cavity. The tumour is encapsulated and the capsule contains the blood vessels supplying the tumour. As it grows, the centre of the tumour becomes less vascular and liable to degenerative change.

Multiple fibroids may be present, giving the uterus an irregular shape (see Fig. 7.7). The fibroids may cause displacement of the uterus and uterine vessels.

Common presenting symptoms. Menstruation becomes heavier and is prolonged when there are fibroids in the uterus. If the tumours are submucous then menstruation may become irregular and there may be bleeding between periods, but this is not common. Uterine pain may result as the uterus strongly contracts to attempt expulsion of the fibroid. Pressure upon pelvic nerves may cause back or leg pain, or pressure on pelvic organs may lead to:

- frequency of micturition
- retention of urine
- obstruction of the gastrointestinal system
- oedema of a leg.

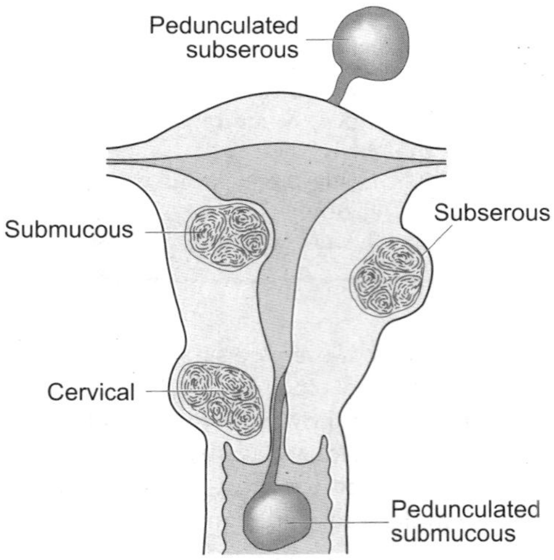

Fig. 7.7 Common sites of fibromyomata in the uterus.

A fibroid may become infected and necrotic, causing a purulent vaginal discharge.

The most noticeable change that the woman may talk about is that of increasing girth of the abdomen. Rapid increase in the size of the abdomen may indicate that malignant change has taken place in the fibroid. Polycythaemia is associated with uterine fibroids but is a rare condition.

MEDICAL MANAGEMENT

On abdominal and vaginal examination, the uterus is usually found to be symmetrically enlarged. It feels harder than it does in pregnancy, unless there is some degeneration of the fibroid(s), as occurs after the menopause. The uterus may feel nodular due to the presence of multiple tumours. The lower part of a tumour may be felt through the cervix and the difference between fibroid and carcinoma of cervix may be difficult to ascertain.

Investigations. Pelvic X-ray and ultrasound scan may assist with diagnosis of fibroids. Diagnostic curettage may be performed to exclude endometrial carcinoma. An examination under anaesthetic is helpful in diagnosis. Carcinoma of the bowel may have to be excluded if a hard mass of tumour exists. A sigmoidoscopy or barium enema may be performed.

Treatment. Small fibroids may not be treated and any symptoms should disappear with the menopause. Medical treatment may be prescribed in the interim to relieve symptoms. Zoladex, a gonadotrophin-releasing hormone analogue, may be prescribed. In a woman who desires a future pregnancy it may be suitable to shell out the fibroids from the myometrium (myomectomy). An older woman may best be treated by hysterectomy. If the fibroids are small, a vaginal hysterectomy may be possible. Any anaemia experienced by the patient is rectified by blood transfusion before surgery.

Embolisation of uterine arteries is a new technique introduced in a few centres as an alternative treatment to hysterectomy (Thomas 1997). This involves cannulating the right femoral artery after administration of a local anaesthetic to the inguinal region. Under screening control, a catheter is passed through the arterial system and eventually to the right and then left uterine arteries which are individually embolised with polyvinyl alcohol solution. Contrast medium is injected to ensure effective arterial occlusion. Thomas (1997) stresses that patients require good opiate pain control following this procedure, but once pain is controlled patients can be discharged.

Fibroids and pregnancy

A woman with a fibroid in the uterus may become pregnant. The pregnancy may be maintained but with increased risks to the fetus. The endometrium may fail to develop adequately to support the fetus, the placenta may be weakly attached and the pregnancy may be aborted. The fibroid may cause retroversion of the uterus (see Fig 7.8, p. 253), which will complicate early developmental stages of the pregnancy and possibly result in abortion. The fibroid may begin to degenerate due to an obstructed venous blood supply, and haemorrhage may occur into the fibroid, giving it a red discoloration.

In pregnancy, the uterus increases in size and moves upwards out of the pelvis, but the fibroid may remain in the pelvis and obstruct labour and the normal delivery of the infant. Caesarean section will be necessary for the birth.

Fibroids may disturb the normal contraction of the uterus after delivery of the child. The placenta may fail to separate and cause postpartum haemorrhage. The fibroids may become involved in a puerperal uterine infection and complicate the mother's recovery.

NURSING PRIORITIES AND MANAGEMENT: FIBROMYOMATA

Nursing care will be prioritised depending upon the type of surgery completed. The maintenance of a safe environment will be important after myomectomy. Observations of pulse, blood pressure and vaginal blood loss are recorded to monitor internal bleeding from the operation site.

Care following hysterectomy will be similar to that described on page 242, but the patient will not have the worry of having a malignant disease that may continue to cause problems. Fibromyomata may recur in some women (Fedele et al 1995).

BENIGN TUMOURS OF THE OVARY

Benign cystic teratoma or dermoid cyst

Dermoid cysts may develop in women of all ages. They comprise 25% of all ovarian tumours. There is a 3% possibility of such cysts becoming malignant.

PATHOPHYSIOLOGY

The dermoid cyst is believed to develop from the aberrant division of an unfertilised oocyte, but the cause is not known (Lewis & Chamberlain 1995). It is formed from accumulated sebaceous material from the glands of the neoplasm. It is a thick-walled cyst, whitish-yellow in colour, lined with skin, hair follicles, hair and sweat glands. Teeth may be found emerging from primitive sockets, and bone cartilage, lung and intestinal epithelium can be identified within the cyst.

MEDICAL MANAGEMENT

The patient may visit her GP because of abdominal pain. Following an abdominal and vaginal examination, she is referred to a gynaecologist for assessment.

Pain may be caused by peritoneal irritation from the cyst. Peritonitis may result from rupture of the cyst contents into the abdomen. The cyst may become infected if salpingitis, appendicitis or diverticulitis are present. Dense adhesions may occur between an infected cyst and the peritoneum or bowel. Torsion or twisting of the pedicle or stalk of the cyst may develop and this may reduce the blood supply, particularly the venous return, to the cyst and cause pain. Malignant change may occur in any of the primitive tissues of the cyst.

Investigations. A Pap cervical smear test may be completed at the time of vaginal examination by the GP. Any malignant cells present might be associated with an ovarian cancer. An ultrasound scan can identify the ovarian cyst.

Treatment. Surgery will be undertaken by laparoscopy or laparotomy. The extent of surgery will vary according to the age of the woman. In younger women, with child-bearing years ahead of them, the benign cyst alone may be shelled out of the ovary, leaving the normal ovarian tissue to continue functioning. Both ovaries will be assessed, as the cysts are often bilateral.

Women who already have a family or who are over 50 years of age would be advised to have the ovary removed. In the event of malignancy of the dermoid cyst, both ovaries and the uterus would be removed. Involvement of the peritoneum in the spread of malignancy would necessitate the installation of a cytotoxic agent, such as thiotepa, into the abdominal cavity at the time of surgery.

NURSING PRIORITIES AND MANAGEMENT: DERMOID CYST

Nursing care will depend upon the extent of the surgery undertaken and has already been described in the section on ovarian cancer (p. 247).

TROPHOBLASTIC TUMOURS

Trophoblastic tumours arise from the primitive tissues destined to develop into the placenta. They may be benign or malignant.

Hydatidiform mole (vesicular mole)

The hydatidiform mole results from hydropic degeneration and vesicle formation of the chorionic villi. These project from the outer mass of cells forming the trophoblast and are destined to become the placenta when the fertilised ovum settles into the endometrium. The uterus fills with grape-like vesicles which produce large quantities of chorionic gonadotrophin. The chromosomal pattern is 46, XX, but all the chromosomal material is derived from the sperm, which doubles its chromosomes and takes over the ovum. No fetus develops.

PATHOPHYSIOLOGY

A hydatidiform mole is a benign tumour mass of chorionic cells in the uterus, which exists as though it were a developing pregnancy. Ovarian follicles are enlarged and there is an increase in blood and urine levels of chorionic gonadotrophin (hCG). The uterus increases in size, sometimes faster than in a pregnancy. The villi of the trophoblast become swollen and the villi or vesicles cluster together like a bunch of grapes.

Common presenting symptoms. A woman may visit her doctor complaining of a vaginal discharge of fresh or altered blood which does not seem like normal menstruation. She may have noticed that some jelly-like mole vesicles have been expelled. She may be feeling unwell with some nausea and vomiting that resembles early pregnancy. Pelvic pain is not usually a problem.

MEDICAL MANAGEMENT

The doctor will complete a general physical and vaginal examination. The uterus may be increased in size. A 'blighted ovum' might be suspected but the watery vesicles of the mole, if identified or reported, will alert the doctor to the condition.

Investigations. A series of pregnancy tests will be completed. Pregnancy tests are positive, although there is no fetus present. The urine is diluted 1:10, 1:100 and 1:1000 — a positive pregnancy test in the 1:100 dilution is strongly suggestive of the mole. The diagnosis is confirmed by ultrasound investigation and by the finding of high levels of hCG in urine or serum. Choriocarcinoma is a serious complication following hydatidiform mole in 1 in 30 cases.

Treatment. The uterus may be stimulated to contract by administration of oxytocin, in order to expel the mole, or it may be evacuated vaginally by suction apparatus. The uterus is in a soft, delicate state and is gently curetted to prevent perforation. A hysterectomy may be advised for a woman who has a family or is past child-bearing age. Thorough follow-up of the patient is necessary if hysterectomy has not been performed. At weekly or 2-weekly intervals for 2 years there must be measurement of urinary output of hCG by radioimmunoassay.

Complications. A rising level of hCG with negative curettings of the uterine cavity suggests that the mole has become invasive of the muscle of the uterus and may even erode through the uterine wall. Deposits of molar tissue may be found in other parts of the body, in the peritoneum or in the lungs, and may cause death.

Choriocarcinoma

Choriocarcinoma of the uterine wall, in 50% of cases, occurs after hydatidiform mole. The malignant condition may appear to arise spontaneously from the ovary but it is more likely to be associated with other neoplastic tissues, such as a teratoma. It may follow a normal pregnancy, an abortion or an ectopic pregnancy.

PATHOPHYSIOLOGY

The uterus becomes ulcerated and causes an offensive, blood-stained vaginal discharge. Metastatic spread of the cancer is speedy and extensive; the brain, lung, liver and other organs may be involved. Early deterioration to death is expected if the condition is not treated early.

Diagnosis is difficult but is confirmed by hCG estimations in urine and plasma. The tissues contain malignant syncytioblast and cytotrophoblast cells.

MEDICAL MANAGEMENT

The patient may have experienced persistent vaginal bleeding after evacuation of a hydatidiform mole or after a termination of pregnancy. Follow-up arrangements after mole removal are usually stringent and early signs of development of the malignant tumour should become obvious, but there are greater risks in other cases if a woman delays visiting the GP.

Investigations. The tumour produces large amounts of hCG, which is used as a tumour marker. Urine and venous blood specimens are tested. Persistently raised hCG levels are diagnostic. Uterine curettings provide histological evidence that also confirms diagnosis and excludes a very rare ovarian teratoma. hCG levels are also used to monitor the response to therapy.

Treatment. Choriocarcinoma is a rare, highly malignant tumour but is also highly sensitive to single-agent chemotherapy. If the tumour is confined to the uterus then intensive cytotoxic drug treatment is given using the drug methotrexate, toxic to the decidua, with almost 100% successful results. Folinic acid is given to protect the bone marrow. Special facilities are needed to protect patients who have a lowered resistance to infection because of diminished white blood cells in the circulation.

If there is metastatic disease, methotrexate may be combined with other cytotoxic agents. The drugs induce marked side-effects during the treatment period and cardiac toxicity may occur. Early detection and treatment of the condition are advised, the disease being known to be curable even after systemic spread. Eighty per cent of patients may make a complete recovery if the disease is identified within 6 months of onset. Good prognosis from metastatic disease is associated with hCG titre levels of less than 40 000 mIU/mL before chemotherapy. hCG levels above 40 000 mIU/mL give a poor prognosis.

Some women may need a hysterectomy before treatment is complete but, as the condition occurs in child-bearing years, conservation of the uterus is of concern. Women may wish to become pregnant after a lapse of 2 years from recovery.

NURSING PRIORITIES AND MANAGEMENT: HYDATIDIFORM MOLE/CHORIOCARCINOMA

Hydatidiform mole

Nursing care following evacuation of hydatidiform mole will be similar to that following curettage of the uterus. Recovery from anaesthetic should be speedy and the patient will become self-caring very soon after returning to the ward. In addition to routine observations following an anaesthetic, the nurse should check on the level of vaginal blood loss, which should be minimal within 24 h, diminishing quickly. Persistent bleeding should be reported to the doctor.

Minimal abdominal discomfort should be experienced by the patient. A mild analgesic will be prescribed, if necessary. If a patient experiences more severe pain, she should be closely observed and have vital signs recorded. Intensive curetting of the uterus might, in rare cases, result in perforation of the uterus and even damage to the bowel. Any cause for concern should be reported to the doctor.

A series of postoperative urine and blood specimens will be required to estimate hCG levels. Specimens may need to be sent to one of the specialised centres in the UK, where there is greater experience in assessing the significance of the hCG levels and reporting results.

Choriocarcinoma

In the event of persistently high levels of hCG, a diagnosis of choriocarcinoma would require transfer of the patient to a specialised centre for chemotherapy. The patient will be very anxious about her condition, having to face up to the seriousness of her illness and the urgency of treatment. The nurse will plan to reinforce the information already given to the patient by the doctor, by emphasising the positive aspects of the care and the expertise of the staff at the specialised centre. The patient must be given time to talk about any worries she might have, and the nurse must be prepared to cope with any outpouring of emotion and to facilitate any special wishes the patient may have. Her partner can be fully involved in the events and can accompany her to the treatment centre.

Intensive nursing care will be planned for the patient at the specialised centre. Special facilities are available for reverse barrier nursing of the patient, to protect her from infection as chemotherapy progresses and her immune system is suppressed (see Ch. 16).

Physical, psychological and social aspects of nursing care will be of primary concern. Many weeks of treatment may be involved before recovery is achieved and the patient returns to normal family life. Follow-up and further hCG monitoring will be essential.

SALPINGITIS

Infection of the fallopian tubes is known as salpingitis and usually affects both tubes simultaneously. It may result from an ascending infection from the vagina, cervix or uterus or it can occur directly from appendicitis, a pelvic abscess or bowel inflammatory disease such as diverticulitis. The ovaries may also be involved in the inflammatory process. Salpingitis may be part of generalised pelvic inflammatory disease (PID).

Acute salpingitis may follow childbirth, abortion, diagnostic or operative procedures involving the uterus, or the insertion of intrauterine devices.

PATHOPHYSIOLOGY

Ascending infection of the fallopian tubes through the vagina, cervix and uterus is most commonly caused by the organism *Chlamydia trachomatis*. More than one infecting agent may be involved. Gonococcal infection, which is sexually transmitted, may be the cause. Streptococcal and staphylococcal organisms are associated with salpingitis following abortion, childbirth or the insertion of an intrauterine device. These causes are rarer and may reflect reactivation of pre-existing disease. Intestinal tract commensals, *Escherichia coli* or *Streptococcus faecalis* may be involved if the infection is linked to appendicitis or bowel infection. The blood-borne tubercle bacillus may unobtrusively inflame the reproductive organs.

The fallopian tubes become engorged and swollen, possibly being filled with a seropurulent exudate. Epithelium cells are shed, damaging the delicate ciliated, transporting function of the tubes.

Common presenting symptoms. The patient experiences a generalised feeling of being unwell, with:

- raised body temperature and associated sweating
- nausea
- vomiting
- aching joints
- severe pelvic and abdominal pain
- dyspareunia.

MEDICAL MANAGEMENT

Salpingitis may be identified for the first time at laparoscopic surgery, the tubes being observed as red, oedematous, distended and blocked. Adhesions may form between the fallopian tubes and other pelvic structures and peritonitis may be evident.

Abdominal and vaginal examinations identify tenderness over the cornua of the uterus. Vaginal discharge may not be observable if the salpingitis has been from lymphatic spread and the muscle of the fallopian tube is mainly involved in the inflammatory process. Infection spread via the mucous membrane of the genital tract will affect the lumen of the fallopian tube, creating a purulent, foul discharge that is drained through the vagina. Scar tissue may form, causing narrowing or closure of the fallopian tube and the severe complication of sterility may result. Adhesions may form between the inflamed tubes and the peritoneum. Peritonitis may occur if pus leaks out of the tubes into the peritoneal cavity. Rarely, a pelvic abscess may form in the rectovaginal pouch or abscesses may form on the ovaries.

Investigations. High vaginal or cervical swabs of discharge are pathologically investigated. Throat, urethral and rectal swabs may be taken. During surgery, exudates from the fallopian tubes or the pouch of Douglas may be obtained. Causative organisms are identified by cell culture or antigen detection, using immunofluorescence or enzyme immunoassay. Examination for specific antibody may assist in diagnosis. The drug sensitivities of organisms are established.

Diagnosis may be confirmed by laparoscopy.

Treatment. Appropriate antibiotic therapy is administered at the earliest opportunity. Analgesic drugs will be necessary for the patient's physical comfort. Pain will be assessed to estimate the most suitable drug. Paracetamol, pentazocine or pethidine may be used at different levels of pain severity.

Patients appreciate rest in bed in the acute phase of the illness. An upright position is considered helpful to promote simple downward drainage within the abdominal cavity, towards the utero-colonic pouch of Douglas, reducing the possible spread of infection to structures nearer to the diaphragm. Salpingitis may follow a chronic course and surgical removal of fallopian tubes, ovaries and uterus may be necessary.

NURSING PRIORITIES AND MANAGEMENT: SALPINGITIS

Nursing care will be organised to relieve the patient's pain, pyrexia and associated sweating, nausea, vomiting and potential dehydration. Analgesics and antibiotic drugs are administered as prescribed. Increased amounts of fluid, 3–4 L in 24 h, will require to be taken orally, or intravenously if vomiting is a problem. When the patient's pain is more tolerable, she will appreciate tepid sponging and a change of linen as a general comfort measure and to reduce body temperature. An electric fan at the bedside and a reduced room temperature should be helpful. The doctor will usually explain to the patient the extent of her problem and the treatment given. In addition to giving information, a counselling approach may be helpful in giving support while encouraging the woman to look to the future. Information will need to be shared with her about the prevention of infection, the risk of infertility and the possibility of an ectopic pregnancy following salpingitis.

ECTOPIC PREGNANCY

A pregnancy that develops outside the uterus is referred to as an 'ectopic' pregnancy. It is possible for a pregnancy to develop in the pouch of Douglas, the omentum, the broad ligament or the ovary. The most common site for an ectopic pregnancy is the fallopian tube — hence the term tubal pregnancy is often used.

Chronic salpingitis is the most common condition associated with a tubal pregnancy. At greater risk of an ectopic pregnancy are women who:

- have experienced an abortion
- wear an intrauterine contraceptive device
- are of older child-bearing age
- have given birth to many children.

PATHOPHYSIOLOGY

A fallopian tube may fail in its usual function of transporting a fertilised ovum to the uterus, and the ovum will then implant in the tube. This delayed passage of the ovum, or obstruction, may be due to a deficiency in peristaltic movement, damage to the ciliated epithelium, a developmental abnormality or adhesions from an earlier inflammation. The trophoblast erodes through the epithelium and connective tissue, embedding itself in the muscle wall of the tube, where the pregnancy develops and erodes into blood vessels, causing bleeding around the embryo and into the muscle wall. Increased tension in the tube may lead to rupture.

Common presenting symptoms. The woman experiences the early indications of pregnancy: amenorrhoea, breast changes, early-morning sickness and frequency of micturition. Amenorrhoea may not occur in one-third of women with a tubal pregnancy and this may result in delayed diagnosis.

The trophoblast slowly erodes the tubal wall, which results in gradual or sudden rupture of the tube before the 10th week of gestation. The woman complains of spasms of abdominal pain that are not too severe at first. Shoulder pain may be experienced. This is referred pain from the diaphragm, which is irritated by blood in the abdominal cavity.

Tubal rupture causes severe localised pain, which is followed by intense, more generalised abdominal pain. The products of conception are expelled into the peritoneal cavity and there is haemorrhage from the tubal placental site. Uterine bleeding may occur at this time. The patient is in a state of shock, with rapid, feeble pulse rate, lowered blood pressure, sighing respirations and pallor — an acute abdominal emergency exists. Diagnosis of the condition is difficult because similar symptoms and signs may occur in other abdominal emergencies such as perforation of a peptic ulcer or torsion of an ovarian tumour.

MEDICAL MANAGEMENT

Investigations are as follows:

Pregnancy tests. Standard immunological pregnancy tests are not helpful as a tubal pregnancy may not produce enough hCG to give a positive result. Estimation of the β subunit of hCG in the serum is of greater value. Absence of β-hCG excludes pregnancy. A level of 6000 mIU/L suggests a normal pregnancy in the uterus, whereas a level below 6000 mIU/L suggests a tubal pregnancy or a missed abortion.

Ultrasound scanning. By the sixth or seventh week of pregnancy, a gestational sac can be identified within the uterus on ultrasound scanning. From the sixth week onwards, it may be possible to show a gestational sac and fetal cardiac echoes outside the normal uterus, directly confirming an ectopic pregnancy.

Laparoscopy. Direct vision of the fallopian tubes using a laparoscope allows diagnosis of an ectopic pregnancy when there is uncertainty in clinical diagnosis. Laparoscopy involves giving the patient a general anaesthetic, which should be avoided if there is the possibility that a pregnancy exists in the uterus. The use of HCG estimations and ultrasound scanning may reduce the need for patients to undergo laparoscopy.

Treatment. An ectopic pregnancy always requires urgent surgical intervention. The damaged tube is usually removed. An unruptured ectopic pregnancy may be removed from a linear incision in the tube, ensuring conservation.

A ruptured ectopic pregnancy quickly produces a state of hypovolaemia in the patient and a blood transfusion is necessary. This will sustain the patient through surgery and partially relieve the hypotensive symptoms. Immediate surgery is essential even though the patient is in a poor physical condition. Improvement is speedy once the intraperitoneal bleeding is controlled.

The ruptured fallopian tube is removed but the ovary is conserved if possible. Recovery after salpingectomy is usually rapid and uncomplicated. Prompt surgery ensures a low mortality rate from a ruptured ectopic pregnancy. A woman who has suffered one ectopic pregnancy is at risk of developing a similar pregnancy in the second fallopian tube. It is usual for the patient to be encouraged to be optimistic about the future and having a normal pregnancy by means of the remaining fallopian tube.

NURSING PRIORITIES AND MANAGEMENT: ECTOPIC PREGNANCY

Preoperative care

Risk of hypovolaemia

The nurse assesses and monitors the patient's physical state intensively from the time of admission to the ward. There are life-threatening concerns as the patient is at risk of hypovolaemic shock and cardiac arrest if the tubal pregnancy ruptures. Vital signs are recorded every 15 minutes. Problems of increased pulse rate, lowered blood pressure and the patient's pain experience are communicated to the doctor. A state of readiness is maintained to resuscitate the patient if necessary.

Pain

Pain is a major problem for the patient. It may be moderate but may become intense and intolerable if the pregnancy ruptures through the tube, with bleeding and spillage of gestational sac fluid into the peritoneal cavity. Analgesia is given as prescribed.

Preparation for general anaesthesia

Emergency surgery will be planned. Fasting from food and fluid by mouth prior to laparotomy will be as described in Chapter 26. In the case of emergency surgery it is important for the anaesthetist to know the last time the patient ate or drank and of any vomiting. It may be necessary to introduce a nasogastric tube prior to surgery to reduce the risk of regurgitation and inhalation of gastric contents when the patient is anaesthetised.

Anxiety and the need for information

The patient may be fearful about the operation to come and distressed about losing a pregnancy. She will need information about the surgery and postoperative care, and needs to be encouraged to talk about any worries she may have. It is possible that she may be too weak to talk and the nurse must show empathy and understanding of the patient's feelings and concerns. The nurse may indicate that she will talk with the patient some time after the operation and that she will accompany her to the operating theatre and be responsible for her care when she returns to the ward.

Postoperative care

Postoperative care will be individualised according to patient need, but will follow the general principles of postoperative care described in Chapter 26. Her condition will begin to stabilise as soon as the ectopic pregnancy is removed and bleeding is controlled. Her main problems will be similar to those of other patients who have had abdominal surgery, when organs and the peritoneum have been handled by the surgeon and tissues have been cut through, as follows:

Change in vital signs. The nurse monitors pulse rate, blood pressure and body temperature. Wound, drainage tube and blood loss from the vagina are observed for more than minimal drainage. Primary and secondary haemorrhages are risks. Wound dehiscence may occur. Any causes for concern will be shared with the doctor.

Postoperative pain. The level of pain can be assessed using a verbal rating scale (VRS 1–10). Analgesics are prescribed and administered to control pain.

Post-anaesthetic nausea. This problem may be prevented or treated by giving an antiemetic drug with analgesics as prescribed.

Fluid and electrolyte imbalance. Intravenous fluid and electrolyte replacement therapy is administered as prescribed, until oral intake is resumed. Fluid intake and output are recorded.
Venous stasis and pressure-area damage. The patient is actively encouraged to exercise her legs hourly whilst confined to bed. Assistance is given to change the patient's position every 2 hours to protect pressure areas. A programme of early mobilisation will be introduced.
Personal care. Whilst intravenous therapy is in situ, assistance will be given to maintain her preferred standard of personal care until fully mobile.
Loss and grieving. Time is planned for counselling the patient. She needs to know that she can talk about her feelings and express emotion freely. Information should be shared about the possibility of future pregnancies. Details of local support groups for those who suffer loss should be given.

Further considerations

Psychological support

A woman who is suffering a second ectopic pregnancy will become infertile. She may become emotionally distressed at any time during her hospital stay and may show behaviour associated with a crisis of loss and a grief reaction. She will need support whilst expressing her feelings of regret and possibly guilt. Both the nurse and the patient's partner may be helpful in assisting the woman to be realistic about future options and limitations. Some reorganisation of the woman's life will emerge as she accepts her inevitable situation.

Special services

As a result of media coverage, the public are now aware of techniques such as in vitro fertilisation (IVF) and embryo transfer into the uterus (ET) and the possibility of surrogacy for infertile couples. Nurses need to know about such special services and policies within their own units, so that they are informed and can respond to the patient with appropriate caution and discretion and refer enquiries to the patient's doctor.

DISPLACEMENTS OF THE UTERUS

The basic criterion of uterine normality is mobility rather than position. The cervix is laterally anchored but the fundus is free to move widely in an anteroposterior position. If the long axis of the endometrial cavity is hinged forwards in relation to the cervical canal, the body of the uterus is anteflexed in relation to the cervix. Similarly, if the long axis of the endometrial cavity is hinged backwards in relation to the axis of the cervical canal, then the body of the uterus is retroflexed in relation to the cervix (see Fig. 7.8).

Careful assessment of the position of the uterus is necessary to prevent perforation of the uterus during diagnostic or therapeutic curettage.

Cervicovaginal prolapse

The cervix can become prolapsed and elongated by the opposing forces of pull of the transverse and uterosacral ligaments against prolapsed vaginal walls. The cervix prolapses but the uterus stays in the pelvis.

Anterior vaginal wall prolapse

Cystocele. The upper part of the vaginal wall prolapses due to underlying failure of the fascia and the bladder base descends.

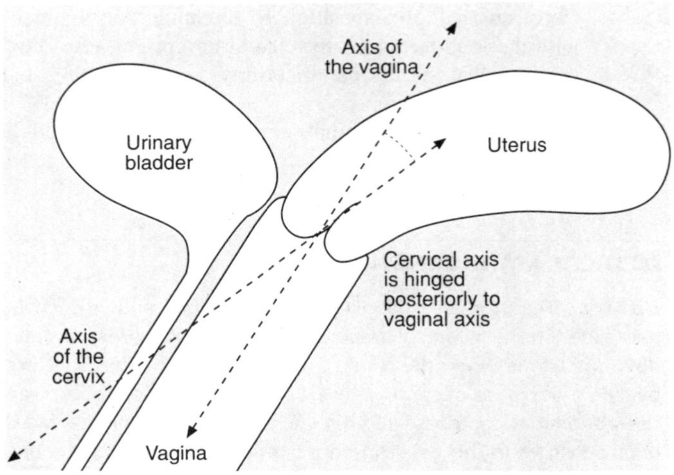

Fig. 7.8 The retroverted uterus.

Urethrocele. The lower part of the vaginal wall prolapses and the urethra descends. This is caused by stretching of the urogenital diaphragm, which holds the urethra to the pubic bone.

Posterior vaginal wall prolapse

Rectocele. If the prolapse is at the level of the middle third of the vagina, the retrovaginal septum is involved and the rectum prolapses with the vaginal wall. If the lowest part of the vaginal wall prolapses, the perineal body is involved rather than the rectum.
Enterocele. If the upper part of the posterior vaginal wall prolapses, the pouch of Douglas is elongated and the small bowel or omentum may descend.

Both anterior and posterior vaginal walls may be involved in the prolapse. When a cystocele is present, bladder emptying tends to be incomplete, causing hypertrophy of the bladder. The uterus may become distorted, leading to reflux of urine and, ultimately, hydronephrosis. Urinary tract infection is inevitable and this contributes to hypertension and raised blood urea levels in women with prolapse.

Uterovaginal prolapse

When the ligaments and muscles supporting the uterus and vagina become ineffective, the genital tract descends, prolapses or herniates through the gap between the muscles of the pelvic floor. The uterus descends in the axis of the vagina taking the vaginal wall with it. This prolapse is essentially but not exclusively a postmenopausal condition.

Three degrees of uterine prolapse are described:

- *first degree* — the cervix is still within the vagina
- *second degree* — the cervix appears at the introitus
- *third degree* — the uterus and vagina are completely prolapsed and lie outside the vulva. Rectal prolapse may also occur. This is sometimes called complete 'procidentia' or 'vault prolapse'. The vaginal rugae are smoothed out, and the epithelium becomes thickened and keratinised. The uterus becomes dry, sore, swollen, inflamed, congested and ulcerated from contact with clothing. Contributing factors are:
  — Stretching of muscle and fibrous tissue from repeated child-bearing. It is suggested that it is due to the action of progesterone relaxing muscles during pregnancy

— Injury to the muscles of the pelvic floor during childbirth
— Constitutional predisposition to stretching of ligaments with the long-term maintenance of an upright, erect body position that strains the transverse ligaments (the chief support of the uterus)
— Increased intra-abdominal pressure, as experienced by obese women with a chronic cough or those engaged in heavy industrial work.

MEDICAL MANAGEMENT

History. The woman is likely to be overweight and suffer from backache. She is aware of feelings of the internal organs coming down at a time when she is in an upright position. This is relieved by lying down or resting. Pelvic venous congestion occurs and the abdominal contents exert pressure on the inadequate, weakened pelvic floor. There is frequency of micturition, incomplete bladder emptying and the residual urine is a focus for infection. Stress incontinence may be a major problem for some women (see Ch. 24). There may be difficulty in voiding urine and in defaecation. The cystocele or rectocele may have to be supported or pushed upwards vaginally before urine can be passed or the bowel evacuated. Physical movements become difficult and uncomfortable.

Examination. Severe prolapse may be diagnosed by inspecting the vulva with the patient lying on her back and straining downwards. A vaginal speculum is used to allow direct vision of a prolapsed anterior vaginal wall and any rectocele or enterocele formed by a prolapsed posterior vaginal wall. A rectal examination is needed to confirm the latter type of displacement. The degree of uterine prolapse is usually assessed before surgery when the patient is anaesthetised. Volsella forceps can be attached to the cervix, which is pulled downwards to show the prolapse level.

Investigations. Apart from an examination under anaesthetic, no routine procedures are necessary to assist with diagnosis of uterine displacement. Preoperative assessment will usually involve a full blood count, a dipstick urinalysis, and a midstream specimen of urine for culture and sensitivity. Other procedures, such as a chest X-ray, ECG or blood chemistry estimation, may be necessary to assess the patient's general medical fitness for surgery.

Treatment. Surgical treatment is curative for prolapse but a small number of women may be unfit for surgery due to advanced age or poor physical condition. The uterus may be supported by the use of a ring pessary made from polyethylene or flexible vinyl. Such pessaries may have the disadvantage of acting as a foreign body in the vagina, causing some local inflammation. Pessaries are changed every 4–6 months when the vaginal walls can be examined for inflammation or ulceration. A course of vaginal oestrogen may be prescribed from time to time to diminish atrophic changes, inflammation, infection and discharge.

Surgery to conserve the uterus. If there is only a first-degree descent of the uterus or if the woman prefers to retain her uterus, although prolapsed, then the Manchester (Fothergill) operation is performed. This involves partial amputation of the elongated cervix and the joining of the cut transverse cervical ligaments to the stump of the cervix. The shortened ligaments antevert and elevate the uterus. The vaginal walls are repaired as necessary.

Repair of uterovaginal prolapse. Reconstruction of the pelvic floor involves restoring the pelvic aperture to its previous competent state. This is achieved by bringing together skeletal muscle between the anus, vagina and bladder, and approximating the medial borders of the pubococcygeus muscles. Childbirth can result in supporting structures being torn, separated and overstretched. These structures are identified at operation and reconstructed. An elongated cervix may be amputated. The fascia supporting the bladder and bladder neck is tightened across the midline. The parametrial tissues supporting the uterus are shortened to raise the uterus to its normal position.

Repair of cystocele is known as anterior colporrhaphy, which includes supporting the urethra and urethrovesical junction. A rectocele is repaired by a posterior colpoperineorrhaphy, which includes the repair of the perineal body. Bladder, perineum and vulva have an excellent capacity for repair, related to a rich blood supply and good venous drainage. Surgery is usually very successful.

A complete uterine prolapse will usually be treated by hysterectomy.

NURSING PRIORITIES AND MANAGEMENT: DISPLACEMENTS OF THE UTERUS

Preoperative care

Preoperative assessment and care of patients for gynaecological operations has been fully described earlier in the chapter. Care is always individualised according to needs, but some problems and interventions are similar.

Information. Needs exist for information about procedures before and after the operation, in order to increase patient understanding and cooperation and to reduce anxiety and risk of venous stasis.

Potential embarrassment. A woman admitted for repair of prolapse may experience embarrassment in having to identify that she has a problem of stress incontinence that requires her to wear some form of protection. The nurse will ensure that her special requirements are met discreetly.

Evacuating the lower bowel before surgery. According to the surgeon's requirements, the patient will be given two rectal suppositories or an evacuant enema on the evening before the operation day.

Preparing the operation site. As required by the surgical protocol, an antiseptic vaginal douche can reduce the numbers of bacteria inhabiting the area and inhibit their multiplication. This should allow healing of the vaginal wounds without infection.

Postoperative care

Risk of strain on internal suture lines from a full bladder. An indwelling catheter is required and a continuous urinary drainage system is maintained. Precautions are taken to prevent the introduction of infection when collecting specimens or changing drainage bags.

Loss of bladder tone. This is possible after catheter removal. Catheterisation is completed after the patient has passed urine once daily to assess the level of urine retained in the bladder. A residual urine of less than 60 mL is satisfactory.

Risk of wound infection. The patient can use the bidet for perineal toilet twice daily to minimise the risk of infection.

Constipation. This will potentially cause strain on the repaired posterior vaginal wall. A stool-softening agent, as prescribed, can be administered to promote easy bowel actions.

Strain on healing ligaments and muscles. The patient is advised to avoid jarring or lifting activities for 2 months.

Pre-discharge counselling. An opportunity is created for the patient to discuss her feelings and any worries about her level of recovery from surgery, bladder functioning, future return to sexual activity and work. An appointment is given for a medical follow-up in the outpatient department. The patient is given the name of the nurse to contact in the ward if she needs further advice.

FAMILY PLANNING SERVICES

Birth control was considered 'social' medicine prior to 1950 and responsibility for family planning advice was established within the Family Planning Association (FPA) and its clinics. The National Health Service Reorganisation Act of 1973 made provision for free family planning advice within the National Health Service. The FPA clinics and domiciliary services were merged into the NHS in 1974, when a completely free contraceptive service became available at clinics and hospitals and was extended into primary care in July 1975 (Loudon 1985).

Free contraceptive services are now available from general practitioners, family planning clinics in hospitals and the community, and voluntary organisations such as the FPA and Brook Advisory Centres. The voluntary groups receive grants from central government or from purchasing health authorities.

All contraceptive supplies are available free of charge from family planning clinics, and GPs provide prescriptions, except for condoms. Male and female sterilisations are available free in NHS hospitals. Vasectomies may be performed in some large family planning clinics and by some GPs in the surgery. Item-of-service payments are made to GPs and hospital staff.

Postnatally, midwives, health visitors and GPs routinely discuss birth control methods with the new mother. This is invaluable in reminding women of their fertility and the possibility of another early pregnancy if precautions are not taken when resuming sexual activities.

Women who discontinue attending the GP or Family Planning Clinic may do so because they have changed their birth control method. Women who have completed their family may have chosen sterilisation or their partners may have chosen vasectomy for a permanent form of birth control. Others may be abandoning contraception because the time is favourable for them to begin a family.

The contraceptive needs of young people

Provision of extra contraceptive services for young people after puberty, under 16 years and up to 20 years of age, is controversial and, in the past, was given a low priority. With more recent concern about AIDS and HIV transmission, young people have been specially targeted for health education and advice about their sexual behaviour. Grimley & Lee (1997), in a study of 15- to 19-year-old American females, found that subjects perceived the male condom to be acceptable for both prevention of pregnancy and sexually transmitted diseases. The Contraceptive Choices Survey (Family Planning Today 1996) commissioned by the Contraceptive Education Service showed condoms to be the second most popular method of birth control. The most popular method of contraception, especially for younger women, is still the contraceptive pill, used by 43% of those aged 16–24 years. The combined pill of progestogen and low oestrogen is favoured for high contraceptive protection and ease of use.

ABORTION

The term 'abortion' refers to the premature delivery of a non-viable fetus, spontaneously or by induction. The term 'miscarriage' is sometimes used when the pregnancy loss is spontaneous and is a term generally considered to be more acceptable to women who lose a wanted pregnancy. Debate surrounds the issue of 'non-viability' and the accepted stage at which a fetus is considered viable or capable of independent existence varies between different countries. In the UK, a fetus is considered viable from the 24th week of pregnancy. This viability is recognised and safeguarded in the Infant Life (Preservation) Act 1929 and its amendment under the Human Fertilisation and Embryology Act 1990. It has been proposed that the fetus should be deemed viable as early as 18–20 weeks because of the possibility that life-support equipment can maintain the vital functions of such a small fetus and it has been argued that technological advances in medicine have the potential for saving the life of an infant weighing as little as 500 g. Such debates continue, reflecting different social attitudes and the scientific developments.

Abortion may be discussed in terms of:

- the level of certainty of the abortion occurring
  —threatened
  —inevitable
  —missed
  —induced
- the cause or relative incidence of the abortion
  —spontaneous
  —habitual (recurrent)
- the degree of success in expulsion of the products of the pregnancy
  —incomplete
  —complete.

Threatened abortion

PATHOPHYSIOLOGY

An abortion is presumed to threaten when a woman known to be pregnant develops vaginal bleeding during the first 24 weeks of pregnancy. Some lower abdominal pain related to uterine muscle contractions may be experienced at the time of bleeding, but there may be no uterine contractions and no pain. The blood loss may be brown or red.

It is not unusual for a show of blood to coincide with the woman's regular date of menstruation. This type of bleeding is due to the fertilised ovum becoming more deeply implanted in the uterine wall. There is little risk of loss of the pregnancy if the bleeding settles quickly (see Fig. 7.9A).

MEDICAL MANAGEMENT

The presence of bleeding, slight uterine contractions and a closed cervical os established by medical examination assist in identifying threatened abortion; 70–80% can be expected to continue to full-term pregnancies and give birth to a healthy infant.

Treatment. While the woman is continuing to lose blood vaginally, rest in bed is prescribed to ensure that the best possible adjustments can be made within the uterus and to allow a better blood flow to the uterus. Bed rest is usually maintained as long as the blood loss is bright red. One week of bed rest may result in considerable improvement for the patient.

NURSING PRIORITIES AND MANAGEMENT: THREATENED ABORTION

The patient will be very concerned about the possible loss of the pregnancy. This may result in tearfulness, anxiety, irritability and feelings of frustration. The immediate and long-term future may be feared. The patient may be apprehensive of pain and uncertain of what to expect. Small doses of anxiolytic-sedative drugs and progesterone may be prescribed to encourage rest and to help sustain the pregnancy.

Nursing care will be planned with the goal of reducing anxiety and inducing relaxation in the patient. Vaginal bleeding will be observed and quantified. The patient's experience of abdominal discomfort or pain will be assessed and recorded. The supportive, counselling contact time with the nurse will be appreciated by the patient and her partner. When talking with the patient and partner, both doctor and nurse will usually refer to a threatened miscarriage of the pregnancy rather than using the term abortion.

Inevitable abortion

PATHOPHYSIOLOGY

A threatened abortion can progress to an inevitable abortion if bleeding continues. Inevitable abortions occur in 20% of all pregnancies. An abortion becomes inevitable, with no possibility of saving the pregnancy, when the following are present:

- vaginal blood loss
- strong uterine contractions
- pain
- dilatation of the cervix.

Contractions will increase, the fetal sac membranes will rupture and the uterine contents move through the cervical os. Part or all of the products of conception will be voided from the uterus (see Fig. 7.9B). An inevitable abortion may be complete if all products of conception are voided, or incomplete if some products are retained.

MEDICAL MANAGEMENT

The aborting process will involve blood loss that will need to be evaluated. Estimation of blood loss and assessment of pulse rate, blood pressure readings, and appearance of the patient will indicate whether a state of shock is developing. Blood replacement therapy may become essential. Pain from strong contractions of the uterus can be relieved by analgesic drugs as necessary.

The fetus that has been expelled is retained and examined to assess whether the fetal sac and contents are intact or whether remnants of placenta or membranes have been retained. Ergometrine maleate 125–500 mg will be given intramuscularly or intravenously according to blood loss. This drug will induce strong contraction of the myometrium, which will exert and sustain pressure on the multiple open-ended blood vessels to the placental bed in the wall of the uterus. Thus, bleeding will be controlled until the uterus itself reduces size gradually.

If any of the products of conception are thought to have been retained then evacuation of the uterus will be performed under a general anaesthetic in theatre.

NURSING PRIORITIES AND MANAGEMENT: INEVITABLE ABORTION

Assessments of vaginal blood loss may need to be maintained for a further period of 12 h in the event of further heavy bleeding, when the effects of ergometrine diminish and the uterine muscle relaxes, blood vessels open up and bleeding and blood clots continue as problems. Further doses of ergometrine, in tablet form, may then be prescribed to control the bleeding and expel blood clots. The blood clots will cause further pain for the patient until they are finally voided from the vagina.

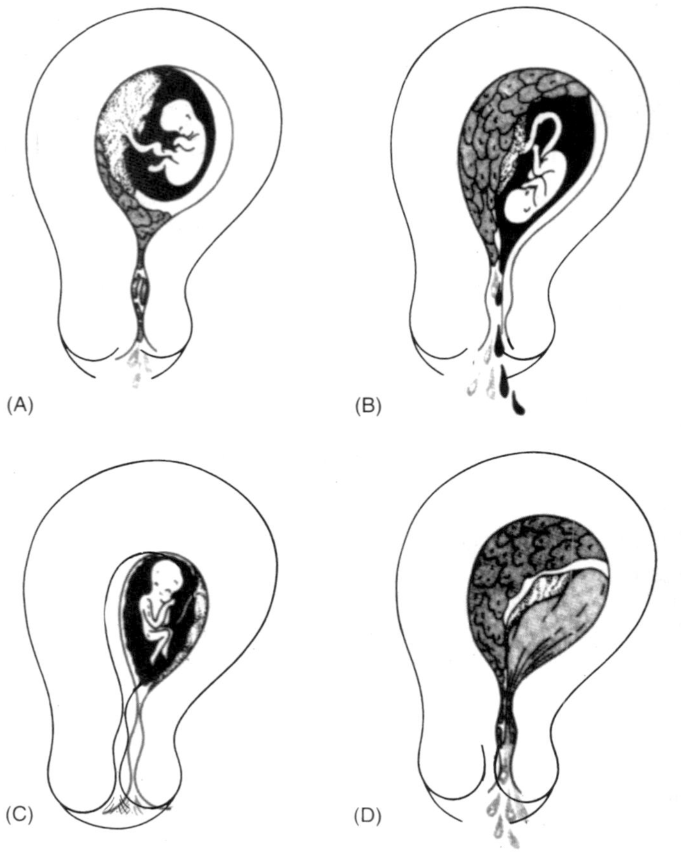

Fig. 7.9 The types of abortion that may be seen. A: Threatened abortion. B: Inevitable abortion. C: Missed abortion. D: Incomplete abortion.

The patient may be distressed by the blood loss, pain, sight of the fetus and the anguish of losing a pregnancy to which she had become emotionally attached. She is likely to experience considerable physical and emotional distress and will need the nurse to be readily available to support, reassure, comfort and assist her through the procedures and experience of pregnancy loss. The patient will need to have the opportunity to talk about her feelings of loss. In this respect, time and empathy from the nurse will be appreciated (Leask 1991, Nazarko 1992). It may be that she has already had a previous miscarriage and will also be recalling that experience as part of her grieving process. The patient's sadness may be sustained for many months after the abortion occurs. To plan some continued support, the nurse in hospital can refer the patient to the community midwife, who is able to provide bereavement counselling until resolution of the grief reaction takes place.

Missed abortion

PATHOPHYSIOLOGY

The term 'missed abortion' describes the intrauterine death of a fetus that has not been expelled. The size of the uterus fails to increase over a 2-month period and the expected signs of a normally developing pregnancy will be missing. The death of the fetus may occur at any week of gestation. Some placental tissue survives to produce progesterone and prevent expulsion (see Fig. 7.9C.)

MEDICAL MANAGEMENT

The woman may have experienced movements of the fetus in the uterus, but later reports that she has not felt the baby kicking for some time. The doctor will no longer be able to hear the fetal heart beat on auscultation of the abdomen. The uterus may seem to have increased in size but this is due to increased fluid level in the uterus, known as 'hydramnios'. The patient may state that she feels empty and has lost her feelings of being pregnant. She is asked to record on a chart any sensation she has of the baby moving or kicking.

Investigations. An ultrasound scan of the uterus and a cardiotocograph reading will assess the status of the fetus and the position of the placenta.

Treatment. The diagnosis of a missed abortion will require the doctor to decide whether to allow some time for the fetus to be aborted spontaneously as a natural labour response or whether to evacuate the uterus immediately after diagnosis. The decision may be to let nature take its course and wait for labour to begin. However, the doctor is also likely to take account of the preference of the woman, who has already had to adjust to the loss of the pregnancy and may be further distressed by brooding about the dead baby within her. This may cause anxiety and depression.

A risk exists, with missed abortion, that hypofibrinogenaemia will occur. One-third of patients may develop defective blood coagulation due to lowering of fibrinogen levels. Death of the fetus leads to major utilisation of clotting factors at the placental site, and this reduces clotting factors in the woman's blood. Disseminated intravascular coagulation is the mechanism that is said to bring about the change in the woman's systemic circulation from the release of thromboplastins at the site of the damaged placental tissue.

The missed abortion may be evacuated from the uterus by vacuum extraction under general anaesthetic if the pregnancy was less than 12 weeks. Otherwise, induction of labour by the use of drugs such as an antiprogesterone or prostaglandin, either alone or in combination, would be appropriate.

NURSING PRIORITIES AND MANAGEMENT: MISSED ABORTION

The nursing care of the patient with a missed abortion will focus on the patient's need for information about her condition and planned treatment, while responding to the sense of loss and sadness that has replaced the joy of pregnancy and anticipated childbirth. A counselling approach will be necessary to provide the patient with opportunities to express her needs and feelings freely.

If evacuation of the uterus under general anaesthetic is planned, the patient will need the usual pre-anaesthetic care in terms of fasting, taking a shower, and precautions against mis-identification and maintenance of personal safety. Following surgery, observations of vaginal blood loss, temperature, pulse rate and blood pressure will be required to assess recovery.

If the products of conception are to be evacuated by inducing labour with drug treatments, the patient may be given a dose of mifepristone while still an outpatient and be admitted to hospital 36–48 h later. A drug such as misoprostol is then administered in divided doses. The products of pregnancy should be expelled 4 h later. The nurse must be readily available to observe the patient's temperature, pulse and blood pressure regularly and to assess the need for pain relief. The patient may experience drug side-effects of nausea, vomiting or diarrhoea, but these are usually transitory rather than prolonged. The very presence of the nurse can be comforting to the patient, reducing feelings of isolation while treatment progresses.

The way in which individual patients cope emotionally is unpredictable, but the nurse can anticipate that any patient will feel sad and angry about the lost pregnancy. Follow-up counselling can be arranged by the nurse with the community midwife or health visitor, when the woman's level of adjustment can be assessed.

Spontaneous abortion

PATHOPHYSIOLOGY

A spontaneous abortion is a response to a naturally occurring phenomenon such as hormonal problems, uterine abnormality, incompetence of the cervix, a genetic malformation in the fetus or psychological factors. Pearce (1991) estimated that 25% of all pregnancies terminate in miscarriage in the first trimester; reasons include both fetal and maternal factors. Some women may not be aware that they have aborted a blighted ovum. Congenital abnormalities of the reproductive tract or long-standing medical problems may have an unfavourable influence on the pregnancy. Abortions in the early weeks of the second trimester of pregnancy are often found to be due to an incompetent cervix that responds to the increasing weight of the fetus. The cervical os dilates, the membranes rupture and the pregnancy is lost.

MEDICAL MANAGEMENT

To counteract recurrence of abortion, it is necessary to identify the pregnancy and any incompetence of the cervix at an early stage. In the case of cervical incompetence, a Shirodker's suture can be inserted surgically, closing the internal os, to increase the resistance of the cervix until the pregnancy reaches full term. When the patient goes into labour, the suture is removed to enable delivery to occur.

NURSING PRIORITIES AND MANAGEMENT: SPONTANEOUS ABORTION

The physical care of the patient with a spontaneous abortion is similar to that of the patient with an inevitable abortion. The patient will be distressed by the loss of the pregnancy and will need psychological support from the nurse. A counselling approach to communication will encourage the expression of feelings. Continued support should be arranged by referral to the community midwife.

Habitual (recurrent) abortion

Recurrent abortion refers to a spontaneous abortion that occurs in three or more successive pregnancies. Many factors may contribute to recurrent abortions.

PATHOPHYSIOLOGY

Genetic, hormonal, anatomical, infectious and immunological factors have been implicated in the causation of recurrent abortion. In explaining immunological factors, Taylor & Faulk (1981) suggested that:

- Couples share more HLA antigens than usual. If the union results in many shared HLA antigens from the parents, this may result in failure to stimulate maternal protecting or blocking factors, culminating in rejection of the blastocyst.

- Women lack the inhibitors of cell-mediated immunity usually produced during pregnancy.
- Human trophoblast membranes have discrete antigens that could form the basis for a maternal immune reaction against the fetus, and they lack transplantation antigens.

MEDICAL MANAGEMENT

Treatment. Patients with immunological problems have been treated with leucocyte transfusions with successful results. Identified hormonal deficiencies are treated by replacement hormones, thyroid preparations and progesterone. Vaginal suppositories of progesterone 25 mg, twice daily, beginning 3 days after ovulation, are given and continued throughout the luteal phase, until the 10th week of gestation. At this time the placenta should be sufficient to maintain the pregnancy.

The administration of antibiotic drugs is routine, where culture and sensitivity of organisms are known. Otherwise, drugs of the tetracycline group are given to offset an infective focus that might disrupt the pregnancy. Reconstruction surgery has achieved considerable success in treating structural abnormalities of the uterus and eventual successful pregnancies.

NURSING PRIORITIES AND MANAGEMENT: RECURRENT ABORTION

Physical and psychological care are paramount at the time that the abortion occurs. Sensitivity in responding to the woman's needs is central. Potential for future assisted maintenance of a pregnancy will be fully discussed by the doctor and reinforced by the nurse. The patient who is anxious can be helped to learn relaxation techniques that may be used for self-induction of relaxation as an everyday activity, and one that can be practised in future pregnancies.

Incomplete abortion

An incomplete abortion is one in which only part of the products of conception are expelled from the uterus (see Fig. 7.9D).

PATHOPHYSIOLOGY

Portions of placenta and membranes are retained, some bleeding continues and could possibly be heavy.

MEDICAL MANAGEMENT

The residual products may be voided spontaneously by the patient but usually a dilatation and curettage is required to clear away the retained remnants of the pregnancy. Ergometrine 500 mg is administered intravenously to control uterine bleeding. Heavy blood loss will necessitate blood replacement by transfusion.

NURSING PRIORITIES AND MANAGEMENT: INCOMPLETE ABORTION

The patient may experience continuous abdominal pain while the uterus retains products of conception. Nursing care involves the administration of analgesia as prescribed to reduce the discomfort, which may continue until the curettage is complete. Vaginal blood loss will need to be observed. Heavy, continuous blood loss may reduce the patient's circulating blood volume, resulting in signs of shock. Observations of the pulse and blood pressure, half-hourly, will facilitate early recognition of shock and prompt correction of the condition by transfusion.

The patient will be worried about her condition and the operation planned and will feel very upset about the miscarriage. Adjustment to the loss will be gradual over time. Counselling time spent with the nurse may help to begin the adjustment process, and continuity may be gained by follow-up support from the community midwife or health visitor.

Induced abortion: termination (voluntary) of pregnancy

An unwanted pregnancy creates anguish and acute difficulties for a woman. She may experience feelings of conflict about both wanting and rejecting the pregnancy. She may fear having to explain it to her family and so admit to sexual activities and to her incompetence in contraceptive methods. Family standards of behaviour, cultural norms and religious beliefs may appear to be violated both by the pregnancy and by the possibility of an abortion. The woman may feel very alone, may have perhaps only one person to confide in, may be indecisive and be under pressure from a partner who rejects the pregnancy. The conditions of the Abortion Act require decision-making to be completed early in the pregnancy.

The Abortion Act 1967 and 1990 amendments

In the UK, the Abortion Act 1967 became operative in 1968 and applies to England, Wales and Scotland but not to Northern Ireland. The Act states that the termination of pregnancy by a registered practitioner is not illegal under certain conditions. Notification of a termination must be given on a prescribed form to the Chief Medical Officer of the Department of Health within 7 days of the termination.

The Human Fertilisation and Embryology Act 1990 has amended the Abortion Act 1967, recognising viability of the fetus at 24 weeks.

Conditions of the Act and statutory grounds. A legally induced abortion must be:

- performed by a registered medical practitioner
- performed, except in an emergency, in a National Health Service Hospital or in a place for the time being approved for the purpose of the Act
- certified by two registered medical practitioners as necessary on any of the following grounds:
  —the continuance of the pregnancy would involve risk to the life of the pregnant woman greater than if the pregnancy were terminated
  —the continuance of the pregnancy would involve risk of injury to the physical or mental health of the pregnant woman greater than if the pregnancy were terminated
  —the continuance of the pregnancy would involve risk of injury to the physical or mental health of any existing child(ren) in the family of the pregnant woman greater than if the pregnancy were terminated
  —there is a substantial risk that if the child were born it would suffer from such physical or mental abnormalities as to be seriously handicapped
- in emergency, certified by the operating practitioner as immediately necessary:
  —to save the life of the pregnant woman
  —to prevent grave permanent injury to the physical or mental health of the pregnant woman.

The conscience clause of the Abortion Act (1967). The Act states that no-one shall be under any legal obligation to participate in any treatment authorised by the Act to which he or she has a conscientious objection unless the treatment is necessary to save the life or prevent grave permanent injury to the physical or mental health of a pregnant woman.

The conscience clause does not only apply to members of a particular religion or faith. In England and Wales, a person must prove conscientious objection in the event of any legal proceedings. The clause also makes it explicit that the conscientious objector is not exempt from participation in the emergency care of the patient should such a situation arise. This is affirmed by the United Kingdom Central Council for Nursing, Midwifery and Health Visiting (UKCC) in *Guidelines for Professional Practice* (UKCC 1996).

Counselling of the pregnant woman requesting termination

In many hospitals the woman who requests a termination of pregnancy is referred to the Assessment and Counselling Service. The social worker seeks to understand what the pregnancy and termination mean to the woman, identifies any contraindications to termination and provides evidence for the final decision-making and the best solution.

It is valuable to interview couples together for counselling. Adolescent girls are often accompanied by parents who may be angry and rejecting of their daughter's pregnancy. The risk is then that the girl passively acts in accordance with the parents' wishes. The counsellor would usually speak with them together and then separately.

Counselling clarifies the woman's conflicting feelings about the pregnancy and strengthens her capacity to face up to her responsibilities. She may be more confident in making a decision in an unpressured atmosphere. The counsellor may have established that contraindications to the termination exist or that the request for termination be supported. In either case the information is made available to the gynaecologist. The counselling service ensures that adequate assessment and advice are provided for the woman who seeks a termination. It is suggested that in this way she will experience less regret, guilt or long-term psychological problems.

MEDICAL MANAGEMENT

Vacuum aspiration (suction curettage). This is the most commonly used abortion method for early termination of pregnancy. It may be performed with a general anaesthetic or a paracervical nerve block with lignocaine hydrochloride 0.5%. The cervix is dilated, a flexible cannula is inserted and the contents of the uterus are aspirated by suction. The uterus is then curetted to ensure total removal of the products of conception, and to reduce haemorrhage and the possibility of infection. Ergometrine 0.5 mg is administered intravenously to promote contraction and involution of the uterus.

Medical termination. A combination of Mifegyne, a potent antiprogesterone, and prostaglandin has been approved for termination of early pregnancy (up to 63 days amenorrhoea) in the UK. Mifegyne is taken in the form of three tablets (600 mg). The patient swallows these tablets in the hospital/clinic under clinical supervision and thereafter may go home but must return 36–48 h later for prostaglandin administration of gemeprost 1 mg in the form of a vaginal pessary. The latter softens the cervix, allows it to dilate and stimulates uterine contractions. The patient remains under observation for a further 6 h. The nurse monitors pulse, blood pressure, blood loss and other signs and symptoms experienced by the patient. The medical abortion is usually complete within 4–6 h. Anti-D Rhesus immunisation is given before discharge and an appointment is made for the patient to return in 5–9 days to assess the outcome.

While this method of terminating a pregnancy has its advantages — the woman can carry on her daily activities following administration of the tablets and there is no anaesthetic or surgical intervention — there are also potential problems of which the woman should be made aware. These include:

- a 5% chance that the termination will be unsuccessful/incomplete, resulting in the need for surgical abortion
- possibility of pain following administration of gemeprost, necessitating powerful analgesics
- possible psychological distress for the woman seeing the expelled fetus.

Dilatation and evacuation of contents. Abortion that is induced in the second trimester of pregnancy may be completed by dilatation of the cervix with graduated dilators. (Preoperatively the patient may have a prostaglandin pessary to soften the cervix and facilitate easier dilatation.) A curette is introduced into the uterus and the products of conception and the superficial layer of endometrium are curetted or scraped from the walls of the uterus. Care is taken to avoid damage to the pregnant uterus. Ergometrine 0.5 mg is administered and few side-effects to the procedure are expected. Patients are followed up at the clinic.

Prostaglandin abortion. Prostaglandin may be used in young women in the second trimester of pregnancy (13–18 weeks), when the cervix is soft and more easily damaged, or in older women when the pregnancy is beyond 18 weeks. Prostaglandin can be administered intravenously, extra-amniotically, intra-amniotically or in the form of pessaries. If pessaries are used these can be administered 4-hourly (maximum five doses). Abortion can take place within 12–20 h but this varies. Observations of pulse, blood pressure, blood loss, uterine contractions, cervical dilatation and any side-effects of the drug are noted and treated as appropriate. This more prolonged procedure causes more side-effects and can be more traumatic for patients. Psychological care and emotional support constitute an important part of their care.

Intra-amniotic injection. The instillation of prostaglandins or other substances into the amniotic sac to induce labour and expulsion of the fetus may be used between the 14th and 20th week of pregnancy but this method carries a higher risk of complications.

NURSING PRIORITIES AND MANAGEMENT: TERMINATION OF PREGNANCY

Preoperative care

In many units a qualified nurse undertakes the nursing care of patients presenting for a termination of pregnancy, rather than the student nurse becoming involved in a potentially stressful event. The procedure is generally completed on an outpatient basis or as a day patient in hospital. There is only a short time available for the nurse to build a relationship with the patient whilst documentation is completed. The usual appraisal of the patient's needs will be made and information must be given as to what procedures are to occur before and after surgery. Every effort must be made to show acceptance of the woman and understanding of the difficulties she has been experiencing. Opportunities must be created for her to express her feelings as she wishes and the nurse should be available to listen. A consent form is signed for the termination and consent for anaesthetic is given. Blood tests such as haemoglobin and haematocrit, ABO grouping and the Rhesus factor are necessary precautions prior to the procedure.

Postoperative care

Vital signs related to bleeding and abdominal cramping pain must be observed by the nurse. Inspection of vulval pads will indicate the degree of blood loss, which can range from slight to moderate. Heavy bleeding will usually require further administration of ergometrine to sustain contraction of the uterus and to evacuate blood clots. Pyrexia may indicate the onset of infection. Mild analgesics may be ordered to relieve cramping pain and also for their antipyretic properties. Women with Rhesus-negative blood require an injection of anti-D immunoglobulin.

The patient is advised to avoid the use of tampons, douching, strenuous activities or sexual intercourse for 2 weeks, to reduce the risk of infection and aid healing. The patient's contraception methods are reviewed with her so that any changes needed are understood and appropriate decisions made. A follow-up outpatient examination is completed 2–3 weeks after the abortion to exclude the possibility of a failed abortion, an ectopic pregnancy or other complications. It also allows for an assessment of the patient's acceptance of and comfort with her decision to terminate. Relief is often expressed. Sadness, regret and depression are sometimes short-lasting but at other times prolonged. The patient's relationship with her sexual partner may also be discussed; it may have been strengthened or weakened by the abortion experience. Referral to a post-abortion support group may be helpful, if there is one active in the area.

Complications of abortion

- Pelvic infection — inflammation of the endometrium (endometritis) and fallopian tubes (salpingitis) may occur
- Perforation of the uterus — may occur accidentally during insertion of cannula or use of the curette
- Haemorrhage — bleeding should not be more than a normal menstrual period
- Laceration of cervix, cervical incompetence and recurrent abortion
- Ectopic pregnancy — related to previous salpingitis
- Incomplete removal of uterine contents
- Hydatidiform mole
- Delayed menstruation
- A live fetus at the time of delivery
- Possible susceptibility to subsequent pregnancy loss and premature births
- Infertility.

With improved services the numbers of complications to abortion can be greatly reduced. Effective networks of outpatient facilities with good access, to avoid delays in uptake of services and reduced travel for women in need, should be the aim of authorities responsible for service provision.

CHILDLESSNESS

While some couples living together choose not to have children, the majority clearly do raise a family. For many people this is an important role, and when childlessness is a reality it brings disappointment. In addition, many other feelings, associated with social and cultural expectations and religious beliefs, may be experienced.

Barbour (1997) suggests that, until recently, much attention relating to treatment and counselling in this area has been directed towards women. Her experience with infertile couples, however, suggests that the feelings and reactions of men require also to be addressed. Mason (1994) also recognises the significance of fatherhood in the context of male infertility.

Some couples choose not to have children in the early years of their relationship but later may experience difficulty in conceiving. It is well documented that one in six couples will seek specialist help for a fertility problem (Winston 1991, Templeton 1992). It is usually the woman who first questions her own physical capacity to become pregnant and who will seek medical advice and submit to multiple investigations. In one-third of couples experiencing subfertility, the problem lies with the woman, in one-third with the man and in the remaining third both the man and the woman contribute some causative factor (see Tables 7.1 and 7.2).

The provision of general facilities to investigate and treat subfertility and to assist in conception are well established at the endocrinology and gynaecological surgery level in the NHS, but the specialist in vitro fertilisation services have been slow to develop, hampered by lack of finance. The need for subfertility services is expected to grow due to the trend towards later first pregnancies and an increasing number of remarriages. Demand is increased due to raised public awareness of treatment possibilities (Effective Health Care Consortium 1992).

Childlessness is deliberately maintained in women who use birth control methods. This is regarded as voluntary childlessness. Sterility refers to an absolute factor preventing procreation in either the man or woman. The condition may be induced by ligation and separation of the fallopian tubes or by vasectomy.

Subfertility

A couple is said to be subfertile if there is a lack of conception after a 12-month period of unprotected sexual intercourse (Mueller & Darling 1989, Thonneau et al 1991). Primary subfertility refers to those cases where a pregnancy has never occurred, and secondary subfertility to those cases where there has been a previous pregnancy, irrespective of the outcome. The literature suggests that one in seven women experience subfertility (Hull et al 1985, Thonneau et al 1991).

The principal causes of subfertility are shown in Tables 7.1 and 7.2. In some couples there will be more than one cause of subfertility. As diagnostic testing becomes more accurate, the proportion of unexplained cases of subfertility may decrease. The contribution of psychological factors to prolonged subfertility is not yet clearly established by research. A small proportion of cases of subfertility may be preventable, particularly tubal damage associated with sexually transmitted diseases.

MEDICAL MANAGEMENT

The diagnosis and management of subfertility is complex. The couple may require to undergo a variety of tests and investigations which can cause embarrassment and stress (see Tables 7.1 and 7.2).

Female subfertility

Female subfertility may be due to failure to ovulate, irregular egg release from the ovary, obstructed fallopian tubes, hostile cervical mucus, endometriosis or uterine conditions which inhibit implantation.

Table 7.1 Subfertility: summary of causes, investigations and treatment in women

Causes	*Investigations*	*Treatment*
Disorders of ovulation Stein–Leventhal syndrome Failure of one or both pituitary gonadotrophins (trauma or vascular disorder) Failure of hypothalamic releasing factor (stress, anorexia nervosa) Primary ovarian failure Tumours of ovary Cysts of ovary Endometrial hyperplasia (causing upset ovarian function) XO karyotype Drugs — post-pill amenorrhoea, phenothiazines, tricyclic antidepressants Adrenal dysfunction Thyroid, hyper- and hypothyroidism	• History • Examination (bimanual) • Skull X-ray • Endometrial biopsy, histology and culture • Plasma progesterone level • Urinary oestrogens level • Ovarian biopsy • Cervical mucus specimen (can be used as a parameter of ovulation) • Full blood count and ESR (erythrocyte sedimentation rate) • Thyroid function tests • Chromosome studies	• Clomiphene • Bromocriptine — for raised prolactin only • LH releasing hormone (LHRH) by pump injection • Pergonal and human chorionic gonadotrophin (hCG) • Buserelin with human menopausal gonadotrophin (hMG) is useful for those with polycystic ovaries • Surgical wedge resection of ovary under laparoscopy. May be effective when drug treatment failed • GIFT — gamete intrafallopian transfer
Disorders of fallopian tubes Congenital absence Blocked due to infection —tuberculosis —recurrent appendicitis —gonococcal infection —septic abortion Hydrosalpinx Disturbance of tubal secretions	• History • Examination • Hysterosalpingogram • Laparoscopy • Biopsy of fallopian tube • Hormone studies (no oestrogen surge)	• Salpingolysis • Salpingostomy • Tubal reconstruction — by microscopy • Tubal excision and transplantation • Oral oestrogens • IVF and ET — in vitro fertilisation and embryo transfer
Endometrium lining of the uterus Not prepared due to disorder of ovulation Endometriosis Endometritis Fibroids Endometrial hyperplasia Endocervicitis	• History • Examination (bimanual) • Hysterosalpingogram • Endometrial biopsy • Evidence of discharge	• Treatment of disorders of ovulation • Dilatation and curettage • Myomectomy • Endometriosis IVF-ET/GIFT
Factors in the cervical mucus Hostile mucus Cervical mucus not prepared due to deficiency of oestrogen as a result of disorders of ovulation Sperm antibodies in cervical mucus	• Postcoital test • Mucus/sperm match test • Spinnbarkheit test • Fern test • Sperm invasion test	• Deficient oestrogen — clomiphene • Ethinyl oestradiol (0.01 u daily for a 3-day period before ovulation) • Refrain from intercourse for a set period or use condom during intercourse. At the end of this time, there may be a decrease in antibodies
Psychosexual problems Frigidity Vaginismus Stress-affecting hypothalamic function Decreased sexual libido	• History and interview	• Psychological referral • Use of vaginal dilators
Others Congenital abnormalities (e.g. bicornate uterus) Obesity Retroverted uterus Hirsutism and virilism (disorders of ovarian or adrenal function, also by certain drugs)	• Examination • Hysterosalpingogram	• Lose weight • Ventro-suspension surgery • Surgical restructuring of genital organs as possible

Table 7.2 Subfertility: summary of causes, investigations and treatment in men

Causes	*Investigations*	*Treatment*
Testes Congenital absence of both Klinefelter's syndrome Cryptorchidism Trauma Testicular failure —torsion —infections —unrestricted pituitary output	• History • Examination • Testicular biopsy • Urinary gonadotrophins • Chromosome investigations	• Cryptorchidism should be detected early in school career and requires surgical intervention • Hormone therapy
Vas deferens and epididymis Congenital absence of both Blockage due to infections —partial —complete Venereal disease Vasitis Epididymitis	• History • Vasogram • Semen analysis • Postcoital test	• No treatment for congenital absence • Vaso-epididymostomy • Microsurgery — removal of blocked section of vas
Spermatozoa Oligospermia (less than 20 million in 1 mL) Varicocele Hernia Physical exhaustion and overwork Aspermia Factors in the testes, vas deferens and epididymis (see above) Endocrine abnormalities, failure of pituitary, adrenal and thyroid glands	• History • Examination — consistency of testicles, presence/absence of varicocele • Semen analysis • Postcoital test • Seminal plasma analysis for fructose content and its glycerol phospherol choline • Interstitial cell-stimulating hormone, follicle-stimulating hormone and testosterone levels • Testicular biopsy • Thyroid tests • Urine analysis — gonadotrophins, ketosteroids • Vasogram	• Surgical treatment of varicocele or hernia • Moderation with alcohol, tobacco and work • Wearing loose underpants • Intrauterine insemination by donor • Vaso-epididymostomy • Assisted conception techniques using partner sperm
Semen volume Too low — sperms fail to contact cervical os Too high — overdilution Quality	• Semen analysis • Postcoital test	• Pooling of two or more semen samples and intrauterine insemination by partner • High doses of gonadotrophins • Split ejaculate and intrauterine insemination by partner
Agglutination of spermatozoa Sperm autoantibodies. Hostile mucus. Sperm antibodies in cervical mucus (penetrate the mucus but become agglutinated and immobilised and die)	• Seminal fluid analysis • Rosette formation of head-to-head clumping, or a wheatsheaf formation of tail-to-tail clumping in seminal fluid • No sperm invasion is seen	• It may be possible to wash the antibodies off these sperm and then, after centrifuging, produce a concentrated specimen; they can be inseminated directly into the cervix • Corticosteroid therapy
Ejaculatory disorders Hypospadias Epispadias Retrograde ejaculation	• History • Examination	• Collection of semen and artificial insemination by partner • Surgical treatment
Sexual problems Impotence Premature ejaculation Stress Decreased sexual libido	• History • Interview	• Psychological referral • Help regain self-confidence • Apply local anaesthetic to penis before coitus. Treatment for premature ejaculation • Monoamine oxidase inhibitor drugs
Others Poor general health Febrile illness Emotional shock Acute allergic response	• History • Examination • Erythrocyte sedimentation rate	• Full recovery ensues naturally

Ovulation disorders

These are among the commonest causes of subfertility (Spira 1986, Thonneau et al 1991). Failure to ovulate is linked with the functioning of hormones from the hypothalamus, pituitary and ovary (HPO axis). Anovulation is categorised into five groups:

- *Hypergonadotrophic hypogonadism* — elevated FSH and LH to within the accepted menopausal range; no response to ovulation induction.
- *Hypogonadotrophic hypogonadism* — hypothalamic suppression of gonadotrophin-releasing hormone (GnRH) release causes very low levels of pituitary gonadotrophin and results in suppression of ovulation.
- *Eugonadotrophic hypogonadism* — functional disturbance of the HPO axis, generally with oligomenorrhoea.
- *Polycystic ovarian disease* — small cysts on the ovarian surface coupled with hormonal imbalance. Multiple small follicles partly develop but none reaches maturity.
- *Hyperprolactinaemia* — high levels of prolactin suppress pulsatile secretion of GnRH and oestradiol production mediated by LH.

Treatment seeks to remedy problems arising from imbalances in the HPO axis. Ovulation induction is aimed at encouraging development of one follicle, leading to a single pregnancy. Clomiphene citrate can be used in women with eugonadotrophic hypogonadism or polycystic ovaries. This anti-oestrogen stimulates gonadotrophin release by inhibiting the negative feedback of gonadal steroids on the hypothalamus.

Treatment should commence in the early follicular phase. In amenorrhoeic women or those with severe oligomenorrhoea, treatment begins after an induced withdrawal bleed. Generally 50 mg of clomiphine is administered daily for 5 days. Ovulation is expected 5–10 days after the last clomiphene tablet and intercourse is best timed between days 10 and 16. In successive anovulary cycles, clomiphine can be increased by 50 mg/day to a maximum of 200 mg/day.

For women who do not respond to clomiphene therapy, human menopausal gonadotrophin (hMG) may be used for direct ovarian stimulation. Careful monitoring of the dose is required to reduce the risk of multiple pregnancy.

Pulsile GnRH is a suitable therapy for women with hypogonadotrophic hypogonadism. This is administered as a pulse dose via an infusion device and stimulates pituitary gonadotrophin release, resulting in the menstrual cycle with positive and negative feedback loops.

Elevated prolactin levels can result in chronic anovulation by inhibiting GnRH release and LH-mediated oestradiol production. Bromocriptine, a powerful dopamine agonist, inhibits prolactin release and may therefore be a therapy considered for such patients.

Tubal disorders

Where tubal factors are the cause of the subfertility, tubal surgery may be advised but this depends upon the nature, site and severity of the condition of the tube, the presence and extent of adhesions, and the skill of the surgeon. Diagnostic procedures will include laparoscopy and hysterosalpingography for full assessment of the condition.

Treatment. Surgical procedures used to treat tubal infertility include fimbrioplasty, salpingostomy, salpingo-ovariolysis, tubotubal anastomosis, uterotubal anastomosis and tubal cannulation. Results of such reconstructive surgery show great variation depending on the degree of tubal damage and the adequacy of the surgery performed; for example, the pregnancy rates following fimbrioplasty reported by Gomel & Taylor (1992) are between 26 and 50%.

The World Health Organization (WHO) cautions against quoting statistics to patients since the 'success' rates reported in studies are often not defined in terms of achieving an intrauterine pregnancy and delivery of a live baby. Reversal of sterilisation, however, is more likely to be sucessful if the occlusive technique used for sterilisation caused minimal damage to the tubes. Clips, for example, generally have minimal traumatic effect and are associated with the highest proportion of intrauterine pregnancies following reversal. Successful reversal can also depend on the site of occlusion (WHO 1997).

Endometriosis

The relationship between endometriosis and subfertility is unclear. Many women with the condition conceive successfully without intervention.

Treatment. There is controversy over the treatment of infertile women with endometriosis without distortion of the pelvic viscera. Chong et al (1990) and Seibel et al (1992) found that, in such cases, surgical treatments appear to confer no benefits. Martin (1995) suggested that surgery should only be performed where symptoms such as pain and deep dyspareunia are attributable to endometriosis. Surgery, however, is recommended in cases of distortion of pelvic tissues. Surgery to remove endometrial tissue, correct anatomical relationships and enhance the possibility of fertility can be successful by laparotomy or laparoscopic techniques (Candiani et al 1991, Redwine 1991). Other options for women with endometriosis include in vitro fertilisation, embryo transfer (ET) and gamete intrafallopian transfer (GIFT) (Effective Health Care Report 1992).

Male subfertility

Male fertility problems can be categorised into three therapeutic groups: untreatable sterility, treatable conditions and subfertility. Subfertility is the most common (Baker 1995). Impaired semen quality and sperm dysfunction can occur as a result of many factors. The cause may be unknown, but it may be associated with a previous infection or factors such as stress, excessive smoking or alcohol intake. Obstruction of the vas deferens will result in ejaculate without sperm. Anti-sperm antibodies which attack sperm or inhibit their motility may be present in semen. Common presentations are:

- oligozoospermia — reduced number of sperm
- asthenozoospermia — reduced motility
- tetratozoospermia — abnormal morphology
- oligoaesthenotetratozoospermia — a combination of the above three
- azoospermia — absence of sperm.

Semen analysis includes an assessment of volume; sperm concentration, motility and morphology; and the number of white cells present. Sperm mucus interaction can be examined in a postcoital test.

Men presenting with subfertility should be fully investigated to ascertain the type of subfertility and identify any related health issues requiring independent treatment.

Treatment should be aimed at achieving natural conception. If male antibodies to spermatozoa are produced, prednisolone has been shown to be effective as an immunosuppressant (Hendry et al 1990). When natural conception is not possible, assisted reproductive techniques (ARTs) offer another possibility. ARTs involve the collection of sperm and eggs and either the immediate placement of the gametes into the fallopian tubes (GIFT) where fertilisation takes place or in vitro fertilisation (IVF) and subsequent transfer of the embryos (ET). Microinsemination techniques such as partial zona dissection (PZD) or subzonal insemination (SUZI) may be appropriate in, for example, oligozoospermia or tetratozoospermia (Fishel et al 1993). Green et al (1997) suggest that almost all cases of male infertility can be treated by intracytoplasmic injection (ICSI) if viable sperm can be obtained.

While ARTs allow many subfertile men to father children, these techniques do not meet the needs of men who do not produce sperm. Donor insemination (DI) may be an option in such cases. DI may also be considered by couples where the man is known to be a carrier of a genetic disease or where couples do not wish to take the risk of having a child born with a genetic disorder transmitted by recessive genes. Kovacs (1997) suggests that a reasonable conception rate from DI in most units is about 10% per cycle. The cumulative conception rate increases to approximately 40% over five treatment cycles.

Provision of information and counselling

The stressful nature of investigations and treatment of subfertility and the psychological impact of the condition on couples require an information-providing service that is sensitive to their needs. They will wish to know about the nature of investigations, the implications of and alternatives to treatment. Emotional support and therapeutic counselling should be easily available to the couple. The Committee of Inquiry into Human Fertilisation and Embryology (1984) recommended that 'counselling should be available to all infertile couples and third parties at any stage of the treatment'. Infertility counselling is recognised by counsellors as a specialised area (Jennings 1995). Anderson & Aleisi (1997) believe that infertility counselling is necessary to help patients deal with the psychological implications and consequences of infertility.

In vitro fertilisation and embryo transfer (IVF-ET)

The work of Edwards & Steptoe in 1978 (summarised in Edwards & Steptoe 1983) led to the birth of the first human infant after conception in vitro. In the intervening decades improvements have been made and the success rate has improved as a result of fertility drugs and the prematuration of oocytes before fertilisation (Trounson et al 1981). However, the success rate, measured by the end result of live healthy babies, depends on many factors, including the age of the woman and the existing fertility problem(s) of the couple (Power 1997) (see Box 7.9). While the chances of achieving a pregnancy may be around 33%, it is recognised that the actual delivery rate can be lower (22%) (Power 1997), since some pregnancies terminate with spontaneous abortion or ectopic pregnancy (Talbot & Lawrence 1997).

Ovarian stimulation. Various protocols are use to achieve controlled hyperstimulation of the ovaries. Agents used include clomiphene citrate, purified FSH, exogenous gonadotrophin and gonadotrophin-releasing hormone agonists (GnRHAs). Modifications to protocols depend on the patient's response.

Clomiphene citrate acts in a negative feedback system to increase endogenous gonadotrophin. A hypothalamic site of action has been reported with increased pulsile release of GnRH. Clomiphene results in synchronous development of multiple follicles, allowing many oocytes to be retrieved. A disadvantage can be a premature rise in LH, resulting in premature ovulation. To avoid the patient's spontaneous ovulation, hCG is used to induce timed ovulation for ovum retrieval.

Box 7.9 Indications for selection into IVF programmes

- Husband and wife are generally healthy
- Ovaries are accessible
- The uterus is functioning normally
- Menstrual function is normal or correctable
- Age preferred below 40 years but a flexible individual approach is taken
- The couple have an uncorrected problem, e.g.:
  —tubal
  —inadequate sperm for normal reproduction
  —endometriosis
  —cervical hostility
  —immunological
  —anovulation
  —undiagnosed by available methods

While purified FSH has the theoretical advantage of enhancing synchronous follicular development, this has not been supported in clinical trials comparing hMG with FSH (Lavy et al 1988), but lowering of the LH surge in patients having purified FSH has been significant.

A dose of exogenous gonadotrophin is determined on the basis of the patient's age and history.

GnRHAs have increased pregnancy rates per cycle (Hughes et al 1992). GnRHAs can be used in combination with hMG for improved folliculogenesis.

Harvesting of eggs. Eggs (oocytes) for fertilisation can be recovered from mature ovarian follicles by:

- ultrasound scanner-guided follicle needle puncture and aspiration
- laparoscopy and needle aspiration.

The laparoscopy method requires a general anaesthetic. The ultrasound method can be completed with either a light general anaesthetic or with the patient sedated. The vaginal ultrasound probe is introduced into the vagina and the pelvis is inspected, noting the position of viscera and blood vessels. An appropriate pathway for the aspirating needle through the pelvis is selected. The laparoscopic method may be used when it is difficult to access the ovaries vaginally. Aspirated oocytes are transfered to the embryologist.

Laboratory procedures. For maximum efficiency and effectiveness there must be close proximity between the operating theatre and the embryology laboratory. There must also be ease of communication between the surgeon and the embryologist; direct verbal and visual contact between the two is needed. Theatre time is usually booked in advance, with 24 h notice, but sometimes egg recovery may need to be done at short notice because of the patient's endogenous LH surge.

The embryologist examines the follicular aspirate for oocytes. The eggs are examined for the level of maturity, washed in clean culture medium and transferred to the culture container. On completion of the oocycte collection, they are placed in an incubator until insemination. This may be 3–6 h later for IVF. (In GIFT the oocytes and prepared sperm are placed into a catheter to be inserted into the fimbrial end of the fallopian tube, where the gametes are deposited for fertilisation.)

Collection of semen can be a stressful experience for the man, who needs to be assured of a secure private environment to produce a specimen of semen by masturbation. Jackson & Burden (1997) indicate that this should be a room specially dedicated for this purpose. A toilet and hand basin should be available. Erotic video and literature may be helpful. However, some couples may wish to be together for this procedure, so a bed with washable covers should be in the room. Men may be able to produce a semen sample in their own home if they are able to deliver it to the laboratory within 1 h.

Insemination involves mixing of sperm, prepared by the embryologist, and eggs in the appropriate concentration. Sixteen to 20 h later the oocytes are examined for fertilisation and once normal fertilisation has been established the embryos are returned to culture in fresh medium for another 24 h.

Embryo replacement. This is usually performed 2–3 days after oocyte retrieval or about 48 h after insemination when the embryos are at the two-cell or four-cell stage. Placement of the embryos in the uterus is a delicate procedure that does not necessarily result in successful implantation and pregnancy. In some centres nurses are taught to perform this procedure, following a specified protocol, as part of their extended role (Peddie 1998). The incidence of pregnancy increases with the number of embryos replaced, but an attempt is made to reduce the risk of multiple pregnancy with the possibility of premature births. Usually two or three embryos are transferred. This is a painless procedure for the patient, requiring no anaesthetic.

On discharge from hospital the patient is given instructions to send samples of urine to the unit on the eighth and 11th days after replacement so that pregnancy tests can be completed. She is also asked to notify the unit if menstruation occurs so that she can be advised about future treatment and her records can be maintained. If her pregnancy is confirmed and develops, the unit will maintain an interest in the pregnancy and will want to celebrate the success of childbirth.

Transport IVF

While there is an increasing demand for IVF treatment in the UK, a lack of funding limits the number of clinics able to offer IVF treatment. Transport IVF, however, makes this treatment more widely available to infertile couples. Here gynaecologists in local communities make arrangements with regional specialist IVF units to share the care of the patients (Kingsland et al 1992). The ways in which the services required at different stages of IVF are organised between the two centres vary. One possibility is for ovulation stimulation and oocyte retrieval to be undertaken at the satellite centre, with subsequent transfer of the oocytes to the central unit for insemination, fertilisation and embryo transfer.

Treatment of low-powered sperm in IVF-ET

Such treatments involve manipulating ovum and sperm together to improve penetration of the ovum by sperm in cases of sperm dysfunction such as poor motility. A deliberate injection of a single sperm into an ovum can be achieved using a sophisticated microscope and special instruments. The human embryos so formed have led to successful pregnancies for a few women.

See Green (1997) for further information regarding intracytoplasmic sperm injection.

Prenatal analysis of DNA for genetic abnormality

Prenatal diagnosis of genetic abnormalities is now possible by analysing DNA for a known gene defect (see 'Genetics', p. 200). A single cell is removed from a 4–16 cell embryo. Information regarding a genetic defect can become available within a few hours, soon enough to allow the embryo to be implanted when it is known to be healthy. Diseases such as cystic fibrosis and Duchenne muscular dystrophy can thus be avoided. Some women have already been treated in this way, but long-term information is needed on whether the loss of a single cell from an embryo is likely to have any adverse effect.

Gamete intrafallopian transfer (GIFT)

GIFT offers an alternative treatment to IVF when women have at least one patent fallopian tube. It is primarily used in patients who have unexplained subfertility and cervical hostility. It is contraindicated in women with stage III and IV endometriosis, active infection and intrauterine abnormalities. GIFT can be performed in hospitals that do not have IVF facilities. However, where such facilities exist, surplus oocytes can be fertilised in vitro and cryopreserved. Thus IVF and later ET may be an option if GIFT is unsuccessful. Wood (1997) shows that between 1990 and 1993 the live birth rate from GIFT was double that from IVF.

The technique involves giving follicle-stimulating drugs to stimulate the ovaries. Retrieval of eggs follows, as in IVF. The eggs are then mixed with the freshly donated sperm and transferred into the fimbriated ends of the fallopian tube(s) (see Fig. 7.10). GIFT is normally performed laparoscopically but it can be achieved vaginally or by means of a colposcope. The eggs, being placed directly in the fallopian tube, have the opportunity to become fertilised more naturally and continue along the tube to implant in the uterus.

Zygote intrafallopian transfer (ZIFT)

This is a similar procedure to that described above, but here the gametes are fertilised before transfer to the fallopian tube. In this treatment, therefore, fertilisation is known to have occurred and embryos have the opportunity to benefit from the tubal environment and to enter the uterine cavity naturally.

NURSING PRIORITIES AND MANAGEMENT: IVF

The patient admitted to an IVF unit will have lived with her state of known subfertility for some years and will have experienced, with her partner, many tests, investigations and surgical interventions before being offered the opportunity to seek pregnancy by the IVF method. The couple will be hopeful for success but must recognise that this is not guaranteed.

Pre-laparoscopy care

Reducing anxiety

Anxiety will be experienced as the treatment cycle is approached with great hope, but pre-treatment counselling should have given a realistic picture of the chances of cumulative success rather than encouraging the couple to focus on success of the first cycle (Anderson & Alesi 1997).

The nurse will need to prepare a plan of care that will minimise the stress level and help the patient to relax. High stress levels are well known to disturb hormone levels and their activity. Planned counselling sessions may be needed to allow the patient to express any concerns. Similarly, information-giving sessions will need to be planned. Slides and videotapes can be invaluable supplements for group work when the special needs of individuals can be identified and met within a supportive group.

The patient will become very knowledgeable about the detailed steps of the programme but may still have questions that need to be answered. She will need truthful information about results of

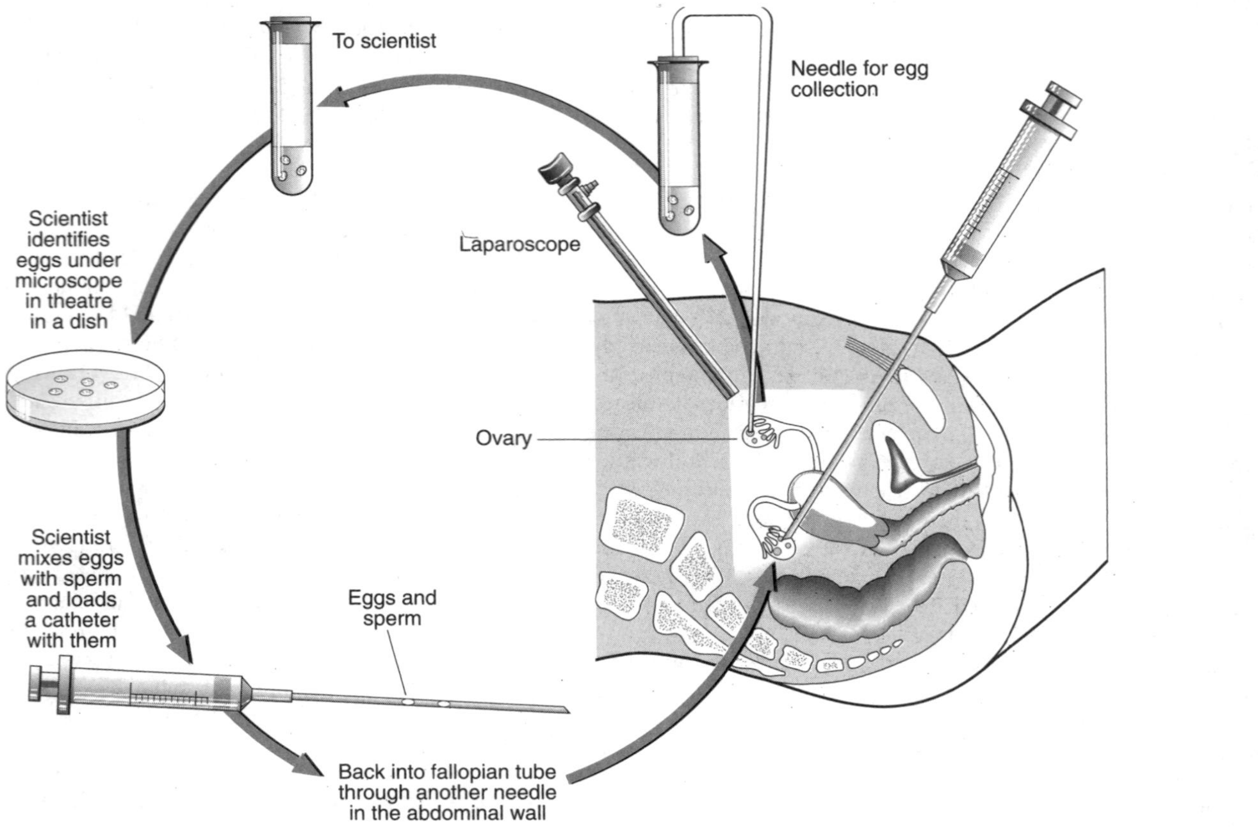

Fig. 7.10 The GIFT treatment.

hormonal assays, the number of eggs available for recovery and the progress of the embryos. A system of open communication is important, whether the information is favourable or disappointing.

Self-care in the follicular stage

The nurse should facilitate the patient's orientation to the comfortable surroundings of the IVF unit. The patient is not ill and her role in maintaining self-care can be explained. She will need to learn how to collect her urine and record the time and amount passed. Verbal instructions can be complemented by a written explanation available in the toilet area. A patient whose first language is not English will need written instructions in her own language.

Blood and urine samples will be required for laboratory testing. Ovarian stimulants are given according to the individual patient's needs. Patients should understand that there are differences in need between individual women and the nurse's explanations can alleviate concerns.

Preparation for egg cell recovery

The procedure of ultrasound scanning should be explained in terms of checking the number of follicles maturing and their stage of development. Once the estimated time of ovulation is known, preparation for theatre begins. Blood is taken for haemoglobin estimation. Skin is prepared according to the policy of the unit; some surgeons still prefer the pubic area to be shaved prior to laparoscopy and oocyte recovery. Fasting arrangements are maintained according to protocol, in preparation for a general anaesthetic. No premedication drugs are prescribed, to avoid compromise of the patient's physiological balance and that of the ripened follicles.

The patient is likely to be excited at this time in anticipation of a successful harvesting of eggs. The nurse should encourage her to relax and be calm for transfer to theatre. The eggs may be recovered vaginally with ultrasound guidance or via a laparoscope. Each mature follicle is carefully aspirated and the eggs are collected in the culture tube. The aspirate is immediately passed to the laboratory for examination and identification of oocytes.

Post-laparoscopy care

Recovery from the laparoscopy is rapid. Rest in bed for a maximum of 8 h is usually necessary to avoid referred pain in the shoulder from retention of residual gas in the abdomen. Mild analgesics such as paracetamol may be prescribed for relief of pain. The patient will be keen to know whether the laparoscopy was successful and how many eggs were recovered.

Unfortunately, sometimes the time of ovulation has been misjudged and the follicles have already ruptured prior to laparoscopy or the recovered eggs are too immature to be viable. During laparoscopy, adhesions may be seen to obscure the ovarian tissue, thus negating the procedure.

The nurse should adopt a counselling, sensitive approach when giving news of the failure of the procedure. The surgeon concerned may prefer to explain his difficulties to the patient and her partner. The nurse may have to repeat the information for the patient together with possible details of re-entry into the programme at a later date.

Preparation for embryo transfer

When a patient's eggs have been successfully recovered, there is a wait of 2–3 days while the eggs are matured in vitro, if this is necessary, and then they are fertilised with the specially prepared semen of her partner. As the fertilised eggs divide and develop, they are closely observed in the laboratory for their readiness for transfer back into the patient's uterus. Failures may also occur at this delicate laboratory stage and this is a further worrying time for the patient.

As soon as a positive decision is made for embryo transfer, the patient takes a shower and dresses in a clean gown. A bath is avoided to ensure there is no water in the vagina. The bed is prepared with clean linen and taken to the theatre. Once there, the patient is positioned in the modified lithotomy in the Trendelenburg position for the procedure of embryo transfer.

Once the fertilised egg is successfully introduced into the uterus, the woman is moved gently. The prone, supine or lateral position may be utilised for the next 2 h of undisturbed rest, still with the head of the bed tilted downwards. After 2 h, the head of the bed is returned to a normal position and the patient can eat and drink. Thereafter she continues to rest, spending the following day quietly and avoiding strenuous activity. Discharge usually takes place 36 h after embryo transfer with the mother anticipating a positive pregnancy outcome.

Q

7.1 Think about how the patient will feel if failure occurs at any of the stages of the IVF treatment programme.
7.2 Write down the patient's possible thoughts about failure:
- during the follicular stage
- at the oocyte recovery stage
- at the embryo development stage in the laboratory
- after embryo transfer into the uterus.

7.3 Write down a few sentences of what you might say to the patient at each of the above stages.
7.4 Discuss with your mentor whether what you have written down could be used as a guide to communication with the patient, with allowances made for differences between patients and their partners.

Continuing need for support and counselling

Nurses working in hospital or in the community must be prepared to use their counselling skills with clients who wish to enter, are involved in, or have terminated a programme of subfertility treatment. Community midwives may participate in the care of women who are pregnant following subfertility treatment and others who have experienced a miscarriage. Health visitors also have a role in counselling following the loss of a pregnancy or an infant after subfertility treatment. Couples may continue to need to talk about their feelings of inadequacy or failure and to be allowed to grieve for their losses, as if they have experienced a bereavement (see Case History 7.1).

For some couples, treatment options for subfertility will not prove successful and it may be necessary for them to accept that they will not have children of their own. Other possibilities can be sensitively discussed. Attitudes and lifestyles may require some readjustment if the couple are to continue with a satisfying life and a supportive relationship.

Case History 7.1 K

K achieved a pregnancy during her programme of subfertility treatments. Unfortunately, she aborted a twin-boy pregnancy and was devastated by the loss. She returned to the programme and became a mother with the birth of quadruplets: three girls and a boy. Unfortunately the boy subsequently died. K visits the unit with her lovely girls in a triple buggy but still grieves over the boys. She has asked to re-enter the programme because she still wants a boy. K has been referred to an independent counsellor.

EMBRYO RESEARCH

The main aim of human embryo research has been the prevention of genetically transferred diseases. Embryo research improves the understanding and management of genetic diseases.

Pre-implantation diagnosis in embryos is possible by removing and examining a single cell, although it is not known whether this cell removal might cause a defect in the child. The treatment offers hope to those who carry genetic defects that can affect the well-being of the child. Further embryo research may help with the understanding of miscarriage of pregnancies, which involve 100 000 women per year, with consequent effects on health and future fertility. Further understanding of the way embryos implant might shed more light on contraception, miscarriages and ectopic pregnancies. It is also expected that embryo research will improve the understanding and treatment of cancer by the study of 'oncogenes' which control cell division and growth.

The Human Fertilisation and Embryology Act 1990

A consequence of reproductive technology and in vitro fertilisation is the production of surplus embryos. This has created public concern about the potential for undesirable experimental work on embryos.

The Human Fertilisation and Embryology Act 1990 prohibits certain practices and has established the Human Fertilisation and Embryology Authority (HFEA) to license and regulate the activities of IVF centres. The Act applies only to the creation of embryos outside the human body. The embryo is not to be kept or used after the appearance of the primitive streak, at the end of 14 days. The primitive streak, or groove, is formed by invagination from the ectoderm, in the formation of the mesoderm between the ectoderm and the endoderm of the embryo. Identification of this structure is used to denote the beginning of human life (Morgan & Lee 1991). Frozen embryos may be stored for a period not exceeding 5 years. Gametes may be stored for 10 years. All centres involved in IVF must prepare a code of practice, which is subject to inspection, and are required to send 12-monthly reports to the HFEA. The Act has a conscientious objection clause. Nurses therefore have 'the right to refuse to participate in technological procedures to achieve conception and pregnancy' (UKCC 1996) on the basis of a conscientious objection.

Surrogate motherhood

The HFE Act defines the woman who carries the embryo as the mother of the child. If the woman then gives the baby to a married couple in a surrogacy agreement, a parental order can be made by a competent court (in private) to make the couple the child's legal parents, providing specified criteria are met (Human Fertilisation and Embryology Act 1990). Regardless of any prior agreement regarding the surrogacy, the Human Fertilisation and Embryology Act renders surrogacy contracts unenforceable.

The right of any childless couple to have a child is generally accepted, but after infertility treatments fail to help the woman to conceive, there may be less support for her seeking another fertile woman to assist in developing a pregnancy. Financial inducement and contractual arrangements cannot guarantee that the surrogate mother will be prepared to hand over the newborn baby to the infertile couple. If the intended parents do not wish to accept the child the surrogate (legal) mother is responsible for its welfare. In the event of the child being rejected by the birth mother and the intended parents the child can be placed for adoption or fostering.

DISORDERS OF THE MALE REPRODUCTIVE ORGANS

The anatomy and physiology of the male reproductive system is described in Chapter 8.

MALDESCENT OF THE TESTES (CRYPTORCHIDISM)

PATHOPHYSIOLOGY

Cryptorchidism is a condition in which one or both testes have not descended into the scrotum before birth. It is a common condition seen in approximately 1% of boys after their first year and may be self-correcting or require surgery in the form of orchidopexy. Normal descent keeps the testes cooler in the scrotum and avoids the germ cell degeneration that is possible in the higher temperature of the abdomen, which carries a risk of malignancy. Three different grades of maldescent are described:

- *a retractile testicle* is normally found in the scrotum but on stimulation is pulled up into the superficial inguinal pouch by an active cremaster muscle
- *an ectopic testicle* is prevented, by tissue structures, from descending from the inguinal canal into the scrotum
- *an undescended testicle* is possibly abnormal: it remains in the abdomen and fails to enter the inguinal canal and pass into the scrotum.

MEDICAL MANAGEMENT

The aim of treatment is to promote normal function of the testicle. Treatment should be completed by the boy's eighth year, before the testicle starts functioning. Untreated cryptorchidism results in sterility, since the cells involved in the initial development of sperm cells are destroyed by the higher body termperature in the pelvis. The testicle may migrate spontaneously, or hormone treatment may be prescribed to stimulate migration. Otherwise, an orchidopexy is performed to bring down the testicle into the scrotum. It is held there by means of a suture passing through the wall of the scrotum and into the thigh. The suture is removed 7–10 days postoperatively.

More extensive surgery may be needed with actual removal of the abnormal testicle and repair of an inguinal hernia if this has occurred. In addition to the risk of infertility, there is also a high risk of malignancy if the testes are left in the abdomen.

NURSING PRIORITIES AND MANAGEMENT: MALDESCENT OF THE TESTES

Pre- and postoperative care is routine (see Ch. 26), with particular emphasis on hygiene and wound care. The nurse should fill in any gaps in the patient's understanding of his condition and the operation performed. The patient who is still a child may feel embarrassed about asking questions and the nurse must judge where to begin and end when giving information and a health education programme. The facts of sexual life may need to be explained to the child with a parent present, or the parent may prefer to be the one to give the child the information. In some cases, the nurse may find it more relevant to focus on the parents' need for education, information and advice.

TORSION OF THE TESTES

Testicular torsion is an acutely painful condition caused by the twisting of the testis on its spermatic cord. It may occur spontaneously or as the result of strenuous exertion. It commonly occurs in adolescents aged 12–18 years, but can occur in adults as well. This condition is classified as a surgical emergency requiring immediate treatment.

PATHOPHYSIOLOGY

Testicular torsion results when an abnormality of the tunica vaginalis allows increased mobility of the testis and axial rotation of the spermatic cord above. The resulting ischaemia can lead to cell damage and infection within approximately 6 h.

Extravaginal torsion, a rare form, can occur in utero or in the newborn. In this case the testis is not painful but on examination is found to be a firm, large mass in the scrotum.

Common presenting symptoms. The patient will present with sudden onset of acute pain in the groin, often radiating to the scrotum and abdomen. Exercise may be the precipitating factor, but the onset of pain can also occur at rest. Nausea and vomiting are common.

MEDICAL MANAGEMENT

The patient may give a history of previous, less severe episodes which resolved spontaneously. Examination of the testis may be hampered by the severity of the pain. The affected testis will be elevated, but abnormality of mobility ('bellclapper' deformity) may be present in the other testis.

Treatment. Treatment is by immediate surgery to relieve the torsion and secure testicular fixation. However, if the torsion is detected at an earlier stage, it may be possible by gentle external manipulation to rotate the twisted testis in the appropriate direction. This may immediately resolve the emergency, but the testes should later be surgically secured to prevent recurrence.

NURSING PRIORITIES AND MANAGEMENT: TORSION OF THE TESTES

The patient will normally be young and fit and his stay in hospital brief. Although the surgery is not considered major, the acute onset of pain and the nature of the problem may give rise to considerable anxiety and perhaps embarrassment. Giving the patient adequate information will help to relieve anxiety and promote recovery. He should be informed that analgesics can be given immediately and that the acute pain will go away once the operation has been performed.

The patient's stay in hospital will normally be for 24 h. Postoperatively, he will have a small inguinal wound and perhaps some scrotal swelling. He will normally be able to return to school or to work in about 2 weeks, at which point he should feel comfortable walking and sitting. Lifting, heavy work and sports involving running, jumping or stretching should be avoided for about 6 weeks. An athletic support should always be worn when sports activities are resumed.

The patient who has received treatment in good time should also be reassured that blood supply to the testes was not interrupted to the degree that any impairment to sexual function or fertility will result.

Q

7.5 Write a care plan for a patient following surgery for fixation of the testes. Consider what problems the patient might have. The care plan should include:

- checking the wound for oozing, swelling and infection
- ensuring the wearing of a scrotal support to prevent swelling
- relieving pain by bed rest and analgesia
- ensuring that the patient passes urine within a specific time postoperatively (it may take him up to 24 h)
- checking temperature, pulse and blood pressure
- informing the patient when he may eat and drink again
- giving discharge advice.

HYDROCELE

PATHOPHYSIOLOGY

A hydrocele is a collection of serous fluid in the membranous sac (the tunica vaginalis) that surrounds the testes. It may occur spontaneously without any cause or it may be secondary to an acute or chronic inflammatory condition of the testis or epididymis. The hydrocele usually occurs on one side only, is painless, and can swell to a considerable size. It may accompany a condition that causes oedema of tissues, such as congestive heart failure or nephrotic syndrome.

Common presenting symptoms. Hydrocele is usually asymptomatic, but an increase in scrotal size and associated discomfort will often prompt the patient to seek advice. The embarrassment caused by the swelling may be such that the individual curtails social activities, swimming, sunshine holidays and sexual relations.

MEDICAL MANAGEMENT

The presence of fluid within the scrotal sac provides a red glow on transillumination. It is dull to percussion whereas a hernia is usually resonant (Cotton & Lafferty 1986). A tense hydrocele can be differentiated from a tumour in that the latter does not illuminate (Gillespie et al 1992). As a hydrocele can form around a testicular tumour, the possibility of cancer should be excluded.

Treatment. The condition may be reducible by the wearing of a scrotal support, but it is often necessary to introduce a fine trochar and cannula to drain off the fluid. Bleeding and infection are common as complications, and recurrence at 6–15 weeks is common.

VARICOCELE

A varicocele occurs when the veins draining the testes become distended and tortuous. This may cause enlargement of the spermatic cord. Palpation of the scrotum will reveal a mass of enlarged varicose veins. The condition most commonly occurs in men aged 15–30 years and sometimes resolves without intervention when there is regular sexual intercourse. A persistent varicocele may induce a raised temperature within the scrotum due to the increased blood supply and contribute to a subfertile state.

MEDICAL MANAGEMENT

Medical intervention may be conservative or surgical. The patient who complains of a dragging discomfort in the scrotum may find that this is relieved by the wearing of a scrotal support. If the condition is more severe, ligation of the veins may be needed. A small length of vein may be removed.

TESTICULAR CANCER

Testicular cancer is an uncommon condition accounting for 1–2% of all cancers in men. It is, however, the commonest malignancy in men aged 20–34 years (Peate 1997). In the last 50 years, the condition has become more common among white racial groups but has remained only one-third as common among black racial groups. Its incidence is highest in Scandinavian countries and lowest in Asian and African countries. In Denmark testicular cancer accounts for 6.7% of all cancers. In Japan it accounts for 0.8%. Cryptorchidism (undescended testicle) and exogenous oestrogens have been linked with an increased incidence of testicular cancer. Exogenous oestrogens are used by women in birth control pills or in medication to prevent miscarriage. While exposure to exogenous oestrogens, in utero, can increase the risk of testicular cancer, Vessey (1989) indicated that such findings are not conclusive.

As survival depends on early detection and treatment, Peate (1997) recommends that men should be encouraged to practise testicular self-examination at least every 6 months. The value of screening programmes for testicular cancer remains a matter for debate (see Research Abstract 7.6).

PATHOPHYSIOLOGY

The cell types of testicular cancer are classified in terms of embryonal tissue rather than adult testes tissue. Almost all the cancers arise from the primordial germ cell, the multipotent cell found in the yolk sac of the embryo. This multipotent cell will have many varieties of cell types as offspring, and a primary testicular tumour may have a wide variety of cell types. The normal cells of the testis have high proliferative potential and can become malignant under the influence of an abnormal environment.

Research Abstract 7.6
Testicular cancer screening

A report of a working party of the Royal College of Physicians (1991) concluded that as testicular self-examination has never been evaluated and because chemotherapy now achieves cure rates of 90% or more, even in advanced cases of testicular cancer, screening is probably unnecessary. Moreover, because there is no identifiable pre-invasive stage, screening cannot reduce the incidence but might even increase it by overdiagnosis of borderline tumours. Thus screening for testicular cancer is not indicated.

Royal College of Physicians 1991 Report on preventive medicine. Royal College of Physicians, London

Testicular cancers are grouped as:

- *Originating from germinal tissue (97%):*
  —seminoma (typical, anaplastic or spermocytic)
  —non-seminomatous:
  —embryonal
  —teratocarcinoma
  —teratoma
  —choriocarcinoma
- *Arising from stromal tissue (3%):*
  —interstitial cell tumour
  —gonadal stromal tumour.

Germinal testicular cancer

The germinal cancer types may develop from a single cell or a multifocus. The malignant growth is fairly rapid in one testis. Metastases may occur by extension locally or via the lymphatics to the retroperitoneal lymph nodes. Lymph node invasion may cause displacement of the ureters or kidneys. The ureters may become obstructed. By direct extension the tumour may invade the epididymis, extend up the spermatic cord or extend through the tunica vaginalis to the scrotum. Late metastases may be found in the lung, liver, adrenal gland or bone.

Common presenting symptoms. The first sign of testicular tumour is painless enlargement of the testicle. This may be discovered by accident or by self-examination (see Box 7.10). A dragging sensation may be felt in the scrotum from the weight of the tumour.

MEDICAL MANAGEMENT

There is usually a lack of pain on palpation of the testis. Any painless lump in the testis that does not respond promptly to antibiotics should be thought of as cancer until proven otherwise. Metastases may cause lumbar pain and abdominal or supraclavicular lymph node masses.

Investigations. Laboratory studies of serum alpha-fetoprotein (AFP) and serum beta-human chorionic gonadotrophin (hCG) help in the diagnosis of germ cell cancer as tumour markers. AFP is high in aggressive non-seminomatous tumours; hCG is elevated in 30% of seminomas. These markers corroborate diagnosis but are also useful in monitoring treatment. Chest X-ray, chest CT scan, tomography, lymphangiography, abdominal CT scan, abdominal ultrasonography and intravenous pyelography may all be used diagnostically.

Treatment is by surgery with adjuvant radiotherapy and chemotherapy.

Surgical intervention. A high radical inguinal orchidectomy is performed. The testis, epididymis, a portion of the vas and parts of the gonadal lymphatics and blood vessels are removed. The remaining testis will undergo hyperplasia and produces enough testosterone to maintain sexual capacity, male characteristics and libido. The semen, however, may be of poor quality. Ejaculatory ability may be reduced.

Radiotherapy. Following surgery, radiotherapy is recommended for lymph node areas. Fatigue, bone marrow depression and diarrhoea may be experienced as side-effects. There may be scatter radiation to the other testicle despite the use of a protective shell during therapy. Sperm recovery is slow, variable and dose-related.

Chemotherapy. A number of cytotoxic drugs are used as an adjunct to surgery and radiotherapy. Cyclophosphamide and chlorambucil may be used with vincristine and actinomycin D in cyclical treatments, every 2 months for 1 year and every 3 months for the second year. Where there is extended disease, vinblastine and bleomycin are the drugs of choice. If the disease is disseminated, the drug cisplatin may be added to the previous two.

Radiotherapy and chemotherapy following sugery can have significant side-effects, such as azoospermia, nephrotoxicity, bone marrow suppression and neurotoxicity (Hawkins & Miaskowski 1996, Hilkens et al 1997). Reduced sexual function and infertility are possible persisting side-effects following treatment for testicular cancer (Arai et al 1997, Jonker-Pool et al 1997).

Box 7.10 Teaching testicular self-examination

The nurse can make a valuable contribution to health promotion by teaching testicular self-examination. An effective teaching plan will explain the reasons for self-examination of the testes, the best time to perform self-examination, the steps to follow in self-examination and the types of abnormality that should be reported to a doctor.

Teaching plan

- Enquire about any previous information the patient may have gained about examination of the testes
- Respond to what the patient says about the topic and build on that knowledge. Give the patient the opportunity to ask questions and seek clarification regularly
- Use a simple diagram of the scrotum and testes to describe the structures involved
- Explain that it is necessary to be aware of the normal condition of the testes so that any later change can be recognised at an early stage
- Advise that the best time to perform self-examination is immediately after taking a shower or bath, when the body tissues are warm, the scrotum is relaxed and the testes easy to feel
- Emphasise the need to look at the scrotum for its colour, texture, any change in shape or any swelling that may be noticeable
- Instruct the patient that it is necessary to hold the scrotum in the palm of the hand and to examine each testicle by rolling the testis between his thumb and fingers:
  —each testicle should feel smooth and be about the size of a small hen's egg
  —the epididymis, which lies behind each testicle, should also be felt and should feel soft and slightly spongy to the touch.
  —the spermatic cords, which extend upwards from the epididymis, should feel like round, firm tubes
- Explain that any abnormality in the shape of the testicle and any lump or swelling should be investigated by a doctor irrespective of how trivial it may seem
- Check that the patient knows why he is completing the self-examination. Help him to understand that a cancerous lump can now be successfully treated

NURSING PRIORITIES AND MANAGEMENT: TESTICULAR CANCER

The preoperative and postoperative needs of a patient having orchidectomy are similar to those of other patients requiring major surgery (see Ch. 26). The need for information, relief of anxiety, pain relief and protection from wound infection are primary. The young adult patient with insight into his cancer condition will undoubtedly be worried about the future, the course of the illness, his family responsibilities and his career.

Postoperatively the patient will require a short period of fully compensatory care whilst recovering from the anaesthetic. A short period of partially assisted care will follow. In the long term the patient will need planned educative and supportive care. (See Case History 7.2.)

7.6 Mr W had his left testis removed 48 h ago. He has extensive lymphatic gland metastases. The medical plan includes radiotherapy and chemotherapy over the coming months.

Consider the circumstances of the family described in Case History 7.2 and:

(a) Identify Mr W's needs for education and support.
(b) Prepare a teaching plan.
(c) List the ways in which you as the nurse can provide support for Mr W during the postoperative period.
(d) Explain the ways that Mr W can continue to be supported after discharge from hospital.
(e) Identify the needs of the family in the short and long term.

Case History 7.2 Mr W

Mr W is 32 years of age. He is married and has two young daughters aged 2 and 4. His wife looks after the children well but has always been very dependent on him for organising the family and helping with domestic chores and the shopping. They have usually enjoyed an average social life, babysitters permitting. Mr W works as a computer engineer. He likes to leave work promptly so that his wife isn't left too long on her own at home. She has had episodes when she has become reliant on alcohol, particularly when she is worried about the children.

For further information, see Bassett (1993).

VASECTOMY

Couples who have used a range of birth control methods over the years may decide that permanent sterilisation by surgical means would now be preferable.

Preoperative counselling

Before such a decision is taken the couple should meet with their GP or family planning counsellor to discuss their needs and circumstances and their reasons for considering sterilisation as a birth control method. The counsellor should provide information about both female and male sterilisation and the risks, side-effects and failure rates of the procedures available. The long-term effects and prospects for reversal of the sterilisation should be explained. The couple should also be encouraged to consider the implications of a breakdown of their marriage or partnership, or the loss by death of one of the couple or of their children.

A man contemplating vasectomy may have particular anxieties about the effect of the procedure on his masculinity and sex drive. He must be assured that, as the testes will not be removed, his hormone production, virility and sex drive will be unaffected. The nature of the operation should be described with the aid of a simple diagram. It should be explained that the ejaculation fluid will be free from sperm and that unused sperm will be broken down and reabsorbed. Further information that the patient will require is summarised in Box 7.11.

Box 7.11 Information for the patient undergoing vasectomy

Every patient undergoing vasectomy should be given an information leaflet containing the following information:

- The type of anaesthesia that will be given (i.e. general or local)
- The operation will be completed via the scrotal sac
- Between 1–5 cm of vas will be removed on each side
- A dressing will be applied to the wound and a scrotal support will be applied and should be worn for 2 weeks
- Some swelling and bruising will occur around the operation site. This may extend down over the thighs or up towards the umbilicus
- Some pain will be experienced, but this can be relieved by paracetamol or codeine tablets
- Skin sutures will dissolve spontaneously within approximately 1 week of the operation
- Strenuous exercise should be avoided for 2 days
- The patient will not become infertile immediately after the operation due to sperm being stored upstream of the operative site. Therefore, he must continue to take contraceptive precautions until two successive sperm samples are proved to be free of sperm
- Normal sexual intercourse can take place from the third postoperative day. As the operation site may be tender, the individual may prefer to wait longer than this
- At least 12 ejaculations should have occurred before the first semen test to clear sperm. A second semen test will be completed 2 weeks later. In a small proportion of cases, sperm persists in the seminal fluid for many months
- There is a 0.5–1.0% failure rate associated with the operation:
  —the ends of a vas may join up again early or late after operation
  —the surgeon may remove some structure other than the vas
  —some men have anatomical abnormalities, such as a double vas that is not fully removed
- Reappearance of fertility after two negative semen tests may mean that the tests were not accurately completed or the ends of a vas have reunited
- Severe, prolonged pain may indicate some slow seepage of blood into tissues from a small blood vessel. A haematoma may have formed, causing the scrotum to swell. Rest in bed should ease the condition. Otherwise the site may need to be drained at the clinic
- The wound may become infected, in which case the GP will prescribe antibiotics
- There is a reasonable chance that the operation can be reversed should this be desired. Reversibility cannot be guaranteed, however, and a return to the previous level of fertility may not be achieved

MEDICAL MANAGEMENT

The surgical procedure. Vasectomy is the ligation or division of the vasa deferens, the genital ducts that store and transport sperm to the urethra in the process of ejaculation (see Ch. 8), and is performed under either general or local anaesthetic. The vas is

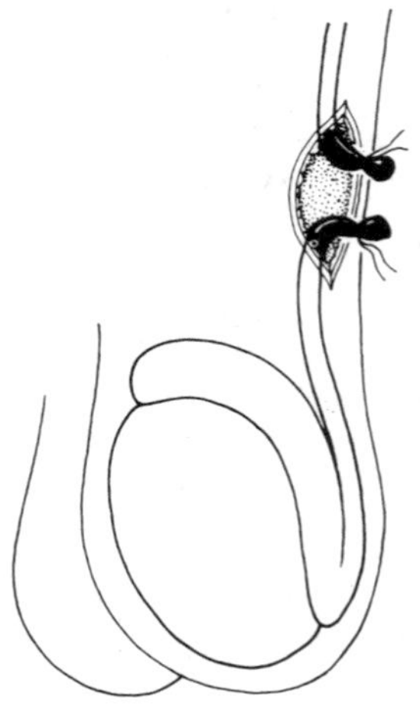

Fig. 7.11 The vas divided.

palpated in the upper scrotum and an incision of 1 cm is made over the vas. The fascia around the vas is incised and the vas drawn out and ligated in two places.

The vas is then simply divided or a small segment is excised (see Fig. 7.11). One end of the vas is enclosed again in the fascia envelope. The other end of the vas is repositioned outside the fascia. Alternatively, the cut ends of the vas may first be cauterised or the cut ends looped back on themselves. The skin is closed with absorbable sutures and the procedure is repeated on the opposite side. The possibility for reversal of the operation is retained.

Outcome. The majority of men are pleased with the vasectomy operation. They usually consider it to have been minor surgery and to have caused no ill effects. They can approach sexual intercourse with greater relaxation and increased enjoyment.

A minority experience regret after the operation, feeling that their sexual drive and performance have been reduced. Others who have taken new partners or remarried may regret being unable to have another child within the new relationship. A new wife who has no child may feel deprived and frustrated.

Reversal. An increasing number of men are requesting reversal of their vasectomy. Surgeons are now attaining 70–90% success rates with such reversals, which are technically feasible, but the pregnancy rate achieved is disappointingly low: only one-third of the reversed vasectomies lead to pregnancy. This low rate may be due to the formation of sperm antibodies.

NURSING PRIORITIES AND MANAGEMENT: VASECTOMY

Preparation for the procedure

The nurse working in a day care facility may be responsible, jointly with the surgeon, for ensuring that the individual undergoing vasectomy and his partner understand what the procedure will entail and its anticipated results.

Postoperative care

Postoperatively, the nurse on the ward or in the GP surgery may be involved in pain management and wound care. The nurse will have an important contribution to make in instructing the patient in postoperative self-care and in informing him about procedures for follow-up and assessment. She should also alert him to the possible complications or problems that should be reported (see Box 7.12).

Box 7.12 Inflammatory conditions of the male reproductive organs

Balanitis and balanoposthitis

The term balanitis refers to inflammation of the glans penis. The term balanoposthitis refers to inflammation of the prepuce or foreskin as well as the glans penis. Both conditions are the result of bacterial infection. They are painful, irritating and produce a discharge. They may be associated with inadequate hygiene and phimosis. A swab from the inflamed area is sent for pathological culture and sensitivity tests. Specific antibiotic therapy can be prescribed. Local treatment will involve bathing the affected areas with normal saline to relieve discomfort.

Epididymo-orchitis

In this condition, infection and inflammation of the testis and epididymis occur together. It may be caused by prostatitis, a urinary tract infection or a sexually transmitted disease. The testes are swollen, tender and painful. The patient is pyrexial and suffers from aches and pains. He may experience nausea and vomiting. Bed rest, extra fluids, analgesics and antibiotics are necessary. Cold packs applied locally to the scrotum and the wearing of a scrotal support will help to relieve discomfort and swelling.

Orchitis

This condition is most often caused by mumps occurring after puberty. It may result in atrophy of the testes and sterility. Males who have not had mumps in childhood should try to avoid contact with the disease. Early administration of gammaglobulin may reduce the severity of mumps in those who have been exposed.

Prostatitis

This is an acute or chronic inflammation of the prostate gland and is usually bacterial in origin. Urgency, frequency and pain with micturition are experienced. Acute retention of urine, cystitis, low back pain, chills and haematuria may occur. The prostate gland is enlarged and tender when examined. Midstream urine specimens are sent to the laboratory for culture and sensitivity. Antibiotics, analgesics and a high fluid intake are prescribed. The condition is liable to recur.

Although information will have been provided preoperatively, many men are concerned about the development of scrotal swelling and haematoma in the postoperative period. Scrotal support, rest and analgesics are necessary for general comfort and to improve the condition over time. Any bleeding from the wounds may be relieved by the use of butterfly sutures to pull the wound edges together. Psychological after-effects of vasectomy should be few if preoperative counselling and information-giving have been adequate. Some men complain of an adverse effect on sexual performance after vasectomy, but they are usually those who have had similar difficulties before surgery.

Some long-term physical complications of vasectomy have been suggested but have not been supported by research. There is, however, some question about vasectomy precipitating development of testicular cancer from a pre-invasive lesion and the possibility of an association between vasectomy and the development of testicular tumours (see Research Abstract 7.7).

The nurse should take the opportunity to check whether the patient understands how to self-examine the testes for the

Research Abstract 7.7
Vasectomy and testicular tumours

In the past 10 years an increased incidence of testicular cancer has been recorded in Scotland. Vasectomy has become a more popular form of contraception, and a retrospective research study by Cale et al (1990) has suggested that there may be an association between vasectomy and subsequent testicular tumours. It is queried whether some immunological and pathophysiological effects may occur following vasectomy, or whether such tumours in fact developed before vasectomy.

The importance of testicular examinations before and after vasectomy is recognised. Men should be screened by an examination at 12–18 months after vasectomy. A large prospective research study is needed to fully establish whether vasectomy contributes to testicular malignancy.

Cale A J R et al 1990 Does vasectomy accelerate testicular tumour? Importance of testicular examinations before and after vasectomy. British Medical Journal 300: 370

development of a lump (see Box 7.10). When the principles are understood, the patient should accept the need to complete a self-examination at appropriate intervals. However, it would be inappropriate to associate the risk of tumour with vasectomy until more research data are available.

Occupational health nurses can take a significant role in promoting testicular self-examination in the working male population, the majority of whom seldom need to visit their general practitioner.

IMPOTENCE OR ERECTILE DYSFUNCTION

Impotence is the persistent inability, due to organic causes, to obtain an erection sufficient for sexual intercourse. The word impotence has wide social and psychological connotations and it is recommended that the use of this term is discouraged with patients and the disorder referred to as erectile dysfunction or another appropriate descriptive expression (Bancroft 1993). It is difficult to show the true prevalence of erectile dysfunction because of the nature of this disorder and the shame, guilt or embarrassment associated with it, but Bancroft (1993) suggests 7–8% of men may be affected and the incidence increases with age.

PATHOPHYSIOLOGY

Impotence may be a primary or secondary condition. The term 'primary impotence' implies that the patient has never had an erection. This is rare and is usually associated with gross abnormality of the penis or with hormone deficiency from childhood. Secondary impotence is much more common and may be due to psychological or organic factors, or to a combination of both.

Most men will occasionally fail to gain or maintain an erection. This can be attributed to stress, overwork or some other reason.

Causes. Psychological factors causing secondary impotence have been categorised by Kolodny et al (1979) as follows:

- *Developmental*
  —maternal or paternal factors
  —conflict in parent–child relationship
  —severe negative family attitude to sex
  —traumatic childhood sexual experience
  —gender identity conflict
  —traumatic first coital experience
  —homosexuality
- *Affective*
  —anxiety about performance
  —guilt
  —depression
  —poor self-esteem
  —hypochondria
  —mania
  —fear of causing pregnancy
  —fear of venereal disease
- *Interpersonal*
  —poor communication
  —hostility towards partner
  —distrust of partner
  —lack of physical attraction to partner
  —sex role conflict
  —divergent sexual preference, or sex value systems, e.g. time, place, type
- *Cognitive*
  —sexual ignorance
  —acceptance of cultural myths
  —performance demands
- *Miscellaneous*
  —premature ejaculation
  —isolated episode of erectile failure
  —iatrogenic influences.

Organic causes of secondary impotence include:

- poor arterial inflow caused by atherosclerosis and aneurysm
- venous leaks between the corpora and venous system
- neurological diseases
- endocrine dysfunction
- drugs, including antihypertensives, narcotics and alcohol
- major surgery — cystectomy, radical prostatectomy (see Ch. 8).

For further information, see Bennett (1994).

MEDICAL MANAGEMENT

Therapy will depend upon diagnosis of the underlying cause of the impotence.

Investigations are carried out to provide an understanding of the problem (Gregoire & Pryor 1993):

- clinical interview to explore the nature of the problem, sexual behaviours and attitudes, relationship with a partner, personal and family history, medical history, psychiatric history and current therapy or medications
- physical assessment, including examination of penis, testes, prostate and seminal vesicles; neurological examination; vascular examination
- blood screen for evidence of endocrine imbalance, diabetes mellitus, renal failure
- assessment of penile blood flow by Doppler studies and angiography
- assessment of neurogenic factors by monitoring nocturnal penile tumescence (NPT), response to visual erotic stimuli, assessment of autonomic nerve function and neurophysiological studies
- psychological testing.

***Treatment* options:**

Local injection. A local injection at the base of the penis using the α-adrenergic receptor blocking agents, papaverine or a combination of papaverine and phentolamine can cause an erection. The action is by vasodilatation and vasocongestion within the spongy tissue of the penis. An erection can be maintained for a period of about 30 min. Patients can be taught to self-inject at home. Complications include fibrosis at the base of the penis and priapism requiring emergency hospital treatment. Priapism is persistent, painful erection of the penis, unrelieved by sexual intercourse or masturbation. Priapism lasting more than 4–6 h can result in necrosis and fibrosis of the cavernosal tissue as a consequence of ischaemia (King et al 1994).

Penile prosthesis. There are various types of penile prosthesis available, ranging from semi-rigid, non-inflatable devices to multicomponent, inflatable implants. A full discussion with the patient (and his partner as appropriate) prior to surgery should include an explanation of the various types, the patient's expectations and possible complications.

The semi-rigid prosthesis consists of two semi-rigid silicone-covered or malleable rods inserted into the shaft of the penis, in the corpora cavernosum. It is important that the correct size is used by the surgeon if the prosthesis is to be effective. They give a permanent erection which is firm enough to allow the patient to have intercourse. A hinged prosthesis allows movement into the upward or downward position. Flaccidity and erection are possible with mechanical and inflatable prostheses.

Individual factors such as motivation, intelligence, dexterity and strength require to be considered in choosing an appropriate prosthesis, to avoid implanting a device that the patient cannot operate (Montague & Lakin 1994).

Infection and erosion are possible complications and usually require removal of the device. The probability of mechanical failure usually relates to the complexity of the device and failure generally requires reoperation.

Revascularisation of the penis. This advance in surgery can help patients who have arterial problems. It involves anastomosing an abdominal artery to the penile vein to improve the blood supply. Although not considered major surgery, it does leave the patient with a fairly large abdominal scar. Infection may be a postoperative problem. This procedure has the advantage of restoring normality. Success rate is reported to vary from 50 to 81% (Sharlip 1994), depending on the selection of patients and the surgical procedure adopted.

Vacuum suction machine. These machines have been available for some time from sex shops and magazines but have only recently been recognised as a valuable treatment for patients with impotence. The machine produces a partial vacuum around the penis, causing it to engorge. An elastic band is then placed around the base of the penis to maintain the erection for a maximum of 15 minutes. The advantage of this treatment is that the patient can control the erection, but the duration of the erection is limited by the ischaemic effect of the tourniquet.

Psychotherapy. Impotence judged to be psychological in origin may be helped by psychotherapy for the patient and his partner.

NURSING PRIORITIES AND MANAGEMENT: IMPOTENCE

Psychological considerations

A man who realises that he has become impotent is likely to be shocked and dismayed. He may be reluctant to talk about the problem, even to his partner. This can become a very complex matter, not only for the individual but also for his partner and family. Failure to accept or understand the problem can lead to the break-up of a marriage or partnership. Moreover, organic causes of impotence, such as multiple sclerosis, diabetes and circulatory problems, may have already caused the patient to change his lifestyle and placed the family under stress.

The patient may be very reluctant to discuss the problem openly with a doctor or nurse. He may present to his GP ostensibly with another problem, only managing with difficulty to mention his real concern. Occasionally it is at an outpatient appointment such as a diabetic clinic that the subject is brought up.

Medical and nursing staff must treat the patient with empathy and sensitivity. While the condition is not life-threatening and may not be considered urgent, once the patient presents he will want something done quickly.

Practical considerations for the patient receiving a penile implant

The nurse should ensure that the patient is given sufficient information about the procedure and the recovery period. He should be told that his hospital stay will be 4–7 days, and that, while there will be some pain, regular analgesics will be given. Catheterisation will be required for at least 24 h. Complete bed rest will not be required, but the patient should not spend too much time walking around or sitting in a chair for the first few days, to encourage healing and reduce discomfort. He must wear a scrotal support for a few weeks, to help prevent swelling and to minimise discomfort.

The consultant will discuss with the patient how soon the prosthesis may be used, but it is likely that he will recommend that it is not used until after the first outpatient appointment in 6 weeks. Sutures will not normally require removal, as they will dissolve on their own. It is helpful to assure the patient that visitors or other patients on the ward will not know what procedure he is undergoing unless he tells them himself. Nor will other people know that he has a prosthesis, although it may be necessary to avoid wearing tight trousers or swimming trunks.

OTHER DISORDERS OF THE MALE REPRODUCTIVE ORGANS

Inflammatory disorders of the male reproductive organs are briefly described in Box 7.12, p. 272. Disorders affecting the prostate, urethra and urinary function are described in Chapter 8.

CULTURAL AWARENESS IN REPRODUCTIVE HEALTH

Sociological change and economic progress have contributed to the integration of immigrants into the UK and some have been in this country for generations. Inevitably, when people move from their particular culture to another, they bring with them their beliefs and values, reflecting their background. Some of these will remain with them, giving direction to their life and practices. Older members of a family tend to rely on tradition and are reluctant to take on board new ideas, whereas younger generations growing up in a new environment may be more influenced by different cultural perspectives and are more likely to adapt to or adopt some of the dominant views of the indigenous population around them. This can cause tension within families as views associated with sex, marriage and family affairs come into conflict.

If health care workers are to provide sensitive care and counselling to patients or clients from various cultural backgrounds, they need to be aware that the beliefs and values associated with a particular culture and upbringing can have profound effects on patients' or clients' perspectives and attitudes towards health, sexuality and family life. While some views of others will conflict with those held by the nurse, a non-judgemental approach is required. In this respect, item 7, in the nurses' *Code of Professional Conduct* (UKCC 1992) states that nurses, midwives and health visitors must:

> *recognise and respect the uniqueness and dignity of each patient and client and respect their need for care, irrespective of their ethnic origin, religious beliefs, personal attributes, the nature of their health problems or any other factor.*

It is not expected that nurses will have a wide knowledge of all cultural and religious beliefs but it is appropriate to find out about the customs relevant to the cultural groups presenting in clinical practice. Much can be learned from patients by showing an interest in them as social beings in their own context.

In some cases, problems with communication can be exacerbated in cross-cultural interactions, not only because English may not be the first language of immigrants, but also because they may feel embarrassed to ask for clarification or further explanation. The possibility of obtaining leaflets with information in different languages should be explored when this is a potential problem. Younger members of a family may be more fluent in English than their older relatives and effective communication may be achieved by sensitively incorporating them for translation and clarification. The services of an interpreter may need to be employed.

While, in British culture, reproductive functioning, sexuality and health disorders affecting the reproductive systems are felt to be very personal and intimate issues, this attitude may in fact be much more exaggerated in some other cultures. Open communication, required for the sharing of information and the giving of health care advice, may therefore be made more difficult. The performance of a necessary vaginal examination, for example, may be seen as a major procedure with significant emotional implications.

While it has been suggested that treatment of fertility problems should incorporate the couple, Muslim or Sikh men may be extremely reluctant to attend a fertility clinic with their wife and can feel humiliated or angry at the suggestion that they might be responsible for the fertility problem. The beliefs held about fertility and the sanctity of semen in its life-giving potential can have important implications in the way men and women view contraception and the options available to them for regulating their family. While the nurse may not be conversant with specific options acceptable in different cultures, an awareness of the existence of such restrictions on individual choice allows a more sensitive, exploratory approach with clients.

Different cultural and religious perspectives view marriage and the production of offspring in different ways. Similarly, family networks vary and the extended family may have a significant influence on younger members showing a sense of responsibility with regard to provision of information and support.

Thus, both culture and religion can have a powerful influence on sexual practices, family support networks and how individuals perceive and feel about their own sexuality and self-concept. In introductory interactions with patients — taking a history and building up a rapport — the nurse can learn much from them by showing an interest in their beliefs and their perspective on life and encouraging them to discuss these. This knowledge can then help nurses to be more aware and sensitive to cultural influences in health care and facilitate more individualised nursing.

Male circumcision — excision of the foreskin — is a procedure with religious connotations for Jews and Muslims. This can be performed by a Jewish rabbi or by a family doctor. Harbinson (1997) indicates that circumcision is carried out in the USA for hygienic and social reasons, but in the UK the operation is only performed within the NHS for medical reasons.

Female circumcision is widely practised in some African and Egyptian ethnic groups in parts of the Middle East and in South East Asia. In the UK, female circumcision is considered to be female genital mutilation, the consequences of which the female has to live with throughout her entire lifetime. Female genital mutilation is a term used to refer to procedures resulting in different degrees of mutilation of the external genitalia of females (Royal College of Nursing 1996) and has been illegal in the UK since 1985. However, immigrant families can return to their home country to have this procedure carried out on their daughter (usually from the early days of birth to 16 years of age). The effects of the procedure are also seen in the UK amongst women who have been mutilated prior to arrival. Within the culture valuing this procedure, there may be difficulty in securing a husband for a female who has not been so treated.

Female mutilation can take various forms:

- *Female circumcision* involves excision of the hood of the clitoris.
- *Clitoral excision* may be performed with or without removal of the labia minora.
- *Infibulation* is a more extensive procedure involving removal of the clitoris, labia minora and some of the labia majora. The vulva is sutured together leaving only a small orifice for passage of urine and menstrual blood.

Although the risk of infection after these procedures is high, women may not present with problems until later in life. Problems may include, for example, recurrent urinary tract infections, vaginal infections, non-consummation, infertility and psychosexual problems. During pregnancy the women require sensitive care. Special antenatal care may be available to allow women to express their fears about labour and childbirth and for the provision of information and counselling. For some women a vaginal delivery will be feasible and deinfibulation may be possible to avoid a caesarean section (Toubin 1994). Deinfibulation can be performed during a pregnancy or during labour but Omer-Hashi (1994) suggests that the earlier this is performed the better the outcome in terms of decreased pain during labour and a shorter recovery time after delivery.

Educating, advising and counselling people who have quite different beliefs, values and attitudes concerning health issues from those of the health professionals providing help and support requires tact and sensitivity. Understanding and empathy can help nurses to appreciate what others consider to be important. A balance is required between giving sound advice and respecting the social, cultural and religious views of others.

REFERENCES

Abernethy K 1997 The menopause. In: Andrews G (ed) Women's sexual health. Baillière Tindall, London, pp 336–364

Abraham G E 1987 Premenstrual tension: current problems in obstetrics and gynaecology. In: O'Brien P M S (ed) Premenstrual syndrome. Blackwell Scientific Publications, London, pp 1–39

Allan P, Jolley M (eds) 1982 Nursing midwifery and health visiting since 1900. Faber, London

Anderson J, Alesi R 1997 Infertility counselling. In: Kovacs G (ed) The subfertility handbook. Cambridge University Press, Cambridge, pp 249–268

Arai Y, Kawakita M, Okada Y, Yoshida O 1997 Sexuality and fertility in long-term survivors of testicular cancer. Journal of Clinical Oncology 15(4): 1444–1448

Baggish M S, Dorsey J H, Adelson M 1989 A ten year experience treating cervical intraepithelial neoplasia with the CO2 laser. American Journal Obstetrics Gynaecology 161: 60–68

Baker H W G (1995) Male infertility. In: de Grost L J (ed) Endocrinology, 2nd edn. WB Saunders, Philadelphia, pp 2404–2433

Bancroft J 1993 Impotence in perspective. In: Gregoire A, Pryor J P (eds) Impotence: an integrated approach to clinical practice. Churchill Livingstone, Edinburgh, pp 3–13

Barbour D 1997 How does infertility affect men? Fertility Nurses' Newsletter 20, 2–5

Bassett C 1993 Pay attention to the testes. Practice Nurse 5(14): 957–958

Bennett A H (ed) 1994 Impotence diagnosis and management of erectile dysfunction. WB Saunders, Philadelphia

Blake P, Lambert H, Crawford R (eds) 1998 Gynaecological oncology: a guide to clinical management. Oxford University Press, Oxford

Brown M A, Woods N F 1984 Correlates of dysmenorrhoea: a challenge to past stereotypes. Journal of Obstetric, Gynaecological and Neonatal Nursing 13(4): 259–266

Budeiri D, Li Wan Po A, Doran J C 1996 Is evening primrose oil of value in the treatment of premenstrual syndrome? Controlled Clinical Trials 17(1): 60–68

Cale A J R, Farouk M, Prestcot R J, Wallace I W 1990 Does vasectomy accelerate testicular tumour? Importance of testicular examinations before and after vasectomy. British Medical Journal 300: 370

Campbell E M, Peterkin D, O'Grady K, Sanson-Fisher R 1997 Premenstrual symptoms in general practice patients. Prevalence and treatment. Journal of Reproductive Medicine 42(10): 637–646

Campbell S, Whitehead M I 1977 Oestrogen therapy and the menopausal syndrome. In: Greenblatt R, Studd J (eds) The menopause: clinics in obstetrics and gynaecology. WB Saunders, London, pp 31–47

Cancer Research Campaign 1994 Cervical cancer (factsheet 12); cervical screening (factsheet 13). CRC, London

Candiani G B, Vercellini P, Fedele L, Bianchi S, Vendola N, Candiani N 1991 Conservative surgical treatment for severe endometriosis in infertile women: are we making progress? Obstetrical and Gynaecological Survey 46: 490–498

Charles E H, Savage E W 1980 Cryosurgical treatment of intra-epithelial neoplasia: a review of the literature. Obstetric Gynaecological Survey 35: 359–548

Chong A P, Keene M E, Thornton N C 1990 Comparison of three modes of treatment for infertility patients with minimal pelvic endometriosis. Fertility and Sterility 53: 407–410

Chow S N, Huang C C, Lee Y T 1997 Demographic characteristics and medical aspects of menopausal women in Taiwan. Journal of Formosan Medical Association 96(10): 806–811

Chuong C J, Coulam C B, Kao P C, Bergstalh E J, Go V L W 1985 Neuropeptide levels in premenstrual syndrome. Fertility and Sterility 44(6): 760–765

Colditz G A, Hankinson S E, Hunter D J et al 1995 The use of oestrogens and progestins and the risk of breast cancer in post-menopausal women. New England Journal of Medicine 332: 1589–1593

Committee of Inquiry into Human Fertilisation and Embryology (Chairman, Dame Mary Warnock) 1984 Report. HMSO, London

Cotton L, Lafferty K 1986 A new short textbook of surgery. Hodder and Stoughton, London

Day N 1989 Screening for cancer of the cervix. Journal of Epidemiology and Community Health 43(2): 103–106

Deeney M, Hawthorn R, McKay Hart D 1991 Low dose danazol treatment of the premenstrual syndrome. Postgraduate Medical Journal 67: 450–454

Department of Health and Social Security 1985 Cervical cancer screening [HC(85)8]. DHSS, London

Department of Health and Social Security 1988 Cervical cancer screening [HC(88)1]. DHSS, London

Edwards R G, Steptoe P C 1983 Current status of in vitro fertilisation and implantation of human embryos. Lancet ii: 1265–1269

Effective Health Care Consortium 1992 The management of subfertility. Effective Health Care 3. University of Leeds

Eluf-Neto J, Booth M, Munoz N et al 1994 Human papilloma virus and invasive cervical cancer in Brazil. British Journal of Cancer 69: 114

Everett S 1997 Contraception. In: Andrews G (ed) Women's sexual health. Baillière Tindall, London, pp 173–217

Facchinetti F, Martignoni E, Petraglia F, Sances M G, Nappi G, Genazzani A R 1987 Premenstrual fall of plasma beta-endorphin in patients with premenstrual syndrome. Fertility and Sterility 47(4): 570–573

Family Planning Today 1996 Contraceptive choices survey: how women decide (editorial). Family Planning Today, First Quarter, UNIPATH, London

Farrer H 1990 Maternity care. Churchill Livingstone, Edinburgh

Fedele L, Parazzini F, Luchini L, Mezzopane R, Tozzi L, Villa L 1995 Recurrence of fibroids after myomectomy: a transvaginal ultrasonographic study. Human Reproduction 10(7): 1795–1796

Finucane F F, Madans J, Bush T, Wolfe P H, Kleinman J C 1993 Decreased risk of stroke among postmenopausal hormone users. Results from a national cohort. Archives of International Medicine 153(1): 73–79

Gangar E, Penny J 1995 Advances in hormone replacement therapy. Nursing Standard 9(50): 23–25

Gasperino J 1996 Ethnic differences in body composition and their relation to health and disease in women. Ethnicity and Health 1(4): 337–347

Giannini A J, Price W A, Loiselle R H 1984 Beta-endorphin withdrawal: a possible cause of premenstrual tension syndrome. International Journal of Psychophysiology 1(4): 341–343

Gillespie I E, Nasim A, Zawawi A R 1992 A guide to surgical principles and practice. Churchill Livingstone, Edinburgh

Glaser B, Strauss A L 1965 Awareness of dying. Aldine, Chicago

Gomel V, Taylor P J 1992 In vitro fertilisation versus reconstructive tubal surgery. Journal of Assisted Reproduction and Genetics 9: 306–309

Gordon H K, Duncan I D 1991 Effective destruction of cervical intra-epithelial neoplasia (CIN) 3 at 100°C using the Semur cold coagulator: 14 years' experience. British Journal Obstetric Gynaecology 98: 14–20

Green S, Fishel S, Stoddart N, Garrett L 1997 Microinsemination for the treatment of male factor infertility. In: O'Brien P M S (ed) The yearbook of obstetrics and gynaecology, vol 5. RCOG Press, London, pp 80–92

Gregoire A, Pryor J P (eds) 1993 Impotence an integrated approach to clinical practice. Churchill Livingstone, Edinburgh

Halbreich U, Rojansky N, Palter S 1991 Elimination of ovulation and menstrual acyclicity (with danazol) improves dysphoric premenstrual syndrome. Fertility and Sterility 56: 1066

Hall G, Spector T D 1992 Hormone replacement therapy and coronary heart disease: a qualitative assessment of the epidemiological evidence. Preventive Medicine 21: 47–63

Harbinson M 1997 The arguments for and against circumcision. Nursing Standard 11(32): 42–47

Harris R E, Namboodiri K K, Wynder E L 1992 Breast cancer risk: effects of estrogen replacement and body mass. Journal of Cancer Institute 84: 1575–1582

Hartmann P E 1991 The breast and breastfeeding. In: Philipp E, Setchell M (eds) Scientific foundations of obstetrics and gynaecology, 4th edn. Butterworth-Heinemann, London

Hawkins C, Miaskowski C 1996 Testicular cancer: a review. Oncology Nursing Forum 23(8): 1203–1213

Health Departments of Great Britain 1989 General pracrice in the national health service. The 1990 contract. HMSO, London

Health Education Board for Scotland (HEBS) Booklets: The time of your life: A fresh look at the menopause; Eat to your heart's content; Look after yourself; Well woman. HEBS, Edinburgh

Helman C G 1997 Culture, health and illness, 3rd edn. Butterworth-Heinemann, Oxford

Hendry W F, Hughes L, Scammell G 1990 Comparison of prednisolone and placebo in sub fertile men with antibodies to spermatazoa. Lancet 335: 85–88

Hildesheim A, Mann V, Brinton L A, Szklo M, Reeves W C, Rawls W E 1991 Herpes simplex virus type 2: a possible interaction with human papilloma virus types 16/18 in the development of invasive cervical cancer. International Journal of Cancer 49(3): 335–340
Hilkens P H, Pronk L C, Verweij J, Vecht C J, Van Putten W L, Van Den Bent M J 1997 Peripheral neuropathy induced by combination chemotherapy of docetaxel and cisplatin. British Journal of Cancer 75(3): 417–422
Hinton J 1980 Whom do dying patients tell? British Medical Journal 218: 1328–1330
Hopwood J 1990 Background to colposcopy and the treatment of the cervix. Schering Health Care, Burgess Hill
Hoshiai H, Ishikawa M, Sawatari Y 1993 Laparoscopic evaluation of the onset and progression of endometriosis. Americal Journal of Obstetrics and Gynaecology 169: 714
Hughes E G, Federkow D M, Daya S, Sagle M, Dekoppel P, Collins J 1992 The routine use of gonadotrophin-releasing hormone agonists prior to in vitro fertilisation and gamete intrafallopian transfer: a meta-analysis of randomised controlled trials. Fertility and Sterility 58: 888–896
Hull M G R, Glazener C M A, Kelly N J et al 1985 Population study of causes, treatment and outcome of infertility. British Medical Journal 291: 1693–1697
Human Fertilisation and Embryology Act 1990 HMSO, London
Hunt K, Vassey M, McPherson K 1990 Morbidity in a cohort of long-term users of hormone replacement: an update analysis. British Journal of Obstetrics and Gynaecology 97: 1080–1086
Ibbotson T, Wyke S 1995 A review of cervical cancer and cervical screening: implications for nursing practice. Journal of Advanced Nursing 22(4): 745–752
Jackson P, Burden J 1997 Laboratory techniques. In: Kovacs G (ed) The subfertility handbook. Cambridge University Press, Cambridge, pp 220–234
Jacobs H, Loeffler F 1992 Postmenopausal HRT. British Medical Journal 305: 1403–1408
Jennings S E 1995 Infertility counselling. Blackwell Science, Oxford
Joint Report of the Council on Scientific Affairs and the Council on Medical Science 1992 Technology Assessment in Medicine, Archives of Internal Medicine 152(1): 46–50
Jones C 1995 Cervical cancer: is herpes simplex virus type III a cofactor? Clinical Microbiological Review 8(4): 549–556
Jonker-Pool G, Van Basten J P, Hoekstra H J, Van Driel M F, Sleijfer D T Koops H S, Van De Wiel H B 1997 Sexual functioning after treatment for testicular cancer: comparison of treatment modalities. Cancer 80(3): 454–464
Khoo S K, Munro C, Battistutta D 1990 Evening primrose oil and treatment of premenstrual syndrome. Medical Journal of Australia 153(4): 189–192
King B F, Lewis R W, Mckusick M A 1994 Radiologic evaluation of impotence. In: Bennett A H (ed) Impotence, diagnosis and management of erectile dysfunction. WB Saunders, Philadelphia, pp 52–91
Kingsland C, Aziz N, Taylor C, Manasse P, Haddan N, Richmond D 1992 Transport in vitro fertilisation – a novel scheme for community based treatment. Fertility and Sterility 58: 153–158
Kjorstad J E, Orjasaester H 1984 The prognostic value of CEA determinations in the plasma of patients with squamous cell cancer of the cervix. Gynaecologic Oncology 19: 284–289
Knight M, Field D 1981 A silent conspiracy: coping with dying cancer patients on an acute surgical ward. Journal of Advanced Nursing 6: 221–229
Kolodny R G, Masters W H, Johnston V E 1979 Textbook of human sexuality for nurses. Little Brown, Boston
Kovacs G T 1997 The use of donor insemination. In: Kovacs G (ed) The subfertility handbook. Cambridge University Press, Cambridge, pp 139–150
Lambert H E, Blake P R, Coulter C, Dawson T, Mason P, Soutter P (eds) 1992 Gynaecological oncology. Oxford University Press, Oxford
Lavy G, Pellicer A, Diamond M, De Cherney A 1988 Ovarian stimulation for the in vitro fertilisation and embryo transfer, human menopausal gonadotrophin versus pure human follicle stimulating hormone: a random prospective study. Fertility and Sterility 50: 74–78
Leask R 1991 Too common a story? Nursing Times 87(2): 22–23
Leather A T, Holland E F N, Andrews G D et al 1993 A study of the referral patterns and therapeutic experiences of 100 women attending a specialist premenstual syndrome clinic. Journal of the Royal Society of Medicine 86(4): 199–201
Lewis T L T, Chamberlain G V P (eds) 1995 Gynaecology by ten teachers, 16th edn. Edward Arnold, London
Lock M 1994 Menopause in culture context. Experimental Gerontology 29(4): 307–317
Loudon J D O 1985 Family planning in the United Kingdom: services and training. In: Loudon N (ed) Handbook of family planning. Churchill Livingstone, Edinburgh
Lumsden M A 1985 Dysmenorrhoea. In: Studd J (ed) Progress in obstetrics and gynaecology, vol 5. Churchill Livingstone, Edinburgh, pp 276–292
Lundstrom V 1981 Uterine activity during normal cycle and dysmenorrhoea. In: Darwood M Y (ed) Dysmenorrhoea. Williams and Wilkins, Baltimore, pp 53–74
Lunn P G 1992 Breast feeding patterns, maternal milk output and lactational infecundity. Journal of Biosocial Science 24(3): 317–324
Lunn P G, Prentice A M, Austin S, Whitehead R G 1980 Influence of maternal diet on plasma-prolactin levels during lactation. Lancet i: 623
Lunn P G, Watkinson M, Prentice A M, Morrell P, Austin S, Whitehead R G 1981 Maternal nutrition and lactational amenorrhoea. Lancet i: 1428
MacIntyre I, Stevenson J C, Whitehead M I, Wimalawansa S J, Banks L M, Healy M J 1988 Calcitonin for prevention of postmenopausal bone loss. Lancet 1(8591): 900–902
Marteau T M, Walker P, Giles G, Smail M 1990 Anxieties in women undergoing colposcopy. British Journal Obstetric Gynaecology 97: 859–861
Martin D C 1995 Pain and infertility – a rationale for different treatment approaches. British Journal of Obstetrics and Gynaecology 102(suppl 12): 2–3
Maruo T, Shibata K, Kimura A, Hoshina M, Mochizuki M 1985 Tumour associated antigen, TA-4, in the monitoring of the effects of therapy for squamous cell carcinoma of the uterine cervix: serial determinations and tissue localization. Cancer 56: 302–308
Mason M C 1994 Male infertility – men talking. Routledge, London
Masood S 1997 Why women still die from cervical cancer. Journal of Florida Medical Association 84(6): 379–383
McQueen A 1995 Gynaecological nursing: nurses' perceptions of their work. MPhil thesis, University of Edinburgh (unpublished)
McQueen A 1997 The emotional work of caring, with a focus on gynaecological nursing. Journal of Clinical Nursing 6: 233–240
Menkes D B, Taghavi E, Mason P A Spears G F S, Howard R C 1992 Fluoxetine treatment of severe menopausal syndrome. British Medical Journal 305: 346–347
Montague D K, Lakin M M 1994 Penile prostheses. In: Bennett A H (ed) Impotence diagnosis and management of erectile dysfunction. WB Saunders, Philadelphia, pp 257–295
Morgan D, Lee R G 1991 Blackstone's guide to Human Fertilisation and Embryology Act 1990. Blackstone Press, London
Mueller B A, Darling J R 1989 Epidemiology of infertility. Extent of the problem – risk factors and associated social changes. In: Soules M R (ed) Controversies in reproductive endocrinology and infertility. Elsevier, New York, pp 1–13
Muse K, Cetel N, Futterman L, Yen S 1984 The premenstrual syndrome. Effects of 'medical ovariectomy'. New England Journal of Medicine 311: 1345–1349
Nabulsi A A, Folsom A R, White A et al 1993 Association of hormone replacement therapy with various cardiovascular risk factors in postmenopausal women. New England Journal of Medicine 328: 1069–1075
National Opinion Poll 1992 Market research survey commissioned by Ciba-Geigy Pharmaceuticals, Horsham, Surrey
Nazarko L 1992 Miscarriage and injustice. Nursing Standard 7(12): 44–45
Ngan H Y, Cheung A N, Lauder I J, Wong L C, Ma H K 1996 Prognostic significance of serum tumour markers in carcinoma of the cervix. European Journal of Gynaecological Oncology 17(6): 512–517
Notelovitz M 1986 Menopause and climacteric. In: Philipp E E, Barnes J, Newton M (eds) Obstetrics and gynaecology, 3rd edn. Heinemann, London, p 201
O'Brien P M S 1987 Premenstrual syndrome. Blackwell Scientific Publications, London, p 115
Omer-Hashi K H 1994 Commentary – female genital mutilation: perspectives of a Somalian midwife. Birth 21(4): 224
Orem D 1991 Nursing: concepts of practice, 4th edn. McGraw-Hill, New York
Overgaard K, Riis B J, Christiansen C, Popenphant J, Johansen J S 1989 Nasal calcitonin in treatment of established osteoporosis. Clinical Edocrinology 30: 435–442
Pearce J M 1991 Spontaneous abortion. In: Varma T R (ed) Clinical gynaecology. Edward Arnold, London
Peate I 1997 Testicular cancer: the importance of effective health education. British Journal of Nursing 6(6): 311–316

Peddie V L 1998 A prospective analysis of embryo transfer; performed by nurses in training. Report of a paper (presented by Barbour D) at British Andrology Society, British Fertility Society and The Society for the Study of Fertility Annual Conference in July 1997. Fertility Nurses' Newsletter 21: 9

Phillips A N, Smith G D 1994 Cigarette smoking as a potential cause of cervical cancer: has confounding been controlled? International Journal of Epidemiology 23(1): 42–49

Power M 1997 Fertility problems. In: Andrews G (ed) Women's sexual health. Baillière Tindall, London, pp 152–172

Purdie D W 1990 Hormone replacement therapy and prevention of osteoporosis. In: Bonnar J (ed) Recent advances in obstetrics and gynaecology 16. Churchill Livingstone, Edinburgh, pp 235–251

Redwine D B 1991 Conservative laparoscopic excision of endometriosis by sharp dissection. Life table analysis of reoperation and persistent or recurrent disease. Fertility and Sterility 58: 628–634

Rees M C P 1988 Recent progress in the aetiology of dysmenorrhoea and menorrhagia. In: Brush M G, Goudsmit E M (eds) Functional disorders of the menstrual cycle. John Wiley, Chichester

Reginster J Y, Deroisy R, Denis R et al 1989 One year controlled randomised trial of prevention of early menopausal bone loss by tiludronate. Lancet 2: 1469–1471

Reid R L 1991 Premenstrual syndrome. Current problems in Obstetrics and Gynaecology and Fertility 8: 1–57

Reid R L, Greenaway-Coate A, Hahn P M 1986 Oral glucose tolerance during the menstrual cycle in normal women and women with alleged premenstrual 'hypoglycaemic' attacks: effects of nazalone. Journal Clinical Endocrinology Metabolism 62: 1167

Reid R L, Yen S S C 1981 Premenstrual syndrome. Americal Journal of Obstetrics and Gynaecology 139: 85–104

Rich P 1996 Practical aromatherapy. Parragon, Bristol

Robinson G 1996 Cross-cultural perspectives in the menopause. Journal of Nervous and Mental Disease 184(8): 453–458

Robinson G E, Garfinkel P E 1990 Problems in the treatment of premenstrual syndrome. Canadian Journal of Psychiatry 35(3): 199–206

Rosano G M, Chierchia S L, Leonardo F, Beale C M, Collins P 1996 Cardiovascular effects of ovarian hormones. European Heart Journal 17(suppl D): 15–19

Rosenberg S, Kroll M, Pastijn A, Vandromme J 1995 Osteoporosis prevention and treatment with sex hormone replacement therapy. Clinical Rheumatology 14(suppl 3): 14–17

Royal College of Nursing 1994 Cervical screening guidelines for good practice. Issues in nursing and health, factsheet 28. RCN, London

Royal College of Nursing 1996 Female genital mutilation. The unspoken issue. RCN, London

Royal College of Physicians 1991 Report on preventive medicine. Royal College of Physicians, London

Sawada M, Okudaira Y, Matsui Y 1984 Immunosuppressive acidic protein in patients with gynecologic cancer. Cancer 54: 652–656

Seibel M M, Berger M J, Weinstein F G, Taymen M D 1982 The effectiveness of danazol on subsequent fertility in minimal endometriosis. Fertility and Sterility 38: 534–537

Sharlip I D 1994 Vasculogenic inpotence secondary to atherosclerosis/dysplasia. In: Bennett A H (ed) Impotence diagnosis and management of erectile dysfunction. WB Saunders, Philadelphia, pp 205–212

Shingleton H M, Orr J W (eds) 1987 Cancer of the cervix: diagnosis and treatment. Churchill Livingstone, Edinburgh

Sliutz G, Tempfer C, Hanzal E, Reinthaller A, Koelbl H, Zeillinger R, Kainz C 1997 Serum M3/M21 in cervical cancer patients. European Journal of Cancer 33(6): 973–975

Smithson A 1992 Girls will be women. Nursing Times 88(6): 46–48

Sondheimer S J, Freeman E, Rickels K 1988 Gynaecologic PMS program: hormonal influences on symptom manifestation. In: Gise L H, Kase N G, Berkowitz (eds) The premenstrual syndromes. Churchill Livingstone, New York, p 69

Spira A 1986 Epidemiology of human reproduction. Human Reproduction 1: 111–115

Stacey M 1988 The sociology of health and healing. Unwin Hyman, London

Stampfer M J, Colditz G A 1991 Oestrogen replacement therapy and coronary heart disease: a qualitative assessment of the epidemiological evidence. Preventive Medicine 20: 47–63

Stevenson J C 1996 Metabolic effects of the menopause and oestrogen replacement. Baillière's Clinical Obstetrics and Gynaecology 10(3): 449–467

Stevenson J C, Cust M P, Ganger K F, Hillard T C, Lees B, Whitehead M I et al 1990 Effects of transdermal versus oral hormone replacement therapy on bone density in spine and proximal femur in post menopausal women. The Lancet 336: 265–269

Sundblad C, Modigh K, Anderson B et al 1992 Clomipramine effectively reduces premenstrual irritability and dysphoria: a placebo controlled trial. Acta Psychiatrica Scandinavica 85(1): 39–47

Szarewski A, Jarvis M J, Sasiem P et al 1996 Effects of smoking cessation on cervical lesion size. Lancet 347(9006): 941–943

Talbot J McK, Lawrence M 1997 In-vitro fertilisation: indications, stimulation and clinical techniques. In: Kovacs G T (ed) The subfertility handbook. Cambridge University Press, Cambridge, pp 88–108

Taylor C, Faulk W P 1981 Prevention of recurrent abortion with leucocyte transfusions. Lancet ii: 68

Templeton A A 1992 The epidemiology of infertility. In: Templeton A A, Drife J O (eds) Infertility. Springer, London

Thomas S 1997 Embolisation of uterine fibroids. Nursing Standard 11(44): 27

Thonneau P, Marchard S, Talle A et al 1991 Incidences and main courses of infertility in a resident population (1 850 000) of three French regions (1988–1989). Human Reproduction 6: 811–816

Thurlow P 1992 Not in front of the students. Nursing Standard 6(48): 54

Tita P, Spina A, Briguglia G et al 1996 Clinical features and hormonal characteristics in a case of ovarian arrhenoblastoma. Journal of Endocrinological Investigations 19(7): 484–487

Toubin N 1994 Female circumcision as a public health issue. New England Journal of Medicine 331(11): 712

Trounce J 1994 Clinical pharmacology for nurses, 15th edn. Churchill Livingstone, Edinburgh

Trounson A O, Leeton J F, Wood E C, Webb J, Wood J 1981 Pregnancies in humans by fertilisation in vitro and embryo transfer in controlled ovulatory cycles. Science 212: 681–682

United Kingdom Central Council for Nursing Midwifery and Health Visiting 1992 Code of professional conduct. UKCC, London

United Kingdom Central Council for Nursing Midwifery and Health Visiting 1996 Guidelines for professional practice. UKCC, London

Vessey M P 1989 Epidemiological studies of the effects of diethylstilboestrol. IARC Publication No. 96. IARC, Lyon, pp 335–348

Webb C, Wilson-Barnett J 1983 Self concept, social support and hysterectomy. International Journal of Nursing Studies 20(2): 97–107

Whitehead M I, Fraser D, Schenkel L, Crook D, Stevenson J C 1990 Transdermal administration of oestrogen/progestogen hormone replacement therapy. Lancet 335: 310–312

Whitehead M I, Godfree V 1992 Replacement therapy – your questions answered. Churchill Livingstone, Edinburgh

Whitehead M I, Hillard T C, Cook D 1990 The role and use of progestogens. Obstetrics and Gynaecology 75: 598–676s

Williams C 1995 Healthy eating: clarifying the advice about fruit and vegetables. British Medical Journal 5992(310): 1453–1455

Wilson K J W, Waugh A (eds) 1996 Ross & Wilson anatomy and physiology in health and illness, 8th edn. Churchill Livingstone, Edinburgh

Winston R M C 1991 Resources for infertility treatment. Baillière's Clinical Obstetrics and Gynaecology 5(3): 551–573

Wood C 1997 The role of gamete intrafallopian transfer. In Kovacs G (ed) The subfertility handbook. Cambridge University Press, Cambridge, pp 109–123

Woodman C B J, Jordan J A, Mylotte M J, Gustafeson R, Wade-Evans T 1985 The management of cervical intra-epithelial neoplasia by coagulation electrodiathermy. British Journal of Obstetrics and Gynaecology 10: 362

World Health Organization 1996 Research on the menopause in the 1990s. Report of a scientific group. WHO, Geneva

World Health Organization 1997 Female sterilisation. WHO, Geneva

Xue P, Fa Y 1989 Microsurgical reversal of female sterilisation. Journal of Reproductive Medicine 34: 451–455

Yang C P et al 1992 Non-contraceptive hormone use and risk of breast cancer. Cancer Causes and Control 3: 475–479

PART 2
THE BREAST

INTRODUCTION

The breast is the human organ of lactation which develops in puberty to enable a mother to feed her offspring. In Western society the breasts are strongly associated with femininity and sexuality as well as with motherhood. The images of femininity and sexuality presented in advertising and other media use breasts, often large and perfectly formed, as symbols of sexual desirability promoting an idealised beauty which few women can attain. It is not surprising, therefore, that breast disease often has profound implications not only for a woman's physical health but also for her social and familial roles, body image and self-confidence. Women who suffer any alteration or disfigurement of the breast often experience anxiety, depression and loss of sexual satisfaction.

This chapter will begin by discussing the anatomy and physiology of the healthy breast before considering the benign disorders of the breast, mammary dysplasia, fibroadenomas, breast pain and breast infections. In addition, the rare condition of gynaecomastia will be described in view of its important psychological implications for the individual.

Breast cancer and a number of new treatments such as high-dose chemotherapy will then be considered. Related health care issues such as breast reconstruction, care of the fungating breast lesion and the management of lymphoedema will be given particular attention, as breast cancers are among the most common malignant conditions among women in the UK. Consideration will also be given to measures for the prevention or early detection of breast cancer.

Finally, the significance of diseases of the breast for a woman's psychological well-being will be discussed. Patient education will be considered in relation to promoting breast health and the early detection of disease. The importance of involving the patient and her family in making informed treatment choices and in carrying out subsequent self-care will also be considered.

ANATOMY AND PHYSIOLOGY OF THE BREAST

Structure of the breast

The breast is made up of glandular, fatty and fibrous tissue and is covered by skin. Men and women both have breast tissue, but in the male it remains rudimentary and does not develop in puberty.

The glandular tissue of each breast is divided into 12–20 lobes or segments (see Fig. 7.12). Each is made up of hundreds of lobules which are activated during pregnancy to produce milk. They are connected by terminal ducts which join to form lactiferous ducts before ending in around 10 openings in the nipple. Breast tissue is supported by Cooper's ligaments, which may contract when affected by tumour causing dimpling of the skin (peau d'orange). With increasing age and weight, these ligaments stretch, causing the breasts to droop, which is otherwise known as ptosis.

The nipple contains smooth muscle and becomes erect when stimulated, allowing a baby to suck more easily. It is surrounded by the areola, on the surface of which are Montgomery's tubercles. These lubricate the nipple during breast feeding.

Blood and lymph vessels

The breast is highly vascularised. It is supplied by thoracic branches of the axillary arteries laterally, and by branches of the internal mammary artery medially. Venous drainage follows arterial supply, and the lymphatic channels follow the main blood vessels outwards, branching out to the regional lymph nodes. Most lymph drainage of the breast is via the axillary lymph nodes, proceeding from there to the supraclavicular lymph nodes. Drainage from the medial part of the breast is via the internal mammary nodes which lie beneath the ribs and lateral to the sternum.

Nerve supply

Branches of the 4th, 5th and 6th thoracic nerves, containing sympathetic fibres, supply the breast. Many sensory nerve endings exist around the nipple, when touched, these cause reflex erection and, after childbirth, the release of milk.

Associated muscles (see Fig. 7.13)

Behind the breast and overlying the rib cage is the pectoralis major muscle. This large triangular muscle, which attaches to the clavicle, sternum and upper six costal cartilages and is used to adduct the arm. Behind the pectoralis major lies the pectoralis minor. This muscle attaches to the third, fourth and fifth ribs and the front of the scapula. Its function is to stabilise the shoulder girdle, serratus anterior and the latissimus dorsi muscle from the base and back of the axilla, respectively. These structures and their nerve supply are important considerations when axillary surgery is performed.

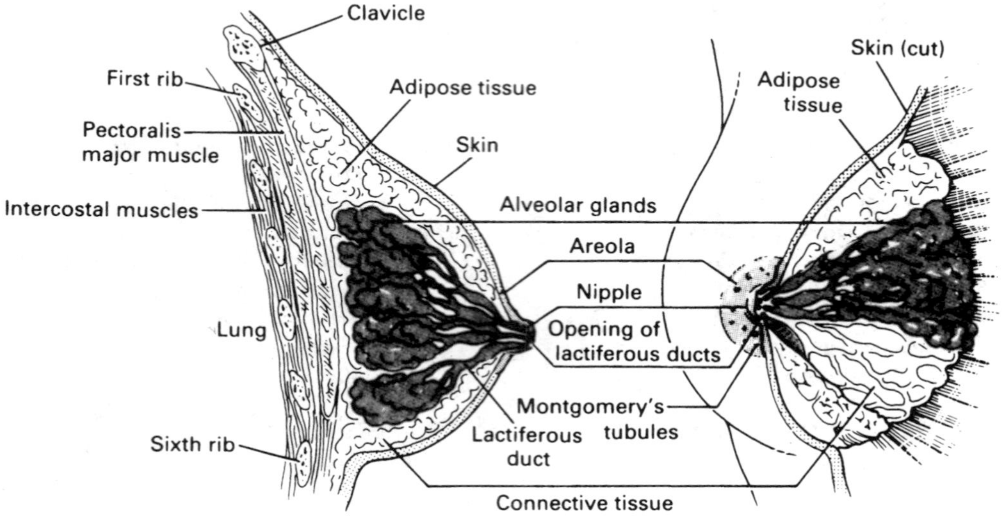

Fig. 7.12 Lateral cross-section of the breast.

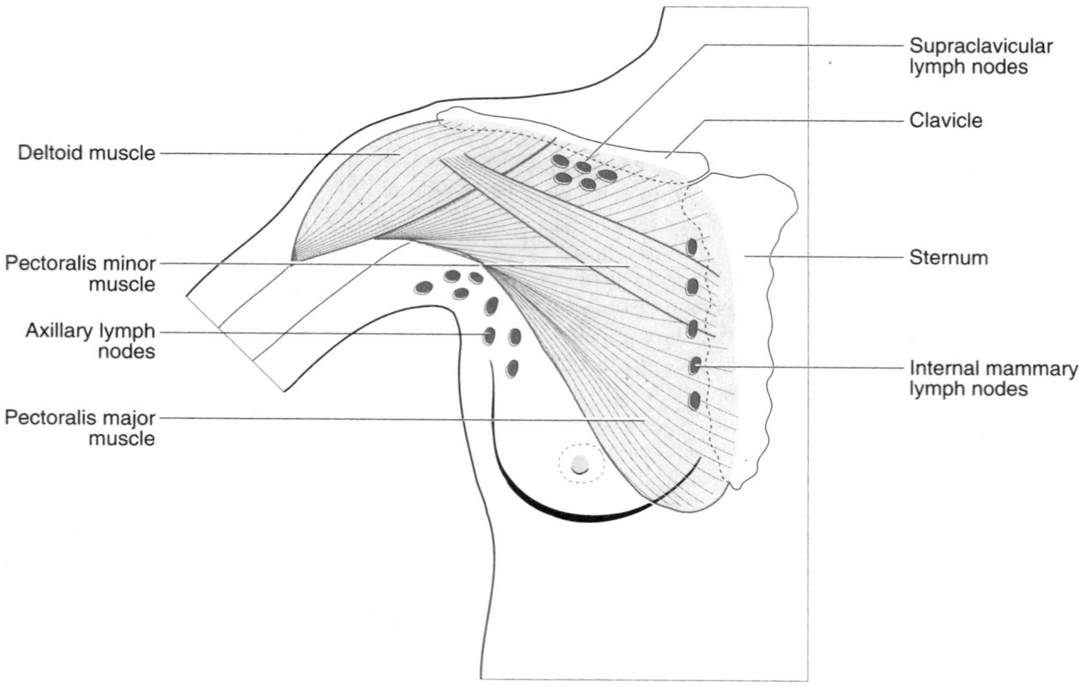

Fig. 7.13 The breast and associated structures.

Normal breast changes

The breasts constantly change as a normal consequence of ageing. Natural changes also occur with menstruation, pregnancy and lactation.

Puberty

A girl's breasts will begin to develop at puberty. The pituitary gland in the brain begins to produce the gonadotrophins, follicle-stimulating hormone (FSH) and luteinising hormone (LH). As the level of these hormones increases, egg follicles within the ovaries are stimulated to release oestrogens, which in turn stimulate an increase in the breast connective tissue, a lengthening of the ducts in the breast and the formation of the breast lobules.

Menstruation

At the start of each monthly cycle, blood oestrogen levels rise, causing the breast ducts and lobules to enlarge. After ovulation, the corpus luteum produces progesterone which causes further breast changes. At this time, tenderness and heaviness may be noticed. If pregnancy does not occur, the hormone levels fall, the ducts and lobules regress, and the breasts lose their tenderness and swollen feeling. This usually precedes the onset of menstruation.

Pregnancy

If pregnancy does occur, the levels of oestrogen and progesterone continue to rise, causing the ducts and lobules to increase in size and number in order to prepare for lactation. The enzymes necessary for milk production are stimulated by prolactin (produced by the anterior pituitary) and by placental lactogen, but milk production is suppressed during pregnancy by high progesterone levels.

Milk production

After birth, progesterone levels drop and milk synthesis can begin. As the baby sucks, prolactin is released (from the anterior pituitary), initiating milk synthesis, and oxytocin is released (from the posterior pituitary), causing milk to be emptied from the ducts. The more the baby sucks, the more milk is produced. Sucking also inhibits the release of FSH and luteinising hormone by the pituitary gland, so blocking ovulation. However, this effect is usually short-lived and cannot be relied upon for contraception. When breast feeding stops, the ducts and lobules start to regress, and milk production slows and then ceases.

Once the baby is born, the breasts produce colostrum for 2 or 3 days before the true breast milk production begins. Colostrum is a yellowish fluid with a lower lactose content than milk and contains very little fat, but more vitamin A, protein and minerals. Like milk, colostrum is rich in IgA antibodies which protect the baby's gastrointestinal tract against bacteria and viruses (Newman 1995). Breast milk contains all that is necessary for an infant in the first few months of its life. Cells of the breast lobules extract amino acids, fatty acids, glycerol and glucose from the blood and build them into proteins, fats and lactose. Milk also contains calcium, phosphorus, vitamins A, B, C and D, and small amounts of iron, but the exact composition depends on the mother's dietary intake.

Menopause

As a woman approaches the menopause, changes in ovarian function, and hence in hormone levels, cause glandular breast tissue to atrophy. This is replaced by fatty tissue so the breasts become softer and less lumpy; consequently, they are easier to examine and assess by mammography.

BENIGN BREAST DISORDERS

Benign breast disorders probably account for 90% of all breast problems. Among the most common, abnormal breast development, benign mammary dysplasia, breast pain, breast infection and structural disorders are considered here. Gynaecomastia is also mentioned because, although rare, it is the most common breast disorder in men.

ABNORMAL BREAST DEVELOPMENT

Aberrations of normal breast development can cause the absence or hypoplasia (underdevelopment) of one breast. This can occur in conjunction with a defect in the pectoral muscle and the upper limbs (Poland's syndrome). There is usually some difference in breast size for a woman, with the left breast being larger than the right, but the difference should not be extreme. If the problem is marked then surgical intervention involving augmentation of one breast and reduction of the other breast is offered by many plastic surgeons (Reshef et al 1996).

Juvenile or virginal hypertrophy

Prepubertal breast enlargement is quite common and only requires investigation if it is associated with other signs of premature sexual development. The overgrowth of breast tissue can occur in adolescent girls whose breasts develop during puberty but then continue to grow. Usually no hormone abnormality can be detected. The treatment of choice for these women is a reduction mammoplasty, i.e. surgical removal of breast tissue from each breast (Dixon & Mansel 1995).

BENIGN MAMMARY DYSPLASIA

PATHOPHYSIOLOGY

This is a common condition amongst women of all ages but particularly affects women between the ages of 30 and 55. It is often called fibrocystic disease, but this term is misleading in that it is really not a disease but a natural occurrence in women as they approach menopause. It is thought to be caused by the incomplete involution of breast tissue during each menstrual cycle, causing an increase in the number of cells lining the terminal duct lobular unit. This, in turn, leads to cystic changes, fibrosis and nodularity. Mammary dysplasia is usually a completely benign condition which does not predispose a woman to breast cancer. If biopsied, the cells show hyperplasia, but with no alteration in the cellular appearance. However, where atypical hyperplasia is present, the risk of breast cancer developing in the breast is raised, and regular screening may be advised.

Benign mammary dysplasia may present as areas of diffuse nodularity or thickening of the breast tissue which may contain single or multiple cysts. Commonly, it is bilateral, although it may occur in only one breast. Premenstrual tenderness is often experienced coinciding with an increase in nodularity. Cysts usually develop as a woman is nearing her menopause and they present as tender, fluctuant entities which, when examined under ultrasound, are shown to be fluid-filled. They may increase in size or stay the same and sometimes they disperse by themselves.

MEDICAL MANAGEMENT

Investigations. Assessment of a woman who complains of a lump or lumpiness within her breasts will involve clinical examination, mammography, ultrasound and sometimes fine-needle aspiration cytology. Cystic fluid is usually sent for examination if the fluid is bloodstained, as this may indicate cancer.

Whenever a cyst or area of nodularity is slightly suspicious in its presentation, excision biopsy will sometimes be recommended to exclude cancer (see p. 283). Follow-up examinations are not usually required unless histology reveals atypical hyperplasia in a younger woman or there is a family history of breast cancer.

Benign mammary dysplasia is sometimes aggravated by oral contraceptive pills. If this appears to be the case, a change of pill may be recommended.

Fibroadenomas

Fibroadenomas are considered as aberrations of normal breast growth and are composed of both fibrous and glandular breast tissue. Under the same hormonal influences as the rest of the breast, a fibroadenoma grows as a centrifugal small nodule that is usually well circumscribed and freely movable within the surrounding breast tissue. They are very common, accounting for 13% of all palpable breast lesions, and in woman aged 20 years or less, they account for 60% of breast masses. Most fibroadenomas occur in the upper outer quadrant of the breast and can vary in size up to 10 cm (Dixon & Mansel 1995).

NURSING PRIORITIES AND MANAGEMENT: BENIGN MAMMARY DYSPLASIA AND FIBROADENOMAS

Major considerations

Assessment

Nursing assessment should include the presenting symptoms of the problem and, in particular, the presence of any discomfort and any aggravating or alleviating factors. The nurse should determine the patient's knowledge about her condition, her fears and concerns, and the ways in which the condition is affecting her normal life.

Perioperative care

General pre- and postoperative nursing practices are discussed in Chapter 26. Surgery is usually minor, involving excision of a small area of nodularity or a cyst, but the presence of a lump may give rise to great anxiety. Reassurance that this is not cancer may be needed. However, the nurse should not give false reassurance where doubt exists as to the nature of the lump. As postoperative recovery is usually rapid, surgery is frequently performed on a day-case basis or may require a 1-night stay in hospital. Postoperatively, the priority of nursing will be wound management and pain control. Because the breast is very vascular, there may be large amounts of bruising and wound drainage even though the surgery is minor. A wound drain is sometimes needed, but is usually removed the following morning.

The breast is likely to be very sore for several days. Paracetamol is usually sufficient for pain relief, but if bruising and oedema are very extensive, stronger medication may be required. Wearing a supportive bra is usually advised for the first 2 weeks postoperatively to improve comfort and avoid strain being placed on the wound.

Patient education

The nurse can take the opportunity to promote breast health by discussing breast screening and breast awareness. It may be appropriate to discuss how breast comfort can be enhanced by a correctly fitting bra. Women who have premenstrual breast discomfort may find reducing salt or omitting caffeine from their diet helpful. Others find that a course of evening primrose oil brings relief.

BREAST PAIN

Breast pain (mastalgia) has been reported in over 50% of women who attend benign breast clinics (Mansel 1995). For most women, some breast discomfort is accepted as a part of the normal changes that their breasts go through each month. However, some women suffer more intense pain which affects their quality of life, usually from mid-cycle onwards, and is often relieved by menstruation. The pain can differ from cycle to cycle and can continue for many years. Evening primrose oil, the oral contraceptive pill, bromocriptine and danazol, have all been found to be of benefit for some patients. Such drug interventions should be medically supervised at a benign breast disease clinic where the clinicians are used to dealing with such problems.

Non-cyclical breast pain, usually experienced in women over 40, is the main type of mastalgia. Often localised within the breast, this type of pain can be helped by infiltrating the area with a local anaesthetic and steroid.

For both cyclical and non-cyclical mastalgia, wearing a firm and well-fitted bra can help (Mansel 1995).

BREAST INFECTIONS

PATHOPHYSIOLOGY

Breast infections, such as mastitis, are relatively common, causing swelling, tenderness and pain, which may be associated with a breast abscess or nipple discharge. Breast abscesses are most commonly seen during or following lactation. Infection may arise from a cracked nipple but often there is no apparent cause. Staphyloccocal organisms are the most common causes.

MEDICAL MANAGEMENT

Systemic broad-spectrum antibiotics are the usual treatment. However, a persistent abscess may require surgical drainage and excision of the surrounding capsule. A persistent nipple discharge may be treated by a microductectomy, which involves removing one of the major ducts behind the nipple, or a Hadfield's procedure, which involves removing the major duct system behind the nipple. Surgery is usually through a circumareolar incision, and an overnight stay in hospital is generally required.

Duct ectasia

Duct ectasia occurs during involution when the major subareolar ducts dilate and shorten. Normal breast secretions are retained behind these blocked ducts. Women with duct ectasia present with nipple discharge, nipple retraction, inflammation or a palpable mass. Surgery is indicated if the discharge is a problem (Curling & Tierney 1997).

NURSING MANAGEMENT AND PRIORITIES: BREAST INFECTIONS

Giving psychological support

Until the presence of infection has been established, fear of a more serious problem, particularly cancer, may remain. An explanation of the nature and possible cause of infection may be necessary to reassure the patient, particularly as recurrent infections are quite common and may cause frustration and distress.

Reducing discomfort

The discomfort and pain accompanying a breast infection are usually the most distressing features of the condition. A supportive bra, applications of heat or cold 'packs' and padding to protect a sore nipple may all reduce discomfort, but mild to moderate analgesic medication is usually necessary to achieve a satisfactory level of comfort.

Surgical management

Where surgical excision of the abscess is required, nursing management will be similar to that for a woman undergoing an excision biopsy (see p. 287). The nurse must be particularly vigilant in observing for signs of wound infection.

OTHER DISORDERS OF BREAST STRUCTURE

Duct papillomas

Duct papillomas are benign lesions which form in the lactiferous duct wall. Most of these occur beneath the areola. Papillomas present with pain or bloody discharge and are usually soft and difficult to locate. Surgical resection is usually the treatment of choice (Blackwell & Grotting 1996).

Lipomas

When examined these fatty lumps can be mistaken for cysts within the breast tissue. They do not cause major problems and diagnosis by ultrasound and cytology should be all the treatment that is needed.

Mondor's disease

Caused by a superficial thrombosis of a vein in the breast, this condition is usually very painful. Malignancy should always be excluded, but no other treatment should be necessary and the condition usually resolves in 6 months (Curling & Tierney 1997).

Galactocele

This is a cystic lesion which occurs in the breasts of pregnant or lactating women. Once diagnosed, treatment is by aspiration. This may have to be performed on several occasions to allow the walls of the cyst to adhere (Curling & Tierney 1997).

Fat necrosis

Presenting as a painful mass, fat necrosis can imitate breast cancer and should be diagnosed with care. About half of the cases of fat necrosis are caused by a blow to the breast, although the other cases have no history of trauma. The treatment is surgical excision to be absolutely sure that the area is not malignant (Blackwell & Grotting 1996).

GYNAECOMASTIA

This is a rare benign disorder which occurs in men and involves overdevelopment of male breast tissue as a result of oestrogen production either in puberty (30–60% of boys aged 10–16 years) or at a later age. This may be due to idiopathic excess oestrogen, e.g. in choriocarcinomatous teratoma or cirrhosis, decreased testosterone, e.g. in Klinefelter's syndrome (see Ch. 6), or drugs, e.g. amphetamines, antidepressants, certain antihypertensives, digoxin, spironolactone or oestrogen administration.

MEDICAL MANAGEMENT

Surgery is not usually recommended, as 80% of cases resolve within 2 years, unless the gynaecomastia is mistaken for a possible carcinoma; in such instances a biopsy may be advised. If the condition has arisen following the administration of a particular drug, modification of that medication can be considered. Hormone manipulation may be of benefit where gynaecomastia is due to the oversecretion of oestrogen (Dixon & Mansel 1995).

NURSING PRIORITIES AND MANAGEMENT: GYNAECOMASTIA

Giving psychological support

Breasts are considered to be a female characteristic, and for this reason the overdevelopment of breast tissue in a man may cause an altered body image and emotional distress. Some men with gynaecomastia believe they have lost their masculinity and experience anxiety and depression as a result. When gynaecomastia occurs in adolescence, such feelings may be particularly acute.

The nurse must be sensitive to such feelings and show an understanding of them. It may be difficult for a man to express these feelings to a female nurse, especially if she is relatively young, but he is more likely to do so within a professional relationship where trust exists. A clear explanation of why the breast tissue has developed and of any treatment that may be given is essential.

It is not appropriate within the context of this chapter to go into greater detail about benign breast conditions. For more information, see Dixon (1995).

MALIGNANT DISORDERS OF THE BREAST AND THEIR SEQUELAE

BREAST CANCER

Incidence and mortality

Breast cancer is the most common malignancy in women, accounting for 20% of female cancers (CRC 1996a). Approximately 1 in 12 women in the UK will develop breast cancer at some time in their lives. There are 25 000 new cases of breast cancer and 15 000 deaths due to breast cancer each year. Approximately 1% of all breast cancers occur in men. It is important for nurses to be aware of the special problems that men may experience when they are diagnosed with a disease that almost exclusively affects women.

Risk factors

The main risk factors associated with breast cancer are listed in Box 7.13. Of these, only increasing age is known to be of any substantial significance.

Increasing age. Breast cancer in women is very rare below the age of 35 years, but incidence rates increase steadily from then, reaching over 300 per 100 000 of the population by the time women are 85 years old. The greatest number of women are diagnosed between the ages of 45 and 75 years (see Fig. 7.14). Breast cancer in men is almost always seen beyond the age of 65 years (CRC 1996a).

Box 7.13 Factors increasing the risk of developing breast cancer

- Early menarche
- Increasing age
- Family history of breast cancer
- First child after age 30
- Geographical location (e.g. UK has higher mortality than Japan)
- Late menopause
- Nulliparity (no pregnancies)
- Social class (class I has highest risk)

Other possible factors under evaluation

- High alcohol intake
- High-fat diet
- Stress

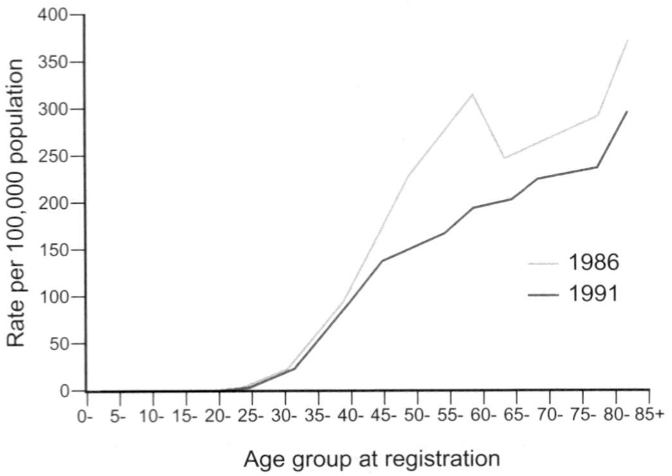

Fig. 7.14 Age-specific rates for 1991 compared with the pre-screening rates of 1986. The increase in incidence for the screened groups (50–64) is clearly shown. Breast cancer is the most common type of cancer in women. (Reproduced with kind permission from Cancer Research Campaign 1996.)

Geography. England and Wales have the highest standardised mortality figures per 100 000 for breast cancer in the world, followed by Scotland and Denmark, Northern Ireland and the Netherlands, Canada and the United States of America (McPherson et al 1995). Generally, incidence in western Europe, North America and Australia is about five times higher than in Asia and Africa. Japanese women have low rates of breast cancer, but incidence rates are seen to rise by the second generation among Japanese-Americans. This suggests that environmental and social risk factors may exist.

Diet. Populations with a high rate of breast cancer generally have a diet high in fat. Obesity has also been found to be associated with a slightly increased risk of breast cancer. However, a clear link between diet and the risk of breast cancer has not been established.

Social class. Breast cancer is slightly more common amongst women in social class 1, suggesting that breast cancer is a disease of affluent societies.

Hormone-related factors. Women who have their first child after the age of 35, those who experience early menarche, and those who have a late menopause are all found to have a slightly increased rate of breast cancer. This has led to the belief that the hormone oestrogen may be implicated in the development of breast cancer. In recent years, there has been much speculation as to the effects of the contraceptive pill and hormone replacement therapy on the incidence of breast cancer. Studies do not give a clear picture yet as oral contraceptive use was not common until the early 1970s and any effect is thought to be a long-term one. There is no increased risk for women in their early 20s who have used oral contraceptives to space their pregnancies. However, use of oral contraceptives for 4 years or more by younger women before their first pregnancy may increase the risk of pre-menopausal breast cancer. Much more research is needed, particularly as today's contraceptive pills contain lower levels of oestrogen or none at all (Hemminki 1996).

Family history. Up to 10% of breast cancers are due to genetic predisposition. The likelihood of a woman carrying a genetic abnormality is higher if:

- there are several cases of breast cancer in a single family
- the relatives in that family have an early onset of cancer
- there is the occurrence of a different epithelial cancer in one family, e.g. bilateral breast cancer, ovarian cancer, colon and prostate cancer. The combination of ovarian and breast cancer is particularly common in families who carry a particular cancer gene (Page et al 1995).

In families that are suspected to have a particular cancer gene, it is important to get a family history, or pedigree, going back several generations to assess who developed cancer and the type of cancer it was. This information is usually taken by a geneticist who is working in a specialised genetics clinic (see Ch. 6, p. 201). These details will usually allow the geneticist to confirm that a cancer gene is present and to estimate the likelihood that any member of the family has the gene. Family histories are often difficult to recall and sometimes it is necessary to extend and verify details of family histories by using public records of births, deaths and marriages, pathology reports and hospital records. Patterns in the family pedigree can then be recognised and the breast cancer predisposing genes BRCA1 or BRCA2 can be identified by genetic linkage analysis. This involves taking tissue or blood samples from affected family members and using specialised genetic techniques to search for the problematic gene.

Women who are at an increased risk of developing cancer because of a genetic predisposition will be offered genetic counselling and psychological support by the geneticist and specialist nurses who work in the clinic.

If the chance of the woman developing cancer is very high, this will be discussed with the woman and her future care will be considered. Interventions are very much under evaluation at the moment because this is a new area of cancer care. Instituting regular mammographic screening 5–10 years younger than the youngest relative already to have developed the disease is a current recommendation. Studies in the USA using the oestrogen-blocking agent tamoxifen for women at risk are ongoing, but the long-term results of these trials will not be available for several years (Powles et al 1998). Finally, some women will have the BRCA1 or BRCA2 gene confirmed by DNA analysis and may then be offered bilateral subcutaneous mastectomy as a preventive treatment, although this is clearly a serious undertaking (see p. 287). Research into this area of cancer care will continue far into the next millennium. The implications for breast care are potentially very exciting, as women who are likely to develop breast cancer could be identified and treated prophylactically (McPherson et al 1995, Page et al 1995).

Prevention in the present

Over the last 30 years, advances in treatments for breast cancer have failed to significantly reduce mortality from the disease. Research has been unable to identify clear causative factors that would enable the implementation of a primary prevention programme. However, we know that if women are diagnosed at an early stage in their disease, treatment is likely to be more effective (see Fig. 7.15). Therefore, taking measures to detect breast cancer earlier would appear to be the best way of reducing breast cancer mortality.

Breast self-examination

In recent years there has been much debate as to the value of monthly breast self-examination in the diagnosis of early breast cancer. Research has been unable to demonstrate that it alters survival from the disease. However, a woman who examines her breasts regularly is more likely to notice any changes. This encourages diagnosis when a cancer is small, so enabling a wider

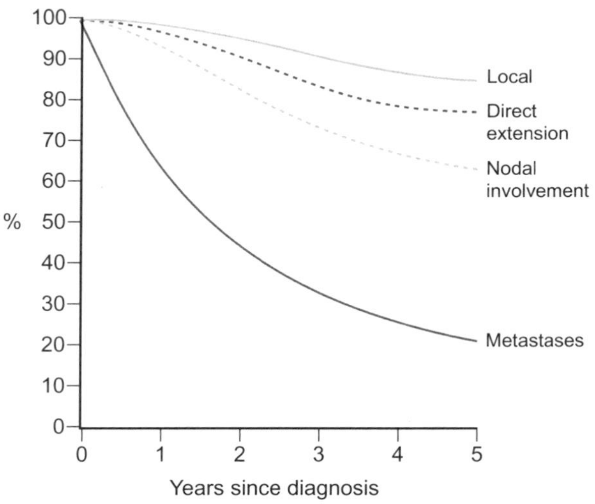

Fig. 7.15 The majority of women diagnosed in south-east England between 1986 and 1989 had early breast cancer: 43% were staged as 'local' and 12% as having 'direct extension'. For women with local disease, 5-year relative survival rates were in the region of 85%, compared with 78% for women in the 'direct extension' category. Only 10% of staged patients were in the metastatic group and their 5-year survival was 21%. (Reproduced with kind permission from the Cancer Research Campaign 1996).

choice of surgical treatment options to be offered. It also allows an individual to participate in her own health care.

A woman should examine her breasts once each month, just after menstruation (e.g. day 8 of her cycle). At this time, the breasts will be least lumpy and easiest to examine. If no longer menstruating, the woman should examine her breasts on the same day each month. Breasts are normally lumpy and so each woman will need to become used to how they feel and to identify her ribs, which are often mistaken for lumps.

To carry out self-examination the woman should sit in front of a mirror and lift her arms above her head, noticing the shape and size of her breasts and any changes from the previous month. She should examine her skin for dimpling and discoloration and the nipple for discharge, crusting and any new inversion.

Lying flat on a bed with one arm behind her head, she should then examine every area of her breast using the flat of her fingers of the opposite hand. Breast tissue is very extensive, running from the clavicle to the costal margin and the sternum to the axilla, and breast examination should cover all these areas systematically. Usually a hollow is noticed beneath each nipple. The upper outer quadrant of each breast will feel firmer as there is much breast tissue located there.

The axilla should be examined by bringing the arm back almost to the side and using the fingers of the opposite hand to feel deep into the armpit. If any lumps, thickening or other changes are noticed, the woman should contact her GP immediately for an examination and advice.

Leaflets are very useful in teaching breast self-examination, but are not as effective as demonstrative teaching. Leaflets and videos can be obtained from several sources (see 'Useful addresses', p. 311).

Breast cancer screening

In 1986, the Forrest report (DHSS 1986) recommended the introduction of a national breast screening programme. Screening units are now in operation around the country, inviting women between 50 and 64 years to attend for screening using mammography, i.e. X-ray examination of the breast.

The aim of breast cancer screening by means of mammography is to detect breast cancer at an earlier stage than is possible by clinical examination or breast self-examination, i.e. before a lump is palpable in the breast. In particular, it is hoped that more women will be detected with pre-invasive (in situ) cancer before the cancer cells have shown any evidence of spreading. A recent meta-analysis of the important research studies conducted on the efficacy of mammographic screening by age showed that mammographic screening significantly reduced breast cancer mortality in women aged 50–70 years (Kerlikowske et al 1995). However, a newly published research study by Sjönell & Ståhle (1999) questions the mammography and screening programme in Sweden and has stirred up some doubts about the breast screening programme in this country. There has been a lot of criticism of the research methodology used in this particular study and the arguments will go on until long-term follow-up of the effectiveness of the breast screening programme provides a definitive answer. There is much less evidence to support the screening of women aged 40–49 years, which is why, for now, the screening programme will only screen women over the age of 50 (Kerlikowske et al 1995).

With good technique and reading, mammography will pick up 85–90% of all breast cancers in the breasts examined. It is most effective in postmenopausal women in whom breast tissue has been largely replaced by fat. For young women, in whom breast tissue is more dense, and detection of abnormalities therefore more difficult, mammography is frequently used in conjunction with breast ultrasound.

The success of the national screening programme will depend on a high uptake of the service. The Tabar et al (1985) study in Sweden had an uptake rate of 70%; this will have to be matched in the UK if the hoped for 30% reduction in mortality is to be achieved. If fewer women participate in the programme, the cost per life saved increases and, although some women will clearly benefit, the cost-effectiveness of the programme will be called into question. Poor attendance at screening units may result from various factors, such as family practitioner committee registers not being up to date, fears of discomfort or radiation, or a lack of understanding of the value of mammography.

Procedures. Screening may take place in static or mobile units. The screening itself is by a mediolateral-view mammogram and, in many screening units, a cranial-caudal view is also taken. Mammograms are repeated every 3 years and, although the screening starts from 50 years, a woman may not be called until she is 53 years old. The woman is notified by letter of the mammogram result. If an abnormality is detected, the letter will ask her to attend for re-screening at an assessment centre (see Fig. 7.16). Here, a fresh two-view mammogram may show the detected lesion to be merely an overlapping of normal structures or a benign lesion requiring no intervention. In some instances, further assessment using ultrasound and a fine-needle aspiration cytology or a core biopsy of the suspicious area will be indicated.

Psychological considerations. Most women who present for breast screening are asymptomatic, apparently healthy people who, on the whole, come to be reassured that all is well. Inevitably, screening reminds the individual that breast cancer is a potential threat. It is therefore important that within the screening programme efforts are made to reduce anxiety where possible. It is particularly important that results are sent quickly. If the first

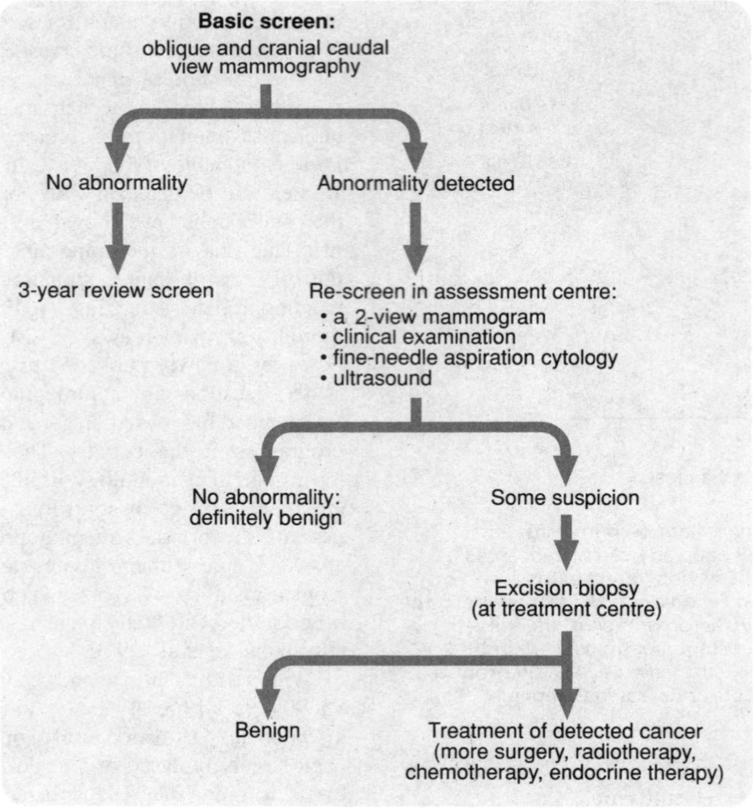

Fig. 7.16 Flow diagram of breast cancer screening procedure.

screening is a positive experience, the woman will be more likely to attend 3 years later and may urge her friends to do the same.

The nurse's role. The Forrest report (DHSS 1986) recommended that trained nurses should be available to support women who are undergoing screening. The report stressed the importance of having specialist nurses with an in-depth knowledge of breast disease and its treatment and with some training in counselling to give support to women recalled to assessment centres following the detection of an apparent abnormality.

However, all nurses have a role in health education and should take every appropriate opportunity to raise women's awareness of the availability and benefits of screening programmes. Community nurses, in particular, can encourage women to attend for screening and can answer queries or discuss worries about breast screening as part of their general health promotion on an individual basis or through group discussion, e.g. in well woman clinics.

PATHOPHYSIOLOGY

Common presenting symptoms (see Table 7.3). Discovery of a non-tender, hard, usually irregular lump or thickening in the breast is the most common presentation of breast cancer. Increasingly, it is also diagnosed after a mass or microcalcifications are seen on a mammogram during routine breast screening.

Pain is not usually a presenting feature, but sometimes a sharp, pricking pain is the first symptom experienced. A change in breast size or shape may be noticed. Signs of inflammation and tissue oedema may also be present, and superficial veins may dilate and become more visible if partially obstructed by a tumour. If the tumour is advanced at the time of presentation, it may be fixed to the muscles beneath the breast. There may also be large palpable axillary lymph nodes or ulceration of the tumour through the skin, causing an infected, weeping, malodorous wound. Oedema of the arm will result if the cancer in the axilla is blocking the drainage of blood and lymph from the arm.

Histology. Breast cancers may be classified according to the type of tissue from which they arise and their appearance under the microscope. The histological type of a cancer is often relevant to the choice of treatment.

Carcinomas arising from the epithelial cells of ducts are known as ductal carcinomas and account for a majority of all breast cancers (Sainsbury et al 1995). Medullary, colloidal and tubular carcinomas are all types of breast cancer arising from ductal tissue. They usually arise in one area of the breast, but they can be multifocal; they are rarely bilateral. Cancers arising from cells of the breast lobules are known as lobular carcinomas. These account for around 15% of breast cancers and are more commonly multifocal and bilateral than ductal carcinomas (Crowe & Lampejo 1996).

In Paget's disease of the nipple, malignant cells are found in the epidermis of the nipple and are usually associated with small multifocal areas of ductal cancer behind the nipple and deep in the breast. Other breast cancer types, such as squamous cell or inflammatory carcinomas, are less common. Sarcomas and lymphomas may also arise in the breast, as may (rarely) secondary cancer tumours.

Table 7.3 Signs and symptoms of breast cancer

Sign/symptom	*Comment*
Breast lump	Usually hard and irregular
Change in breast size or shape	
Impalpable mammographic abnormality	Mass/microcalcifications
Pain	Sometimes
Skin dimpling	Retraction of Cooper's ligaments
Peau d'orange	Thickening and oedema of skin
Nipple discharge	Usually bloodstained
Nipple retraction	Due to disease in main ducts
Nipple crusting	Usually Paget's disease of nipple
Dilatation of superficial veins	Result of partial obstruction of veins by tumour
Palpable axillary lymph nodes	Usually in advanced cancer
Ulceration of skin	Usually in advanced cancer

Breast cancers may also be classified as non-invasive (located only in the ducts or lobules, i.e. 'in situ') or invasive (having the ability to invade the basement membrane of the duct or lobule). This distinction has a bearing on prognosis and treatment. Ductal carcinoma in situ represents a very early stage of breast cancer which is often seen as microcalcifications on a mammogram. It cannot be predicted when, or if, a non-invasive breast cancer will become invasive.

Cellular differentiation, i.e. the degree to which cancer cells resemble their tissue of origin, is another important histological factor in determining prognosis. Cells are described as well, moderate or poorly differentiated, or grades I, II or III. Poorly differentiated cancers tend to be more aggressive, with the ability to metastasise at an earlier stage, and hence carry a poorer prognosis (see p. 296).

More detailed information on the histology of breast cancers in Dixon (1995).

MEDICAL MANAGEMENT

Investigations. Once a breast abnormality has been detected, further diagnostic investigation will be carried out following referral to a specialist. This may involve:

- clinical examination of the breast
- mammography (see p. 285)
- ultrasound to distinguish solid from cystic lesions
- fine-needle aspiration to drain cysts and to obtain samples for cytological study
- biopsy.

Fine-needle aspiration cytology of the breast. In this procedure, a syringe with a small-bore needle is inserted into the breast mass and suction is applied. The contents are withdrawn, placed on a slide and sent to the laboratory for cytological studies. Where a mass is found to be a cyst and a large amount of fluid is aspirated, it is usually discarded, unless it is found to be bloodstained, in which case a sample will be sent for examination. Cytological results will be graded C0–C5: C0 represents an insufficient specimen; C1 and C2, benign cells; C3 and C4, suspicious of carcinoma; and C5, carcinoma. Fine-needle aspiration cytology is a useful diagnostic tool but is not conclusive on its own. A benign result may simply indicate that the needle missed the target; where other signs are suspicious, a biopsy will still be recommended.

Biopsy. On the basis of the investigations listed above, a decision is made as to whether a biopsy should be performed to confirm diagnosis. Biopsy may be of the following types:

- A core or Trucut biopsy — removal of a core of tissue using a special large-bore needle. This is often undertaken in the outpatient department using a local anaesthetic.
- Excision biopsy — excision of the lump in its entirety, usually with general anaesthesia, requiring a 1- or 2-day hospital stay.
- Localisation biopsy — where a mammographic abnormality has been detected but there is no associated palpable mass, a wire may be inserted into the abnormal area under X-ray or ultrasound control. This tissue, once removed from the body, will be X-rayed to ensure that the surgeon has removed the area of abnormality.

Treatment. The choice of treatment in breast cancer will depend on several factors, including:

- the size, position and type of tumour (see Box 7.14)
- the spread of the disease
- the woman's general health
- the woman's priorities and wishes.

Surgical intervention. Surgery is still considered to be the most effective treatment for early breast cancer. Formerly, radical mastectomy was the treatment of choice, but for many women, less extensive surgery followed by radiotherapy can be just as successful (Veronesi et al 1981, Fisher et al 1989, Veronesi et al 1995).

Surgical procedures that may be used are as follows:

- *Lumpectomy.* Removal of the breast lump with very little surrounding tissue. May be equivalent to an excision biopsy.
- *Wide local excision.* Removal of the abnormal areas together with a 1–2 cm margin of apparently normal tissue to reduce the possibility of incompletely excising the cancer. When the pathologist indicates that excision may be incomplete, re-excision is usually recommended. The amount of tissue removed in this operation can be considerable.
- *Partial or segmental mastectomy or quadrantectomy.* Removal of a portion of the breast. Invariably the breast is left smaller and its contour is changed.
- *Radical or Halsted's mastectomy.* This is rarely used today and involves the removal of the pectoralis major and minor muscles,

Box 7.14 Staging of breast cancer tumours

Stage I	Tumour ≤ 2 cm, not fixed, no axillary node involvement
Stage II	Tumour ≤ 5 cm, with/without axillary node involvement
Stage IIIa	Tumour >5 cm or fixed axillary node involvement
Stage IIIb	Any tumour with supraclavicular node involvement, fixation to the chest wall, inflammation, ulceration
Stage IV	Any size tumour and presence of distant metastatic disease

as well as the breast tissue and overlying skin, the nipple and the axillary lymph nodes. A long, oblique scar remains. The axillary skin fold is usually removed and the chest wall can sometimes appear concave with the ribs prominent.

- *Modified radical or Patey mastectomy*. Removal of all the breast tissue, overlying skin and the nipple. The pectoralis major and minor remain, covering the ribs, and the axillary skin fold remains intact. The scar is oblique but less extensive than with a radical mastectomy.
- *Simple mastectomy*. Removal of the breast tissue and overlying skin and nipple; all muscles are left intact and the scar is horizontal.
- *Axillary dissection*. Usually performed with any of the above operations to determine whether the cancer has spread to the lymph glands. The presence of cancer cells in these glands indicates that micrometastatic spread is likely and hence adjuvant drug therapy is indicated. Where possible, axillary dissection, removing some or all of the lymph glands, will be undertaken through the same incision as that made for the breast surgery.

Primary or neoadjuvant chemotherapy. If a woman presents with a large breast cancer, one treatment option will be a mastectomy. However, many breast units across the country are now offering primary chemotherapy, sometimes called neoadjuvant chemotherapy, to shrink the tumour. This treatment can provide a further option for women who cannot tolerate the thought of a mastectomy or whose health precludes an operation (Mansi et al 1989, Richards & Smith 1995). In rare circumstances, often for the elderly patient, hormone therapy is used to achieve the same result. Any micrometastases that may have spread from the original tumour in the breast are systemically treated by the chemotherapy.

Throughout the treatment, which can be up to six courses of chemotherapy, the tumour will be assessed by clinical measurement, or radiologically by ultrasound and mammogram. When the maximum response to the drug has been achieved, surgery is considered. It may be that the tumour has shrunk down sufficiently to allow a quadrantectomy, but if this is not the case a mastectomy should still be the surgery of choice. Sometimes, at the end of the chemotherapy, the tumour is no longer detectable radiologically, but limited surgery in the previous location of the tumour is recommended as small lesions are not always seen radiologically. Radiotherapy is then given to the breast or the chest wall to complete the local treatment.

Radiotherapy. This form of treatment is usually advised following a wide local excision or partial mastectomy to reduce the risk of cancer recurrence in the remaining tissue and to protect the woman from the disease recurring systemically. Recently published research from Denmark and Canada has shown that women with high-risk breast cancer survived significantly longer if they were treated with both chemotherapy and radiotherapy, so there is good evidence to support the use of radiotherapy as a local treatment (Overgaard et al 1997). If the axillary lymph nodes are not all removed and are found to contain cancer, they are also commonly irradiated. The supraclavicular region may also be irradiated. Radiotherapy is not always considered necessary following a mastectomy.

A total of 40–60 Gy of external radiotherapy is usually given to the breast over a period of 3–6 weeks, three to five times a week. The radiotherapy is given at different angles to protect the delicate lung tissue and the heart from receiving high doses of radiation. The immediate common side-effects are erythema and soreness of the treated area, and a general tiredness towards the end of the treatment period. Psychologically it can be quite hard for the woman to attend an oncology/radiotherapy department several times a week, as this is a continual reminder of why she is undergoing treatment. Tiredness seems to be the most reported symptom of women who are undergoing breast radiotherapy (Graydon 1994).

Alternatively, radiotherapy may be administered wholly or partly by iridium wire implants. The patient may be nursed in an isolated room for around 5 days until the required dose of radiotherapy is given. The radioactive wires are then removed. The main advantage of this method is its ability to deliver high doses of radiotherapy to the area from which the tumour was removed. Radiotherapy is discussed in more detail in Chapter 31.

Adjuvant chemotherapy. Over half of the women who present with an invasive breast cancer will already have micrometastatic spread, so adjuvant systemic medical therapy should be given with the aim of destroying the cancer cells that have escaped from the original tumour (Powles & Smith 1991). When breast cancer is present in the axillary lymph nodes, the chance of a woman developing distant metastases is high. Systemic drug therapies circulating to all areas of the body have been shown to reduce the chance of metastases developing or to increase the length of time before metastases become apparent.

Premenopausal women who have positive axillary lymph nodes are likely to benefit from cytotoxic chemotherapy. A commonly used regimen is CMF (cyclophosphamide, methotrexate, 5-fluorouracil). Six courses of this chemotherapy are given over a period of 6 months, usually requiring the woman to attend the outpatient department twice a month.

Administration is by slow i.v. injection, but cyclophosphamide may be given as tablets for 14 days. Other regimens using an anthracycline drug, such as epirubicin, Adriamycin or mitozantrone, are being compared with the CMF regimen to assess whether or not adding an anthracycline confers any survival advantage to the women who receive the treatment (Buzzoni et al 1991, Bonadonna et al 1995, EBCTCG 1998b). A close study is being made of the side-effects and toxicities of such treatments. More detailed information on chemotherapy and its management is given in Chapter 31. The common side-effects of chemotherapy for breast cancer are listed in Table 7.4.

Table 7.4 Common side-effects of chemotherapy regimens used in the treatment of breast cancer

Side-effect	*Comment*
Lethargy	All drugs to some degree, but especially Adriamycin, VAC (vincristine, Adriamycin, cyclophosphamide)
Anorexia/altered taste	Usually only temporary with most regimens
Nausea and vomiting	More common with Adriamycin
Mouth ulceration	Particularly methotrexate
Diarrhoea	Rarely, but more commonly with 5-fluorouracil
Bone marrow depression	Greater where Adriamycin used
Alopecia	CMF: some (Adriamycin: complete, but scalp cooling may reduce this)
Red urine	Adriamycin
Green urine	Mitozantrone
Reactivation of radiotherapy sites	Adriamycin
Nail pigmentation	Adriamycin and 5FU

Premenopausal women whose axillary lymph glands are free of cancer have traditionally not received adjuvant drug therapy. However, some doctors are now advising adjuvant chemotherapy or endocrine therapy, as recent studies have indicated that these might have a preventive effect in some women (EBCTCG 1998b).

High-dose chemotherapy. In some solid tumours there is a direct correlation between the dose of chemotherapy and the response of the tumour. Giving higher doses of chemotherapy means greater tumour cell kill, but it will also mean more side-effects and toxicities, the most serious of which is bone marrow suppression.

For women who have a large number of axillary nodes positive to breast cancer and in whom the breast cancer is very likely to return, clinicians have started to use this high-dose approach to treating such cancer. In the UK, this method of giving chemotherapy is very new and is only offered as part of a randomised trial in a few of the breast units.

The woman's haematopoietic stem cells are mobilised from the bone marrow by small doses of chemotherapy and they enter the peripheral bloodstream. These cells are removed by a cell separator and then processed and frozen for storage. The woman is then given very high-dose chemotherapy and, when her blood counts are at their lowest, the stem cells are reinfused to replenish the haematopoietic cells. This process of giving chemotherapy is very intensive and the woman is often cared for on a haematological ward for medical support. This treatment has many side-effects, caused by a profoundly low white cell count, but it is over relatively quickly and provides another treatment choice for some women with a poor prognosis (Ayash et al 1994). Further research will be necessary to demonstrate if this treatment provides a real survival advantage to such women.

Endocrine therapies. Many breast cancers are thought to be stimulated by female sex hormones, particularly oestrogen. Endocrine therapies act by interfering with the synthesis of oestrogen or preventing it from exerting an effect on cells.

The drug tamoxifen, which competes with oestrogen receptors in the cytoplasm of the cell and so blocks oestrogen from stimulating breast cancer cell growth, has been found to be effective in many women with breast cancer. Tamoxifen is generally more effective in women who are postmenopausal and who have high levels of oestrogen receptors. When the woman's tumour is biopsied or removed, it is stained immunocytochemically for oestrogen receptors. A percentage value is given for the number of receptors that stain positive, e.g. 75%, and this indicates whether the tumour is particularly sensitive to oestrogen. Because of its low toxicity, tamoxifen is given to most postmenopausal women as an adjuvant therapy, regardless of cancer involvement in the lymph nodes.

A new aromatase inhibitor called Arimidex is being given to women as part of a trial in combination with tamoxifen or on its own. As a selective inhibitor of the aromatase enzymes involved in the synthesis of oestrogen, Arimidex prevents the body forming oestrogen and thus reduces the levels of circulating oestrogen (Harvey 1998).

For women who are still menstruating and who are taking tamoxifen, luteinising hormone releasing hormone (LHRH) analogues such as Zoladex are often suggested as an additional hormone therapy. The monthly subcutaneous injections stop the ovaries producing oestrogen, but once the injections are stopped, the effect is reversed. In the younger woman, this may be a more acceptable way of stopping the ovaries producing oestrogen, especially if the woman wants to have a family after her treatment for the breast cancer has finished.

Q **7.7** When is a woman likely to be advised that a mastectomy would be the best treatment for her?

NURSING PRIORITIES AND MANAGEMENT: BREAST CANCER

The pretreatment phase

The period prior to admission to hospital is usually characterised by anxiety and uncertainty. Diagnosis often cannot be confirmed before biopsy and so the patient's hope that everything will be all right will be mixed with fears of cancer and its treatment. Nursing intervention at this time will focus on assessing the patient's situation, helping her to cope with anxiety, providing education and psychological support and assisting her in making informed choices with regard to treatment options.

Assessment

There may be limited time available for assessment at this stage, but where possible the nurse should try to identify the following:

- The woman's reaction, and that of her family, to the diagnosis or potential diagnosis of breast cancer.
- The major fears and concerns of the woman and her family.
- The woman's feelings about body image changes that may result from any proposed surgery.
- The woman's knowledge of breast cancer and cancer generally; how much information she has been given by medical staff; how much she has understood; and how much she wants to know.
- Whether the woman has any previous experience of another member of her family having breast cancer or any other kind of cancer.
- The kind and degree of support available to the woman through family and friends. Northouse et al (1995) found that patients and their partners who reported high levels of social support also reported fewer adjustment difficulties after surgery. Husbands consistently reported that they received less support than their wives from friends, nurses and doctors.
- Concurrent stressors, e.g. recent bereavements, divorce, financial difficulties.
- Previous anxiety/depression. Morris et al (1977) found that women who had experienced previous anxiety/depression were more likely to re-experience it following diagnosis and treatment.

The treatment phase

Assessment

On the patient's admission to hospital, the nurse should undertake a more comprehensive assessment, including medical history, family history and a full physical and psychological assessment. In particular, the factors relevant in the pretreatment phase should be reassessed to determine if the woman's needs and concerns have changed. Particular note should be made of preoperative shoulder function if axillary surgery is to be performed.

Preoperative preparation

The reader is referred to Chapter 26 for a detailed discussion of clinical considerations in preoperative care.

Giving psychological support

The nurse should give each patient the opportunity to discuss her fears but must respect her wishes if she prefers not to disclose her feelings. Where possible, a quiet, private room should be set aside for patients to spend some time in solitude or to talk privately with a nurse, doctor or family member.

Relaxation tapes or gentle massage, particularly of the neck, shoulders, back or face, can be comforting at a time when the patient may feel isolated and insecure. A relaxed but professional atmosphere on the ward will also help, as will allowing women to remain in their day clothes, open visiting and permitting them to go out for meals or a walk.

Patient education

The nurse must ensure that the woman knows what operation she is to undergo and that she has been given as much information about this as she wishes. Where deficits exist, the nurse should try to provide information or refer the woman back to the medical staff or a breast care nurse for further discussion.

The preoperative routine should be explained, including the approximate time of surgery and the timing and type of premedication to be administered.

The patient should be told that she will have drainage tubes in situ on return from theatre (usually one to the breast wound and one to the axilla to prevent the collection of blood and serous fluid beneath the suture line). She should know that she can pick the drains up and walk around with them and that it is difficult to dislodge the tubing as it is sutured in place. Usually, a light dressing is used to cover the breast scar, although surgeons may have their own dressing preferences. It is worth telling the woman what sort of dressing to expect as she may think that the breast wound will be exposed on her return from theatre, which might be distressing.

Anyone undergoing axillary dissection should be warned that she will experience discomfort on moving her arm for a few weeks postoperatively. The nurse should stress the importance of postoperative exercises and, where possible, should refer the patient to a physiotherapist who can assess shoulder function preoperatively and teach exercises that can be used following surgery. Written information about the arm exercises should be provided so that the woman can continue with them after she has been discharged home.

The possibility of a saline or blood i.v. infusion should also be explained so that the patient does not become alarmed at finding one in place.

Patients often find it helpful to be told of the expected appearance of the surgical scar. Wound size and position, and the type of suturing to be used can be mentioned. Drawings and photographs may be helpful aids. It is important to warn the patient that, because the breast is so vascular, bruising and swelling are expected postoperatively. She should be reminded of this when she first looks at the scar.

Postoperative care

The nursing care of patients following surgical intervention is discussed in detail in Chapter 26. The following discussion will focus on considerations that are particularly relevant to breast surgery. The reader is also referred to Nursing Care Plan 7.2.

Wound management (see also Ch. 23). The size and position of the wound will depend on the operation performed. Generally, a low-suction drain is placed beneath the breast wound and another to the axillary region to reduce the likelihood of haematoma or seroma. Initially, the drains and the wound dressing should be observed frequently for signs of excessive blood loss. Undue blood loss should be reported to medical staff immediately.

The wound drains will remain in situ for 2–5 days until the wound drainage is minimal. The nurse should ensure that the drains are patent and that suction is maintained and should record drainage volume. Removal of the drains can be painful; this should be explained to the patient and removal should be preceded by oral analgesics.

Some breast units are allowing women to go home with the axillary drain still in situ. The woman and a member of her family are given instructions on management of the wound drain and are also given written information on wound care. Close contact is usually maintained with the hospital and patients are asked to notify the hospital should the drain become loose or blocked or cause pain. Once the fluid drained has reduced to an acceptable level (usually less than 50 mL/day) the woman returns to the ward to have the drain removed, or the district nurse, if able and trained, removes it at home. Early discharge with the axillary drain still in situ is a new area of research. The work that has been done shows that, with good back-up support, it is safe and does not cause any greater psychological distress for patients (Bundred et al 1998).

The wound should also be observed for signs of infection, i.e. redness, swelling, pain and discharge. Temperature and pulse should be monitored 4- to 6-hourly and a raised temperature brought to the attention of the medical staff.

Wound dressings should be changed only if they are being saturated by wound exudate. Unnecessary dressing changes reduce the rate of wound healing and increase the risk of infection. Frequently a transparent wound dressing covered with gauze (which allows for ready observation of signs of infection) may be left in situ until the sutures are removed from the wound after 10–14 days.

The nurse must also consider other factors, such as nutritional intake, medication, stress and concurrent illness (e.g. diabetes), which affect the rate of wound healing and resistance to infection (see Ch. 23).

Alleviating discomfort. Pain from the wound will always be experienced to some degree, but pain on shoulder movement is often more of a problem. Pain is sometimes more intense a day or so after the operation when the initial numbness has faded. Every patient should be encouraged to take analgesics regularly for the first 48 h, but many women find that the wound is less painful than they had expected and require oral analgesics infrequently beyond this period. It should be stressed, in any event, that it is preferable to have analgesics and continue arm exercises than to avoid the exercises and take no analgesics.

The experience of pain is influenced by many factors, such as anxiety and emotional distress (see Ch. 19). These must be considered by the nurse in her efforts to promote the patient's comfort after surgery. Massage, by reducing muscle tension, may help to reduce pain; at the same time, the use of touch may promote a feeling of self-acceptance within a woman who feels vulnerable after losing her breast.

Women who have had a mastectomy may experience phantom breast and nipple sensations at some point following surgery. This may be very distressing and requires the nurse to reassure her that it will not continue for long.

Promotion of shoulder movement. Women who have undergone surgery involving dissection of the axillary lymph nodes are at risk of developing problems with shoulder movement. This risk is greater if radiotherapy to the axilla is given postoperatively (Lichter 1998). Postoperative exercises will help to ensure that a full range of shoulder movement is attained within 4 weeks following surgery.

Ideally, exercises should be taught by a physiotherapist. The nurse must know what they involve, however, so that she can encourage the patient to practise them. Written information is very

Nursing Care Plan 7.2 Care for a woman who has undergone a mastectomy

Nursing considerations	*Action*	*Rationale*	*Expected outcome*
1. Potential problem of wound complications (infection, haematoma, seroma) and delayed wound healing January 10	❐ Check drains half-hourly for blood loss. Change drainage bottle daily and record volume of drainage. Check wound for swelling	Haemorrhage may occur, compromising patient's health, and may necessitate return to theatre	Prevention of infection where possible and early detection of problems and promotion of wound healing
	❐ Observe wound for signs of infection (erythema, oedema, heat, pain, discharge)	Infection may delay wound healing and compromise general health. Medical treatment may be needed to control infection	There will be no signs of infection or bleeding
	❐ 4-hourly temperature and pulse	Increased temperature and pulse may indicate infection	
	❐ Aseptic dressing change only when absolutely necessary	Wound will heal more quickly if undisturbed, providing drainage is not excessive and there is no infection	
	❐ Assess nutritional intake and encourage balanced diet with plenty of vitamin C and protein	Vitamin C and protein are particularly important in wound healing	Patient will eat a balanced diet while in hospital
	❐ Assess amount of sleep and rest patient has had postoperatively. Where inadequate, consider anxiety reduction, pain control, night sedation to promote rest	Adequate sleep and rest are important in promoting wound healing	She will have at least 6 h sleep each night and report feeling stronger each day

Evaluation

January 11
Returned from theatre 12.30 h. All vital signs stable, now checked 4-hourly. Wound drainage 40 mL in last 4 h. Wound covered by Tegaderm dressing.

January 12
Slight pyrexia of 37.4°C, but no other sign of infection. Wound discharge was 100 mL in 24 h (axilla 60 mL; breast, 40 mL). Not sleeping well at night but managed to sleep a little today and does not wish for night sedation to be given.

January 13
Apyrexial and wound drainage reduced to 40 mL in 24 h. Slept better last night.

January 14
Both wound drains removed today and wound dressing replaced. Wound is moist close to axilla and has oozed a little serous fluid but temperature remains normal.

January 15
Wound still a little moist close to axilla. Going home today so discussed signs of infection and advised visit to GP if they occur. Also advised that a seroma could form in axilla and to contact ward if this happens and arrange for an aspiration. Patient stated that she was worried about anything happening to her wound, particularly that it would open up, but said she was reassured following our discussion.

DISCHARGED

Nursing considerations	*Action*	*Rationale*	*Expected outcome*
2. Anxiety/distress due to altered body image as a result of mastectomy and diagnosis of cancer (Salter 1988) January 12	❐ Give patient time and opportunity to express and explore feelings concerning cancer diagnosis and breast loss	Expression of feelings may help patient to clarify how she feels and relieve anxiety	Some anxiety will be alleviated
	❐ Encourage patient to discuss feelings with partner where appropriate	Partner may then be more easily able to understand and support and give reassurance that she is still attractive	Patient will have more acceptance of changed body image
	❐ Give information about scarring, e.g. bruising, sutures, position (photos shown pre-op may help)	May help to have realistic expectations of wound and know that bruising etc. will fade	

(cont'd)

Nursing Care Plan 7.2 *(cont'd)*

Nursing considerations	***Action***	***Rationale***	***Expected outcome***
	❒ Offer to remain with patient when she first looks at wound, assess reaction and give support in discussing feelings afterwards	Moral support may help patient to sum up courage to look at the wound	Patient will be able to look at scar before discharge
	❒ Fit temporary prosthesis after removal of the drains and show how to use. Show silicone prosthesis if desired and make fitting appointment	A prosthesis may increase a woman's confidence to face the outside world and regain a healthy body image	Patient will be able to fit temporary prosthesis into bra before discharge
	❒ Discuss possibility of breast reconstruction if not previously mentioned	Breast reconstruction is known to be helpful for some women in coping with breast loss. Woman herself is best one to judge value for her	Patient will understand types of reconstruction possible
	❒ Refer to specialist nurse if one exists	Specialist nurses have been shown to aid rehabilitation and may lower anxiety and depression postoperatively	
	❒ Offer written information on breast cancer, prostheses, clothing, etc.	Practical help may increase a woman's confidence to take up her usual social activities and feel she is still the same as ever	
	❒ Ask if she would like voluntary visitor to be put in touch and arrange if desired	Some women find others who have had similar operations a great help and encouragement	

Evaluation

January

Stated that she is very frightened that cancer may recur in the future. Her friend died 2 years ago from breast cancer metastases and this fills her with fear.

Temporary prosthesis fitted today and appointment made for 6 weeks after the wound drains removed. Mrs X also looked at her scar for the first time. She found it was better than she imagined. She has asked that the nurse stay with her tomorrow whilst she shows her husband before she goes home.

Mrs X showed her husband the scar today. He also told her it was much better than he had imagined and that having her was much more important than her having two breasts. Breast reconstruction was mentioned again but Mrs X is sure she will not want this. To be followed up by clinical nurse specialist who saw her again today and gave her a booklet from Breast Cancer Care.

Nursing considerations	***Action***	***Rationale***	***Expected outcome***
3. Difficulty moving arm due to discomfort following axillary dissection	❒ Refer to physiotherapist ❒ Analgesics before physiotherapy ❒ Encourage to practise arm exercises four times a day	Shoulder exercises are known to decrease the problems of reduced shoulder functioning that can result after an axillary dissection	To achieve and maintain full shoulder movement in 4 weeks and prevent 'frozen shoulder'
January 11	❒ Give written information sheets to reinforce what exercises to do and when	Written information will reinforce that given verbally and serve as a reminder after discharge home from hospital	Will be able to demonstrate physiotherapy exercises and perform four times each day
4. Pain January 10	❒ Regular analgesics initially postop. Assess effectiveness. Particularly important prior to physiotherapy	Regular analgesics more likely to be effective than PRN medication	Patient will report that pain is under control
	❒ Use pillow to support arm on affected side postop	Pillow provides a soft, comfortable support and encourages drainage of fluid back from arm	
	❒ Consider relaxation techniques and massage to relieve tension	Tension is known to increase experience of pain	

Nursing Care Plan 7.2 ***(cont'd)***

Evaluation

January 14
Seen by physiotherapist and commenced exercises. Patient says that she is able to move arm quite freely without much discomfort.

January 15
Has been practising arm exercises but a little more uncomfortable today and requested paracetamol prior to exercises this afternoon. She said this helped.

January 10
I.V. analgesic had been given in recovery but Mrs X has declined any further analgesics since returning to the ward.

January 11
Particularly uncomfortable when moving her arm. Had declined analgesics this morning but was persuaded that regular paracetamol for 2 or 3 days will not harm her and will help her move her arm, which is important.

January 14
Much more comfortable today and has again refused analgesics.

January 15
Requested analgesics prior to exercises today as arm feeling stiff and sore.

Nursing considerations	***Action***	***Rationale***	***Expected outcome***
5. Potential problem of lymphoedema of the arm, postoperatively or at some time in the future January 11	❒ Explain what lymphoedema is, how it is caused and when it may occur ❒ Explain signs of lymphoedema and encourage to report to doctor as soon as it occurs ❒ Discuss hand and arm care:	Information will help the patient to understand the pathological basis of lymphoedema and encourage early detection of lymphoedema should it occur	Risk of lymphoedema occurring will be reduced The patient will understand what lymphoedema is, and what to do if it occurs She will be able to recount how to look after her hand and arm
	• Avoid lifting heavy objects with affected arm • Avoid injections, blood tests, blood pressure recordings in affected arm • Use gardening gloves when gardening, kitchen gloves with abrasive cleaners, thimbles when sewing • Clean any cut on hand or arm very thoroughly and apply antiseptic. If any signs of infection appear see GP for antibiotics • Use depilatory creams to remove hair under arm, rather than a razor • Elevate arm whenever possible, particularly initially after surgery • Use a gentle moisturising cream on arm to prevent cracking if skin is dry	Following removal of lymph nodes by surgery and radiotherapy, there is an increased risk of infection in the arm. These precautions reduce the risk of infection, and also the risk of infection precipitating lymphoedema	
	❒ Encourage arm and shoulder exercises	Exercise is thought to reduce the possibility of lymphoedema occurring	

Evaluation

January 14
Long discussion in preparation for discharge. Her friend had lymphoedema so she is very concerned this shouldn't happen to her. Very keen to have advice on hand and arm care and has been given a leaflet about this. Stressed that she can contact clinical nurse specialist at any time if she is concerned that her arm is swollen.

helpful to remind the patient of what exercises should be performed and how often. Generally, gentle exercises are begun on the second or third postoperative day and gradually increased in extent and frequency as drainage from the wound diminishes.

Preparing the patient for discharge

Looking at a mastectomy scar for the first time is often very difficult and may confirm a woman's fears about breast loss and intensify her grief. However, others find the scar neater and less distressing than they had imagined. Women who have lumpectomies may have a similar range of reactions.

The nurse should encourage a woman to look at her scar before she goes home, as this represents a significant step in rehabilitation (Denton & Baum 1983). The woman may wish to be accompanied by her partner or a nurse and this can be the first time she talks about the loss or alteration of her breast. The woman must never be forced to look at her wound and it may not be until the first postoperative outpatient visit that she is able to take this step.

Rehabilitation proceeds at different rates, but the nurse should warn each woman that it may take several months before she feels that her energy has returned to normal. Persistent fatigue may cause frustration and may give rise to anxiety that the cancer has returned. Fatigue is more likely if chemotherapy or radiotherapy are given postoperatively, but where it is profound, depression should also be considered as a possible contributing factor.

Most women can begin driving again in 2–3 weeks, providing they feel confident and their arm movement is not too uncomfortable. Light household duties can be undertaken when the woman feels well enough, usually 2–3 weeks postoperatively, and she may return to work at around 6 weeks. This will, of course, depend on the extent of the surgery, the particular individual and the type of work she does.

Pain and discomfort from the wound will steadily reduce, but some discomfort often remains for 2–3 months. Paraesthesia around the scar and axilla may fade over several months, but some may always remain and can be made a little worse by local radiotherapy.

Swelling of the breast tissue or axilla following surgery will also occur and may take 2–3 months to resolve fully. Some women believe that the large lump they can feel is cancer that has suddenly grown after surgery. Prior explanation of this and the possibility of seroma formation is likely to reduce any anxiety.

Lymphoedema is a possible long-term complication that can occur in anyone who has axillary surgery or radiotherapy. Women should be advised to contact their GP or hospital if they notice any swelling, and not to leave it until it becomes a problem. Lymphoedema following breast surgery is discussed on pages 300–302.

Prior to discharge, any woman who has had a mastectomy or a large lumpectomy should be given a temporary prosthesis, shown how to position it in her bra and alter its shape, and told how to wash it (see Box 7.15).

Q

7.8 Simpson's (1985) survey of prosthetic services suggested that in many areas these were inadequate and did not meet the needs of women with breast cancer. What services are available in your area? Are they adequate, in your view?

7.9 Prepare a 10 min teaching session for your ward colleagues or fellow students on the subject of breast prostheses, including what types are available and why they are important for the patient.

Box 7.15 Breast prostheses

The fitting of a breast prosthesis is an integral part of the rehabilitation of a woman who has had a mastectomy or partial mastectomy. The aim of the prosthesis is to match as closely as possible the woman's other breast in terms of size, shape, weight and feel, so that she may look normal and feel confident in clothing. This is important in helping her to resume her normal social activities and regain a healthy body image.

Temporary prostheses

A temporary prosthesis is fitted as soon as the wound drains have been removed and is worn until a permanent prosthesis can be fitted. It is soft, light and washable, and can be pinned securely into the cup of a bra. If a bra cannot be worn because of discomfort, the prosthesis can be pinned into a camisole or slip. The woman may find that wearing loose clothing helps to achieve an even appearance. However, it is important that the nurse spends time fitting this prosthesis well, as it is with this that the woman will first face the outside world again.

Permanent prostheses

A permanent prosthesis is usually fitted 5 weeks after surgery or 2 weeks after the completion of radiotherapy, when the wound is well healed. Every woman should be given a fitting appointment prior to leaving hospital. The fitting may be undertaken by a specialist nurse, surgical appliance officer or visiting prosthesis company fitter. A private room with a full-length mirror is necessary and it is essential that each woman is treated with respect and sensitivity.

Today most permanent prostheses are made of silicone gel which feels soft and comfortable next to the skin and takes on the body's temperature. Many shapes and sizes are available; it should be possible for all women to be fitted with a prosthesis that gives a balanced appearance in a bra. Partial prostheses are available for women who have breast conservation. Silicone prostheses generally last for 2–3 years, but a woman is entitled to a replacement whenever it begins to show signs of wear and tear or if she loses or gains weight or changes shape.

Special 'mastectomy bras' are not necessary, but the bra does need to be supportive and of the correct cup size, covering all of the tissue of the remaining breast. It is helpful if the nurse can give basic advice about bras and instruct a woman where she may be fitted for a bra locally, if her previous bras are now inappropriate. Volunteer organisations such as Breast Cancer Care give helpful advice about bras, swimwear and other clothing (see 'Useful addresses', p. 311).

Adjuvant therapy

Postoperatively, the woman will probably attend a surgical outpatient clinic where she will hear the results of her surgery, i.e. the number of nodes involved with cancer, the size of the tumour, the grade of the tumour and the oestrogen status, all factors that will determine the need for adjuvant treatment. Many more women are now being offered adjuvant hormone and chemotherapy treatment, following two 'meta-analyses' published in *The Lancet*. The first analysis showed that chemotherapy given to a woman with early breast cancer meant a longer (statistically significant) time to recurrence and a small but significant increase in survival (EBCTCG 1992). The second analysis showed that premenopausal women

Table 7.5 Possible side-effects of adjuvant radiotherapy used in the treatment of breast cancer

Side-effect	*Comment*
Redness and soreness of the area treated	Not easily predictable
General tiredness	Especially toward the end of the treatment period
Photosensitivity	See Chapter 12; sun barrier creams should be worn for a year after therapy
Moist desquamation	Now rare because of the fractionation of radiotherapy
Nausea	Rare; radiotherapy affects only the area to which it is administered
Breast becomes firmer to the touch	Long-term effect due to fibrosis of tissue
Narrowing or blockage of lymph vessels	Increases risk of lymphoedema

who are treated for an early breast cancer can have a 7–11% absolute improvement in 10-year survival (EBCTCG 1998b).

Information on adjuvant radiotherapy and drug therapies should be given, as relevant, both verbally and in writing. The patient should understand why adjuvant treatment has been advised, for what period and at what intervals it will be administered, and what the side-effects may be. At this point the woman may be invited to join a trial, as there are several national trials looking at the effectiveness of different types of chemotherapy and hormone therapy.

Radiotherapy. The common side-effects of adjuvant radiotherapy in breast cancer are listed in Table 7.5. The nurse should also give advice on skin care for women undergoing radiotherapy.

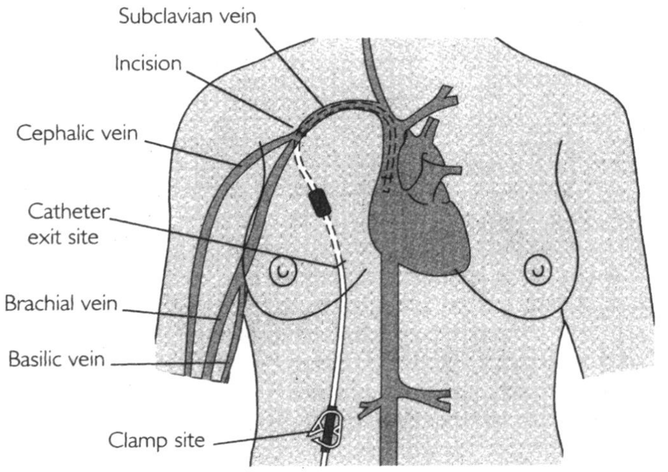

Fig. 7.17 Central line insertion. (Reproduced with kind permission, Andrews 1997.)

Chemotherapy. A variety of chemotherapy regimens are used and the woman may have already received chemotherapy treatment prior to her surgery. The nursing care for patients on chemotherapy regimens will be discussed separately.

Neoadjuvant or primary chemotherapy. This treatment often contains an anthracycline-type drug (see p. 930) and sometimes involves a continuous infusion of 5-fluorouracil via a pliable central venous catheter (sometimes known as a central line). This central line is inserted through the chest wall and into the subclavian vein whilst the woman is under a light anaesthetic. This line allows easy venous access or blood sampling and ensures that prolonged chemotherapy administration via a portable pump does not damage peripheral veins (see Fig. 7.17 and Box 7.16).

Peripherally inserted central catheters (PICC lines) are also becoming a popular way of administering chemotherapy (see Ch. 31). The central line can represent another assault on the woman's

Box 7.16 The central venous catheter in neoadjuvant chemotherapy for breast cancer

Insertion of the central line usually involves the woman having a light anaesthetic and staying overnight in hospital. The line is usually inserted by an anaesthetist in the operating suite and then the woman will be returned to the ward. The line is X-rayed after the operation to ensure that it is positioned correctly. The incision wounds will be covered with a light gauze dressing or an occlusive plastic dressing according to the anaesthetist's wishes. The wound site must be cleaned and dressed regularly either by the woman herself or by the practice or community nurse; the frequency of the dressings is decided locally. The stitches should be removed from the incision site 7–10 days after the line has been inserted and from the exit site 6–8 weeks after insertion, but only if the central line was cuffed. This timing allows scar tissue to form around the line and to anchor it within the subclavian vein. If the line is uncuffed, the exit site stitches remain in for the duration of treatment.

The woman (and often another member of her family or a close friend) will have been taught how to care for her central line while in hospital. Community back-up is essential to continue the care that has been started in the hospital and to assist with the central line dressing. Infection of the exit site of the central line is common and this should be recognised quickly and treated with antibiotics, as septicaemia can develop. If this occurs, the line should be removed and the woman should be treated with i.v. antibiotics. Thromboses forming around the central line in the subclavian vein can be a problem and are indicated by blockage of the line, sometimes swelling of the arm on the side of the line and pain at the site of the thrombosis or referred into the side of the neck. An ultrasound scan or X-ray will be taken of the line for a definitive diagnosis and the woman will be started on anticoagulants. The line will be kept in situ unless the woman does not respond to the anticoagulants in which case it will have to be removed.

Provided that the site has completely healed, the woman can continue with some of her physical activities, e.g. playing golf. She can lightly shower over the central line site but, if receiving chemotherapy via a portable pump, should not get the pump wet. The line should be long enough with an extension to leave the pump outside the shower. Written instructions are often given by the hospital, including contact numbers should any problems occur.

body image as it protrudes out of the chest wall and as hair loss often occurs with this type of chemotherapy. The whole experience can be very stressful and the woman often requires in-depth emotional support. Because this type of chemotherapy treatment is an area of current research, women who are eligible are often asked to take part in a trial. The timing of this decision may put yet another strain on a woman who is already facing up to having cancer, so the support and information she receives from her oncologist, ward nurse and breast care nurse will be crucial at this time. (See Ch. 31 for the nursing care of patients receiving chemotherapy and p. 450 for disorders of white blood cells and lymphoid tissue.)

Adjuvant chemotherapy. The patient should be reassured that the adjuvant chemotherapy regimens used in breast cancer tend to have milder side-effects than those used in the treatment of other cancers and can usually be managed by the outpatient department.

Nausea is commonly experienced but is normally mild and can be controlled by the range of antiemetics, including 5-HT3 antagonists, that are now available. Vomiting is rare.

Thinning of the hair is to be expected in at least three-quarters of patients receiving CMF (Fisher et al 1990), whilst other breast cancer chemotherapy regimens containing an anthracycline such as Adriamycin or epirubicin will cause total hair loss unless scalp cooling is used. Cooling the scalp with the use of ice caps can restrict the amount of chemotherapy reaching the hair follicles in the scalp and so may prevent complete hair loss, although the hair may thin and become drier and of poorer quality. Gentle shampoos should be used, and perms and the use of heated rollers and tongs should be avoided.

Bone marrow depression occurs with all cytotoxic drugs, but it is rare for neutropenia to be severe or for septicaemia to result. Nevertheless, every patient should be advised about good oral hygiene and the avoidance of obvious sources of infection. Usually a contact number is given for the hospital in case the woman's temperature rises above normal. She is usually advised to contact the hospital and to have a full blood count taken to ensure that her white cells are at an acceptable level. If the white cells are low and she is neutropenic, she may be prescribed oral antibiotics or, if necessary, admitted to hospital for i.v. antibiotics.

Fatigue is the most common problem and can be quite debilitating for the woman. Generally it is worst in the middle of a month's treatment cycle, when blood counts are at their lowest level.

A sore mouth and a susceptibility to mouth ulcers can be helped by using a soft toothbrush, salt water or medicated mouth washes.

Menstruation is usually affected, with periods becoming irregular or stopping, and is yet another assault on the woman's body. Menopausal symptoms, e.g. hot flushes, may be experienced, but if the woman is in her early 30s, menstruation has a 90% chance of returning after chemotherapy finishes. Women in their early 40s are much more likely to go into early menopause.

Endocrine therapy. Adjuvant tamoxifen is very widely given in view of its relatively few side-effects and its proven efficacy (EBCTCG 1998a). However, premenopausal women will usually experience menopausal symptoms, which can be very distressing for them. There are vitamin and mineral preparations, often containing evening primrose oil (gamolenic acid), that can be bought over the counter at larger chemists and can help with such symptoms; otherwise the woman's consultant or GP can prescribe drugs to reduce the hot flushes. Unfortunately, these drugs do not come without side-effects and many women prefer to manage without such intervention.

Gastric upsets are uncommon but may occur, particularly if the tamoxifen tablets are not taken with food. Very occasionally, thrombocytopenia is a problem. The individual should be advised to report increased bruising or bleeding from her gums.

Many women complain about an increase in weight, particularly around the abdomen, soon after starting the tablets. This may be due in part to fluid retention and in part to a reduction in physical activity following surgery.

Other, rarer and more serious side-effects include endometrial cancer and cataracts. Any abnormal bleeding should be investigated as well as any rapid deterioration in eyesight (Bruzzi 1998).

METASTATIC BREAST CANCER

Metastatic disease is sometimes obvious at the time of diagnosis but can occur months or many years later. Women in whom axillary lymph nodes are involved at the time of diagnosis are known to be at a high risk of developing metastases at a later date. Often these metastases are too small to be detected by scans or other investigations. The rate at which breast cancer grows and metastasises to other areas of the body varies and it is difficult to assess the long-term prognosis of an individual woman or to say that she is cured of the disease. It is estimated that over 50% of women who present with a breast lump already have metastatic spread (Smith & Richards 1995).

Once breast cancer has metastasised systemically, the oncologists will be aiming to put the disease into remission and to improve survival for the woman. The disease is no longer considered curable and the challenge for the oncologist is to give the woman prolonged life without too many side-effects. The decision to treat should be considered carefully with the woman and her partner.

PATHOPHYSIOLOGY

It seems that the spread of breast cancer is by direct invasion into the surrounding tissue and via the lymphatic and arteriovenous systems to distant areas, although this has not been proven absolutely. If untreated, local invasion of the breast cancer will cause ulceration, fixation to the chest wall and oedema of the arm. It may also erode blood vessels, causing haemorrhage, and invade the ribs or lungs and pleura, causing pleural effusion. Invasion of the brachial plexus can cause severe pain with functional and sensory loss in the arm. Invasion of the cutaneous nerves causes irritation and burning pain in the affected area. Because such aggressive local disease is not necessarily accompanied by metastatic spread, a woman may survive for many years with these problems.

Spread of breast cancer to distant sites is a common occurrence but may not become apparent for months or many years after the initial diagnosis and treatment. Metastases can occur anywhere and do not follow a systematic course. However, metastatic spread may be first discernible in the axillary and then supraclavicular lymph nodes, following the pattern of lymphatic drainage from the breast. The most common sites of metastases are the bones, lungs, liver and brain. Less frequently, they occur in the ovaries and mediastinum and, rarely, in the stomach, oesophagus and intestine. The problems most commonly caused by metastasised breast cancer are listed in Table 7.6.

MEDICAL MANAGEMENT

Surgery rarely has a part to play in the management of metastatic breast cancer but can help with locally recurrent disease.

Table 7.6 Common problems caused by metastatic disease in patients with breast cancer

Site of disease	*Problem*	*Treatment*
Bone	Bone pain Hypercalcaemia Spinal cord compression	Non-steroidal anti-inflammatory drugs, opiates, radiotherapy to site, chemotherapy Emergency: hydration, bisphosphonates, chemotherapy Emergency: radiotherapy and steroids
Bone marrow	Pancytopenia	Supportive blood + platelet transfusions. Chemotherapy (may cause further problems)
Lung/pleura	Pleural effusion Reduced expansion/shortness of breath with persistent cough	Pleural aspiration ± pleurodhesis Low-dose morphine, codeine cough suppressant. Chemotherapy/ endocrine therapy
Liver	Liver pain Ascites	Opiates, steroids, chemotherapy Paracentesis, chemotherapy
Skin	Ulceration/fungation Pain/irritation	Radiotherapy, chemotherapy, endocrine therapy, dressings, analgesia. For nerve pain, steroids and anti-inflammatory drugs
Brain/CNS	Confusion, headaches, nausea, vomiting, altered behaviour, convulsions	Emergency: radiotherapy and steroids Intrathecal methotrexate
Mediastinum	Superior vena cava obstruction	Emergency: radiotherapy and steroids
Axilla/supraclavicular fossa	Lymphoedema Brachial plexus pain and paraesthesia/paralysis of arm	Chemotherapy, endocrine therapy, radiotherapy Anticonvulsants, steroids and non-steroidal anti-inflammatories

Chemotherapy and endocrine therapy are the treatments of choice given their systemic effectiveness. Radiotherapy plays an important role in the relief of bone pain and in the oncological emergencies of spinal cord compression, cerebral metastases and superior vena cava obstruction, where tumour pressure must be reduced quickly. In these contingencies, steroids are used in conjunction with radiotherapy to reduce the oedema in tissues surrounding the tumour and hence relieve pressure further.

The menopausal status of the patient, the site of the metastatic spread and the apparent aggressiveness of the tumour will determine which drug therapies are considered most appropriate.

Chemotherapy. Disease that appears to be advancing rapidly or which involves the liver is most likely to be treated by chemotherapy. Regimens such as CMF are most commonly used if they have not previously been given as an adjuvant therapy. Side-effects are described in Table 7.4 (p. 288). The anthracyclines, alkylating agents, antimetabolites and vinca alkaloids are all effective at treating metastatic breast cancer and can all be given as single agents or in combination, depending on the previous treatment the woman has received. A new group of drugs, the taxanes, are currently receiving attention for the treatment of metastatic disease. The taxanes paclitaxel (Taxol) or docetaxel (Taxotere) are given as outpatient infusions in conjunction with a premedication of steroids and piriton to prevent hypersensitivity reactions. Both are being trialled as single agents or in combination with other chemotherapy agents and the short-term results are promising (Hortobagyi & Holmes 1996).

Endocrine therapy. Disease that is progressing more slowly may respond to endocrine therapies. These work more slowly but have fewer side-effects. Endocrine agents that may be used include the following:

Tamoxifen (see p. 296). This can be used in both pre- and postmenopausal women.

Luteinising hormone releasing hormone (LHRH) analogues (e.g. Zoladex). These interfere with the production of luteinising hormone and therefore oestrogen. Side-effects are the symptoms of menopause, e.g. amenorrhoea and hot flushes. These drugs are administered by subcutaneous injection every month and are only used for pre-menopausal women.

Aminoglutethimide. This drug inhibits the synthesis of aromatase, an enzyme needed to convert androgens produced by the adrenal glands to oestrogen. Allergic rashes are common but usually resolve if treatment continues. This drug is given only to postmenopausal women.

Arimidex. This drug inhibits aromatase enzymes that help to convert androgens to oestrogen and thus prevents the production of oestrogen.

Progestogens (e.g. medroxyprogesterone acetate and megestrol acetate). These drugs are usually used as a third-line treatment when others have failed. Side-effects include an increase in appetite and euphoria; this can be helpful if a patient is depressed, nauseated and has lost her appetite, however the steroid-type 'moon face' can develop. Weight gain is a problem, as is fluid retention, making this a drug to be given with caution to any patient who has a history of cardiac disease.

NURSING PRIORITIES AND MANAGEMENT: METASTATIC BREAST CANCER

Major nursing considerations

Assessment

Nursing assessment should address the physical, psychological and social impact of the disease, with particular consideration of the patient's own perception of these problems. The difficulties faced by the patient are likely to be determined in part by the site or sites of cancer spread. It should be remembered that medical priorities will not necessarily match the personal priorities of the patient and the decision to treat should be discussed carefully.

The reaction of the patient and her family to the news of progressive disease should be sensitively explored, and the nurse needs to assess how well they are coping. For many, the diagnosis of metastatic disease is more devastating than the original diagnosis of breast cancer, as the realisation dawns that treatment is now aimed at controlling rather than curing the illness. The patient and her family may once again experience shock, anger, denial, depression and despair as they try to come to terms with the implications of the diagnosis. They may feel that they had 'paid the price' at the time of the original diagnosis and that disease recurrence is very unfair (see Case History 7.3).

Even where cure is no longer possible, the philosophy of rehabilitation will remain at the centre of care, so that the highest quality of life can be maintained for as long as possible.

Palliative care

For a fuller discussion of the various aspects of long-term and palliative care that will be relevant to the patient with metastatic breast cancer, the reader is referred to Chapters 31 and 33. The important contribution of the nurse in controlling and managing symptoms such as pain, nausea and vomiting, fatigue, sexual problems, anxiety and shortness of breath is described in Chapters 3, 19 and 33.

Q **7.10** Consider the following questions with reference to Case History 7.3:

(a) Mrs J has extensive metastatic disease of her lumbar vertebrae. What implications does this have for nursing care?
(b) What side-effects is Mrs J likely to experience with Adriamycin chemotherapy?
(c) What information should the nurse give to Mrs J to prepare her for her first course of chemotherapy?
(d) Discuss other ways in which the nurse can help to allay Mrs J's anxiety about chemotherapy.

Case History 7.3 Mrs J

Mrs J is a 54-year-old married woman with two adult children. She has a part-time job in a school, but spends a large part of each day looking after her elderly mother, who is disabled with rheumatoid arthritis and is unable to move around.

Mrs J was diagnosed as having cancer of the right breast 4 years ago. This was treated by a wide excision of the tumour with axillary clearance. Adjuvant radiotherapy was also given. At this time four axillary nodes were found to contain cancer, and Mrs J was prescribed six courses of CMF chemotherapy and subsequently tamoxifen 20 mg, which she has been taking ever since. She was well until a month ago, when she began to experience pain in her back; this has since increased in intensity. On admission to hospital, a bone scan revealed extensive metastatic cancer in her lumbar spine, and a chest X-ray showed pulmonary metastases. Doctors have advised a course of Adriamycin chemotherapy, to which she has agreed, but she is 'devastated' by the news of cancer recurrence and is extremely frightened by the thought of chemotherapy. Her other major concern is how she will manage to continue to look after her mother.

BREAST RECONSTRUCTION

Breast reconstruction may be achieved by several surgical methods but frequently includes the insertion of silicone breast implants. It may be undertaken for cosmetic reasons when women feel their breasts are too small, where one breast has failed to develop at puberty, or following breast cancer surgery which has removed part or all of a woman's breast. However, only the latter will be considered here.

The aim of breast reconstruction following breast cancer surgery is to create a breast form which resembles the woman's other breast as closely as possible in terms of size, shape and consistency. Complete symmetry when naked is not possible to achieve but any differences should be slight when wearing a bra.

The King's Fund Forum (1986) consensus committee statement on breast cancer treatments suggested that 'the possibility of reconstructive surgery should be discussed with all women in whom a significant loss of breast tissue will be necessary'. Breast reconstruction may help to reduce the psychological or emotional problems experienced by women after surgery or it may enable a woman to undergo a mastectomy which she would have otherwise found intolerable (Dean et al 1983, Hart 1996).

Only uncontrolled metastatic breast cancer is considered an absolute contraindication in breast reconstruction. The presence of bone metastases should not prohibit a woman from having reconstructive surgery if she perceives that this will improve her quality of life and she is generally well enough to undergo surgery.

MEDICAL MANAGEMENT

Routine surgical preparation involving blood tests, chest X-rays and ECGs will be undertaken prior to surgery.

Several surgical techniques can be used to achieve breast reconstruction. The most common are described below.

Submuscular implant. This involves inserting a silicone implant beneath the muscle overlying the chest wall. Generally this can be done only where the remaining breast is small and droops very little.

Tissue expansion. An inflatable double-lumen silicone bag is inserted beneath the muscle overlying the chest wall and gradually inflated with sterile saline over a period of several weeks via a port valve and connecting tube which lie just beneath the skin. The aim of this is to slowly stretch the skin until the tissue expander is larger than the other breast. It is left overexpanded for several months and then some fluid is removed to create the natural ptosis of a breast. The port and the connecting tube are surgically removed, leaving a sealed prosthesis.

Tissue expansion methods are generally used where the skin of the chest wall is of good quality but inadequate quantity.

There has been much debate about the side-effects of using silicone because of recent claims that silicone prostheses can cause connective tissue disorders such as rheumatoid arthritis. Because of the uncertainty surrounding the use of silicone, many surgeons in the UK favour implants that contain sterile saline rather than silicone gel. Research into the use of silicone implants has been implemented and a recent study conducted in Sweden using a large nationwide cohort showed no association between breast implants and connective tissue disease (Nyren et al 1998). The debate still continues.

Myocutaneous flap. This involves transposing part of the latissimus dorsi muscle and overlying skin from the back, or the rectus abdominus muscle and overlying skin from the abdomen, to the chest wall. If necessary, an implant can then be placed behind this. Oval scarring on the breast form results, as well as scarring on the abdomen or back.

These methods are generally used where a larger breast form is desired, following a radical mastectomy in which all chest wall muscle has been removed, or where radiotherapy has been given to the chest wall, causing the skin to lose its elasticity.

Reduction mammoplasty. Surgery to the remaining breast may be advised if it is very large or pendulous in order to achieve as much symmetry as possible. Scarring following this procedure may be extensive and nipple sensation may be lost. These effects must be discussed with the woman beforehand.

Nipple areola reconstruction. Sometimes the surgeon is able to do a subcutaneous mastectomy and leave the nipple intact. More often the nipple is not saved because of fear of cancer being present there. If this is so, a nipple areola reconstruction can be undertaken. Generally, this is done around 3 months after the initial reconstruction. The nipple may be created from the skin overlying the reconstruction, saved from the other nipple or a graft taken from the labia. The areola is usually created from an upper inner thigh skin graft. Some women do not want to undergo further surgery and opt for adhesive silicone nipples.

Breast augmentation following partial mastectomy. This is usually carried out, if desired, at the time of the original surgery as it is more difficult after radiotherapy has been given. The implant is inserted into the area where tissue has been removed, to reduce any alteration in breast size and shape and hence problems associated with altered body image.

Potential postoperative complications

Seroma/haematoma formation. This is more likely to occur after an immediate reconstruction than it is if reconstruction is delayed. Serous fluid and blood may build up behind the implant in spite of the presence of wound drains, increasing discomfort and the risk of infection. Aspiration may be necessary and, occasionally, removal of the prosthesis.

Wound infection. If wound infection occurs, antibiotics will be prescribed. If the infection fails to respond to these, it may be necessary to remove the prosthesis and attempt insertion after a 3-month recovery period. To try to avoid infection, prophylactic antibiotics may be prescribed at the time of surgery.

Necrosis. This uncommon problem occurs where blood perfusion of the skin flap is inadequate and some of the tissue dies. It is more likely to occur when myocutaneous flaps are used.

Potential long-term complications

Capsular contracture. A fibrous band of tissue forms around the implant and, over time, will contract. If this contracture is severe, the implant will become hard to the touch, uncomfortable and cause the reconstructed breast to change in shape. Manual compression under local anaesthetic may break the capsule; the only alternative is to remove the implant and scar tissue and insert a replacement prosthesis. The incidence of capsular contracture requiring removal is difficult to ascertain but is likely to be around 15%; this figure increases significantly if radiotherapy is given to the breast after the reconstruction. There is some evidence that new textured implants result in a lower incidence of capsular contracture (Coleman et al 1991).

Abdominal herniation. This infrequent problem may follow a rectus abdominis myocutaneous flap reconstruction. The weakness in the abdominal wall resulting from this surgery is strengthened by the insertion of surgical mesh to reduce the possibility of herniation.

NURSING PRIORITIES AND MANAGEMENT: BREAST RECONSTRUCTION

Preoperative considerations

Assessment

Nursing assessment prior to breast reconstruction should address the following points:

- The woman's reasons for wanting a breast reconstruction. These may include wanting to eliminate the need for an external prosthesis, a desire to improve self-confidence and self-esteem or to 'feel more whole', and a desire to have greater freedom in choice of clothing (Goldberg et al 1984, Watson et al 1995).
- The woman's expectations of breast reconstruction. A woman who has realistic expectations is more likely to be satisfied with the overall result of her reconstruction. Expectations for both physical appearance and quality of life should be assessed as, however good the reconstruction is, it will not be an identical replacement for the breast that has been lost.
- The woman's knowledge of breast reconstruction and her understanding of what the surgeon has told her about the procedure and possible complications.

Giving information

The nurse has an important role in promoting realistic expectations of breast reconstruction. Showing photographs of breast reconstructions is one way of helping women to imagine what it will be like. Photographs that show the effect of the reconstruction unclothed, in a bra and under clothing are useful, but photographs should not show only the very best results.

It may also help to arrange for the patient to talk to another woman who has undergone a reconstruction, preferably by a similar method. Breast Cancer Care may be able to put the patient in touch with someone in her area if no-one is known to the nurse or consultant. Some women may also like to see an implant.

Giving psychological support

The woman who is undergoing breast reconstruction at the same time as her breast cancer surgery will be dealing with her recent diagnosis of cancer as well as with the idea of reconstruction. It may be particularly difficult for her to come to a decision about reconstruction at this time and so it should be made clear to her that refusing an immediate reconstruction does not prohibit surgery at a later date. The woman needs to have time to make her decision and should have access to a specialist nurse to go over what has been discussed (Reaby 1998).

Women considering a delayed reconstruction frequently have second thoughts about undergoing further surgery. The nurse can help by taking time to clarify with the patient her worries and concerns and her desire for reconstruction. Concurrent stresses and the woman's family situation should also be assessed and discussed, as these may influence how she feels about undergoing reconstruction and how she will cope postoperatively.

Postoperative considerations

Wound management

The aims and principles of wound management are described in detail in Chapter 23. The following points are of particular relevance to wound healing following breast reconstruction.

The nurse should observe the wound for signs of haematoma, seroma, infection or necrosis. Wound drainage should be observed and the volume recorded every 30 min for the first 2 h after return from theatre and then at gradually increasing intervals. Circulatory perfusion of skin flaps should be checked with the same frequency. The skin flap should be gently prodded using a blunt instrument or finger; it should go white and then quickly return to a pink colour once the pressure is released. This is particularly important where a myocutaneous flap has been used in reconstruction and where tissue expansion is placing the wound under some tension. Where the colour returns slowly, the flap looks blue or feels cold to the touch, the doctor should be informed in case it is necessary to take the patient back to theatre.

Temperature and pulse should be recorded 4-hourly. Dressings should be changed only if they become saturated with wound exudate or if it becomes essential to view the wound. Frequently, pressure dressings are applied in theatre and remain in place for 1–3 days. When these are removed, transparent dressings such as Tegaderm or OpSite are useful. Subcutaneous sutures are normally used and remain in situ for 10–14 days unless they are of the dissolvable variety. Discomfort from wounds will vary. Immediate reconstructions involving the removal of axillary lymph glands and/or abdominal myocutaneous flap procedures will be the most uncomfortable. Opiate analgesics may be required by i.v. injection or continuous infusion pump for the first 2 days; after this time, oral analgesics are usually sufficient. Promoting comfort will increase rest and sleep and so encourage healing and general rehabilitation.

Patient education

Postoperative exercises should be taught, preferably by a physiotherapist, to all patients who have undergone breast reconstruction. Some surgeons prefer shoulder movement to be restricted to 90° flexion and abduction for 2–3 weeks, particularly if the scar is very tight or if they fear movement of the implant. Because the silicone implant is usually placed behind muscle, as the muscle contracts, tightening or discomfort may be experienced. This should disappear as the muscle accommodates the implant.

Advice about bras is commonly sought. Some support is likely to increase comfort, but underwired bras should usually be avoided for the first few months. Surgical breast supports may be recommended for a few weeks, whilst sports bras which give firm support without bra cups may be the best option. A partial prosthesis will need to be fitted to obtain a symmetrical appearance during tissue expansion and sometimes following reconstruction.

Giving psychological support

Although having a reconstruction after a mastectomy may help a woman to cope and foster rehabilitation, research indicates that many women mourn the loss of their breast and suffer from anxiety and depression following surgery (Meyer & Ringberg 1986, Dorval et al 1998). The nurse should not assume that a woman who has had an immediate reconstruction will have no problems related to a changed body image.

Women undergoing tissue expansion often experience frustration at the length of time the process takes to complete reconstruction. Some find it difficult to cope with an inequality in breast size and shape during this time (Goin & Goin 1988). Acknowledgement of these feelings, adequate opportunity to discuss them and access to counselling may help the woman to cope.

When complications do occur and an implant has to be removed, the individual may suffer further psychological distress. A wait of about 3 months is generally required before another implant can be inserted; during this time the woman will have to cope with another alteration in body image. Anxiety, depression and feelings of anger or despair may result. Some women may decide that they do not wish to undergo a further attempt at reconstruction. The nurse should support the patient whatever her decision and give her the opportunity to express her feelings.

LYMPHOEDEMA IN BREAST CANCER

Lymphoedema is the accumulation of a high-protein fluid in the interstitial spaces between cells in the tissue of a limb or other area. It is the result of a defective mechanism of lymph drainage due to tissue fibrosis, disease or a congenital disorder.

Approximately 25% of women with breast cancer will develop some degree of lymphoedema, characterised by a swollen arm, often with some swelling of the adjacent chest and back. This condition can cause considerable physical and psychological distress.

PATHOPHYSIOLOGY

All women with breast cancer who have axillary surgery to remove some or all of their lymph glands, or those who receive radiotherapy to the axillary region, are at risk of developing lymphoedema of the limb on the affected side. Scarring from these treatments will result in the closure or narrowing of many lymph vessels and so reduce the efficiency of lymphatic drainage from the arm. For most women, the drainage remains adequate and collateral vessels may develop to increase the pathways for drainage. However, lymphoedema may develop weeks, months or years after surgery or radiotherapy, sometimes following an infection or injury, but often without an obvious reason. It may remain mild or gradually progress until the arm is so heavy that it is difficult to lift and impossible to use. Over time, fibrosis within the tissue of the arm may occur, causing hardness. There is also a higher risk of infection and cellulitis, as the high-protein fluid is an ideal breeding ground for bacteria.

Disease within the axillary area which causes an obstruction to lymph flow will also cause lymphoedema. This may be seen when cancer has recurred or when a woman presents with an advanced carcinoma of the breast. Signs of venous obstruction are sometimes seen. These are commonly a pink colouring of the arm and distended veins visible on the upper arm and chest wall.

Brachial plexus nerve damage is rarely seen, but may also result from radiation fibrosis or cancer infiltration of the nerve plexus, causing weakness, paraesthesia or nerve pain.

MEDICAL MANAGEMENT

Treatment. Options for medical management are at present limited. The choice of treatment depends on whether the lymphoedema has been caused by fibrosis or by axillary disease. Assessment may include CT scanning and colour Doppler ultrasound to determine the amount of scarring, venous obstruction or disease present.

Attempts to reduce the size and weight of the arm by surgically removing a large amount of tissue have had very little success and have frequently caused further problems with infection, swelling and pain as well as extensive scarring.

Diuretics have a part to play only if generalised fluid retention is exacerbating the lymphoedema. Where venous obstruction is due to a thrombosis, anticoagulation therapy with warfarin may be used.

In the case of axillary disease, surgery to remove as much of the cancer as possible may be of use by reducing the obstruction of lymph and venous flow. However, chemotherapy or endocrine therapies, which have the advantage of not causing the same disruption to normal structures as surgery, are more likely to be used.

Pain relief. Analgesics ranging from paracetamol to opiates will be used as required. If, however, the pain is due to brachial plexus damage by disease or radiotherapy, it is unlikely to respond adequately to opiates since nerve pain is only partly opiate-responsive. Anticonvulsants, serotonin re-uptake inhibitor antidepressants, steroidal and non-steroidal anti-inflammatory drugs and, in some cases, antiarrhythmics may be effective. These should be used under the guidance of the palliative care team (Twycross 1996).

Cellulitis. The risk of infection in a swollen limb is high. A small cut or insect bite may provide an entry point for infection and result in severe cellulitis requiring treatment by antibiotics. If cellulitis is recurrent, patients are often given a prescription to have on hand so that they can obtain an antibiotic as soon as infection occurs.

NURSING PRIORITIES AND MANAGEMENT: LYMPHOEDEMA

Major considerations

Treatment effectiveness is measured in terms of the reduction in size and weight of the arm, and for most people this is possible. However, sometimes all that can be done is to increase the softness and movement of the arm and to reduce the discomfort, but these improvements can represent a substantial increase in the quality of life for the patient.

Assessment

Nursing interventions must be preceded by an assessment to identify the physical and psychosocial needs of the individual patient.

Physical assessment should address the following areas:

- Medical history, particularly of any surgery or radiotherapy, disease in the axilla
- The condition of the skin of the arm: colouring, presence of cuts/infection, previous cellulitis
- The size of the arm. Both arms should be measured at 4 cm intervals from a fixed point at the wrist to the root of the limb so that a comparison can be made and the severity of the oedema estimated to form a baseline for treatment. There is a computerised imaging system available which can take several views of a limb. These pictures can be measured and stored in the computer database for comparison at the woman's next visit
- The duration of the oedema and any precipitating or aggravating factors
- Presence of oedema in the adjacent tissue of the chest wall
- Any previous treatment for lymphoedema
- The type and severity of any discomfort experienced
- The individual's range of shoulder movement and ability to use the arm in activities of daily living.

Psychosocial assessment should include:

- how the lymphoedema has affected the woman's self-esteem and body image
- how the lymphoedema has altered the woman's lifestyle, work and social role and how she feels about this
- whether the swelling has affected the type of clothing she can wear.

Nursing interventions

The aim of nursing interventions in the management of lymphoedema are:

- to reduce arm size
- to improve the use of the arm
- to improve the comfort of the arm
- to improve the shape of the arm.

All treatments involve compression of the limb to try to push more fluid back into the lymph vessels that are patent.

Past treatments included the use of compression pumps attached to inflatable sleeves that were placed on the affected limb. Air was pumped intermittently into the sleeve, increasing pressure on the limb, stimulating the lymphatic system and squeezing the lymphoedema out of the arm and into the circulatory system. This method significantly reduced limb volume by fluid displacement, but unless the lymphatic drainage was permanently stimulated by the inflated sleeve, the displaced fluid reaccumulated (Foldi et al 1985). For the woman who was attached to the inflatable sleeve, this was not a practical solution.

For this reason, elasticated compression sleeves, bandaging, massage and exercises have become the treatments of choice. It is very important to explain clearly the aim of each treatment regimen and to promote a realistic expectation of outcome. Although therapy is aimed at control rather than cure, the patient who is given sufficient information and is encouraged to participate in treatment is likely to adopt a more positive attitude towards her situation.

The main treatment methods are related to the degree of severity of the lymphoedema:

- mild oedema — gentle exercise of the limb and positioning of the limb at rest
- moderate oedema — all of the above plus an elasticated compression sleeve
- severe oedema (or if there is lymphorrhoea) — all of the above plus compression bandaging for 2–3 weeks, after which the patient wears a compression sleeve.

Compression sleeves are at the centre of treatment for lymphoedema. Several specialised ready-made varieties are available, e.g. Medi, Pan-Med and Sigva. Compression needs to be fairly strong (around 40 mmHg) if it is to be effective. Supports such as Tubigrip are not adequate.

Sleeves may be difficult to put on but should be supportive and comfortable. They should be worn all day but not at night, and should not be allowed to form creases, as this will cause ridging in the swollen tissue. The sleeve will need to be worn over many months, during which time the patient must be monitored regularly to assess the effect. The patient should be warned that progress will be slow.

If the oedema is modest, it may be possible for the arm to return to its normal size. At this point the sleeve may be removed, but the patient should be reminded that the oedema may return, in which case the sleeve should be reapplied.

Compression bandaging. For women with severe lymphoedema, lymphorrhoea, skin problems or difficulty using a sleeve compression, bandaging is the treatment of choice. Low-stretch bandages are used to bandage the fingers and hand before the arm is encased. The pressure applied should be graduated, greater pressure being applied at the lower end of the limb.

The bandages should be reapplied daily; due to the large size of the arm and of the bandages required, this may need to be undertaken on an in-patient basis. Although expensive, this also affords an opportunity for the provision of physiotherapy, occupational therapy and psychological support. However, community nurses practised in this technique could undertake compression bandaging in the patient's home. This is particularly helpful for those who have advanced disease and are unwell. Bandaging of a large arm may provide great comfort and relief from pain even if there is no hope of reducing arm size.

Although this bandaging technique is not difficult once learned, it does require practice and guidance.

Regnard et al (1988) may be useful for nurses wishing to learn how to bandage a patient's swollen arm appropriately.

Patient education

Massage. This has long been used in mainland Europe to treat lymphoedema but is only now being recognised in the UK. The type of massage used is light, aiming to stimulate the lymphatic vessels in the skin. Deeper massage would cause increased blood flow to the muscles; this would cause more fluid to accumulate in the tissues and would thus be counterproductive.

The patient can be shown how to massage the affected limb and adjacent part of the chest and back, where some degree of swelling may also occur. Indeed, massage is really the only way of treating oedema in the tissues of the chest and back. Using the hand or an electric massager, the chest and back are massaged by applying light pressure in a direction away from the arm. Next, the arm should be massaged, starting at the top of the arm and working down — but always applying pressure upwards.

It is a good idea to show relatives how to perform therapeutic massage.

Exercise. Muscle contraction exercises and shoulder exercises should be taught to improve and maintain movement and to encourage the return of lymph and venous fluid in the arm. Appropriate exercises include:

- clenching and relaxing the hand
- full circular movement of the wrist
- extension and flexion of the elbow joint
- clasping hands in front of the body and raising the arms, held straight, above the head.

A combination of these exercises should be performed for 5 min, four times a day.

Self-care. Patients should be given advice on how to care for their arm, in order to reduce the risk of infection and to avoid straining it (both of which are likely to increase swelling). Ideally, this advice should be given to all women undergoing surgery or radiotherapy involving the axilla; this will help to prevent lymphoedema occurring and encourage early detection where it does occur.

MALIGNANT FUNGATING BREAST TUMOURS

Breast cancer is the most common cancer to cause ulceration. The result can be an unpleasant, weeping, malodorous, infected wound which is psychologically very difficult to cope with. Women often express feelings of disgust and revulsion and curtail social activities because of their embarrassment. An altered body image may lead to anxiety, depression and sexual problems.

Nurses have an important role to play in supporting women with fungating tumours. By rising to the challenge of wound management and controlling symptoms such as odour and excessive wound exudate, they can help to improve the quality of life for these women. Frequently it is the community nurse who has the greatest involvement with these women and their families (see Case History 7.4).

Case History 7.4 Mrs S

Mrs S has been referred by her GP to the community nurse for management of a large ulcerating left breast carcinoma and for psychological support. She is 65 years old and a retired civil servant. She lives with her husband in a large house, which they own. She visited her GP ostensibly to have her blood pressure checked but broke down in tears and told him that she had had a breast lump for 3 years. She hadn't told anyone, including her husband, because she 'feared the worst'. Now the lump was smelly and oozing and she could no longer hide it from her husband, who had made her visit the GP.

On visiting Mrs S for the first time, the nurse finds a withdrawn and depressed lady who has stopped going out. She is embarrassed to show the nurse her breast, which is a large ulcerating mass with nodules extending to the surrounding tissue on the chest wall. The wound is malodorous, with a large amount of necrotic tissue and a profuse discharge. Mrs S has been covering it with gauze pads but has not cleaned it for some time, as she cannot bear to look at it.

Mrs S describes her husband as supportive and loving, but she will not allow him near her any more because she feels that she is 'disgusting'. She has taken to sleeping in a separate room and avoiding him when she can.

The nurse is able to speak very briefly to Mr S, who appears caring but very anxious about his wife's condition. He is not allowed by his wife to be present during her discussion with the nurse.

PATHOPHYSIOLOGY

Ulceration occurs when breast cancer infiltrates the epithelium and causes a breakdown of the skin. The resulting wound may be superficial or deep; it may affect a small area of the breast or may be very extensive, involving all of the chest wall. Frequently, as a tumour grows, its blood supply becomes inadequate, causing central tissue death and necrosis. When such a tumour ulcerates, a large necrotic mass is revealed, providing an ideal environment for infection to develop. This in turn will increase exudate and cause odour.

As the disease progresses, ulceration becomes more extensive and may erode blood vessels, causing haemorrhage. The severity of bleeding will depend on the size of the blood vessel. Capillary bleeding causing a slow loss of blood is commonly seen, but blood loss may be life-threatening if a large vessel is eroded.

Tumour involvement of the cutaneous nerves can cause pain and irritation. There is often tenderness due to inflammation in the surrounding tissues. Whilst many women have remarkably little pain from these wounds, some have severe pain.

MEDICAL MANAGEMENT

Treatment will depend on the extent and position of the tumour and on what therapy for breast cancer, if any, the woman has previously received. Management may be considered in terms of treatments to try to control the disease and interventions aimed at symptom control.

Surgery. For women who have an ulcerating tumour that appears confined to the breast region, it may be possible to remove the tumour surgically by performing a mastectomy (sometimes, unfortunately, called a toilet mastectomy). Where the tumour extends to the chest wall or a large area of skin, the surgery will be more extensive and surgical closure will require a skin graft or the use of a muscle and skin flap from the abdomen or back. These have been successfully used in some women to increase their quality of life, but careful discussion with the patient beforehand is important to ensure that she understands what the surgery entails, what benefits can be expected and what risks are involved. If the woman's general health is reasonable and she has a life expectancy of more than a few months, she may feel that this approach is the best for her even if recovery is protracted.

Radiotherapy can be used with great success in controlling some breast tumours. Complete remissions are occasionally seen, but more commonly radiotherapy achieves a reduction in tumour size and in the wound symptoms.

Chemotherapy and endocrine therapy may also be used, sometimes in combination with radiotherapy. Systemic drug therapies have the added advantage of treating disease elsewhere in the body as well as in the breast.

Symptom control measures are as follows:

- *Analgesics* may need to be provided frequently to alleviate constant pain or to make dressing changes more comfortable. The choice of analgesic will depend on the type and severity of the pain (see Ch. 19).
- *Antibiotics* may be required in the fight against infection.
- *Supportive transfusion* may be indicated where blood loss has caused anaemia.
- *Surgical debridement* may be very useful in removing necrotic tissue from the wound, but it is often not possible to carry out in view of the risk of haemorrhage.
- *Diathermy* can be helpful in controlling bleeding points but should be used with caution given the necrosis it causes. In severe cases of bleeding, topical adrenaline may also be applied; this too should be used with caution.

NURSING PRIORITIES AND MANAGEMENT: FUNGATING BREAST TUMOURS

Major considerations

Assessment

The nursing assessment of a woman with a fungating breast tumour must include far more than an assessment of the wound itself. It must consider factors such as age, marital status, concurrent disease and disabilities, drug therapies and pain. All of these factors may influence the possibility of wound healing or infection.

The woman's psychological state, her reaction to the wound, her ability to cope with it and the way it has affected her life and her family are all equally important. The nurse should bear in mind that anxiety and depression can have a significant impact on treatment outcome. Frequently it is the community nurse who has the greatest involvement with these women and their families, as hospitalisation is rarely required. Women often live for many years with a slowly progressing fungating tumour, which makes it all the more important that every effort is made to improve their quality of life.

Wound management (see also Ch. 23)

Malignant breast lesions have a pathological cause, i.e. cancer. Unless this cause is being treated, wound healing is unlikely to occur. It is important that the nurse promotes realistic expectations in the patient, so that she is not hoping for complete healing of the wound if she is not receiving treatment for breast cancer.

The general aims of wound management are:

- to control the symptoms produced by the wound
- to minimise possible complications, e.g. infection
- to maximise comfort and minimise discomfort
- to promote healing where possible.

Many types of wound dressings are available. In order to choose products which are likely to be most effective for a given wound, the nurse must first identify the problems that are present. The most common problems associated with ulcerating lesions are discussed below (see also Nursing Care Plan 7.3).

Tissue necrosis. Where tissue necrosis exists it is likely to increase the risk of infection. Debriding the wound of dead tissue will reduce this risk. Although it may be possible to remove the bulk of necrotic tissue by surgical debridement, the risk of haemorrhage sometimes prohibits this, making chemical debridement the preferred treatment even though it is a slower process. Products such as Varidase, Sorbsan, Debrisan and Granuflex may be useful as chemical debriding agents.

Infection is suspected where there is a purulent wound discharge, odour, inflammation and a raised body temperature. A wound swab should be taken by the nurse so that the appropriate systemic antibiotic can be prescribed. Preparations such as metronidazole gel may be applied topically to help fight infection. The pharmacist and the infection control team will advise about the use of particular cleaning solutions when there is wound contamination by particular organisms such as *Pseudomonas*.

Excessive wound exudate is often due to a wound infection. Hence the first action would be to treat the infection and to debride the wound as necessary. The aim of wound dressing is to absorb the maximum volume of exudate with the minimum bulk of dressing. This requires the use of a high-absorbency primary dressing, e.g. Sorbsan, an alginate hydrofibre and a high-absorbency secondary dressing, e.g. CliniSorb, which has the added benefit of containing charcoal to reduce odour from the wound.

It is important to remember that once there is 'strike-through' of the secondary dressing (i.e. saturation of the dressing) a pathway exists for bacteria to move from the outside through the dressing into the wound. This should be prevented by frequent changes of the outer dressing. Waterproofing is also important. Dressings such as OpSite or Tegaderm may sometimes be used as a tertiary dressing. Disposable nappies are effectively used by some nurses where great absorbency is needed.

Odour. Despite the lack of research to legitimise the use of natural live yoghurt in reducing wound odour, it is in fact widely used and appears to be effective. It is thought that the application of yoghurt creates an acid medium in which bacteria find it difficult to live, and that the lactobacilli in the yoghurt also act directly on the bacteria within the wound.

Yoghurt is usually applied thickly for around 20 min before it is removed with saline or gently showered off in the bath. A further dressing such as Sorbsan or Kaltostat can then be used on the wound. Where odour is a severe problem, yoghurt can be applied three or four times a day to try to reduce the odour as quickly as possible. A secondary dressing containing charcoal can also be used.

Metronidazole gel is also effective, but the problem of bacterial resistance to antibiotics must be considered.

External deodorisers may be helpful, e.g. Ozium, Neutradol, Nilodor, but sometimes the smell of air fresheners or deodorisers is unacceptable to the patient or her family, or may even cause nausea. Fresh air is probably the most effective agent for removing

Nursing Care Plan 7.3 Caring for a woman with an ulcerating breast tumour (See Case History 7.4)

Nursing considerations	*Action*	*Rationale*	*Expected outcome*
April 6			By April 13:
1. Ulcerating left breast cancer: the wound is malodorous, necrotic, and has a profuse discharge	❒ Take wound swab for culture and sensitivity ❒ Twice a day:	Odour and discharge may be due to infection in wound	A reduction in wound odour
	• Cleanse wound with saline using syringe and quill • Remove any areas of *loose* necrotic tissue with forceps and sterile scissors • Apply thick layer of natural live yoghurt and leave for 15 min, covering patient with sterile towel • Remove yoghurt using saline in syringe again	Quill allows gentle but thorough cleansing (no cotton wool fibres may be left which act as focus for infection). This will increase speed of debridement but should only be done on loose dead tissue and should not be painful Natural *live* yoghurt very good at deodorising but need to leave 15 min to work	Reduction in necrotic tissue Amount of wound drainage will be reduced and controlled by wound dressings Mrs S will state that she finds her dressing comfortable and that the symptoms have improved
	❒ Apply Hydrogel wound dressing ❒ Cover with dressing, taking care to protect sore and friable areas with Vaseline	Dressing necessary to ensure Hydrogel is kept in place	
	❒ Apply absorbent secondary dressing containing charcoal, e.g. CliniSorb	Absorbent secondary dressing used because of profuse discharge. Charcoal helps to deodorise	
	❒ Keep in place with Netelast	Using Netelast reduces trauma to friable skin on chest wall	
	❒ Suggest change bedclothes frequently and open windows each day	These measures will help to prevent the odour lingering in the house	
April 10	❒ Apply Sorbsan instead of Hydrogel. Continue with rest of dressing	Sorbsan has a haemostatic action. Though more gentle than Varidase, it is also very absorbent	

Evaluation

April 10
Hydrogel debriding wound well but wound bleeding close to medial edge. Using Sorbsan to stop bleeding. Will continue with yoghurt.

April 13
Discharge reduced and now controlled by Sorbsan dressing. Odour much less obvious but still present, therefore will continue with yoghurt, Sorbsan and charcoal dressings.

Wound swab indicates *Staph. aureus* infection. GP will visit tomorrow and prescribe a course of antibiotics.

smells from a room, and changing clothes daily will help to prevent odours from penetrating clothing.

Haemorrhage/capillary bleeding. Capillary bleeding is commonly seen in malignant wounds and is often difficult to stop. Dressings such as Kaltostat, an alginate hydrofibre, have a haemostatic property and are particularly useful where capillary bleeding exists.

It is extremely important that dry dressings are not applied to wounds that bleed, as removal is likely to cause further bleeding. To reduce trauma, adherent dressings should be removed only after soaking. Dressings such as Kaltostat and Sorbsan absorb exudate and turn to a gel which is then easily removed by syringing the wound with saline. Where possible, wounds which are liable to bleed should be irrigated, for even the gentle use of cotton wool may be enough to cause bleeding.

Silver nitrate and Flamazine also have haemostatic properties. The use of pressure and ice may help to control bleeding, but if a major vessel is eroded, bleeding may be very difficult to control and alarming to the patient.

Weak solutions of adrenaline may be advised by medical staff in such a situation, but these should be used with caution because of the possibility of systemic absorption.

Care must also be taken when using tapes to hold dressings in place. The skin around an ulceration is often inflamed, tender and delicate. As tapes may cause trauma, it is a good idea to rotate the sites to which tape is applied. In fact, it is preferable for dressings to be held in place by net body bandages such as Netelast, which obviates the need for tape.

Pain. Wound pain can range from very slight to severe. The nurse must assess the severity and type of pain being experienced

Nursing Care Plan 7.3 (*cont'd*)

Nursing considerations	*Action*	*Rationale*	*Expected outcome*
April 6 **2. Embarrassment and disgust at wound causing:** (a) Difficulty in communicating with husband (b) Social isolation (c) Reduced self-esteem	❐ Dress wound to control symptoms of odour and discharge	If symptoms of odour and discharge are controlled Mrs S will be more likely to go out again and not feel so self-conscious	
	❐ Encourage Mrs S to express her feelings about her wound and the way it is affecting her life	This may help Mrs S to 'let go' of tension, to see her situation more clearly and to allow her to accept support from the nurse. It will also help the nurse to identify specific problems/concerns	Mrs S will verbalise her feelings about her wound
	❐ Encourage her to talk about her relationship with her husband and how it has altered	This will help the nurse to understand how they used to communicate and how close their relationship was. This will help her to plan intervention which may improve communication and mutual support	She will identify how her relationship with her husband has changed
	❐ Assess her social support and what sort of activities she used to do	This will indicate what the norm was for Mrs S and how things have changed. It will allow the nurse to know what activities and relationships she might encourage Mrs S to take up again	
April 10	❐ Suggest that Mr and Mrs S sit down together and discuss how they feel about the cancer, the wound and how it has altered their life	This would allow Mr and Mrs S to begin communicating again and to break down barriers so that they can support each other	Mr and Mrs S will discuss together how they both feel about Mrs S having breast cancer and an ulcerating lesion
April 13	❐ Suggest Mrs S should go out to her daughter's next week for tea	Mrs S is close to her daughter. As her wound is improving, this is an appropriate first step in taking up her social life again	She will arrange to go out to visit her daughter by April 20
	❐ Arrange for Mrs S to visit hospital for partial prosthesis to be fitted	Mrs S has voiced concern about her appearance in clothes. A partial prosthesis will enable her to regain a balanced appearance	
	❐ Discuss the choice of loose clothing to minimise the altered shape due to the dressings		

Evaluation

April 10
Mrs S says she feels very down today. Expressed feelings of guilt that she hadn't sought help before and believes she has let her husband down. She knows that he loves her but believes he cannot possibly want to be near her because of her wound's odour. She describes her marriage as previously very strong. They used to talk about most things but both find it difficult to express their feelings to each other and have not spoken of the cancer diagnosis or what will happen now. She has spoken to her daughter, who has said they should all talk about it. She would like to but doesn't feel she can. I reinforced that I felt it would be a good idea and offered to be present if that would help. She will think about it.

April 13
Mrs S is feeling better. She is very pleased that her wound is more manageable and particularly that it is less smelly. I suggested she might consider going out. She is hesitant about this but I suggested perhaps a couple of hours with her daughter. She is still conscious of the wound and feels everyone will know something is wrong because her appearance is not balanced due to the dressings and tumour itself distorting her breast shape. I suggested partial prostheses may help this and she is very keen on this idea.

(*cont'd*)

Nursing Care Plan 7.3 (*cont'd*)

Nursing considerations	*Action*	*Rationale*	*Expected outcome*
April 6 **3. Fear of breast cancer**	❒ Assess Mrs S's information needs by finding out what her knowledge of breast cancer is and identifying misconceptions she may have ❒ Encourage Mrs S to express and explore her feelings concerning breast cancer ❒ Offer literature about breast cancer	Providing appropriate information may help to allay anxiety and remove misconceptions This is often therapeutic in itself but also allows the nurse to more accurately identify her fears Written information reinforces verbal information	Mrs S will specify the fears she has about breast cancer She will define her information needs concerning breast cancer and its treatment
April 7 **4. Fear of dying in pain. Fear of nausea and vomiting**	❒ Reassure Mrs S that effective pain control is available. (Discuss worries about taking opiates if this is a problem for her.) Stress that nausea and vomiting can normally be controlled by medication		Mrs S will understand that pain from cancer can be effectively controlled and that nausea and vomiting, if they occur, can also be controlled by medication

Evaluation

April 7
Very upset today. Feels very guilty that she didn't go to the GP before. Feels she has let her husband down. Has always been frightened of having breast cancer, although she doesn't know anyone who has had breast cancer. She knows that it is likely that she will die from this, in spite of any treatment she may be given, and she is frightened about how this will happen. She equates cancer with a painful death and cannot bear the thought of pain or feeling nauseated.

April 10
Given booklet by Breast Cancer Care. Suggested that she should let her husband read it too. Also wanted to know about possible treatments for breast cancer of this stage. Discussed chemotherapy, radiotherapy and hormone therapy.

Nursing considerations	*Action*	*Rationale*	*Expected outcome*
April 6 **5. Anxiety of Mr S due to Mrs S's condition and withdrawn behaviour**	❒ Arrange a time to sit down and talk to Mr S ❒ Encourage him to express and explore his feelings and define the particular anxieties he has regarding his wife and any other areas of stress ❒ Assess the support systems that Mr S has and emphasise that the nurse is concerned for his welfare as well as his wife's ❒ Provide information about breast cancer and its treatment	This will ensure the nurse has time specifically with Mr S Expression and exploration of feeling are therapeutic in reducing anxiety and will enable the nurse to assess the home situation more fully Many carers do not consider their own needs and consider the nurse only as a support for the patient Appropriate information may help to reduce anxiety by enabling Mr S to feel more involved and more in control of the situation	By April 13, Mr S will define areas of anxiety Mr S will discuss his feelings concerning Mrs S's illness, behaviour and the ulcerating cancer

Evaluation

April 6
Arranged to speak to Mr S tomorrow following visit to his wife.

April 7
Reluctant to discuss his feelings about his wife, preferring to dwell on his wife's problem and her feelings. Fought back tears when discussing the future. However, he did say he feels angry with himself and his wife that the cancer got to this stage before medical help was sought. He feels guilty he didn't know about it and frustrated with his wife's withdrawn behaviour as he believes she will just give up and die. We discussed how control of the wound problems may give her the confidence to go out again, and how she will require his support, which he appears very willing to give.

Mr S appears to have very little support, only talking to his daughter on rare occasions about his wife. He used to talk over everything with his wife but now she won't allow this.

April 13
Seen briefly. Looks more relaxed. Has talked to GP re. possible treatments and appointment to see consultant oncologist has been made for next week. Also believes that his wife is brighter because her wound has improved.

and whether it is always present or affects the patient only during dressing changes. Pain assessment should be ongoing so that the effectiveness of pain control measures can be evaluated (see Ch. 19). Where dressing changes cause discomfort, analgesics should be offered to the woman at least 30 min before each change. The use of Entonox during the dressing procedure may also be helpful. The use of non-adherent dressings and, where possible, cleansing of the wound by irrigation will also reduce discomfort.

Patient education

Wound care. As much information as the woman requires concerning her wound, dressings and general condition should be given. The degree to which the patient and her family are involved in wound management will depend largely on their own wishes and sensitivities. Some women prefer to be taught how to dress their own wounds completely at home, with only minimum supervisory involvement by the community or hospital nurse. This may originate in a desire to be independent or it may be prompted by embarrassment. Some patients feel unable to have anything to do with their wound and do not want family members to intervene either. No-one should be made to look at her wound if this is intolerable to her; to do so may destroy the only way in which she knows how to cope.

Diet. Dietary advice may be appropriate if a woman is malnourished, has an infection, is anorexic or is considering starting a 'cancer diet'. The nurse should be able to give basic advice about a balanced diet (see Ch. 21) but may wish to refer the patient to a dietician for further advice. The decision to go on to a cancer diet rests with the patient. There are many such diets: some are reasonably well balanced, but others are likely to cause extreme weight loss. Where this is likely to be detrimental to the individual, the nurse should discuss this with her. Ultimately, however, the nurse should support the patient in whatever decision she makes.

Prostheses and clothing. Practical advice about clothing may be appreciated if the disease has radically altered the contour of the chest or where a large amount of absorbent dressing is necessary to control the wound exudate. The use of partial prostheses fitted over the dressings may restore a more normal breast contour. A larger soft bra may enable the dressing to be held in place comfortably but securely whilst maintaining a normal appearance in clothing. Where a bra cannot be worn due to discomfort, loose clothing will help to disguise any altered shape without causing any restrictions around the wound.

Q

7.11 Consider the following questions with reference to Case History 7.4:

(a) Identify the main problems that Mrs S has.
(b) Consider the effects a fungating lesion might have on a woman's body image.
(c) It is important that Mrs S does not feel that her nurse is disgusted by her wound. Consider how the nurse might demonstrate both verbally and non-verbally that this is not the case.
(d) How might the nurse endeavour to reduce Mr S's anxiety about his wife?
(e) What properties should the wound dressing have? Can you suggest any appropriate products for such a wound?

THE PSYCHOLOGICAL IMPACT OF BREAST DISEASE

Nurses have a particularly important role to play in supporting patients through the traumatic experience of breast disease. Although many women with breast cancer, will face similar problems, no two individuals will respond to their diagnosis and treatment in exactly the same way. As this chapter stresses, ongoing assessment is the key to providing psychological and emotional support that is genuinely responsive to each woman's needs and priorities.

For most women, a diagnosis of breast cancer is devastating. They may have to cope with the prospect of mutilating surgery to a part of the body associated with femininity, sexuality and motherhood, the prospect of several months of intensive medical treatment and the possibility that they may eventually die of the disease. Most women with breast cancer discover a lump by accident, often when washing or during self-examination. Symptoms of acute anxiety, panic, palpitations, tachycardia, loss of concentration and insomnia may be experienced in the period when a medical opinion is sought and a diagnosis awaited. Some women describe this time of flux as the most agonising period of their illness. For some women, the fear of cancer or its treatment is so great that they deny the presence of a lump or delay seeking medical help.

Some of this fear may be based on misconceptions about the nature of cancer treatments. It is important for nurses, especially those in community practice, to dispel myths about cancer therapy, to raise awareness of the success rate of breast cancer treatment, and to emphasise the importance of early detection.

Some women who undergo surgery for breast cancer initially experience euphoria that the cancer has been removed. Others deny the removal of their breast or find themselves unable to talk about it or to look at the scar. Much research has been carried out into the psychosocial sequelae of breast surgery. Maguire et al (1978) found that 25% of women experience anxiety, depression or sexual problems in the first year after a mastectomy. Morris et al (1977) found similar incidences of anxiety and depression. It was thought that this was related mainly to the altered body image of mastectomy, but Fallowfield et al (1986) found that women who had a lumpectomy and radiotherapy had levels of anxiety and depression similar to those experienced by women who had undergone mastectomy (see Research Abstract 7.8). In their study, Dorval et al (1998) found that having a partial or total mastectomy did not significantly affect quality of life but that the individual's response to the surgery was affected by her age. Their study suggested that having a partial mastectomy may have lessened the negative effect of breast cancer for younger women.

Following diagnosis and surgery, a period of adjustment occurs which is characterised by fluctuating emotions. Northouse (1989) found that following mastectomy the major concern for most women and their partners surrounded issues of survival, in particular the extent of the cancer and the possibility of recurrence. Patients may also be worried about changes in lifestyle, treatment regimens and altered appearance.

For the majority of women who have undergone breast surgery, anxiety begins to reduce after about 3 months and the activities of normal life will be resumed. Some women, however, will continue to experience great anxiety, show signs of depression, withdraw from social contact or have sexual problems. These women are likely to benefit from more in-depth counselling and psychological support. Nurses, particularly those in the community and in

Research Abstract 7.8

In a study by Fallowfield et al (1986), 101 women being treated for early breast cancer (stages T0, T1, T2, N0, N1 and M0) were assessed for psychiatric morbidity, sexual functioning and social adjustment. Of the group, 53 were treated by mastectomy and 48 by lumpectomy and radiotherapy.

The study found that 33% of the women following mastectomy and 38% following lumpectomy experienced anxiety and/or depression; 38% in each group reported reduced sexual interest.

Reasons given for anxiety and depression varied between the two subgroups. Both were worried by the diagnosis and prognosis of breast cancer. The women who had undergone lumpectomy were concerned about the recurrence of cancer in the breast operated on and were worried about radiotherapy and its after-effects. They were also more commonly worried that they had opted for the wrong procedure. The women who had undergone mastectomy voiced more concern about the effect of surgery on their appearance and personal relationships.

This study suggests that women who undergo lumpectomy and radiotherapy do not experience less psychosocial distress than those who undergo mastectomy and therefore require as much support and counselling as those who undergo more extensive surgery.

Fallowfield L J, Baum M, Maguire G P 1986 Effects of breast conservation on psychological morbidity associated with diagnosis and treatment of early breast cancer. British Medical Journal 293: 1331–1335.

outpatient departments, should be able to recognise emotional problems and, where necessary, suggest referral to a counsellor, psychiatrist or psychologist via the GP or hospital medical staff.

PATIENT EDUCATION

Being a recipient of the bewildering treatments for breast cancer can take control away from the woman and this lack of control can lead to psychological morbidity (Morris et al 1977). Research has shown that many patients find that information helps them to make sense of their situation, and hence to feel more in control, less vulnerable and less anxious (Boore 1978). Information may also help to reduce the pain and complications experienced postoperatively (Hayward 1975). Most women have some general knowledge of breast cancer, but will not be familiar with the details of the tests or treatments they are to undergo. Many will, in fact, have misconceptions about breast cancer and its prognosis because of the misinformation that is found in the media.

The nurse must bear in mind that the amount of information each woman wants about her disease or proposed treatment will vary. As too much information is likely to cause confusion and anxiety, it is important for the nurse to find out what each individual wants to know, and to clarify what has been understood. It is also important to remember that, in times of stress, information is more difficult to assimilate. It is therefore often necessary for the nurse to repeat information.

If the nurse feels unable to answer any questions, she should either find someone who can or arrange a further consultation with medical staff. The nurse may be able to facilitate communication by helping the patient to articulate her concerns and by clarifying concepts or terminology unfamiliar to the patient.

Areas of information that are likely to be relevant include:

- how breast cancer is and is not caused, e.g. it is not caused by a knock on the breast
- the aim of treatment and what outcome may realistically be expected
- the nature and likely cosmetic effect of any proposed surgery
- the possibility of breast reconstructive surgery if all, or a large part, of the breast is removed
- if axillary lymph node removal is advised, the effects of removal and the postoperative exercises necessary to ensure the return of full shoulder movement (see p. 290)
- staging tests that will need to be performed prior to or following surgery
- the availability of prostheses, when this is appropriate.

The nurse should ensure that the patient understands what the operation involves and the likely pre- and postoperative experiences, including the presence of wound drains, i.v. infusions, pain, scarring and any possible short- or long-term complications. Photographs or diagrams may be useful to demonstrate likely scarring or alteration in breast shape or size, and patient videos are becoming a popular way of reinforcing what has already been said.

Information given verbally may be reinforced in written form. Booklets on breast surgery and breast cancer can be obtained from the British Association of Cancer United Patients (BACUP) and Breast Cancer Care (BCC) or The Royal Marsden Hospital, if local literature is not available (see 'Useful addresses', p. 311). These publications can also be useful for family and friends to read. Admission booklets providing information about the hospital, its facilities and visiting hours are also helpful.

Women who wish to have more in-depth knowledge may find Baum et al (1994) useful. This book is written for the informed lay public.

THE ISSUE OF INFORMED CONSENT

The patient's rights

In order to give informed consent to an operation or treatment, a patient must be told what the procedure or therapy entails and its consequences, and must understand the information that she is given.

A woman who is diagnosed as having breast cancer has the right to be told of all the possible medical options and to decide which, if any, of these options she will take. She may wish to seek a second opinion from another specialist and to gather information to help her make a decision as to which is the best treatment for her.

The increasing recognition of the patient's right to informed consent has led to the virtual abolition of the all-in-one procedure of excision biopsy of a breast lump for frozen section pathology followed immediately by mastectomy if cancer is found.

The nurse's role

The issue of informed consent is an important one for all nurses who aim to give truly patient-centred care. Doctors have the responsibility for obtaining informed consent, but nurses can help to ensure that this occurs by asking patients to state what they understand is to happen to them and by providing any additional information that is desired. Often patients feel very vulnerable when consulting a doctor and a nurse may act as advocate by representing the patient or support her in meetings with the doctor.

Where a nurse feels she does not have the necessary information or communication skills, she may be able to contact a specialist breast care nurse, now employed by many hospitals to support women from the time of breast cancer diagnosis.

Explaining the choices

For many women with breast cancer, the consultant will be able to give two treatment options which are equally promising, e.g. a mastectomy or a wide excision of the tumour and axillary dissection followed by radiotherapy. In order for the woman to make a decision, she needs to understand what each operation or treatment involves, and any side-effects which may result.

Most women find the thought of losing a breast very distressing and will prefer a wide excision of the cancer or a segmentectomy, if this is a safe option. However, mastectomy may be a better choice in some instances. The King's Fund consensus statement on breast cancer (King's Fund Forum 1986) reads:

> *...for tumours which are multi-focal, or involve a large portion of the breast, mastectomy will often be the best surgical treatment. Mastectomy may also be preferred by women with small tumours to reduce the risks of local recurrence, and the need for adjuvant radiotherapy.*

A tumour that is multifocal (i.e. occurs in several areas of the breast) cannot safely be removed by conservative surgery as the risk of local recurrence would be unacceptably high. The cosmetic result of removing a large tumour from a small breast or removing a tumour that is centrally sited beneath the nipple could be so poor that a mastectomy would be more acceptable, although only the individual woman will know how she feels about this.

Some women facing breast surgery are not aware of the possibility of reconstructive surgery. In part, this reflects the lack of facilities and skills in many areas to undertake such surgery. The long waiting lists at centres where breast reconstructions are done may cause professionals to hesitate in disclosing the possibility of this surgery. Nonetheless, in fairness to the woman, all options should be explained so that she can decide whether breast reconstruction is right for her in light of the benefits and the possible complications.

THE ROLE OF THE CLINICAL NURSE SPECIALIST IN BREAST CARE

The role of the clinical nurse specialist in breast care has developed largely in response to the recognition that women with breast cancer benefit from the support and expertise of nurses specialising in this area (Maguire et al 1980, Watson et al 1988, Maguire 1995, McArdle et al 1996). It must be stressed that the clinical nurse specialist provides an additional service to that provided by hospital and community nursing staff, and not an alternative to that service. The clinical nurse specialist functions as a resource for patients, their families and other nurses.

Ideally, the clinical involvement of the nurse specialist with the patient will begin at the time of diagnosis and prior to hospital admission. This may involve meeting patients in screening assessment units, and requires the cooperation of outpatient nurses and doctors in informing the nurse specialist of new patients. Many specialist nurses follow a limited intervention strategy of seeing patients in hospital before and after their surgery and then visiting them once or twice at home in the first 4 months postoperatively to assess how they are coping. Where problems arise, referral for more in-depth psychological support can be made, but the nurse is likely to continue her involvement with the patient and her family. Because of the increasing complexity of the treatments available, the larger breast units may employ more than one nurse specialist, and each is then able to focus her expertise on different aspects of the woman's care.

The nurse specialist also provides a contact point for patients and their family should they require advice or support at any time. She will also resume contact with patients should metastatic breast cancer develop. Many breast care nurse specialists also provide prosthetic and lymphoedema services.

REFERENCES

Andrews G (ed) 1997 Women's sexual health. Baillière Tindall, London

Ayash L, Elias A, Wheeler C et al 1994 Double dose intensive chemotherapy with autologous marrow and peripheral – blood progenitor – cell support for metastatic breast cancer: a feasibility study. Journal of Clinical Oncology 12(1): 37–44

Blackwell R E, Grotting J C 1996 Diagnosis and management of breast disease. Blackwell Science, Oxford

Bonadonna G, Zambetti M, Valagussa P 1995 Sequential or alternating doxorubicin and CMF regimes in breast cancer with more than three positive nodes. Ten year results. Journal of the American Medical Association 273(7): 542–547

Boore J R R 1978 Prescription for recovery. Royal College of Nursing, London

Bundred N, Maguire P, Reynolds J et al 1998 Randomised control effects of early discharge after surgery for breast cancer. British Medical Journal 317: 1275–1279

Bruzzi P 1998 Tamoxifen for the prevention of breast cancer. British Medical Journal 316: 1181–1182

Buzzoni R, Bonadonna G, Valagussa P et al 1991Adjuvant chemotherapy with doxorubicin plus cyclophosphamide, methotrexate and fluorouracil in the treatment of resectable breast cancer with more than three positive axillary nodes. Journal of Clinical Oncology 9: 2134–2140

Cancer Research Campaign 1996a Factsheets 6.1 to 6.6 CRC, UK

Cancer Research Campaign 1996b Factsheet 6.2 Breast Cancer. CRU, UK

Coleman D J, Foo I T H, Sharpe D T 1991 Textured or smooth implants for breast reconstruction? A prospective controlled trial. British Journal of Plastic Surgery 44: 444–448

Crowe D R, Lampejo O T 1996 Malignant tumours of the breast. In: Blackwell R E, Grotting J C (eds) Diagnosis and management of breast disease. Blackwell Science, Oxford

Curling G, Tierney K L 1997 Breast screening and breast disorders. In: Andrews G (ed) Women's sexual health. Baillière Tindall, London

Dean A, Chelty N, Forrest A P M 1983 Effects of immediate breast reconstruction on psychosocial morbidity after mastectomy. Lancet i: 459–462

Denton S, Baum M 1983 Psychosocial aspects of breast cancer. In: Margolese R (ed) Breast cancer. Churchill Livingstone, Edinburgh

DHSS 1986 Breast cancer screening: The Forrest report. HMSO, London

Dixon J, Mansel R 1995 Congenital problems and aberrations of normal breast development. In: Dixon J (ed) The ABC of breast diseases. BMJ Publishing Group, London

Dorval M, Maunsell E, Deschenes L, Brisson J 1998 Type of mastectomy and quality of life for long term survivors. Cancer 15(10): 2130–2138

Early Breast Cancer Trialists' Collaborative Group (EBCTCG) 1992 Systemic treatment of early breast cancer by hormonal, cytotoxic, or immune therapy. The Lancet 339: 1–15

Early Breast Cancer Trialists' Collaborative Group (EBCTCG) 1998a Tamoxifen for early breast cancer: an overview of the randomised trials. The Lancet 351: 1451–1467

Early Breast Cancer Trialists' Collaborative Group (EBCTCG) 1998b Polychemotherapy for early breast cancer: an overview of the randomised trials. The Lancet 352: 930–942

Fallowfield L J, Baum M, Maguire G P 1986 Effects of breast conservation on psychological morbidity associated with diagnosis and treatment of early breast cancer. British Medical Journal 293: 1331–1335
Fisher B, Brown A M, Dimitrov N V et al 1990 Two months of doxorubicin-cyclophosphamide with and without interval reinduction therapy compared with 6 months of cyclophosphamide, methotrexate, and fluorouracil in positive-node breast cancer patients with tamoxifen-non-responsive tumours: results from the National Surgical Adjuvant Breast and Bowel project B-15. Journal of Clinical Oncology 8(9): 1483–1496
Foldi E, Foldi M, Weissleder H 1985 Conservative treatment of lymphoedema of the limbs. Angiology. Journal of Vascular Diseases 31: 171–180
Goin M K, Goin J M 1988 Growing pains: the psychological experience of breast reconstruction with tissue expansion. Annals of Plastic Surgery 21(3): 217–222
Goldberg P, Stolzmann M, Goldberg H M 1984 Psychological considerations in breast reconstruction. Annals of Plastic Surgery 13(1): 38–43
Graydon J E 1994 Women with breast cancer: their quality of life following a course of radiation therapy. Journal of Advanced Nursing 19: 617–622
Hart D 1996 The psychological outcome of breast reconstruction. Plastic Surgical Nursing 16(3): 167–171
Harvey H A 1998 Emerging role of aromatase inhibitors in the treatment of breast cancer. Oncology-Huntington 12(3 suppl. 5): 32–35
Hayward J 1975 Information: a prescription against pain. RCN, London
Hemminki E 1996 Oral contraceptives and breast cancer. British Medical Journal 313: 63–64
Hortobagyi G N, Holmes F A 1996 Single agent paclitaxel for the treatment of cancer: an overview. Seminars in Oncology 23(suppl. 1): 4–9
Kerlikowske K, Grady D, Rubin S M, Sandrock C, Ernster V L 1995 Efficacy of screening mammography. A meta analysis. Journal of the American Medical Association 273: 149–154
King's Fund Forum 1986 Consensus development conference: treatment of primary breast cancer. British Medical Journal 293: 946–947
Lichter A S 1998 Breast cancer. In: Leibel S A, Phillips T L (ed) Textbook of radiation biology. WB Saunders, Philadelphia
McArdle J, George W D, McArdle C S, Smith D C, Moodie A R, Hughson A V M, Murray G D 1996 Psychological support for patients undergoing breast cancer surgery: a randomised study. British Medical Journal 312: 813–816
McPherson K 1995 Breast cancer – epidemiology, risk factors and genetics. In: Dixon J (ed) ABC of breast diseases. BMJ Publishing Group, London
Maguire P, Lee E G, Bevington D J, Kuchemann C S, Crabtree R J, Cornell C E 1978 Psychiatric problems in the first year after mastectomy. British Medical Journal 1(6118): 963–965
Maguire P, Tait A, Brooke M, Thomas C, Sellwood R 1980 Effect of counselling on the psychiatric morbidity associated with mastectomy. British Medical Journal 281: 1454–1456
Maguire P 1995 Psychological aspects. In: Dixon J (ed) The ABC of breast diseases. BMJ Publishing Group, London
Mansel R E 1995 Breast pain. In: Dixon J (ed) The ABC of breast diseases. BMJ Publishing Group, London
Mansi J L, Smith I E, Walsh G E et al 1989 Primary medical therapy for operable breast cancer. European Journal of Cancer Clinical Oncology 25(11): 1623–1627
Meyer L, Ringberg A 1996 A prospective study of psychiatric and psychosocial sequelae of bilateral subcutaneous mastectomy. Scandinavian Journal of Plastic Reconstructive Surgery 20: 101–107
Morris T M, Greer H S, White P 1977 Psychological and social adjustment to mastectomy: a two-year follow-up study. Cancer 40: 2381–2387
Newman J 1995 How breast milk protects newborns. Scientific American December: 58–61
Northouse L 1989 The impact of breast cancer on patients and husbands. Cancer Nursing 12(5): 276–284
Northouse L, Dorris G, Charron–Moore C 1995 Factors affecting couple's adjustment to recurrent breast cancer. Social Science Medicine 41(1): 69–76
Nyren O, Yin L, Josefsson S et al 1998 Risk of connective tissue disease and related disorders among women with implants: a nationwide retrospective cohort study in Sweden. British Medical Journal 316: 417–422
Overgaard M, Hansen P S, Overgaard J, Rose C et al 1997 Post-operative radiotherapy in high risk premenopausal women with breast cancer who receive adjuvant chemotherapy. New England Journal of Medicine 337: 949–954
Page D L, Steel C M, Dixon J M 1995 Carcinoma in situ and patients at high risk of breast cancer. In: Dixon J (ed) The ABC of breast diseases. BMJ Publishing Group, London
Powles T J, Smith I E (eds) 1991 Medical management of breast cancer. Martin Dunitz, London
Powles T, Eeles R, Ashley S et al 1998 Interim analysis of breast cancer in the Royal Marsden Hospital tamoxifen chemoprevention trial. The Lancet 352: 98–101
Reaby L L 1998 Breast restoration decision making: enhancing the process. Cancer Nursing 21(3): 196–204
Reshef E, Sanfilippo J S, Levine N S 1996 Breast dysfunction: congenital abnormalities of the breast. In: Blackwell R E, Grotting J C (eds) Diagnosis and management of breast disease. Blackwell Science, Oxford
Richards M, Smith I E 1995 Role of systemic treatment for primary operable breast cancer. In: Dixon J (ed) The ABC of breast disease. BMJ Publishing Group, London
Sainsbury J R C, Anderson T J, Morgan D A L 1995 Breast cancer. In: Dixon J (ed) The ABC of breast disease. BMJ Publishing Group, London
Salter M 1988 Altered body image: the nurse's role. Wiley, Chichester
Simpson G 1985 Are you being served? Senior Nurse 2(6): 14–16
Sjönell G, Ståhle L 1999 Hälsokontroller med mammografi minskar inte dödlighet i bröstcancer. Läkartiningen 96: 904–913
Tabar L, Gad A, Holmberg L H et al 1995 Efficacy of breast cancer screening by age. New results of the Swedish two-counties trial. Cancer 75: 2507–2517
Twycross R 1996 Symptom management in advanced cancer. Radcliffe Medical Press, Oxford
Veronesi U, Saccozi R, Del Vecchio M et al 1981 Comparing radical mastectomy with quadrantectomy, axillary dissection and radiotherapy in patients with small cancer of the breast. New England Journal of Medicine 305(1): 6–12
Veronesi U, Salvadori B, Luini M et al 1995 Breast conservation is a safe method in patients with small cancer of the breast. Long term results of three randomised trials on 1,973 patients. European Journal of Cancer 31A: 1574–1579
Watson M, Denton S, Baum M, Greer S 1988 Counselling breast cancer patients: a specialist nurse service. Counselling Psychology Quarterly 1(1): 25–34
Watson J D, Sainsbury J R C, Dixon J M 1995 Breast reconstruction. In: Dixon J (ed) The ABC of breast disease. BMJ Publishing Group, London

FURTHER READING

Andrews G (ed) 1997 Women's sexual health. Baillière Tindall, London
Blamey R W 1986 Complications in the management of breast disease. Baillière Tindall, London
Baum M 1988 Breast cancer: the facts. Oxford University Press, Oxford
Bostwick J 1987 Breast reconstruction after mastectomy. In: Harris J R et al (eds) Breast diseases. Lippincott, Philadelphia
Baum M, Saunders C, Meredith S 1994 Breast Cancer: A guide for every woman. Oxford Medical, Oxford
Cancer Research Campaign 1997b Factsheets 7.1–7.5: Breast cancer screening. CRC, UK
Dixon J (ed) 1995 The ABC of breast diseases. BMJ Publishing Group, London
Faulder C 1985 Whose body is it? Virago Press, London
Gateley C A, Mansel R E 1990 Management of cyclical breast pain. British Journal of Hospital Medicine 43: 330–332
Lamb M A, Woods N F 1984 Sexuality and the cancer patient. Cancer Nursing 4: 137–144
Margolese R (ed) 1983 Breast cancer. Churchill Livingstone, Edinburgh
Marks-Maran D J, Pope B M 1985 Breast cancer nursing and counselling. Blackwell Scientific, Oxford
Pfeiffer C H, Mulliken B 1984 Caring for the patient with breast cancer. Reston Publishing, Reston
Regnard C, Badger C, Mortimer P 1988 Lymphoedema: advice and treatment. Beaconsfield Publishers, Beaconsfield

Sims R, Fitzgerald V 1985 Community nursing management of the patient with ulcerating fungating malignant breast disease. Royal College of Nursing, London

Tiffany R, Borley D (eds) 1989 Oncology for nurses and health care professionals, 2nd edn. Vol. 3: Cancer nursing. Harper & Row, Beaconsfield

Tabar L, Gad A, Holmberg L H et al 1985 Reduction in mortality from breast cancer after mass screening with mammography: randomized trial from breast cancer screening working group of Swedish National Board of Health and Welfare. Lancet i: 829–832

USEFUL ADDRESSES

CancerBACUP (British Association of Cancer United Patients)
3 Bath Place
Rivington Street
London EC2A 3DR

Breast Care and Mastectomy Association of Great Britain
15–19 Britten Street
London SW3 3TZ
Helpline: 0171 867 1103
Publications: *Living with Breast Surgery*, *Coping with Cancer*, *Looking Good after Breast Surgery*
Cassette tape: Coping with Breast Surgery

The Royal Marsden Hospital
Fulham Road
London SW3 6JJ

Womens Nationwide Cancer Control Campaign (WNCCC)
Suna House
128–130 Curtain Road
London EC2A 3AR
(videos available on breast awareness)

THE URINARY SYSTEM

Lesley Selfe

8

INTRODUCTION

The practice of urology as a speciality in its own right is now commonplace in many general hospitals. Many patients who once would have been treated by a general surgeon are now referred to consultants in urology. This has come about partly in response to advances in technology, especially in the field of endoscopic and laser surgery. It has also become an accepted view that patients with urological disorders deserve the same level of understanding and sensitivity as those with gynaecological problems.

The movement within nursing towards patient-centred care in combination with the evolution of new, less traumatic and non-invasive treatments has allowed more individuals to be treated as outpatients or day cases. The appointment of clinical nurse specialists, including stoma care nurses and continence advisors, has also done much to improve standards of care.

It is important for nurses to bear in mind that patients with urological disorders often suffer from intense psychological distress. Nurses in this area of practice must develop good interpersonal skills so that they can discuss problems openly, sensitively and non-judgementally.

This chapter begins with a brief overview of the anatomy and physiology of the urinary system and of the male reproductive organs. With respect to the latter, this chapter complements the anatomy and physiology described in Chapter 7. Common disorders of the urinary tract and their treatment are then described, including infections, obstructive disorders, disorders of the bladder and some of the more important renal disorders. With regard to the male urinary system and reproductive organs, only prostatic disorders and conditions primarily affecting the urethra are considered here. Conditions more directly affecting reproductive and sexual function, such as testicular cancer and impotence, are discussed in Chapter 7.

ANATOMY AND PHYSIOLOGY

The urinary system comprises the kidneys, the ureters, the urinary bladder and the urethra. Its function is to excrete in the form of urine the waste products of metabolism.

The kidneys

Structure

The kidneys are a pair of slightly lobulated organs which lie on the posterior abdominal wall. Because of the position of the liver, the right kidney is normally slightly lower than the left. Anteriorly, the kidneys are covered by the peritoneum and the contents of the

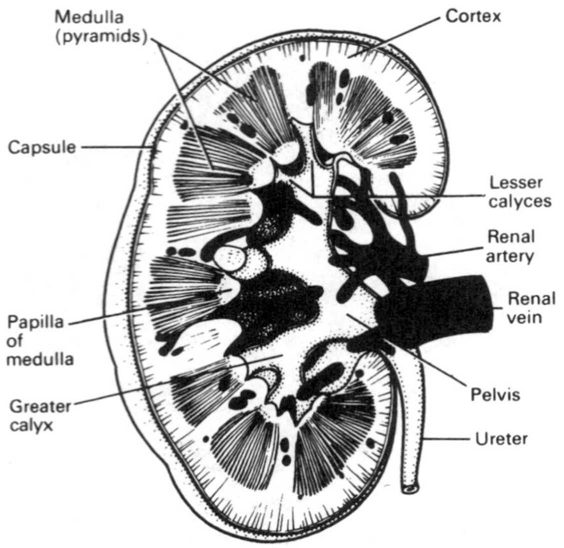

Fig. 8.1 Longitudinal section of the right kidney. (Reproduced with permission from Wilson & Waugh 1996.)

abdominal cavity. Three layers of supportive tissue surround each kidney: an inner fibrous layer, a middle fatty layer and an outer fascia. This fatty encasement is necessary for maintaining the kidneys in their normal position. Beneath this, a dark outer cortex surrounds a paler medulla, which consists of pale conical striations called the renal pyramids (see Fig. 8.1).

At the hilus, i.e. the concave medial border of the kidney, blood vessels, lymph vessels and nerves enter and leave the organ. Medial to the hilus is the flat, funnel-shaped renal pelvis, which is continuous with the ureter leaving the hilus. Extending from the pelvis into the medulla are the cup-shaped calyces; these receive from the renal papillae the urine that has been formed in the nephrons and has passed through the collecting tubules. From the calyces the urine passes into the renal pelvis, which acts as a reservoir.

The nephron. Each kidney is composed of about 1 million functional units called nephrons, which channel urine into collecting tubules. A nephron consists of a convoluted tubular system and a tuft of capillaries known as the glomerulus. The glomerulus is enclosed in the cup-shaped upper end of the tubule (Bowman's capsule; see Fig. 8.2).

The tubule has three sections: the proximal convoluted tubule, which is the longest segment; the loop of Henle, which forms a hairpin-shaped curve; and the distal convoluted tubule. The distal convoluted tubules merge to form straight collecting tubules; these ultimately terminate at the renal papillae. Some nephrons lie entirely within the cortex; others lie further within the organ such that the tubules extend deep into the medulla.

Blood supply. The kidney is supplied with blood by renal arteries arising directly from either side of the abdominal aorta immediately below the superior mesenteric artery. The renal arteries branch into smaller and smaller vessels, ultimately becoming afferent arterioles which lead into the nephrons. Each afferent arteriole subdivides further into a glomerulus. These capillaries then merge again to form an efferent arteriole which leaves the capsule and subdivides into a second network of peritubular capillaries which supplies the proximal and distal tubules, the loop of Henle and the collecting ducts. The capillaries merge into venules and then veins, eventually joining the renal vein, which in turn flows into the vena cava.

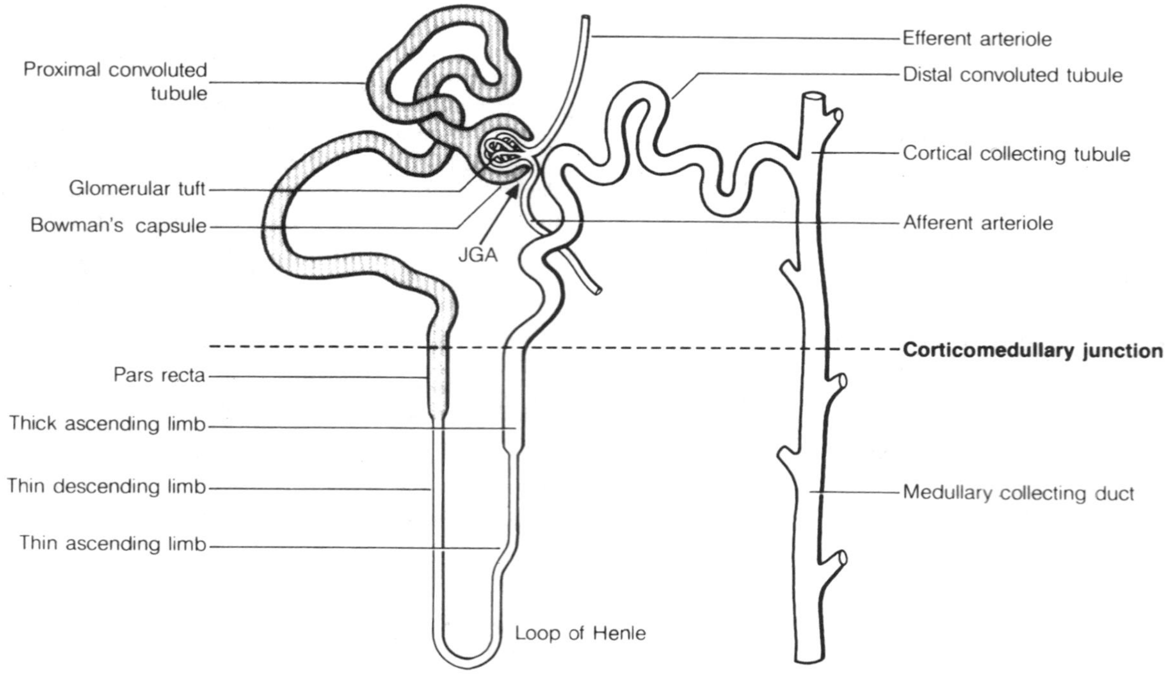

Fig. 8.2 Nephron with long loop of Henle (deep nephron). (Reproduced with permission from Edwards et al 1995.)

Box 8.1 Physical characteristics of urine. (Adapted from Anthony & Thibodeau 1983)

Volume (24 h)	1500 mL, but varies greatly according to fluid intake and insensible losses
Clarity	Transparent or clear; on standing, becomes cloudy
Colour	Amber or straw-coloured; varies according to amount voided; diet may change colour (e.g. reddish colour from eating beetroot)
Odour	'Characteristic'; on standing, develops pungent odour from formation of ammonium carbonate
Reaction	Acid, but may become alkaline if diet consists largely of vegetables. A high-protein diet increases acidity. Stale urine has alkaline reaction from decomposition of urea forming ammonium carbonate. Normal range for urine pH is 4.8–7.5, with the average about 6; it rarely becomes more acid than 4.5 or more alkaline than 8
Specific gravity	1.015–1.020; highest in morning specimen

Chemical composition

Urine is approximately 95% water, in which is dissolved several kinds of substances. The most important of these are:

- Nitrogenous wastes from protein metabolism such as urea (most abundant solute in urine), uric acid, ammonia and creatinine
- Electrolytes, mainly the following ions: sodium, potassium, ammonium, chloride, bicarbonate, phosphate and sulphate — the amounts vary according to diet and other factors
- Toxins. During disease, bacterial poisons leave the body in the urine; this is an important reason for 'pushing' fluids on patients suffering from infectious diseases, as a high fluid intake dilutes the toxins that might damage the kidney cells if they were eliminated in a concentrated form
- Pigments
- Hormones
- Abnormal constituents such as glucose, albumin, blood, casts or calculi are sometimes found

Function

The kidneys process about 180 L of blood-derived fluid daily. Of this, only about 1–2 L actually leave the body as urine; the remainder is returned to the blood. The kidney's basic function of producing urine takes place in the nephron. Here, the processes of glomerular filtration, tubular reabsorption and tubular secretion result in the removal of wastes and toxins from the blood as it passes through the kidney and in the maintenance of fluid and electrolyte balance (Marieb 1995). The characteristics of normal urine are summarised in Box 8.1.

Glomerular filtration. The initial filtration of blood takes place across a semi-permeable membrane in which fluid, electrolytes and certain non-electrolytes pass into the Bowman's capsule. Filtrate formation is a passive process and follows the same principles that account for all tissue fluid formation (see Ch. 20). However, the renal corpuscle is much more efficient because the filtration membrane is highly permeable and the glomerular pressure much higher than in other capillary beds. Hence the kidneys are able to filter 180 L of fluid daily, as compared with the 3 L/day produced by other capillary beds in the body.

The chemical composition of the glomerular filtrate is identical to that of plasma, with the following exceptions:

- the formed elements of blood are absent, i.e. red and white blood cells and platelets
- plasma proteins are absent (the presence of protein in the urine can therefore be an indication of abnormality).

In order for glomerular filtration to take place, there must be adequate blood volume in the intravascular space and sufficient glomerular hydrostatic pressure. It is the glomerular hydrostatic pressure that essentially forces the water and solutes across the filtration membrane. This pressure (55 mmHg) is opposed by the colloid osmotic pressure exerted by the glomerular plasma proteins (30 mmHg) and the capsular hydrostatic pressure (15 mmHg). Thus the net filtration pressure responsible for filtrate formation is 10 mmHg. The rate at which fluid filters from the blood to the glomerular capsule is directly proportional to the net filtration pressure. The normal filtration rate is 120–125 mL/min.

Tubular reabsorption. The greater part of reabsorption takes place in the proximal convoluted tubule. Sodium, chloride, bicarbonate and potassium are returned to the blood by passive or active transport. Glucose is actively reabsorbed. Normally, all of the glucose is reabsorbed such that none appears in the urine. However, if blood levels of glucose are too high, some will be excreted in the urine.

About 99% of the water in the filtrate is reabsorbed. The continuous removal of sodium, chloride, bicarbonate, glucose and other materials from the tubule increases the osmotic forces such that water follows the dissolved materials. This is often referred to as obligatory water reabsorption.

One of the major functions of the kidney is to maintain a constant concentration of body fluids by regulating urine concentration. It is still uncertain exactly how this is achieved, but it would seem to be the result of the function of the loop of Henle, which may act as a 'counter-current multiplying system' in which the concentrations of sodium and negative ions move through a gradient, being greatest at the base of the loop. This allows the urine to be more dilute leaving the loop of Henle than when it left the proximal tubule. This urine remains essentially unaltered unless the need to conserve fluid results in the release of antidiuretic hormone (vasopressin) by the posterior pituitary.

For further information, see Marieb (1998).

Tubular secretion. In the distal convoluted tubule and the collecting duct, sodium is reabsorbed from the tubular fluid while hydrogen and potassium ions are secreted into the fluid. This helps to regulate acid–base balance and rid the body of excessive potassium. In addition, tubular secretion can eliminate substances such as urea and uric acid, which may have been returned to the blood by passive processes, and can also dispose of substances not already in the filtrate, e.g. certain drugs.

Hormonal control of the kidney

Two hormones, antidiuretic hormone (vasopressin) and aldosterone, are important regulators of renal function.

Antidiuretic hormone (ADH) (vasopressin) is produced in the hypothalamus and stored and secreted by the posterior lobe of the pituitary gland. It affects water permeability in the distal convoluted tubule and the collecting ducts, allowing sodium, other ions and water to be reabsorbed, making the urine more concentrated. In the absence of ADH, sodium and other ions are reabsorbed, but not water. This makes the urine more dilute.

Pain, exercise, emotion and the use of narcotics or barbiturates can increase the secretion of ADH. Factors that decrease output are low plasma osmotic pressure, venous distension and alcohol consumption.

Aldosterone is produced in the outermost layer of the adrenal cortex. It acts on the distal tubule, where it increases the reabsorption of sodium (see Ch. 5, p. 150).

Other functions of the kidney

In addition to its role in removing waste products from the blood, the kidney has the following functions:

- It helps to regulate blood pressure through the maintenance of fluid volume.
- It produces the hormones renin, erythropoietin and 1,25-dihydroxycholecalciferol.

Renin is liberated through the juxtaglomerular cells and acts on angiotensinogen (a glycoprotein made in the liver and normally found in plasma), converting it into angiotensin I. Another enzyme in the pulmonary capillary bed acts on angiotensin I to convert it into angiotensin II. Angiotensin II has the following functions:

- It stimulates the release of aldosterone, which helps to enable sodium reabsorption and therefore water reabsorption. This in turn helps to maintain plasma volume.
- It has a powerful vasoconstricting effect, acting on the arterioles and precapillary sphincters to shut down the capillaries, allowing blood volume to be maintained.

Erythropoietin is produced in response to lowered O_2 in the blood. It acts on the bone marrow, stimulating the production of red blood cells (erythropoiesis; see Ch. 11, p. 431).

1,25-dihydroxycholecalciferol is synthesised in the renal tubule cells and is the active form of vitamin D which enables calcium uptake from the small intestine (see Box 5.2, p. 149).

The ureters (see Fig. 8.3)

Urine is conveyed from the pelvis of each kidney to the bladder via the ureters. The ureters are tubular structures approximately 30 cm long, ranging in diameter from 2 to 8 cm at various points along their length.

Each ureter descends behind the peritoneum from the renal hilus to the level of the bladder and comes obliquely through the bladder wall before opening into the bladder cavity on its posterior inner surface. This arrangement is such that, when the bladder fills or empties, it is compressed, closing the distal ends of the ureters; in this way, there is no back-flow into the ureters.

Each ureter is composed of three layers of tissue:

- an outer fibrous layer which is continuous with the fibrous renal capsule
- a middle layer consisting of muscle fibres spiralling clockwise and anticlockwise; contraction of the muscle layer produces peristaltic movement of urine along the ureter into the bladder
- an inner mucosa of transitional epithelium.

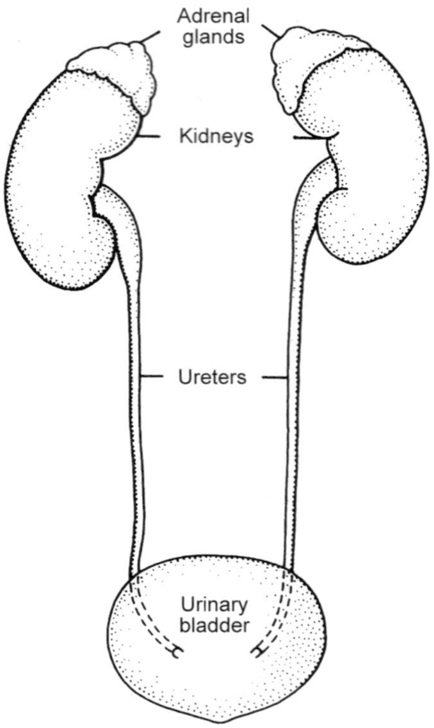

Fig. 8.3 The ureters and their relationship to the kidneys and the bladder. (Reproduced with permission from Wilson & Waugh 1996.)

The urinary bladder

The bladder is a muscular sac which acts as a reservoir for urine before it is expelled from the body. It lies behind the peritoneum in the pelvic cavity, with its anterior surface located just behind the symphysis pubis. In males, the bladder lies in front of the rectum, inferiorly to the urethra and the prostate gland. In females, it lies just anterior to the ureters and the superior section of the vagina.

Structure

The bladder is composed of four layers: an outer fibrous adventitia (except where the peritoneum covers the superior surface); a muscular layer; a submucosal layer of connective tissue; and a mucosal layer of transitional epithelium. The muscle layer consists of intermingled smooth muscle arranged in inner and outer longitudinal layers and a middle circular layer and is called the detrusor muscle.

The interior of the bladder has three orifices, two for the ureters and one for the opening of the urethra. This forms a triangle called the trigone (see Fig. 8.4).

Nerve supply to the bladder is both sensory and motor. Sympathetic nerves arise from T9 to L2 and parasympathetic and somatic nerves from S2 to S4. The motor innervation involves the parasympathetic supply to the detrusor muscle and the sympathetic supply to the trigone. Pudendal nerves under voluntary control supply the external sphincter and muscles of the perineum.

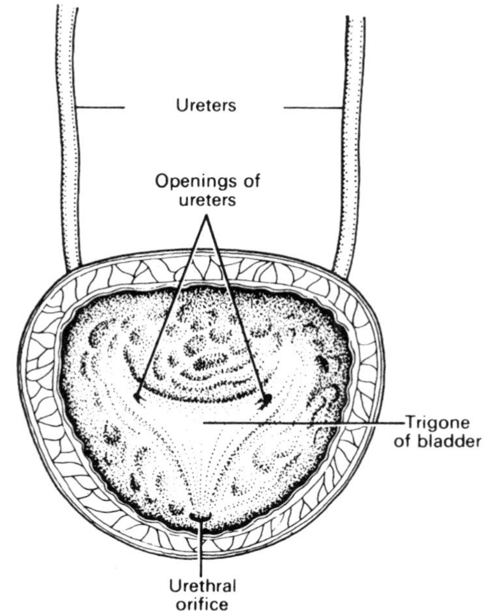

Fig. 8.4 The trigone. (Reproduced with permission from Wilson & Waugh 1996.)

The urethra

The urethra is a tube 8–9 mm in diameter which extends from the neck of the bladder to the exterior. In males, it is about 21 cm long and in females about 4 cm long. It has an outer layer of smooth muscle continuous with that of the bladder. Beneath this lies a thin, spongy layer supplied with blood vessels, lymph vessels and nerves. The innermost layer is a lining of mucous membrane continuous with that of the bladder.

The male urethra is a shared pathway by which both urine and semen reach the exterior. Originating at the urethral orifice in the bladder neck, it is surrounded by the prostate gland and ends at the tip of the glans penis. It is lined with a large number of small mucus-producing glands (Littre's glands). It has an internal sphincter composed of smooth muscle which responds to parasympathetic and sympathetic stimulation. The external urethral sphincter lies at the point where the urethra leaves the prostate; this sphincter is composed of skeletal muscle and is hence under voluntary control.

The female urethra runs behind the symphysis pubis, opening at the external urethral orifice (the meatus) just in front of the vagina. The passage of urine from the bladder through the urethra is governed by two sphincter muscles. At the opening from the bladder is an internal sphincter composed mainly of elastic tissue and smooth muscle and controlled by autonomic nerves. Near the external urethral orifice the smooth muscle is replaced by striated muscle to form an external sphincter under voluntary control.

Micturition

Micturition, the act of passing urine, is a complex physiological process governed by a number of neural controls. The bladder is very distensible, as is necessary for the storing of urine. When empty, the bladder is no more than 5–8 cm long, and its walls are thick, falling into folds. As urine fills the bladder, it expands to accommodate the increasing quantity of fluid. The muscle walls stretch and become thinner such that the bladder can comfortably hold 500 mL of urine. In extremis the bladder could hold more than 1 L. If this occurs it can be palpated above the symphysis pubis.

When the bladder contains 300–400 mL of urine, nerve fibres in the wall which are sensitive to stretch are stimulated (Wilson & Waugh 1996). In the infant or young child, this triggers a spinal reflex which results in contraction of the bladder muscle and relaxation of the internal urethral sphincter. When the nervous system is more mature, the individual is aware of a desire to pass urine and can inhibit the reflex action for a time.

Micturition is normally a painless function that occurs four to six times during the day. Decreased bladder capacity and weakened sphincter and detrusor muscles can, in elderly people and others, necessitate voiding once or twice during the night.

The composition of urine is given in Box 8.1.

Q

8.1 Keep a fluid balance chart for yourself over a 24-h period. Record all your fluid intake and the amount and frequency of all urine output. In addition, record your activities for this period. Then compare your results with those of your colleagues. If possible, also compare your results with a patient's fluid balance chart.

The male reproductive organs

The male reproductive organs are those structures responsible for the production, maturation, and delivery into the female reproductive tract of spermatozoa necessary for the fertilisation of ova. The essential organs of this system are the two testes, in which spermatogenesis occurs. The accessory organs which support the reproductive process include:

- the genital ducts — the epididymis (2), vas deferens (2), ejaculatory ducts (2) and urethra, which convey sperm to the exterior
- the glands — the seminal vesicles (2), the prostate gland and the bulbourethral (Cowper's) glands (2), which produce fluid as a vehicle for sperm
- the supporting structures — the scrotum, penis and spermatic cords.

The essential organs

The testes are oval organs 4–5 cm in length weighing 10–15 g each. They are suspended in the scrotum by the spermatic cords and are encased in three layers of tissue, as follows:

- the tunica vaginalis, or outer layer — a down-growth of the abdominal and pelvic peritoneum
- the tunica albuginea — a layer beneath the tunica vaginalis which consists of fibroelastic connective tissue containing some smooth muscle cells
- the tunica vasculosa — an inner layer made up of delicate connective tissue supplied by a network of capillaries.

Each testis contains 200–300 lobes, within which are tightly coiled seminiferous tubules. It is here that the primitive sex cells (spermatagonia) present in male babies at birth become transformed into spermatozoa (spermatogenesis). This process starts at puberty and continues throughout life.

A spermatozoon provides one-half of the genetic material required to create a new life. Each spermatozoon has a head, neck, body and tail, each with a specialised function. The head contains a highly compact package of genetic material encased in a specialised covering, called the acrosome, which contains digestive enzymes that can penetrate the ovum during fertilisation. The body contains mitochondria and the tail adenosine triphosphate (ATP); these provide energy for sperm locomotion.

The testes also produce androgens (masculinising hormones), the most important of which is testosterone, which is produced by interstitial cells (Leydig's cells). Testosterone promotes:

- maleness and male sexual behaviour
- the development and maintenance of male secondary sex characteristics and the functions of the accessory organs
- protein anabolism
- growth of bone and skeletal muscle and closure of the bony epiphyses
- a mild stimulant effect on the kidney tubule, with reabsorption of sodium and water and excretion of potassium
- inhibition of anterior pituitary secretion of the gonadotrophins follicle-stimulating hormone (FSH) and interstitial cell-stimulating hormone (ICSH). FSH stimulates the seminiferous tubules of the testes to produce spermatozoa. A negative feedback mechanism operates whereby, when testosterone levels are high, FSH and ICSH production is inhibited.

At the upper pole of the testis, the tubules combine to form the rete testis and then penetrate the tunica vaginalis to empty into the epididymis. The epididymis leaves the scrotum as the deferent duct (vas deferens) through the spermatic cords. The testes are well supplied with blood, lymph vessels and nerves from both divisions of the autonomic nervous system.

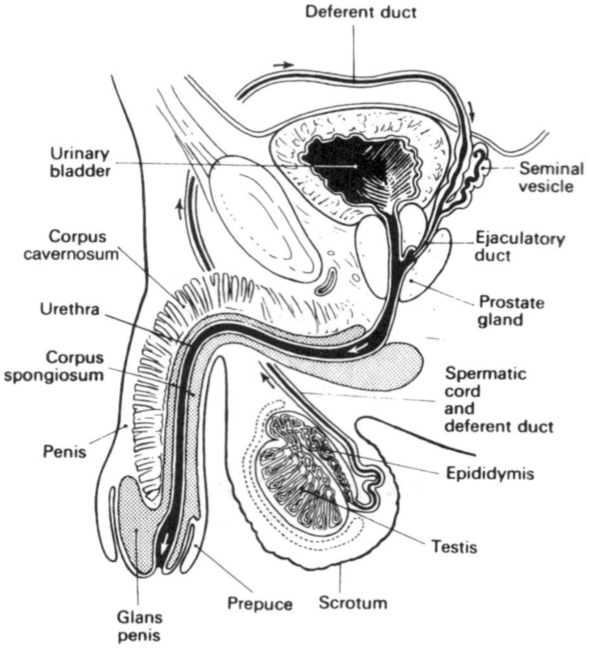

Fig. 8.5 Section of male reproductive organs. Arrows show the structures through which the spermatozoa pass. (Reproduced with permission from Wilson & Waugh 1996.)

The ductal system

The epididymis is the first part of the ductal system and forms a collection of tubules arising from the testis. The vas deferens, which is continuous with the epididymis, loops through the inguinal canal and joins the ejaculatory ducts, which pass through the prostate gland and lead into the urethra (see Fig. 8.5).

Sperm undergo a ripening process as they pass through the ductal system before ejaculation. They remain in the vas deferens for varying periods of time, depending upon the individual's degree of sexual activity. Sperm may remain in storage in the vas deferens for more than a month with no loss of fertility.

The accessory glands

The seminal vesicles are small, lobulated glands lined with secretory epithelium which lie to the posterior of the bladder at the base of the prostate. The lower end of each vesicle opens into a short duct, which joins with the deferent duct to form the ejaculatory duct.

The seminal vesicles secrete a thick, nutritive alkaline fluid that mixes with sperm on ejaculation. This fluid accounts for 30% of the volume of the seminal fluid and contains fructose and protein, which are essential to sperm motility and metabolism.

The prostate gland is a lobulated structure which lies in the pelvic cavity in front of the rectum and behind the symphysis pubis, surrounding the uppermost part of the urethra. It is palpable on rectal examination. The prostate gland secretes a thin, milky, alkaline fluid that makes up 60% of the seminal fluid; this fluid creates an environment more hospitable to sperm by giving protection from the normally acidic environment of the male urethra and female vagina. A neutral or slightly alkaline medium also increases sperm motility.

The prostate is susceptible to hyperplasia, which, because of its proximity to the urethra, can lead to urinary problems.

The bulbourethral glands are two pea-sized glands opening onto either side of the urethra. They produce a lubricating alkaline mucus that is expressed into the urethra during ejaculation, reducing its typically acidic state, and contribute less than 5% to the volume of seminal fluid.

The supporting structures

The penis is a pendulous, soft tissue structure with a root and a body. The root lies in the perineum and is attached to the anterior and lateral walls of the pubic arch. The body, which surrounds the urethra, consists of three elongated masses of erectile tissue and involuntary muscle.

The erectile tissue is supported by fibrous tissue and covered with skin. The three elongated masses, which are longitudinal in shape, consist of an encompassing central column (the corpus spongiosum) containing the urethra, and two parallel columns (the corpora cavernosa) which provide the organ's main structural support. These structures are richly supplied with blood vessels.

At the distal end of the penis, the corpus spongiosum and the corpora cavernosa expand to become the glans penis, which surrounds the urethral meatus. The covering of skin folds upon itself at the glans penis to form a movable double layer called the prepuce.

Coitus and fertilisation. The penis is supplied by autonomic and somatic nerves. Tactile, visual or mental stimulation causes a parasympathetic reflex leading to engorgement of the penis with blood and consequent erection. In the next phase, emission, sperm and secretions from the accessory glands are deposited in the posterior urethra. Finally, during ejaculation, the bladder neck closes and is followed by relaxation of the distal sphincter mechanism and spasmodic contraction of the bulbourethral muscles. This forces semen out through the urethra in spurts and is accompanied by the intensely pleasurable sensation of orgasm. Once ejaculation has taken place, the corpora cavernosa and the corpus spongiosum empty their excess of blood and the penis resumes its flaccid state.

The sperm, although anatomically complete and highly motile, undergo a further maturation process referred to as capacitation after introduction into the vagina. This enables the head of the sperm to use its hydrolytic (splitting) enzymes to penetrate the encasing membrane (the zona pellucida) of the ovum.

The millions of sperm ejaculated act collectively to produce hyaluronidase to liquefy the intracellular substance surrounding the ovum. This mass action is necessary for a single sperm to penetrate the ovum and bring about fertilisation.

The scrotum is a thin-walled pouch continuous with the abdominal wall. It is deeply pigmented and divided into two compartments, each of which contains one testis, one epididymis and the testicular end of the spermatic cord. The temperature of the testes is 2–3°C below body temperature, which helps to preserve sperm viability.

The spermatic cords. Leading from each testis is a spermatic cord consisting of a testicular artery, a testicular venous plexus, lymph vessels, a deferent duct (vas deferens) and nerves; these are all surrounded by a fibrous connective sheath.

DISORDERS OF THE URINARY SYSTEM

URINARY TRACT INFECTIONS

Urinary tract infections are second only to respiratory infections in incidence. Infection can occur in both the upper and lower urinary tracts. The risk of developing a urinary tract infection varies throughout life. In childhood and adulthood, urinary infections are common in females; in women, infections are often precipitated by sexual intercourse (Bullock et al 1994). In healthy individuals, bacteriuria of the lower urinary tract increases transiently following sexual intercourse. In the over-60 age group, urinary infections are more common in men (Whitworth & Lawrence 1994), and are often associated with bladder outflow obstruction and with the presence of a urinary catheter.

PATHOPHYSIOLOGY

Normally, the anterior urethra and, in women, the entrance to the vagina contain microorganisms. The posterior urethra and the urinary tract are sterile. The urethral mucosa has antibacterial properties and is frequently washed by sterile urine, which discourages the passage of bacteria up the urethra to the bladder, ureters and kidneys. The female ureter is short, wide and straight, and allows the passage of organisms into the urinary tract more readily than does the longer male ureter.

The predisposing factors for urinary tract infections are as follows.

Vesico-ureteric reflux. This can be:

- *Congenital primary reflux.* This occurs when there is a defect of the muscles around the vesico-ureteric junction (i.e. junction of the bladder and ureter). Abnormalities such as duplication and ectopic ureters can give rise to vesico-ureteric reflux and are one of the major causes of primary and recurrent infections in children (Laker 1994).
- *Acquired reflux.* This may be seen in patients with neuropathic dysfunction, urethral valves and (more rarely) in those with bladder outflow obstruction due to strictures. Injury to the ureteric orifice during surgery may also result in reflux. Tuberculosis and interstitial cystitis are other causes.

Obstruction. Stones or strictures can prevent the free flow of urine and interfere with the ability of the kidneys to decontaminate themselves of organisms:

- *Tumours* of the prostate, bladder and kidney can give rise to urinary tract infections.
- *Pregnancy.* Hydroureter (distension of the ureter with urine) and hydronephrosis (distension of the kidney pelvis) can occur during pregnancy and persist for some months after childbirth. It is caused by relaxation of the muscles due to the high level of progesterone and by the obstruction of the ureters by the uterus.
- *Intubation.* Nephrostomy tubes inserted into the kidney pelvis, urethral or suprapubic catheters and other drainage tubes that communicate with the urinary tract predispose the individual to infection.

Fistulae. Abnormal communication between the urinary tract and other structures (especially between the bladder and the colon) will allow organisms to enter the urinary tract.

Sexual trauma. During sexual intercourse the female urethra can be traumatised. The movement of the penis in the vagina may also milk organisms along it into the bladder and cause infection. Varied sexual practices, inadequate personal hygiene and the use of foreign bodies can all play a part.

Iatrogenic factors. Surgical and diagnostic procedures such as urethral and ureteric catheterisation, cystoscopy and other endoscopic instrumentations may exacerbate existing infections or send infection further up the urinary tract.

Pyelonephritis

Pyelonephritis, or inflammation of the renal pelvis, may occur in one or both kidneys. Bacteria may enter the urinary tract, especially the kidneys, via the bloodstream, or more commonly the bladder. Most organisms causing urinary tract infection are found in the bowel and the perineum. They are *Escherichia coli*, *Klebsiella*, *Proteus*, *Pseudomonas*, *Streptococcus faecali* and *Staphylococcus albus*.

Acute pyelonephritis

PATHOPHYSIOLOGY

In acute pyelonephritis, the kidney is usually swollen and soft and the pelvis and calyces may contain pus. The mucosal lining of the pelvis may be congested and oedematous.

Common presenting symptoms. The patient typically experiences a sudden onset of severe pain in the loin (the area of the back immediately above the buttocks) radiating to the iliac fossa. Other common features are pyrexia, rigor, nausea and vomiting.

Where cystitis (inflammation of the bladder) coexists, dysuria, frequency of micturition and discoloured urine will be noted.

MEDICAL MANAGEMENT

Investigations. Procedures will include the following:

- The collection of a midstream specimen of urine (MSU) to be cultured for evidence of a causative organism and antibiotic sensitivity. The specimen must be collected in clean conditions to prevent the introduction of contaminants (Jamieson et al 1992).

Box 8.2 Intravenous urogram or pyelogram (IVU or IVP)

This investigation, which involves the i.v. injection of an iodine-based contrast medium which is then excreted by the kidneys, allows a series of X-ray pictures of the kidneys, ureters and bladder to be taken.

Prior to the IVU, a control X-ray of the kidneys, ureters and bladder (KUB) is taken. The patient is requested to abstain from food and fluids several hours before the start of the X-rays. This helps the contrast medium to be excreted more quickly. The patient is also given an aperient to clear the bowel and thus ensure a clear image of the contrast medium on the X-ray.

Following the investigation, the patient is allowed to eat and drink again. The contrast medium will be passed when the patient voids urine, with no after-effects or change in the colour of the urine.

The IVU X-rays may show:

- absence of kidney
- obstruction of kidney
- obstruction of the ureter
- irregularities of the bladder wall — this finding may indicate the presence of a bladder tumour, diverticulum, calculi or foreign body.

- A full blood count and urea and electrolyte estimation. A raised white blood cell count and erythrocyte sedimentation rate (ESR) may be revealed in response to infection.
- An intravenous urogram (IVU) to locate any obstruction in the urinary tract (see Box 8.2). An ultrasound scan may also be performed for the same purpose.

Q **8.2** While the patient is undergoing investigations, what might the nurse do or say to reduce anxiety and help him to understand the reasons for the tests?

Treatment. The main aim of treatment is to eradicate the infection by means of antibiotic therapy. This may be commenced even before organism sensitivities are known. A more specific antibiotic can then be used following urine culture results. Analgesics, antiemetics and antipyretics may be prescribed. Oral fluids are recommended, up to 3 L/24 h.

In addition, the doctor will endeavour to determine and resolve any predisposing cause. Urine cultures will be repeated at 7 days to ensure that the infection has been eradicated.

NURSING PRIORITIES AND MANAGEMENT: ACUTE PYELONEPHRITIS

Major considerations

The patient with acute pyelonephritis of sudden onset is likely to require nursing on bed rest; she will feel lethargic and may be unable to care for herself fully.

In the acute phase, nursing priorities will include the administration of prescribed antibiotics and other medications. Attention should be given to the patient's personal hygiene and comfort, as well as to maintaining an accurate fluid balance record. Increasing fluid intake to as much as 3 L/24 h is to be encouraged as this may reduce the osmotic pressure in the renal medulla and thereby decrease the proliferation of bacteria (Pitt 1989).

As the patient recovers, the nurse should focus on giving advice regarding hygiene. The importance of attendance at outpatient appointments for assessment of renal function and investigation of further urine infection should be stressed. Follow-up may be particularly problematic if the patient feels well and is symptom-free.

Q **8.3** Mrs V is 6 months pregnant and has been admitted to the antenatal ward for investigation and monitoring of a raised blood pressure. Early one evening she complains of feeling very unwell and feverish and is visibly shivering. She is known to have a history of recurrent urinary tract infection. Refer now to Chapter 22. What would be your priorities for Mrs V's immediate care?

Chronic pyelonephritis

Chronic pyelonephritis results from recurrent urinary tract infection. In children, vesicoureteric reflux is often present.

PATHOPHYSIOLOGY

Chronic pyelonephritis is focal and irregular and may affect both kidneys. Progressive infection causes fibrosis and scarring, which gradually destroy the parenchyma. Eventually, the kidney becomes small, granular and infected.

Common presenting symptoms. This condition may be asymptomatic until the patient finally presents with features associated with renal failure. These include uraemia, lethargy, hypertension and proteinuria. Urinary frequency and dysuria may be reported.

MEDICAL MANAGEMENT

Investigations. As with acute pyelonephritis, diagnosis can be made by IVU. Urine culture should be performed and urinary tract obstruction excluded.

Treatment. Antibiotic treatment can be administered as either a short course in response to organism sensitivities or a long-term course where chronic infection proves difficult to eradicate. Where inflammation persists, renal impairment may progress to end-stage renal failure requiring treatment by dialysis (see p. 146).

NURSING PRIORITIES AND MANAGEMENT: CHRONIC PYELONEPHRITIS

Major considerations

Where the patient experiences acute episodes of inflammation, priorities may be the same as for patients with acute pyelonephritis. However, some individuals with chronic pyelonephritis only experience feelings of tiredness or of being 'under the weather'. Nevertheless, recurrence of infection is common and disturbances of renal function and end-stage renal failure are possibilities that must be taken seriously. The nurse should educate the patient regarding the condition, treatment and potential long-term complications and should emphasise the importance of attending outpatient clinics for assessment even when there are no symptoms. Where long-term antibiotic therapy is required the patient may have concerns about the necessity for such treatment and the chronic nature of her condition. The nurse should provide the opportunity for the patient to ask questions and voice concerns.

In the event that progressive renal failure occurs, the nurse should help to prepare the patient and her family for the treatment options available and for the lifestyle adjustments that will need to be made.

For further information, see Preshloch (1989).

Cystitis

Cystitis may be chronic or acute and is characterised by severe inflammation of the bladder walls. More commonly affecting women, cystitis may result from predisposing factors such as the presence of foreign bodies or stones, obstruction, tuberculosis, carcinoma in situ, chronic urinary infection and schistosomiasis.

PATHOPHYSIOLOGY

Common presenting features are scalding pain on micturition, often followed by bladder spasm resulting in an urge to pass urine a second time. Frequency, urgency, nocturia and incontinence may also be present. The patient may have a fever and complain of fatigue and abdominal discomfort.

MEDICAL MANAGEMENT

Investigations. Urine culture will identify the causative organism, although antibiotic therapy may be commenced before sensitivities are known.

Treatment. Repeat urinary cultures should be examined. Persistent infection may require long-term antibiotic treatment. The patient should be encouraged to maintain a fluid intake of at least 3 L/24 h (Pitt 1989) and to void urine frequently. This may help to wash out contaminating bacteria. The measurement and recording of fluid balance, temperature and pulse are necessary until the patient's clinical symptoms are eradicated.

Many people, however, suffer from recurrent cystitis over several years and attempt to manage the associated problems, often depending on such things as lemon barley water, over-the-counter preparations and advice found in popular magazines. This is an example of a condition for which self-help often plays an important role.

For further information, see Kilmartin (1989).

OBSTRUCTIVE DISORDERS OF THE URINARY TRACT

Disorders that cause obstruction to the flow of urine (see Fig. 8.6) are not uncommon. Although the early stages may cause only mild symptoms which are easily ignored, the progressive damage caused by abnormal pressure, infection and stone formation can lead to renal failure. The importance of early detection and intervention cannot be overemphasised.

Urinary stones (renal calculi)

The formation of stones or calculi in the urinary tract is common in Europe, North America and Japan. Worldwide, however, the incidence varies between 45 and 80/100 000. In the UK, the incidence of stone formation is about 2–3% of the population. Stone formation is more common in men than in women (M:F = 3:1), but when associated with urinary tract infection it is more frequently found in women (Hanno & Wein 1994). Children and people of black African extraction are rarely affected.

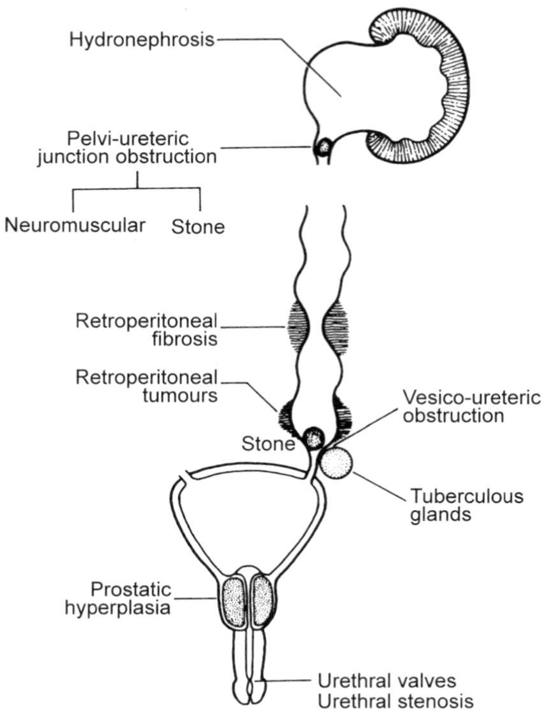

Fig. 8.6 Disorders causing obstruction to the urinary tract. (Reproduced with permission from Haslett et al 1999.)

PATHOPHYSIOLOGY

Table 8.1 summarises the features of the main types of stone that can form. In the majority of cases, however, unless there is an underlying disorder, no cause is evident. Box 8.3 identifies the predisposing factors.

Clinical features. Stone formation may occur at any point in the urinary tract. Presenting symptoms and features will depend on the stone site:

- Stones that have formed in the renal calyces are often asymptomatic, but obstruction can occur at the calyx neck, resulting in infection and giving rise to pyrexia and pain. Scarring, renal atrophy and pyocalyx can occur.
- Stones found in the calyx can travel to the renal pelvis, causing pyrexia, nausea, vomiting and renal colic.
- The main presenting symptom of upper ureteric stones is colicky pain extending across the abdomen. Haematuria (gross and microscopic) may also be noted.
- The main presenting feature of mid-ureteric and lower ureteric stones is colicky pain radiating towards the scrotum, together with urgency, frequency and abdominal distension.
- The main presenting symptoms of stone formation in the bladder are pain, dysuria, frequency and urgency.

MEDICAL MANAGEMENT

Treatment. Small calculi may pass unobstructed through the urinary tract and be excreted in the urine. Intervention is indicated if there is evidence of anaemia, infection or hydronephrosis.

Table 8.1 Chemical composition, clinical features and aetiology of urinary tract stones. (Reproduced with permission from Burkitt et al 1996)

Chemical composition	*%*	*Clinical features*	*Aetiology*
Calcium oxalate	40	Three types of stone are described: —small smooth 'hempseed' stones —small irregular 'mulberry' stones —small spiculate 'jack' stones	Most cases are idiopathic; predisposing factors include urinary stasis, infection and foreign bodies. Some are due to metabolic disorders: — hyperparathyroidism causing hypercalcaemia rather than hypercalciuria — hyperoxaluria (rare inherited disorder)
Mixed calcium oxalate and phosphate stones	15		Some are due to disorders associated with hypercalcaemia, e.g. sarcoidosis, multiple metastases, multiple myeloma, milk-alkali syndrome, overtreatment with vitamin D
Calcium and phosphate (hydroxyapatite)	15		Some patients excrete abnormally large amounts of calcium (idiopathic hypercalciuria, but without hypercalcaemia)
Magnesium ammonium phosphate	15	Typical of large 'staghorn' calculi of the pelvicalyceal system and some bladder stones	Caused by chronic infection by organisms capable of producing urease. This enzyme splits urea, forming ammonia if the urine is alkaline
Uric acid	8	Stones tend to absorb yellow and brown pigments. Pure stones are radiolucent	Occur in primary gout and also hyperuricaemia following chemotherapy for leukaemias and myeloproliferative disorders. Childhood urate bladder stones occur in some underdeveloped countries when urine pH is low
Cystine or xanthine	2	Excess urinary excretion of cystine or xanthine. Pure stones are radiolucent	Autosomal recessive inherited disorders

Box 8.3 Predisposing factors in stone formation. (Reproduced with permission from Burkitt et al 1996)

- Idiopathic (most common)
- Stasis of urine, e.g. congenital abnormalities, chronic obstruction
- Chronic urinary infection (urea-splitting organisms, e.g. *Proteus*, cause alkaline urine and the development of magnesium-ammonium-phosphate stones, typically the 'staghorn' calculi of the renal pelvis)
- Excess urinary excretion of stone-forming substances, e.g. idiopathic hypercalciuria (calcium stones), hyperparathyroidism (calcium stones), hyperoxaluria (oxalate stones), gout (uric acid stones), cysteinuria (cysteine stones), xanthinuria (xanthine stones)
- Foreign bodies, e.g. fragments of catheter tubing, self-inserted artefacts, parasites (*Schistosoma* ova)
- Diseased tissue, e.g. renal papillary necrosis
- Multifactorial, e.g. prolonged immobility, children in developing countries

Conservative management. Calcium-chelating agents and avoidance of calcium-rich foods may be indicated where increased absorption of calcium is responsible for calculi formation. Acidification or alkalination of urine may prevent stones which form in these conditions. Fluid intake should be enough to ensure a urine output of 2 L/24 h. The drinking of large quantities of fluid serves no useful purpose. The rationale behind this practice is to produce sufficient urine flow to flush out the stone, but in practice the presence of a continued obstruction will simply result in further distension of the collecting system and make matters worse. Normal hydration is therefore recommended.

For further information, see Bullock et al (1994).

MANAGEMENT OF ACUTE RENAL COLIC

Investigations. Procedures are listed in Table 8.2.

Treatment. The patient with renal stones may be acutely ill, suffering from excruciating, spasmodic pain arising in the loin region and radiating to the groin. Pain is caused by small calculi being moved along the ureter by peristaltic movements, by impaction and by obstruction of urine. Bed rest and analgesia are the first line of treatment.

Medications include i.m. pethidine (50–100 mg given 3- to 4-hourly), which produces prompt but short-acting relief as well as an antispasmodic effect. Diclofenac sodium (100 mg given per rectum, usually at night) is a prostaglandin synthetase inhibitor which reduces renal blood flow and urination. It has an antispasmodic and anti-inflammatory effect and is long-acting. Nausea may be relieved by an antiemetic such as i.m. prochlorperazine (12.5 mg) (Trounce & Gould 1997).

Flush-back of calculi and stenting. This procedure affords temporary relief when a small calculus causes obstruction and pain in the ureter. The stone is flushed back to the pelvis of the kidney. A small silicone tube, called a stent, is positioned in the ureter from the pelvi-ureteric junction to the bladder. This stent is left in position to hold the stone in place. Further treatment to remove the stone can now be planned. The stent should not be left for more than 6 weeks. If the planned treatment cannot be carried out by the end of this period, it should be changed.

Insertion of a nephrostomy tube is indicated when obstruction in the kidney or the ureter cannot be relieved by flush-back and stenting (see Fig. 8.7, Box 8.4). This is carried out under X-ray control, usually with a local anaesthetic. A small silicone tube is placed

Table 8.2 Some investigations used for patients with renal calculi. (Adapted from Haslett et al 1999, with permission)

Type of investigation	*Test*	*Purpose*
Investigation of urinary tract	Examination of urine for protein, RBC, WBC	Indicates abnormality of urinary tract
	MSU	Urinary infection
	Plain film abdomen	Shows opaque calculi, nephrocalcinosis
	IVU	Shows all calculi obstruction and abnormalities of urinary tract
Investigation of renal function	Blood urea, plasma creatinine	
	Creatinine clearance	
Investigation to determine underlying cause	Chemical analysis of calculus	Provides information as to what investigations to pursue
	Plasma calcium, phosphate	Hypercalcaemia
	Plasma parathyroid hormone	If hypercalcaemia is present to investigate possible hyperparathyroidism
	24 h urine calcium (× 2)	Hypercalciuria
	Plasma urate, 24 h urine urate (× 2)	In patients with urate stones or calcium stones
	24 h urine cystine (× 2)	In patients with cystine stones
	24 h urine oxalate (× 2)	Hyperoxaluria

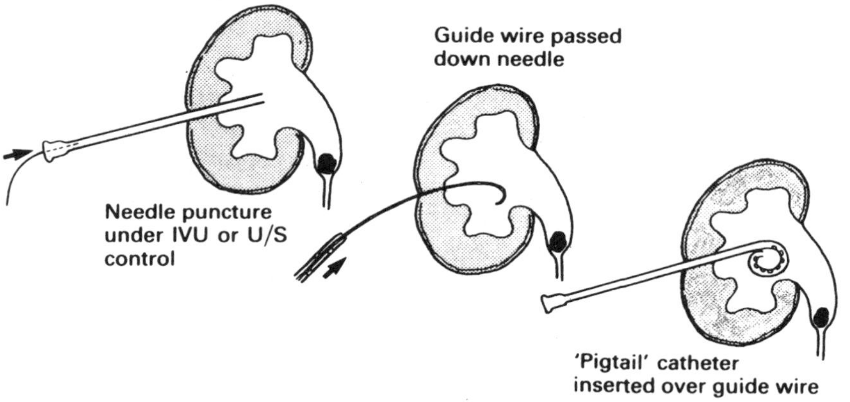

Fig. 8.7 Percutaneous nephrostomy. (Reproduced with permission from Bullock et al 1994.)

percutaneously into the collecting system of the kidney. The tube is held in place by a suture and connected to a closed-system drainage bag.

Ureteroscopic removal of calculi. This procedure is suitable in the treatment of small calculi in the ureter. The ureteric orifice is dilated cystoscopically and a ureteroscope, to which a 'stone basket' is attached, is introduced into the ureter. The basket is opened out to ensnare the stone. The basket and stone are then withdrawn.

Rigid ureteroscopes are now available which can be inserted under direct vision. The surgeon is able to see the stone and can disintegrate it in situ before removing the smaller fragments in a 'basket' (see Burkitt et al 1996).

Extracorporeal shock wave lithotripsy (ESWL). This procedure is the treatment of choice for the majority of calculi, both renal and ureteric (Dawson & Whitfield 1994). It effectively treats 70–80% of cases (Hanno & Wein 1994). Large calculi are broken up by means of this technique before percutaneous removal.

There are several lithotripsy centres in the UK, but some patients have to travel some distance for this treatment. Second-generation lithotripsers allow most patients to be treated without anaesthetic. However, sometimes the patient's age, the degree of pain or the size and position of the stone make general anaesthetic necessary. Some patients may require more than one treatment.

Box 8.4 Stenting

The stents used by most surgeons are called 'double-J' or 'pigtail' stents and have small holes down most of the length of their tubing. These stents are self-retaining and must be removed endoscopically.

Some surgeons use an infant feeding tube as a stent following pyeloplasty, pyelolithotomy or ureterolithotomy. Infant feeding tubes are self-retaining to a degree, but the patient will need a urethral catheter in situ to keep the tube in place. When the catheter is removed the patient may pass the feeding tube without intervention. If this does not happen within 24 h, endoscopic removal will be required.

The patient lies on a special table, with the area to be treated over a special dish containing water. This dish produces shock waves from a spark generator, which are then reflected to focus on the kidney stone, causing it to disintegrate. The whole procedure is performed under specialised X-ray and ultrasonic control. The disintegrated or powdered calculus is then allowed to pass down the ureter over the next few days.

Percutaneous nephrolithotomy (PCNL). This procedure is used to remove calculi lying within the kidney. Large staghorn calculi may need breaking up by ESWL first.

PCNL is performed under X-ray and ultrasound control. The patient will normally have a general anaesthetic. The kidney is punctured and the tract into the kidney is dilated to allow the nephroscope and a variety of grasping instruments to be inserted. The stone can then be removed or broken down into fine powder by ultrasonic probes (see Fig. 8.8). This powder can be aspirated through the centre of the probe.

Sometimes an electrohydraulic probe is used. This produces shock waves in the irrigating fluid to the kidney and results in the stone splitting into several fragments.

At the end of the procedure, a large nephrostomy tube with a smaller tube running down its centre is left in position to allow drainage and to prevent haematoma formation. This also allows access for a nephrogram 24–48 h postoperatively to assess the effectiveness of treatment.

Nephrogram. No anaesthetic is required for this procedure. A contrast medium is injected down the smaller tube of a nephrostomy tube into the kidney. X-rays can then be taken and any fragments of calculi identified. Provided that there are no fragments left, the tubes can be removed.

Ureterolithotomy. This open surgery is appropriate in the treatment of calculi occurring mid-ureter and causing obstruction that cannot be dealt with any other way. An X-ray to identify the position of the stone will determine the incision to be made. The ureter is exposed and opened and the stone removed. The ureter is repaired either by removing a small section or by suturing the opening. A stent is usually left in place, positioned along the length of the ureter. This allows the ureter to heal and prevents leakage. A wound drain will be left in position in the normal way to prevent haematoma formation. The stent will normally be removed after 7 days.

Pyelolithotomy. This open surgery can be used for calculi in the pelvis of the kidney which are causing an obstruction that cannot be removed in any other way. The procedure involves first exposing the affected kidney and then opening the pelvis of the kidney to remove the stone. Sometimes it is not possible to remove all of a staghorn calculus (see Table 8.1) in this way, in which case further incisions into the surrounding renal tissue (nephrolithotomy) are necessary. A stent will be left in place for 7 days.

NURSING PRIORITIES AND MANAGEMENT: ACUTE RENAL COLIC

Major considerations

A patient admitted with renal colic can often do little more than cope with the pain, and is often unable to answer questions or to follow advice and instructions until the pain is relieved. Once the acute attack has subsided, the patient should be allowed to rest. Only then will she feel able to attend to all the necessary explanations relating to investigations and treatment. Nursing Care Plan 8.1 outlines the priorities of nursing care for a patient admitted with acute renal colic.

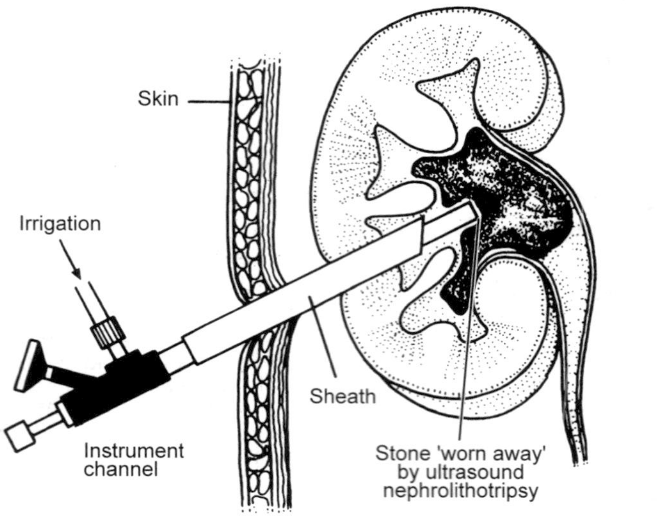

Fig. 8.8 Percutaneous stone removal. (Reproduced with permission from Bullock et al 1994.)

Following specific interventions

Flush-back and stenting

The patient should be prepared for a general anaesthetic as discussed in Chapter 26. Normally, only a short-acting anaesthetic is required. Priorities in postoperative nursing care are as follows:

- To record observations, temperature, pulse and blood pressure and to watch for signs of infection.
- To monitor urine output and record volume and colour of urine on the fluid chart. A decrease in volume may indicate obstruction. Haematuria may indicate trauma, but some haematuria is to be expected.
- To encourage a fluid intake of 3 L to prevent infection.
- To administer analgesics if the patient is in pain. Severe pain must be reported to medical staff, as this may indicate trauma, a misplaced stent, or return of obstruction.

Discharge advice. The patient should be advised:

- to continue to drink 3 L daily
- to take mild analgesics such as paracetamol or co-proxamol if in pain
- to seek help from the GP if urine output is bloodstained or 'burning'.

The patient should also be advised when follow-up treatment will take place and what this will entail. If treatment is not within 6 weeks, it must be impressed upon the patient that it is very important to have the stent changed. If it is not changed sediment and crystals will build up around it and form more calculi.

Extracorporeal shock wave lithotripsy (ESWL)

The role of the nurse in the ESWL unit includes giving reassurance to the patient and her family, explaining what to expect, administering any prescribed medication, encouraging the patient to drink following the procedure and giving discharge advice.

Nursing Care Plan 8.1 Nursing care for a patient admitted with acute renal colic

Potential problem	*Action*	*Desired outcome*
1. Pain of a potentially excruciating nature	❒ Administer prescribed analgesics ❒ Evaluate effect of analgesics: return to patient in 30 min: • ask if she is pain-free • observe for evidence of pain, e.g. raised pulse rate, sweating and evidence of neurogenic shock (see Ch. 18)	Pain is relieved
2. Frequency and urgency of micturition	❒ Locate urinal within reach of patient	Sensations decline as pain is relieved
3. Nausea and vomiting	❒ Administer prescribed antiemetics ❒ Evaluate effect of treatment: return to patient in 30 min ❒ Locate vomit bowl within patient's reach	Patient obtains relief from feelings of nausea and from vomiting
4. Fluid and electrolyte imbalance	❒ Institute i.v. fluids if patient is unable to take adequate fluid orally	Fluid and electrolytes are maintained at satisfactory levels
5. Ureteric obstruction	❒ Check and record blood pressure ❒ Observe BP trends and report elevations ❒ Measure urine output; report reduction in volume ❒ Observe for haematuria and passage of stones	Any obstruction is recognised immediately
6. Urinary tract infection	❒ Check and record temperature; report pyrexia ❒ Check and record pulse rate; observe trends and report elevations	Infection is prevented or immediately recognised
7. Non-passage of small calculi	❒ Encourage normal volumes of fluid intake ❒ Alleviate nausea and vomiting ❒ Check urine for presence of calculi (use plastic urinal to prevent sticking of calculi)	Passage and collection for analysis of small calculi
8. Inability to perform personal hygiene	❒ Offer wash and change of bed gown as required, particularly if sweating is profuse	Patient is clean and comfortable Self-esteem is maintained
9. Difficulty in finding a comfortable position in bed	❒ Assist patient to find a comfortable position ❒ Evaluate position regularly; ask the patient if she is comfortable	Patient is relaxed and comfortable
10. Anxiety	❒ Give patient the opportunity to voice concerns ❒ Provide information about the condition, investigations and treatment ❒ Ensure the nurse call system is close at hand at all times	Patient has an understanding of the condition and has reduced anxiety about outcome

The patient may receive an oral premedication such as diazepam or temazepam prior to treatment. The treatment is not normally painful. Anxiety may be experienced due to the noise from the shock waves and the requirement to lie still for 1–1.5 h. Playing recorded music may help to alleviate anxiety and boredom.

Following treatment, frusemide may be given orally to increase diuresis and help the stone fragments to pass. The patient will normally stay in the lithotripsy unit until urine has been passed. Prophylactic antibiotics and analgesics may also be given.

Most patients will be able to return home and continue with their normal daily activities. However, a small percentage will need hospital admission during the first week post-treatment because of colicky pain, oedema and, occasionally, obstruction of the ureter. This will sometimes settle with no further treatment, but a stent may need to be inserted to allow the oedema to settle down.

Discharge advice. The patient should be advised:

- to drink 3 L of fluid a day, to help prevent infection and to help the gravel to pass down the urinary system
- to expect some haematuria and gravel when passing urine
- to take prescribed analgesics, but if pain increases to see the GP or report back to the hospital
- to attend a follow-up appointment about 6 weeks later to have further X-rays taken to assess the effect of the treatment.

Percutaneous nephrolithotomy (PCNL)

Preoperatively, the patient should be prepared for a general anaesthetic (see Ch. 26). Postoperatively, the patient is likely to return to the ward with:

- a urethral catheter in situ
- an i.v. infusion of clear fluids
- a nephrostomy tube in the affected kidney.

The latter will be a large-bore tube with a narrower tube running down its centre. These tubes will normally be sutured into position and enclosed in a System-2 urostomy drainage bag attached to a large 2 L drainage bag.

Priorities in the management of the nephrostomy tube are to maintain a closed drainage system in order to prevent infection, and to monitor drainage. The nurse responsible must:

- check the position and the placement of the nephrostomy tube
- help the patient into a position that is comfortable and allows the tube to drain
- empty the drainage bag when necessary and record the volume and colour of output
- remember that the urine will take the path of least resistance, so most of the output from the affected kidney will discharge via the nephrostomy tube.

The urethral catheter is normally removed 24 h following surgery. The i.v. infusion is discontinued at the same time, if the patient is able to drink normally. A nephrogram is carried out 48 h following surgery, and the nephrostomy tube removed if treatment has been successful. Following removal of the nephrostomy tube, the patient may continue to pass urine via the puncture site. This will normally cease after 12–24 h.

The patient may have colicky pain following the removal of the tube, as the urine must now redirect itself via the correct route. Analgesia can be given, and the patient should be asked to lie on the affected side. This will take the pressure off the affected kidney, and the drainage will pass via the puncture site.

Once the drainage has ceased from the puncture site, a small, dry dressing can be applied and the patient discharged home. Occasionally the nephrostomy tube may need to be left in situ for a prolonged period because further treatment may be necessary. In this case, the patient may be discharged home into the care of the GP and community nurse.

Ureterolithotomy or pyelolithotomy

Preoperative preparation is as normal, including skin preparation and shaving of the area to be operated upon (see Ch. 26).

If the patient has an uneventful 2- or 3-day postoperative period, and a double-J stent or pigtail stent has been used, she may be discharged home into the care of the GP and community nurse, returning as a day case to the hospital for removal of the stent. The community nurse will check the wound and take note of the patient's temperature and urine output. Sutures are removed from the wound at 7–10 days. If an infant feeding tube has been used as a stent (see Box 8.4), then the urethral catheter will remain in situ for 5–6 days. In this case, the patient may need to stay in hospital until the stent and sutures have been removed.

Urethral strictures

PATHOPHYSIOLOGY

A stricture is a narrowing within a structure which may arise from inflammation, muscular spasm or neoplastic occlusion. Most urethral strictures are caused by trauma, as in pelvic fracture, self-inflicted introduction of foreign bodies, investigative instrumentation of the urethra (e.g. cystoscopy) or the presence of an indwelling urethral catheter (see Fig. 8.9). Infections such as non-specific urethritis and gonorrhoea may result in stricture formation. In women, inflammation caused by endometriosis and the trauma of pregnancy may, in some cases, result in strictures.

Common presenting symptoms which can prove to be both distressing and frustrating are poor urinary flow, a feeling of incomplete bladder emptying, frequency, dysuria or haematuria, and dribbling incontinence secondary to chronic urinary retention.

MEDICAL MANAGEMENT

Tests and investigation required are flow rate studies, urethrography, urethroscopy, IVP, renogram and full blood screening.

Treatment options include the following:

Urethrotomy. The optical urethrotome allows the surgeon to divide the urethral stricture under direct vision. A silicone catheter would normally be left in place for up to 48 h postoperatively.

Stenting. The stricture is held open by the stent. Over time the stent is gradually covered with epithelial tissue, rendering it continuous with urethral tissue (Laker 1994).

Self-dilatation. Often used in conjunction with urethrotomy, this technique involves using a self-lubricating urethral catheter on a regular basis to increase the urethral diameter and keep the urethral passage open.

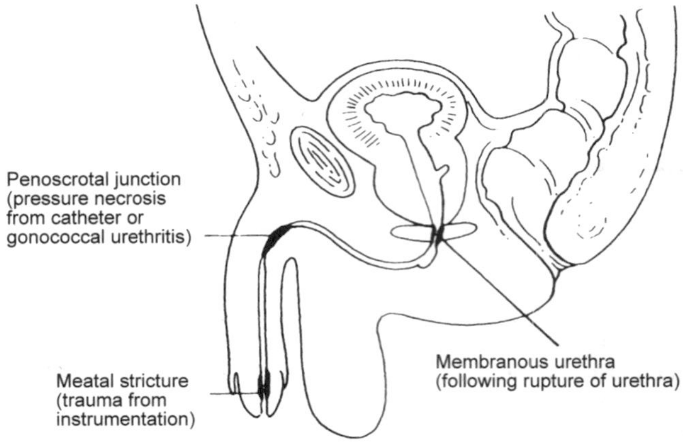

Fig. 8.9 Common sites and causes of urethral stricture. (Reproduced with permission from Forrest et al 1995.)

Urethroplasty. Usually performed in two stages, this procedure aims to open the narrowed urethra by insertion of a split-skin graft. This surgery requires a longer stay in hospital and is normally performed only after other treatments have failed.

NURSING PRIORITIES AND MANAGEMENT: URETHRAL STRICTURES

Q

8.4 As a nurse looking after Mr E (see Case History 8.1), what could you do to help him come to terms with the idea of performing self-dilatation and to feel more positive about it?

Major patient problems

Urethral strictures can cause lifelong disability (Burkitt et al 1996), and when any catheterisation or instrumentation of the urinary tract is necessary, great delicacy is required. Catheterisation should be performed only when absolutely necessary and, as Burkitt et al (1996) put it, urological instruments should be 'hammered into place with a feather'.

Self-dilatation

The patient faced with the prospect of needing to perform self-dilatation on an ongoing basis will need moral support and encouragement from the health care team. A specialist nurse will explain the procedure initially and guide the patient through it. He will also ensure that the patient receives continuing support as needed. It will also be helpful for the named nurse to emphasise the following points:

- No-one need know that the individual is using this technique.
- Although the idea is not very appealing, this treatment will minimise the risk of further admission to hospital and time off work.
- There is always a risk of infection, but this can be minimised with good hygiene, washing of hands and meatus, and adequate intake of fluids.
- Dilatation will be necessary once a day at first, but as time goes on it can normally be reduced to once a week.
- Irregular working schedules should not pose a problem; the patient can work out a routine that is convenient for her.

Fibrosis

PATHOPHYSIOLOGY

Fibrosis is the formation of excessive fibrous connective tissue within a structure. Fibrosis around the ureters predisposes them to obstruction; the cause of the fibrosis is often unknown. This condition, known as retroperitoneal fibrosis, is not neoplastic but can result in damage to renal function. Other external causes of fibrosis are post-radiotherapy treatment, scarring arising from other surgical procedures, and aortic aneurysm. Fibrosis within structures (e.g. ureters/urethra) is usually secondary to traumatic procedures.

Case History 8.1 Mr E

Mr E, a 35-year-old fireman, was having difficulty in passing urine. Two years previously, he had been involved in an accident in which he suffered crush injuries to his pelvis and urethra. At that time he had had a suprapubic catheter (i.e. a catheter inserted into the bladder via the abdominal wall) for 6 weeks.

On the more recent occasion, he was referred to the urologist by his GP for two reasons. Firstly, Mr E had had repeated urinary tract infections over the last year. Secondly, he had noticed that for the last 6 months there was a difference in the time it took him to pass urine and that the stream was thinner than normal.

After a full investigation, the surgeon decided that the best course of action would be to perform an optical urethrotomy, followed by the patient being taught to perform self-dilatation. Mr E agreed to have the operation, although he did not like the idea of performing self-dilatation. When given the opportunity to discuss this, he expressed the following concerns:

- 'What if my friends and relatives find out?'
- 'I don't want to put a tube up there. How do I do it?'
- 'What about infection?'
- 'How often will I need to do this?'
- 'I work shifts. How can I do this?'

DISORDERS OF THE PENIS AND MALE URETHRA

Phimosis

In this condition, the foreskin or prepuce of the penis is too tight to be retracted over the glans penis. It may be caused by early attempts to draw back the foreskin before it has naturally separated or developed fully in size. Retraction before separation is complete tears the surfaces that are still adhered. These will heal, forming scar tissue, but may later cause difficulty with retraction and hygiene.

A poorly performed circumcision operation may also contribute to a phimosis. The scar tissue will need to be separated and a recircumcision performed. Phimosis is very rarely a congenital defect.

PATHOPHYSIOLOGY

The natural separation of the two layers of skin from the glans penis normally occurs by about the age of 2 years. Following separation, the prepuce should be retracted to permit daily hygiene. Retained smegma (the white collection) which results from poor personal hygiene can give rise to inflammation and infection and has been implicated as a cause for carcinoma of the penis.

Common presenting symptoms. Phimosis often causes balanoposthitis, which is an inflammation of both the glans penis (balanitis) and the prepuce (posthitis). Presenting features include itching, a white discharge, pain, discomfort and bleeding at sexual intercourse, and sometimes urinary retention.

MEDICAL MANAGEMENT

Treatment. Initial treatment may be with antibiotics or anticandidal agents. If the individual is sexually active, he and his partner will both require treatment to prevent the infection being passed back and forth. Circumcision is the treatment of choice and may have to be performed as an emergency if urinary retention has occurred (see Box 8.5 and Case Histories 8.2 and 8.3).

Box 8.5 Circumcision

Circumcision, the surgical removal of the prepuce (foreskin), may be indicated for penile carcinoma (Hanno & Wein 1994), balanitis or posthitis (which usually occur simultaneously), candidal infection, phimosis or adherent prepuce; these conditions generally affect adults. Circumcision may also be performed in accordance with religious beliefs, in which case the procedure is usually performed in childhood.

The main complications of circumcision are infection and bleeding. Painful erections in the immediate postoperative period can usually be relieved by the application of a local anaesthetic gel. Postoperative swelling or oedema may make micturition difficult. Dribbling or urinary leakage to the wound area can delay or prevent wound healing and cause secondary infection. The insertion of a urethral catheter may be necessary to relieve this problem in order that wound healing may take place.

NURSING PRIORITIES AND MANAGEMENT: PHIMOSIS

Prevention

Health education of the parents is important in the early years. It should be stressed that retraction of the foreskin for cleansing is unnecessary before puberty. Normal bathing or showering routines should suffice. After puberty the boy will need to pull back the foreskin to clean away smegma that accumulates around the glans penis.

Promoting wound healing after circumcision

The nurse can promote wound healing by the following means:

- teaching good personal hygiene to the newly circumcised person
- washing the wound area daily with soap and water and applying a protective, non-adhesive dressing to prevent clothing disturbing wound healing
- providing more frequent washing and dressing changes should urine leakage onto the wound or dressing occur
- counselling the sexually active patient to refrain from sexual intercourse until the wound is well healed.

Q **8.5** How would your discharge advice to Mr A in Case History 8.2 compare with that given to Mr C in Case History 8.3? Would you make any changes, omissions or additions in your advice to the older man? What assumptions would prompt such changes? Are all of these assumptions fair?

Case History 8.2 Mr A

Mr A, aged 20, presented to his GP with bleeding from the foreskin following sexual intercourse. He was concerned as this was the sixth occurrence.

On examination the foreskin was found to be very tight, and the GP advised circumcision. Referral was made to the local consultant urologist, and Mr A was put on the waiting list. After only a few weeks he was admitted as a day case for circumcision.

Before discharge, he was given the following advice verbally and in written form by nursing staff:

- Take daily baths
- Do not go straight back to work. Avoid walking around for the next few days
- Change underwear daily. Do not wear anything tight until the wound has healed
- You must be able to pass urine before leaving hospital, and you should drink at least 3 L of fluids in 24 h to prevent urinary tract infection
- If you have pain, take a simple analgesia such as paracetamol every 4–6 h for the first 48 h
- At any sign of swelling, redness or fever, go and see your GP
- Sexual intercourse should be avoided until the skin is healed and feels normal
- Should any other problems arise, report to your GP or, if necessary, return to the hospital
- Change the dressing if it becomes wet with urine. Use a non-stick dressing.

Case History 8.3 Mr C

Mr C, a 70-year-old widower, was referred by his GP to a urologist as an emergency, because he was in pain and having difficulty passing urine. On examination it was found that he had a tight foreskin and it was difficult to see the meatus. On abdominal examination he appeared to be retaining urine. Ultrasound confirmed that there was approximately 500 mL in his bladder.

Mr C was admitted to the ward with instructions that he would be operated on within the next 2 h for circumcision and urethral catheterisation. He was told that the catheter may need to stay in position for 24–48 h, depending on his general condition, and that his stay in hospital would be between 48 h and 1 week.

Paraphimosis

Paraphimosis is a condition in which a foreskin that has been retracted over the glans penis cannot be returned to its usual position. The swollen band of foreskin obstructs the circulation to the glans, which in turn becomes swollen and painful. The condition may subside in a few hours, with general relief gained from taking a mild analgesic.

Cold compresses applied to the penis may help to relieve the swelling and pain. The doctor or nurse may be able to manipulate the glans back under the foreskin with or without anaesthesia. If this is unsuccessful, a dorsal slit may be made in the foreskin. There remains a risk of recurrence of the paraphimosis and a circumcision may be advisable at a later date.

Congenital disorders of the urethra and penis

At birth, an infant is examined to confirm its sex and to make sure that expected bodily structures are present. In boys the urethral meatus is normally seen at the anterior tip of the glans penis. Occasionally a malformation of the urethra is identified as a congenital defect.

Hypospadias

In the condition of hypospadias, the meatus of the urethra is found in a position on the undersurface of the glans penis. The condition is usually treated quite effectively by enlargement of the meatus by plastic surgery. In some cases the urethral orifice is positioned further back on the lower surface of the penis, and this will complicate treatment. To allow a series of operations to take place, a temporary perineal urethrostomy may be formed, so creating a urinary diversion. Time is gained for the promotion of wound healing as a new urethral meatus is created.

Epispadias

The condition of epispadias is one in which the urethra opens onto the upper surface, or dorsum, of the penis. The meatus of the urethra may be positioned anywhere along the length of the penile surface. The epispadias may coexist with other serious congenital abnormality involving a poorly developed anterior section of the urinary bladder and abdominal wall. Surgical reconstruction is likely to be complex and may involve transplantation of ureters.

DISORDERS OF THE PROSTATE

Benign prostatic hyperplasia

The prostate gland increases in size with age, reaching about 20–25 g by the time the individual is 20 years old. In individuals over the age of 45, the smooth muscle segments atrophy and are replaced by collagen fibres. As ageing progresses, connective tissue accumulates, resulting in benign prostatic hyperplasia. The latter condition is the most common neoplastic growth in men. Studies suggest that one in three men in the UK over 50 will develop benign prostatic hyperplasia and that this incidence will continue to rise with the increasing age of the population (Webb & Simpson 1997). The cause of benign prostatic hyperplasia is unknown, but it is thought that it may be associated with reduced androgen secretions.

Bladder outflow obstruction can occur for a number of reasons (see Box 8.6), but the most common cause is benign prostate hyperplasia.

PATHOPHYSIOLOGY

Stasis of the urine in the bladder and a build-up of pressure in the bladder and ureters predispose the individual to infection, the formation of stones and possible renal failure. The bladder becomes enlarged, forming bundles called trabeculae. Diverticula may also be noted. If left untreated, obstructive effects will develop (see Fig. 8.10).

Common presenting symptoms. The enlargement of the gland may be asymptomatic, perhaps noted only on a routine rectal examination. However, as the hyperplasia increasingly distorts and compresses the urethra and even the bladder, an inability to void normally will become obvious. Many men tolerate symptoms indefinitely, seeing them as just 'old men's problems' that have to be accepted. Presenting symptoms include:

- difficulty in starting micturition
- difficulty in stopping micturition
- frequency and urgency
- poor flow and force in the urine passed
- dribbling and incontinence
- a feeling that the bladder is never completely emptied.

In addition, a history of recurrent urinary tract infections may be given. Increasing pressure due to obstruction can eventually result in renal impairment.

Acute urinary retention may be the single presenting feature, particularly if the prostate gland suddenly increases in size or if infection occurs. Some patients present with chronic urinary retention, sometimes associated with haematuria and urethral bleeding. Abnormal voiding patterns and disruption of daytime activities or sleep patterns can affect the individual's ability to work and interact normally with colleagues, partners and family. Bedwetting or

Box 8.6 Bladder outflow obstruction

Causes
- Benign prostatic hyperplasia
- Bladder calculi
- Bladder tumour
- Diuretics
- Neurological disturbances
- Phimosis
- Prostatic carcinoma
- Urethral strictures, stenosis, trauma

Common symptoms
- Double voiding
- Dribbling post-voiding
- Dysuria
- Force of urine flow/stream
- Frequency
- Hesitancy
- Haematuria (occasional)
- Nocturia
- Incontinence
- Interrupted stream
- Urgency
- Urinary retention

Inadequate emptying of the bladder can result in a build-up of residual urine, increasing the risk of urinary tract infection and the incidence of bladder stone formation.

Diagnosis
Diagnosis of bladder flow obstruction may be assisted by:
- Blood screen of urea, electrolytes and creatinine
- Endoscopy — urethroscopy and cystoscopy
- History of symptoms
- Physical examination
- Ultrasound scan — residual urine volume and upper urinary tract
- Urinalysis
- Urine culture
- Urodynamic evaluation
- Voiding cystometrogram

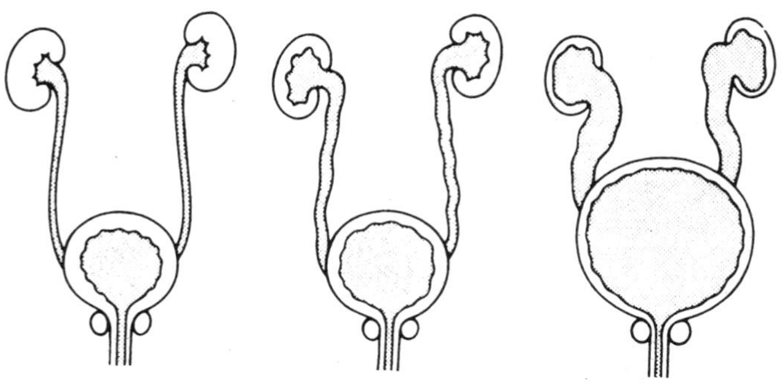

Fig. 8.10 The progressive effects of obstruction from an enlarged prostate gland. The bladder, ureters and kidneys all become affected. (Reproduced with permission from Charlton 1984.)

urinary incontinence may cause embarrassment and distress. Embarrassment about such symptoms may also result in failure to seek professional help until the condition becomes unbearable.

MEDICAL MANAGEMENT

Investigations. Diagnosis can be made by rectal examination; the prostate gland will feel large, elastic and uniform (Haslett et al 1999). Investigations will include:

- IVU (see Box 8.2)
- urinary flow rates
- renal function tests
- full blood count
- serum acid phosphatase or serum prostate-specific antigen (PSA) to eliminate diagnosis of carcinoma
- MSU
- transurethral ultrasound scan and/or biopsy (see Box 8.7).

Treatment. Prostatectomy is indicated if there is significant outflow obstruction. Transurethral resection of the prostate gland (TURP) is the operation of choice. Where the gland is too large to resect transurethrally, an open procedure is used, most commonly taking the retropubic or transvesical approach. Other treatments include (Downey 1997):

- drug therapies
- laser therapy
- transurethral needle obliteration
- transwave thermotherapy
- prostatic stent insertion.

For further information, see Willis (1992), Garraway & Alexander (1997) and Webb & Simpson (1997).

TURP. Prior to commencing the resection, a cystoscope is passed to view the bladder (see Box 8.7). A resectoscope is then passed and small sections are chipped away from the prostatic lobes, removing the material that had been intruding into the urethra and bladder neck. Irrigation fluid of a non-electrolyte solution, glycine, constantly flushes out the bladder during the procedure (an electrolyte solution is contraindicated in the presence of diathermy). Most commonly, irrigation continues postoperatively, as the operative bed can give rise to considerable bleeding and clots could lead to obstruction.

Potential postoperative complications of TURP are:

- haemorrhage — evident as haematuria
- clot retention
- extravasation — escape of urine into surrounding tissue due to bladder or urethral drainage
- infection — urinary tract, epididymis or testis
- deep vein thrombosis and pulmonary embolism.

Possible late complications are:

- urethral stricture
- incontinence
- impotence
- retrograde ejaculation
- bladder neck stenosis.

For further information, see Hanno & Wein (1994) and Laker (1994).

Box 8.7 Cystoscopy

This procedure allows the surgeon to visualise the interior of the bladder and to take biopsies where suspicious lesions are evident. It may be carried out either under general anaesthetic with a rigid cystoscope or under local anaesthetic with a flexible cystoscope. The method selected will depend on the condition of the patient.

Cystoscopy under general anaesthetic

The standard procedures for preparing a patient for general anaesthesia will apply. The lower bowel should be free of faeces so that insertion of the cystoscope is not impeded or the view restricted.

Once recovered from the anaesthetic, the patient should be encouraged to drink. He should be able to pass urine within 6 h of the procedure. The nurse should collect the first specimen passed and record its colour and amount.

Upon discharge, the patient should be advised that he may experience some frequency of desire to pass urine. He should watch for blood in the urine, and should this appear, increase his fluid intake. If the frequency does not settle, or if any bleeding continues, the patient should contact his GP or the hospital.

Cystoscopy under local anaesthetic

There is no restriction on the taking of food or fluids prior to this procedure, but the lower bowels should be free of faeces. The local anaesthetic is placed directly into the urethra in the form of lignocaine gel. In a male patient, a penile clamp is applied to the penis to allow the gel to move along the urethra. A period of 10–20 minutes should normally be allowed for the local anaesthetic to take effect.

Following the procedure, the patient will normally pass urine sooner than under general anaesthetic, as there will have been no restriction applied on fluid intake prior to the operation.

NURSING PRIORITIES AND MANAGEMENT: BENIGN PROSTATIC HYPERPLASIA

General considerations

Patients with acute retention

Those men who present with acute urinary retention as a result of prostatism will normally be catheterised and referred to hospital care for prostatectomy. There is no urgency to perform surgery once the obstruction is relieved; therefore treatment of any associated medical conditions should be undertaken first and, when appropriate, the patient can be placed on the operating list. Should social conditions or hospital resources not permit this, the individual may be discharged to community care with the catheter in situ until a mutually convenient date can be set for surgery. Normal procedure would, however, be for the patient to have his operation on the next available list.

Patients with chronic retention

Chronic urinary retention is usually the result of a crescendo of symptoms of prostatism. These men do not always complain of symptoms of bladder outflow obstruction, but mainly of urge incontinence, dribbling urine or wet beds at night. They usually have no pain and, although they have a large amount of residual urine, their bladder distension is not always obvious to the eye or palpable on physical examination.

Because of the large amount of residual urine, these patients are at risk of developing upper urinary tract dilatation and impaired renal function. However, if there is no renal impairment, it is not essential that these individuals are catheterised. It is urgent to make a diagnosis and proceed to prostatectomy once rehydration and renal function have returned to normal.

Catheterisation will permit bladder drainage and allow renal function recovery (see Boxes 8.8 and 8.9). Once catheterised, the patient may have a huge diuresis. His thirst mechanism will not allow adequate fluid replacement, making parenteral fluid replacement necessary. Large fluid replacement volumes put the patient at risk of heart failure and it should be borne in mind that renal function may have precipitated anaemia.

Box 8.8 The use of catheters

Indications for catheterisation

- Acute or chronic retention of urine
- Diagnostic investigations of the bladder function
- Pre- and postoperative needs
- Following trauma, burns, road traffic accidents or any trauma to the lower urinary tract
- Therapeutic instillations of medication specifically prescribed
- Intractable incontinence where all other methods have failed
- Protracted loss of consciousness

Choice of catheter

Points to consider when choosing a catheter are:

- The purpose of the catheterisation
- The length of time the catheter must remain in situ
- Whether a self-retaining catheter is necessary
- The sex of the patient

Features of the catheter

- The smallest catheter which will adequately drain the bladder should be used: size 12–16 Fg for adults with clear urine; size 18–22 Fg for adults with haematuria
- The lumen of the catheter will vary depending on the material used. A latex catheter is made up of several layers of material, often coated inside with silicone, and its lumen will be smaller than that of a silicone catheter, which is extruded from one piece of material (Pomfret 1996)
- Balloon size: the larger the balloon, the higher the drainage eye lies in the bladder. This can impair drainage and cause more irritation to the sensitive trigone of the bladder. The balloon should be just large enough to stop the catheter falling out or being pushed out if the patient bears down. The recommended balloon size for routine use is 5–10 mL. A 30 mL balloon should be used only following surgery on the prostate gland.

  Note that underinflation of a large-capacity balloon causes distortion of the tip of the catheter and occlusion of the drainage eye. Therefore a large balloon should be filled with at least 20 mL of water. A smaller-ballooned catheter, because the water must reach the balloon, should be filled with at least 10 mL
- Short-term catheters are made of a latex material that can cause irritation of the urethra and build-up of crystals in the bladder. Therefore it is not recommended to use this type of catheter for longer than 2 or 3 weeks
- Long-term catheters are made of 100% silicone material; they are less irritating, softer, and cause less build-up of crystals

Once the patient has been catheterised, his renal function restored and any anaemia corrected, there is no urgency to proceed to surgery. The individual may in fact benefit from a period of recuperation and bladder rest with the catheter in place. Depending upon the general well-being of the individual and upon community resources, care may be given in hospital or in the patient's home.

A trial without the catheter should not be made, as this would again lead to chronic retention followed by renal failure.

Whilst receiving community care, pending hospital referral or surgery, some patients will develop acute or acute-on-chronic urinary retention. Hospital admission must be expedited to permit urgent or emergency hospital treatment.

For those with milder symptoms, it is a matter of discussion between the patient and his doctor as to whether symptoms are interfering with the individual's lifestyle sufficiently to warrant an operation and whether he stands a good chance of improvement from surgery. In rare cases where there is poor life expectancy or the patient is too unfit for surgery, prostatectomy may not be offered and a permanent indwelling catheter may be considered the best management.

Specific considerations for the patient undergoing TURP

Informed consent

The patient must be given a clear explanation of the after-effects of TURP, so that he can give his informed consent prior to the procedure. Since almost all men have retrograde ejaculation after prostatectomy, it is essential that they are counselled adequately beforehand. Retrograde ejaculation does not cause impotence, but a patient who has not been given adequate reassurance on this point could suffer psychological upset resulting in impotence. Retrograde ejaculation will not render the patient sterile, but neither will it necessarily permit him to father children easily. It should not be presumed that all elderly men are not sexually active, and all patients are entitled to preoperative information (see Case History 8.4, Box 8.10 and Research Abstract 8.1).

Q **8.6** Identify and consider all the information that it will be necessary to give to Mr M in Case History 8.4. How could this information best be given to ensure he can really understand and remember the details?

Major patient problems

Patients who have undergone TURP may have the following problems and concerns postoperatively:

- anxiety
  - —about the success of the surgery and the outlook for recovery
  - —about bleeding from the prostatic bed
  - —feelings of embarrassment about having a catheter
- pain
  - —from the raw area in the bladder
  - —from clots forming in the prostatic bed, blocking the catheter
  - —from the catheter itself
  - —from bladder extravasation

Box 8.9 Principles of catheter management

Performing catheterisation

The nurse performing catheterisation must introduce the catheter into the bladder using aseptic technique, without causing trauma and with minimum discomfort to the patient. The following considerations are essential:

- Adequate cleaning of the genital area
- Working under good light, especially when catheterising females
- Positioning the patient correctly
- Ensuring the patient's privacy
- Providing adequate anaesthetisation of the urethra for both male and female patients. An anaesthetic-containing antiseptic should be instilled and left to take effect for a minimum of 5 min

Management of the indwelling catheter

The main priorities of catheter care are to prevent infection and to safeguard the dignity of the patient. To minimise the risk of infection the nurse should:

- Establish and maintain a closed system of drainage
- Promote good personal hygiene
- Provide catheter toilets once a day and after each bowel movement, with soap and water
- Encourage a fluid intake of 2–4 L daily, according to the individual's needs
- Encourage maximum mobility
- Change the catheter only when necessary, rather than routinely
- Avoid causing trauma to the urethra and bladder neck
- Give bladder washouts only when absolutely necessary, i.e. when the catheter is blocked or when washouts have been prescribed as a treatment. Bladder washouts should not be employed as a prophylactic treatment for urine infections (Roe 1990)

Maintaining the dignity of the patient

The following measures will help to preserve the patient's dignity and self-esteem:

- Providing education and promoting self-care where possible in catheter toilet, the use of a bidet, emptying and changing bags
- Using a female length catheter for a female patient to allow her to wear skirts
- Encouraging the use of leg bags so the catheter is not in view
- Encouraging maximum mobility to promote confidence and give better drainage

Problems and possible interventions

The nurse should be prepared for the following potential problems:

Bypassing

- Check to see if the catheter or drainage tube is blocked or kinked
- Consider reducing the water in the balloon or changing to a smaller catheter. It is a misconception that if the catheter bypasses, a larger catheter is required
- Check whether or not drugs which can cause spasm have been prescribed
- Exclude constipation — relieve constipation immediately and emphasise the importance of a high-fibre diet
- Check with the doctor about the possibility of prescribing anticholinergic drugs if the bypassing still persists

Balloon not deflating

- Attach syringe to the valve in position without aspiration. It may self-deflate
- The balloon may be burst by injecting 2–5 mL of dilute ether via the balloon inflating channel
- A fine sterile wire may be passed up the inflating channel and the balloon burst
- Never cut off the end of the inflation channel of the catheter

Blockage

- This may be caused by drugs, e.g. aperients causing phosphatic debris in the urine — change or stop the drug, encourage the patient to take a high-fibre diet and encourage more exercise
- Infection will need to be treated with the correct antibiotic. Check the amount of fluid intake and where possible try to increase this. Check the standard of personal hygiene
- If clots occur, perform a bladder washout with normal saline

Urethral discharge

- Normal secretion of the urethral mucosa is increased with the presence of a foreign body, i.e. the catheter. To prevent this becoming troublesome to the patient adequate meatal toilet should be instituted from the first day of catheterisation

- immobility
  —due to inability to get out of bed because of the surgery
  —because of irrigation
  —due to fear of moving
  —due to i.v. infusion
- difficulty eating and drinking
  —due to nausea
  —due to immobility
- disturbed sleep
  —due to irrigation changes, checks on temperature, pulse, blood pressure
  —due to pain
  —due to noise in the ward.

Major nursing considerations

Risk of haemorrhage. Since bleeding or haemorrhage is a major risk after prostatectomy, preoperative care should involve determining baseline haematological values. Careful consideration must be given to those individuals receiving oral anticoagulants for other disease, since the risk of haemorrhage is so great. It may be necessary to discontinue oral therapy preoperatively and to use i.v. heparin postoperatively until the oral regimen can be

Case History 8.4 Mr M

Mr M was admitted for a TURP. He was 73 years old and had been suffering from the miserable symptoms of an enlarged prostate gland for some time. He was glad to be in hospital but did not feel well. His joints and bones ached from long-standing osteoarthritis. His chest was not good and his feet and hands were always cold. He knew smoking did not help and he had been cutting down.

The surgeon and anaesthetist visited him and explained the surgery and that he would have an epidural anaesthetic. The physiotherapist visited him and discussed breathing techniques and encouraged him with giving up smoking. Nursing staff were always at hand. They explained all the tests and procedures involved in preparation for surgery as well as how he could expect to feel after the procedure.

recommenced and stabilised. This may take some weeks to achieve and will require the patient to make additional visits to the hospital or GP surgery.

Anaemia. Preoperative anaemia should be corrected and blood transfusion given postoperatively to replace blood loss. It would be normal to cross-match two units of blood for each patient so that should transfusion be required postoperatively the blood will be available on demand. Future trends may change this protocol, since protein and plasma products are now more readily available.

Fluid and electrolyte balance. Preoperative determination of urea and electrolyte levels will provide baseline measurements and permit correction before surgery if required. This may involve urethral catheterisation to permit adequate bladder drainage, the use of i.v. fluid to achieve hydration and, if necessary, the provision of saline.

Box 8.10 Information for patients undergoing prostatectomy. (Reproduced with kind permission from the Department of Urology, The Freeman Hospital, Newcastle upon Tyne)

Your doctor has already explained to you that you require an operation on your prostate gland. The prostate is situated at the base of the bladder and it is quite common in older men for the prostate to enlarge, causing the symptoms which you have been experiencing. In order to relieve these symptoms it is necessary to remove that part of the prostate gland which is causing a blockage to the flow of the urine from the bladder.

The anaesthetic

The operation may be performed under a general anaesthetic, when you will be completely asleep, or a spinal anaesthetic, which involves an injection in your back and makes the lower half of your body completely numb. This decision is usually made by the anaesthetist. If you wish, you may have something else to make you relaxed or sleepy. The power and feeling of your legs recover within a few hours and by the morning after the spinal anaesthetic you will be completely normal.

The operation

There are two ways of removing the prostate gland. Generally it is possible to do the operation through a telescopic instrument which is passed up through the penis. This operation is known as a transurethral resection of the prostate (TURP). The prostate tissue is cut away in small pieces which are washed out of the bladder and any bleeding is stopped using a special electrocautery probe.

Alternatively, it is sometimes necessary to remove the prostate by an open operation through an incision in the lower part of the abdomen. The same amount of tissue is removed by both operations and the end result is the same. Your surgeon will naturally try to remove your prostate with the tele-endoscopic instrument but it may be necessary to perform the 'cutting' operation, especially if the prostate is unusually large.

After the operation you will have a tube (catheter) draining the urine from your bladder into a bag which will be emptied regularly by the nursing staff. Immediately after the operation the catheter will contain blood, so the bladder, prostate and catheter are washed continuously with fluid that runs through an extra tube attached to the catheter. This is disconnected when the urine is clear, usually the morning after the operation. After the operation you will also have an infusion into a vein for about 24 h to provide extra fluid or blood if necessary.

After the operation

As soon as possible after the operation we like you to start drinking large quantities of tea, squash, fruit juice or water, but fizzy drinks are not recommended. An occasional can of beer is permissible. This will speed up your recovery by producing more urine to wash away the blood in the catheter and prevent infection. The catheter will be removed between 2 and 5 days after the operation. This is not painful. After it has been removed you should continue to drink as much as possible and pass urine every 2–3 h. This may be uncomfortable to start with and you may have to hurry or experience some dribbling but these minor symptoms improve rapidly. Once you are satisfied that you are passing urine well and your surgeon is satisfied with your progress, you may return home, usually 1–2 days after removal of the catheter.

At home

When you get home you should continue to drink well and avoid constipation, strenuous exercise and heavy lifting. You should not drive a car for 1 week or play golf or go jogging for at least 3 weeks. Sometimes you may see some blood in your urine 7–10 days after the operation. This is rarely serious and if you drink plenty of fluids and rest it should disappear. If bleeding persists you should contact your family doctor. Infection and other problems are unusual. The bladder may be 'irritable' for several weeks after a prostate operation with frequency and urgency, but any remaining symptoms should disappear within 12 weeks.

You will be seen again in the urology outpatient clinic about 2 months after your operation. You can return to light work at that time or even sooner, if you feel able to do so.

Sexual activity after prostatectomy

This operation will alter your sex life but it is unlikely that there will be any change in the quality of the erections or climax. Sexual intercourse can take place 5–6 weeks after the operation. During sexual climax, however, you will not emit any semen from your penis. The ejaculation (semen) may flow into the bladder instead of down the penis and the first time you pass urine after intercourse it will be cloudy. This is not harmful. You are unlikely to produce any children following this operation but this should not be relied on as safe contraception.

Research Abstract 8.1
Preoperative information-giving

However commonplace certain surgical procedures might become to medical and nursing staff, they will never be so for the actual patient, who will wish to know about the operation. Understanding illness and surgery can help in the recovery process and reduce stress (Argyle 1981). However, the giving of information and support is not always as effective as the doctor or nurse may believe. A small research study in Edinburgh assessed the quality of the perioperative information given to patients undergoing a TURP. In a two-phase study the researchers were able to show that the use of a booklet both complemented and enhanced verbal communication (Brewster 1992).

Brewster J 1992 Operations explained. Nursing Times 88(39): 50–52

During TURP the bladder is irrigated with fluid to provide a clear view for the surgeon. Some of this fluid is usually absorbed, and if there is an interruption in the venous system during the resection, the fluid absorbed can be excessive. The fluid used in irrigation is usually isotonic glycine, excessive absorption of which can cause the patient to become hyponatraemic. This can cause confusion, a restless mental state and, in some cases, unconsciousness. This imbalance can be corrected by restricting fluid intake and encouraging the patient to increase the amount of salt in his diet.

Water is not used for irrigation because it can be readily absorbed and cause haemolysis. Saline interferes with the use of diathermy, and so is also unsuitable for irrigation during surgery. It is, however, the solution of choice for postoperative bladder washouts.

Urinary infection. Men who have an indwelling urethral catheter preoperatively are at a high risk of developing infective complications. The effectiveness of prophylactic antibiotics is uncertain, but it would seem that those who do not receive systemic therapy at the time of operation followed by a postoperative course will be likely to develop bacteraemia and become unwell.

Urinary infection is common after prostatectomy, even in those who had sterile urine preoperatively. About one-third of men who have bacteria in their urine postoperatively are asymptomatic but should receive the appropriate oral therapy. This reduces the incidence of secondary haemorrhage caused by infection.

Management of irrigation

An irrigation set with a Y-connection will be used to allow two 3 L bags of normal saline to be erected at any one time, with one bag running at a time. The irrigation runs into the bladder via the irrigating channel of the catheter, and then out through the outlet channel from a classic system drainage bag, thus preventing the introduction of infection.

The irrigation is regulated via a clamp to run at a speed sufficient to keep the bladder clear of blood clots. The bags are numbered and the amount of irrigation fluid recorded on a fluid chart. The patient's total output, i.e. urine and irrigation fluid, should be measured and recorded. The amount of irrigation fluid used should be subtracted from the measured output to give the urine output volume.

Specific assessment points are as follows:

- Observe and feel the size of the patient's lower abdomen. Abdominal distension may indicate clot retention or extravasation. Clot retention is a common complication in the first 12–24 h. Bladder washout or deflation and reinflation of the catheter balloon may be required.
- Note the colour of the irrigation fluid. A bright red colour may indicate fresh bleeding. A dark red colour would suggest old blood.
- In an uncircumcised male patient, check that the foreskin is over the glans penis to prevent paraphimosis.

The morning following surgery, the irrigation will be discontinued provided that the patient is able to drink large quantities of fluid to help flush the prostatic bed of any further bleeding or clots.

Pain relief should be adequate to allow the patient to rest and feel comfortable. Opiate analgesics such as morphine or oral co-proxamol may be prescribed.

Catheter care (see also Boxes 8.8 and 8.9). A common problem while the catheter is in situ is the bypassing of urine around it. This is sometimes difficult to resolve, and the nurse should take the following preventive measures:

- Check that the catheter is not blocked by clots or debris and that it is in the bladder.
- Check the amount of water in the balloon. If it is 30 mL, then reduce it to 20 mL or so, but not less than 15 mL.
- Give anticholinergic medication as prescribed.
- Encourage the patient to continue to drink large quantities of fluid.

The catheter will stay in position for 2–3 days following surgery or until the output is clear. Before removing it, the nurse should ensure that the patient's bowels have moved, as straining following catheter removal can lead to further urethral bleeding. Following removal, the patient may experience urgency and frequency as before. He should be reassured that this is normal and that it may take up to 8 weeks for a normal voiding pattern to be established. The patient should be educated to tighten the sphincter muscle and to hold on as long as possible before passing urine.

Patients who had chronic retention before surgery often fail to void postoperatively. A long-term catheter will normally be inserted in such cases, and the patient allowed home for several weeks (usually 6). This time allows the bladder to rest and regain its elasticity.

Patient involvement

The patient's dependence on nursing care will gradually decrease as blood loss and hence the need for irrigation lessens. Involvement of the patient in aspects of his own care is to be encouraged and may include:

- Making entries in his own fluid chart; drinking at least 3 L in 24 h; emptying own drainage bag; recording amount and colour (most patients will be happy to do this but may need guidance on colour and amount).
- Attending to own personal hygiene; this would include cleaning the urethral catheter once or twice a day using soap and water (Falkiner 1993).
- Taking regular, if somewhat gentle, exercise (it should be remembered, however, that some patients feel embarrassed about carrying around a urinary drainage bag).

Discharge

Once the urine is clear, the catheter can normally be removed. This is usually done in the morning to allow the patient to establish a normal voiding pattern before retiring to bed. Provided the patient is able to pass urine without difficulty, he may be discharged from hospital the following day.

For further information, see Roe (1991), Barnett (1991) and Pomfret (1996).

Many patients feel after the operation that they have gained no relief from their problems. It must be understood that it will take about 6 weeks for healing of the prostatic bed to occur such that full urinary control is possible. During the early postoperative weeks, the patient should refrain from vigorous exercise. He should drink plenty of fluids and avoid becoming constipated. The community nurse will give advice and support should urinary problems occur.

It should be noted that at about 14 days postoperatively, when desiccated tissue has sloughed off the prostatic bed, haemorrhage can occur (secondary haemorrhage; see Ch. 26, p. 817).

Occasionally, urethral stricture occurs as the urethral mucosa in the prostatic region heals.

For further information, see Sueppel (1992) and Reynolds (1993).

Cancer of the prostate

Cancer of the prostate gland is the second most common malignancy among the Western male population (Dean & Downey 1997). The incidence of prostatic cancer increases with age and postmortem studies have shown that about 30% of asymptomatic men over the age of 50, and 90% over the age of 90, have microscopic foci, evident only on histological examination. About 10% of men thought to have benign prostates on examination are later found by histological examination to have prostatic cancer.

PATHOPHYSIOLOGY

The cause of prostatic cancer is not clear, but there is some evidence to show that hormonal activity plays a part in the transformation of certain normal cells into cancerous ones. Benign hyperplasia and carcinoma arise in different parts of the gland. Carcinoma occurs in the peripheral gland. Metastases often move to bone, where they are associated with severe pain. In cases of extreme bony destruction, pathological fractures may occur. It has been known for spinal destruction to cause paraplegia.

Common presenting symptoms. Diagnosis of this disease is difficult because the patient is often asymptomatic. The GP is likely to see patients who present with advanced disease which is already beyond cure. Patients with locally advanced disease are likely to complain of bladder outflow obstruction, a sudden onset of urgency to void urine, and possibly haematuria.

Chronic urinary retention secondary to bladder outflow obstruction may cause renal damage by dilating the upper renal tracts. The patient may present with a palpable bladder or with renal failure; he is likely to be generally unwell and losing weight. Renal failure may also be caused by ureteric infiltration of tumour or by para-aortic lymph node obstruction causing ureteric obstruction. Those who feel unwell and are anaemic are likely to have suffered bone marrow infiltration and/or renal failure. A complaint of persistent backache may suggest bone metastases.

An irregular, enlarged, hard prostate gland does not prove diagnosis, although most advanced carcinomas will be felt as such on rectal examination. However, prostatitis or prostatic stone disease may feel similar on rectal examination. Moreover, if there is a tumour within the anterior part of the gland, rectal examination will reveal no abnormality.

MEDICAL MANAGEMENT

Tests and investigations. The only certain means of making a diagnosis is by histological examination. Fine-needle transrectal prostatic biopsy can be done without anaesthetic for this purpose. Specimens (prostatic chips) resected at the time of transurethral or open prostatectomy should be sent for histological examination. However, this may yield a false negative if the sample is not taken from the peripheral part of the gland. Prostatic cancer is graded histologically to assess malignant potential.

Additional investigations to provide evidence of local and metastatic spread include IVU, CT scanning, magnetic resonance imaging (MRI), ultrasound scanning, skeletal X-rays and lymphangiography.

Treatment. The nature of the treatment offered and whether it is given on an outpatient or an in-patient basis will depend upon the extent of the disease and on how the patient presents symptomatically and clinically. Transurethral resection of the prostate gland (TURP) is normally carried out to relieve urinary symptoms and retention. This does not, however, afford a cure.

In a small number of cases, radical prostatectomy and clearance of any pelvic lymphatic involvement are performed in the hope of achieving a cure. The patient should be counselled preoperatively about his disease and the almost certain complication of urinary incontinence.

Radical radiotherapy. If the patient is generally fit and quite well, he will probably attend for daily treatment as an outpatient. Should the patient or medical team prefer, in-patient treatment may be given.

The side-effects of treatment vary from person to person. Liaison with the patient's relatives and with the community health care team will help to ensure that the patient is given optimum support in dealing with these (see Ch. 31, p. 924). In some cases, the side-effects will necessitate hospitalisation, e.g. when nausea, vomiting and diarrhoea cause dehydration or when urinary frequency or incontinence cause severe physical and psychological distress.

Treating advanced disease. The aims of treatment in advanced disease are to provide symptomatic relief and to preserve an acceptable quality of life for the individual. The outlook for improvement will depend upon various factors; those with renal failure, anaemia or urinary retention and metastases have a poor prognosis.

Those who have metastatic disease and are symptomatic are normally offered hormonal treatment. Hormonal manipulation can be achieved by bilateral orchidectomy (excision of the testes) or by the administration of oestrogens or of LHRH (luteinising hormone-releasing hormone) agonists. Of patients given hormonal treatment, 70% will experience symptomatic relief for a period but will have recurrent symptoms in the long term.

The treatment of those with metastatic disease who are not symptomatic will usually be deferred until symptoms develop. Once hormonal treatment has been given and relapse occurs, the outlook is very poor.

It would appear that chemotherapy is ineffective in treating advanced prostatic carcinoma. However, radiotherapy is sometimes beneficial in the relief of bony pain caused by metastases. Vertebral collapse caused by metastatic disease of the spinal cord requires emergency radiotherapy or laminectomy and hormonal manipulation. If effective, these measures may prevent neurological symptoms and/or paraplegia from developing.

Pain control by means of opiate analgesics may cause secondary constipation; this in turn can cause urinary retention. It may be more appropriate to administer non-steroidal anti-inflammatory medication to avoid this side-effect. Should analgesics be required, they should be given in doses which prevent pain occurring (see Ch. 19, p. 661). Sustained or slow-release drugs are often very useful.

NURSING PRIORITIES AND MANAGEMENT: CARCINOMA OF THE PROSTATE

General considerations

The nursing management of prostatic cancer is very much influenced by the particular presentation of the disease in each individual. The nurse should take a problem-solving approach to care, and promote independence and self-care for as long as possible. The nurse should bear in mind that constipation and urinary retention or urinary incontinence are commonly encountered and can be very distressing both for the individual and for his family. Ongoing liaison between hospital and community teams will help to ensure that care is effective and genuinely responsive to the individual's unique situation (see Ch. 33).

A range of medical interventions may be necessary at different stages in the disease process. Nursing involvement will then include assisting with procedures such as:

- correction of anaemia by blood transfusion
- TURP to relieve retention
- bilateral subcapsular orchidectomy to reduce the hormone level, help prevent the spread of metastases and reduce pain.

In many cases, medical intervention can offer only temporary improvement, and the emphasis of care will turn to palliation. Treatment of advanced disease is usually shared between hospital and home, and the patient and his family will need a great deal of moral support in both settings. It is important to convey a sense of optimism so that life can continue to be enjoyed to the fullest degree possible. In the last stages of the illness, however, it should not be seen as a defeat or failure to help the patient to let go of life and face death with dignity (see Ch. 33).

Marsh (1992) examines early detection and treatment and discusses the management of local and advanced disease, highlighting the importance of patient education and family support.
Gledhill (1996) is also recommended.

DISORDERS OF THE BLADDER

Cancer of the bladder

Tumours of the bladder (usually transitional cell carcinoma) occur more commonly in men than in women (M:F = 4:1). About 8000 new cases of bladder cancer are registered each year. The peak incidence of bladder cancer in the UK occurs at around 65 years of age. Bladder tumours are histologically similar to tumours of the renal pelvis and ureter. About 95% are malignant, and benign tumours often recur after apparently successful treatment.

There are geographical variations in incidence — tumours are more common in industrialised regions than in underdeveloped regions. Possible causative agents or factors include:

- occupational exposure (industrial dyes, solvents)
- cigarette smoking
- calculi
- diverticula
- chronic inflammation due to indwelling catheterisation.

Screening of those in high-risk groups may help to reduce incidence. Controls do exist to monitor factors associated with bladder cancer, but as many years may elapse between exposure to a carcinogen and the development of cancer, direct connections are difficult to establish.

8.7 What part can the occupational health nurse play in prevention?
Refer to RCN (1991).

PATHOPHYSIOLOGY

Tumour growth usually commences in the epithelial lining of the bladder, often as a papillary growth. (Papillae are minute nipple-shaped projections.) Benign growth will without treatment usually progress to malignancy and then by stages from superficial to deep muscle tissue involvement, eventually spreading locally into surrounding tissue or organs. Metastatic spread to other parts of the urinary tract will also occur.

Common presenting symptoms (see Table 8.3). About 80% of people with bladder cancer will notice haematuria. This may be the only presenting feature of the disease. Dysuria, frequency, symptoms of obstruction and infection may also be noticed, but embarrassment may prevent the individual from visiting the GP's surgery. Symptoms may not persist following initial presentation, e.g. if associated infection is resolved by a course of antibiotics. Investigations should, however, be undertaken if the cause of haematuria is unclear.

8.8 A 35-year-old man notices blood in his urine each morning. He has no discomfort and is otherwise well. Unless the haematuria persists this man may decide not to visit his GP. How might you encourage him to report the haematuria? What anxieties might he have about reporting to his GP?

MEDICAL MANAGEMENT

Investigations. Diagnosis may be aided by physical examination, a full blood count, urea and electrolyte estimation and other biochemical assays. Examination of an MSU specimen will exclude evidence of infection. Table 8.4 lists the principal diagnostic investigations; in many respects these will be similar to those used in diagnosing prostatic disorders.

Staging. The staging of bladder tumours is illustrated in Figure 8.11 (see also Ch. 31). In addition to staging according to the actual tumour, the pathologist will grade transitional cell tumours according to invasion differentiation of the lesion (Burkitt et al 1996).

Table 8.3 Presenting features of bladder cancer

Sign/symptom	*Reason*
Haematuria, urine retention	Tumour growth Tumour spread
Dysuria, urgency, hesitancy, frequency	Stimulation of reflex micturition arc Secondary infection
Urinary incontinence	Irritability of bladder
Chills and cystitis	Obstruction/infection
Backache, pain	Ureteric obstruction Dependent upon the stage: infiltration Symptoms of cystitis or burning
Lower limb oedema	Venous obstruction Lymphatic obstruction
Infection	Obstruction Tumour necrosis
Malaise, anaemia	Frequency causing lack of rest or sleep Bleeding
Suprapubic mass, abnormal mass on rectal examination	Tumour size Tumour spread

Treatment. The choice of treatment will depend on the type of tumour and the degree of invasion of local tissue, as determined by cystoscopy (see Table 8.5). Superficial lesions without muscle invasion can be treated by excision of the tumour through the urethra — transurethral resection of tumour (TURT) or cysto-diathermy. Irrigation of the bladder may be used to keep the bladder clear of blood clots following transurethral resection (see p. 334).

For invasive bladder tumours a combination of surgery (i.e. total cystectomy), radiotherapy and chemotherapy may be used.

Total cystectomy involves removing the lower ureters, bladder, prostate, urethra and lymphatics in men, and also, in women, the gynaecological organs. Urinary diversion is required and is most commonly ileal conduit and stoma formation (see Fig. 8.12). With this type of diversion, the ureters are anastomosed to an isolated section of the bowel (ileum with blood supply) and the loop brought to the abdominal surface as a stoma. This is a major procedure which will fundamentally affect the lifestyle of both the patient and family members.

Recent developments in reconstructive surgery have led to the use of bladder substitutes in place of urinary diversion. Part of the intestine is anastomosed directly to the membranous urethra which provides a reservoir for urine; however, this technique is not appropriate for everyone.

For further information, see Laker (1994), Leaver (1994) and Dickson (1995).

Radiotherapy is normally given as an external treatment for bladder carcinoma over a 6-week period. It may be used as a palliative measure or in conjunction with surgery and/or chemotherapy, pre- or post-treatment. The age and general condition of the patient will determine whether treatment is given on an outpatient or in-patient basis. Sometimes the severity of the symptoms encountered leads to conversion from outpatient to in-patient care and a rest in the treatment plan to allow the patient to recuperate before progressing to the next treatment.

Chemotherapy. Treatment of invasive bladder cancer with systemic chemotherapy is under investigation. Regimens of treatment vary. Some patients receive care on a day-care basis, receiving i.v. injections, while others attend for in-patient hospital care involving 2–3 days in hospital for each cycle of treatment. (For further details on systemic chemotherapy, refer to Chapter 31.)

Intravesical chemotherapy may be offered in some cases. The recurrence of superficial bladder tumours resected endoscopically is about 65%. Recurrent tumours are usually of the same type and stage as those previously resected. Further endoscopic resection may be the treatment of choice, but sometimes intravesical chemotherapy is also given. This involves the introduction of a variety of drugs via a urethral catheter. Treatment may be weekly, monthly or bimonthly, depending upon the type of tumour and the drug used. A urethral catheter is inserted and the chosen drug instilled via the catheter. The catheter can then be removed. The patient is requested to avoid passing urine for an hour and is asked to turn from back to front to sides every 15 min, in order to wash the drug around the bladder.

The nurse administering the treatment should bear in mind that this patient may have difficulty in postponing the passing of urine for up to 1 h because of symptoms of frequency, irritability and so on. The patient should be reassured that an inability to comply with this request is not a sign of 'failure'.

The side-effects of the drugs used in this treatment vary, but chemical cystitis leading to inflammation and bladder irritability, urgency and frequency is common. Sensitivity rashes are seen less commonly, as are more severe effects such as systemic toxicity and bone marrow suppression.

Table 8.4 Principal diagnostic investigations for tumours of the bladder

Investigation	*Reason*
Intravenous urogram (IVU)	If presenting feature is haematuria, IVU may exclude renal pelvic carcinoma
Cystoscopy and biopsy	Suspicious lesions can be examined for abnormal cells
CT scan	If local spread of tumour is suspected
Chest X-ray	If metastatic spread is suspected
Bone scan	
Liver function tests	

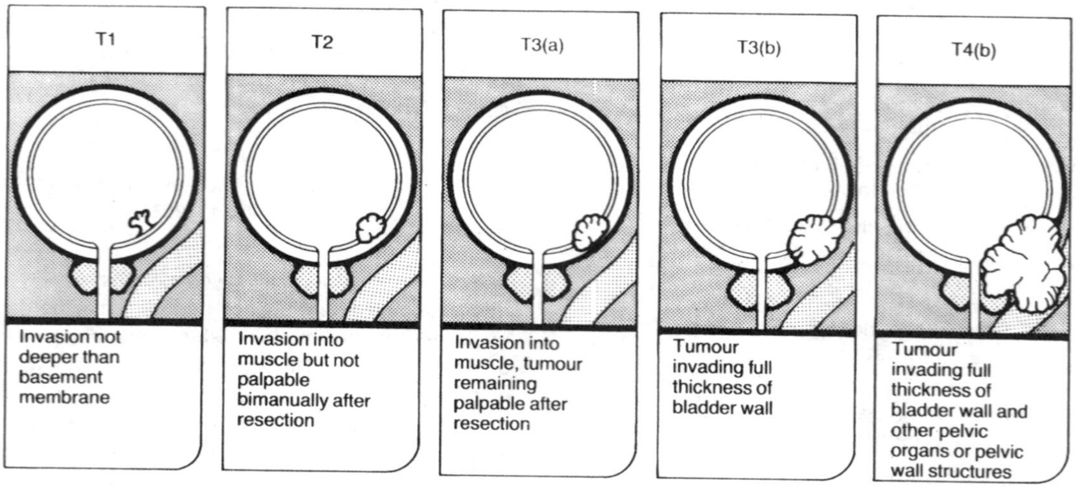

Fig. 8.11 System for staging bladder tumours. Note: stage T3(b) indicates tumour invasion of prostate gland. (Reproduced with permission from Burkitt et al 1996.)

Table 8.5 Treatment choices in tumours of the bladder

Tumour	*Treatment*	*Comment*
Localised, well-differentiated tumour	Diathermy	Annual cystoscopy to check for recurrence
Histologically malignant tumours —extensive superficial —locally invasive	Chemotherapy: intravenal Radiotherapy TURT	Annual cystoscopy to assess effect and check for recurrence
Failure to control tumour spread/severe symptoms	Cystectomy and ureter transplant to ileal conduit (urinary diversion)	Radiotherapy may be used to reduce size of tumour prior to surgery
Inoperable tumour	Analgesia Palliative radiotherapy	
Metastatic spread	Systemic chemotherapy	An option although success is limited

Since the drugs used are toxic agents, precautions such as wearing protective goggles, gloves and gowns should be taken when preparing and administering treatments and when discarding used equipment.

After the treatment is completed, the patient should be advised that urine passed will contain chemical substances that will irritate the skin and that leakages or dribbles should be washed off immediately.

Effectiveness of treatment with intravesical chemotherapy varies considerably from individual to individual.

NURSING PRIORITIES AND MANAGEMENT: TOTAL CYSTECTOMY AND URINARY DIVERSION

Preoperative care

Psychological preparation (see Case History 8.5)

The patient admitted for cystectomy and urinary diversion may already know the nursing and medical staff on the ward from a previous admission. Staff should try to build upon this rapport and provide information both verbally and in written form to prepare the patient for the physical effects of the operation, particularly the formation of a stoma. Considerable psychological adjustment may be required on the part of the patient to come to terms with the lifestyle changes that will be necessary and with the alteration in body image that may occur.

The patient is likely to have concerns relating to any pain that will be experienced; whether the operation will effect a 'cure'; how his family will cope in his absence and after his return home; and how he will appear to other people. The contribution of the named nurse and the stoma therapist in answering questions and allaying fears in the preoperative period is invaluable. It may be helpful to arrange for the patient and his family to meet with someone who has a stoma.

It should be noted that patients rarely ask about the effect surgery may have on sexual function. However, one of the side-effects for male patients of this life-saving procedure is impotence. This important matter must be discussed with male patients and their partners prior to the surgery in order to help them return to and lead a normal life (Black 1994a).

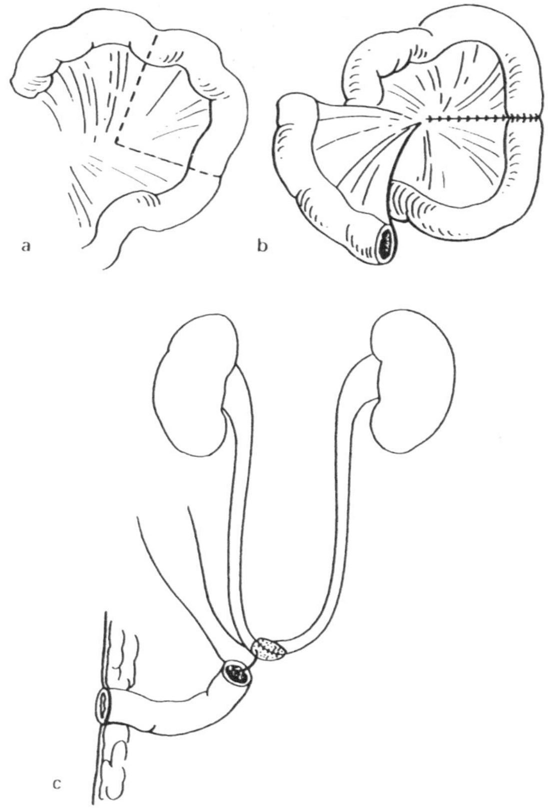

Fig. 8.12 Ileal conduit urinary diversion. (a, b) Isolation of segment of ileum. (c) Ureteroileal anastomosis. (Reproduced with permission from Forrest et al 1995.)

The patient may gain confidence from the knowledge that his community nurse and GP as well as a stoma nurse are available to support him. He should be given a contact telephone number to use in the event of difficulty. He should be reassured that any problems and concerns, however small, can be discussed as he makes the challenging adjustment from hospital to home.

For further information see Black (1994b) and Myers (1996).

8.9 How can the nurse help Mr L in Case History 8.5 to come to terms with his disappointing news and the prospect of total cystectomy?
8.10 Mr L is provided with an indwelling catheter which will remain in situ until he can be admitted to hospital. What advice and support could you offer to Mr L and his wife to ensure that no catheter-related problems develop? What part can the community nurse play? Review Boxes 8.8 and 8.9.

Physical preparation

The stoma will be sited on the abdomen below the waist, normally on the right-hand side. Considerations in choosing the exact site include:

- the patient's build
- access for the surgeon
- previous surgery
- access for the patient following surgery
- type of clothing to be worn after the surgery.

Case History 8.5 — Mr L

Mr L, a 58-year-old married man employed as a bus driver, was diagnosed 5 years ago with cancer of the bladder. He was treated with regular cystoscopies and transurethral resections of tumour. Six months ago the tumour was found to be stage T2, and a course of chemotherapy was prescribed. Recent cystoscopy showed that this treatment had not been successful. Total cystectomy is now being considered for this patient.

The following procedures are carried out in preparation for surgery:

1. The patient is kept on a fluid-only or low-residue diet at commencement of bowel preparation.
2. The bowel is cleared of faeces. This may be by means of an enema or a high colonic washout and is carried out 2 days prior to the operation. Bowel sterilisation with systemic and local antibiotics may be prescribed.
3. Prophylactic antibiotic therapy is commenced preoperatively (and continued postoperatively).
4. The skin is shaved from nipple to knee, or according to the surgeon's wishes (see Ch. 26).
5. The patient is assisted to take a shower on the day of the operation.
6. The chosen site for the stoma is marked.

Postoperative care

Return from theatre (see Nursing Care Plan 8.2)

Following surgery and recovery from anaesthetic, the patient will return to the ward. A nasogastric (NG) tube will be in place for aspiration of gastric contents. Examination will reveal a midline incision, covered by a surgical dressing, and a wound drain. The stoma, in the pre-marked position, should have a moist, red appearance and be covered by a collection bag fitted with a drainage tap and autoreflux valve to prevent back-flow of urine when the patient is lying flat.

Infant feeding tubes which form temporary splints across the ureteroilial anastomosis may be seen protruding from the stoma. The splints, one for each ureter and inserted at surgery, pass through the ileal loop and along the ureters across the junction of the anastomosis. The support provided by the splints reduces the risk of urine leakage from the anastomosis before healing has taken place.

The recovery period

The NG tube will be in place for 24–48 h, or until bowel sounds have returned. Drains may be removed when discharge is less than 50 mL/24 h; this is usually at 4–5 days postoperatively. Removal of splints from the stoma can usually be done at 10–14 days, and removal of sutures at 10 days. Assessment by the dietician and provision of a diet plan may aid wound healing and recovery by ensuring an adequate nutritional intake.

During this time, the stoma nurse will visit. Working with the named nurse, she will teach the patient how to clean the stoma and change the bag and flange on a daily basis. The patient should be shown how to cut the flange to shape and fit it in position with the bag.

Nursing Care Plan 8.2 Nursing care in the first 24 h following total cystectomy and urinary diversion

Potential problem	*Action*	*Desired outcome*
1. Cardiovascular instability and hypovolaemic shock due to haemorrhage and pain	❒ Record vital signs and report any deviations from normal range ❒ Monitor and mark extent of blood loss evident on wound dressing ❒ Record blood loss in drains and report if in excess of 100 mL/h	Cardiovascular stability Minimal blood loss Minimal pain
2. Pain	❒ Observe patient for distress (NB — generalised abdominal pain may indicate peritonitis caused by leakage from anastomosis) ❒ Administer prescribed analgesics ❒ Evaluate effect after 30 min by asking patient if pain has been relieved	Patient is pain-free
3. Fluid and electrolyte imbalance	❒ Measure and record hourly urine output (NB — output <30 mL could indicate obstruction or possible leakage from ureteroilial anastomosis leading to peritonitis ❒ Balance all fluid output against all fluid input in 24 h ❒ Observe for evidence of dyspnoea and dehydration, e.g. dry skin and mouth ❒ Observe for vomiting	Fluid and electrolytes maintained at satisfactory levels
4. Paralytic ileus	❒ Allow nil by mouth ❒ Perform NG aspirations hourly/free drainage ❒ Administer antiemetics as necessary	Comfort is maintained until return of bowel sounds
5. Deep vein thrombosis (DVT) and/or pulmonary embolism (PE)	❒ Supply anti-embolic stockings preoperatively ❒ Encourage movement of lower limbs ❒ Observe for evidence of DVT or PE	Circulatory integrity is maintained
6. Chest infection	❒ Encourage deep breathing and coughing ❒ Refer to physiotherapist ❒ Position patient as upright as possible	Chest is clear with no evidence of infection
7. Wound infection	❒ Observe wound for leakage, check drains hourly ❒ Record temperature and report pyrexia ❒ Leave dressings undisturbed for 48 h if dry	Wound heals without infection
8. Development of pressure sores	❒ Change patient's position regularly and observe for reddening ❒ Use a risk assessment scale to assess patient's needs ❒ Ensure skin is clean and dry ❒ Use Spenco mattress if necessary	Skin integrity is maintained
9. Inability to perform personal hygiene tasks	❒ Provide bedbath and mouth care	Patient is clean and comfortable
10. Anxiety	❒ Ensure the nurse call system is close at hand at all times ❒ Discuss patient's concerns with her. Provide information, but take post-anaesthetic drowsiness into account ❒ Evaluate patient's understanding of information given. Return next day and ask if there are further questions or concerns	Patient understands what is happening and feels secure in the care provided

Patients differ in the time it takes them to come to terms with management of their stoma. Some show no interest at first in looking after the stoma and need a lot of encouragement. Planning a programme with the patient, identifying goals to be attained and involving close relatives/carers will help to ensure successful self-care. A second visit with an individual who has already made the adjustment to life with a stoma may also help.

Discharge

Provided no complications have arisen, by 10–14 days after the operation the patient and nurse should be planning for discharge home. The first follow-up appointment will usually be scheduled for 6–8 weeks after the operation. Thereafter, outpatient appointments will be arranged at longer intervals, but will continue for life. To ensure optimal function and prevent long-term complications

Box 8.11 Complications following total cystectomy

Specific complications post-cystectomy
- Breakdown of anastomosis
- Breakdown of blood supply to stoma (necrosis)
- Pelvic abscess
- Poor wound healing post-radiotherapy
- Prolapse of stoma
- Renal failure
- Retraction of stoma
- Urinary infection

Later complications
- Depression
- Prolapse of stoma
- Recurrence of tumour
- Retraction of stoma
- Stenosis of stoma
- Stone formation
- Urinary infection
- Urinary reflux

Box 8.12 Causes of glomerulonephritis

Primary causes
- Minimal change glomerular disease
- Proliferative glomerulonephritis
  —mesangial
  —diffuse capillary
  —focal
  —IgA nephropathy
  —mesangiocapillary
  —crescentic (Goodpasture's syndrome)
  —membranous glomerulonephritis
  —focal segmental glomerulonephritis

Common secondary causes
- Systemic lupus erythematosus
- Polyarteritis
- Diabetes mellitus
- Amyloidosis
- Henoch–Schönlein purpura
- Malarial nephropathy

(see Box 8.11), periodic i.v. urograms or loopograms may be performed. A loopogram is the radiological examination of the bowel segment used to form the urinary diversion; this investigation may reveal any disorder of filling or capacity (Hanno & Wein 1994).

RENAL DISORDERS

Glomerulonephritis

The term 'glomerulonephritis' refers to a group of disorders characterised by the presence of a lesion in the glomerulus of the kidney. The disease may be primary to the glomerulus or secondary to a systemic disorder. Box 8.12 lists primary and secondary causes.

Proteinaemia, haematuria, hypertension and renal impairment characterise this disease but the severity of these effects will vary between individuals. Presentation is usually described in terms of a range of clinical syndromes, but accurate diagnosis requires histological investigation.

PATHOPHYSIOLOGY

Histological examination of renal tissue will demonstrate inflammation in the majority of cases, but it is also possible to find minimal change and no evidence of an inflammatory process. The disease process results from a defect in the immune response, such as a hypersensitivity to an exogenous antigen. The antigen–antibody reaction results in the formation of insoluble immune complexes that circulate in the blood and, instead of being ingested by macrophages, reach the kidney, where they become 'trapped' and set up a damaging inflammatory reaction in the delicate filtration structure. As a result of this:

- protein and red blood cells pass through the filtration fenestration
- the osmotic pressure of the blood plasma falls, leading to oedema
- sodium and water are retained, as are waste products and potentially toxic substances.

It would seem that most cases of acute glomerulonephritis occur 1–3 weeks after an 'innocent' streptococcal infection such as tonsillitis or otitis media; this most commonly occurs in children or adolescents, however only 5% of these infections lead to glomerulonephritis. In recent years, there has been a significant reduction in the incidence of post-streptococcal glomerulonephritis, as a result of better hygiene and the use of antibiotics. The disease can range from a mild, transitory, asymptomatic condition to a very severe form that precipitates acute renal failure, cardiac failure and convulsions.

Common presenting symptoms are exemplified in Case History 8.6.

For further information, see Whitworth & Lawrence (1994), Smith (1997) and Haslett et al (1999).

MEDICAL MANAGEMENT

Tests and investigations. A patient such as T (see Case History 8.6) would probably be admitted to hospital, where investigations would confirm the diagnosis. This would be especially likely if there

Case History 8.6 T

T was an active 15-year-old schoolgirl. In September she developed a sore throat which completely robbed her of her voice for several days. It didn't last long and she was used to such minor ailments. In early October she began to notice a feeling of weariness that was quite uncharacteristic. She found herself longing for her bed as the day progressed and declined evening invitations for the usual lively events. On waking one morning, she noticed that her face appeared rather puffy and, on close inspection, found she had puffy ankles. Her parents became concerned and T made an appointment to see her doctor. She now began to consider other problems. She had lost her appetite, often felt rather sick and had noticed that her urine had been rather smoky and darker in hue.

T's GP identified significant proteinuria and haematuria, an elevated blood pressure and marked oedema. A diagnosis of acute glomerulonephritis was made.

were symptoms of breathlessness or a risk of convulsions, which would indicate cardiac or cerebral complications. Investigations would include:

- urinalysis
- MSU
- full blood count and urea and electrolyte estimation
- throat swab
- chest X-ray
- ECG
- ultrasound scan
- biopsy.

Treatment. There is no cure as such for glomerulonephritis. The aim of treatment is to reduce renal workload, restore and maintain fluid and electrolyte status and prevent uraemia. Thus management aims to prevent serious complications from occurring (see Box 8.13).

NURSING PRIORITIES AND MANAGEMENT: GLOMERULONEPHRITIS

Major nursing considerations

Promoting rest

Bed rest is a necessity, especially in the early period, to reduce the workload of both the kidneys and the heart. This can pose quite a challenge in the care of younger patients. Time needs to be spent with the patient, explaining why rest is so important.

Maintaining fluid and electrolyte balance

While renal function is impaired and fluid overload poses a very real problem, fluid and sodium intake must be restricted. Potassium levels in the blood must be closely monitored and, if necessary, dietary modification made or ion exchange resins given. If hypertension is marked, anti-hypertensive medication may be required.

Preventing uraemia

While the kidney is impaired, the waste products of metabolism will build up in the blood. To prevent this, a protein-restricted diet will be necessary. Calorie intake can be maintained with carbohydrates, and vitamin supplements can be given. This diet must also be low in salt and many patients find meals unpalatable. The dietician can contribute tremendously to the patient's well-being by ensuring that the restricted diet includes at least some favourite foods.

Preventing infection

If a streptococcal link is confirmed, penicillin may be prescribed. All patients with renal impairment are prone to infection. All procedures necessary for the prevention of cross-infection must be adhered to (see Ch. 16, p. 586).

Promoting convalescence and the maintenance of health

Most patients make a full recovery, but convalescence may take as long as 2 years. The acute condition can resolve fairly rapidly, and the majority of people recover normal renal function within a couple of months. Such patients often feel better quite quickly and it can be hard to persuade them that restrictions are still needed. Proteinuria can persist and regular monitoring will be necessary. After discharge, support for the patient and family will ensure that necessary lifestyle adjustments are made for the initial months. Exercise should be gentle and energetic sports activities avoided. Any infection should be treated seriously and medical advice sought.

Box 8.13 Life-threatening complications of glomerulonephritis

Acute hypertensive encephalitis leading to convulsions (see Ch. 9)

Management
- Maintain airway
- Monitor level of consciousness (e.g. with Glasgow Coma Scale)
- Give anticonvulsant therapy, e.g. i.v. diazepam
- Give hypotensive agents

Pulmonary oedema/cardiac failure (see Chs 2 and 3)

Management
- Give oxygen therapy
- Monitor cardiovascular status
- Give diuretic therapy, e.g. i.v. frusemide
- Give opiate analgesics, e.g. i.v. morphine combined with an antiemetic

Acute renal failure

Management
- Dialysis

Incomplete resolution and permanent glomerular damage can result in chronic glomerulonephritis and all the associated symptoms of renal impairment. Failure of function may be such that dialysis is required (see p. 346).

Nephrotic syndrome (see Case History 8.7)

Nephrotic syndrome encompasses a group of symptoms including proteinuria, oedema and lipidaemia. It can be a manifestation of certain forms of glomerulonephritis but may also result as a complication of diabetes mellitus or amyloid disease whereby insoluble starch-like deposits occur in kidney tissue. Often no cause can be found.

PATHOPHYSIOLOGY

In the normal kidney, protein molecules passing across the glomerulomembrane are reabsorbed in the kidney tubules. However, where increased glomerular permeability occurs, increased numbers of protein molecules enter the tubules. When the capacity of the tubule to reabsorb protein is exceeded, protein is lost in the urine. Further protein is lost following catabolism of protein reabsorbed in the tubule, resulting in hypoproteinaemia. Muscle wasting can result from the catabolism of muscle protein as the body tries to maintain normal plasma protein levels. A low plasma protein reduces plasma osmotic pressure and fluid leaks into the extracellular areas. The resultant oedema occurs in dependent areas and may give rise to ascites in severe cases. Intravascular volume is maintained in many cases. How this occurs is not fully understood, but activation of the renin–angiotensin–aldosterone mechanism is thought likely.

Clinical features. This syndrome is characterised by heavy proteinuria and hypoproteinaemia and by oedema. These patients generally have a low urine output and low urine sodium. Derangement of lipoproteins is evident and loss of fibrinogen in the urine can occur. Infection and thrombosis are common complications.

Case History 8.7 Mrs Y

Mrs Y, aged 29, presented to her GP with a 3-week history of anorexia and tiredness. Examination revealed no muscle wasting but did show a moderate degree of ankle and sacral oedema. Mrs Y said that her complexion was naturally pale but that her face seemed to have become puffy in the last week or so. Urine testing showed heavy proteinuria. Blood samples were taken for biochemical analysis.

A clinical diagnosis of nephrotic syndrome was made and she was prescribed 80 mg of frusemide daily and a diet with no added salt. Mrs Y was advised that a renal biopsy may be necessary. She resisted immediate admission to hospital and the GP and district nurse arranged to attend Mrs Y's home on alternate days.

Mrs Y wished to stay at home as she had a 3-year-old son and a 6-month-old daughter to care for. On weekday mornings she took her son to a nursery half a mile away and collected him at midday. The family were dependent financially on Mr Y, who worked 200 miles away and was able to return home only at weekends.

One of the major difficulties Mrs Y will face is dealing with the increased diuresis that results from diuretic therapy. A heavy diuresis will occur for about 4 h following each dose. This may make it virtually impossible for Mrs Y to leave the house. Taking her son to the nursery and shopping for household necessities may become difficult. Confined to the house with two small children and a husband 200 miles away, Mrs Y may become socially isolated. The 'no-added-salt diet' may also pose a problem for Mrs Y, particularly if she enjoys salty foods.

The symptoms that Mrs Y has experienced are uncomfortable and frightening. It has been suggested to her that she might need a renal biopsy to determine the cause of her symptoms. It is likely that she will be worried and may need time to voice her concerns and perhaps obtain information and reassurance about her physical condition. It is possible that she may feel unable to carry out all the care for her children and require assistance at some times during the day.

MEDICAL MANAGEMENT

Treatment. The main aim of treatment is to reduce oedema. Diuretic therapy can be adjusted according to the severity of the oedema and small maintenance doses can be administered when the oedema is under control. Severe oedema may also be treated by the administration of salt-poor albumin to temporarily increase plasma osmotic pressure. Patients are advised to adhere to a diet free from added salt.

Identification of the underlying disease process, possibly by renal biopsy and histological examination, will dictate the nature of ongoing treatment. In many patients, chronic renal failure will eventually develop.

8.11 Since Mrs Y in Case History 8.7 has young children, the health visitor will already know this family well. The effectiveness of intervention will depend on the quality of communication between members of the primary health care team. What are the essential features of teamwork that will contribute to the well-being of Mrs Y and her family? Draw from the following references as you consider these issues in a discussion group.

For further information, see Gregson et al (1991), Pearson (1992) and Waine (1992).

Acute renal failure (ARF)

Acute renal failure, the sudden and severe reduction in previously normal renal function, may result from primary renal disease but is more frequently associated with other organ failure. Failure is often reversible, but should the kidneys fail to recover, permanent treatment will be required.

A mortality rate of 50% is associated with acute renal failure, the actual risk depending on the type of patient, the cause of failure and other organ involvement (Morgan 1996). Where death occurs, renal failure is often not the primary cause.

PATHOPHYSIOLOGY

Causes. The causes of acute renal failure may be classified into pre-renal, renal and post-renal.

Pre-renal causes are those in which a loss or decrease in renal perfusion results in renal ischaemia. They include:

- extracellular depletion, e.g. large GI loss such as vomiting, diarrhoea or NG aspiration; urinary loss due to polyuria or diuresis; loss from the skin, e.g. sweating or burns
- circulating volume loss, as in haemorrhage or hypoalbuminaemia
- reduced cardiac output, as in cardiac arrest, valvular disease, cardiac tamponade
- vascular disease, e.g. renal artery thrombosis or embolism.

Renal causes include conditions that impair renal function by damaging the structure of the kidney (tubules, interstitium, glomeruli or capillaries). If tubular damage occurs, this is termed acute tubular necrosis (ATN), although microscopically the tubules usually show dilatation rather than necrosis. Pre-renal causes can also cause the destruction of the renal parenchyma.

Nephrotoxic substances can also result in acute failure. These include:

- drugs, e.g. the antibiotics kanamycin and gentamicin
- exogenous chemicals, e.g. heavy metals, phenols, carbon tetrachloride, chlorates, ethyl glycol
- bacterial toxins, particularly those released in Gram-negative septicaemia (see Ch. 18, p. 640).

Post-renal causes are mainly attributed to obstruction. The most common of these is bladder output obstruction which may be due to prostatic hypertrophy, tumours or calculi.

Clinical features. Acute renal failure proceeds through three phases: the oliguric stage, the diuretic stage and the recovery stage. If oliguria persists for more than 48 h, major metabolic problems can arise.

Oliguria and abnormal plasma levels of creatinine, urea and electrolytes are the principal features of presentation. The effects of acute fluid overload and hyperkalaemia (K^+ >6 mmol/L) can result in sudden death.

The patient may complain of anorexia, nausea and vomiting. Increased respiration due to pulmonary oedema and acidosis can occur. Drowsiness, confusion and coma may follow.

MEDICAL MANAGEMENT

Tests and investigations will depend on the suspected cause and on the immediacy of the presentation but may include:

- full blood count and urea and electrolyte estimation
- urinalysis, MSU, 24-h collections of urine for creatinine clearance
- X-ray of kidneys, ureters and bladder
- ultrasound
- renal biopsy.

Treatment. The goal is to restore biochemical balance and prevent ARF progressing. The onset of renal failure must be identified early to minimise damage and, if possible, prevent the necessity for dialysis. The priorities of treatment are as follows.
Treating the cause, e.g. correcting hypovolaemia and increasing renal perfusion; managing sepsis; relieving any urinary obstruction.
Reversing, restoring and maintaining fluid and electrolyte status:

- *Hyperkalaemia.* Immediate measures may be required to correct hyperkalaemia, which could cause lethal dysrhythmias. Cardiac monitoring is essential and particular attention must be paid to the T wave (Hampton 1992). Hyperkalaemia can be corrected in the short term by i.v. insulin–glucose infusion or sodium bicarbonate, either of which will shift potassium into the cells. Other measures include the administration of ion exchange resins, which when administered orally or rectally remove potassium ions.
- *Hyponatraemia and hypernatraemia.* In the oliguric state there is a real danger of hyponatraemia, due to the very real risk of fluid overload and to the failure of the damaged tubules to reabsorb sodium. However, hypernatraemia can also be a problem in pre-renal ARF, as mechanisms instituted retain sodium in order to restore blood volume. Fluid intake must be restricted to the equivalent of insensible loss plus the previous day's urinary output. Sodium intake must be monitored closely.
- *Uraemia.* The inability to excrete the waste products of metabolism is managed by restricting protein intake and maintaining a high-calorie intake in the form of carbohydrates. Parenteral nutrition may be necessary and potassium intake will be restricted (see Ch. 21, p. 713).
- *Metabolic acidosis.* The loss of the kidneys' buffering function, the electrolyte imbalance and the increased anaerobic respiration by damaged renal cells all result in acidosis. In the short term, this is managed by i.v. sodium bicarbonate.

If acute renal failure is very severe, persists or worsens, dialysis will be necessary.

NURSING PRIORITIES AND MANAGEMENT: ACUTE RENAL FAILURE

Major nursing considerations

The care of patients with ARF may involve a large multidisciplinary team and be carried out in an intensive care setting. However, many may be nursed in a general ward and require close monitoring and support by the nursing staff. Priorities of nursing intervention will be as follows:

- to reduce the patient's very real anxieties and recognise the risk of altered consciousness due to uraemia and electrolyte imbalance
- to control fluid and electrolyte balance by:
  —monitoring cardiac status for signs of dysrhythmias
  —monitoring pulse, respiration and blood pressure for signs of overload and hypertension
  —restricting fluid intake and measuring and recording urine output and other losses; daily weighing may be required
  —administering prescribed medication and carrying out urinary assays as required
- to maintain nutritional status within the necessary limitations by the oral or parenteral route and to monitor the nutritional status of the patient
- to prevent infection due to uraemia by strict asepsis with regard to infusion sites and catheter management and by close monitoring of temperature and the patient's reported symptoms
- to manage anaemia by the safe administration of blood transfusions, if required
- to promote comfort at all times.

8.12 Reconsider the care of T, who had acute glomerulonephritis (see Case History 8.6). Severe forms can result in acute tubular necrosis and acute renal failure. Draw up a care plan that would have met T's needs should ARF have developed.

The diuretic and recovery stages

So far we have considered the oliguric stage of renal failure. This may last 1–3 weeks and is followed by the diuretic stage, which indicates that renal function is returning. This is often a time of relief, but because the kidneys will not yet have regained their capacity for selective reabsorption, urine output can be as much as 4 L/day. This, in itself, could potentiate dehydration and electrolyte imbalances. Close monitoring must therefore continue. The recovery phase that follows can last several months and will require close medical follow-up of renal function. Convalescence in the form of rest, restricted activity, the avoidance of infections and alertness to any symptoms that might indicate renal problems may be a source of considerable stress to the patient, who may also be concerned about fulfilling family and work responsibilities.

For further information see Joynes (1996).

8.13 What community support services might help to alleviate such stress?

Chronic renal failure

Chronic renal failure is the gradual and progressive reduction in renal function. Failure may occur over weeks, months or even years. Each year, approximately 55 new patients per million of the population require renal replacement therapy to maintain life. The available treatments are dialysis or transplantation.

PATHOPHYSIOLOGY

Any disorder which damages kidney function can result in renal failure (see Box 8.14).
Clinical features. In the initial stages of failure the patient may be asymptomatic. Proteinuria, hypertension, anaemia or an elevated blood urea are, however, common presenting features.

As renal failure progresses, the patient may complain of fatigue, lethargy, pruritus, nausea, vomiting and indigestion. Breathlessness on exertion, headaches, visual disturbances, pallor and loss of libido may also be noted. A reduced immune response occurs, making the patient prone to infection, particularly of the urinary tract (see Ch. 16).

Metabolic bone disease, generalised myopathy, neuropathy and metabolic acidosis can be seen in advanced stages of renal

Box 8.14 Aetiology of chronic renal failure. (Reproduced with permission from Haslett et al 1999)

Congenital and inherited diseases
- Polycystic kidney disease (infantile or adult)
- Alport's syndrome
- Fabry's disease

Vascular disease
- Arteriosclerosis
- Vasculitis (polyarteritis nodosa [PAN], systemic lupus erythematosus [SLE], scleroderma)

Glomerular disease
- Proliferative GN
- Crescentic GN
- Membranous GN
- Mesangiocapillary GN
- Glomerulosclerosis
- Secondary GN (PAN, SLE, amyloidosis, diabetic glomerulosclerosis)

Interstitial disease
- Chronic infective interstitial nephritis (chronic pyelonephritis)
- Vesicoureteric reflux
- Tuberculosis
- Analgesic nephropathy
- Nephrocalcinosis
- Schistosomiasis
- Unknown origin

Obstructive uropathy
- Calculus
- Retroperitoneal fibrosis
- Prostatic hypertrophy
- Pelvic tumours
- Other causes

impairment. Atherosclerosis due to altered lipid and carbohydrate metabolism and hypertension may also occur. Vascular calcification and pericarditis may also be identified.

MEDICAL MANAGEMENT

Treatment aims to identify the cause, extent and complications of the renal failure and to preserve useful renal function for as long as possible.

Where hypertension is evident, anti-hypertensive drugs may be used to gradually reduce and control blood pressure.

Fluid restriction may be required if the glomerulofiltration rate is less than 5 mL/min. Poor concentration can, however, result in a urine output of more than 2.5 L/24 h, in which case an intake of about 3 L is required.

Dietary restrictions are likely to include protein restriction to about 40 g daily if the serum creatinine is greater than 300 mmol/L. Sodium restriction is not indicated unless there is evidence of oedema, hypertension or cardiac failure. In the case of salt-losing conditions, sodium supplements may be required. A diet with no added salt may be appropriate in some cases.

Regular monitoring of biochemistry and assessment of symptoms allow treatment to be readjusted and progression of the disease to be assessed.

Dialysis in the form of haemodialysis or continuous ambulatory peritoneal dialysis are the treatments available to replace the excretory functions of the kidneys (see Box 8.15). At present, transplantation is restricted by a lack of available cadaver donor kidneys. In some cases it may be possible to consider a close family member as a live donor.

NURSING PRIORITIES AND MANAGEMENT: CHRONIC RENAL FAILURE

General considerations

Nursing management requires a strategy to help the patient and her family come to terms with an illness for which there is no cure and in which sudden death can occur. Nursing intervention should aim to help the patient develop a way to cope with the constraints of the available treatments and the possibility of other disorders associated with the renal failure occurring, e.g. bone disease.

Compliance

Patient beliefs about the value and benefit of a treatment may differ markedly when compared with the priority given to the same treatment by the nurse. Non-compliance with diet and fluid restrictions is a suggestion that the patient has an underlying problem and is not coping with some aspect of the treatment. An understanding of the patient's social and cultural background can give insight into her behaviour with regard to a particular treatment.

Major patient problems

Fatigue and lethargy characteristic of chronic renal failure can reduce both ability and performance at work. Absence from work due to sickness or attendance at hospital may result in unemployment or reduction of income. Feelings of helplessness, hopelessness and depression are often expressed by patients with a chronic illness (Killingworth 1993). Loss of control over many aspects of life and low self-esteem are likely to influence family relationships. Transplantation may be seen as a cure or an escape from dialysis, and indeed a more normal lifestyle and a feeling of physical well-being can follow transplant. The patient may be poorly prepared to deal with graft failure and the need to return to dialysis, or with inadequate graft function and the need for continued restrictions. The need to return regularly to hospital for check-ups, and continued problems associated with complications of renal failure or a second disease process such as diabetes can contribute to disappointment in transplantation as a treatment. On the other hand, some patients who undergo a successful transplant have difficulty abandoning the sick role (see Ch. 32).

For further information, see Locking-Cusolito (1990), Holecheck et al (1991) and Beckman et al (1992).

Living with CAPD

Continuous ambulatory peritoneal dialysis offers patients a degree of control over their treatment. While the number of fluid exchanges per day will be prescribed by the doctor, the timing of each exchange can be decided by the patient to fit in with family life or work commitments. In addition, freedom to be away from home for visits or holidays is possible. For holidays abroad, the dialysate manufacturer may be able to deliver fluid requirements to the holiday destination.

The need for regular fluid exchanges and aseptic technique can be limiting for some patients. Performing the exchange in a designated area at home can give confidence and reassure patients that

Box 8.15 Dialysis

Principles
Dialysis requires a semi-permeable membrane to combine three principles — diffusion, osmosis and filtration — in order to permit the removal of metabolic wastes, excess electrolytes and fluids from patients with renal failure.

Diffusion
Diffusion is the movement of molecules from an area of high concentration, across a semi-permeable membrane, to an area of low concentration. This process continues until the concentrations in each compartment are the same.

Osmosis
Osmosis is the movement of a fluid or solvent from a lower concentration to a higher one.

Filtration
Filtration is the movement of both solvent and solute across a semi-permeable membrane under pressure.

Types
Haemodialysis
Haemodialysis requires a means of vascular access, e.g.:
- *Percutaneous access*, including subclavian, femoral and jugular lines which are either temporary or permanent.
- *Arteriovenous fistula and arteriovenous grafts (synthetic).* A fistula involves the anastomosis of an artery and a vein. The increased blood flow causes increased pressure on the vein walls which leads to thickening and dilatation (arterialised); this allows the repeated insertion of needles for dialysis. This developmental stage takes about 12 weeks. The fistula can be seen as well as felt.

The blood is pumped from the patient to an artificial kidney (the dialyser) and back to the patient, having now been cleansed by the dialysate. The artificial kidney is normally a disposable hollow fibre or flat plate dialyser; different dialysers consist of different membranes. The type of membrane used is important as part of the patient's individualised dialysis prescription. Issues to consider are desired clearance, fluid removal and biocompatibility.

Peritoneal dialysis
The peritoneal membrane serves as the semi-permeable membrane for dialysis. A temporary or permanent Tenckhoff catheter is placed into the abdomen. The dialysate is instilled into the abdomen (usually 2 L at each session). A set time elapses and the dialysate is drained out.

Continuing ambulatory peritoneal dialysis (CAPD)
Two litres of dialysate are instilled into the peritoneal cavity and left in place, usually for 6 h, when it is exchanged.

Once patients have been instructed in this method, they can be independent, visiting the hospital only for clinic appointments or when any problems arise; the main potential problems are peritonitis, dehydration and constipation.

Other methods
Other methods of renal replacement therapy are often used in intensive care, including:
- continuous arteriovenous haemofiltration (CAVH)
- continuous arteriovenous haemodiafiltration (CAVHD)
- continuous venovenous haemofiltration (CVVH)
- continuous venovenous haemodiafiltration (CVVHD)

they have done all they can to reduce the risk of peritonitis. There may be a reluctance to perform exchanges in the homes of friends and relatives, particularly if the patient's illness is poorly understood and a source of embarrassment.

Q **8.14** How might you help a patient to gain confidence dealing with her treatment so that she can take advantage of the relative freedom that CAPD offers?

The insertion of a tube and presence of fluid in the abdomen can alter body image and sexuality, thus discouraging those who are conscious of their appearance. A further disadvantage of CAPD is that it presents a constant reminder to the patient of her illness.

For further information, see Galpin (1992) and Smith (1997).

Living with intermittent haemodialysis

For some patients, haemodialysis requiring treatment on an outpatient basis two to three times a week may be the preferred option. This form of treatment does have a number of drawbacks, including the following:

- the need for transport to and from hospital
- the need to be away from home and dependants two or three times a week
- the difficulty of fitting in dialysis sessions with work and family commitments
- the increased fluid load prior to dialysis
- the need to restrict the diet
- the financial implications of lost work time
- the side-effects of dialysis and the continuing feeling of not being fully fit
- living with the uncertain hope of a kidney transplant
- the stress and strain on the family of dealing with the lifestyle constraints imposed by treatment.

Q **8.15** Consider the problems listed above and, for each, suggest ways in which the health care team can help. (A)

Nursing support during dialysis. Assessments to be performed before haemodialysis are:

- Record patient's weight — compare with weight after last dialysis.

- Record temperature, pulse and blood pressure — compare these with values after the last dialysis. Any temperature increase could indicate an infected dialysis site. Raised blood pressure may indicate fluid overloading.
- Enquire if the patient has been encountering any problems.
- Assess any known specific medical problem, e.g. blood sugar level in diabetics.
- Once a month, take blood for urea and electrolyte levels pre- and post-dialysis; a full blood count should be checked every 2 weeks.

During dialysis, the nurse should record the pulse and blood pressure. A drop in blood pressure may mean that the patient needs extra fluid. If necessary, the nurse should check the patient's weight halfway through the session. Some patients may be nursed on weigh beds during haemodialysis.

At the end of dialysis, the patient's temperature, pulse, blood pressure and weight should be recorded in order to assess the effectiveness of the treatment. Any prescribed medications should be administered and the patient should be given the opportunity to raise any further concerns.

REFERENCES

Anthony C P, Thibodeau G A 1983 Textbook of anatomy and physiology, 11th edn. Mosby, St Louis, MO

Argyle M 1981 Social skills and health. Methuen, London

Black P K 1994a Hidden problems of stoma care. British Journal of Nursing 3(14): 707–711

Brewster J 1992 Operations explained. Nursing Times 88(39): 50–52

Bullock N, Sibley G, Whitaker R 1994 Essential urology, 2nd edn. Churchill Livingstone, Edinburgh

Burkitt H G, Quick C R G, Gatt D 1996 Essential surgery: problems, diagnosis and management, 2nd edn. Churchill Livingstone, Edinburgh

Charlton C A C 1984 The urological system. Churchill Livingstone, Edinburgh

Dawson C, Whitfield H N 1994 The long term results of urinary stones. British Journal of Urology 74: 397–404

Dean M, Downey P 1997 Prostate cancer. Professional Nurse 12(10): 722–724

Downey P 1997 Benign prostatic hyperplasia. Professional Nurse 12(7): 501–506

Edwards C R W, Bouchier I A D, Haslett C, Chilvers E R 1995 Davidson's principles and practice of medicine, 17th edn. Churchill Livingstone, Edinburgh

Falkiner F R 1993 The insertion and management of indwelling urethral catheters – minimising the risk of infection. Journal of Hospital Infection 25: 79–83

Forrest A P M, Carter D C, Macleod I B (eds) 1995 Principles and practice of surgery, 3rd edn. Churchill Livingstone, Edinburgh

Hampton J R 1992 The ECG made easy. Churchill Livingstone, Edinburgh

Hanno P M, Wein A J 1994 A clinical manual of urology, 2nd edn. Prentice Hall, London

Haslett C, Chilvers E R, Hunter J A A, Boon N A (eds) 1999 Davidson's principles and practice of medicine, 18th edn. Churchill Livingstone, Edinburgh

Jamieson E M, McCall J M, Blythe R 1992 Guidelines for clinical nursing practice, 2nd edn. Churchill Livingstone, Edinburgh

Killingworth A 1993 Psychological impact of end stage renal disease. British Journal of Nursing 2(18): 905–908

Laker C 1994 Urological nursing. Scutari Press, London

Marieb E N 1995 Human anatomy and physiology, 3rd edn. Benjamin/Cummings Publishing, California

Morgan A G 1996 The management of acute renal failure. British Journal of Hospital Medicine 55(4): 167–170

Pitt M 1989 Fluid balance and urinary tract infection. Nursing Times 85(1): 36–38

Pomfret I 1996 Catheters: design, selection and management. British Journal of Nursing 5(4): 245–250

RCN Society of Occupational Health Nursing 1991 A guide to an occupational nursing service: a handbook for employers and nurses. Scutari Press, Harrow

Roe B 1990 The basis for sound practice. Nursing Standard 14(51): 22–25

Trounce J, Gould D 1997 Clinical pharmacology for nurses. Churchill Livingstone, Edinburgh

Webb V, Simpson R 1997 Older man's burden. Nursing Times 93(5): 77–79

Wilson K J W, Waugh A 1996 Ross & Wilson anatomy and physiology in health and illness, 8th edn. Churchill Livingstone, Edinburgh

FURTHER READING

Barnett J 1991 Catheters: preventative procedures. Nursing Times 87(10): 66–68

Beckman N J, Schell H M, Calixto P R, Sullivan M M 1992 Kidney transplantation: a therapy option. Clinical Issues in Critical Care Nursing 3(3): 570–584

Black P K 1994b Management of patients undergoing stoma surgery. British Journal of Nursing 3(5): 211–216

Bullock N, Sibley G, Whitaker R 1994 Essential urology, 2nd edn. Churchill Livingstone, Edinburgh

Dickson C 1995 The bladder: cystectomy and ileal conduit to treat cancer. Nursing Times 91(42): 34–35

Galpin C 1992 Body image in end stage renal failure. British Journal of Nursing April/May: 21–23

Garraway W M, Alexander F E 1997 Prostatic disease: epidemiology, natural history and demographic shifts. British Journal of Urology 79(suppl 2): 3–8

Gledhill E 1996 The potential of shared care. British Journal of Healthcare Management 2(2): 71–73

Gregson B A, Cartlidge A, Bond J 1991 Interprofessional collaboration in primary health care organisations. Occasional paper 52. Royal College of General Practitioners, London

Hanno P M, Wein A J 1994 A clinical manual of urolog. Prentice Hall, London

Holecheck M J, Burrell-Diggs D, Navarro N O 1991 Renal transplantation: an option for end stage renal disease patients. Critical Care Nursing Quarterly 13(4): 62–77

Joynes J 1996 An analysis of the component parts of advanced nursing practice in relation to acute renal care in intensive care. Intensive and Critical Care Nursing 12: 113–119

Kilmartin A 1989 Understanding cystitis: the complete self-help guide. Arrow Books, London

Laker C 1994 Urological Nursing. Scutari Press, London

Leaver R 1994 The mitrofanoff pouch: a continent urinary diversion. Professional Nurse Aug: 748–753

Locking-Cusolito H 1990 Renal transplant and uncertainty. Canadian Nurse 86(7): 27–28

Marieb E N 1998 Human anatomy and physiology. Benjamin/Cummings Publishing, California

Marsh M 1992 Malignant disease of the prostate gland. Nursing Standard 6(36): 28–31

Myers C 1996 Stoma care nursing. A patient centred approach. Arnold, London

Pearson P 1992 Defining the primary health care team. Health Visitor 65(10): 358–361

Pomfret I 1996 Catheters, design, selection and management. British Journal of Nursing 5(4): 245–250

Preshloch K 1989 Detecting the hidden urinary tract infection. Registered Nurse 52(1): 65–69
Reynolds R 1993 Coping successfully with prostate problems. Sheldon Press, London
Roe B H 1991 Catheters: looking at the evidence. Nursing Times 87(33): 72–74
Royal College of Nursing 1991 A guide to an occupational health nursing service: a handbook for employers and nurses. Scutari Press, London
Smith T (ed) (1997) Renal nursing. Baillière Tindall, London
Sueppel C 1992 Prostate poundage perks. Urologic Nursing 12(4): 147
Waine C 1992 The primary care team (editorial). The British Journal of General Practice 42(365): 498–499
Webb V, Simpson R 1997 Older man's burden. Nursing Times 93(5): 77–79
Whitworth J A, Lawrence J R 1994 Textbook of renal disease, 2nd edn. Churchill Livingstone, Edinburgh
Willis D 1992 Taming the overgrown prostate. American Journal of Nursing 92(2): 39–40

THE NERVOUS SYSTEM

9

Douglas Allan

INTRODUCTION

Many nurses will have only brief contact with patients suffering from neurological disorders, either while they are waiting to be transferred to a specialist neurological unit or following their return from such a unit. Community staff are increasingly involved with patients recovering at home from acute neurosurgical interventions and long-term neurological disorders requiring supportive therapies, where the disorder cannot be cured. The last few years have also witnessed a growth in the number of specialised liaison or support nurses for patients with disorders such as epilepsy and multiple sclerosis.

This chapter covers the more common neurological and neurosurgical disorders and, where appropriate, makes reference to the more uncommon disorders. The specialised neuroscience textbooks listed at the end of the chapter provide more detailed information. It is hoped that the information contained here will help to alleviate any apprehension that the student may have regarding this specialised field of nursing, and that it will stimulate further discussion as to how best to meet the needs of the neurologically impaired patient and his family.

ANATOMY AND PHYSIOLOGY

The nervous system is a complex, interrelated body system responsible for many functions including communication, coordination, behaviour and intelligence. It constantly receives data from the external and internal environment, interprets this and then makes adjustments to cope with this.

The nervous system can be considered in two distinct parts, namely the central nervous system (CNS), comprising the brain and spinal cord, and the peripheral nervous system (PNS), consisting of the cranial and spinal nerves. The peripheral nervous system has two functional parts:

- the sensory division
- the motor division; this is further divided into:
  —the somatic nervous system, which conducts impulses from the CNS to skeletal muscles
  —the autonomic nervous system, which conducts impulses from the CNS to smooth muscle, cardiac muscle and glands.

Basic tissue structure

Nervous tissue consists of neuroglia (or 'glial cells') and neurones (or 'nerve cells'). The neuroglia markedly outnumber the neurones and form a supportive and protective network for the nervous system, e.g. by attaching neurones to their blood vessels and protecting the nervous system through phagocytic action, as the white cells do elsewhere in the body. In the peripheral nervous system, supporting cells, called 'Schwann cells', form the myelin sheath as well as having a phagocytic role.

Myelin protects and electrically insulates nerve fibres from one another, and speeds up nerve impulse transmission. Myelinated nerve impulses are transmitted by saltatory conduction, whereby the impulse jumps from one node of Ranvier to the next. Impulses in myelinated nerves are therefore transmitted very much faster than in unmyelinated nerves and require very much less energy. The

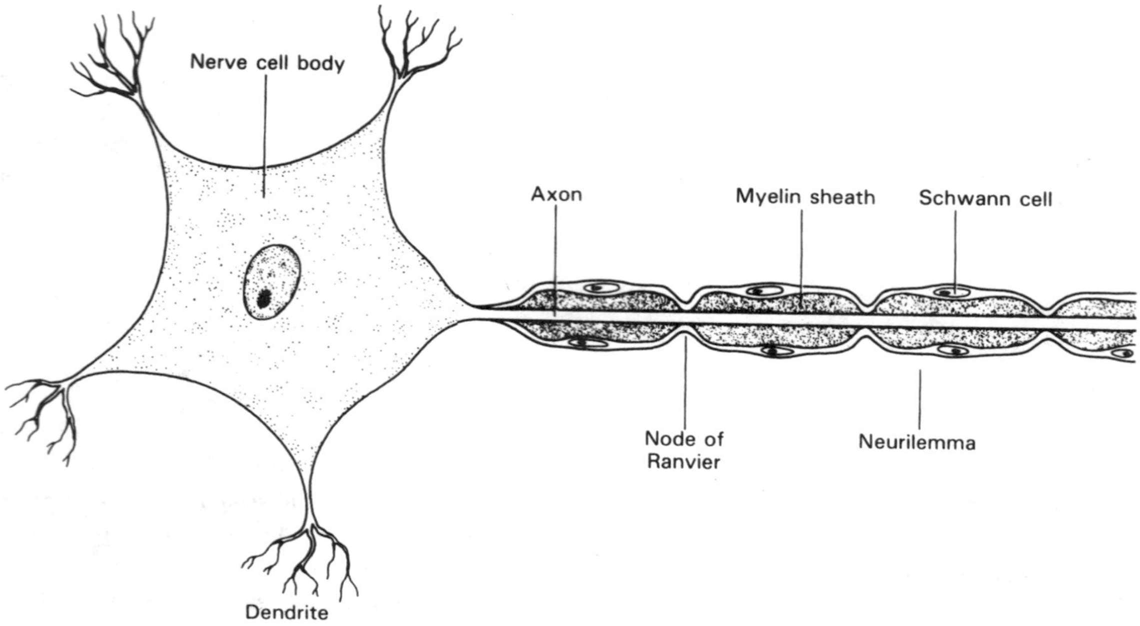

Fig. 9.1 Structure of a multipolar neurone. It consists of three parts: (1) *The nerve cell body*, which is grey in colour. Each cell body is enclosed in a selectively permeable membrane, which also extends along the cell processes. The cell body contains a nucleus surrounded by cytoplasm which also contains other structures called organelles. (2) *The dendrites* are thread-like extensions of the cell body which increase the surface area available to receive signals from other neurones. (3) *The axon* is a single long process that conducts impulses away from the cell body. In many large peripheral axons, the axolemma is surrounded by another covering called the myelin sheath. This is a multiple-layered covering of fatty material which is white in colour. Its function is to insulate the neurone electrically and thus speed up the conduction of the nerve impulse, by segmentation. Each interruption of the sheath is known as a node of Ranvier and the speed of the impulse is increased by its 'jumping' from node to node. The axon and its collaterals branch into axon terminals, the ends of which form a bulb-like structure. These help to transmit an impulse from one neurone to another across the gap (synapse) between them or at the junctions with effector cells.

importance of myelin in nerve impulse transmission is painfully clear to those suffering from demyelinating diseases such as multiple sclerosis. In this condition, the myelin sheath is destroyed, impulse conduction ceases and the affected individual loses the ability to control voluntary muscle movement (p. 381).

Neurones

Although fewer in number, neurones form the basis of the structural and functional unit of the nervous system. They are capable of conducting impulses throughout the nervous system and to other excitable tissues, including the muscles and glands. The structure of a typical multipolar neurone is shown in Figure 9.1.

The axons of sensory and motor neurones constitute the nerve fibres. They are bundled together in the peripheral nervous system by connective tissue to form the peripheral nerves (see Fig. 9.2). In the CNS, the axons of connector neurones are held in distinct tracts by the glial cells.

Classification of neurones. Neurones are classified according to their function and structure. The functional classification is determined by the direction in which the impulse travels and the structural classification is based on the number of poles on the cell body.

Sensory or afferent neurones transmit impulses from receptors in the skin, sense organs and viscera to the brain and spinal cord. Structurally these are unipolar, i.e. cells with processes projecting from one pole, or bipolar, where processes project from two poles at opposite ends of the cell. Bipolar neurones are only found in special sense organs, e.g. the retina of the eye.

Motor or efferent neurones transmit impulses in the opposite direction, from the brain and spinal cord to muscles and glands in the body (the effectors). Typically, these are multipolar, i.e. cells with processes projecting from many points all over the cell body (see Fig. 9.1).

Connector neurones or interneurones convey impulses within the CNS. Typically, these are also multipolar.

The nerve impulse

A nerve impulse can be initiated by a stimulus such as a change in temperature, pressure or the chemical environment, or impulses can be generated spontaneously by pacemaker cells. The impulse is described as a self-propagating wave of electrical charge along the membrane of the neurone, effecting changes crucial to the conduction of the impulse.

At rest, the nerve cell has an unequal distribution of ions on either side of the plasma membrane. This chemical difference also produces an electrical difference: the inside of the cell is negatively charged in relation to the outside. This has been measured at –70 mV and this is termed the resting membrane potential. The cell is maintained in this condition by a system whereby ions are exchanged between the intracellular and extracellular fluids. A property of all nerve cells is their ability to respond to stimuli by producing an impulse when the stimulus is sufficient to initiate certain electrical and chemical changes within the cell membrane. These positive–negative changes occur in rapid succession, spreading to the end of the axon.

Other more subtle and complex changes also occur.

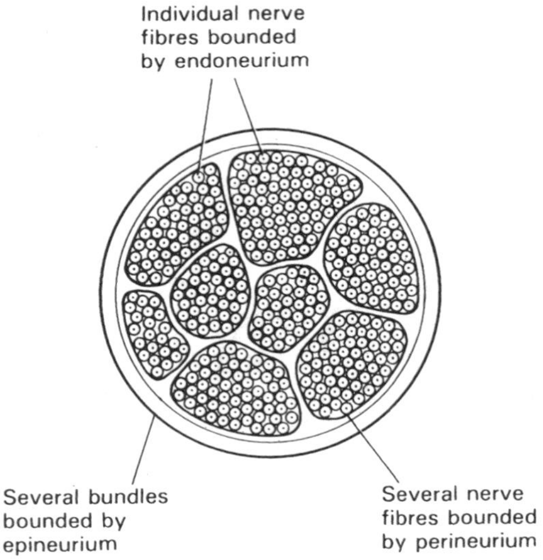

Fig. 9.2 Transverse section, peripheral nerve. The nerve fibres are surrounded by a fine connective tissue covering called the endoneurium. Several nerve fibres are bound together by another connective tissue covering called the perineurium and a number of these bundles may be surrounded by another covering called the epineurium.

Generally, the larger the diameter of the axon, the quicker the nerve impulse travels, but the alternative device of saltatory conduction is found in myelinated neurones, as shown in Figure 9.3.

Neurotransmitters

The junctions between one neurone and another, and between neurones and muscles or glands, are known as synapses. Nerve impulses are transmitted across the gap at these synapses by chemical transmitters (neurotransmitters). The chemical is stored in vesicles in the expanded end of the axon and is released when the nerve impulse reaches this point. Several chemical transmitters have been identified, the most common ones being acetylcholine and noradrenaline. Many of these neurotransmitters are excitatory, resulting in the nerve impulse being transmitted to the receiving tissue and thus producing an effect such as contraction of muscle cells. Some, however, have an inhibiting effect and prevent the onward transmission of impulses, allowing, for example, muscle cells to relax. The effect of the neurotransmitter is terminated when it is destroyed by enzymes or reabsorbed into the neurone.

Detailed information appears in Rutishauser (1994).

The central nervous system

The central nervous system consists of the brain and spinal cord.

The brain

The cerebrum, the largest constituent of the nervous system, forms the bulk of the brain. The outer surface, the cortex, is of grey matter and consists of nerve cell bodies. The surface area of the cerebral cortex is increased by a series of grooves (sulci) and ridges (gyri). The deeper grooves are termed fissures and some form landmarks, e.g. the longitudinal fissure which almost splits the brain into two hemispheres (see Fig. 9.4).

Each hemisphere is subdivided into four lobes, and each lobe is named according to the skull bones it underlies:

- frontal
- temporal
- parietal
- occipital.

The cerebral cortex is responsible for three main functions:

- receiving and interpreting a mass of sensory information from various sources in the internal and external environment
- initiating and controlling voluntary movement in response to the sensory information received
- integrating crucial functions such as memory and consciousness.

Certain areas of the cerebral cortex have been identified as being responsible for these functions, and these areas form a map, as illustrated in Figure 9.5.

Relative size. The lips, thumbs and face use more receptors than the trunk and legs. Similarly, the thumbs, fingers, lips, tongue and vocal cords are more sensitive than the trunk due to the greater number of receptors found in them. The size of the represented area is determined by its functional importance and the need for sensitivity.

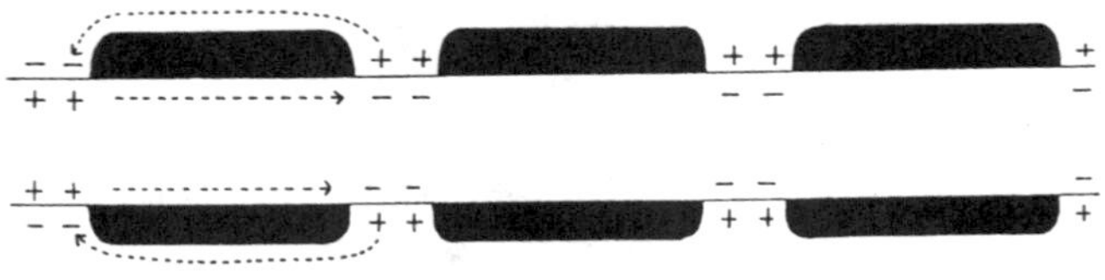

Fig. 9.3 Saltatory conduction in a myelinated nerve.

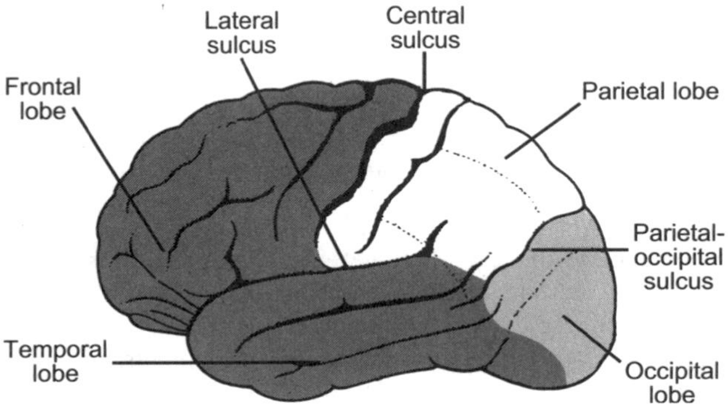

Fig. 9.4 The lobes and sulci of the cerebrum. Each of the lobes is bounded by 'landmark' fissures: the frontal lobe is separated from the parietal lobe by the central sulcus; the temporal lobe is separated from the frontal and parietal lobes by the lateral sulcus; and the occipital lobe is separated from the temporal and parietal lobes by the parietal-occipital sulcus.

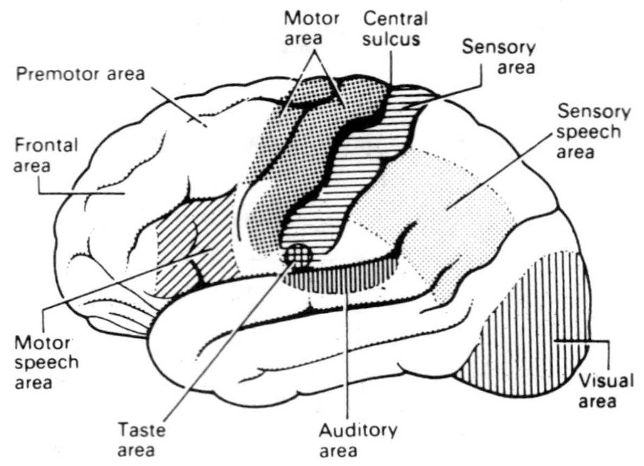

Fig. 9.5 The cerebrum showing the functional areas.

The concept of dominance. The functions of speech and motor control are usually more highly developed in one cerebral hemisphere than in the other. This is referred to as dominance. Approximately 95% of the population are dominant in the left hemisphere and, as most of the spinal pathways cross over, they are right-handed. However, if the dominant hemisphere is damaged, the opposite hemisphere can take over and assume a dominant role.
Association areas. Some areas remain unmapped (see Fig. 9.5). These are called 'association areas' and are thought to be responsible for complex functions such as integration of the senses, memory, learning, thought processes, behaviour and emotion.
Connecting pathways. Below the outer cortical layer can be found areas of white matter (myelinated nerve fibres) that form connections between the cerebral cortex and other areas of grey matter in the CNS. Three types of connecting pathways (Fig. 9.6) have been identified:

- association fibres — these connect between gyri in the same hemisphere
- commissural fibres — these connect between gyri in different hemispheres; one important group of commissural fibres is the corpus callosum
- projection fibres — these provide connections between the brain and spinal cord in ascending and descending pathways; one example is the internal capsule.

Further details on these interconnecting pathways can be found in Hinchliff et al (1996).

Basal ganglia. Within the white matter of the cerebrum are paired islands of grey matter called the 'basal ganglia'. They control large subconscious movements, such as swinging the arms while walking and regulating muscle tone for specific body movements, a function that is lost in Parkinson's disease.

Other structures closely associated with the cerebrum are the cerebellum and the pituitary gland.
The cerebellum is located below the posterior part of the cerebrum and is separated from it by a fold of dura mater. It consists of two hemispheres separated by a narrow strip called the 'vermis'. The cortex of the cerebellum consists of grey matter which has many folds to increase its surface area. The interior comprises white matter presented in a branching configuration termed the arbor vitae or 'tree of life'. There are three connections, called the 'cerebellar peduncles', which link the cerebellum to the rest of the brain and spinal cord. These allow the cerebellum to receive sensory information and thereby to maintain equilibrium and modify voluntary movement, making it smooth and coordinated.

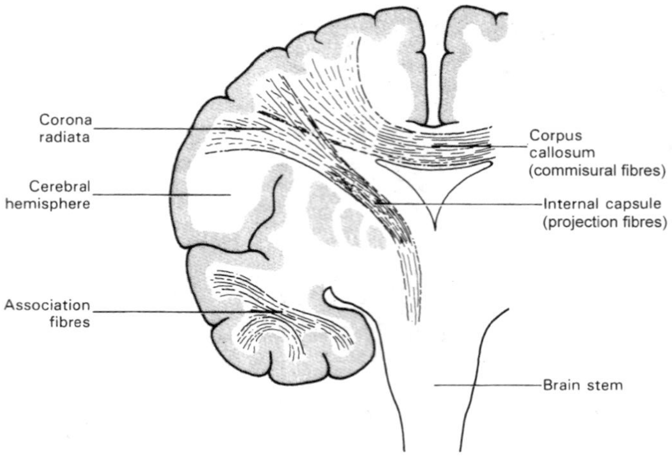

Fig. 9.6 White matter of the cerebrum.

Further detail can be found in Rutishauser (1994).

Pituitary gland. The pituitary gland is situated at the base of the brain in a depression in the sphenoid bone called the 'sella turcica'. It is attached to the brain via a stalk which is continuous with the hypothalamus and communication is by means of nerve fibres and blood vessels. It has three lobes, an anterior, middle and posterior lobe, which secrete hormones that exert an influence on other parts of the body (see Ch. 5 for details of the actions of pituitary hormones).
Diencephalon. Three bilaterally symmetrical structures comprise the diencephalon:

- the thalamus
- the hypothalamus
- the epithalamus.

Collectively, these three structures enclose and form the boundaries of the third ventricle.
Thalamus. The thalamus consists of two oval-shaped masses (thalami), mainly consisting of grey matter with some white matter, and is situated within the cerebral hemispheres just below the corpus callosum. Sensory impulses associated with pain, temperature, pressure and touch are conveyed to the thalamus, which acts as a 'filter'. Chaos would reign if all the sensory information flooding into the nervous system were allowed to reach the sensory cortex.
Hypothalamus. The hypothalamus is situated below the thalamus and forms the walls and floor of the third ventricle. It controls the output of the hormones from the pituitary gland and is located directly above it. Other functions include controlling hunger, thirst and body temperature (see Ch. 22). The latter function is significant for patients with a hypothalamic disturbance following head injury.

The complex control of body temperature is explained in more detail in Rutishauser (1994).

Epithalamus. The epithalamus is the most dorsal part of the diencephalon and forms the roof of the third ventricle. Extending from its posterior border is the pineal gland, thought to be concerned with body rhythms, acting as some sort of biological clock and concerned with melatonin synthesis, although the function is as yet obscure for both melatonin and the pineal body.

The brain stem. This is the collective name given to three structures: the medulla, the pons and the midbrain. Inferiorly, the medulla is continuous with the upper spinal cord and connects with the pons above. The pons is continuous with the midbrain, which connects with the lower portion of the diencephalon.

The medulla. All the spinal pathways pass through the medulla, constituting its white matter. Some of these cross to the opposite side in triangular-shaped structures called the 'pyramids', a process known as 'decussation' (the purpose of this has never been established).

- It contains the reticular formation, a diffuse area of grey and white matter that has connections with the rest of the brain stem and cerebral cortex, forming a structure known as the reticular activating system. It is responsible for consciousness and arousal.
- It accommodates three reflex centres, which control vital functions; these include:
  —the cardiac centre, which regulates heartbeat and force of contraction
  —the medullary rhythmicity area, which adjusts the basic rhythm of breathing
  —the vasomotor centre, which regulates the diameter of blood vessels (important in control of blood pressure).
  Other non-vital centres include those responsible for coordinating swallowing, vomiting, coughing, sneezing and hiccupping.
- It also contains the nuclei of cranial nerves VIII to XII (see Table 9.1).

The pons. The pons acts as a bridge between the medulla and the midbrain. It comprises fibres and nuclei; the fibres run in two directions. The transverse fibres connect with the cerebellum and the longitudinal fibres maintain the vital link between the spinal cord and the brain. The nuclei are the origins of cranial nerves V–VIII inclusive (see Table 9.1). Other important nuclei also exert an influence on respiration.

The midbrain. The third component of the brain stem is the midbrain, which contains the central centres for visual, auditory and postural reflexes. It is located above the pons and is the origin of the nuclei of cranial nerves III and IV (see Table 9.1). Cranial nerves I and II originate in the cerebrum.

The meninges

The brain and spinal cord are surrounded and protected by three meninges:

- the outer layer, the dura mater
- the middle layer, the arachnoid mater
- the innermost layer, the pia mater.

The dura mater is a double layer of dense fibrous tissue. The outer, periosteal layer adheres closely to the underside of the cranial bones, whilst the inner, meningeal layer is much thinner. The spinal dura mater has only one layer, which corresponds to the meningeal layer of the cranium. The two layers of the dura mater separate at several locations and these spaces contain the venous sinuses, e.g. the falx cerebri and the tentorium cerebelli. The former forms an incomplete division dipping down between the two cerebral hemispheres and is attached to the ethmoid bone at the front and the occipital protuberance at the back (see Fig. 9.7).

The tentorium cerebelli forms a division between the occipital lobes of the cerebrum and the cerebellum. It is attached along the midline to the falx cerebri, which draws it upwards to produce a tent-like appearance.

The arachnoid mater consists of collagenous and elastic fibres, covered by squamous epithelium. Fine strands of connective tissue connect the arachnoid with the pia below. The arachnoid mater projects into the sinuses as arachnoid villi, which are the structures responsible for the absorption of cerebrospinal fluid, and at certain points it joins the linings of the ventricles to form the choroid plexus, where cerebrospinal fluid is produced.

The pia mater is of the same structure as the arachnoid, except that it has its own blood supply. The pia closely follows and adheres to the contours of the brain and spinal cord.

The ventricular system

The ventricular system consists of four fluid-filled irregular cavities (ventricles) interconnected by narrow pathways (see Fig. 9.8) and is connected with the central canal of the spinal cord and the cranial subarachnoid space. There are two lateral ventricles, one in each cerebral hemisphere, one ventricle (the third) located in the diencephalic region and another located in the medulla, called the fourth ventricle.

Cerebrospinal fluid (CSF) circulates within the closed ventricular system. Healthy cerebrospinal fluid is crystal clear and colourless and its normal features are as outlined in Box 9.1 (p. 356).

The CSF production–absorption cycle is continuous, and a fairly constant volume of 120–150 mL is maintained. When this process is interrupted and the volume is increased beyond normal limits, hydrocephalus occurs.

The main source of production is the choroid plexus, a collection of specialised capillaries located within the internal lining of the ventricles, the largest amount being produced in the lateral ventricles. From here, the CSF passes through two interventricular foramina (foramen of Monro) to the third ventricle; then via the single cerebral aqueduct (aqueduct of Sylvius) to the fourth ventricle. Some CSF passes down into the central canal of the spinal cord but most passes up through the two lateral and one medial foramina in the roof of the fourth ventricle, to circulate round the brain and spinal cord in the subarachnoid space before being reabsorbed into the blood via the arachnoid villi.

The functions of cerebrospinal fluid are:

- protection and cushioning of the brain and spinal cord
- provision of nourishment
- maintenance of a uniform intracranial pressure
- removal of waste products.

Blood supply and drainage

The supply of blood to the head arises from the left and right common carotid arteries, which subdivide to form the internal and external carotid arteries. These supply blood to the anterior part of the brain, and the vertebral arteries supply the posterior part.

The greater part of the brain is supplied with blood by the circle of Willis, an unusual configuration of anastomosed blood vessels located in the base of the brain (see Fig. 9.9).

Table 9.1 Cranial nerves (Allan 1988)

Nerve	*Origin*	*Termination*	*Functions*
I Olfactory	Olfactory mucosa	Olfactory cortex	Sensory: Smell
II Optic	Retina	Visual cortex (synapses in lateral geniculate body)	Sensory: Vision
III Oculomotor	Midbrain	Upper eyelid muscle Extrinsic eye muscles (superior, medial and inferior recti, inferior oblique) Ciliary muscles Sphincter muscle of iris	Motor: Eyelid movement Eyeball movement Accommodation of lens Pupillary constriction
	Proprioceptors in extrinsic eye muscles	Midbrain	Sensory: Proprioception
IV Trochlear	Midbrain	Extrinsic eye muscle (superior oblique)	Motor: Eyeball movement
	Proprioceptors in extrinsic eye muscle (superior oblique)	Midbrain	Sensory: Proprioception
V Trigeminal	Pons Ophthalmic branch takes sensory fibres from skin of upper eyelid, eyeball, lacrimal glands, nasal cavity, side of nose, forehead and anterior half of scalp Maxillary branch takes sensory fibres from mucosa of nose, palate, parts of pharynx, upper teeth, upper lip, cheek and lower eyelid Mandibular branch takes sensory fibres from anterior two-thirds of tongue, lower teeth, skin over mandible and side of head in front of ear	Muscles of mastication Midbrain, pons and medulla	Motor: Chewing Sensory: Touch, pain, temperature, proprioception
VI Abducens	Pons Proprioceptors in lateral rectus	Extrinsic eye muscle (lateral rectus) Pons	Motor: Eyeball movement Sensory: Proprioception
VII Facial	Pons	Facial, scalp and neck muscles Lacrimal and salivary glands (sublingual and submandibular)	Motor: Facial expression Salivation Lacrimation
	Taste buds on anterior two-thirds of tongue	Gustatory cortex (synapses in pons and thalamus)	Sensory: Taste
	Proprioceptors in muscles of face and scalp		Proprioception
VIII Vestibulocochlear	Cochlear and vestibular portions of the ear	Cochlear nuclei in pons Vestibular nuclei in medulla	Sensory: Hearing Equilibrium
IX Glossopharyngeal	Medulla	Swallowing muscles in pharynx Parotid gland	Motor: Swallowing Salivation
	Taste buds on posterior one-third of tongue	Gustatory cortex (synapses in medulla and thalamus)	Sensory: Taste
	Carotid sinus		Regulation of blood pressure
	Proprioceptors in swallowing muscles		Proprioception
X Vagus	Medulla	Visceral muscles (muscles of pharynx, larynx, respiratory tract, oesophagus, heart, stomach, small intestine, proximal half of large intestine, gall bladder, liver, pancreas)	Motor: Swallowing, digestive movements and secretions
	Receptors in the same structures that the motor portions innervate	Medulla and pons	Sensory: Range of sensory inputs from organs supplied and proprioception from muscle
XI Accessory	Bulbar portion: medulla	Muscles of pharynx, larynx, soft palate	Motor: Swallowing
	Spinal portion: cervical spinal cord	Sternocleidomastoid and trapezius muscles	Head movements
	Proprioceptors in muscles supplied by motor fibres	Medulla	Sensory: Proprioception
XII Hypoglossal	Medulla Proprioceptors in tongue	Muscles of tongue Medulla	Motor: Tongue movements Sensory: Proprioception

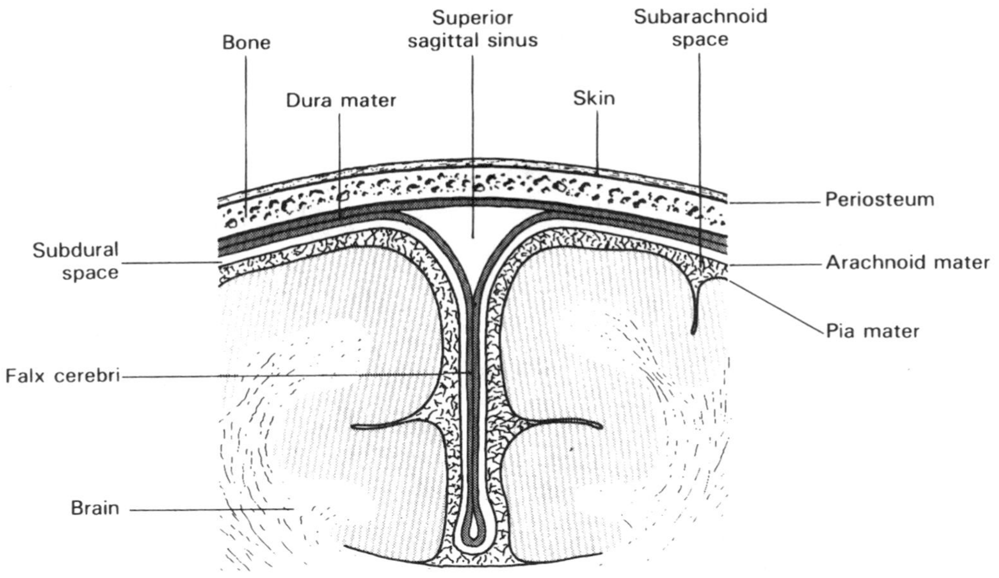

Fig. 9.7 Meninges of the brain.

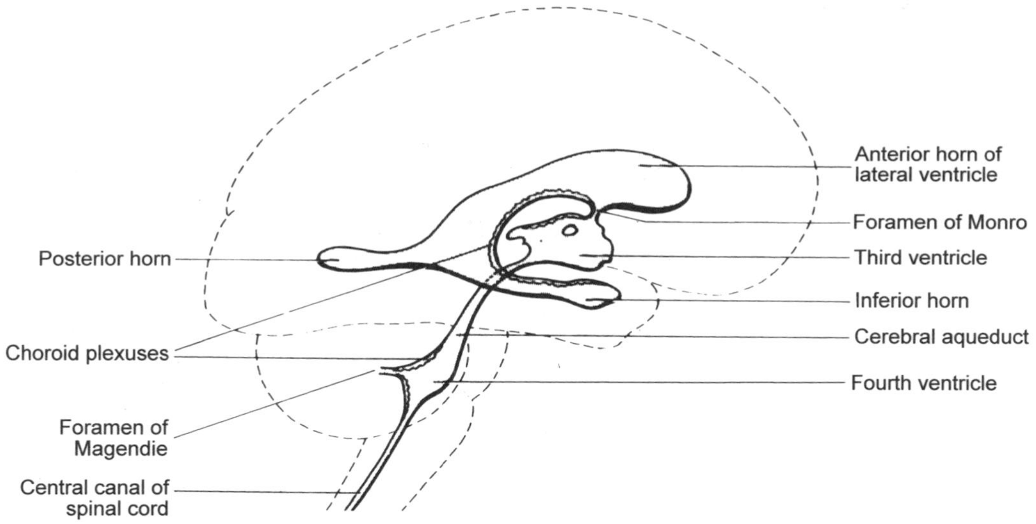

Fig. 9.8 Ventricular system.

More detailed information on the areas of the brain supplied by the cerebral circulation can be found in Hinchliff et al (1996).

Venous drainage is by small veins in the brain stem and cerebellum, and external and internal veins draining the cerebrum. Some of the external and internal veins empty into one large vein called the vein of Galen (great cerebral vein). Unlike other parts of the body, these veins do not correspond with their arterial supply. All these veins empty directly into a system of venous sinuses, which is shown in Figure 9.10.

The principal sinuses are the superior and inferior sagittal, the straight, transverse, sigmoid and cavernous sinuses.

The limbic system

The limbic system comprises an interconnected complex of structures, including the hypothalamus. These are thought to be responsible for special types of behaviour associated with emotions, subconscious motor and sensory drives and the intrinsic feelings of pain and pleasure.

Further information is given in Tortora & Grabowski (1996).

The blood–brain barrier. The capillaries supplying the brain consist of endothelial cells with very tight junctions, which make their permeability relatively low. This means that some substances

Box 9.1 Normal features of cerebrospinal fluid

Colour: crystal clear
Pressure: 80–160 mmH_2O
Volume: 120–150 mL
Cells:
- red blood — none
- white blood
  —polymorphonuclear leucocytes — none
  —lymphocytes 0–5/mm^3

Protein: 0.2–0.4 g/L
Gamma globulin (IgG): less than 13% of total protein
Sugar: 3.6–5.0 mmol
Wassermann reaction: negative

are prevented or hindered from gaining access to the brain, as a protective mechanism. This is termed the 'blood–brain barrier'.

For further details see Rutishauser (1994).

The spinal cord

The spinal cord is an oval cylinder that lies within the spinal cavity of the vertebral column. In adults, it is approximately 45 cm in length and extends from the medulla above to the first or second lumbar vertebrae at its lower end. Beyond this, the spinal nerves from the lumbar and sacral segments of the cord form the cauda equina, or 'horse's tail'. The cord is surrounded by the three meninges and cerebrospinal fluid circulates in the subarachnoid space. The lower part of the cord is attached to the coccyx by the filum terminale and is tapered in shape (see Fig. 9.11).

The cord is segmented into five parts or regions, each corresponding to a specific number of vertebrae (in brackets):

- cervical (7)
- thoracic (12)
- lumbar (5)
- sacral (5)
- coccyx (1).

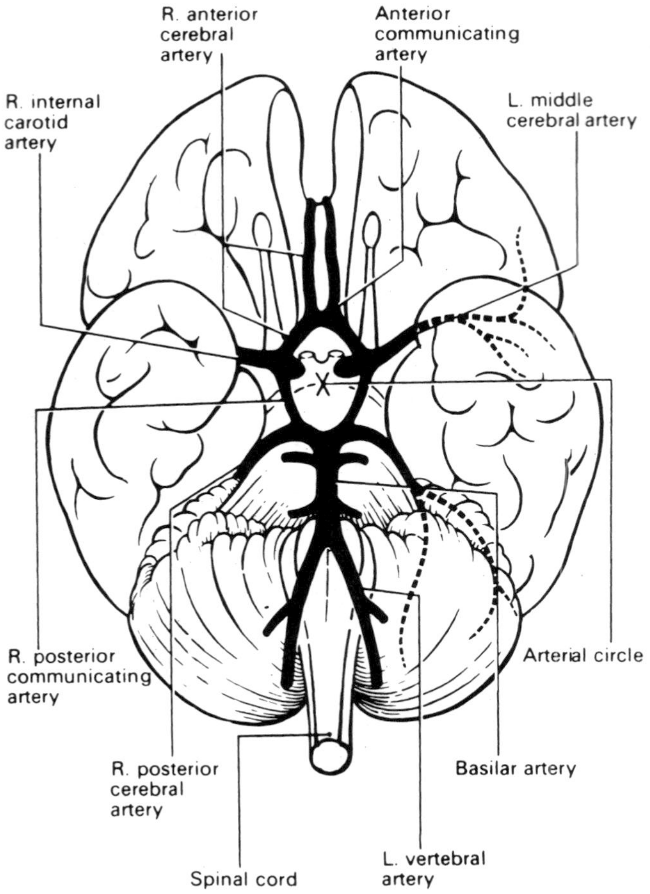

Fig. 9.9 Blood supply to the brain.

A shorthand labelling system has evolved to identify different levels within the spinal cord and vertebrae. For example, the third cervical vertebra becomes C3 and the fourth lumbar vertebra becomes L4 and so on.

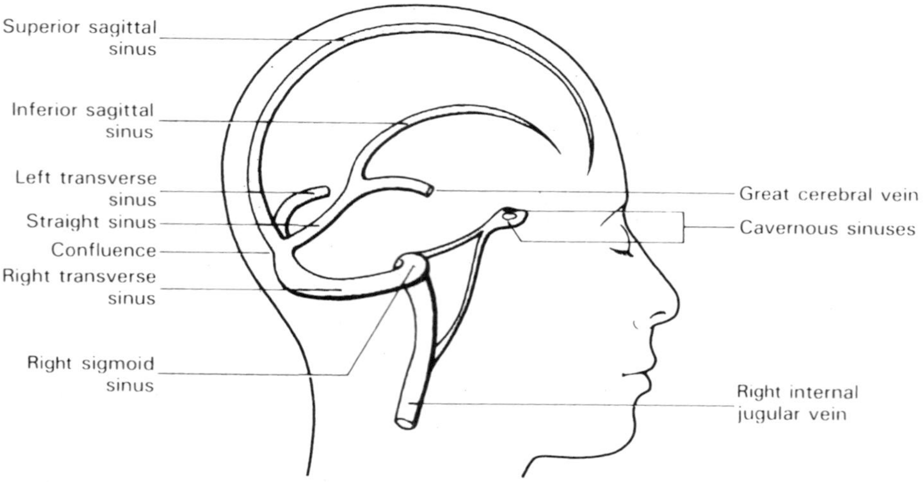

Fig. 9.10 Venous drainage of the brain.

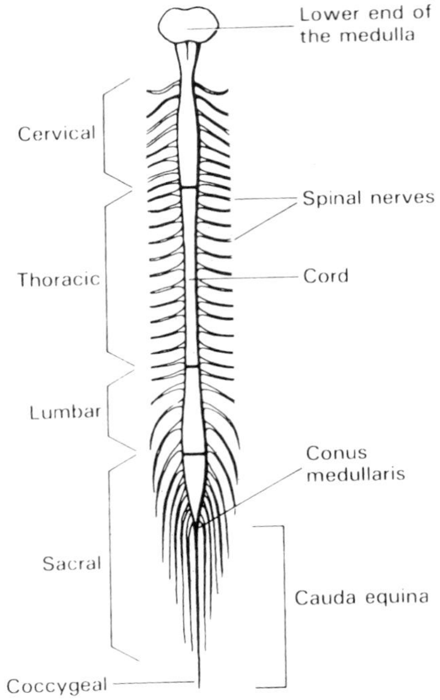

Fig. 9.11 Spinal cord.

Two enlargements of the spinal cord can be noted. The first is in the cervical region, extending between C4 and T1 and containing the nerve supply for the upper limbs. The second enlargement is lower in the lumbar region and is called the 'lumbosacral enlargement'. It extends from L2 to S3 and supplies innervation to the lower limbs. The spinal nerves (which are considered to be part of the peripheral nervous system) are attached by two short roots to the cord. There is a pair of spinal nerves equivalent to each of the vertebrae outlined above and these are labelled and numbered in a similar way. More detail on the spinal nerves can be found in the section on the peripheral nervous system (p. 359).

The structure of the spinal cord is illustrated in cross-section in Figure 9.12.

The spinal pathways are described as:

- sensory — these ascend from the periphery of the body, e.g. cutaneous receptors in the hand, and are conveyed to the sensory cortex for interpretation
- motor — these descend from the brain down to the periphery of the body, e.g. to skeletal muscles, where they initiate a motor response.

Each pathway has a name, derived from the white column in which it travels, the origin of the cell bodies and the termination of the axon. For example, the anterior spinothalamic tract is located in the anterior white column, originates in the spinal cord and terminates in the thalamus.

The sensory pathways consist of:

- the posterior column pathway
- the spinothalamic pathway
- the cerebellar pathway.

The posterior column pathway. Each pathway consists of a chain of three neurones, which transmit information such as discriminative touch and vibration sense from the appropriate receptors to the sensory cortex (see Fig. 9.13).

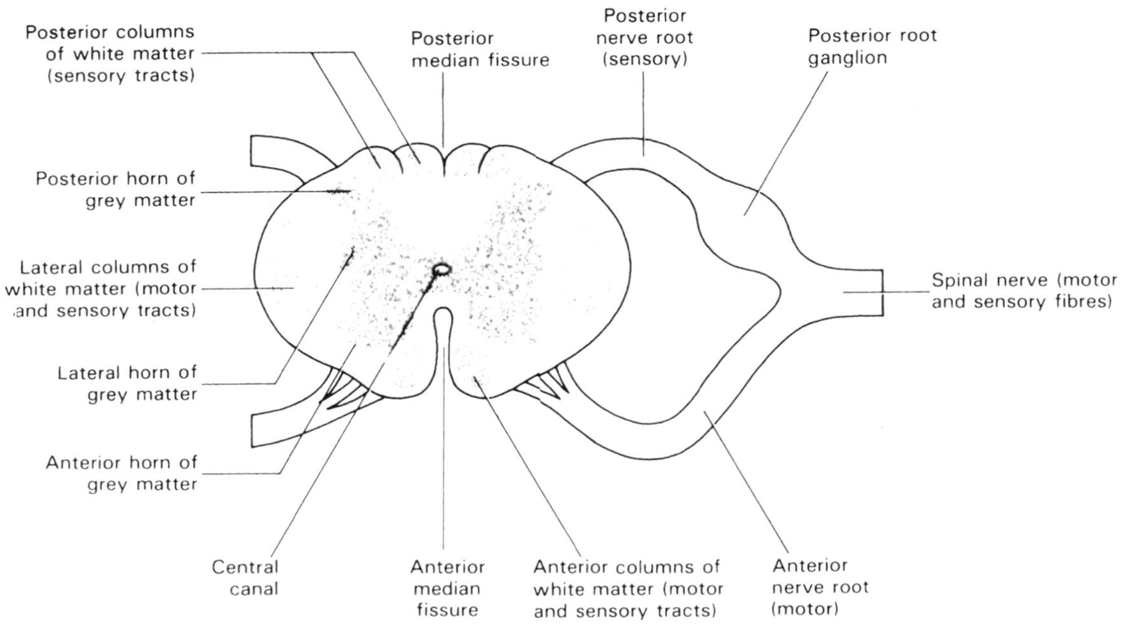

Fig. 9.12 Cross-section of spinal cord. It can be seen that the cord is incompletely divided into right and left halves by the posterior and anterior median fissures. In the centre is the central canal which contains cerebrospinal fluid originating from the fourth ventricle. Extending the entire length of the cord, this is located within an H-shaped area of grey matter with posterior and anterior and, at some levels, lateral horns. The remainder of the cord is made up of white matter organised in columns in the posterior, lateral and anterior segments.

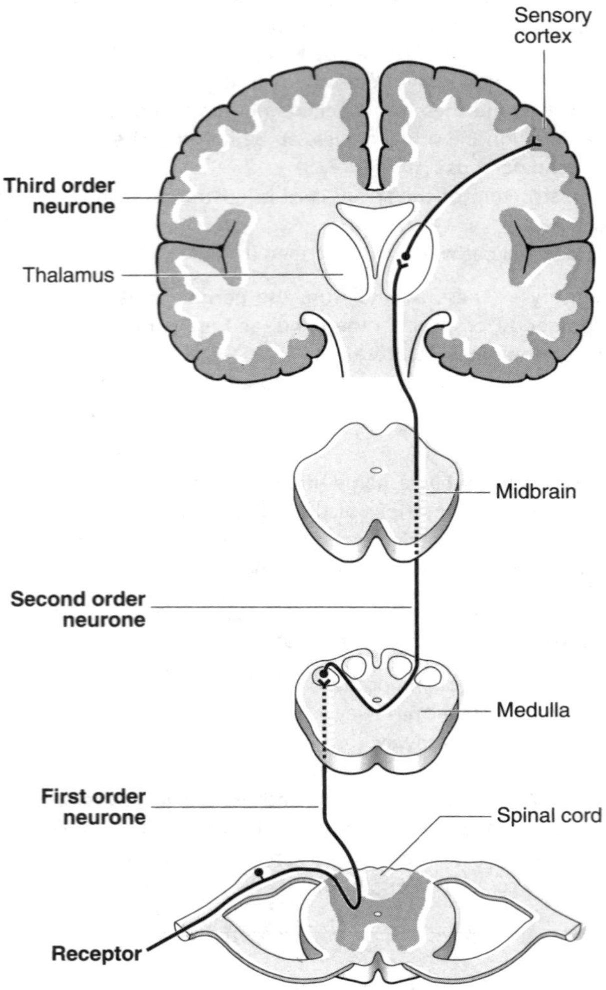

Fig. 9.13 The posterior column pathway. The first order neurone connects the receptor with the spinal cord and medulla on the same side of the body. In the medulla, the first order neurone synapses with the second order neurone, which decussates and then passes upwards to the thalamus where it synapses with a third order neurone which completes the sensory pathway, terminating in the sensory cortex.

The spinothalamic pathways are:

- the lateral spinothalamic tract
- the anterior spinothalamic tract.

The first order neurone in both pathways connects the receptor with the spinal cord where it synapses with the second order neurone in the posterior grey horn. The pathway crosses over to the opposite side of the cord and ascends in either the lateral or anterior spinothalamic tract to the thalamus. The second order neurone synapses with the third order neurone, which then continues, terminating in the sensory cortex. The lateral tract is responsible for conveying information about pain and temperature, and the anterior tract conveys light touch and pressure (further information on pain can be found in Ch. 19).
The cerebellar tracts are:

- the posterior spinocerebellar tract
- the anterior spinocerebellar tract.

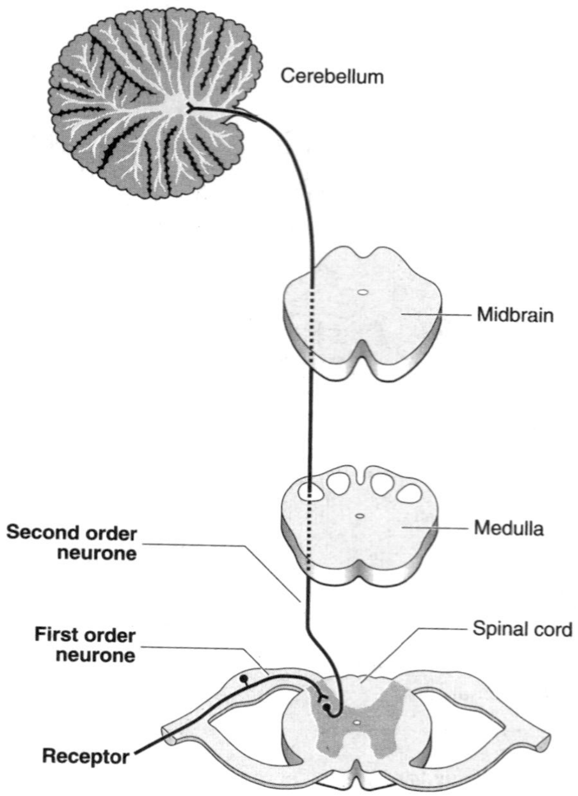

Fig. 9.14 The spinocerebellar tracts.

Both tracts are concerned with conveying impulses about subconscious muscle sense. Proprioceptors in the muscles and joints convey information via the spinal pathways, terminating in the cerebellum instead of the cerebral cortex. This time there are only two neurones involved, synapsing in the posterior grey horn (see Fig. 9.14).

The sensory pathways are responsible for conveying a mass of information into the central nervous system. This information forms part of a large pool and decisions are made regarding the response to a given situation. The response is manifested by the motor system via its own set of pathways; this is described as 'integration'.

Motor pathways. Once the motor process is initiated within the motor area of the cortex, the impulses descend via two main motor pathways, classified as:

- pyramidal — this indicates that the pathway passes through the pyramids in the medulla
- extrapyramidal.

It is important to clarify the terms upper and lower motor neurones. These are the functional units of the motor system and they convey motor impulses. Damage to one or the other will result in very different functional impairment. An example of lower motor neurone disease is poliomyelitis.

Q **9.1** Can you find some examples of upper motor neurone disease?

The upper motor neurones extend from the motor cortex of the brain and pass down the pathways to end at the cranial nerve nuclei in the brain stem and the anterior horn of the spinal cord. This means that the upper motor neurone is contained entirely within the central nervous system. These are described in Box 9.2.
The lower motor neurones start at the anterior horn of the spinal cord and pass via the anterior nerve roots of the spinal nerves and the motor end-plate of muscles. Some start in the brain stem and are contained in the cranial nerves.

Peripheral nervous system

The peripheral nervous system has two functional parts:

- the motor division — this is further divided into:
  —the somatic nervous system, which conducts impulses from the CNS to skeletal muscles
  —the autonomic nervous system, which conducts impulses from the CNS to smooth muscle, cardiac muscle and glands
- the sensory division.

The cranial nerves

The cranial nerves pass from their origin, principally from the brain stem, out via small openings in the skull to innervate the appropriate structures. Each pair of nerves is named according to its distribution or function and is also numbered I–XII (see Table 9.1). Cranial nerves were formerly described as either motor or sensory, or a mixture of both, but more recently, most motor nerves are considered to be mixed, but with a dominance of motor fibres.

Spinal nerves

There are 31 pairs of spinal nerves, named and grouped according to the vertebrae with which they are associated (no. of nerves in brackets):

- cervical (8)
- thoracic (12)
- lumbar (5)
- sacral (5)
- coccygeal (1).

Note that there is one more cervical spinal nerve than there are vertebrae. This is because the first pair leave the vertebral canal between the occipital bone and the atlas, and the eighth pair leave below the last cervical vertebra. Thereafter, the spinal nerves are named and numbered according to the vertebra immediately above.

As can be seen from Figure 9.12, each spinal nerve has an anterior and posterior root. The anterior root consists of motor nerve fibres, whilst the posterior roots are sensory. The posterior root can be distinguished by its root ganglion, a cluster of nerve cell bodies.

Shortly after leaving the intervertebral foramina, both roots join together to form a mixed nerve. From here the spinal nerves continue to form a complex network all over the body, carrying motor signals to effectors such as the skeletal muscles and conveying sensory information such as touch to the CNS for interpretation.

Further details of this complex network can be found in Tortora & Grabowski (1996).

The autonomic nervous system

The autonomic nervous system is the most complex and perhaps least understood part of the nervous system. Its involvement in, and effect upon, everyday activities is vague until its delicate mechanisms are upset. The effects are then readily felt by the individual.

The autonomic nervous system consists only of the nerves carrying motor impulses to the internal organs; thus it is exclusively peripheral and motor. Its activity is influenced by many factors, including sensory information from the internal organs, numerous peptides and hormones, and signals from higher control centres such as the hypothalamus. It is described as having two divisions, the sympathetic and parasympathetic, each imposing different effects (see Figs 9.15 and 9.16).

For more detailed information, see Rutishauser (1994).

Box 9.2 The motor pathways

Pyramidal tracts
The pyramidal pathway comprises three main tracts:

- lateral corticospinal
- anterior corticospinal
- corticobulbar.

The lateral corticospinal tract
This is the actual pyramidal tract. It originates in the motor cortex and descends to the medulla where 85% of the fibres decussate. They continue downwards in the lateral white column of the corticospinal tract. Most synapse in the anterior grey horn with the lower motor neurone, which then exits the spinal cord via the spinal nerves to terminate on the appropriate skeletal muscle.

The anterior corticospinal pathway
These fibres follow a similar pathway to the lateral, except that they travel in the anterior white column and most of the fibres do not decussate.

The corticobulbar tracts
These are important in that they terminate in the nuclei of the cranial nerves in the medulla. They follow the same pathway as the corticospinal pathway.

Extrapyramidal tracts
These consist of all the descending motor pathways that do not pass through the pyramids. They are concerned with functions of tone and posture such as control of head movement and maintaining balance.

There are three of these pathways:

- *The rubrospinal tract*, which originates in the midbrain, decussates and descends in the lateral white column. It is concerned with tone and posture.
- *The tectospinal tract* also originates in the midbrain, decussates and descends in the anterior white column and enters the anterior grey horns of the cervical cord.
- *The vestibulospinal tract* originates in the vestibular nucleus of the medulla and descends on the same side in the anterior white column and terminates in the anterior grey horn at the cervical and lumbosacral levels of the cord. It is concerned with regulating muscle tone in response to movements of the head and therefore has an important part to play in maintaining equilibrium.

HEAD INJURY (INCORPORATING RAISED INTRACRANIAL PRESSURE)

Head injury is difficult to quantify and estimates suggest that 1 million people in the UK each year are affected. It predominates

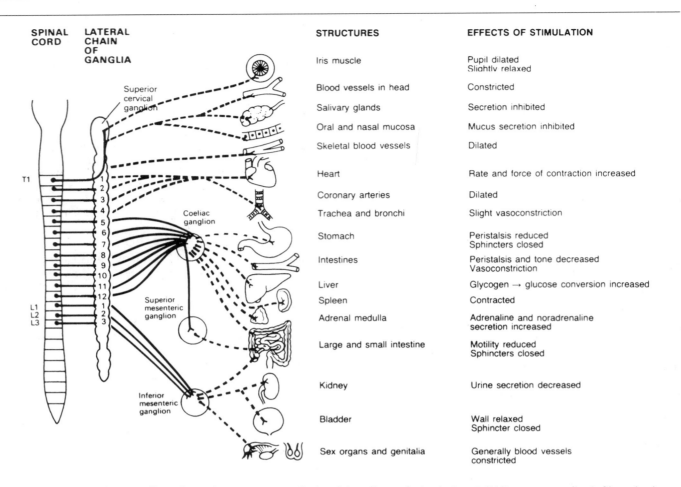

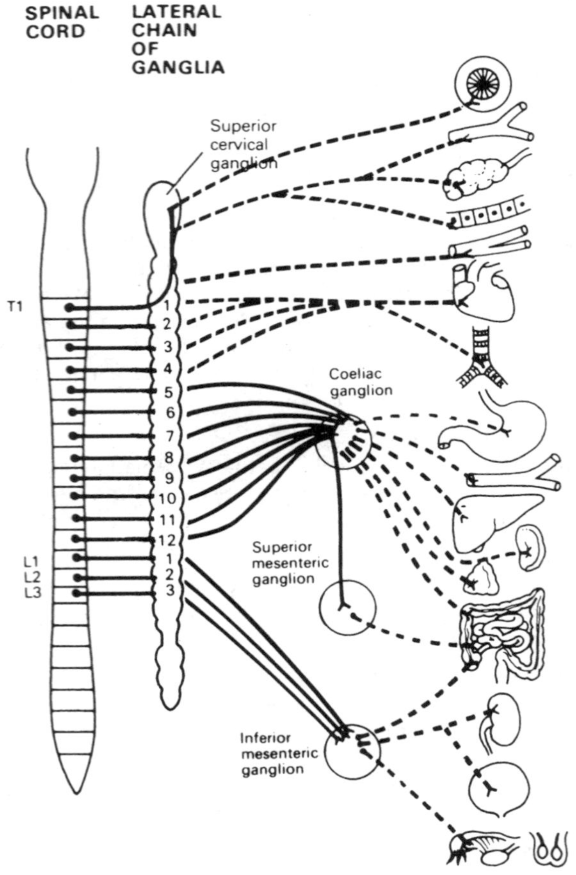

STRUCTURES	EFFECTS OF STIMULATION
Iris muscle	Pupil dilated Slightly relaxed
Blood vessels in head	Constricted
Salivary glands	Secretion inhibited
Oral and nasal mucosa	Mucus secretion inhibited
Skeletal blood vessels	Dilated
Heart	Rate and force of contraction increased
Coronary arteries	Dilated
Trachea and bronchi	Slight vasoconstriction
Stomach	Peristalsis reduced Sphincters closed
Intestines	Peristalsis and tone decreased Vasoconstriction
Liver	Glycogen → glucose conversion increased
Spleen	Contracted
Adrenal medulla	Adrenaline and noradrenaline secretion increased
Large and small intestine	Motility reduced Sphincters closed
Kidney	Urine secretion decreased
Bladder	Wall relaxed Sphincter closed
Sex organs and genitalia	Generally blood vessels constricted

Fig. 9.15 The sympathetic outflow, the main structures supplied and the effects of stimulation. Solid lines, preganglionic fibres; broken lines, postganglionic fibres. (Reproduced with kind permission from Wilson & Waugh 1996.)

in the 16–35 year age group and has a distinct male bias of 3:1. Over 1 million people attend accident and emergency departments each year as a result of head injury and 150 000 are admitted to hospital (Treadwell & Mendelow 1994). Head injury accounts for a quarter of trauma deaths, and almost half of those are caused by road traffic accidents. The financial cost is inestimable and this is of major significance, particularly as it is preventable. This is an area in which nurses could exercise their health education skills, e.g. by emphasising the dangers associated with head injury and its detrimental effects when communicating with those patients and their families who have suffered a minor head injury and made a good recovery. Depending on the original cause, this may include consideration of driver behaviour or unsafe work practices. The use of seatbelts for the driver and all car passengers has led to a reduction in head injuries, as has the use of protective headgear for motorcyclists and horse riders (Lee 1993). A common contributing factor in head injury is overindulgence in alcohol and, where appropriate, the patient can be encouraged to consider his personal lifestyle and the consumption of alcohol. This section describes the effects of moderate to severe head injury. However, not all head-injured patients sustain a serious injury. Some will experience the post-concussion syndrome following a minor injury (Jackson 1995).

PATHOPHYSIOLOGY

The adult skull can be considered as a rigid box divided into two major compartments, containing non-compressible components. A uniform pressure, called 'intracranial' pressure (ICP), is maintained. It is defined as the pressure exerted within the cerebral ventricular system. When an individual sustains a head injury or there is some abnormal pathology, e.g. a tumour, it can alter this delicate balance. When an increase in ICP occurs, the pressure in one compartment is higher than that in its counterpart, and abnormal movement of tissue from an area of high pressure to one of low pressure occurs, a process known as 'herniation' or 'coning'.

Three intracranial components are involved in the process of maintaining ICP:

- the brain
- the cerebrospinal fluid
- blood.

The brain is the largest of these, occupying 80% of the content. The remaining 20% is taken up in equal proportion by the cerebrospinal fluid and the blood. Under normal circumstances, ICP is maintained within normal limits, but when there is an alteration to

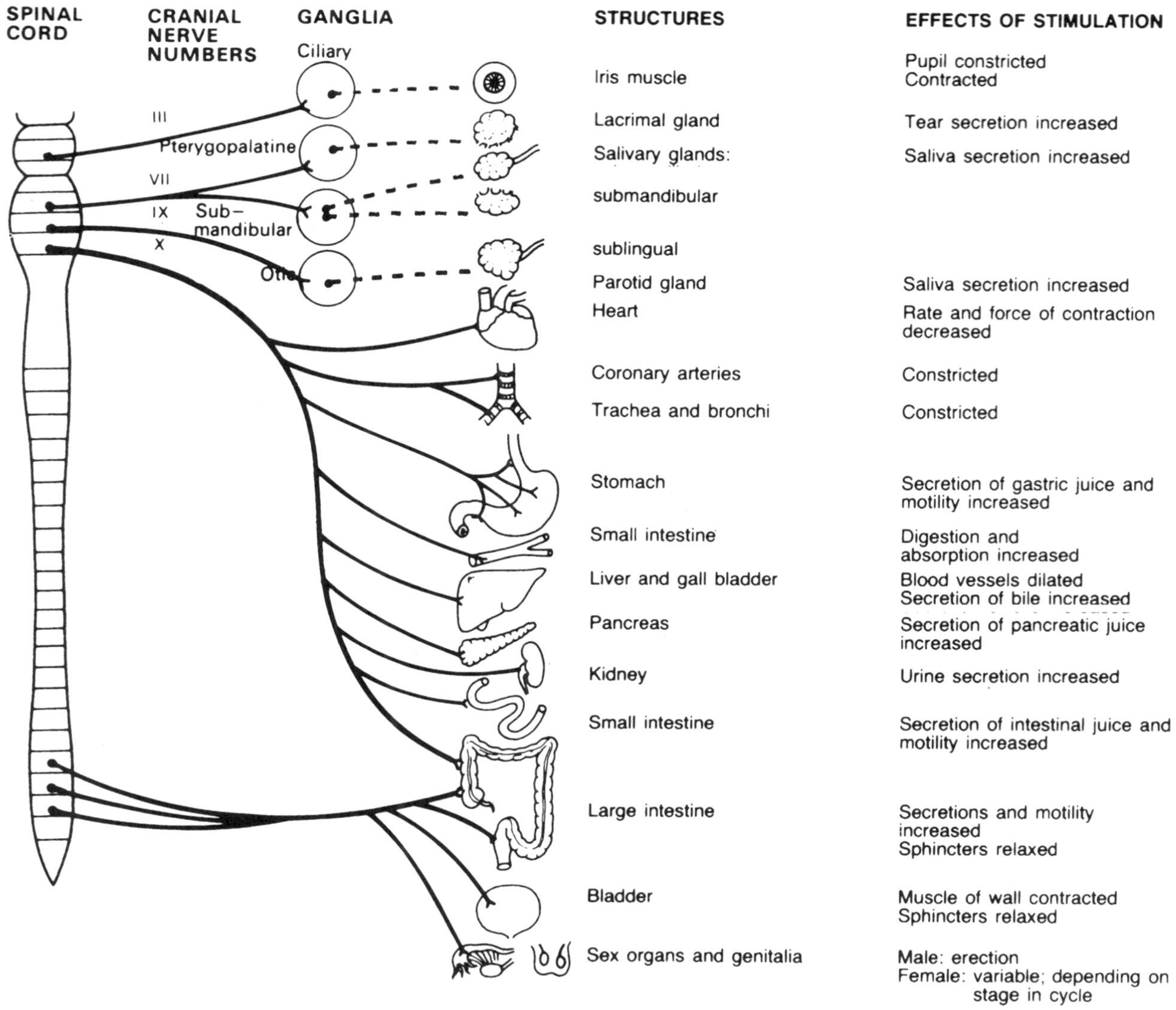

Fig. 9.16 The parasympathetic outflow, the main structures supplied and the effects of stimulation. Solid lines, preganglionic fibres; broken lines, postganglionic fibres. Where there are no broken lines, the second neurone is in the wall of the structure. (Reproduced with kind permission from Wilson & Waugh 1996.)

the volume of one of these components within the confined space of the skull, the other two are compressed, resulting in a rise in ICP. The normal range of ICP is 0–15 mmHg and anything over 15 mmHg is considered abnormal. Transient rises in pressure occur with activities such as coughing or sneezing and this is a normal physiological response.

Changes to the brain and its associated structures following trauma may cause ICP to rise to a dangerous level, resulting in coma and leading to permanent brain damage.

The causes and presenting symptoms of raised ICP

Causes of raised ICP can be classified according to the intracranial components involved.

- *Brain.* Brain tissue volume can be increased due to the presence of an expanding intracranial lesion, such as a brain tumour or a haematoma following head injury.
- *CSF.* Increased production, decreased absorption or blockage of a CSF pathway will result in an abnormal accumulation of CSF within the cerebral ventricular system. This is a condition known as hydrocephalus.
- *Blood.* Cerebral blood flow can be increased principally as a result of an abnormally high level of carbon dioxide in the blood (hypercapnia) and to a lesser extent due to a lack of oxygen in the tissues (hypoxia). These lead to congestion within the cerebral circulation, culminating in a raised ICP. Such a situation can be precipitated by neglect of the patient's airway during the postoperative period following neurosurgery or following head injury.

A rise in ICP can develop over a variable period of time. It can occur over a number of years in a slow-growing brain tumour, with the patient hardly noticing any symptoms, or it can occur in a matter of minutes following severe head injury, when the patient

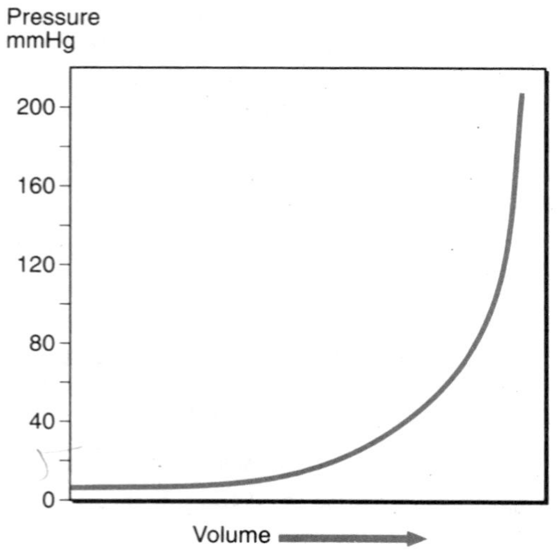

Fig. 9.17 Volume–pressure curve.

Box 9.3 Stages of the volume–pressure relationship in raised intracranial pressure

Stage 1 The compensation phase: there is no rise in ICP, and conscious level remains unaltered.

Stage 2 The early phase of reversible decompensation: a slight increase in brain mass will produce an elevated ICP. Early signs of deterioration in conscious level are noted.

Stage 3 The late phase of reversible decompensation: ICP is now very high and conscious level is deteriorating rapidly. Detrimental changes occur in the respiratory rate and pattern. ICP will soon equal mean arterial pressure with, ultimately, cessation of cerebral blood flow.

Stage 4 The irreversible decompensation phase: in which further deterioration leading to death will occur if intervention is not initiated.

becomes profoundly unconscious. The underlying principle remains the same and is centred on the volume–pressure relationship curve (Fig. 9.17).

A distinct correlation exists between ICP and conscious level. As ICP rises, conscious level deteriorates.

During the initial rise in ICP, compensatory mechanisms come into play, principally the ability of the cerebral ventricular system to reduce the volume of CSF by displacing it into a distensible spinal dural sac. A reduction in cerebral blood volume also occurs as a result of autoregulation, the ability of blood vessels to alter their diameter according to local conditions. This is represented by the flattened part of the curve. However, this is only a temporary measure and, as the volume of the expanding lesion increases, compensation is overcome and the steep part of the curve is entered. The addition of the same volume to that which was added previously and produced very little change in ICP now results in dramatic increases. This process has four identifiable stages, as described in Box 9.3.

Other factors which have an influence on this complex process include cerebral blood flow and cerebral oedema.

Further information on influencing factors can be found in Hickey (1997).

Herniation

Herniation is the process by which tissue in a high-pressure compartment is compressed and forced through an available opening into an adjoining low-pressure compartment. Such a situation can exist in the patient with raised ICP. The skull has two compartments: the supratentorial, i.e. the region above the tentorium; and the infratentorial, i.e. the region below the tentorium. The opening that permits supratentorial herniation is the tentorial notch, and that which permits infratentorial herniation is the foramen magnum.

Supratentorial herniation is either central tentorial herniation or lateral transtentorial herniation.

Central tentorial herniation is when symmetrical herniation is produced by a midline expanding lesion or generalised swelling of brain tissue. It involves the downward displacement of the cerebral hemispheres, diencephalon and midbrain. The nerves and posterior cerebral arteries are stretched and compression of the oculomotor nerve (third cranial nerve) occurs. These and other structures are displaced into the posterior fossa.

Lateral transtentorial herniation occurs in the presence of an expanding lesion located close to the temporal lobe. The medial part of the temporal lobe (the uncus) is forced downwards. This type of herniation can inflict pressure on the reticular activating system, resulting in a decrease in conscious level (see Ch. 28). Lateral transtentorial herniation can subsequently develop into a central herniation (Fig. 9.18).

Infratentorial herniation is the downward displacement of the lower part of the cerebellum (the cerebellar tonsils) through the foramen magnum where compression of the medulla results. The offending lesion is located in the posterior fossa and this type of herniation is less common.

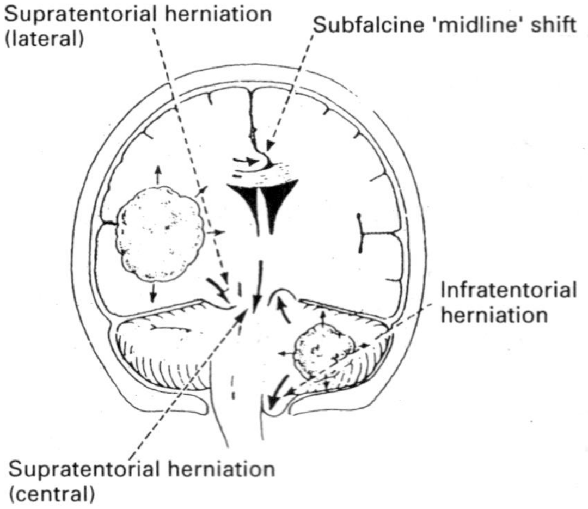

Fig. 9.18 Types of herniation. (Adapted from Lindsay & Bone 1997.)

Table 9.2 Signs and symptoms of raised intracranial pressure. (Adapted from Allan 1988.)

Clinical parameter	*Signs/symptoms*	*Reasons*
Conscious level	Deterioration in conscious level	Raised intracranial pressure will reduce the amount of oxygen received by the oxygen-sensitive cells of the cerebral cortex.
Respiration	Deterioration in respiratory pattern	A particular respiratory pattern will be seen in relation to the non-functioning area in the medulla and pons. *Breathing pattern* — *Non-functioning area* Cheyne–Stokes — Affects various areas Apneustic — Pons varolii Ataxic — Medulla Central neurogenic — Lower midbrain Hyperventilation — Upper pons Cluster breathing — Medulla
Pupils	(a) Alteration in pupil size (b) Reaction to light (c) Blurring of vision/diplopia (d) Ocular muscle paresis/paralysis	All the pupillary and eye movement responses to raised intracranial pressure are as a result of compression of the 3rd cranial nerve (oculomotor). The ipsilateral pupil is usually affected first, followed by the other one.
Blood pressure	(a) An increase in systolic blood pressure followed by (b) a fall	The increase in blood pressure occurs as a result of ischaemia (due to raised intracranial pressure) of the vasomotor centre. Implicated in this is a widening pulse pressure. If this is not corrected, the intracranial pressure continues to rise and the blood pressure then begins to fall dramatically until it is unrecordable.
Pulse	Initially bradycardia (<60 beats/min) develops with a full and bounding pulse. In the later stages the pulse becomes weak and thready	This is brought about as a result of increased workload on the heart which is attempting to overcome cerebral blood vessel resistance by pushing more blood into the cerebral circulation.
Motor function	Contralateral hemiparesis/hemiplegia	The raised intracranial pressure affects pyramidal tract function, and continued deterioration will ensue until the limbs are unresponsive to deep painful stimuli.
	Headache usually in the early morning	Headache due to raised intracranial pressure is thought to be the result of displacement of the cerebrospinal fluid cushion producing dilatation of cerebral blood vessels, stretching of arteries at the base of the brain and traction of bridging veins. Intracranial pressure will be adversely affected following REM sleep and by the retention of carbon dioxide during sleep resulting in exacerbation of intracranial pressure in early morning.
'Cushing's triad'	Headache, becoming more severe or persistent	This indicates that the ICP is rising and the intracranial contents are being compressed; 'herniation' may occur.
	Vomiting: may occur with early morning headache	The mechanism involved is not well understood.
	Projectile vomiting and problems with swallowing	These indicate that there is increasing pressure on the brain stem, where the control centres for these functions are located.
	Papilloedema	Occurs as a result of raised intracranial pressure being transmitted down the optic nerve to produce a swollen nerve head. This may be seen on direct fundoscopy. An unreliable sign, which is not constantly seen in all patients with raised intracranial pressure.
	Problems with speech or comprehension	These may indicate that ICP is rising and that there is pressure on the cerebral cortex.

No order is implied within the above set of signs and symptoms. Any combination in varying degrees can occur in each patient. Individually, each of the signs and symptoms can be caused by other pathology, including extracranially.

MEDICAL MANAGEMENT

Common presenting symptoms. The head-injured patient with raised ICP may be fully alert and orientated or may range from experiencing drowsiness to being deeply unconscious. Neurological deficits can usually be found, e.g. alteration of conscious level, occurrence of a seizure or onset of confusion. Answers to the questions listed below should be obtained as they bear an influence on the management and outcome:

- *How long has the patient been unconscious?* The period of unconsciousness relates to the severity of brain damage, i.e. the longer the patient is unconscious, the more severe the damage.
- *Does post-traumatic amnesia (PTA) exist and for how long?* The patient's memory for events following injury are an indicator of the severity of brain damage, i.e. the longer the period of PTA, the worse the brain damage.
- *What were the cause and circumstances of the injury?* This may indicate if other extracranial injuries exist.
- *Does the patient have any headache or vomiting?* These would indicate the possibility of intracranial haemorrhage.

Table 9.2 lists the signs and symptoms of raised ICP.

Investigations. Following the taking of the patient's history and examination, investigations will be conducted. In the head-injured patient, skull X-ray may reveal a fracture and computed tomography (CT) or magnetic resonance imaging (MRI) may demonstrate cerebral contusions or lacerations and/or an intracranial haematoma (Hickey 1997). Box 9.4 gives a description of the types of injury the brain may suffer.

ICP monitoring. One of the most important diagnostic measures is the monitoring of ICP. This is an invasive technique involving direct measurement of ICP. A typical system comprises a fibreoptic transducer-tipped catheter, which can be placed in the lateral ventricle, subdural space or extradural space. The level of ICP is then transmitted to a digital data display or as a waveform. A pulsatile waveform will be demonstrated along with a pressure level indicating if the patient's ICP is within normal limits (≤15 mmHg) (see Fig. 9.19).

Treatment. In the past, the treatment of head injury focused primarily on the interventions required to reduce ICP. However, greater emphasis is now placed on maintaining cerebral perfusion pressure (CPP) at more than 70 mmHg. This is because it has been shown that those patients with a high ICP, low blood pressure and low CPP make a poorer recovery. The means by which this is achieved is varied according to circumstances, however the methods described here must not be used indiscriminately.

Hyperosmolar agents. An intravenous infusion of 100 mL of 20% mannitol over 15 min will reduce ICP by establishing an osmotic gradient between the plasma and brain tissue, thus removing water from the oedematous brain tissue to the blood. This will 'buy' time to allow the patient to be prepared for transfer to a specialist unit or for surgery. However, if repeated boluses are administered, its effect is neutralised, leading to a rebound increase in ICP.

Davies & Lucatorto (1994) offer a useful review of its use.

Controlled hyperventilation. Reducing the P_aCO_2 causes vasoconstriction, thus reducing cerebral blood volume and ICP. To achieve this, the patient requires to be paralysed, intubated and mechanically ventilated. It is suggested by Lindsay & Bone (1997) that the resultant reduction in cerebral blood flow may itself cause brain damage. Maintaining the blood pressure and CPP appears to be as important, if not more important, than lowering ICP. It is necessary to measure the amount of oxygen extracted from the brain to determine whether or not the brain can withstand further vasoconstriction.

Fluid management. Views on the management of fluids have been contentious for some time. Some advocate restricting fluid in order to induce slight dehydration. By controlling intake, the extracellular fluid, including that of the brain, is decreased, thus reducing ICP. The intake may be set at 1–2.5 L per 24 h. However, some now advocate achieving normovolaemia or increasing fluids. Doing this increases cerebral blood flow and thus improves oxygen delivery to the brain.

Sedatives. After years of advocating that patients with a head injury should never be sedated as this would impede assessment of conscious level, there are now special circumstances under which sedation may be used. If ICP fails to respond to standard measures then sedation may help under carefully controlled conditions (Lindsay & Bone 1997). Drugs that may be used include propofol and etomidate, however each has associated ill-effects that require to be countered. Propofol causes vasodilatation that may require to be counteracted to prevent blood pressure from falling and a reduction in cerebral perfusion. Etomidate inhibits steroid synthesis, and thus steroid cover will be required.

Box 9.4 Description of injury to the brain

Contusions
Described as a bruising of the cerebral tissue. Most commonly affects the frontal, occipital and undersurface of the temporal lobes. There are two types:

- coup — indicates haemorrhage and oedema immediately under the injury site
- contrecoup — damage occurs directly opposite the injury site. This is caused by the rapid acceleration or deceleration movement of the brain within the skull following severe trauma. Contused brain tissue affects the blood supply to that area, resulting in swelling of the brain which will raise ICP.

Lacerations
Brain tissue is lacerated as a result of, for example, a skull fracture, resulting in disruption to cellular activity which will produce focal neurological deficits such as hemiparesis. Contusions and cerebral oedema may also occur.

Haematoma
A localised collection of blood. These are named according to their location:

- extradural — situated or occurring outside the dura mater
- subdural — between the dura mater and the arachnoid
- intracerebral — within the brain substance.

Diffuse brain injury
Here, there is no specific focal pathology. Shearing of the white matter occurs, causing disruption and tearing of the axons.

Surgical intervention. Surgery may be performed to remove a focal mass lesion such as an expanding haematoma and this may be combined with decompression. Withdrawal of small aliquots of CSF via a ventricular catheter results in a reduction of ICP, but this only provides temporary relief. To be effective, drainage would require to be continuous, but this is often impractical. Examples of neurosurgical approaches are given in Box 9.5.

NURSING PRIORITIES AND MANAGEMENT: HEAD INJURY

Head-injured patients with raised ICP can present in different ways on admission to hospital. The person may appear to have sustained no injury initially but can become drowsy or confused, or develop speech problems or limb deficits. Epileptic fits may occur.

Immediate priorities

The immediate nursing aim is to prevent further damaging rises in ICP and the first priority is to identify any alteration in respiratory function due to an obstructed airway or an absent cough or gag reflex. The appropriate interventions are described in Box 9.6.

The nurse should be aware of the presence of other injuries, e.g. multiple injuries if the patient has been in a road traffic accident. Elaboration of the assessment and appropriate interventions for this can be found in Chapters 18 and 27.

Assessment of neurological status

This is performed in order to:

- make an initial assessment of the patient, which may influence any immediate action that needs to be taken
- have a baseline with which to compare the patient's condition, in order to facilitate observation of changes in his condition.

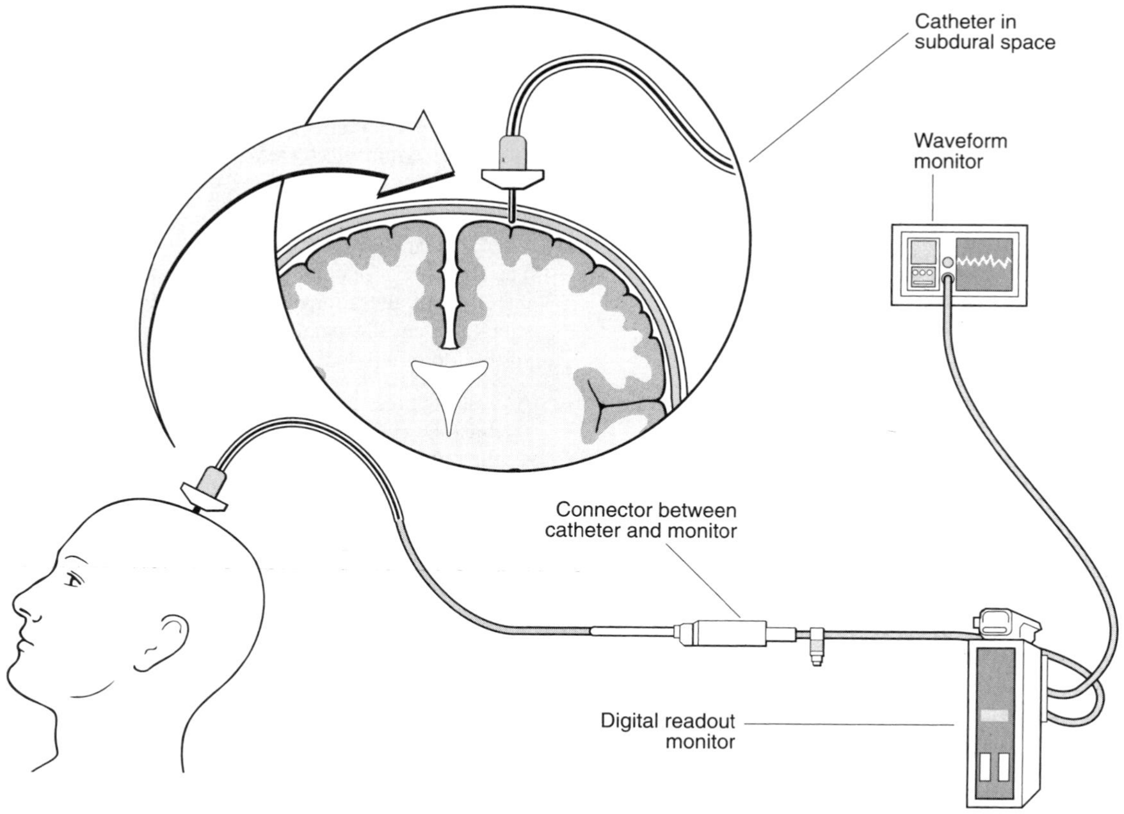

Fig. 9.19 The fibreoptic transducer-tipped catheter system for monitoring intracranial pressure (Camino system). (Adapted from Hickey 1997.)

Box 9.5 Neurosurgical approaches

Burr hole
A burr hole is a hole drilled through the cranium to allow access to the brain, usually to obtain a biopsy of tumour tissue.

Craniotomy
Access is gained to the brain via the formation of a bone flap, which is fashioned by several burr holes in a circular formation. The bone between the burr holes is cut with a wire saw and usually replaced at the close of surgery.

Craniectomy
This is a hole made in the skull by chipping away the bone, which means that it cannot be replaced. Usually used in the posterior fossa approach where the bone is particularly thick.

Trans-sphenoidal approach
This approach gains access to the pituitary gland and the incision is upper submucosa. This allows easier access to the pituitary gland (Allan 1988).

An additional surgical technique is the transoral route. To gain access to the base of the brain and upper cervical spinal cord, an approach via the patient's mouth has been successfully used. This particular approach is not usually indicated for tumour removal.

Box 9.6 Respiratory care priorities in a patient with raised intracranial pressure

1. Assess the rate, depth and pattern of respirations to indicate the patency of the airway. Report if the rate is less than 14 and more than 24, and any irregularities in rate or rhythm, as these would indicate a rise in ICP.
2. Assess the skin for cyanosis, which would indicate inadequate respiration.
3. Apply oropharyngeal and tracheal suctioning only as required to remove secretions. Suction for no more than 15 s and consider pre-oxygenation prior to suctioning with 100% oxygen to prevent a build-up of carbon dioxide in the blood, resulting in further elevation of ICP.
4. Institute measures to achieve optimal respiratory status including insertion of a Guedal airway, positioning the patient on his side with a 30° head-up tilt, and administer oxygen as prescribed.
5. Assist with monitoring arterial blood gases and mechanical ventilation as required.

Research Abstract 9.1

The interrater reliability of the Glasgow Coma Scale (GCS) was tested using a videotape of seven patients with various neurological impairments; 57 nurses and physicians used the GCS to score each of the patients. The responses were then compared for consensus and against an agreed criterion. The comparison showed a low disagreement rating and a moderate to high agreement rating, demonstrating that this tool had good interrater reliability. The authors concluded that nurses may use this tool with confidence as one measure of assessment in evaluating neurologically impaired patients.

Juarez V J, Lyons M 1995 Interrater reliability of the Glasgow Coma Scale. Journal of Neuroscience Nursing 27(5): 283–286

Any deterioration in neurological status may be an early indication that ICP is rising further, thus increasing the likelihood of herniation. Neurological assessment is important, as this may be the only indication that the patient's condition is deteriorating and a standardised method of monitoring neurological status will enhance this process. One commonly used method is the Glasgow Coma Scale (Rowley & Fielding 1991). This is described in Chapter 29 (see Research Abstract 9.1).

The frequency of observations is determined by the patient's condition, ranging from intervals of 15 min to 4 h. Medical staff should be promptly informed of any changes in the patient's neurological status.

The nurse is normally the health care professional who spends most time with the patient and she should learn to observe changes in the patient's behaviour which may herald an impending change in neurological status. These may include the patient who does not answer questions so readily or who is becoming more agitated and restless.

The expert neurosurgical nurse (Benner 1984) will be alert to the early warning signs which are so important to recognise, so that either surgical or conservative treatment can be carried out as soon as possible (see p. 363). Quite subtle changes in the patient's condition may be the only initial indication that ICP is rising.

9.2 Explore, as a group, your experience of caring for patients with raised ICP. What range of signs and symptoms have you and your fellow students noted?

Cardiovascular assessment

The final life-threatening concern in a patient with a rising ICP is the effect of alterations to systemic and cerebral circulation due to shock and cardiovascular instability. Unless requested by medical staff to do otherwise, the nurse should always report if:

- systolic pressure is less than 90 or more than 170 mmHg
- diastolic pressure is less than 50 or more than 100 mmHg
- the pulse rate is less than 50 or more than 100 beats/min.

Readings which exceed these parameters will render the patient more susceptible to brain damage as a result of raised ICP and a lowered cerebral perfusion pressure.

Surgery

Preoperative. Urgent surgery may be indicated shortly after admission or in response to subsequent deterioration. The nurse will need to prepare the patient in a very short time and also to provide adequate explanation and reassurance (see Ch. 26).

The approaches used in surgery are as outlined in Box 9.5.

Postoperative. The overall goals of care for patients following neurosurgery are:

- continuous assessment of the patient's neurological status (see Ch. 28 p. 856.)
- instituting measures to avoid secondary brain damage
- administration of appropriate therapies.

The main complications of neurosurgery are outlined in Table 9.3.

As the patient progresses, his needs will require to be reassessed and the nursing interventions adjusted accordingly.

Table 9.3 Complications of neurosurgery

Complications	*Cause*	*Interventions*
Altered conscious level	Increased ICP due to cerebral haemorrhage/oedema	Frequent assessment of neurological status
Onset of seizures	Cerebral irritation	Observation of seizures. Appropriate interventions if they occur (see p. 378).
Limb weakness	Increased ICP due to cerebral haemorrhage/oedema	Frequent assessment of limb movements
Speech problems	Increased ICP due to cerebral haemorrhage/oedema	Frequent assessment of verbal responses
Respiratory problems	Increased ICP due to cerebral haemorrhage/oedema	Frequent assessment of respiratory status
Loss of swallowing reflex	Increased ICP due to cerebral haemorrhage/oedema	Frequent assessment of swallowing reflex
Loss of corneal reflex	Increased ICP due to cerebral haemorrhage/oedema	Frequent assessment of corneal reflex
Periorbital oedema	Direct result of surgery	Observe for swollen/bruised periorbital tissues

Each patient will progress at a different rate, so continuing assessment and meeting the identified needs on an individual basis are important. The aim of care is to ensure that optimum function is obtained and early detection of complications.

Subsequent considerations

All of the nursing interventions identified in Chapter 26 will apply. Only those interventions specific to the patient who is unconscious due to raised ICP are included here. The main aim of care remains that of preventing further rises in ICP.

Rising (1993) offers a useful review of this.

The patient care outlined in the following sections uses the Roper et al (1996) framework of the activities of daily living (ADLs).

Communicating

Unpleasant stimuli are known to cause a rise in ICP, so the nurse should take a calm, reassuring approach. Relatives should be encouraged to talk to the patient and, although they may feel rather foolish at first, they will be encouraged if they see the nurse talking to him. They should, however, be warned to avoid discussing upsetting topics. Everyone should be made aware that the unconscious patient may still be able to hear (Hickey 1997) and that they should therefore be careful what they discuss in his presence.

Non-verbal communication, particularly touch, has been shown to decrease ICP, so relatives should be encouraged to touch the patient, e.g. by holding hands or gently stroking the patient's arm, despite the extensive equipment which may surround him.

Any investigations that are to be performed should be explained to the patient and his family, who will be anxious and distressed at this time, particularly as there may be uncertainty about the likely outcome for the patient.

Breathing

Respiratory assessment and appropriate intervention, as outlined in the previous section, will continue as long as the ICP remains elevated. In addition, the patient's position should be changed every 2 h or as the need arises, and physiotherapy should be instituted as this helps to prevent pooling of secretions in the lungs and the development of atelectasis. The patient, if able, should be encouraged to undertake deep-breathing exercises.

Maintaining a safe environment

The patient should be positioned in the ward where he can be easily observed. If the patient is restless or agitated, the nurse should attempt to find out why. Adequate non-narcotic analgesics such as codeine phosphate and dihydrocodeine can relieve a headache and are the first choice as they do not mask conscious level and will minimise the risk of raising ICP. If the patient is confused, he may attempt to climb out of bed, despite explanations as to why he should not do so. He may not appreciate that he has a limb deficit and may attempt to walk, thus endangering himself. If appropriate, relatives can help to persuade him to stay in bed and, as a last resort, sedation may be used. The use of side rails should be considered, but the correct precautions must be taken. If the patient proves very difficult to manage, it may be necessary to place a mattress on the floor and to nurse the patient on it; however, this should be fully explained to relatives beforehand. Some patients may respond to sitting up in a chair with a table secured in front.

The nurse should always be aware of the possibility of a seizure. The appropriate first aid action as outlined in the section on epilepsy (see p. 378) should be adopted.

Controlling body temperature

Each 1°C rise in body temperature increases the metabolic demand of the brain by 10% (Hickey 1997). This increases blood pressure and encourages vasodilatation, which will increase ICP. Body temperature should be recorded at least 4-hourly. Pyrexia may indicate hypothalamic damage or the presence of infection. Any source of potential infection, such as CSF rhinorrhoea, should be identified and reported. Leakage of CSF from the patient's ears (otorrhoea) or nose (rhinorrhoea) may occur from a base-of-skull or anterior-fossa fracture. Confirmation is obtained by testing the fluid for the presence of glucose using a reagent strip. A positive result indicates the presence of CSF, although it is not absolutely conclusive. The identification of a fracture on the skull X-ray will confirm the evidence. If CSF leakage is left undetected, the patient will be at risk of developing meningitis.

Measures to reduce the patient's temperature should be adopted. These might include tepid sponging, cool fanning or medication such as paracetamol suppositories.

Mobilising

The patient will require frequent positional changes to avoid developing pressure sores. Semi-prone and lateral positions are both suitable. Moving the patient also encourages expansion of the lungs and prevents pooling of secretions. A slight head-up tilt of 30° will not only reduce ICP but will aid respiration, thus helping to prevent chest infection. The patient's body should be maintained in neutral alignment, avoiding neck flexion and rotation. The hips should be carefully positioned, avoiding flexion over 90°. These positions aid venous drainage as they minimise intra-abdominal and intrathoracic pressure, which will help to decrease ICP (see Research Abstract 9.2).

Passive movement exercises should be performed to prevent muscle wasting and limb contractures as these will hinder rehabilitation. Isometric exercising (see Ch. 10) should be avoided as this raises ICP. Anti-embolism stockings should be used to minimise the risk of deep venous thrombosis.

As the patient's condition improves, he should be encouraged to move around more. The physiotherapist will provide specialised exercises if there is a limb deficit (Hickey 1997). Sitting in a chair will help to reduce respiratory complications and encourage limb

Research Abstract 9.2

This study described changes in intracranial pressure (ICP) during 74 nurse-initiated repositionings of 30 patients who either had raised ICP or had the potential for it. Measures were recorded of ICP, body position, heart rate and mean arterial blood pressure prior to, during and 5 min after repositioning. Grouped data showed that a rise in mean ICP occurred during each of the position changes and that the mean pressure was close to or below the baseline observation of 5 min after each position change. The author then discusses the nursing implications of these findings.

Jones B 1994 The effects of patient repositioning on intracranial pressure. Australian Journal of Advanced Nursing 12(2): 32–39 movements. It may also act as an important psychological boost for the patient and his family as they will view this as progress.

Eating and drinking

As soon as the patient is able, an oral fluid intake and diet should be encouraged. Intravenous fluids may be required, however, and any fluid restrictions should be carefully observed and the intake recorded to avoid inadvertent increases in ICP due to worsening cerebral oedema. Some patients will require nasogastric or intragastric feeding and this should be facilitated by the nurse observing all the usual precautions, as detailed in Chapter 4. The patient with a basal skull fracture must not have the tube passed nasally as there is a danger of further damage and infection.

Eliminating

Observation of output should be monitored, in line with any restricted intake. Some patients require urinary catheterisation. The precautions and associated nursing care for this can be found in Chapter 8. As the patient regains consciousness, he may attempt to remove the catheter, an indication that normal functioning is returning.

Constipation should be avoided to minimise rises in ICP caused by straining at stool.

Q

9.3 Choose an alternative nursing model and, using the information you now have, create a nursing care plan for a patient with a head injury using that model.

Which model do you now feel is more appropriate to the care of the unconscious patient?

Rehabilitation

This forms a crucial part of the recovery process and the principles outlined in Chapter 34 apply. The aim is to maintain and promote function, improve or prevent further deterioration and also to prevent further complications occurring.

The neurological deficits which can impede progress during the rehabilitation process are described in Box 9.7.

The patient with a head injury may experience neurological deficits including limb weaknesses, speech problems and visual problems. He may also experience changes in personality, memory and intellect, and a combination of all these factors makes full rehabilitation very difficult to achieve.

Box 9.7 Neurological deficits that can impede rehabilitation

- Motor impairment, e.g. spasticity or ataxia
- Sensory impairment, e.g. loss of sense of pain or touch
- Communication disability, e.g. dysphasia
- Psychological disability
  —cognitive intelligence, e.g. memory loss
  —perceptual, e.g. eye–hand coordination
  —emotional, e.g. irritability
  —behaviour or personality, e.g. poor self-image
- Social disability, e.g. social withdrawal
- Educational or vocational disability

All the above have an effect on the patient's ability to resume educational or vocational activities.

The ward team, with the help of the patient's family and friends, should aim to assess the patient's needs and provide the optimal care and support to achieve these. Grant & Grinspun (1994) highlight the need for a safe and predictable environment for rehabilitation. Realistic goals are set and the rehabilitative process may take months or years to achieve, or the patient may remain in a persistent vegetative state requiring constant nursing care in an institution.

Often, the patient's role within the family changes. He may previously have been the provider within a family and may now have to revert to being dependent on others. Employment prospects may alter and, for some, a return to work is impossible. This can affect the family's long-term plans and will also have financial implications. An alteration to the patient's personality may affect relationships within a family, resulting in much stress and disagreement. Some families will report that the person has completely changed and is now different from the person they knew before. A family support programme to assist families of head-injured survivors is described by Acorn (1995) (see also Ch. 34).

Very often, repeated explanations of the patient's change in behaviour towards members of his family are required, as they find this change distressing. The reaction of the family can range from apparent calm acceptance to rudeness and verbal aggression towards nursing staff. This should be accepted and seen as the family's method of coping.

The multidisciplinary approach

Early and close liaison between the many health care professionals involved in hospital and community work is essential. The resources of the voluntary sector and self-help groups should be brought in, as well as the patient's family and friends. Hemingway (1995) describes the role of the community psychiatric nurse in terms of therapeutic support.

Preparation for discharge

Many patients and their families will be particularly anxious as the time for discharge approaches. Much of this anxiety can be allayed if adequate preparation and reassurance are provided, along with an effective plan for discharge. The residual problems that may persist vary widely, ranging from headache to major behavioural changes, with or without neurological deficits. The degree of residual difficulty will determine what action is required in the discharge plan. Other influences may include whether the patient requires further surgery or other therapies, necessitating attendance at a hospital or rehabilitation centre. A home assessment can be performed by the occupational therapist and district nurse. Brief pre-discharge visits home may be considered and will help to identify potential problems. If there is a community liaison nurse, a referral should be made for assessment and support within the community, and if not, referral should be made to the primary health care team.

Despite these preparations, it is not usually until the patient is at home that the family members fully appreciate the difficulties before them. Much of the home routine requires to be adjusted, and whilst this may be easy in the early stages, it becomes more difficult to accept in the long term. Other members of the family will often view the disruption to their personal lives negatively and eventually much of the early support gradually disappears. If the patient is still at a stage in which he requires support, this withdrawal can be catastrophic. Very often the patient's partner can be left to shoulder the burden alone, and in this situation, a support group such as Headway (see 'Useful addresses', p. 392) may help. This organisation seeks to provide help and assistance to patients and their families. Regular meetings and other special outings are arranged, along with helpful literature. Relatives can be provided with a forum for discussion of the problems that they face and many appreciate sharing their problems with others who are similarly placed. Some families have to acknowledge a sense of failure should the patient require to be admitted for institutional care in either the short or long term. They may feel that they have let the patient down and do not like to admit that they are unable to cope.

Q **9.4** Using the information on care of the head-injured patient, select a nursing model other than Roper et al (1996) and write a nursing care plan for the first postoperative day following craniotomy (see also Ch. 28).

CEREBROVASCULAR DISEASE

'Cerebrovascular disease' can be defined as brain disease occurring secondarily to a pathological disorder of the blood vessels or of the blood supply. This section considers:

- cerebrovascular accident, the most common cerebrovascular disorder
- subarachnoid haemorrhage, an uncommon but major life-threatening situation that demands acute neurosurgical intervention.

Cerebrovascular accident

The term 'cerebrovascular accident' (CVA) is often used interchangeably with 'stroke', although, clinically, stroke refers to the sudden dramatic development of focal neurological deficits.

CVA can occur at any time during adult life but is uncommon in children. Thrombotic CVA is seen in the 60–90 year age group, and embolic and haemorrhagic CVA in the 25–60 year age group.

CVA is the third commonest cause of death in developed countries: 200 per 100 000 will have a CVA each year. Age increases the risk. Most CVAs occur in the 65–75 year age group and are more common in men. In the UK, 100 000–120 000 CVAs occur per annum, of which 70 000 result in death. The mortality rate rises in proportion to the length of time the patient is unconscious. Of patients unconscious for 48 h or more, 98% will die, compared with 12% where there is no loss of consciousness (Lindsay & Bone 1997).

Subarachnoid haemorrhage

Subarachnoid haemorrhage is often wrongly referred to as 'cerebral' or 'brain haemorrhage'. A subarachnoid haemorrhage is experienced by 10 000–15 000 people per year, with 15% dying before they reach hospital. It has a male bias in the under-40s, but this reverts to a female bias in the over-40s (Lindsay & Bone 1997).

PATHOPHYSIOLOGY

Causes of cerebrovascular accidents

There are three main causes of CVA:

- cerebral thrombosis
- cerebral embolus
- cerebral haemorrhage.

As a result of the rise in substance abuse, an increasing cause of stroke in the under-45s is the pharmacological action of drugs such as crack and crack cocaine (Blank-Reid 1996).

Cerebral thrombosis. This is the most common cause of CVA, in which atherosclerosis causes narrowing of the lumen of the affected blood vessels (Lindsay & Bone 1997) (see Ch. 2). It occurs either during sleep or shortly after waking and is thought to be due to the older person's poorer reflex response to changes in position (postural hypotension). As the atheroma builds up, it initially only partially occludes the blood vessel until the blood supply is suddenly disrupted. During the 24–48 h following this, neurological deficits frequently worsen.

Cerebral embolus. An embolus may lodge in the narrowed lumen of a bifurcation in the cerebral circulation. The usual origin of the embolus is a cardiac thrombus, in the presence of cardiac disease such as myocardial infarction. Air or fat, e.g. from a fractured femur, can also act as an embolus. Embolic stroke can occur at any time.

Cerebral haemorrhage. Haemorrhage can occur into:

- the cerebral tissues — intracerebral haemorrhage
- the subarachnoid space — subarachnoid haemorrhage.

The most common cause of subarachnoid haemorrhage is a weakness in the wall of a cerebral blood vessel, which causes a dilatation (an 'aneurysm'). Other causes include arteriovenous malformations (AVMs), but in some patients no cause is identified. Hypertension, although seen in some patients, is not always present, but damage caused by arteriosclerotic changes is common. Cerebral aneurysms may be described as 'berry' or 'saccular'. Most aneurysms form on the anterior part of the circle of Willis (see Ch. 2). Some patients have multiple aneurysms.

The exact cause of aneurysm formation remains unknown and some remain silent, causing no symptoms. Some bleeding can occur through the very thin aneurysmal wall and produce mild signs and symptoms of subarachnoid haemorrhage without rupture occurring.

Risk factors

Certain predisposing contributory factors increase the likelihood of cerebrovascular disease (see p. 14).

The effects of a CVA

The occurrence of a CVA, for whatever reason, will result in an interruption of the cerebral blood supply, diminishing the essential oxygen and glucose levels of the brain. Within hours, oedema occurs at the site of the main lesion. This gradually worsens, peaking between the fifth and seventh day and then gradually resolving.

A classification system of CVA is given in Box 9.8.

The damage caused by a stroke is due largely to the extent of ischaemia that occurs. It has been established that there is a reduction in global cerebral blood flow following stroke. In and around the immediate area of the infarction, more subtle changes are detected in regional cerebral blood flow. These comprise areas of reduced blood flow bordered by areas of increased flow due to vasodilatation of the arteriolar bed. Progression from reversible ischaemia to infarction depends on the degree and duration of the reduced blood flow (Lindsay & Bone 1997). The affected area of the brain loses its ability to carry out its function, e.g.:

- controlling movement in a specific part of the body
- controlling mental or emotional processes, speech or language
- experiencing sight, sound, taste or touch.

Another influence on the course of events is the occurrence of cerebral oedema. As the oedema starts to subside, cells begin to

Box 9.8 Classification of cerebrovascular accident

Transient ischaemic attacks
- Onset and disappearance of a neurological deficit within 24 h due to temporary disturbance of blood supply to the brain
- No residual neurological deficit
- Symptoms commonly last from several minutes to 2–3 h, but may last up to 24 h

Reversible ischaemic neurological deficit
- Neurological deficit persists longer than 12–24 h
- Symptoms may last days or weeks
- Minimal, partial or no residual neurological deficit

Stroke in evolution
- Symptoms persist beyond 24 h with an associated progressive deterioration of neurological status
- Residual neurological deficits
- Probably due to a failure of collateral circulation

Completed stroke
- Condition stabilises and neurological deficit remains

function again, causing rapid progress to be made in the first 2–3 weeks.

After this initial period, recovery is slower and is due partly to other cells taking over the functions of the permanently damaged cells. At this stage, the patient also learns ways of handling his disability and regains his self-confidence and interest in general affairs.

Generally speaking, if a patient shows marked improvement within the first week, then minimal deficit will result and, conversely, if little or no improvement is made during this time, the outcome is likely to be poorer. The most common types of disability are listed in Box 9.9.

Common presenting symptoms. The true onset of cerebrovascular disease can be difficult to pinpoint. In thrombotic and embolic stroke, the patient usually seeks medical intervention after a major episode. Earlier symptoms will not have been noticed by the patient. Early symptoms, e.g. tingling and weakness of a limb, are the result of mild transient interruptions of neurological function. Major episodes requiring medical intervention include loss of consciousness, speech difficulties and hemiplegia, which may be accompanied by loss of vision on the affected side.

Subarachnoid haemorrhage typically causes sudden, severe headache, often accompanied by vomiting. The patient may be alert and orientated and may feel intense fear at what he is experiencing. Alternatively, there may be loss of consciousness, seizures and evidence of neurological deficits such as third nerve palsy, hemiplegia or hemiparesis. Many of these symptoms are related to the effects of raised ICP (see p. 363).

The patient may still have a residual headache and neck stiffness which may be confirmed by passive neck flexion. This indicates meningism, caused by the presence of blood in the subarachnoid space irritating the sensitive tissue of the meninges. Kernig's sign, extending the knee to stretch the nerve roots, thus causing the patient some pain, is another indicator of meningism. Conscious level may be depressed and there may be evidence of epilepsy. Other findings may include hypertension and pyrexia. Signs and symptoms will depend on a variety of factors and can occur according to the area of the brain affected (see Fig. 9.5).

Box 9.9 Common types of disability caused by stroke

Motor deficits
- Speech difficulties, such as:
  —loss of movement in the limbs on one side of the body (hemiplegia)
  —weakness in the arms and legs (hemiparesis)
  —dysarthria, where the patient has distorted and indistinct speech but is able to understand what is said to him and can still read and write
  —dysphasia, i.e. loss of the ability to talk, read and write
- Facial paralysis on the affected side, causing drooling, indistinct speech and difficulty in chewing and swallowing

Sensory deficits
- Visual deficits
  —partial loss of the visual field
  —double vision
  —poorer vision than previously
- Poor response to superficial sensation, e.g. heat and cold
- Perceptual deficits, such as correct perception of the environment or loss of sense of smell
- Lack of awareness of the disabled part of the body

Loss of consciousness
- From mild impairment to coma
- Loss of memory or shortened attention span

Emotional deficits
- Emotional disturbances, e.g. change of personality, from quiet and pleasant to surly and aggressive, or vice versa
- Loss of self-control or inhibitions
- Confusion
- Depression

Bladder/bowel dysfunction
- Loss of bladder and/or bowel control (incontinence)
- Frequency
- Urgency

Q **9.5** Think of two patients you have cared for, who have had a stroke. For each patient, write a short word picture of how you recall them, then compare your notes with the common presenting symptoms you have just read about. How similar were they?

MEDICAL MANAGEMENT

Investigations will be as follows:

CT scan may be performed to determine the location and type of CVA and to ensure that there is no other, potentially treatable, lesion to account for the stroke. If a subarachnoid haemorrhage is diagnosed and the patient is alert, obeying commands and has no focal neurological deficits, lumbar puncture is indicated (Jamieson et al 1997). Confirmation of the subarachnoid haemorrhage will result when examination of the CSF reveals uniform bloodstaining or, if 6 h have elapsed since the original bleed, straw-coloured CSF, called 'xanthachromia'. This colour is due to the breakdown of haemoglobin.

If the patient is displaying any signs of raised ICP, e.g. he is in coma or has a neurological deficit, lumbar puncture is contraindicated because of the risk of coning (see p. 363). The safe alternative of CT is used which may reveal the presence of blood in a variety of locations such as the surface of the cerebral hemispheres or in the ventricular system.

Angiography. If blood is detected either by lumbar puncture or CT scan, angiography is indicated (see Appendix 1). The presence and location of aneurysms and other blood vessel anomalies such as stenosis will be demonstrated. Angiography is not without risk and its performance may be delayed if the patient is in a poor clinical condition. Four-vessel angiography is most commonly performed. Digital subtraction angiography produces a clearer image, as surrounding anatomical structures do not show up.

Electroencephalography (see Appendix 1) may assist in differentiating between a haemorrhagic stroke, which has high-voltage slow waves, and thrombotic stroke, which has low-voltage slow waves.

In addition, electrocardiography may be performed to exclude or confirm cardiac disease.

Treatment. Approaches in stroke vary widely because of the huge variety of presentations. They will depend on:

- the site of the occlusion or aneurysmal rupture
- the degree and extent of the ischaemia or haemorrhage
- the effectiveness of medical and nursing intervention
- the patient's response.

The aims are to prevent further brain damage, reduce the risk factors, provide supportive care and regain functional independence.

Treatment can be conservative or surgical.

Conservative management is as follows.

- Anticoagulant therapy has been used in an attempt to halt further deterioration and to improve the patient's recovery; however, some doubt has now been cast on its usefulness, as a risk of further haemorrhage into the infarcted brain has been identified. One example of an anticoagulant is warfarin.
- The use of thrombolytic agents, especially recombinant tissue plasminogen activator (rTPA), has been investigated recently. Early indications are that its use within a few hours of infarction produces a sustained, significant neurological improvement (Lindsay & Bone 1997).

An overview of the use of this approach can be found in Donnarumma et al (1997).

- Antifibrinolytic agents have been used in patients following subarachnoid haemorrhage. Their use is thought to prevent rebleeding by delaying dissolution of the clot around the aneurysm, but their effect on the overall outcome is questionable.
- Antiplatelet agents. The use of aspirin as an antiplatelet agent has received attention in recent years and research into its use continues. The patient suffering from transient ischaemic attacks may benefit from its use.
- Other factors. Pre-existing contributory disorders may be treated with drug therapy, e.g. antihypertensive agents and diuretics may be used in the patient with raised blood pressure.

Surgical management uses two techniques:

- carotid endarterectomy, which involves the removal of stenosing or ulcerating atheromatous lesions at the bifurcation of the common carotid arteries
- a superficial temporal to middle-cerebral artery anastomosis (ST–MCA bypass), which provides an artificial collateral blood supply to the affected part of the brain.

Aims of treatment in subarachnoid haemorrhage. The main aim of treatment is to avoid potentially fatal recurrence of bleeding. In untreated patients, 30% will bleed again within 28 days, and 70% of these will die.

Preventing rebleeding. An effective way to prevent rebleeding is to place a metal clip across the neck of the aneurysm. This entails a craniotomy, a major neurosurgical procedure. This procedure is not suitable for all patients, owing either to their general condition or to the location of the aneurysm. Alternative surgical procedures include wrapping, which involves the application of muslin gauze around the fundus of the aneurysm. Wrapping may be combined with clipping in some patients. A third technique, known as 'trapping', may be indicated. This involves clipping the feeding vessels supplying a large aneurysm. A new technique involves the insertion of helical platinum coils into the aneurysmal sac to induce thrombosis (Coleman & Sifri-Steele 1994).

The timing of surgery is crucial and opinions vary with regard to this. When surgery is carried out as soon as possible to avoid the risk of rebleeding, there are higher morbidity and mortality rates during the operation. Delayed surgery decreases the operative risks but increases the risk of rebleeding. Antifibrinolytic therapy may be used in an attempt to prevent this.

There are now well-established grading systems to identify the patient most at risk from deterioration after subarachnoid haemorrhage. The best known of these is the Hunt and Hess scale which is described in Hickey (1997).

Complications of subarachnoid haemorrhage that may influence treatment are as follows.

Rebleed. This is a risk which peaks between days 7 and 10 following the original bleed. This is due to the process of fibrinolysis, which dissolves the clot that formed over the ruptured vessel (Rusy 1996).

Cerebral ischaemia. Reduction of the blood supply to any part of the brain can have serious consequences for the patient. The extent of its effects will depend on the site and extent of the ischaemia. About half of the patients who develop ischaemia will be left with a permanent deficit. Arterial narrowing (vasospasm) is common following subarachnoid haemorrhage and can have similar results (Armstrong 1994, Rusy 1996).

Hydrocephalus. The normal drainage of cerebrospinal fluid may be impaired by the presence of a haematoma or by-products of blood in the cerebrospinal fluid. About one-fifth of patients are affected, although only one-third require treatment (see Box 9.10).

Box 9.10 Hydrocephalus

This is a condition in which there is a progressive dilatation of the cerebral ventricular system due to a production of CSF which exceeds the absorption rate. This may be brought about by an obstruction of one of the pathways by, for example, a tumour. Other causes include congenital stenosis and infection.

It can occur at all ages; it may be congenital in the newborn or secondary to some other intracranial pathology in the older child and adult.

Treatment is by insertion of a ventriculoperitoneal shunt. This is a long narrow plastic tubing, valve and reservoir device. One end is inserted into the lateral ventricle and the other end is sutured into the child's peritoneum via a subcutaneous route. The excess CSF is now 'shunted' from the ventricles into the peritoneum, from where it then returns to the bloodstream.

Intracerebral haematoma. Bleeding during a subarachnoid haemorrhage may result in a localised collection or haematoma. This will contribute to a rise in intracranial pressure and may demand treatment.
Epilepsy. Seizures may occur, necessitating treatment with anticonvulsants (see p. 378).

NURSING PRIORITIES AND MANAGEMENT: STROKE

Prevention

One of the most important aspects of stroke management is prevention, by identifying at-risk individuals and dealing with early predisposing factors such as hypertension.

Transient ischaemic attack

If the sufferer or a relative notices the symptoms of a mild transitory ischaemic attack (TIA), they should contact a doctor immediately, as TIAs can be treated. A TIA is caused by insufficient blood reaching the brain, for a brief period. It is similar to a stroke but the symptoms last for only a few minutes (The Stroke Association 1992). These are:

- weakness of one side of the body
- tingling and twisting of the mouth
- loss of speech
- disturbance of vision.

Reducing the risk of stroke

The following factors put people at greater risk of having a stroke, but action can be taken to reduce the likelihood of stroke occurring.
High blood pressure. Using drugs to reduce high blood pressure does reduce the risk of a stroke. Blood pressure should be checked periodically, e.g. every 4 years until the age of 40, and every 2 years after that. Drinking alcohol raises blood pressure. The recommended sensible limit is up to 21 units a week for men and up to 14 units a week for women, with one or two drink-free days per week (HEBS 1994).
Cigarette smoking. In people who smoke 20 cigarettes a day or more, the risk of having a stroke is three times greater than that for people who do not smoke (Hopkins 1992). Smokers should therefore be encouraged to stop smoking, and young people discouraged from starting to smoke.
High blood cholesterol may lead to coronary heart disease. Patients with high blood cholesterol can reduce the amount of cholesterol-rich foods they take, by the following measures:

- using spread which is high in polyunsaturates rather than saturates, and using vegetable oil for cooking
- using skimmed milk, not full-cream milk
- avoiding cream and cheese, and cutting down on the number of eggs eaten
- choosing lean cuts of meat or removing the fat.

Being overweight may increase the likelihood of high blood pressure, so at-risk patients should control their weight.
Diabetic patients are more likely to have a stroke, so the level of sugar in the blood and urine should be checked regularly.
The contraceptive pill increases the risk of stroke in younger women, particularly if there is a family history of arterial disease. Other forms of contraception are therefore more suitable.

Nursing care following a stroke

Often the immediate priorities and follow-up care overlap, and they are separated here for the purposes of explanation only. A successful outcome is more likely when the optimum techniques and resources are utilised, encompassing every member of the multidisciplinary team. The outcome can also be influenced by other factors such as recognising the need to start the rehabilitative process as soon as possible.

Immediate priorities

Airway. Techniques for maintaining a patent airway and adequate ventilation, outlined in Box 9.6, are a priority (see Ch. 28).
Safety and comfort. Hemiplegia is often caused by stroke, so the care of paralysed limbs and avoiding the hazards of immobility are important.

Similarly, the patient with a decreased level of consciousness will require to have his safety needs met and this is dealt with in Chapter 28. This includes an accurate assessment of conscious level. Raised intracranial pressure will pose a number of dangers for the patient (see the interventions outlined on p. 364 for care of a patient with a head injury).

The patient who has experienced a haemorrhage will be assessed for headache and an analgesic administered if required. The drugs of choice are codeine phosphate and dihydrocodeine, which do not mask conscious level. Patients often have a sore neck which can be alleviated by cold packs and a position in bed which avoids extreme flexion and sudden movement of the neck. A quiet darkened room will also relieve discomfort, particularly if the patient is photophobic. An antiemetic may also be prescribed for nausea and vomiting.

Patient safety and comfort are greatly enhanced when consideration is given to the patient's ability to communicate and to his emotional well-being, as well as that of his family.
Communicating. Speech impairment or loss can be a frightening experience for the patient and his family. Early referral to a speech therapist is important in order that an expert assessment can be performed and a strategy identified. It is crucial to ascertain the type and nature of the speech deficit, e.g. whether the patient's difficulties are related to expression or to comprehension. The nurse should encourage the patient to perform the prescribed exercises, with her help, between sessions with the speech therapist.

Powerful emotions are often displayed by the patient following stroke. Many of these patients display anger at or frustration with the frightening situation in which they find themselves. This can be vented onto the nurse and can manifest itself as lack of cooperation or physical abuse. Patients who are unable to communicate their feelings verbally may feel trapped inside a body that refuses to do as they want. Some patients are convinced that their words are properly formed and fail to realise that what the nurse or family is hearing is indistinct or jumbled. The patient needs to be repeatedly reminded of what has happened to him and why he feels the way he does, in order to try to reassure him. Patients and their friends and family can become very distressed when they meet and this needs to be handled with sensitivity. Some patients experience denial (see Research Abstract 9.3).
Mobilising. Patients with walking difficulties require a clutter-free environment and this may necessitate rearrangement of furniture. The nurse should ensure that any obstacles likely to pose a danger are removed and that the patient is wearing appropriate clothing and footwear, e.g. outdoor shoes rather than loose-fitting slippers.

Visual impairment may also be dangerous for the patient (see Box 9.9). Simple interventions that may help include providing an eye patch to eliminate double vision and approaching the patient from the side with the intact field of vision. These interventions

Research Abstract 9.3

A denial assessment tool was used by interdisciplinary rater teams to identify and differentiate types of denial in stroke patients. It was found that right hemispheric CVA patients were more likely to be in denial than those with left hemispheric CVA. The suggestion is that use of the tool can provide a means for ongoing assessment to support precise nursing diagnoses and promote effective patient-focused care planning throughout the rehabilitation process.

Christensen J M, Cook E A, Martin B C 1997 Identifying denial in stroke patients. Clinical Nursing Research 6(1): 105–118

should also be explained to the patient's family, who should be advised about basic safety precautions at home following discharge, e.g. removal of loose rugs and any necessary rearrangement of furniture.

Differences of opinion exist with regard to mobility following subarachnoid haemorrhage. One approach advocates that patients should have strict bed rest and that their visitors should be restricted; however, this approach can heighten the patient's anxiety, particularly when he feels well. An alternative approach is to allow the patient up to the toilet provided he is symptom-free. The patient with a neurological deficit or alteration to his conscious level should be nursed in an easily observable bed with cot sides if required. Seizure precautions should also be adopted as outlined on page 378.

Eating and drinking. Initially the patient's fluid intake is likely to be via an intravenous infusion and the nurse will be responsible for maintaining this at the correct rate. A patient who has had a subarachnoid haemorrhage may be prescribed a fluid regimen of 2.5–3 L/day. This helps to maintain arterial blood pressure, which encourages adequate cerebral perfusion and, in turn, prevents cerebral ischaemia and infarction. An accurate record of fluid balance should be maintained. As the patient progresses, an oral diet may gradually be introduced, providing that swallowing and cough reflexes are intact. The patient may need help with feeding, or can be given adapted eating utensils which allow him to feed himself. Being spoon-fed can be embarrassing and sensitivity is required on the nurse's part to preserve the patient's dignity and self-esteem. The nurse should determine what the patient is capable of; for example, hemiplegia may prevent him from cutting up his own food but not stop him from feeding himself. The patient with a facial paralysis should be instructed to chew food on the unaffected side only.

Dysphagia will hinder this progress. If the patient experiences swallowing difficulties, these should be assessed to determine the extent of the difficulty before attempting oral feeding. A combined assessment may be performed by the dietician and speech therapist. Recommendations may include the use of a nasogastric feeding tube and a prescribed proprietary liquid diet, and the use of specialised exercises and techniques. Increased oral hygiene is important in both instances. The patient with dysphagia receiving nasogastric feeding will be more prone to a dry mouth and the patient on an oral diet may leave food debris in the mouth, particularly on the affected side, so regular oral inspection and oral hygiene should be carried out (see Ch. 15).

Eliminating. Interruption of the patient's usual elimination pattern is due to loss of consciousness and enforced immobility. Urinary incontinence is best dealt with by retraining the patient to use bedpans or urinals at specified intervals, rather than resorting to catheterisation. Condom-type urinary appliances may be suitable for male patients, but no successful female equivalent is yet available.

Rehabilitation

The overall aim of rehabilitation, as outlined in Chapter 34, is the active promotion and restoration of independence, and this applies equally to all patients following a stroke, whether they are at home, in hospital or in a rehabilitation centre (see Case History 9.1).

Lindsay & Bone (1997) describe the common complications following a stroke and provide advice on how to deal with these.

Q **9.6** Can you seek out an example of such a multidisciplinary approach in support of a patient and his family from your own placement experience of nursing in the community?

Therapy. Different types of therapy can aid rehabilitation. These are not necessary immediately, as many people recover spontaneously, but can be of help once it is apparent that specific problems remain.

Physiotherapists can assist people to walk again and suggest suitable aids such as canes, Zimmer frames or foot splints. They can also help the patient to regain movement in paralysed arms.

Occupational therapists can teach patients to dress and cook for themselves, and can suggest suitable home aids.

Case History 9.1 Mrs F

Mrs F had her stroke on May 21st. She was completely paralysed on the right side and had lost all power of speech. A CT scan on May 25th showed a large area of brain loss on the left side. By June 1 her speech was normal, yet she still could not walk at all or use her right arm. She took her first steps on June 21st, and 1 month later was walking alone using a tripod. Her arm also developed a little movement 6 weeks after her stroke. She returned home on July 16th, and by early November she was walking to the local shops, talking normally and was able to use her right hand and arm for holding cans.

Mrs F's story is not unusual, and illustrates several points:

- There was a rapid recovery over the first month, when her speech returned and leg movements started
- Her recovery continued, although slowly, for about 6 months
- This happened despite the scan showing that Mrs F had lost a lot of brain tissue.

Dead brain cannot regenerate, yet people known to have brain loss can recover quite well. How is this?

Processes of recovery

1. Learning new ways of coping
2. Use of other parts of the brain
3. Possible growth of nerve axons
4. Reduction of brain swelling around the stroke area
5. Adaptation by others to the person who has had a stroke.

Behind this success story must be close collaboration between community nurses and other members of the health care professions.

Box 9.11 Some dos and don'ts for home carers. (Adapted from Mulley 1990)

- Do not overprotect him
- Do encourage him to exercise
- Do not accuse him of 'not trying'
- Do not pull his weak arm
- Do encourage his friends to visit him
- Do not become gloomy and pessimistic
- Do think twice before selling the double bed
- Do continue a normal sex life

Speech therapists help patients to overcome problems with speech, often involving the patient in attending speech therapy sessions at the hospital.

The nursing interventions identified during the acute period will often be continued during the rehabilitative phase, e.g. care of the paralysed limbs must be maintained. Other areas of nursing will include attention to speech difficulties and sensory deficits and preparing the patient for discharge home with adequate support and advice. Involvement of the patient's family in the recovery phase is crucial as their cooperation can result in the increased likelihood of success (see Box 9.11).

The use of self-help leaflets from the Chest, Heart and Stroke Association should be considered along with help and support from appropriate community groups.

The patient will have been referred to the local primary health care team for assessment and support. Once home, the patient's ability to live independently can be enhanced by aids such as handrails in the bathroom and adapted cutlery. Advice on re-arranging the patient's furniture at home may facilitate easier mobility and reduce the likelihood of an accident.

9.7 How many people in the UK suffer from stroke every year?

Have you looked after a stroke patient with severe physical and behavioural problems? If not, ask a fellow student to help you with this question. How many different members of the hospital and primary care teams do you think were involved in the patient's care? Consider each team member's role, then try to draw a circle with the patient and his spouse, partner or main carer in the middle, surrounded by each team member. What might be their feelings about having to meet so many people?

INTRACRANIAL TUMOURS

Brain tumour is the best-known disorder affecting the nervous system, and primary brain tumour occurs in 6 per 100 000 of the population (Lindsay & Bone 1997).

Astrocytoma, a malignant tumour, occurs twice as often in males as in females and is most common in the 40–60 year age group (Armstrong & Gilbert 1996). Up to 50% of brain tumours are multiple. Approximately 2250 people die from a brain tumour every year. The cause of primary brain tumours is unknown. Some appear to be congenital while others are related to hereditary factors (Hickey 1997).

There are two age peaks for intracranial tumours: the first decade of life, and the 50s and 60s. There is a slight male preponderance, except for meningiomas and neurilemmomas (Armstrong & Gilbert 1996).

PATHOPHYSIOLOGY

Intracranial tumours can be classified according to their pathology as outlined in Table 9.4, but the presence of a benign tumour in a crucial location, such as a confined space, can prove fatal. Intracranial tumours can grow in one of two ways: they may encapsulate, or spread and infiltrate surrounding tissue. Their rate of growth can be very slow or extremely rapid.

The pathological phenomena of tumours are:

- cerebral oedema
- raised ICP
- focal neurological deficits
- seizures
- altered pituitary function
- hydrocephalus.

Common presenting symptoms are extremely variable. Presentation will be determined by the location, type, size and speed of growth of the tumour and its effect on surrounding structures.

The neurological symptoms of brain tumours may occur alone or in combination. There may be general symptoms, e.g. epilepsy, focal symptoms such as hemiparesis or cranial nerve deficits, and signs of raised ICP such as headache.

MEDICAL MANAGEMENT

Investigations. CT scanning is likely to be the investigation of first choice. In the absence of this, skull X-ray, EEG and isotope scanning may be performed. These investigations may suggest a lesion but may be unable to identify the pathology. Other investigations may include MRI scanning and cerebral angiography. Additional investigations include measuring the ESR and taking a chest X-ray to establish the presence of a primary lesion. If a pituitary tumour is suspected, endocrine studies and visual field testing will be performed. If acoustic neuroma is suspected, audiometric studies will be performed.

Exploratory surgical procedure. Burr hole biopsy, in which a small piece of tissue is removed for pathological examination, may confirm the diagnosis. This technique relies upon the ability of the operator to remove a specimen of tumour tissue which reflects the true extent and pathology of the growth.

Treatment. This may be with surgery, radiotherapy and/or chemotherapy.

Surgery. The tumour is removed (if possible) using one of four different approaches, as outlined in Box 9.5.

Radiotherapy may be indicated for malignant tumours and pituitary tumours, in combination with surgery.

Chemotherapy has been used for some time, but the clinical benefits remain uncertain (Lindsay & Bone 1997).

NURSING PRIORITIES AND MANAGEMENT: INTRACRANIAL TUMOURS

Assessment should be made of the patient's and his family's understanding of the reason for admission. The doctor may suspect a brain tumour but may wish to perform the investigations to confirm this before telling the patient and his family.

Someone with an intracranial tumour can usually carry out his normal daily activities, unless there is a rise in ICP caused by

Table 9.4 Classification of tumours (Allan 1988)

Tumour	*Description*	*Usual sites*	*Incidence (% of total)*	*Remarks*
Tumours of neuroepithelial tissue				
Astrocytoma Grade 1 Intermediate astrocytoma Grades II & III	Well differentiated, insidiously invasive, relatively benign Will possess some of the characteristics of grade 1 astrocytomas but cell differentiation less well defined	Cerebral hemispheres of adults; most commonly the frontal lobes followed by the temporal and parietal sites (Occipital lobe astrocytoma is rare)	10%	A cystic type of astrocytoma is sometimes located in the cerebellum. A childhood tumour of the first decade of life
Glioblastoma multiforme (anaplastic astrocytoma) Grade IV	Rapidly growing, undifferentiated cells, extremely malignant and highly vascular. Infiltrates brain tissue extensively. Peak age is 48–52 years with a male bias. Can produce extensive brain swelling while still relatively small in size	Grade IV shown to spread into the white matter of both hemispheres via the anterior corpus callosum	18%	
Oligodendroglioma	Rare, slow-growing tumour, age of onset = 40 years. Relatively benign — minor signs and symptoms can be present for a number of years before diagnosis is confirmed. Shows a marked tendency to calcify (May be seen on skull X-ray)	Demonstrates a predilection to grow in close proximity to the ventricular wall and commissural midline structures in the frontal region of the cerebral hemispheres. Can also be found in the temporal lobes	4%	Can 'mimic' a meningioma upon presentation. Unlike many tumours, raised ICP is a late sign in the patient with an oligodendroglioma. Sudden deterioration can occur, thought to be due to spontaneous haemorrhage and cystic degeneration within the tumour body
Ependymoma	Rare undifferentiated slow-growing glioma. Often seen in childhood and young adult	Arises from the ependymal layer of the ventricular system; therefore may be found in any of four lobes	5%	Due to involvement of the CSF pathways, hydrocephalus and raised ICP are early common features
Optic nerve glioma	Occurs mainly before the age of 20 years. Follows a relatively benign course, remaining localised to the optic nerve and chiasma	Optic nerve and chiasma	4%	Approximately 60% of patients have an associated neurofibromatosis called a spongioblastoma
Medulloblastoma	Rapidly growing, malignant tumour of childhood. Composed of round, undifferentiated cells. Commonest intracranial neoplasm of childhood. Usually occurs before the age of 10 years	Cerebellar vermis or 4th ventricle roof	3%	Can 'seed' throughout the subarachnoid space. Slight male bias. Hydrocephalus is common
Tumours of nerve sheath cells				
Neurilemma/ Schwannoma	Slow-growing, benign tumour. Well encapsulated. Usually unilateral, predilection for females, occurs in the middle years of life	The Schwann cell sheath of cranial nerves VIII, V & VII located within the confined cerebellopontine angle		A tumour of the sheath of the VIII nerve. Referred to as an acoustic neuroma. Other tumour types may be seen in this location, e.g. meningioma, but a differential diagnosis may not be made until surgery
Neuroma (neurofibroma)	A complex familial disorder characterised by widespread benign tumours throughout the nervous system. Inherited as an autosomal dominant trait. Known as Recklinghausen's disease. Manifests itself in young adulthood	The neurilemma of nerves; therefore tumours may appear intracranially, i.e. VIIth nerve, acoustic neuroma or extra-cranially, i.e. spinal roots and peripheral nerves	10%	Patient will present with cutaneous pigmentation of the skin termed 'café au lait' spots. Some of these patients will also have a meningioma or glioma as well

(cont'd)

Table 9.4 *(cont'd)*

Tumour	*Description*	*Usual sites*	*Incidence (% of total)*	*Remarks*
Tumours of meningeal and related tissues				
Meningioma	Benign, slow-growing tumour arising from the arachnoid cells of the arachnoid villi. An irregular single mass usually well encapsulated	Intracranial venous sinuses — most common, superior sagittal sinus known as a parasagittal meningioma. Other sites include sphenoid ridge convexity of hemispheres and suprasellar region and olfactory groove	15%	Can become very large before signs and symptoms appear. Predilection for females in 40–60 year age group. Do not show any malignant change
Tumours of blood vessel origin				
Haemangio-blastoma	Slow-growing, vascular tumour of developmental origin. Single or multiple lesions occur. Manifests in children and young adults, male bias. May be familial	Cerebellar hemisphere	2%	May be associated angiomatosis of the retina or abnormal organs. von Hippel–Lindau disease
Germ cell tumours				
Teratoma	Rare tumour of childhood and young adulthood	Pineal parenchymal cells; therefore located around the pineal gland		The terms pinealoma and teratoma are often interchanged
Local extensions from regional tumours				
Chordoma	Soft tumour with a jelly-like consistency	Arise extradurally at the base of the skull		
Metastatic tumours				
Metastatic tumour	Well defined, usually multiple secondary deposits of a primary growth elsewhere in the body. Common primary sites are bronchus and breast	As lesions are often multiple, can occur anywhere in the cerebrum or cerebellum	12%	The symptoms and signs of a secondary intracranial growth may precede those of the original growth
Other malformative tumours				
Craniopharyn-gioma	A tumour of developmental origin, may be cystic or solid. Does not usually present until adolescence. May calcify	Arises from embryological remnants of the cranio-pharyngeal duct (Rathke's pouch) into the suprasellar region and the posterior fossa	3%	Sometimes referred to as cholesteatoma
Epidermoid cyst	Congenital fluid-filled cyst of the ectodermal layer. May contain keratin and cholesterol. Occurs in childhood	Posterior fossa		
Dermoid cyst	Similar to epidermoid cyst; arises from the ectodermal layer but contains more solid material such as hair, sebaceous glands or even teeth	Posterior fossa		Difficult to differentiate from other posterior fossa tumours until direct visualisation at surgery
Colloid cyst of the third ventricle	Rounded cystic tumour of childhood	Choroid plexus within the third ventricle		Often presents with an acute, sometimes intermittent hydrocephalus
Vascular malformations				
Angioma	Arterial and/or venous congenital abnormality comprising enlarged and tortuous vessels. Usually have a 'feeder' artery and a 'draining' vein	Anywhere in the cerebral cortex, most commonly in the region of the middle cerebral artery		A unilateral capillary-venous malformation and the presence of a facial naevus is termed the Sturge–Weber syndrome. Hamartomas are small vascular malformations
Angioblastoma	Cystic tumour comprised of angioblasts	Cerebellum		The patient may also exhibit an angioblastoma of the retina

Table 9.4 ***(cont'd)***

Tumour	*Description*	*Usual sites*	*Incidence (% of total)*	*Remarks*
Tumour of the anterior pituitary				
Pituitary adenoma	Benign, slow-growing, well encapsulated tumour. Classified by the clinical syndrome, i.e. the hormone produced. Three types of hypersecreting adenomas: prolactin-secreting (prolactinoma); excess growth hormone (acromegaly); ACTH-secreting (Cushing's disease). Hyposecreting tumours are very rare	Anterior lobe of the pituitary gland	8%	Hyposecreting tumours will produce panhypopituitarism and chiasmal compression

swelling or by the tumour becoming larger. The onset of symptoms can be slow and progressive or almost immediate, in which case the person's condition deteriorates rapidly.

Immediate priorities

The patient should be assessed for increasing ICP, and the nurse should observe for any deterioration in the patient's condition. If the patient has experienced seizures before admission, this should be carefully noted and the nurse should be prepared should a seizure occur.

If the patient has speech problems, e.g. dysphasia, time should be taken to give careful explanations.

Subsequent considerations

After neurological and physical assessment, the speech therapist, physiotherapist and occupational therapist should be involved in assessing the patient and offering advice and assistance.

Support during investigations

The patient will be anxious to know the results of investigations but will also be worried about the diagnosis. The investigations can confirm the diagnosis or identify the type of tumour and the patient should be encouraged to discuss his fears and anxieties (Amato 1991). He may be aware of the possibility of neurological deficits or even death. The nurse should be aware of the grieving process and accept the patient's reactions. Some of the fears and anxieties may be unfounded and the nurse may be able to alleviate some of these.

Non-surgical interventions

Medication. Steroids are prescribed once a tumour is diagnosed. The drug of choice is dexamethasone, which helps to reduce swelling around the tumour, decreasing the overall mass of the brain and therefore ICP. The patient can feel better after 1 day of steroids, finding relief from headache, nausea, vomiting and from the improvement of neurological deficits. However, there are side-effects from steroid medication:

- irritation of the lining of the stomach — antacids are routinely prescribed to counteract this
- glycosuria — urine is routinely tested for glucose and ketones
- adrenal insufficiency, which will occur if medication is withdrawn suddenly.

Radiotherapy. The radiotherapist can assess the patient in the ward or the patient can attend as an outpatient. If the patient requires urgent radiotherapy, this will be discussed by the radiotherapist, but the nurse should be available if the patient wants to discuss his feelings about the treatment (see Ch. 32).

Inoperable tumours

A tumour may be inoperable due to inaccessibility or because of its type and size. Surgery could involve great risk of neurological deficits postoperatively. This situation offers a great challenge to the nurse: to be able to communicate effectively and offer adequate support (see Chs 31 and 33).

Ongoing care

Major deficits

The patient's condition may be very poor and the doctor may advise the family that his condition will not improve. The nurse should ensure that the relatives are made welcome in the ward at any time of the day or night and reassure them that they are not 'in the way'.

It is important to tell the relatives that the patient is as comfortable as possible and that adequate pain relief is being administered.

Preparation for discharge

The patient may have no neurological deficits or only slight deficits such as limb weakness and may decide to go home and try to continue a normal life.

If the patient has a severe neurological deficit and requires a lot of assistance with the activities of daily living, the situation should be discussed with both patient and family.

If the family members are anxious to have the patient at home, their wishes should be discussed with the ward team, community nurses and the patient's GP in order to ensure adequate support is available and in place prior to the patient's discharge.

Hospice care should be discussed prior to discharge and, if the patient and family wish, further information on this can be obtained by the nurse.

A home visit by the occupational therapist or physiotherapist may be advisable to assess the patient's requirements when he is at home.

EPILEPSY

Epilepsy can be a symptom, e.g. of head injury, or a disorder with no identifiable cause. Five per cent of the population will have a seizure in their lifetime, but with recurrence in only 0.5% (Lindsay & Bone 1997). Box 9.12 shows causes at different stages of life. Lannon (1993) describes the particular problems of epilepsy in the elderly. For some, the cause will prove to be psychogenic (Benbadis et al 1994).

Box 9.12 Causes of epilepsy at different stages of life

Newborn
- Hypocalcaemia
- Hypoglycaemia
- Asphyxia
- Hyperbilirubinaemia
- Water intoxication
- Inborn errors of metabolism
- Trauma
- Intracranial haemorrhage (vitamin K deficiency, thrombocytopenia)

Infancy
- Febrile convulsions
- Inborn errors of metabolism
- Congenital defects
- CNS infection

Childhood
- Trauma
- Congenital defects
- Arteriovenous malformation
- CNS infection

Adolescence and adulthood
- Trauma
- Neoplasm
- Withdrawal from drugs or alcohol
- Arteriovenous malformation
- CNS infection

Late adult
- Trauma
- Neoplasm
- Drug/alcohol withdrawal
- Vascular disease
- Degenerative disease
- CNS infection

Epileptic seizures can occur at any age, although the age of onset can provide a clue as to the cause, e.g. in childhood it may be due to pyrexia, whereas in the middle years of life, a brain tumour is more likely (Hickey 1997). The occurrence of an isolated seizure does not mean that the person is 'epileptic'.

PATHOPHYSIOLOGY

An intermittent, uncontrolled discharge of neurones within the central nervous system results in a seizure. It can range from a major motor convulsion to a brief period of lack of awareness and can occur in any individual at any time, even in an apparently healthy nervous system. Each individual is susceptible to seizure if a threshold level, which is different for everyone, is breached. In some instances, the cause is obvious, e.g. a seizure can be secondary to structural damage to the brain; in others, no apparent cause can be detected and it is described as an 'idiopathic' or 'primary' seizure.

Common presenting symptoms depend on when the person is examined. During certain types of seizure, the patient may be unconscious, apnoeic and incontinent of urine, whilst in others, changes are barely noticeable. Between seizures, the patient may show no neurological impairment or deficit. Seizures are classified as outlined in Box 9.13.

MEDICAL MANAGEMENT

Investigations. Electroencephalography (EEG) will be carried out. Other investigations such as CT scanning and MRI may also be considered in order to identify possible causes.

The most reliable diagnostic tool is a reliable eyewitness account of the seizure.

Treatment. The mainstay of therapy is medication, which is effective in keeping many people free from seizures. Anti-epileptic drugs such as phenytoin sodium and sodium valproate are given.

A small number of patients who have an identifiable focus which is amenable to surgery may be offered this option. The most commonly employed technique is temporal or other cortical area resection. Over half of the patients treated become free from seizure or acquire easier control (Hodges & Root 1991, Rusy 1991).

NURSING PRIORITIES AND MANAGEMENT: EPILEPTIC SEIZURES

Most individuals with seizures live in their own home, with regular monitoring by their GP or at an epilepsy outpatient clinic. However, occasionally treatment is no longer effective and the patient requires to be admitted to hospital for reassessment.

Immediate priorities

Once notification is received at the ward that a patient is to be admitted due to a worsening of his seizures, the following essential equipment should be assembled and be readily available:

- oxygen and suction in good working order
- a selection of various sizes of artificial airways
- charts for recording neurological status, vital signs and seizures
- bedside rails should be in place (may be padded for additional safety)
- supplies of anticonvulsant medication, particularly in the intravenous or intramuscular form.

If the patient is having a seizure, the following actions must always be carried out:

- use suction if necessary to prevent aspiration of secretions
- ensure privacy is provided for the patient
- ensure bedside rails are in place, using pillows as padding if required
- if the patient is on the floor, ensure safety by removing any objects or furniture likely to cause harm
- loosen any restrictive clothing
- insert an airway only when teeth have unclenched (after the tonic stage); any attempts to insert objects into the patient's mouth prior to this serve no purpose and may endanger the nurse (bitten fingers) or the patient (broken teeth)
- record pupillary activity — pupils will begin to react as the patient recovers.

Immediately following a seizure the nurse should:

- turn the patient on his side to facilitate the drainage of secretions
- allow the patient to sleep
- allow time for the patient to wake up and provide reassurance and assistance to encourage reorientation
- record a description of what happened on the seizure observation chart.

The nurse's record should include a note of (Allan 1988):

- the time at which the seizure occurred
- what the patient was doing at the time

Box 9.13 Classification of seizures

Partial seizures

Focal seizure
Localised twitching, usually of the face and hands. Consciousness is maintained and the duration is brief.

Jacksonian seizure
As for focal seizure, except that the seizure activity spreads to affect other parts of the body, e.g. twitching of the finger may spread to involve the hand, arm and side of face.

Psychomotor seizure
The origin is usually the temporal lobe and these seizures are characterised by subjective symptoms, e.g. the patient may experience hallucinations prior to its onset. The patient will exhibit altered behaviour for which he is amnesic, followed by a period of automatism. Consciousness may be lost and the seizure may last 1–4 min.

Generalised seizures

Absence seizure
Affects children. There is a brief lapse of consciousness lasting 5–10 s following which the child will continue what he was doing prior to the attack. Can easily go undetected. During the attack the child will appear blank and the eyes become vacant. Can occur repeatedly in 1 day.

Tonic–clonic seizure
Has several stages which are characteristic of this type of seizure:

- *Aura*. A warning of the impending seizure. May be a smell or other feeling which the patient can learn to recognise. Not all patients experience an aura.
- *Tonic phase*. Loss of consciousness occurs, with stiffening of the body's limbs. If the patient is standing, he will fall to the ground and may bite his tongue. The muscular contraction will expel air via the vocal cords and thus a shrill cry may be heard. Both bladder and bowel may empty. The patient will become apnoeic and cyanosed for a period of 15–30 s. During this period, the patient is unresponsive.
- *Clonic phase*. The phase of stiffness passes to give way to clonus in which there is a violent rhythmical jerking of the limbs, accompanied by hyperventilation and the production of excess saliva. The pulse is rapid and the patient is sweating profusely. This phase can last for several minutes.
- *Coma*. Once the clonic phase subsides, the patient will lapse into coma and be difficult to rouse. This can last for 1 h or longer. If the patient wakes up at this stage, he may complain of headache and tiredness and will appear confused.

Tonic seizure
This is the tonic phase as described in the tonic–clonic seizure above. Usually occurs in children.

Clonic seizure
This is the clonic phase as described in the tonic–clonic seizure above.

Myoclonic seizure
Characterised by sudden jerky movements, usually of the limbs, accompanied by a brief lapse of consciousness. Usually occur in clusters and, following these, the patient can become confused.

Atonic seizure
Characterised by sudden loss of postural tone with alterations of consciousness.

Akinetic seizure
Characterised by sudden loss of postural muscle tone and sometimes called 'drop attacks'.

- any aura or crying out prior to the seizure
- any loss of consciousness
- which parts of the body were affected
- any stiffening or jerky movements and the length of each phase
- any urinary or faecal incontinence
- the length of the recovery period
- the patient's behaviour after the seizure
- any weakness in part of the limbs.

The doctor should be informed about the seizure and any prescribed anticonvulsant medication should be administered.

Further considerations

The patient should be allowed to express his feelings and fears and he and his family should be given adequate explanations and support. Explanation about the medication prescribed will encourage compliance by the patient. Side-effects should be discussed. Blood-level monitoring of drug serum levels will be carried out and it should be explained to the patient that this test will indicate if there is an adequate or inadequate dosage of the drug. It will also indicate if the blood levels are too high. If too high, the patient may be experiencing side-effects of the drugs; and if too low, it will indicate that seizures will occur again. Common side-effects of anticonvulsant drugs are:

- drowsiness
- dizziness
- gastric upset
- diplopia
- ataxia.

The patient should be allowed time to come to terms with the diagnosis of epilepsy. He may experience feelings of anger and grief.

Q **9.8** What information does your local library have about self-help groups for people with epilepsy?

The nurse should discuss with both the patient and his family the social implications of epilepsy and encourage a positive outlook.

The patient should be told that he may experience an aura (see Box 9.13) prior to a seizure and that it may be advisable to use the time available to ensure his personal safety.

It is important for the patient to recognise certain 'triggers' that may induce a seizure, such as:

- lack of food and sleep
- excessive heat
- constipation
- menstruation
- alcohol
- anxiety or stress.

Medical opinion varies as to whether someone with epilepsy should drink alcohol, as it can interfere with anti-epileptic drugs, preventing them from reaching the levels that control seizures. Large amounts of any liquid can trigger a seizure; heavy drinking is often associated with late night, irregular eating habits and forgotten tablets (Gumnit 1995). This is an individual decision, bearing in mind medical advice on the particular case.

It may be suggested to the patient that he consider carrying a card or wearing a Medic-Alert to inform strangers about his condition should a seizure occur.

Advice should be given prior to discharge about safety in the home (see Box 9.14) and the patient should be made aware that an occupational therapist can be invited to become involved, especially if the patient is elderly or lives alone.

Employment

The patient's employment situation should be discussed, especially if it entails driving or operating machinery. The patient must be told that he is required to inform the DVLA of his liability to have seizures and should be advised to stop driving in the meantime. This may present major problems to the patient, as he may have to look for alternative employment, and it will not help his self-esteem or his outlook for the future.

9.9 Discuss with your fellow students what may be some of the social implications of epilepsy (see Case History 9.2). Try to find out whether someone with epilepsy is permitted to drive a car.

Box 9.14 Safety measures at home

- Fireguards are essential and should be securely fixed to the wall.
- Smokers should consider the dangers of smoking in an armchair or in bed.
- Cordless kettles and irons are safer than trailing flexes.
- Pot handles should point to the back of the cooker. Hot food or liquid should not be carried.
- Sharp corners can be covered by rounded plastic pieces; available from supermarkets, children's departments and ironmongers.
- Glass doors should either use safety glass or be covered in safety film; available from children's departments.
- If seizures are frequent and unpredictable, the patient should let someone know when he is taking a bath or shower. The water should not be very hot and the depth should only be a few inches. The patient should turn the taps off before getting in. A shower is more suitable, particularly if the patient can sit, unless the shower tray has a high lip where water can gather.
- If the toilet door can be hung to open outwards, the person will not block it if he falls. Locks should not be used, except for special safety locks that can be opened in an emergency. An 'engaged' sign can be used instead.
- Soft pillows can be dangerous. It is best to avoid pillows or to obtain special safety pillows.
- In a small proportion of people with epilepsy, a seizure may be triggered by flickering light. These people should place the television set at eye level, at least 3 m away, with a small, lit lamp on top.
- An epileptic parent should ensure that garden gates have locks, to prevent children from wandering off during a seizure.

The patient must realise that some employers may not be prepared to employ someone with epilepsy and that his current position may have to be reviewed. Epilepsy is common in adolescents and it may be necessary to warn them that they may experience a change in outlook for the future or that they may have to consider a change to their career structure.

Physical activity

The patient should be encouraged to continue normal physical activities, with some emphasis being placed on the need to take adequate precautions, e.g. when swimming. It should be suggested that the patient lets someone know or takes a friend who can deal with a seizure when he is considering some physical activity.

Involving the patient's family

The patient's family should be given time and the opportunity to express their fears and worries, and the nurse should be prepared to provide advice and explanations when necessary. The nurse should explain about the type of seizure the patient is experiencing, e.g. a generalised seizure. Family members should be told what to expect if a seizure occurs, e.g. that the patient will have sudden uncontrolled movements and will appear to be holding his breath. They should know exactly what to do and why they are doing it. The Epilepsy Association issues helpful factsheets, helping lay people, including those with epilepsy, to understand more about the condition (see 'Useful addresses', p. 392). Consideration needs to be given to meeting the needs of children whose parents have epilepsy (Lannon 1992). Advice should include the following:

- Ensuring the safety of the patient, which can involve removing harmful objects and ensuring that all restrictive clothing is loosened.
- After the seizure the patient should be placed on his side and allowed to sleep. He should be given adequate time to wake up and reorientate himself.
- The family should know that they should seek medical advice if a seizure lasts longer than usual or if seizures continue without time for the patient to recover.
- The family should be aware that the patient may have feelings of shock, anger and lack of self-esteem and should allow time for him to come to terms with these feelings.

Case History 9.2 Epilepsy: a teenager's viewpoint

I am 18 years old and in my last year at school. My friends are all making plans to go to college in the autumn and for most it will mean leaving home for the first time. I have had epilepsy since the age of 7 and my parents have always accompanied me everywhere. Even now, I am not allowed to go to the shops on my own in case something happens.

Since having my treatment reviewed 2 years ago, my attacks are under much better control and I cannot understand why I am not allowed more freedom. They do not seem to have noticed either the improvement or my age.

My friends ask me what I plan to do when I finish school and I have told them that I want to go away to college. I know that I will have to discuss this with my parents, who will be upset and angry when they find out. They will think of all sorts of reasons why I cannot go and I know they worry about me, but I feel they don't think about what I want for myself. How can I convince them to let me go?

Gumnit (1995) provides useful advice to help women and their husbands or partners to understand the precautions to be taken when pregnant or when looking after their children.

The ward team should work together to give the patient and his family encouragement and advice about being at home. Sadler (1996) highlights the provision of support for clients in the community who have epilepsy. It may be helpful to explain that one person in every 200 has epilepsy, so that they can recognise that they are not alone. Involvement in groups for people with epilepsy provides advice and support.

For further information, see Chadwick & Usiskin (1991).

MULTIPLE SCLEROSIS (DISSEMINATED SCLEROSIS)

The occurrence of multiple sclerosis is not consistent in different parts of the world. Its incidence in the Orkney and Shetland Islands of the UK is 309 per 100 000, whereas in Italy, it is 13 per 100 000. It is therefore described as a disorder of temperate climates. Those who move from an area of high risk to one of low risk do not lessen the chance of the disease occurring. Multiple sclerosis is not hereditary, but the risk of a child developing multiple sclerosis where the parent is afflicted is approximately 15 times greater than in the unaffected population (Lindsay & Bone 1997).

The age of onset is 20–50 years and it is slightly more common in females. The cause is unknown and the disorder typically follows a pattern of relapses and remissions (Lindsay & Bone 1997).

Definitive diagnosis is usually very difficult because demyelination develops over a varying period of time. To be conclusive, there must be dissemination over a period of time and in several locations within the nervous system. In Stubbs (1992), a nurse suffering from multiple sclerosis describes her vague but often frightening symptoms and their almost random occurrence, and how it took 11 years for her own suspicions that she had the disease to be confirmed by a neurologist.

PATHOPHYSIOLOGY

It is thought that a viral infection affects the white matter of the brain and spinal cord, producing demyelinated lesions that prevent normal conduction of nerve impulses. The demyelination results in sclerotic patches or scarring, and the remission, typical in multiple sclerosis, is the result of healing of these areas. However, in time, these lesions degenerate to a point where recovery is unlikely and the resultant disruption of function becomes permanent.

Common presenting symptoms. Clinical features vary considerably, depending on which nerves are affected, but may include:

- blurring of vision or double vision
- weakness and dragging of limbs and extreme fatigue
- slurred speech
- nystagmus
- loss of sensation in a specific area of the body, e.g. part of the arm
- difficulty in determining the position of limbs in space
- 'stiff limbs'
- intention tremor
- clumsiness/difficulty with movement
- incontinence/retention of urine.

Sometimes fatigue will override all these symptoms.

MEDICAL MANAGEMENT

Investigations

Lumbar puncture. Examination of the CSF may reveal:

- a mild rise in cell count
- an elevated total protein and gamma globulin fraction (in 60% of cases)
- oligoclonal bands in the gamma globulin in 80% of cases.

Visual evoked responses. A delay in conduction is noted in the pathways.

MRI identifies areas of demyelination.

CT scan excludes other disorders (see Appendix 1).

Treatment. There is still no specific treatment. Steroid therapy may be helpful in acute exacerbations and physiotherapy is helpful to the rehabilitation of numb limbs. Many complementary therapies exist and are used with varying degrees of success, e.g. special diets and hyperbaric oxygen. More recently, studies have explored the use of interferons, which appear to decrease the frequency and severity of exacerbations in the relapsing-remitting type of multiple sclerosis (Leith-Kelley 1996). Research continues to establish the usefulness of these drugs.

Essentially, care consists of supporting the patient and his family and alleviating the symptoms.

NURSING PRIORITIES AND MANAGEMENT: MULTIPLE SCLEROSIS

The extensive tests involved in obtaining a diagnosis may necessitate admission to hospital.

Many patients with multiple sclerosis lead a normal lifestyle at home, requiring admission to hospital only if they are experiencing a deterioration in their condition. Many have made adjustments to their home and lifestyle in order to lead as independent a life as possible.

For the patient who is experiencing difficulties, hospitalisation will not only provide an opportunity for nursing and other health care staff to help the patient and his family to deal with problems that are disrupting the patient's daily life, but often enable the nurse to learn more from the patient about the experience of living with multiple sclerosis (see Case History 9.3).

Immediate priorities

Communicating

The patient admitted for investigations is likely to be fearful and will require adequate explanation about the tests and examinations to be carried out. Frequently, the nurse is asked about these tests and she should be prepared to answer questions or, if unable to do so, should try to find the answer for the patient. It is important that she is aware of the patient's knowledge regarding his condition, as the patient will either fear the worst, often with only a partial understanding of what the diagnosis may be, or may not be aware of the possibility of having multiple sclerosis until the diagnosis is confirmed.

It is advisable for the nurse to be present when the doctor is speaking to the patient as this allows the nurse to know what information the patient has received. Often the patient wishes to discuss certain points and will find it reassuring to speak to the nurse when the doctor has left.

The patient will require time to consider his condition and what effects it will have on his outlook for the future. Patients often experience the range of feelings and emotions related to the loss of self-esteem and body image and may worry about how the condition will eventually affect them. Expressed feelings may include

Case History 9.3 Multiple sclerosis: a carer's view

'It's the "not knowing" what I'll be like tomorrow that I find so difficult to cope with,' was the heartfelt cry of one MS sufferer. Caught up in the turmoil of wanting desperately to make plans for the following day, she was weary of the continual conflict between her desire to be independent and her body's limitations. The uncertainty and unpredictability of MS make it particularly wearing and difficult to come to terms with. As both a nurse and the relative of an MS sufferer, it would appear to me that coping with frustration becomes a major part of everyday life:

- frustration at having to rely heavily on family and friends
- frustration at loss of bodily function
- frustration at some members of society who don't seem to understand
- frustration at feeling a burden.

Coming to terms with limitations is only one aspect of living with MS; making the most of life within the confines of such restrictions is another. When caring for someone with MS, whether in hospital or in the community, the most important part we can play is in helping the patient to maintain his or her integrity and to adapt to changes imposed by further degeneration.

shock, denial, depression and anger. The nurse requires to accept these feelings and provide adequate support to facilitate coping mechanisms. Providing information about support groups, e.g. The MS Society (see 'Useful addresses', p. 392), may be helpful.

The patient's family must also be included and will require explanations about their relative's condition. They should be provided with opportunities to discuss their feelings and fears.

A deterioration in the patient's physical condition can cause major psychological and social problems. Carers may experience difficulties in coping and may require help and advice.

Admission to hospital can cause considerable stress, especially for the patient who has a set routine at home that allows him to maintain his independence. The nurse should encourage the patient to continue to be independent and to follow his daily routine as far as possible when in hospital. People often have well-developed coping mechanisms, and if nurses think they know best, it can cause patients frustration and anger. They can then seem difficult to look after and a vicious circle develops, where patients dread even more having to come into hospital.

Subsequent considerations

Problems with communication

Communication impairments in the patient with multiple sclerosis can include difficulties in pronouncing words, slow, slurred speech and poor concentration. This can create major problems with everyday communication for the patient. People do not understand that, although the person has speech problems, his intellectual capabilities are not affected and their reactions towards the patient may cause him to lose confidence in his ability to communicate.

The speech therapist should be involved in the patient's care as she can give advice on how to improve the patient's ability to express himself. Useful techniques to help the patient communicate are:

- to ensure that an erect posture is maintained, as this aids breathing and assists with speech
- to reduce background noise as much as possible
- to encourage the patient to express the most important points at the beginning of a sentence, when energy and concentration are greatest
- to use communication aids such as picture boards or computer boards.

Maintaining a safe environment

The patient with multiple sclerosis can experience difficulties with:

- movement, e.g. ataxia, unintentional tremors or paralysis
- vision, e.g. diplopia
- sensory disturbance, e.g. detection of pain and temperature.

Account needs to be taken of the patient's immediate environment both at home and in hospital in order to avoid accidents.

The patient may already be aware of the potential dangers at home and may take care to avoid them, or may be experiencing a deterioration in his condition and realise that adaptations are required in order to maintain safety.

Some patients may be unable to accept that their condition is deteriorating and that they are not able to perform certain tasks safely. When in hospital, an accurate assessment of the patient's condition, his level of understanding and, if necessary, his home conditions should be made. This will involve assessments by the community team, including the community nurse, occupational therapist, physiotherapist and social worker.

In hospital, the nurse should involve the patient in making any necessary changes to his new surroundings, as he will know best what suits him, e.g. the location and height of the bed, depending on his ability to mobilise. Ensure there is adequate space to manoeuvre a wheelchair properly. The nurse-call system should be within easy reach and the patient should be instructed in its use. The patient with clumsiness of movement or tremor may require assistance with some activities, e.g. at mealtimes, when there is a risk of spilling liquid and food, possibly risking a burn.

Mobility

Maintaining independence and mobility plays a large part in being independent. A problem for the patient with multiple sclerosis is the uncertainty of the rate at which deterioration in mobility will occur. The patient's family should be aware of any limitations that are necessary and also encourage the proper use of any mobility aids required when at home.

The attitude of the ward team is very important; the members should work together to encourage a positive outlook for the patient, while making time to understand his and his family's feelings and fears.

If the patient uses mobility aids at home, they should also be used when he is admitted to hospital. This enables the patient to maintain independence and also allows the physiotherapist to assess the effectiveness of any aids. For example, if the patient's mobility is deteriorating, is a walking stick sufficient to maintain safety? Common problems may include ataxia, limb weakness and lack of coordination. Techniques which may be useful in helping these problems are:

- maintaining a good posture
- when walking, making contact with the ground with the heel of the foot first
- taking care to place feet firmly in the direction of travel
- looking straight ahead rather than down at the ground
- relaxing and trying not to feel self-conscious.

The physiotherapist may suggest exercises to maintain the function of a limb and to prevent muscle wastage. The nurse and the patient's family can give encouragement for the exercises to be practised.

Skin care

The patient and his family should be taught the importance of regular skin inspection, e.g. to observe the sacrum and heels closely and to look for redness or blanching of the skin. If this occurs, the patient should be aware of the importance of relieving the pressure from the problem area, e.g. by lying on his side in bed.

Using a wheelchair

The physiotherapist and occupational therapist may advise that the patient requires a wheelchair in order to maintain mobility. It can be very distressing for the patient to realise that he has reached such a stage. It must be emphasised that this does not mean that the patient becomes totally reliant on the wheelchair and is unable to maintain his independence. He may require to use the wheelchair outside the house only if required to walk a long distance, or around the house only when he is feeling tired.

The patient may have become unable to stand and be able to weight-bear for short periods only. In this case, he is dependent on the wheelchair for mobility, but he should be encouraged to continue to perform tasks involving his hands, e.g. shaving and washing, in order to maintain a degree of independence.

If the patient requires physiotherapy when at home, advice and support can be obtained from the community physiotherapist. Some local multiple sclerosis societies also offer a physiotherapy service.

Advice should be given to the patient about when to use the wheelchair, what in particular to look for, and why:

- The wheelchair should be used only when necessary, so that the patient utilises any residual walking ability, thus helping to prevent muscle weakness.
- The importance of relieving pressure, especially on the sacral area, should be discussed, as the immobile patient may lie or sit in the same position for a period of time.
- Careful positioning of limbs should be ensured, taking into account any weakness or paraesthesia.
- The footrest on the wheelchair should always be used; care should also be taken that no part of the foot or ankle is rubbing against the footrest or wheel.
- The legs should be placed in proper alignment and the patient should check regularly that the limbs are safely in position on the footrest.

Balance of rest and exercise

The patient should be advised about the importance of rest periods to avoid becoming overtired or overstressed, which will exacerbate the condition. Relaxation techniques and a specific rest/exercise programme may be beneficial for the patient and should be discussed with him and his family.

Fatigue is a symptom of multiple sclerosis and can enforce changes to the patient's existing lifestyle. The patient may have to learn to ask for help when feeling very tired and this can be difficult for someone who normally leads an active, independent life.

Although rest is very important for the patient with multiple sclerosis, exercise is also vital to maintain muscle strength and help reduce spasticity. It will also improve circulation and prevent pressure sores and joint stiffness. Exercise will contribute to maintaining the patient's independence.

Employment

If the patient's current employment involves a lot of physical exertion, this may prove problematic with regard to returning to work. He may have to consider how his disorder will affect current employment and think about finding alternative work, although in many cases this may prove impossible. Stubbs (1992) gives a sensitive account of her sheer determination to stay at work and fulfil normal duties, driving herself to overwork and severe exacerbation, with resulting numbness and inability to walk.

Eliminating

The patient may experience incontinence, urinary frequency or urine retention, and problems with constipation. The urinary problems are due to the reflex action of the bladder having been disturbed due to damage to the nerve pathways in the lower spine.

The social implications of incontinence can be enormous and some patients will avoid going out for fear of embarrassment (see Ch. 24). The patient should be encouraged to take his time when passing urine and to ensure that the bladder is completely empty. Journeys can be planned to take account of the availability of toilets and this will reassure the patient. If a urine infection is suspected, a specimen should be sent to bacteriology for culture and sensitivity.

The patient may find it necessary and useful to use aids such as protective pants and pads (see Ch. 24).

Urinary catheterisation may be required if the patient experiences persistent urinary retention. Some patients will prefer self-catheterisation at set intervals and many become very competent at performing this procedure. Adequate instruction on hygienic technique can facilitate this (see Ch. 8). Advice from a continence advisor may also be useful.

Some patients will require an indwelling catheter, and support should be provided to enable them to come to terms with this alteration to body image. The community nurse can provide support at home.

The importance of an adequate fluid intake of 2–2.5 L/day should be stressed. Many patients mistakenly think that if they stop drinking they will no longer be incontinent.

The immobile patient will be especially prone to constipation, which will aggravate coexisting urinary problems. The patient and his family should be taught how constipation can be avoided by means of an appropriate diet, an adequate fluid intake and by maintaining mobility. Regular aperients may be required and the occasional use of enemas and suppositories may be indicated.

Expressing sexuality

The patient may experience a change in body image, and the nurse should try to encourage a positive attitude in order to improve the patient's self-esteem.

Sexual counselling may be beneficial for both partners. Men may experience impotence due to neurological damage and women may experience diminished libido. The patient may be too embarrassed or worried to discuss such difficulties with a nurse or doctor, and external counselling services such as SPOD (Sexual and Personal Relationships of people with a Disability) (see Ch. 34) and marriage guidance services may be a good alternative. (See Useful Addresses p. 392).

Q **9.10** Find out where the marriage guidance and SPOD counselling services are in your area.

Advice on contraception may be required, especially by women, as some oral contraceptives may interfere with existing medication. Pregnancy should be avoided during active stages of the disease as this may exacerbate the symptoms, although successful pregnancy is not completely ruled out.

Eating and drinking

There has been considerable research into the link between diet and multiple sclerosis, and a number of specialised diets have been identified (Swank & Dugan 1990). It has been shown that people with multiple sclerosis have higher levels of saturated fats and lower levels of polyunsaturated fats in the myelin sheath and the dietary advice outlined below may be useful to patients. They should:

- decrease the intake of saturated fats and increase the intake of unsaturated fats
- try to include more chicken and white fish in the diet
- when cooking red meat, ensure that visible fat is trimmed off prior to cooking
- note that liver contains vitamin B_{12} and arachidonic acid, an essential fatty acid (see Ch. 21)
- use semi-skimmed or skimmed milk
- ensure a high-fibre content, i.e. wholemeal and wheaten bread, pulses and cereals, and eat plenty of fruit and fresh vegetables.

The speech therapist and dietician may be able to offer assistance and advice if the patient has swallowing difficulties. The nurse can assist by encouraging the patient to:

- sit up straight with the head supported, if necessary
- eat in a quiet, relaxed atmosphere and not speak while eating
- take his time when eating to avoid choking
- eat certain types of food that are easier to swallow, e.g. semi-solid or liquidised foods.

Personal cleansing and dressing

In hospital and at home, the patient should be encouraged to maintain independence with regard to washing and dressing. It may seem to the patient, and at times to the nurse or to the patient's family, that it would be quicker and easier for the nurse to do these activities for the patient. The patient may feel under stress to hurry in order to release the nurse to go and attend to other patients. The nurse should explain that there is no hurry to have everything finished for a set time.

9.11 Many people with multiple sclerosis develop particular patterns of behaviour over the years. Have you or any of your fellow students observed this in such patients, either at home or in hospital? If so, can you describe them? How did you adapt your work to fit in with these routines?

The carer should be encouraged to allow the patient to perform these activities at home to allow the patient to have some degree of independence. The occupational therapist can assess the patient when in hospital and give advice regarding washing and dressing. She can offer a range of dressing aids and suggest specially adapted clothing, e.g. with Velcro instead of buttons and zips. The patient can be referred to the community occupational therapist if further difficulties are expected to arise in the future due to the possible deterioration in the patient's condition.

Patient education

The patient and his family should be as well informed as possible about the diagnosis of multiple sclerosis. They should be aware of the most successful methods of maintaining independence. They should know their primary care team and know that they can increasingly call on the community services, e.g. the community nurse, physiotherapist or general practitioner, as the patient's condition worsens.

The patient and his family should be aware of the possibility of the occurrence of behaviour and mood changes, as this can help them to cope with these problems when they arise, and help both the patient and his family to understand his behaviour. Euphoria, depression, apathy and emotional lability are common.

For a study of the impact of multiple sclerosis on care-givers, see Dewis & Niskala (1992).

Preparation for discharge

Episodic hospitalisation may become necessary as the multiple sclerosis condition becomes more widespread, and the patient and his family should be given the opportunity to voice any worries or fears to allow adequate preparation for discharge on each occasion. A comprehensive assessment of the patient's home situation should be performed if possible, well before there is any mobility problem, and should involve all members of the multidisciplinary team in order to gauge the suitability and likely success of discharge.

In cases where there is decreasing ability to perform the activities of daily living, a home visit for the patient involving the nurse, occupational therapist, social worker and physiotherapist may be indicated. Assessment of the patient's home situation, layout and the patient's ability to adapt, while maintaining safety and maximal independence, can be carried out. Some adjustments may be required in the house, e.g. bath aids and rearrangement of furniture. If the patient depends on a wheelchair for mobility, the doorways may have to be widened, cupboards may have to be lowered, and a shower may be required instead of a bath.

The patient may have to be rehoused to be at ground floor level in order to accommodate access to and from the house in a wheelchair. This involves major changes not only for the patient but also for the family and can be very traumatic if they have to leave a district they have lived in for a long time, and to leave good friends and neighbours.

Advice regarding income and benefits available, e.g. mobility and attendance allowance, can be given by the social worker. Outpatient appointments can be arranged for physiotherapy, occupational or speech therapy, if necessary.

Some doctors advocate discussing the possibility of relapse so that the patient is better prepared when it occurs. On the other hand, some patients may not have a period of relapse for up to 20 years and may worry unnecessarily if the subject is broached too soon.

Some patients may benefit from being informed of the availability of support groups. It may even be possible for the patient to be seen by a member of a support group prior to discharge. Such groups may offer a range of services, including general advice, physiotherapy and counselling.

PARKINSON'S DISEASE (PARALYSIS AGITANS)

Chronic neurological disorders typically run an unremitting course, often resulting in premature death. Parkinson's disease is not usually seen prior to the age of 50 years, affects both sexes and afflicts one individual in every 1000. It is a chronic degenerative disorder of the basal ganglia, with a slow onset that progresses gradually (Lindsay & Bone 1997). A disorder indistinguishable from Parkinson's disease is now emerging in some drug abusers. Some 'designer' drugs contain a substance called MPTP (1-methyl-4-phenyl-1,2,3,6,tetrahydrapyridine) which, when injected into animals, has resulted in typical Parkinsonian features. It is thought that this breakthrough may lead to further developments in the treatment of this disorder (Lindsay & Bone 1997).

PATHOPHYSIOLOGY

The Parkinsonian patient is known to have degenerative changes in the substantia nigra which forms part of the basal ganglia. Depletion of the dopaminergic neurones in the substantia nigra results in a decrease in the levels of dopamine. This is a neurotransmitter essential for the control of movement, coordination and posture. Several causes have been identified, including drug-induced Parkinsonism with, for example, the use of phenothiazines. Another unusual cause was an outbreak of encephalitis lethargica in 1916–28, and those afflicted, now 80–90+ years old, developed Parkinson's disease. No new such outbreaks have occurred in the UK.

Common presenting symptoms. The clinical features may include:

- a triad of symptoms: tremor, rigidity and dyskinesia
- muscle rigidity
- tremor
- a mask-like face
- disturbance in free-flowing movement
- loss of postural reflexes
- autonomic manifestations, e.g. excessive perspiration
- general weakness and increased fatigue.

MEDICAL MANAGEMENT

Investigations such as CT scanning may be considered to eliminate other disorders. There is no specific diagnostic test for Parkinson's disease. Diagnosis is usually based on clinical presentation.

Treatment. Drug therapy is the mainstay of treatment and the aim is to maintain the patient at the lowest effective level of medication (McGuire 1997). Treatment is symptomatic and does not halt the pathological process. Drugs can be divided into different categories and their prescription and use in particular combinations or on their own requires careful management and monitoring. Dopaminergic preparations such as levodopa are administered to replace the depleted dopamine. In older people, levodopa with a decarboxylase inhibitor is often used; however, it is only used once the symptoms of the disease compromise the individual's normal functioning. In younger patients, dopa-agonists, e.g. pergolide, are given to stimulate the surviving dopamine receptors in the basal ganglia. Anticholinergic agents such as benzhexol may be considered to treat the cramps, tremor and rigidity associated with Parkinsonism, but their use does appear to be receding (McGuire 1997). The enzymes monoamine oxidase A and B play a key role in the breakdown of dopamine. Selegiline is a drug which inhibits this process and appears to have a symptomatic effect. Amantadine acts by allowing the dopamine to stay longer at its site of action without being used up by other cells. It may be useful in the control of tremor but helps only a small proportion of patients. Patients who experience sudden fluctuations in their symptoms in spite of careful management of their drugs may be prescribed apomorphine. This is a potent dopa-agonist and is sometimes given as a 'rescue' drug in advanced states. It produces a direct effect at the sites where dopamine is active in the brain. It is usually given by intermittent subcutaneous injection, but continuous infusion may be considered.

Many of the drugs have variable side-effects, and accurate titration usually necessitates admission to hospital. Another curious aspect is an 'on–off' phenomenon, whereby, at certain times of the day, the patient loses the benefit of the dopamine and becomes rigid and immobile for a period of time. It is important to recognise this, as alteration to the drug regimen can reduce the likelihood of this happening.

Surgery may be indicated for some patients. This comprises pallidotomy to relieve contralateral dyskinesia (Gilbert et al 1996).

NURSING PRIORITIES AND MANAGEMENT: PARKINSON'S DISEASE

Parkinson's disease has an insidious onset. Some of its effects may be attributed by the patient and his family to old age. The progressive nature of the disease, combined with the potential embarrassment of many of its symptoms, can result in a patient who is aware of what is happening but at a loss to know how to obtain help (see Case History 9.4).

The importance of the role taken by the patient's family cannot be overstressed. Their ability to cope with the mobility and other problems associated with Parkinson's disease can make the difference between a level of independence, with the patient living in his own home, and enforced, frequent hospitalisation or long-term care with total dependence on others for everything. Mobility aids may be of limited use. The use of self-assessment is significant for the accurate evaluation of needs (see Research Abstract 9.4).

Immediate priorities

Typically, many of the early symptoms of Parkinson's disease may be treated by the family doctor, with the patient and his family making necessary adjustments to their home, e.g. removal of rugs and other obstacles over which the patient may trip.

As the patient's condition worsens, admission to hospital becomes necessary in order to confirm the diagnosis and establish

Case History 9.4 — Parkinson's disease: the family's perspective

We are 7 years into living with Father's Parkinson's disease. There have been so many challenges for him and for us over the years, and the challenges keep changing as the disease progresses. Here are just three of them;

- *'They didn't know him as he was.'*
  With each new admission to care, we are having to work harder to make sure that staff understand that the painfully slow speech from an expressionless face still conveys humour, awareness of world events, kindness and insight.
- *'Food goes everywhere, from face to shoelaces.'*
  It is hard to accept that it is probably now right to use that large bib at mealtimes. It lets him enjoy his meals independently and keeps his clothes clean, which matters a lot to him...but I still don't like it.
- *'He's changing.'*
  We knew it would happen, but it's been a shock to watch the first signs of mental change. It is painful to listen patiently to his attempts to sort out delusion from reality.

Research Abstract 9.4

This study examined the frequency and severity of symptoms reported by 39 patients with Parkinson's disease and compared them with symptoms suggested by the literature and by specialists. Four categories of symptoms were examined: (a) motor disability or activity loss, (b) mental change, (c) psychosocial difficulties, and (d) non-specific symptoms. The findings showed correspondence between expert judgement and subjects' reports on dyskinesia/tremor as well as walking, freezing gait and changing position. Symptoms such as dressing self, getting in/out of bed, morning stiffness and deficit in cognitive sequencing, which experts described as characteristics of Parkinson's disease patients, bothered subjects less. In general, patients' mental and psychosocial symptoms were higher in their frequencies and perceived severity than problems of performing activities of daily living. It was concluded that self-assessment is significant for the accurate evaluation of patients' needs.

Abudi S et al 1997 Parkinson's disease symptoms – patients' perceptions. Journal of Advanced Nursing 25(1): 54–59

the patient's medication regimen where appropriate. Hospitalisation will also provide an opportunity for nursing and other health care staff (such as the physiotherapist, speech therapist and occupational therapist) to advise the patient and his family on how to deal with the problems which are interfering with the patient's daily life.

Once stabilised, and if the home circumstances permit, the patient is discharged. Re-admission to hospital will only become necessary should further problems arise, such as worsening of symptoms. The stabilised patient is nursed in his own home until this is no longer possible; therefore, much of the care and advice which the patient receives during hospitalisation is directed towards maintaining his independence, dignity and self-esteem in what is a profoundly distressing disorder.

Mobility

Problems for the patient can include initiating walking, shuffling, tottering, being unable to stop walking, 'freezing' and stiffness.

Many of the techniques employed to assist the patient can be used by the relatives in the patient's home. The patient's strength and range of motion need to be improved in conjunction with the drug therapy programme. Warm relaxing baths and passive and active range of movement exercises are a good starting point. Relatives should be advised to continue this activity at home. Effort should also be directed towards improving the patient's gait, with the assistance of the physiotherapist. Useful tips to consider are given in Box 9.15.

If the patient experiences difficulty in rolling over in bed or getting in and out of bed, he can be advised to use a low bed with a firm mattress or to place a board under his existing mattress. Additional techniques are given in Box 9.15 (Lieberman & Williams 1995).

Exercise

Some patients may benefit from an exercise programme to assist mobility and improve posture. It is important that this programme is performed under supervision initially, until the patient and his helper are conversant with the techniques. Again, the importance of continuing these at home should be stressed to both the patient and his family.

Eating and drinking

The patient with Parkinson's disease may have difficulty with eating and drinking due to abnormal posture, tremor, poor swallowing and excessive saliva. The patient will be embarrassed by his untidiness when eating, and the length of time it takes him to eat often results in food going cold. People will often choose to eat alone rather than endure the social embarrassment of seeing others watching them eat. Families may adapt mealtimes creatively; for example, two small servings may mean that food stays hot and portion size is less daunting. Staff in some restaurants, following discussion, may be sensitive to such difficulties and very helpful.

The speech therapist may be asked to assess the patient's swallowing ability and to draw up a programme of swallowing management. This could include facial exercises and techniques to encourage swallowing, e.g. taking a sip of iced water to stimulate the swallowing reflex.

The dietician's advice should also be sought. It is usual to establish what kind of foods the patient likes best. A review of his current dietary intake will alert the nurse to any deficiencies or inappropriate foods; for example, it is easier to swallow semi-solid food than lumpy food. If tremor is a problem, the patient can be taught to hold his arm close in to his body, using his elbow as a pivot. Bendable straws could be used and cups containing hot liquids should only be filled halfway to avoid spillage or scalding.

It is important for the patient's self-esteem to resist the temptation to feed him before this is absolutely necessary. Many patients may still be able to feed themselves if their food is cut up for them. Feeding the patient for the convenience of speed is to be condemned.

Some of the swallowing difficulties which the patient may experience (Oxtoby & Williams 1995) are as follows:

- coughing within a few seconds of the act of swallowing
- food sticking in the throat
- nasal regurgitation
- fear of swallowing
- drooling
- food which remains in the mouth once the meal is completed.

The Parkinsonian patient who wears dentures should have these checked frequently to ensure that they fit properly. The importance of good oral hygiene should be emphasised. Patients should check their body weight weekly and keep a record of this, as weight loss may occur. Some hospitalised patients need to have suctioning equipment readily available while they are eating, in case they choke.

Communication

The communication impairments seen in the Parkinsonian patient include a mask-like facial appearance, which often leads to the assumption that the patient is stupid, and loss of eye contact and normal body language due to the abnormal stooping posture.

The speech therapist should be involved in the care of the patient at a very early stage, if communication problems arise. A programme of exercises and therapy should be instituted as quickly as possible. Facial exercises encourage the patient to pronounce sounds more clearly, e.g. by mouthing words slowly and clearly. Imagining that someone else is trying to lip read his words can help the patient. There are also exercises for breathing, strengthening the voice and controlling the speed of speech. Many can be continued in the patient's home. Other simple measures include reading out loud or singing in the bath. Alternatively, the patient could stand in front of a mirror, watching his lips as he talks.

Box 9.15 Useful tips to encourage mobility

General tips

- Gently rocking the patient to and fro encourages initiation of walking when he 'freezes'.
- Instruct the patient to consciously lift each foot as he is walking and to place his heel on the ground first. To encourage this, tell the patient to think that he has a series of imaginary steps to climb. These techniques help to counteract the usual propulsive movement.
- Remind the patient to swing his arms when walking.
- Teach the patient to broaden his stance to provide a more stable base.
- Remind the patient to think about his posture and to stand erect.
- If the patient starts to shuffle, tell him to stop and start again.
- Tell the patient to adopt the habit of taking small steps when he is turning and to turn only in a forward direction.

Rolling over in bed

1. The patient is advised to bend his knees so that his feet are flat on the mattress and then swing the knees in the direction that he wishes to turn.
2. The next move involves gripping the hands and lifting them straight up, straightening the elbows as they do so, then turning the head and swinging the arms in the same direction as the legs.
3. The patient then grips the edge of the mattress and adjusts his position until comfortable.

To turn in the opposite direction, the process is reversed.

Some patients find a 'monkey pole' helpful. Whilst this is easy to attach to a hospital bed it is not usually possible in the home; however, an alternative the patient may consider is tying a stout rope to the bottom of the bed and ensuring that the free end of the rope is within the patient's reach. This may allow the patient to alter his position in bed without help.

Getting into and out of bed independently

1. To get into bed, the patient sits on the edge of the bed near the pillow so that when he lies down, his head is in the correct position on the pillow.
2. Once this manoeuvre has been mastered, the patient only has to lift his legs onto the bed and then adjust himself into a comfortable position.

Finding the correct spot to sit on the mattress may take some practice, but once mastered the patient will find this a convenient way to get into bed.

Getting out of bed is more complicated and several techniques can be suggested. One example is as follows:

1. The patient lies on his back with his arms at his side.
2. He then lifts his head, tucking his chin into his chest, and sits up supported by the elbows.
3. The patient then sits up, pushing the trunk so that he is leaning forward, bent at the hips.
4. Support is now achieved by using his outstretched arms behind him.
5. He should now move his legs towards the edge of the bed until he is sitting up and ready to stand up.

Rising from a chair

The patient should avoid low chairs, choosing instead firm, high-backed chairs. In the home, the height of a low chair can be increased with blocks under the legs and it will help to raise the back of the chair slightly higher than the front. Cushions or a spring-ejector seat will also help. Placing a sturdy armchair in a frequently used location within the home is ideal. The patient can use the arms of the chair to assist him to rise from it.

Eventually the voice may become so weak that meaningful communication is impossible and an alternative means of communication becomes necessary. Communication aids must be appropriate to the patient's needs, and advice regarding their use should be taken from the speech therapist. Aids can range from a simple picture board through to sophisticated computer devices.

More simply, it may be possible for the patient to write down messages using pen and paper. However, the ability to write also deteriorates progressively and the writing becomes smaller and smaller as muscle stiffness increases. An alternative device which may be useful for some patients is a portable amplifier which will make a weak voice sound louder, but this will not improve slurred speech (Disabled Living Foundation/Parkinson's Disease Society 1992). Reading books and newspapers also becomes difficult when muscle rigidity interferes with the ability to hold them and to turn pages.

Q **9.12** Work out how many day-to-day abilities need to be considered in helping a person with advanced Parkinson's disease to continue to enjoy watching television.

Elimination

The impairment of mobility in conjunction with urinary frequency or hesitancy can lead to embarrassing episodes of incontinence. This can be difficult to deal with and initially the patient is encouraged to visit the toilet regularly. The use of continence aids may be indicated (see Ch. 24). The advice of a continence advisor should be sought.

Eventually catheterisation of the bladder may be unavoidable. Many patients and their families reach a stage where they would prefer to have a catheter inserted rather than suffer the continual embarrassment of incontinence and odour. For some, the increasing expense associated with laundering clothes and sheets may become overwhelming. It is important that patients are encouraged to maintain a fluid intake of 2.5–3 L/day.

Constipation is a common accompaniment to Parkinson's disease, so the patient and his family should be taught preventive action. A high-fibre diet and plenty of fluids will encourage regular bowel motions. Failing this, it will be necessary to administer faecal softeners or bulking agents regularly. Some patients may require an enema from time to time.

Personal cleansing and dressing

The oily skin and excessive perspiration seen in patients with Parkinson's disease demand more frequent washing and bathing. If tremor is present, men will find an electric or battery-operated shaver easier to use.

Slowness in performing voluntary movement (bradykinesia) can make dressing difficult for the patient. For example, buttoning clothes and tying shoelaces may become impossible. Adaptations to clothing and the use of appropriate aids will allow the patient to continue to dress himself for as long as possible, thus maintaining his independence. Fastenings can be replaced by Velcro and cardigans are sometimes easier to take off and on than pullovers. A change of style may be indicated, e.g. pull-on tracksuit trousers and front-opening skirts with an elasticated waistband. Slip-on shoes or elastic shoelaces are also easier to manage.

Discharge

Every opportunity should be taken to teach the patient and his family the best way to manage the disorder at home. Each of the areas already outlined should be included in the discharge plan.

Additional points to consider if the patient has been hospitalised are as follows:

- The names and times of the medicines to be taken should be written down. The importance of maintaining the correct dosage is emphasised and some indication of the possible side-effects should be given.
- A daily exercise programme should be devised for the patient, along with instructions about how much the patient should do.
- Contact should be established with the appropriate community services, such as nursing, social services, physiotherapy, occupational therapy and speech therapy, who may be providing the patient and his family with support at home.
- Advice on dietary aspects along with sample menus should be provided.
- Advice on safety should be provided. The removal of loose rugs and identification of other similar dangers in the home should be highlighted.

The patient should be encouraged to remain as active as possible for as long as possible, but should also be warned to pace himself. Each individual patient will approach this situation in his own unique way and this has to be taken into account when proffering advice. The attitude and approach of the patient's family (where appropriate) can be crucial to the patient's progress towards maintaining his independence for as long as possible.

INFECTIONS OF THE CENTRAL NERVOUS SYSTEM

There are many infections of the central nervous system, of which the following are considered: bacterial meningitis (infection of the meninges), viral encephalitis (infection of the brain) and brain abscess.

A serious outbreak of bacterial meningitis occurred in Stroud, Gloucestershire, in 1985 (Cartwright et al 1986) and since then sporadic outbreaks have occurred in other parts of the UK. Many of the victims are young children and teenagers. It is estimated that there are about 5000 cases per year in England and Wales, with 500 deaths and approximately 1000 patients being left permanently disabled. Approximately 10 000 people contract viral meningitis annually. As a result of this, the National Meningitis Trust (see 'Useful addresses', p. 392) was set up with the following aims:

- to raise funds for research into all aspects of meningitis
- to provide help and support for the victims and families
- to educate the public about the disease and its symptoms in the hope that awareness and early diagnosis will save lives.

PATHOPHYSIOLOGY

In bacterial meningitis, purulent exudate is found in the subarachnoid space. The most likely route of entry is via the bloodstream, which can carry microorganisms from, for example, an infected middle ear. Other routes of entry include direct extension from a skull or facial fracture, via the cerebrospinal fluid, and extensions along cranial and spinal nerves. The circulating CSF acts as an effective means of spreading the microorganisms. Causative organisms in adults include *Streptococcus pneumoniae*, *Haemophilus influenzae* and *Neisseria meningitidis*.

Viral encephalitis may accompany viral infections elsewhere in the body, e.g. the respiratory tract. The commonest virus in the UK is the herpes simplex virus. Some viruses, such as in Creutzfeldt–Jakob disease, appear to be latent for many years and are called 'slow viruses' (Lindsay & Bone 1997).

Cerebral abscess most commonly occurs following middle ear and mastoid infections. Pus accumulates in the brain, its location depending on the source and method of spread of infection. Other related conditions are extradural abscesses (pus accumulates in the extradural space) and subdural empyema (pus accumulates in the subdural space). The offending organisms include the *Streptococcus* and *Staphylococcus aureus*. Once formed, the abscess comprises a mature capsule containing necrotic tissue, inflammatory cells and necrotic debris. The presence of an intracranial abscess can result in raised ICP.

Common presenting symptoms. A patient with meningitis may have had some predisposing infection and be receiving treatment for it, e.g. antibiotics and ear drops for an ear infection, or may have experienced a head injury and have a compound skull fracture, a fractured base of skull or a facial fracture (see 'Head injury', p. 359).

The patient may not have realised the extent of his injury, initially deferring medical attention after the accident, but may begin to feel unwell over a period of time. His GP may suspect a serious problem as the patient's condition deteriorates. Admission to hospital will be necessary and, if the patient's condition is serious, referral to a neurosurgeon will be made, as the condition can rapidly become fatal, especially in children.

Infections of the central nervous system affect all age groups. Common symptoms are described in Box 9.16.

MEDICAL MANAGEMENT

Examination. Typically, the patient, often a child, is pyrexial, complaining of headache and may be disoriented and drowsy. This is highly distressing for the parents. The patient's reaction to interference is often aggressive and they find all external environmental stimuli, such as strong light (photophobia), painful (see Box 9.16).

For information relating particularly to children, see Robinson (1994).

Investigations. The patient in coma or with any focal neurological signs should have a CT scan performed to exclude an intracranial mass, such as an abscess. A lumbar puncture may be performed to identify the offending organism. A moderate increase in lumbar CSF pressure may be noted. The changes seen in the CSF are outlined in Table 9.5.

Other investigations include blood cultures and X-rays to detect the source of infection. In the patient with a cerebral abscess, there may be a rise in the ESR. This may be confirmed by the identification of the organism on CSF analysis or of a lesion, such as an abscess, on CT scanning. Brain biopsy guided by CT scan may be helpful. When an abscess is suspected, the CT scan should be enhanced with contrast medium to highlight small lesions which may otherwise be missed.

Box 9.16 Features of presentation in CNS infections

Bacterial meningitis (abrupt onset)

Infants

Non-specific:

- Drowsiness
- Irritability
- Off feeds
- Distress on handling
- Vomiting or diarrhoea
- Fever

More specific:

- Neck stiffness
- Tense or bulging fontanelle
- Purpuric or petechial rash that does not blanch under pressure

Late:

- High-pitched or moaning cry
- Coma
- Neck retraction
- Shock
- Widespread haemorrhagic rash

Older children and adults

Non-specific:

- Vomiting
- Fever
- Back or joint pains
- Headache

More specific:

- Neck stiffness
- Photophobia
- Confusion
- Purpuric or petechial rash that does not blanch under pressure

Late:

- Coma
- Neck retraction (in severe cases this, in combination with spasm, causing the heels to bend backwards, produces opisthotonos)
- Shock
- Widespread haemorrhagic rash

Viral encephalitis (insidious onset)

- Headache and fever are both present
- Consciousness level deteriorates gradually. Confusion is common
- Moderate neck stiffness
- Seizures can occur
- ICP may be elevated as a result of cerebral oedema
- Cranial nerve deficits and focal neurological signs may be present.

Cerebral abscess (insidious onset, 2–3 weeks or more)

- Headache is recurrent and fever is usually present
- Patient becomes confused and drowsy
- Neck stiffness is indicative of circulating CSF infection
- Partial or generalised seizures occur in 30% of patients
- ICP is elevated as abscess expands
- Cranial nerve deficits occur and focal neurological signs include speech disorders, motor and sensory deficits and ataxia

Table 9.5 Changes in cerebrospinal fluid which is infected

CSF	*Acute bacterial meningitis*	*Viral encephalitis*
Appearance	Yellow	Clear
Cells	Polymorphs 1000–2000 per cubic mm or more	Mononuclear 50–1500 per cubic mm
Protein	Increased 1.0–5.0 g/L	Mildly elevated
Chloride	110–115 mmol/L	Normal
Glucose	Much reduced or absent	Normal
Organisms	Present on culture	Absent on culture. Require specialist virological testing to identify.
Pressure	Increased	Increased.

Treatment. The patient with bacterial meningitis or a cerebral abscess requires to commence antibiotics as soon as possible. Penicillin is the antibiotic of choice and is usually given intravenously in high doses, such as penicillin 24 million units over 24 h, but it should be remembered that a significant proportion of the population is allergic to this drug and so other antibiotics may be used. Surgery will be performed if the presence of a cerebral abscess is confirmed and adequate explanations should be given to the patient and his family of what is involved in this course of treatment (see Hickey 1997 for complications). This may involve burr hole aspiration (repeated, if necessary), primary excision of the whole abscess or evacuation of the abscess contents leaving the capsule intact (this avoids damaging the surrounding brain).

When there are signs of high ICP, the patient may be taken to theatre immediately to drain the abscess. This will relieve the ICP and will prevent coning and herniation of cerebral contents (see 'Head injury', p. 359).

The patient may be in a coma or have a focal neurological deficit (see Ch. 28).

NURSING PRIORITIES AND MANAGEMENT: INFECTIONS

Pre- and postoperative care

For those patients who require surgery, the general pre- and post-operative care is as given in Chapter 26. The nurse should observe the patient for signs of the abscess re-collecting: this will present as raised ICP.

Care of the dying patient

The patient's condition may deteriorate rapidly after admission, if medication and surgery have not treated the cause of the infection successfully. In these circumstances, all of the patient's needs should be attended to. Adequate pain relief should be given and the patient should be comforted (see Ch. 28).

The patient's family will also require explanations, support and comfort (see Ch. 33).

Immediate priorities

Neurological status and vital signs

Because the patient with an intracranial infection may have a decreased conscious level and because this may deteriorate rapidly, observations should be recorded, reporting any change in condition immediately. Vital signs are very important as the patient may be pyrexial, and as the infection continues, the patient's temperature can increase further. Pulse, blood pressure and respirations may be high when recorded, owing to infection: any changes in these observations should be reported. There may be signs of raised ICP (see p. 363).

Breathing

The patient's respiratory pattern should be observed for rate, depth and frequency, as a change may indicate a rising ICP. Any respiratory distress should be reported immediately. Oxygen may already have been prescribed and the nurse should encourage the patient to tolerate it, giving explanations when necessary. Nursing the patient in a bed with a head-up tilt of 30° will not only help to decrease ICP, but also encourage lung expansion. The nurse should be aware of the risk of a chest infection developing.

Controlling body temperature

In order to reduce pyrexia, the patient's temperature should be recorded frequently and any further rise reported immediately, as this may indicate that the antibiotics are not controlling the infection and that the patient's condition could deteriorate. Each 1°C increase in temperature increases the body's demand for oxygen by 10%, which encourages vasodilatation and increases ICP.

Nursing measures to reduce pyrexia include tepid sponging, use of a fan and the administration of paracetamol, either per rectum or orally. The effects of these measures should be evaluated.

Seizure activity

If seizures are observed, they should be recorded, noting the type of seizure, its duration and exactly what happened (see section on 'Seizures', p. 378). An airway, oxygen and suction should be at hand.

Communication

Communication can be difficult, as the patient may be experiencing severe headache, nausea and vomiting, have photophobia and be disorientated and drowsy. A calm darkened environment will comfort the patient, who will be distressed about his condition and what is happening to him.

Explanations should be given to the patient about what is happening and why, and the patient should be given time to ask questions and express his feelings.

His family will also require reassurance and explanations, but they should be advised not to overstimulate the patient, although touch could be suggested as this can be comforting to the patient.

Maintaining a safe environment

Bed rails should be placed in position to prevent the patient falling out of bed due to restlessness or confusion.

Medication

In order to give the patient adequate relief from pain, analgesics should be administered.

The nurse should ensure that prescribed antibiotics are given, or taken at the correct time by the patient, to ensure maintenance of the drug at a therapeutic level in the bloodstream. An accurate fluid balance chart should be maintained, as the patient can become dehydrated due to pyrexia, nausea and vomiting. Signs of dehydration include dry skin or mouth or a diminishing urinary output and these should be reported. Intravenous fluids will be prescribed until the patient is able to tolerate adequate oral fluids.

Personal cleansing and dressing

Once an assessment of the patient's needs has been carried out, he should be assisted with personal cleansing and dressing. If the patient has a decreased conscious level, care should be exercised in meeting his needs and, as his condition improves, independence should be encouraged.

Mobility

The patient should be as mobile as his condition allows. Initially, bed rest may be necessary and all care should be taken to ensure that his position is changed 2-hourly. Examination of the skin should be carried out at frequent intervals in order to detect signs of pressure, such as redness.

Preparation for discharge home

If the source of the infection has been identified, it will be treated or, if necessary, further investigations carried out. If it has been treated successfully, e.g. in sinusitis or an ear infection, the patient should be informed that he should contact his GP if there is a recurrence of the infection. The need to continue medication on discharge should be fully explained, with emphasis on the importance of completion of the course of antibiotics.

Further investigations may be required to ensure proper healing, if the reason for the introduction of the infection was an injury, such as a skull or facial fracture.

The patient will have been assessed by the ward team while rehabilitating in the ward. Maintenance of optimum function of the patient is a priority, both physically and mentally, and outpatient appointments may be required, e.g. for physiotherapy. The patient's family should be involved in the patient's rehabilitation programme and planned discharge home. Advice and encouragement for this should be given by the ward team. Advice should also be given on employment, driving and other activities, especially if the patient has experienced seizures (see p. 380).

Coping after meningitis

The Meningitis Trust offer a comprehensive support system for those affected by meningitis. This includes a 24 h support and information line, home and hospital emotional support visits, provision of financial support, grant funding and a rehabilitation advisory service. The Trust emphasises that complete recovery takes time and they provide guidance on how to deal with a range of minor after-effects, e.g. general tiredness, headaches and difficulty in concentration.

REFERENCES

Abudi S, Bar Tal Y, Ziv L, Fish M 1997 Parkinson's disease symptoms – patient's perceptions. Journal of Advanced Nursing 25(1): 54–59

Acorn S 1995 Assisting families of head injured survivors through a family support programme. Journal of Advanced Nursing 21(5): 872–877

Allan D 1988 Nursing and the neurosciences. Churchill Livingstone, Edinburgh

Amato C A 1991 Malignant glioma: coping with a devastating illness. Journal of Neuroscience Nursing 23(1): 20–23

Armstrong S L 1994 Cerebral vasospasm: early detection and intervention. Critical Care Nursing 14(4): 33–37

Armstrong T S, Gilbert M R 1996 Glial neoplasms: classification, treatment, and pathways for the future. Oncology Nursing Forum 23(4): 615–625

Benbadis S R, Stagno S J, Kosalko J, Friedman A L 1994 Psychogenic seizures: a guide for patients and families. Journal of Neuroscience Nursing 26(5): 306–308

Benner P 1984 From novice to expert: excellence and power in nursing practice. Addison Wesley, London

Blank-Reid C 1996 How to have a stroke at an early age: the effects of crack, cocaine and other illicit drugs. Journal of Neuroscience Nursing 28(1): 19–27

Cartwright K A V, Stuart S M, Noah N D 1986 An outbreak of meningococcal diseases in Gloucestershire. Lancet 2: 558–561

Christensen J M, Cook E A, Martin B C 1997 Identifying denial in stroke patients. Clinical Nursing Research 6(1): 105–118

Coleman R, Sifri-Steele C 1994 Treatment of posterior circulation aneurysms using platinum coils. Journal of Neuroscience Nursing 26(6): 367–370

Disabled Living Foundation/Parkinson's Disease Society 1992 Resource paper. Advice notes for people with Parkinson's disease. Disabled Living Foundation, London

Gilbert M, Counsell C M, Snively C 1996 Pallidotomy: a surgical intervention for the control of Parkinson's disease. Journal of Neuroscience Nursing 28(4): 215–216

Grant A M, Grinspun D R 1994 The road home from traumatic brain injury. Canadian Nurse 90(4): 22–27

Gumnit R J 1995 The epilepsy handbook: the practical management of seizures, 2nd edn. Raven Press, New York

Health Education Board for Scotland (HEBS) 1994 That's the limit. HEBS, Edinburgh

Hemingway S 1995 Rehabilitation of people with traumatic head injury. Mental Health Nursing 15(3): 9–11

Hickey J V 1997 The clinical practice of neurological and neurosurgical nursing, 4th edn. Lippincott, Philadelphia

Hodges K, Root L 1991 Surgical management of intractable seizures. Journal of Neuroscience Nursing 23(2): 93–100

Hopkins A 1992 Reducing the risk of a stroke. Copyright Stroke Series Leaflet S3. The Stroke Association, London

Jackson S 1995 Not so minor head injuries? Emergency Nurse 3(1): 19–22

Jamieson E M, McCall J M, Blythe R, Whyte L A 1997 Guidelines for clinical nursing practice, 3rd edn. Churchill Livingstone, Edinburgh

Jones B 1994 The effects of patient repositioning on intracranial pressure. Australian Journal of Advanced Nursing 12(2): 32–39

Juarez V J, Lyons M 1995 Interrater reliability of the Glasgow Coma Scale. Journal of Neuroscience Nursing 27(5): 283–286

Lannon S L 1993 Epilepsy in the elderly. Journal of Neuroscience Nursing 25(5): 273–285

Lannon S L 1992 Meeting the needs of children whose parents have epilepsy. Journal of Neuroscience Nursing 24(1): 14–18

Lee A 1993 Peer pressure in cycle helmet use. Paediatric Nursing 5(4): 12–15

Leith-Kelley C 1996 The role of interferons in the treatment of multiple sclerosis. Journal of Neuroscience Nursing 28(2): 114–120

Lieberman A N, Williams F 1995 Parkinson's disease – the complete guide for patients and carers. Thorsons, London

Lindsay K, Bone I 1997 Neurology and neurosurgery illustrated, 3rd edn. Churchill Livingstone, Edinburgh

McGuire R 1997 Parkinson's disease. Professional Nurse 13(1): 33–37

Mulley G 1990 Stroke: a handbook for the patient's family. CHSA Stroke Series, Booklet S7. The Stroke Association, London

Oxtoby M, Williams A 1995 Parkinson's at your fingertips. Class, London

Robinson M J (ed) 1994 Practical paediatrics, 3rd edn. Churchill Livingstone, Edinburgh

Roper N, Logan W, Tierney A J 1996 The elements of nursing: a model of nursing, based on a model of living, 4th edn. Churchill Livingstone, Edinburgh

Rowley G, Fielding K 1991 Reliability and accuracy of the Glasgow Coma Scale with experienced and inexperienced users. Lancet 337(8740): 535–538

Rusy K L 1991 Temporal lobectomy: a promising alternative. Journal of Neuroscience Nursing 23(5): 320–324

Rusy K L 1996 Rebleeding and vasospasm following subarachnoid haemorrhage: a critical care challenge. Critical Care Nursing 16(1): 41–50

Sadler C 1996 Giving support. Community Nurse 2(4): 12

The Stroke Association 1992 Stroke: questions and the answers. Copyright Stroke Series Leaflet S1. The Stroke Association, London

Stubbs C 1992 Facing up to MS. Nursing Times 88(8): 34–36

Swank R L, Dugan B B 1990 Effect of low saturated fat diet in early and late cases of multiple sclerosis. Lancet 336(8706): 37–39

Treadwell L, Mendelow D 1994 Audit of head injury management in the northern region. British Journal of Nursing 3(3): 136–140

Wilson K J W, Waugh A 1996 Ross and Wilson's anatomy and physiology in health and illness, 8th edn. Churchill Livingstone, Edinburgh

FURTHER READING

Aldenkamp A P, Suurmeijer T P, Bijvoet M E, Heisen T W 1990 Emotional and social reactions of children to epilepsy in a parent. Family Practice 7(2): 110–115

Barch C, Spilker J, Bratina P et al 1997 Nursing management of acute complications following rt-PA in acute ischemic stroke. Journal of Neuroscience Nursing 29(6): 367–372

Barker E 1994 Neuroscience nursing. Mosby, St Louis

Barron M 1992 Life after stroke. Nursing Times 88(10): 32–34

Benz C 1993 Coping with multiple sclerosis. Optima, London

Braimach J, Kongable G, Rapp K et al 1997 Nursing care of acute stroke patients after receiving rt-PA therapy. Journal of Neuroscience Nursing 29(6): 373–383

Bratina P, Rapp K, Barch C et al 1997 Pathophysiology and mechanisms of acute ischaemic stroke. Journal of Neuroscience Nursing 29(6): 356–360

Byers V L 1993 Novel antiepileptic drugs: nursing implications. Journal of Neuroscience Nursing 25(6): 375–379

Campion K 1996 Meeting multiple needs – multiple sclerosis. Nursing Times 92(24): 28–30

Chadwick D, Usiskin S 1991 Living with epilepsy. Macdonald Optima, London

Coyne P, Mares P 1995 Caring for someone who has had a stroke. Age Concern, London

Davies M, Lucatorto M 1994 Mannitol revisited. Journal of Neuroscience Nursing 26(3): 170–174

Dewis M E, Niskala H 1992 Nurturing a valuable resource: family caregivers in multiple sclerosis. Axon 13(3): 87–94

Donnarumma R, Kongable G, Barch C et al 1997 Overview: hyperacute rt-PA stroke treatment. Journal of Neuroscience Nursing 29(6): 351–355

Gibbon B 1991 Measuring stroke recovery. Nursing Times 87(44): 32–34
Greenwood R, Chew S, Powell J 1996 Stroke in younger adults. The Stroke Association, London
Handler B S, Patterson J B 1995 Driving after brain injury. Journal of Rehabilitation 61(2): 43–49
Hartshorn J C, Byers V L 1992 Impact of epilepsy on quality of life. Journal of Neuroscience Nursing 24(1): 24–29
Hickey J V 1997 The clinical practice of neurological and neurosurgical nursing, 4th edn. Lippincott, Philadelphia
Hinchliff S, Montague S E, Watson R 1996 Physiology for nursing practice, 2nd edn. Baillière Tindall, London
Holloway N 1993 Medical surgical care plans. Springhouse, Pennsylvania
Isaacs B 1992 Understanding stroke illness. Copyright Booklet S5. The Stroke Association, London
Jacoby A 1992 Epilepsy and the quality of everyday life: findings from a study of people with well-controlled epilepsy. Social Science and Medicine 34(6): 657–666
Kaplan P W, Loiseau P, Fisher R S, Jallon P 1995 Epilepsy A–Z. A glossary of epilepsy terminology. Demos Vermande, New York
Kelly M 1995 Emergency! Status epilepticus. American Journal of Nursing 95(8): 50
Laidler P 1994 Stroke rehabilitation. Chapman & Hall, London
Lechtenberg R 1995 Multiple sclerosis fact book, 2nd edn. Davis, Philadelphia
Long L, McAuley J W 1996 Epilepsy: a review of seizure types, aetiologies, diagnosis, treatment and nursing implications. Critical Care Nursing 16(4): 83–92
Oxtoby M, Williams A 1995 Parkinson's at your fingertips. Glass, London
Rapp K, Bratina P, Barch C et al 1997 Code stroke: rapid transport, triage and treatment using rt-PA therapy. Journal of Neuroscience Nursing 29(6): 361–366
Rising C J 1993 The relationship of selected nursing activities to ICP. Journal of Neuroscience Nursing 25(2): 302–308
Rose F D, Johnson D A 1996 Brain injury and after. Wiley, London
Rutishauser S 1994 Physiology & anatomy. Churchill Livingstone, Edinburgh
Specht D M 1995 Cerebral oedema. Nursing 25(11): 34–38, 45–46
Swaffield L 1996 Stroke: the complete guide to recovery and rehabilitation. Thorsons, London
Tortora G J, Grabowski S R 1996 Principles of anatomy and physiology, 8th edn. Harper Collins, London
Weber C E 1995 Stroke: brain attack, time to react. Advanced Practice in Acute and Clinical Care 6(4): 562–575
Whitney Jess L 1987 Assessing your patient for increased ICP. Nursing 87 17(6): 34–41

USEFUL ADDRESSES

Headway
7 King Edward Court
King Edward Street
Nottingham NG1 1EW

British Epilepsy Association
Anstey House
40 Hanover Square
Leeds LS3 1BE

The Stroke Association
CHSA House
123/127 Whitecross Street
London EC1Y 8JJ

The Multiple Sclerosis (MS) Society of Great Britain
25 Effie Road
Fulham
London SW6 1EE

The National Meningitis Trust
Fern House
Bath Road
Stroud GL5 3TJ

Parkinson's Disease Society
22 Upper Woburn Place
London WC1H 0RA

Sexual and Personal Relationships of People with a Disability (SPOD)
286 Camden Road
London N7 0BJ

Relate — National Marriage Guidance Council
Herbert Gray College
Little Church Street
Rugby
Warwickshire CV21 3AP

Disabled Living Foundation
390–384 Harrow Road
London W9 2HU

Action for Dysphasic Adults
Canterbury Adults
Canterbury House
1 Royal Street
London

British Brain and Spine Foundation
Royal College of Surgeons
35–43 Lincoln's Inn Fields
London WC2A 3PN

THE MUSCULOSKELETAL SYSTEM

10

Liz Jamieson   Cath M. McFarlane
Joyce M. Brown

INTRODUCTION

A fully functioning musculoskeletal system is fundamental to optimal health in the normal active human being. Injury or disease involving this system can have a profound effect on an individual's ability to perform the activities of daily living and can result in either temporary or permanent disability, one of the main problems usually being in the degree of decreased mobility. The overall aim of nursing care is to prevent further injury, reduce the risk of complications, promote healing, maximise independence within individual constraints of the existing condition and promote optimal rehabilitation.

This chapter will describe some of the more common disorders of the musculoskeletal system that are caused by either trauma or disease and will outline relevant principles of nursing management.

Epidemiology

The main causes of musculoskeletal trauma or disease in the UK mirror cultural influences, changing patterns of social activity and the prevailing climatic conditions. They include road traffic accidents (RTAs), industrial and other work-related accidents, sporting accidents and damage due to underlying disease.

Road traffic accidents

In 1996, 3598 people died following road traffic accidents in the UK, the lowest recorded level of deaths in the last 10 years (Office for National Statistics 1998). The incidence of RTAs reached an all time high in 1990, at a rate of 341 141, and although there was a reduction (30 000) in 1991, the figures have started to rise again, with the 1996 figures standing at 320 302 (Office for National Statistics 1998), which may be due to the increasing number of motor vehicles on the roads (Office for National Statistics 1997). RTAs account for a significant proportion of the workload in A&E departments throughout the country, the main contributing factor being drivers whose blood alcohol level is above the legal limit. It should be emphasised that it is often the immediate treatment of injury or suspected fracture that determines the ultimate outcome of an RTA; this applies particularly to injuries of the spinal column and fractures of major long bones.

Work-related injuries

The construction, agriculture, forestry and fishing industries have the highest proportion of injuries which are sustained at work (Health and Safety Commission 1995). This is occurring in spite of government legislation such as the Health and Safety at Work Act 1974, Manual Handling of Loads 1992 and the Control of Substances Hazardous to Health Act 1989.

Back pain is common in all industrialised societies and is now one of the most rapidly increasing causes of work days lost, demand for health care and need for state benefit (Clinical Standards Advisory Group 1995).

Occupational health nurses have an increasingly important role to play in the education of workers and employers regarding accident prevention. Most nursing roles, in fact, offer the opportunity to raise public awareness of risks and preventive measures available.

Sporting injuries

With increased leisure time and facilities and the many health campaigns promoting the benefits of exercise, more time is being spent in sporting activities, with a resultant increase in sporting injuries. In many cases these are minor, but they can also be serious and result in permanent disability: diving into shallow water can cause serious injury to the cervical spine; knee and lower limb injuries are common in football and skiing; and shoulder and upper limb injuries often result from horse riding accidents.

There is increasing emphasis in sports medicine on the importance of initial correct treatment and thorough rehabilitation. This often involves major physiotherapy input and can significantly affect the degree of residual musculoskeletal damage (McLatchie et al 1995).

Damage due to underlying disease

Relatively minor trauma may also serve to highlight a previously undiagnosed underlying disease process. For example, osteoporosis in a postmenopausal woman may only be diagnosed when she presents with a fractured wrist or neck of femur. Osteoporosis is loss of bone mass leading to increased porosity and brittleness and is due to an imbalance between calcium reabsorption and bone formation (Dandy 1993). Its presence may also indicate endocrine disturbances or inadequate exercise.

Rheumatoid arthritis is a chronic or subacute disease of the musculoskeletal joints and is one of the most common rheumatic diseases in the UK. It usually affects more than one joint (polyarthritic) and can be extremely disabling. It is estimated that 1.5% of the population will develop rheumatoid arthritis, with the sex ratio (F:M) being 3:1 (Adams & Hamblen 1995).

Osteoarthritis (degenerative arthritis) is mainly due to wear and tear on the articular cartilage of the larger weight-bearing joints and to the degenerative changes associated with the ageing process. When it is associated with old injury or strenuous sport or work, it can affect any age group and both sexes, but it has a higher incidence in women over 55 years old. Prevalence increases with age until the condition is almost universal, in varying degrees, in people aged over 75 years (Walsh 1997).

The contribution of the science of bioengineering

Musculoskeletal conditions involve, or are caused by, disruption of the mechanics of the human body. Through research, bioengineers are making vital contributions to the understanding of these mechanics and, with the availability of more biologically compatible materials, are able to design a wider and more refined range of replacement joints and limbs. Joint replacement surgery is now a common procedure and has revolutionised the quality of life for thousands of post-injured or elderly people.

ANATOMY AND PHYSIOLOGY OF THE MUSCULOSKELETAL SYSTEM

This section gives a brief overview of the anatomy and physiology of the musculoskeletal system. For detailed information, refer to anatomy and physiology textbooks and become familiar with the model skeleton in your classroom.

For further information, see Marieb (1998).

For ease of reference, the skeletal system and the muscular system will be outlined separately.

The skeletal system

The skeleton is a supportive framework of bones bound together by ligaments. It can be divided into an axial part (the bones of the head and trunk, excluding the pectoral and pelvic girdles) and an appendicular part (the bones of the limbs, including the bones of pectoral and pelvic girdles). Its main functions are to provide the basis for the mechanics of movement and to protect the internal organs and vital structures.

Bones store the body's supply of calcium and release it to maintain the constant level in body fluids that is necessary for normal nervous and muscular activity, heart action and blood clotting. Red bone marrow also plays an essential role in the manufacture of blood cells.

Structurally, the skeletal system consists of two types of connective tissue: bone and cartilage.

Bone

10.1 Look up the factors involved in the development and growth of healthy bone. Describe them.

Unlike other connective tissue, bone contains large amounts of mineral salts (mainly tricalcium phosphate and calcium carbonate) which, when deposited on the collagen fibres, results in hardening. There are two types of bone tissue: compact and cancellous.

The hard outer layer of a bone is compact bone tissue (cortical bone), while cancellous tissue fills the inside. Cancellous tissue is spongier in appearance and the larger spaces contain the highly vascular red bone marrow and the fatty yellow bone marrow. The thickness of each type of tissue varies, depending on the type and function of the particular bone. In long bones such as the femur, the shaft (diaphysis) is enclosed by a thick layer of cortical tissue which gives strength for weight-bearing, while at each end (epiphyses) the cortical tissue is thinner and encloses a greater mass of cancellous tissue.

Flat bones, such as the sternum and the pelvis, have a thinner layer of cortical tissue and a relatively greater amount of cancellous tissue. This is the reason why they are chosen for bone marrow biopsy.

Tissue renewal. Like the skin, bone tissue is constantly being replaced, but at variable rates in different parts of the body. The cancellous bone at the epiphyses, e.g. in the upper end of the femur, is replaced about every 4 months in an adult, in contrast to the compact bone in the shaft of the femur which will never be completely replaced during a lifetime. This process of growth and repair is dependent on balanced activity between the three types of bone cell: osteoblasts, osteocytes and osteoclasts (see Fig. 10.1).

10.2 Referring to an anatomy and physiology text, define the function of each type of bone cell.

For further information on bone, see Wilson & Waugh (1996), pp. 371–395.

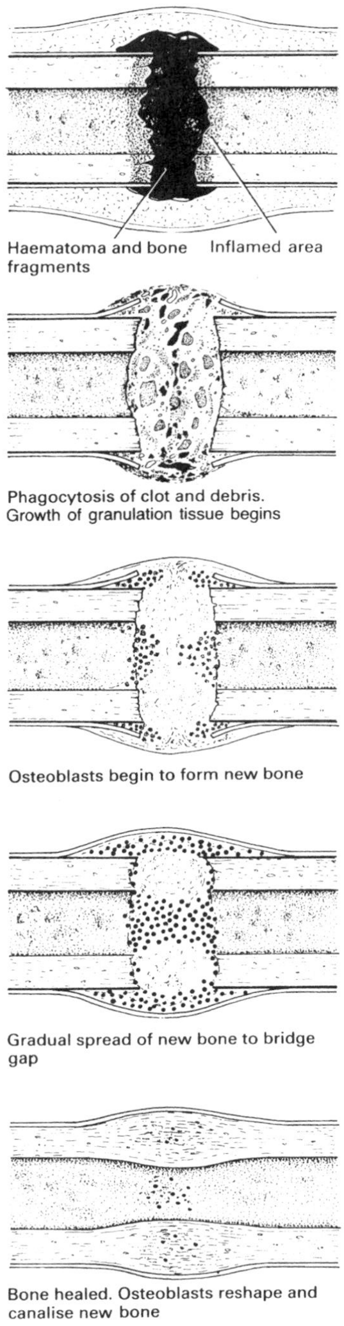

Fig. 10.1 Stages in bone healing. (Reproduced with kind permission from Wilson & Waugh 1996.)

Cartilage

This is a form of connective tissue which is tough, flexible, avascular and devoid of nerve fibres. It forms part of the support mechanism of the body.

There are three types of cartilage:

- hyaline cartilage — firm yet pliable and forms the articular cartilage that covers the articulating surfaces of synovial joints
- fibrocartilage — strong, compressible and tension-resistant and is found in areas such as the intervertebral discs

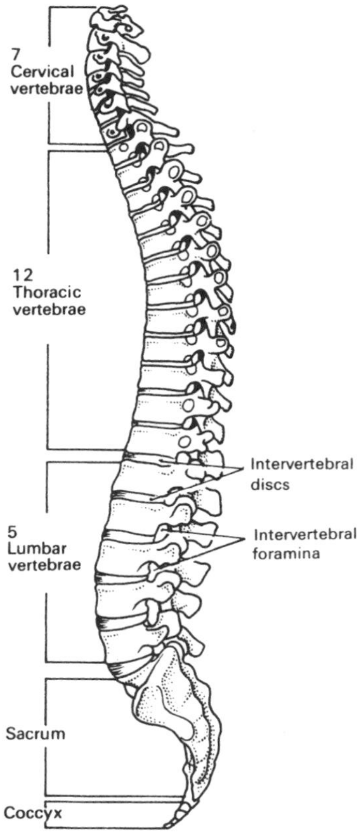

Fig. 10.2 The vertebral column — lateral view. (Reproduced with kind permission from Wilson & Waugh 1996.)

- elastic cartilage — contains more elastin fibres than the others and therefore has a greater ability to stretch whilst retaining its strength; it is found in the external ear and the epiglottis.

The axial skeletal system

The skull and vertebral column form the central axis of the skeletal system. It is a strong, flexible column of 33 bones, 24 of which are 'true' vertebrae — the cervical, thoracic and lumbar — the remainder being fused to form the sacrum and coccyx (see Fig. 10.2). Between each of the vertebrae from C2 to S1 is a strong joint created by the fibrocartilaginous intervertebral discs, which allow flexibility and act as shock absorbers when the spine is exposed to vertical forces.

The spinal column functions to protect the spinal cord, support the skull and act as a point of attachment for the ribs and muscles of the back.

The appendicular skeletal system

The bones of the upper and lower limbs and their girdles are the main parts of the appendicular skeletal system and are characterised by the presence of synovial joints which connect the articular surfaces of adjoining bones (see Fig. 10.3). The bones that make up the joint are held within a fibrous capsule, which consists of two layers.

The outer layer is of dense connective tissue which allows movement but resists dislocation. In some joints the fibres of this connective tissue are arranged parallel to each other and in bundles and

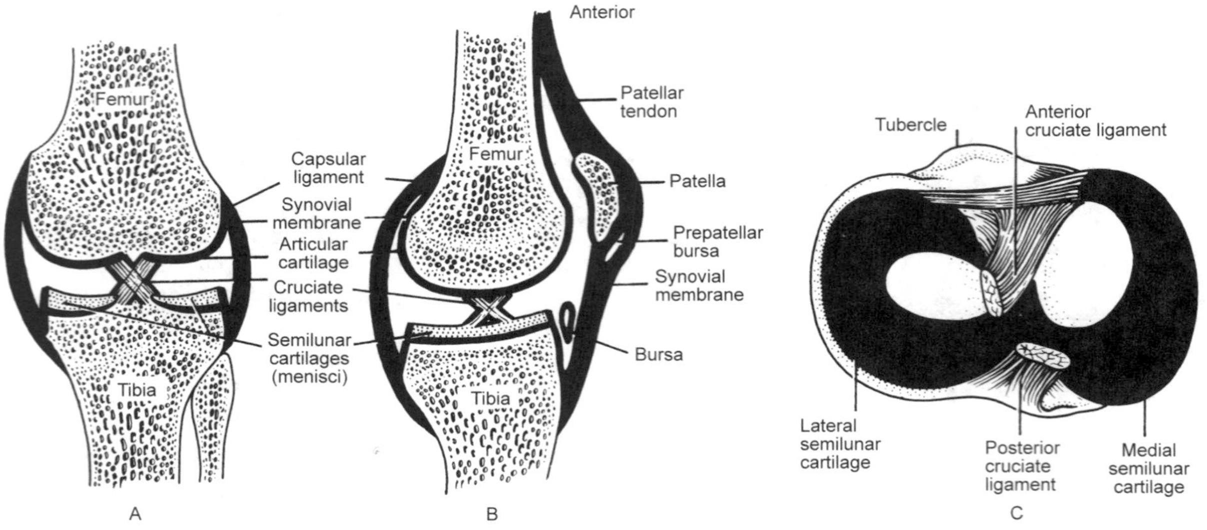

Fig. 10.3 The knee joint. A: Section viewed from front. B: Section viewed from side. C: Superior surface of the tibia showing the semilunar cartilages and cruciate ligament. (Reproduced with kind permission from Wilson & Waugh 1996.)

are known as ligaments. The inner layer of the fibrous capsule is lined with synovial membrane which secretes synovial fluid. This provides nourishment and lubrication. The articular surfaces of the bones involved are covered in hyaline cartilage — articular cartilage. Many synovial joints contain extracapsular and/or intracapsular ligaments which help to increase their stability.

The muscular system

Skeletal muscle tissue is composed of multinucleated muscle cells which are long and cylindrical in appearance. Each muscle is made up of muscle fibres and connective tissue and is attached to periosteum or other muscles by aponeuroses. A good blood and nerve supply is essential for muscle function and the mechanics of movement.

10.3 Find a chart or model of the muscular system. Identify and name the main muscle groups.

Information on the muscular system can be found in Wilson & and Waugh (1996), Ch 17.

Aspects of the musculoskeletal system

There are a number of variables involved in the discussion of musculoskeletal injuries and disease, i.e. skeletal, joint, muscle, skin, neurovascular, and the patient's perception of cause and abnormal sensation and pain. These interacting components, although often present at the same time in varying degrees, will be addressed under the following headings: skeletal disorders, joint disorders and soft tissue disorders.

Assessment

Assessment of the condition and function of the musculoskeletal system is by:

- patient history
- visual inspection
- palpation
- measurement
- radiological and imaging studies (see Box 10.1).

GENERAL PRINCIPLES OF NURSING MANAGEMENT OF MUSCULOSKELETAL DISORDERS

Nursing assessment

This will involve general observation and taking a nursing history. The selected philosophy and model of nursing will influence the focus of care planning. Orem's (1995) model is often suggested as being particularly useful because of the emphasis on promoting self-care, maximising independence and the progression towards the supportive educative role of the nurse.

Observations are made on life-threatening problems, such as the presence of severe bleeding or shock (see Ch. 27), and on:

- abnormal position or appearance of limbs or affected part with loss of function (compare with contralateral side)
- report of, or signs of, pain
- abnormal posture or gait
- use of walking aids or prostheses.

The nursing history includes:

- comprehensive cover of universal health care requisites, concurrent health problems, allergies and medications
- patient's perception of the cause of the primary problem and the impact on activities of living (ALs) (Roper et al 1996), especially relating to impaired mobility
- patient's description of pain and other symptoms
- patient's and her family's expectations, coping strategies, alteration to normal roles and educability.

Problems and strengths (actual and potential) are identified in the following categories:

- life-threatening problems
- shock
- pain
- impaired mobility

Box 10.1 Investigations for musculoskeletal abnormalities

Radiological and imaging studies

- X-ray — to detect abnormal position, fractures, bone density and presence of fluid or abnormalities in joint capsules
- Tomogram — X-ray technique for detail of specific plane (slice) of bone
- Computed tomogram (CT scan) — makes use of the fact that different tissues have varying radiodensities. A series of radiographs are made at different angles and planes and the computer integrates the information to produce pictorial slices (sometimes 3D) which can be used to detect soft tissue injuries or tumours and inflammatory or metastatic skeletal disease or fracture
- Magnetic resonance imaging (MRI) — magnetic fields used to show the difference in hydrogen density of various muscle and soft tissues, indicating the presence of abnormalities
- DEXTA scan — scan for bone densimetry
- Arthrogram — injection of a radio-opaque substance or air into a joint followed by X-ray to identify abnormalities of joint structures
- Myelogram — a contrast medium is injected into the subarachnoid space of the lumbar spine in order to visualise disc herniation or tumours

Joint examination

- Arthroscopy — endoscopic visualisation of structures inside a joint. May also involve withdrawal of synovial fluid for analysis

Muscle and nerve studies

- Electromyography (EMG) — measures electrical potential of muscle during rest and activity
- Nerve conduction velocities (NCVs) — measures speed of nerve impulse conduction

Other tests

- These include bone biopsy, densimetry, total body calcium and various haematological studies for hormone and mineral levels

- potential for further injury — physical safety and neurovascular complications
- psychosocial consequences
- rehabilitation
- patient and family strengths — these should be defined and used constructively.

Nursing interventions

- Treat life-threatening problems — ABC of resuscitation
- Monitor and treat shock
- Relieve pain
- Maintain an appropriate degree of therapeutic splintage and mobility
- Constantly monitor and reduce the risk of neurovascular complications
- Maintain a safe environment
- Coordinate multidisciplinary intervention for psychosocial problems
- Prevent the boredom of greatly reduced mobility
- Facilitate rehabilitation
- Promote patient and family strengths to support adaptation and rehabilitation.

SKELETAL DISORDERS

This section will focus firstly on fractures and their management and then more briefly on tumours and infections of the bone.

FRACTURES

PATHOPHYSIOLOGY

Paton (1992) defines a fracture as loss of normal bone continuity, which can be caused by direct or indirect violence, weakening of the bone due to underlying disease (pathological fracture) or repeated bending stresses on a bone (stress fracture).

Classification of fractures. A simple or closed fracture is one where there is no communication between the external environment and the fracture site. When direct contact between the fracture site and the external environment occurs, it is known as a compound or open fracture.

A fracture may be described as 'stable' when the bone ends are lying in a position from which they are unlikely to move, or as 'unstable' when the bone ends are displaced or have the potential to be displaced.

Common fracture patterns are shown in Figure 10.4 (Dandy 1993).

MEDICAL MANAGEMENT

Priorities of treatment. A fracture is often associated with some degree of general trauma and first aid is very important, as mishandling can add to the severity of the injury. Priorities are established: the ABC of resuscitation is attended to and accompanying shock, which may be severe owing to pain and blood loss, is treated (see Ch. 27).

The irregular edges of broken bones can cause further major injury if they penetrate or sever internal organs, nerves or blood vessels. Immobilisation will also reduce shock and assist in pain management. Immediate immobilisation and maintenance of alignment are imperative until the full extent of the fracture has been established. This is especially important when spinal injury is suspected, as irreparable damage may be done to the spinal cord.

Once the patient's physical condition has been stabilised, specific treatment of the injuries will continue.

Reduction of fractures. Fractures are said to be reduced when displaced bone fragments are pulled into their normal anatomical position. In many cases, a general anaesthetic will be necessary to overcome the protective muscle spasm and severe pain.

Splintage or reduced mobility. It is important, following reduction, that the fracture is held in the correct anatomical position until bony union occurs. Various methods are used, depending on the site and type of the fracture. These include external splintage using plaster of Paris (POP) or synthetic casts, which is the simplest means of immobilisation, skin or skeletal traction, or an external fixator frame. Operative reduction with internal fixation by metal pins, plates, screws and nails may also be used to hold the bony fragments in position. When the supply of nutrients is grossly affected, it may be necessary to implant prostheses to replace the affected bone, e.g. in some cases of fractured neck of femur.

Maintenance and restoration of function. When one part of a limb is immobilised, there is a tendency for related joints and muscles to become stiff and weak; for example, during splintage of a wrist fracture, the finger and shoulder joints can be affected. Appropriate physiotherapy is essential.

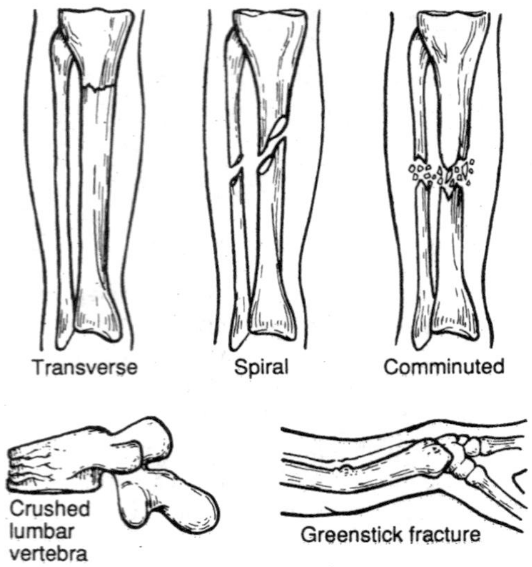

Fig. 10.4 Patterns of fracture. (Reproduced with kind permission from Dandy 1993.)

Rehabilitation. Patients require varying degrees of rehabilitation, which involves a multidisciplinary team approach (see Ch. 34).

Traction

Traction is force applied in a specific direction by a variety of systems in order to maintain anatomical alignment and overcome the natural pull of muscles (Footner 1992). It is used in the following circumstances:

- to reduce and immobilise fractures/dislocations and maintain normal alignment of all injured tissues
- to prevent and correct deformity
- to reduce muscle spasm
- to relieve pain
- to immobilise an injured or inflamed joint
- to keep joint surfaces apart.

Types of traction

Balanced or sliding traction. This uses weights and pulleys as mobile counterbalancing forces, and skeletal pins and external slings as suspensory devices. For example, in order to achieve the degree of traction needed to maintain reduction of a fractured femur, a Steinmann or Denham pin is inserted through the upper end of the tibia to provide a firm point of attachment for the stirrup, ropes and pulley and the required weight (see Fig. 10.5). The extremity may be suspended within the apparatus and a fairly constant line of pull maintained even when the patient changes position. Together with an overhead trapeze, this allows greater freedom of movement. The patient in balanced or sliding traction may lift herself up and move up and down the bed (see Fig. 10.6).

Fixed traction. This is traction between two points with the pull exerted in one plane. Skin or skeletal traction may be used (Fig. 10.7). Methods used to establish skin traction are outlined in Box 10.2.

For further information, see Davis (1994).

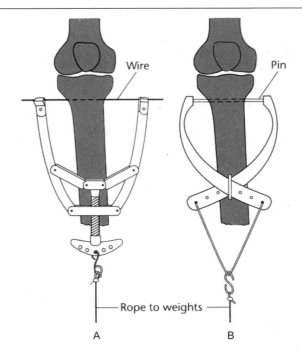

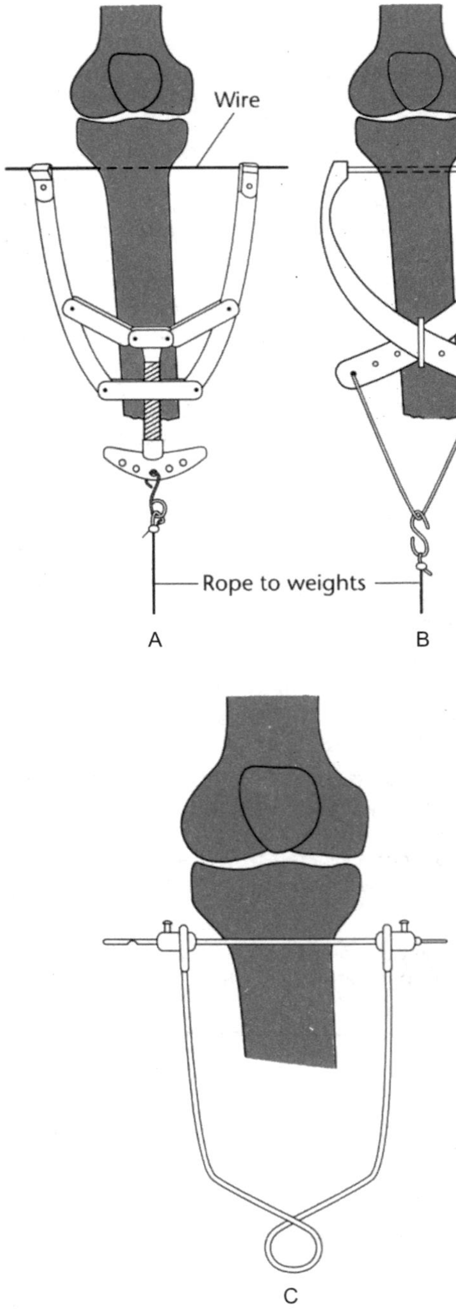

Fig. 10.5 Skeletal traction may be applied by — A: a Kirschner wire and traction stirrup; B: a Steinmann pin and traction stirrup; or C: Steinmann pin and Böhler stirrup. (Reproduced with kind permission from Walsh 1997.)

PRINCIPLES OF NURSING MANAGEMENT: TRACTION

In addition to the general principles outlined earlier for management of musculoskeletal injuries, the following are specific to a patient in traction.

Traction equipment and purpose

The nurse should have a thorough understanding of the type and purpose of the particular traction in use and explain these simply

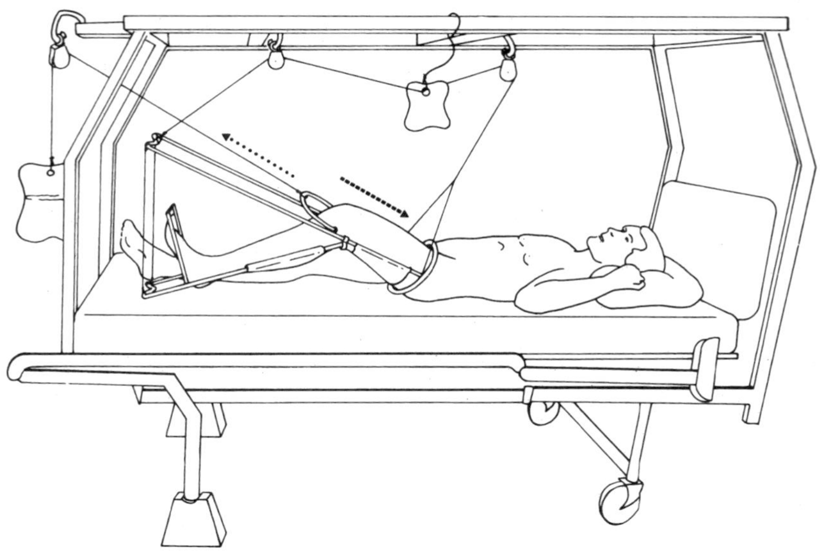

Fig. 10.6 Skeletal traction in balanced suspension in Thomas' splint. Countertraction is achieved by elevating the foot of the bed. (Reproduced with kind permission from Taylor 1990.)

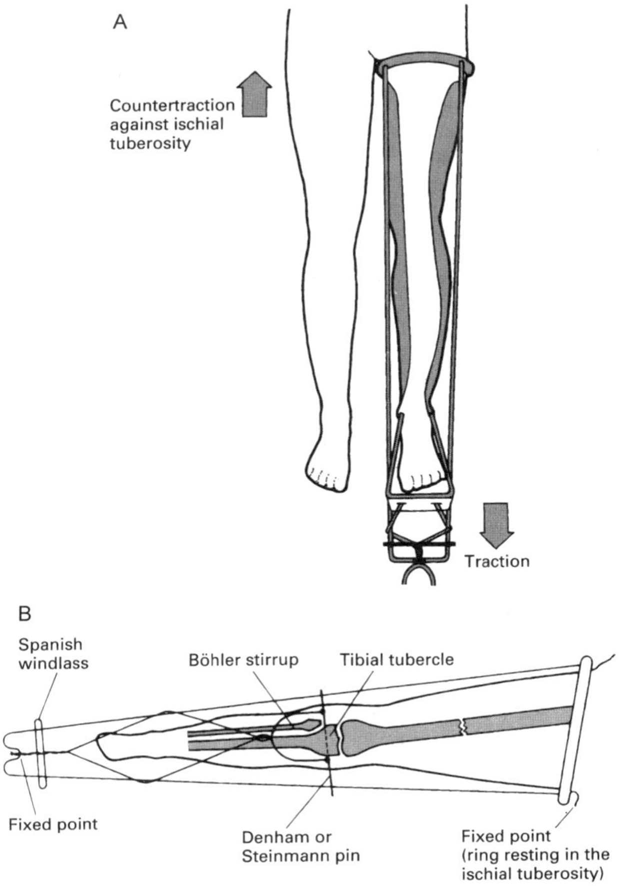

Fig. 10.7 A: Fixed traction using skin traction and Thomas' splint. B: Fixed traction using skeletal pin and Thomas' splint. (Reproduced with kind permission from Walsh 1997.)

Box 10.2 Application of skin traction

Skin traction can be applied using a ready prepared skin traction kit made of either Elastoplast or Venfoam.

Elastoplast kit
First ensure that the patient is not allergic to tincture of benzoin compound by doing a patch test. Then prepare the skin carefully by shaving, drying gently and spraying with tincture of benzoin compound. This protects the skin and gives added adhesion. The Elastoplast strips are then applied directly to the skin on either side of the injured limb with the spreader parallel to, and a few inches away from, the sole of the foot. The Elastoplast is bandaged with crepe bandages to give added strength. Pulleys are attached to the foot of the bed and ropes and weights attached; 15 kg is the maximum that can be applied without causing damage to the skin. The foot of the bed is elevated to provide traction counterbalance.

Venfoam kit
Made of non-adhesive, soft foam padding, this can be applied directly to the skin and held in position with a crepe bandage. It will take approximately 2–3 kg of weight and is often used as a method of pain relief for patients with fractured neck of femur or in paediatric fractures. It must be reapplied twice a day because of loss of bandage pressure.

and clearly to the patient in order to get her active participation in overall treatment, rehabilitation and prevention of complications. All patients in traction should be assessed by the nurse for their moving and handling needs with particular reference to the equipment required. Patients are taught how to lift themselves up using the overhead lifting aid and also which movements are safe. All parts of frames, pulleys, ropes and slings should be inspected at regular intervals every day to ensure that they are correctly positioned and in good working order.

Observation of neurovascular status and prevention of complications

Keen and constant observation of colour, sensation and movement of the injured limb must be carried out throughout the patient's stay in hospital. Her involvement in this is essential and she should be helped and encouraged to describe changes in sensation and levels of pain. Any complaint of discomfort, pain or paraesthesia must be thoroughly investigated (Davis 1994).

External pressure can come from any part of the traction or be caused by restricted movement. Internal pressure may be the result of tissue damage and swelling.

Nursing staff must be alert for:

- Increased risk of pressure sores and skin reactions due to the patient's reduced mobility and/or the traction equipment
- Drop foot caused by excessive pressure on the common peroneal nerve located around the head of the fibula
- Compartment syndrome (CS) — a compartment consists of muscles surrounded by inelastic fascial tissue. CS occurs when there is increased tissue pressure resulting in inadequate tissue perfusion and anoxia within the compartment (Tucker 1998). This results in tissue death and permanent loss of function can occur within 6–8 h.

It is vital to be aware that compartment syndrome is a hazard of the complex nature of musculoskeletal trauma, surgery and immobilisation (Maher et al 1994) that can occur even when a pulse is present and there is capillary refill (see Box 10.3).

Box 10.3 Impending compartment syndrome — dialogue between student (S) and mentor (M)

S You've explained what compartment syndrome is but how do I know that it is actually happening, especially when I can still feel a pulse and the capillary refill appears to be normal?

M Well, the first thing to keep in mind is that there is always a possibility of it happening where there is fairly extensive musculoskeletal trauma and constricting devices or traction are in use. Also don't depend solely on observation of capillary refill and pulse — they can give a false sense of security. Obviously, degree of swelling, colour, pulse and capillary refill are very important and you may be able to feel a tight and tense muscle mass on palpation — but what the patient feels and can describe to you will be the deciding factor.

S I've noticed that you spend a lot of time talking to the patients about how things feel and really pursuing their answers — but what are the critical clues that you're looking for?

M I get red alerts when they describe deep throbbing pain inappropriate to the injury and a persistent sensation of pressure or pain on stretch, or if they complain of abnormal sensations such as numbness, tingling, loss of sensation, increased sensitivity or weakness.

S How can we prevent compartment syndrome?

M Attention to all the basic principles of treatment such as correct tissue alignment, splinting the affected part but encouraging normal movement of other parts, elevations, keen and constant observation of neurovascular status, assessment of major nerve function such as in the peroneal, ulnar and median nerves, prompt action to relieve constriction from bandages, slings and plaster casts, educating the patient to detect adverse signs and symptoms and possibly anticipating fasciectomy, i.e. surgically opening the skin and fascia to allow the tissues to expand and relieve pressure.

S What action should we take if we suspect impending compartment syndrome?

M Report signs and symptoms immediately to a member of the surgical team and take any necessary nursing action, such as reassuring the patient, elevating and supporting the affected part, checking and possibly reapplying the traction, relieving the constriction and continuing to monitor changes. It is possible to measure tissue pressure with a direct needle measurement device — and anything above 30 mmHg needs action.

Prevention of infection at skeletal pin sites

- The pin should be immobile in the bone and the insertion sites kept clean and free from infection. They may be dressed initially with sterile dressings around the pin and left open when dry.
- The pin ends are cleansed as prescribed by local policy. This may, for example, be done regularly, using sterile applicators and a prescribed agent, and keeping the pin ends dry. The sharp ends of pins should be covered with pin guards.
- The site is inspected regularly for signs of localised infection such as heat, redness or oozing. Be alert for pyrexia.

Maintaining normal body system functions

Traction with its accompanying degree of restriction on movement and positioning can create special problems and the following interventions are important:

- Assessment and planning of care together with a physiotherapist, to coordinate and encourage breathing exercises, active and passive exercises to maintain joint mobility and prevent muscle wasting and deep vein thrombosis (DVT). In particular, encourage regular dorsiflexion to counteract foot drop. Local policy may determine the prophylactic measures to be implemented with the aim of preventing the complication of DVT.
- Ensure adequate fluid intake (2 L or more daily) and a balanced diet with plenty of fibre.
- Assessment and planning of care to prevent constipation; treat if present.
- Awkwardness in using bedpans and urinals and fear of soiling the bed should be dealt with sympathetically. Initially, adequate protective covering for the bed and appliances, such as the leather ring of the Thomas splint, will help to allay this anxiety.
- Normal sleep position and pattern will be disturbed and every attempt should be made to make the patient comfortable and relaxed before resorting to the use of regular hypnotic medication.
- Often patients are in traction for a long time and will feel the need for close physical contact with their partners. Ensure undisturbed privacy for them.
- Boredom is a hazard of lengthy hospitalisation, particularly when movement is restricted.
- An issue that occurs more frequently on orthopaedic wards than others, because the patients are often young men and women, is that a strong attraction may develop between a patient and a nurse. This will require sensitive discussion between the staff member and the ward manager to seek an agreed resolution. The *Code of Professional Conduct* (UKCC 1992a) outlines the appropriate action to be taken by registered practitioners when this type of situation arises. If the nurse is transferred to another ward, the relationship can continue normally.

10.4 Discuss ways in which you can help relieve the boredom of a patient who is in traction. Which other health professionals could you call upon to help in this respect?

10.5 Ask the physiotherapist in your clinical area to show you how to measure a patient for crutches and how to use them. Try walking with crutches yourself.

10.6 How many different kinds of walking aids can you identify in your clinical area? Discuss each with the physiotherapist.

Casts

A cast is a splinting device consisting of layers of bandages impregnated with plaster of Paris (POP), fibreglass or resin, some of which are applied wet and solidify as they dry out. Their main uses are to immobilise and hold bone fragments in reduction and to support and stabilise weak joints.

There are different methods of application, and the manufacturer's instructions should be followed. The advantages and disadvantages of the main categories of casting types are summarised below.

Plaster of Paris. POP takes 48 h to become completely dry, and therefore no weight can be placed on the cast during this period. It requires several layers to ensure adequate strength and, as such, can become very heavy. POP is most commonly used for patients who have just received their injuries, as it is relatively easy to mould into the shape of the limb and will, if well padded, allow for a certain amount of swelling before interfering with circulation and sensation. It is relatively inexpensive.

Synthetic casts. These casts set within 20 min and allow early weight-bearing. They are stronger than POP due to the fibreglass content; thus, fewer layers are required and they are lighter. As they do not allow for swelling, this material is frequently not used as the initial method of cast immobilisation following trauma, but if used, regular assessment of the neurovascular status of the limb should be implemented. Synthetic casts are ideal for use in the older patient, because they are lightweight and allow early mobilisation. A disadvantage is that they are more expensive than POP.

Cast bracing

All fractures of a long bone of the upper or lower limb can be immobilised in a cast brace to permit early mobilisation. In some centres, a patient with a fracture of the shaft of femur may have a cast brace applied within days of the initial injury.

The top cast is applied snugly to the femur and moulded carefully to the shape of the limb (Morgan 1989). Minimal padding is used — usually stockinette and a cast sock. The ischium will take the weight load. A cast is also applied to the lower part of the leg and may include the foot. The casts are joined by a set of hinges which can be left free or locked at the knee in various degrees of flexion (Dandy 1993). The patient is encouraged to be mobile and usually fully weight-bearing, initially with the help of a walking aid.

Advantages of using a cast brace include early mobilisation and discharge home, and immobilisation of the fracture site with free movement of the joints above and below.

PRINCIPLES OF NURSING MANAGEMENT: CASTS

In addition to the general principles of nursing management for musculoskeletal disorders (p. 396), the following will also apply.

Potential for neurovascular problems

Although padding such as 'Velband' will allow for some swelling within the restricting cast, tissue pressure may build up and result in pain, tingling and discoloration. Unexplained pain is an important indicator that something is wrong, and therefore careful assessment and investigation of the cause while alleviating the patient's discomfort are essential. If not attended to immediately, pressure could lead to tissue necrosis and nerve palsy, the signs and symptoms of which include severe pain, odour and discoloration on the cast.

Always be alert for signs of thromboembolic complications in patients with trauma and reduced mobility.

Prevention of neurovascular complications

- Elevate the limb above the level of the heart on cloth-covered pillows.
- Avoid denting a moist cast by handling it only with the palms of the hands and not allowing it to rest on a flat, hard or sharp surface.
- Ensure that physiotherapy is carried out regularly.
- If signs and symptoms of neurovascular compromise do occur, have plaster cutting equipment ready and bivalve the cast — i.e. split it down both sides into two halves. Spread it enough to relieve pressure and remember to cut the padding, which may have shrunk due to drying blood and exudates.
- An inspection and treatment window can be cut if pressure sore symptoms occur. The window must be replaced so that swelling does not rise into the space and cause more problems.
- Use of an appropriate bed aid, such as a bed cage, to allow adequate air circulation which aids in the drying process.

Care of the cast

Avoid getting the cast wet. Do not cover a leg plaster for any prolonged period with plastic or rubber boots because of condensation; however, synthetic protective covers can be bought to permit the patient to take a shower. Teach the patient how to protect the cast when washing and when using bedpans and urinals. Casts can be cleaned by wiping with a damp cloth.

Many patients will go home wearing casts, so be sure to give them clear verbal and written instructions specific to their cast (e.g. see Box 10.4). Ensure that they can read English or provide a translation.

Removal of a cast

Application of a cast should be carried out only by experienced nurses or other health professionals, but all nurses need to be aware of the procedure for removal of a cast, to be familiar with the equipment used and to know where it is located.

Casts may need to be removed and renewed if they become too loose or are damaged in any way. Where serious signs and symptoms of neurovascular compromise have developed, splitting and removal will be required as an emergency procedure.

Guidelines for removal of a cast are given in Box 10.5.

External fixation

With this kind of fixation, the bone fragments are held in position by skeletal pins inserted into the bone on either side of the fracture and held in alignment by external rods (Dandy 1993).

PRINCIPLES OF NURSING MANAGEMENT: EXTERNAL FIXATION

In addition to the general principles relating to altered neurovascular status, positioning and potential for pin site infection that have

Box 10.4 Advice to patient with hand to elbow plaster

The plaster holds all the broken bones firmly in place to allow them to heal in the correct position. To prevent your fingers swelling, support your arm in the sling provided during the day and on pillows at night. It is important that you exercise the finger, elbow and shoulder joints of your injured arm at regular intervals, otherwise they will become stiff and painful to move.

The following exercises should be carried out at least four times each day:

- make a firm fist then stretch the fingers as wide as possible
- try to touch each fingertip with the thumb of that hand
- bend and stretch the elbow joint
- lift your arm high above your head — use the other arm to help
- move your arm behind your back as if you wanted to scratch between your shoulder blades.

Do not wet, heat or otherwise interfere with the plaster and do not insert sharp objects between the plaster and the skin to scratch — this could cause skin damage and infection.

Report to the doctor or A&E department AT ONCE if:

- the plaster cracks, becomes loose or uncomfortable
- there is pain
- the fingers become numb or difficult to move
- the fingers become more swollen, blue or very pale
- there is discharge
- you have any other problems.

already been stated, the following is specific to external fixation. As this device allows for early discharge of a patient, the nurse must ensure that the patient, carers and community staff are familiar with and confident in the care required (Calcraft 1995).

Appearance

The appearance of the appliance may cause the patient some concern. Full explanation and support in managing it will often help her to gain confidence. Early assisted weight-bearing and mobilisation, together with information about the beneficial effect this has in reducing the potential for complications, will also reinforce a positive attitude.

Internal fixation

Fractures may also be stabilised by surgical intervention where various nails, plates, wires, screws and rods hold the bone fragments in place (Fig. 10.8). Again this permits earlier mobilisation and reduces the potential for complications. All perioperative principles of nursing management apply in this instance (see Ch. 26).

For further information, see Dandy (1993).

FRACTURES OF SPECIFIC SITES

Fracture of the femoral shaft

Femoral shaft fractures are most commonly seen in young men following motorcycle or car accidents.

Box 10.5 Guidelines for removal of a cast

Equipment

- Plaster cutter — a small electric saw with a circular oscillating blade
- Plaster spreader
- Large flat-bladed bandage scissors
- Plaster shears
- Plaster knife

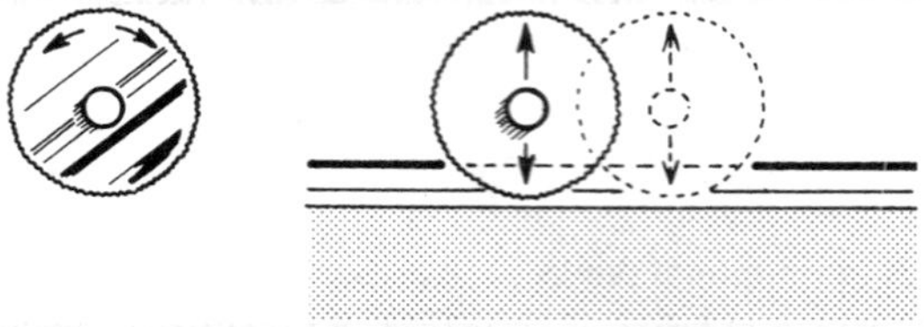

Procedure

- Explain to the patient what the procedure entails and, if the cast is padded, demonstrate the plaster cutter by turning it on and explaining its action (the electric cutter is not used on plasters that are not padded). Shears will be used on unpadded casts. Instruct the patient to shield her eyes as the saw could throw off fragments of plaster. Give reassurance that the saw will not cut the skin because of its oscillating action and the depth of padding.
- Mark where the cutting line will be with a felt pen and dampen it to reduce plaster dust. This line should avoid bony prominences; it is usually in front of the lateral malleolus and behind the medial malleolus in the lower limb, and along the ulnar or flexor surface in the upper limb.
- Grasp the electric cutter.
- Dust extractor apparatus should be used to comply with health and safety regulations.
- Turn on the cutter and push the blade firmly and gently through the cast, at the same time allowing the thumb to contact the cast as the blade oscillates. When you feel a 'give' or lack of resistance, you know you are through.
- Lift the cutter blade up a degree but not out of the groove and repeat until the line of cut is complete. The movement is one of alternating pressure on the oscillating blade and lifting slightly, at right-angles to the plaster within the groove of the cut. It is wise to get the 'feel' of this by practical experience with discarded plasters and then in actual practice under the guidance of an expert.
- Cut the cast down both sides.
- Insert the blades of the plaster spreader at several sites along the line of cut then separate the cast with the hands.
- Cut the padding with the bandage scissors.
- Lift the limb carefully out of the posterior portion of the cast, maintaining the same position.
- After removal of the cast, wash the skin gently with pure soap and water, pat dry and apply skin cream. Expect a scaly appearance, some muscle atrophy, pain and stiffness. Reassure the patient that prescribed exercise will help to regain normal feeling, appearance and function.

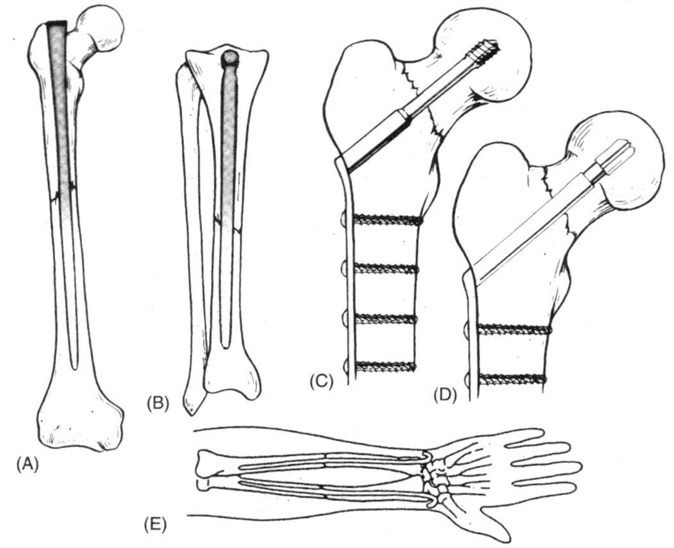

Fig. 10.8 Types of internal fixation. A, B: Intramedullary nails. C: Compression nail for fixation of femoral neck. D: Sliding nail fixation of the femoral neck. E: Rush nails to radius and ulna. (Reproduced with kind permission from Dandy 1989.)

MEDICAL MANAGEMENT

Following X-ray to confirm the diagnosis:

- Operative treatment may consist of either internal fixation (usually the preferred option) as described earlier or, rarely, external fixation.
- The fracture may be reduced under general anaesthetic and skeletal traction applied. Any accompanying wounds are debrided or sutured at the same time. If there is adequate callus formation within 2–6 weeks, a cast brace may be applied.
- Blood samples will be taken for various types of haematological analysis.

NURSING PRIORITIES AND MANAGEMENT: FRACTURE OF THE FEMORAL SHAFT

In addition to the principles of management relating to a fracture, operative intervention and traction, the following are specific to fracture of the shaft of femur.

Haemorrhage. An early complication may be damage to the femoral artery from bone fragments, in addition to bleeding from other damaged tissues and the bone marrow. As much as a litre of blood can be contained within the thigh, and this hidden haemorrhage can result in hypovolaemic shock (see Ch. 18).

Be alert for signs of haemorrhage and shock and ensure that i.v. replacement therapy is ready and that blood is sent for cross-matching.

Fat emboli. Fat emboli are a particular hazard following fracture of the shaft of the femur but can occur following fracture of any long bone (McRae 1994). There are two theories relating to the cause. One is that fat cells from damaged tissue migrate into ruptured veins, and the second is that catecholamines released through the stress of trauma mobilise lipids from fatty tissue. In the lung these droplets are converted into free fatty acids which are toxic to lung tissue and disrupt alveolar function. Additionally, the droplets may become enmeshed in the capillary network of the alveoli and

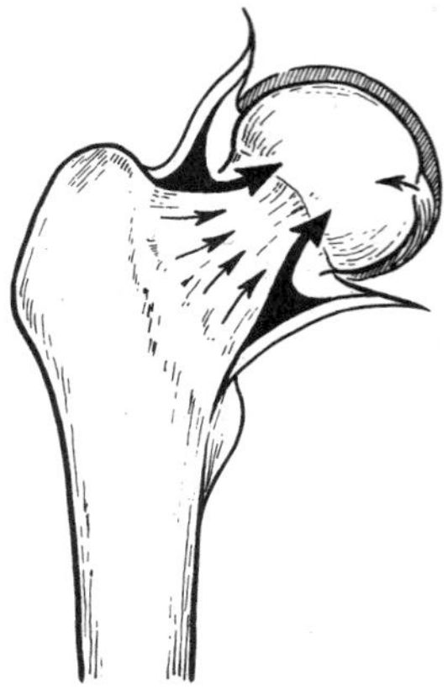

Fig. 10.9 Blood supply of the femoral head via the capsule. Intramedullary vessels and ligamentum teres. (Reproduced with kind permission from Dandy 1993.)

disrupt gas exchange. This can lead to cerebral hypoxia and, if large vessels in the pulmonary system are involved, to respiratory failure and death. Early signs of fatty emboli are increased respiratory rate, anxiety, transient petechial haemorrhage and confusion. The latter two are the classic and most important clinical signs.

Be alert for early signs of altered mental status — anxiety, irritability and especially confusion. Report this immediately and be prepared to deal with respiratory failure and arrest and to transfer the patient to intensive care. Have equipment ready for blood gas analysis.

Collaborative care

The contributions of different health professionals to the care of a patient with fracture of the femoral shaft are summarised in Table 10.1. The nurse has an important role in coordinating the care provided.

Q **10.7** Complete Table 10.1, giving the rationale for your interventions. Say how you would evaluate them. You may refer to the text.

Fracture of neck of femur

The Audit Commission (1995) has estimated that 60 000 people anually will sustain a fracture of the neck of the femur (hip fracture), the majority of whom will be women. It may be associated with a fall and/or the presence of bone disease or thinning of the bones due to osteoporosis (see Research Abstract 10.1).

MEDICAL MANAGEMENT

History and examination. The patient may have been found on the floor following a fall and, if living alone, could have been there for some time and be suffering from hypothermia and dehydration. Careful assessment to identify other reasons which led to the fall, such as a cerebrovascular accident or myocardial infarction, should be made. She will complain of severe pain in the hip or knee and there will be visible shortening and external rotation. Diagnosis will be confirmed by X-ray.

Treatment. Depending on the site of the fracture, and the age and condition of the patient, the treatment will be either internal

Table 10.1 Collaborative care of 18-year-old man with closed, comminuted fracture of femoral shaft that has been reduced under general anaesthetic

Problem focus	*Surgical*	*Nursing*	*Physiotherapy*	*Social work*	*Occupational therapy*
Maintain reduction and alignment of fractured left femoral shaft Balanced, sliding skeletal traction Steinmann tibial pin 6 kg weight	• X-ray Check reduction alignment • Check traction equipment — adjust weight prn • Check skeletal pin	• Assist radiographer • Reassure patient • Monitor and maintain traction • Explain principles and aims in lay terms, gain patient's cooperation • Reinforce physiotherapy	• Explain and demonstrate safe movements within limits of traction apparatus		
Pain/anxiety	• Answer questions • Assess level/cause • Prescribe analgesics	• Reassure • Assess level/cause • Give analgesics	• Teach smooth movements	• Contact visit	
Prevent complications • Shock • Further haemorrhage into thigh • Neurovascular compromise (compartment syndrome)	• Maintain IVT • Blood cross-matched • Repeat Hb • Inspect swelling • Check vital signs • Check: distal pulses colour sensation movement tissue pressure dorsiflexion	• Monitor IVT • * • * • * • * • *	• Deep-breathing and coughing exercises • Active and passive limb and joint exercise regimen • Teach regular dorsiflexion of foot on affected limb	• Contact visit Deal with pressing issues Reassure continuing contact to deal with insurance, family or work-related issues	Admission noted — to visit when acute symptoms resolve
• Cardiopulmonary complications (Pulmonary embolus, fat embolus)	• Examine: respiratory function, blood gases, mental state	• *			
• Infection	• i.v. antibiotics	• *			

*See Question 10.7. p. 403

fixation with a plate and screws or replacement of the head of femur with a metal prosthesis. Intracapsular fractures high in the neck of the femur have a serious effect on the blood supply to the femur head (Fig. 10.9) which would certainly need operative replacement.

NURSING PRIORITIES AND MANAGEMENT: FRACTURE OF NECK OF FEMUR

In addition to the general principles relating to musculoskeletal injury and fractures, the following priorities need to be addressed.

Complications. As a result of age and general physical condition when found, the patient may be confused and fearful and need a great deal of comfort and reassurance. Measures will be taken to reverse any hypothermia and dehydration. Risk assessment of the patient for skin breakdown using an approved scale such as the Waterlow scale should be recorded (Bridel 1993), and the use of a therapeutic bed may be implemented. Vital signs will be monitored at 4-hourly intervals to detect early signs of complications.

Pain. There is often extensive bruising with an extracapsular fracture which adds to the severe pain. When the cause has been established, this may be treated by repositioning and supporting the body and limbs, and administering prescribed analgesics. Local policy regarding pain assessment and pain relief should be implemented (see Ch. 19).

Increased risk of multisystem complications. For an elderly patient, such acute trauma and associated surgery may lead to

Research Abstract 10.1
Osteoporosis: delaying the onset. (Reproduced with kind permission from Roper et al 1996)

From the Hospital Inpatient Enquiry data for England (quoted in Law et al 1991) it can be seen that 37 600 people aged 65 years or more fractured a hip. In all, 82% of those aged 65 and over were women, of whom 83% were aged 75 or over. With serious potential complications such as failure to regain mobility, pressure sores, pneumonia and the precipitation of confusional states and dementia, hip fracture is a major cause of morbidity and institutional care in elderly people; it contributes considerably to the cost of health care.

Reviewing data from numerous studies, Law et al suggest several strategies to reduce or delay the loss of bone density which underlies fracture:

- regular exercise — a substantial body of evidence indicates that physical activity is a method of prevention which can be both enjoyable and social
- post-menopausal oestrogen replacement — it can more than halve the risk
- stopping smoking — if done before the menopause it can reduce risk by a quarter
- calcium supplementation — it is of some benefit.

Murphy et al (1994) conclude from their cross-sectional study that frequent milk consumption before the age of 25 years favourably influences hip bone mass in middle-aged and older women.

multisystem failure (see Ch. 18). It is widely recognised in the UK that mortality rates are high following hip surgery compared with other forms of surgery (Audit Commission 1995).

Fracture of the tibia and fibula

Fracture of the tibia and fibula is one of the most common injuries dealt with by orthopaedic surgeons. These fractures usually result from direct violence to the limb, and extensive skin and soft tissue damage may be present. RTAs and sports injuries are a common cause.

MEDICAL MANAGEMENT

Treatment. There are three choices of treatment.

Cast immobilisation. This is the treatment of choice for closed stable injuries. If the fracture requires manipulation, the patient will receive a general anaesthetic which will necessitate a stay in hospital; otherwise she may be discharged home from the A&E department. Following reduction of the fracture, a long leg plaster cast will be applied and plain radiographs taken to confirm the position of the fracture. Repeat X-rays will be taken at 1 week, 2 weeks and then at monthly intervals following reduction. The patient will not be allowed to bear weight on the injured leg for at least 1 month following injury. At this point in time a Sarmiento type plaster (patellar tendon bearing) may be applied (McRae 1994) and the patient allowed to bear weight through the injured limb. The average length of stay in plaster for this type of injury is 12–16 weeks.

Internal fixation. Fractures which are closed but unstable will benefit from internal fixation using a nail. On occasions, the patient will be placed in a plaster cast for 6–8 weeks following surgery. Routine postoperative care as discussed in Chapter 26, and cast care (see p. 401) will be required. The patient will be able to be up on crutches once fully recovered from the effects of surgery.

External fixation. If there is skin loss or a contaminated wound at the fracture site, the choice of treatment is commonly an external fixator. This enables frequent observation of the wounds and easy access for wound dressing changes. An external fixator is applied under a general anaesthetic in an operating theatre.

This type of fixator holds the fracture in position and the patient can be up walking, weight-bearing or not, dependent on the injury and the stability of the fixation of the injured limb, and discharged home to allow the community nurse and general practitioner (GP) to attend to the wounds. The patient would be reviewed at regular intervals at the outpatient clinic (see Case History 10.1).

NURSING PRIORITIES AND MANAGEMENT: FRACTURE OF THE TIBIA AND FIBULA

The principles of nursing management for each type of treatment are given on pages 398, 401 and 401.

> **10.8** Jot down the complications associated with fractures. Discuss with colleagues the causes of each complication and say how you can prevent it. Check your findings with Table 10.2.

Case History 10.1 Mr K

Mr K is a 40-year-old man who lives alone. He sustained a compound fracture to his left tibia and fibula while skiing with friends in the Highlands of Scotland. One friend stayed with him on the mountain side while the other alerted the emergency services, who arrived within an hour. The paramedical team applied a clean dressing over the open wound and splinted his leg. On arrival at the hospital, Mr K was in obvious pain, although he had been using the analgesic gas Entonox, so the doctor administered intravenous analgesia.

In the A&E department, his named nurse, Bill, noted his temperature, pulse, blood pressure and respirations, and the colour, sensation and movement of the injured limb, all of which were within normal limits. A clean sterile dressing was applied to the wound following inspection by the doctor.

Confirmation of the diagnosis was made by radiography and it was decided to take Mr K to the operating theatre for application of an external fixator to his left leg. This was explained to him and a picture of an external fixator in position was shown to him and the two friends who had accompanied him. His first reaction was revulsion at all the metal pins and scaffolding, but as his friends joked about his 'bionic parts' his anxiety subsided.

After an uneventful postoperative period, Mr K was allowed to sit in an armchair on day 1 with his leg elevated on a stool to reduce the swelling. The wound had been dressed in theatre following the local dressing policy of the institution. The physiotherapist gradually mobilised Mr K to walk with the help of crutches without bearing weight on his left leg, and showed him how to manage the awkward appliance to avoid injuring himself. He was helped to widen two pairs of trousers below the knee so that he could cover the external fixator.

As Mr K lived on his own, the social worker made arrangements for a home help to be provided on discharge. His two friends agreed to visit him and provide him with food and other provisions at the weekends.

The nurse contacted the community nurse attached to Mr K's GP practice with background treatment information, proposed discharge date and continuing care needs. All of this information was confirmed in writing and sent by fax to the community nurse. Mr K was discharged home 6 days after his accident with a return appointment for 2 weeks later.

Fracture of neck of humerus

Fracture of the neck of the humerus commonly occurs in elderly adults with osteoporosis after a fall on an outstretched hand. Often the bone is not displaced or badly impacted and normally heals well, depending on its stability. The major complication is of shoulder and elbow stiffness.

MEDICAL MANAGEMENT

Treatment. This injury can usually be treated at home following the initial visit to the A&E department, providing there is no gross displacement or neurovascular complications. The arm is supported in a shoulder immobiliser, broad arm sling or collar 'n' cuff for approximately 2 weeks. Movement is gradually introduced, followed by outpatient physiotherapy in order to avoid the major complication, which is development of a stiff shoulder joint.

NURSING PRIORITIES AND MANAGEMENT: FRACTURE OF NECK OF HUMERUS

Assessment of ability to carry out normal activities of daily living. This is done before the patient is discharged home from the A&E department. Home nursing and home help are arranged accordingly.

Skin care of injured arm. It is wise to have the community nurse attend to washing the injured arm two or three times a week, taking particular care of the axilla. The sling is reapplied and

Table 10.2 Prevention of complications of fractures

Complication	*Cause*	*Prevention*
Damage to soft tissue — neurovascular compromise	Trauma Sharp fragments/edge of bone	Monitor neurovascular function regularly — report abnormalities
Complications associated with immobility		
Diminished function of all body systems	Decreased physical stimulation	Encourage active and passive exercise
Muscle atrophy — decreased range of movement — contractures	Lack of normal exercise	Coordinate physiotherapy programme
Altered psychological processes	Decreased social stimulation	Provide social and mental stimulation
Pressure sores	Casts — prolonged pressure	Regular pressure area care and position change
Infection	Open wound postoperatively Skeletal pin sites	Principles of infection control
Malunion	Mal-apposition of bony fragments Inadequate mobilisation (e.g. swelling subsides — cast becomes loose)	Meticulous and regular monitoring of cast fit and traction alignment
Delayed union	Unstable fracture Poor blood supply	Maintain adequate circulation and splintage
Non-union	Infection Soft tissue intrusion	Infection control
Fat embolus — emergency	Fat globules released into circulation from bone marrow at fracture site — usually associated with fractured femur or multiple fractures	Early reduction and splintage Report confusion, chest pain, dyspnoea immediately (see p. 403)
Osteoarthritis	Extension of fracture into joint surface	Early physiotherapy

Case History 10.2 Mrs L

Mrs L is a 70-year-old lady living alone in sheltered housing. She was admitted to hospital overnight following treatment for fractured neck of humerus. As the evening progressed, she became more steady when walking, obviously recovering from the initial shock of her fall. An oral analgesic was given for pain relief. When in bed, she found the most comfortable position was sitting up, well supported with pillows. The following day she was discharged with arrangements having been made for a community nurse to call to see her. The social worker would arrange a suitable social care package to provide the support Mrs L would require.

When the community nurse called, she washed and dried the skin around Mrs L's injured shoulder, inspecting it for any signs of friction or pressure. Extensive bruising was noted all over the shoulder region. The broad arm sling was reapplied. The nurse checked that Mrs L was moving her joints as instructed and that no joint stiffness was present. On identifying where Mrs L had slipped, the nurse found a bath mat lying over a shiny floor covering in the toilet. She advised Mrs L to remove the mat in order to reduce the chance of further accidents, and suggested a non-slip mat for the base of the bath. She checked whether Mrs L needed a further prescription for the analgesic and arranged to call on alternate days.

Mrs L was to attend the hospital outpatient department 10 days later when she would be seen by an orthopaedic specialist. Her GP would then be contacted to arrange physiotherapy at her local health centre.

neurovascular status and degree of mobility monitored. Case History 10.2 outlines the continuing care of an elderly lady with fractured neck of humerus.

Q **10.9** After initial instruction from your tutor or mentor and with a fellow student, practise applying a broad arm sling, a high sling and a collar 'n' cuff.

Colles' fracture

This is one of the most common fractures seen at the A&E department and is often found in elderly women after a fall on an outstretched hand. It is frequently associated with the subsequent diagnosis of osteoporosis. The fracture usually involves the lower end of the radius within 2.5 cm of the wrist joint and there may be an associated fracture of the ulnar styloid. The obvious feature of a Colles' fracture is the classic 'dinner fork' deformity (Fig. 10.10).

MEDICAL MANAGEMENT

Examination. Diagnosis will be confirmed by the appearance of the patient's wrist and by plain X-rays.

Treatment. A regional anaesthetic is advisable in order to reduce the fracture. A Bier's block, which is a form of regional anaesthetic, is usually performed and, as this involves a degree of risk of reactive cardiac arrest, it must only be performed where resuscitation facilities are available (McRae 1994). The patient is fasted from the time of admission to the A&E department in case the nerve block is unsuccessful and a general anaesthetic is needed.

Prevention. This fracture is more often seen in the winter months, and elderly people should be advised to avoid slippery surfaces.

NURSING PRIORITIES AND MANAGEMENT: COLLES' FRACTURE

In addition to the management principles already discussed which relate to musculoskeletal trauma, fractures and plaster casts, the following priorities should be noted.

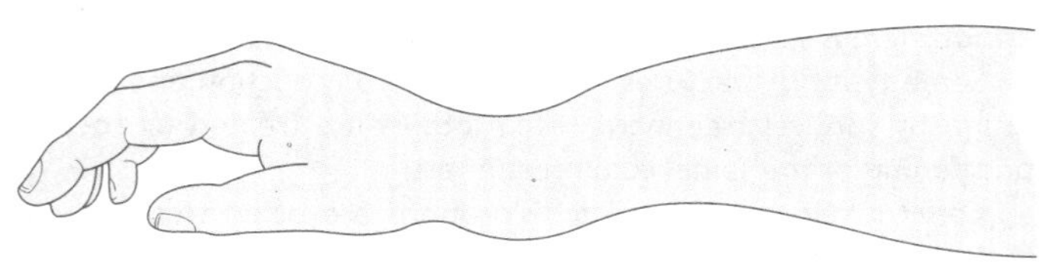

Fig. 10.10 The 'dinner fork' deformity of Colles' fracture.

Removal of rings. Marked swelling of the fingers is likely to occur and it is important to remove all rings and bracelets from the injured hand as soon as possible. If swelling has already made this impossible, it will be necessary to obtain the patient's permission to cut the rings off using the special ring cutter found in all A&E departments.

The arm should be kept elevated to reduce swelling.

Splinting. Following successful reduction, a POP back (dorsal) slab is usually applied and the POP will be completed when the swelling has subsided — around 24–48 h later.

Advice. Ensure that the patient is given written and verbal advice as described for a hand to elbow plaster in Box 10.4 (p. 402).

Fracture of the clavicle

This fracture is given brief mention because it is a common sporting injury (see Fig. 10.11).

NURSING PRIORITIES AND MANAGEMENT: FRACTURE OF THE CLAVICLE

Treatment is usually managed at home and the GP practice nurse or community nurse may be called upon to assist with hygiene to the axilla and reapplication of the special shoulder brace or arm support. The aim is to maintain comfortable alignment and supervise exercise of distal joints.

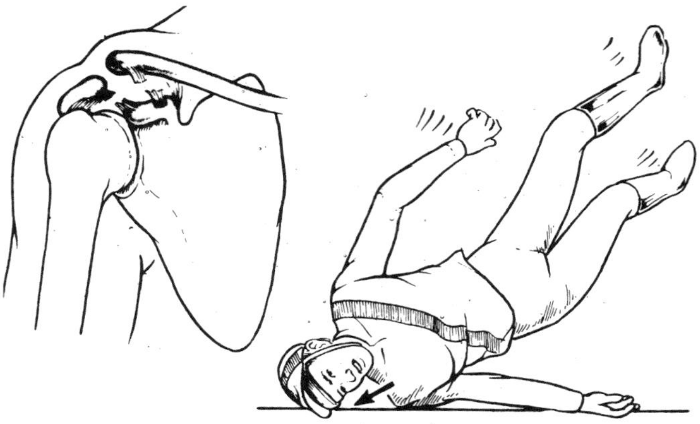

Fig. 10.11 Fracture of the acromioclavicular joint. (Reproduced with kind permission from Dandy 1993.)

SPINAL INJURIES

PATHOPHYSIOLOGY

Fracture, dislocation, whiplash or any other injury to the spine is potentially serious because of the danger of injury to the spinal cord.

The main causes of spinal injury are motor vehicle, motorcycle and sporting accidents. However, inflammatory and degenerative disease, and pathological conditions such as metastatic disease can result in spinal trauma. The resultant damage can involve transection, compression, contusion or interference to the spinal cord, accompanied by varying degrees of paralysis and sensory deficit below the level of the lesion. In some cases the paraplegia or quadriplegia that results is permanent because of the inability of the adult spinal cord to regenerate, although recent research indicates that there is room for guarded optimism in this respect (see Research Abstract 10.2).

Research Abstract 10.2
International spinal research

Until recently, it was thought that damaged spinal cord nerves, unlike peripheral nerves, could not regenerate. A report from the International Spinal Research Trust (ISRT), however, gives new hope that it may eventually be possible to overcome the hostile conditions preventing regrowth and provide conditions that encourage it (ISRT 1993).

It is known that the mechanism that gives fetal CNS cells the ability to grow long connecting fibres is weakened in adult CNS cells, and although injured adult nerves sprout new fibres, they lack the ability to continue this growth over a distance long enough to repair the lesion.

Researchers have isolated two kinds of glial cells that act to block the regenerative process:

- oligodendrocytes, which form the insulating sheath
- astrocytes, which form almost impenetrable scarring at the site of the injury.

By introducing CNS nerve fibres into a culture medium that contains a high density of astrocytes and behaves in a similar way to glial scarring, several factors in blocking regrowth have been defined and are influencing the direction of research:

- Whereas adult nerve cells sprouted but soon lost impetus, embryonic nerve cells continued to grow strongly through the glial tissue. This suggested that an alternative to disarming astrocytes may be to implant embryonic nerve cells to help the repair process.
- Growing nerve fibres produce enzymes to break down proteins and make a pathway through the hostile CNS tissue. The balance of enzyme and inhibitory proteins can be altered by using nerve-growth factors, thus increasing the permeability of the glial tissue and the possibility of useful growth.
- Genetically engineered cells with growth-enhancing properties could be used to knock out and replace the hostile properties of the glial cells.

Other projects are also under way. One involves use of an antibody to the inhibitory factors in the CNS, and another the use of growth-enhancing proteins identified within the body and able to be reproduced in the laboratory. By combining these two approaches in the laboratory, it is possible to get some adult CNS nerve fibres to grow over a long distance.

Eventually a combination of several of these research findings should bring success in the actual repair process of the adult spinal cord. The task will then be to find out whether these fibres can successfully reactivate appropriate target areas to restore body movement, feeling and function. There is guarded optimism in this respect.

International Spinal Research Trust 1993 Review. Burnet Associates, London.

Injury to the spine and surrounding structures need not always involve spinal cord damage; in many instances damage can be prevented by correct handling. The basic principles are to suspect spinal injury until proven otherwise and to maintain anatomical alignment and immobilise the spine immediately.

MEDICAL MANAGEMENT

Management of spinal injury is critical throughout, with immediate immobilisation, early reduction and stabilisation, full assessment of the extent of the injury and its consequences, and ongoing specialist treatment and rehabilitation. For this reason, following initial treatment in the receiving A&E department, it is vital to transfer the patient to a spinal injuries or neurology unit as soon as possible (refer to Ch. 27 for reception and handling of the patient in the A&E department).

Investigations. History, loss of function and sensation, X-rays, CT or MRI scanning will confirm the diagnosis and indicate the extent of the injury.

Treatment depends on the type and level of injury and whether or not there is spinal cord involvement (see Fig. 10.12).

Some types of fractures are amenable to reduction and stabilisation by surgical treatment, while others are treated by specific positioning of the spinal column and rest.

Cervical spine fractures or dislocations are often treated with skeletal traction attached to the skull by a halo device, Crutchfield or Gardner–Wells tongs or halter (see Fig. 10.13).

The damage that can be done following injury in which the spinal ligaments are torn or stretched should never be underestimated as this can leave a potentially dangerous unstable spine. Cervical whiplash injury is a prime example of this (see Fig. 10.14), where an injury originates from a combined extension–flexion injury to the neck (Dandy 1993). This usually occurs from a RTA when the car in which the patient is travelling is hit from behind causing the head to be thrown backwards (hyperextended). As the car decelerates, the head is thrown into flexion causing damage to the ligaments and soft tissues of the spine (Duckworth 1995).

Some fractures, especially lower thoracic and lumbar fractures, can be treated by bed rest on a firm base.

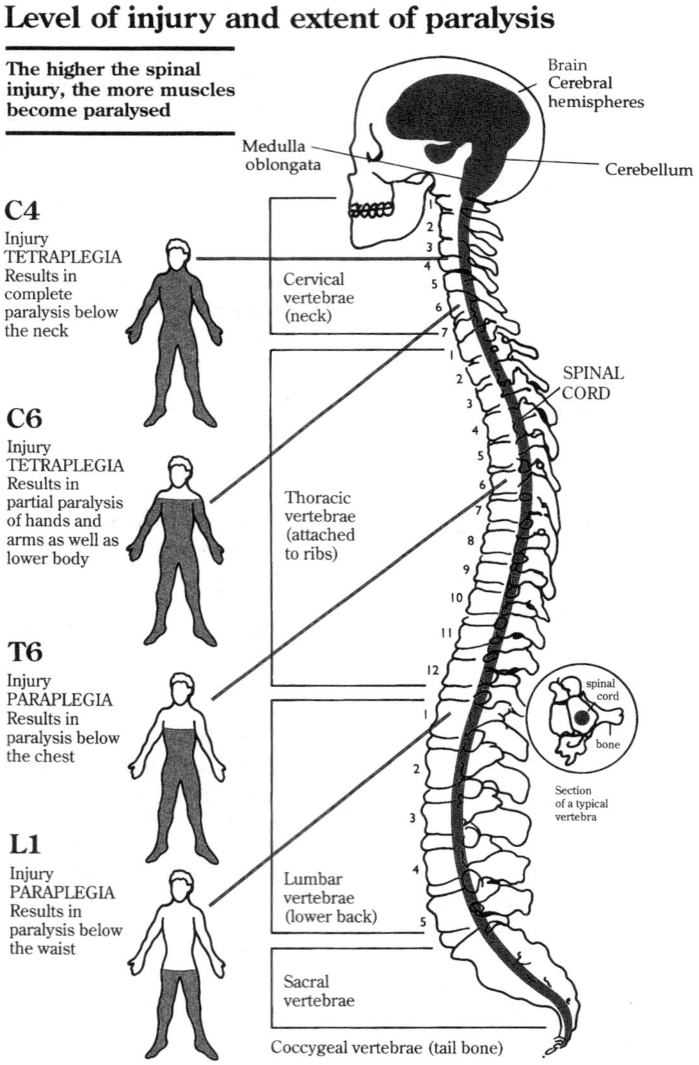

Fig. 10.12 Level of injury and extent of paralysis. (Reproduced with kind permission from the Spinal Injuries Association 1993) (See Useful Addresses p. 427)

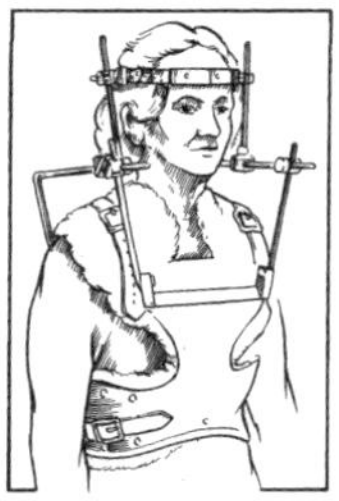

Fig. 10.13 'Halo-vest' traction. A halo fixed to the skull — attached to bars mounted on a chest (Reproduced with kind permission from Dandy 1993.)

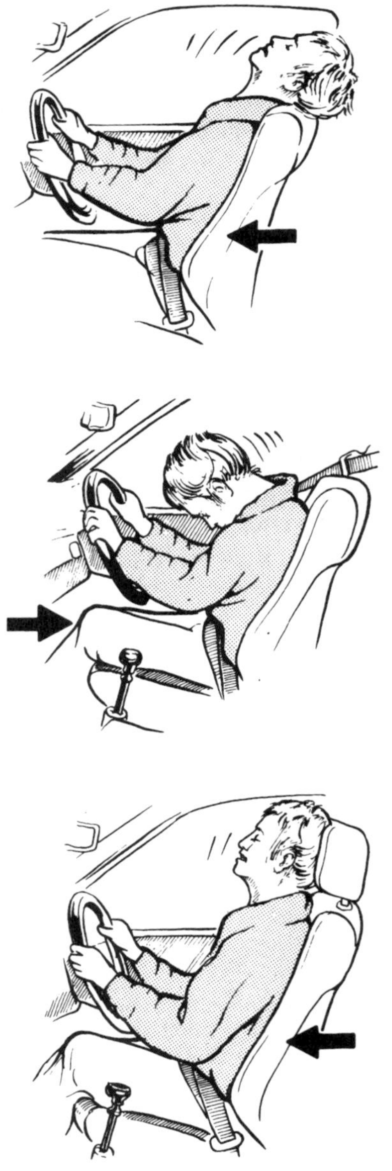

Fig. 10.14 Combined flexion/extension (whiplash) injury of the cervical spine. Movement of the head is limited by a head restraint. (Reproduced with kind permission from Dandy 1993.)

NURSING PRIORITIES AND MANAGEMENT: SPINAL INJURIES

In addition to principles of nursing management for musculoskeletal disorders and perioperative care, the following specific points are of importance here.

First aid. Knowledge and application of the basic principles of first aid for spinal injuries are essential in many areas of nursing practice.

For information on first aid principles, see Webb et al (1997).

Additionally, nurses in the community have the opportunity to teach the general public the basic principles of first aid management in order to prevent the potentially serious consequences of spinal cord injury (see Case History 10.3).

10.10 What do you suspect are the main reasons for such different outcomes for the accident victims described in Case History 10.3?

Basic principles of positioning and moving patients with spinal injury. As indicated earlier, it is vital to maintain anatomical alignment and fracture reduction. Manoeuvres such as log rolling the patient, pelvic twists and using special beds (e.g. an electric turning bed) are best, initially practised under expert guidance.

Spinal shock. Be aware of the phenomenon of spinal shock, which is a response to sudden loss of continuity between the spinal cord and higher centres of the brain caused by trauma to the spine. This involves a complete loss of all motor, sensory, reflex and autonomic activity below the level of the lesion, whatever the actual damage consists of. Main features involve falling blood pressure with bradycardia, paralysis below the level of the injury and of bladder and bowel function. It can therefore be life-threatening, especially in cervical spine injury where respiratory function is compromised. It is temporary but may last for weeks. As the hypotension associated with spinal shock is not due to a lack of circulating blood volume, care must be taken not to overhydrate the patient (see Ch. 28).

Adaptation to paraplegia or quadriplegia. This adaptation is particularly long and painful for most people especially if they are young. The Spinal Injuries Association and the International Spinal Research Trust publish reports and newsletters which often include in-depth perspectives of how different people learn to cope.

10.11 You are a community nurse who has been asked to teach first aid. Outline the key points you would cover in a teaching session relating to first aid in spinal injury.

BONE TUMOURS

A satisfactory classification of primary bone tumours is difficult to achieve. A bone tumour can consist of many different cells; therefore classification by the original cell type may not be accurate. However, separating the tumours into benign and malignant categories can be helpful, provided that one is aware that benign tumours can undergo cell change and become malignant (see Table 10.3).

Metastatic bone disease is malignant bone disease due to secondary deposits in bone tissue from a primary neoplastic site elsewhere (see Ch. 31).

Case History 10.3 First aid for accident victims — the effect on outcome

Two 18-year-old men were brought into the A&E department on the same night. They had both sustained multiple injuries to the head and body in similar RTAs. P had been moved from his overturned vehicle by well-meaning people at the scene of the accident whilst waiting for the ambulance to arrive. T was supported in the position in which he was found until the ambulance men arrived. They applied a neck collar and maintained skeletal alignment whilst transferring him to the ambulance and at all times subsequently. Spinal X-rays showed that the men had identical injuries to the cervical spine.

Two months later, T walked out of the spinal injuries unit. Many months later, P was wheeled out of the same unit as a quadriplegic.

PATHOPHYSIOLOGY

Primary bone tumours are known to occur in specific age groups and in certain sites of bone tissue. Osteosarcoma, for example, is most often seen in people under the age of 20 and usually occurs in the metaphyseal region of the lower end of the femur, upper end of the tibia and upper end of the humerus.

As the bone tumour grows, eruption into the surrounding tissues can occur, which may be noted as a warm swelling of the affected area. The tumour will originate from a specific cell type within the bone tissue, but may then involve a variety of bone cells.

The secondary malignant bone growth of metastatic bone disease normally occurs in the later stages of neoplastic disease. Bony metastases are usually transmitted by the blood and tend to occur in sites where red bone marrow is present, such as the vertebrae, pelvis and upper ends of the humerus or femur.

MEDICAL MANAGEMENT

History. The patient may present complaining of a warm swelling over the affected bone, which may be painful when palpated. Swelling and restriction of the neighbouring joint may also be evident. Some patients may initially present with a pathological fracture as the first indication.

Investigations. Plain radiographs of the affected area will highlight changes in the normal radiological appearance of the bone tissue. This may be in the form of increased or decreased bone density and/or distortion of the normal bone outline. Imaging studies may also be performed and a biopsy of the tumour taken to obtain cells for examination.

Diagnosis will be confirmed by the appearance of the tumour on X-ray and positive pathology. Each bone tumour has a typical radiological appearance, such as that found in a Ewing's tumour when the radiograph will show alternating layers of bone destruction and new bone growth.

Treatment. This is usually dependent on the type of bone tumour.

Benign bone tumours. These are usually treated by excision or curettage, followed by insertion of a bone graft into the subsequent bony defect (Russell 1994).

Malignant bone tumours. A patient with a confirmed malignant tumour will usually be screened for metastatic deposits. This may be performed by radioisotope skeletal survey and other scanning techniques. If no metastatic deposits are found, the method of treatment may involve amputation of the affected limb or total replacement of the affected bone with a custom-built artificial implant, thus avoiding the mutilation of an amputation. A course of chemotherapy is usually given preoperatively and is always given postoperatively.

When a metastatic deposit is found, the patient may be given a course of chemotherapy and/or radiation, but seldom would an amputation be carried out as the prognosis is very poor.

Metastatic bone disease. The treatment of a patient with metastatic bone disease tends to be symptomatic. The major problem for the patient is pain, which can be severe and debilitating. Pain assessment is crucial in facilitating good pain control and frequently a course of radiotherapy may be prescribed as adjuvant therapy (Havard 1997) (See Ch. 19).

NURSING PRIORITIES AND MANAGEMENT: PRIMARY BONE TUMOURS

Certain bone tumours are known to affect particular age ranges of patient, and therefore the nurse may care for a young child, adolescent or adult.

Once the patient has seen her GP, immediate hospitalisation will ensue (see Ch. 31). The care of a patient undergoing chemotherapy and/or radiotherapy is described on pages 921–933.

Table 10.3 Common bone tumours

Tumour type	*Cell origin*	*Comments*
Benign tumours		
Osteochondroma	Osteocyte	Most common benign tumour — bony outgrowth with cartilage cap. Symptoms depend on impingement. Common sites: distal end femur, proximal end tibia and humerus
Osteoclastoma	Osteocyte	Rarefaction of bone occurs. Femur, tibia and humerus. Young adults. Treat: curettage, resection and bone graft. May become malignant. Treat with chemotherapy and amputation
Malignant tumours (primary)		
Chondrosarcoma	Chondrocyte	Age group 30–40 years. Sites: femur, scapula, pelvis, humerus. Treat: excision, amputation or chemotherapy and endoprosthetic replacement
Osteosarcoma	Osteocyte	Destroys medullary and cortical bone tissue. Sites: end of long bones — 50% knee joint. Severe pain, swelling, tenderness. Treat: amputation and chemotherapy or chemotherapy and endoprosthetic replacement

The care of a patient who has a custom-built prosthetic implant can be specialised but the principles of postoperative care are similar to the care of a patient following joint arthroplasty (see p. 423).

Amputation of the affected limb may be a necessity.

AMPUTATION OF A LIMB

Amputation of a limb may be carried out for any of a number of reasons:

- primary malignant bone tumour
- trauma, such as a crushing injury
- vascular insufficiency, such as peripheral vascular disease
- congenital anomaly
- severe infection, such as chronic osteomyelitis with systemic manifestations.

It has been estimated that a large number of the patients who undergo amputation of a limb, or part of a limb, in the Western world do so due to the effects of peripheral vascular disease, while trauma remains the commonest reason in the developing countries.

Sites for amputation

The aim of surgery is to provide a useful, functional, healthy, well-moulded stump which will permit the application of a prosthesis. Factors taken into account when deciding on the site are:

- total excision of all diseased tissue
- maintenance of an adequate blood supply to the tissue around the stump
- provision of a stump which is of an appropriate length to allow fitting of a prosthesis with optimum function.

As the stump will be exposed to some friction and (if a lower limb) to weight-bearing, the surgeon must ensure adequate cover and padding of the bone end with the surrounding tissues, otherwise breakdown of the skin tissue could occur.

NURSING PRIORITIES AND MANAGEMENT: AMPUTATION OF A LIMB

Counselling and support when surgery is planned

The patient who has been diagnosed as suffering from a malignant bone tumour will be devastated by the information on two counts: firstly that she has cancer of the bone; secondly that treatment may involve amputation of the affected limb, which appears to her to be totally healthy (Russell 1994).

Coping with loss. Loss of a limb through amputation is like any other major loss. If the surgery is performed as an elective procedure, the patient, her family and other relatives will need support and understanding from the health care team to help them accept and adjust to the altered body image. The impending loss may cause the patient to display some of the initial characteristics of the bereavement process as described by Kubler Ross (1973) (see Ch. 33).

As the majority of amputations are carried out as elective procedures, the nurse will be able to make physiological, psychological and social assessments of the patient, and therefore plan care which will assist in the adjustment and adaptation process for the patient (Donohue 1997).

Occasionally a patient may undergo an amputation as an emergency procedure following a severe crushing injury. In this case, the psychological preparation of the patient and family can only be very limited. They are very likely to require extra support and understanding during the postoperative period.

A visit to the local prosthetic department should be arranged and/or an introduction to a previous amputee who is of similar age and gender. This will help the patient to be aware of the level of mobility and lifestyle that can still be achieved after surgery, and hopefully to begin the process of accepting her altered body image. If time permits, these visits should be arranged before the patient is admitted to hospital.

The details of specific pre- and postoperative care that follow are as for a patient undergoing a mid-thigh amputation.

Preoperative care

Standard preoperative care as outlined in Chapter 26 should be delivered.

Specific care

Mobilising. Information regarding the initial change in mobility level should be given. The physiotherapist will usually teach the patient to use crutches or other form of walking aid. When a lower limb amputation is planned, attention will be paid to maintaining the muscle power of the other limbs as the arms and remaining lower limb will be used to support the patient during the early days of postoperative mobilisation. The patient should experience lying prone as this position will need to be adopted at least twice a day postoperatively to minimise the risk of flexion contracture. A patient with respiratory problems may not be able to tolerate lying prone, as this position reduces the usual level of respiratory ventilation.

The surgeon will usually mark the limb for amputation with a waterproof marker pen the day before the patient's operation, thus reducing the risk of amputating the wrong limb.

Postoperative care

A standard postoperative care plan may be utilised (see Ch. 26) with additional specific care on an individualised basis.

Specific care

Comfort measures. A bed cage should be utilised to relieve pressure on the stump during the immediate postoperative period. The stump should be maintained in the neutral position, lying parallel to the other limb in a non-flexed and non-abducted orientation.

Wound dressing. Most commonly, this is in the form of a soft dressing and stump bandage. The bandage will need to be reapplied at regular intervals, commencing usually within 72 h. Pain medication should be given at an appropriate time prior to the dressing change. After the initial postoperative period, a special stump bandage, such as an 'Elset' or a shrinker sock, both of which have better elastic properties and are lighter than a crepe bandage, is used to maintain uniform compression on the wound, thereby reducing oedema, promoting wound healing and beginning to shape the stump, which eases the fitting of the prosthesis (Fig. 10.15). Stump bandaging requires practice to achieve a skilled technique. One or two vacuum wound drains will usually be in position and these are removed within 48 h unless the drainage is excessive.

Alternatively, the patient's stump may be encased in a plaster cast dressing, which helps healing by maintaining the stump in a neutral position and reducing swelling and oedema. The main disadvantage of this type of dressing is that regular assessment of the wound for signs of infection cannot be undertaken; therefore any rise in temperature, offensive odour and/or complaint of pain must be reported as this may indicate wound infection or tissue breakdown. If such circumstances arise, the plaster cast will be removed, the wound inspected and a stump bandage applied and regularly reviewed.

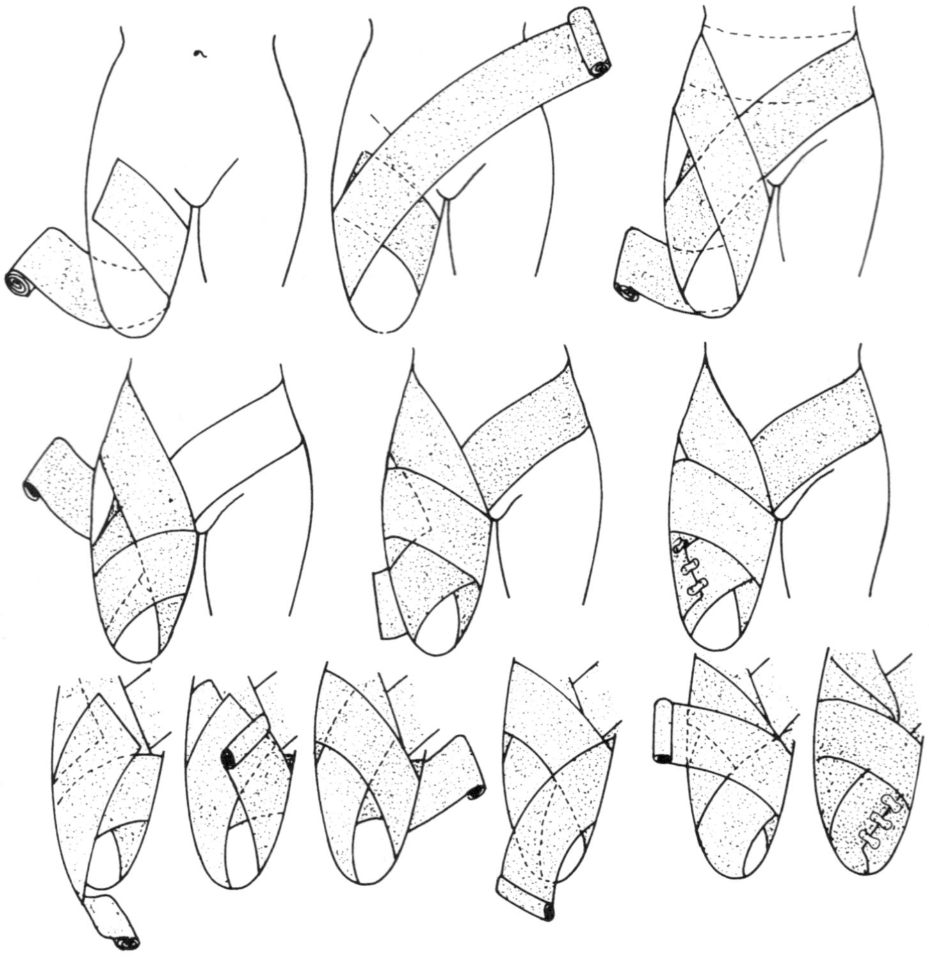

Fig. 10.15 Stump bandage. (Reproduced with kind permission from Smith Suddarth 1991.)

Phantom sensation (phantom limb). This is the name given to the painful sensation experienced by some patients following an amputation and can develop into a form of non-malignant pain, the causal mechanism of which is still not fully understood (McCaffery & Beebe 1994). The sensation can be very distressing for the patient as, for many, not only is the preoperative pain still felt but the full limb seems still to be present. These perceptions may continue for many months after surgery. Regular, effective analgesics in the immediate postoperative period are thought to reduce the incidence of phantom pain (Nikolejsen et al 1997). If it becomes a chronic problem, treatment in the form of transcutaneous nerve stimulation (TENS), ultrasound, local nerve blocks, relaxation therapy or medication such as carbamazepine has been shown to be effective (Judd 1997). Some patients may find benefit from the use of one of the many alternative complementary therapies that are available.

Preventing flexion contracture. Where possible, the patient should lie prone at regular intervals commencing from the first postoperative day to prevent the development of a flexion contracture of the stump. The patient who normally sleeps lying prone can return to this position.

Mobilisation. The patient will normally sit out of bed within 12 h of surgery and may use a wheelchair initially to assist with mobilisation. Practice in standing, and transferring from bed to chair and from wheelchair to toilet will be given. This increases the patient's independence and improves her morale. The physiotherapist will supervise walking. The patient may find that her sense of balance has been temporarily altered, but with advice and support this problem will be overcome.

Pneumatic post-amputation mobility aid. Some centres use a prosthesis known as a pneumatic post-amputation mobility (PPAM) aid to help the patient regain balance, reduce oedema of the stump and encourage early walking. The aid consists of an inflatable plastic tube which is placed around the patient's stump. The tube is encased in a metal frame with a rocker foot. The use of the PPAM aid can help the patient adjust to the change in body image as the time without an artificial limb is reduced.

Clothing. The patient's clothing may need to be adapted temporarily until the prosthesis is supplied. The tucking of an empty arm of a jacket or the leg of a pair of trousers into the body of the garment is an apparent detail, but failure to do this can often be the last straw for a patient who, until then, has been coping well.

Promoting independence. The patient should be taught how to care for the stump once the sutures are removed, by maintaining skin hygiene, moisturising the skin surface if required and, twice daily, inspecting the whole stump for any skin discoloration, which may indicate the potential development of a pressure sore. This care will be reinforced during visits to the prosthetic department where information about care of the prosthesis will be given.

The patient or a relative should be taught to apply the stump bandage so that necessary compression is maintained, to help mould and firm the tissue in preparation for fitting the definitive prosthesis. Should the patient for any reason be unable to wear her prosthesis at a later date, she must be advised to apply the stump bandage in order to maintain the shape of the stump.

Social adaptation. The amputation of a limb can markedly affect a person's ability to continue her previous pattern of work and leisure activities. The nurse should encourage the patient to voice anxieties that relate to this and, if necessary, refer her to a social worker.

Discharge. Prior to discharge, the patient's home will be assessed by the occupational therapist to define any need for aids to assist with activities of living. Referral to the local occupational retraining officer may be needed if the amputation makes it impossible for the patient to continue in her former occupation. The patient will attend the prosthetic centre at regular intervals following discharge until she has achieved a safe, correct walking pattern. Thereafter, the patient may attend annually or as the need arises should any problem with the prosthesis develop. Some patients may be supplied with more than one definitive limb, depending on their age and the level of use/abuse of the prosthesis. Outpatient attendance for review by the surgeon will continue during the period of rehabilitation.

BONE INFECTIONS

In order to raise awareness of infective bone conditions and the problems associated with them, a brief outline of osteomyelitis, joint infection and tuberculosis will be given below.

Osteomyelitis

PATHOPHYSIOLOGY

This disease is more common in children and adolescents. It often follows minor trauma which probably causes a small haematoma at the epiphyseal plate in which blood-borne bacteria proliferate and infection develops. It is the marrow that is primarily involved. As the infection spreads, the patient develops pyrexia and severe pain and the affected part is hot and swollen (Dandy 1993). If untreated, the infection spreads through the marrow, erodes the cortex and the periosteum and an abscess forms, which will eventually discharge through the skin. By this stage it has become chronic osteomyelitis. A serious complication of osteomyelitis in a child could be the permanent damage to the epiphyseal cartilage resulting in stunted growth of the affected bone. The separate condition of septic arthritis is of infection present within a joint, and this has the potential of leading to the destruction of the joint surfaces.

MEDICAL MANAGEMENT

Investigations. The patient is hospitalised, the limb elevated and blood is sent for culture and to estimate the erythrocyte sedimentation rate (ESR), C-reactive protein (CRP) and white cell count, which confirms the presence of an inflammatory process, and haemoglobin level. Plain radiographs and bone scanning will show destructive bone changes. The infective lesion may be aspirated to identify the organism and its sensitivity, so that appropriate antibiotic therapy can be prescribed.

Treatment. Antibiotic therapy must be commenced immediately. When the culture sensitivity is known, the antibiotic may need to be altered specific to the causative agent.

If there is no response to the antibiotic treatment, the infected area may be opened surgically and the pus drained.

NURSING PRIORITIES AND MANAGEMENT: OSTEOMYELITIS

This condition is very distressing for the patient and the parents. Potentially the patient may be extremely unwell due to the sepsis and can rapidly develop septic shock (see Ch. 18).

Early detection. Community nurses need to be alert to the condition so that early referral and treatment can be instituted to prevent progression.

Elevation of the affected part. Pillows or bed elevation can be used.

Pain and comfort. Rest, gentle handling, use of bed cradles to relieve pressure of bedclothes, prompt administration of analgesics and antipyretics, reassurance and distracting activity will all help to relieve pain to some extent.

Antibiotic therapy. Initially antibiotics will be administered intravenously. Once evidence of the therapeutic action of the antibiotics is noted by a reduction in the patient's pyrexia, pain and swelling and the ability to tolerate oral fluids and food, the medication will usually be given orally.

Joint infection

Septic arthritis

PATHOPHYSIOLOGY

Septic arthritis can be caused by osteomyelitis, infection from a penetrating wound or bacteraemia. It should be suspected in systemic conditions, especially diabetes, which present with swollen and painful joints. In bacteraemia it is part of a potentially fatal condition. In every case, if untreated, it destroys articular cartilage and eventually the joint becomes ankylosed (fused).

MEDICAL MANAGEMENT

Treatment consists of arthroscopic joint lavage and division of adhesions, together with aggressive antibiotic therapy.

NURSING PRIORITIES AND MANAGEMENT: SEPTIC ARTHRITIS

Emphasis is on early detection, promotion of comfort, support, rehabilitation and specific management of arthroscopic procedures.

Tuberculosis

Tuberculosis, previously rare in developed countries, is now on the increase in Western societies and is rampant in underdeveloped countries. It affects all age groups. The course of the disease is similar to that of osteomyelitis although the pace is much slower. Treatment is by antitubercular drugs and addressing the symptoms. Tuberculosis may be a secondary infection in the immunosuppressed patient, such as in AIDS.

NURSING PRIORITIES AND MANAGEMENT: TUBERCULOSIS

Management involves implementation of the principles of infection control, health education and comfort measures to alleviate symptoms.

The *Tubercle and Lung Disease Journal* is a useful source of additional information.

DISORDERS OF JOINTS

Review the anatomy and physiology of joints.

For further information, see Wilson & Waugh (1996), pp. 397–411.

This section gives examples of the management of disorders of the knee and the lumbar spine, shoulder dislocation, rheumatoid arthritis and osteoarthritis.

DISORDERS OF THE KNEE

There are many disorders of the knee. Only the more common are outlined below.

Meniscus lesions

PATHOPHYSIOLOGY

The menisci are part of the load-bearing mechanism in the knee joint and absorb much of the weight of the femoral condyles. They can be torn or injured in relatively minor sporting accidents which include a twisting force (Duckworth 1995) and, when not intact, cause mechanical problems as loose gristly fragments move around within the joint.

MEDICAL MANAGEMENT

Diagnosis is confirmed by arthroscopy or MRI scan.
Treatment. Loose fragments are excised arthroscopically — arthroscopic meniscectomy (removal of the menisci). This is a minimally invasive technique which permits visualisation of the fragments and preservation of as much healthy tissue as possible. This is important because meniscectomy exposes the articular cartilage to the full downward thrust of body weight. In spite of surgical intervention, damage to the menisci may eventually lead to degenerative osteoarthritis in about 75% of patients 10 years after total meniscectomy (Dandy 1993).

NURSING PRIORITIES AND MANAGEMENT: MENISCUS LESIONS

These follow the principles for all musculoskeletal injuries and orthopaedic surgery. The majority of patients receiving this form of surgery will attend day surgery units, and therefore community and practice nurses should be aware of the background procedures and processes because they will advise the patient and follow up her treatment.

DISORDERS OF THE LUMBAR SPINE — BACK PAIN

Disorders of the lumbar spine and 'back pain' are responsible for more human suffering and time lost from work in any one year than any other medical condition (Dandy 1993). It has been estimated that 20–25% of referrals to an orthopaedic outpatient department are of people with low back pain (Paton 1992).

PATHOPHYSIOLOGY

Back pain in itself need not be an orthopaedic problem; rather it is a symptom, and once the cause has been determined it is best managed by the appropriate speciality. For example, it may be related to rheumatoid, gynaecological or urological conditions; to poor posture, obesity, lack of exercise; to metastatic or infectious bone disease; or to degenerative disc disease. However, often it is classified as musculoskeletal and brought within the orthopaedic remit. This section will focus on management of acute back strain, recurrent back strain and management of prolapsed intervertebral disc.

Acute back pain

This is associated with a sudden sharp movement or an attempt to lift a heavy object from an extended position, or it may occur when people with sedentary occupations indulge in bursts of excessive exercise. It may be manifest by sudden severe pain radiating from the lumbar region to the back of the knee. There are no other neurological symptoms and it is usually due to an acute muscle or ligament strain in the lumbar spine.

MEDICAL MANAGEMENT

The history indicates the cause, and differential diagnosis excludes two similar but serious conditions:

- lumbar disc protrusion — which would be accompanied by pain extending below the knee in the presence of other neurological symptoms
- metastatic spinal tumours — which can be excluded by imaging studies.

Treatment:

- Rest for 24 h maximum in the most comfortable position
- Analgesics, non-steroidal anti-inflammatory drugs (NSAIDs) and/or antispasmodics
- Refer to physiotherapist
- Gradual mobilisation
- Advice on application of heat.

NURSING PRIORITIES AND MANAGEMENT: ACUTE BACK PAIN

Prevention through health education. Nurses have many opportunities in the workplace, community and hospital to teach people how to organise their environment and activities in order to avoid acute back strain. Much research has gone into the ergonomics of correct lifting techniques (see Fig. 10.16) and many teaching aids such as videos and leaflets are available.

Prevention of back injury in the workplace has been given greater emphasis with the Health and Safety at Work Regulations (Health and Safety Commission 1992) on Manual Handling of Loads. It is important that both workers and employers are kept aware of their responsibilities in this respect.

Nurses, in particular, are a high-risk group for back injury and a code of practice has been published by the RCN Advisory Panel for Back Pain in Nurses (1996). Both employer and employee responsibilities are set out and there are specific guidelines for assessment and planning of patient care (see Box 10.6).

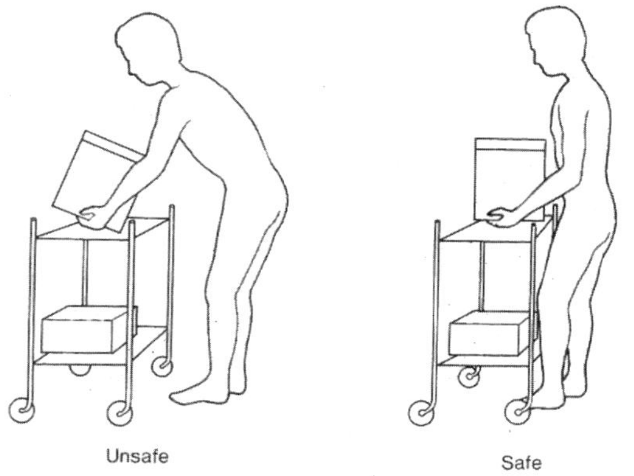

Fig. 10.16 Examples of safe and unsafe lifting. (Reproduced with kind permission from Jamieson et al 1997.)

For information about lifting practices, see National Back Pain Association and the Royal College of Nursing (1996) and Jamieson et al (1997), pp. 219–226.

10.12 Find out what lifting aids are available in the clinical area to which you are currently attached. How often are they used? What different techniques for lifting and handling patients have you personally used?

Box 10.6 The management of patients/clients (RCN Advisory Panel for Back Pain in Nurses 1996)

Assessment and planning

1. Particularly heavy patients, or helpless patients with no ability to assist nurses, need to be individually assessed by a competent patient handling team. Nurses in training and support workers should not be expected to undertake these assessments without competent supervision.
2. The care plan or profile should include the following information:
   - The current weight of the patient
   - The extent of the patient's ability to assist and weight-bear, and any other relevant information
   - The technique to be employed to handle that particular patient which should be consistent with the activity undertaken. This should be based upon:
     —the task
     —the patient
     —the environment
     —the equipment
     —the lifters.
3. Where the patient weighs 50 kg (8 stones) or more, or the conditions are less than ideal, mechanical handling devices must be used.
4. Mechanical handling devices or equipment should be used for moving totally dependent patients from bed to chair, trolley, toilet, etc. Sliding equipment should be used for moving totally dependent patients in bed.

Recurrent back pain/strain

A patient who suffers recurrent back strain should be fully investigated and if no significant pathology is discovered, education about safe lifting and movement practices should be given, together with advice and support to assist the individual to adapt her lifestyle in order to cope with this chronic health problem. Complementary therapists may be found to be helpful with these people.

Prolapsed intervertebral disc

PATHOPHYSIOLOGY

The intervertebral discs consist of a firm nucleus pulposus surrounded by a ring of fibrocartilage and fibrous tissue which links two vertebrae together. Disturbance of fluid physiology within the disc, which is partly but not wholly due to the ageing process, causes the disc to lose its elasticity and ability to act as a shock absorber (Duckworth 1995). The disc space becomes narrowed and distorted leading to increased stress on the spine and intervertebral discs. Eventually the disc may rupture and the soft contents, the pulposus, will prolapse, causing compression and stretching of nerve roots or fibres. Dandy (1993) states that 90% of lumbar disc protrusions involve L4–5 or L5–S1 (Fig. 10.17).

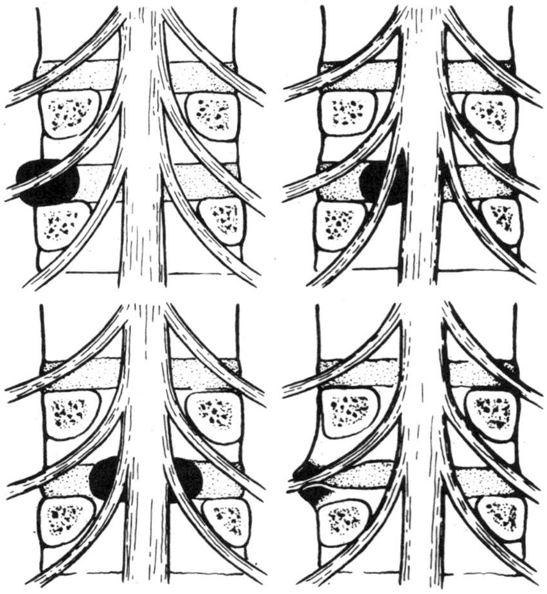

Fig. 10.17 Disc prolapse and root compression in the lumbar spine. A laterally placed prolapse may compress the L4 root, a more central prolapse will compress L5, and a central prolapse will compress the cauda equina. Osteophytes in the lateral canal will also produce root compression. (Reproduced with kind permission from Dandy 1993.)

MEDICAL MANAGEMENT

History. The classic presentation is of a patient with acute lumbar pain radiating down the thigh and lower leg; the precise position is dependent on the spinal nerve root affected, but a few patients may present with only leg symptoms. The patient may also be 'locked' in the classic bent position. There may be a history of dull lower back pain.

Examination. Muscle spasm and an intense focal area of pain may be identified. The straight leg raising test will indicate restriction of movement well below 90° of hip flexion and there may be neurological signs such as numbness, tingling or diminished motor function. If necessary, a MRI scan will confirm the diagnosis.

Treatment. Current orthopaedic opinion suggests that conservative treatment should always be attempted before surgical intervention. This would consist of analgesics, NSAIDs, muscle relaxants and minimal rest. The patient should then be mobilised having first been given general back care advice. Manipulation of a spine with acute disc prolapse is said to be dangerous as it could lead to a spinal cord injury (Dandy 1993).

The indication for disc excision is when there is proven disc protrusion with accompanying neurological signs and no improvement after 6 weeks of conservative treatment, or if any neurological deficit worsens. Intervention will comprise either of the following:

- *Disc excision* involves excision of the ligamentum flavum and inferior portion of the lamina (laminectomy) overlying the affected nerve root. The herniated portion of the disc and all disc material is excised, relieving the pressure on the nerve root. Symptoms are relieved in approximately 75% of patients (Dandy 1993).
- *Chemonucleolysis* is injection of an enzyme (chymopapain) into the prolapsed disc which breaks down the disc material, thus relieving pressure on the nerve root (Duckworth 1995). This procedure is done under image intensifier control and appropriate analgesic cover to prevent/relieve the accompanying pain which can be severe. There is a small possibility of anaphylactic shock. Symptoms are relieved in approximately 70% of patients.

As in both procedures some disc tissue will have been removed, there will be a reduction in its shock-absorbing function, and unnatural stresses may trigger degenerative reactions with the result that between 30 and 60% of patients may suffer permanent, though varying degrees of stiffness and back pain (Dandy 1993).

NURSING PRIORITIES AND MANAGEMENT: PROLAPSED INTERVERTEBRAL DISC

A patient who presents with a central disc prolapse is an orthopaedic emergency as the prolapsed disc causes pressure directly on the spinal cord. Without prompt surgical decompression, the presenting neurological manifestations will result in permanent disability.

Myelography. For care of a patient undergoing myelography, see Box 10.7.

Box 10.7 Care of a patient undergoing myelography

This investigation is used to provide clear radiological detail of the spinal cord, nerve roots and nerve root sheaths.

The patient will usually be admitted to hospital for 24–48 h when myelography is carried out. As it is an invasive procedure performed under local anaesthetic, preoperative preparation should be implemented. The patient may have a light snack before the investigation. The radiopaque contrast medium is injected into the subarachnoid space through a lumbar puncture. An adverse reaction to the contrast medium may occur during the procedure, such as anaphylactic shock, convulsions, hypotension or cardiac arrest. All emergency equipment should be present in the radiological department and the staff should be skilled in emergency patient care.

Care following the procedure depends on the type of contrast medium used. This should be clearly defined in the patient's notes, along with specific instructions for positioning. For example, if a water-based solution is used (Amipaque), the patient will need to sit up for at least 6 h until the remaining contrast medium has been absorbed. If she lies flat, the medium will move towards the brain and act as an irritant which may cause chemical meningitis or convulsing.

Twenty per cent of patients are said to suffer from headache and some experience nausea for 24 h after a myelogram (Powell 1986). A mild analgesic and antiemetic may be prescribed to alleviate these symptoms. Pulse, blood pressure and respiration rate are monitored at regular intervals until the patient is fully ambulant. If the headache persists for longer than 48–72 h after discharge from hospital, the patient should be advised to contact her GP.

Conservative treatment

As most of the conservative treatment can be carried out at home, it is the community nurse who will have responsibility for advising and supporting the patient and her family in all comfort measures. The care that might be given by the community nurse is described in Nursing Care Plan 10.1. Case History 10.4 provides background information about the patient.

Operative treatment

In addition to the general principles for perioperative care, the following points are specific to postoperative management of patients having a discectomy/laminectomy and chemonucleolysis.

Pain. This can be expected to be severe following chemonucleolysis, but it may be complicated by the development of neurological deficit — therefore neurological status should be monitored carefully and prescribed pain relief administered promptly when indicated.

Positioning and mobilising. Frequent position changes should be encouraged, always maintaining spinal alignment. The patient can be mobilised as soon as her general condition permits. Slight flexion of the knees using the knee rest or a pillow for support while in the supine position will allow spinal muscles to relax. A pillow between the knees will provide comfortable alignment when in the lateral position.

Early mobilisation is usually prescribed. The bed should be lowered and the patient taught to roll herself to the edge, swing her legs to the floor and stand up in one smooth movement.

DISLOCATED SHOULDER

Shoulder dislocation is addressed here because it is a fairly common sporting injury. It is a very painful condition with associated muscle spasm and usually requires i.v. sedation and analgesics, or possibly a general anaesthetic during reduction of the dislocation.

NURSING PRIORITIES AND MANAGEMENT: DISLOCATED SHOULDER

The arm should be supported in a sling until it can be manipulated following analgesic and muscle relaxant drugs. The colour, sensation and movement of the patient's injured arm should be monitored at regular intervals.

Nursing Care Plan 10.1 Community nursing care of patient with prolapsed intervertebral disc (see Case History 10.4)

Problem ***A, actual P, potential***	***Goal***	***Nursing intervention***	***Evaluation***
Communication **Pain (A) related to disc prolapse**	Improvement and control	Advise on: ❒ Self-administering medication ❒ Self-assessment on pain chart	Significant reduction in level of experienced pain
Anxiety (A) related to chidren's welfare and reduced mother role	Reduce anxiety by addressing causes	❒ Define problems — discuss with Mrs S and husband ❒ Neighbour willing to help Mon./Wed./Fri., husband at weekend ❒ Arrange nursery care for Emma Tues. and Thur. (social worker)	Mrs S will report satisfaction with arrangements Enquire daily Children and husband adapting and appear happy
Reduced mobility related to rest (A)	Maintain Mrs S in limited mobility — ensure comfort	❒ When lying in bed, advise to lie supine on a well supported mattress ❒ Mr S to assist with shower ❒ Ensure radio, TV, telephone, magazines available	Mrs S states she is more comfortable Adequate diversional therapy observed
Maintaining a safe environment (P)	Prevent accidental ingestion of Mrs S's medication by children Prevent other accidents	❒ Discuss problem with Mrs S, husband and neighbour ❒ Locate safe place ❒ Ensure child-proof medication cap ❒ Discuss potential home accidents — give Royal Society for Prevention of Accidents (RoSPA) leaflet	There are no preventable incidents or accidents Family and friends demonstrate raised awareness of safety — discuss leaflet
Nutrition (P)	Maintain balanced diet to prevent constipation	❒ Arrange friend to assist with food preparation ❒ Home help Tuesdays and Thursdays ❒ Mrs S to sit well supported when eating	Mrs S will report no constipation

Case History 10.4 Mrs S

Mrs S is 30 years old and married to a builder. The couple have two children, 7-year-old Tim and 4-year-old Emma. Mrs S is being treated at home for a prolapsed intervertebral disc, her prescribed treatment being pain control and neurological assessment. The community nurse plans to visit Mrs S until her condition begins to improve. She has already ascertained that Mrs S's next door neighbour is also a friend.

INFLAMMATORY AND DEGENERATIVE JOINT DISORDERS

This section focuses on two common joint diseases: rheumatoid arthritis and osteoarthritis (see Fig. 10.18).

Rheumatoid arthritis

PATHOPHYSIOLOGY

Rheumatoid arthritis (RA) is a systemic disease of connective tissue, characterised by a chronic/subacute non-bacterial inflammation of synovial joints and the surrounding tendons and their sheaths (Adams & Hamblen 1995). The disease also has extra-articular features.

The joints are acutely inflamed due to inflammatory changes in the synovial membrane. The synovium becomes thicker, very vascular and the site of increased cell infiltration which may cause an effusion within the joint that manifests as a swollen joint. As the proliferative tissue spreads as a 'pannus' over the articular cartilage, the cartilage is slowly eroded. Research has not yet identified the causal agent(s) of RA, although current work on the involvement of the autoimmune system has increased our understanding of the complexities of this disease (Duckworth 1995) (see Ch. 16).

MEDICAL MANAGEMENT

History. The disease may start gradually or acutely, often affecting the small joints of the hands and feet in the early stages.

The person with gradual onset of RA may present to her GP complaining of loss of appetite and weight, mild pyrexia, characteristics of anaemia and warm painful stiff joints, especially marked in the morning. As the RA progresses, more joints may be involved, with inflammation, swelling and progressive loss of function. The acute form of RA is characterised by multiple joint involvement from the onset with rapid progress to loss of function.

Examination. The affected joints will appear swollen, be warm to the touch, and the patient will complain of pain when the normal range of movement is attempted. If the joint is severely affected, some crepitus may be heard.

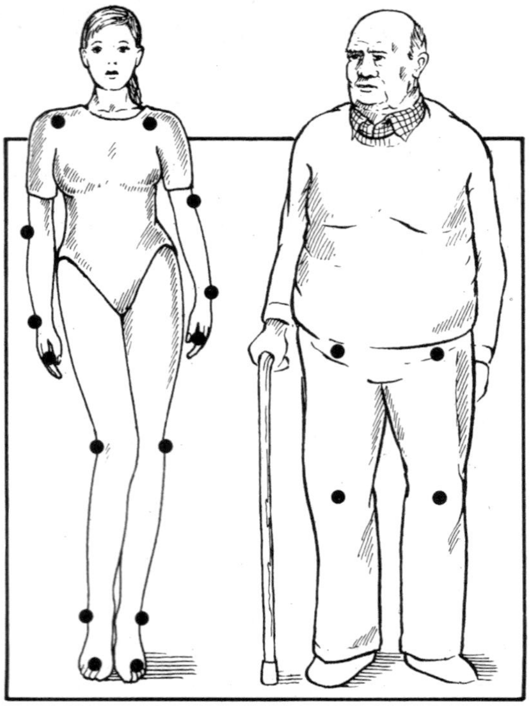

Fig. 10.18 Some differences between rheumatoid arthritis and osteoarthritis. Rheumatoid arthritis affects small joints, is symmetrical and is commonest in young women. Osteoarthritis mainly affects the weight-bearing joints and is more common in elderly and heavyweight people. (Reproduced with kind permission from Dandy 1993.)

Investigations. X-rays of both hands and feet will usually be sufficient to confirm the diagnosis. A blood specimen will be taken for assessment of the level of haemoglobin, number of white blood cells, erythrocyte sedimentation rate (ESR) , C-reactive protein (CRP) and the presence of rheumatoid factor.

Diagnosis. The diagnosis may be confirmed by the patient's history of pain and morning stiffness, radiological changes showing bone erosion, a raised ESR and CRP level and possibly a positive test for rheumatoid factor. Rheumatoid factor may be detected in the majority of patients who suffer from RA, but in some cases definitive diagnosis by haematological investigations is difficult, and therefore the medical practitioner may make a diagnosis purely from the patient's history and presentation (Dandy 1993).

Treatment. There is no known cure for RA, and therefore intervention is directed towards treatment of the disease characteristics. This will be the primary responsibility of a consultant rheumatologist in conjunction with an orthopaedic surgeon. The patient may receive non-operative and operative treatment.

The objectives of the rheumatologist's care are to:

- reduce the patient's pain with the use of analgesics and NSAIDs
- reduce joint destruction by curtailing the inflammatory process within the joint with the use of NSAIDs and/or early short-term use of local or systemic steroid therapy
- prevent or minimise deformity of a joint by splinting damaged or painful joints (see Fig. 10.19)
- assist the patient to adapt her lifestyle
- correct anaemia.

The orthopaedic surgeon will manage any surgical procedures which may be required during the course of the disease, such as:

- synovectomy — removal of excess synovial membrane from within the joint capsule of the affected joint
- osteotomy — division of a bone, which may be done to alter the weight distribution within a joint
- arthroplasty — remodelling of an affected joint using synthetic materials and/or metal
- arthrodesis — surgical fusion of a joint, which will reduce/eliminate the joint pain but create a stiff immovable joint.

NURSING PRIORITIES AND MANAGEMENT: RHEUMATOID ARTHRITIS (RA)

The aim of care is to maintain independence as long as possible and provide comfort and support. A multidisciplinary approach is essential, but coordination of care and implementation of major comfort measures are mainly nursing responsibilities which span both hospital and home. For this reason, these are given in detail below.

Controlling pain

Pain is the overriding and chronic problem and requires accurate assessment using an appropriate pain assessment tool. The National Medical Advisory Committee (1994) suggested that GPs and rheumatologists have the major contribution to make to the relief of arthritic pain, and the use of analgesics and NSAIDs will help to control such pain. When corticosteroids are used, the nurse should be aware of the serious side-effects, which can be life-threatening (see Ch. 5). Nurses need to be alert to these and should educate patients and their carers about this type of medication (UKCC 1992b). Due to the chronic nature of arthritic pain, narcotics are not normally used as a first-line medication and are usually avoided until all other medications have been tried and have failed to control the pain.

In an acute exacerbation of RA, the patient's affected joint(s) will be rested until the pain and inflammation process subside. This may require the use of a lightweight splint to hold the joint in the optimal position (Fig. 10.19). The splint will be removed for gentle physiotherapy, which will be increased as the inflammation subsides.

The patient should avoid cold environments, as low temperature has an adverse effect on joint stiffness. Where possible, the patient with RA should be helped into a warm immersion bath in the morning to ease pain and stiffness. At home, she may require bathing aids, such as a non-slip bath mat and a bath stool, which can be supplied by the occupational therapist. Cold packs placed over warm swollen joints and wax baths for the hand joints can give effective pain relief.

Maintaining independence and fostering well-being

Exercise and mobility. The patient will be involved in a daily programme of isometric and resistive exercises under the supervision of a physiotherapist (see Ch. 9). This will enable full joint movement to be maintained. If possible, the programme should include a routine of lying prone at least twice a day to prevent formation of joint contractures which can further reduce mobility. Alternately sitting and standing, i.e. regularly changing position, will also reduce development of joint contractures.

When handling an inflamed joint, the nurse should avoid grasping movements. The limb should be supported above and below the joint using an open-handed technique.

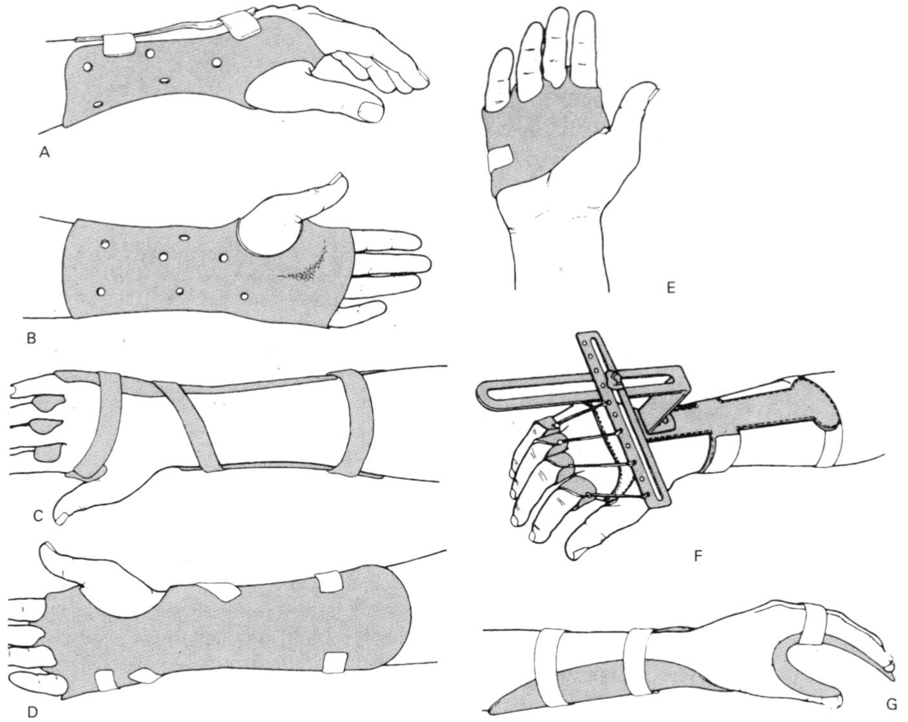

Fig. 10.19 Different types of splint. A–E: Resting splints. F: Functional splint used to stabilise a joint during activity. G: Corrective splint to immobilise a joint, realign soft tissue or correct contracture or deformities. (Reproduced with kind permission from Walsh 1997.)

The muscle power of the patient with RA is reduced, and therefore the use of aids such as a variable-height bed, raised chair and an ejector chair may be of assistance.

Walking aids, such as a stick or elbow crutches, may help to retain the patient's level of mobility by reducing the weight load placed on specific joints. The hand pieces of the aids may need to be adapted to accommodate the finger and wrist deformities that are common features of the disease.

The patient should be reminded not to carry heavy objects as this will increase the load on the affected joints. Stress and strain on small joints such as the fingers should also be avoided.

Safety. The nurse should assist the patient to identify potential hazards in the home and workplace, such as the storage of medications and the suitability of floor coverings. The hospital environment should be hazard-free.

Diet. A patient with RA is likely to develop anaemia due to the chronic inflammatory process of the disease and drug therapy. Iron supplements may be prescribed. Advice about dietary iron supplements should be given.

A number of NSAIDs have the common side-effect of constipation. This should be explained to the patient and an increased dietary intake of fibre advised. The patient with RA may require assistance in maintaining her nutritional status due to anorexia and/or difficulty in using eating and drinking utensils. Frequent, light, appetising meals should be served. The occupational therapist can supply a variety of utensils, such as large-handled cutlery and a tilting kettle stand, which will help the patient to retain independence.

Clothing. The fastenings of clothing may need to be adapted; the use of Velcro is of great benefit to patients with RA.

The patient may suffer from a prolonged mild pyrexia due to the chronic inflammatory process, resulting in the need for frequent attention to personal hygiene and changes of clothing.

Skin care. The patient's skin can be extremely fragile due to the disease and/or side-effects of some of the medications, particularly corticosteroids. Ongoing risk assessment of skin breakdown caused by restriction of movement and the effects of equipment is necessary. Preventive measures should be taken, such as regular position changes and the use of pressure-relieving aids.

Eliminating. The use of a raised toilet seat will be beneficial, as this prevents the necessity to flex the hips and knees to 90°. A grab rail on the wall next to the toilet will also help when attempting to sit or stand.

Sleep. The physical and psychological recuperative benefits of sleep are such that the patient should be advised and encouraged to maintain as regular a sleep pattern as the painful nature of the disease will allow (see Ch. 25). In order to facilitate beneficial rest, pain, so detrimental to sleep, must be relieved using conventional or alternative therapies. With more severe cases, it may be necessary to fit night-resting splints, which will prevent painful muscle spasm. The patient may require assistance to position, secure and remove these splints.

Patient education. The patient should be alerted to possible side-effects of the drugs she is taking and told what action to take should they occur. Information about the disease and the various treatment regimens should be freely available because this tends to help reduce anxiety. There are numerous information booklets that can be used by patients; some will have been written by local staff, while others are supplied by national charity organisations such as the Arthritis and Rheumatism Council (ARC) (see p. 427).

Counselling and support

It may be necessary for patients with RA to modify or change their jobs due to limitations of mobility. Long periods of illness and absence from the workplace may cause employment to be problematic. The disablement resettlement officer's assistance in finding appropriate employment may be of benefit. Some patients will reach a stage where full-time employment is impossible. When this happens, the patient will become a registered disabled person who is eligible for various benefits and allowances, available from the Department of Social Security.

Modification of the structure and content of the home may also be required when the patient's disability increases. This may involve minor additions, such as extra handrails to external and internal stairs, or major changes such as the instalment of toilet facilities at ground level. Frequently a patient may need to move to more suitable housing.

Self-image. As RA progresses, the joints may become so distorted that the patient may develop a negative body image. Helping the patient to maintain individuality and self-esteem will help to create a more positive body image. The nurse can help by suggesting alterations to the style of clothing, such as wearing a longer skirt over swollen knees in order to camouflage them.

Due to the nature of the disease and the effects RA has on a person's quality of life, the patient may suffer from periods of depression which may necessitate the use of antidepressive medication.

Sexual activity. Counselling regarding sexual activity may be required. The Arthritis and Rheumatism Council and the Association to Aid the Sexual and Personal Relationships of People with a Disability (SPOD) have both produced booklets containing useful information for RA patients and their partners (see p. 427).

Social contact. It is important that every effort is made to maintain social contact, even when the patient may be house-bound. Family, friends and RA self-help groups will assist in this sphere.

Rheumatoid arthritis inevitably affects the lives of the patient's family members; they too will have a need for counselling and support (see Research Abstract 10.3).

Research Abstract 10.3
Rheumatoid arthritis — effects on the family

Prior to this study there has been little research into the impact of rheumatoid arthritis (RA) on the families of people with this crippling and painful disease.

A qualitative study was undertaken on 22 patients with RA, their well partners and their 40 children.

The findings suggest that the disease has wide-ranging effects on work patterns and family roles depending on personality types, pre-existing relationships and ability to adapt to increasing restrictions. The frustration of not being able to go out and do 'useful' work was more evident in men than in women. Lack of social support networks and professional awareness of the total impact of the disease on both the patient's and the partner's work patterns, along with the impact of altered financial status on the family, was perceived to be problematic.

Sexual relationships were affected by physical symptoms and changed body image, but this was seldom discussed between the partners and for the majority did not result in a real threat to the marriage, although it added to the stresses of coping.

For most children, the effects of living with a parent with a chronic and disabling disease were not detrimental, although a minority did suffer physical and verbal abuse as a result; many expressed fear of getting the disease but most said they themselves would like to have children. Very few took on extra duties within the home, because the partner usually compensated for the patient's role. Stresses were evident but in some instances family bonds were strengthened by the increased awareness of relationships and everyday values.

Recommendations coming from the families were that they should have ready access to more information about the disease and earlier involvement in caring for the patient's changing needs. This information is actually available, as are support groups, but does not appear to reach many families. There was an obvious need for counselling and support at two critical points: firstly with initial diagnosis, and secondly when work patterns for both partners become radically changed. The role of the community nurse and the specialist rheumatology nurse is obvious here.

Le Gallez P 1993 Rheumatoid arthritis: effects on the family. Nursing Standard 7(39): 30–34.

Osteoarthritis

PATHOPHYSIOLOGY

Osteoarthritis is a non-inflammatory degenerative condition affecting the hyaline cartilage of synovial joints. This is the most common musculoskeletal condition causing disability in the UK, with the large weight-bearing joints of the lower limb, such as the hips and knees, being the most commonly affected (Footner 1992).

People with osteoarthritis do not normally feel ill. The disease may be classified as primary or secondary, the former being a progressive condition of unknown origin due to degeneration of the cartilage and changes in the underlying bone. It is more common in the older person, and females are more frequently affected (Dandy 1993). Secondary osteoarthritis can affect people of any age or sex and is usually associated with a previous injury/condition of the joint.

MEDICAL MANAGEMENT

History and examination. The first indication a patient with osteoarthritis of a hip joint may have that something is wrong is a dull nagging pain, most commonly felt when bearing weight on or moving the affected joint, but which can also manifest itself during periods of rest or sleep. The patient may suffer from referred pain in the knee or thigh and may visit her GP erroneously complaining of a knee problem when in fact it is a hip joint that is affected. Loss of function and movement of a joint may occur if the pain is severe. The patient may not be aware of a shortening of the limb which may cause a limp.

The normal range of movement of a joint will be reduced. A fixed flexion deformity and wasting of the hip muscles may be present.

Investigations. Plain radiographs (X-ray) of the affected joint will be taken.

Diagnosis. This is confirmed by the patient history and the appearance of the joint on the X-ray showing narrowing of the joint space and possible osteophyte formation.

Treatment. This can be classified into non-operative and surgical (Box 10.8).

Radiological evidence can be misleading in relation to the level of pain and disability experienced by the patient, and therefore the

Box 10.8 Treatment of the patient with osteoarthritis

Non-operative
- Explanation
- Analgesics and NSAIDs
- Physiotherapy
- Walking aids
- Occupational therapy
- Shoe raise
- Modification of life

Surgical (Fig. 10.20)
- Osteotomy — removing parts of a bone to correct line of weight-bearing
- Arthrodesis — fusion of a joint
- Arthroplasty — creation of a joint

orthopaedic surgeon will listen carefully and usually be guided by the patient regarding the decision as to which form of treatment is most suitable. There are many facts to be considered before coming to this decision, such as the age of the person, general medical status, home and family circumstances, level of disability and, most importantly, the level of pain the person is experiencing and how disruptive it is to normal life.

Examples are as follows:

- An overweight 50-year-old male patient who has a physically demanding occupation which causes stress and strain to his joints would benefit initially from conservative treatment. He may require surgical intervention at a later date.
- An elderly lady who places less stress and strain on her joints would benefit greatly from an arthroplasty. The incidence of complications arising following an arthroplasty is increased when the patient is under 60 years of age, obese or physically highly active (Dandy 1993).

Operative treatment. There are many variations on surgical procedures for osteoarthritis which usually involve either partial or total joint replacement (see Fig. 10.20).

Joint replacement has revolutionised the lifestyle of thousands of patients who have suffered severe chronic pain and the disabling effects of this degenerative condition.

Hip replacements are now a common procedure, although there are still problems associated with loosening of prostheses and failure due to infection which can lead to dislocation of the replacement. Research continues into technical and material improvements. Figure 10.21 illustrates types of prostheses used in hip replacement (see Case History 10.5).

Postoperative complications

Dislocation of the femoral component. O'Brien et al (1997a) suggest that a number of factors will influence dislocation, such as age, gender, care immediately following surgery and type of lifestyle activities in the months after hip replacement. Many of these factors have implications for nursing care.

To help prevent dislocation, some orthopaedic surgeons request that the patient is nursed sitting with no more than 45° of flexion at the hip joint. A Charnley wedge or foam troughs in which the patient's lower legs rest may also be used to reduce excessive adduction which can increase the incidence of dislocation of the hip joint replacement. These two measures are thought to decrease the physical strain placed on the operation site and thus prevent the development of laxity of the hip joint by stabilising tissues following the trauma of surgery.

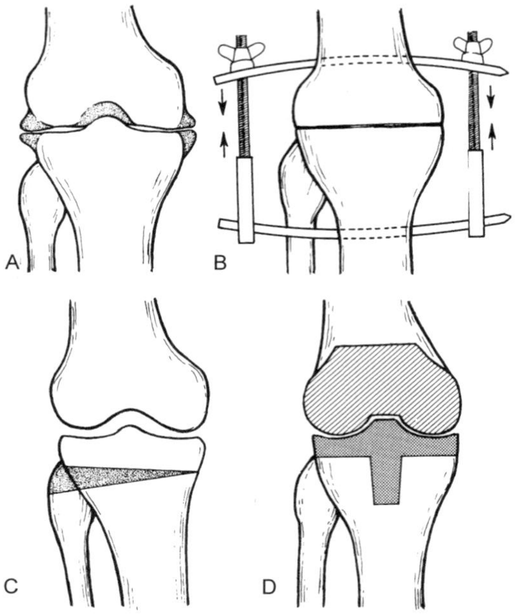

Fig. 10.20 Operations for osteoarthritis. A: Debridement and removal of osteophytes. B: Arthrodesis. C: Osteotomy to correct alignment. D: Total joint replacement. (Reproduced with kind permission from Dandy 1993.)

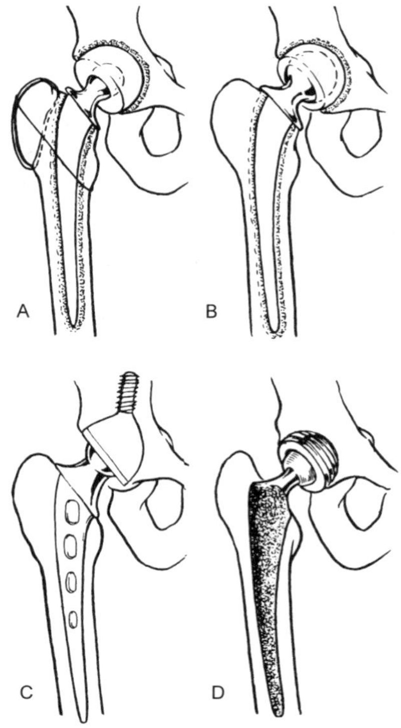

Fig. 10.21 Types of total hip replacement. A: Charnley hip replacement with greater trochanter reattachment. B: Müller-type replacement with larger femoral head. C: Ring-type replacement using a long threaded acetabular component, without cement. D: Uncemented prosthesis with sintered surfaces and screw-in acetabular prosthesis. (Reproduced with kind permission from Dandy 1993.)

Case History 10.5 The patient's perceptions of an experience surrounding total hip replacement

Two months after an operation for hip replacement I am trying to record my experiences, but one thought predominates to such an extent that everything else fades into insignificance. I can think of nothing other than the fact that I have no pain: no pain walking, no pain sitting, no pain lying in bed, no pain at all. Two ideas arise from this: one, that it does not seem at all healthy to be so conscious of the absence of pain. The hope must be that sooner or later being pain-free will become the normal unobserved fact of life. The other is a retrospective awareness of the debilitating effect of continuous chronic pain, the insidious way in which everything developed. People now keep exclaiming that I look so well, that my colour has improved so much. They never in the past told me that I looked old and grey. This must have been as unremarkable to others as the experience of continuous pain was to me.

There were many different kinds of pain. The worst in intensity was probably the pain on weight-bearing, but somehow it did not bother me so very much, I felt I could anticipate it, control it by leaning on a stick or furniture, or by refraining from walking altogether. There were sudden and very acute bouts of pain, sharp like toothache, on sudden movements or jolts, but these passed and did not matter much. There was the impossibility of ever sitting or lying in comfort — much less severe pain, but the most difficult to bear. It was when that particular pain suddenly got much worse that I first told the GP how I felt. When, in spite of anti-inflammatory painkillers, even the weight of the sheet became intolerable and lack of sleep became difficult to cope with, an appointment was made with the Orthopaedic Specialist Services. The nature of the worst of the continuous pain, however, was none of these; it was almost not experienced as pain at all. It was a deep nagging, dragging, twisting sensation which was nauseating and depressing, not responding to analgesics at all, analgesics which I took in maximal dosage and which added to the feeling of nausea, depression and apathy. Neither the GP nor I myself was keen on the thought of surgery, the GP no doubt because he was conscious of obesity being a contraindication for surgical intervention, I myself because I knew of many cases when no great improvement followed hip replacement. As soon as my friends had heard that I had been put on the waiting list, example after example was related to me of how wonderful Mr or Mrs X, Y, Z were as a result of this operation — 'a new lease of life', 'years younger', 'never looked back'. But my own attention focused, not on their reassurance, but on those people I had met who had developed infections, whose prosthesis had broken down, who had to have a second operation. It was no help to see a television programme and read a newspaper article about the inferior quality of the prostheses which were coming on the market at that time.

Now after the operation I have joined the ranks of those who extol its virtue, but even the most enthusiastic supporters had not prepared me for the speed with which it would be possible to lead a normal life: walking within 48 h, discharged from hospital within 2 weeks, fully independent by the time of the follow-up outpatient appointment 6 weeks after operation. Here, in summary, are the events which I now believe made the whole experience entirely positive: on first appointment at the orthopaedic outpatient clinic the thorough examination, the fact that the surgeon appeared to understand how much pain I had — perhaps even better than I did — and did not belittle what I was saying. The fact that he arranged immediately, before the operation, to start physiotherapy and that he promised an operation as soon as possible. I was on the waiting list for only 4 months. A week before the operation there was a day of tests and examinations in the ward to which I was to be admitted, giving a good opportunity to allay anxiety. I was glad that I had explanations of the operation, the anaesthetic and the possible risks. I appreciated the time taken to answer my questions and the sensitivity of the staff, though I do not think I could have entered into any decision-making in spite of the explanations. My anxiety about the postoperative phase, about living alone, upstairs, in a relatively large flat was well understood and arrangements were made by the occupational therapist, at that early stage, for various pieces of helpful equipment to be delivered to the house. I was assured that I would be fully rehabilitated by the time of discharge which was anticipated to be after about 2 weeks, but I found this difficult to believe.

On admission I was immediately aware of the cordiality and friendliness of the nursing staff and of the community spirit of the patients who made me feel welcome and who augmented the very adequate information given to me by the staff, both in print and in discussion.

Preoperative relief of anxiety and postoperative pain control were superb; after the initial intravenous analgesic cover, painkillers were offered every 4 h, but not really needed, except before physiotherapy, after the first few days. It was interesting to observe that all patients who had hip operations went through the same progression of skill acquisition and setbacks, learning how to get in and out of bed, how to turn in bed, how to walk, first with a Zimmer frame, then with two sticks, and later one stick, how to pick things up off the floor, to put on stockings and shoes, to shower independently, to dress and undress, to climb stairs and to get in and out of a car. It was evident that all the nurses knew exactly what each patient was capable of doing. All were willing to help but clearly expected and encouraged independence. Primary nursing was not practical. It would have made no sense to deploy the skills of the most highly trained and most experienced nurse on a patient approaching discharge, when newly operated patients needed them so much more. But their awareness of patients' progress and the supervision of the activities of less highly qualified staff were always in evidence. It was reassuring to notice that there was vigilance in case deep vein thrombosis arose and to see the speed with which one patient was advised to go to bed, the foot of which was raised, and how speedily support stockings were offered. With the emphasis throughout on what one can do by oneself and encouragement to get moving, it was a boost to self-confidence to know that nurses were vigilant for complications and setbacks. I found it helpful to have been shown the X-ray of the new hip as it makes it possible to visualise what the joint is doing during various activities, and to understand why one is advised never to cross the legs, to get on all fours or to pick things up off the floor from the sitting position. A pillow between the legs during sleep helps prevent crossing the legs accidentally.

There were 12 women in the ward, most of them in for hip or knee operations. The impression gained on admission of a friendly, supportive group spirit was reinforced throughout. What a wealth of experience, what a reservoir of knowledge, what abundance of empathy, goodwill and helpfulness. There was also a tremendous amount of fun and humour, perhaps enhanced by the experience all had of being pain-free all of a sudden.

I learned a lot, not only about health and illness, but also about emotional, social and economic stress, and about coping strategies. The importance of the patient community and its therapeutic potential is seldom recognised in general nursing but it should never be underestimated.

The patient will usually have one or more wound drains of the closed vacuum type in position postoperatively, although a recent survey has demonstrated that wound drains offer little advantage in the outcome of primary total hip replacements (O'Brien et al 1997b). The femoral bone tissue has an excellent blood supply; therefore blood drainage can be excessive compared with other forms of surgery. Accurate recording of the drainage volume is essential and, if excessive, the patient may need a blood transfusion. If a wound drain is used the nurse must ensure that contamination of the drainage system does not occur when emptying the collecting chamber(s). Autotransfusion is becoming a more frequent practice within orthopaedic surgery (see Ch. 18).

NURSING PRIORITIES AND MANAGEMENT: JOINT REPLACEMENT

Perioperative care

Perioperative care will follow the basic principles outlined in Chapter 26 with the following additions.

Prevention of infection. Bacterial infection of the bone around the prosthesis can have a severe debilitating effect and the prosthesis may have to be removed, leaving a grossly unstable joint; therefore prophylactic therapy is essential. In addition to basic attention to infection control, especially when undertaking invasive procedures, and attention to clearing up any septic foci, i.v. antibiotic therapy is commenced perioperatively and continued.

Communication and information. A full explanation of hip replacement procedures and pre- and postoperative care, which may require information pertaining to spinal anaesthesia, should be given and the patient's questions answered. In many centres, the patient will be assessed at a nurse-led preoperative screening clinic. A full explanation of the hip replacement procedure is given at this time and the prosthesis is demonstrated, unless the patient expresses a wish not to see it at this stage.

Deep vein thrombosis (DVT). Hip and pelvic surgery have the highest incidence of DVT, and therefore local policy to prevent this complication should be implemented. This will usually involve the fitting of anti-embolic stockings preoperatively. They should be removed and replaced twice daily for skin inspection and hygiene. An exercise programme will be supervised by the physiotherapist.

Urinary retention is a potential problem. If all purely nursing measures fail then intermittent catheterisation may be advised. The insertion of a self-retaining catheter should be avoided because of the risk of creating a septic focus. In some orthopaedic centres, oral or i.v. antibiotics may be administered prior to and after catheterisation, but as the research evidence is inconclusive this practice remains a debatable issue.

Mobility and rehabilitation. The patient may begin to mobilise as soon as her condition permits, which is usually on the first day postoperatively. This will be supervised by the physiotherapist and the nurse. A hydraulic bed is essential for correct manoeuvring as care must be taken not to flex the hip more than 45° when helping the patient out of bed or while sitting; therefore a high armchair should be used.

A walking frame may be used at first and the physiotherapist will re-educate the patient to use a normal walking gait. Depending on progress, the patient should practise using crutches or walking sticks before discharge.

Aids to living. The occupational therapist will provide aids for dressing such as tights or a stocking applicator and any other aids found to be necessary after an assessment of the home environment and the patient's capabilities.

Discharge planning

Discharge planning should begin preoperatively, and in some centres patients will be identified as suitable for an early supported discharge scheme where a hospital at home environment is provided (Black 1997).

The patient will be given a letter for the GP and one for the community nurse should that be necessary. The continuing medication regimen will be clarified. Written instructions on adapting to the artificial hip will be given to the patient and discussed in detail. These will include restrictions to normal mobility such as avoiding rotational movements, extreme adduction and hip flexion, leg crossing and any activity that puts stress on the new joint. Counselling regarding sexual activity should be included in the pre-discharge discussions. It is a subject often avoided by doctors and nurses, but it must be addressed because of the possibility of hip dislocation if the correct advice is not given, i.e. that sexual activity should be avoided for 6–8 weeks and that, once resumed, any position involving extreme hip flexion should be avoided.

Physiotherapy may be continued and a gradual return to a more active lifestyle than was possible preoperatively. (Read Case History 10.5 again.)

Q **10.13** From the information provided above, write a concise discharge plan for a patient who has undergone an uncomplicated total hip replacement.

SOFT TISSUE INJURIES

LIGAMENT INJURIES

PATHOPHYSIOLOGY

Excessive extension, flexion and/or rotation of a joint may result in a partial or complete rupture of a ligament. Whiplash injury is the term used to describe a ligamentous injury to the cervical spine area often occurring after a RTA (see Fig. 10.14, p. 409). This injury is due to excessive flexion and extension movements to the neck. A sportsman's knee joint can often be subjected to extreme rotational force which results in a severe ligamentous injury with often permanent disability.

MEDICAL MANAGEMENT

History and examination. People who suffer these injuries are often young and will complain of severe pain around the injured area after feeling or hearing something snap or tear. Pain may be increased when the person's body weight is exerted through the injured limb. Frequently, if other serious injuries have been sustained, this injury may be overlooked until the patient complains of pain from the ligamentous injury at a later time.

Limitation of normal joint movement may be found with swelling of the injured part. Joint instability may be noted during the physical examination.

Investigations. Plain radiographs are taken to rule out a bony injury to the area. A MRI scan or examination of the joint under general anaesthesia may be undertaken.

Treatment. Non-operative management is the usual mode of treatment. If bleeding into the injured joint (haemarthrosis) has occurred, this may be aspirated under local anaesthesia. The injured area will be supported, e.g. using a cervical collar for a whiplash injury (Fig. 10.22) or a POP cylinder/knee brace for a knee injury. Surgical intervention is usually needed only when the injury affects the knee joint or where there is damage to more than one ligament and/or gross instability of the joint.

NURSING PRIORITIES AND MANAGEMENT: LIGAMENT INJURIES

The patient may arrive at the A&E department within a few hours of injury (see Ch. 27). In other cases, the patient may present 12–24 h after injury when the pain and swelling have greatly increased. If no other injury has been sustained, the patient may be treated and discharged to attend as an outpatient.

Pain. This will be the major patient problem on presentation at hospital. Such pain should be assessed (see Ch. 19, p. 665) and an effective analgesic prescribed. As ligamentous injuries are sustained following severe trauma to the body part, the surrounding soft tissues will also be involved, causing further bleeding which will increase the swelling and irritate the surrounding tissues, thus increasing the patient's pain. The use of NSAIDs will be of value to reduce the inflammatory process.

Muscle spasm. This is a common sign of soft tissue irritation and, if severe, the patient may need a mild antispasmodic to be prescribed as well as an analgesic.

Support/immobilisation. Refer to priorities and management of patients in casts (see p. 401). In addition, when a cervical collar is worn, it can usually be removed to allow daily skin care. Men should be advised to shave regularly, in order to keep the skin under the mandibular and neck regions stubble-free and thereby prevent irritation.

MUSCLE AND TENDON INJURIES

PATHOPHYSIOLOGY

These injuries are most often caused either by direct trauma at the site of the injury or by a sudden sharp movement of the joint associated with sports such as tennis and squash.

The large tendons and muscles of the lower limb are the most common sites of injury.

MEDICAL MANAGEMENT

History and examination. The patient will experience a distressing tearing sensation or a kick at the site of the injury and possibly an inability to put the foot down. Swelling and tenderness will develop within a few hours following the injury. Bruising will appear later and may be extensive and alarming for the patient.

On examination, a gap between the ends of the muscle or tendon may be felt.

Treatment. Initial treatment is by a cold compress and elevation to reduce the extent of the swelling. Contraction of the muscle should be avoided during the first few days following the injury as this will increase the extent of the swelling. Rest in the most comfortable position is advisable initially. A padded crepe bandage may be applied to help reduce the swelling and provide some gentle compression. The physiotherapist may use ultrasound therapy to help disperse the haematoma. The injury may take 6 weeks or more to heal.

Surgical intervention is seldom indicated in muscle injuries. Complete muscle tears and tendon injuries will require total immobilisation in a cast or splint until healed. A ruptured tendon may require surgical repair, especially following accidental or self-inflicted hand or wrist injuries.

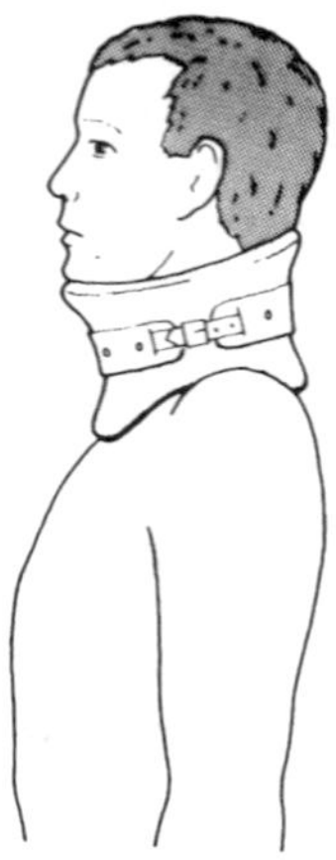

Fig. 10.22 Cervical collar. (Reproduced with kind permission from Allan 1988.)

NURSING PRIORITIES AND MANAGEMENT: MUSCLE AND TENDON INJURIES

Comfort. General principles relating to comfort and support will be implemented as required.

Swelling. Cold compresses using commercial cold packs or specially manufactured systems allowing ice therapy will help to reduce this. Care must be taken to protect the patient's skin from a cold burn, and the cold pack must be wrapped in a towel or similar material before it is applied to the skin surface. The injured limb should be kept elevated as much as possible.

Mobility. Once mobilisation is commenced, the physiotherapist will teach the patient to use the most appropriate walking aid, which is usually a pair of crutches. Assessment of the patient's home circumstances with regard to her mobility will be required. It is unlikely that any active physiotherapy will be given over the first 6 weeks following injury; thereafter the patient will attend as an outpatient. An ambulance may be required to transport the patient to and from hospital for these appointments.

Should the patient have a cast applied, advice and information about cast care will be given (see p. 401).

PERIPHERAL NERVE INJURIES

Nerves can be damaged due to underlying disease or following trauma. In this section, the focus will be on injuries following trauma.

PATHOPHYSIOLOGY

A single nerve or group of nerves may be damaged depending on the site of injury. Nerve injuries can be due to either direct or indirect force.

MEDICAL MANAGEMENT

History and examination. Following an accident, a patient may become aware of tingling (paraesthesia), numbness and/or loss of movement of the affected part. A common cause of a severed nerve is a cut from a sharp knife, a piece of glass or bone fragment. RTAs are frequently the cause of a crushing or stretching nerve injury.

Examination of the distribution of the loss of sensation and movement will assist the medical practitioner in making a diagnosis as to the extent of the injury.

Investigations. Plain radiographs are useful to assess bony injury and the presence of any foreign material, such as glass fragments, which may have caused the injury.
Diagnosis is confirmed by the absence or alteration of neurological function and sensation of the affected part. The specific nerve(s) can often be identified due to the distribution of the change in movement and/or feeling.
Treatment. Primary surgical repair is indicated only when a nerve has been cleanly divided. Secondary repair may include suturing and grafting of nerve tissue from a less important nerve within the patient's body. Non-operative management involves immobilisation of the affected part in the anatomical position, using a lightweight cast or splint. Peripheral nerves are capable of regenerating at a rate of 2–3 cm/month (Adams & Hamblen 1995). It is possible to calculate roughly the length of time of recovery although there is no guarantee that each nerve cell will heal.

NURSING PRIORITIES AND MANAGEMENT: PERIPHERAL NERVE INJURIES

A patient who suffers a nerve injury may come to hospital immediately after being injured or there may be a time delay before the full extent of the injury is realised.

As the patient will have been involved in some form of trauma, nursing care as outlined in Chapter 27 will apply.

Should the patient require surgery, general perioperative care will be as described in Chapter 26.

Preventing further injury

The major problem will be loss of function and sensation of the body area supplied by the injured nerve. As the patient will have partial or complete loss of the protective mechanisms of touch and pain, care must be taken to prevent further injury to the affected part. Movement of the injured limb must be through the normal range of passive joint movements; otherwise joints, muscles, tendons, ligaments and other nerves could be damaged further. To prevent the development of joint contracture and deformity, the patient will be fitted with a lightweight splint which holds the joints in their anatomical position. This may be needed for a long period. Exposure to extremes of temperature should be avoided, thus preventing the development of a skin burn. Loss of function and/or sensation of any part of the body is extremely frightening. The members of the health care team need to give easily understood explanations to the patient and her relatives during the period of treatment and rehabilitation to help reduce anxiety.

Subsequent considerations

Pain. Sharp shooting pain and a constant tingling sensation can be very troublesome and the patient may need prolonged use of analgesics. Antidepressants such as amitriptyline are known to be beneficial as a supplementary medication in the relief of neuropathic pain. Diversional therapy as organised by both the physiotherapist and the occupational therapist can be helpful should the acute pain become a chronic problem.

The nurse may also wish to suggest as an adjunct the use of one of the many alternative therapies that are widely available.
Washing and dressing. The patient will need advice and information to assist in adapting her usual mode of personal cleansing and dressing. For instance, a patient with a median nerve injury due to a laceration of the wrist of her dominant hand may have difficulty in brushing her teeth or combing her hair. The occupational therapist can provide advice and appropriate aids.
Splints. If a splint is used, the patient will need information and advice about the correct method of application and removal. The patient with sensitive skin has to be taught to inspect it for signs of pressure by removing the splint at regular intervals throughout the day.
Exercise. The physiotherapist will exercise the joints of the injured limb passively to prevent stiffness and muscle wasting. The patient may be able to use her own hands to exercise her joints, or a relative can be taught the skill of passive exercises. Not only will this assist physical recovery but it can also be of psychological benefit.
Support. As a peripheral nerve injury may take many weeks to recover, the patient will require support and understanding from family, friends and the members of the health care team to relieve boredom and prevent the development of depression. Group sessions for patients with similar injuries who are receiving physiotherapy, occupational therapy and/or diversional therapy can create an excellent psychological support mechanism for all concerned. The social worker can assist with any social and/or financial problems which may develop due to the possible lengthy absence from employment.
Permanent disability. If the nerve injury prevents the patient from returning to her previous occupation, it will be necessary for the local occupational resettlement officer to be contacted. For example, a butcher who sustains a severe injury to the nerves of the dominant hand, which leaves a permanent paralysis, will not be able to continue with his previous employment. With retraining, he could be employed, for example, as a driver of an automatic vehicle with a slightly altered steering wheel.

In some instances, alteration to body image could have a severe psychological effect. Nurses should be aware of this and provide support and counselling as needed by the patient.

CONCLUSION

This chapter has outlined the basic principles of nursing management that relate to the more common musculoskeletal disorders and has focused on some of the critical factors that influence management and care in specific disorders. It has stressed that the focus of care is the patient and her family, and that the challenge to nursing increases with changing trends in health orientation, care in the community, early discharge home and an ageing population whose lifestyle has been revolutionised by joint replacement surgery and multidisciplinary care and support.

Trauma is a constant in human societies and musculoskeletal injuries will always be a fact of life. However, continuing research and more attention to health screening and health promotion have shown that many accidents and conditions are preventable and many diseases amenable to treatment.

A wide knowledge of musculoskeletal disorders is essential for both hospital- and community-based nurses, to enable them to respond to the needs of patients and their families, to work actively to prevent accidents and complications, and to give appropriate information and advice.

REFERENCES

Adams J, Hamblen D 1995 Outline of orthopaedics. Churchill Livingstone, Edinburgh
Audit Commission 1995 United they stand. HMSO, London
Allan D 1988 Nursing and the neurosciences. Churchill Livingstone, Edinburgh
Black C 1997 An evaluation of setting up an orthopaedic early discharge scheme. Journal of Orthopaedic Nursing 1(3): 119–122
Bridel J 1993 Assessing the risk of pressure sores. Nursing Standard 7(25): 32–35
Calcraft D 1995 Nursing input in Ilizarov fixation. Nursing Times 91(13): 26–28
Clinical Standards Advisory Group 1995 Back pain. HMSO, London
Dandy D 1989 Essential orthopaedics and trauma. Churchill Livingstone, Edinburgh
Dandy D 1993 Essential orthopaedics and trauma, 2nd edn. Churchill Livingstone, Edinburgh
Davis P 1994 Nursing the orthopaedic patient. Churchill Livingstone, Edinburgh
Donohue S 1997 Lower limb amputation 3: the role of the nurse. British Journal of Nursing 6(20): 1171–1174, 1187–1191
Duckworth T 1995 Lecture notes on orthopaedics and fractures, 3rd edn. Blackwell Science, Oxford
Footner A 1992 Orthopaedic nursing, 2nd edn. Baillière Tindall, London
Havard C 1997 Caring for the patient with cancer. In: Walsh M (ed) Watson's clinical nursing and related sciences, 5th edn. Baillière Tindall, London
Health and Safety Commission 1992 A guide to the Health and Safety at Work Act, 5th edn. HMSO, London
Health and Safety Commission 1995 Health and safety statistics 1994/95. HMSO, London
Health and Safety Executive 1992 Approved codes of practice for manual handling operations regulations EC 90 269. HMSO, London
International Spinal Research Trust 1993 Review. Burnet Associates, London
Jamieson E M, McCall J M, Blythe R, Whyte L A 1997 Guidelines for clinical nursing practice, 3rd edn. Churchill Livingstone, Edinburgh
Judd M 1997 Caring for the patient with musculoskeletal trauma. In: Walsh M (ed) Watson's clinical nursing and related sciences, 5th edn. Baillière Tindall, London
Kubler Ross E 1973 On death and dying. Tavistock, London
Law M, Wald N, Meade T 1991 Strategies for the prevention of osteoporosis and hip fracture. British Medical Journal 303(6800): 453–459
Le Gallez P 1993 Rheumatoid arthritis: effects on the family. Nursing Standard 7(39): 30–34
McCaffery M, Beebe A 1994 Pain: clinical manual for nursing practice. Mosby, London
McLatchie G, Harries M, King J, Williams C (eds) 1995 ABC of sports medicine. BMJ Publishing Group, London
McRae R 1994 Practical fracture treatment, 3rd edn. Churchill Livingstone, Edinburgh
Maher A, Salmond S, Pellino T 1994 Orthopaedic nursing. WB Saunders, Philadelphia
Morgan S 1989 Plaster casting. Heinemann Nursing, Oxford
Murphy S, Khaw K, May H, Compston J 1994 Milk consumption and bone mineral density in middle-aged and elderly women. British Medical Journal 308(6934): 939–941
National Medical Advisory Committee 1994 The management of patients with chronic pain. HMSO, Edinburgh
Nikolejsen L, Iikjaer S, Karsten K, Jorgan K, Jensen T 1997 Influence of pre-amputation pain on post-amputation stump and phantom pain. Pain Journal 72: 393–405
O'Brien S, Engela D, Leonard S, Kernohan G, Beverland D 1997a Prosthetic dislocation in customized total hip replacement: a clinical and radiographic review. Journal of Orthopaedic Nursing 1(1): 4–10
O'Brien S, Gallagher P, Engela D et al 1997b The use of wound drains in total hip replacement surgery. Journal of Orthopaedic Nursing 1(2): 77–83
Office for National Statistics 1997 General household survey. Stationery Office, London
Office for National Statistics 1998 Annual abstract of statistics. Stationery Office, London
Orem D 1995 Nursing: concepts of practice, 5th edn. Mosby, New York
Paton D 1992 Fractures and orthopaedics. Churchill Livingstone, Edinburgh
Powell M 1986 Orthopaedic nursing and rehabilitation. Churchill Livingstone, Edinburgh
Roper N, Logan W W, Tierney A J 1996 The elements of nursing, 4th edn. Churchill Livingstone, Edinburgh
Royal College of Nursing Advisory Panel for Back Pain in Nurses 1996 Code of practice for the handling of patients. RCN, London
Russell L 1994 Bone tumours. In: Davis P (ed) Nursing the orthopaedic patient. Churchill Livingstone, Edinburgh
Smith Suddarth D (ed) 1991 The Lippincott manual of nursing practice, 5th edn. Lippincott, Philadelphia
Spinal Injuries Association 1993 Annual Review. Spinal Injuries Association, London
Taylor I 1990 Ward manual of orthopaedic traction, 2nd edn. Churchill Livingstone, Edinburgh
Tucker K 1998 Compartment syndrome: the orthopaedic nurse's vital role. Journal of Orthopaedic Nursing 2(1): 33–36
UKCC 1992a Code of professional conduct for the nurse, midwife and health visitor. UKCC, London
UKCC 1992b Standards for the administration of medicines. UKCC, London
Walsh M (ed) 1997 Watson's clinical nursing and related sciences, 5th edn. Baillière Tindall, London
Wilson K J W, Waugh A 1996 Ross & Wilson anatomy and physiology in health and illness, 8th edn. Churchill Livingstone, Edinburgh

FURTHER READING

Bode P 1995 Imaging in multiple trauma: a concept. Current Orthopaedics 9(1): 49–55
Boore J 1978 Prescription for recovery. RCN, London
Dandy D 1993 Essential orthopaedics and trauma, 2nd edn. Churchill Livingstone, Edinburgh
Davis P 1994 Nursing the orthopaedic patient. Churchill Livingstone, Edinburgh
Hayward J 1975 Information — a prescription against pain. RCN, London
Jamieson E M, McCall J M, Blythe R, Whyte L A 1997 Guidelines for clinical nursing practice, 3rd edn. Churchill Livingstone, Edinburgh
McRae R 1990 Clinical orthopaedic examination, 3rd edn. Churchill Livingstone, Edinburgh
Marieb E 1998 Human anatomy and physiology, 4th edn. Benjamin Cummings, California
Robertson S 1993 Disability rights handbook April 1993–1994. Educational and Research Association, London
Royal College of Nursing 1992 Avoiding low back pain injury among nurses. RCN, London
Scottish Intercollegiate Guidelines Network 1997 Management of elderly people with fractured hip. SIGN, Edinburgh
Trounce J 1988 Clinical pharmacology for nurses. Churchill Livingstone, Edinburgh
Webb M, Scott R, Beale P 1997 First aid manual: the authorised manual of St John's Ambulance, St Andrew's Ambulance Association, the British Red Cross Society. Dorling Kindersley, London
Wilson K J W, Waugh A 1996 Ross & Wilson anatomy and physiology in health and illness, 8th edn. Churchill Livingstone, Edinburgh

USEFUL ADDRESSES

Arthritis Care
18 Stephenson Way
London NW1 2HD

The Arthritis and Rheumatism Council
Copeman House
St Mary's Gate
Chesterfield
Derbyshire S41 7TD

The Association to Aid the Sexual and Personal Relationships of People with a Disability (SPOD)
286 Camden Road
London N7 0BJ

Disabled Living Foundation
380–384 Harrow Road
London W9 2HU

National Osteoporosis Society
PO Box 10
Radstock
Bath BA3 3YB

RCN Orthopaedic Forum
20 Cavendish Square
London W1M 0AB

Spinal Injuries Association
Newpoint House
76 St James Lane
Muswell Hill
London N10 3DF

BLOOD DISORDERS

Fiona M. Duke

11

INTRODUCTION

Blood is a vital body fluid which, via the cardiovascular system, reaches all body organs and tissues. Its three primary functions are:

- to transport oxygen, nutrients and other substances
- to protect the body against microorganisms and other foreign materials
- to regulate homeostatic systems.

Disorders of the blood are diverse and may be acute or chronic. All age groups may be affected, although some disorders are more common in certain age bands than in others. Some disorders, such as haemophilia, are sex-linked. Others, such as sickle cell disease and thalassaemia, are more prevalent among certain ethnic groups; still others, such as nutritional anaemia, occur worldwide.

Causes of blood disorders

Contributing factors in the development of blood disorders can be divided into nine types:

- *Developmental*. Infants and elderly people can be predisposed to anaemia, the former group because of increased nutritional requirements for growth and development, and the latter because of poor eating habits resulting from such factors as depression and reduced mobility.
- *Genetic*. Inherited disorders include certain abnormalities of the red blood cells (e.g. spherocytosis), haemoglobin abnormalities (e.g. thalassaemia and sickle cell anaemia) and the lack of a clotting factor (haemophilia and von Willebrand's disease).

- *Dietary.* Nutritional deficiencies can be related to poverty, lack of knowledge about nutrition and healthy cooking methods, and to overriding political and economic circumstances.
- *Sociocultural.* Dietary habits leading to nutritional deficiency may be related to values and beliefs. Strict vegetarians, for example, may develop vitamin B_{12} deficiency anaemia. Lifestyle factors, such as a reliance on fast foods or a habit of skipping meals, can also lead to nutritional anaemias. Other social factors such as homelessness and unemployment can contribute to poor nutrition, leading to the development of blood disorders.
- *Environmental.* Exposure to industrial chemicals (e.g. benzene, lead, sodium chlorate) and to ionising radiation has been linked to the development of blood disorders such as aplastic anaemia, agranulocytosis and leukaemia.
- *Pharmacological.* Some over-the-counter and prescription drugs are known to cause several blood disorders (Firkin 1995). Agranulocytosis can be caused by dapsone (an anti-leprotic) and by some antithyroid drugs (e.g. carbimazole). Quinine, quinidine and heparin can cause thrombocytopenia by damaging the platelets. Prolonged use of aspirin and non-steroidal anti-inflammatory drugs (NSAIDs) can lead to iron deficiency anaemia. Most cancer chemotherapy agents cause myelosuppression and thus anaemia, neutropenia and thrombocytopenia.
- *Iatrogenic.* Surgical interventions that cause blood disorders include the use of prosthetic heart valves, which can damage red blood cells, and total gastrectomy which, through the resulting lack of intrinsic factor, leads to vitamin B_{12} anaemia.
- *Pathological.* Diseases which can cause blood disorders, particularly anaemia, include inflammatory diseases, malabsorption syndromes, cancers and infections.
- *Idiopathic.* In some cases of anaemia, especially aplastic anaemia, no cause may be discovered.

The nurse's role in the treatment of blood disorders

The nurse's role in caring for patients with blood disorders in a community, hospital or occupational setting will include the following functions:

- promoting health, e.g. by encouraging good dietary habits
- detecting early signs of illness such as fatigue, pallor, frequent absence from work
- assisting with medical investigations, e.g. bone marrow aspiration, dietary history-taking
- explaining tests, diagnoses, treatments and prognoses to patients
- educating patients about lifestyle, diet and medication
- providing emotional support to patients and their families
- referring patients to other professionals such as genetic counsellors.

Depending upon their work setting and specialism, nurses will play a variety of roles in the care of patients with blood disorders. Primary health care nurses, e.g. district nurses, health visitors and practice nurses, may be involved in health screening and may be the individual's first point of contact with the health care team. Hospital nurses may come across anaemic patients in all types of wards and units. Specialist nurses may work as sickle cell disease counsellors or in a haemophilia centre. Macmillan nurses may provide care at home for patients with leukaemia.

The particular needs of patients with blood disorders will vary in accordance with the nature of their illness. Some patients may present with one very acute episode of illness, e.g. massive haemorrhage, and then return to full health after treatment. More commonly, patients are diagnosed with blood disorders after a prolonged period of malaise.

ANATOMY AND PHYSIOLOGY

Blood is red viscous fluid which is pumped from the heart via the arteries to the capillaries in the tissues and returns via the veins to the heart. Its central role is to help maintain an optimal environment for the functioning of the body cells. It fulfils this role by performing the following functions:

- transporting oxygen, essential nutrients and other important substances (e.g. hormones, enzymes, chemicals) to all cells
- removing carbon dioxide and other waste products from the cell
- haemostasis
- protecting the body from microorganisms and antigens
- regulating water, electrolyte and acid–base balance
- regulating body temperature.

The total volume of blood circulating in an average adult is 5 L. Blood consists of cellular and fluid components, the main constituents of which are:

- water
- plasma proteins
- electrolytes
- nutrients
- hormones
- enzymes
- waste products.

Cellular components of blood

There are three different cellular components of blood:

- erythrocytes
- leucocytes
- thrombocytes.

These cellular components are developed in the active bone marrow found in the medullary cavity of certain bones of the adult. The sites of the active bone marrow are:

- ends of the long bones (e.g. humerus)
- ribs
- sternum
- ilia of the pelvis
- vertebrae
- skull.

These sites can be extended when there is an increased demand for blood cells. There is evidence that all types of blood cell are derived from a common pluripotent stem cell (Montague 1996).

Erythrocytes (red blood cells)

Red blood cells are biconcave discs. Haemoglobin (the molecule involved in the transport of oxygen within the red cell) makes up 33% of the red cell weight and gives blood its characteristic red colour. The thin cell membrane allows gaseous exchange between the cell and surrounding tissues. The cell is also soft and pliable, allowing it to pass along the capillary lumen easily. During maturation, the red blood cell extrudes its nucleus. The mature cell therefore has no capacity to reproduce, repair, grow or make haemoglobin.

Function. Oxygen is carried in the form of oxyhaemoglobin by the red blood cells from the lungs to the tissues. Carbon dioxide, as carboxyhaemoglobin, is transported from the tissues to the lungs.

Maturation (see Fig. 11.1). The total number of circulating red blood cells remains fairly constant at $4.5–5.4 \times 10^{12}$ cells/L to ensure that the optimum amount of oxygen is available to the tissues. To ensure this number, the body has to maintain a balance between the number of cells produced and the number broken down.

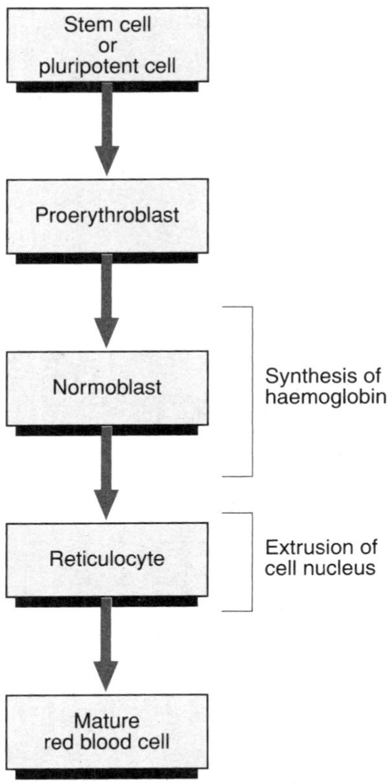

Fig. 11.1 Maturation of red blood cell.

The reticulocyte numbers are increased when there is a greater demand for red blood cells. Therefore, a reticulocyte count can be used as a measure of response to treatment for anaemia (a deficiency of haemoglobin in the blood due to a lack of red blood cells and/or haemoglobin content). Treatment should stimulate production of more reticulocytes.

The essential factors required for red cell production are:

- erythropoietin
- iron — part of haemoglobin molecule (see below)
- amino acids
- vitamins B_{12} and folic acid (both for DNA synthesis)
- vitamins B_6, thiamine, riboflavin, C and E
- intrinsic factor — for absorption of vitamin B_{12} from the gut
- thyroxine
- androgens
- adrenocortical steroids
- human growth hormone.

Haemoglobin is a complex molecule of haem and globin. The haem fraction is a combination of porphyrin and iron. The globin complex is composed of four polypeptide chains.

Destruction. The average life span of a red blood cell is 120 days. At the end of its life span, the cell is broken down in the bone marrow, spleen and liver by macrophages. The haemoglobin molecule is split into its major components: haem and globin. The globin is further split into amino acids, which are then stored in the body's amino acid pool. The haem is split into iron (which is stored in the liver and reused by the marrow) and porphyrin (which is converted to bilirubin). The bilirubin (insoluble in water and bound to albumin) is transported to the liver, converted into soluble bilirubin and excreted into the small intestine as a constituent of bile. From there, some is reabsorbed and excreted by the kidneys as urobilinogen. The majority of the bilirubin is excreted in the faeces as stercobilirubin.

White blood cells (leucocytes)

There are three types of white blood cells:

- granulocytes
- lymphocytes
- monocytes.

Granulocytes are characterised by the presence of granules in the cytoplasm and are divided into three subtypes: neutrophils, eosinophils and basophils. Lymphocytes are subdivided into T lymphocytes and B lymphocytes.

Normal numbers and percentages of each type and subtype are given in Table 11.1.

Function. The white blood cells are involved in the defence of the body against microbes and other foreign antigens (for further details of their functions, see Ch. 16).

Maturation. All white blood cells develop from the pluripotent stem cell in the bone marrow and mature through several stages as illustrated in Figure 11.2. Leucocyte maturation is regulated by several haemopoietic growth factors.

Lymphocytes mature in either bone marrow (B lymphocytes) or the thymus (T lymphocytes) (see Ch. 16).

Life span. The different types of white blood cells have variable life spans. Neutrophils, once they enter the blood, circulate for about 7 h and then migrate into the tissues, where they die after a few days. Lymphocytes have a variable life span, ranging from 100 days to several years. Monocytes, which mature into macrophages (scavenger cells) in the tissues, can survive for many years.

Table 11.1 Normal number of different subtypes of white blood cells

Type	*Subtype*	*Normal value (cells/L)*	*% of total*	
Granulocytes		$2.5–8.0 \times 10^9$	40–75%	
	Neutrophils	$2.0–7.5 \times 10^9$	40–70%	% of total white blood cell count
	Eosinophils	Up to 0.4×10^9	1–6%	
	Basophils	$<0.1 \times 10^9$	<1%	
Lymphocytes		$1.5–4.0 \times 10^9$	20–50%	
	B lymphocytes		15–30%	% of total lymphocytes
	T lymphocytes		40–80%	
Monocytes		$0.2–0.8 \times 10^9$	2–10%	

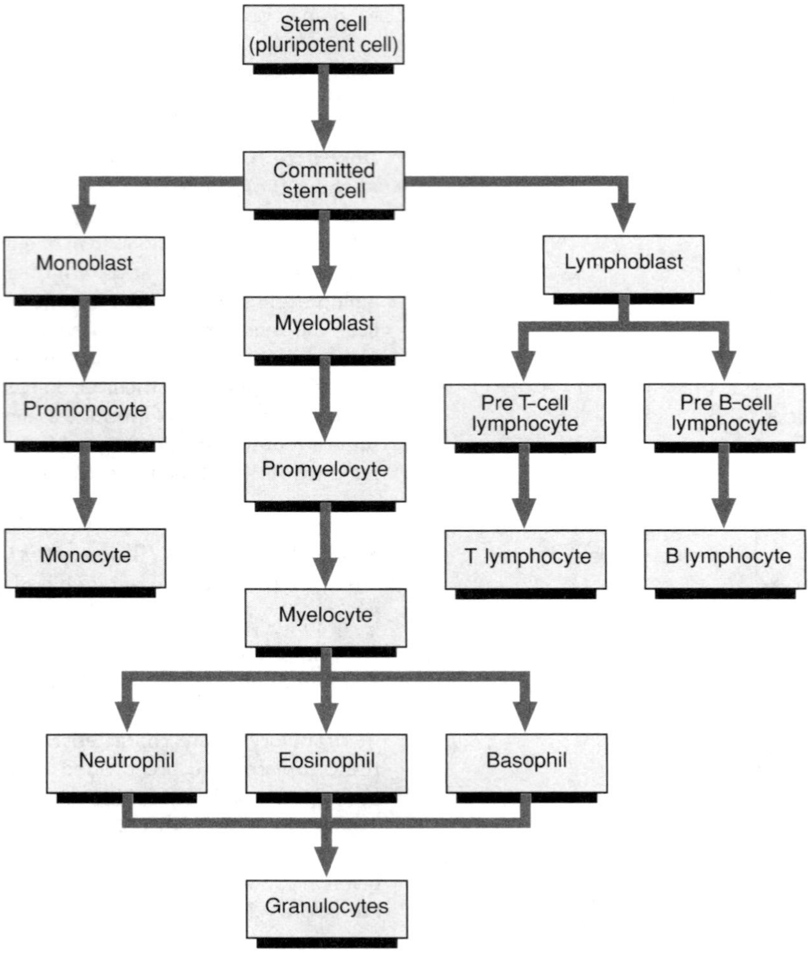

Fig. 11.2 Development of different types of leucocytes.

Platelets (thrombocytes)

Platelets are small, granular, non-nucleated blood cells that play a vital role in haemostasis (the arrest of bleeding).

Function. Platelets are involved in the first three phases of haemostasis:

- phase 1 — vasoconstriction of an injured vessel
- phase 2 — formation of platelet plug
- phase 3 — formation of fibrin clot.

The fourth and final stage, fibrinolysis (dissolution of the fibrin clot), does not involve platelets.

During phase 1 of haemostasis, narrowing of the damaged blood vessel occurs in response to the release of powerful vasoconstrictors — serotonin and thromboxane A — by the platelets. This reduces blood flow and thus decreases the likelihood of the platelet plug being sloughed off. In phase 2, platelets adhere to the site of the damage and release adenosine diphosphate (ADP), which causes the platelets to adopt a spherical shape conducive to aggregation. In phase 3, a fibrin clot is formed. This involves the conversion of prothrombin to thrombin, which then acts on fibrinogen (a plasma protein) to form fibrin. This fibrin clot is soluble at first but becomes insoluble in the presence of calcium and clotting factor XIII (fibrin-stabilising factor).

The formation of fibrin in stage 3 is made possible by two cascades of events known as the extrinsic pathway (events outside the damaged blood vessel) and the intrinsic pathway (events inside the vessel) (see Fig. 11.3). The extrinsic pathway is activated by the tissue damage. The intrinsic pathway is activated by exposed collagen. Each stage in the intrinsic pathway is regulated by a particular clotting factor. Together, the two cascades act on clotting factor X, which then activates the prothrombin.

Vitamin K, a fat-soluble vitamin, is required for the synthesis in the liver of the following clotting factors (Montague 1996):

- factor II (prothrombin)
- factor VII
- factor IX (Christmas factor)
- factor X (Stuart factor).

Q

11.1 What foods contain vitamin K? A

11.2 Where is vitamin K synthesised in the body?

11.3 Which patients are likely to have a prolonged clotting time because of vitamin K deficiency?

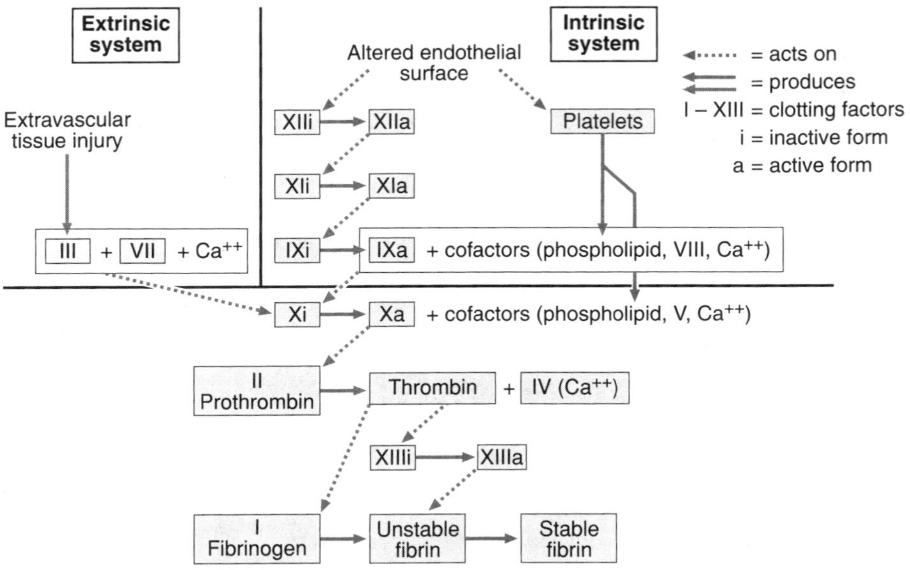

Fig. 11.3 Blood coagulation.

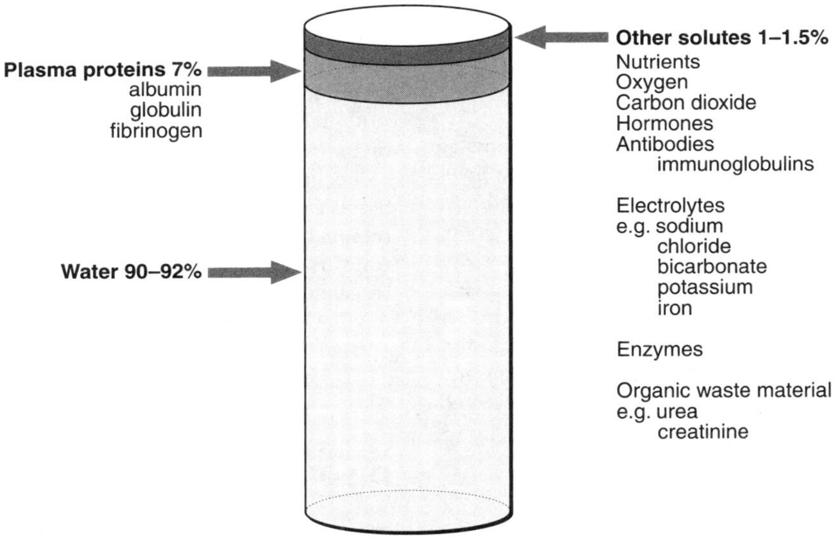

Fig. 11.4 The main constituents of plasma.

Plasma

Plasma is the straw-coloured fluid part of the blood which is left after the cellular components are removed. It contains blood clotting factors. Serum is the term for the fluid which separates from blood when it coagulates. It contains none of the blood clotting factors. The main constituents of plasma are shown in Figure 11.4.

Further details on the anatomy and physiology of blood can be found in Montague (1996) and Tortora & Grabowski (1996).

Blood groups

ABO blood groups

Red blood cells have specific antigens, called agglutinogens, on the red cell membrane. These agglutinogens are referred to in terms of the ABO blood group system. A person can have either the A or B agglutinogen on the red blood membrane, or neither, or both. Agglutinogens are inherited and are present from birth.

The importance of these agglutinogens is apparent when one person is given blood from another person. A person with the agglutinogen A (blood group A) has anti-B antibodies in his serum (antibodies are substances that cause clumping to occur when attached

Table 11.2 Antigens and antibodies present in different blood groups

Blood group	*Agglutinogen present on red cell membrane*	*Agglutinin present in serum*
A	A	Anti-B
B	B	Anti-A
AB	AB	None
O	O	Anti-A and anti-B

to particular antigens). A person with agglutinogen B (blood group B) has the anti-A agglutinin (or antibody). A person with both agglutinogens A and B (blood group AB) has no agglutinins, whilst a person with neither A nor B agglutinogens (blood group O) has both anti-A and anti-B agglutinins (see Table 11.2). Therefore, if a person is given a transfusion of blood of a different group from his own, the red cells will clump together and haemolyse (break down). In a blood transfusion, it is the reaction between the donor's red cells and the recipient's serum (i.e. between the introduced agglutinogen and the agglutinin already present) that causes an adverse reaction which can be fatal. Thus, if the recipient's serum has anti-B agglutinin present, the donor's cells must be either blood group A or O.

Not only the red cells but also the white blood cells and platelets have ABO agglutinogens. Therefore, if a patient is to receive a transfusion of other cellular components, the correct blood group should be used.

The Rhesus factor

In the UK, 85% of the population have a second important class of antigen present on their red cells: the Rhesus (Rh) factor (Campbell 1993). A person is either Rh-positive or Rh-negative. The antibody, anti-D, does not occur naturally in the plasma of Rh-negative blood, but stimulation to produce it can occur if a person receives a Rh-positive blood transfusion or if, during childbirth, red blood cells from a Rh-positive baby cross the placental barrier into the circulation of a Rh-negative mother. In either of these cases, if the person is later exposed to Rh-positive red blood cells, agglutination and haemolysis of the red blood cells will occur. Blood to be transfused must therefore be carefully cross-matched for the Rh factor.

The Rh factor is only carried on the red blood cells.

Other blood groups

The ABO and Rh factor blood groupings are the most important blood classifications, but there are more than 12 other blood group systems which normally do not cause agglutination unless the patient requires multiple blood transfusions, e.g. patients who have had a massive haemorrhage or who have leukaemia; in such cases it may be necessary to ensure the donor's blood is compatible with other known antibodies in the recipient's serum.

Blood transfusion

A blood transfusion is the administration to one individual of blood donated by another individual. The practice of blood transfusion makes it possible to save lives when severe haemorrhage has occurred, when major surgery is required or when there is failure of the bone marrow to produce blood cells. Transfusion does, however, expose patients to the risk of potentially fatal complications, e.g. infection and haemolytic reactions (see p. 441). The blood transfusion products available are given in Table 11.3.

11.4 Attend a blood donor session to find out about:

(a) the categories of people who are allowed to donate blood
(b) the screening process for blood donations
(c) the process of donating a unit of blood
(d) the care of the donor before, during and after the procedure
(e) how the blood is stored after donation.

Cross-matching

Before a unit of blood or blood component is transfused into another person, the blood from the donated unit must be cross-matched with that of the recipient's serum, i.e. the blood from the donated unit is mixed in the laboratory with a sample of the recipient's serum. The donor's blood should be of the same ABO blood group to prevent a potentially fatal agglutination reaction. A Rh-negative recipient should receive Rh-negative blood. Details of the results of the cross-matching are recorded along with the blood unit number on the documentation sent with the unit of blood when the blood transfusion is given. This documentation is retained after the unit of blood has been used in case of any transfusion reactions (see p. 441 for the nursing care of patients receiving transfusions).

For further details on blood groups consult Tortora & Grabowski (1996).

DISORDERS OF RED BLOOD CELLS

These disorders can be divided into:

- disorders in which there is a deficiency of haemoglobin in the blood due to lack of red cells and/or reduced haemoglobin content
- disorders due to blood loss
- disorders due to excessive production of the red blood cells.

ANAEMIAS

Anaemias are those disorders in which the blood has a reduced oxygen-carrying capacity. There are three main types of anaemia (see Fig. 11.5):

- anaemia due to decreased red cell production, resulting from:
  —reduced bone marrow function
  —lack of essential factors for cell maturation
- anaemia due to blood loss
- haemolytic anaemia — due to excessive destruction of the red cells.

Table 11.3 Blood transfusion products available

Product	*Indications for use*	*Special points*
Whole blood	Acute, severe bleeding requiring replacement of red blood cells and plasma and clotting factors	Stored at 4°C Remains viable for 35 days Platelets and clotting factors have much reduced viability
Fresh whole blood	As above	Blood <24 h old, therefore more likely to contain viable clotting factors
Red cell concentrate	Replacement of red blood cells only. Therefore used when haemoglobin level is low	Up to 200 mL plasma removed per 500 mL blood
Leucocyte-poor red cells	Indicated for patients who have had febrile reactions during previous transfusions: • patients undergoing transplant • prevention of cytomegalovirus transmission	White blood cells and platelets removed to minimise the risk of an incompatible reaction. Cytomegalovirus (CMV) could be transmitted to a person who has no CMV antibodies. This could be fatal in a patient who is immunocompromised (see Ch. 16)
Washed red cells	As for red cell concentrate. Specially prepared to remove antigens	Prevents anaphylactic transfusion reactions
Frozen red cells	As for red cell concentrate	Storage life span lengthened, therefore useful for rare blood groups
Platelet concentrate	Patients with platelet count <20×10^9 cells/L but not actively bleeding	Platelet units from blood banks contain platelets from many units of blood, therefore there are frequent reactions. Patient may require i.v. hydrocortisone + i.v. chlorpheniramine prior to transfusion. Stored at 20°C. Viability of platelet concentrate only 24 h
Granulocyte concentrate	Aplastic anaemia or other severe bone marrow depression + septicaemia not responding to antibiotics and antifungal agents. White cell count <0.2×10^9 cells/L	Rarely used. Must be tissue-typed (see Ch. 16) and therefore few compatible donors available Prophylactic i.v. hydrocortisone and chlorpheniramine given
Other blood components		
Fresh frozen plasma	Hereditary or acquired bleeding disorder Volume replacement Liver disease Disseminated intravascular coagulation	Frozen within 6 h of cell separation and viable for 1 year. Once thawed, use within 30 min
Dried plasma	As above	Advantage that it can be stored at room temperature and therefore is readily available
Cryoprecipitate (factor VIII, fibrinogen)	Haemophilia	From fresh frozen plasma. Last part to thaw is cryoprecipitate
Factor VIII	Haemophilia A	From fresh frozen powder (half-life 12 h)
Factor IX	Christmas disease	
Human immunoglobulin	Passive immunity, especially immunosuppressed patients	
Albumin solution	Hypoproteinaemic oedema, ascites, acute volume replacement	

Anaemia is extremely common worldwide; the overall incidence of iron deficiency is 20% of the world population (Barnard et al 1989). The World Health Organization (WHO 1972) defines anaemia as a haemoglobin level of less than 130 g/L blood for men and less than 120 g/L for women.

The anaemias are a complex group of red blood cell disorders, which may be:

- primary, i.e. the presenting illness
- secondary to another disease, e.g. infection, cancer, gastrointestinal malabsorption syndrome, chronic renal failure, or an inherited disorder of haemoglobin synthesis or formation
- acquired:
  —iatrogenic, e.g. drug-induced
  —environmental, e.g. benzene exposure
  —nutritional, e.g. iron, protein, vitamin B_{12} or folate deficiency.

Anaemia is found in all age groups. At each developmental

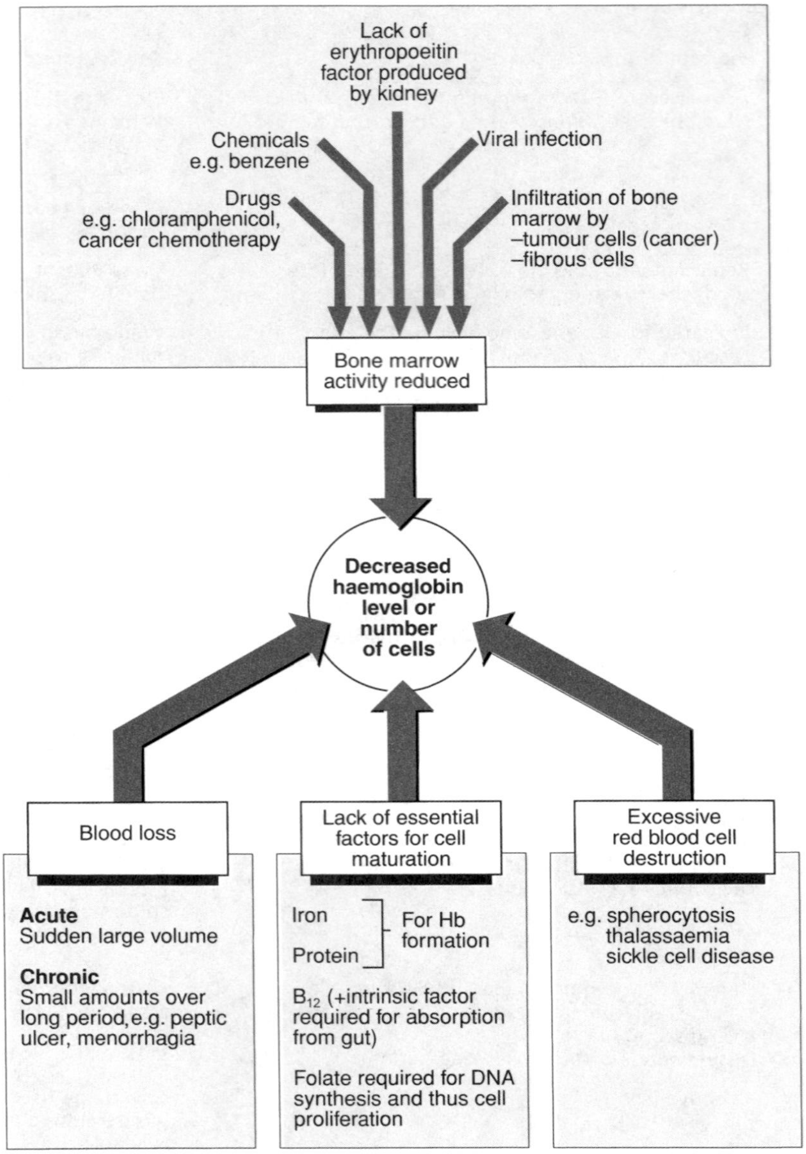

Fig. 11.5 Main types of anaemia.

stage there are potential dietary reasons for the occurrence of anaemia, as follows (Davies 1990):

- In infancy, anaemia can occur if a poor diet is provided, especially at the time of weaning
- In adolescence, a growth spurt may cause anaemia, particularly if during this period 'fad eating' leads to an inadequate intake of the essential nutrients for red cell formation (see Ch. 21)
- Women of child-bearing age may become anaemic due to menstrual blood loss for which inadequate dietary compensation is made
- In pregnant women, extra demands for red cell synthesis may lead to the development of anaemia
- In elderly people, poor eating habits resulting from difficulty in shopping, reduction in income, depression, poor dental hygiene or badly fitting dentures can all lead to a reduced intake of essential nutrients for red blood cell formation.

Q **11.5** In a group, discuss the social, cultural and environmental factors which might contribute to the development of anaemia.

Many people are diagnosed as anaemic only by chance when they seek medical advice for an unrelated symptom or attend a health clinic (e.g. antenatal or occupational health) for a routine medical examination. It is therefore likely that nurses working in any area of community or hospital nursing will care for people with anaemia.

PATHOPHYSIOLOGY

Anaemia occurs when the oxygen-carrying capacity of the red blood cells is reduced. Its symptoms all stem from a lack of oxygen in the tissues. Their severity depends on two main factors:

- haemoglobin concentration, i.e. oxygen-carrying capacity of the red blood cell
- ability of the person to adapt to lower oxygen concentration — some patients with chronic anaemia live very active lives with a haemoglobin level that in other people would cause severe symptoms.

Common presenting symptoms. The clinical features of anaemia are diverse. Each type of anaemia has specific clinical features but there are common presenting symptoms, as follows:

- Tiredness and lethargy — a very subjective symptom for which the person is unlikely to consult his general practitioner (GP). Some people have a variety of explanations for tiredness, e.g. the season, social life, stress and workload
- Breathlessness — a compensatory mechanism to overcome low oxygen concentration, which may be present only on exertion. The person may dismiss this symptom, thinking he is just 'not fit'
- Palpitations due to the heart increasing its rate to increase blood flow to tissues
- Loss of appetite — often an unexplained feature but may be due to dysphagia, sore mouth or sheer fatigue
- Dysphagia (difficulty in swallowing) and sore mouth due to epithelial lining fragility
- Oedema of ankles, especially at the end of the day — due to a degree of heart failure
- Dizziness, fainting and dimness of vision due to lack of oxygen to the brain
- Headache and lack of concentration — resulting from insufficient oxygen supply to the brain
- Angina and/or intermittent claudication because of impaired blood flow to peripheral and/or coronary arteries; this is especially likely in older people
- Bleeding, e.g. rectal bleeding, haematuria, haemoptysis or menorrhagia.

MEDICAL MANAGEMENT

To diagnose anaemia and establish its cause, it is necessary to clarify the patient's symptoms and discover if he has any other symptoms he may not consider significant or does not wish to volunteer.

History and examination. Careful questioning about the patient's state of health in the present and recent past and about his use of medication (e.g. aspirin, which causes bleeding, or phenytoin, which causes folate deficiency) may help to uncover the cause of the anaemia. A determination of the person's social circumstances and dietary intake may also be important.

An accurate and detailed dietary history is often difficult to obtain but may reveal deficiencies in iron, folic acid or vitamin B_{12}. This history may be taken by the GP, practice nurse or dietician. Questioning about social background should include consideration of:

- financial circumstances
- home circumstances
- work environment, including exposure to harmful substances.

Clinical examination may reveal:

- evidence of paleness of skin and mucous membranes (e.g. conjunctiva, palms of hands, buccal cavity) — this may be difficult to assess as many people are pale but not anaemic; assessment of pallor in dark-skinned people will be especially difficult
- signs of an underlying disease, e.g. cancer, hypothyroidism or infection
- signs of complications of anaemia, e.g. cardiac failure, glossitis, stomatitis, jaundice (due to haemolytic breakdown) (see p. 447)
- signs of pregnancy.

Investigations used in the diagnosis of anaemia include the following:

Blood tests. Not all of the following will be relevant for all patients:

- Full blood count — to establish total number of red cells, white cells and platelets. The result is compared with normal values (see Appendix 2).
- Blood film — examination of blood cells under the microscope to detect any abnormality in size or shape.
- Haemoglobin concentration — a level 10% below normal is usually considered a sign of anaemia.
- Haematocrit or packed cell volume (PCV) — proportion of total blood volume which consists of red cells. Dehydrated patients have a high PCV as the plasma volume is reduced.
- Reticulocyte count — a small percentage of reticulocytes are normally present in blood. A larger percentage may indicate increased bone marrow activity if the red blood cell count is low (see p. 431 on maturation of red cells).
- Mean corpuscular volume (MCV) — measures the average red cell volume.
- Mean corpuscular haemoglobin concentration (MCHC) — measures the average concentration of haemoglobin in each red cell. A low MCHC may be found when haemoglobin is low.
- Erythrocyte sedimentation rate (ESR) — measures the speed at which red cells settle in uncoagulated blood left standing for 1 h. The height of the plasma column above the sedimented blood cells is measured (in mm) and compared with normal height. ESR may be raised because of an underlying problem causing the anaemia, e.g. infection.

Bone marrow aspiration. This is the removal with a special needle of a small quantity of bone marrow which can then be mounted on slides and stained for examination under a microscope. This is not done routinely but is indicated if the anaemia is severe or has no apparent cause, or if there is evidence of another blood disorder such as aplastic anaemia or leukaemia (see Box 11.1).

Treatment. The type of treatment given for anaemia will depend on the cause and severity of the condition. A few patients will need to be hospitalised but most can be treated in the community by their GP. The treatment may involve medication and health education. Blood transfusions may be needed either initially or repeatedly over a period of time. Intervention will also include treatment of the underlying cause of the anaemia.

Treatment may be short-term (a few weeks), long-term (months or years) or, as in the case of pernicious anaemia, lifelong. Follow-up care for all anaemic patients is important to encourage compliance with medication and to prevent recurrence and long-term effects. This care may be provided by the GP or at an outpatient clinic.

NURSING PRIORITIES AND MANAGEMENT: ANAEMIAS

As the anaemias are such a diverse group of disorders, nursing intervention can take a variety of forms. It is vital that the patient is considered as an individual and that psychological, social and

Box 11.1 Bone marrow aspiration

Purposes
- Diagnosis — to examine cell populations and thus determine type of anaemia, leukaemia or lymphoma
- Monitoring — to assess progress of disease and response to treatment.

Sites
Red bone marrow is found in the cavities of the flat bones of the adult, e.g. skull, clavicle, scapula and iliac crest. The sites which are usually chosen (for ease of access to minimise trauma to nearby structures) are:

- Iliac crest — left and right, anterior and posterior
- Sternum — care is required to avoid cardiac tamponade (pressure on heart caused by pericardial haemorrhage).

The nurse's role
The patient may be anxious about this investigation, especially if he knows that the results may show that he has a malignant condition. This anxiety may be heightened if the patient has been talking with others who have undergone the procedure.

Providing the patient with information on all aspects of the test — the use of premedication and local anaesthetic, the site to be used, the degree of discomfort to be expected, the time that it will take, and when the results will be reported — will help to reduce his anxiety.

It is the policy of some doctors, especially where repeated aspiration will be required, to give a sedative such as lorazepam or a light general anaesthetic.

The individual may undergo the procedure as an outpatient, in-patient or in a day ward. Whatever the setting, the nurse's role will include:

- Assessing the patient's understanding of the test and providing more information if necessary
- Preparing the equipment
- Ensuring that the patient is comfortable and is positioned correctly
- Observing the patient throughout the procedure and drawing attention to any change in his condition
- Assisting the doctor
- Applying a pressure dressing and making the patient comfortable after the procedure
- Inspecting the aspiration site frequently for haemorrhage or haematoma formation
- Documenting the patient's response to the procedure
- Preparing the patient for discharge by explaining care of puncture site, what discomfort may be expected, whom to contact if ill effects arise, when results will be available and timing of the next appointment.

Possible complications
- Haemorrhage — patient's platelet count should be checked before aspiration
- Infection
- Cardiac tamponade if sternum site used — the needle should be fitted with a guard to prevent overpenetration.

environmental concerns are taken into account along with the medical considerations pertinent to his specific form of anaemia.

Certain nursing interventions will be common to all cases. The first task to be carried out is an assessment of the patient's background, illness, needs and goals. Following assessment, a treatment plan will be agreed between the patient and the health care team.

Life-threatening complications

The patient may present with any of the following potentially life-threatening problems:

- cardiac failure
- breathlessness
- shock.

These complications may arise if there has been severe blood loss over a short period of time or if a chronic condition suddenly enters an acute phase. This is more likely to occur in individuals who have other conditions such as hypertension, chronic obstructive airways disease (COAD) and/or pre-existing chronic blood loss (see Chs 2, 3 and 18).

Major problems of nursing anaemic patients

Tiredness

Anaemic patients will tire easily because of poor oxygenation of cells and tissues. Patients with severe anaemia will be exhausted after even the slightest exertion. It is important that their daily routine in hospital or at home ensures periods of rest. If cardiac failure is evident, they will need to be nursed in bed or in a chair. The nurse should be aware of the potential problems of immobility, paying particular attention to pressure areas. Such patients may require assistance with personal hygiene and dressing. They should be reassured that their tiredness is not imaginary but is part of the anaemia and that it will lessen as treatment progresses.

Breathlessness (see Ch. 3)

This problem will not be present unless the anaemia is severe (haemoglobin level below 8 g/100 mL of blood). The breathlessness may be mild, arising only on exertion, or it may be a major problem causing great distress.

The most important aspects of nursing the breathless patient are to ensure good perfusion of oxygen to the tissues and to reduce the patient's distress. This can be achieved by nursing the patient in an upright position (to allow maximum lung expansion and use of accessory respiratory muscles), administering oxygen as prescribed, explaining to the patient the reason for his breathlessness and reassuring him that it will lessen as the anaemia improves.

Breathlessness, if incapacitating, will require the nurse to assist the patient with personal hygiene, changing position in bed and mobilisation.

Nutrition

The anaemic patient will require a high-protein diet which includes all the nutrients necessary for red cell production (see p. 431). Breathlessness, a lack of energy to shop and prepare food, a sore mouth and dysphagia may all contribute to anorexia. A sore mouth can be especially distressing and the nurse will need to carry out an initial evaluation using an assessment tool such as that described in Eilers et al (1988) (see p. 458). Care should include not only that which will improve and heal the mouth but also relevant health education about oral hygiene and care of dentures, e.g. use of a soft toothbrush, regular mouthwashes and prevention of dry and cracking lips (Leach 1991).

It will be necessary for anaemic patients who have a low income and/or a poor understanding of nutrition to receive guidance in budgeting and the components of a balanced diet as well as advice about social security allowances. The multidisciplinary team may therefore include a dietician and a social worker.

Other important considerations include dietary restrictions deriving from the patient's cultural background and/or spiritual beliefs. Dietary restrictions may also be imposed by a pre-existing medical disorder such as diabetes mellitus. Elderly patients may have ill-fitting dentures which lead them to rely on a poorly balanced 'soft' diet. In such cases, referral to a dentist may be appropriate.

Safety

Giddiness, faintness, lightheadedness and reduced sensitivity to cold may make the anaemic patient prone to injury. Since the body responds to poor oxygenation by preserving the blood supply to the essential organs, anaemic patients will have poor peripheral circulation and, consequently, fragile skin. The reduced attention span typical of anaemic patients will also make them vulnerable to falls, minor injuries and hypothermia. Anaemic patients should be warned against changing position suddenly (especially from lying to standing) and should be given instruction on first aid for minor injuries and on the prevention of hypothermia (see Ch. 22).

Skin integrity (see Chs 12 and 23)

The anaemic patient's reduced oxygen and nutrient supply to the skin will make him susceptible to pressure sores. Hypoxic skin will not necessarily break down quickly, but if damaged it will take longer than usual to heal. When the patient's mobility has been impaired, either as a result of the anaemia or because of a concurrent condition (e.g. arthritis), the nurse must be alert to the importance of maintaining skin integrity.

An initial assessment of all pressure points should be made using such tools as the Norton scale or the Waterlow scale (see pp. 753–754). Once the patient's level of risk of developing pressure sores has been determined, an appropriate intervention should be planned. Prevention of pressure sores is likely to include ensuring that the patient's position is changed 2-hourly, the use of appropriate medical aids (e.g. silicone-filled mattresses and cushions, sheepskin pads, alternating pressure beds) and instructing the patient about the importance of regularly changing position.

Communication

Anxiety and fear may present a barrier to communication by preventing the patient from asking for information about diagnosis, prognosis and treatment. The patient's physical condition (e.g. breathlessness, sore mouth) may also impede communication. The nurse caring for anaemic patients must be aware of these potential difficulties and of the effect that they can have upon patient–staff relationships.

The nurse should assess actual and potential communication difficulties and help the patient and the health care team to anticipate and overcome obstacles. The patient should be allowed the opportunity to voice his fears and should be given the appropriate reassurance and information. Here, the nurse should try to involve other relevant members of the team. The nurse should be receptive to the patient's non-verbal as well as verbal messages and, in doing so, anticipate those times when he will need support and reassurance.

Anxiety

Prior to diagnosis the anaemic patient may fear that he has a life-threatening illness, particularly if he has been experiencing symptoms such as breathlessness, palpitations and chronic headaches.

The disorientation, confusion and general slowing of intellectual responses arising from cerebral hypoxia can be especially distressing. Explanation of the causes of these symptoms and reassurance that they should improve as the anaemia responds to treatment will help to reduce the anxiety suffered by the patient and his family.

Iron deficiency anaemia

Iron deficiency anaemia is the most common anaemia worldwide. It affects an estimated 500 million people (Pippard & Heppleston 1996) and is recognised as one of the most prevalent diseases of nutritional origin (Davies 1990). The onset of this form of anaemia is usually insidious, taking place over a period of months. This may be explained by the fact that iron stored in the body is usually re-used after the breakdown of red blood cells and only a very small proportion is lost (less than 1 mg/day) through urine, faeces and sweat (Torrance & Jordan 1995).

PATHOPHYSIOLOGY

Iron is part of the haem component of the haemoglobin molecule: each haemoglobin molecule is composed of four molecules of haem with one ferrous ion, which is the oxygen carrier that transports oxygen from the lungs to the tissues (Tortora & Grabowski 1996).

A typical Western diet contains 16–25 mg of iron/day, but only 5–10% is absorbed (Frewin et al 1997). The ferrous form is more soluble than the ferric form; a low pH in the duodenum maintains iron in ferrous form — the form in which it can be absorbed from the gut.

Iron deficiency anaemia may be caused by:

- inadequate intake, i.e. poor diet
- increased iron requirement, e.g. in pregnancy
- lack of gastric acid, e.g. following total gastrectomy or gastric atrophy
- duodenal or jejunal malabsorption.

Common presenting symptoms. As the onset of iron deficiency anaemia is usually very gradual, the patient may not consult his doctor until some time after symptoms have begun to appear. The most common presenting symptoms are tiredness and pallor, but any of the other general symptoms of anaemia (see p. 437) may be apparent. Symptoms specific to iron deficiency anaemia include:

- painless glossitis — smooth, raw tongue
- angular stomatitis
- koilonychia — brittle spoon-shaped nails
- dysphagia and glossitis; with the formation of a pharyngeal web (5–15% of cases), also called Plummer–Vinson syndrome
- atrophic gastritis and achlorhydria
- pica — a strong desire to eat unusual substances, e.g. coal.

MEDICAL MANAGEMENT

History and examination. The patient may give a history suggesting chronic blood loss (e.g. menorrhagia) and examination may reveal general signs of anaemia.

Investigations. Blood samples will be taken for such tests as full blood count, haemoglobin level, blood film, MCV, MCHC and total iron-binding capacity (TIBC) (see Appendix 1). Estimates will also be made of plasma iron levels and plasma TIBC; this can be done in a GP's surgery. Other investigations, e.g. faecal occult blood, barium examinations and endoscopy, may be undertaken to establish the cause of the deficiency. Such tests will be selected according to the patient's symptoms and medical history.

Bone marrow aspiration is rarely performed but will show a bone marrow with no iron stores (see p. 438) if iron deficiency anaemia is present.

Treatment. If dietary adjustment is insufficient to correct the anaemia, medication is given and, in very severe cases, blood transfusion is carried out.

Medication. Iron supplements will be prescribed, usually in the following forms:

- *Oral iron supplements* — usually ferrous sulphate 200 mg three times a day after food (to prevent gastric irritation). Ideally, medication should be continued for 6 months after the haemoglobin level is normal to build up iron stores (Pippard & Heppleston 1996). Side-effects, which include constipation, nausea, abdominal pain and diarrhoea, often lead to poor compliance. Alternative iron preparations which may be better tolerated, but which are more expensive, include ferrous gluconate and ferrous fumarate.
- *Intramuscular iron injections.* These are given only where there is proven malabsorption syndrome or poor compliance. Administration of i.m. iron via the 'Z track' technique prevents or minimises back-tracking of iron and skin discoloration.

Blood transfusion. If the anaemia is very severe (less than 7 g/dL), a slow infusion of red cell concentrate will be administered. However, there is a danger, particularly in elderly or very young patients, of blood volume overload leading to cardiac failure.

Q **11.6** What accounts for this risk of cardiac overload? Ⓐ

NURSING PRIORITIES AND MANAGEMENT: IRON DEFICIENCY ANAEMIA

Many of the general nursing considerations for the care of anaemic patients (see pp. 438–439) are relevant to the treatment of iron deficiency anaemia. Patients with this condition will most likely be cared for by a community nurse.

Nursing considerations

Blood transfusions

A few patients with iron deficiency anaemia will require a blood transfusion (see Case History 11.1). This measure may be interpreted by the patient and his family as a sign that the condition is very grave; therefore, it is important that the nurse clarifies the reason for the transfusion, explains what is involved, and gives reassurance that the procedure is safe. Many people fear being infected with a transmittable disease, especially AIDS, and it may be necessary to explain the screening procedures performed on all blood donations (Linch 1997). Practising Jehovah's Witnesses will refuse blood transfusions (see Box 11.2). Some Muslims may be reluctant to accept a blood transfusion and may wish to consult their families or a religious leader before agreeing to the procedure.

Case History 11.1 — Mrs B (see Nursing Care Plan 11.1)

Mrs B, a frail lady aged 82 years, has been admitted to hospital as an emergency after collapsing at home. She used to enjoy an active social life until her husband died a year ago. Since then her family and friends have noticed that she has become withdrawn and depressed and rarely goes out except to shop.

Mrs B has always enjoyed good health, until recently. On admission to hospital she admitted that over the past few months she has become increasingly tired and breathless when she climbs stairs or walks uphill. She has noticed that her ankles tend to swell, especially in the evening. She also finds that she has become forgetful; her neighbours have noticed that she appears confused at times.

A blood test has revealed that Mrs B has a haemoglobin level of 7 g/100 mL blood, and other blood test results have proved that she has an iron deficiency anaemia. Mrs B has been prescribed three units of red cell concentrate to be given prior to any further investigations of the iron deficiency anaemia.

Box 11.2 Jehovah's Witnesses and blood transfusions

Devout Jehovah's Witnesses believe that it is against God's law to receive transfusions of blood or blood products. This belief is based on three biblical references: Genesis 9: 4; Leviticus 17: 14; and Acts 15: 28–29. Members of the faith consider that those who disregard God's law will be deprived of eternal salvation (Clark 1982).

If a Jehovah's Witness requires a blood transfusion as an urgent or essential part of treatment, he or his next of kin will need to be approached by the medical practitioners and informed of the gravity of the situation. If the treatment is refused, this must be documented.

The nurse must be familiar with local policies for prescribing and checking blood products prior to transfusion to minimise the risk of administering incompatible blood. Any doubt about the unit of blood to be given should be referred to the haematology laboratory medical staff.

Each unit of blood must be administered at the prescribed rate and correct temperature. Close observation of the patient in the initial hour of each unit is essential as this is when transfusion reactions are most likely to occur (see Nursing Care Plan 11.1).

Patient education

By helping the patient to understand the nature of his disorder and come to terms with the fact that, although the anaemia is not a life-threatening illness, it may become very severe if left untreated, the nurse will encourage him to comply with treatment.

The patient will need to learn which foods are rich in iron and may need advice on budgeting for a well-balanced diet. By assessing the patient's perception of the problem, his level of knowledge and his sociocultural background, the nurse can ensure that the advice she offers is relevant and comprehensible. Referral to a social worker (e.g. for advice about social security benefits) may be appropriate.

Careful and clear instruction should be given to reinforce the doctor's and pharmacist's directions regarding medication.

Nursing Care Plan 11.1 Care of Mrs B during blood transfusion (See Case History 11.1)

Nursing considerations	***Action***	***Rationale***	***Expected outcome***
1. Anxiety (a) About cause of anaemia	❐ Reduce anxiety and stress of receiving blood transfusion by explaining and clarifying information given	Information given about procedures and care reduces anxiety and discomfort	Appear calm, not anxious
(b) About safety of blood transfusion	❐ Reassure Mrs B by explaining screening and cross-matching of blood	Mrs B may fear receiving infection from donor, especially HIV, AIDS or hepatitis B virus. Fear of receiving wrong blood group	Accept blood transfusion
(c) About possibility of complications	❐ Reassure Mrs B she will be observed and monitored frequently for any signs of complications. Tell her she must inform nurses of any new symptoms		
2. Correct blood given to correct patient	❐ Check blood unit details against blood transfusion cross-matching form, prescription and patient's details with a registered nurse as per local policy. Document blood unit transfused	Prevention of wrong blood being given to wrong patient, with possible incompatible reaction	Correct blood given to correct patient as detailed on prescription sheet
3. Condition of blood to be transfused is optimal	❐ Ensure blood stored at correct temperature prior to commencing transfusion. Blood is commenced within 30 min of removal from special refrigerator. Blood is not artificially warmed (unless directed by doctor because of special antibodies)	Blood not stored at correct temperature may undergo haemolysis (red cell breakdown) Risk of microorganism contamination increased	Blood is given at correct temperature
4. Early detection of blood transfusion incompatibility	❐ Record Mrs B's temperature and pulse quarter-hourly during first hour of each unit of blood and then hourly until completion of each unit ❐ Observe Mrs B for any restlessness ❐ Record and report any nausea or vomiting	Signs and symptoms of blood transfusion incompatibility usually occur very soon after the unit of blood is commenced	Any symptoms or signs of incompatibility are detected immediately
	❐ Observe and record any complaints of: • burning sensation in arm above cannula • chest tightness or pain • dyspnoea • loin pain • lumbar pain ❐ Report any signs or symptoms to doctor	Symptoms of pain in arm, chest, lumbar region and loin and dyspnoea are due to agglutination of red blood cells in blood vessels, causing obstruction to blood flow	
	❐ Summon doctor immediately if Mrs B develops circulatory collapse ❐ Stop blood transfusion if any signs or symptoms of incompatibility occur	Incompatible blood transfusion rarely causes sudden collapse	
	❐ Keep unit of blood and infusion-giving set if incompatibility occurs Return both to haematology laboratory	Blood will be further tested for cause of incompatibility. Mrs B's unit of blood may have been wrongly cross-matched or labelled or her red blood cells may have other rare antibodies which require special cross-matching	

(cont'd)

Nursing Care Plan 11.1 *(cont'd)*

Nursing considerations	*Action*	*Rationale*	*Expected outcome*
5. Circulatory overload	❒ Monitor Mrs B's pulse, respiratory rate and blood pressure. Report any abnormal measurements ❒ Observe and report to medical staff any dyspnoea or wheezing ❒ Ensure transfusion is regulated at prescribed rate ❒ Measure urinary output ❒ Give frusemide as prescribed and monitor urinary output	Mrs B has developed some cardiac failure due to her anaemia and the transfusion could increase her blood volume to a level at which the cardiac failure deteriorates. It is important that signs of cardiac failure and pulmonary oedema are detected early Frusemide, as a diuretic, will increase fluid output and thus reduce circulatory volume	Any signs of cardiac overload are detected immediately
6. Pyrexia	❒ Monitor temperature and pulse as in 4 ❒ Report any abnormal temperature and pulse recordings to doctor	Fever can occur for unknown cause at start of each unit. Temperature falls if transfusion slowed. High fever with rigors may be due to white cell antibodies. May occur 1.0–1.5 h after transfusion. Subnormal temperature which rises later may be a sign of infection	All episodes of abnormal temperature are recorded and reported. Any further action requested by doctor is implemented immediately
	❒ Report any chest pain or sign of infections ❒ Ensure blood used has been out of special blood fridge for maximum 30 min ❒ Do not continue transfusion of a unit of blood after 8 h ❒ Report if transfusion rate becomes slow ❒ Administer any drugs as prescribed, e.g. antipyretics, antibiotics	To prevent blood temperature rise with the increased risk of growth of organisms Greater risk of contamination by microorganisms	Blood unit always commenced within 30 min of removal from special blood fridge
7. Allergic reactions	❒ Observations of temperature and pulse as in 4 ❒ Observe for any skin rashes ❒ Observe for any oedema around eyes ❒ Observe for any signs of laryngeal oedema (see Ch. 3) ❒ Observe for shortness of breath ❒ Record and report any of above signs to doctor immediately. If symptoms are mild, slow transfusion. If severe, stop transfusion, treat patient for shock (see Ch. 18)	Allergic response to protein in the plasma	Any signs of allergic reaction are detected immediately and the appropriate action implemented

Important points to emphasise are:

- how frequently the medication should be taken
- that it is to be taken with food
- the possible side-effects of constipation and indigestion and how to overcome them; to avoid undue alarm, the patient should be warned that oral iron supplements will turn his stools black
- safe storage
- the importance of the continuation of medication and the importance of follow-up.

If, for any reason, the patient is unable to take oral iron preparations, then for a period of about a week, daily administration of i.m. iron may be necessary. The patient needs to trust both the virtue of this short-term therapy and the skill of the practitioner, as the possible side-effects of an unpleasant taste in the mouth, palpitations and potential pain on administration could easily result in non-compliance.

Discharge planning

If the person has been hospitalised for treatment, the following considerations should be discussed before discharge:

- socioeconomic conditions at home
- social services available (e.g. home helps, lunch clubs) if family members are unable to help

- the importance of a follow-up appointment with the consultant or GP
- the importance of taking the prescribed medication.

In older people, there is often a link between recent bereavement (i.e. in the last 6–12 months) and the onset of iron deficiency anaemia, as grief and depression may lead to self-neglect. This problem may be accentuated if the bereaved person is also physically unable to look after himself. Care needs to be taken that such patients are not returned to their former social circumstances without the necessary follow-up and support by the GP, health visitor, social worker or grief counsellor.

Q **11.7** A 72-year-old widower is admitted to hospital with general tiredness, breathlessness and mild congestive heart failure. He is diagnosed as having iron deficiency anaemia. His wife died 6 months ago and his only daughter, who is married and has two young children, lives a considerable distance away. A

With regard to the patient's discharge:
(a) identify potential problems
(b) discuss how these might be resolved
(c) identify what community services might be required.

Megaloblastic anaemias

These anaemias stem from a lack of one or more of the essential factors for the synthesis of DNA, resulting in a reduction in red blood cell proliferation. There are two types of megaloblastic anaemia (see Table 11.4):

- folate deficiency
- vitamin B_{12} deficiency.

In the UK, 60% of megaloblastic anaemias are due to folate deficiency (Mackie & Ludlam 1995), and 1 in 100 people over the age of 60 have pernicious anaemia.

PATHOPHYSIOLOGY

Red blood cells are produced continually and have a life span of approximately 120 days (see p. 430). Folate and vitamin B_{12} are essential factors for the synthesis of DNA required by each cell (see Figs 11.6 and 11.7). If DNA synthesis is reduced (because of lack of folate or vitamin B_{12}), the time between each cell division will be prolonged. This results in the normoblasts (see p. 431) becoming larger than normal (macrocytic). While macrocytes may contain a greater amount of haemoglobin than normoblasts, the total amount of haemoglobin will be reduced as the total number of red blood cells is reduced. There may also be large, primitive nucleated red cells (megaloblasts) in the peripheral blood.

Common presenting symptoms. Vitamin B_{12} is required by rapidly dividing cells. A deficiency of vitamin B_{12} affects the gastrointestinal epithelium, giving rise to glossitis, anorexia, diarrhoea and malabsorption. It also causes spinal cord and peripheral nerve damage which can give rise to the following symptoms:

- paraesthesia (pins and needles or tingling)
- coldness or numbness in limbs
- ataxia (lack of coordination of movement, staggering)
- paralysis.

MEDICAL MANAGEMENT

History and examination. Medical investigation is similar to that for iron deficiency anaemia. However, in suspected megaloblastic anaemia the doctor will be alert to the following specific features:

- Folate deficiency — underlying causes such as pregnancy, malabsorption, malignancy
- Vitamin B_{12} intrinsic factor deficiency:
  —slow, insidious onset (especially in older person)
  —glossitis
  —lemon-yellow skin pallor with possible skin irritation (megaloblastic red blood cells are fragile and may be misshapen, resulting in haemolysis.
  —paraesthesia (pins and needles) in fingers and toes
  —symptoms of subacute combined degeneration of the spinal cord resulting in muscular weakness, loss of muscular coordination and paralysis; these symptoms, which may arise before any others, occur in approximately 10% of all cases of pernicious anaemia
  —weight loss
  —excess urobilinogen in urine (because of increased haemolysis).

Investigations. The following diagnostic blood tests are performed in cases of suspected megaloblastic anaemia: full blood count, haemoglobin level, blood film, MCV, serum B_{12} levels and red cell folate level. Other investigations include:

- assessment of gastric parietal cell antibodies
- Schilling test (see Appendix 1)
- endoscopy

Table 11.4 Causes of the megaloblastic anaemias

Type	*Causes*
Folate deficiency	Inadequate dietary intake Disease of upper small bowel (malabsorption or extensive surgical resection of small bowel) Increasing body demands because of: • very active cell proliferation, e.g. in haemolytic anaemia or leukaemia (see pp. 446 and 451) • pregnancy Interference with folate metabolism by drugs (e.g. methotrexate; see Ch. 31) Unexplained mechanisms, e.g. ingestion of alcohol and anti-epileptic drugs (e.g. phenytoin and primidone)
Vitamin B_{12} — pernicious anaemia	Inadequate vitamin B_{12} in diet (especially vegans) Gastric surgery, gastric atrophy or intrinsic factor deficiency Disease of terminal ileum (where vitamin B_{12} is absorbed, e.g. Crohn's disease; see Ch. 4)

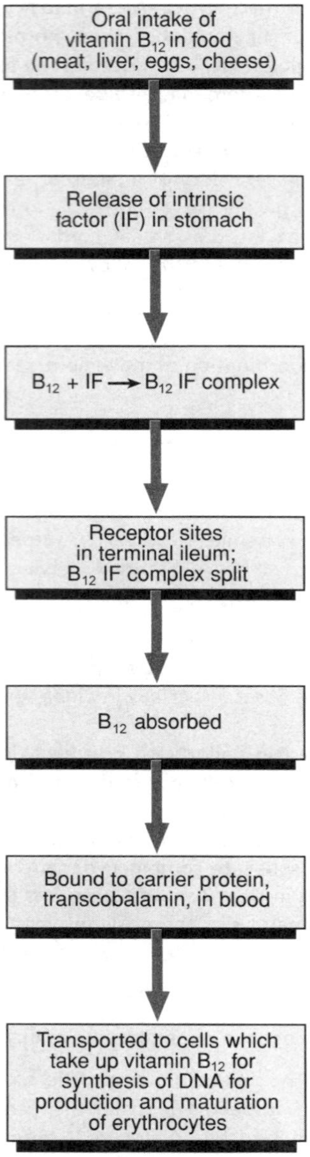

Fig. 11.6 Vitamin B_{12} absorption and transport.

- bone marrow aspiration (see p. 438)
- neurological examination (see Ch. 9)
- past medical history for gastric or intestinal surgery, alcohol abuse or epilepsy.

Treatment for megaloblastic anaemia is as follows:

- Folate deficiency — 5 mg folic acid daily until anaemia is corrected, followed by 5 mg maintenance dose weekly
- Vitamin B_{12} and intrinsic factor deficiency:
  —injection of hydroxocobalamin 1000 μg (1 mg) i.m. twice during first week, then weekly until blood count is normal
  —maintenance dose of hydroxocobalamin 1000 μg (1 mg) i.m. every 3 months for life.

For further information about folate deficiency in pregnancy, see DoH (1992).

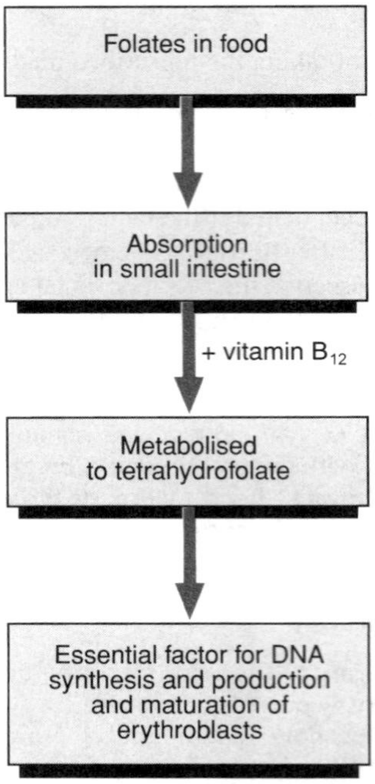

Fig. 11.7 Absorption and utilisation of folates.

11.8 What might be the implications for the patient of the lifelong necessity for 3-monthly injections?

NURSING PRIORITIES AND MANAGEMENT: MEGALOBLASTIC ANAEMIAS

Folate deficiency

Individuals with folate deficiency are usually diagnosed and treated by a GP or at an antenatal clinic and are referred to a haematology outpatient department only if further tests are necessary (e.g. bone marrow aspiration). The setting for nursing intervention will therefore be a community health centre or the patient's home. Patient education with regard to diet and acceptance of medication will be the most important aspect of nursing care.

A patient with folate anaemia will need to know which foods contain folic acid, how to budget for these if his income is low and how to avoid destroying folic acid in food preparation. He will also need to understand how to take folic acid supplements correctly. The nurse should also emphasise the importance of follow-up check-ups with the consultant or GP.

Nurses must be on the alert for patients who may be susceptible to folic acid deficiency (i.e. those whose diet is inadequate, those with extensive disease of the small intestine and those with increased folic acid requirements) and advise them as to how to prevent its occurrence.

11.9 Which foods contain folic acid?

11.10 How can the destruction of folic acid in food preparation be prevented?

For further information on the role of folic acid in health, see Fox & Cameron (1989).

Vitamin B_{12} and intrinsic factor deficiency

Many patients will need to be admitted to hospital for diagnosis and treatment in the initial stages. Others will have been diagnosed by their GP. If the anaemia is not yet acute, treatment can be commenced immediately by a community or practice nurse, who will administer prescribed vitamin B_{12} injections. The nurse should bear in mind that the patient may be very breathless at first and will need some degree of assistance with personal care tasks (see p. 438).

He will also need support in adjusting to the illness and to a regimen of regular injections. The patient and his family should be encouraged to participate in the management of the anaemia, possibly by learning how to administer the hydroxocobalamin injections themselves.

Patients in the advanced stages of pernicious anaemia are rarely seen today. If cardiac failure and severe neurological problems do develop, major nursing interventions will be required (see Chs 2 and 9).

Aplastic anaemia

This form of anaemia results from the failure of bone marrow stem cells to mature and proliferate. In 20–50% of all cases of this very rare disease, onset can be connected with exposure to one of the following:

- chemical compounds, i.e. industrial chemicals, especially benzene
- drugs, e.g. chloramphenicol, therapeutic cytotoxins, phenothiazines, anti-epileptics
- ionising radiation, whether therapeutic or industrial
- viral infection, notably hepatitis
- bone marrow infiltration by disease, e.g. multiple myeloma, metastases from primary tumours.

The remaining 50–70% of cases are idiopathic, having no detectable cause.

PATHOPHYSIOLOGY

Bone marrow failure causes:

- lack of red blood cells: anaemia
- lack of white cells: leucopenia
- lack of platelets: thrombocytopenia.

These three conditions together are referred to as pancytopenia. In aplastic anaemia, the degree of anaemia, leucopenia and thrombocytopenia (and therefore the severity of the disorder) is variable.

Common presenting symptoms. The onset of aplastic anaemia is often insidious. One or two months may elapse between the individual's exposure to the causal agent and the development of symptoms. The presenting symptoms are the result of pancytopenia and include:

- bleeding, e.g. in the skin and mucous membranes, especially the gums
- epistaxis
- infections of the throat, upper respiratory tract, etc.
- general symptoms of anaemia.

MEDICAL MANAGEMENT

History and examination. Medical investigation may uncover no abnormality other than the presenting symptoms; for example, careful examination will reveal no enlarged liver or spleen. However, questioning might bring to light the patient's exposure to chemicals or the use of over-the-counter medication. It may require very careful and extensive questioning to uncover the causative factor, which may have seemed trivial to the patient at the time. The recollections of family and friends may be of help.

Investigations will include:

- blood film and blood count to reveal pancytopenia
- bone marrow aspiration to reveal the degree of stem cell failure. This procedure gives a definitive diagnosis.

Treatment. If the patient was not admitted to hospital on presentation, he will be hospitalised immediately if a diagnosis of aplastic anaemia is made.

In mild to moderately severe cases, supportive therapy with blood and platelet transfusion will be given. Antibiotic therapy will be essential to treat any infections. Steroids are thought to stimulate bone marrow cell synthesis (e.g. oxymetholone orally or high-dose methylprednisolone) and may be tried (see Ch. 5). Other possible drugs are antilymphocyte or antithymocyte globulin or cyclosporin. However, the side-effects of these drugs may cause problems, e.g. pyrexia, rashes, hypotension or hypertension, and nephrotoxicity (Howard & Hamilton 1997).

If the aplastic anaemia is severe or the above treatment is unsuccessful, allogeneic bone marrow transplantation will be considered as an urgent treatment.

NURSING PRIORITIES AND MANAGEMENT: APLASTIC ANAEMIA

Life-threatening complications

The nurse must be on the alert for the development of grave complications of aplastic anaemia. The nurse's role will therefore include:

- prevention of infections
- early detection of infections
- immediate implementation of nursing care of septicaemic patients when infection is confirmed
- prevention and early treatment of bleeding.

Nursing considerations

Psychological state

The patient or his family and friends may experience feelings of guilt if and when the causative agent of the anaemia is identified; they may believe that they were to blame for the patient's contact with the toxin. The nurse must be sensitive to the patient's concerns as he assimilates information about his diagnosis and prognosis (some patients will not survive a year) and as he copes with the sudden transfer to hospital and, possibly, with being nursed in protective isolation (see Ch. 16).

Patient education

It is vital to inform the patient how to prevent and detect the signs of injury, bleeding and infection. He should be warned to avoid overexertion. The teaching programme will depend on the severity of the disorder and the patient's response to treatment and should include not only the patient but also his family, friends and carers.

The nurse should also assess the patient's understanding of the reason for and importance of all medication, what action to take if any is omitted by chance and how to get new supplies in good time. A patient prescribed steroids (e.g. prednisolone) should understand that it is most important to continue taking them even when he feels ill. He should also be advised to inform any doctor or dentist treating him that he is taking steroids and always to carry a card giving details of his medication.

The nurse will also need to instruct the patient, his family and any members of staff unfamiliar with caring for pancytopenic patients about reducing the risk of infection and haemorrhage. Information leaflets are invaluable in reinforcing all details given, as patients and carers will find it hard to remember everything.

Test coordination

The nurse will act as coordinator in the programme of diagnostic tests and will prepare the patient for bone marrow graft if this is to be performed. Further details on caring for profoundly pancytopenic patients are given in the section on nursing management of acute leukaemia (p. 453).

Rehabilitation

Rehabilitation commences even before the patient's discharge from hospital and must be planned in response to his potential for recovery, motivation and needs (see Ch. 34). The multidisciplinary team involved may include a physiotherapist, occupational therapist, dietician, social worker, district nurse, health visitor, counsellor and psychologist.

Realistic goals must be set in discussion with the patient. Consideration must be given to avoiding the causative agent of the anaemia in the future. It may be necessary for the patient to change his job. This may require liaison between medical staff, the patient's employer and a social worker.

Discharge planning

Before discharge it will be important to discuss with the patient any fears or apprehensions he may have, to clarify details of whom to contact if he has any further episodes of illness and to go over with him any written information which has been provided.

Haemolytic anaemias

These anaemias result from the premature destruction of red blood cells, in response to either an inherited or an acquired defect. Many of the haemolytic anaemias are rare or very rare. The most common inherited anaemias are sickle cell disease and thalassaemia. The most common acquired forms result from direct cell injury following infection or medical treatment. Causes of haemolytic anaemias are listed in Box 11.3.

Box 11.3 Causes of haemolytic anaemias

Inherited

- Red cell membrane fragility, e.g. spherocytosis
- Haemoglobin defects:
  —structure: sickle cell
  —synthesis: thalassaemia
- Red cell metabolism defect, e.g. glucose-6-phosphate dehydrogenase deficiency

Acquired

- Antibody attack, e.g. mismatched blood transfusion
- Direct cell injury:
  —traumatic, e.g. prosthetic heart valve
  —chemical or drug-induced, e.g. sodium chlorate, vitamin K analogues, Salazopyrin, nitrates
  —infection, e.g. bacterial, DIC
- Paroxysmal nocturnal haemoglobinuria

PATHOPHYSIOLOGY

In this type of anaemia, the life span of the red blood cells is reduced because of a condition called red blood cell fragility, leading to excessive breakdown of these cells. This results in a reduced oxygen-carrying capacity in the blood and thus hypoxia in the tissues. This causes stimulation of the production of erythropoietin, which stimulates the bone marrow to increase erythropoiesis (see p. 431). A healthy person with mild haemolytic anaemia will not experience symptoms. However, if the red cell life span is greatly reduced (<15 days) the bone marrow will not be able to compensate adequately and the person will experience symptoms of haemolytic anaemia. This will occur more quickly if for any reason the bone marrow is not healthy. The resulting haemolytic anaemia gives rise to increased bilirubin and urobilinogen (see Fig. 11.8).

MEDICAL AND NURSING MANAGEMENT

The medical and nursing care provided will vary according to the specific type of haemolytic anaemia. This chapter will discuss only the management of sickle cell anaemia.

Sickle cell anaemia

The sickle cell anaemias are a group of haemolytic anaemias in which there is an inherited structural abnormality in the haemoglobin molecule (HbS). This abnormality is the result of the substitution of one amino acid in the haemoglobin molecule for another. The abnormal haemoglobin causes a characteristic sickle-like shaping of the red blood cell when it is in the deoxygenated state (France-Dawson 1994). It is a recessively inherited blood disorder of which there is a homozygous and a heterozygous variant (see Ch. 6). In the heterozygous variant, the person inherits the abnormal haemoglobin gene (HbS) from one parent and the normal (HbA) gene from the other parent. This person has the sickle cell trait (HbSA) and will usually be unaware of the abnormality unless he is tested for the trait or develops symptoms when exposed to hypoxic conditions (e.g. anaesthesia or unpressurised aircraft) (Pallister 1992). The trait will be passed on to any children. In the homozygous variant, the abnormal gene is inherited from both parents and the person will suffer from sickle cell anaemia.

This inherited sickle cell trait or sickle cell anaemia occurs among people of African, Caribbean, East Mediterranean, Middle Eastern, Indian and Pakistani origin. It is thought that this geographical distribution might be explained by the fact that sickle cell trait (not sickle cell anaemia) offers some protection against malaria (Pallister 1992).

Of people with sickle cell anaemia, 80% lead normal lives; 20% will have severe complications and die early.

PATHOPHYSIOLOGY

The normal pattern of the amino acids in the beta chains of the globin part of haemoglobin (see p. 431) is altered in the sickle cell haemoglobin by the substitution of a different amino acid for the normal one (HbS). HbS has certain properties which distinguish it from normal HbA haemoglobin. It is less soluble, especially when

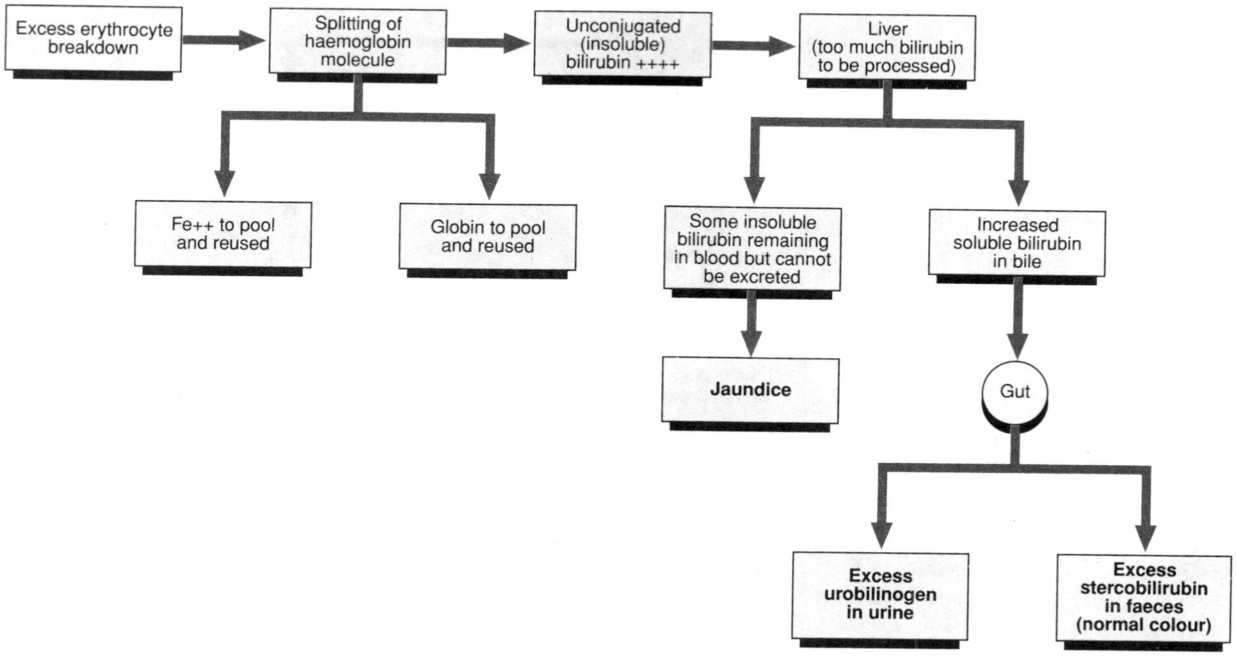

Fig. 11.8 Development of symptoms of haemolytic anaemia.

in a deoxygenated state and when the blood pH is below normal. Under these conditions crystals are formed within the red blood cell, making it more rigid and distorting it into a sickle shape (Pallister 1992). The effects of this abnormal cell are shown in Figure 11.9.

Common presenting symptoms. Sickle cell anaemia normally presents in childhood but might not become apparent until adulthood. Often the presenting symptoms are those of haemolytic anaemia (see Fig. 11.8) or of a painful 'sickle cell crisis' in response to a triggering factor (see Box 11.4). The clinical features of a crisis are:

- Pain caused by the obstruction of small blood vessels in the tissues. Characteristics of the pain are the acuteness of the onset and its unresponsiveness to mild analgesia. The location of the pain depends on the location of the obstruction.
- Anaemia — although these patients are usually anaemic, the body often compensates so that the symptoms of anaemia occur only as the result of a very severe crisis.
- Infection — there is an increased incidence of minor infections, septicaemia, pneumococcal meningitis and osteomyelitis.

MEDICAL MANAGEMENT

Investigations. A blood film will demonstrate the presence of the sickle-shaped red blood cells. The presence of HbS can be demonstrated when the red blood cells are mixed with a special solution of sodium metabisulphite and left for 20 min.

The screening test for sickle cell anaemia and sickle cell trait uses electrophoretic analysis to measure the rates of movement of the different haemoglobins in an electrical field.

Treatment. There is no cure for sickle cell disease. Management is based on alleviation of symptoms and promotion of a lifestyle that minimises crisis events and includes the following elements:

- early treatment of any infections, even minor ones
- avoiding situations in which the person could become chilled
- avoiding dehydration
- managing crisis situations with prescribed analgesics (opiates are often required during crises)
- prophylactic folic acid, penicillin and pneumococcal vaccination
- alerting other practitioners, e.g. surgeons and anaesthetists, to the condition
- obtaining support from sickle cell centres and social work departments in improving home conditions
- learning to recognise complications of sickle cell disease, including bone and joint pains, leg ulcers, priapism in males, gallstones, blurred vision, kidney disease (in patients over 50 years old) and peptic ulcers
- frequent follow-up in special clinics to monitor disease
- genetic counselling
- good antenatal care
- education on general health and nutrition
- possible trial of hydroxyurea, a cytotoxic drug.

NURSING PRIORITIES AND MANAGEMENT: SICKLE CELL ANAEMIA

Life-threatening concerns

Patients in sickle cell crisis admitted as emergencies to hospital may be very frightened. The nurse needs to appreciate the severity of the pain and the need for the administration of opiates. These should not be withheld and addiction problems rarely occur (France-Dawson 1994). The severe pain of a crisis does not respond to mild analgesics. Some hospitals within areas with a population in which sickle cell anaemia is relatively common have set up protocols for the management of patients admitted with sickle cell anaemia crisis in order to minimise the trauma of admission and to ensure the appropriate management of care.

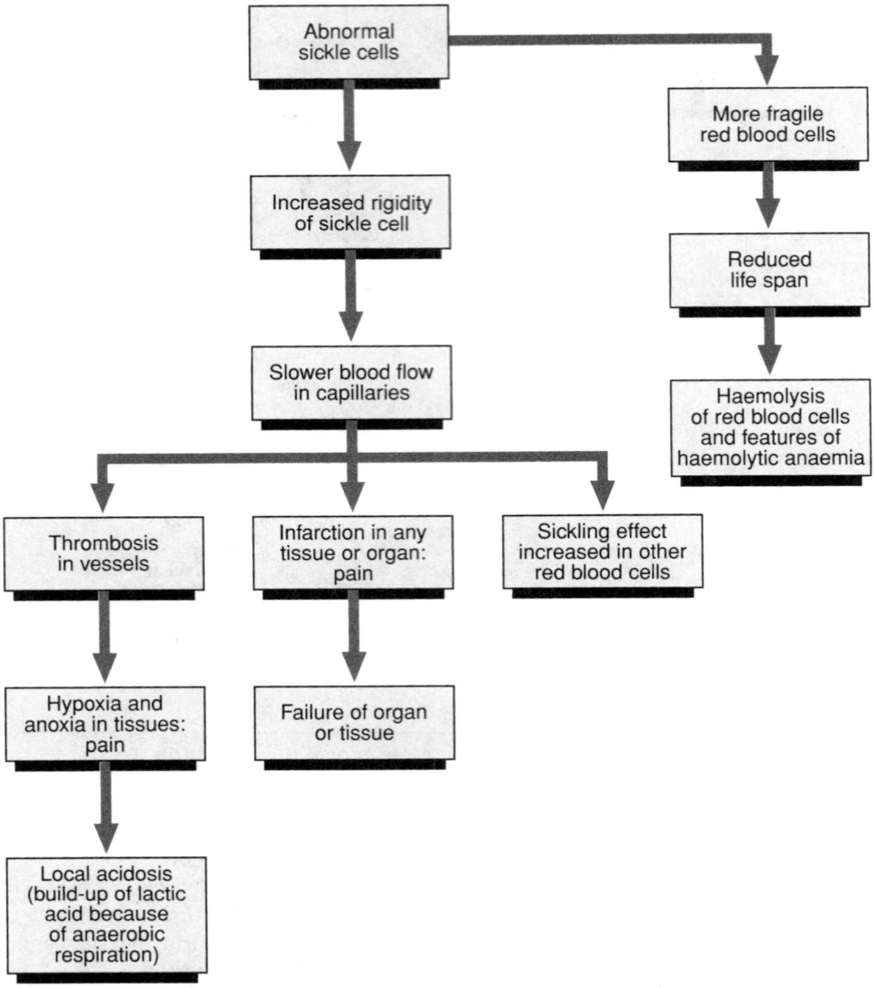

Fig. 11.9 Pathophysiology of sickle cell anaemia.

Box 11.4 Trigger factors in sickle cell anaemia

- Reduced oxygen, e.g. during strenuous exercise
- Anaesthetics
- Dehydration
- Infection
- Fever
- Pregnancy
- Sudden change in temperature
- Alcohol — possibly because of dehydration
- Emotional stress

Of equal importance to the alleviation of pain in sickle cell crisis is the management of the underlying cause of the crisis. An i.v. infusion will be commenced to maintain good hydration and to administer drugs (e.g. antibiotics).

Patients admitted in a crisis require vigilant observation and monitoring. It must be realised that the underlying cause may not be apparent at first and therefore monitoring of the patient may alert nurses to signs and symptoms of the cause as well as to changes in the patient's condition.

Oxygen therapy (see Ch. 3) and blood transfusion (see p. 441) may be necessary.

Nursing considerations

Because these patients are often frightened, the nurse should listen carefully to their concerns. Since they may have had several previous episodes, such patients often know the best way that they should be treated when in a crisis.

Q **11.11** It may not always be appropriate to ask a family member to act as interpreter. Why?

Men may be admitted with a particularly embarrassing condition, priapism (prolonged penile erection due to thrombosis in the corpus cavernosa). This requires not only the administration of analgesia but also i.v. hydration and possibly exchange blood transfusion (to reduce the percentage of sickle cells). Chronic priapism can occur and the patient's sexual function may be impaired (Midence & Elander 1996).

Before the patient is discharged from hospital, he should be made aware of the importance of recognising and avoiding situations that may cause a sickle cell crisis and of the need to seek medical advice at the onset of a painful episode, especially if it is accompanied by symptoms of another illness (including minor ailments).

A newly diagnosed patient will require a comprehensive education programme about the disorder, the ways to minimise complications, and any adaptations to be made to lifestyle. Arrangements should be made for the screening of all members of the family if this has not been done previously. Genetic counselling should be offered. Some areas with a high incidence of sickle cell disease employ special nurse counsellors to carry out screening and to advise patients and their families about the disorder and its consequences (see Ch. 6).

The emphasis in caring for a person with sickle cell anaemia is on promoting health and minimising ill-health.

Q

11.12 What is the difference between sickle cell disease and β-thalassaemia? A

11.13 What is the treatment for β-thalassaemia?

11.14 What are the possible complications of this treatment and how are these minimised?

Anaemia resulting from blood loss

The blood loss responsible for these anaemias may be:

- acute — loss of large volume of blood over a short period of time, as in haemorrhage (for pathophysiology, medical management, and nursing priorities and management, see Chs 18, 20 and 28)
- chronic — loss of a small, even microscopic, amount of blood over a long period of time.

Chronic blood loss is very common and is the form that will be considered here.

There are a number of disorders in which there is a constant or intermittent loss of small amounts of blood. Thus, this type of anaemia is secondary to another disorder, although it may be the presenting illness. Frequently, it is only when a diagnosis of anaemia has been established that the causative illness is suspected. The most common causes of chronic blood loss are listed in Box 11.5. Some patients realise that they have been bleeding but are too afraid to seek advice and discover what the cause of the bleeding may be.

PATHOPHYSIOLOGY

No ill effects will be felt until the blood loss has caused depletion of the body's iron stores. Thus the pathophysiology is similar to that of iron deficiency anaemia.

Common presenting symptoms are as for iron deficiency anaemia. There may be additional symptoms according to the underlying disorder, e.g. stomach pains, heavy menstruation, weight loss or blood in stools (either fresh or digested resulting in black tarry stools known as melaena). The patient may be known to have an underlying illness, e.g. peptic ulceration.

MEDICAL MANAGEMENT

History and examination are as for the diagnosis of iron deficiency anaemia. Detailed and careful questioning may uncover symptoms that the patient considers insignificant or is afraid to report.

Box 11.5 Common causes of chronic blood loss

- Peptic ulceration, including side-effects of steroid therapy
- Gastric irritation — side-effect of alcohol and some drugs, e.g. aspirin
- Menorrhagia — excessive regular menstrual flow
- Genitourinary bleeding, e.g. with bladder carcinoma
- Liver disease
- Chronic inflammatory disease
- Oesophageal varices (blood loss may be acute)
- Malignancy

Investigations are as for the diagnosis of iron deficiency anaemia. Other tests may be required according to clinical features presented. Common investigations include barium meal and barium enema, rectal examination and endoscopy.

Treatment will depend on the specific cause of the blood loss. Possibilities for treatment include oral iron therapy and blood transfusion.

NURSING PRIORITIES AND MANAGEMENT: ANAEMIAS RESULTING FROM BLOOD LOSS

Life-threatening concerns

If anaemia is very severe, the nursing care will be implemented according to the complications that arise (see Chs 2, 3 and 18). If immediate transfusion is required, nursing care will be as on page 431. The nurse will need to monitor the patient very closely for possible cardiac failure and pulmonary oedema.

Nursing considerations

In her initial interactions with a patient who presents with unexplained bleeding, the nurse should bear in mind that he is likely to be feeling apprehensive about receiving a diagnosis. He may also be feeling guilty about not seeking medical advice earlier. Giving the patient clear information about the tests and investigations to be done will help to allay anxiety. If the patient is to undergo tests at an outpatient department he should be given a clear explanation about any pre-investigative preparation, how long the tests will take and what they will involve, and whether he will be fit to return home unaccompanied afterwards.

Thorough nursing assessment can be invaluable in establishing the cause of bleeding and will include questioning, observation, monitoring of vital signs and discussion with the patient's family and friends.

The patient should be informed about the implications of the diagnosis and the proposed treatment. In planning care, the nurse must attempt to prioritise the patient's needs and problems; in so doing, she must be sensitive to individual values and perceptions. Counselling may help the patient, especially if the diagnosis is cancer or any other chronic disorder that will affect the patient's lifestyle. Counselling may also be appropriate if the patient has a self-inflicted disorder, e.g. alcohol-induced gastritis.

The patient with anaemia caused by blood loss may be treated in hospital, in an outpatient clinic or health centre, or at home. Good liaison among all staff involved in the various stages of treatment is vital in ensuring continuity of care. Whether the patient's care is long- or short-term, follow-up must be emphasised to ensure that the disorder has been cured or is being adequately monitored.

DISORDERS CAUSED BY OVERPRODUCTION OF RED BLOOD CELLS: ERYTHROCYTOSIS

A raised haemoglobin level usually indicates an absolute increase in the number of circulating red blood cells. This may be a false finding if the plasma volume is reduced, as in dehydration.

There are three situations in which the number of red blood cells is increased:

- Pathological proliferation of red blood cells with no erythropoietin stimulus — this is called primary proliferative polycythaemia or polycythaemia rubra vera
- Physiological response due to hypoxia, e.g. at high altitudes or with pulmonary disease — a secondary polycythaemia
- Inappropriate production of erythropoietin (or similar substance) in certain pathological conditions, e.g. malignant tumours — a secondary polycythaemia.

Polycythaemia vera

This disease, often characterised by high facial colour and suffused conjunctiva, occurs most commonly in men over the age of 40 years. If the disorder is well controlled, survival for 20 years is possible. There is usually an increased white cell and platelet count as well as a high red cell count.

PATHOPHYSIOLOGY

The raised red cell, leucocyte and platelet count and haemoglobin level have a number of consequences, including hyperviscosity of the blood, thrombosis and hypertension, all of which could precipitate cardiac failure. Thrombosis and sluggish circulation may precipitate peripheral vascular disease. Splenomegaly develops in 75% of all patients due to the increase in the number of red blood cells to be broken down.

Common presenting symptoms. Hyperviscosity of the blood can give rise to symptoms associated with a sluggish circulation and arterial and venous thrombosis. The patient may therefore present with symptoms of cerebral vascular disease (headaches, dizziness, blackouts, stroke and lack of concentration), peripheral vascular disease (intermittent claudication), hypertension (headaches, epistaxis, dyspnoea), angina and cardiac failure. Gout may also be a feature due to the increased cell turnover and raised uric acid levels. Excess histamine production released from basophils can cause gastric ulceration and pruritus (especially on exposure to extremes of temperature).

MEDICAL MANAGEMENT

History and examination. The patient may not present to the doctor with any symptoms but may attend for a health check-up and be found to have hypertension. He may have a ruddy complexion and the palms of the hands and the oral mucosal membrane may be a deep red colour. An enlarged spleen is found in 75% of patients.

Investigations. Blood analysis will include full blood count, haemoglobin level, PCV and blood viscosity. Estimation of the red blood cell mass will be made using radioactive chromium-51. Bone marrow aspiration will be performed and usually demonstrates a hypercellular state and an increased number of megakaryocytes (large nucleated cells of the marrow that produce platelets).

Treatment. Venesection (the removal of whole blood) is the simplest form of treatment. It is repeated until the PCV is reduced to below 0.50 and leads to a dramatic alleviation of symptoms.

Once the diagnosis is established, radioactive phosphorus (^{32}P) may be given by i.v. injection. This treatment is given in an outpatient department, as the radioactive level within the body will not be high enough to present a risk to other people within the community provided the patient complies with certain guidelines. This treatment takes up to 3 months to be effective.

Myelosuppressive drugs (e.g. busulphan, melphalan) may be given orally until the disorder is controlled (see Ch. 31).

All patients will require frequent monitoring to minimise the effects of the disorder. Possible complications are thrombosis, haemorrhage, myelofibrosis (fibrosis of bone marrow tissue which interferes with all blood cell production) and acute leukaemia.

NURSING PRIORITIES AND MANAGEMENT: POLYCYTHAEMIA VERA

The main aims of nursing care are:

- to support the patient during diagnostic tests
- to help the patient understand diagnosis, treatment and possible long-term effects
- to teach the patient how to detect the onset of complications.

Nursing considerations

The patient and his family will need to come to terms with a chronic disorder that may alter the patient's lifestyle and shorten his life. The patient will probably undergo tests as an outpatient or day patient. The nurse should provide the patient with information about all investigations. She will be required to assist the doctor in performing a bone marrow aspiration (see p. 438).

The patient undergoing venesection (which will be commenced by the doctor) must be monitored for signs and symptoms of shock (see Ch. 18). One complication of venesection in patients with polycythaemia vera is difficulty in maintaining flow because of the hyperviscosity of the blood.

Patient education

If the patient is to receive ^{32}P he must be given, preferably in writing, clear instructions regarding limitations of activities or contact with people (e.g. children or pregnant women) in view of the fact he is radioactive. If this care is impossible at home, arrangements will have to be made to admit the patient to a single room in a ward. If admission is required, the need for isolation to protect patients, visitors and staff must be tactfully explained to the patient (see Ch. 31).

Once treatment has begun, it is important to teach the patient to monitor himself for any signs of thrombosis, e.g. pain. If medication has been prescribed, he will need detailed instructions about taking oral cytotoxins (see Ch. 31). The importance of continued monitoring via blood tests and outpatient appointments should be emphasised.

DISORDERS OF WHITE BLOOD CELLS AND LYMPHOID TISSUE

The following sections will consider the nurse's role in the treatment of the following disorders:

- leukaemia
- lymphoma
- multiple myeloma
- agranulocytosis.

LEUKAEMIA

The leukaemias are a group of disorders in which there is an abnormal proliferation of immature white cells, usually confined to one specific subtype of white cell, i.e. granulocyte, lymphocyte or monocyte.

The leukaemias are divided into two types: acute and chronic. Acute leukaemia is characterised by the malignant proliferation occurring at the 'blast' level of maturity of the cell (see p. 432). In the chronic form, the malignant proliferation occurs probably at a later, but still immature, stage of development.

Leukaemia occurs in all age groups, in both sexes and in all races. The total number of new cases in England and Wales of all types of leukaemia is approximately 5000 per year, or 19 new cases per 100 000 of the population per year (OPCS 1994).

Within the UK, the incidence of leukaemia has been increasing by 5–10% every 5 years and varies from region to region. This variance might be explained by certain of the aetiological factors listed below.

Aetiology

The aetiology of leukaemia is not understood but certain factors are associated with an increased incidence. These factors include ionising radiation, viruses, chemicals (especially benzene, toluene and other petroleum derivatives) and alkylating cytotoxic drugs; in addition, heredity e.g. Down's syndrome, or congenital factors, may link to damage to certain chromosomes. There is also an association between acute myeloblastic leukaemia and multiple myeloma (see p. 461) and lymphoma (see p. 461) (Greaves 1997).

PATHOPHYSIOLOGY

The leukaemias, like the lymphomas and myelomas, are thought to arise from a genetic alteration in a single bone marrow cell. From this single abnormal cell, a clone of identical cells arises. Myeloblastic or myeloid leukaemia begins in the myeloid stem cells and lymphoblastic leukaemia begins in the lymphoid stem cells (see Fig. 11.2). However, the two types can coexist (Haslett et al 1999). As leukaemic cells proliferate they gradually crowd out the bone marrow, which therefore produces fewer and fewer normal blood cells. In acute leukaemia, there is an abnormal and excessive proliferation of immature (and therefore ineffective) white blood cells. In adults, acute myeloblastic leukaemia (AML) is four times more common than acute lymphoblastic leukaemia (ALL). In children, ALL accounts for 80% of cases (Souhami & Tobias 1995). In chronic leukaemia, the proliferation may occur in the stem cell (chronic myeloid leukaemia, see p. 459) or at a later stage in white cell development (chronic lymphocytic leukaemia, see p. 459), but the leukaemic cells still serve a less useful function. Chronic leukaemia can develop into acute leukaemia.

The results of the leukaemic process are:

- anaemia
- leucopenia, especially neutropenia
- thrombocytopenia.

Acute leukaemia

PATHOPHYSIOLOGY

Common presenting symptoms (see Table 11.5). The most common symptoms, which derive from the effects of the disease on bone marrow function, are:

- acute infections (associated with fevers), e.g. upper respiratory infections, influenza, dental abscesses, oral *Candida albicans* and skin infections — more than one infection may occur at once, or there may be a succession of acute infections
- bleeding of gums, epistaxis, purpura
- symptoms of anaemia (see p. 438).

Q **11.15** How can these symptoms be explained in terms of blood cell function?

Other symptoms may occur because leukaemic cells infiltrate tissues or organs. Common tissues and organs infiltrated are the bones (giving rise to bone pain), the liver and spleen (hepatosplenomegaly — resulting in abdominal pain), the gums (causing gum swelling), the meninges (causing headaches) and the testes (causing swelling and pain).

MEDICAL MANAGEMENT

History and examination. The patient usually describes an abrupt onset of symptoms — sometimes less than 72 h history of being unwell. He is usually pyrexial, tachycardic and often tachypnoeic with signs and symptoms of acute infection. He may be pale and often has cold sores on his lips (see Case History 11.2). On examination, evidence may be found of lymphadenopathy (enlarged lymph glands), petechiae, purpura and bruising.

Investigations. Diagnosis can be established on examination of a blood film, which usually shows a picture of:

- high white blood cell count (mainly blast cells)
- low red blood cell count
- low haemoglobin
- low platelet count
- raised MCV.

A bone marrow aspiration and biopsy are always required to establish the exact type of acute leukaemia (myeloblastic, lymphoblastic or some other, rarer, form). The bone marrow will show replacement of normal marrow by leukaemic cells. This examination is important as a baseline measurement; further aspirations are done during and after treatment to show response to treatment, which will also help to indicate prognosis.

A lumbar puncture (see Ch. 9) will be performed if the patient has ALL, as there is a high risk of central nervous system involvement, especially in the cerebrospinal fluid.

Table 11.5 Summary of symptoms of acute leukaemia

Result of leukaemic process	*Symptoms*
Anaemia	Pallor Dyspnoea on exertion Palpitations
Leucopenia	Fever Malaise Joint pain Sore throat Mouth infection
Thrombocytopenia	Bleeding gums Petechiae Purpura Bruising

Case History 11.2 Mrs D

Mrs D, aged 40 years, is a housewife. She and her husband have two sons, aged 12 and 14. Mrs D's husband often works overtime so she is kept busy looking after the household. She enjoys gardening, keep-fit classes and reading.

Over the past 2 or 3 months she has been excessively tired. Although she sleeps well at night, she does not feel rested in the morning. She has had mouth ulcers, cold sores and a persistent sore throat. At first, she attributed these symptoms to being run down. Finally, she sought her GP's opinion about the sore throat. He prescribed antibiotics but, because of her other symptoms, took a blood sample for a full blood count in case she was anaemic. He advised her to contact the surgery in a few days for the blood test results and to return to see him if the sore throat continued.

Mrs D was very shocked when the next day the GP telephoned to tell her she was very anaemic and that he had arranged an emergency appointment the next day at the local hospital for her to see the haematology consultant. At that appointment, Mrs D was advised that she needed urgent investigation into her abnormal blood count; arrangements were made for her immediate admission to hospital.

Further investigation confirmed a diagnosis of acute myeloid (myeloblastic) leukaemia. After further discussion with the consultant and her husband, Mrs D has consented to chemotherapy.

A central infusion long line (Hickman catheter) has been inserted to provide long-term access for repeated drug administration, blood specimen collection, blood product transfusion and possible parenteral nutrition. Mrs D has received a blood transfusion so that her haemoglobin level immediately prior to the first course of treatment is 11 g/100 mL. She is neutropenic and thrombocytopenic.

Her nursing care for day 2 of her first course of chemotherapy is given in Nursing Care Plan 11.2. The chemotherapy drugs she is receiving are i.v. daunorubicin, cytosine arabinoside and oral 6-thioguanine.

Careful examination of the testes will also be carried out in male patients with ALL, as this is another region where leukaemia often spreads (Howard & Hamilton 1997).

Treatment

Treatment is directed towards controlling the disease process by means of powerful chemotherapeutic agents and, by so doing, bringing the leukaemia into remission. The initial treatment (induction phase) is aimed at achieving remission (indicated by a reduction of blast cells to <5% of the total white cell count in the bone marrow). Remission is then consolidated (consolidation phase) with the aim of eliminating all leukaemic cells. If remission continues, treatment may be in the form of maintenance therapy for up to 3 years.

Chemotherapy

The aim of chemotherapy is to suppress the abnormal cell production and prevent the major complications of infection and bleeding. Nursing care during treatment aims to support the patient both physiologically and psychologically during the rigours of the chemotherapeutic programme.

The major drawback of this form of treatment is that, as well as destroying abnormal cells, the chemotherapeutic agents used can be highly toxic to normal cells, especially those that, like the neoplastic cells, divide rapidly, e.g. those in the hair and the gastrointestinal tract.

Although chemotherapy is discussed in detail in Chapter 31, for the purposes of the present chapter it is important to understand how the various drugs used are classified and how they act on both leukaemic and healthy cells.

The stages of chemotherapy may be briefly described as follows:

1. Induction chemotherapy. A combination of chemotherapeutic agents is given until remission is achieved. An additional two cycles are then normally given. The common chemotherapy agents used are:

- ALL:
  - —vincristine
  - —daunorubicin
  - —L-asparaginase
  - —prednisolone
- AML:
  - —daunorubicin
  - —6-thioguanine
  - —cytosine arabinoside.

2. Consolidation chemotherapy. At this stage, some change in chemotherapeutic agents may be made, or a single drug at a high dose (e.g. cytosine arabinoside) may be given. Radiotherapy to the cranium may be given during consolidation therapy as part of central nervous system prophylaxis.

3. Maintenance therapy. Oral drugs may be given, but i.v. or intrathecal chemotherapy drugs may also be administered as part of central nervous system prophylaxis. Patients with AML who are under the age of 50 and whose leukaemia goes into complete remission usually have a bone marrow transplant at that stage. Patients of a similar age group with ALL whose leukaemia goes into complete remission may not have a bone marrow transplant at this stage, but if the ALL recurs and further chemotherapy achieves a second remission, they are usually given a bone marrow transplant at that time. This difference in timing is based on the finding that there is a higher rate of maintenance of complete remission in ALL than in AML.

The transplanted bone marrow may be allogeneic, i.e. from a donor (usually with matched human leucocyte antigen, HLA), or autologous, i.e. from the patient himself, collected and stored while he is in complete remission.

Preventing infection and promoting healing

The failure of white blood cells and platelets in the leukaemic patient may require the following medical interventions.

Transfusions. Blood transfusions to minimise the effects of anaemia may be needed. Platelet transfusion will be required if the platelet count is $<10 \times 10^9$ cells/L; it may also be required with a higher count if the patient is having bleeding problems. Platelet transfusions should be cross-matched for ABO blood group.

Platelet transfusions may be required daily and can cause allergic reactions to foreign antibodies. Consequently, i.v. hydrocortisone and i.v. chlorpheniramine are given to minimise this risk.

Antibiotic therapy. In such a vulnerable patient, a pyrexia of 38°C or over and lasting for more than an hour can indicate possible septicaemia. Intravenous antibiotics, given according to an agreed protocol, and immediate blood cultures are essential. The antibiotic regimen can be adjusted according to the blood results.

To reduce the incidence of endogenous infection (i.e. arising from a bacterial source already present in the body, such as commensal organisms in the gut), oral antibiotics that will not be absorbed through the gut wall may be prescribed.

Antifungal and antiviral agents will be administered to minimise the incidence of infection, e.g. from *Candida albicans*, herpes simplex and herpes zoster. These agents will also be used as part of an oral hygiene regimen.

Protective isolation will be necessary to reduce the incidence of septicaemia (see Ch. 16).

Monitoring. A central venous catheter (CVC, e.g. Hickman line) will be inserted prior to treatment. This long-line i.v. catheter, the tip of which lies in the right atrium of the heart, can be left in situ for many weeks, allowing easy access to obtain the many blood samples that will be required to monitor the patient's haematological profile and electrolyte balance and to administer i.v. drugs.

Prevention of tumour lysis syndrome. Oral allopurinol (which slows the production of uric acid) will be prescribed from the commencement of treatment to prevent the development of tumour lysis syndrome, i.e. metabolic upset caused by the rapid breakdown of tumour cells during the induction phase of treatment. This syndrome can lead to renal failure.

If, despite prophylaxis, tumour lysis syndrome does occur, i.v. normal saline should be given to improve diuresis; the urine should be kept alkaline by the administration of sodium bicarbonate and chemotherapy should be discontinued.

For further details on the medical care of patients with malignant blood disorders, see Souhami & Tobias (1995).

NURSING PRIORITIES AND MANAGEMENT: ACUTE LEUKAEMIA (see Nursing Care Plan 11.2)

The aims of nursing care for the patient undergoing chemotherapy are:

- to help the patient cope with the diagnosis
- to support the patient as complications of the disease arise
- to support the patient during the therapy and while he experiences side-effects.

During the diagnostic process the nurse's role will be to keep the patient and his family informed about the tests to be performed and any necessary preparations, and to discuss the implications of the results once they are known. Particular reassurance should be given prior to and during bone marrow aspiration, as this procedure will need to be repeated frequently in the course of treatment.

Psychological support is vital for patients who are faced with a serious diagnosis that demands immediate and prolonged treatment and which is likely to give rise to life-threatening complications. The nurse must exercise good communication skills and show a sympathetic understanding of the patient's emotional state.

Nursing considerations

Preventing infection

The overwhelming concern of nursing care for patients undergoing chemotherapy will be to minimise the incidence and effects of septicaemia (see Chs 16 and 18). The nurse must be aware of potential infective agents (e.g. *Pseudomonas aeruginosa*, *Escherichia coli*, *Candida albicans*) and of their source, routes of transmission and portals of entry.

Of key importance in the prevention of cross-infection is good handwashing technique and the use of protective isolation (see Ch. 16). Also of crucial importance is the strict aseptic management of the central i.v. infusion.

For research findings and discussion about handwashing techniques and aseptic i.v. management, see Mallet & Bailey (1996).

Vigilant and accurate monitoring of vital signs, fluid balance and consciousness level may give the first indication of septicaemia. The nurse must bear in mind that in immunosuppression there are few symptoms of infection; close monitoring is therefore crucial. Moreover, it is only by virtue of early detection that potentially fatal septic shock can be avoided (see Ch. 18, p. 640).

It is essential to realise that an infected mouth can be the cause of septicaemia and that frequent mouth inspection is consequently extremely important. An objective oral assessment tool such as that described by Eilers et al (1988) may be useful (see Table 11.6).

The patient should be given instruction in maintaining a high standard of oral hygiene. He should be advised to use a very soft toothbrush and a bactericidal mouthwash (e.g. chlorhexidine); he may also need to use a topical antifungal agent (e.g. nystatin) along with an antiviral ointment (e.g. acyclovir). If the mouth is very sore, the patient may find a local anaesthetic solution (e.g. Difflam) or lozenges (e.g. Merocaine) helpful (Crosby 1989).

Chest infection, should it occur, may cause considerable distress arising from breathlessness and (due to weakness) difficulty expectorating sputum. The patient should be taught breathing exercises to ensure good lung expansion. If an infection occurs, he may need oxygen therapy, administration of bronchodilators and chest physiotherapy. Haemoptysis, should it occur, may be particularly frightening for the patient.

Preventing haemorrhage

Careful observation and monitoring must be practised to detect any bleeding. This should include:

- at least 4-hourly pulse and blood pressure readings — the nurse should be aware of the risk of bruising from the sphygmomanometer cuff in thrombocytopenic patients; the frequency of blood pressure readings may have to be reduced
- daily urinalysis for visible and occult blood
- testing of all stools for visible or occult blood
- observation of changes in conscious level or development of headaches (signs of cerebral haemorrhage)
- observation of sputum and vomit for blood
- daily inspection of skin for purpura
- observation for pain, especially in the abdomen, as this may be an indication of haemorrhage.

All signs and symptoms of bleeding must be reported immediately to the doctor. At no time should i.m. or s.c. injections be given.

Platelet transfusion will also be given to minimise the risk of haemorrhage. The transfusion units must be stored at 20°C and therefore must never be kept in a refrigerator. Each unit must be checked for the same details as for a blood transfusion. Particular note should be made of the expiry date, as platelet transfusions have a short life span. The transfusion will normally be administered over 30 min. The patient must be closely observed for allergic reactions (see p. 442).

Nursing Care Plan 11.2 Care of Mrs D during chemotherapy for myeloid leukaemia (See Case History 11.2)

Nursing considerations	*Action*	*Rationale*	*Evaluation*
1. Risk of infection (because of neutropenia and chemotherapy)	❐ Wash hands using antiseptic solution before giving any nursing care, with scrupulous attention to wrists and between fingers and careful drying	To remove commensal bacterial skin flora that may cause infection in patient; single most important preventive action against cross-infection	All symptoms and signs of infection are noted and reported immediately and thus treatment for any infection commences early
	❐ Instruct and assist with personal hygiene using antiseptic solution	To reduce skin bacterial flora and risk of endogenous septicaemia	
	❐ Inspect skin daily for infection, especially folds of buttocks, axilla, perineum, breasts, puncture sites, skin breakdown, skin lesions and rashes	To detect any skin infection early	
	❐ Explain mouth care regimen: • use of chlorhexidine 0.4% solution after meals and at bedtime • use of antifungal agent in mouth care as prescribed by doctor (after all meals and at bedtime)	To prevent bacterial and fungal infections of mouth and reduce risk of septicaemia	
	• gentle brushing of teeth using a soft toothbrush	To reduce risk of bacterial infection	
	• application of antiviral cream to lips as prescribed	To reduce risk of viral infection	
	Inspect mouth daily for signs of infection using Oral Assessment Guide (see p. 458). Take swabs from any new lesions	Early detection of mouth infection	
	Record of axillary temperature, pulse and BP 4-hourly (unless patient is receiving blood products)	Early detection of infection. Axillary route used because of sore mouth and risk of infection	
	Report any elevation of temperature to doctor immediately	To ensure any infection is treated appropriately and immediately	
	❐ Take nasal, throat and skin swabs from axilla, groin, umbilicus	To detect any microorganisms that might cause skin infections and septicaemia	
	❐ Inform patient and visitors of the restrictions re. plants and flowers	Earth is a source of *Serratia murcesens*, stagnant water a medium for *Pseudomonas aeruginosa*	
	❐ Advise Mrs D about dietary restrictions: no raw unpeeled fruit or raw vegetables	Raw, unpeeled fruit and raw vegetables may be contaminated with *Pseudomonas aeruginosa*, *Klebsiella* species and *Escherichia coli* and cause septicaemia	
	❐ Administer no drugs rectally or evacuant enemas or suppositories	Can cause rectal abscesses and septicaemia in immunosuppressed patient	
	❐ Report any symptoms, e.g. dysuria, to doctor immediately.	To commence appropriate antibacterial/antifungal or antiviral treatment immediately	
	Report any change in patient's condition, especially increased drowsiness, headache, irritability or restlessness	Changes in central nervous system may be first indication of septicaemia	
2. Inadequate oxygenation of tissues due to anaemia	❐ Assist with all activities of living as appropriate	To conserve energy and reduce oxygen requirements	Patient is not unduly tired
	❐ Observe pressure areas twice daily	To detect any skin breakdown due to hypoxia of skin	Any pressure sore is detected at first sign, if not prevented
	❐ Organise nursing care or assistance to allow periods of rest	To conserve energy	
	❐ Use Spenco mattress on bed	To reduce risk of pressure sores	

Nursing Care Plan 11.2 *(cont'd)*

Nursing considerations	*Action*	*Rationale*	*Evaluation*
3. Easy bleeding due to thrombocytopenia	❒ Inspect skin daily for signs of new bruises, petechiae, purpura	To detect any bleeding immediately	Bleeding is detected early and prompt treatment is given
	❒ Inspect mouth daily for bleeding ❒ Test urine daily for protein and blood ❒ Test and inspect all stools for blood ❒ Observe any vomit for blood ❒ Observe any headache and/or change in conscious level ❒ Observe any other overt episodes of bleeding, e.g. epistaxis		
	❒ Report to doctor immediately any signs or symptoms of bleeding	To ensure treatment is given as soon as possible	
	❒ Record pulse and BP 4-hourly	To detect any hidden bleeding suspected because of tachycardia and hypotension	
	❒ Administer platelets as prescribed, ensuring compatibility of donor blood, observing and monitoring for any allergic or other reaction by recording quarter-hourly pulse and BP and asking patient about any complaints	To ensure platelets are given safely	
	❒ Ensure i.v. chlorpheniramine and hydrocortisone are given prior to platelet transfusion		
4. Side-effects of chemotherapy			
a. Bone marrow suppression	See 1, 2, 3		All side-effects of chemotherapy agents are observed and prompt relevant nursing care is implemented so that Mrs D experiences as few side-effects as possible
b. Extravasation of chemotherapeutic agents especially daunorubicin	❒ Observe cannula site vigilantly for signs of extravasation Report any soreness at cannula site to doctor		
c. Nausea and vomiting	❒ Reassure patient that nausea will stop when chemotherapy course has been completed	Patient already aware of possibility but symptoms can be very depressing	
	❒ Record all episodes of and measure all vomit electrolyte imbalance	To assess possibility of dehydration and possible	
	❒ Administer antiemetics according to prescription	To prevent or minimise nausea and vomiting	
	❒ Report to doctor nausea and vomiting not controlled by antiemetics	So that antiemetic regimen can be reviewed	
	❒ Encourage patient to try alternative measures of controlling nausea and vomiting, e.g. relaxation tapes	To prevent or minimise episodes of nausea and vomiting	
d. Stomatitis	❒ As for mouth regimen in 1		
e. Flu-like symptoms due to cytosine arabinoside	❒ Observe and report any symptoms to doctor immediately of shivering, headache or pyrexia Monitor temperature 4-hourly	Early detection	
f. Conjunctivitis due to high doses of cytosine arabinoside	❒ Administration of prednisolone eye drops as prescribed by doctor	To reduce conjunctivitis inflammation	

(cont'd)

Nursing Care Plan 11.2 *(cont'd)*

Nursing considerations	***Action***	***Rationale***	***Evaluation***
4. Side-effects of chemotherapy *(cont'd)*			
g. Red urine after i.v. daunorubicin	❒ Reassure patient that red urine is temporary consequence of i.v. daunorubicin ❒ Test all urine for blood during and immediately after bolus injection of daunorubicin	Difficult to differentiate between red colouring and bleeding due to thrombocytopenia	
h. Hyperuricaemia because of rapid breakdown of tumour cells following chemotherapy	❒ Observe and measure output. Encourage oral fluid intake especially between administration of chemotherapy drugs ❒ Administer allopurinol as prescribed	To reduce uric acid crystal formation and possible renal failure; to prevent or minimise high uric acid levels	
5. Anxiety about diagnosis, treatment, side-effects, prognosis	❒ Be prepared to listen to any anxieties ❒ Answer questions honestly and ensure, by reporting in writing, that all members of the multidisciplinary team know what information was given and what anxieties Mrs D is voicing ❒ Request further discussion with doctor or registered nurse as required ❒ Arrange for support from other relevant personnel if appropriate, e.g. social worker, chaplain, special organisations, e.g. CancerBACUP, Cancerlink	May require reiteration of information previously given by doctors, nurses or other members of the team, because of mental adjustment to diagnosis	Mrs D feels able to talk with staff and feels she fully understands as much as she wishes to know about her disorder, its treatment and the consequences
6. Altered body image **a. Alopecia**	❒ Reassure Mrs D that hair loss is temporary: reinforce information given about when hair loss will occur, likely duration and rate of regrowth	To try to reduce emotional trauma of alopecia. Accurate information will help her to adjust and explain to her husband and her children	Mrs D is able to feel she is still attractive to her husband and that her appearance is acceptable to her children
	❒ Advise Mrs D to reduce handling of hair but encourage her to keep hairstyle attractive	To reduce trauma to weak hair and minimise loss	
	❒ Discuss ways of enhancing her appearance once hair loss starts, e.g. wearing a wig, turban or scarf	To help her to feel as attractive as possible when alopecia is complete	
b. Herpes	❒ Give written information to read	To help her understand information given and a basis to ask further questions	Mrs D will feel staff understand the disfigurement of the herpes and that she is helping herself
	❒ Educate and assist Mrs D to carry out mouth care regimen as in 1		
c. Sexuality	❒ Be sensitive to possible worries about sexuality ❒ Listen to worries; give truthful answers to any questions about sexual functioning ❒ Offer written information for her to read	To help her explore feelings about changes in sexual functioning and help her discuss this with her husband when she feels able	Mrs D will feel she received relevant information and is able to discuss this topic

Nursing Care Plan 11.2 *(cont'd)*

Nursing considerations	***Action***	***Rationale***	***Evaluation***
7. Inadequate nutrition and hydration			
a. Anorexia	❒ Ensure oral hygiene regimen continued as in 1	To maintain infection-free mouth and because absence of blood improves taste	Weigh weekly: Mrs D should maintain admission weight
b. Nausea and vomiting	❒ Administer antiemetics as prescribed by doctor	To prevent or minimise nausea and vomiting	
c. Hypermetabolic state	❒ Help her choose a high-protein/high-carbohydrate diet from menu	To reduce or minimise effects of malnutrition, minimise weight loss and maintain protein intake	
	❒ Arrange for dietician to talk to her daily to help meet dietary needs ❒ Discuss with Mrs D and her husband the possibility of him bringing certain foods she particularly wishes within restrictions (see 1) ❒ Encourage high-protein/high-energy drinks between meals ❒ Ensure meals are attractively served and in small portions if appropriate	To improve or minimise effects of malnutrition and immunosuppression	
	❒ Ensure 2–3 L fluid intake (see 4)	To prevent hyperuricaemia	Fluid balance assessed daily: Mrs D does not develop negative fluid balance

Minimising the side-effects of therapy

The side-effects of chemotherapy may include nausea and vomiting, which in turn may cause dehydration and electrolyte imbalance. Stomatitis may also develop. Each cytotoxic chemotherapeutic agent will have characteristic side-effects; the nurse should be well informed about these (see Ch. 31).

During the induction and consolidation phases of chemotherapy, the patient may feel very lethargic and ill; it will be important for the nurse to assist him with personal hygiene in order to help minimise infection. Special skin cleansing solutions (e.g. povidone-iodine) may be advised. If the patient is very weak, preventive measures should be taken against the complications of immobility. Of particular importance is the observation of pressure areas. A rating scale (e.g. Norton, Waterlow) should be used as a basis for estimating pressure sore risk and planning appropriate intervention. The Waterlow scale (Waterlow 1988) considers risk factors additional to those addressed by the earlier Norton scale (Norton et al 1975); these include medication (e.g. steroid and cytotoxic therapy), nutritional states and skin condition. Any pressure sore that does develop must be carefully assessed. Intervention must be carried out without delay as the sore can become infected and, in a debilitated patient, lead to septicaemia.

The patient may lose his appetite, especially if he has a sore mouth (from infection or stomatitis) or suffers from nausea and vomiting (from cytotoxic and other medication). A high-protein, high-carbohydrate diet is recommended. The dietician will be able to suggest supplementary high-protein drinks. It may be possible to involve the family as well in providing food that the patient might find tempting. Nonetheless, it may be necessary to give parenteral nutrition (PN) for a time. If this is the case the patient will require special monitoring to ensure that his optimum weight is maintained (see Ch. 21).

Altered body image may pose major difficulties for the patient. Weight loss, alopecia (as a result of cytotoxic chemotherapy), herpes lesions on lips and bleeding gums may all contribute to him feeling unhappy about his appearance. Central i.v. infusions can accentuate the problem, especially if PN is required. Loss of libido, fears of sterility and anxiety about losing the affection of a partner may result in low self-esteem and depression (Holmes 1997). The topic of sexuality will need to be explored sensitively and the help of a psychologist or special counsellor might be required.

Communication may be difficult for the patient because of his mood, sore mouth and debilitated state. It is important for staff to listen to his anxieties, fears and wishes. He should be given as much autonomy in lifestyle choices as possible, especially if he feels he has lost control of his life. He should also be encouraged to be responsible for as much of his own care as is feasible. If he is being nursed in an isolation unit, the staff should ensure they spend time interacting with him so that he does not feel cut off (Mallet & Bailey 1996).

Patient education

Teaching the patient about his illness and its management right from the start of treatment may help him to feel that, even when very ill, he is able to retain some control. This information will

Table 11.6 Oral assessment guide (reproduced with kind permission from Eilers et al 1988). This assessment tool, based on clinical experience and research, requires the nurse to score, on a scale of 1–3, eight different indicators of mouth hygiene and health, thus obtaining a total score of between 8 and 24. If a score of 8–10 is obtained, assessment should be repeated morning and evening. For scores >10, assessment should be carried out 8-hourly

Category	*Tools for assessment*	*Methods of measurement*	*Numerical and descriptive ratings*		
			1	*2*	*3*
Voice	Auditory	Converse with patient	Normal	Deeper or raspy	Difficulty talking or painful
Swallow	Observation	Ask patient to swallow	Normal swallowing	Some pain on swallowing	Unable to swallow
Lips	Visual/palpatory	Observe and feel tissue	Smooth, pink and moist	Dry or cracked	Ulcerated or bleeding
Tongue	Visual/palpatory	Feel and observe appearance of tissue	Pink and moist; papillae present	Coated or loss of papillae with a shiny appearance with or without redness	Blistered or cracked
Saliva	Tongue blade	Insert blade into mouth, touching the centre of the tongue and the floor of the mouth	Watery	Thick or ropey	Absent
Mucous membranes	Visual	Observe appearance of tissue	Pink and moist	Reddened or coated (increased whiteness) without ulcerations	Ulceration with or without bleeding
Gingiva	Tongue blade and visual	Gently press tissue with tip of blade	Pink, stippled and firm	Oedematous with or without redness	Spontaneous bleeding or bleeding with pressure
Teeth or dentures (or denture-bearing area)	Visual	Observe appearance of teeth or denture-bearing area	Clean and no debris	Plaque or debris in localised areas between teeth (if present)	Plaque or debris generalised along gumline or denture-bearing area

also equip him to cope during periods at home. The active involvement of the family should be encouraged as the patient is given instruction in the following areas:

- monitoring body temperature
- recognising the symptoms of infection
- maintaining a high standard of oral hygiene
- managing the CVC such as the Hickman line and administering i.v. drugs and/or parenteral nutrition
- responding to symptoms of infection or bleeding
- taking oral medication: which drugs, how much, how often.

Discharge planning

Before the patient's discharge, arrangements must be made with his GP and district nurse regarding continuing care and a plan of action should complications arise. It may be necessary to prearrange special emergency care (e.g. platelet transfusion) with a local hospital. Other professionals who will be involved in discharge planning include:

- the social worker — for help with housing, financial problems, home help arrangements and social security benefit claims
- the occupational therapist — to assess the patient's ability to cope with everyday activities and to determine what adaptations might be needed to the home environment
- the physiotherapist — to assess the patient's mobility and help him to achieve and maintain optimal fitness
- the dietician — to advise on nutrition, supplementary foods and, if necessary, parenteral nutrition.

Sadly, many patients will require frequent readmission after their initial discharge, and their condition may deteriorate despite the therapeutic team's best efforts. These patients and their families will need support from team members in hospital and in the community as they come to terms with their situation. Well coordinated support can help families to care competently for their loved ones and to have confidence in the professional team (see Ch. 33).

Q **11.16** A 21-year-old woman who is engaged to be married in 6 months is diagnosed as having acute leukaemia. She has undergone chemotherapy and is in remission (i.e. there is no evidence of the leukaemia in the peripheral blood film or in the bone marrow). She has been in hospital for 3 months and is now about to be discharged. She has experienced a degree of alopecia, has lost a great deal of weight and is sensitive about her appearance. Discuss the following: A

(a) What do you think her main fears and anxieties might be?
(b) How could you help her to enhance her appearance?
(c) What support services are available in the community for the patient, her fiancé and her family?
(d) What practical advice should she be given prior to discharge?

Chronic leukaemia

PATHOPHYSIOLOGY

Unlike that of acute leukaemia, the onset of chronic leukaemia is insidious and the disease may be present for some time before the nature of the patient's symptoms prompt him to seek medical advice. Indeed, a proportion of patients are diagnosed as the result of blood tests done for some other medical reason.

Common presenting symptoms. These may be similar to those of acute leukaemia and include:

- tiredness, lethargy
- anorexia, weight loss
- abdominal discomfort (caused by grossly enlarged spleen)
- visual defects and priapism (due to increased blood viscosity and slower blood flow).

MEDICAL MANAGEMENT

History and examination. In addition to the above symptoms, the patient may have a history of persistent low-grade infections. On examination, he is often pale and has an enlarged spleen and liver. Purpura may be found. In patients with chronic lymphocytic leukaemia, enlarged, rubbery lymph glands may be palpable.

Investigations. Diagnosis is based on blood count and blood film results (see Appendix 1). Results indicating the presence of leukaemia include:

- low haemoglobin
- abnormal white cell count — may be extremely high (100×10^9 cells/L) or very low
- low platelet count.

Bone marrow aspiration is performed to determine what specific type of chronic leukaemia the patient has.

Treatment. Patients with chronic leukaemia are rarely admitted to hospital unless their symptoms make it impossible for them to cope at home. The aim of treatment is to control the disease, usually by means of oral chemotherapy. The treatment regimen employed will depend on whether the leukaemia is of the chronic lymphocytic or chronic myeloid type.

Chronic lymphocytic leukaemia is a malignant disorder of the B-lymphocyte (or occasionally T-lymphocyte) white blood cells. Chronic myeloid leukaemia is a malignant transformation of the peripheral blood stem cells, notably neutrophils and monocytes. Ninety-five per cent of the leukaemic cells have an abnormal chromosome — the Philadelphia chromosome — resulting from a translocation of part of the long arm of chromosomes 22 and 9 (Hoffbrand & Pettit 1993). Treatment for these two conditions is as follows:

- *Chronic lymphocytic leukaemia* — oral chlorambucil or cyclophosphamide is administered until control is achieved. Fludarabine may also be used.
- *Chronic myeloid leukaemia* — hydroxyurea with or without interferon is given to control the disease. Alternatively, busulphan may be used. Allogeneic bone marrow transplant may be considered if the patient is under 55 years old. Splenectomy may be required. Chronic myeloid leukaemia can transform into acute leukaemia; treatment would then be as for acute leukaemia.

Patients with chronic leukaemia may require blood transfusions to maintain a satisfactory haemoglobin level. Platelet transfusions, however, are rarely required and in chronic myeloid leukaemia, due to the presence of some normal functioning granulocytes, infections are not as common as with acute leukaemia.

NURSING PRIORITIES AND MANAGEMENT: CHRONIC LEUKAEMIA

These patients may well remain at home. Some require little nursing care but others may need considerable support. In either case, it is likely therefore that community nurses rather than hospital nurses will be involved. However, hospital nurses may be involved in assisting with diagnostic procedures and/or the administration of blood transfusions.

The nursing care required will include:

- giving information about tests, diagnosis and treatment
- providing psychological support to help the patient come to terms with a chronic and potentially life-threatening disease
- educating the patient about medication, including the importance of continuing with intermittent courses of chemotherapy, perhaps over several years
- supporting the patient as he experiences concurrent symptoms, e.g. tiredness and abdominal discomfort
- giving advice about the level of work and activity that can realistically be attempted
- stressing the importance of follow-up in outpatient clinics.

In the terminal stages of the disease, the patient and his family will require especially sensitive care (see Ch. 33).

LYMPHOMA

The lymphomas are a group of malignant disorders with clonal expansion of B, or more rarely T, lymphocytes. They are divided into two types:

- Hodgkin's lymphoma (Hodgkin's disease)
- non-Hodgkin's lymphoma.

Hodgkin's lymphoma is the more common form. Its incidence in the UK is 4–5 new cases per year per 100 000 of the population (OPCS 1994). It is most common among people aged 15–35 or over 50 years of age. It is more common among men than among women in the ratio of 1.5:1 (Gupta 1995). Non-Hodgkin's lymphoma is most prevalent among people aged 50–80 and has an overall incidence in the UK of 22 new cases per year per 100 000 of the population (OPCS 1994).

PATHOPHYSIOLOGY

Cells in the affected lymph tissue (usually lymph nodes) show a disruption of their normal structure or architecture. In Hodgkin's lymphoma, abnormal, giant, multinucleate cells known as Reed–Sternberg cells are usually present.

In non-Hodgkin's lymphoma, these structural abnormalities are very varied. There may be a close resemblance to the normal architecture — called follicular or nodular non-Hodgkin's lymphoma — or a complete loss of architecture, called diffuse non-Hodgkin's lymphoma.

Another frequently used classification of non-Hodgkin's lymphoma is according to complex grading criteria. The grading names used are high, intermediate or low grade. Low-grade lymphomas have the best prognosis, as they run an indolent course, whilst high-grade lymphomas are aggressive with an acute clinical onset.

However, a high-grade lymphoma may respond better to treatment and achieve long-term remission, whilst a low-grade lymphoma may initially respond to treatment but relapse repeatedly (Howard & Hamilton 1997).

For further details on the pathophysiology of lymphomas, see Gupta (1995) and Price (1995).

Common presenting symptoms. Patients with Hodgkin's lymphoma often feel well but have accidentally found a painless, enlarged lymph gland that they may describe as 'rubbery'. Such glands are often found in the cervical, axillary or inguinal regions.

Patients with non-Hodgkin's lymphoma may present with a wide variety of symptoms, including:

- breathlessness — as a result of enlarged mediastinal lymph nodes or obstruction of the superior vena cava, affecting respiratory function
- oedema — especially of limbs, due to lymph node obstruction
- backache — due to retroperitoneal lymph node enlargement
- acute or subacute bowel obstruction — due to small bowel lymphoma
- nausea, anorexia and upper abdominal discomfort — due to lymphoma of stomach
- bone pain — due to bone involvement
- symptoms of anaemia — due to bone marrow involvement
- weakness or paralysis of one or more limbs (often involving both legs) — due to compression of spinal nerve roots.

Some patients, more commonly those with Hodgkin's lymphoma, also present with some or all of the following symptoms:

- low-grade fever (this may sometimes be a swinging fever)
- drenching night sweats (requiring patient to change bed linen and night clothes)
- weight loss (>10% of body weight).

The above symptoms are referred to as B symptoms and are significant in staging the lymphoma (see 'Staging', below). Other possible symptoms include pruritus and pain on consuming alcohol. The reason for all of these symptoms is not entirely clear. They may be due to the secretion of a cytokine by malignant cells.

MEDICAL MANAGEMENT

History and examination. As it is very difficult to palpate certain lymph nodes, clinical examination must be very thorough. Careful examination will also detect any other signs of the disease, e.g. oedema, muscle weakness, splenomegaly and hepatomegaly.

Investigations. Diagnosis is by means of lymph node biopsy. The patient typically undergoes this procedure as a day patient under local anaesthesia. Blood tests include:

- full blood count and differential count
- serum biochemical estimations
- tests to exclude infections that also cause enlarged lymph nodes, e.g. glandular fever, tuberculosis, toxoplasmosis.

Other tests include:

- bone marrow aspiration and trephine
- chest X-ray
- computed tomography (CT scan).

Box 11.6 Staging of lymphomas

Stage I	One lymph node involved or one extralymphatic site (e.g. stomach, Peyer's patches, thyroid)
Stage II	Two or more lymph nodes involved but on the same side of the diaphragm or an extralymphatic site plus lymph nodes on the same side
Stage III	Lymph node involvement on both sides of the diaphragm with or without extralymphatic sites
Stage IV	Diffuse involvement of extralymphatic sites, e.g. bone marrow, liver

Staging. After all the results of the investigations are known, the lymphoma is staged, i.e. the extent of the disease is classified according to the number and location of involved lymph nodes or extralymphatic sites (see Box 11.6). B symptoms are also taken into account. The staging of the disease provides a basis for making a prognosis and planning care.

Treatment: Hodgkin's lymphoma

Stages I and II. As the disease is localised to one or the other side of the diaphragm, it is treated with radiotherapy (see Ch. 31). Disease localised in lymph nodes above the diaphragm is usually treated using a mantle-shaped field. If involvement is confined to below the diaphragm, an inverted-Y technique of radiotherapy is usually used (Souhami & Tobias 1995). Chemotherapy may be given in stage II or if B symptoms are present.

If the lymphoma appears to be in either advanced stage I or advanced stage II, this may be confirmed by a staging laparotomy, whereby biopsies are taken from the spleen, the liver and from lymph nodes (Souhami & Tobias 1995).

Stages III and IV. As the disease is present both above and below the diaphragm, combination chemotherapy (see Ch. 31) with or without radiotherapy is usually the treatment of choice.

Since it is delivered via the blood, chemotherapy will treat a greater volume of disease than will radiotherapy. Radiotherapy is either directed at specific affected nodes or applied more extensively in a 'mantle' or 'inverted Y' field.

Drugs employed in the treatment of stage III and IV lymphomas include combinations of at least three of the following:

- chlorambucil tablets
- prednisolone tablets
- procarbazine capsules
- i.v. vinblastine
- i.v. daunorubicin
- i.v. bleomycin
- i.v. doxorubicin.

The drugs are often given in 2-week 'pulses' every 4 weeks for 6–12 pulses, depending on how the disease responds. If there is no response or if relapse occurs during the course of chemotherapy, the combination of drugs will be changed (see Ch. 31).

Most of these treatments can be given in a day ward. The patient need never be admitted to hospital unless side-effects of therapy occur, or unless he lives too far away to attend hospital as a day patient. If relapse occurs, high-dose chemotherapy with autologous peripheral stem cell transplant may be given.

Prognosis. In localised Hodgkin's lymphoma, 85% of patients will be alive and well 5 years after treatment. Many of these can be considered cured. In advanced Hodgkin's lymphoma, 70% will be alive and well 5 years after treatment (Howard & Hamilton 1997).

Patients who are ineligible for radiotherapy and/or chemotherapy because their disease is too extensive on first assessment or because they are too frail will receive palliative single-agent chemotherapy (see Ch. 31).

Treatment: non-Hodgkin's lymphoma. The type of treatment chosen will depend upon the type of lymphoma as well as on the stage of the disease. Specific chemotherapy regimens are prescribed according to the type of lymphoma and are constantly being refined as clinical understanding of these lymphomas improves.

The general outline of treatment for non-Hodgkin's lymphoma is as follows:

Low-grade lymphoma. A low-grade lymphoma is one which follows an indolent course. The median survival is in excess of 8 years. A partial or complete regression of the disease may be achieved with the use of the cytotoxic chemotherapy drugs chlorambucil or cyclophosphamide. An autologous peripheral blood stem cell transplantation may be considered in young patients, in whom low-grade lymphoma can be fatal.

High-grade lymphoma is an aggressive disease for which the prognosis varies widely. It tends to be associated with high mortality, but there is a 70% response rate to treatment. A small number of patients with localised disease may be cured (Hoffbrand & Pettit 1993).

In the early stages of the disease, a combination of chemotherapy and radiotherapy is used. If complete remission is achieved, further high-dose chemotherapy is given with autologous peripheral blood stem cell transplantation. Transplantation may also be considered if relapse occurs and complete remission is obtained again.

In a more advanced stage of the disease, combination chemotherapy is used.

NURSING PRIORITIES AND MANAGEMENT: LYMPHOMA

Many patients with lymphoma do not need to be admitted to hospital, even for original diagnosis and staging, unless they require a staging laparotomy.

Patients who are to receive radiotherapy using one of the extended fields (mantle or inverted Y) may need to be admitted, as they may experience considerable tiredness, nausea, vomiting, dysphagia and diarrhoea.

The effects of treatment are in fact very variable. Some individuals are able to attend as outpatients and manage to carry on with their jobs with minimal side-effects. The distance that the patient must travel for treatment may be a consideration, as daily travel for up to 6 weeks can prove to be exhausting. The patient's age is also likely to have a bearing on arrangement for hospitalisation, as older people generally do not cope as well with treatment as younger patients (Lichtman 1995).

Nursing considerations

During diagnosis, staging and planning, the nurse should explain all tests and investigations to the patient and his family. Testing should be coordinated to minimise delay. Some tests, such as bone marrow aspiration, will require the direct involvement of the nurse.

The patient may have previously considered himself fit and well and may be shocked to find himself faced with the possibility of serious illness. He will need to be prepared for an unfavourable diagnosis and for a course of treatment that may last for up to 9 months. The nurse should be prepared to cope with a range of emotional responses and should be sensitive to the patient's changes of mood, allowing him time to absorb the implications of his situation, to voice his feelings and concerns, and to seek clarification as needed.

The specific nursing care required will depend upon whether radiotherapy or chemotherapy is the prescribed treatment. For a detailed description of patient care during either of these therapies, see Chapter 31.

After the initial course of treatment, the patient and his family should be given detailed, individualised advice on post-radiotherapy or post-chemotherapy care. The patient should be given the name of someone to contact when he is in need of advice (see Ch. 31). Preparation for coping after therapy should address the following areas:

- medication — how to take it and for how long; how to obtain prescription refills
- diet
- level of activity; return to work
- self-monitoring for signs of infection or bleeding; whom to contact should either of these occur
- the importance of attending follow-up clinics for check-ups and assessment
- appropriate self-help groups
- sexual counselling as appropriate
- referral to district nurse, social worker and GP.

As the lymphomas are such a diverse group of blood disorders, and their treatment is so varied, nursing care cannot be definitively prescribed. Some patients will remain independent of any nursing assistance, whilst others will be hospitalised throughout the course of the disease. After the course of treatment, nursing care may be required continually or intermittently. For some patients, palliative care will be required from an early stage. The key to providing high-quality nursing care lies in recognising the needs, values and concerns that are unique to each individual.

MULTIPLE MYELOMA

Multiple myeloma, or myeloma, is a rare haematological disorder in which there is a malignant proliferation of the plasma cells which develop from the B lymphocytes.

The incidence of multiple myeloma is 3.5 new cases per 100 000 of the population per year in Europe. About 50% of cases are under 65 years, but the average age on diagnosis is 60 years. There are only 0.1 new cases per 100 000 of the population per year aged 23–34 years, but 21 per 100 000 of the population per year aged 75 and over (Selby & McVerry 1995).

There is no known cause or factor associated with the occurrence of myeloma.

PATHOPHYSIOLOGY

Normal plasma cells develop from B lymphocytes following antigen stimulation. Each plasma cell releases a specific immunoglobulin with a special immune function. In myeloma there is a malignant proliferation of plasma cells, which then release an immunoglobulin, or paraprotein as it is called, which is incapable of normal function.

The paraprotein has a number of effects on the body which can be summarised as:

- bone marrow infiltration
- skeletal destruction
- production of the abnormal protein, with subsequent effects in the blood, kidneys and other tissues
- depression of production of normal immunoglobulins.

Each of these effects has pathophysiological consequences. The bone marrow infiltration will lead to pancytopenia. The skeletal destruction can lead to characteristic lesions in the bone, bone pain, hypercalcaemia and pathological fractures. The abnormal protein may cause renal failure (due to its deposition in the renal tubules). Depending on its specific properties, the paraprotein may cause hyperviscosity of the blood, bleeding disorders and the presence of cryoglobulins (abnormal proteins which are insoluble at low temperatures and therefore cause obstruction in small blood vessels). If the abnormal protein is deposited in the tissues, the formation of amyloid tissue (an abnormal material which accumulates and is deposited in an organ, e.g. kidney or liver, causing failure) can result. Reduction in immunoglobulin levels will lead to the patient becoming immunocompromised.

Common presenting features. The most common presenting symptoms (Sheridan 1996) are:

- pain in the lumbar or thoracic spine due to the myeloma deposits, pathological fractures, demineralisation, muscle spasm or periosteal pressure (80% of patients on first presentation)
- tiredness, lethargy, cardiac failure and other symptoms of anaemia (74%).

Other presenting features are:

- weight loss
- bone tenderness and pathological fractures
- infections
- spinal cord compression.

MEDICAL MANAGEMENT

History and examination. The patient may have had symptoms for a number of months but may not have considered them significant enough to report to a doctor. Back pain, for example, is often not reported until it becomes incapacitating. Alternatively, the patient may have been receiving treatment by a GP and/or physiotherapist for a condition which did not improve or even became worse.

Some patients have a history of sudden-onset bone pain caused by pathological fracture. Others present with pneumonia due to neutropenia and lowered immunoglobulin levels. Some patients may have noticed lumps on their forehead, or extreme bone tenderness throughout the body.

Patients may present with clinical features of renal failure and/or hypercalcaemia. There may be abnormal neurological symptoms such as reduced sensation and muscle power.

Investigations. Tests and investigations are aimed at establishing the diagnosis, staging the disease and assessing the effects of the disease on the body.

To confirm a diagnosis of myeloma and determine its stage, evidence of two of the following three features is required:

- presence of paraprotein
- bone lesion
- bone marrow infiltration.

Evidence of the paraprotein is established by means of electrophoresis examination of serum and urine. Serum electrophoresis reveals the unique patterning of the different immunoglobulins. It is then determined whether this patterning is normal and, if it is not, which paraprotein is involved. Urine electrophoresis will show whether paraprotein is present. The paraprotein present in urine is called Bence–Jones' protein.

A skeletal survey and isotope bone scan will demonstrate the presence and extent of any bone lesions. On X-ray these appear as circular lesions resembling punched-out holes. They are often seen in the skull, long bones and vertebrae (Howard & Hamilton 1997).

Bone marrow aspiration and trephine biopsy are performed to establish any bone marrow infiltration.

To establish the systemic effect of multiple myeloma on the body, the following tests are performed:

- full blood, differential white blood cell count and ESR
- serum urea and electrolytes
- serum calcium and alkaline phosphatase levels
- uric acid levels
- plasma viscosity.

Treatment. If the patient presents with severe complications of the disease, these must be treated first.

Specific treatment of the myeloma will include chemotherapy with or without radiotherapy. Radiotherapy will target specific bony lesions to reduce bone deposits, prevent fractures and reduce pain.

The chemotherapeutic agents commonly used are melphalan, cyclophosphamide, prednisolone, doxorubicin and vincristine. These are used usually in a combination regimen intermittently over several months (see Ch. 31). Certain patients under 50 years of age may be considered for high-dose chemotherapy and autologous peripheral blood stem cell transplantation.

Plasmapheresis (the removal of blood from the patient followed by removal of the plasma fraction and the return of the blood cells with donated plasma) may be used to reduce a high blood viscosity, as the removal of the patient's plasma will also reduce the paraprotein level. This is done only as a temporary measure whilst other treatment is given.

NURSING PRIORITIES AND MANAGEMENT: MULTIPLE MYELOMA

Myeloma is a serious disorder with multisystemic effects, some of which are potentially life-threatening. The most serious of these are:

- renal failure — due to myeloma paraproteins causing degeneration, blood hyperviscosity, hyperuricaemia, hypercalcaemia, dehydration and anaemia
- spinal cord compression — due to vertebral collapse
- hypercalcaemia — due to bone destruction
- severe cardiac failure — due to anaemia and hyperviscosity
- immunosuppression — due to reduced normal immunoglobulin formation.

For the patient, the most distressing symptom may be bone pain. As the disorder is insidious in onset, bone pain may have existed for some time but may have been ignored or rationalised until it became too much to bear. Assessment must take this into account as the patient may well be exhausted and depressed by chronic pain (see Ch. 19). Pain management strategies will depend on the cause of and level of distress associated with the pain. Strategies include the use of radiotherapy to local bone lesions and the use of analgesics (usually NSAIDs and opioids). The patient's distress will be compounded if spontaneous fractures occur, severely curtailing activity (which may already be impaired). Frequent and debilitating infections may also be experienced, along with fatigue, anaemia and bleeding tendencies, such that every daily activity becomes an effort. Many patients are in their middle years and have considerable family and financial responsibilities. For them, the stress of ill-health and of coming to terms with the diagnosis of a malignant disease will be keenly felt.

Close monitoring by health professionals in the community will be required to ensure that activity is maximised and pain kept to a minimum. Hospital admission may not be necessary until the more serious effects of the disease become apparent. Of these, renal failure can cause the most concern. Optimal hydration is crucial in preventing renal failure and hypercalcaemia, the requirement often being as much as 4–5 L/day. Sensitive and creative nursing strategies will help the patient to maintain a good fluid intake; even then, the renal impairment may still progress and perhaps necessitate haemodialysis.

Nursing considerations

Communication

As always, good communication skills will be vital to effective nursing intervention. On admission, the patient may or may not know his diagnosis and may be trying to cope with debilitating symptoms, e.g. paralysis, severe pain and immobility. The nurse should be sensitive to the patient's anxieties and should bear in mind that individuals with myeloma often have a reduced attention span as a result of fatigue, weakness and pain. The patient will need clear explanations of the reasons for investigations, the implications of diagnosis and the options for treatment. He and his family should be given honest and accurate answers to their questions and requests for clarification. Written information which the patient can read at his own pace and discuss with the nurse later is often helpful.

Back pain often prompts patients to enquire about complementary forms of treatment such as osteopathy or homeopathy. The nurse should be able to provide enough background information to enable the patient to make up his own mind about these and other therapies.

Mobility

The nurse will work alongside the physiotherapist and occupational therapist in helping the patient to attain an optimal level of mobility. In setting goals for rehabilitation, a balance must be struck between the need to reduce the risk of hypercalcaemia (which is increased with immobility) and the danger of fracturing weak bones. As pain will be a restricting factor, the assessment and constant evaluation of pain levels will form an integral part of the therapeutic process.

For a patient on bed rest, mobilisation may need to commence with passive movement of joints and limbs, progressing to gentle muscle-strengthening exercises. The next step will be for the patient to practise getting out of bed with the appropriate aids and assistance. Before the patient is discharged, it will be necessary for his home to be assessed for any adaptations needed to facilitate access and accommodate the use of aids.

Patient education

Acquiring knowledge about his disease and its management will help the patient to feel that he is in control of his life. In preparation for discharge, he should be fully briefed on the following:

- self-monitoring for side-effects of chemotherapy (see Ch. 31)
- the importance of continued follow-up with the GP for medication and blood tests, as well as attendance at outpatient clinics
- safe techniques for lifting and carrying
- preventing or minimising complications, e.g. taking extra fluids
- reducing muscle weakness.

Discharge planning

The nature of arrangements for discharge will depend on the patient's physical and psychological state, the type of treatment he is receiving and the availability of carers at home or in the community. Important aspects to consider in planning are:

- How dependent is the patient and how willing is he to participate in his own care?
- Who are his family carers and what type and degree of support will they need (e.g. Macmillan nurses, Marie Curie nurses)?
- What skills will carers need to learn (e.g. handling and moving the patient)?

Prognosis

Myeloma is a progressive, debilitating condition for which palliative care will eventually be the only treatment option. However, 90% of patients show a response to treatment of up to a 75% reduction in tumour mass. Many patients will be able to enjoy an acceptable quality of life for some time; some who enter hospital immobile and in considerable pain return home able to walk and be independent in all activities of daily living.

AGRANULOCYTOSIS

This rare disease is caused by the partial or complete absence of neutrophils, resulting in susceptibility to infection, septicaemia and death. The causal factor may be unknown (idiopathic agranulocytosis). Known factors include drugs (e.g. antithyroid drugs, rarer chemotherapy drugs, allopurinol, gold salts, phenothiazines, tricyclic antidepressants) and excess exposure to ionising radiation. Agranulocytosis may also be part of pancytopenia following bone marrow failure.

PATHOPHYSIOLOGY

Agranulocytosis differs from other bone marrow failure in that it is only the granulocytes that are involved, in contrast to aplastic anaemia (in which there is pancytopenia), thrombocytopenia (in which only the platelets are involved) and the pancytopenia caused by myelofibrosis, leukaemia and bone marrow infiltration. Therefore, the patient with agranulocytosis will have a problem with infection but not the additional problems of anaemia and thrombocytopenia. However, anaemia and thrombocytopenia may both occur as the result of septicaemia.

Common presenting symptoms. Onset may be acute or chronic. The common presenting features of the acute-onset form include a history of sore throat, often progressing rapidly to necrotic throat ulceration with no pus formation (because of an absence of phagocytes) and septicaemia. The patient is very ill, hyperpyrexial, and often has rigors.

Onset of chronic agranulocytosis is insidious. The patient complains of vague general symptoms of malaise and weakness; sore throat follows but the progression of the disease is much less dramatic.

MEDICAL MANAGEMENT

Investigations. Diagnosis is based on the results of full blood count, white blood cell differential, blood film and bone marrow aspiration. These tests will confirm a very low neutrophil count or a complete absence of neutrophils. They may also point to an underlying cause, e.g. leukaemia or cancer metastases. A careful and detailed clinical history may reveal exposure to a possible cause of the agranulocytosis, e.g. medication.

Treatment is aimed at removing the cause of the illness (if this is known) and establishing control over the disease process by means of antibiotic therapy. If the bone marrow has not been significantly impaired, the prognosis is good and neutrophil production will resume.

NURSING PRIORITIES AND MANAGEMENT: AGRANULOCYTOSIS

The nursing management is the same as that required for any patient with severe infection and risk of septicaemia. It must be remembered, of course, that because of the absence of neutrophils, the patient's response to infection will be atypical and, as with patients with acute leukaemia, endogenous infection may well occur. Progression to a state of septicaemia may be rapid and vigilance is required to prevent and detect early signs of potentially serious infection (see Nursing Care Plan 11.2).

The disease is indeed life-threatening and, as has been said, may arise suddenly. Newly diagnosed patients are often frightened and disbelieving, and need to be given time and support as they adjust to the diagnosis and learn to cope with treatment. Information and counselling are of a multidisciplinary nature and should involve other family members and possibly friends. If the patient survives the acute phase, rehabilitation will take time and patience. Lifestyle issues will have to be addressed in order to ensure that any identified cause is avoided in the future and that the patient understands how to avoid infections and when to seek medical advice. Such constraints can be unwelcome and advice should always be framed positively. This is especially important if fundamental changes are required, e.g. a change in occupation to avoid a causative agent. The support and advice of the community nursing team can do much to make necessary adjustments acceptable to the patient and to ensure his future health.

DISORDERS OF PLATELETS AND COAGULATION

Disorders of coagulation can be subdivided into three types:

- disorders due to lack of clotting factors
- platelet disorders
- disorders due to another cause, e.g liver disorders.

These disorders may be inherited or acquired. All age groups are affected, but some coagulation disorders are sex-linked; for example, haemophilia occurs only in males but is genetically carried by females.

CLOTTING FACTOR DISORDERS

These disorders all involve a deficiency in one or more of the blood factors required for haemostasis. Inherited clotting disorders result from the lack of specific clotting factors. The acquired disorders involve the failure of certain clotting factors to be activated usually as a result of vitamin K deficiency or liver disease.

Haemophilia

The haemophilias are a group of inherited disorders in which there is a lifelong deficiency of one of the substances necessary to blood clotting. These deficiencies include:

- haemophilia A — lack of factor VIII (see Ch. 6)
- haemophilia B or Christmas disease — lack of factor IX
- von Willebrand's disease — lack of von Willebrand factor, which is necessary for normal platelet adhesion and factor VII production; it is not sex-linked.

Box 11.7 Causes of acquired thrombocytopenia

- Decrease in platelet production
- Aplastic anaemia
- Vitamin B_{12}, folic acid deficiency
- Bone marrow infiltration
  - —leukaemia and lymphoma
  - —carcinoma
  - —myelofibrosis: formation of fibrous tissue within the bone marrow cavity
- Other disorders
  - —viral infection
  - —bacterial infection
- platelet destruction
- idiopathic autoimmune disorder
- idiopathic thrombocytopenic purpura (ITCP)
- large-volume blood transfusion — due to the short life span of platelets, there may be no viable platelets in the blood transfusion units and the patient will, if requiring a large volume of blood, have insufficient platelets
- disseminated intravascular coagulation (DIC) (see Ch. 29)

PLATELET DISORDERS

Thrombocytopenic purpura (TCP)

Any disturbance in the number or function of circulating platelets will affect the normal coagulation process (see p. 464). The condition thrombocytopenia implies a reduction in the number of platelets and may be either inherited or acquired.

PATHOPHYSIOLOGY

Inherited TCP is fortunately rare. Acquired TCP may occur as a result of factors which either decrease normal platelet production or increase platelet destruction (see Box 11.7). Decreased production is usually caused by drugs or some other agent whereby the bone marrow is suppressed. The most common form of TCP due to increased platelet destruction is idiopathic thrombocytopenic purpura (ITCP). This commonly affects individuals in their teens or early 20s and is thought to be autoimmune in origin. Whatever the cause, TCP will result in a prolonged bleeding time, which may give rise to bruising, purpura or petechiae. Less obviously, visceral bleeding can also occur.

Common presenting symptoms include a history of bleeding episodes, e.g. bleeding gums, epistaxis, melaena and haematuria. In contrast to haemophilia, if pressure is applied to the bleeding point, bleeding will stop and not recur unless further trauma occurs. As with leukaemia, symptoms of anaemia may be presenting features in chronic thrombocytopenia.

MEDICAL MANAGEMENT

History and examination. A careful clinical history is required, especially to pinpoint any recent minor illness or drug therapy (including medicines bought at a pharmacy). Thorough clinical examination is made for any signs of bruising, petechiae, purpura or any underlying disorder.

Investigations. These will include:

- full blood count to identify low platelet count or anaemia and exclude any other blood disorder
- coagulation screen to exclude other coagulation disorders.

Treatment. Many cases of thrombocytopenia (acute or chronic) resolve spontaneously, possibly because the formation of antibodies against the person's own platelet membrane antigens is transient. In cases where an exacerbating factor such as a drug or chemical is withdrawn, spontaneous remission may also occur.

Steroid therapy may be given until resolution occurs, as steroids improve platelet survival. Response to steroid therapy is usually seen within days or weeks; however, thrombocytopenia may recur when the steroids are withdrawn.

Immunoglobulin G i.v. may be given for 3–5 days (see Ch. 16). Splenectomy may be required, as the spleen is a major site of platelet destruction.

NURSING PRIORITIES AND MANAGEMENT: THROMBOCYTOPENIC PURPURA (TCP)

Nursing considerations

In hospital

Nursing priorities during the patient's stay in hospital will include:

- Controlling superficial bleeding by application of external pressure. The bleeding tendency is not generally life-threatening.
- Observing the patient for evidence of bleeding, and determining severity of bleeding by means of:
  —regular monitoring of patient's pulse during diagnostic stage and initial treatment. Blood pressure is not usually measured as this may cause bruising and petechiae
  —daily inspection of the skin for petechiae, purpura and bruises, and of the mouth for bleeding and infection. Precautions must be taken to minimise the occurrence of infection in soft tissue which has been damaged
  —regular testing of urine, stools and vomit for less obvious sources of blood loss.
- Being alert to complaints of headaches and drowsiness, as these may indicate cerebral bleeding.
- Ensuring that the patient is protected from injuring himself by advising him on environmental hazards and making him aware that feelings of faintness may indicate anaemia or low blood pressure.
- Giving explanations and support during tests and treatment, and looking and listening for indications of anxiety.

Discharge planning

The aim of discharge planning is to enable the patient to make the transition from dependence upon the nurse to monitor his condition to becoming competent and confident in monitoring himself. The importance of monitoring all bleeding episodes must be stressed, along with the need for regular follow-up to monitor platelet levels.

Q **11.17** What adjustments might be required to enable the individual to lead a fulfilling life without risk to health?

Precautions which the patient should be advised to take include:

- taking medicines as prescribed
- avoiding aspirin preparations
- avoiding i.m. injections
- carrying identification, e.g. Medic-Alert bracelet
- minimising potential for soft tissue injury
- avoiding contact sports.

The family should be included in the patient's education programme to ensure that all members of the household understand the necessity of certain restrictions upon lifestyle. However, it should also be stressed that it is important for the patient to maintain a balance between being overcautious on the one hand and taking unnecessary risks on the other.

The aim of rehabilitation is to allow the patient to achieve an optimal level of function until his spontaneous recovery or throughout the remainder of his life.

REFERENCES

Barnard D L, McVerry B A, Norfolk D R 1989 Clinical haematology. Heinemann Medical, Oxford

Clark J M F 1982 Surgery in Jehovah's Witnesses. British Hospital Journal of Medicine 27(5): 497

Campbell J 1993 Making sense of blood groups. Nursing Times 89(22): 36–38

Crosby C 1989 Methods in mouthcare. Nursing Times 85(35): 38–41

Davies J 1990 Anaemias of nutritional origin. Nutrition and Food Science 300: 5–7

Eilers J, Berger A M, Peterson M C 1988 Development, testing and application of the oral assessment guide. Oncology Nursing Forum 15(3): 325–330

Firkin F 1995 Haematological side effects of drugs. Medicine 23(12): 534–536

France-Dawson M 1994 Painful crises in sickle cell conditions. Nursing Standard 8(45): 25–28

Fox B A, Cameron A G 1989 Food science, nutrition and health, 5th edn. Edward Arnold, London

Frewin R, Henson A, Provan D 1997 ABC of clinical haematology – iron deficiency anaemia. British Medical Journal 314: 360–363

Greaves M F 1997 Aetiology of acute leukaemia. Lancet 349: 344–349

Gupta R K 1995 Hodgkin's disease. Medicine 23(12): 482–484

Haslett C, Chilvers E R, Hunter J A A, Boon N A 1999 Davidson's principles and practice of medicine, 18th edn. Churchill Livingstone, Edinburgh

Hoffbrand A, Pettit J E 1993 Essential haematology, 3rd edn. Blackwell Scientific Publications, London

Holmes S 1997 Cancer chemotherapy, 2nd edn. Asset Books, Dorking

Howard M R, Hamilton P J 1997 Haematology. Churchill Livingstone, Edinburgh

Leach M 1991 Anaemia – the nursing care and intervention. Professional Nurse 6(8): 454–456

Lichtman S M 1995 Lymphomas in the older patient. Seminars in Oncology 22(1): S25–28

Linch D C 1997 Haematological disorders. In: Souhami R L, Moxham J (eds) Textbook of medicine, 3rd edn. Churchill Livingstone, Edinburgh

Mackie M, Ludlam C 1995 Diseases of the blood. In: Edwards C R W, Bouchier I A D, Haslett C, Chilvers E R (eds) Davidson's principles and practice of medicine, 17th edn. Churchill Livingstone, Edinburgh

Mallet J, Bailey C 1996 Royal Marsden NHS Trust manual of clinical nursing procedures, 4th edn. Blackwell Scientific Publications, Oxford

Midence K, Elander J 1996 Adjustment and coping in adults with sickle cell disease: an assessment of research evidence. British Journal of Health Psychology 1: 95–111

Montague S E 1996 The blood. In: Hinchliff S M, Montague S E, Watson R (eds) Physiology for nursing practice, 2nd edn. Baillière Tindall, London

Norton D, McLaren R, Exton-Smith A N 1975 An investigation of geriatric nursing problems in hospital. Churchill Livingstone, Edinburgh

Office of Populations Censuses and Surveys 1994 Cancer statistics registrations: Registrations of cancer: diagnosed in 1989. HMSO, London

Pallister C J 1992 A crisis that can be overcome: management of sickle cell disease. Professional Nurse 7(8): 509–513
Pippard M J, Heppleston A D 1996 Microcytic and macrocytic anaemias. Medicine International 24(1): 4–10
Selby P, McVerry B A 1995 Multiple myeloma and related diseases. Medicine 23(12): 485–488
Sheridan C A 1996 Multiple myeloma. Seminars in Oncology Nursing 12(1): 59–69
Souhami R, Tobias J 1995 Cancer and its management, 2nd edn. Blackwell Scientific Publications, Oxford
Torrance C, Jordan S 1995 Bionursing: signs of iron deficiency. Nursing Standard 10(12–14): 29–31
Tortora G J, Grabowski S R 1996 Principles of anatomy and physiology, 8th edn. Harper & Row, London
Waterlow J 1988 The Waterlow card for the prevention and management of pressure sores: towards a pocket policy. Care: Science and Practice 6(1): 8–11
World Health Organization 1972 Nutritional anaemias. Technical report series no. 503. WHO, Geneva

FURTHER READING

Alkire K, Collingwood J 1990 Physiology of blood and bone marrow. Seminars in Oncology Nursing 6(2): 99–108
Bassett C 1996 Caring for surgical patients with sickle cell disease. Nursing Standard 10(33): 38–39
Belcher A E (ed) 1993 Blood disorders. Mosby clinical nursing series. Mosby, St Louis
Borley D (ed) Cancer nursing, 2nd edn. Oncology for nurses and health care professionals, vol 3. Harper & Row, London
Contreras M 1992 ABC of transfusion, 2nd edn. BMJ Publishing, London
Department of Health 1992 Folic acid and the prevention of neural tube defects: report from an expert advisory group. HMSO, London
Fox B A, Cameron A G 1989 Food science, nutrition and health, 5th edn. Edward Arnold, London
Freedman S, Halsford M E, McGuire D B et al 1990 Nursing considerations in the administration of blood component therapy. Seminars in Oncology Nursing 6(2): 155–162
Gupta R K 1995 Hodgkin's disease. Medicine 23(12): 482–484
Levenson J A, Lesko L M 1990 Psychiatric aspects of adult leukaemia. Seminars in Oncology Nursing 6(1): 76–83
Mallet J, Bailey C 1996 Royal Marsden NHS Trust manual of clinical nursing procedures, 4th edn. Blackwell Scientific Publications, Oxford
Montague S E 1996 The blood. In: Hinchliff S M, Montague S E, Watson R (eds) Physiology for nursing practice, 2nd edn. Baillière Tindall, London
Oniboni A C 1990 Infection in the neutropenic patient. Seminars in Oncology Nursing 6(1): 50–60
Price C G A 1995 Non-Hodgkin's lymphoma. Medicine 23(12): 478–481
Souhami R, Tobias J 1995 Cancer and its management, 2nd edn. Blackwell Scientific Publications, Oxford
Tortora G J, Grabowski S R 1996 Principles of anatomy and physiology, 8th edn. Harper & Row, London
Waters J, Thomas V 1995 Pain from sickle cell crisis. Nursing Times 91(16): 29–31
Webb P (ed) 1988 Care and support. Oncology for nurses and health care professionals, vol 2. Harper & Row, London
Wujcik D 1990 Options for post-remission therapy in acute leukaemia. Seminars in Oncology Nursing 6(1): 25–30

USEFUL ADDRESSES

CancerBACUP
3 Bath Place
Rivington Street
London EC2A 3JR

Leukaemia Research Fund
43 Great Ormond Street
London WC1N 3JJ

Leukaemia Care Society
14 Kingfisher Court
Vinny Bridge
Pinhoe
Exeter
Devon EX4 8JN

OSCAR (Organisation for Sickle Cell Anaemia Research)
4th Floor
Cambridge House
109 Mayes Road
Wood Green
London N22 6U

Sickle Cell Society
54 Station Road
London NW10 4UA

SKIN DISORDERS

Christine Docherty   *Rhoda Hodgson*

12

INTRODUCTION

Intact skin is vital to health and well-being. As the biggest organ in the body, comprising 16% of body weight and having a surface area of 1.8 m^2, the skin has many vital functions (Gawkrodger 1997):

- sensation
- temperature regulation
- synthesis of vitamin D
- insulation and protection of internal organs
- barrier to harmful external factors.

Skin disorders range from minor conditions resolved with over-the-counter (OTC) preparations to potentially life-threatening skin conditions requiring intensive treatment in specialist units. Many conditions are of a cyclical long-term nature with patients requiring care in different settings: ward, outpatient treatment centre and community. This chapter aims to introduce the student to dermatology nursing by discussing the commonest conditions encountered. Dermatology as a visual speciality may require the reader to consult a colour atlas.

Nurses in every specialism encounter individuals with skin disorders, creating opportunities to detect early disease, give knowledgeable treatment advice and provide emotional support to patients and family members coping with chronic conditions. A good knowledge base helps the nurse to dispel myths about the contagious nature of skin disorders, as the social and emotional implications of skin disease should not be dismissed lightly. Success, power and achievement are often dependent on appearance and 'image'. The media support images of the soft-skinned baby, blemish-free teenager, the smooth sophisticated adult and such images are reflected in money spent by both sexes to achieve cosmetic perfection. Dermatology research has investigated the quality of life of patients with skin disorders and has recorded the impact of skin disease on an individual's life (see Research Abstract 12.1).

Research Abstract 12.1

The effect of a skin disorder on a patient's quality of life is often of greater importance than the discomfort of having abnormal skin. Quality of life is of central concern with an improved quality of life probably the most desirable outcome of health care policies. A survey of the social and psychological effects of psoriasis reported the high social and emotional morbidity present for many patients despite access to modern treatment facilities. A questionnaire response from 104 patients highlighted that the social and psychological effects of a skin disorder were being forgotten or actively ignored mainly because they were too time-consuming or too difficult to deal with during a routine consultation. The researchers challenged dermatologists to acknowledge and address the holistic needs identified by the client group and to ensure hospital services were constantly evaluated.

If skin disease is acknowledged as having a detrimental effect on quality of life, then focusing on the psychosocial problems experienced has major implications in optimal management of the patient with a skin disorder. By incorporating simple quality of life assessments into routine management, information is gained about the impact of the skin disorder on all aspects of the patient's life. This knowledge will be relevant when making risk–benefit analysis in therapeutic decisions. It may also help patients and professionals to work in partnership to address the needs and concerns that are relevant to improving or maintaining the desired level of quality of life.

Ramsay B, O'Reagan M 1988 A survey of the social and psychological effects of psoriasis. British Journal of Dermatology 118: 195–201

Patients can restrict social, professional and personal activities with a resultant impact on careers and relationships. Problems with sexuality and relationships can be linked to low self-esteem and the self-concept of an altered body image associated with having a skin condition (Poorman & Webb 1992). The psychological morbidity of skin disease is often unrecognised by professionals (Lewis-Jones 1999) despite patients actively reporting their experiences of ostracism, stigmatisation and isolation — the 'unclean' leper status of having a skin disorder. The person with a skin disorder has to cope with the physical problem and its associated complex therapies while being confronted with psychological, social and cultural rejection.

Q **12.1** Before reading further, try this exercise. You are in a communal changing room in a busy clothes shop when you realise the person trying on clothes next to you has a generalised rash. It appears to be very itchy, and as the person scratches, numerous flakes of skin are shed. Stop now and write down your immediate reaction to this scenario. Ask your colleagues to join you in this exercise.

Repeat this exercise when you have read through this chapter. Evaluate any changes in your answer.

Epidemiology

Skin disease is common and its prevalence is such that approximately 20% of the UK population have a skin disorder meriting medical management. The type, incidence and prevalence of skin disorders depend on social, economic, geographical, racial and cultural factors (Gawkrodger 1997). Internal and external factors contributing to skin disorders are summarised in Figure 12.1. The economic implications of skin disease can be considerable for individuals, families and employers. Skin diseases are the commonest group of occupational health problems leading to absence from work. Industrial-acquired dermatoses lead to lost working time and often to compensation claims for work-induced disorders.

Age is an important factor in diagnosing disorders, with some conditions being exclusive to a particular age group, and others persisting throughout life. Atopic eczema, for example, is most common in infancy, while acne develops in adolescence and normally wanes by the late 20s. Middle age brings pemphigus and malignant melanoma. The elderly show expected degenerative skin changes, with 27% having malignant skin lesions. Psoriasis and eczema occur in all age groups and can be cyclical in nature throughout life.

Research confirms malignant melanoma as a significant health problem in the white adult population, affecting 3% of the population and accounting for two-thirds of deaths from skin cancer (p. 489). In 1992, in response to the rise in skin cancer, the government defined a target and key actions to be taken to 'halt the year on year increase in the incidence of skin cancer by the year 2005' (Department of Health 1992). Current UK campaigns aim to change social behaviour in relation to sunlight by educating the public that a suntan is a sign of damaged skin rather than a desirable fashion statement. In Australia, a shift in public attitude towards skin protection was achieved by the 'slip, slap, slop' campaign in which an animated seagull persuaded sun-lovers to slip on a T-shirt, slop on some sunscreen and slap on a hat. UK initiatives have used an amiable mole called 'Monty' to convert us into a nation of 'mole watchers', able to identify changes in our skin vital to early detection and treatment (see p. 489). Travel leaflets promote sun screens and avoidance of sunburn.

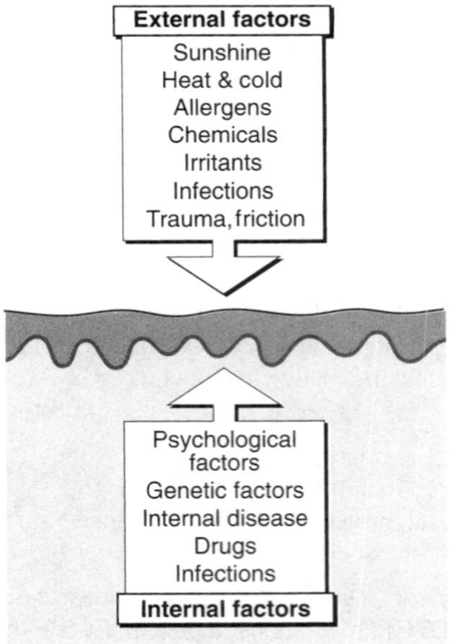

Fig. 12.1 Internal and external factors causing skin disease. (Adapted from Hunter et al 1995, with kind permission from Blackwell Science Ltd.)

Genetic or hereditary factors can be relevant to the diagnosis, and a family history should be part of the assessment. Patients with skin disorders report stress as a contributory factor in creating or exacerbating their condition, e.g. divorce, trauma, bereavement, exams. Psychological stress is common, but while psychological problems can make conditions worse, most skin disorders are stressful conditions in their own right. Certain skin disorders are recognised as being entirely of psychogenic origin, e.g. dermatitis artefacta, trichotillomania and dysmorphobia. Social factors are relevant to skin disorders, and improvements in standards of living, personal hygiene and nutrition have reduced the rate of infectious diseases and infant mortality (Gawkrodger 1997). The current rise in the number of patients with asthma and eczema appears to be associated with increasing affluence and these might now be considered as diseases of the advantaged. High unemployment and low wages restrict job mobility and the patient with acquired industrial skin disease may have difficulty in making appropriate job changes to alleviate the condition. Continuing rises in prescription charges force patients into decisions about which of the prescribed medications they can afford. Skin care prescriptions often involve combinations of preparations, and anecdotal evidence suggests that patients choose those parts of the prescription they can best afford, thus preventing full management of a skin disorder. Homelessness and poor housing create problems in maintaining skin care, the former often resulting in limited access to medical care. Nurses working with vulnerable client groups need to be aware of this issue and intervene appropriately.

The nurse's role

Following publication of the *Patients' Charter* (Department of Health 1991), patients with skin disorders and associated support groups asserted their right to access specialist staff and be nursed in specialist areas (National Eczema Society 1991). In-patient hospital management is an effective method of targeting, educating and training the patient in skin management techniques. Cure is not a word widely used in dermatology due to the cyclical nature of many conditions, so nurses involved in care often forge long-term relationships with patients. Dermatological nursing skills, reflected within holistic practice, can revitalise patients who require sympathy, empathy and guidance from specialist practitioners with the time, knowledge and willingness to share clinical skills with this motivated client group. Kurwa & Findlay (1995) report in-patient management as improving quality of life for dermatology patients, while peer group interaction between patients in dermatology wards is recognised as a beneficial adjunct to therapy (Price et al 1991).

Standards of care for dermatology nursing, addressing the complexity of caring for people with skin disorders (Royal College of Nursing 1995), aim to promote good practice and improve communication between professionals and patients.

The role of the dermatology liaison nurse is now well established (Venables 1996). The liaison role focuses on the sharing of specialist knowledge and skills, resulting in a seamless transition of care and the removal of arbitrary barriers that used to coexist between care settings (Ruane-Morris et al 1995). The supportive role of nurses in primary care is vital. Patients referred to dermatologists reflect a small minority of people with skin disorders. Self-medication, over-the-counter therapies from pharmacists (Nathan 1996) and nurse prescribing mean that community teams are the first point of contact for most patients. The liaison nurse uses educational input to support the primary care team in providing information and therapies that are valid, accurate and up to date. This independent role means availablity to visit patients' homes, nursing homes, schools and places of work and provides expertise to reduce the fragmented care that sometimes exists in primary care settings. The *Scope of Professional Practice* (UKCC 1992) supported dermatology nurse practitioners in extending nurse-led initiatives in many areas of clinical practice, including (Legge 1997):

- nurse-led clinics — leg ulcers, cryotherapy, skin biopsy
- laser therapy
- nurse counselling
- nurse-led phototherapy
- patient education programmes
- nurse prescribing.

Nurses are an important group within the dermatology team, playing a vital role in the provision of direct specialised care. The move towards care in the community encourages the provision of primary care, thus reducing the cost of hospitalisation and minimising disruption for patients. The dermatology nurse can liaise with primary care colleagues and is available as a specialist resource in an advisory and consultative capacity, helping to sustain continuity of care (Stone 1997a).

ANATOMY AND PHYSIOLOGY

Structure of the skin

Originally formed from the embryonic ectoderm and mesoderm, skin is composed of two layers: epidermis and dermis. Beneath these layers, a bed of subcutaneous fat protects and insulates the underlying organs. In adults, the surface area of skin is 1.5–2.0 m^2 and it weighs approximately 9 kg.

The epidermis

The epidermis is composed of stratified epithelium and varies in thickness between different parts of the body, e.g. the skin on the palms and soles is thicker than that on the face or back. There are no blood vessels in the epidermis and the cells are nourished by diffusion of materials. Structures tracking through the epidermis include hair follicles and sweat and sebaceous glands (see Fig. 12.2A). The epidermis is composed of several layers, and its health depends on three factors involving these layers (Wilson & Waugh 1996):

- regular division and migration of epidermal cells to the skin surface
- gradual keratinisation of these cells
- desquamation or rubbing away of these cells.

The layers of the epidermis are as follows (see Fig. 12.2B):

Basal layer (stratum basale). The cells lying nearest the dermis form the germinative layer where cell division occurs. Cells migrate upwards from this layer, becoming keratinised over a period of 21–28 days before being shed.

Prickle cell layer (stratum spinosum). Cells in this layer appear to be connected by fine processes or prickles. These intercellular connections act as protection against shearing forces or trauma to the skin.

Granular layer (stratum granulosum). Within this layer, fine granules form in the cells. This granular substance, keratohyalin, is a precursor of keratin, which gradually replaces the cytoplasm of the cells.

Clear cell layer (stratum lucidum). This layer is present only where the skin is thickened, e.g. the soles of feet. The cells exhibit nuclear degeneration and contain large amounts of keratin. Injury or friction to the skin increases the production of these cells, resulting in a callus or corn.

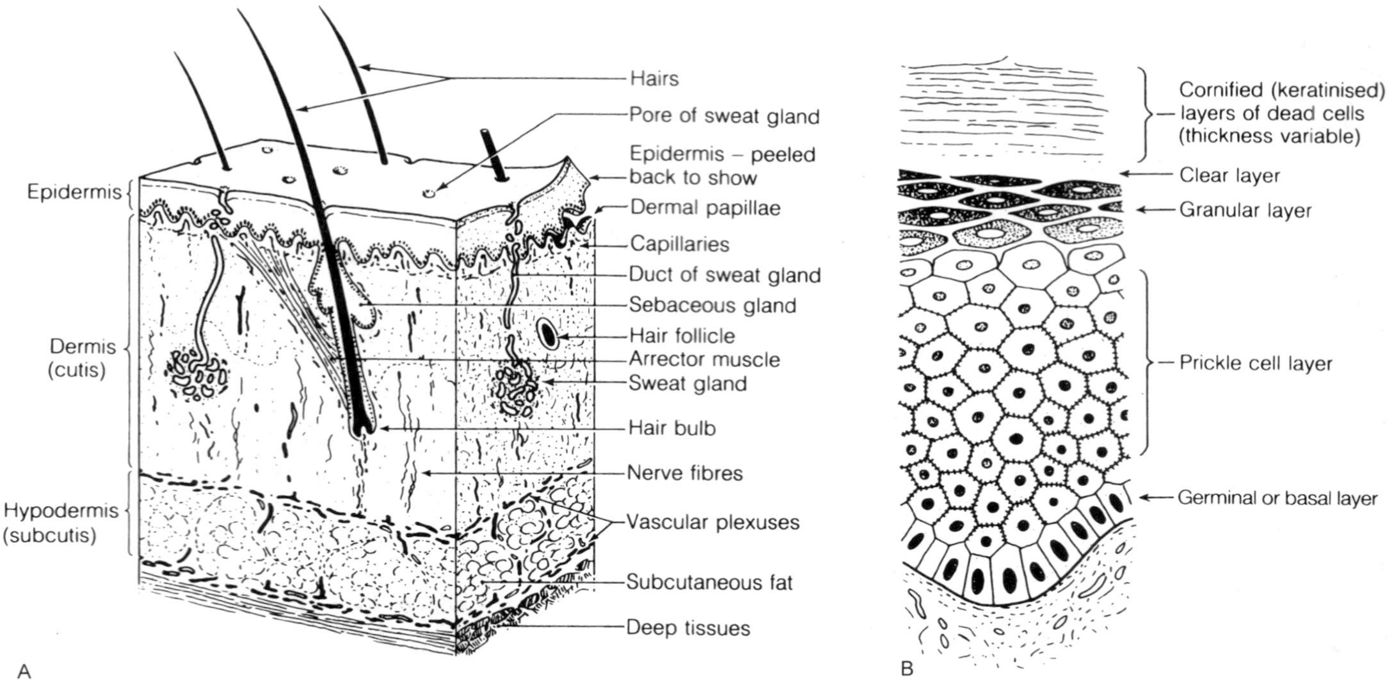

Fig. 12.2 A: The structure of the skin. B: The layers of the epidermis. (Reproduced with kind permission from Hinchliff et al 1996.)

Horny layer (stratum corneum). This layer is composed of thin, flat, non-nucleated cells, the cytoplasm of which has been lysed and totally replaced by keratin.

The epidermal/dermal junction is convoluted into dips and ridges called rete pegs, which help to prevent damage to the skin from shearing forces. The configuration of these ridges is visible at the epidermal surface as corresponding characteristic patterns, e.g. at the fingertips.

The dermis

The dermis is composed of fibrous connective tissue and provides a supportive meshwork for the structures and organs within. The papillary layer has many capillaries and lies next to the basal layer of the epidermis. The reticular layer, lying above the subcutaneous fat layer, has fewer blood vessels and is less reactive.

The ground substance of the dermis is a jelly-like material acting as a support and a transport medium. It functions as a water reservoir which may be utilised by the body in an emergency (e.g. during haemorrhage).

Tissue mast cells are often found near hair follicles and blood vessels, producing heparin and histamine when damaged.

Tissue macrophages. These cells have the protective function of engulfing foreign particles within the dermis.

Collagen fibres. Ascorbic acid is required by fibroblasts to generate these strong fibres, which have the property of binding with water molecules to give skin its tight, 'plump' appearance; 40–80% of the total body water is thought to be accommodated within the dermis. Wrinkling is thought to occur when collagen fibres lose their water-binding properties. They may also rupture during growth spurts, pregnancy or obesity, leaving fine white scar-like striae.

Elastin fibres. These yellow fibres, also formed by fibroblasts, are bound loosely around bundles of collagen and, in combination with the ground substance and collagen, help the dermis to maintain its characteristic properties.

Lymph vessels play a major role in draining excess tissue fluid and plasma proteins from the dermis, thereby maintaining correct volume and composition of tissue fluids.

Nerve endings. Specialised sensory receptors present in the dermis and basal layer of the epidermis detect mechanical and thermal changes (see Ch. 22).

Glands

Sweat glands are coiled tubes of epithelial tissue opening as pores onto the skin surface. They have individual nerve and blood supplies and secrete a slightly acid fluid containing excess excretory products (water and salts). Sweat also helps to keep keratin supple. Sweat glands are of two types. Eccrine glands are controlled by the sympathetic nervous system, producing secretions in response to temperature elevation or fear (release of latent heat by the evaporation of sweat helps to lower body temperature). Apocrine glands in the pubic and axillary areas are not functional until puberty. They are thought to secrete pheromones, chemical signals released into the external environment.

The sebaceous glands are lined with epidermal tissue, secreting sebum, a greasy, slightly acid substance which helps to form a waterproof covering over the skin and (like sweat) to keep the keratin supple. The acid sebum has antibacterial and antifungal properties. Most sebaceous glands open into hair follicles. Sebum production is influenced by sex hormone levels.

Functions of the skin

Protection

The skin has several protective properties. The greasy horny layer forms a waterproof seal against undue entry or loss of water. The skin surface protects against microorganisms (through its acidity) and acts as a barrier to chemicals, gases and gamma and beta rays. Internal organs are shielded by the skin from minor mechanical blows, and repeated pressure or friction stimulates an increase in cell division, producing thickened areas of skin, e.g. corns and calluses. Melanin produced in the basal layer of the epidermis screens the dermis from ultraviolet rays.

Sensation

Nerve endings present throughout the dermis and basal epidermis continually monitor the environment and are most highly concentrated in areas such as the fingertips and lips. Innervated hair follicles help the individual to avoid injury by stimulating reflex action in response to touch.

Formation of vitamin D

Epidermal cells synthesise 7-dehydrocholesterol, which is slowly converted to vitamin D when skin is exposed to ultraviolet rays. Circulatory vitamin D, in combination with phosphorus and calcium, is essential to the formation of healthy bone. Deficiencies can lead to the development of disorders such as rickets and osteomalacia. Excess vitamin D is stored in the liver.

Temperature regulation (see Ch. 22)

Core body temperature is usually static at around 37°C. Heat is produced in the body by the metabolic processes of the liver, muscles and digestive system. Temperature is controlled by the heat-regulating centre in the hypothalamus, which responds to changes in the temperature of circulating blood and influences cardiovascular centres in the medulla oblongata. These centres control the size of the lumen of the arteries and arterioles and thereby control the rate of blood flow through the capillary beds in the dermis.

In cold conditions heat is retained by vasoconstriction and generated by the involuntary muscular action of shivering. During overheating, sweating is induced and vasodilatation occurs. As sweat evaporates from the skin, latent heat is lost from the skin surface, causing it to cool. Vasodilatation allows large quantities of blood to circulate in the uppermost layers of the dermis. Heat is then lost through convection, radiation and conduction. Blood flow is controlled by precapillary sphincters directing blood either to the capillary bed closer to the skin surface (resulting in maximum heat loss) or to the deeper tissues of the skin (minimising heat loss).

Other functions

During starvation, subcutaneous fat is utilised both as an energy source and as a water reserve. Water can also be mobilised from the dermis during haemorrhage or shock. The skin also has an excretory function, with urea and salts being excreted in small amounts through sweat.

SKIN ASSESSMENT

In completing a comprehensive skin assessment, it is important to obtain a full history, which should include:

- onset and duration of the condition
- associated symptoms, e.g. itch, redness
- actions that worsen the condition, e.g. sunlight exposure
- family history, e.g. genetic predisposition, allergies
- associated systemic disorders, e.g. asthma, hay fever
- current medication — oral and topical therapies (prescribed and OTC)
- social history — occupation, hobbies, housing, alcohol/drug intake
- impact of the disorder on daily life — personal coping strategies, self-esteem and self-image.

The history should reveal the person's description and understanding of the disorder as well as her perception of living with it. An effective assessment should determine the impact of the skin disorder on those around the patient. Skin disease, with all its social implications, has a major cultural impact that varies tremendously within our multicultural society. In Asian society, skin disease may impact on arranged marriages or payment of dowries for brides (Barker 1995). Cultural beliefs need to be identified if treatment programmes are to be adapted to acknowledge such issues. It is always pertinent to ask patients what they have already used to treat their skin. Many OTC preparations or treatments borrowed from well meaning friends can exacerbate an existing skin condition. When examining skin, the nurse needs a knowledge of 'normal' skin to be able to identify the abnormal. The entire skin surface is examined to determine the extent of the disorder. Palpation of skin lesions will determine changes in skin texture with associated crusting or scaling.

Refer to Gawkrodger (1997), pp. 14–15, for a diagrammatic representation of, and terminology associated with, dermatological lesions.

The term 'lesion' describes a small area of disease, while an 'eruption' or 'rash' describes widespread skin involvement. Skin assessment includes routine examination of the hair and nails, as changes can aid diagnosis, e.g. nail changes in psoriasis. The distribution of lesions can vary. Psoriasis tends to localise on the outer aspects of elbows and knees, while eczema is commonest in the flexural areas.

During assessment, the nurse should recognise that systemic disorders can manifest with skin changes, e.g. T-cell lymphoma (see Ch. 11). Baxter (1992) also reminds the nurse to recognise the wide diversity of skin colour in our multiracial society. The physiology of the disorder will be the same, but differences in pigmentation can influence skin changes during illness (Talbot & Curtis 1996). Skin assessment methods must be pertinent to racial groups. Communication with patients is important for accurate assessment, as a patient's description of symptoms is relevant to diagnosis and management. Initial nursing management involves alleviation of distressing symptoms while awaiting diagnosis. The nurse should also recognise that the effect of a skin disorder on quality of life is often viewed by the patient as being of greater importance than the discomfort of having abnormal skin (Salek et al 1993).

PRINCIPLES OF THERAPY IN SKIN DISORDERS

This section looks briefly at the available therapies and the basic principles of application.

Topical therapy

The skin as the target organ of treatment is readily accessible and the pathology of many skin disorders requires topical therapy as the first line of management. Topical therapy describes all treatments applied directly to skin. The classification of topical preparations is outlined in Box 12.1, and the advantages and disadvantages in using topical therapies are outlined in Box 12.2.

Box 12.1 Classification of topical preparations

- Creams — have a light effect due to high water content. They rub in easily and cool the skin
- Lotions — used if skin is 'weeping'. Good for scalp treatment as they are not greasy to apply
- Ointments — greasy preparations used as a base for the drug being applied. They last for 6–8 h on the skin, encouraging absorption by a barrier effect
- Pastes — ointments applied to medicated bandages for occlusive use or used in combination as a stiffer paste to apply treatment directly to lesions. This permits a slower, more effective absorption on the target sites

Box 12.2 Advantages and disadvantages of topical therapy

Advantages
- Drug delivered directly to target area
- Reduces systemic absorption
- Patient can view improvement
- Side-effects easily identified

Disadvantages
- Time-consuming
- Messy
- Preparations smell or stain the skin
- Patient can see deterioration or lack of improvement

Emollients — agents that moisturise and lubricate the skin — are the mainstay of dermatology treatment. They can be used in skin maintenance programmes and are vital in preparing the skin for the specific therapies available for different disorders, e.g. tar, steroids. The choice of emollient depends on the disorder:

- dry, hyperkeratotic skin — use oily occlusive ointments
- flaky rough excoriated skin — use grease-based preparations
- erythematous, inflamed skin — benefits from the cooling effect of water-soluble creams.

Patients may use a combination of emollients for different areas, e.g. cream for the face and ointment for the body.

For further reading on the application of emollients, see Dawkes (1997).

The commitment needed to maintain treatment cannot be underestimated as topical therapies can be messy, time-consuming and smelly. Treatment programmes often have to be customised because of the unique therapeutic response of each patient.

Regular nursing assessment will identify any improvement or deterioration and allow treatment to be amended appropriately. In order to achieve the desired outcome, the skilled practitioner needs a sound knowledge of dermatology therapies balanced with clinical nursing abilities to educate, support and motivate the patient to complete lengthy treatment programmes.

Phototherapy (ultraviolet light B)

Patients with certain skin disorders can be treated with ultraviolet light B (UVB) in measured doses. UVB is the wavelength in natural sunlight responsible for sunburn. Treatment requires outpatient attendance two to three times weekly over a period of weeks. A test dose administered to the patient's back determines a safe starting dose. This dose is gradually increased over the treatment period. Phototherapy is given in a cabinet with fluorescent lamps emitting UVB. The skin disorder most commonly treated is psoriasis, but eczema can also improve with phototherapy.

Photochemotherapy (psoralen and ultraviolet light A)

The treatment combination of psoralen and ultraviolet light A (PUVA) requires the patient to take oral psoralen (a natural plant extract in tablet form) 2 h before exposure to UVA. Photochemotherapy is given in a cabinet with fluorescent lamps emitting UVA. Bath PUVA (methoxypsoralen lotion) is a treatment in which a measured amount of psoralen is added to 150 L of bath water. Patients soak for a specific time, pat the skin dry and then treatment is given in a UVA light cabinet. Psoriasis and eczema can both be treated with PUVA. A test dose is administered to determine a safe starting dose and treatment is given in twice weekly sessions.

Patients having light therapy wear protective eyeglasses during UVB/PUVA exposure. After PUVA they must also wear dark glasses for 24 h to protect the lens of the eye. UVB/PUVA is administered in specialist units to ensure accurate recording of the amount of light therapy given, as guidelines exist that restrict the amount a patient may receive. Patient education prior to initiating treatment, combined with effective nursing support during therapy, empowers the patient with the skills and knowledge needed to undergo therapy and may sustain the commitment to complete treatment (Galloway & Lawson 1995).

Complementary therapies

The increasing interest in complementary therapies to treat skin disorders reflects a rise in public awareness of non-traditional approaches to treatment, perhaps stimulated by the failure of orthodox medicine to provide 'cures'. The nurse is ideally placed to discuss both the orthodox and complementary options available. Discussion should focus on the safe use of complementary therapies initiated by referral to a licensed practitioner who has undergone accredited training. Frost (1994) stresses that complementary therapy should be viewed as a useful adjunct and not as a full alternative to routine therapies. As orthodox medicine cannot provide a cure, nurses need some knowledge of complementary therapies in order to help their patients in decision-making regarding the use of such therapies as positive adjuncts to conventional management.

DISORDERS OF THE SKIN

PSORIASIS

Psoriasis is a chronic, non-infectious inflammatory skin disorder characterised by well demarcated erythematous plaques with adherent silver scales. The epidermal cell proliferation rate increases greatly, while epidermal turnover time is reduced. During normal skin production, epidermal cells mature in transit through the skin layers and are eventually shed as keratin. In psoriasis, increased cell production and transit time mean that cells do not keratinise completely and so cannot be shed. This causes the build-up of a white, waxy silver scale as immature skin cells remain adherent to the skin. Psoriasis is prevalent in 2% of the UK population, yet the cause remains unknown. It can occur in any age group and is an unpredictable skin disorder with exacerbations and remissions. Genetic influences predispose to the condition, with 35% of patients showing a family history.

Precipitating factors include:

- infection — streptococcal throat infection
- drugs — can exacerbate or trigger psoriasis
- sunlight — in some patients, psoriasis improves during the summer and relapses during the winter; however, others report that sunlight aggravates the condition
- hormonal — psoriasis can get better or worse during pregnancy
- psychological stress — can exacerbate psoriasis, but the condition itself is recognised as a stressful condition
- trauma — creates the 'Koebner effect' where psoriasis is triggered in damaged skin, e.g. surgical scar.

Psoriasis varies from mild forms, with plaques localised to the knees and elbows, to severe forms which are potentially life-threatening. Classification of psoriasis is made on clinical presentation (Hunter et al 1995).

Guttate psoriasis (see Fig. 12.3) presents as drop-like symmetrical lesions on the trunk and limbs. It is most common in adolescents and young adults and is often triggered by a streptococcal throat infection. It responds well to therapy.

Plaque psoriasis (see Fig. 12.4) presents as well demarcated erythematous plaques covered in dry, white waxy scale often localised to the knees and elbows. Removal of this build-up of keratin leaves small bleeding points. Plaques vary considerably in size and can extend to cover the trunk and scalp. Plaque psoriasis tends to be chronic, with exacerbations and remissions.

Flexural psoriasis affects the axillae, submammary and anogenital areas and looks different from typical psoriasis. Plaques are sharply defined but the skin has a thin glistening redness, often with painful fissures in the skin folds.

Pustular psoriasis (palmoplantar pustulosis) is a localised form of psoriasis affecting the hands and feet. It is characterised by yellow/brown pustules which dry into brown scaly macules. It is a painful and difficult condition to treat.

Generalised pustular psoriasis is a rare yet serious form of the disease. Sheets of sterile pustules develop, merging on an erythematous background. These areas of skin shear and the patient will be unwell. It is often triggered when attempts are made to withdraw oral or topical steroids, or may just reflect the instability of the condition.

Scalp psoriasis can often be the sole manifestation of the disorder. Thick scale adheres to the scalp and can extend to the edges of the scalp margin and behind the ears.

Nail changes in psoriasis can involve pitting of nails and onycholysis, where the distal edge of the nail separates from the nail bed. Treatment is difficult and unsatisfactory.

Erythrodermic psoriasis is a rare but severe form. The skin becomes uniformly red with high blood volume flushing it. The patient feels unwell and temperature control is difficult. It can be triggered by the irritant effects of therapies (e.g. dithranol, tars), by withdrawal of oral/systemic steroids or by a drug reaction. Erythrodermic psoriasis is an unstable state that is potentially life-threatening and warrants urgent hospital admission. The condition can progress to a generalised pustular psoriasis.

Psoriatic arthropathy. Psoriasis can be complicated by psoriatic arthropathy. Psoriatic joint disease occurs in about 5% of psoriasis patients. Joint changes occur in hands, feet, spine and sacroiliac joints. Rheumatoid factor tests are negative. Psoriatic arthropathy is a difficult combination to treat, meriting the combined expertise of a rheumatologist and a dermatologist.

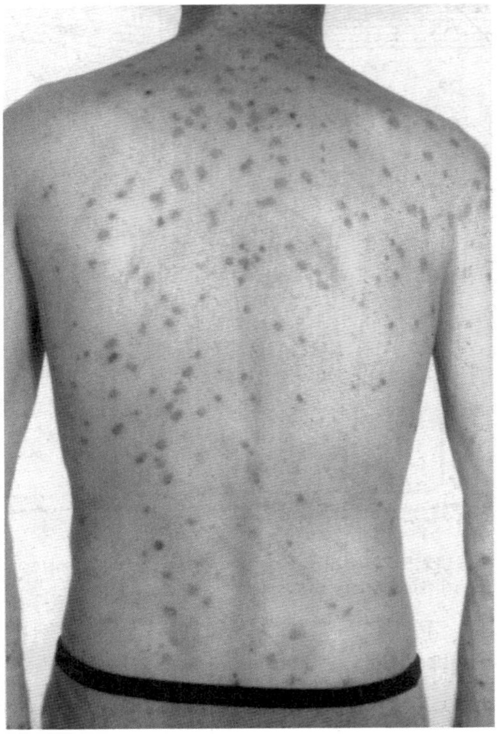

Fig 12.3 Guttate psoriasis. (Reproduced with kind permission from Dr Graham Lowe, Ninewells Hospital, Dundee.)

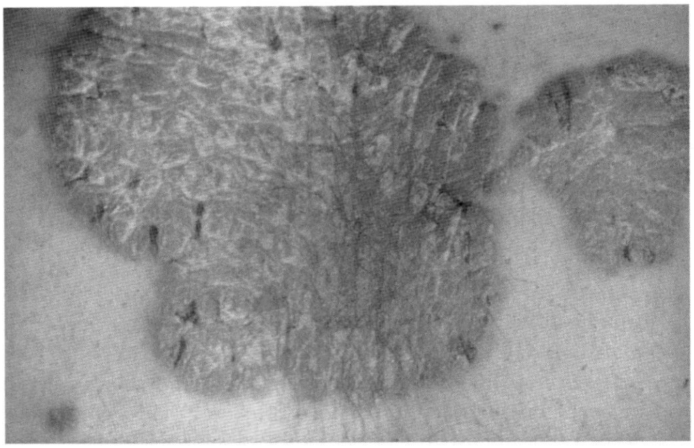

Fig. 12.4 Plaque psoriasis. (Reproduced with kind permission from Dr Graham Lowe, Ninewells Hospital, Dundee.)

PATHOPHYSIOLOGY

The pathophysiology of psoriasis is characterised by certain general processes (see Fig. 12.5). The epidermis thickens, becoming raised to accommodate skin changes. The epidermal cell proliferation rate increases. The transit time of epidermal cells maturing through normal skin is about 27 days, whereas in psoriasis it is 4 days. This suggests that psoriasis results from an increase in activity of dividing cells associated with an increase in their rate of reproduction, with trigger factors as yet unidentified.

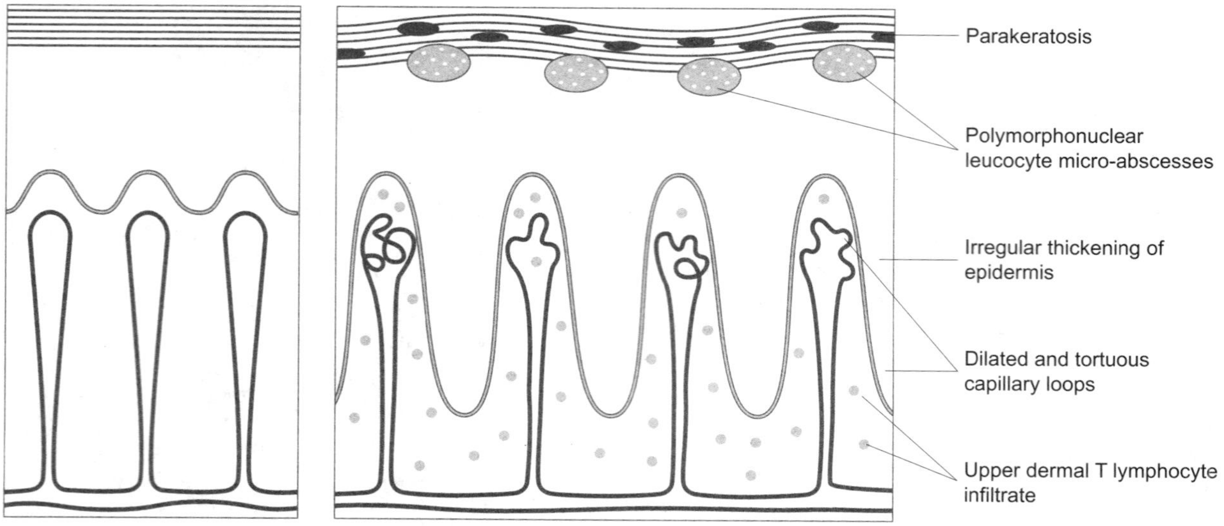

Fig. 12.5 Histology of psoriasis (right) compared with normal skin (left). (Reproduced from Hunter et al 1995, with kind permission from Blackwell Science Ltd.)

Common presenting symptoms are as follows:

- *Pain* due to fissures which form, particularly on hands and feet, because of loss of flexibility in the thickened epidermis.
- *Erythema*. Within the dermis, blood vessels dilate and increase blood flow to skin, causing generalised redness and heat loss.
- *Scaling*. The horny layer of the epidermis sheds easily in normal skin, but in psoriasis the cells become 'sticky' and build up, creating the silver-scale appearance diagnostic of psoriasis.
- *Pustules*. In inflammatory conditions, an infiltration of white blood cells is normal. Increased infiltration in pustular psoriasis accumulates as microabscesses in the outer layer of the skin.
- *Itch*. Many textbooks describe psoriasis as non-itchy, but patients often report itch to be troublesome.

MEDICAL MANAGEMENT

Where possible, psoriasis is managed on an outpatient basis, but the severity of activity in erythrodermic/pustular psoriasis may warrant hospital admission to prevent potential life-threatening complications of an unstable psoriatic state (see p. 473).

Investigations. Diagnosis can be made from the clinical picture and relevant history. Diagnosis and subsequent management may require all or a combination of the following examinations and tests:

- skin biopsy
- skin swab for flexural psoriasis
- throat swab
- Auspitz sign — gentle removal of the silvery scale from a plaque reveals pinpoint bleeding from the dilated superficial capillaries
- routine blood tests — viral check and full blood count.

Treatment may involve topical and systemic drug therapy and phototherapy. PUVA/UVB are effective therapies for psoriasis. The combination of therapies chosen depends on diagnosis and severity of the disorder. Topical prescribed therapies remain the mainstay of psoriasis treatment.

Drug therapy. Combined systemic and topical medication is useful in the management of psoriasis. Drugs used include:

- antihistamines — to alleviate itch and promote sleep and rest
- analgesics — to reduce discomfort of inflamed skin
- antibiotics — to treat streptococcal throat infections.

Drug therapy in the treatment of psoriasis should be carefully monitored. The majority of psoriatic patients respond to topical therapies, but the more extensive forms of psoriasis may require a systemic approach (Hunter et al 1995). Drugs that are particularly important in this regard are methotrexate and retinoids (p. 476).

NURSING PRIORITIES AND MANAGEMENT: PSORIASIS

General nursing considerations

The goals of nursing management will vary depending on the type and severity of the psoriasis. For example, erythrodermic or pustular psoriasis will merit skilful clinical in-patient management. However, many psoriasis patients will be treated as outpatients in a combination of settings, e.g. a specialist centre, the GP practice or at home. Education, support and empathy are vital to underpin the practical management of psoriasis. The nurse involved in outpatient management needs dermatology skills to support the patient through treatment regimens which can be messy and long-term. Decision-making regarding appropriate therapies should involve the patient and establish a partnership addressing the physical, social and emotional rehabilitation inherent in a successful outcome. Treatment sessions provide ideal opportunities for the nurse to educate the patient about her psoriasis and the rationale for using topical therapies.

Psychological support

During skin assessment and nursing review, it often becomes apparent how the patient's psoriasis is affecting her quality of life. Sharing clinical skills with the patient and using the nurse as educator can lead to therapeutic partnerships providing a supportive framework for care. The patient with a skin disorder is very vulnerable and treatment sessions provide a private time between nurse and patient during which routine conversation can reveal the true effect of the impact of the skin disorder on daily life

Box 12.3 Problems reported by patients with skin disorders

Emotional problems
- Low self-esteem
- Feel body is 'unclean'
- Relationships can be problematic
- Feel people stare — real and imagined
- Regarded as infectious or contagious

Clothing restrictions
- Avoid short sleeves
- Avoid dark clothes due to skin shedding
- Avoid summer clothes where skin is exposed
- Clothes get stained or ruined due to messy creams

Social restrictions
- Skin gets itchy in hot pubs/clubs
- Avoid swimming or sports as people stare
- Avoid communal changing rooms when shopping

Financial implications
- Routine prescriptions are expensive but essential
- No allowances available to replace clothing or bedding
- No allowances available for fuel bills due to extra laundering and bathing, etc.

Box 12.4 Examples of topical therapies used in psoriasis management

- Emollients — emulsifying ointment, aqueous cream, 50/50 (white soft paraffin/liquid paraffin)
- Bath oils — Oilatum, Hydromol
- Soap substitute — emulsifying ointment
- Coal tar ointments — coal tar solution, crude coal tar solution, Carbo-dome, Alphosyl
- Dithranol — Miconal, Dithrocream, Psoradrate, Dithranol in Lassar's paste
- Calcipotriol — synthetic vitamin D analogue, e.g. Dovonex, Curatoderm
- Scalp therapy — olive oil, Cocois scalp application, Capasal shampoo, Polytar liquid, Alphosyl shampoo
- Phototherapy — ultraviolet light B (UVB)
- Photochemotherapy
  —oral: Psoralen tablets + ultraviolet light A (UVA)
  —bath: Trimethyl-psoralen + UVA

(Box 12.3). Psoriasis is a condition requiring long-term management, and it is through the collaboration of patient, carer and professional that the right blend of therapies for effective treatment can be found. Clinical psychologists in dermatology units work closely with the patient. Body image, sexuality, quality of life and personal coping strategies are all linked to management, and effective counselling can enhance the therapeutic effect. The Psoriasis Association (see 'Useful addresses', p. 491) is a nationwide patient support group with local groups highly active in raising public awareness, supporting the patient and family, and raising funds for research.

Nursing considerations in outpatient treatment

Management of topical therapy

A range of topical therapies is used in the outpatient management of psoriasis (see Box 12.4). The nurse should encourage patients to attend regularly for treatment, stressing the importance of meticulous adherence to prescribed treatment regimens. The nurse should also explain the different preparations used, giving advice on correct application and potential side-effects. Most prescribed topical therapies are not appropriate for use on the face. By providing clear information and ongoing psychological support, the nurse can help to ensure the patient's compliance with treatment. Specific considerations in using topical preparations are as follows:

Emollients. The application of emollients is fundamental in the management of psoriasis. Bland emollients moisturise and lubricate the skin, helping to ease scaling and promote patient comfort. Regular applications seal the stratum corneum, thus reducing transdermal heat and fluid loss, which is particularly relevant in erythrodermic psoriasis.

Patients with unstable psoriasis are often treated with emollients initially to allow fiery skin to 'settle' before the next line of treatment is introduced.

Coal tar ointments are distilled from coal in the production of gas. They are usually blended with white soft paraffin and have an antipruritic, anti-inflammatory and keratolytic effect. Treatment starts with low concentrations, which are gradually increased according to the tolerance of the skin. Tar applications are messy and smelly and they stain, and so tend to be used for in-patient treatment. Proprietary blends of tar creams are available for outpatient therapy.

Tar is never applied to the face or to flexures. Patients must be advised that if ointment irritates or burns the skin, it should be removed immediately in an emollient bath and advice sought.

Dithranol is a potent plant extract that suppresses cell proliferation. It is available in many forms, but it stains skin and clothing and tends not to be popular among patients.

Dithranol is applied by spatula to affected skin, dusted with maize starch to let it set, and then covered with stockinette gauze to prevent the ointment spreading to surrounding skin. This procedure is time-consuming and messy but effective. For outpatient therapy, short-contact treatment is available. Cream is applied to the plaque after protecting the surrounding skin with Vaseline and removed 30 min later.

Calcipotriol is a synthetic vitamin D analogue applied as a cream or ointment directly to plaques. It is non-messy, non-staining and well tolerated. Calcipotriol inhibits cell proliferation and stimulates epidermal cell differentiation, correcting the increased cell turnover time associated with psoriasis. Due to potential systemic absorption, there is a restriction on the quantities prescribed, e.g. Dovonex 100 g over 7 days, Curatoderm 60 g over 12 days. The restriction will relate to the extent and severity of the psoriasis and it is important that patients are aware of the prescriptive guidelines.

PUVA/UVB (see p. 472). Both therapies are available to patients on an in-patient and outpatient basis. The treatment programme varies for each individual after identification of skin type and tolerance of sunlight. In PUVA therapy, 8-methoxypsoralen taken orally 2 h before ultraviolet exposure is photoactivated, causing cross-linkage between DNA and inhibiting cell division. Retinoids (see p. 476) can be given with PUVA to stimulate more rapid skin clearance at lower total doses of ultraviolet light. Phototherapy is a pleasant treatment, and acquiring a gentle, safe tan will boost the morale of many patients.

Goeckerman regimen. This is a long-established and effective combination treatment in which the patient takes tar baths prior to exposure to ultraviolet light (Williams 1985).
Ingram regimen. This is a combination therapy involving tar baths, ultraviolet exposure and dithranol applications.
Cocois ointment is a blend of tar, emulsifying ointment and salicylic acid used to treat scalp psoriasis. It is gently massaged into the scalp, left overnight and removed with shampoo.
Olive oil can be used in maintenance therapy to reduce the build-up of scale on the scalp. Patients are advised to warm the oil before applying it to the scalp for maximum benefit.

Nursing considerations in in-patient care

Generalised pustular psoriasis and erythrodermic psoriasis can be life-threatening conditions requiring skilled nursing management.

Monitoring vital signs

Body temperature. The patient will have difficulty in adapting to changes in environmental temperature. Body temperature must be monitored regularly, as skin temperature will fluctuate and may mask subnormal core temperature (see Ch. 22).
Blood pressure should be checked regularly. Hypotension may develop due to the shunt of blood to the peripheral circulation, leading to reduced cardiac output and potential cardiac and renal failure.

Maintaining fluid balance

Rehydration is important due to the insensible fluid loss from the skin. The majority of patients will maintain a balance if encouraged to supplement their oral intake. The liberal use of topical emollients will help to reduce fluid loss.

For further reading on the management of erythroderma, see Kerrigan (1993).

Other fundamentals of care

Basic hygiene. Soothing emollient baths are ideal in psoriatic conditions to lubricate the skin and prevent further heat and fluid loss. In severe cases, however, bathing may be prohibited due to the disruption in the patient's thermoregulatory control caused by a high blood volume flushing the skin. Regular and liberal use of emollients will suffice until the patient's condition is stable enough to permit bathing.
Rest is of paramount importance to the patient's recovery.
Diet. The possibility of protein loss through the skin dictates an adequate, nutritious diet. Dieticians can advise the patient on appropriate food choices and supplementary protein drinks.
Physiotherapy will help to minimise the side-effects of bed rest. Patients with psoriatic arthropathy will benefit from joint preservation exercises to maintain mobility and flexibility.

Systemic drug therapy

The severe nature of pustular and erythrodermic psoriasis usually merits systemic drug therapy, e.g. methotrexate and etretinate.
Methotrexate. This cytotoxic drug is a folic acid antagonist with an anti-inflammatory effect inhibiting mitosis. It is given once weekly via the oral, intramuscular or intravenous route. Careful monitoring of liver and bone marrow function is carried out and the patient on long-term methotrexate will have a liver biopsy to monitor the potential side-effect of liver fibrosis or cirrhosis. Improvement can usually be seen in 2–4 weeks. The patient should be advised to avoid alcohol and certain drugs that can interact with methotrexate, e.g. aspirin. Antiemetics should be available in case nausea is a problem.
Etretinate. This retinoid is a vitamin A derivative (Acitretin) which is very effective in pustular and plaque psoriasis. The drug is given on a daily basis in a dosage related to body weight. Etretinate influences the activity of the epidermis, normalising the plaques by thinning down hyperkeratotic lesions. A fasting blood lipid level is checked before starting the drug and the patient is monitored for hyperlipidaemia during therapy, with referral to a dietician for advice on a low-cholesterol diet if necessary. Patients may report side-effects persisting until the dose is reduced (as the psoriasis improves). Dryness of the mouth, lips and nose are common and unpleasant. Patients should be advised to use basic emollients and lip salves to ease discomfort. Reassurance that side-effects will abate once treatment is reduced or discontinued may help the patient to persevere with treatment.

Female patients taking etretinate require counselling to take adequate contraceptive measures during treatment as this drug can be harmful to the fetus.

Complementary therapies

Many 'cures' are offered in psoriasis. For example, treatment programmes involving holidays in Israel are advertised, where therapy takes the form of skin exfoliation with Dead Sea salt during natural exposure to sunlight. Acupuncture, hypnotherapy and aromatherapy are also treatment options which have varying degrees of success. The best advice the nurse can offer is that the patient considering complementary therapy consults a recognised licensed practitioner. Combined complementary and conventional therapies can provide an active and beneficial treatment programme.

The contribution of the nurse

The nurse's role in assisting the patient to manage her psoriasis will be varied and invaluable. Education, empathy and skilful clinical nursing must underpin practical management and psychological support (Penzer 1996). Psoriasis can have a major impact on quality of life. In a survey of 127 patients with psoriasis, 10% reported a wish to die and 6% reported active suicidal intent (Gupta et al 1993). This study reinforces the importance of assessing the psychological impact of the skin disorder. The range of topical therapies can be bewildering, so the nurse must utilise clinical skills, supported by information leaflets, to ensure that the patient fully understands the treatment and methods of application. This practical support can enhance treatment compliance and have an impact on successful treatment outcomes.

ECZEMA

The word 'eczema' comes from the ancient Greek for 'to boil out of' and is the term applied to a range of inflammatory skin disorders. The aetiology of eczema is unknown. Most classifications of eczematous skin disorders use the term 'eczema' synonymously with 'dermatitis', as both terms apply to the inflammatory skin changes provoked by either internal (endogenous) or external (exogenous) factors. Eczema may occur as a result of one or both types of factors (Gawkrodger 1997).

Priorities of medical and nursing management are similar for all classifications of eczema.

Endogenous eczema

Atopic eczema (see Fig. 12.6)

Atopic eczema is a common inflammatory cutaneous skin disorder affecting 1–3% of infants in the UK; there are associated genetic

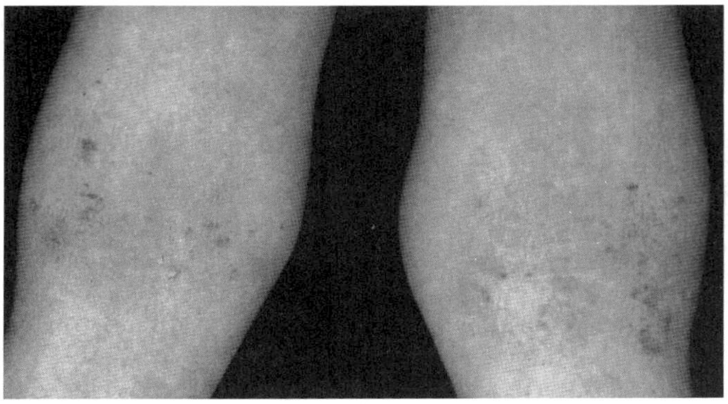

Fig. 12.6 Atopic eczema. (Reproduced with kind permission from Dr Graham Lowe, Ninewells Hospital, Dundee.)

and environmental factors. The word 'atopy' covers the classification of related disorders, e.g. asthma, eczema and hay fever. Atopic eczema can be a chronic itchy distressing disorder having a major impact on the child's behaviour and quality of life and causing severe disruption to family life. Infantile eczema can resolve spontaneously but sometimes progresses to a chronic pattern of episodic exacerbations. Sites affected are the flexural aspects of knees and elbows with involvement of the face and wrists. The prevalence of atopic eczema continues to rise and there is a significant social class gradient, with higher rates of the condition occurring in socioeconomically advantaged groups and small families (Williams et al 1994).

For further information on the impact of atopic eczema on the family, see Lawson et al (1995) and Venables (1995).

Pompholyx eczema

This is a blistering eczema localised to palms of the hands and soles of the feet. It develops rapidly, causes acute discomfort and the hands and feet can develop secondary infections. The cause is unknown and outbreaks do not appear to be related to any external factors.

Asteatotic eczema

This condition mainly affects the elderly and appears to be associated with a deficiency of sebaceous secreting glands, resulting in excessive dryness and scaling of the skin. Central heating, diuretic therapy and over-frequent washing are also implicated as possible causes. The stratum corneum develops a 'crazy paving' appearance due to a network of fine red superficial fissures. Asteatotic eczema is readily treatable at the early stages with liberal use of emollients and bath oils. Scratching of a persistent itch creates a more resistant eczema which may merit topical steroid therapy.

Varicose eczema

This usually presents as chronic patchy eczema of the legs with or without the presence of a varicose ulcer (see Ch. 23). The eczema arises due to associated chronic venous stasis and the area involved may become itchy. Scratching and tissue necrosis will lead to ulceration. The eczema is often accompanied by the presence of varicose veins, oedema and pigmentation of the skin, the latter occurring due to haemosiderin from the blood leaking through capillary vessels under elevated venous pressure (Morison & Moffat 1994). Patients often develop a secondary response to this initial area of eczema and may produce associated eczematous areas on other parts of the body.

Exogenous eczema

Irritant eczema is very common, especially in industrial settings. The eczema usually erupts at the maximum point of contact. Presentation varies according to the nature of the irritant contact. The epidermis may be damaged by abrasion, and the effect of the irritant (coal dust, cement, etc.) exacerbated by rubbing against clothing. Epidermal necrosis may occur within hours of contact with strong chemicals, while eczema triggered by milder substances (e.g. detergents) may take longer to evolve. Many patients with atopic eczema appear prone to irritant eczema and should be advised to avoid work where exposure to irritants could be problematic.

Allergic contact dermatitis

Allergic contact dermatitis is a condition in which the skin develops a specific immunological hypersensitivity. The most common allergic response of this type, particularly amongst women, is to nickel as found in inexpensive jewellery. Continued exposure to the allergen will result in an eczematous response, ranging from mild to severe. Allergic contact dermatitis may be triggered by, for example, rubber, certain plants and cosmetics, and in many cases a change of job or avoidance of the allergen will help (Williams 1993). The most difficult cases to treat are those in which allergic contact dermatitis is suspected but no definitive triggering factor can be proven.

PATHOPHYSIOLOGY OF ECZEMA (See Fig. 12.7)

Acute eczema presents with redness and swelling caused by increased vasodilatation and generalised oedema of the skin. The erythema may be generalised over the body. Acute eczema exacerbated by scratching will extend to an exudative, scaling and crusting phase.

In chronic eczema involving recurrent exacerbations, the skin is scaly, excoriated, thickened and pigmented. The eczematous areas will be localised to more defined parts of the body and lichenification will be apparent. Lichenification is a skin response to repeated scratching in which the affected areas become thickened and toughened and show a marked exaggeration of normal skin markings. Chronic scratching and thickened skin in combination allow deep, painful fissures to develop as the skin loses its normal elasticity.

Common presenting symptoms are as follows:

Itch (pruritus), which accompanies most eczematous conditions, can be acute and distressing. The itch–scratch–itch cycle quickly becomes established. The skin is well supplied with sensory nerves that respond quickly to the mechanical stimulation of scratching (or any external stimulation). Itch has two components because of the manner in which sensory impulses are transported: a quick, localised prickly sensation will be followed by a slow and diffuse burning itch.

Redness. Blood supply to the skin is prolific and is normally only required to function at low volume. Inflammatory skin diseases alter this balance by causing dilatation of blood vessels feeding the skin, leading to a generalised total body redness (erythroderma). In atopic eczema, white dermographism can be evoked due to the abnormal response of the skin's vascular change. Firm strokes of the skin normally produce a 'weal and flare' response, but in atopic patients a simple white line arises, leaving the pressure site with no erythema.

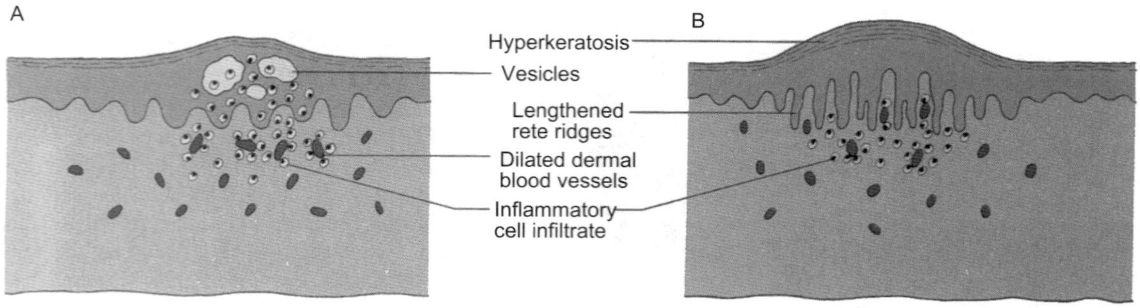

Fig. 12.7 The histology of acute (A) and chronic (B) dermatitis. (Reproduced with kind permission from Gawkrodger 1997.)

Fissures/lichenification. Chronic stages of eczema create a thickening of skin over flexures or any area traumatised by scratching. Open fissures are painful and slow to heal. In the chronic stages, there is also a generalised thickening of the prickle cell and horny layers of the skin.

Summary. Eczematous conditions present with varying degrees of severity. An acute phase of eczema may present as a weeping, inflamed response, while a chronic condition gives rise to fissures and clearly defined excoriated areas. Patients will describe itch, pain and tenderness. Loss of the normal barrier of intact skin has associated fluid and heat loss. Excoriations may lead to secondary infections, which contribute to keeping the eczema active, and patients with atopic eczema tend to be more susceptible to viral infections, e.g. herpes simplex virus and eczema herpeticum (see p. 484).

MEDICAL MANAGEMENT

Initial diagnosis is from the clinical picture of the disease process and the patient's history. Many of the exogenous conditions are managed in an outpatient setting; however, severe exacerbations warrant hospital admission.

Investigations. Precise diagnosis may require all or a combination of the following.

Laboratory investigations will include:

- Skin swabs — excoriated lesions contribute to secondary infection
- Skin scrapings — to identify bacterial, fungal or viral involvement
- Skin biopsy — for immunohistological examination (when diagnosis is in doubt).

Patch testing may be carried out to confirm allergic dermatitis. A range of patch tests is available in which suspected allergens (e.g. hairdressing products, plant material, rubber) are made up in a concentration which would normally produce no reaction unless the patient is sensitive. Allergens are applied to the back, left in situ for 48 h and then removed. The site of the test is 'read' at 96 h. Positive results vary from mild erythema to small blisters. Patch tests should not be carried out while the patient is in the acute phase of eczema or using a topical steroid, to avoid exacerbating the condition or obtaining misleading results.

Blood tests may indicate the presence of specific antibodies which can confirm an eczematous response to external factors, e.g. dust mite, cat /dog hair, certain foods.

For further reading on patch testing, see Ratcliffe (1998).

Treatment is either systemic or topical.

Systemic drug therapy includes the use of:

- antihistamines — reduce itch by blocking histamine receptors; side-effect of drowsiness aids sleep and rest
- antibiotics — bacterial infection due to excoriation is treated with broad-spectrum antibiotics
- analgesics (e.g. paracetamol) — may ease heat, tenderness and localised pain.

Topical therapies are a priority in the management of eczema (see Box 12.5). Eczema also improves in some patients on exposure to natural sunlight.

NURSING PRIORITIES AND MANAGEMENT: ECZEMA

General nursing considerations

Nursing management is of central importance in the treatment of eczema, and patients and their families must be involved in setting goals for care. The short-term priority of management is to alleviate discomfort. A tired, hot, itchy patient is not in an ideal state to absorb information and learn self-care techniques.

Ongoing support and reassurance are fundamental to achieving long-term goals. Informing the patient about eczema creates greater understanding of the condition and its outlook. Treatment sessions present the ideal opportunity to familiarise the patient with topical therapies, their effects and the rationale for their use.

Box 12.5 Examples of topical therapies used in the management of eczematous conditions

- Emollients — 50/50 white soft paraffin/liquid paraffin, emulsifying ointment, aqueous cream, Epaderm, Diprobase cream, Lipobase
- Bath oils — Oilatum, Oilatum + Stersac
- Soap substitute — emulsifying ointment, Epaderm
- Steroids — Dermovate, Betnovate, Eumovate
- Steroids/antibiotics — Dermovate-NN, Betnovate-C
- Bandages — Icthopaste, Quinaband, Coltapaste, wet wrap dressings
- UVB

Giving psychological support

Collaboration of patient, carer and health professional is vital to a successful treatment outcome. Substantial time and effort can be required to motivate, educate and empower the patient to share the process of managing the condition. Sharing of clinical skills blends into a background of psychological support that permits patient and nurse to develop a therapeutic partnership that can enhance care. The National Eczema Society is an active patient support group offering a wide range of information, skin education road shows and peer group support essential to raising self-awareness and self-esteem (Jeyasingham 1997).

Nursing considerations in topical therapy

Emollients

These moisturisers, used to make dry and scaly skin smoother, take the form of bath oils, creams and ointments and are the mainstay of treatment. Itch, heat and dryness all respond promptly to lubrication. Many emollients create a barrier for inflamed skin, preventing further fluid and heat loss. Eczema is a condition in which the skin is chronically dry, so long-term use of emollients maintains good skin tone. Patients should avoid perfumed products and use prescribed bath oils and soap substitutes. Continued use of emollients throughout the day is a major adjunct to therapy.

In hospital, the patient will use very greasy moisturisers and emollients, but these products may be totally unsuitable for use at home or in the workplace. For community use, there are bland emollients which are effective, non-messy and non-staining. Many of these are available in pump dispensers and are attractively packaged to encourage compliance.

Steroids

The application of steroid creams and ointments constitutes the next line of management in inflammatory skin disorders. These preparations are absorbed into the skin to dampen down the inflammatory response mechanism. Because steroid therapy will have a major impact on the eczematous skin, it is important that the patient understands the correct methods of application. Absorption of topical steroid and the volume of cream used will be greater if the skin is dry and excoriated (Morris 1998). Thus the skin must be regularly moisturised with emollient as an adjunct to steroid therapy, and steroids should be applied to freshly bathed skin or at least 20 min after the application of an emollient. Using the 'fingertip method', measured amounts of cream (Fig. 12.8) are gently massaged into the affected areas for maximum effect (Finlay et al 1989).

Although the best treatment advice is to start with the lowest strength of steroid possible to treat the skin, many eczematous conditions require a potent steroid to switch off the inflammatory process. Treatment programmes involve starting with a medium to strong steroid applied twice daily, gradually reducing the strength of the creams used as the condition improves. Many patients are aware of the side-effects of topical steroids, e.g. systemic absorption, striae, loss of subcutaneous fat and fragile skin. The nurse must emphasise that it is prolonged use of strong topical steroids with inadequate use of emollients that produces chronic side-effects. In eczema, secondary bacterial infection may be present and treatment may include a combined steroid antibiotic cream.

Bandaging

A variety of occlusive, medicated bandages is available for dermatological therapy (see Box 12.5). Applied overnight they provide a cooling effect and their occlusive action creates a moist environment, which aids the absorption of topical therapy. They also provide a mechanical barrier, preventing damage to the skin from scratching. The use of wet wrap dressings is a well established therapy in managing the child or adult with eczema. The technique involves the initial application of emollient, or steroid and emollient, followed by covering with, first, a wet layer of Tubifast bandage, and then a dry layer of Tubifast. Water in the moist bandages evaporates, creating a cooling effect that markedly reduces pruritus (Turnbull 1994). This is a simple procedure that is quick to apply, well tolerated and effective. The skilled community nurse who can teach bandaging techniques to parents can help to restore harmony to a family when a child with eczema is distressed by itch, particularly during the night.

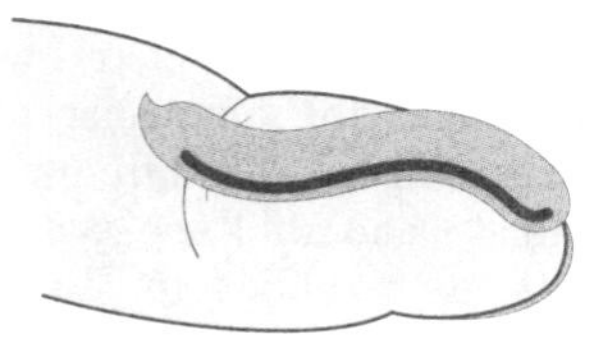

Fig. 12.8 Fingertip unit measures about 0.5 g of ointment. (Reproduced from Hunter et al 1995, with kind permission from Blackwell Science Ltd.)

Other considerations

Rest

Rest is imperative for recovery in more severe eczematous conditions. In hospital, the patient is afforded the opportunity to suspend activities of socialisation, taking time out to allow the skin to heal. In the home or school, disruptive, manipulative behaviour is often described in the child with atopic eczema, who may merely be distraught by itch and inadequate sleep (Reid & Lewis-Jones 1995). The nurse must give clear information and reassurance on the safe use of antihistamine drugs in children. Many parents are not keen to give their child drugs, but the judicious use of antihistamines will provide rest and relief for the eczema sufferer and her family (Bysshe 1996).

Diet

Diet is implicated in some forms of infantile eczema where the child is allergic to milk or milk products. The best advice to give to patients is to maintain a well-balanced diet while avoiding foods known to cause irritation (Bacon 1995). Exclusion diets to identify food allergy are difficult and should be attempted only under the supervision of a dietician. Research to identify whether breast feeding reduces the incidence of infantile eczema is ongoing. Parents are advised to choose feeding methods appropriate to them and their baby.

Complementary therapies

The stress of having a skin disorder applies particularly to eczema, where patients can be distraught with physical symptoms and altered body image. Conventional medicine with its potential side-effects cannot offer a cure, and so the nurse working with patients with skin disorders should be aware of the diverse range of complementary therapies available.

These include:

- evening primrose oil
- homeopathy
- herbalism — Chinese herbal drinks
- aromatherapy.

Complementary therapy should not be viewed as a total alternative to conventional medicine and referral to a trained recognised practitioner is essential for safe management (Frost 1994). Eastern techniques using self-help tools from energy-based therapies, e.g. Dru Yoga, Shiatsu and Chi Kung, can blend with Western techniques to reduce stress and boost the body's natural healing capacity. Habit reversal methods are available that focus on breaking the itch–scratch–itch cycle of eczema (Bridgett 1996). The main aim of habit reversal is to create awareness in the patient of when and how often she scratches her skin. Treatment methods vary for each age group so specialist help must be sought before undertaking such techniques.

The contribution of the nurse

The specific role of the nurse depends on the severity of the condition and the treatment setting. Current moves to maximise outpatient management put the primary care team at the forefront of skin care, and therefore their clinical skills and educational abilities must address the identified need. Much of dermatology nursing focuses on the child with atopic eczema and her family, due to the acknowledged impact this condition has on quality of life. Planned nursing care must be committed to the sharing of clinical skills and education of carers. Coordinated care and holistic practice can be achieved through a multidisciplinary team approach (Lynn et al 1997).

The primary care of children with eczema must reflect the specific needs of the child and her family. School nurses can support and motivate the child to maintain skin care at school while educating teachers about the physical and psychosocial impact of eczema. Health visitors should be involved in regular monitoring to ensure therapies are not inhibiting the child's development.

In the workplace, the occupational health nurse advises on changes in work practice to reduce risk factors and the incidence of industrial-acquired skin disorders (Payling 1996). In every setting, the nurse practitioner should utilise all available resources and refer patients appropriately to the relevant agencies and support groups.

Q

12.2 Ms H is the single parent of three children aged 1, 3 and 5 years. She is unemployed and lives in rented one-bedroom accommodation while on a council house waiting list. Her 3-year-old son has severe eczema. He is kept awake at night by severe itch and disrupts the household.

Discuss with a health visitor how this mother might be helped to cope with this situation.

SKIN INFECTIONS AND INFESTATIONS

This section describes infections and infestations commonly encountered in the community, and an awareness of them is thus particularly relevant to the community practitioner. Many of these conditions cause consternation among sufferers because of their real or perceived social implications. Sound common sense, the ability to dispel myths, and practical skill in identifying, assessing and treating the conditions described are fundamental to care.

Fungal infections

The commonest fungal infections are caused by the dermatophyte or yeast-like fungus *Candida albicans*, which is responsible for superficial infections confined to the skin and mucous membranes. Deep fungal infections can remain localised or cause systemic disease.

Dermatophyte infections

Dermatophytes are botanically related fungi responsible for ringworm infections. Some dermatophyte infections are confined to humans, while others principally affect animals, although transfer of fungal infections from animal to humans does occur, causing severe inflammatory skin reactions. Dermatophytes grow in keratin, i.e. stratum corneum, hair and nails, and these superficial infections are usually indirectly acquired by contact with keratin debris carrying fungal hyphae (Graham-Brown & Burns 1990).

The term 'tinea' is the generic description given to these fungal infections.

Tinea pedis or athlete's foot is the commonest of the dermatophyte infections. The patient complains of itchy, scaling skin between the toe webs and this is commonly acquired through contact with infected keratin on the floors of swimming pools or showers.

Tinea cruris affects young males, presenting as scaly erythematous lesions on the inner thighs and spreading to the perineum and buttocks. The source of infection is usually athlete's foot and the fungus is transferred to the groins on fingers or towels.

Tinea unguim is the term for fungal dystrophy of the toenails in which the nail thickens, discolours and becomes very friable.

Cattle ringworm (tinea corporis) is common amongst farm workers or visitors to farms. The fungus is picked up from gates or fences where cattle have left keratin debris containing the organism. The face and forearm tend to be affected and the fungus provokes a severe inflammatory reaction.

MEDICAL MANAGEMENT

Skin scrapings taken for examination under the microscope confirm the diagnosis. Topical treatments are broad-spectrum antifungal creams, e.g. miconazole (Daktarin) and clotrimazole (Canestan), which are available over the counter. Topical therapy for dystrophic nails is ineffective. Oral therapy is available for scalp and skin ringworm. Griseofulvin is a fungistatic and prevents proximal spread of the fungus.

NURSING PRIORITIES AND MANAGEMENT: DERMATOPHYTE INFECTIONS

Nursing management focuses on containment of infection and promotion of basic hygiene (White 1991). Avoidance of shared face cloths/towels etc. prevents further spread. The nurse can advise on prescribed and OTC therapies and their correct method of application. Treatment programmes may involve combined oral and topical therapies, and patients should be advised to persevere where therapies take time to resolve the condition. Conditions can recur, so educating the patient in management of the condition is beneficial in preventing this.

Candida infection

Candidiasis (thrush) is the term applied to infections of the skin and mucous membranes by *Candida albicans*. This fungus is a normal commensal of the human digestive system, only becoming pathogenic if the opportunity presents itself. Immunosuppressed patients, diabetics, patients on broad-spectrum antibiotics or on topical and systemic steroid therapies are all at risk from this opportunistic infection.

Buccal mucosal candidiasis refers to oral thrush presenting as milky curd-like spots on the tongue and inner cheeks. It often affects babies, the elderly and patients on broad-spectrum antibiotics (see Ch. 15).

Candida vulvovaginitis describes vaginal thrush, which presents with a creamy vaginal discharge and itchy erythema of the vulva. This condition tends to be associated with pregnancy, use of oral contraceptives and diabetes.

Candida balanitis is a thrush infection of the foreskin and glans. It tends to be commoner in uncircumcised males and may be associated with poor hygiene or diabetes. It can recur if a sexual partner also has vaginal thrush.

Chronic paronychia is a candidal infection of the nail plate which is common in people whose occupation involves repeated immersion of the hands in water, e.g. hairdressers, bartenders. The nails become distorted and the nail base is painful, red and swollen.

Intertrigo is the term given to candidal infection of the skin folds. Where two skin folds are in opposition, such as the groins, axillae and submammary regions, there is increased heat and humidity and thrush infections are common, e.g. nappy rash. Obesity and poor hygiene exacerbate the problem. The skin displays erythematous, well demarcated erosive lesions and is tender, moist and painful in these areas.

Angular cheilitis is a common condition of the elderly where the deep grooves at the side of the mouth tend to be moist with saliva; a *Candida* infection exacerbates the problem. It is common in denture wearers but can also be a feature of iron or vitamin B_{12} deficiency.

MEDICAL MANAGEMENT

Skin swabs, scrapings or nail clippings are taken to confirm diagnosis. Urinalysis should be performed to exclude diabetes. A full blood count must be carried out in the elderly with angular cheilitis.

Treatment is specific to the area affected. Antifungals in the form of creams, ointments and pessaries are very effective. Oral antifungal drugs are indicated in the treatment of nail infections. A combined mild steroid/antifungal, e.g. Trimovate, is appropriate to treat intertrigo, reducing both inflammation and infection. Combination packs of vaginal pessary and cream are available for vaginal thrush, e.g. clotrimazole, and these are usually single applications, depending on the dose/strength of the preparation. Newer OTC preparations include a single dose of the antifungal drug fluconazole (Diflucan).

NURSING PRIORITIES AND MANAGEMENT: *CANDIDA* INFECTION

Providing advice on basic skin hygiene and information about therapies available is an important nursing role. The nurse must be able to identify clients at risk of opportunistic infection, e.g. the elderly, babies, patients having chemotherapy, etc. The nurse's role as counsellor is vital in the treatment of genital thrush and he should respect confidential information when sexual partners are treated concurrently to prevent reinfection. Again, as many of the preparations are available over the counter, the nurse should be aware of current therapies and their application and of their efficacy in the different forms of candidal infection.

Infestations

Scabies

Scabies is a skin infestation caused by the mite *Sarcoptes scabiei* and acquired by prolonged close physical contact. The female scabies mite burrows approximately 1 cm into the stratum corneum, is fertilised by the male mite and begins to lay eggs along the burrow. Initially the patient will not notice anything, but 4–6 weeks after contact the affected person will describe intense itch, particularly at night — this is thought to be due to a hypersensitive response to mite faeces (Graham-Brown & Burns 1990). Skin examination usually reveals burrows, principally on the hands and feet, the sides of fingers/toes, between finger and toe webs, the wrists and the insteps. Burrows also present on the genitalia of males. A scabies 'rash' can be found in the axillae, umbilicus and thighs. Due to itching and scratching, burrows can become excoriated, eczematised and infected, which can confuse diagnosis.

Norwegian scabies is the term given to the form of scabies presenting in patients who have sensory deficits where the sensation of itch is absent, e.g. in spinal injuries, or in patients who are immunosuppressed because of either disease or treatment of disease, e.g. AIDS, lymphoma, systemic steroids or transplantation. Absence of scratching leads to large numbers of mites remaining on the skin in crusted lesions. During skin shedding, mites are shed into the environment, and therefore any person in contact is at considerable risk of developing scabies from the patient with Norwegian scabies.

MEDICAL MANAGEMENT

Diagnosis can be confirmed by using a needle to remove a mite from a burrow and examining it microscopically. Topical therapy is dependent on Department of Health guidelines, as therapy is prescribed on a rotational basis to reduce the probability of producing a 'supermite' resistant to conventional therapy. Current topical therapies are Lyclear and Derbac M (see Box 12.6 for treatment advice and guidelines for application). Once the infestation is treated, further therapy with a combined steroid/antibiotic cream may be necessary to reduce itch and treat excoriated lesions until the skin is fully healed. Antihistamine tablets are appropriate if itch disturbs sleep. Soothing topical preparations, e.g. Eurax cream, can be useful until residual itch disappears.

NURSING PRIORITIES AND MANAGEMENT: SCABIES

The priority is to treat the patient and identify close contacts requiring treatment. The nurse blends practical advice with psychological support, recognising the social embarrassment that infestation creates. Outpatient management is ideal and the nurse must identify current treatments and their correct method of application. As recurrent scabies is often due to poorly applied treatments, both patient and nurse should read the advice leaflets provided with topical scabicides carefully. Transient contact with the patient is unlikely to cause transmission and the nurse should reassure himself and colleagues about this. However, the patient with Norwegian scabies is highly contagious and should be isolated while treatment is ongoing. Local infection control policies should be followed regarding linen etc., and the patient may require repeated applications of scabicide until the condition resolves.

Q **12.3** A family of five (two adults and three children, aged 15, 6 and 3 years) have to treat themselves for a scabies infestation. Their GP suggests that a leaflet could be given to them to ensure they follow the correct advice. Devise a printed sheet with treatment advice for this family.

Box 12.6 Patient advice sheet for the self-treatment of scabies

How to apply a scabicide

1. Read the advice leaflet thoroughly before starting treatment
2. The skin should be cool and dry. Avoid bathing immediately before applying cream
3. Apply the cream as prescribed from the neck down — avoid the face
4. Pay particular attention to the finger/toe webs, soles of the feet, skin folds (axillae/groin), under finger- and toenails
5. Put on clean nightwear and change bed linen — normal laundering is adequate
6. Leave the cream for 8–12 h as the prescription states (overnight is ideal)
7. Bathe or shower at the end of the 8–12 h period

Points to note

- It is important that all family members/contacts are treated at exactly the same time. If there is any delay in treatment, avoid further contact with the person until they are treated
- If hands are washed during the treatment period of 8–12 h ensure cream is reapplied to the hands
- Weaker strengths of cream are available for pregnant women or infants
- Treatment can be repeated but your doctor will decide if this is needed

Head lice (pediculosis capitis)

Head lice are transmitted by close contact. The adult female louse lays eggs cemented to the hair about 0.5 cm from the root. Scalp irritation and itch are due to the saliva produced as the louse bites the scalp. The 'nit' is the empty case left once the larvae have hatched — the case becomes white and is more easily detected. Head lice is an emotive topic, as it continues to be endemic amongst schoolchildren and causes great consternation to parents.

NURSING PRIORITIES AND MANAGEMENT: HEAD LICE

The initial priority is to treat the patient and appropriate contacts. Treatment usually consists of a lotion applied to the scalp, e.g. Malathion and Prioderm, which is left on for a number of hours and then shampooed out. Treatment may need to be repeated. Gently combing with a fine-tooth comb assists in the final removal of nits. Department of Health guidelines rotate scalp therapies to prevent the development of treatment-resistant head lice.

Carbonyl, a product found in head lice treatments, was highlighted as carcinogenic in animals and many scalp preparations were restricted to prescription-only availability. Department of Health guidelines identified a theoretical risk to humans but acted in response to public alarm. There has also been recent media controversy implicating head lice preparations in myalgic encephalitis (ME) in children. At present the nurse should continue to reassure parents that compliance with treatment is preferable to an increased uncontrollable rise in head lice infestation. Current scalp therapies are constantly reviewed and their safe use is to be encouraged, following the treatment guidelines issued with each product. These preparations cannot be used as prophylactic treatment to prevent infestation. The school nurse is ideally placed to target and educate students, teachers and parents in the treatment, preventive strategies and environmental measures that will assist in the reduction and control of head lice.

For further reading on diagnosis, treatment, screening and prevention programmes, see Clore (1990). The comprehensive text includes diagrams and flow charts to assist students in completing a study guide.

Bacterial infections

Streptococcal infection: cellulitis

Cellulitis is an acute, spreading and potentially serious infection of dermal and subcutaneous tissue, characterised by red, tender skin at the site of bacterial entry. Organisms isolated in cellulitis include *Staphylococcus aureus* and *Streptococcus pyogenes*. Cellulitis is a common condition in the elderly, who tend to suffer from lower limb oedema. Infection enters the skin in a variety of ways, including surgical lesions, stasis eczema or leg ulcers, minor abrasions and i.v. drug injection sites. Erysipelas is the name given to a superficial streptococcal infection of the skin.

In adults, the most common presentation is cellulitis of the lower limbs, with the point of entry of infection usually being a fissure between the toes. The site affected will be oedematous, red, hot and painful. An associated general malaise with rigors and fever develops. Enlarged lymph nodes are evident due to the severity of the infection.

MEDICAL MANAGEMENT

Treatment concentrates on diagnosis, isolation of the organism by blood cultures and relevant oral or i.v. antibiotic therapy. Analgesics reduce the pain of inflammation.

NURSING PRIORITIES AND MANAGEMENT: CELLULITIS

Bed rest, monitoring of temperature and appropriate action if rigors occurs are the first line of nursing management. Pain assessment and administration of regular analgesics will ease discomfort.

Cellulitis of the lower limbs requires bed rest and elevation of the affected limb to reduce oedema. Encouragement in passive exercising reduces the complications of prolonged bed rest. Once the condition resolves, general advice on basic skin care and avoidance of predisposing factors is helpful. Patients can have recurrent cellulitis and may be prescribed prophylactic antibiotic therapy to prevent future episodes.

Staphylococcal infections: impetigo

Impetigo is a superficial bacterial infection of the skin caused by *Staphylococcus aureus* often combined with haemolytic streptococci. The head and neck are the commonest sites. The condition starts as a small but gradually enlarging pustule that ruptures to leave a raw exuding surface. The exudate dries and forms the yellow golden crust typical of impetigo. It can occur as a secondary infection, e.g. associated with eczema and scabies.

Staphylococcal infections: folliculitis

Folliculitis, an infection of superficial hair follicles by *Staphylococcus aureus*, presents as a small pustule on an erythematous base centred around the follicle. In dermatological conditions, folliculitis may be exacerbated by the use of greasy ointments, occlusive bandages and tar therapies.

MEDICAL MANAGEMENT

In all bacterial infections, treatment is by the use of topical and oral antibiotic therapies (Ritchie & Thompson 1992).

NURSING PRIORITIES AND MANAGEMENT: BACTERIAL INFECTIONS

The nurse should give guidance about each infection and its transmission. Guidelines on personal hygiene and the avoidance of communal use of towels/cloths can reduce the spread of infection. Practical management includes the gentle application of mild topical antiseptics to remove crusted lesions. Correctly applying creams and ointments in the direction of the hair growth can reduce the incidence of folliculitis and patients should be advised to complete their course of systemic or topical antibiotics to ensure treatment efficacy. The nurse must recognise and acknowledge the profound psychological impact of having a skin infection, as the social stigma of impetigo and the public perception that these conditions are associated with poor hygiene create major worries for the patient and her family. Good clinical practice, enhanced with practical information and sympathetic support, will help to address the patient's physical and psychological needs.

Viral infections

Warts (see Fig. 12.9)

Infection by the human papilloma virus affects the DNA in epidermal cells, creating warts. Different clinical manifestations are specific to different viruses (Fitzpatrick et al 1992).

Warts are benign, highly contagious and can be cosmetically unacceptable. Group transmission is the mode of contact, e.g. in gyms, swimming baths or schools. The classification of warts is outlined in Box 12.7.

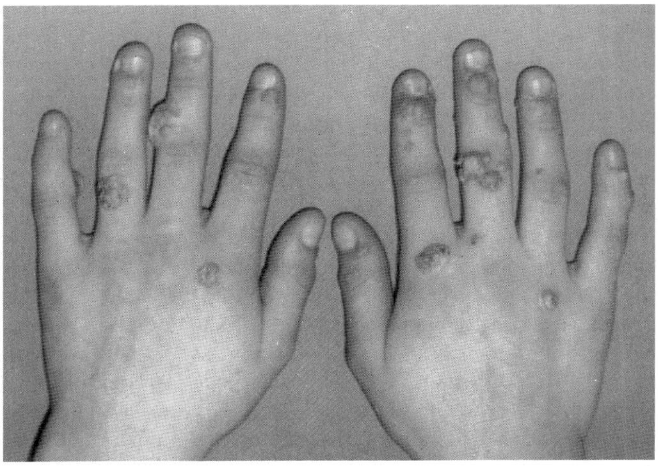

Fig. 12.9 Hand warts. (Reproduced with kind permission from Dr Graham Lowe, Ninewells Hospital, Dundee.)

Box 12.7 Classification of warts

- **Common warts** — hyperkeratotic nodules occurring on the hands and feet of children. These often resolve spontaneously
- **Plane warts** — smooth flat-topped warts appearing on the face and hands
- **Plantar warts** — commonly known as veruccae where the papilloma virus is pressured into the dermis, creating a callus. The commonest sites are the feet
- **Genital warts** — a mass of warts with a cauliflower-like appearance present on the perianal and genital areas

MEDICAL MANAGEMENT

Diagnosis is by history and clinical appearance. Histological examination of curetted lesions confirms this. Treatment may involve topical application of ointments or premedicated plasters containing salicylic acid to soften and remove the wart, curettage under local anaesthetic, or cryotherapy.

The nurse should explain virus transmission and encourage the meticulous continuation of treatment. Many patients become disheartened by the slow resolution of the problem and discontinue treatment. Regular assessment by the practice nurse may encourage treatment compliance.

Molluscum contagiosum

This is a pox virus producing solid, skin-coloured or pearly-white papules on the skin. It affects both adults and children, arising over a period of 2–3 months. The lesions may be single or multiple, occurring on the neck and trunk. In adults this condition can be a sexually transmitted disease.

MEDICAL MANAGEMENT

Initial diagnosis is by history and clinical appearance, and removal and microscopic examination of the molluscum provide confirmation. If the condition does not resolve spontaneously, freezing with local applications of liquid nitrogen may be carried out. When the condition occurs in children, parents require explanation and reassurance that the condition tends to be self-limiting. Normal basic hygiene rules prevent further spread.

Herpes simplex virus (HSV)

There are two types of herpes simplex virus: type 1 causes cold sores on the lip and face, and type 2 is associated with genital herpes. Initial contact with the herpes simplex virus is usually in childhood and often goes unnoticed. However, development of primary cutaneous herpes simplex can occur and, in a child with atopic eczema, can be a severe life-threatening condition. Following primary infection, the virus can establish itself in sensory ganglia and be reactivated by, for example, sunlight, stress and colds. Reactivation of the virus is preceded by a tingling sensation before a cluster of small vesicles develops. The vesicles burst and lesions then crust, usually resolving in 10–14 days. Genital herpes is a sexually transmitted disease affecting the penis, vulva, perianal area and rectum. Following the primary episode, the virus persists in the presacral ganglion and can recur. This is a serious condition, particularly in pregnant women because of the risk of transmitting the virus to the baby during labour.

MEDICAL MANAGEMENT

Recurrent herpes simplex is treated with oral acyclovir (Zovirax) which is now available without prescription. It must be used immediately the sufferer is aware of the tingling sensation and applied five times daily for 5 days to inhibit vesicle eruption. Patients with genital herpes should be referred to genitourinary medicine for further investigation, appropriate management and expert counselling.

NURSING PRIORITIES AND MANAGEMENT: HERPES SIMPLEX

The nurse can advise patients at risk of recurrent episodes of primary herpes simplex on the use of topical Zovirax and should recommend its continued use until course completion. The patient should be reminded of basic hygiene standards to avoid further transmission of the virus during the active phase. The patient with genital herpes may require support and counselling from specialist genitourinary services. The pregnant woman with genital herpes requires good liaison among patient, nurse, obstetrician and midwife, to acknowledge the condition and its potential complications and to initiate appropriate action to minimise virus transfer during delivery (Beardsley 1993).

Eczema herpeticum (complication of HSV)

Eczema herpeticum is a widespread cutaneous herpes simplex infection occurring in patients with atopic eczema. In children it can be life-threatening and the patient will be systemically unwell. Vesicles erupt rapidly over the face and neck and can extend to the body. The skin is taut, red and painful. As vesicles erupt and rupture, the patient becomes susceptible to secondary bacterial infection, e.g. impetigo (see p. 483).

MEDICAL MANAGEMENT

Treatment depends on the severity of illness and is a combination of antiviral and antibiotic therapies. The patient who is pyrexial and systemically unwell should be hospitalised. A side room to ensure source isolation is ideal, but good infection control procedures using hospital universal precautions will reduce the infection risk to other susceptible patients. Oral acyclovir (Zovirax) is adequate in minor cases, but if the patient is unwell then Zovirax is given by the i.v. route. The patient with eczema using topical steroids must discontinue these immediately until the virus resolves. Any secondary bacterial infection should be treated with topical antibiotic cream and oral antibiotic therapy, e.g. fucidin cream and oral flucloxacillin capsules.

NURSING MANAGEMENT AND PRIORITIES: ECZEMA HERPETICUM

The nurse's role in hospital is to maintain infection control policies to reduce the transmission of infection. The patient who is systemically unwell requires regular observations of temperature, adequate fluid intake and rest until infection resolves. The nurse should assist in topical applications of prescribed creams as the patient may feel too unwell or too distressed by pain to manage independently. Once the viral infection resolves, the nurse can advise the patient on restarting topical steroids for the eczema. Patients who are at risk of cold sores should keep Zovirax in reserve to use promptly if one develops. As Zovirax is now an OTC preparation, this advice is easier to follow as a few days' delay in getting an appointment with a GP can be detrimental in this condition which erupts quickly.

Herpes zoster (shingles)

Herpes zoster is caused by the varicella zoster virus. After an attack of childhood chickenpox, the virus remains dormant in the dorsal root ganglia of the spinal cord but can be reactivated later as shingles. The trigger factor is unknown, but the condition is common in immunosuppressed patients (see Ch. 16) and tends to affect the elderly and middle-aged.

PATHOPHYSIOLOGY

Once reactivated, the virus multiplies by invading host cells and utilising the replicatory mechanisms of the host cell to produce new DNA. The cell is lysed and virus particles are released to invade another cell. The virus particles migrate along the nerve fibres towards the skin surface, causing nerve damage and consequent pain. Balloon degeneration of the prickle cell layer of the epidermis results in the formation of fluid-filled vesicles (Gawkrodger 1997), which erupt across the thoracic and/or cranial dermatome with a characteristic unilateral band-like distribution. Fluid taken from vesicles will contain virus particles. Pain and tenderness often precede the vesicular erosions, and patients may have fever and will feel generally unwell. As the vesicles crust over, the infective risk resolves, which takes 2–3 weeks. The lesions can be erosive and may take longer to heal in the elderly.

MEDICAL MANAGEMENT

Diagnosis is confirmed by clinical history and viral culture. Treatment is by topical antiviral agent if lesions are still erupting, e.g. acyclovir. Oral or i.v. acyclovir is essential management in immunosuppressed patients. The potential complications of herpes zoster are:

- herpes zoster ophthalmicus
- postherpetic neuralgia — merits the attention of the specialist pain team.

NURSING PRIORITIES AND MANAGEMENT: SHINGLES

In an acute attack of shingles, the patient should be hospitalised. Hospital infection control policies will give guidelines for isolation of the patient until the infectious stage resolves. The patient should be nursed by staff who have had chickenpox, to reduce the contact problem. In the early stages of shingles, topical applications of antiviral cream, e.g. acyclovir, can shorten duration of the illness. The more seriously ill patient will require oral or i.v. acyclovir. Prompt referral to an ophthalmologist is vital for the patient with any eye involvement (see Ch. 13).

Certain groups of people are particularly susceptible to the transmission of herpes zoster, e.g. patients having radiotherapy and/or chemotherapy, immunocompromised patients on oral or topical steroids. Community nursing staff should be aware of the long-term problems associated with shingles. A small proportion of patients report persistent pain (postherpetic neuralgia) continuing for many years. Chronic pain has a major impact on daily living and requires full assessment. Treatment options available for postherpetic neuralgia include transcutaneous electrical nerve stimulation (TENS), ultrasound and antidepressants and/or anticonvulsant therapy. Referral to a pain control clinic is advisable for the patient with intractable pain (see Ch. 19).

For further reading on skin infections, see Gawkrodger (1997), pp. 44–47, 48–51, 54–55.

BULLOUS DISORDERS

The term 'bullous disorders' covers those skin conditions in which large watery blisters (bullae) arising within or immediately under the epidermis are a presenting feature (Hunter et al 1995). There are many causes of bullae (see Fig. 12.10) and histological location influences the classification of the disorder.

Early detection and treatment are essential, as many of the bullous conditions are severe and potentially life-threatening. The toxic effect of therapy in itself may prove fatal.

This section will highlight the bullous conditions most commonly encountered.

Pemphigus (intraepidermal bullae)

PATHOPHYSIOLOGY

This is an autoimmune disease occurring in adults. It is characterised by the development of autoantibodies against epidermal cell surface molecules creating superficial erosions and blisters on epidermal and mucosal surfaces.

Common presenting symptoms. The main presenting feature is the presence of superficial fluid-filled blisters within the epidermis. These blisters are flaccid, thin-roofed and offer little resistance; consequently they shear, leaving raw, denuded skin. Pain from the exposed sites is a major factor in management. Oral lesions are common.

Clinical diagnosis is confirmed by a positive Nikolsky's sign, such that when lateral pressure is applied to the skin surface with a thumb, the epidermis shears and appears to slide over the dermis (MacKie 1991).

Pemphigoid (subepidermal bullae)

PATHOPHYSIOLOGY

This is a common condition among elderly people; 80% of patients presenting are usually aged 60 and over (Graham-Brown & Burns 1990). Like pemphigus, pemphigoid is an autoimmune disease. Antibodies bind to the junction between dermis and epidermis, and blisters are formed in response to enzymes released from inflammatory cells.

Common presenting symptoms. The patient reports generalised intense itch, followed by erythematous plaques on the skin (pre-pemphigoid stage), followed by the development of tense blisters affecting any area of the body. Nikolsky's sign is negative.

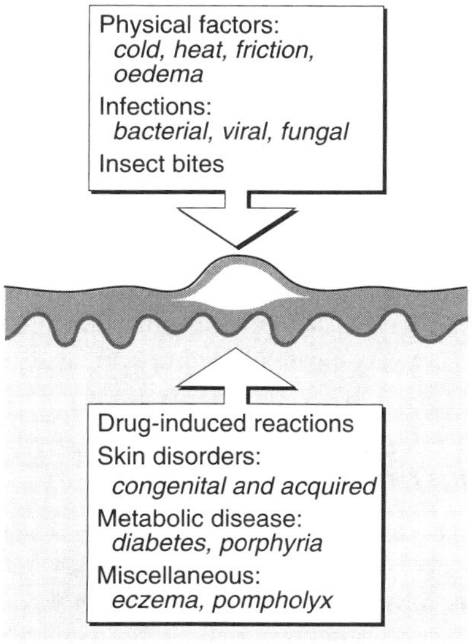

Fig. 12.10 Causes of blisters (bullae).

Toxic epidermal necrolysis (subepidermal)

PATHOPHYSIOLOGY

This condition presents as a dermatological emergency and is often precipitated by a drug hypersensitivity. The skin split is subepidermal and the entire epidermis shears off in layers, leaving raw, denuded areas. A review of the patient's drug therapy and removal of the causative factor are essential to management.

Common presenting symptoms. The skin is erythrodermic and painful, with the skin shearing off in sheets. Nikolsky's sign is positive. The patient will be distressed by pain and may have erosions in the mouth, oesophagus and bronchus.

MEDICAL MANAGEMENT OF BULLOUS DISORDERS

Early diagnosis is imperative due to the life-threatening potential of bullous disorders. Hospitalisation is a major aspect of treatment and management.

Investigations will include the following:

- Skin biopsy — to identify the type of skin split and exclude other bullous disorders
- Blood tests — to monitor urea and electrolytes in view of the associated fluid loss from eroded skin. In pemphigus the serum contains antibodies binding to the intracellular areas of the epidermis; titration of these antibodies is relevant to building a picture of the disease activity
- Skin swab — to define the bacteriological status of skin exposed to secondary infection.

Treatment will involve drug therapy with the following:

- Antibiotics — to treat secondary infection
- Steroids — in pemphigus and pemphigoid, high-dose oral steroids (prednisolone 60–100 mg daily) are the first line of management and are maintained until blistering stops. A gradual reduction in dosage is then commenced, aiming for low-dose maintenance therapy
- Analgesics — to alleviate pain from eroded skin lesions; choice is dependent on patient need and disease activity
- Antihistamines — to reduce itch and aid rest
- Immunosuppressants (e.g. cyclophosphamide, azathioprine) — used in combination with oral steroids to control the disease process of pemphigus and pemphigoid.

Plasmapheresis is considered in severe cases and allows monitoring of circulating pemphigus antibodies. Topical therapy is non-specific, aiming for patient comfort.

NURSING PRIORITIES AND MANAGEMENT: BULLOUS DISORDERS

This section focuses on general nursing care of the three disorders described. Although rare, they are commonly seen in dermatology units. It may help the reader to understand the rationale behind nursing priorities to note that these patients have similar needs to patients with severe burn injuries (see Ch. 30).

Major nursing considerations

Analgesia

Analgesia must be effective and consistent. Pemphigus and toxic epidermal necrolysis are distressing, painful conditions when shearing of the skin is active. Pain assessment tools (see Ch. 19) permit the nurse and patient to determine pain control needs, ensure accurate delivery of analgesics, and evaluate their efficacy, which is particularly relevant prior to dressing changes. Pain clinics are a specialist service to assist in prescribing appropriate analgesics by the most effective route for this type of pain.

Bed rest

Patients must rest to avoid further trauma to the skin. Special beds are available which are helpful in nursing patients with these conditions.

Hygiene

The maintenance of good personal hygiene and the prevention of cross-infection are extremely important. Gentle washing or the application of soaks, i.e. potassium permanganate, for their mild antiseptic/antipruritic effect can be soothing and help to minimise further trauma.

Isolation nursing may be necessary due to skin loss. The patient will be susceptible to infection and the use of immunosuppressants will increase this susceptibility. In severe cases, barrier nursing may be required (see Ch. 16).

Diet

Approximately 20% of an adult's dietary protein is used for skin repair and growth in normal health. Therefore, an increased intake of dietary protein is advisable in bullous conditions. Referral to a hospital dietician will ensure the prescription of any necessary supplements. Constipation induced by fluid loss, or as a side-effect of analgesics, is an associated problem. Mild laxatives may be indicated to prevent added discomfort.

Monitoring vital signs

Temperature. Regular observation of body temperature is required, as fluctuations may occur due to fluid and heat loss from the skin. Variations in environmental temperature can be reduced by nursing the patient in a side room.
Blood pressure is checked regularly if there is associated fluid loss, steroid-induced hypertension or rehydration by i.v. fluids.

Monitoring electrolyte and fluid balance

This is imperative in any condition associated with skin loss. Rehydration may initially be achievable by increasing the patient's oral intake and monitoring output. An i.v. infusion will be appropriate in severe cases. If skin loss presents problems in siting a peripheral infusion, a central line can be inserted, with monitoring of central venous pressure providing an accurate assessment of fluid requirements.

Urinalysis should be monitored for a potential diabetic state induced by oral steroid therapy.

Dressings and topical therapy

A dressing procedure provides the best opportunity to complete a skin assessment and evaluate disease activity. In pemphigus and toxic epidermal necrolysis, raw areas are recorded and dressed. The tense bullae of pemphigoid are identified and left intact to permit reabsorption of blister fluid, thereby minimising further trauma. Blisters restricting movement are uncomfortable for the patient and can be aspirated using a sterile alcohol swab, syringe and needle, leaving the blister roof intact (Stone et al 1989). Administration of analgesics prior to the application of topical therapy is important to reduce the patient's apprehension about dressing changes. Each patient's needs and disease severity determine dressing requirements, but the main aims of management are to:

- keep dressing changes to a minimum
- maximise patient comfort
- ensure dressings are easily removable.

By following these guidelines, the nurse minimises further trauma and promotes skin healing. Simple applications of soothing emollients or a non-adherent dressing secured by gauze stockinette will possibly be all that is tolerated. Heavier pads and bandaging create constriction and pain. The skilled practitioner will be guided by the patient's comments and adjust dressings appropriately.

Special care beds/pressure-relieving equipment

Facilitating rest and comfort is a primary aim in care. The use of low-pressure, air-fluidised beds has enhanced comfort and reduced the need for positional changes which contribute to shearing forces on the skin. The temperature regulator in these beds maintains an appropriately warm environment, helping the patient to maintain body temperature. This warm environment also increases the amount of insensible fluid loss, so the patient's fluid intake must be increased to compensate. Most patients achieve this by increasing oral intake, but i.v. supplements are a consideration. Dressings are kept to a minimum and remain moist with the use of these beds, and so tend to be easily removed.

Care in the community

Although these conditions are rare, as our elderly population increases, their incidence will rise. The community nurse has a dual role: firstly, in identifying disorders and coordinating referral for specialist help; and secondly, after discharge from hospital, in ensuring the patient understands the rationale behind long-term maintenance drug therapy, encouraging patient compliance and monitoring side-effects of systemic therapies.

ACNE

Acne is a disorder of the pilosebaceous glands. It is a common condition usually developing during adolescence. The psychological impact of acne should not be underestimated, as its onset during the years when visual impact is important to developing new relationships can have a devastating effect on the young adult. Dermatologists are very aware of the impact that acne can have on quality of life.

PATHOPHYSIOLOGY (Fig. 12.11)

During puberty, circulating androgens stimulate sebum production. Hyperkeratosis occurs at the mouth of the hair follicle and the dilated chamber fills with sebum. The organism *Propionibacterium acnes* grows in large numbers creating the comedone. *Propionibacterium acnes* breaks down the sebum into inflammatory chemicals which leak into the surrounding dermis or pour out through a rupture in the follicle wall (Gawkrodger 1997).

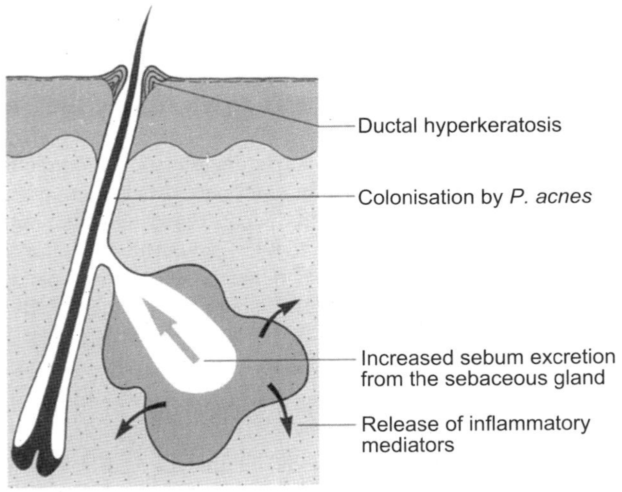

Fig. 12.11 Aetiopathogenesis of acne. (Reproduced with kind permission from Gawkrodger 1997.)

Common presenting symptoms. Acne targets the face, neck, upper back and front of the chest. In more severe cases, these lesions will spread further. Lesions can include comedones, papules, pustules, nodules, cysts and residual scars.

MEDICAL MANAGEMENT

Treatment relates to the severity of the condition. Mild acne should respond to topical therapies, antiseptic washes and antibiotic preparations used daily, while moderate/severe acne will merit combined topical and systemic therapies (Layton 1995), as follows:

- Antibiotics — oral tetracycline given over a 6-month period reduces the inflammatory process. If the patient is intolerant of tetracyclines, the drug of choice is erythromycin.
- Isotretinoin — a drug derived from vitamin A that reduces sebum production. It does have side-effects and careful monitoring of liver function and blood fat levels are indicated. The drug is teratogenic and female patients must use effective contraception. Isotretinoin has been shown to clear acne in 90% of patients with no recurrence. At present it is only available by prescription from hospital dermatology departments (James 1996).

NURSING PRIORITIES AND MANAGEMENT: ACNE

The role of the nurse is to educate and dispel the many myths of acne (Black 1995). The patient should be reassured that acne is not linked to poor diet, an excess of sweets or chocolate, or poor hygiene. Indeed, most acne sufferers are overzealous in personal hygiene. The nurse should encourage continuation of topical and oral therapies for the full treatment course. The female patient starting isotretinoin needs counselling and referral to family planning services to ensure adequate contraceptive measures are established from 1 month before starting treatment until 3 months after completion. The nurse must respond sympathetically to the acne sufferer. The degree of distress may not always equate with the severity of disease, and care must address the social and psychological impact of acne. Skin disease has been known to provoke suicide, and the nurse working with acne patients should recognise that individuals can become so disturbed by their perceived problem that they are pushed to this extreme (Cotteril & Cunliffe 1997). It is imperative that the impact of acne is not underestimated, and prompt referral to a dermatologist will initiate effective treatment.

Q **12.4** You are asked to provide a series of health talks for a group of school students. Acne is one of the topics requested. Devise a plan for your talk with relevant aims for this age group. Consider answers to the questions you may be asked on diet, cosmetics, infection and social impact.

PHOTODERMATOSES

This term applies to skin disorders that are induced or aggravated by sunlight. These disorders are relatively common and can impose severe limitations on daily life. This section will highlight specific disorders and briefly describe diagnostic techniques and treatment options. The discussion on nursing management focuses on assisting the patient to maintain independent living within the limitations imposed by photosensitivity.

Sunlight

Sunlight is composed of different wavelengths of ultraviolet light, divided into ultraviolet A (UVA), ultraviolet B (UVB) and visible light. UVA can produce erythema in larger doses, passes through window glass and is less variable in intensity. UVB is well recognised as the cause of sunburn. Visible light consists of longer wavelengths and easily penetrates the epidermis with minimal significance. Some conditions, however, demonstrate an abnormal sensitivity to visible light. Certain factors affect the intensity of sunlight:

- time of day (strongest between 11.00 and 15.00 h)
- geography
- season (UVB less intensive in winter months)
- reflective effect of snow, water and sand.

Note that clouds do not protect against sunburn as UVB penetrates cloud cover.

Types of photodermatosis

PATHOPHYSIOLOGY

Polymorphic light eruption (PLE) is the most common of the photodermatoses (Ferguson 1990a), affecting around 10% of the population. It affects patients in early spring, disappearing in autumn. Several hours after exposure to sunlight, the patient develops an itchy papular rash, which persists for 7–10 days. The rash can be provoked by UVB or UVA wavelengths, and it should be remembered that UVA also penetrates window glass and thin clothing. The rash heals without scarring (Proby 1993).

Solar urticaria is very rare and appears as itchy red patches which may be swollen and resemble nettlerash or weals. This reaction occurs almost immediately (within 10 min) after sunlight exposure and subsides within 1 h of sunlight avoidance, with no residual damage to skin.

Photo-aggravated dermatoses. Some pre-existing skin conditions, e.g. atopic eczema, psoriasis, rosacea and herpes simplex, can be exacerbated by sunlight exposure.

Photo-contact dermatitis refers to disorders in which direct contact of the skin with a substance (e.g. tars, sunscreens) followed by exposure to ultraviolet light provokes a dermatitis. Certain genetic disorders, e.g. xeroderma pigmentosum, also produce a photosensitive reaction.

Photosensitive dermatitis/actinic reticuloid syndrome. This condition particularly affects men over the age of 50 years but can occur in women as well (Ferguson 1990b). Patients are sensitive to sunlight (UVB, UVA, visible light) and artificial light sources and have many allergies to substances in direct contact with their skin, e.g. plants, flowers, wood, perfumes, sunscreens and rubber. Sparing of the shaded skin can be present, e.g. behind ears, eyelids, under a watch strap, and there may be marked differences between skin covered by clothing and exposed skin, particularly the neck and arms. The condition presents with marked erythema, eczema and thickening of the skin of the face, neck and hands. Skin changes may be evident in areas covered by clothing, e.g. the arms.

MEDICAL MANAGEMENT

Management begins with a full history and assessment of related factors and presenting symptoms (see Box 12.8).

Investigations required are as follows:

Phototesting provides an objective assessment of photosensitivity disorders and is available in specialist photobiology/dermatology units. Phototesting is performed with the use of a monochromator (Frain-Bell 1985) to identify if abnormal light sensitivity is present and establish which wavelengths are responsible, i.e. UVA, UVB or visible light. The patient's back is the test site used. Varying doses at different wavelengths are irradiated to small areas and delayed erythema is noted at 7 and 24 h. These responses are compared with known responses of a control group, thus helping to determine the degree of photosensitivity and wavelengths responsible.

Patch testing is used to identify contact allergies causing an exacerbation of the disorder. Patients may have multiple allergies which are relevant to diagnosis and subsequent management.

Treatment involves systemic and topical therapy and sometimes UVB and PUVA therapy. Drug therapy may include antihistamines, immunosuppressants and oral and topical steroids. Sunscreens offer a sun protection factor (SPF) either by chemically absorbing and filtering ultraviolet light or by physically reflecting and scattering ultraviolet rays to protect the skin. A combination sunscreen creates a more effective sun block. Some light-sensitive conditions (e.g. PLE) can be treated with a course of phototherapy (UVB/PUVA) and patients should be encouraged to continue exposure to maintain their new tolerance level. Unfortunately, this is lost during winter and the phototherapy has to be repeated the following spring.

Box 12.8 Influencing factors and common presenting symptoms of photosensitive conditions

Influencing factors
- Drug history
- Family history
- Hobbies
- Allergies
- Occupation
- Sites involved
- Skin type

Common presenting symptoms
- Eczema
- Erythema
- Heat
- Itch
- Oedema
- Pain
- Urticaria

NURSING PRIORITIES AND MANAGEMENT: PHOTODERMATOSES

Patients with diagnosed photosensitive disorders require practical help and support from nursing practitioners. Many patients are relieved that investigations have produced a diagnosis rather than a dismissal of symptoms as merely 'a bit of sunburn'. Factual information from nursing staff is vital if the patient is to cope with lifestyle changes imposed by the diagnosis. General advice includes:

- regular use of emollients
- meticulous, regular (every 2 h) application of prescribed sunscreens to exposed sites
- treatment with a reducing steroid ointment/cream regimen if the condition flares
- sun avoidance between the hours of 11.00 and 15.00 h
- protective clothing (closely woven) to provide a further effective barrier to sunlight; in severe cases, a wide brimmed hat, scarf and gloves may prove helpful
- use of clear museum film applied to house windows and car windows (Dawe et al 1996).

Giving psychological support

Social isolation is a major problem for individuals with severe photosensitive disorders. Many patients, distressed by their diagnosis and the restrictions it entails, reject management regimens, finding the maintenance of topical therapies to be time-consuming, messy and cosmetically unacceptable. Others stoically accept the limitations and persevere with the use of sunscreens to permit them freedom to continue a restricted form of daily living. The nurse must display a sympathetic understanding of the psychological trauma associated with the restrictions imposed by such a diagnosis. The overall aim of nursing support should be for the patient to control skin management in an informed and motivated manner, with instant access to professional help as needed.

URTICARIA, ALLERGY AND ANAPHYLAXIS

Urticaria is a common condition and lesions are described as 'hives' or nettlerash. The skin feels irritable and produces white raised weals that turn pink with a bordered edge. The weals can be extensive over the body. There are many causes, but the condition often resolves spontaneously. In some cases the condition can extend, creating swelling around the eyes, mouth and throat known as angioedema (see Ch. 16). In severe attacks, breathing can be compromised, so angioedema must be treated promptly (Mygind et al 1996).

PATHOPHYSIOLOGY

In response to the initial trigger factor, the dermis becomes oedematous with dilatation of blood vessels and degranulation of mast cells and the release of histamine. The weal of urticaria is oedema of the dermis, which can extend rapidly into the subcutaneous tissues causing angioedema.

Classification of urticaria (see Box 12.9). Acute urticaria can be related to contact factors, e.g. animal fur, plants, insect stings. Extensive urticaria associated with angioedema is usually related to the ingestion of food or drugs, e.g. strawberries, nuts, aspirin and penicillin. Urticaria is common in individuals with atopic eczema.

Box 12.9 Classification of urticaria. (Reproduced with permission from Gawkrodger 1997)

- Chronic — idiopathic
- Acute — IgE-mediated, e.g. food allergy, drug reaction
- Physical — dermographism, cholinergic, cold, solar, heat, delayed pressure
- Contact — immune (e.g. animal saliva) or non-immune (e.g. nettle sting)
- Pharmacological — aspirin, opiates, non-steroidal drugs, food additives
- Systemic cause — systemic lupus erythematosus, lymphoma, thyrotoxicosis, infection, infestation
- Inherited — hereditary angioedema
- Other — urticarial vasculitis, papular (insect bites), mastocytosis, pregnancy

Cold, heat, sun, pressure and water can all induce physical urticarias. Sweating in response to physical exercise or eating spicy food may also induce urticaria. Hereditary angioedema is a rare and potentially fatal autosomal dominant condition. It presents in childhood and requires skilful long-term management during acute attacks and in establishing prophylactic therapy.

MEDICAL MANAGEMENT

Clinical history and skin examination will help to determine the provoking factors. Further investigation may be required to exclude systemic conditions. Antihistamines are essential in the management of urticaria. These H_1 antagonists block histamine release and the newer preparations have a non-sedative effect. In acute attacks, the patient requires oral antihistamines until the condition resolves (usually a few days). In chronic urticaria, the patient will remain on a maintenance antihistamine for a few months before stopping the drug. In an acute attack of angioedema, the use of i.v. antihistamines may be necessary. Urticaria can be associated with anaphylaxis (see Ch. 16), and adrenaline and antihistamine drugs will be used in combination. Severe urticaria may also require short-term use of systemic steroids. Patients with identified severe reactions to foodstuffs are trained to administer i.m. or s.c. adrenaline at the onset of attacks (Lawlor 1998).

NURSING PRIORITIES AND MANAGEMENT: URTICARIA, ALLERGY AND ANAPHYLAXIS

The nurse in every setting will encounter the patient with allergies. Angioedema and anaphylactic reaction can prove fatal so professionals must recognise the urgency of the situation and be fully trained in initiating emergency action (McGeary 1997). The role of the nurse during an acute attack is to assist with medical management of urticaria until the acute phase stabilises. Afterwards, the nurse's role as provider of factual information and management of the condition begins.

Dieticians provide dietary advice to assist in the avoidance of foods that trigger urticaria. Dietary exclusion is difficult as food labelling is not always helpful. Public pressure has persuaded food companies and supermarkets to focus on the importance of accurate food labelling, as the incidence of food allergy, and in particular peanut allergy, seems to be increasing (Ministry of Agriculture, Fisheries and Food 1996). Peanut allergy and sensitisation can lead to severe anaphylactic shock and death, so accurate food labelling is vital. Expectant mothers are advised to avoid eating nuts to prevent sensitisation in children. However, as our knowledge of the mechanisms of food allergy improves, diagnosis and management will also improve. The link between breast feeding, weaning and allergy is still being researched (Obeid 1996).

The patient who has severe allergic reactions should be trained in the use of adrenaline pens (Epipen). The nurse can help the patient and family in relation to all aspects of the allergy, in particular to recognise warning symptoms and to use the adrenaline pen promptly whilst seeking medical assistance. It will be necessary for those involved in caring for the child with an allergy, e.g. school teachers, to be aware of potential problems and to be given instruction on using the Epipen (Keen & Comer 1995).

The nurse has a positive role in raising awareness of allergies, giving informed advice to patients, carers and fellow professionals, and providing the empathy and support that clients require to improve and maintain their quality of life.

SKIN TUMOURS

The skin, as a complex organ system, produces many tumours, both benign and malignant, within the epidermis and dermis. The reader should refer to a colour atlas of dermatology to fully appreciate the wide diversity of skin tumours (Fitzpatrick et al 1992). Skin biopsy and histology are necessary in the diagnosis, prognosis and management of skin tumours.

Malignant melanoma is the most serious of the skin tumours and its incidence is rising. Melanoma accounts for only 3% of cutaneous tumours but is responsible for two-thirds of deaths attributable to skin cancers. UK figures suggest that 65% of patients with melanoma have a survival rate of 5 years (MacKie 1991). Melanoma commonly arises in a naevus (mole), involves the pigment producing melanocytes and can metastasise rapidly via the circulatory and lymphatic systems. This differentiates it from other skin tumours. Prognosis depends on tumour thickness (Breslow 1970). Early detection and excision of thin tumours (less than 0.78 mm thick) carries an excellent prognosis and potential cure. Late-stage untreated melanoma with secondary deposits has a poorer outcome and treatment is often palliative, e.g. radiotherapy, chemotherapy, laser therapy (see Ch. 31).

Research is producing evidence that excessive childhood sun exposure is an important factor in the aetiology of melanoma. The general perception, furthered by the media, that 'tans' are fashionable and that sunshine generates psychological and physical well-being is now being challenged. During the 1990s, Imperial Cancer Research Fund campaigns targeted young children and adolescents, e.g. 'Sun Cool' and 'Monty Mole's Marvellous Mission', aiming to increase public awareness of the dangers of excessive sun exposure and the importance of regular skin checks to ascertain changes in moles at an early stage (Box 12.10). Nurses can assist in promoting health education that sanctions 'safe sun' and encourages behavioural and social changes that might prevent or reduce the incidence of melanoma. Advice includes:

- avoidance of direct sun during the hours of 11.00–15.00 h
- use of high sun protection factor (SPF) creams
- use of T-shirts/sun hats.

Nurses in contact with any group of people can encourage regular checking of 'moles' as a preventive strategy which could have a profound impact on the early detection and incidence and mortality rates of malignant melanoma.

For further reading, see Perkins (1992), Van Der Weyden (1996) and Chapter 11 of the present text.

Box 12.10 Mole watching — warning signs of melanoma

- Are new or existing moles changing in size or getting larger?
- Changes in the normal smooth edge of the mole to a more irregular shape
- Changes in colour of the mole
- Is the mole itchy or painful?
- Is there any surrounding or underlying inflammation?
- Is there any bleeding, oozing or crusting?

CONCLUSION

This chapter has focused on some of the more common skin disorders encountered in hospital and in the community, but there are many more that could have been included. Further reference to a specialist textbook will reveal the full scope of dermatology as a major speciality. In raising the profile of dermatological nursing, the British Dermatology Nursing Group (BDNG) has developed educational initiatives addressing the needs of nurses working with patients with skin disorders. The Royal College of Nursing document *Standards of Care for Dermatology Nursing* (RCN 1995) was developed to provide an established level of requirement on which to base specialist practice (Stone 1997b). The role of the nurse in primary and secondary care settings cannot be underestimated. Nurse prescribing (Bowman 1998) and the development of care systems (Gradwell & Haynes 1999) are practice initiatives enhancing communication with patients by empowering them to be involved in care delivery. Incorporating quality of life indices into nursing assessment provides subjective measurement of the impact skin disorders have on life (Thoms 1997). The role of the named nurse is invaluable as assessor and in planning care that is patient-focused and need-centred. Education, counselling and sharing of clinical skills underpin a supportive partnership that may enhance treatment compliance. Advice leaflets reinforcing verbal instructions are simple to prepare and beneficial to the patient overwhelmed by the bewildering array of ointments and lotions prescribed for her skin disorder.

Further innovations in health screening and primary prevention campaigns will ensure nurses working with patients with skin disorders are a major link between primary and secondary care, with an active role in reappraising, developing and adapting practice to directly meet the needs of the client group.

REFERENCES

Bacon P 1995 Nutrition and skin care. Community Nurse 1(7): 34
Barker D 1995 More than skin deep. Practice Nurse 8(13): 761–767
Baxter C 1992 Observing skin. Community Outlook 2(9): 29–31
Beardsley J 1993 Understanding herpes simplex virus. Professional Nurse 8(5): 322–328
Black P A 1995 Acne vulgaris. Professional Nurse 11(3): 181–183
Bowman J 1998 Changing roles – should nurses prescribe? Dermatology in Practice 6(3): 14–16
Breslow A 1970 Thickness, cross sectional area and depth of invasion in the prognosis of cutaneous melanoma. Annals of Surgery 172: 902–908
Bridgett C 1996 Behavioural approaches to treating atopic eczema. Health Visitor 69(7): 284–285
Bysshe J 1996 Eczema: making an unpleasant condition more bearable. Professional Care of Mother and Child 6(3): 59–61
Cotterill J A, Cunliffe W J 1997 Suicide in dermatology patients. British Journal of Dermatology 137: 246–250
Dawe R J, Russell S, Ferguson J 1996 Borrowing from museum and industry – two photoprotective devices. British Journal of Dermatology 135: 1016–1017
Department of Health 1991 The patients' charter. HMSO, London
Department of Health 1992 Health of the nation. HMSO, London
Ferguson J 1990a Photosensitive dermatitis and actinic reticuloid syndrome (chronic actinic dermatitis). Seminars in Dermatology 9(1): 47–54
Ferguson J 1990b Polymorphic light eruption and actinic prurigo. Current Problems in Dermatology 11(5): 127–147
Finlay A Y, Edwards P H, Harding K G 1989 'Fingertip unit' in dermatology. Lancet 2: 155
Fitzpatrick T, Johnson R, Polana M, Suurmound D, Wolff K 1992 Colour atlas and synopsis of clinical dermatology, 2nd edn. McGraw-Hill, New York
Frain-Bell W 1985 Investigation of cutaneous photosensitivity. Cutaneous photobiology. Oxford University Press, Oxford
Frost J 1994 Complementary treatments for eczema in children. Professional Nurse 9(5): 330–332
Galloway G A, Lawson G B 1995 Photochemotherapy (PUVA) protocol. Dermatology Nursing 7(6): 348–351
Gawkrodger D J 1997 Dermatology: an illustrated colour text, 2nd edn. Churchill Livingstone, Edinburgh
Gradwell C, Haynes M 1999 Developing a care system for dermatology patients. Professional Nurse14(12): 821–823
Graham-Brown R, Burns T 1990 Lecture notes on dermatology, 6th edn. Blackwell, Oxford
Gupta M A, Schork N J, Gupta A K et al 1993 Suicidal ideation in psoriasis. International Journal of Dermatology 32: 188–190
Hinchliff S M, Montague S E, Watson R (eds) 1996 Physiology for nursing practice. Baillière Tindall, London
Hunter J, Savin J, Dahl M 1995 Clinical dermatology, 2nd edn. Blackwell Science, Oxford
James M 1996 Isotretinoin for severe acne. Lancet 347: 1749–1750
Jeyasingham M 1997 National Eczema Society – 21 years of patient advice and support. British Journal of Dermatology Nursing 1(1): 10–12
Keen S, Comer L 1995 Subcutaneous administration of adrenaline for anaphylaxis. Nursing Times 5(91): 36–37
Kurwa H A, Finlay A Y 1995 Dermatology inpatient management greatly improves life quality. British Journal of Dermatology 113: 575–578
Lawlor F 1998 Diagnosing and treating common urticaria. Dermatology in Practice 6(3): 18–20
Layton A 1995 Acne: assessment and treatment. Community 1(7): 36
Legge A 1997 Skin care: take three experts. Nursing Times 93(44): 70–71
Lewis-Jones S 1999 Quality of life – skin disease and disability. Dermatology in Practice 7(3): 8–10
Lynn S, Lawton S, Newham S 1997 Managing atopic eczema: the needs of children. Professional Nurse 12(9): 622–625
MacKie R M 1991 Clinical dermatology: an illustrated textbook, 3rd edn. Oxford Medical, Oxford
McGeary T 1997 Fatal reaction. Nursing Times 20(93): 26
Ministry of Agriculture, Fisheries and Food 1996 Food safety information bulletin 78, pp 1–2
Morison M J, Moffat C J 1994 A colour guide to the assessment and management of leg ulcers, 2nd edn. Mosby, London
Morris A 1998 Effects of long-term topical corticosteroids. Dermatology in Practice 6(3): 5–8
Mygind N, Dahl R, Pederson S et al 1996 Essential allergy. Blackwell Science, Oxford
Nathan A 1996 Over the counter treatments. Primary Health Care 6(5): 16–17

National Eczema Society 1991 A statement of guiding principles on the needs of people with eczema. National Eczema Society, London
Obeid A 1996 Infant feeding and allergy – a critical review. Paediatric Nurse 8(9): 17–22
Payling K J 1996 Occupational skin disorders. Professional Nurse 11(6): 393–395
Penzer R 1996 Psoriasis. Nursing Standard 10(29): 49–55
Poorman S G, Webb C A 1992 Sexuality and self concept: issues in skin disease. Dermatology Nursing 4(4): 279–284
Price M, Mottahedin I, Mayo P R 1991 Can psychotherapy help patients with psoriasis. Clinical and Experimental Dermatology 16: 114–117
Proby C 1993 Starting from scratch – polymorphic light eruption. Nursing Times 89(29): 54–55
Ramsay B, O'Reagan M 1988 A survey of the social and psychological effect of psoriasis. British Journal of Dermatology 118: 195–201
Reid P, Lewis-Jones M S 1995 Sleep difficulties and their management in preschoolers with atopic eczema. Clinical and Experimental Dermatology 20: 38–41
Ritchie S R, Thompson P J 1992 Primary bacterial skin infections. Dermatology Nursing 4(4): 261–268
Royal College of Nursing 1995 Standards of care for dermatology. Scutari Press, Middlesex
Ruane-Morris M, Thomson G, Lawton S 1995 Community liaison in dermatology. Professional Nurse 10(11): 687–688
Salek M, Finlay A Y, Luscombe D K 1993 Cyclosporin greatly improves the quality of life in adults with severe atopic dermatitis – a randomised, double blind placebo controlled trial. British Journal of Dermatology 129: 422–430
Stone L 1997a Dermatology nursing: planning for the future. Nursing Standard 11(49): 39–41
Stone L 1997b Education and training in dermatology nursing. British Journal of Dermatology Nursing 1(1): 5–7
Stone L A, Lindfield E M, Robertson S J 1989 A colour atlas of nursing procedures in skin disorders. Wolfe, London
Talbot L, Curtis L 1996 The challenges of assessing skin indicators in people of color. Home Healthcare Nurse 14(3): 167–173
Thoms H 1997 Quality of life in psoriasis. British Journal of Dermatology Nursing 1(3): 5–7
Turnbull R 1994 Use of wet wrap dressing in atopic eczema. Paediatric Nursing 6(2): 22–26
UKCC 1992 The scope of professional practice. UKCC, London
Venables J 1996 Skin graft…dermatology, liaison nursing. Nursing Times 92(7): 42–43
White G 1991 Management of fungal infections. Nursing Standard 6(9): 38–40
Williams H C, Strachan D P, Hay R J 1994 Childhood eczema: disease of the advantaged. British Journal of Dermatology 308: 1132–1135
Williams N 1993 Recognising occupational skin diseases. Practice Nurse 5(1): 593–596
Williams R 1985 PUVA therapy vs. Goekerman therapy in the treatment of psoriasis. Physiotherapy Canada 37(6): 361–366
Wilson K J W, Waugh A (eds) 1996 Ross and Wilson anatomy, physiology in health and illness, 8th edn. Churchill Livingstone, Edinburgh

FURTHER READING

Absolon C M, Cottrell D, Eldridge S M, Glover M T 1997 Psychological disturbance in atopic eczema: the extent of the problem in school aged children. British Journal of Dermatology 137: 241–245
Bridgett C, Noren P, Staughton R 1996 Atopic skin disease – a manual for practitioners. Wrightson Biomedical, Petersfield
Clore E 1990 Pediculosis screening and treatment. School Nurse 6(3): 20–25
Cox N, Walton Y, Bowan J 1995 Evaluation of nurse prescribing in a dermatology unit. British Journal of Dermatology 133(2): 340–341
Dawkes K 1997 How to apply emollients effectively. British Journal of Dermatology Nursing 1(2): 8–9
Farquar M 1995 Definitions of quality of life: a taxonomy. Journal of Advanced Nursing 22: 502–508
Finlay A Y, Khan G K 1994 Dermatology life quality index DLQI – a simple practical measure for routine clinical use. Clinical and Experimental Dermatology 19: 210–216
Forsdyke H 1993 Treatment for life. Nursing Times 89(32): 34–36
Gawkrodger D J 1997 Dermatology: an illustrated colour text, 2nd edn. Churchill Livingstone, Edinburgh
Imperial Cancer Research Fund 1990 Sun Cool: sun, skin, moles and melanoma. ICRF, London
Kerrigan K 1993 Chronic generalised erythroderma – a guide for nurses. Dermatology Nursing 5(4): 257–262
Lawson V, Lewis-Jones M S, Reid P 1995 Family impact of childhood atopic eczema. British Journal of Dermatology 133(45): 19
Perkins P 1992 Malignant melanoma: mole watching and the adolescent. Professional Nurse 7(10): 678–680
Poyner T 1995 The role of infection in skin diseases. Community Nurse 1(11): 16–18
Ratcliffe J 1998 How to conduct a patch test. British Journal of Dermatology Nursing 2(4): 8–9
Sarkany R 1999 World wide web – the impact of the internet on dermatology. Dermatology in Practice 7(3): 16–18
Van Der Weyden R 1996 Changing attitudes to sun exposure. British Journal of Nursing 3(5): 765–769
Venables J 1995 Management of children with atopic eczema in the community. Dermatology in Practice 3(5): 1–4
Walsh D 1996 Aromatherapy in the management of psoriasis. Nursing Standard 11(13): 53–56
Wessex Cancer Trust 1990 Monty mole's marvellous mission. Wessex Cancer Trust, Southampton

USEFUL ADDRESSES

Acne Support Group
16 Dufour Place
Broadwick Street
London W1V 1FE

CancerBACUP
British Association of Cancer United Patients
3 Bath Place
Rivington Street
London EC2A 3JR

British Dermatology Nursing Group
19 Fitzroy Square
London W1P 5H

Marie Curie Cancer Care
Education Department
28 Belgrave Square
London SW1X 8QG

National Eczema Society
163 Eversholt Street
London NW1 1BU

Shingles Support Society
41 North Road
London N7 9DP

The Psoriasis Association
Milton House
7 Milton Street
Northampton NN2 7JG

DISORDERS OF THE EYE

13

Ruth F. M. Gardner   Margaret A. Studley

INTRODUCTION

The aim of this chapter is to equip nurses with a sound understanding of the causes and treatment of common eye disorders. It is also intended to raise awareness of the importance of vision to all activities of daily living and of the disabling effects, both physical and psychological, of visual impairment. In outlining the principles of ophthalmic nursing practice, it also acknowledges the need for individualised care and encourages a patient-centred approach.

Although most serious ophthalmic disorders are treated in specialist hospitals, many conditions are encountered and treated in other contexts. The trend towards early discharge and outpatient department treatment has resulted in the increasing involvement of community nurses in supporting, educating and caring for the perioperative patient and for patients with chronic or age-related eye conditions. In taking on this expanded role it is important for nurses in the community to be able to recognise adverse signs and symptoms and to ensure early referral for specialised care.

Nurses in the community are also responsible for first aid and for health promotion and screening, and should bear in mind that the eye is a sensitive indicator of health and health breakdown. Many eye conditions are diagnostic of systemic disease and are intercurrent with other conditions treated in medical, surgical, care of the elderly and/or ITU wards. A good ophthalmic knowledge base is therefore an essential component of a nurse's preparation for practice.

Incidence of blindness

Although it is difficult to quantify the incidence of blindness in the world with any degree of accuracy, it is estimated that it affects 38 million people. World Health Organization statistics (WHO/World Bank 1993) indicate that 80% of blind people live in the developing countries and that there are approximately 21 million blind people in Asia and roughly 7 million in Africa. The risk of blindness in developing countries is 10–14 times higher than in developed countries. It is estimated that about 80% of cases of blindness in poorer countries would be preventable, given appropriate resources and improved environmental conditions (Riordan-Eva 1995).

The main causes of blindness worldwide include:

- cataract (opacity of the lens) — the leading cause, responsible for approximately 50% of all blindness
- trachoma — corneal opacity caused by repeated infection of the cornea and conjunctiva by *Chlamydia trachomatis*
- glaucoma — raised intraocular pressure causing retinal and optic nerve damage
- xerophthalmia — dryness and ulceration of the cornea associated with vitamin A deficiency
- onchocerciasis — a microfilarial infestation transmitted by a fly; it can invade and eventually destroy all the structures of the eye, causing 'river blindness' (Perry & Tullo 1995).

In developed countries such as the UK, where the necessary resources are available, cataract extraction and lens implantation is a common surgical procedure which prevents all but a few people with cataracts from progressing to blindness (see p. 504). In these countries the main causes of blindness are age-related maculopathy, diabetic retinopathy and glaucoma, which so far are not preventable (Perry & Tullo 1995).

Q **13.1** Using library resources such as CD-ROM, investigate the present epidemiological trends in relation to blindness and its causes.

ANATOMY AND PHYSIOLOGY

The components of the sensory mechanisms responsible for sight are the eyes, the optic nerves and tracts, and the visual cortex and association areas of the brain.

Accessory structures play a vital role in enabling the eyes to scan and focus on objects in the environment and in protecting and maintaining the optical properties of the eyes.

The eye

The eyeball (see Fig. 13.1)

With minor individual variations, the eyeball is spherical in shape, with the cornea on the anterior aspect being slightly more steeply curved. The length of an adult eye is approximately 24 mm.

The eyeball or globe is a hollow structure composed of three main layers of tissue:

- *The outer layer* of the globe consists of the fibrous white sclera posteriorly and the transparent cornea anteriorly. The junction of the two is called the limbus. The cornea is transparent due to its avascularity and the regular arrangement of its fibres. It is well supplied with nerve endings from the trigeminal nerve.
- *The middle vascular layer*, known as the uveal tract, consists of the choroid, the ciliary body and the iris. The choroid lines the sclera in the posterior compartment of the eye and continues into the muscular ciliary body, into which are inserted the suspensory ligaments. These ligaments extend to the lens and hold it in position. This diaphragm-like ligamentous structure is known as the zonule. The contraction/relaxation of the ciliary body changes the shape of the lens and controls its refractive and focusing power. The iris is the pigmented anterior portion of the uveal tract. It contains both circular and radial muscle fibres which control the size of the pupil.
- *The inner layer* of the eyeball is the retina. It contains several million photoreceptive cells which are responsible for converting light into electrical impulses. The retina arises just behind the equator of the eyeball in an area known as the ora serrata. This leaves a small anterior section of the choroid — the pars plana — exposed. This is important because it allows surgical access without retinal damage.

The retina consists of two layers: the pigmented outer layer, which lines the choroid, and the innermost neural layer, which is in contact with the vitreous humor. Rod cells predominate in the periphery and function best in dim light. Cone cells predominate

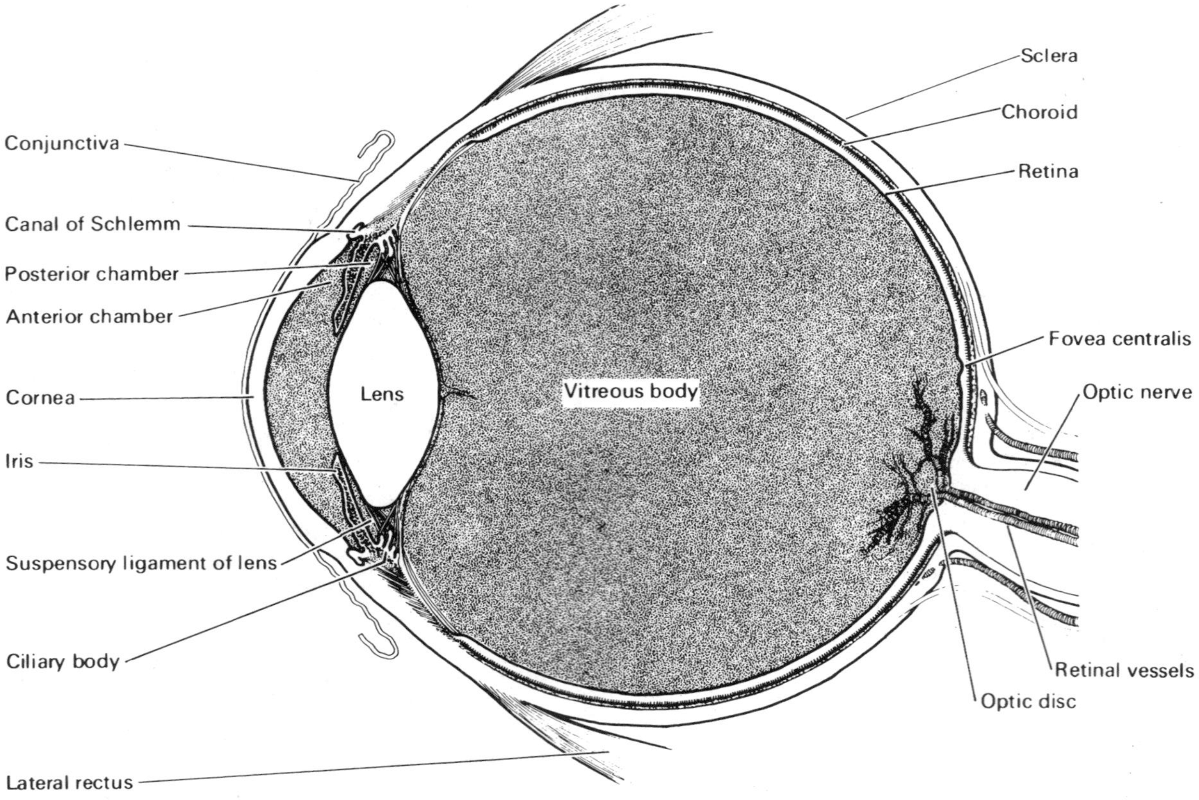

Fig. 13.1 Section through eyeball. (Adapted from Peattie & Walker 1995.)

near the centre of the retina and are adapted for bright light and colour vision. The greatest concentration of cone cells is at the macula, a small area in the centre of the retina which has as its mid-point the fovea centralis, the most vital part of the retina for high-definition vision. These photoreceptor cells are linked through a series of synapses to ganglion cells whose axons run together to form the optic nerve.

The two compartments and three chambers of the eye

Inside the globe, the lens, suspended by the zonule, divides the eye into two main compartments. The anterior compartment is itself divided into two chambers, the anterior chamber in front of the iris and the posterior chamber behind the iris. The compartment behind the lens is sometimes referred to as the third chamber of the eye, or the vitreous chamber, as it contains the clear jelly-like substance called the vitreous humor. The boundaries of each chamber are defined by the three tissue layers described above.

Internal environment and intraocular pressure (IOP). The anterior compartment is bathed in a clear fluid called the aqueous humor, or simply aqueous, which is produced by the ciliary body and provides nutrients to the lens and cornea. Aqueous flows from the posterior chamber through the pupil to the anterior chamber and drains away through the sieve-like fibrous trabecular meshwork located in the angle between the iris and cornea around the circumference of the eye (see Fig. 13.2). This in turn drains into the vascular canal of Schlemm and thereby into the systemic venous circulation. The production and drainage of aqueous must be constant in order to maintain a normal IOP, which is variable over a 24-h period within the range of 12–20 mmHg (Perry & Tullo 1995).

The shape of the eye can, by determining the depth of the anterior chamber and the angle between the cornea and iris, affect the functioning of the drainage system. The larger, elongated eye of the myope (short-sighted person) has a naturally occurring deep anterior chamber with an open angle, whilst the small eye of the hypermetrope (long-sighted person) has a shallow anterior chamber with a narrow angle. Any interference with normal production or drainage of the aqueous humor raises the IOP, leading to the decreased blood supply, pain and impaired vision associated with conditions such as glaucoma and postoperative or traumatic complications. IOP can be measured by tonometry techniques (see p. 505).

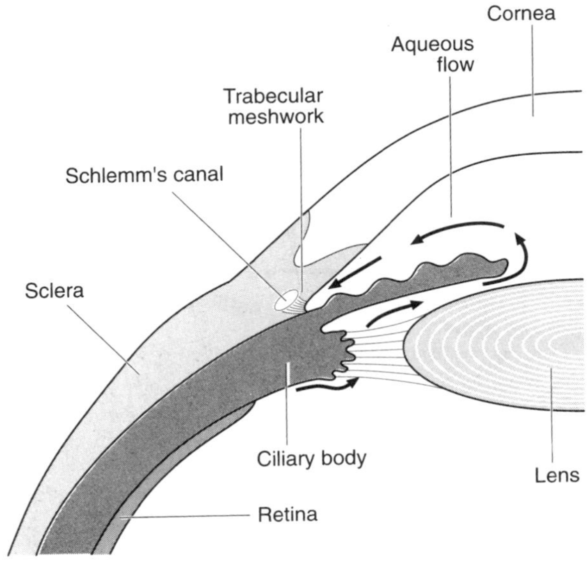

Fig. 13.2 Flow of aqueous humor from the posterior to the anterior chamber of the eye.

The visual pathways and interpretative centres

The optic nerve runs from the posterior aspect of the globe and enters the cranial cavity via the optic foramen. The medial nerve fibres cross over to the opposite side at the optic chiasma (see Fig. 13.3) to join with the lateral fibres and form the optic tract before synapsing in the lateral geniculate body of the thalamus. From the lateral geniculate body, the fibres run in the optic radiations to the occipital cerebral cortex of the brain.

The main blood supply to the eye is via the ophthalmic artery, a branch of the internal carotid artery, which runs alongside the optic nerve.

Accessory structures

The exposed anterior aspect of the eyeball is protected by the eyebrow, eyelids and eyelashes. To facilitate free movement over the globe, the lids are lined with the conjunctiva, a mucous membrane which is reflected back on itself to cover the exposed sclera. At the limbus, the conjunctiva is modified to form the epithelial layer of the cornea. This fold forms the conjunctival sac or fornix and is an ideal site for the instillation of topical drugs.

The exposed surface of the eye is also covered by a three-layered film of tear fluid. Mucous secretion from conjunctival goblet cells forms the first layer of the tear film and ensures an even spread of tears over the cornea. The second (middle) layer of the tear film is the watery fluid secreted by the lacrimal glands (situated under the

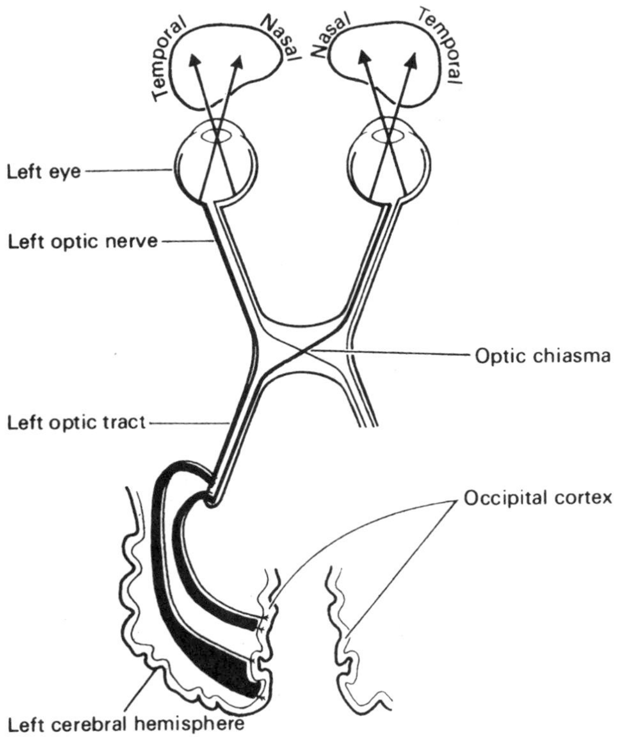

Fig. 13.3 The visual pathways from the eye. (Reproduced with kind permission from Peattie & Walker 1995.)

outer aspect of the upper orbital rim) and by the accessory glands in the conjunctiva. The third (outer) oily layer of tear film is secreted by the Meibomian glands of the lids. This is thought to reduce the evaporation rate of tears and to prevent the lids sticking together during sleep. The main functions of tear fluid are to lubricate the eye, to facilitate O_2 and CO_2 exchange, to provide an optically smooth corneal surface and to cleanse the eye with a bacteriostatic enzyme, lysozyme.

Excess tears are drained from the eye via the lacrimal apparatus at the inner canthus (nasal end of the lid margins) into the lacrimal sac and thence into the nose through the nasolacrimal duct (see Fig. 13.4).

Posteriorly and laterally the globe is protected by the bony orbit, the extraocular recti and oblique muscles (responsible for tracking movements) and by orbital fat.

The physiology of vision

Light rays are bent (refracted) as they pass through the varying densities of the clear media of the eye to focus on the retina. The cornea is responsible for about two-thirds of the refractive power of the eye and is constant. However, by virtue of its elasticity, the lens has the ability to change shape and thereby vary the amount of refraction for clarity of focus. This is known as accommodation and is necessary in order for objects at different distances to be visualised with equal clarity.

The normal eye in its relaxed state brings rays of light from distant objects into sharp focus. However, for clear focusing on near objects, an autonomic reflex known as the synkinetic near reflex comes into play. This reflex involves accommodation, miosis and convergence, as follows:

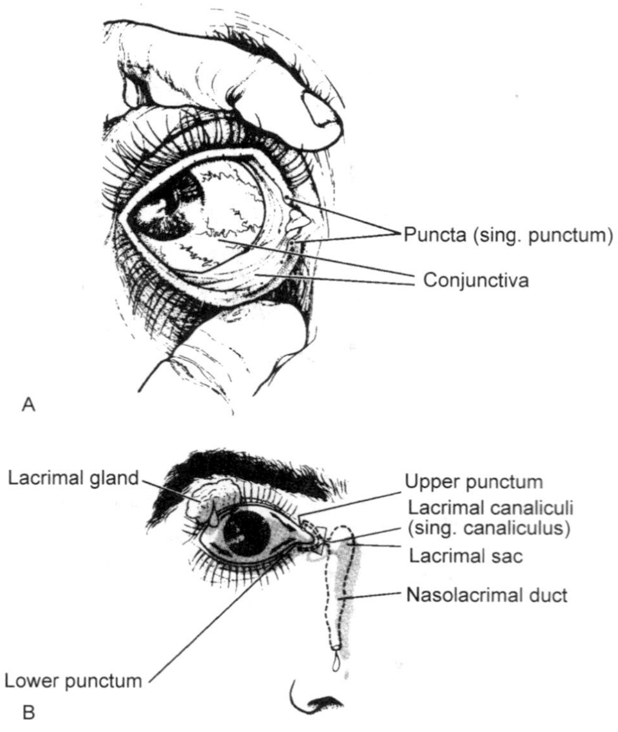

Fig. 13.4 A: The eyelids and conjunctiva. B: The lacrimal apparatus. (Reproduced with kind permission from Peattie & Walker 1995.)

- *Accommodation*, the ciliary body contracts and changes shape, thus releasing tension on the zonular fibres and allowing the lens to thicken and increase its refractive power
- *Miosis*, or constriction of the pupil, accompanies accommodation and ensures that light rays are concentrated to pass through the centre of the lens and focus on the macula
- *Convergence*, or in-turning of the eyes, seeks out the object to be focused on.

Failure to focus may be described as ametropia, or refractive error (see Box 13.1).

Once the rays of light are focused on the retina, their energy is converted into neuroelectrical energy by the photoreceptor cells. These nerve impulses are transmitted via other neural cells in the retina to the optic nerve and so by the visual pathway to the visual cortex. Here, they are interpreted as sensations of light, form and colour and are processed into images of objects which are given meaning by other cerebral areas through correlation with information stored as memory in the association areas of the brain.

ASSESSING THE EYE AND VISUAL FUNCTION

Examination of structure

It is vital for nurses working with ophthalmic patients to learn to examine the eye in a systematic and meticulous way and to be able to recognise abnormalities and their significance. In order to do so, it is necessary to know what a normal eye looks like and what normal expectations are for an eye recovering from surgery or disease. It is essential to work in good light using a pen torch and to proceed systematically, examining all ocular structures from outermost to innermost as follows:

- lids — observe position, closure, bruising, discharge
- conjunctiva — observe degree of injection (visible blood vessels), chemosis (thickening due to oedema), discharge, wounds
- cornea — observe clarity, type and extent of any opacity, shape, suture lines, wounds
- anterior chamber (AC) — observe depth, clarity, presence of hyphaema (blood in AC), hypopyon (pus in AC)
- iris — observe colour, position, appearance
- pupil — observe size, shape, position, colour of reflection from lens
- intraocular lens (IOL) — if appropriate, observe position
- retina — examine through dilated pupil using ophthalmoscope.

The possible implications of clinical features that may be found in the course of an eye examination are listed in Table 13.1.

Box 13.1 Terms associated with visual acuity and refractive errors

- Emmetropia — normal sight; light rays focus on the retina
- Ametropia — defective sight due to refractive error
- Myopia — short-sightedness; light rays focus in front of the retina
- Hypermetropia — long-sightedness; light rays focus behind the retina
- Presbyopia — loss of focused reading/near-vision capacity, resulting from loss of lens elasticity due to ageing
- Astigmatism — irregular curvature of the cornea which prevents light rays from focusing at a single point

Table 13.1 Significance of clinical features found on eye examination

Structure	*Clinical features*	*Possible significance*
Lids	Bruising (ecchymosis) Swelling Drooping Increased lacrimation Discharge	Surgical handling Trauma Infection
Conjunctiva	Redness (injection) Swelling (chemosis) Allergy Infection	Surgical handling Trauma
Cornea	Cloudy Crinkled Fluorescein staining Suture line not intact Penetrating injury	Increased IOP Infection Loss of AC Ulceration
Anterior chamber (AC)	Hyphaema (blood in AC) Hypopyon (pus in AC) Shallow AC	Hyphaema due to surgery should gradually resolve Increasing IOP = bleeding/inflammation Hypopyon = infection Shallow = ? aqueous loss
Iris	Muddy	Inflammation
Pupil	Irregular shape	Iris prolapse Adhesions Trauma

Testing visual function

Visual acuity

Visual acuity (VA) assessment is frequently carried out by nurses and is the mathematical estimation of visual function for different distances.

Distance vision. This is tested using test-type charts. These charts display letters or pictures arranged in rows of diminishing size (see Fig. 13.5). A patient with normal VA would be able to see the top letter (i.e. the 60 m line) at a distance of 60 m and successive lines at progressively shorter distances. Each eye should be tested separately, because if both eyes are used the result will be that of the better eye. In normal testing, the patient is positioned 6 m away from the chart and asked to read each line aloud until he can no longer make out the letters. The result is recorded as a fraction of the distance from the chart in metres over the normal reading distance of the last complete line read, plus the number of extra letters read from the line below or minus the number of letters read incorrectly, e.g. 6/9 – 2 is the same as 6/12 + 4 (see Fig 13.5). If glasses or contact lenses are worn, this is recorded as i/c gl. or i/c CL, respectively.

Normal distance acuity is accepted as 6/6 (see Fig. 13.6). The patient may be asked to read the chart again, looking through a pinhole disc. A pure refractive error should improve by two lines with this simple method of sharpening focus. The improved acuity would be recorded as 6/9 i/c PH (see Fig. 13.7).

If the patient cannot read the test letters even when he stands closer to the chart, his ability to count fingers (CF), detect hand movements (HM) or perceive light (PL) is tested. Awareness of direction of a light source may also be noted (projection).

Near vision is tested in a similar fashion by asking the patient to read text in various sizes of standard print, all graded and prefixed with the letter N. N5 is accepted as normal reading acuity.

Binocular vision involves simultaneous perception of an image by both eyes and fusion of the two images in the visual cortex to form a single image. Binocular vision is thought to play a role in depth perception. Having two eyes also widens the field of vision and counters gaps in the visual field caused by natural blind spots.

Q **13.2** Look carefully straight ahead and note what you see. Now close one eye. What do you not see? Now repeat with the other eye. What do you no longer see?

The visual field. The range of what the eye can see with respect to angle of view (rather than distance) is called the visual field. Normally this is about 60° nasally, 90° temporally, 50° superiorly and 70° inferiorly. Assessment of the integrity of the visual field is an important aid to diagnosis of retinal detachment and neurological disease and is essential in the management of open-angle glaucoma. Visual field testing can be carried out in the following ways:

- *Simple confrontation test*. The examiner compares the patient's field of vision with her own. Facing the patient, who is asked to maintain a fixed gaze on the examiner's face, she moves a finger from various points on her own periphery of vision and asks the patient to indicate when it appears in his field of vision.
- *Field analyser systems*, e.g. Henson, Friedmann or Goldmann, give accurate measurements of visual field defects known as scotoma.
- *The Bjerrum screen*. This is used for greater refinement in testing the central 30° of field.

Colour-blindness

Colour vision depends on the normal functioning of the retinal cones. A colour-blind person is unable to distinguish between some colours — usually red and green. While approximately 7% of the male population are born with defective colour vision, this

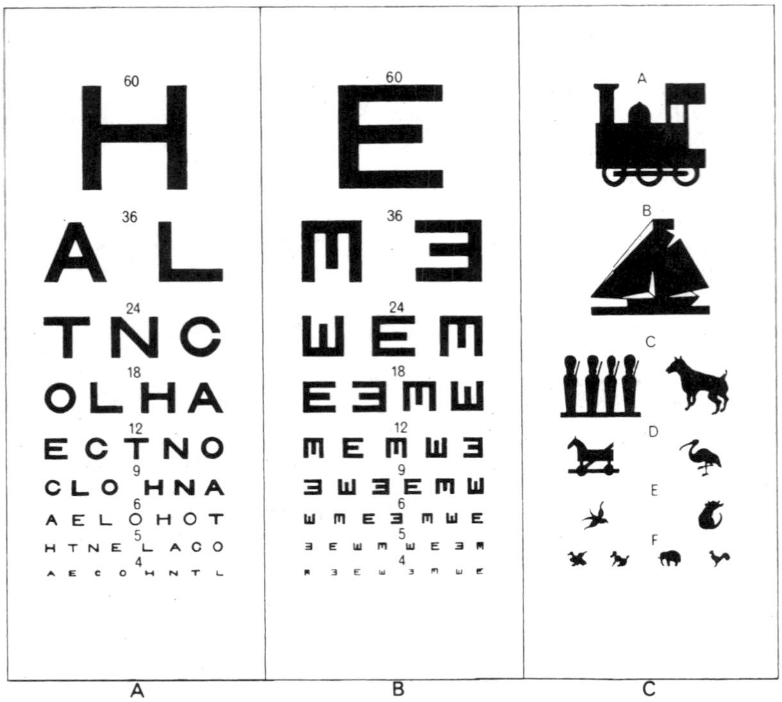

Fig. 13.5 Eye testing charts. A: Snellen test-type chart. B: 'E' chart for children, non-English speakers, etc. The person is given a wooden E which he moves to indicate the positions he 'reads' on the chart. C: Object recognition chart. (Reproduced with kind permission from Peattie & Walker 1995.)

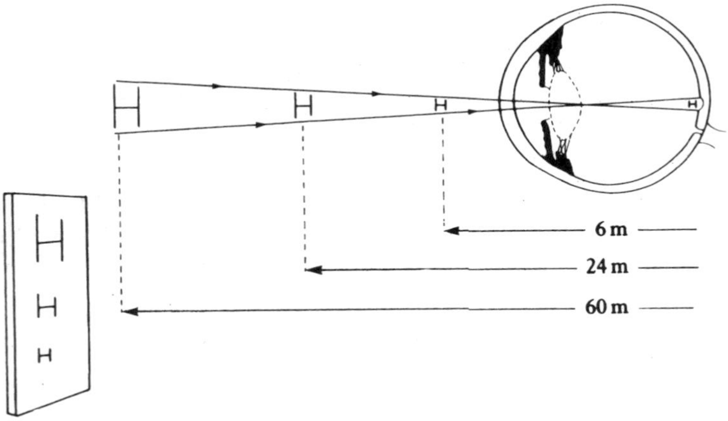

Fig. 13.6 Normal vision. The 6 m letter at 6 m and the 60 m letter at 60 m appear the same to the eye. The nearer the larger one approaches the eye, the bigger it will appear, because it throws an angle of increasing size at the macula. (Reproduced with kind permission from Chawla 1999.)

problem is rare in females (Perry & Tullo 1995). Colour-blindness can also be acquired; it is characteristic of certain disease processes such as optic neuritis and some macular disorders, and may develop in people with a drug dependency.

The most common method of testing for colour blindness is by means of Ishihara colour plates. These are a series of cards on which numbers composed of red and green dots have been printed against a background of different coloured dots. A person with defective colour vision would be unable to distinguish the numbers from the surrounding background.

Some occupations require normal colour vision, usually for reasons of safety. For example, an electrician needs to be able to distinguish between coloured wires and an airline pilot between the coloured lights on his instrument panel. Applicants for positions

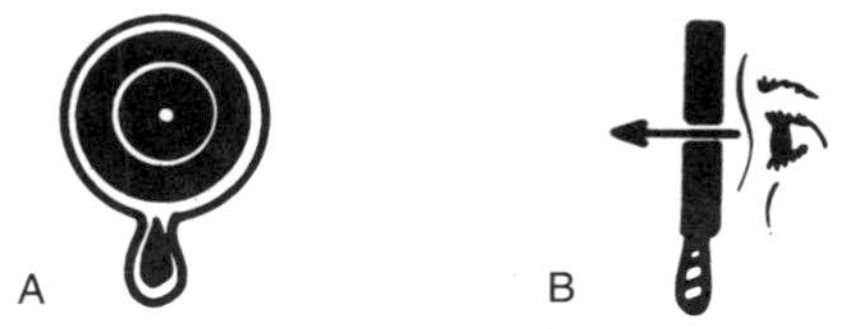

Fig. 13.7 The pinhole disk. A: By omitting all but the central ray of light reaching the macula, this simple apparatus demonstrates whether or not poor central vision is due to refractive error. B: How the apparatus works. (Reproduced with kind permission from McKenzie et al 1986.)

such as these will be tested for colour vision. There are no restrictions on driving cars, lorries or buses, as traffic lights have a fixed sequence and can be recognised by position rather than colour.

13.3 What other occupations can you think of that require normal colour vision?

Eye changes with ageing

By age 70, most people will need some form of visual aid, since with advancing years the ability of the lens to accommodate decreases as it becomes less elastic. Focusing is affected as the cornea flattens, causing astigmatism (see Box 13.1). A decrease in pupil size reduces the amount of light entering the eye, and retinal cells become less efficient due to deposits laid down by ageing pigment epithelial cells. Tear film is reduced in volume and altered in structure, with the result that tears evaporate more quickly, leading to dryness and irritation of the eye. However, some elderly patients complain of watering eyes, e.g. due to malposition of eyelids (see p. 519). The corneal periphery often develops a marked grey ring at its junction with the sclera — known as arcus senilis.

For further information, see Goodrich (1993).

PRESERVATION OF VISION

Nurses can do a great deal through health education and active intervention to help people preserve their vision. The following list suggests how nurses working in a range of specialisms can make an important contribution to this aspect of health promotion:

- Nurses in every area of practice should take all appropriate opportunities to promote general health and a well-balanced diet.
- The community nurse's observation of changes in appearance or behaviour in her patients can often bring ophthalmic problems to light and result in early diagnosis and treatment. Prompt referral to the appropriate community health team professional is essential.

13.4 What behaviours would lead you to suspect that a person's sight is deteriorating?

- Regular eye examination and sight testing should be encouraged — especially in children, people over 40 years of age and those belonging to high-risk groups (e.g. diabetics). The NHS provides free sight testing to those over the age of 60 and, every two years, to certain high-risk and socially deprived groups.

13.5 On your next community placement, talk to the practice nurse about free sight testing and benefits for visually impaired people.

- Nurses can give advice regarding the use and cleanliness of spectacles and contact lenses. In particular, contact lenses should be cared for properly and used strictly in accordance with the optometrist's instructions. There is a danger of corneal ulceration if such instructions are not followed.
- Care in monitoring oxygen therapy in babies can prevent retinal damage.
- Prompt treatment of eye infections can often prevent residual damage.
- Work- and leisure-related eye injuries can be prevented by appropriate eye protection (see Box 13.2). Statutory health and safety regulations and better supervision by occupational health nurses have helped to reduce the number of industrial eye injuries (Burlew 1991). Non-compliance is, however, still a problem.
- Individuals should be urged in the workplace and at home to heed the labels on chemical products indicating whether they are harmful to the eyes; careful note should also be taken of first aid instructions in case of accidental splashing.
- The increasing use of visual display units (VDUs) carries potential for eye damage. The Health and Safety Executive recommends short, frequent rest periods to prevent eye fatigue (Health & Safety Executive 1993).

THE VISUALLY IMPAIRED PERSON

Sometimes it is difficult for sighted persons to appreciate fully the importance of vision to carrying out the activities of living (ALs).

13.6 Working through the following activities may help you to gain some understanding of the daily experience of visually impaired people. Ask a colleague to blindfold you, using a sleep shade, and then to assist you through as many of the activities of living as possible. Try to include basic hygiene, eating a meal, going into a busy room and travelling on public transport. Exchange roles. Then, using a structured framework such as Roper et al's (1996) ALs, discuss how being visually impaired affected each activity. Additionally, ask yourself how it affected the essential 'you'. Did you feel any less intelligent? How great was the potential loss? Did it change the way others reacted to you? How did it feel to be the helper? Share your experiences and insights with the other members of your student group.

Registration of blindness and partial sight

There are few totally blind people, as most visually impaired people have some residual sight or perception of light. An ophthalmologist will certify the degree of impairment. Rehabilitation support can be obtained without registration.

Registration, which is completely voluntary, entitles the individual to many local and national benefits. These will be explained by the social worker, who visits eligible individuals in their homes and helps to arrange for additional support. Some areas also have the benefit of a mobility or rehabilitation officer who is specially trained to help newly registered individuals to relearn living skills and to move about safely in their own environment. This may involve the use of special canes or guide dogs. Rehabilitation

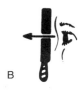

Box 13.2 Preventing eye injury

Protective eyewear should always be worn during any prolonged exposure to strong sunlight or snow, as well as for the following activities:

- Chipping masonry
- Chopping wood
- Drilling
- Laying insulation
- Playing squash
- Pruning trees or shrubbery
- Stripping paint
- Sunbed bathing
- Welding
- Working under the chassis of a car

officers also teach communication and information technology skills, and advise on retraining for employment. Their overall aim is to enable the visually impaired person to function as independently as possible.

People with impaired vision may be referred to a low-vision clinic and provided with aids, which can help them to make the most of residual sight, and with information and advice on adaptation or retraining for employment. Employers can also be advised by various agencies, including the Royal National Institute for the Blind (RNIB) (see 'Useful addresses', p. 523) on the sophisticated electronic equipment now available for visually impaired employees.

Considering the needs of the visually impaired person

All nursing care should be planned using a structured approach to assessment and implemented using an agreed care pathway. This approach facilitates accountability and audit mechanisms.

Rowell (1995) suggests an adaptation of Orem's model (Orem 1995), which takes account of universal needs but focuses on specific areas of self-care deficit, builds on the individual's strengths and promotes personal responsibility for health maintenance. Education and counselling are also essential components of this model.

Some general principles of care for the visually impaired person are outlined below:

- *Orientation to place*. If the person is at home, he will know his own environment and it is therefore important to keep things in their usual place. Every assistance should be given to help him to move around the community and workplace until he is confident to do so on his own. Appropriate visual aids should be used. If he is admitted to hospital, it is the nurse's responsibility to orientate him adequately. Old people, in particular, can become very confused and are likely to need constant guidance.
- *Maintaining a safe environment*. In organising the environment it is essential to remove objects that the person might fall over or bump into. Doors should be fully open or closed properly. Fires should have guards. People who smoke should be warned about the high inflammability of eye pads.

13.7 Look at a ward in your hospital and identify problems that a patient with impaired vision might have. How could you make it safer? Consider also problems encountered by a person in the community in buying, preparing and eating food.

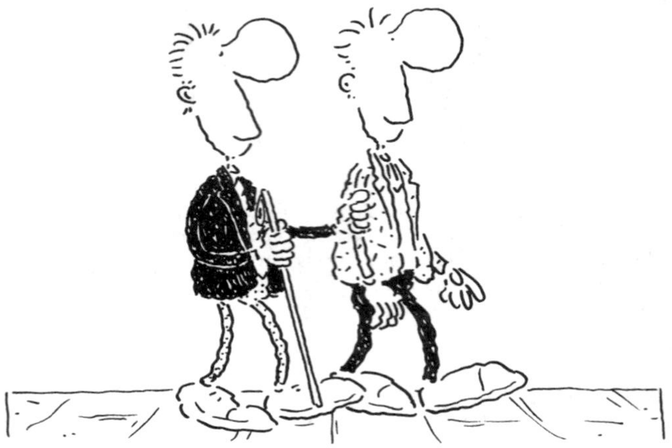

Fig. 13.8 Guiding a blind person. The blind person grasps the helper's arm firmly just above the elbow. The helper then walks beside and half a pace in front of him. In this way, the blind person can sense any manoeuvre or turning of the helper's body and can walk more confidently. (Reproduced with kind permission from RNIB 1995.)

- *Communication*. A visually impaired person will develop heightened perception in his other senses — especially hearing and touch — and it is important to provide additional sensory input to facilitate this. Make sure the person has access to radios, talking books and other more sophisticated means of communication if he wants them. When you approach the person, address him by name and identify yourself. Describe what you are doing so that he feels involved. It is equally important to inform the person of your intention to leave so that he is not embarrassed by being left talking to himself.
- *Eating and drinking*. In hospital, food should be placed close to the patient, bearing in mind his functioning visual field, and the position of what is on the plate should be described using a clock-face analogy. Plate guards, non-slip mats and other aids may be offered. Many safety devices are available for use in the home to help with cooking. After proper training, a good degree of independence can be achieved.
- *Personal hygiene and grooming*. After initial orientation and help, the individual should be encouraged to carry out personal self-care tasks for himself.
- *Mobility*. When other factors permit, early mobilisation should be encouraged in hospital and every assistance given. The preferred method of guiding a person with visual impairment is illustrated in Figure 13.8.

The RNIB (1995) leaflet *How to Guide a Blind Person* gives valuable advice.

With good rehabilitation training and family support, the visually impaired person should be able to get around in his environment safely and effectively. It will take courage, time and patience to achieve this level of competence, however, and the person will require understanding and unflagging moral support.

DISORDERS OF THE EYE

The more common eye disorders and their management are described in the sections which follow. The coverage is by no means exhaustive and the reader is urged to consult specialist ophthalmic texts as the need arises.

For further information, see Perry & Tullo (1995) and Kanski (1997).

The present survey of common eye disorders and their management will begin, however, by setting out the basic principles that must be followed when carrying out ophthalmic nursing procedures.

NURSING PRIORITIES AND MANAGEMENT: GENERAL OPHTHALMIC PROCEDURES

The eye is a delicate organ which can be easily damaged — even in the course of treatment. The nurse must be scrupulous in observing the following principles in any situation in which she provides ophthalmic care.

Asepsis

Strict asepsis must be observed by the nurse and taught to patients and relatives. Each eye should be treated separately. Drops and ointments should only be used in the eye for which they are prescribed. In hospital, topical medication should be dated upon opening and discarded after 1 week (after 4 weeks in the community). These precautions will reduce the risk of eye infection, which can quickly destroy vision.

Handling

Gentle handling is essential. Pressure on the eyeball must be avoided at all times. This applies particularly to the cleansing of the upper eyelids. A sterile, moist swab is used to wipe from inner to outer canthus along the eyelash line and is discarded after a single use. Patients should be cautioned against rubbing their eyes. The cornea is particularly sensitive and vulnerable to abrasion injuries.

Irrigation

When irrigating the eye, the warmed solution should be directed onto the nasal side of the sclera. This will wash harmful foreign material away from the lacrimal duct to the side of the cheek, where it can be received in a kidney dish.

Examination

Both eyes should be examined systematically (see p. 496) before and after any treatment, using a good pen torch. Any abnormality must be reported immediately to the ophthalmologist. Visual acuity should be assessed and any significant change reported at once. The patient should be asked how each eye feels. Severe pain must be reported immediately. Systematic examination will ensure that no detail is overlooked. As eye complications can develop rapidly, it is vital to refer patients immediately to avoid permanent damage. Both eyes should be examined, because the unaffected eye may react in sympathy with the affected one (sympathetic ophthalmitis). Photophobia is to be expected postoperatively and following trauma.

Instilling eye drops and ointments

Eye drops are inserted into the middle to outer third of the lower conjunctival sac. To facilitate this, the patient is asked to tilt his head back and look up while the lower lid is gently pulled down (see Fig. 13.9). Dropping the solution onto the sensitive cornea will cause discomfort and trigger a reflexive squeezing shut of the eye. After drop instillation the patient is asked to close his eyes gently for 30 s to maximise absorption.

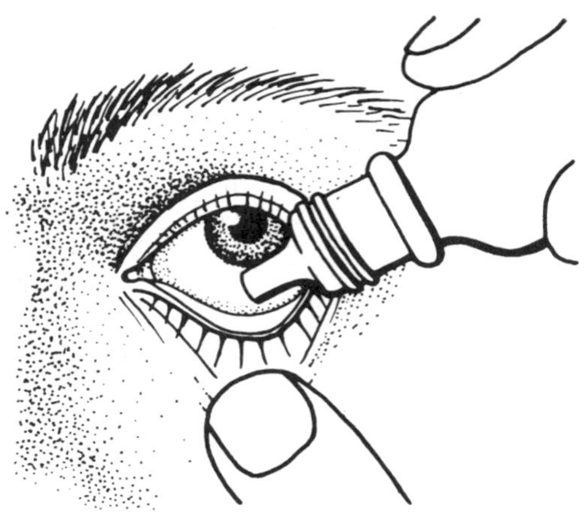

Fig. 13.9 Instilling eye drops. (Reproduced with kind permission from McKenzie et al 1986.)

Eye ointment is instilled into the lower conjunctival sac with the patient's head tilted back as described above. Contact of the tube with the eye should be carefully avoided.

Topical drugs used in ophthalmology are listed in Table 13.2.

Padding the eye

Eyepads are applied to promote healing or to apply pressure to the eye and occasionally for comfort, when photophobia or lacrimation is excessive. It is important to appreciate that the term 'double padding' does not mean that both eyes are covered but that two pads are applied to the treated eye.

Eyepads are applied after eyes have been cleansed (if required), examined and treatment instilled. Ensure that the eye is closed underneath the pad at all times to prevent corneal damage.

The eyepad is held in position and non-allergenic tape is applied by first attaching one end lightly to the forehead, then diagonally across the eyepad towards the lateral aspect of the cheek, before the end is secured with light pressure. The downward movement maintains lid closure. The diagonal position of the tape facilitates comfort, permitting facial muscle movement. To facilitate removal, the tape is cut below the eyebrow, the pad is folded down and the skin of the cheek supported to ensure there is no pressure on the eyeball. The skin of the forehead is supported in a similar method for the removal of the remaining tape. Pads must be inspected for signs of infection or haemorrhage before discarding.

When the eye cannot be closed voluntarily, e.g. in the unconscious patient, care should be taken to avoid corneal abrasion from bedclothes or other articles when turning or attending to the patient. The cornea must be kept moist by the instillation of artificial tears.

NURSING PRIORITIES AND MANAGEMENT: CONDITIONS REQUIRING SURGICAL INTERVENTION

The term 'intraocular surgery' describes procedures that are carried out inside the globe of the eye and which may involve structures in the anterior, posterior or vitreous chambers. Although there are many ophthalmic conditions which require operative intervention, the present discussion will focus on some of the more common of these, including cataract, retinal detachment, glaucoma and perforating injuries. These conditions will have in common certain general priorities for ophthalmic and perioperative nursing management along with specific priorities relating to each condition. The general

Table 13.2 Classification by usage of topical drugs utilised in ophthalmology (Mauger & Craig 1996, Gandham 1997)

Drug	*Strength*	*Specific action and usage*
Dilation of the pupil		
Drugs in this group act on the autonomic nervous system to induce mydriasis (dilatation of the pupil by acting on the iris muscles) or cycloplegia (contraction of the ciliary muscles). Some drugs (*) have a combined mydriatic cycloplegic action. All examples given have rapid onset (within 20 min) and short duration of action (4–24 h). They are frequently used in combination to facilitate refraction (cycloplegia required), ophthalmoscopy, fundal photography, cataract and retinal surgery, and the laser treatment of diabetic retinopathy.		
Cyclopentolate (G)*	0.5% and 1%	Treatment of anterior uveitis
Tropicamide (G)*	0.5% and 1%	
Phenylephrine (G)	2.5%	
Glaucoma medication		
Pilocarpine (G)	0.5%–4%	Constricts the ciliary muscle and increases the aqueous outflow via the trabecular meshwork (action is accompanied by pupil constriction—miosis) More commonly used in the management of acute glaucoma or as an adjunct treatment for chronic glaucoma
Timoptol (G)	0.25% and 0.5%	A non-selective beta-blocker which reduces aqueous production Used for the treatment of chronic and secondary glaucoma
Betopic (G)	0.5%	A β_1-blocker used as above
Alphagan (G) (Brimonidine tartrate 0.2%)		An α_2-blocker which reduces aqueous production and increases aqueous outflow via the uveoscleral outflow system Used for the treatment of chronic and secondary glaucoma
Latanoprost (G)	0.005%	A prostaglandin analogue which increases aqueous outflow via the uveoscleral outflow system Used as an adjunct treatment for chronic glaucoma
Trusopt (G)	2%	A carbonic anhydrase inhibitor which reduces the production of aqueous Used for the treatment of chronic and secondary glaucoma
Anti-inflammatory		
Betamethazone (G) or (Oc)	1%	Steroid Used to treat anterior segment inflammations May be combined with the antibiotic neomycin
Ocufen (G)	0.03%	Non-steroidal Used to inhibit intraoperative pupil miosis
Antibacterial		
Chloramphenicol (G) or (Oc)	0.5%	Broad-spectrum bacteriostat
Fucithalmic (G)	1% viscous eye drop	Broad-spectrum bactericidal
Antiviral		
Zovirax (Oc)	3%	Disrupts the synthesis of viral DNA in the treatment of herpes simplex keratitis
Anaesthetic agents		
Surface active anaesthetics which have rapid onset (30 s) and short duration of action (20 min). Used to facilitate the removal of conjunctival and corneal foreign bodies, investigative procedures which require surface anaesthesia, and selectively as pain relief.		
Benoxinate (G)	0.4%	Used in combination with G fluorescein for tonometry
Amethocaine (G)	1%	
Staining agents		
Fluorescein (G)	1% and 2%	Stains damaged living tissue Facilitates the detection of corneal surface damage, i.e. abrasions and leaking corneal wounds
Rose Bengal (G)	1%	Stains dead devitalised tissue Facilitates the diagnosis of keratoconjunctivitis sicca (xerophthalmia)
Lubricating agents		
Tear replacement solutions — surface contact time is improved by the choice of viscous bases.		
Liquifilm (G)	1.4%	Viscosity from polyvinyl alcohol
Viscotears (G)	0.2%	Viscosity from polyacrylic acid
Lacri-Lube (Oc)		Viscosity from white soft paraffin Useful overnight

G, guttae — drops; Oc, oculentum — ointment.

principles of perioperative ophthalmic nursing care are outlined below, followed by a discussion of nursing care specific to particular conditions. To facilitate shorter patient admission periods, patient assessment and education are increasingly undertaken in pre-admission clinics which may be nurse-run. The reader is also referred to Chapter 26 for the principles of pre- and postoperative nursing management.

General nursing considerations

Assessing visual status

The patient's visual acuity and functional status are determined following his admission to the ward, through formal testing and interview. It is important to establish the patient's normal visual status so that he can retain his self-respect and independence and is not demeaned by inappropriate restrictions. It is equally important to determine any deficits, in order to ensure that a safe environment is maintained for him.

The patient should be oriented to the ward area with a view to maintaining his normal degree of independence as far as possible. His dependency level will fluctuate during the perioperative period, e.g. owing to anaesthesia, treatment and/or padding. The potential difficulties should be discussed fully with the patient.

Alleviating stress

Anxiety levels are normally high for patients admitted to hospital and this may be exacerbated in ophthalmic patients by fear of blindness and loss of independence. The patient should be given the opportunity to discuss particular fears and should be provided with clear and realistic information. Care should be taken not to raise false expectations about operative results and the patient should be referred for counselling if the need is identified. Realistic expectations will provide a more functional base for adaptation to any remaining disability. The patient may have practical concerns about managing the activities of living following the operation. These should be addressed and the individual should be reassured that he will be able to receive continuing guidance and support from the health care team and community organisations.

Giving information

Most patients are anxious to know the time of their surgery and how long it will take. If a local anaesthetic is to be used, they may be concerned about their level of awareness during the procedure and about whether they will be able to cooperate (see Research Abstract 13.1). Depending on the patient's visual acuity, it is often helpful to discuss the operation using a model of the eye. It is important to anticipate and dispel any misconceptions that the patient may have about eye surgery. However, not everyone will want to know the details of the surgery and the individual's wishes in this regard should be respected.

Procedures for preoperative eye preparation should be explained. If the patient is able to carry out self-medication, instruction in the instillation of drops can provide a good opportunity to begin a teaching programme for postoperative self-care.

For further information see Norlet & Kelly (1996).

Managing positioning and activity

As a general rule, any position or activity that increases venous pressure in the head should be avoided in ophthalmic patients. It is usually recommended that they are nursed with the head slightly raised, with the patient either semi-recumbent or lying on the unoperated side. Exceptions to this are:

- in cases of retinal detachment — the surgeon will prescribe both pre- and postoperative positions, depending on the site of the detachment
- following vitrectomy — the surgeon may prescribe the position.

It is vital that such instructions for positioning are followed precisely.

Postoperative vomiting should be prevented by ensuring that an antiemetic is prescribed and given promptly if the patient complains of nausea. The patient should also avoid bending down and lifting heavy items. Increased blood flow caused by a head-down position or straining will raise IOP and can result in damage to optical structures or suture lines. Many patients go home shortly after surgery and some restrictions on activity and positioning may be applicable. The reason for these activity and positioning regimens, and for their duration, should be carefully explained to the patient to encourage compliance.

> **Research Abstract 13.1**
> Local versus general anaesthesia in eye surgery
>
> There is a growing trend towards the use of local anaesthesia in eye surgery and early discharge from hospital, which is significant for nurses involved in community care (see Ch. 1).
>
> Cheng et al (1992) conducted a study to compare the morbidity and length of hospital stay associated with retrobulbar neuromuscular blockade (local anaesthesia) with that associated with general anaesthesia for monocular strabismus (squint) surgery in adults.
>
> Results indicated that there was no significant difference in postoperative nausea and vomiting between the two groups. However, patients who had received local anaesthesia experienced significantly less postoperative discomfort, had higher activity levels and were discharged from hospital sooner than patients in the other group, allowing more efficient use of hospital resources.
>
> Cheng K P, Larson C E, Biglan A W, D'Antonio J A 1992 A prospective, randomized, controlled experiment of retrobulbar and general anaesthesia for strabismus surgery. Ophthalmic Surgery 23(9): 585–590.

Examining the eye

The eye should be examined systematically, using a pen torch, both preoperatively and postoperatively, to check for signs of infection, and postoperatively to ensure that normal healing occurs. Early recognition of abnormalities is critical, as irreversible damage resulting in loss of sight can occur if action is not taken immediately.

Haemorrhage is abnormal. If bleeding into the anterior chamber (hyphaema) is present, it will be recorded and a diagram indicating size relative to the anterior chamber entered in the medical and nursing notes. Postoperative expectations may include some degree of lid bruising and swelling, especially following local anaesthesia. Conjunctival redness (injection) and oedema (chemosis) should be confined to the wound site. The cornea and anterior chamber (AC) should be clear. A fine suture line may be evident. The depth of the AC should be noted, as this may relate to the disease process, the surgery or a leaking wound.

A systematic approach to eye examination will help to ensure that no detail is missed.

Managing dressings

The eye is protected by a plastic Cartella shield for the first night postoperatively. Dark glasses may be worn to reduce the discomfort of glare. The patient should be taught to put the glasses on over his forehead to avoid accidentally poking the earpieces into his eye. If desired the Cartella shield may be worn at night for the first week post-surgery to protect the eye.

PAINLESS LOSS OF VISION

Cataract

Any opacity of the lens can be defined as a cataract. Cataracts can develop as part of the ageing process. They can also be congenital or develop following trauma, as sequelae to inflammatory and degenerative disease, or as a result of the prolonged use of some drugs, e.g. corticosteroids.

PATHOPHYSIOLOGY

The lens of the eye is normally transparent due to the regular arrangement of its crystalline fibres and the nature of the proteins inside them. These fibres, which originate in the epithelium of the lens capsule, continue to be laid down throughout life. This results in thickening and a loss of elasticity. Opacity may eventually develop with ageing.

Clinical features. The main feature of a mature cataract is that it reflects as a grey or milky white lens behind the pupil, which normally appears black.

Common presenting symptoms. The nature of the symptoms experienced by the patient will depend upon the cause of the cataract, as follows:

- *Age-related cataract*
  —gradually decreasing acuity affecting distance vision more than near vision
  —general dimming of vision because of the reduced amount of light reaching the retina
  —more frequent refractive errors because of reduced elasticity of the lens
  —increased dazzle and glare in bright light and haloes around lights at night
  —monocular diplopia (double vision in one eye)
  —alteration in colour and depth perception
- *Cataract related to inflammation or trauma*
  —pain due to an acute inflammatory response in which the lens swells, causing acute closed-angle glaucoma
  —opacity following trauma.

Whatever the combination of early presenting symptoms, the patient will eventually experience greatly reduced visual acuity and may describe this as 'like looking through ground glass'.

Q **13.8** Wrap several layers of clear adhesive tape around both lenses of a pair of glasses. Alternatively, smear both lenses with petroleum jelly. Wear them for a while to experience something of what it feels like to have bilateral cataracts. Then try this with vision totally occluded in one lens and the other lens wrapped in just a few layers of tape or smeared with a thin film of jelly. How would this affect your daily activities? Discuss the experience with your colleagues.

MEDICAL MANAGEMENT

During the developmental stages of cataract, spectacles may provide a degree of improvement in visual acuity. It is impossible, however, to reverse the opacification process. Surgical removal of the cataract will ultimately be the only effective treatment. Cataract removal is one of the increasing number of surgical procedures now performed as day surgery, provided the ophthalmic surgeon, general practitioner and patient agree there are no contraindications to this (Audit Commission 1997).

The retinal function is examined and, although there may be age-related maculopathy, cataract removal will still be considered, with a guarded prognosis, to give 'walking sight'.

Surgical procedures. Cataract removal is performed when the cataract interferes with activities of living (ALs).

Several methods of cataract extraction are in common use, most of which are performed with only local anaesthesia. Before the operation, the pupil is dilated to facilitate lens delivery and to reduce the risk of damage to the iris. An incision is then made into the globe at the limbus. Methods of lens removal include:

- phaco-emulsification, i.e. ultrasonic fragmentation to break up the nucleus and aspirate soft lens material
- extracapsular extraction — removal of the nucleus and cortex, leaving the posterior capsule intact
- intracapsular extraction — total removal of the lens and capsule (rarely carried out now).

Intraocular lens implantation. The best visual correction is achieved by the insertion of an intraocular lens (IOL) at the time of cataract removal. This is possible in approximately 99% of cases. Unforeseen surgical complications are the main contraindication to non-insertion of an IOL.

IOLs may be inserted as a secondary procedure. It is important to know which kind of lens is in situ, in order to ensure appropriate postoperative care. In the rare situation when no IOL is inserted, a contact lens or corrective spectacle may be issued.

Postoperative medication. The inflammatory response which accompanies all healing is controlled postoperatively by a combination of topical steroids and antibiotics. It is vital that the patient understands the reasons for compliance with the regular instillation of drops.

NURSING PRIORITIES AND MANAGEMENT: CATARACT EXTRACTION AND IMPLANTATION OF AN INTRAOCULAR LENS (IOL)

Using an agreed nursing model, an individual care plan is drawn up for each patient by the nursing team, taking into account the basic perioperative management principles covered in Chapter 26 and those relating to intraocular surgery on page 506. Additionally, the following points specific to cataract extraction and IOL implantation should be noted.

Major nursing considerations

IOL management

It is important for the nurse to find out which method has been used for extraction and whether or not an IOL has been implanted. If an IOL is in situ, its position must be checked at each eye examination.

The most common problems which may arise following IOL implantation are displacement, corneal endothelial damage and the 'UGH' syndrome, i.e. uveitis + glaucoma + hyphaema. Should any of these be present, instant action is required in order to circumvent permanent eye damage. Severe pain is an important symptom of raised IOP.

It should be explained to the patient that there will be a period of adaptation as the brain adjusts to changes in visual perception. During this time the patient can expect a certain amount of visual distortion resulting in central field magnification and peripheral blurring and rounding. This will affect distance and depth perception and the individual should be cautioned to take care on steps and stairs and to turn his head more, in order to scan the whole visual field.

Nursing Care Plan 13.1 outlines some considerations that might arise in the care of a patient undergoing cataract extraction and IOL implantation.

Q

13.9 One of your patients has undergone a cataract extraction and IOL implantation. As you systematically examine the eye, you note the following clinical signs:

- eyelids — slightly bruised and swollen
- conjunctiva — pink
- cornea — cloudy, suture line intact
- anterior chamber — formed, hyphaema noted and more extensive than at previous dressing
- iris — muddy
- pupil — dilated and round
- posterior chamber IOL — in situ and reflecting.

Which of these clinical signs are within normal expectations and which would alert you to a problem that demands immediate attention? What could this problem be? What action will you take?

Glaucoma

Glaucoma can be defined as a disease process with a characteristic pattern of cupping of the optic disc and reproducible field loss. The IOP may be raised or normal. The condition may be acquired or genetic in origin. Acquired glaucoma can be further classified as primary open-angle glaucoma (POAG), primary closed-angle glaucoma (PCAG — both acute and chronic), and glaucoma secondary to pathological processes (secondary glaucoma).

Q

13.10 Revise your knowledge of aqueous dynamics within the eye.

Primary open-angle glaucoma

This type of glaucoma (also known as chronic simple glaucoma) causes progressive and irreversible loss of the peripheral visual field, with the central 10% being spared until a later stage. It is initially symptomless.

PATHOPHYSIOLOGY

The normal range of IOP is 12–20 mmHg. This varies throughout a 24-h period, being lower during the day than at night when the individual is lying down. In POAG, the pressure is persistently elevated and the diurnal variation is greater than normal (Spalton et al 1994).

Raised IOP decreases the blood flow in the optic disc capillaries with resultant excavation and atrophy of the optic nerve head and subsequent loss of nerve fibres passing through it (cupping). A progressive loss of the visual field results from damage to nerve fibre bundles as they enter the optic disc.

Clinical features. The outward appearance of the eye is normal. On examination, if there is cupping of the optic disc, peripheral visual field loss and possible raised IOP, a diagnosis of glaucoma may be made.

Common presenting symptoms. There is usually a gradual and painless loss of peripheral vision. The patient rarely notices this deterioration until considerable damage has been done. This loss of vision is irreversible. The glaucoma is often discovered by an optometrist during a routine eye examination. The normal diurnal variation of IOP may in some instances have caused this vision loss.

MEDICAL MANAGEMENT

The main aim of treatment is to reduce IOP to allow better capillary perfusion at the optic nerve head. This involves improving the aqueous drainage system or decreasing the production of aqueous, or a combination of both. Medical treatment is the mainstay in the majority of cases, although there is a growing trend towards early surgical or laser intervention.

Tests and investigations. Diagnosis and medical assessment of the nature and severity of the condition will rely on the following:

- tonometry — measurement of IOP by specialised instruments
- visual field analysis
- ophthalmoscopy to examine the optic nerve head and estimate the degree of cupping
- gonioscopy — examination of the state and depth of the angle of the eye
- phasing — measurement of IOP by tonometry at different times of the day.

Treatment. Whether the medical regimen is implemented alone or in combination with a surgical procedure, it is important to maintain monitoring of the efficiency of treatment indefinitely. The regimen may include the administration of some combination of the following medications:

- Topical beta-blockers, and topical carbonic anhydrase inhibitors to reduce aqueous production (see Table 13.2). Topical regimens may be prescribed for long-term continuous use; systemic drugs are generally prescribed for short-term or intermittent use.
- Topical miotic drops to constrict the pupil and stretch open the trabecular meshwork, thus facilitating aqueous drainage.

Surgical treatment for POAG is usually performed when conservative management has failed (progression of visual field loss and persistent elevation of IOP) or when drug compliance is unsatisfactory.

The principle of surgery is to create a fistula between the anterior chamber and the subconjunctival space in order to bypass the existing drainage system and increase the outflow of aqueous. The most commonly used procedure is trabeculectomy.

Postoperatively a small bleb under the conjunctival flap will be visible. A small V-shaped hole in the iris may be noted if a peripheral iridectomy has been performed.

The success of surgery is measured by whether the IOP remains within normal limits, but there can be no actual improvement in visual acuity. If a trabeculectomy drains well, topical treatment may be discontinued.

Nursing Care Plan 13.1 A patient undergoing intraocular surgery

Nursing considerations	***Action***	***Rationale***	***Expected outcome***
Preoperative preparation			
1. Anxiety relating to local anaesthetic; being awake during the procedure; draping procedure in theatre; communication with staff during procedure	❒ Explain that local anaesthetic (LA) ensures painless procedure, reduces postoperative discomfort of GA, and enables earlier discharge (see Research Abstract 13.1, p. 503) ❒ Explain that draping and skin cleansing are carried out to reduce the risk of infection ❒ Explain that the unoperated eye needs to be closed to protect the cornea from accidental damage and reduce eye movement	Information given about procedures reduces patient anxiety and discomfort	Patient is able to recall details of preparation and appears more relaxed
	❒ Explain that whilst the eye is anaesthetised it is possible to overcome muscle activity and position the eye in the orbit so as to permit easy access to most surgical sites ❒ Explain that some patients may experience periods of 'seeing lights' during the procedure	Patients commonly express a fear that the eye will be placed on the cheek to facilitate surgery. Placing the eye on the cheek is impossible without total destruction of the optic nerve, which, together with the extraocular muscles and cheek ligaments, tethers the eye securely within the orbital cavity	
	❒ Explain that throughout the patient's time in theatre one nurse will hold his hand and that they will agree on a signalling system so that if he has any discomfort or pain he can communicate this; remedial measures will be taken immediately	An agreed communication system reduces anxiety and increases well-being	He communicates appropriately during the procedure and tolerates the operation well
Discharge considerations			
1. Anxiety about visual function following surgery	❒ Explain that visual recovery is not complete until the eye is fully healed ❒ Visual function is to be assessed at first dressing within 48 h ❒ Explain that 'floaters', which occur following discharge, and the experiencing of flashing lights may precede the development of complications and urgent review in OPD should be sought	Improved knowledge reduces anxiety	Patient is able to recall information given Patient can demonstrate procedure used Patient states arrangements he would make to obtain urgent OPD review
2. The patient has a Parkinsonian tremor and is unable to instil his own eye drops	❒ Teach carer(s) to instil eye drops prior to surgery. If there is no carer (or neighbour), the community nurse should visit and instil eye drops twice daily	Rehabilitation and discharge planning should begin at pre-admission clinic or first hospital attendance. Early liaison with the community nurse will help to ensure that treatment continues and that the nurse is fully informed of individual aspects of the case. It will also reassure the patient that a supportive health care team exists	

For further information, see Perry & Tullo (1995), Chapter 18

Laser treatment. This involves applying short bursts of a laser beam through a lens resembling a gonioscopy lens, targeting selected areas of the trabecular meshwork. Application of argon laser burns to the trabecular meshwork (argon laser trabeculoplasty) has been found to be effective in selected cases in reducing IOP. The scarring caused by the laser burns appears to stretch the tissues between the burns, thus opening up spaces in the trabecular meshwork and facilitating drainage of aqueous.

NURSING PRIORITIES AND MANAGEMENT: PRIMARY OPEN-ANGLE GLAUCOMA (POAG)

Major nursing considerations

Screening

Measurement of IOP and visual field testing may be carried out in the community by the optometry service or hospital-based screening clinics.

Patient compliance with treatment

This is a major concern, especially in the outpatient department and the community setting where most cases of glaucoma will be seen. It is a nursing responsibility to assess the patient's understanding of his condition and the rationale for treatment and his ability to instil his own drops and comply with other aspects of treatment.

Self-administration of drops may be difficult and requires arm and neck flexibility and hand dexterity to successfully manage the drop dispenser bottle. Various appliances are available to help with the procedure but it still requires skilful instruction and demonstration to ensure success. In some cases, relatives or carers must be taught to carry out the treatment regimens. Where deficits occur, additional follow-up and nursing support must be organised.

13.11 How could you encourage compliance in a patient who is prescribed topical anti-glaucoma treatment?

Postoperative observation and monitoring

Depth of AC. Postoperatively, the depth of the AC in the operated eye should be equal to that of the unoperated eye. Variations must be reported. It is possible for over-drainage to result in a shallow AC or for under-drainage to result in a deeper AC.

Signs of raised IOP. Severe postoperative pain, accompanied by a cloudy cornea and flat AC, is abnormal and must be investigated. Raised IOP must be suspected in the presence of these symptoms.

Administering laser treatment

Fully explaining what is involved and reassuring the patient that he will be supported throughout the procedure, and carefully monitored afterwards, will help to ensure compliance. Protective goggles are mandatory for all staff in attendance.

During application of laser treatment, it is necessary for the nurse to understand the potential hazards to the patient and to staff. (see Nursing Care Plan 13.2).

For further information, see Frost (1993).

Retinal detachment

Retinal detachment describes a separation between the neural and pigmented layers of the retina.

PATHOPHYSIOLOGY

The light-sensitive cells in the neural layer are detached from the essential pigments in the pigment layer as fluid effusion between

Nursing Care Plan 13.2 Ensuring patient cooperation in laser treatment

Nursing considerations	*Action*	*Rationale*	*Expected outcome*
1. Anxiety due to **• Lack of understanding of laser treatment** **• Fear of pain and discomfort during procedure**	❐ Explain to the patient that he will be asked to sit as for gonioscopy and that a similar lens will be applied to his eye ❐ Describe the anatomy of the eye, how the laser beam is targeted on the problem areas and what the expected outcome will be ❐ Explain the importance of maintaining a steady position and gaze ❐ Reassure the patient that the treatment may be uncomfortable but should not be painful. He will experience bright flashes of light and there may be a slight headache afterwards ❐ Reassure him that the procedure is well controlled and that there will be careful follow-up	The patient will have experienced gonioscopy as part of his earlier examination and will therefore be familiar with the procedure Expectations of a positive outcome will reduce anxiety The patient's cooperation is necessary in order to ensure that only targeted areas are exposed to the laser Information given about procedures reduces patient anxiety and discomfort	The patient can demonstrate awareness of what the procedure entails and has confidence in the medical and nursing team. He is cooperative during the treatment, keeps a steady direction of gaze and does not appear unduly anxious. Accidental burns are avoided

the layers gradually causes more separation. Retinal detachments are most frequently associated with holes or tears in the retina. These occur as a consequence of vitreous traction, degenerative disease or vitreous loss, which may be traumatic or postoperative. Predisposing factors include myopia, aphakia, trauma or retinal/choroidal tumour. If one eye is affected, the other is also at risk (see p. 500).

Common presenting symptoms. The patient may present at various stages with painless visual disturbances or loss of vision. The external appearance of the eye is unchanged, unless recent traumatic injury or surgical intervention has taken place. During the early stages the rods and cones are falsely activated, causing sensations of flashing light. As flakes of pigment are shed into the vitreous, the patient may see showers of floating shapes and strands in the vitreous field. Later, he may describe an impression of a curtain coming down or drifting smoke passing across his line of vision.

MEDICAL MANAGEMENT

Treatment. The exact nature and extent of the retinal detachment and the presence of retinal fluid will dictate the specific procedure for repair that is used.

Surgical procedures. The aim of surgery is to produce a controlled inflammatory response to seal the detachment, release the subretinal fluid and bring the retinal layers into normal apposition. Surgery should be undertaken at the earliest opportunity to give the best possible visual outcome.

A carbon dioxide (CO_2) freezing probe is applied to the sclera behind the detached retina, producing the required inflammatory response (cryosurgery). This is often explained to patients as 'spot welding'. Release of subretinal fluid aids repositioning of the layers, which may be supported by internal tamponade, created by intravitreal air or volume-expanding gases. A silicone explant may be temporarily sutured into position on the outside of the eye. Once it is seen to be in the correct position and of the correct size, it is permanently tied with non-absorbable sutures. Complex cases may require more extensive intraocular surgery such as vitrectomy (removal of the vitreous humor from the vitreous chamber) and replacing with balanced salt solution.

Outpatient treatment with argon laser and volume-expanding gases may be satisfactory in cases of dry retinal detachments. Here, the inflammatory response is controlled by mydriatic and steroid eye drops.

For further information, see Chawla (1998).

NURSING PRIORITIES AND MANAGEMENT: RETINAL DETACHMENT

Major nursing considerations

Patient positioning

Correct positioning is a vital adjunct to the management of retinal detachment. Individualised regimens determined by medical staff and prescribed in the case notes must be strictly observed. The positioning that is prescribed will depend on the site of the retinal hole and on the nature of the surgical repair procedure. The patient must be fully informed of the reasons for positioning, as his compliance is very important to the success of the treatment. Normal functional positions are usually allowed at mealtimes and for toilet purposes. 'Bed-fast' positioning is seldom necessary for longer than 24 h postoperatively, after which mobilisation is permitted with the patient following an individualised regimen of head positioning if intravitreal air or gas is used (see Nursing Care Plan 13.1).

The overall aim is to help the detached area fall back into position preoperatively and to maintain normal apposition postoperatively. Generally, if the patient has a superior detachment he will be nursed lying flat with one pillow, and if the detachment is inferior he will be nursed sitting up in bed or in a chair. In the case of a temporal or nasal detachment, the patient will be nursed on the opposite side to the affected area. These positions are reversed postoperatively if surgery has included internal tamponade, i.e. intravitreal air. Nursing actions that can help to encourage patient compliance with positioning regimens are described in Nursing Care Plan 13.3.

Postoperative pain

Postoperative pain can be expected to be fairly severe, depending on the complexity and the duration of the surgery. Narcotic analgesics may be necessary for effective pain control, but if severe pain persists it must be reported and investigated immediately. In some units, patient-controlled analgesia (PCA) may be used (see Ch. 19). An acute rise in IOP can be precipitated by retinal surgery. To avoid permanent damage, action must be taken immediately to reduce raised IOP. If severe pain persists and the IOP is within normal limits, some problem with the explant must be suspected.

Postoperative appearance of the eye

In retinal surgery, the conjunctival incision is encircling, there is extensive handling of the globe and, if vitrectomy instruments have been used, there may be considerable trauma to the conjunctiva. The nurse can therefore expect to observe marked chemosis with bruising and swelling of the eyelids. Pressure dressings or regular cold compresses may be applied postoperatively. The eye must be monitored closely to ensure that the conjunctival incision heals cleanly and that there is no evidence of rejection or extrusion of the silicone explant.

Corneal transplant (keratoplasty)

Indications for corneal transplant include destruction of the cornea by injury or disease, some cases of advanced keratoconus (conical cornea) and corneal opacity. Transplants may be full thickness or partial thickness. Keratoplasty is primarily an elective procedure with donor material supplied by the National Eye Bank in Bristol. The donor eyes are screened to ensure no underlying infection or corneal disorder is present before being harvested within 10 h of death. The donor eye should be accompanied by blood samples which are tested for HIV and tissue-matched. However, because of the avascularity of the cornea, it is not absolutely essential to use a tissue-matched cornea.

NURSING PRIORITIES AND MANAGEMENT: CORNEAL TRANSPLANT

The perioperative period is managed as for other intraocular surgery.

Special considerations

The use of donated tissue

Recipients rarely ask questions regarding the source of a donated cornea, but nurses must be prepared to give a carefully worded answer to those who do. They must also be ready to give reassurance and support, as the use of donor corneas can be an emotive

Nursing Care Plan 13.3 Positioning of a patient with retinal detachment

Nursing considerations	*Action*	*Rationale*	*Expected outcome*
The patient has knowledge deficit re enforced positional bed rest to prevent further detachment of retina and help postoperative recovery	❒ Establish knowledge base by preparing and presenting a teaching session using a model of an eye. Include a family member if patient has significant visual loss. Include: • description of normal retina and its function • possible cause of detachment • description of surgical procedure • positioning before and after surgery to help retina fall back into place. Explain that this will be prescribed by the specialist and that every attempt must be made to observe it	Misconceptions about eye surgery are often lurid and frightening. Understanding what really happens will reduce fear and make compliance with instructions more likely. The informed patient experiences a significant reduction in anxiety levels and is more likely to comply	The patient is able to describe what happens in retinal detachment, how it can be repaired, and asks questions which indicate an acceptable level of knowledge He appears more relaxed about the need for positioning and is very cooperative
	❒ Encourage questions	Given time and encouragement, patients may express a variety of questions and individual concerns	
	❒ Reinforce explanations frequently	Due to blocking effect of anxiety, patients do not always absorb information and it may be necessary to repeat or rephrase it	

issue. Sometimes the donor's relatives ask if the tissue has been used. Confirmation is usually given by medical staff but nurses may also be involved. Care should be taken not to violate confidentiality whilst still providing adequate information. Ideally, the entire team caring for the patient should invest time in preparing and delivering relevant, individualised information.

Postoperative examination

Following surgery, the degree of conjunctival redness (injection) may be considerable. This should lessen progressively. If the conjunctiva does not soon return to the 'white eye' state, the cause may be (1) raised IOP, (2) failure of the transplant, (3) transplant rejection. These three possibilities must also be considered when inspection of the cornea reveals a loss of clarity, a finding which must be reported immediately. The wound should be examined to ensure the suture line remains intact and the corneal disc (transplant) has stayed in position, as disruption of either may affect the optical power of the transplant.

Patient involvement and cooperation

The patient and his family should be made aware that corneal transplant requires a lengthy follow-up period. The cornea is an avascular structure, and therefore healing will be slow. The corneal suture will remain in situ for several months or, if a good optical result has been obtained, it may be decided to leave the sutures in indefinitely rather than risk disturbing the transplant.

It must also be emphasised that it is vital to continue any topical medication prescribed to avoid rejection of the transplant and to prevent infection. The patient should be warned that optimum visual recovery cannot be expected until some months after surgery. Some may be disappointed by the initial outcome, when vision may seem to be poorer than before transplant. These patients should be advised of realistic visual expectations.

Prior to discharge, patient and carer teaching should ensure that the importance of early recognition of symptoms of transplant rejection is understood. These symptoms could include:

- increased redness of the conjunctiva
- cloudiness of the cornea
- reduction of visual function, and/or
- discomfort.

Temporal arteritis (giant cell arteritis, cranial arteritis)

This is a progressive disease process affecting the over-60 age group, in which the middle layer of medium-sized arteries becomes inflamed. When the external carotid system is involved, ocular damage results with sudden loss of vision, which may be preceded by, or accompany, polymyalgia rheumatica (stiff aching muscles, especially around the shoulders).

PATHOPHYSIOLOGY

There is degeneration of the retina, which results from thrombosis or occlusion of the ophthalmic artery, secondary to necrotic inflammatory changes in the middle layer of the temporal and cranial arteries. The cells in the destroyed middle layer are replaced by collagen. During the active phase of this process, there is a raised erythrocyte sedimentation rate (ESR) (see Ch. 11).

Clinical features. Patients often complain of general malaise, loss of weight and lethargy, or a 'flu-like' illness which may last for a few days or weeks and which precedes a sustained visual disturbance. This is in contrast to the prodromal phase, in which fleeting episodes of blurred vision may occur, accompanied by unilateral temporal or occipital headache. The loss of vision is sudden in onset, usually affecting one eye before the other. The length of time between both eyes being affected is extremely variable, ranging from several hours to several days.

MEDICAL MANAGEMENT

Diagnosis is made following ophthalmoscopy and the discovery of a raised ESR. It has to be remembered that the ESR may not be high in the early stages of the disease and repeat tests may be necessary. The diagnosis may be confirmed by carrying out a temporal artery biopsy.

Treatment may be instigated in the community or in hospital and consists of systemic corticosteroid therapy which reduces the ESR to within normal limits. The initial dose may be given intramuscularly (i.m.) to achieve the effective therapeutic level. The starting high-dosage rate, i.e. 80–120 mg daily, is reduced to a maintenance oral dose, which will be administered for at least 2 years. Topical treatment is not usually prescribed unless a secondary condition, e.g. iritis, develops.

NURSING PRIORITIES AND MANAGEMENT: TEMPORAL ARTERITIS

Nursing effort is directed towards the care of a patient undergoing corticosteroid therapy. In particular, monitoring and recording regimens, e.g. of blood pressure, urinalysis and body weight, will be required to give warning of any complication arising from the therapy. If vision deficit is severe, help and support will be necessary and blind or partially sighted registration will become inevitable. This entails a multidisciplinary approach to rehabilitation care, in which the nursing staff participate fully.

RED EYE

Primary closed-angle glaucoma (PCAG)

Closed-angle glaucoma usually presents as an acute episode affecting one eye, although it may be subacute or chronic. It is an ophthalmic emergency and needs specialist attention within 24 h to prevent permanent visual damage. It is also necessary to initiate early prophylactic treatment in the other eye.

PATHOPHYSIOLOGY

Raised IOP develops as a result of disruption of the circulation of aqueous humor in a narrow anterior chamber, which is often associated with hypermetropia. Pupil dilatation is accompanied by forward displacement of the iris which occludes the trabecular meshwork, blocking the flow of aqueous to the canal of Schlemm. The pupillary margin of the iris also comes into contact with the lens, causing the pupil to become semi-dilated and fixed, further impeding the flow of aqueous and increasing forward displacement of the iris. Aqueous build-up results in corneal oedema and disturbance of sensory nerve fibres.

Common presenting symptoms are as follows:

- Onset is usually sudden, with severe pain in one eye accompanied by frontotemporal headache on the affected side
- The patient often complains of nausea and may vomit
- Vision is reduced
- The individual is photophobic and experiences increased lacrimation
- The eye is red, particularly around the limbus (due to marked ciliary injection)
- The cornea is hazy due to oedema
- The pupil is semi-dilated and does not react to light
- Iris details are poorly defined (muddy in appearance)
- On palpation over a closed lid, the eye feels hard because of raised IOP.

MEDICAL MANAGEMENT

Tests and investigations include medical history, systematic structural examination, slit-lamp and gonioscopy examination of the angle of the eye (see Appendix 1), and measurement of IOP. (A slit lamp illuminates the eye with a narrow band of light which allows particular structures, e.g. cornea, lens and anterior chamber, to be examined through a binocular microscope.)

Treatment. Acute signs and symptoms will be controlled by the following means:

- Pain relief by analgesics, including opiates i.m.
- Control of nausea and vomiting with i.m. antiemetics
- Increase in outflow of aqueous humor by freeing the iris angle. To achieve this, a regimen of intensive topical miotic therapy is commenced to constrict the pupil rapidly and draw the iris away from the angle. Prophylactic therapy is also prescribed for the other eye to prevent an acute attack
- Reduction in production of aqueous humor by administration of carbonic anhydrase inhibitors such as acetazolamide (Diamox). If the response to this is unsatisfactory, osmotic diuretics such as oral glycerol or i.v. mannitol can be used.

Surgical intervention. Once the acute signs and symptoms have been controlled, surgical intervention may be decided upon. The method depends on the appearance of the angle and may be any of the following:

- laser iridotomies (small holes in the iris) to both eyes
- surgical iridectomy or trabeculectomy to the acute eye, and laser iridotomy to the other eye.

Following laser iridotomies, topical steroid treatment may be given to reduce tissue irritability and ensure normal IOP.

For surgical procedures such as peripheral iridectomies or trabeculectomies, the preparation and perioperative care are as for glaucoma (see p. 506).

NURSING PRIORITIES AND MANAGEMENT: PRIMARY CLOSED-ANGLE GLAUCOMA (PCAG)

Screening

The nurse working in a general practice, community or emergency department setting frequently has to assume a screening role and prioritise patients' needs for specialist attention in ophthalmic conditions. Awareness of the significance of various signs and symptoms, such as severe pain in one or both eyes, a hazy cornea and a significant deterioration in vision, will prevent the patient suffering unnecessary loss of vision.

In PCAG, priority is given to the immediate control of acute signs and symptoms and to the delivery of prescribed intensive therapy regimens. Otherwise, nursing priorities and management are as for POAG (see p. 507). The initial pain and distress experienced by patients with PCAG will be severe. A satisfactory pupillary miosis with resolution of corneal oedema generally occurs about 4 h after commencement of treatment and can be maintained thereafter by medical management or surgical intervention or a combination of both. Some aspects of the nursing support that can be given to patients undergoing laser treatment are described in Nursing Care Plan 13.2.

Uveitis

PATHOPHYSIOLOGY

Uveitis is inflammation of the uveal tract. Anterior uveitis (or iritis) can involve the iris or the ciliary body, or both. Posterior uveitis involves the choroid (choroiditis). It is an acute condition, the precise cause of which is unknown, although it is often associated with rheumatoid conditions, ankylosing spondylitis and sarcoidosis. Recurrent episodes are relatively common; they usually respond to prompt treatment and carry a fairly good prognosis. Secondary iritis may accompany other eye infections or trauma.

Clinical features are as follows:

- pain, probably due to pupillary spasm, may mark the onset of iritis and may be severe
- a red eye due to vascular congestion in the conjunctival vessels at the limbus
- photophobia
- cloudy aqueous due to the increase in aqueous protein content and presence of white blood cells (the debris floating in the aqueous is known as 'flare and cells')
- reduced vision, proportional to the severity of the attack
- cellular exudate (keratic precipitates, KPs) may be present on the posterior surface of the cornea
- loss of iris details (muddy iris)
- swelling of the iris may cause it to adhere to the anterior surface of the lens (synechia formation); this will interfere with aqueous flow
- IOP may be raised and, if untreated, may progress to secondary glaucoma.

MEDICAL MANAGEMENT

Patients with acute iritis are treated on an outpatient basis whenever possible. Inflammatory episodes are controlled using a combination of topical and systemic drugs. Steroids and mydriatics are administered as eye drops or by subconjunctival injection. Steroids may be prescribed systemically when the response to topical medication is poor. In some complicated cases, immunosuppressive drugs may be necessary. In addition, when the intraocular pressure is raised, oral or topical acetazolamide or topical beta-blockers will be prescribed. Pain-relieving drugs are given as required. Dark glasses are supplied to relieve the discomfort of photophobia.

NURSING PRIORITIES AND MANAGEMENT: UVEITIS

Major nursing considerations

Setting priorities

Screening for potential health problems and prioritising patients' needs are two interrelated aspects of the nurse's role in the community. It is vital that community nurses are able to recognise ophthalmic conditions which need urgent medical attention. Uveitis is one such condition, as raised IOP and/or severe infection will quickly cause irreparable damage if treatment is delayed.

Q **13.12** State the ophthalmic conditions that must receive the most urgent attention.

Providing instruction

Once the diagnosis is confirmed and treatment has been commenced, the nurse's role will include providing guidance and support for the patient and his family to ensure compliance with the treatment regimen. If a pattern of recurrence emerges, it may be advantageous to explain the importance of early initiation of self-medication. This will reduce the severity of the attack and the risk of complications.

Ensuring a safe environment

Dilated pupils allow an increased amount of light to enter the eye, causing photophobia. Patients experience dazzle when in bright sunlight or when facing car headlights from oncoming traffic at night. Appropriate adjustments to lifestyle may be required for the duration of the treatment.

Keratitis

The term keratitis refers to inflammatory conditions of the cornea. These may be caused by certain bacteria, viruses or fungi and result in corneal ulceration. If the superficial layer (epithelium) alone is affected, there is minimal damage with little visual loss. If the middle portion (stroma) is involved, loss of transparency and altered corneal curvature may lead to significant loss of vision. Severe inflammation may result in inflammatory debris being shed into the anterior chamber and settling as a collection of cells (hypopyon).

PATHOPHYSIOLOGY

Bacterial keratitis

Causative agents of bacterial keratitis include *Pneumococcus*, *Streptococcus* and *Pseudomonas*, which invade the cornea and cause an inflammatory reaction. The condition tends to be recurrent. Severe, deep ulceration erodes the middle portion of the cornea (stroma) to the level called Descemet's membrane, which herniates to form a descemetocele due to the pressure of the aqueous humor. Corneal perforation will occur if the descemetocele ruptures.

Clinical features. The lesion appears as a grey circular area on the surface of the cornea, with oedema of the surrounding epithelium which dulls the corneal reflex. Other features include:

- a painful red eye
- photophobia with spasm of the eyelid (blepharospasm)
- excessive lacrimation in most cases, although there are some instances of dry eye presentation.

Viral keratitis

The most common form of viral keratitis is dendritic (herpetic) ulcer, which is caused by the herpes simplex virus. Its distinguishing feature is the branching, tree-like pattern it forms on the cornea, which is visible only on corneal staining with fluorescein.

Fungal keratitis

Fungal infections of the eye are an increasing problem presenting to eye departments. The damage they cause is severe, and specific antifungal treatment agents are few. Complications can develop

Research Abstract 13.2
Contact lenses and keratitis risk

Disposable soft contact lenses have been marketed as a safer alternative to conventional soft lenses. A study of patients in the casualty department at Moorfields Eye Hospital (Matthews et al 1992) set out to investigate the validity of this claim and to establish patterns of use (*n* = 242).

The results did not support the claim but indicated that keratitis — microbial and sterile — was the most common complication found in disposable lens users and that disposable lenses were associated with a significantly higher risk and incidence of keratitis than any other lens type. Matthews et al concluded that lens type, poor hygiene and failure to follow instructions for cleansing and use could account for these statistically significant trends.

Matthews T D, Frazer D G, Minassian D C, Radford C F, Dart J K G 1992 Risks of keratitis and patterns of use with disposable contact lenses. Archives of Ophthalmology 110(11): 1559–1562.

rapidly. The distinguishing feature of this kind of ulceration is that it appears as fluffy, feathery extensions over the cornea. Often it can be associated with minor trauma from vegetation or with contact lenses (see also Research Abstract 13.2).

Acanthamoeba

Acanthamoeba keratitis is a rare but serious chronic infection of the cornea, associated with corneal trauma, contact lens wear or exposure to polluted water. Acanthamoeba inhabit polluted water and swimming pools worldwide (Radford 1995). Poor compliance with the handling, cleansing or storage of both contact lenses and lens cases, and ignoring the guidelines for contact lens wear contribute greatly to the worldwide increase of this form of keratitis. Characteristic corneal clinical features include ring abscess formation and corneal melt. If the response to treatment, given intensively, is poor, then blindness is the end result.

For further information, see Cotgreave et al (1989).

MEDICAL MANAGEMENT

Diagnosis can be confirmed by conjunctival and corneal swabs and fluorescein staining. The fluorescein fixes to damaged corneal tissue and turns the affected area a bright fluorescent green, indicating the extent of the damage. Topical antibiotic, antiviral or antifungal therapy, e.g. Zenica Pharma 0.2% and Brolene 0.1%, is usually commenced immediately to avoid rapid development of complications. Any accompanying iritis or rise in IOP is treated as necessary. It is important to note that steroids are generally contraindicated for keratitis. There are some exceptions to this rule, but these can only be determined by an ophthalmic specialist.

NURSING PRIORITIES AND MANAGEMENT: KERATITIS

Management may be on an in-patient or outpatient basis and follows the principles outlined earlier for uveitis, with the following additions:

- The patient should be taught not to touch or rub his eye as this may extend the ulceration.
- Careful hygiene is essential to prevent cross-infection. Tears should be wiped from the cheek only. A clean disposable tissue should be used on each occasion. Principles of isolation and infection control will be observed in the hospital situation (see Ch. 16).
- With regard to dendritic ulcer, it is important to note that anyone who has an outbreak of herpes simplex — commonly known as 'cold sores' — should be advised to guard against touching the sores and then rubbing their eyes. Nursing staff with active sores should not have contact with ophthalmic patients.

Conjunctivitis

Conjunctivitis, i.e. inflammation of the conjunctiva, is a common condition, which may be acute, subacute or chronic. It can be unilateral or bilateral in presentation, the latter form often being due to cross-infection. Causative agents are bacteria, viruses, fungi, parasites, toxins, chemicals, foreign bodies and allergies.

PATHOPHYSIOLOGY

The activating agent causes vascular dilatation (injection) of the palpebral and bulbar conjunctiva, cellular infiltration leading to formation of papillae and follicles, and serous exudation. In severe cases, oedema of the conjunctiva (chemosis) may occur.

Clinical features include:

- brick-red appearance
- gritty feeling and varying degrees of pain
- in bacterial conjunctivitis, often mucopurulent discharge and sticking together of the eyelids at night.

The eye is not usually photophobic, nor is vision affected. Eversion of the lids may reveal follicle formation, which is the cause of the gritty sensation.

MEDICAL AND NURSING MANAGEMENT

This entails treating the cause, educating the patient in eye hygiene and self-medication, and monitoring for complications. Conjunctivitis is highly infectious and family members, peers and other patients should be advised about the prevention of cross-infection. Scrupulous handwashing and the use of individual towels should be emphasised.

Herpes zoster ophthalmicus (ophthalmic shingles)

This is an acute unilateral infection of the trigeminal ganglion which extends from the scalp to the nose and includes the eye. It is caused by the chickenpox virus and is fairly common in people over 50 years of age (see Ch. 16).

PATHOPHYSIOLOGY

Common presenting symptoms are as follows:

- the manifestation of the disease is usually preceded by pain, regional adenopathy and general malaise
- the eyelids swell on the affected side
- the skin of the forehead above the eye becomes red

- characteristic vesicular eruptions occur over the course of the nerve
- there may be serious ocular complications, including uveitis, keratitis, conjunctivitis and visual impairment.

MEDICAL MANAGEMENT

Treatment with systemic antiviral agents should begin immediately. Ocular involvement should be treated symptomatically and with equal vigour. Prevention of cross-infection is a priority.

Allergy to topical medication

Allergic reaction to topical eye medication manifests as inflammation of the eyelids extending to the cheeks. The lids become red and oedematous and may be moist in the acute stage, drying to form light crusts later. There is intense itching, which may result in excoriation. Common causative agents are atropine and neomycin eye drops.

Management consists of reviewing medication, suspending all medication for 24 h if possible and substituting an alternative agent. Cortisone lotion may be prescribed for the affected skin area to relieve itching and oedema.

Stye (hordeolum)

A stye is a staphylococcal infection of the eyelash follicle or its associated sebaceous gland. It may be treated by hot spoon bathing (see Box 13.3) and application of an antibiotic ointment. Principles of prevention of cross-infection should be observed.

Box 13.3 Hot spoon bathing

This is a method of applying moist heat locally to the eye or abscess site, in order to relieve pain, improve the effectiveness of local treatment and assist in the 'pointing' of abscesses.

Requirements

- A wooden spoon, cotton wool to pad the bowl of the spoon, a gauze swab to cover the cotton wool and a rubber band or muslin bandage to secure the padding
- A jug containing nearly boiling water standing in a tray or a basin large enough to contain the volume of water if accidentally spilt
- A plastic cape or towel to protect the patient's clothing

Method

The procedure is explained to the patient and he is positioned comfortably with his legs beneath a table. The bowl or tray containing the filled jug is placed within easy reach on the table, which should be checked for stability. The patient is instructed to soak the spoon in the hot water, to remove excess water by pressing it against the rim of the jug, which must be held firmly during this part of the procedure. The steaming spoon is then held close to the *closed* eyelid to provide comfortable heat without skin contact in order to avoid any possibility of a scald. As the spoon cools, it is re-dipped to maintain an effective temperature. The process is continued for 10–15 min and is usually carried out four times daily. All patients require supervision during the procedure. The frail, the handicapped and children must always have assistance in order to prevent accidents.

DIPLOPIA (DOUBLE VISION)

Diplopia refers to a person's experience of seeing the same object in two different areas of his visual field. If this occurs with one eye closed it usually means that the light entering the eye is broken up, as in the presence of a cataract. If it occurs with both eyes open, it is caused by an imbalance in the extraocular muscles (a squint). In adults this is usually acquired and is associated with systemic disorders or trauma. These include meningitis, multiple sclerosis, cerebral aneurysm, myasthenia gravis, neoplasm, hypertension, thyrotoxicosis, diabetes and head injury. Different factors are involved in childhood squints and for further information reference should be made to paediatric texts.

NURSING PRIORITIES AND MANAGEMENT: DIPLOPIA

Symptomatic treatment in the community. Diplopia caused by a squint can be alleviated by occluding one eye with an eye patch. This can be initiated by the nurse until the patient is seen by a specialist or, in the case of paralytic squint, during treatment of the underlying disease. If one eye is occluded there is no conflict of images in the visual cortex. This reduces the dizziness and nausea often associated with the sense of imbalance caused by diplopia.

MEDICAL MANAGEMENT

Treatment of the underlying cause will be ongoing. Treatment specific to the double vision includes:

- occlusion of one eye
- the use of prism spectacles
- surgical squint correction — this would not be contemplated for at least 6 months after stabilisation of the squint as spontaneous improvement is possible
- injection of botulinum toxin to the overacting muscle which gives temporary flaccid paralysis (approximately 3 months) during which the opposing muscle undergoes contraction, reducing the angle of deviation. The botulinum blocks the transmission of the nerve impulses at the neuromuscular junction by interfering with release of the neurotransmitter acetylcholine (see Ch. 9).

EYE INJURIES

The eye is susceptible to many types of injury, most of which are frightening and painful. A careful history (Table 13.3), which must include a record of visual acuity and a systematic eye examination (Table 13.1), is taken to establish a diagnosis and for medicolegal reasons. Chemical burns are the only exception to this where the main priority is first aid treatment. A triage system for ophthalmic injuries is outlined in Box 13.4 (see also Ch. 27, p. 834).

Careful history-taking is especially important if it is suspected that a particle may have entered the eye at a high velocity. In such a case there could well be no external evidence of injury and no pain, and if the particle were left in situ it could result in blindness many years later. Some of the more commonly occurring types of eye injury are described below.

Hyphaema

The term 'hyphaema' refers to a haemorrhage into the anterior chamber of the eye.

PATHOPHYSIOLOGY

A primary hyphaema is usually caused by a direct blow to the eye, e.g. a clenched fist, golf ball or champagne cork, causing rupture of the small iris blood vessels. It may be microscopic with diffuse red

Table 13.3 Systematic approach to history-taking

Assessment	*Question*	*Rationale*
History of injury	How did the accident occur? When did the accident occur? Where did the accident occur? Which eye is affected? Is the injury unilateral/bilateral? Were safety goggles worn?	To aid diagnosis For medicolegal reasons
Ophthalmic history	Are glasses or contact lenses worn? Has a similar accident occurred before? Has patient attended eye hospital before?	To ascertain if preventive lessons are learnt
Medical history	Does patient have a general health problem? Has patient had previous surgery?	Some systemic disorders may affect the eye, e.g. diabetes Patient may require surgery and may have had a reaction to an anaesthetic previously
Medications	Is patient taking medication at present?	Some drugs may affect the eye, e.g. aspirin and the contraceptive pill Patient may have an allergy to a drug
Allergies	Is patient allergic to any substance, e.g. drugs, Sellotape, Elastoplast?	Patient may be inadvertently given a substance to which he is allergic

cells visible only with the aid of a slit lamp, or severe with a level of blood seen. Rarely, the blood can completely fill the AC.

The degree of pain and reduction in vision depend upon the severity of the bleeding.

A secondary hyphaema may occur after intraocular surgery or an eye injury.

MEDICAL MANAGEMENT

A systematic approach to history-taking is carried out as outlined in Table 13.3.

A patient with a microscopic hyphaema or moderate hyphaema will not be admitted but advised to rest at home for several days. These hyphaemas rarely re-bleed.

A patient with a severe hyphaema may be admitted for observation as there could be an associated rise in IOP. Quiet activity will be allowed. If a re-bleed occurs, it usually happens between the third and fifth day.

NURSING PRIORITIES AND MANAGEMENT: HYPHAEMA

Observation of the level of hyphaema is made 2–4 times daily. Any increase in pain or discomfort may be caused by raised IOP or a re-bleed.

The patient is advised to bend at the knees to reach things from below waist height and not to lift or strain.

Topical antibiotic and/or steroid eye drops may be prescribed. On discharge, the patient will be advised to avoid active or contact sports until the first follow-up appointment. He will be told to assess visual function in the injured eye, daily, to detect possible complications, e.g. retinal detachment (see p. 507 and Nursing Care Plan 13.1). Protective eyewear may be necessary in the future, e.g. whilst playing squash, to prevent a similar injury again (see Box 13.2).

Penetrating injuries

Whatever the apparent extent of a penetrating injury, it must always be treated as an emergency and thoroughly investigated. Depending on the results of history-taking and examination, X-rays and ultrasound scanning may be necessary to confirm the presence, location and type of a foreign body.

Box 13.4 Ophthalmic triage

Ophthalmic patients attending an A&E department are placed in one of three categories depending on the severity of their disorder (York 1990).

Category 1
True emergencies requiring immediate specialist attention:
- Chemical burns (initiate first aid immediately)
- Penetrating injuries
- Intraocular foreign body
- Acute glaucoma
- Extensive retinal detachment
- Sudden loss of vision in one eye (initiate first aid immediately)

Category 2
Specialist attention required as soon as possible:
- Hyphaema
- Corneal foreign body, abrasion or ulcer
- Radiation and welding burns
- All acute infections or allergies
- Recent in-patient who suspects complications

Category 3
Minor irritations and long-standing visual disturbances

MEDICAL MANAGEMENT

Treatment will depend on the cause of the injury and on the extent of involvement of ocular structures. It will usually include the administration of mydriatic, steroid and antibiotic eye drops, and possibly of systemic antibiotics to reduce the risk of complications from inflammation and infection. In addition, the measures described below will be taken.

Perforating injuries. The patient will be admitted to hospital for surgical repair of the wound and possible excision of iris prolapse. If the lens is damaged it may be removed at the same time. If facial or other injuries are present these will be repaired by the appropriate specialists (see Ch. 15).

Small puncture wounds. These may seal themselves, but the patient is admitted to ensure that the wound stays closed and that

Table 13.4 Possible complications following penetrating eye injury

Structure	*Complication*	*Cause*	*Onset*	*Treatment*
Cornea	Astigmatism Scarring	Sutures and scarring Wound	After surgery After surgery	Remove sutures Contact lens in future Corneal transplant in future
Anterior chamber	Hypopyon — sterile Hypopyon — infected Hyphaema	Iritis Infection Bleeding iris vessels	1–3 days 1–7 days 1–7 days	Intensive steroids Intensive antibiotics Treat as secondary hyphaema
	Raised IOP	Damage to drainage angle	Immediate/weeks later	Beta-blocker eye drops and acetazolamide
Iris	Prolapse through wound	Original injury or loose suture	1–7 days	Excision of prolapse and resuturing
Lens	Cataract	Original trauma	Immediate/weeks later	Intra/extracapsular lens extraction
	Dislocation	Original trauma to suspensory ligaments	Immediate	Lens extraction or no treatment
Vitreous chamber	Haemorrhage Fibrous bands	Bleeding into vitreous humor	Immediate Weeks later	Vitrectomy Vitrectomy
Retina	Retinal tears Detachment	Original trauma Original injury Fluid vitreous	Immediate/weeks later Immediate/weeks later Immediate/weeks later	Cryotherapy Surgical repair Surgical repair

intraocular infection does not develop. If the wound is not completely sealed, acrylic glue may be instilled onto the cornea to seal the wound, or a contact lens may be applied.

Intraocular foreign bodies. Admission is essential for surgical removal of the foreign body, which could be embedded in the iris, vitreous humor or lens. If the foreign body is metallic, it may be removed with the aid of a magnet. If it is found in the lens, a lens extraction is carried out (see p. 504). Vitrectomy may be necessary if there has been vitreous haemorrhage.

Complications following penetrating injury. Many complications can occur after a penetrating injury — some immediately, others months later (see Table 13.4). Severe infections can occur in any injury, making intensive treatment with antibiotic eye drops and systemic antibiotics necessary.

It is always very important to examine the uninjured eye regularly for signs of a rare complication known as 'sympathetic ophthalmitis', which presents as a low-grade iritis. The cause of the sympathetic inflammatory process is thought to involve an immune response to damaged uveal tissue. The use of topical steroids has reduced the occurrence of this potentially sight-threatening condition, which was formerly managed by enucleating the injured eye.

A severely damaged eye with no prospect of useful vision may become very painful and unresponsive to analgesics. It may be necessary to remove the eye to give relief to the patient.

Following repair of large penetrating injuries (or severe infections), the eye may collapse entirely and become a shrunken mass in the orbit. This wasting of the globe (phthisis bulbii) can be unsightly and the patient may wish the eye to be removed.

NURSING PRIORITIES AND MANAGEMENT: PENETRATING INJURIES

Major patient problems

Anxiety

Many injuries are severe and mutilating and pose a grave danger to sight. Fear of becoming blind will heighten the patient's anxiety. Comforting the distressed patient and his relatives is a nursing priority. Enabling the patient and his carers to express their feelings and fears is an important part of the comforting process. All questions must be answered honestly, with a uniformity of approach, so that no false or unrealistic expectations are raised.

Postoperatively, the patient's main concern will be to know how severely affected his vision will be and the duration of the visual loss.

Fears about body image, work and lifestyle will be paramount. The patient and his relatives may approach different members of staff for answers to their questions. This may reflect their high level of anxiety or it may indicate that explanations have been inadequate. Discussion and good communication among staff are vital to prevent misunderstanding. Where the prognosis is poor, clear and consistent information will dispel false expectations and help the patient and his family to adapt to the reality of the situation. The loss of sight is like any other significant human loss and will be accompanied by a process akin to grieving.

Return to the community

If the eye is damaged to the extent that no useful vision is retained, the patient will need continuing support in the community. This should be arranged before his discharge. Patients in this situation are particularly susceptible to depression when they return home and begin to grapple with the full implications of their disability. They will need practical and psychological support through the grieving and adaptation period. There are support groups in some parts of the country.

Chemical burns

Treatment should begin immediately after a chemical has entered the eye. The sooner the eye is irrigated with copious amounts of water, the less damage will be caused. Speed is essential and it may

Box 13.5 Occupational health nurse

Many industries employ an occupational health nurse, who educates staff in the first aid treatment of a chemical entering an eye, which is immediate irrigation of the eye.

This has made a significant reduction in the number and extent of these injuries.

be necessary to plunge the whole head into a basin of water and force the eyelids open or to hold the head under a running tap. Many chemical substances have antidotes but no time should be wasted in finding one. Immediate irrigation is paramount (see Box 13.5).

PATHOPHYSIOLOGY

The burn may be caused by an acid or an alkali. In general, acids cause only superficial burns because coagulation of the tissues prevents further penetration. The structures involved are usually the palpebral (lining the eyelids) and bulbar (covering the eyeball) conjunctivae and the cornea. Alkalis penetrate the eye structures more deeply and, as well as severely damaging the eyelids, conjunctivae, cornea and sclera, readily penetrate the internal structures.

Substances which cause burns are often in aerosol cans, e.g. antifreeze, but car battery acid and cement are frequent culprits. Superglue can be particularly dangerous. The patient is often a manual worker or a DIY enthusiast who has not taken necessary precautions (see Box 13.2).

The patient will complain of severe, burning pain due to the exposure of the pain receptors of the trigeminal nerve. Absence of pain does not mean the burn is mild: the burn may be so severe that it has destroyed the nerve endings. There will be extreme watering of the eyes due to reflex action. The lids will be very swollen and red. Burns to the surrounding skin may be evident.

MEDICAL MANAGEMENT

On arrival in the A&E department the patient is taken for immediate irrigation of the eye. This is one time when visual acuity is not assessed before treatment. Anaesthetic eye drops are instilled to reduce the pain and ensure the patient's cooperation with irrigation. The irrigating fluid will be either sodium chloride 0.9% or a neutralising fluid for alkaline burns, e.g. Limclair (see Box 13.6).

Once the nurse is sure that all traces of the chemical have been removed, a full history can be taken and visual acuity assessed.

After irrigation, the doctor will examine the eyes using a slit lamp to assess the extent of the injury. Many chemical injuries are successfully treated before any lasting damage can occur. Occasionally, however, the burn can cause extensive damage to the cornea and conjunctiva.

Treatment for minor burns. The patient is allowed to return home. He is prescribed an antibiotic ointment. An eye pad is applied, to remain in place for at least 6 h. If both eyes require padding, the better eye is left exposed until the patient arrives at home, where he is instructed to pad the other eye. The antibiotic ointment is prescribed for several days and the patient is given a follow-up appointment.

Treatment for severe burns. The patient is admitted to the ward for intensive treatment and observation. Depending on the severity of the pain, i.m. analgesics are given for at least the first 24 h. An antibiotic ointment is applied at least four times daily to

Box 13.6 Irrigation of an eye

The irrigation can be carried out with an i.v. giving set or a syringe (in an emergency) and should continue for at least 15–30 min to each eye. The patient should be lying down or seated with his head supported. He should be asked to look up, down and from side to side, to ensure that as far as possible the fluid washes over all parts of the eyeball. The upper eyelids should be everted to ensure that any particles (e.g. of lime or cement) have been washed out. If not, they can be removed with a moistened cotton bud or fine forceps.

The irrigation is discontinued once litmus paper shows that the chemical has been neutralised.

In some cases, the patient may require a general anaesthetic while all traces of the chemical are removed.

Box 13.7 Rodding of fornices

This procedure is carried out by a nurse. Local anaesthetic eye drops are instilled. A glass rod is lubricated with antibiotic ointment and inserted under the upper eyelid. The patient is asked to look down and the rod is passed gently but firmly from side to side several times whilst outward pressure is exerted. This breaks down any adhesions already formed and leaves a film of ointment in the fornix to prevent any recurrence.

The process is repeated under the lower eyelid with the patient looking up.

lubricate the fornices, and mydriatic eye drops are instilled to relieve accompanying iris spasm and iritis. To prevent the development of conjunctival adhesions (symblepharon), rodding of the fornices may be required (see Box 13.7).

NURSING PRIORITIES AND MANAGEMENT: CHEMICAL BURNS

Major patient problems

Anxiety

It will be important for the nurse to provide reassurance and emotional support for patients who have suffered chemical burns to the eye, as their anxiety level is likely to be high. The patient may have bilateral eye pads in situ and may find this very stressful. Once the eyepads are removed, dark glasses may be necessary to reduce the photophobia caused by iris spasm and pupil dilatation.

Return to the community

The patient will be advised to maintain prescribed treatment for several weeks and to attend follow-up outpatient appointments.

If there is permanent damage to one or both corneas, a keratoplasty may be carried out (see p. 508).

It may be necessary, in cases of significant sight loss, to ensure that the patient and his carers are fully supported and are offered appropriate advice by special community services for the visually impaired person.

Radiation injuries

Irradiation from ultraviolet, infrared or laser light can cause eye damage.

PATHOPHYSIOLOGY

Ultraviolet radiation causes corneal epithelial damage (arc eye, welders' flash) and most commonly occurs when approved eye goggles with protective sides are not worn during welding or when the individual is using a sunbed or sunlamp (see Box 13.2). Usually the signs and symptoms do not appear until several hours after exposure, when the patient presents with photophobia, pain and excessive lacrimation. The reason that there is this latent period is not fully understood. Fluorescein drops show dot-like staining of the cornea. Treatment is symptomatic and includes pain relief and the use of eye pads or dark glasses. The corneal healing is variable but there should be no long-term effects.

Infrared radiation penetrates the eye through the cornea and can cause cataracts.

Laser radiation can cause irreversible damage to the retina.

NURSING PRIORITIES AND MANAGEMENT: RADIATION INJURIES

Prevention

Health education and accident prevention are major parts of the nurse's role. The need for protective eyewear wherever there is a danger of radiation must be actively stressed. Nurses working in occupational health, general practice, in the community and in A&E and outpatient departments with laser equipment could implement a programme of health education which focuses on this topic. It is also important to stress that other people working in the immediate environment of the radiation source may sustain injuries.

13.13 Can you think of reasons why people might fail to use appropriate eye protection? Is there any legislation governing the provision of protective eyewear? Discuss this issue with your tutor and reflect on how it applies to your own workplace.

Minor eye injuries

Corneal foreign body

The patient can usually give an accurate history of something entering the eye. The eye will be extremely painful, especially on blinking. On examination, a foreign body will be visible on the anterior surface of the cornea. Anaesthetic eye drops are instilled and the foreign body is removed with a moistened cotton bud or a 10G needle. This can be carried out by the doctor or a trained ophthalmic nurse (see Box 13.8 for additional information).

Subtarsal foreign body

The nurse should suspect the presence of a subtarsal foreign body when, despite the patient's complaint of something entering his eye, nothing can be seen on normal inspection. There will be discomfort, especially on blinking. The upper lid should be everted and the foreign body, if present, removed with a moistened cotton bud (see Box 13.9).

Corneal abrasion

This can be caused by a fingernail, a twig or other sharp object. It is an extremely painful condition with profuse lacrimation. Fluorescein eye drops should be instilled in order to determine the extent of the abrasion.

Box 13.8 Rust ring

If a metallic foreign body is left in contact with the cornea for more than 4 h, a rust ring may develop around its perimeter.

It can usually be very easily removed after 1 or 2 days of the application of antibiotic ointment. This is done with a 10G needle or a small battery-powered instrument called a burr.

Box 13.9 Eversion of an eyelid

This procedure is carried out if the presence of a foreign body is suspected under the upper eyelid. With the patient's eyes open and looking down, the upper lid lashes are grasped. At the same time, the upper edge of the tarsal plate (at the crease of the eyelid) is depressed, using a glass rod or cotton bud. This allows the lid to be turned over to expose the subtarsal conjunctiva and facilitates inspection, irrigation and foreign body removal.

An eye pad need not be applied after treatment for abrasion or removal of a foreign body but, if the patient feels more comfortable with the eye closed, a pad may be worn for about 6 h. Antibiotic ointment may be prescribed to prevent infection. A follow-up appointment may be given depending on the severity of the abrasion or the depth at which the foreign body was embedded.

SURGICAL REMOVAL OF AN EYE

There are three methods of removing an eye:

- *Enucleation*. This is surgical removal of the globe. The extraocular muscles are cut at their insertion and the optic nerve severed.
- *Evisceration*. This is the removal of the contents of the globe, leaving the scleral shell.
- *Exenteration*. This is a more extensive operation which involves removing the eye and surrounding tissues.

Special considerations

The choice of operation performed is dependent upon the diagnosis necessitating the removal of an eye. A badly injured eye may be enucleated (see Nursing Care Plan 13.4) whilst an infected eye would require to be eviscerated. Exenteration would be required when a malignant tumour extended beyond the globe.

Maintenance of good cosmetic appearance post-surgery has led to the development of a range of socket and orbital implants, which may reduce the psychological trauma experienced.

Management is as for extensive penetrating injuries. The nurse may find that if a patient has suffered severe pain and blindness in an eye, the relief from pain after it has been removed is often so great that this helps him to cope with the loss. Contact with others who have had an eye removed may help to reassure the patient that it is possible to adapt and to live a full life following this distressing experience. Many areas throughout the country do have support groups.

For further information, see Albiar & Holds (1992).

Nursing Care Plan 13.4 A patient undergoing enucleation: postoperative

Nursing considerations	Action	Rationale	Expected outcome
Anxiety/distress			
• **Due to having eye removed**	❒ Reassure and spend time with the patient. Encourage him to express his feelings and talk about his fears. Reassure him that it is normal to grieve over the loss of an eye	Giving information reduces anxiety and aids recovery	The patient will come to terms with the necessity of having his eye removed
• **Due to altered body image**	❒ Discuss what the wound and socket will look like after surgery, likening it to the inside of the mouth. Discuss after-care of socket and show him an artificial eye, allowing him and his family to handle it, if he wishes ❒ Arrange for someone who has had similar surgery to come and talk with the patient. Suggest dark glasses can be worn until he is fitted with artificial eye	Reduces fear about the after-effects of the operation	The patient will be adjusted to altered body image and will accept the situation of wearing an artificial eye
• **Due to fear of having wrong eye removed**	❒ Eye to be removed is identified and checked with patient, doctor and case notes (some units mark the forehead with an arrow to identify correct eye) ❒ Reassure patient that many checks are made prior to the operation to ensure correct eye is removed	Relieves anxiety and reassures the patient	Correct eye will be removed. Patient will be reassured of this

Artificial eye fitting

The National Artificial Eye Service (NAES) in Blackpool provides training to enable personnel to make and fit artificial eyes. Patient education, support and follow-up services are also provided by technicians in local ocular prosthetic departments.

An artificial eye is individually designed to fit the socket and implant exactly and is painted by an ocular artist to match the patient's other eye. The prosthesis is shell-like in shape and form and not, as anticipated, ball-shaped. If an orbital implant has been inserted, the artificial eye will move in unison with the natural eye because the extraocular muscles have been preserved and attached to the implant.

Unfortunately, lack of information about artificial eyes can cause a great deal of anxiety and often a degree of revulsion. This is usually dispelled by explaining that the appearance of the socket is similar to the inside of the mouth. Anxiety is further reduced by contact with people who have adapted successfully to living with an artificial eye and by an opportunity to see and handle an artificial eye before surgery and thereby gain reassurance that they look quite natural (see Nursing Care Plan 13.4).

Principles of artificial eye care

Nurses should be prepared to assist or advise on the care of an artificial eye. Principles of daily management are as follows.

Removal of an artificial eye

A special extractor is provided by the ocular prosthesis department. The eyelids are opened with the thumb and forefinger, and the lower edge of the eye is gently levered out with the aid of the extractor. If an extractor is not available, then a finger will suffice (see Fig. 13.10A).

Insertion of an artificial eye

The eyelids are opened with the thumb and forefinger. The eye is inserted under the upper lid with the curve of the eye towards the nose. The lower lid is depressed slightly. The eye can then be slipped into position (see Fig. 13.10B).

Care of the artificial eye

An artificial eye should be cleaned at least once a day with ordinary soap in cold or lukewarm water. It should be thoroughly rinsed afterwards under running water. Chemical cleansers or disinfectants must not be used.

The patient is encouraged to wear the eye both day and night. If he prefers not to, the eye should be placed in cold water or a saline solution in a clean, labelled receptacle.

When not in regular use, the eye should be stored in cotton wool or tissue to prevent scratching. Through normal wear the eye may lose its high polish. It can be sent to the nearest ocular prosthetic department for repolishing, free of charge. Replacements can be obtained cost-free (NHS patients) from the same department.

The community nurse may need to prompt elderly patients, in particular, to take advantage of this service, and they may need to approach their GP for initial referral to a consultant.

Care of the socket

The socket should remain healthy if the artificial eye is kept clean in the recommended way. Occasionally, infection or irritation may result from scratches on the eye and lead to ulceration.

The socket can be irrigated with normal saline and treated with an antibiotic ointment for a short period. The artificial eye should not be inserted until the infection or irritation has cleared up.

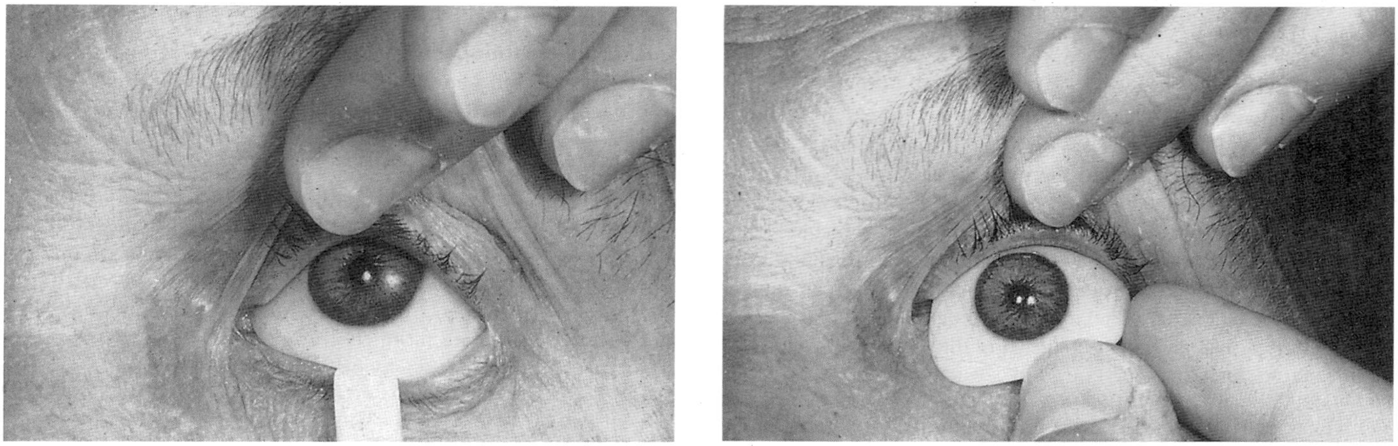

A B

Fig. 13.10 A: Removing an artificial eye. B: Inserting an artificial eye. (Reproduced with kind permission of Blackpool, Wyre and Fylde Community Health Services NHS Trust 1998.)

It is not advisable to leave the eye out for long periods as shrinkage of the socket can occur, causing difficulty and discomfort on re-insertion of the eye.

AGE-RELATED CONDITIONS

Age-related maculopathy

Macular degeneration is the major cause of blindness in the elderly in developed countries.

Sufferers are described as being 'walking sighted – reading blind', as the peripheral retinal function is retained (Woods 1992).

PATHOPHYSIOLOGY

Retinal pigment epithelial cells (RPEs) wear out with age and are never replaced. As they degenerate they deposit material on the underlying membrane which accumulates to form yellowish white spots on the retina. Initially this process does not affect vision but eventually the cell loss will result in atrophy of the RPE layer, which may then disperse pigment into the macula. This condition is called macular degeneration. It affects form and colour vision first and the patient notices difficulty with activities such as reading and sewing, and problems in identifying faces and coins.

In some cases, a new blood vessel membrane may develop and cause lifting of the central retina. This results in distorted and blurred central vision.

Macular degeneration can occur in the presence of other eye conditions such as cataract and glaucoma, and each will complicate the diagnosis and treatment of the other.

MEDICAL MANAGEMENT

There is no treatment, as yet, for RPE degenerative changes but any underlying disease should be diagnosed and treated. If there are early symptoms of new blood vessel membrane formation, krypton or argon laser treatment could be of some benefit. In some cases a degree of vision can be regained following this, although if there is foveal damage there will be a persistent central scotoma (blind spot). Those affected severely will need encouragement to make adjustments to daily living skills to maintain their independence. Advice on the use of low vision aids should be given, and contact with the Macular Disease Society and social work services may be advised, in addition to blind or partially sighted registration (see p. 499).

Case History 13.1 Mrs S

Mr and Mrs S are both 70 years old and live in a bungalow on the outskirts of a large town. Over the past 2 months, Mrs S has noticed a marked reduction in her near vision. Increasingly, she has noticed that she requires help to identify her shopping items correctly and to clean her house. The pleasure obtained from completing the crosswords and reading has been lost. After a visit to her optician, she is referred to her GP and then to the eye hospital. At her appointment, the consultant tells her she has macular degeneration and that, although she will not go blind, her sight will not improve. He recommends that she should consider becoming registered as partially sighted. Mrs S is quite distressed by this and goes home to think about it.

Q **13.14** You are a community nurse who visits Mr S (see Case History 13.1) daily to give him his insulin injection. Mrs S breaks down whilst you are there. What advice would you offer her and where would you advise her to go for assistance?

Entropion

This is a malposition of the eyelid in which the lid margin is turned towards the globe. It most commonly affects the lower lid and is caused by reduced elasticity of the connective tissue, which may be the result of trauma, a badly applied eye pad or the ageing process. The eyelashes irritate the cornea and can cause discomfort and ulceration.

Nursing and medical management. Discomfort can be relieved by the application of tape to the affected lid margin in such a way that downward traction of the tape when applied to the cheek restores the normal position of the lid. If the entropion persists the lid can be repositioned by a simple surgical procedure.

For further information, see Kanski (1997).

Ectropion

This is a malposition of the eyelid in which the lid margin is turned away from the globe, mainly affecting the lower lid, and is associated with atonic tissue around the eyes. Because the punctum of the lacrimal duct is not in position to drain them, tears overflow and run down the cheeks. The sufferer constantly wipes his eyes, drawing the lid even further down and exacerbating the condition.
Nursing and medical management. Minor surgery can reposition the lid if necessary. Cautery to the inner eyelid contracts the tarsal conjunctiva and inverts the lid. Plastic surgery may be required to reposition the eyelid.

Both entropion and ectropion are fairly common conditions in the elderly, who often do not complain because they do not realise that the remedy is so simple or because they feel that they are too old to bother. Both conditions cause great discomfort and it is often the community nurse who is in a position to detect them and to advise on treatment.

SYSTEMIC DISEASE AND DISORDERS OF THE EYE

The eye is a sensitive indicator of systemic disease. Visual disturbance or abnormal appearance of the retina or optic disc may be the first manifestation of health breakdown. In this section, ophthalmic conditions associated with some of the more common systemic diseases will be described to alert the nurse to the possibility of their coexistence within a disease process and to assist her in her screening role. Other conditions are described in Table 13.5.

Nursing priorities and management should be based on the general principles of ophthalmic management as well as the specific principles that pertain to the disease process in question. The reader should refer to relevant chapters in the present text as well as to more specialised ophthalmic texts.

For further information, see Spalton et al (1994).

Diabetes mellitus

Diabetes is a common disorder in developed countries and its incidence is increasing in developing countries as diets include more processed foods and refined sugars. Poorly controlled diabetes can lead to retinopathy, early cataract development, vascularisation of the iris (rubeosis) and a high incidence of minor eye conditions.

Diabetic retinopathy

PATHOPHYSIOLOGY

Elevated blood sugar levels, associated with prolonged poor diabetic control, damage blood vessel basement membrane. In the retina, this leads to leakage and the formation of fatty and haemorrhagic lesions. These changes are given the term 'retinopathy' (see Ch. 5B). The patient will usually complain of gradual and painless loss of vision — unless there is bleeding into the vitreous humor, in which case loss of vision may be sudden and very frightening (Hall & Waterman 1997). The diagnosis and progression of the disease can be confirmed by fluorescein angiography. Diabetic retinopathy is the major cause of blindness in the 20–65 year age group in Western countries (Hamilton et al 1996).

There are two forms of the condition: background and proliferative.
Background retinopathy. The small retinal vessels become fragile, aneurysms form and leakage occurs, causing localised oedema and haemorrhage. Background retinopathy can cause loss of central vision if macular oedema occurs and the hard exudates encroach on the fovea. Peripheral vision will be retained.
Proliferative retinopathy. In this condition there is further deterioration as new blood vessels and fibrous bands form in response to breakdown and occlusion of the normal circulation. The main complications that can arise from this are bleeding into the vitreous humor and traction retinal detachment. Eventually, proliferative vascularisation can affect the angle of the eye, blocking the trabecular meshwork and causing glaucoma.

MEDICAL MANAGEMENT

Early diagnosis is critical, as is good control of blood sugar levels and regular monitoring of ophthalmic status. Complications are treated as they arise. Laser treatment may be used to delay the progress of proliferative retinopathy. This involves bombarding the peripheral retina with laser burns (panretinal ablation) so that the oxygen requirement of retinal tissue is reduced. This in turn reduces the stimulus for new vessel formation. Focal burns may also be used to seal off leaking blood vessels.

Severe vitreous haemorrhage or tractional retinal detachment may be treated by removing the vitreous humor (vitrectomy) and replacing it with clear infusional fluid, gas or silicone oil.

NURSING PRIORITIES AND MANAGEMENT: DIABETIC RETINOPATHY

Patient education

Ongoing education and encouragement to comply with diabetic regimens are important in the attempt to delay the onset or progression of complications and to encourage early awareness of visual changes. The community nurse often has a key role to play here. Explanation and support during laser treatment will be particularly important to encourage the patient's cooperation to prevent accidental burns (see p. 507).

Vitrectomy management

Perioperative care for patients undergoing vitrectomy procedures is as for other intraocular surgery, with a particular emphasis on ensuring that the prescribed postoperative position is maintained. Where vitreous has been removed from the posterior compartment of the eye and the cavity has been filled by fluid, gas or silicone oil, strict positioning is vital. The objective is to ensure continued apposition of the retina and to minimise contact of the gas or silicone oil with the posterior surface of the lens or cornea, as this could lead to opacification of either structure.

Cerebrovascular accident (CVA)

A CVA involves an interruption of the blood supply to a part of the brain and may be caused by blockage or rupture of a blood vessel. CVA results in ischaemia of the affected part and development of neurological defects. If the visual pathways are involved, vision will be affected and the damage may be permanent. When a patient suffers a transient ischaemic attack (TIA), vision may be temporarily affected, but will usually be restored when the attack subsides (see Ch. 9).

Table 13.5 Further eye problems secondary to systemic diseases

Disorder	*Main ophthalmic clinical features*	*Cause*	*Treatment*
Thyroid function imbalance (Graves' disease)	Upper lid retraction	Sympathetic nerve innervation	Lubricating drops during day and antibiotic ointment nightly
	Exposure keratitis	Exposure of eyeball	As above
	Swelling of lids and conjunctiva Exophthalmos Compression of optic nerve	Infiltration of lymphocytes in orbital tissue and associated oedema	Partial tarsorrhaphy Systemic steroids Surgical decompression
	Diplopia	Infiltration of lymphocytes in muscle tissue leading to fibrosis	Prism spectacles Botulinum A neurotoxin injection into the appropriate lid muscle Strabismus surgery
Migraine	Headache with visual disturbances Characteristic aura: multicoloured, jagged shape, firework-like	Idiopathic; possibly chemical changes in the brain caused by various triggers, e.g. stress, or dietary, e.g. eating oranges or chocolate	Feverfew herbal remedy Ergotamine Rest
Multiple sclerosis	Uniocular	Localised demyelinating lesion to the cranial nerves	Symptoms may recover spontaneously but will always recur
	Small unequal pupils: do not react to light but do with accommodation, unable to dilate with atropine	III IV VI	
	Optic neuritis		
	Rapid reduction of central vision		
	Sudden onset of pain especially when looking upwards		Systemic painkillers
	Central scotoma		
	Diplopia		• Prism spectacles • Botulinum A neurotoxin injection • Strabismus surgery
Intracranial aneurysm	Uniocular/binocular Diplopia Blurred vision Ptosis Visual field defects	Pressure on visual pathway Pressure on cranial nerves III IV VI	• Detection and clipping of aneurysm • Botulinum A neurotoxin injection • Strabismus surgery
Nephritis	a) Blurred vision b) Papilloedema c) Retinal haemorrhage d) Retinal detachment	Hypertension	• Reduce hypertension • Laser treatment • Vitrectomy • Surgical repair of detachment

NURSING PRIORITIES AND MANAGEMENT: CEREBROVASCULAR ACCIDENT (CVA)

The extent of the visual deficit must be assessed to facilitate rehabilitation and maintain patient safety. This may be difficult if the patient's ability to communicate has been affected by the CVA. The accuracy of the assessment is dependent upon the nurse's skilled observation.

Q **13.15** You have a patient who has recently suffered a right-sided CVA. He is aphasic (unable to speak) and has left hemiplegia (paralysis of the left side). Discuss how you might go about detecting visual field loss just by observing his activity. Having done this, describe how your findings would affect your care plan.

Central retinal artery occlusion

This condition is an ophthalmic emergency. The compelling reason for seeking medical help is sudden, complete and painless loss of vision in one eye. Obstruction of the central retinal artery is associated with arteriosclerotic emboli, hypertension and cranial arteritis in the elderly. In younger people, it may be a result of a clot being released into the circulation in valvular heart disease. The retinal artery and some of its branches may be obliterated; the damage to retinal cells is irreparable.

MEDICAL MANAGEMENT

Emergency intervention. Treatment must begin within minutes if any degree of visual recovery is to be achieved. The aim is to reduce IOP rapidly by massage of the globe and administration of osmotic medication, e.g. i.v. mannitol, to draw fluid from the eye by osmosis. Paracentesis to release aqueous from the anterior chamber will further reduce the IOP. This should allow the retinal artery to dilate and the clot may be flushed along to a peripheral branch.

Continuing management. Once the emergency stage has passed the patient is given a full examination. The underlying medical condition is diagnosed and treated appropriately. Residual visual impairment is assessed and the patient given all necessary support.

Hypertension

The condition of the retina and optic disc are used to aid the diagnosis of hypertension; fundal examination of the eye is in fact part of the screening process for hypertension (see Ch. 2).

Hypertensive retinopathy in a young adult appears as widespread narrowing of the arteries caused by spasm of the arterial walls. In an older person with arteriosclerosis, the arteries are narrow and rigid. As hypertension increases in severity, haemorrhages and exudates are visible. The haemorrhages are flame-like in appearance and are found close to the disc. The exudates are due to lipids and occur around the macula. Oedema of the retina occurs in malignant hypertension and may also be present in some cases of mild hypertension. The optic disc is swollen and hyperaemic. The patient will complain of varying degrees of visual disturbance. The condition is painless. The outward appearance of the eye remains normal.

The eye condition improves as hypertension is brought under control by appropriate treatment (see Ch. 2).

Acquired immune deficiency syndrome (AIDS)

Ophthalmic complications develop in about 75% of patients with AIDS. They are caused by HIV infection, opportunistic infections and AIDS-related neoplasms, and may affect any part of the eye (Blaustein 1994).

HIV retinopathy

Clinical signs are yellowish-grey, cotton wool-like spots, dot-like haemorrhages and microaneurysms over the retina. Vision remains normal unless the macula is involved. Some patients respond to antiviral agents.

HIV encephalopathy nystagmus

In central nervous system involvement, nystagmus, gaze palsies and visual field defects may occur. No treatment is available at present.

Opportunistic infections

HIV/AIDS patients are prone to all types of eye infections. The most common infections include severe herpes zoster ophthalmicus, herpes simplex, *Candida retinitis*, *Toxoplasma choroidoretinitis* and cytomegalovirus (CMV) retinitis. Some of these infections may respond to prolonged administration of systemic antiviral agents.

CMV retinitis, which develops in the late stages of AIDS, deserves special mention. Fear of blindness is often more distressing for the patient than fear of dying. CMV retinitis, with intraretinal haemorrhages and retinal necrosis, leads to retinal detachments and progressive loss of vision. Palliative treatment by antiviral agents, e.g. ganciclovir, may be offered in an attempt to prevent blindness in the last few months of life. This can be given intravenously or by intravitreal implant.

AIDS-related neoplasms

Kaposi's sarcoma may involve any of the ocular structures. Treatment may include cryotherapy, radiotherapy or the administration of cytotoxic drugs.

NURSING PRIORITIES AND MANAGEMENT: AIDS

The general principles of nursing a patient with AIDS (see Ch. 37), together with the principles of nursing a patient with eye infections, apply in all of the above conditions. Full care and support facilities should be mobilised for both the patient and his family/partner.

CONCLUSION

Eye disorders may be encountered in a wide range of contexts and nurses should be prepared to recognise these conditions and provide appropriate treatment or prompt referral for specialist help. Even where treatment is being carried out in an ophthalmic unit, it is necessary for general and community nurses to have a working knowledge of what is involved, so that they can prepare the patient and his family and/or carers for the necessary procedures and monitor progress and after-care when the patient has returned home.

The impact of visual impairment on everyday life must never be underestimated. This chapter has stressed the importance of recognising the significance of adverse signs and symptoms and the fact that delay can result in irreparable damage and permanent loss of sight. It has emphasised the nurse's responsibility in helping to preserve sight and in supporting the patient and his family and/or carers as they meet the practical and emotional challenges of visual impairment.

REFERENCES

Audit Commission for Local Authorities and the NHS in England and Wales 1997 A short cut to better services: day surgery in England and Wales. HMSO, London

Blackpool, Wyre and Fylde Community Health Services NHS Trust 1998 The use and care of artificial eyes. NAES, Blackpool

Blaustein B H (ed) 1994 Ocular manifestations of systemic diseases. Churchill Livingstone, New York

Burlew J 1991 Preventing eye injuries – the nurse's role. Insight 16(6): 24–28

Chawla H B 1999 Ophthalmology: a symptom-based approach. Butterworth-Heinemann, London

Cheng K P, Larson C E, Biglan A W, D'Antonio J A 1992 A prospective, randomized, controlled comparison of retrobulbar and general anaesthesia for strabismus surgery. Ophthalmic Surgery 23(9): 585–590

Gandham S B 1997 New topical medications in the treatment of glaucoma. Journal of Ophthalmic Nursing and Technology 16(6): 290–291

Hall B, Waterman H 1997 The psychosocial aspects of visual impairment in diabetes. Nursing Standard 11(39): 40–43, 45–46

Hamilton A M P, Ulbig M W, Polkinghorne P 1996 Management of diabetic retinopathy. BMJ Publishing Group, London

Health and Safety Executive 1993 Working with VDUs. HMSO, London

McKenzie G J, Chawla H B, Gordon D 1986 The special senses, 2nd edn. Churchill Livingstone, Edinburgh

Matthews T D, Frazer D G, Minassian D C, Radford C F, Dart J K G 1992 Risks of keratitis and patterns of use with disposable contact lenses. Archives of Ophthalmology 110(11): 1559–1562

Mauger T F, Craig E L 1996 Mosby's ocular drug handbook. Mosby, St Louis

Orem D 1995 Nursing: concepts of practice, 5th edn. Mosby, New York

Peattie P I, Walker S 1995 Understanding nursing care, 4th edn. Churchill Livingstone, Edinburgh

Perry J P, Tullo A (eds) 1995 Care of the ophthalmic patient, 2nd edn. Chapman and Hall, London
Radford C F 1995 Risk factor for acanthamoeba keratitis in contact lens users: a case control study. British Medical Journal 310(699): 1567–1570
Riordan-Eva P 1995 Anatomy and embryology of the eye. In: Vaughan D G, Asbury T, Riordan-Eva P (eds) General ophthalmology, 14th edn. Appleton-Lange, USA, ch 1
Roper N, Logan W W, Tierney A J 1996 The elements of nursing: a model for nursing based on a model of living, 3rd edn. Churchill Livingstone, Edinburgh
Royal National Institute for the Blind (RNIB) 1995 How to guide a blind person. RNIB, London
Rowell M 1995 Models for ophthalmic nursing practice. In: Perry J P, Tullo A (eds) Care of the ophthalmic patient, 2nd edn. Chapman and Hall, London
Spalton D J, Hitchings R A, Hunter P A (eds) 1994 Atlas of clinical ophthalmology, 2nd edn. Wolfe, London
WHO/World Bank 1993 World development report. Investing in health. Oxford University Press, New York
Woods S 1992 Macular degeneration. Nursing Clinics of North America 27(3): 761–765
York S 1990 Ophthalmic triage. Nursing Times 86(8): 40–42

FURTHER READING

Albiar E, Holds J B 1992 Hydroxyapatite orbital implants: indications for use and nursing considerations. Journal of Ophthalmic Nursing and Technology 11(2): 71–76
Allen M, Knight C, Falk C, Strang V 1992 Effectiveness of a pre-operative teaching programme for cataract patients. Journal of Advanced Nursing 17: 303–309
Brady F B 1992 A singular view. Edgemore, Toronto
Burlew J 1991 Preventing eye injuries – the nurse's role. Insight 16(6): 24–28
Caunt H 1992 Preoperative nursing intervention to relieve stress. British Journal of Nursing 1(4): 171–174
Chawla H B 1998 Retinal detachment: diagnosis and management, 2nd edn. Butterworth-Heinemann, London
Cotgreave J T, Patch T M, Perthen C E, Stewart A B, Crutchlow K 1989 Part of your daily routine: teaching good contact lens care. The Professional Nurse 4(9): 446–449
Dodds A 1993 Rehabilitating blind and visually impaired people. Chapman and Hall, London
Donnelly D 1987 Instilling eyedrops: difficulties experienced by patients following cataract surgery. Journal of Advanced Nursing 12: 235–243
Dossey B 1996 Help your patient break free from anxiety. Nursing 96 26(10): 52–54
Dutton J J 1992 Atlas of ophthalmic surgery, vol 2. Oculoplastic, lacrimal and orbital surgery. Mosby, St Louis
Frost J 1993 Clinical application of lasers. Professional Nurse 8(5): 298–303
Goodrich J 1993 The ageing eye. Practitioner 237(1527): 514–518
Henson D B 1983 Visual fields. Oxford University Press, Oxford
Hull J 1990 Touch the rock. SPK Publishers, London
Jones J, Diner B A 1992 A different dimension: adapting to monocular vision. Institute of Maxillofacial Technology, Bristol
Kanski J J 1997 Ophthalmology. Colour guides, 2nd edn. Churchill Livingstone, Edinburgh
Kanski J J, Thomas D J 1990 The eye in systemic diseases, 2nd edn. Butterworth-Heinemann, London
Kerrigan P (ed) 1998 Insight: GP guide to practical ophthalmology (pulse supplement). Ocular hypertension and glaucoma, Miller Freeman, London
McGory A 1997 Eye injuries: a review of the literature with nursing implications. International Journal of Nursing Studies 34(2): 87–92
Mehta V 1987 Sound shadows of the new world. Picador, London
Mehta V 1989 The stolen light. Collins, London
Mudie S 1992 Evaluating day care. Nursing 5(7): 22–23
Norlet N, Kelly M 1996 Improving drop administration by patients. Journal of Ophthalmic Medicine and Technology 15(2): 60–64
Pavan-Langston D 1995 Manual of ocular diagnosis and therapy, 4th edn. Little, Brown, Boston
Perry J P, Tullo A (eds) 1995 Care of the ophthalmic patient, 2nd edn. Chapman and Hall, London
Phelps Brown N A 1993 The morphology of cataract and visual performance. Eye 7: 63–67
Rendall J 1998 Discharge instructions after cataract surgery. Ophthalmic Nursing 2(1): 10–16
Salmon P 1993 The reduction of anxiety in surgical patients: an important nursing task or the medicalisation of preparatory worries. International Journal of Nursing Studies 30(4): 232–330
Sivalingham E 1996 Glaucoma: an overview. Journal of Ophthalmic Nursing and Technology 15(1): 15–18
Smith B 1993 Ophthalmic anaesthesia, 2nd edn. A Practical Handbook. Arnold, London
Smith G, Hamilton R C, Carr C A 1995 Ophthalmic anaesthesia, 2nd edn. Arnold, London
Smith H 1995 The effects of botulinum toxin on ocular tissue. Nursing Times 91(4): 41–43
Spalton D J, Hitchings R A, Hunter P A (eds) 1994 Atlas of clinical ophthalmology, 2nd edn. Wolfe, London
Teich S A, Cheung T W, Freidman A H 1992 Systemic anti-viral drugs in ophthalmology. Journal of Ophthalmic Nursing and Technology 37(1): 19–20

USEFUL ADDRESSES

Royal National Institute for the Blind
224 Great Portland Street
London W1A 6AA

Partially Sighted Society
Queens Road
Doncaster DN1 2NX

International Glaucoma Association
Kings College Hospital
Denmark Hill
London SE5 9RS

Talking Newspaper Association of the UK (TNAUK)
90 High Street
Heathfield
East Sussex TN21 8JD

In Touch
BBC Broadcasting House
London W1A 1AA

Guide Dogs for the Blind Association
Hillfields
Burghfield Common
Reading R97·3YG

Institute of Maxillofacial Technology
MOTA
Maxillofacial Prosthetic Laboratory
1st floor, South Wing
Charing Cross Hospital
Fulham Palace Road
London W6 8RF

Macular Disease Society
P O Box 247
Haywards Heath
West Sussex RH17 5FF

DISORDERS OF THE EAR, NOSE AND THROAT

14

Anna M. Serra Muriel E. Reffin

INTRODUCTION

Some problems of the ear, nose and throat (ENT) are very common. Most people at some time in their lives suffer from nosebleeds, sore throats or earache. Many of these problems will be dealt with successfully at home, often with the advice of a pharmacist or general practitioner (GP). Some ENT problems, however, can be life-threatening, requiring an immediate visit to an accident and emergency (A&E) department, surgery and, in some cases, a period of nursing care at home following discharge.

To nurse ENT patients effectively in a home or hospital setting, a basic knowledge of the anatomy and physiology of the relevant structures along with a thorough understanding of the clinical features of common disorders is essential. The health visitor, district nurse, school nurse or occupational health nurse is often in a position to detect problems before the medical practitioner or even the patient himself is aware of them.

This chapter will describe, in turn, the basic structure and functioning of the ear, nose and throat, describing the most commonly encountered disorders of each, and outlining appropriate medical and nursing interventions. As in every area of nursing care, one of the most important contributions of the nurse will be in the area of communication and education as she provides support and reassurance to the patient and his family and conveys information about the causes of the patient's condition, its treatment and measures to prevent its recurrence.

THE EAR

ANATOMY AND PHYSIOLOGY OF THE EAR

The ear can be divided into three sections: the external ear, the middle ear and the inner ear. The external and middle ears are primarily involved with the transmission of sound. The inner ear contains the organ of hearing as well as structures concerned with body balance (see Fig. 14.1).

The external ear comprises the cartilaginous pinna and the external auditory canal (or external meatus), the inner two-thirds of which is composed of bone rather than cartilage. The purpose of the pinna and canal is to capture sound waves and funnel them to the tympanic membrane, which is located at the end of the external canal and divides the external from the middle ear. The healthy membrane has a pearly sheen and reflects light.

The middle ear is ventilated by the eustachian tube, which communicates with the nasopharynx. Three small bones, called the auditory ossicles or ossicular chain, pass on sound vibrations received by the tympanic membrane to the inner ear. The first of these, the malleus (i.e. 'hammer'), is attached to the tympanic membrane and joins with the incus ('anvil') or middle ossicle. The incus in turn is attached to the stapes ('stirrup'), the 'footplate' of which lies against the membranous oval window or fenestra of the inner ear.

The inner ear houses the cochlea, which is shaped like a snail shell and is the organ of hearing. The cochlea contains the organ of Corti, which consists of cells with hair-like projections on a membranous layer and connects with the terminal ends of the auditory nerve. The canals of the cochlea and the organ of Corti are bathed in endolymph. Perilymph is the fluid contained within the bony (osseous) cavities of the inner ear, whereas endolymph is the fluid within membranous cavities. As sound waves are transmitted by the ossicles they travel along this fluid and disturb the hair cells. This disturbance changes to impulses which travel along the auditory nerve to the brain stem and cortex, where they are interpreted as meaningful sound.

The posterior part of the inner ear is formed by three semicircular canals and by the vestibular apparatus. These assist in the perception of body position against gravity and in the maintenance of balance. The vestibular apparatus consists of the utricle and saccule and is sensitive to linear acceleration. The semicircular canals are sensitive to rotatory acceleration. Balance is maintained by the adjustment of muscles, joints, tendons and ligaments in response to information gathered by the vestibular apparatus and the canals as well as that received by the eyes.

For further information, see Becker et al (1993).

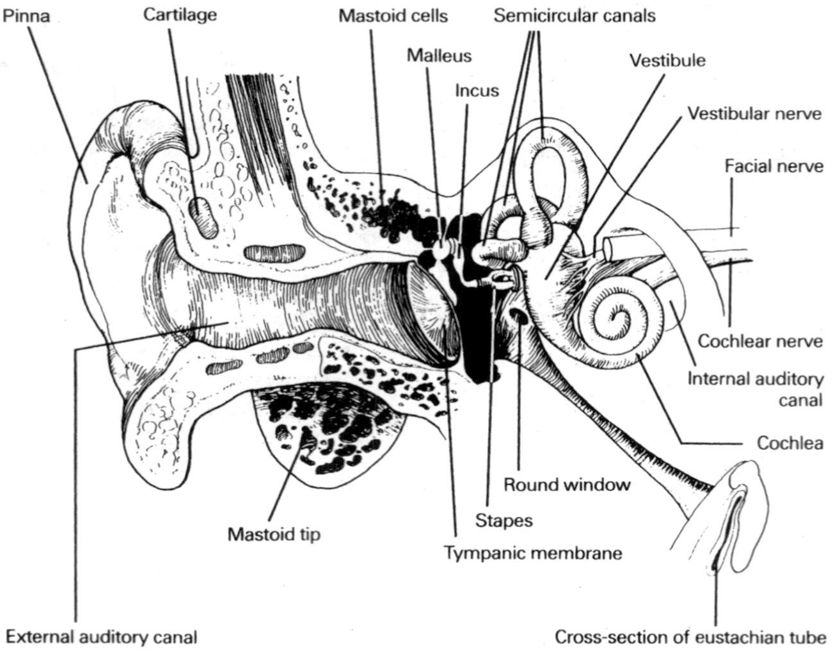

Fig. 14.1 Sagittal section of the ear. (Reproduced with kind permission from McKenzie et al 1986.)

DISORDERS OF THE EXTERNAL EAR

Otitis externa

PATHOPHYSIOLOGY

The most common causes of otitis externa, or inflammation of the external ear, are infection and allergy. Infection may be caused by scratching the ear with contaminated fingernails or other sharp objects. Instruments such as auriscopes or hearing aid earpieces placed in the meatus may cause minor injuries, giving rise to infection if they have been inadequately disinfected (see Ch. 16). Itching is an early symptom of allergy and may be caused by cosmetics or antibiotic preparations. In otitis externa, multiple bacteriological flora are usually present. The condition most commonly occurs in hot, humid climates, where it tends to be recurrent and may be severe.

Common presenting symptoms. The patient usually presents with a history of pain and itching localised to the ear and a burning sensation followed by discharge, which may be watery to begin with and then become thicker. If there is gross oedema of the meatus and a large amount of debris is present, the patient may suffer from conductive deafness (see p. 528).

MEDICAL MANAGEMENT

If a discharge is present in otitis externa, a swab is obtained for culture and sensitivity. Cleansing of the external meatus is performed so that a full inspection can be carried out and to ensure good skin contact for any topical treatments.

NURSING PRIORITIES AND MANAGEMENT: OTITIS EXTERNA

The first priority of the nursing staff when caring for these patients is to clean the external meatus so that an examination can be carried out and any prescribed treatment administered effectively. This procedure is called aural toilet and should only be carried out by an appropriately trained ENT nurse. Cotton wool dressed carriers can be used. Care must be taken not to damage the skin. Gentle pulling of the pinna will straighten the canal and allow easier access. The best light source is a Bulls' eye lamp and head mirror or an operating microscope. Large amounts of discharge and debris are best removed by an appropriately qualified nurse or doctor using suction via a fine-bore tube under an operating microscope in the outpatient department.

It may be necessary to administer an oral analgesic before the external auditory canal can be properly examined as often any movement of the pinna is painful.

Since the vast majority of patients are seen in the community or outpatient department, the nurse's involvement will include demonstrating how to administer topical preparations effectively. This can be quite difficult for the patient to master and will require time and careful attention. The nurse should also teach the patient safe techniques for cleansing the external ear and stress the importance of frequent, thorough cleansing of any appliances, including hearing aids, that are put in the ear.

For further information on nurse-led aural care clinics and courses, see Rogers (1992) and Zeitoun et al (1997).

Cerumen excess

PATHOPHYSIOLOGY

Cerumen is the normal waxy secretion of special glands in the external auditory canal. Along with shed skin scales and hair, the cerumen normally migrates to the external meatus but can be hindered by coarse hair, particularly in the elderly male, or if the individual impacts the material by attempting to clean the ears with cotton wool buds or other instruments. Nurses should provide patients with health education information regarding the normal cleansing mechanism and avoiding the use of cotton buds and other foreign bodies (Hooper 1991).

Common presenting symptoms. The patient usually presents with dulled hearing. Tinnitus may develop, causing the patient distress (see p. 534), and disturbance of balance may result from pressure of the hard material on the tympanic membrane.

MEDICAL MANAGEMENT

Sometimes smaller amounts of soft wax can be removed by instruments or suction under a microscope. If there is an excessive amount, the doctor, district nurse, practice nurse or outpatient nurse will need to remove the material by syringing the external canal. Often, however, the wax is too hard and compacted for this to be carried out immediately and a course of drops containing sodium bicarbonate in glycerol, or warmed olive or almond oil has to be prescribed first for several days to soften the wax. At this stage, written information on the procedure can be taken home by the patient to aid his understanding.

NURSING PRIORITIES AND MANAGEMENT: CERUMEN EXCESS

Individuals with cerumen excess are usually seen in the doctor's surgery or, more rarely, in the outpatient department for removal of the impacted wax. Ear syringing is a potentially harmful procedure and should only be performed by those aware of the dangers.

The nurse will have to teach the patient how to insert the ear drops at home over the required period before the syringing is carried out. The doctor or nurse who performs the syringing should first take a full history to eliminate the presence of a weakened tympanic membrane and should examine the ear for any infection, inflammation or perforation, in order to determine that the tympanic membrane is intact, thus eliminating the danger of the solution being introduced into the middle ear and causing infection and damage. During the procedure the patient sits upright with his clothing protected by a waterproof covering. It is helpful if he can cooperate by holding a container under his ear to receive the returning fluid. Various types of ear syringe are available. Non-disposable varieties must be sterilised after each use. Unless a special solution has been prescribed, tap water or an isotonic solution such as normal saline may be used to irrigate the canal. It is important that the solution is at 37°C, i.e. body temperature, as variations in temperature may cause the patient to experience vertigo (see p. 535).

Before starting, ask the patient to inform you if he experiences any side-effects. After the syringe has been filled and any air expelled, the pinna is pulled gently upwards and backwards to straighten the canal while the solution is introduced from the syringe in an upwards direction so that the wax will be washed out with the return flow (see Fig. 14.2). It is important that the flow of

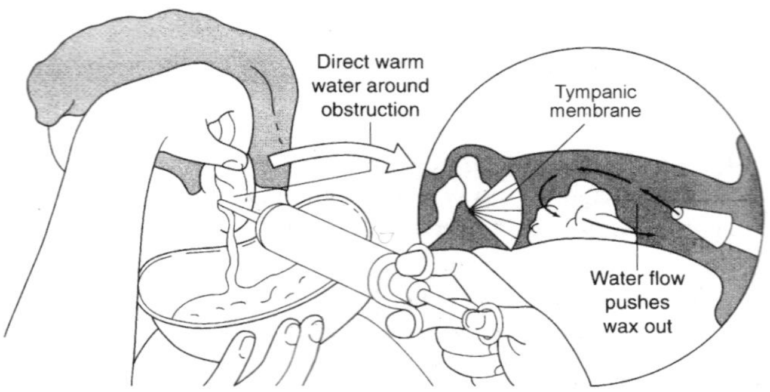

Fig. 14.2 Ear syringing, showing fluid being directed to the roof of the aural canal. The nurse should gently pull the pinna upwards and backwards to straighten the canal and aim the fluid towards the roof, or posterior wall, of the canal. (Reproduced with kind permission from Jamieson et al 1997.)

water is not aimed directly at the tympanic membrane as this could damage it. When the canal is clean or when 2 min have passed (Stilwell 1992), the procedure is discontinued and the canal gently dried and re-examined. To avoid vertigo the patient should be encouraged to remain seated for a few minutes to recover. He should also be advised that, following effective ear syringing, he may be hypersensitive to even quite normal sounds for a short time.

For further information on ear syringing, refer to Thurgood & Thurgood (1995) and Cook (1998).

Foreign bodies in the ear

Small objects may become lodged in the ear by some mishap or, as frequently occurs among children, by accident during play (Denyer 1990). Such objects may lie undetected for years unless they have damaged the tympanic membrane. Sometimes gentle syringing will wash out the foreign body, but if it has become impacted it may be necessary for the patient to be admitted to hospital as a day case and for the object to be removed under general anaesthetic.

Only objects that will not expand when in contact with water should be syringed.

DEAFNESS AND HEARING LOSS

Although total deafness is comparatively rare, many people suffer hearing loss to varying degrees. Deafness can affect adults or children. Many children who are deaf continue to be so for all their lives, but some can be helped to maximise auditory function. The present chapter will concentrate on hearing problems among adults. There are estimated to be 8.4 million deaf and hard of hearing adults in the UK, with 640 000 of them being severely or profoundly deaf and 7.8 million suffering from mild or moderate deafness (Royal National Institute for Deaf People [RNID] 1996).

PATHOPHYSIOLOGY AND MEDICAL MANAGEMENT

Deafness is usually classified into conductive and sensorineural disorders, as follows.

Box 14.1 Hearing tests

Tuning fork tests
These tests are a simple means of determining a patient's basic auditory status. They may be performed in a clinical or home environment.

Rinne Test
Air conduction is tested by holding a vibrating tuning fork first to the front of the ear and then by placing the tuning fork footplate against the mastoid bone. Patients should hear sound clearer to the front of the ear. Result = Rinne positive. Normal hearing.

Weber Test
Bone conduction is tested by placing the vibrating footplate of a tuning fork to the middle of the forehead. This sound should be heard centrally. If conductive hearing loss is present, sound will be lateralised. If sensorineural hearing loss is present then sound will localise to the good ear.

Audiometry
Audiometric tests measure hearing acuity. Relatively simple tests, which include delivering tones of variable frequency and intensity, the spoken word and measuring middle ear pressures, are amongst the methods used to determine the type and source of any hearing loss. Electric response audiometry measures the patient's response to an acoustic stimulus by way of an electroencephalogram and can provide reliable and exact information on the site of a disorder, e.g. the cochlea, auditory nerve tract or brain stem.

Detailed descriptions of these tests can be found in Becker et al (1993).

Diagnosis of the type of hearing loss from which an individual is suffering will be by examination and audiometry (see Box 14.1). Conductive deafness can often be helped by removing any obstruction (cerumen or a foreign body) or by amplifying sounds by means of a hearing aid. Because the external and middle ear are fairly accessible, surgical intervention may also be an option. By contrast, in sensorineural deafness, where the damage is to the organ of Corti or the cochlear portion of the eighth cranial nerve, surgery does not usually have much effect.

Conductive deafness results from a reduced ability of the sound waves to reach the fluid in the cochlea. The sound is quieter but not distorted. This can be due to:

- congenital abnormality
- otitis externa
- foreign bodies
- excessive cerumen
- perforated tympanic membrane
- otitis media (secretory and suppurative)
- damage to the incus, malleus or stapes.

Sensorineural deafness is caused by a defect of the cochlea or its connecting nerves. The sound heard is quieter and also distorted. This is a result of the loss of the high frequencies which register consonant sounds. In severe cases, the patient may not be able to hear the sound of his own voice. This can be due to:

- ageing
- medication
- trauma, including head injury and noise

- infection
- Ménière's disease
- congenital malformation
- ischaemia.

Presbycusis, the most common type of sensorineural deafness, develops as a consequence of ageing and is becoming increasingly prevalent in Western society. In the UK, 55% of people over 60 are deaf or hard of hearing (RNID 1997). Audiometry initially shows loss of ability to hear high tones, but there is gradual deterioration of lower tone hearing as well. Degeneration of the nervous tissue leads to loss of intelligibility in the sounds that are heard. Hearing loss in this disorder is symmetrical (i.e. affects both ears). A hearing aid may be of slight advantage, but distortion and poor discrimination may cancel out any benefit from amplification. When communicating with these patients, it is important to speak a little slower and distinctly and to try to eliminate any background noise. Because the high tones are affected first, the individual may have trouble hearing consonants, as these are usually of higher tone than vowels.

Medication. It has been recognised for some time that salicylates and quinine can cause deafness, but this can be reversed by discontinuing these medications. Other drugs, such as antibiotics of the aminoglycoside group, some diuretics, such as i.v. frusemide, and cytotoxic agents of the nitrogen mustard group can cause irreparable damage.

Trauma. Noise-induced hearing loss is well documented and has become recognised as an industrial disease. Socioacusis, the term used to describe the hearing loss caused by sources of noise outside work, can be as great a risk as loud noise in the workplace (RNID 1999). A single exposure to a loud noise such as an explosion or gunshot can cause permanent deafness, or the injury may be temporary. Tinnitus usually accompanies this injury and often takes longer to improve than any deafness (see p. 534). Exposure to loud noise over a period of time leads to destruction of the hair cells in the organ of Corti. The Noise at Work Regulations (1989) laid down strict standards of noise control and protection for employers, who are liable to be prosecuted if they do not comply (see 'Useful addresses', p. 553, for more information). Occupational health nurses have a role to play in monitoring noise levels and encouraging auditory health through education. Unfortunately many people, particularly the young, willingly subject themselves to high levels of noise, e.g. at rock concerts, discos and dances, where the music is usually amplified. On audiometry, early changes in hearing caused by exposure to noise are seen as a dip which gradually deepens and involves adjacent frequencies. Although personal stereos present less of a risk than rock concerts, it is recommended that only those with a mechanism to limit the volume be used, and children should be prevented from playing with toys that make a loud sound close to their ears (RNID 1999).

Head injuries or trauma resulting in deafness usually involve fractures or penetrating injuries of the temporal bone. Occasionally, concussion (see Ch. 9) can cause deafness due to haemorrhage into the middle ear or cochlea. These injuries are often accompanied by severe vertigo, nausea and vomiting.

Infection leading to deafness is usually viral in origin. The causative viruses are those associated with mumps, measles, chickenpox, rubella, poliomyelitis and influenza types A and B.

Ménière's disease. See page 535.

For information on deafness resulting from congenital malformation, see Serra et al (1986), pp. 102–103.

NURSING PRIORITIES AND MANAGEMENT: DEAFNESS AND HEARING LOSS

In the case of conductive deafness, the nurse's role may be to prepare the patient for surgery and facilitate his postoperative recovery. Some of the surgical procedures that may benefit patients are myringoplasty, ossiculoplasty and stapedectomy. A patient for whom surgery is not feasible may be fitted with a hearing aid and educated in its use by members of the audiology department, including the hearing therapist. In this case the nurse, as a member of the multiprofessional team, should also explain how to obtain the greatest benefit from the aid. Most patients in this situation also benefit from learning how to lip-read. Lip-reading sessions are available as a day or evening class at the audiology department or a local college. It can take many months to become proficient at lip-reading, so the earlier the patient starts the better. Slow progress combined with deteriorating hearing can be very demotivating.

Communicating effectively with a hearing-impaired patient is a very important nursing priority. In the assessment, the nurse should obtain and record information about the patient's preferred method of communicating, e.g. lip-reading, finger-spelling or sign language. For a less profoundly deaf patient it may be that speaking face to face in a distinct voice and eliminating background noise are adequate (see Box 14.2). A study by Wright (1993) suggested that deaf adults who used sign language were dissatisfied with and disadvantaged in their communication with health care staff, including nurses. None of Wright's sample had been offered access to an interpreter, indicating a lack of understanding of communication needs (see Research Abstract 14.1).

It is now recognised that deafness can have a profound psychological impact and that hearing-impaired individuals may require support to help resolve problems. Many deaf people would prefer to have counselling from a counsellor who is deaf, and attempts should be made to find such a professional if preferred (via BAC if necessary, see 'Useful addresses'). According to Ratna (1994), the problems deaf clients bring to counselling include isolation, frustration, discrimination and physical and sexual abuse.

Box 14.2 Talking with someone who has a hearing deficit

- Do not speak until you have the person's attention and he can see your full face
- Never turn your back on the person when you are speaking
- Ask the person if he can lip-read
- Do not exaggerate your lip movements
- Direct your voice to one ear if it has better hearing than the other
- Speak slowly, enunciate clearly and do not shout
- Remember that vowels are heard more easily than consonants
- Check that the person has understood what you have said
- If the person has difficulty in understanding, try rephrasing the sentence
- Do not laugh at misinterpretations
- Have patience. Give the person time to adjust his hearing aid if necessary
- Encourage the person to participate in group conversations when the occasion arises
- If verbal communication is impossible, explore alternative means, e.g. sign language

Research Abstract 14.1
Deaf people's perceptions of communication with nurses

This qualitative study focuses on the nature of deaf people's perceptions of their communication experiences with health care professionals. There is a dearth of British literature about deaf people in relation to nursing practice, and what is available indicates a tendency for nurses to treat deaf people as handicapped rather than acknowledging that it is the lack of communication between people who can hear and people who are deaf that is the handicap. Nurses appear to know no more about deaf people than do the general public.

The sample in Wright's (1993) study conducted in the north of England comprised 23 people who used British Sign Language (BSL) and who had accessed an area of health service provision in the previous 6 months. Data were collected via a questionnaire and, for an unstated number of respondents who needed help in completing the questionnaire, by semi-structured interview, conducted using BSL.

Results indicated that none of the sample had been provided with an interpreter by the health services, and some, who had been accompanied by an interpreter, still experienced problems. The main problems reported were the use of long words which neither the respondent nor the interpreter could understand, poor lip movements, not directing speech to the deaf person, and what was seen as 'avoiding communication'. Such inadequacies clearly make a major contribution to the dissatisfaction which respondents expressed about communication between themselves and health care professionals.

The author acknowledges the small size of the sample and considers that the research should be regarded as a pilot. Although the findings cannot be generalised they do support the existing literature in relation to poor communication with deaf people in health care settings and illustrate the need for nurses to improve their knowledge and skills in this area of care.

Wright D 1993 Deaf people's perceptions of communication with nurses. British Journal of Nursing 2(11): 567–571.

Chan (1997) describes a service he and his team of hearing and deaf health care professionals have developed for deaf people with mental health problems.

Nurses can make a valuable contribution by recognising the problems faced by patients with hearing loss and helping them to obtain the appropriate help. A Commission of Inquiry (National Deaf Children's Society 1992) into human aids in communication found that a number of deaf people were unhappy about the quality of their care in hospital and in outpatient departments. The Commission recommended that nurses should make a greater effort to ascertain what services are available to deaf people in their care.

Q **14.1** How might a person with a severe hearing deficit know that her telephone or doorbell is ringing?

Community nurses can provide tremendous help and support for patients and their relatives when sensorineural deafness is a problem. They should be able to assist their patients to obtain many of the aids available, including a hearing dog for the deaf, which can help to overcome communication difficulties in everyday life. There are many associations, both voluntary and professional, which can provide support and help. The nurse working in the community should be a resource person for her patients and guide them to the support that is available (see 'Useful addresses', p. 553).

Q **14.2** Find out which professional or voluntary support groups there are for deaf people in your area. What services do they offer? Compile a resource list.

Hearing aids

It is estimated that there are 2 million hearing aid users in the UK. In addition, there are thought to be another 2 million people who would benefit from the use of a hearing aid (RNID 1996).

All electronic hearing aids consist of three parts: the microphone, which picks up the sound; the amplifier, which is powered by batteries and which makes the sound louder; and the earpiece, which delivers the amplified sound to the ear via an ear mould. As there are many models on the market, it is important that the most appropriate one is chosen for each person's needs and lifestyle. While most hearing aids enclose all the components in a neat package on or near the ear, they differ in such aspects as frequency response, output and ability to reduce the effects of sudden, loud noise. Hearing aids conduct sound either through air or via the bone behind the ear. Old-fashioned speaking tubes or ear trumpets can still be of surprising benefit to some people.

After the most appropriate model of hearing aid has been identified, the patient will require some training in order to be able to receive maximum benefit from it. The fact that the aid makes all sounds, including background noise, louder for the patient means that he will have to develop the skill of picking out sounds essential to communication. Social interaction may be difficult until this skill is mastered, and if the individual is not given enough information and support, he may abandon his aid as useless.

Q **14.3** Find out how many patients in your ward or on your community caseload have a hearing aid. How much training and support regarding their use did they receive? How many use them? How useful do they find their hearing aids to be? What would you do if you were visiting an elderly person in his own home, and he responded to your questions by showing you a drawer containing several hearing aids and saying, 'None of these are any use'?

All hearing aid models are battery-powered and have an on/off switch which is sometimes combined with the volume control. Many models also have a switch marked 'T' which is for use with telephone and other systems fitted with an induction loop. This loop eliminates some background noise and clarifies incoming speech.

Q **14.4** Where in your area are induction loops fitted? How can you tell?

The ear moulds are individually made to fit each user's ear. They can be disconnected from the aid for cleaning, which should be done frequently. The tube which connects the earpiece to the main aid can also be detached and washed and any blockage removed with a pipe cleaner. If a hearing aid is not working, make sure that:

- the switch is in the 'on' position
- the battery is still good and is of the right type
- the mould is clean and fits properly (check for excessive cerumen)
- the connecting tube is pliable and patent.

If all of the above are in order and the aid is not working, it should be returned to the hearing aid clinic for maintenance. All hearing aids and batteries supplied by the NHS are maintained and replaced free of charge.

DISORDERS OF THE MIDDLE EAR

Secretory otitis media (glue ear)

Glue ear is the most common cause of hearing impairment and the most common reason for elective surgery in children.

For a comprehensive account, see Department of Health (1992).

PATHOPHYSIOLOGY

This disorder is known as glue ear because it is characterised by a thick, tenacious fluid which collects in the middle ear. Normally, the mucosal secretions of the middle ear drain down the eustachian tube into the nasopharynx. It is not certain whether the abnormal accumulation of this fluid is caused by the viscosity of the fluid, congestion of the eustachian tubes, or obstruction caused by enlarged adenoids or a tumour.

Common presenting symptoms. Pain is not usually associated with this condition. The adult patient usually comes to the medical practitioner complaining of hearing loss. A child might never complain, and her condition might be discovered only upon investigation into poor performance at school or school screening audiometry.

MEDICAL MANAGEMENT

Examination of the tympanic membrane by auriscope usually confirms diagnosis, as in this disorder the membrane has a characteristic dull grey or orange appearance. It will also lose its normal translucence and become retracted.

Treatment

Conservative treatment is to prescribe a vasoconstricting nasal preparation or antihistamines to reduce oedema of the nasal mucosa. This is often sufficient to allow the secretions to escape through the eustachian tube. Alternatively, attempts can be made to liquefy the mucus to help it escape, by prescribing mucolytic medicines.

Surgical intervention involves performing a myringotomy, incising the tympanic membrane and suctioning of the glue. If a grommet is not inserted, the delicate tympanic membrane heals within a few days. The fluid may, of course, accumulate again. The insertion of a grommet (see Fig. 14.3) is sometimes considered appropriate, although some specialists think this can lead to scar formation in later years which will impair hearing. If a grommet is inserted, it usually gradually slides out of the membrane over 9–12 months; patients sometimes find it on their pillow when they waken one morning. A grommet allows aeration of the middle ear, thus restoring middle ear air pressure. There is usually a marked improvement in hearing after this procedure, which is maintained in about 75% of patients.

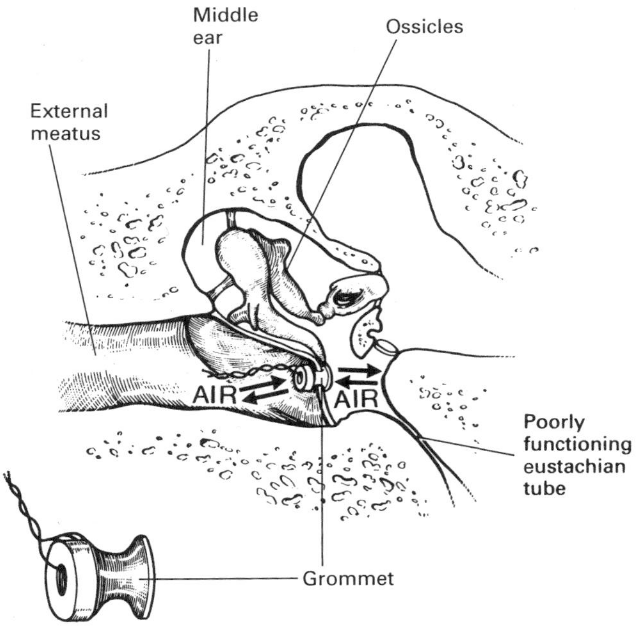

Fig. 14.3 Grommet and grommet in situ. (Reproduced with kind permission from McKenzie et al 1986.)

NURSING PRIORITIES AND MANAGEMENT: SECRETORY OTITIS MEDIA (GLUE EAR)

Only care specific to ENT patients is outlined in this chapter. The reader is referred to Chapter 26 for details of perioperative care.

Preoperative care

The nurse must ensure that the patient and his family are adequately informed about what any surgical procedure will entail. This may involve the use of diagrams and it may be helpful to show a grommet to them if one is to be inserted. As grommet insertion is usually performed on children and young people, it is vital that the appropriate emotional and psychological support is given by suitably qualified staff in a specialist area.

When communicating with the patient preoperatively, the nurse should make allowances for hearing loss (see Box 14.2).

Postoperative care

The anaesthetic for this operation is very light, e.g. ketamine hydrochloride, and so the patient is usually discharged on the day of surgery. Measures to prevent the spread of infection (e.g. washing the hands before and after touching the affected ear), how to change and dispose of cotton wool plugs in the external auditory canal, and specific instructions about whether, and when, it is safe to allow water to enter the ear must be discussed with the patient. Some surgeons allow swimming when a grommet is in place, as long as the patient does not dive or swim underwater. Others prefer their patients not to swim until the grommet has been expelled. Usually, a cotton wool plug moistened with petroleum jelly is inserted in the external canal when the hair is being washed or during a shower. The nurse must ensure that the patient and his family understand this advice, and it is recommended that an information booklet or advice sheets are given. The importance of attending the clinic for a follow-up visit, even if the hearing has improved dramatically, should be stressed. This visit is to ensure that the membrane is healing satisfactorily, to check the position of the grommet and to check for signs of infection. The patient should be told to go to his GP if he experiences any pain or if there is a bloodstained discharge from the ear. Most of these precautions apply to all patients who have undergone aural surgery.

Serra et al (1986) and Sigler & Schuring (1993) give information which the nurse should explain to the patient in relation to postoperative self-care at home.

Otosclerosis

Otosclerosis is a condition in which the ossicles in the middle ear, along with the temporal bone, begin to soften. This spongy bone gradually becomes a dense sclerotic mass; the ossicles may become fixed and less effective in passing on auditory vibrations. The individual with this condition will complain of increasing hearing loss. While this loss is conductive in origin, if the damage extends to the cochlea, sensorineural loss of hearing will also occur. Mild tinnitus (see p. 534) may also be experienced, in which case some people find that they can actually hear better in a noisy environment where their tinnitus is masked.

This disorder commonly begins in adolescence and appears to affect women twice as often as men. Its cause is as yet unknown. Heredity, vitamin deficiency and otitis media have all been cited as significant factors.

Medical management and nursing priorities

Although no cure for otosclerosis is known, surgery can often dramatically improve hearing. The surgery of choice, stapedectomy, involves freeing the stapes and replacing it with a prosthesis. This restores the vibration necessary to permit the transmission of sound waves. The procedure is a very delicate one requiring the use of an operating microscope, as the stapes is one of the smallest bones in the body. Surgery may be performed under local anaesthetic and hospital admission may be no more than 24 h.

Great care must be taken in the early postoperative period, as the patient may take a little while to regain her sense of balance. This short-term vertigo, if discussed and explained in the preoperative period, should cause minimal distress to the patient. Prior to discharge, advice should be given on the prevention of aural infection, the importance of preventing the entry of water into the ear and the need to guard against blowing the nose until the operative site is completely healed. Violent nose blowing can force air up the eustachian tube, increasing middle ear pressure, which can affect the operated area and prosthesis. Follow-up appointments in the outpatient department and appropriate community support by the GP will ensure optimal progress and recovery.

For those for whom the symptoms of otosclerosis are not too severe or for whom surgery is inappropriate, a hearing aid may restore and maintain satisfactory hearing. For others, neither surgery nor a hearing aid will have long-term effectiveness and varying degrees of deafness will result.

Acute suppurative otitis media (ASOM)

PATHOPHYSIOLOGY

This is an acute bacterial infection of the middle ear which is especially common in childhood. The most common causative organisms are *Streptococcus pneumoniae*, *Haemophilus influenzae*, *Streptococcus pyogenes* and *Staphylococcus aureus*. Onset usually follows acute tonsillitis, the common cold or influenza, when infection travels up the eustachian tube to the middle ear. The whole middle ear may be affected, including the mastoid air cells, small air spaces in the posterior portion of the temporal bone, behind the middle ear (see Fig. 14.1).

Common presenting symptoms. The patient usually presents with acute ear pain. There may be deafness, general malaise and pyrexia. On examination, the eardrum is red and bulging due to the collection of pus in the middle ear. The tympanic membrane may rupture, releasing the discharge and dramatically and instantaneously relieving the pain.

MEDICAL MANAGEMENT

Treatment. The patient with ASOM is usually seen and treated by a GP. The exact treatment given will depend on the stage of the infection, as follows.

Early stage. At this stage the tympanic membrane will still look normal. A broad-spectrum antibiotic effective against the most common organisms is usually prescribed. The initial dose may be given intramuscularly (and the rest of the course orally) in order to reduce the time taken for the antibiotic to become effective. Antipyretic analgesics such as paracetamol will be necessary to relieve pain and reduce fever. Vasoconstricting nasal sprays may also be helpful in keeping the eustachian tubes patent and thereby allowing escape of fluid from the middle ear. In severe cases, admission for intravenous (i.v.) antibiotics and pain control may be necessary.

Bulging eardrum. If the infection has reached this stage, a myringotomy may be performed. This involves applying a local anaesthetic before making an incision in the tympanic membrane to allow the pus to escape. If a myringotomy is performed in preference to allowing the eardrum to rupture, the membrane will heal with less scarring and hearing should not be impaired. During this procedure a swab of the discharge will be taken and sent to the laboratory for culture and sensitivity so that the appropriate antibiotic can be prescribed.

Discharging ear. By this stage the tympanic membrane will already have ruptured. A swab of the discharge will be taken and the ear carefully mopped and then dressed with a small plug of cotton wool. Broad-spectrum antibiotics will be prescribed in the first instance while the results of bacteriology are awaited.

The patient will have to visit her GP regularly so that healing of the membrane can be monitored. If necessary, a myringoplasty (reconstruction of the eardrum) will be performed.

NURSING PRIORITIES AND MANAGEMENT: ACUTE SUPPURATIVE OTITIS MEDIA (ASOM)

Early stage

If at this stage a nurse (possibly a practice nurse) is involved, her role will be to ensure that the prescribed course of antibiotics is completed in order to eradicate all the organisms. It may be necessary to teach the patient or a relative how to administer a nasal spray.

Discharging ear

If the disease has reached this stage, the nurse's tasks will include mopping out the external ear as often as required and helping the patient complete his course of antibiotics.

If appropriate treatment is given early enough, ASOM should resolve and hearing return to normal. Occasionally, complications do occur, including chronic suppurative otitis media and acute mastoiditis, which are described below.

Chronic suppurative otitis media (CSOM)

PATHOPHYSIOLOGY

Common presenting symptoms. This condition follows unresolved ASOM. The patient will present with a perforated tympanic membrane, a discharging ear and some degree of conductive deafness. Pain is not usually a complaint. The discharge may be intermittent and is mucoid, becoming purulent in the presence of secondary infection.

MEDICAL MANAGEMENT

The recommended treatment would be to keep the ear dry by the use of topical medication before correcting the hearing loss by performing a tympanoplasty.

For further information on middle ear reconstructive procedures and care, see Waddington et al (1997).

Tympanoplasty. Following removal of diseased tissue, an attempt may be made to reconstruct the sound transmission mechanism in the middle ear by reconstructing the tympanic membrane (myringoplasty) using a connective tissue graft taken from the fascia covering the temporal bone and reconstructing the ossicular chain (ossiculoplasty). This combined reconstruction is known as a tympanoplasty.

NURSING PRIORITIES AND MANAGEMENT: TYMPANOPLASTY

Preoperative care

The patient is usually admitted on the day of surgery. He will have an obvious hearing deficit and therefore the establishment of good communication is very important. To help avoid complications, the ear must be dry and free from infection. Hearing tests will be carried out to confirm the degree of hearing loss. If the patient has been taking aspirin regularly, the dosage should be reduced to minimise the risk of bleeding. If some of the patient's hair has to be removed, this will be done in the operating theatre.

To help alleviate anxiety, the nurse should give the patient information about the procedure and warn him about the sensations that he may experience afterwards, such as dizziness and tinnitus (see p. 534). It is also helpful to describe the very bulky bandage that will be present around the head and affected ear so that this does not alarm the patient and his relatives. Hearing aids should be worn to the operating theatre.

For patients who are having surgery on the ear in which they normally wear a hearing aid, a temporary aid may be fitted to their other ear if appropriate.

Postoperative care

General postoperative care is as described in Chapter 26. The majority of patients undergoing ear surgery are given a hypotensive anaesthetic in order to reduce bleeding and thereby allow the surgeon a clearer view of the tiny operative field. This involves the i.v. administration of a hypotensive agent such as trimetaphan or pentolinium. Frequent blood pressure readings are therefore required until the preoperative baseline levels are regained.

Following the operation the patient should be encouraged to lie with the affected area uppermost and observed for nausea, vomiting and vertigo, all of which might be present due to interference with the semicircular canals during surgery. The aim of the pressure dressing and bandage is to prevent haematoma formation and bleeding, but the nurse should always observe the patient's bandages and pillows for bloodstains.

Following this type of surgery, the patient should be asked to smile, wrinkle his nose and shut his eyes tightly. The ability to perform these movements indicates that there has been no damage to the facial nerve. A record of the time of checking and level of function of the nerve should always be kept for medical and legal reasons. Because of its location the VIIth cranial facial nerve is at risk of damage during surgery to the middle or inner ear.

Most patients are able to be up on the evening of surgery and return home the next day. The patient should be advised that he may experience dizziness during the following 2 or 3 weeks and that he should avoid sudden movements such as quickly turning the head. The patient should return to the ward in 5–7 days to have the sutures removed. Packing is usually present in the external meatus for between 1 and 3 weeks following surgery. The patient will be shown how to change the piece of cotton wool at the entrance to the meatus as required without disturbing the packing.

Patients will naturally be very anxious to know if the graft has taken and if the infection has been completely removed. Offering accurate information and giving specific answers to questions will help to alleviate these anxieties.

CSOM with choleastoma

PATHOPHYSIOLOGY

This potentially dangerous condition is sometimes called attico-antral disease. On examination it may be possible to see the choleastoma, which is an ingrowth of keratinising squamous epithelium from the external ear into the middle ear, usually from the site of a previous perforation. The squamous epithelium growing within the middle ear produces keratin, which has the ability to erode the bony ossicles and may even spread into the inner ear.

Common presenting symptoms. The patient will complain of a foul-smelling discharge from the ear and of deafness.

MEDICAL MANAGEMENT

The treatment of choice is mastoidectomy (see below).

Acute mastoiditis

This condition arises from acute otitis media and is caused by the infection spreading to the bony walls of the cells of the mastoid process.

MEDICAL MANAGEMENT

The conservative medical management is by administration of antibiotics.

Mastoidectomy. A cortical mastoidectomy involves incision, drainage and removal of unhealthy mucosa and bone cells from the mastoid process of the temporal bone, leaving the middle ear structures intact. A modified mastoidectomy may be performed if the disease is confined to the attic and the patient has good hearing.

This is currently the most common surgical procedure for middle ear infection. It involves removal of most of the air cell system within the mastoid cavity, especially in the attic or upper area, and preservation of the remnants of the tympanic membrane and the ossicles, although these are not usually functioning. Every effort is made to preserve the ossicular chain and tympanic membrane in order to retain hearing. The procedure involves extenerating (clearing out) the mastoid cells and removing the outer attic and posterior wall, thus leaving a large cavity to allow air from the meatus to circulate and dry up secretions.

NURSING PRIORITIES AND MANAGEMENT: MASTOIDECTOMY

Nursing care is as for patients undergoing tympanoplasty (see p. 533).

Other complications of middle ear infection

Less common complications of middle ear infection are facial nerve paralysis, meningitis, extradural or subdural abscess, labyrinthitis, lateral sinus thrombosis and brain abscess.

DISORDERS OF THE INNER EAR

Tinnitus

Tinnitus is a little understood but most distressing feature of some ear diseases and disorders. It may also occur spontaneously or as a postoperative complication. Possibly because it is so puzzling, has no known cause and is not a visible symptom, sufferers often feel that they receive very little sympathy.

PATHOPHYSIOLOGY

Tinnitus is usually a subjective sensation of sound in the ear. It is a relatively common complaint which may arise in association with a wide range of conditions, including inner and middle ear disease, overuse of drugs such as aspirin and quinine, abnormalities of the auditory nerve, renal problems, cardiac problems and anaemia. It is often accompanied by vertigo and/or deafness. (The Tinnitus Helpline produces an excellent range of factsheets and a free newsletter for interested professionals, as well as helping sufferers; see 'Useful addresses', p. 553.)

Common presenting symptoms. Tinnitus can vary in severity from an intermittent mild ringing sensation in the ear to an incessant noise loud enough to make life unbearable. The perceived sound varies in volume and character from one individual to another. Some patients are aware of the sound only during their waking hours, while others are aware of it mainly at night or when they are somewhere very quiet. Tinnitus may cause difficulty in sleeping, with irritability, tiredness and lack of concentration following restless nights. The persistent symptoms cause many tinnitus sufferers to feel anxious and depressed (see Box 14.3). The feelings are exacerbated in some by fears that the tinnitus is an indication of a more serious underlying disease or that it will cause an increase in hearing loss.

In the worst cases, individuals with tinnitus may suffer total deafness because the noise in their ear eliminates all other sounds.

For further information on tinnitus and health anxiety, see Heath (1994).

Box 14.3 An experience of tinnitus

I shall never forget the first time I experienced tinnitus. It was in the dead of night when I heard a high-pitched whine in my left ear. I was so taken aback that I got up out of bed and went in search of the source of the noise. Before long, however, I realised that the noise was being carried with me.

The tinnitus had been preceded about a month beforehand by nausea and severe vertigo which I had accepted as transitory. To find that I was left with this noise made me feel very anxious indeed. I had difficulty in coming to terms with the fact that it might always be present. My reaction was 'It can't be! There must be something to combat it and make the noise go away!'

When it became clear to me that I was now a 'tinnitus sufferer' I experienced a phase of reactive depression and felt that life was not worthwhile. Naturally, I searched for a cure and eventually joined the local branch of the Tinnitus Association. This was a move which I made by myself, but the Association proved to be an invaluable source of emotional and practical support and information.

I had no idea early on that things could get worse. With hindsight, I realise that it was just as well, as I do not think I would have had the emotional strength to carry on. Things did get worse and one New Year's night the noise changed to an intermittent, low-pitched, buzzing sound. To say I nearly went insane is putting it mildly. I recall at one point I was banging my head (none too gently) against the wall to try to dislodge the sound. I felt suicidal and realised that if this latest occurrence persisted, the only way I would get peace would be to be dead.

I have been most fortunate because that phase lasted only 2 days and eventually the tinnitus burned itself out. Some of my friends at the Association have not been so lucky and have seriously considered committing suicide.

A hearing therapist has now joined the team at my audiology clinic and is giving tinnitus sufferers like myself a great deal of help in many ways.

MEDICAL MANAGEMENT

To aid diagnosis a careful history must be taken, which includes information about all other symptoms and any medications. This should be done in a tinnitus clinic within an ENT department. A hearing test and careful examination of the ear (including radiography) may help determine the cause. Unfortunately, in many instances, no treatable cause will be found. In certain patients, a hearing aid can give some relief by reducing or masking the tinnitus. A noise generator which looks like a hearing aid can help to cancel out the undesirable sound and can be of help to some. Tinnitus retraining therapy (TRT) aims to reduce the brain's perception of tinnitus and so reduce the problem it is causing. TRT may include counselling, relaxation therapy, the appropriate use of hearing aids, noise alleviators and medication, as well as the treatment of any stress and anxiety.

Sizer (1998) gives an overview of the issues surrounding the use of this new therapy.

NURSING PRIORITIES AND MANAGEMENT: TINNITUS

Very few tinnitus sufferers will be patients in hospital unless their condition has arisen as an early postoperative complication. The majority will attend their GP's surgery or their nearest ENT outpatient department. Wherever nursing staff encounter these patients, high priority should be given to allowing patients to express their fears and to recognising and relieving patient anxiety and depression. Once an ENT specialist has carried out all the tests required to determine a diagnosis, any prescribed treatment and training can be commenced. Where there is no treatment, a planned programme, including counselling, explanations and information-giving (e.g. details of support groups and follow-up outpatient appointments), will be necessary to relieve the patient's worries. There are more than 100 tinnitus support groups in the UK and they can be of enormous help to sufferers by providing ongoing emotional support.

14.5 Find out if there is a tinnitus support group in your area. If there is, try to arrange to attend one of their meetings.

Vertigo

PATHOPHYSIOLOGY

Vertigo is a disturbance of equilibrium in the absence of an external cause which creates a sensation of rotating motion of oneself or one's surroundings. It is usually caused by irritation of the vestibular apparatus and is most frequently associated with disorders of the bony labyrinth and with Ménière's disease. Cardiac, neurological or viral infections and therapeutic drugs such as streptomycin can also cause vertigo.

Common presenting symptoms. Vertigo is a disabling and often frightening sensation which may be transient or recurring. It is not the same as dizziness and may be relatively mild or quite severe. The motion perceived is often described as a whirling sensation, but rocking and swaying sensations are also sometimes reported. Severe attacks of vertigo may be sudden and dramatic, accompanied by pallor, nausea and vomiting.

More information on vertigo management can be found in Lauder (1993).

MEDICAL MANAGEMENT

A careful history is required from the patient and must include any precipitating factors such as head and neck movements. Any other symptoms such as tinnitus or deafness should be ascertained. It is also helpful to know how long the periods of vertigo last. Details of medication and any recent trauma can also aid diagnosis. A neurological and cardiovascular examination and perhaps radiography, hearing tests and blood tests may be advisable.

Occasionally, surgery will be required to treat the particular disorder of which vertigo is a symptom, but treatment is more commonly pharmacological (see Box 14.4). Cooksey Cawthorne head and neck exercises taught by a physiotherapist are often very helpful (Serra et al 1986, Lauder 1993). An occupational therapy assessment of home safety may be beneficial.

NURSING PRIORITIES AND MANAGEMENT: VERTIGO

As is the case with tinnitus sufferers, the majority of individuals who experience vertigo will be distressed and incapacitated by their condition. They will usually be seen in their homes, as they are likely to feel unsafe venturing out. The first nursing priority for these patients is safety. The attacks of vertigo may be unpredictable, or may be associated with a particular head movement. For example, for one individual, a precipitating circumstance might be standing on a stepladder with his head back and to one side in order to change a light bulb; for another, it may be simply a quick movement to bend down and pick up a baby from its cot. The nurse should discuss with the patient and his family how to avoid the particular head and/or other movements in order to eliminate attacks, if this is possible.

Ménière's disease

PATHOPHYSIOLOGY

In Ménière's disease, the membranous labyrinth is distended by an increase in the endolymph at the expense of the perilymph, and the organ of Corti degenerates. The most widely held theory of its cause is that it arises as a result of local ischaemia, although it has been suggested that it may be due to viral infection, biochemical disturbance, vitamin deficiency or local physiological faults.

Common presenting symptoms. Ménière's disease is characterised by four disabling features:

- vertigo
- tinnitus
- sensorineural hearing loss
- nausea and vomiting.

It may arise at any age but is most common among individuals aged 30–50. As it runs its course over a period of many years, deafness increases. Although this hearing loss may initially affect only one ear, it will, in 10% of patients, eventually affect the other as well (Becker et al 1993). Many patients have a warning that an attack is imminent, e.g. there is a feeling of fullness in the ear or the character of the tinnitus changes.

During an attack the patient will have vertigo, nausea and vomiting and will want to lie down and remain as still as possible in order to relieve these distressing symptoms. Nystagmus may be present and, as a consequence of vagal stimulation, sweating, bradycardia and diarrhoea may occur.

MEDICAL MANAGEMENT

It may be difficult to arrive at a conclusive diagnosis of Ménière's disease, as many other disorders (e.g. labyrinthitis, intracranial disease and acoustic neuroma) display similar symptoms. Given that, between attacks, clinical examination may prove negative, diagnosis will rely heavily on careful history-taking and audiological investigations.

Treatment. The most common treatment for the symptoms of Ménière's disease is the prescription of medication (see Box 14.4). This will entail the use of diuretics and adherence to a low-salt diet to reduce the volume of endolymph. Vasodilators may be prescribed to alleviate local ischaemia, antihistamine labyrinthine sedatives to suppress the attacks of vertigo and (in very anxious patients) tranquillisers. The majority of patients respond well to drug therapy and may have long periods of respite from severe symptoms.

Surgery may occasionally help to relieve symptoms. This may take the form of decompression of the endolymphatic sac, the creation of a fistula between the endolymph and perilymph reservoirs, or a vestibular neurectomy.

Box 14.4 Examples of medications used in Ménière's disease

Antihistamine labyrinthine sedatives
- Prochlorperazine maleate
- Cinnarizine

Tranquillisers
- Beta histine
- Hydrochloride

Vasodilators
- Nicotinic acid
- Thymoxamine

NURSING PRIORITIES AND MANAGEMENT: MÉNIÈRE'S DISEASE

The main nursing priority in case of an attack of Ménière's disease is to ensure the patient's safety. Attacks are often so severe that the patient needs to lie as still as possible, and, if in hospital, he may gain a sense of security if the side rails on the bed are raised. Vomiting can be so severe as to cause dehydration. If the patient cannot take fluids orally, i.v. fluids and antiemetic drugs will be necessary until oral medication and feeding can be tolerated.

Patients suffering from Ménière's disease often have to make lifestyle changes in order to cope with some of the symptoms of the disorder. The nurse should be prepared to offer advice on lifestyle adaptations. As an individual faced with the problems associated with Ménière's disease is likely to feel anxiety, it is vital that he be given clear information and explanations, particularly with regard to prognosis.

The involvement of the primary health care team and of the occupational health nurse will be especially important, as it is often not until the patient is back at home following diagnosis that he will begin to consider many questions with regard to participation in sport, driving, safety at home and in the workplace, and so forth.

THE NOSE

ANATOMY AND PHYSIOLOGY OF THE NOSE

The principal function of the nose is to provide a passageway for air entering and leaving the respiratory tract. In so doing, it acts as an 'air conditioner', ensuring that inspired air is humidified, sufficiently warm and free from particulate matter.

The terminal fibres of the olfactory nerve are located in the nasal cavity (see Fig. 14.4). The lower two-thirds of the nose are supported by cartilage and the upper third is enclosed by bone. The cavity is divided in half by the septum which consists of cartilage anteriorly and bone posteriorly. The entrance is lined with stratified squamous epithelium and coarse hairs (termed vibrissae) and the passages are lined with a mucous membrane of ciliated columnar epithelium. These passages are highly vascularised. A branch of the maxillary artery supplies the lower posterior section of the cavity, and the anterior and posterior ethmoidal arteries supply the mucous membrane. All these vessels join at Little's area on each side of the septum (see Fig. 14.5).

For further information, see Becker et al (1993).

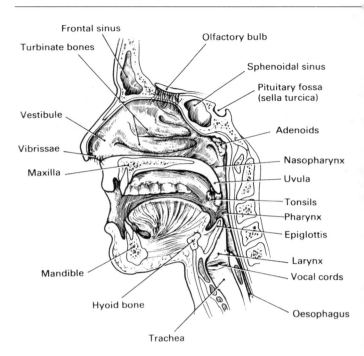

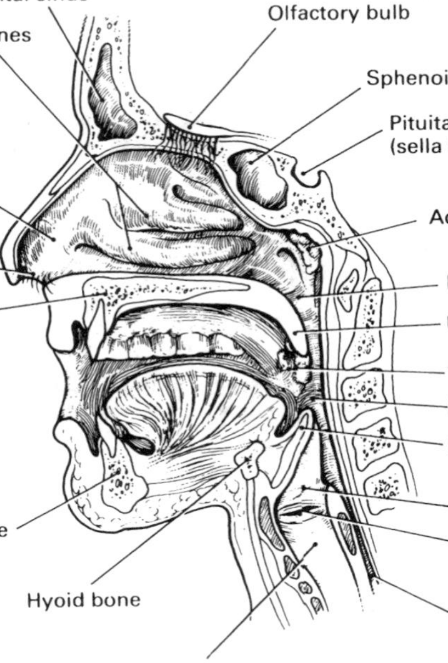

Fig. 14.4 Sagittal section showing lateral walls of nose and pharynx. (Reproduced with kind permission from McKenzie et al 1986.)

DISORDERS OF THE NOSE

Epistaxis

PATHOPHYSIOLOGY

Epistaxis is bleeding from the nose. It is not a disease in itself but a symptom of some other disorder, which may be of a local or general nature. Local causative disorders include idiopathic, trauma caused by nose-picking, foreign bodies, a blow to the nose or surgery. More generalised disorders that sometimes give rise to nosebleeds can be:

- vascular, e.g. hypertension and cardiac failure
- congenital, e.g. haemophilia and hereditary haemorrhagic telangiectasia
- neoplastic, e.g. leukaemia
- drug-induced, e.g. a side-effect of anticoagulant therapy related to infections such as influenza, rhinitis and sinusitis.

Common presenting symptoms. Epistaxis can affect males and females and can occur at any age but is most common in childhood and early adolescence, when it usually occurs in Little's area (see Fig. 14.5) and is often the result of trauma or infection. In middle-aged or elderly individuals, the bleeding can also occur in the posterior part of the nose and may be associated with hypertension. This form of epistaxis may be very frightening and can be life-threatening if it proves difficult to control.

Patients may refer themselves to the local A&E department when they have an active epistaxis. They may then be either admitted to the appropriate hospital ward or given an appointment for the outpatient clinic and sent home with an anterior nasal pack in situ. The latter practice is not widely carried out due to the risk of the pack slipping and being inhaled. One patient's experience of severe epistaxis is recounted in Box 14.5.

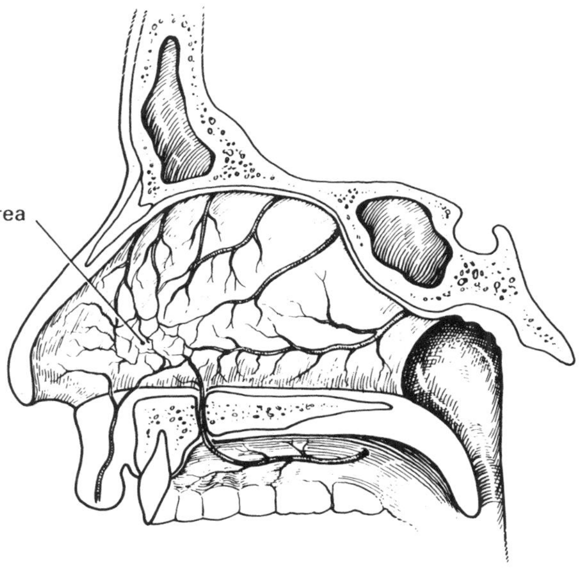

Fig. 14.5 Blood supply to nose (sagittal section). (Reproduced with kind permission from McKenzie et al 1986.)

Patients often present at clinics with a history of recurrent epistaxis, but rarely is a bleed in progress at the clinic visit. On examination, dilated blood vessels may be apparent. The best treatment to prevent the bleeding recurring is cautery by the use of a chemical such as silver nitrate or electrocautery with a red hot wire or diathermy.

MEDICAL MANAGEMENT

The management of epistaxis can be divided into resuscitation of the patient, arrest of the haemorrhage and diagnosis and treatment of any underlying cause (Ell & Parker 1992).

A patient with a severe active epistaxis is usually admitted to hospital as an emergency. Vital signs are recorded to monitor for shock, as bleeding may be severe enough to necessitate blood transfusion. Treatment is by insertion of a nasal pack. This may take the form of a nasal tampon or pneumatic packing with an inflatable balloon. Nasal packs are usually left in place for 24–72 h. Antibiotics are given to prevent any risk of infection developing and spreading to the middle ear if the packs are in longer than 24 h. Occasionally, when these measures fail to control the bleeding, arterial ligation is necessary. If the bleed is the result of some underlying medical condition, this will need to be investigated and treated at the same time.

Box 14.5 An experience of severe epistaxis

Fortunately, I was leaning forward at my desk when it started: a week earlier a nosebleed had doused my waistcoat. The next several hours were spent trying to staunch the flow. A lab technician put a small plug of cotton wool into the offending nostril, which helped for a while, and two students took my blood pressure, which as it happened was normal. When the bleeding worsened towards the end of the afternoon, I resolved to go home via my GP. With a 25-mile drive ahead of me, I donned an old lab coat back to front to protect my clothes and made for my car, leaving a trail of blood behind me. The drive, needless to say, was a strain.

The doctor's surgery was very busy and, after registering, I went over to the pharmacist's window for more cotton wool. My bloodied face evidently shocked the pharmacist; in her panic she could find neither tissues, cotton wool, nor any suitable material. At this point my GP emerged from an adjacent consulting room, took one look at me and said, 'We'd better get you laid down somewhere'. In a spare room he examined me between consultations. I made a terrible mess of his sink when he encouraged me to blow my nose in order to gain a better view of the point of bleeding. He could not find the origin and plugged the nostril with yards of ribbon-like bandage thrust high up into the nasal cavity: an excruciatingly painful procedure, leaving my nostril twice its normal size. As I rose to clean up, the other nostril began bleeding and was also packed; this was equally excruciating.

I arrived home feeling somewhat groggy and bunged up, couldn't eat much and knew I would not sleep much. Breathing constantly through my mouth made it, and my throat, uncomfortably dry. Knowing I wouldn't be able to go to work the following day, I started making the necessary phone calls, during which the bleeding started again, this time going down my throat. After some time my wife felt this couldn't continue overnight and phoned the night service GP at about 23.00 h. He advised keeping very still, was alarmed to hear I had drunk part of a can of beer, and horrified to learn that I was swallowing the blood rather than spitting it out. He said if the bleeding had not abated in 30 min we were to call back. In fact it did let up during that time and, having fixed me a bed downstairs, my wife went to bed around midnight. I passed a miserable few hours of dozing and bleeding, and by 05.00 h I had to wake my wife. She phoned the same GP, who advised us to go to the casualty department of our local hospital. Leaving a note for our sleeping teenagers we drove on icy roads to the hospital, where a young houseman was roused to repack my nose. Although less painful than the first time, this was still quite horrible and left me feeling faint. I was admitted to the ENT ward and given a single room within view of the nurses' desk.

Then followed 6 days of hopes raised and dashed as the doctors required 24 h clear of bleeding before I could be discharged. I needed another two repacks in that time as I had a problem with repeated sneezing, bleeding through the packs and, on two occasions, the fairly revolting experience of the pack unravelling down my throat. Each time the packs were disturbed this stimulated further bleeding and I did become anaemic. The nurses were very attentive and explained that they were relatively helpless if the bleeding continued once the packs were in place. Ice packs were their main remaining option. (One poor chap, discharged during my stay, was readmitted 2 days later with further bleeding.)

On being discharged I was put on a course of iron tablets and told to take a further week off work, advice I was happy to take since in the ensuing week I felt surprisingly weak. Two months later I am well and about to attend a follow-up appointment at the hospital.

NURSING PRIORITIES AND MANAGEMENT: EPISTAXIS

Nursing intervention will vary, depending on the site, severity and cause of the epistaxis, as well as on the patient's age.

Anterior nosebleeds

Most patients with anterior nosebleeds will be children or adolescents and will be treated as outpatients in the doctor's surgery or hospital.

NURSING PRIORITIES AND MANAGEMENT: ANTERIOR NOSEBLEEDS

The first priority of nursing intervention will be to stop the bleeding whilst providing psychological support. The patient should be helped to sit upright with his head slightly forward and asked to mouth breathe and spit out all blood. This helps to estimate the blood loss and prevents the blood from being swallowed and causing nausea. Digital pressure with the thumb and forefinger should be applied to the cartilaginous part of the nose and ice packs to the area above it (Little's area; see Fig. 14.5). This area has many surface arterioles which may have weakened walls. Ten continuous minutes of this pressure is usually sufficient to control an anterior nosebleed. If these first aid measures fail (or if there are recurrent nosebleeds) the patient will probably be transferred to hospital for insertion of a nasal pack or cautery of the area.

Once the bleeding is under control the nurse should explain to the patient and, where appropriate, to the parents how to prevent nosebleeds from recurring. Advice should be given about blowing the nose gently, avoiding picking the nose and trying to keep the nasal mucosa slightly moist by the use of soft petroleum jelly. An explanation of how to cope with and control a nosebleed should also be given.

Hospital treatment

This will be necessary for severe epistaxis which cannot be controlled by the above measures. By providing clear and concise information, the nurse can help alleviate the patient's anxiety and aid recovery. A specialist nurse can pack the nasal cavity or assist the medical practitioner to do so. When a nasal pack is in place, the patient will be able to breathe only through his mouth and may be afraid of suffocation. Frequent oral hygiene and plenty of oral fluids should be offered to prevent the oral mucosa becoming dry. These drinks must not be hot as this can cause local dilatation of blood vessels and exacerbate the problem. Eye care may be necessary as the packing may obstruct the nasolacrimal duct, causing tears to overflow. Nasal packing can also cause hypoxia, with disorientation as well as alterations to vital signs. Oxygen therapy and blood gas monitoring will be needed in this situation. The systemic effects of nasal packing were investigated by Hady et al (1983). Their results suggested that bilateral anterior nasal packs caused hypoxia and hypercapnia due to hypoventilation. This led them to recommend that nasal packs be removed as early as possible and that oxygen therapy be given routinely, especially in the elderly and patients with cardiac disease or inadequate pulmonary function, with appropriate monitoring of arterial blood gases.

Areas that have been cauterised may become encrusted. Soft petroleum jelly should be applied to such areas twice a day for a few weeks until the mucosa has healed.

Some patients admitted as emergencies with uncontrollable nosebleeds will be in hypovolaemic shock (see Ch. 18, p. 643).

For further information on first aid, read Malem & Butler (1993).

14.6 Revise the signs and symptoms of shock so that you can visualise the likely appearance of a patient admitted with severe, uncontrollable epistaxis.

Although anxieties can be reduced by answering the patient's questions and giving information, sedatives may also be prescribed. Following an epistaxis, patients are usually nursed propped up in bed to aid venous return from the area and make it easier for them to spit out any blood. Ice packs may be applied to the nose to help constrict the vessels and control bleeding. The nurse should explain to the patient how to breathe through the mouth and an emesis basin or sputum carton should be to hand. Again, it is important to offer frequent oral hygiene, plenty of cool drinks and eye care as necessary. As these patients often have dysphagia because of the pressure of the nasal pack on the soft palate, a nutritious soft or even liquid diet may be appropriate. Bed rest is usually advised, although patients should be allowed to use the commode at the side of the bed to ease the strain of elimination.

Packing is usually removed in 2 or 3 days. If the bleeding has not been controlled, the patient will have the appropriate arteries ligated in theatre. If a deviated nasal septum (see p. 540) has been a contributory cause, corrective surgery may be performed.

If hypertension or another medical disorder has caused the nosebleed, an appropriate specialist medical opinion is sought and treatment commenced. The nurse may, in the meantime, obtain appropriate patient education booklets or information sheets in relation to the relevant disorder from colleagues working in the ward(s) specialising in the care of such patients, so that they can be given appropriate advice (see Ch. 2).

Community care

To prevent the recurrence of epistaxis, support should continue after the patient has returned home and resumed his normal activities. If the patient is at home, his GP and the practice nurse will be informed of his condition so that they can encourage him to implement the advice received in hospital and monitor hypertension if present.

Information on epistaxis and the elderly can be found in Ell & Parker (1992).

14.7 Using a nursing model familiar to you, prioritise and plan the nursing interventions you think Mrs E (see Case History 14.1) will require over the next 24 h and say how you would evaluate her care. Discuss the plan with your teacher and/or with a qualified member of your nursing team.

DISORDERS OF THE PARANASAL SINUSES

The paranasal sinuses are a group of air spaces surrounding the nose which, it is said, make the skull lighter and add resonance to the voice. They consist of two frontal, two maxillary and two ethmoid sinuses and a single sphenoid sinus divided by a septum. These sinuses all drain into the nose.

Case History 14.1 Mrs E

Mrs E is 58 years old and lives with her husband, who suffers from chronic obstructive airways disease and is unemployed. They have a son and a daughter, both of whom are married and have children. Mrs E works in a television assembly factory and enjoys watching TV, going to bingo and participating in the factory social club. She smokes 20 cigarettes a day and drinks about 14 units of alcohol a week, mainly at the weekend. She often babysits for her son and daughter. She has to do all the housework, cooking and shopping as her husband's breathing problems leave him with little energy.

For the past few months Mrs E has been suffering from nosebleeds, but today's was very severe and could not be controlled even with the help of the occupational health nurse at the factory. She was brought to the local hospital's A&E department by ambulance. By the time she arrived her blood pressure was 90/50 and her pulse 105; she was pale and shivering. She was also very anxious and frightened.

In the A&E department an Epistat catheter was inserted and an intravenous infusion commenced. Mrs E was then transferred to the ward where the staff nurse welcomed her and took her to the bed she had prepared. The staff nurse was given a report by the A&E nurse and after helping Mrs E to transfer from the trolley to bed she planned to observe her infusion closely and to monitor the bleeding and her blood pressure.

On admission, Mrs E was still anxious and distressed. She was a very fastidious lady and the mess her nosebleed had made concerned her. She was also very worried about what her husband would do for his meal and how he would be kept informed of her condition.

In prioritising Mrs E's needs, the staff nurse took into account the details of her medical condition as well as other concerns that the patient herself felt to be important. She helped Mrs E into a hospital nightgown after washing the blood from her skin and put her blouse into cold water to soak. She checked the infusion and Mrs E's blood pressure, then brought the ward phone to the bedside and telephoned Mrs E's husband. As Mrs E had difficulty talking, because of the nasal catheter, the nurse assisted in a three-way conversation in which Mrs E was reassured that her husband was all right. A neighbour had made his tea for him, and Mrs E's daughter was on her way to the hospital, bringing her mother's toiletries and nightclothes. This conversation reassured Mrs E and allowed her to feel more relaxed. This in turn helped the staff nurse to concentrate on monitoring Mrs E's condition and helping to alleviate her problems.

For further information, see Becker et al (1993).

Acute sinusitis

PATHOPHYSIOLOGY

Acute sinusitis is the inflammation of one or more of the paranasal sinuses. It usually develops as an infection secondary to an upper respiratory tract infection or dental disease. Because of the close anatomical connection of the sinuses with the nose, sinus infection is common. It may be acute or chronic.

Common presenting symptoms. Pain is a symptom, and it may be facial, supraorbital or interocular, depending on the sinus involved. Tenderness in the area of pain and nasal obstruction may also be features, and nasal discharge may be present. The patient usually complains of general malaise and is pyrexial.

MEDICAL MANAGEMENT

A nasal swab may be taken for culture and sensitivity. Sinus radiography may also be performed to determine which sinuses are affected. Medical treatment usually consists of the prescription of mild analgesics, antibiotics and nasal decongestant drops.

NURSING PRIORITIES AND MANAGEMENT: ACUTE SINUSITIS

The patient with acute sinusitis is usually nursed at home. He will be advised to rest in bed, to drink plenty of fluids, to take mild analgesics such as paracetamol and to self-administer any prescribed nasal drops. Oral hygiene is also important as the individual will probably be mouth breathing because of the nasal obstruction. Moist steam inhalations can also bring some relief and help to loosen crusting in the nasal cavities. Many sufferers find inhalations very soothing first thing in the morning and last thing at night. After 2 or 3 days the person should have improved sufficiently to be fully active again.

Chronic sinusitis

PATHOPHYSIOLOGY

Chronic sinusitis is common and can be quite debilitating. It can develop for several reasons, including:

- inadequate treatment of an acute episode
- septal deviation or nasal polyps preventing adequate drainage of the sinuses
- pollution, e.g. cigarette smoke
- allergic nasal disease.

Common presenting symptoms. The main symptoms of chronic sinusitis are purulent nasal discharge, postnasal drip, facial pain, headache and recurrent throat infections.

MEDICAL MANAGEMENT

Treatment is usually conservative, consisting of treating any infection with antibiotics and prescribing nasal decongestant drops. It may be necessary to treat polyps or a deviated septum surgically. Surgery may be necessary to remove all of the diseased mucosal lining and widen the opening to the nasal passage to allow more effective drainage. This more radical surgery requires general anaesthesia.

The introduction of functional endoscopic sinus surgery (FESS) has revolutionised the surgical treatment of sinus disease. FESS is the most recent advance in the surgical management of nasal and paranasal sinus disease. By means of nasal endoscopes, the surgeon is able to visualise, diagnose and treat any disease or deformity. CT and/or MRI scans are vital for both diagnostic and intraoperative use. Meticulous postoperative management and follow-up are essential in achieving effective results.

Possible complications of FESS are:

- haemorrhage
- cerebrospinal fluid leak
- visual disturbance/blindness
- periorbital haematoma.

NURSING PRIORITIES AND MANAGEMENT: CHRONIC SINUSITIS

Nursing priorities when caring for these patients are:

- to prepare the patient for surgery and ensure scans are available preoperatively to observe for any possible complications, including haemorrhage and infection
- removal of nasal packing as per the surgeon's instructions
- administration of prescribed analgesics and antibiotics.

On discharge, the patient must be advised on the correct method for installation of nasal drops and the importance of steam inhalations.

See Krouse et al (1997) for fuller details of FESS.

14.8 Discuss with a patient the experience of nasal packing and its removal.

Nasal injury

PATHOPHYSIOLOGY

Injuries to the nose are fairly common and usually occur in sporting activities, falls, accidents and assaults. A blow to one side of the nose may fracture and displace the bone, causing deviation on the other side. A direct blow to the front of the nose can splay out the nasal bones, resulting in a depressed bridge. An injury which is sufficiently severe to fracture the nasal bones will also cause soft tissue swelling and may cause epistaxis.

MEDICAL MANAGEMENT

Investigations will involve a radiographic examination, although this does not always reveal the fracture or may simply reveal a previously undetected fracture. An examination of the nose using a nasal speculum will allow the practitioner to see if the airways are patent and if there is any damage to the septum. Palpation of the nasal bones must be carried out very gently as they will be very tender and painful for up to 3 weeks following a fracture.

Treatment of a broken nose involves manipulating the fractured bones. Occasionally this can be done at the time of the accident, but more commonly it is done a few days later, when the oedema has subsided. The patient is given a light general anaesthetic. The manipulation must be performed within 10 days of injury to prevent calcification of the nasal bones. If the corrected fracture is unstable, a plaster of Paris cast is usually taped in position over the nose for about 10 days to allow the fracture to set correctly.

NURSING PRIORITIES AND MANAGEMENT: NASAL INJURY

If nursing attention is available immediately, treatment of a fractured nose will probably involve first aid measures to stop any epistaxis and to limit the oedema. This involves compressing the end of the nostrils gently between the thumb and forefinger (unfortunately, this will be very painful to the patient) and encouraging the patient to sit with his head slightly forward and to spit out any blood. If ice is available, an ice pack applied to the bridge of the nose can help to control bleeding and swelling. Any epistaxis which results from a blow to the nose is usually short-lived.

Common problems during nasal surgery

Bleeding. This occurs because the nasal mucosa has such a rich blood supply. It can be controlled by the use of ice packs, and if the surgeon suspects that the bleeding might be severe, a nasal pack may be inserted.

Oedema of the mucosa is likely to occur as a consequence of manipulation. Ice packs may help to minimise swelling.

Watery discharge. The irritation of the mucosa which results from surgery will cause the production of an excessive amount of watery discharge known as rhinorrhoea. The nurse should provide an adequate supply of tissues or apply a nasal bolster made of gauze to absorb discharge. This helps to make the problem more manageable.

Pain. As there is a very good nerve supply to the nose, the patient may experience quite severe pain which should be alleviated by means of prescribed analgesics.

DISORDERS OF THE NASAL SEPTUM

Deviation of the nasal septum

The nasal septum separates the nostrils. It is usually thin and quite straight. The upper part is composed of bone and the lower part of cartilage. Deviations of the nasal septum can range from a simple bulge to a marked S-shaped deformity. Most people have some degree of deviation; hence, when introducing a nasogastric tube, the practitioner should always ask the patient which nostril would cause less discomfort.

PATHOPHYSIOLOGY

Developmental problems or trauma may result in a deviated nasal septum. Patients usually complain of nasal obstruction, infection of the sinuses or chronic otitis media due to the inability of the eustachian tubes to function properly. Any combination of these symptoms (including no symptoms) may be present. Simply having a septal deviation is not a reason to operate on it.

MEDICAL MANAGEMENT

An assessment by the medical practitioner of the symptoms, correlated with the degree of the deformity, should be carried out before a treatment plan is agreed. Inspection of the nose with a nasal speculum should reveal the extent of the deviation.

If surgery is the chosen treatment, this is likely to be either a submucous resection or a septoplasty. There is often some confusion as to what these procedures involve. In both operations, access to the bony and cartilaginous parts of the septum is gained by stripping off the nasal mucosa. In a submucous resection, the affected parts of the septum are removed. During a septoplasty the septum is freed, allowing it to be repositioned along the midline of the nose. A nasal pack is usually inserted following these procedures to prevent haemorrhage.

NURSING PRIORITIES AND MANAGEMENT: DEVIATION OF THE NASAL SEPTUM

For up to 24 h after surgery, the patient will have a nasal pack in position. Nursing care in hospital will be similar to that given for epistaxis (see p. 538). Patients are usually fit to return home later in the day after the nasal packing has been removed. There will be a degree of nasal obstruction for 2 or 3 weeks after surgery, until the postsurgical swelling has subsided. Patients are usually advised to stay away from work or crowded places for 10–14 days after surgery to minimise the risk of infection. They are also advised to follow the surgeon's instructions with regard to steam inhalations, nasal douches or decongestant sprays.

Septal haematoma

This usually results from trauma, including surgery, and is a collection of blood beneath the mucoperichondrium of the septum. The patient complains of nasal obstruction and pain. Examination usually reveals a bilateral swelling in the nasal cavities. Antibiotics are given to prevent infection and it is sometimes necessary to incise and drain the haematoma.

Septal perforation

Trauma is usually the cause of a hole in the septum. Although the patient is often symptom-free, excessive crusting or epistaxis may occur. Occasionally the patient complains of whistling on inspiration. If symptoms are troublesome, surgical closure may be attempted.

NASAL OBSTRUCTION

Obstruction of the nasal cavities can result from a number of causes but patients usually present with similar symptoms, the most common of which are obstructed breathing and increased nasal discharge. Some of the most common causes are:

- infection
- allergy
- foreign bodies
- polyps
- neoplasms.

Nasal obstruction resulting from the first two causes does not usually require hospital treatment. The others are described below.

Foreign bodies in the nose

PATHOPHYSIOLOGY

It is usually very young children, aged 2–4 years, or those with learning difficulties, who insert foreign bodies into the nasal cavity. These objects may be organic or inorganic. Inorganic bodies include buttons, beads and small plastic or metal objects which may lie undetected for a long time, only to be found during a routine examination, sometimes as late as when the child reaches adolescence or adulthood. Organic bodies such as peas, wood, paper, cotton wool or sweets cause a local inflammatory reaction which will eventually lead to the formation of granulation tissue. The resulting nasal discharge will eventually become purulent, foul-smelling and bloodstained. Characteristically, the discharge is from only one cavity.

MEDICAL MANAGEMENT

Following a thorough examination, the foreign body is usually removed in the outpatient department. Occasionally it has been in place for such a long time that a general anaesthetic is needed for smooth and safe removal.

NURSING PRIORITIES AND MANAGEMENT: FOREIGN BODIES IN THE NOSE

The care needed is described in the day surgery section (see p. 550). Epistaxis is a possible complication following removal, irrespective of the type of anaesthetic used.

Nasal polyps

PATHOPHYSIOLOGY

Nasal polyps are projections of oedematous mucous membrane and may look like bunches of grapes. They result from prolonged infection or allergy and are usually bilateral and multiple. They occur more commonly in adult males than in women.

Common presenting symptoms. Patients usually complain of nasal obstruction and discharge. Occasionally the size of the polyps may cause broadening of the external nose. The patient may complain of headaches if there is sinus involvement and there may be loss of smell and taste.

MEDICAL MANAGEMENT

On examination, a characteristic glossy, greyish swelling will be visible. If probed it will be found to be soft, insensitive and mobile. Surgical removal is the treatment of choice. This may be carried out under local or general anaesthetic. The patient will require less time in hospital for a local anaesthetic but the decongestant that it contains shrinks the polyps and makes them more difficult to identify and remove. With a general anaesthetic the polyps can be removed at a less hurried pace but bleeding may be more profuse and might therefore obscure some of the smaller polyps. Recurrences are common and an attempt should be made to treat any underlying infection or allergy.

NURSING PRIORITIES AND MANAGEMENT: NASAL POLYPS

Nursing staff should be alert to epistaxis, which is the main postoperative complication of polyp removal. Given that polyps can be associated with allergies, many patients may also suffer from asthma and should be closely observed in this regard.

A nasal pack is usually inserted after the procedure. Appropriate nursing care is detailed on page 538. As it is fairly common for polyps to recur, the importance of attending the outpatient department for follow-up should be explained to the patient.

NEOPLASMS

Nasal and sinus tumours are rare. When they occur, they usually start on one side of the head. Malignant tumours are often infected and ulcerated, in which case they usually produce epistaxis or a profuse purulent discharge. Headache may also be a feature if there is sinus involvement.

Treatment may consist of surgery, radiotherapy, chemotherapy or a combination of these. Patients receiving radiotherapy or chemotherapy are usually treated as outpatients and may be visited by community nurses, including Macmillan nurses, if they experience any side-effects of treatment requiring nursing intervention.

For further information on nasal and sinus neoplasms and treatments, see Sigler & Schuring (1993).

THE THROAT

ANATOMY AND PHYSIOLOGY OF THE THROAT

The throat is usually considered to consist of the pharynx and the larynx (see Fig. 14.4, p. 536). The pharynx may be divided into the nasopharynx and the oropharynx.

The nasopharynx extends from the nasal septum to the eustachian tubes and rests behind and above the soft palate. The oropharynx extends from the posterior boundary of the hard palate to the hyoid bone; it contains the uvula and the tonsils and is surrounded by lymphoid tissue.

The larynx is the organ of voice production and airway protection. It is composed mainly of cartilage and muscle and is lined with a mucosa of stratified squamous epithelium (upper part) and ciliated pseudostratified columnar epithelium (lower part).

For further information see Becker et al (1993).

DISORDERS OF THE THROAT

Benign tumours

These generally arise as a result of voice abuse or overuse and the patient usually presents with continued hoarseness. The tumours are usually attached to the vocal cords and vary greatly in size. Resolution of small nodules may be achieved by voice rest and appropriate speech therapy. Larger nodules may require surgical removal.

For further information on benign and malignant tumours, see Sigler & Schuring (1993).

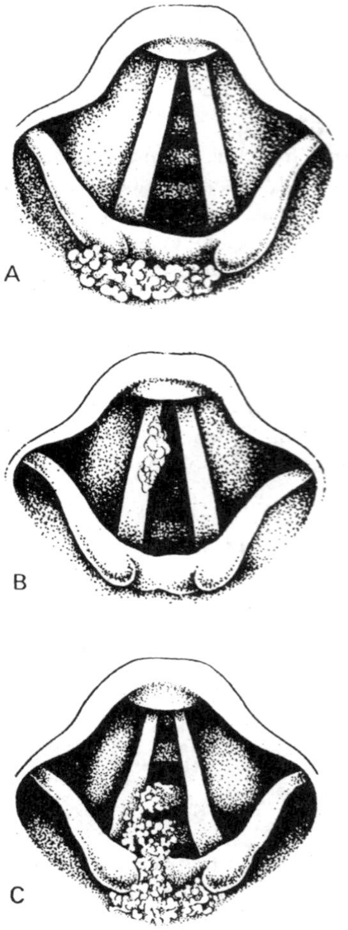

Fig. 14.6 Tumours of the larynx. A: Supraglottic tumour. B: Glottic tumour. C: Subglottic tumour — extensive spread to supraglottic area. (Reproduced with kind permission from McKenzie et al 1986.)

Carcinoma of the larynx

PATHOPHYSIOLOGY

Carcinoma of the larynx is classified according to its location and extent, i.e. glottic (confined to the vocal cords), supraglottic (above the vocal cords) or subglottic (below the vocal cords) (see Fig. 14.6). It accounts for 1% of all malignant disease and is more common in males than in females. The majority of patients have a history of heavy smoking, although the disorder does occasionally occur in non-smokers. It is also thought that high levels of alcohol consumption can be an influencing factor. The most common form of the disease is squamous cell carcinoma. About 10% of all patients with carcinoma of the larynx have a coexisting carcinoma of the bronchus.

Common presenting symptoms. Some patients with laryngeal carcinoma do not consult their medical practitioners until the disease is advanced, having ignored the symptom of hoarseness for some time. Occasionally patients are treated initially for laryngitis and by the time a tumour has been diagnosed it is advanced. Otalgia, dyspnoea, dysphagia, neck lumps and weight loss are all symptoms of advanced laryngeal carcinoma.

MEDICAL MANAGEMENT

Carcinoma of the larynx has a high rate of cure if detected early, but sadly many people dismiss the classic symptom of hoarseness as trivial. The form of treatment offered will depend on the site of the tumour and on how early it has been detected. If the tumour is confined to the vocal cords it is usually diagnosed as a result of the patient consulting his medical practitioner with a history of hoarseness. Patients who have suffered from hoarseness for more than 3 weeks should have a mirror examination of their larynx (indirect laryngoscopy) to investigate the possibility of carcinoma. Diagnosis is confirmed by an examination of the patient's larynx under general anaesthesia (direct laryngoscopy) and a histological examination of a biopsy of the tumour.

The treatment of choice for a glottic tumour is a course of radiotherapy. If the disease is more extensive or the tumour has developed into the supraglottic or subglottic area, or if the vocal cord(s) have become immobile, radiotherapy is not the most effective treatment. The recommended treatment is most likely to be laryngectomy, which involves removal of the larynx, the creation of a permanent tracheostomy (see pp. 547–548) and the closure of the pharyngeal defect. Some tumours may not require a total laryngectomy, but can be effectively managed by a partial or hemi-laryngectomy. Laryngeal surgery may also have to be performed on patients who have a residual or recurrent tumour following radiotherapy. Nursing interventions appropriate to this procedure are outlined in the next section.

Very advanced tumours of the larynx may be considered inoperable, in which case the patient may be given palliative radiotherapy and/or chemotherapy to relieve some of the more distressing symptoms of the disease (see Ch. 31). In addition, a tracheostomy is sometimes performed to relieve any respiratory obstruction.

Laryngectomy

Preoperative preparation

Various members of the multidisciplinary team will spend some time with the patient and his family prior to surgery to explain the operation and its after-effects. This team will consist of medical and nursing staff, speech therapists, physiotherapists, medical social workers, dieticians and, often, former patients who have had a laryngectomy.

Physical preparation. Diagnostic radiography of the neck and chest is usually performed and CT scan or MRI carried out. A full blood analysis is made. Patients who are undergoing total laryngectomy may also require a partial thyroidectomy, in which case thyroid function must be checked pre- and postoperatively (see Ch. 5).

An electrocardiograph (ECG) is usually ordered to check heart function (see Ch. 2). The patient will also be given a dental check-up and receive any necessary dental treatment to help circumvent the risk of pathogenic organisms in the oral cavity. Local preparation of the skin may be required.

NURSING PRIORITIES AND MANAGEMENT: TOTAL LARYNGECTOMY

Preoperative priorities

The nurse's priorities at this stage will centre on providing support and information for the patient and his family and preparing them physically and psychologically for the operation (see Ch. 26; see also Research Abstract 14.2).

Q

14.9 Consider Case History 14.2. What information would you consider it important to obtain during an initial chat with Mr G to help you plan his nursing care?

Discuss this with your colleagues and check your ideas with your teacher or a qualified member of the nursing team.

The patient is usually admitted the day before surgery. It is important for the patient to get to know the team members at this stage, and in some units it is possible to meet the community nurse who will be helping him on his return home.

The patient and his family will need support in adjusting to the diagnosis of cancer and the altered body image which will result from this type of surgery (Price 1992) (see Case History 14.2). The patient will need to be prepared for the fact that he will have a permanent 'hole' in his neck through which he will breathe. He will be unable to talk initially. He will be able to swim only under supervision and after receiving advice and guidance on the use of special stoma devices. The patient will lose his sense of smell because he will take air through the mouth and stoma rather than the nose. In view of these after-effects, some patients will refuse therapy altogether, a decision which may be very difficult for the patient's family and members of the health care team to accept.

Research Abstract 14.2
Laryngectomy: the patient's view

This study of laryngectomy, which looked at the incidence of disability and acceptability, was carried out in Wolverhampton. Data were collected using a 10-question questionnaire. Sixty-five of the 82 patients approached replied, giving a response rate of 79%. Of the 65 who responded, 54 had undergone a total laryngectomy and 11 had this operation combined with a partial pharyngectomy. The average age was 68 years, the male:female ratio was 3:1, and the time since surgery ranged from 6 months to 35 years.

Respondents had experienced a substantial number and range of problems. These included having a worse sense of smell, being unable to blow their noses, experiencing difficulties in swallowing, an increase in chest infections, and stomal crusting or bleeding. None of the respondents reported weight loss and a majority were satisfied with their voice rehabilitation. Communication methods did not include voice prosthesis so one could reasonably expect this satisfaction rate to be higher now. Generally, respondents who felt they had achieved satisfactory rehabilitation indicated no reduction in their social acceptability. Thirty-four of the 54 people who replied to the question about their sexual activity said there was no restriction. Most of those who had enjoyed swimming prior to surgery (29%) expressed their unhappiness at being unable to continue. The availability of stoma swimming aids may help those anxious to swim again. A disappointing 9% of respondents continued to smoke, most having changed from cigarettes to pipe or cigars.

Despite their problems, 91% of respondents considered the operation to have been worthwhile and 78% had found a laryngectomy club to be useful.

These findings can and should be used to better inform patients preoperatively and to act as a focus for postoperative problem identification and education.

Jay S, Ruddy J, Cullen R J 1991 Laryngectomy: the patients' view. Journal of Laryngology and Otology 105: 934–938.

Case History 14.2 Mr G

Mr G is a 64-year-old retired labourer. A widower with no family, he lives alone but has helpful neighbours. He is a keen bowler and enjoys the social side of the bowling club. He also reads a lot and listens to music. He smokes 20 cigarettes a day and consumes about 30 units of alcohol per week. He has been diagnosed as having a subglottic tumour with extensive spread and a total laryngectomy has been recommended.

Mr G arrives at the ward with his friend Mr J and is welcomed by the staff nurse, who takes Mr G to a four-bed room and explains that he will be there until his operation and then in a single room for a few days while he recovers from the surgery. The nurse leaves Mr G and his friend to unpack his things and then returns with a cup of tea for them both. She asks about his activities of living with a view to planning his nursing care. Since Mr G's only relative is his wife's sister, who lives 200 miles away, he gives her name and that of his friend as next of kin. His friend tells the staff nurse that he and his wife will visit and do Mr G's washing for him.

To aid observation, the patient is usually nursed in a single room. He is admitted into this room so that he can familiarise himself with his surroundings. A nasogastric or stomagastric tube will be present postoperatively for feeding, as well as i.v. infusions, oxygen and wound drains. These, along with tracheal suction humidification and practical aspects of care, need to be demonstrated and discussed preoperatively to help reduce anxiety and thereby aid recovery (Feber 1998).

An appropriate means of communication which works for the patient, his family and the multidisciplinary team should be arranged before surgery. For example, a pad and pencil would usually be kept close to hand, but if the patient has literacy difficulties or problems with his sight, other means of communication must be sought. The establishment of a good communication scheme preoperatively will help the patient to regain his confidence postoperatively and should minimise frustration.

The speech therapist will visit the patient preoperatively to introduce herself and to explain her role. She may suggest to the patient that a visit from a previous laryngectomy patient would be of benefit. This visitor must be someone who has developed good speech, is an effective communicator and is well integrated back into the community. During this visit it may be suggested that the patient look at the visitor's stoma, but this issue is not forced. If well planned, these visits can be very reassuring to the patient and his family. Some people refuse the offer of such a visitor and their choice must be respected.

The physiotherapist will also assess the patient prior to surgery, explaining his role in the patient's postoperative care and teaching him deep breathing and leg exercises.

In the period leading up to surgery, it is important that any malnourishment is corrected by enteral or parenteral supplements. The dietician or nursing staff will assess the patient's nutritional state preoperatively and will explain to the patient how he will be fed postoperatively. Kelsey (1997) describes a successful nutritional assessment tool. The duration of parenteral feeding is dependent on the type of surgery performed and the state of the wound.

Postoperative priorities

Immediately following surgery the main nursing priorities will be maintenance of a clear airway (see Box 14.6), observation of the tracheostome, establishment of good communication with the patient, and reassurance and support of the patient and his family.

A nurse will 'special' the patient for the first 24 h in a single room or high-dependency unit. He will be nursed in the semi-recumbent position initially and then gradually encouraged to sit more upright to aid respiration and neck drainage. It is important that the patient's head is flexed slightly forward to ease tension on the suture lines. When the patient is being moved, his head should always be supported by a nurse.

Box 14.6 Resuscitation of a 'neck breathing' patient

The principles of resuscitation of a 'neck breathing' patient are the same as those for any other patient, although a few alterations of technique apply. The ABCs of first aid — airway, breathing and circulation — are given top priority.

Initially, the stoma would be covered by the resuscitator's mouth, but as soon as possible a cuffed tracheal tube should be inserted, and inflated to prevent any leakage of the air which is being introduced by the resuscitator. The tube should then be connected to an Ambu bag and resuscitation continued as normal.

On return to the ward, the patient's vital signs should be recorded at half-hourly intervals; as these become stable within the normal range, recordings can be reduced to 4-hourly.

In the immediate postoperative period the naso/stomagastric tube should be on free drainage, to prevent vomiting. This allows the pharyngeal repair to heal and prevents fistula formation (see Box 14.7). A stomagastric tube is inserted through a created tracheo-oesophageal fistula which is later used for a voice prosthesis.

Once bowel sounds have been detected (usually 24 h postoperatively) the patient can commence oral fluids. Water is given for the first hour and then full-strength feeding gradually established. This gradual progression is necessary to avoid the problems of vomiting and diarrhoea. Before administering each feed, the nurse must check that the naso/stomagastric tube is in the correct position.

Q **14.10** What are the methods for confirming that the naso/stomagastric tubes are correctly positioned in the stomach? (See Ch. 21)

Box 14.7 Potential complications of laryngectomy

Blockage of trachea
This potentially life-threatening complication can occur if the trachea has not been sufficiently humidified. The potential for tracheal blockage should be stressed during the teaching programme, as it tends to occur when patients have returned to the community and have not cared for their stoma (in particular the humidification and cleansing aspects of care) as taught in hospital.

Stenosis of the tracheostome
Like tracheal blockage, this complication is potentially life-threatening and may occur when the patient has returned to the community. It can arise as a result of neglect which has allowed crusting to build up in and around the stoma or it may be the result of fibrosis as healing takes place. Careful and regular toilet of the stoma should prevent its occurrence, and the wearing of a tube or stoma button for part or all of the time can be a useful preventive measure if fibrosis is the problem.

Failure to produce voice
Coltart (1998) discusses why, despite advances including surgical voice restoration and the use of voice prostheses, not all patients learn to speak again but become dependent on non-verbal communication.

Fistula formation
If the pharyngeal repair breaks down, a fistula may form which allows saliva and food to leak from the incision, causing excoriation of the skin and possibly leading to infection. This is usually treated by inserting a feeding tube and not allowing anything to be consumed orally. Reilly (1998) gives a comprehensive overview on enteral feeding, including techniques which can be used in this situation. Healing may take several weeks and antibiotics may be prescribed if infection is present. If the fistula does not heal by itself, surgical closure may be necessary.

Wound breakdown
This may occur in patients who are undergoing a course of radiotherapy following surgery. Careful wound care can help to prevent its occurrence.

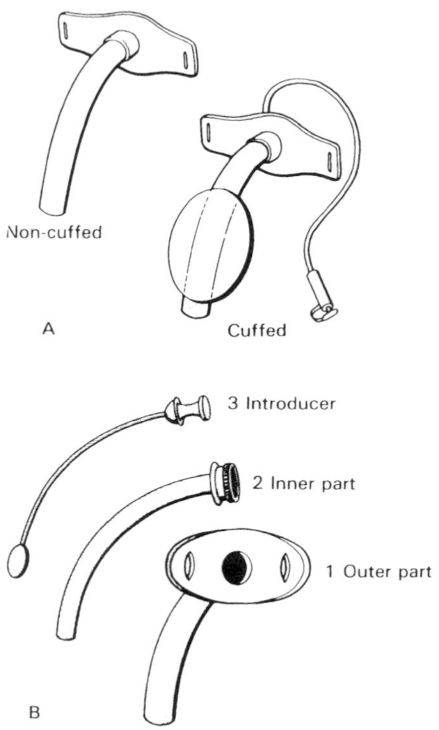

Fig. 14.7 Tracheostomy tubes in common use. A: Disposable. B: Non-disposable. (Reproduced with kind permission from Jamieson et al 1997.)

Once naso/stomagastric feeding has been established the i.v. infusion will be discontinued.

Humidified oxygen is administered to the patient during the immediate postoperative period to help keep the lining of the tracheal mucosa and the inspired gases moist (Baxter et al 1993). On his return to the ward he may have a cuffed (preferably with a low-pressure cuff) tracheostomy tube in position (see Fig. 14.7). The cuff pressure must be recorded and released as soon as possible to prevent damage to the tracheal lining. The tube is usually removed 24–48 h after surgery. Some patients return from theatre without a tube in position; here careful observation of the stoma for swelling or obstruction will be necessary. Normally, excessive secretions are moved into the trachea by ciliary action and expelled by coughing; for the new laryngectomy patient, however, this can be difficult. Tracheal suction is usually necessary in the immediate postoperative period as these secretions can be excessive and the patient able to make only limited coughing movements.

A suction drain will be present on each side of the neck. These drains must be patent and the vacuum maintained at all times. The colour, nature and amount of drainage must be recorded. The wound is usually closed with fine sutures or clips and may be covered by a clear plastic dressing so that it can be easily observed. Stoma care is performed as necessary and usually at least twice daily postoperatively to prevent crusting.

Good pressure area care is necessary in the first 24 h, but care must be taken when moving the patient due to his neck wound. A 2-hourly change of position should be carried out and full use made of special mattresses.

The immediate postoperative period can be very difficult for the patient and his family as they realise the full implications of the surgery. Often the patient is very agitated the first time he is awake enough to ask for something and discovers that he has no voice. The communication skills of the ENT nurse are especially important at this time. The nurse should remind the patient of the prearranged communication plan and display patience and understanding (see Box 14.8). The patient should never be left without any means of communication such as a buzzer or bell. This is very important for the patient's confidence, as he may have the very natural fear of requiring tracheal suction and not being able to attract attention.

Box 14.8 Communication with a person who has lost the ability to speak following head and neck surgery

- As much preoperative explanation and information as possible should be given in the time available.
- Adequate materials, e.g. pen, paper, picture cards or 'magic' slate, should be available (and seen by patient to be available) before surgery and subsequently at all times.
- Be patient, and maintain a calm and unhurried atmosphere.
- Always give encouragement and praise.
- Remember that previous hearing levels have not been altered. There is no need for you to raise your voice or write down information.
- Pay extra special attention to non-verbal communication such as facial expression, hand and body positions and movements.
- Stress that the inability to communicate is temporary; skill levels will considerably improve in almost all patients.
- Communicating by writing only is difficult for most. The following points are worth remembering:
  —some people are unable to read or write, i.e. they are illiterate
  —writing takes much longer than speaking
  —writing can be disruptive of thought processes
  —for most people it is difficult to communicate depth of emotions and feelings by the written word
  —lack of privacy (? use 'magic' slate which can be immediately erased)
  —never read a previously written communication unless invited to do so.
- Do not ask two questions at once.
- On occasions, ask questions that only require a yes or no answer.
- Develop your own lip-reading skills.
- Do not finish sentences for the patient.
- If the person is only able to say the first few words or part of a sentence, repeat what you have understood and ask him to fill in on what you have missed.

Q **14.11** Try not speaking for a minimum of 1 h during an average non-working day. Record how you felt during this time, indicating the number of times you went to speak and the times you actually were unable to stop yourself automatically speaking. Discuss your findings with your mentor or personal tutor.

Mouth care is very important while the nasogastric tube is in position and should be carried out at least 4-hourly, as well as around the time when feeds are due in order to stimulate digestive juices. The specific mouth care given to each patient will be determined by individual assessment.

On the first or second postoperative day, the patient is usually well enough to be helped out of bed and begin walking. Over the following days he should be encouraged to increase his activity until he is fully ambulant.

Naso/stomagastric feeding is continued until the patient's pharyngeal repair is fully healed (usually 10–14 days after surgery). This is tested by giving the patient a drink of dye and observing the wound for any signs of leakage as he swallows. Barium or niopam swallows are alternatives. If the wound appears to have healed, the nasostoma/gastric tube is removed at the surgeon's discretion and the patient is allowed to commence a soft diet. Foods should be of a gradually increasing consistency until a normal diet for that person is tolerated.

Wound drains are removed when drainage is minimal (approximately 3–4 days after surgery). The neck sutures may be removed on approximately the seventh day, although they may remain in position a few days longer if the patient has had previous radiotherapy. Stoma sutures are usually removed after 10 days.

Tracheal suction is given when necessary but the need for this should gradually diminish as the patient's cough reflexes become stronger. Stoma care is continuous; the nurse should encourage the patient to participate in this. Humidification may still be required at certain times and can be administered via a mechanical humidifier. Alternatively, a Buchanan laryngectomy or other protector may be worn. The patient should be taught how to remove any crusting which may form around the stoma. Patients requiring to wear a tube or stoma button must be shown how to use it.

Rehabilitation of the patient should start as soon as possible; ideally, this will involve the supportive participation of the patient's family and of the community nurse. The patient will first need to become accustomed to his altered appearance. If appropriate, he could be given a hand mirror on perhaps the second postoperative day after he has been told about what to expect. The presence of family members at this time might be helpful but the patient should make the decision about this. Progress in wound healing and a decrease in face and neck puffiness over a period of days can be encouraging for the patient. Once he has become accustomed to looking in a mirror, he may be encouraged to wipe away secretions from his stoma, gradually progressing to performing stoma care and changing his stoma tube or button by himself. The patient must be made aware of the importance of wearing a protector for humidification purposes to prevent the formation of crusts which can cause obstruction as well as a predisposition to chest infections.

Voice rehabilitation

Coltart (1998) considers what forms of operative planning will be most appropriate to achieve the best results for the patient. The surgeon will have discussed voice rehabilitation with the patient preoperatively, in conjunction with the speech therapist and other members of the multidisciplinary team. In selecting the most appropriate voice aid, they will have addressed the physical, social and psychological needs of the patient, as not every voice aid is suited to all patients.

Following laryngectomy, voice rehabilitation may only begin when the surgeon is satisfied that the wounds are adequately healed. Some patients will be reviewed in outpatient departments for fitting of a prosthesis. The speech therapist will see patients on a regular basis to teach the use of the aid. It is important to advise patients that it can take time to achieve coherent speech again.

Once the naso/stomagastric tube has been removed, the speech therapist can begin to start voice restoration by means of speaking valves or oesophageal speech. If the patient has mastered a few simple words such as 'yes' and 'no' prior to discharge, his confidence may be increased tremendously. Motivation and support are important factors in the acquisition of speech; again, the participation of the patient's family can be of enormous benefit. Following discharge the patient will continue to attend for speech therapy. Voice restoration methods available for individuals who have undergone laryngectomy are described in Box 14.9.

Box 14.9 Voice restoration after laryngectomy

Oesophageal speech
This used to be the only method available to restore voice after laryngectomy. It requires regular specialised speech therapy over a period of months, at least. Success rates vary dramatically. If a valve has been inserted, most speech therapists will still teach this method alongside the techniques used with valves, as no single method can guarantee success.

Tracheo-oesophageal puncture with voice prosthesis
The voice prosthesis is a valve which can be inserted into a tracheo-oesophageal puncture created at the time of laryngectomy (primary puncture) or later (secondary puncture) if necessary. The patient breathes in, covers his stoma with a finger, thus forcing expired air through the valve and producing voice. Alternatively, a special housing which opens on inspiration and closes on expiration can be used instead of the patient's finger. The speech therapist will teach the patient and nursing staff how to care for the valve. The most commonly used valves are the Blom Singer and Provox.

Electronic Vibrator or Artificial Larynx.
The device produces a tone when applied to the soft tissues of the neck. When the patient articulates, sound is produced. The sound is monotonous, mechanical and somewhat 'Dalek'-like in nature.

Preparation for discharge

By demonstrating patience and understanding and sensitively implementing a planned rehabilitation programme, the multidisciplinary team can help to build up the patient's confidence prior to discharge, to try to ensure that he will be able to cope with any problem that may arise. The patient should feel at ease with his stoma and be confident in caring for it and any voice prosthesis. He should be encouraged to socialise with other patients, perhaps by moving to a multi-bed room. This may be difficult at first but should be seen as a first step to socialising after discharge. Mason et al (1992) describe a stepwise method for teaching self-care to laryngectomy patients prior to discharge, called the Nottingham system. The aim of this system is to identify problems early, assess progress continuously and provide extra support when needed. Tracheostomy care is divided into 10 different aspects of care, e.g. removing the tube, cleaning the stoma and skin care. Each element of care is then broken down into five teaching phases, commencing with the professional performing the task for the patient and ending when the patient is totally self-caring. The date of successful completion of each phase is recorded. Before starting the teaching plan an agreement is reached between patient and professionals on the anticipated number of days required to reach competence. If a patient is found to require a considerably longer time to gain competence in any aspect of self-care, his GP is informed of the likely need for extra support. Although the Nottingham system was devised for laryngectomy patients, it can just as easily be used for those who have had a tracheostomy.

The community nursing services will be involved in preparations for the patient's return home. They will be contacted by ward staff as soon as a discharge date has been decided. The community nurse's main role is one of support and she will withdraw services slowly as the patient becomes increasingly confident at home.

The social worker is often required to help patients and their families with practical difficulties before, during and following surgery. Individuals who have undergone a laryngectomy may be unable to return to their former employment; for example, patients previously employed doing heavy manual labour, being unable to hold their breath and increase intrathoracic pressure, will be unable to resume such work. Negotiation between the social worker and the employer to try to find a feasible job reallocation may allow such a patient to continue working. However, if continued employment is impossible, the social worker will assist patients to receive all the social security benefits to which they are entitled. The social worker may also be able to help patients and their families with travelling expenses during the treatment programme.

Patients will attend the ENT outpatient clinic after discharge to ensure that no problems arise with which they feel unable to cope. The National Association of Laryngectomy Clubs (NALC) circulates a regular newsletter and has branches in most areas of the UK (see 'Useful addresses', p. 553). The support which this association can give is invaluable to many patients, who greatly benefit from the opportunity to share experiences and talk about problems with others in a similar situation. NALC also holds regular national study days for nurses and other health care professionals. Many patients form lasting friendships with the previous laryngectomy patient(s) who visited them preoperatively.

For further information on coping with dysfunction and disfigurement after head and neck cancer surgery, see Dropkin (1989, 1997). For information on promoting self-esteem after laryngectomy, see Feber (1996). More information on rehabilitation is to be found in Baker (1992).

Tracheostomy

The surgical procedure of tracheostomy involves making an opening through the skin and structures of the neck into the trachea. It is one of the earliest operations described; there is evidence that it was performed by the Egyptians in biblical times.

A tracheostomy may be temporary or permanent and may be planned as elective surgery or performed as an emergency procedure.

Indications

The indications for a tracheostomy are as follows:

- *Airway obstruction.* This may be caused by the inhalation and impaction of a foreign body in the larynx. Severe inflammation may also cause obstruction. Laryngeal cancer which is being treated by radiotherapy may also cause obstruction.
- *Bronchial toilet.* After head injury, drug overdose, cerebral vascular accident, coma or certain neurological disorders, the patient may require assistance with respiration and removal of bronchial secretions.
- *Need to improve respiratory efficiency.* When patients with impaired respiration are relying on their own efforts rather than assisted ventilation, the performance of a tracheostomy cuts down dead space and improves respiratory efficiency by 30–50% (Serra 1998).
- *Artificial ventilation.* If artificial ventilation is required for more than 72 h, a tracheostomy may be indicated, as it has been shown that endotracheal intubation for 72 h or longer can cause laryngotracheal damage.
- *Major head and neck surgery.* A tracheostomy will maintain the airway and protect it from haemorrhage and obstruction due to oedema both during and after surgery (see also Ch. 28).

Box 14.10 lists some of the indications for temporary and permanent tracheostomies.

MEDICAL MANAGEMENT

Prior to performing a tracheostomy, the medical staff must explain to the patient what is involved and the effect the procedure will have. In an emergency situation, such as when the patient presents with stridor, the medical and nursing staff will have very little time to prepare the patient preoperatively. Consequently, a planned programme of support and explanation will be required afterwards.

Tracheostomy is usually carried out with the patient under a general anaesthetic, but in emergencies a local anaesthetic may be used. Tracheostomy involves making an incision into the trachea through the third and fourth tracheal rings. The percutaneous or mini-tracheostomy is a recent innovation which is sometimes used in the ENT situation.

For further information on this, see Fisher & Howard (1992) and Nelson (1992).

An appropriately sized tracheostomy tube is then inserted. For the first 24–48 h, a cuffed tracheostomy tube (see Fig. 14.7) is normally used to prevent blood from the wound being aspirated and aspiration pneumonia developing. A permanent tract usually forms 2–3 days postoperatively, at which time it is possible to change the tube. Tracheal dilators must always be to hand in case the tube is expelled accidentally and it is necessary to keep the stoma open. The first tube change should be performed by medical staff or by experienced nursing staff with medical back-up.

Box 14.10 Indications for tracheostomy

Temporary tracheostomy
- Anaphylactic oedema
- Assisted ventilation
- Burns and scalds
- Foreign body lodged in trachea
- Major head and neck surgery
- Severe infection
- Trauma to larynx, face, mouth or oropharynx
- Vocal cord paralysis

Permanent tracheostomy
- Congenital deformity
- Trauma causing permanent damage
- Tumours
- Vocal cord paralysis

There are several types of tracheostomy tube available, and the most appropriate one will be chosen for each patient. As mentioned above, a cuffed tube, preferably with a low-pressure cuff, may be inserted during the operation. Single-use disposable tubes are usually employed and may be cuffed or plain. They have an introducer which is removed immediately on insertion. All have an inner tube which can be removed for cleaning without necessitating removal of the whole tube. Less commonly used now are silver tracheostomy tubes, although they may still be used by a patient who had a tracheostomy performed many years ago.

NURSING PRIORITIES AND MANAGEMENT: TRACHEOSTOMY

Preoperative priorities

The physical and psychological preparation of the individual for a tracheostomy is a priority of preoperative nursing care as the procedure can present him with many difficulties. If the tracheostomy is temporary, at least these problems will be of limited duration, but if it is to be permanent, the patient and his family will require additional information and education in order to be able to cope. They may need help in coming to terms not only with the problems presented by the stoma but also with the diagnosis (e.g. cancer) that necessitated surgery. Patients who have been well prepared for a tracheostomy tend to cope better than those who have not. Unprepared patients may become insecure, withdrawn and depressed. The main problems in the immediate postoperative period for which the patient has to be prepared prior to surgery are as follows:

Temporary loss of voice. Air will bypass the vocal cords following the tracheostomy, making speech impossible unless a tube with a speaking valve is inserted. A system of communication whereby the patient can make herself understood by staff and family members should be worked out beforehand (see p. 545).

Altered body image. Information and education must be offered to the patient to help him and his family adjust to the fact that she will have a tube in his neck. A visit from a patient who has adjusted well to having a tracheostomy may help.

Increased secretions. These are produced because of the irritation caused by the tube and air bypassing the nose. This should be explained to the patient along with the need for suction; it is helpful to show the equipment required for this before the surgery.

Ideally, a patient undergoing tracheostomy should be nursed in a single room initially and his care assigned to one nurse who can gain his confidence and that of his family.

Postoperative priorities

Maintenance of the airway

On his return to the ward the patient should be nursed in a sitting position with his neck well supported; the tapes around his neck, which are fixed to the flange of the tracheostomy tube, must be tied securely in position.

Suction should be carried out when secretions appear to be accumulating and blocking the airway. To prevent infection, it is necessary to perform this procedure with a clean technique (Harris 1984, Harris & Hyman 1984) (see Ch. 29). A sterile catheter should be used each time and should touch only the inside of the tracheostomy tube. The catheter diameter should be no more than half that of the tube to allow adequate flow of gases around it. If it is too wide, it will draw air out of the lungs more quickly than it can be replaced, which can cause atelectasis (Serra et al 1986). Griggs (1998) gives a formula and chart to allow calculation of the correct catheter size.

Suction should be applied only as the catheter is being removed (thumb-control catheters are ideal for this). Since the patient is unable to breathe during suction, it should be performed for no longer than 10–15 s; the patient should be allowed enough time to recover before it is repeated. The amount and type of secretions should be observed and recorded.

The physiotherapist will teach the patient how to cough into a tissue; as the patient becomes competent at this, the need for suction will gradually be eliminated.

Continuous humidification is given immediately postoperatively via a mechanical humidifier. When the patient begins to be up and about, a protector over the stoma will humidify inhaled air. This will also act as a filter and have a cosmetic effect by disguising the tracheostomy tube.

Care of the wound

The stoma into which the tube is inserted will require regular cleansing to prevent crusting and infection. A dressing beneath the tracheostomy tube will help to prevent pressure sores caused by the tube as well as excoriation of the skin from secretions which are expectorated. Some sutures may be present; these will normally be removed according to local policy (see Ch. 23 p. 758).

For further information on adult tracheostomy care, see Serra (1995, 1998).

Complications

The nurse should be on the alert for the following potential complications after tracheostomy.

Blockage of tracheostomy tube. Tracheal dilators and a spare tracheostomy tube must always be kept to hand in case this problem arises. Sometimes the blockage can be relieved by suction or by changing the inner tube. At other times it will be necessary to change the whole tube.

Displacement of the tube. The tube can become displaced into the pretracheal tissue or right out of the stoma if the tapes holding it in place have not been secured adequately. Dilators should be used to keep the stoma open until the tube can be replaced. Tapes should be checked for correct fit at least twice daily. Assessment and management of a patient in this situation are described by Seay & Gay (1997).

Surgical emphysema. Emphysema is the abnormal presence of air in the tissues. Surgical emphysema is iatrogenic, being a result of faulty suturing, and can be corrected by releasing the sutures.

Haemorrhage. The insertion of a cuffed tracheostomy tube can help to control bleeding and prevent aspiration of blood. It is possible, however, for a major blood vessel to be eroded by a badly placed or poorly managed tube, causing a massive haemorrhage.

Dysphagia, nausea, vomiting. If the tracheostomy tube is the wrong shape for the type of tracheostomy and the size of the patient, it may exert pressure on the posterior wall of the trachea and oesophagus, resulting in nausea, dysphagia and vomiting. These effects can be relieved by the insertion of a different tube.

Damage to the tracheal mucosa. This can result from poor suctioning technique, badly chosen or improperly inserted tubes, or prolonged and overinflation of the tube cuff. Ulceration of the anterior wall or a tracheo-oesophageal fistula may result and can lead to tracheal stenosis.

Infection. A wound or respiratory tract infection can result from poor technique when performing stoma toilet, changing the tube or applying suction, or from inadequate maintenance of respiratory status.

Changing the tracheostomy tube

The first tube change should be performed by experienced medical or nursing staff, as it takes 2–3 days for a tract to form and there is a danger of the tube being displaced or inserted into the pretracheal tissues. Two people should always be present for this procedure. One will remove the old tube and the other will immediately insert the new one. The tapes are then securely tied.

Decannulation or removal of the tube

Occasionally the tube can be removed without any preliminaries, but usually the patient is gradually reintroduced to breathing through his nose and mouth. A tube with a speaking valve allows the patient to breathe in through the tube and out through his larynx. Once the patient has become accustomed to this, the tube can be replaced by a 'blocker' so that he has to breathe in through his nose and mouth. When he is able to tolerate this continuously for 24 h and his oxygen saturation levels are satisfactory day and night, the tracheostomy tube can be removed. Another method of achieving decannulation is to insert a smaller tube each time it is changed.

Whichever method is used, after removal of the tube an airtight dressing must be applied to allow the tracheostomy site to heal. This can be a very anxious time for patients and support and encouragement are necessary. The stoma should shrink rapidly and close off in a short time.

Humidification

Humidification will prevent the tracheostomy patient breathing in cold dry air which could cause the secretions of the trachea to become dry and difficult to remove and eventually lead to infection and blockage of the tube. A selection of aesthetically pleasing covers which humidify and filter air are available and the patient should be introduced to these before discharge.

Preparation for discharge

Before discharge can take place, the patient and his family must be well prepared for all foreseeable difficulties and should be proficient in changing the tracheostomy tube. The teaching of self-care techniques can begin with the nurse demonstrating procedures while the patient watches in a mirror. It is wise to teach not only the patient but also his family how to care for the tracheostomy in case the occasion arises when the patient is unable to do this himself (Mason et al 1992). However, some surgeons do prefer their patients to report to the ward or outpatient department for a weekly tube change.

Minsley & Wrenn (1996) outline outpatient nursing care.

The community nurse will be actively involved in the patient's discharge and reintegration into the community. Ideally, she will visit the patient in hospital and arrange for suction apparatus to be installed in his home if necessary. After discharge she should visit the patient regularly to ensure that he is coping with his stoma and altered body image (see Ch. 4 and Serra 1986).

Tonsillitis

The tonsils are composed of lymphoid tissue and lie between the faucial pillars (see Fig. 14.8). During early childhood they enlarge in response to upper respiratory tract infections and in adulthood should become reduced in size. In old age they normally atrophy.

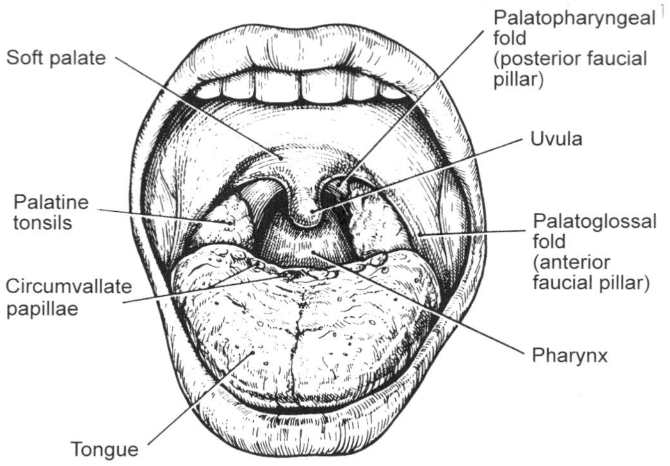

Fig. 14.8 Tonsils and surrounding area.

It is generally agreed that tonsils have a role to play in the body's defence system against infection.

Each year an average of 12 000 people in the UK undergo the surgical procedure of tonsillectomy. The majority of these patients are 14 years of age or younger. Among people aged 15–25, more females seem to require this surgery than males. Among the elderly population the tonsils are usually removed as a treatment for tumour.

PATHOPHYSIOLOGY

Common presenting symptoms. Patients usually present with a history of pain in the throat. This may be due to the many lesions caused by infection or to the presence of a tumour. Tonsil pain increases with swallowing and is often referred to the ear because of the involvement of the trigeminal nerve, which supplies both sites.

Recurrent bouts of infection are the most common reason for the removal of tonsils. Infection may take the form of acute tonsillitis, acute otitis media (see p. 532) or a peritonsillar abscess (see p. 550). Streptococci, staphylococci, and *Haemophilus influenzae* are the organisms most commonly present.

Patients with tonsillar tumours normally present with dysphagia. These patients usually also complain of weight loss and may have speech problems. They may also suffer from facial pain and deafness because of the involvement of cranial nerves. Tonsillar tumours are rare.

MEDICAL MANAGEMENT

There is some controversy among medical practitioners about when tonsil infections should be treated conservatively and when tonsillectomy, with or without adenoidectomy, should be performed. Each surgeon has his own criteria for the removal of a patient's tonsils. The size of the tonsils is not usually the main criterion, but rather the history of the effect of repeated infections on the general health of the patient. Consideration is also given to absence from school or work, loss of appetite, speech defects, nasal catarrh or colds, hearing loss, breathing problems and abdominal pain (a sign of mesenteric adenitis which occurs because of transmission of infection through the lymphatic system).

Tonsillectomy is an elective operation and is not considered in the presence of respiratory tract infections or during the incubation period after contact with an infectious disease or if there is tonsillar inflammation.

There are two methods of carrying out the operation. The guillotine method is very rarely performed nowadays as it puts the patient at risk of potential complications such as mesenteric adenitis. The current method of choice for adults (and children) is tonsil dissection. In this method, bleeding vessels are ligated or diathermy is applied, whereas in the guillotine method the vessels are left to seal themselves by contraction.

NURSING PRIORITIES AND MANAGEMENT: TONSILLECTOMY

Postoperative priorities

Airway

On returning from theatre, patients should be positioned in the post-tonsillectomy position, i.e. semi-prone (Serra et al 1986). This allows any blood or saliva to flow out of the mouth and helps keep the airway clear.

Haemorrhage

Half-hourly recordings of pulse and blood pressure and observations of breathing, pallor, restlessness and frequent swallowing are carried out to permit early diagnosis of haemorrhage. Frequent swallowing is one of the first signs of tonsil haemorrhage and can go unnoticed unless the patient is closely observed. Particular attention must be paid to the sleeping patient.

Chewing and swallowing

Encouraging the patient to eat regularly (Cook et al 1992) and to swallow is important, as the exercising of the throat muscles seems to help keep the tonsil bed free from infection and to prevent the occurrence of secondary haemorrhage.

Infection

Pyrexia is not uncommon on the first postoperative day as part of the general metabolic response to the trauma of surgery, but if it continues antibiotics should be prescribed and the source of infection sought.

Analgesics

Prescribed analgesics should be administered and their effectiveness observed. They should be administered before meals, before going to sleep and first thing in the morning. Good pain management is vital in ensuring the patient has a comfortable and uncomplicated postoperative recovery.

Preparation for discharge

Patients are usually discharged from hospital within 24 h. They are advised to avoid dirty, dusty atmospheres for approximately 2 weeks and to take a similar amount of time away from work or school/college. An advice sheet should be given on discharge with a contact number to ring should any difficulties be experienced at home, including bleeding, pyrexia and otalgia (earache). Research Abstract 14.3 discusses post-tonsillectomy morbidity after discharge.

Post-tonsillectomy pain control and pain relief following discharge and the adequacy and accuracy of preoperative information and advice were the topics of a study by Stone (1996).

Research Abstract 14.3
Early post-tonsillectomy morbidity

This prospective study was undertaken to assess the amount and nature of post-tonsillectomy morbidity within 2 weeks of discharge from hospital. Complete follow-up data were obtained from 149 patients (103 children under 16 years and 46 adults) when they attended a follow-up review with one of the authors.

All patients were admitted on the day of surgery, had their tonsils removed by dissection and, with two exceptions, were discharged within 24 h. The two exceptions were discharged within 36 h when pyrexia had subsided and oral antibiotics had been commenced.

Following verbal advice from medical and nursing staff, all patients were discharged with oral analgesics and a written information sheet, which advised different actions for specific problems. In spite of this, a surprisingly large number of patients contacted their GP. Whether these patients were adults or children is not stated. Forty patients (27%) were responsible for a total of 53 GP consultations, 23 were prescribed antibiotics and two were prescribed mouth washes. Throat pain was the commonest reason for consultation. Two out of five patients who consulted for otalgia were inappropriately prescribed a topical steroid and antibiotic. The responses to secondary haemorrhage were particularly worrying. Nineteen patients had this potentially fatal complication. Despite clear advice to the contrary, only seven patients sought advice or care. The inability to recognise expected symptoms such as throat pain or to seek advice for haemorrhage, despite the information given, led the authors to suggest that all patients who experienced any operation-related problems should telephone the ward in the first instance. The need to improve or reinforce information was recognised, as well as the very real increase in workload for GPs and increase in antibiotic prescriptions. Other suggestions for improvement included routine assessment by a nurse practitioner and giving patients a review appointment which could be cancelled if all was well.

As the number of day-case patients and early discharges continue to rise, the need to provide them with information which can be clearly understood, remembered and accepted, so as to enable patients to recognise problems and act appropriately when they do occur, is essential. General practitioners must also become familiar with normal symptoms and responses to tonsillectomy.

Kuo M, Hegarty D, Johnson A, Stevenson S 1995 Early post-tonsillectomy morbidity following hospital discharge: do patients and GPs know what to expect? Health Trends 27(3): 98 –100.

Peritonsillar abscesses (quinsy)

PATHOPHYSIOLOGY

This is a very painful condition and can be life-threatening. It usually occurs as a complication of acute tonsillitis. Pus forms in the space behind the capsule of the tonsil. The abscess is usually unilateral and affects males more than females.

The patient presents with a pyrexia high enough to cause a rigor. There is usually a history of an episode of acute tonsillitis which has subsided only to return on one side. There is acute pain radiating to the ear on the affected side, trismus (spasm of the jaw muscles) is present and swallowing is so difficult that saliva dribbles out of the mouth. The voice becomes muffled because of the large swelling and affected function of the palate. The neck glands on the affected side will be enlarged and tender.

MEDICAL MANAGEMENT

Antibiotic cover must be prescribed and the abscess may need to be incised and drained. Usually it is necessary to administer i.v. fluids, and antibiotics are always given parenterally for the first 24 h. Analgesics will be required when the pain is severe. Very rarely the swelling will be so severe that it will obstruct the airway; it may then be necessary to perform a tracheostomy to allow the patient to breathe.

NURSING PRIORITIES AND MANAGEMENT: PERITONSILLAR ABSCESS

Nursing care of the patient with peritonsillar abscess will include:

- physical and psychological support of the patient
- administration of analgesics, antipyretics and antibiotics
- administration of prescribed i.v. fluids
- ensuring good oral hygiene
- observation and recording of the patient's airway, temperature, pulse, blood pressure, fluid intake and output
- care of the tracheostomy if this has been performed (see p. 548).

Patients who require admission to hospital will be very anxious, agitated and in pain. They will require explanations, reassurance and swift administration of analgesics. As many will be unable to swallow, observations must be made for signs of dehydration and it will be necessary to administer i.v. fluids as prescribed by medical staff.

Good oral hygiene is important, especially once the abscess has been drained, as the patient will have had to spit out pus and will have a foul taste in his mouth. Once the pain has been relieved by analgesics and drainage of the abscess, the patient will be able to commence oral fluids and gradually begin taking a normal diet. Oral antibiotics will be substituted for the i.v. administration.

The patient is usually discharged once he is able to eat and drink normally and has been apyrexial for 24 h. If the abscess has been severe enough to require a tracheostomy, this would be removed and the patient would be discharged only when the wound had healed. Patients are often sent home before they have finished their course of antibiotics; the importance of completing the course must therefore be clearly explained to them. Most patients are re-admitted in 6–8 weeks to have a tonsillectomy performed (if they have a previous history of tonsillitis) as peritonsillar abscesses have a habit of recurring.

For further details of the management and care of a patient with a peritonsillar abscess, see McCall (1993).

Snoring/obstructive sleep apnoea (OSA)

Over the last few years, the issue of snoring in association with OSA has been addressed as it has been recognised that these individuals may have a contributing anatomical defect.

PATHOPHYSIOLOGY

The patient may show signs of chronic sleep deprivation. The patient's partner and/or family may complain of loud snoring and periods of breath-holding when he is asleep. This may be as a result of the tissues of the soft palate and pharynx collapsing and causing a temporary obstruction of the oropharynx. When the patient breathes, this tissue, including the uvula and possibly large tonsils, may vibrate, resulting in loud snoring. Patients may hold their breath due to this obstructing tissue. This condition can be dangerous, due to the possible development of severe hypoxaemia and systemic and pulmonary hypertension (Shenwell & Wilson 1994).

MEDICAL MANAGEMENT

Investigations. Admission to hospital for a sedation nasendoscopy will be necessary. By means of a nasendoscope the medical staff can view the oropharynx of the sleeping patient and observe the activity and position of the tissues and structures. At this time monitoring of oxygen saturation levels is also possible.

Treatment. A variety of treatments is available. These include weight loss in overweight people, change of sleeping position and the use of nasal decongestants. Continuous positive airway pressure may also be used (see below).

If it is obvious that there is collapse of excess tissues in the oropharynx then the surgical technique of uvulopalatopharyngoplasty, with or without tonsillectomy, may be performed at a later date. This involves tightening of the soft palate and pharyngeal tissue, removal of the uvula and possible tonsillectomy. Correction using a laser or punctate diathermy is an alternative procedure (Macdougald 1994, Whinney et al 1995).

Lasers are used for a wide range of problems in ENT, not only sleep apnoea. See McKennis & Waddington (1993) for fuller details.

NURSING PRIORITIES AND MANAGEMENT: OBSTRUCTIVE SLEEP APNOEA (OSA)

Uvulopalatopharyngoplasty

The priorities and management are the same as for tonsillectomy (see p. 550). Patients may experience nasal regurgitation on swallowing. This will usually resolve over a short period of time.

Continuous positive air pressure (CPAP)

This treatment avoids surgery and can be carried out by the patient in his own home each night. The patient requires a considerable amount of education and supervision during the initial stages and continuous ongoing support. This education and support are usually provided by a specialist nurse who plays a key role in coordinating and implementing continuity of care from the initial sleep investigation stage and throughout.

Nasal CPAP works as a pneumatic splint, as the continuous positive pressure stops the pharynx collapsing and vibrating. At night the patient wears a well-fitting nasal mask which is connected via tubing to a small machine which delivers the positive pressure airflow. The mouth is left uncovered. The nasal cavity needs to be free of obstruction.

Most patients tolerate it well despite occasional problems with nasal and face irritation. It is most commonly used for moderate to severe OSA.

For further information on sleep apnoea see Shenwell & Wilson (1994), Macdougald (1994) and Kendrick (1995).

CONCLUSION

The speciality of ENT care is a constantly evolving one that presents many challenges to the nurse. She will encounter patients of various ages and backgrounds who will have specific needs with respect to the intensity, duration and setting of treatment. The ENT nurse is likely to encounter a wide range of disorders, some of which will have profound implications for the patient's ability to function within his family, work and social spheres and which will require thorough assessment and individualised care planning. As always, the nurse's ability as communicator will do much to determine the effectiveness of her interventions. In this speciality, in which many patients will suffer from disorders that will impair hearing and/or the ability to speak, the need for skill and inventiveness in communication is especially important.

Nurses in various fields can make an important contribution to health education and preventive care as it relates to, for example, smoking and potential and existing ENT disorders. By helping to implement programmes for MMR vaccination, community and school nurses help to prevent the hearing impairment often seen in children whose mothers contract rubella during the early months of their pregnancy. A knowledge of how to evaluate noise levels can help occupational health nurses to protect workers from noise-induced hearing loss, and school nurses can alert young people to the fact that personal stereos are capable of producing the same volume of sound as a pneumatic drill, and thus present a serious risk of hearing impairment. For patients with a chronic condition such as Ménière's disease or tinnitus, hospital and community nurses can provide ongoing psychological support, practical advice on day-to-day coping and information about local support groups. As the causes of certain ENT disorders become better understood, and as pharmacological and surgical treatments make further strides forward, ENT nursing will continue to offer challenges and rewards for nurses in a variety of care settings.

Most large ENT units also care for patients suffering from head and neck cancer. The implementation of the recommendations for cancer units and centres made by Drs Calman and Hine in *A Policy Framework for Commissioning Cancer Services* (HMSO 1995) has implications not only for where these patients should receive their care but also for the education and training needs of the nurses who care for them.

REFERENCES

Baxter K, Nolan K, Winyard J, Roulson C, Goldhill D 1993 Are they getting enough? Meeting the oxygen therapy neeeds of postoperative patients. Professional Nurse 8(5): 310–312

Becker W, Naumann H H, Pfaltz C R 1993 Ear, nose and throat diseases, 2nd edn. Thieme, New York

Chan E 1997 A talent for listening. Nursing Times 51(93): 36–37

Coltart L 1998 Voice restoration after laryngectomy. Nursing Standard 13(12): 36–40

Cook J A, Murrant N J, Evans K L, Lavelle R J 1992 A randomised comparison of three post tonsillectomy diets. Clinical Otolaryngology 17: 28–31

Denyer S 1990 Foreign bodies: where do children put them? Health Visitor 63: 5

Ell S R, Parker A J 1992 A study of epistaxis in the elderly. Care of the Elderly, 4(2): 80–83

Feber T 1998 Design and evaluation of a strategy to provide support and information for people with cancer of the larynx. European Journal of Oncology Nursing 2(2): 106–114

Griggs A 1998 Tracheostomy: suctioning and humidification. Nursing Standard Continuing Education Reader. RCN, London

Hady M R, Kodeira K Z, Nasef A H 1983 The effects of nasal packing on arterial blood gases and acid-base balance and its clinical importance. Journal of Laryngology and Otology 97: 599–604

Harris R B 1984 National survey of aseptic tracheostomy care techniques in hospitals with head and neck/ENT surgical departments. Cancer Nursing, February 7(1): 23–32

Harris R H, Hyman R B 1984 Clean vs. sterile tracheostomy care and level of pulmonary infection. Nursing Research 33(2): 80–85

HMSO 1995 A policy framework for commissioning cancer services. A report by the expert advisory group on comments by the Chief Medical Officers of England and Wales, April 1995. HMSO, London

Hooper M 1991 Aural hygiene and the use of cotton swabs, Nursing Standard 66(12): 38–39

Jamieson E M, McCall J M, Blythe R, Whyte L A 1997 Guidelines for clinical nursing practices, 3rd edn. Churchill Livingstone, Edinburgh

Jay S, Ruddy J, Cullen R J 1991 Laryngectomy: the patients' view. Journal of Laryngology and Otology 105: 934–938

Kelsey A 1997 A nutritional assessment tool for patients with cancer. Journal of Cancer Nursing 2: 95–97

Kuo M, Hegarty D, Johnson A, Stevenson S 1995 Early post-tonsillectomy morbidity following hospital discharge: do patients and GPs know what to expect? Health Trends 27(3): 98–100

Lauder W 1993 Preventative measures to maintain control: management and treatment of vertigo. Professional Nurse 8(8): 506–508

Macdougald I 1994 Laser therapy for OSAS. Nursing Times 90(19): 32–34

McKenzie G, Chawla H, Gordon D 1986 The special senses, 2nd edn. Churchill Livingstone, Edinburgh

Mason J, Murty G, Foster H, Bradley P C 1992 Tracheostomy self care: the Nottingham system. Journal of Laryngology and Otology 106: 723–724

National Deaf Children's Society 1992 Communication is your responsibility. Commission of Inquiry into Human Aids in Communication. (Obtainable through C Shaw, Panel of Four, 48 Gallows Hill Lane, Abbots' Complex, Herts WD5 0BY, England.)

Price B 1992 Living with the altered body image: the cancer experience. British Journal of Nursing 1(13): 641–645

Ratna H 1994 Counselling deaf and hard of hearing clients. Counselling, May 5(2): 128–131

Reilly H 1998 Enteral feeding: an overview of indications and techniques. British Journal of Nursing 7(9): 510–512, 514–516, 518

RNID 1996 Statistics of deafness. RNID Policy Division, London

RNID 1997 Statistics on deafness. RNID Policy Division, London

RNID 1999 Noise exposure and hearing loss. RNID Policy Division, London

Seay S J, Gay S L 1997 Problem in tracheostomy patient care: recognising the patient with a displaced tracheostomy tube. ORL – Head and Neck Nursing 15(2): 10–11

Serra A 1995 Care of an adult patient with a tracheostomy in an ENT setting. Dimensions Mallinckrodt Medical, UK

Serra A M 1998 Tracheostomy care: part one. Nursing Standard Continuing Education Reader. RCN, London

Serra A M, Bailey C M, Jackson P 1986 Ear, nose and throat nursing. Blackwell Scientific Publications, London

Shenwell A, Wilson P 1994 Rest and respiration during obstructive sleep apnoea. Nursing Times 90(19): 30–32

Stilwell B 1992 Ear syringing skills update. Macmillan, London, pp 20–21

Whinney D J, Williamson P A, Bickwell P G 1995 Punctate diathermy of the soft palate: a new approach in the surgical management of snoring. Journal of Laryngology and Otology 109: 849–852

Wright D 1993 Deaf people's perceptions of communication with nurses. British Journal of Nursing 2(11): 567–571

FURTHER READING

Baker C A 1992 Factors associated with rehabilitation in head and neck cancer. Cancer Nursing 15(6): 395–400

Becker W, Naumann H H, Pfaltz C R 1993 Ear, nose and throat diseases, 2nd edn. Thieme, New York

Cook R 1998 Ear syringing. Nursing Standard 13: 56–61

Davis R, Roberts D 1999 Nursing care of the patient with head and neck cancer. Oncology Nurses Today 4(1): 9–15

Department of Health 1992 The treatment of persistent glue ear in children. Effective Health Care, no. 4

Dropkin M J 1989 Coping with disfigurement and dysfunction after head and neck cancer surgery: a conceptual framework. Seminars in Oncology Nursing 5(3): 213–219

Dropkin M J 1997 Coping with disfigurement/dysfunction and length of hospital stay after head and neck cancer surgery. ORL – Head and Neck Nursing 15(1): 22–26

Edward D 1997 Face to face. Patient, family and professional perspectives of head and neck cancer care. King's Fund, London

Ell S R, Parker A J 1992 A study of epistaxis in the elderly. Care of the Elderly, February: 80–83

Feber T 1996 Promoting self-esteem after laryngectomy. Nursing Times 92(30): 37–39

Fiorentini A 1992 Potential hazards of tracheobronchial suctioning. Intensive and Critical Care Nursing 8: 217–226

Fisher E W, Howard D J 1992 Percutaneous tracheostomy in a head and neck unit. Journal of Laryngology and Otology 106: 625–627

Freshwater D 1992 Pre-operative preparation of skin – a review of the literature. Surgical Nurse 5(5): 6, 9–10

Hanger H C, Mulley G 1992 Cerumen: its fascination and clinical importance. Journal of the Royal Society of Medicine 85: 346–349

Heath I 1994 Tinnitus and health anxiety. British Journal of Nursing 3: 10: 502–505

Hung P 1992 Pre-operative fasting. Nursing Times 88(48): 57–60

Jamieson E M, McCall J M, Blythe R, Whyte L 1997 Guidelines for clinical nursing practices, 3rd edn. Churchill Livingstone, Edinburgh

Kane K 1996 Functional endoscopic sinus surgery (FESS). Acorn Journal 9(2): 21–24

Kendrick A H 1995 Sleep apnoea. Professional Nurse 10(10): 624–628

Krouse H J, Krouse J H, Christmas D A 1997 Endoscopic sinus surgery in otolaryngology nursing using powered instrumentation. ORL – Head and Neck Nursing 15(2): 22–26

Lauder W 1993 Preventative measures to maintain control: management and treatment of vertigo. Professional Nurse 8(8): 506–508

McCall M E 1993 It killed George – or managing the peritonsiller abscess patient effectively. ORL – Head and Neck Nursing 11(1): 10–12

Macdougald I 1994 Laser therapy for OSAS. Nursing Times 90(19): 32–34

McKennis A, Waddington C 1993 Lasers: uses in otolaryngology – lighting the way to the future. ORL – Head and Neck Nursing 11(1): 26–32

Malem F, Butler K 1993 Nurse-aid management of ear and nose emergencies 2. British Journal of Nursing 2(18): 926–928

Minsley M A, Wrenn S 1996 Long-term care of the tracheostomy patient from an outpatient nursing perspective. ORL – Head and Neck Nursing 14(4): 18–22

Nelson S 1992 Mini-tracheostomy: the benefits for patient care. British Journal of Nursing 1(10): 492–495

Phillips S 1997 Obstructive sleep apnoea: diagnosis and management. Nursing Standard 11(17): 43–46

Rogers R 1992 Isn't it time we stopped washing out ears? Primary Health Care 2(3): 13, 16, 17

Salmon P 1993 The reduction of anxiety in surgical patients: an important nursing task or the medicalization of preparatory worry? International Journal of Nursing Studies 30(4): 323–330

Serra A 1995 Care of an adult patient with a tracheostomy in an ENT setting. Dimensions Mallinckrodt Medical, UK

Serra A M 1998 Tracheostomy care, part two. Nursing Standard Continuing Education Reader. RCN, London

Serra A M, Bailey C M, Jackson P 1986 Ear, nose and throat nursing. Blackwell Scientific Publications, London

Shenwell A, Wilson P 1994 Rest and respiration during obstructive sleep apnoea. Nursing Times 90(19): 30–32

Sigler B A, Schuring L T 1993 Ear, nose and throat disorders. Mosby's Clinical Nursing Series. Mosby, St Louis

Sizer D 1998 How TRT got NBM-ed (editorial) Online, RNID Tinnitus Helpline Newsletter 19: 1–5

Stilwell B 1992 Ear syringing skills update. Macmillan, London, pp 20–21

Stone C 1996 Post-tonsillectomy pain relief following discharge from hospital. NT Research 1(1): 57–65

Thurgood K, Thurgood G 1995 Ear syringing: a clinical skill. British Journal of Nursing 4(12): 682–687

Thurston-Hookway F, Seddon S 1989 Care of the laryngectomy. Nursing 3(35): 5–10

Waddington C, McKennis A, Goodlett A 1997 Treatment of conductive hearing loss with ossicular chain reconstruction procedures. AORN Journal 65(3): 511–525

Zeitoun H, Demajunder R, Hemmings C, Lee W 1997 Developing a nurse-led aural care clinic. Nursing Times 93(45): 45–46

USEFUL ADDRESSES

British Association of the Hard of Hearing
7–11 Armstrong Road
London W3 7JL

British Deaf Association
3 Worship Street
Moorgate EC2A 2AG

British Association of Counsellors (BAC)
1 Regent Place
Rugby CV21 2PJ

National Deaf Children's Society
31 Gloucester Place
London W1H 4EA

Scottish Association for the Deaf
158 West Regent Street
Glasgow G2 4RL

Hearing Dogs for the Deaf
London Road (A40)
Lawknor
Oxon OX9 5RY

Hearing Dogs for the Deaf (Scottish Branch)
29 Craigiehall Road
Erskine PA8 7DD

Association of Teachers of Lip-reading for Adults (ATLA)
70 Fernway
Kingswood
Watford
Herts WD2 6HQ

Royal National Institute for Deaf People (RNID)
19–23 Featherstone Street
London EC1V 8SL
(The RNID has six regional offices spread across the UK)

Tinnitus Helpline
Castle Cavendish
Norton Street
Nottingham NG7 5PN
(Information and advice on tinnitus and details of services and support groups)

Ear, Nose and Throat Nursing Interest Group
Royal College of Nursing
20 Cavendish Square
London W1M 0AB

Let's Face It (London Office)
62 Fortescue Road
Edgware
Middlesex HA8 0HN
(A national and international group for the facially disfigured, including cancer sufferers)

Changing Faces
1 and 2 Junction Mews
London W2 1PN
(A national group for the facially disfigured)

British Association of Head and Neck Cancer Nurses
Information from:
Secretary, BAHNCN
Macmillan Head & Neck Cancer Nurse Specialist
ENT Outpatient Department
Queen's Medical Centre
Nottingham NG7 2UH

National Association of Laryngectomy Clubs
Ground Floor
6 Rickett Street
Fulham
London
(For laryngectomy patients, but tracheostomy and head and neck cancer patients are also welcome)

HSE Information Services
Health and Safety Laboratory
Broad Lane
Sheffield S3 7HQ
(For more information on The Noise at Work Regulations 1989)

DISORDERS OF THE MOUTH

15

Rosemary Kelly

INTRODUCTION

The mouth is central to many activities of daily living which we often take for granted until some minor but painful problem such as toothache or an aphthous ulcer reminds us of the importance of the condition of the mouth to our general feeling of well-being. The mouth is the source of the infant's first pleasurable activity (the sucking reflex being present at birth) and perhaps, during teething, of his first experience of *dis*-ease. For individuals approaching the end of life, or for anyone who is acutely ill, good mouth care can give much comfort and relief and help to preserve dignity.

Oral health is defined as (The Scottish Office Department of Health 1995):

> *a standard of health of the oral cavity and related tissues without active disease. This state should enable the individual to eat, speak and socialise without discomfort or embarrassment and contribute to general well-being.*

Although this book addresses adult health, it is important to realise that good oral health practices laid down in childhood can only influence adult health in a positive way, and the nurse can help to encourage these (see Box 15.1, p. 559).

The mouth is often the first indicator of generalised systemic disease or disease in adjacent structures. In addition, its immediate visibility gives any dysfunction a particular significance for the individual, who may be acutely aware of any disfigurement, whether cosmetic or functional. This can give rise to many difficulties affecting the person's perception of himself and his quality of life.

Q **15.1** From your own experience, how many activities of daily living (see Roper et al 1996) are affected, and in what ways, after a dental procedure (e.g. a filling or extraction requiring local anaesthesia)? Now consider how much worse it would be for a patient if any of these activities were affected in the long term or even permanently.

ANATOMY AND PHYSIOLOGY

The mouth or oral cavity has evolved as a 'workshop', where much activity associated with chewing (mastication), drinking and speaking takes place (see Fig. 15.1):

- Entrance is between the lips (red, muscular and sensitive) through the vestibule, a small space immediately before the inner entrance which consists of gums (gingivae) covering alveolar ridges of maxillae and mandible, into which are set teeth.
- The opening (parotid duct) from the parotid gland, one of the salivary glands, is into the vestibule.
- The roof of the mouth is formed by bony hard palate (maxilla) and muscular soft palate.

1(A) Oral stage: preparatory phase
(Time taken varies)

Lips open; saliva is stimulated
Liquid or portion of food is taken
↓
Solid material is broken down by teeth, moistened by saliva
↓
Strenuous movements of jaw and cheek muscles and mobile tongue against the hard palate, teeth and alveolar ridges form food into bolus
↓
Tongue tip gathers stray food particles from between lips and teeth and from the floor of the mouth and incorporates them into bolus
↓
The lips must be closed. The soft palate is lowered and bolus or liquid is propelled backwards by strong humping movements and funnelling of the tongue

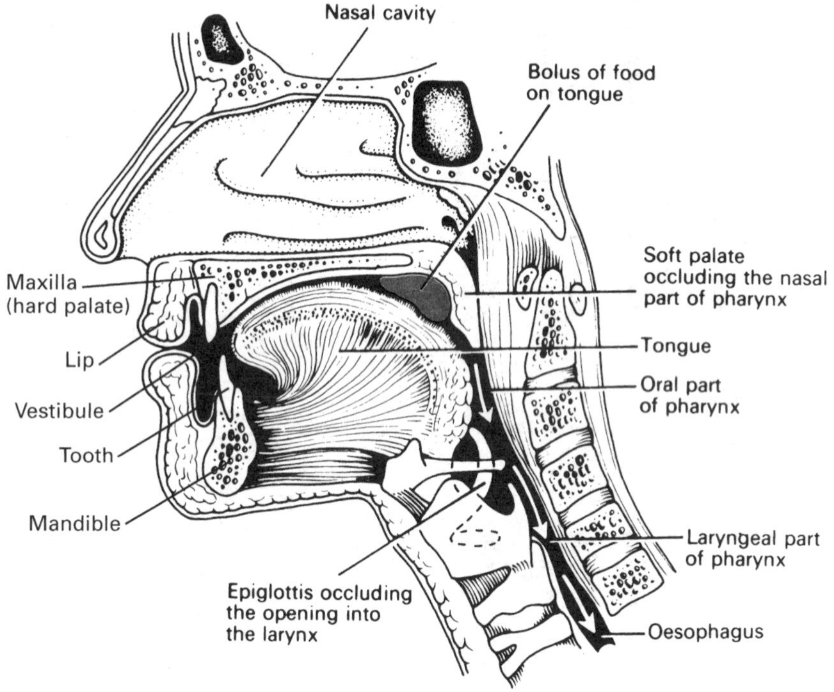

1(B) Oral stage: executive phase
(Time taken should not exceed 1 s)

The bolus of food on the tongue is propelled towards the oropharynx. The soft palate rises to close the nasopharynx and so prevent nasal regurgitation
↓
The bolus must contact pillars of fauces and the posterior oropharyngeal wall to trigger the swallow 'reflex' and initiate:
↓
2 The pharyngeal stage
(Normally lasts 0.75 s)
↓
The bolus passes the laryngeal part of the pharynx, through the open cricopharyngeal sphincter, and so to:
↓
3 The oesophageal stage
(2 s)

Fig. 15.1 The importance of oral competence to the process of feeding, chewing and swallowing.

- Lateral walls are formed by the muscles of the cheeks.
- The floor of the mouth is almost entirely filled by the muscular tongue, which is very mobile and sensitive. Tiny projections on it, called papillae, contain nerve endings of taste. There are also openings from two pairs of salivary glands: submandibular and sublingual.
- The rear exit to the oropharynx is under the border of the soft palate, through two archways (palatoglossal and palatopharyngeal), which enclose the palatine tonsil. The area posterior to the molar teeth is known as the retromolar trigone.
- The entire oral cavity is lined with mucous membrane, much of which is stratified epithelium to cope with 'wear and tear'.

The mouth is situated close to many other structures, and disease or injury of the mouth may also affect, for example, the eye, ear, nose, maxillary sinuses, pharynx, larynx and neck. The face and neck are richly supplied with arteries, veins, nerves, muscles, lymph vessels and nodes, and knowledge of all these is important to understanding the effects of trauma or disease arising in, or affecting, the mouth.

See also Chapter 4 and Wilson & Waugh (1996) and, for a more detailed account, Johnson & Moore (1997).

Functions of the mouth

The stages of normal swallowing

Only in the mouth is there normally any voluntary control over the process of digestion. The first stage (oral) must be accomplished (see Fig. 15.1) so that the swallowing reflex is triggered when the bolus reaches the posterior pharyngeal wall, and the second stage (pharyngeal) then commences. During this and the third stage (oesophageal), swallowing is involuntary.

A deficiency in the mouth may cause difficulty in the later stages of the swallowing mechanism.

Several cranial nerves (CNs) are involved in the acts of swallowing and voice production (see Table 15.1 and Wilson & Waugh 1996).

Normal swallowing is discussed in detail by Langley (1989).

A means of communication

The lips, tongue, hard and soft palate and teeth, together with throat and facial muscles, all manipulate sound to give quality and resonance to speech. The mouth also contributes to other expressions of emotion, e.g. smiling, laughing, whistling and kissing. Thus any disturbance to the norm caused by trauma, cerebrovascular accident or surgery can cause diminution or failure of these very basic functions and so reduce quality of life. Understanding some of the changes that may occur will help the nurse to assist the patient's recovery (see 'Orofacial trauma', p. 568, and 'Tumours', p. 571, and also Ch. 4).

Saliva

This is formed by a combination of secretions from the parotid, submandibular and sublingual glands and from the mucous membrane. It keeps the mouth moist, and without it, oral functions are very difficult. Salivary amylase is the enzyme that assists with digestion of food.

Table 15.1 Cranial nerves involved in stages of swallowing. Damage to any of these nerves may affect the ability to eat. (Adapted from Wilson & Waugh 1996 and Langley 1989)

Nerve	*Type*	*Function*
CN I	Olfactory	Sense of smell
CN V	Trigeminal	Sensory to gums, cheek, lower jaw and muscles of mastication; motor to muscles of mastication
CN VII	Facial	Taste from anterior two-thirds of the tongue; motor to muscles of face
CN IX	Glossopharyngeal	Secretion of saliva; sensory to posterior one-third of tongue, soft palate, pillars of fauces and pharynx; taste from posterior tongue; motor to pharynx
CN X	Vagus	Sensory to larynx; motor to palate, pharynx and larynx
CN XI	Accessory	Motor to laryngeal and pharyngeal muscles, and muscles of head control
CN XII	Hypoglossal	Motor to muscles of tongue

Teeth

Teeth are important structures for biting and chewing food. Children have 20 temporary or deciduous teeth, which are gradually replaced by 32 permanent teeth between the ages of about 6 and 24 years. Time of eruption can be a measure of developmental age.

Overcrowding of teeth may necessitate extraction of third molars (wisdom teeth) during young adulthood. However, impaction of wisdom teeth is now more commonly seen at a later age because fewer molars are now extracted.

The importance of good orodental health throughout life is discussed later in the chapter.

For greater detail see Wilson & Waugh (1996).

Bones of the face (see Fig. 15.2)

Many of these bones are complex and fragile, and hence trauma to the mouth may result in a complicated injury (see 'Orofacial trauma', p. 565).

DISORDERS OF THE MOUTH

Disorders of the mouth can be broadly classified into five categories:

- derangement of orofacial tissues
- orodental disease

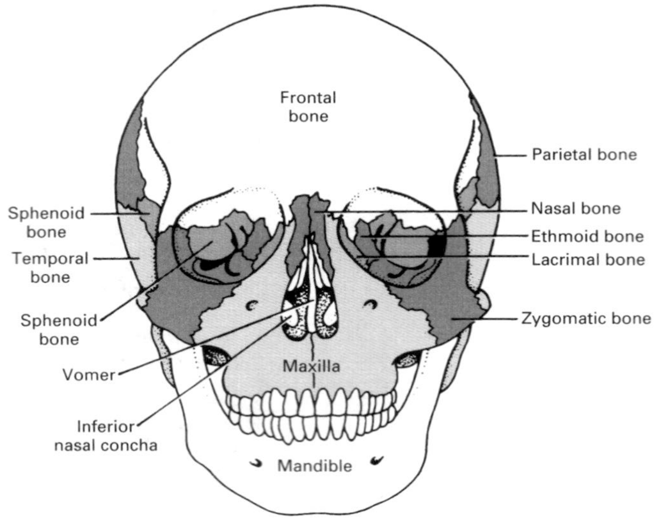

Fig. 15.2 The bones of the face.

- infections and inflammatory conditions (localised or systemic)
- traumatic injury
- tumours.

Each of these categories will be considered in turn in the following sections.

DERANGEMENT OF OROFACIAL TISSUES

Defects involving the mouth may require a series of corrective procedures and may present the individual with physical, social and emotional problems in childhood, young adulthood and maturity. The most commonly occurring congenital malformations of the mouth are dental and jaw disproportion. In a UK survey in 1993, 54% of 9-year-olds examined were assessed as having treatment needs for disproportion varying from moderate to very great (O'Brien 1994). Cleft lip and cleft palate together have an incidence of approximately 1 in 600 live births. Of this number, roughly one-third are cleft lip, one-third cleft palate, and the remaining third cleft lip and cleft palate. Other deformities of the face and mouth are comparatively rare, but can be devastating for the child and his parents.

Problems associated with dental/jaw disproportion, cleft lip/palate and other deformities of the face or mouth may concern the following:

- appearance
- dentition/occlusion
- eating and drinking
- speech
- hearing
- mid-face growth
- psychosocial adjustment.

See Henderson (1985) for information on rarer deformities of the mouth and face.

PATHOPHYSIOLOGY

Cleft lip results from failure of the embryonic maxillary prominence to fuse with the intermaxillary segment and occurs 6–7 weeks after conception. Cleft lip may be unilateral or bilateral and can vary in degree from a slight notch to a complete division of the lip and the alveolar process (gum).

Table 15.2 Treatment of cleft lip and palate

Procedure	*Timing/patient's age*
Lip repair	0–6 months
Palate repair	4–24 months
Bone graft to alveolus	9–11 years
Osteotomy (for correction of defect of hard palate) Rhinoplasty (for nasal defect)	Around 18 years
Pharyngoplasty (to correct the pharynx) Myringotomy revision procedures	As and when necessary
Orthodontic treatment Speech therapy	Throughout childhood and into adulthood if necessary

Cleft palate is caused by a failure of the palatine processes to fuse with each other and with the nasal septum or with the primary palate. This occurs 7–12 weeks after conception. As a result of this failure of fusion, the soft palate is unable to meet the posterior pharyngeal wall and thus to close off the nasopharynx. Because of this, the individual's speech is affected, producing a typically 'nasal' delivery in which certain consonants, particularly C, D, K, P, S and T, cannot be properly enunciated.

MEDICAL MANAGEMENT

Treatment. The medical management of oral defects often requires a multidisciplinary approach extending from infancy to adulthood. Treatment protocol will depend on the extent of the deformity and on the age of the child (for management of cleft lip/palate, see Table 15.2).

Orthognathic surgery (i.e. surgery to correct major facial deformities) is an important and developing area of maxillofacial work and is carried out in only a few units in the UK. It requires a team approach involving neuro-, maxillofacial, plastic and ophthalmic surgeons, and assessment and correction take place throughout life.

NURSING PRIORITIES AND MANAGEMENT: CONGENITAL OROFACIAL DERANGEMENT

Nursing considerations

Referral. A parent's discovery that his or her newborn child has a facial deformity may be very traumatic, and the provision of sensitive and supportive counselling should not be delayed. Parents should be referred within a few days of their child's birth to the relevant specialist professionals (e.g. orofacial consultant, orthodontist, speech therapist, specialist nurse) and should be given information on their local branch of the Cleft Lip and Palate Association (CLAPA) (see 'Useful addresses', p. 579) or other appropriate self-help group. Professional psychological support may also be required as there can be great family stress (Martin 1995).

Oral hygiene. Nurses should emphasise the importance of good dental hygiene to parents as there is a higher risk of caries and infection, and they may mistakenly feel that compared with gross abnormality the loss of a few teeth due to dental caries is inconsequential.

Pre- and postoperative nursing care of patients undergoing major corrective surgery will take into account the general considerations discussed in Chapter 26, incorporating the specialised skills and techniques demanded by each procedure.

See Kemble & Lamb (1984) for the nursing care of cleft lip/palate.

ORAL HEALTH AND ORODENTAL DISEASE

Dental and periodontal disease affects about 95% of the population of the UK in varying degrees and accounts for the largest proportion of disorders of the mouth. Because most of this disease is preventable, this discussion of orodental disease will begin with a consideration of dental health, first with respect to recent trends and then with regard to the promotion of orodental care.

Changing patterns of dental health

From the early 1970s, there was a substantial improvement in dental health in the UK. More people retained their natural teeth into later life, and there was a marked decrease in dental caries in children (Downer 1991). The incidence of dental caries can be measured in terms of the number of decayed, missing and filled deciduous teeth (dmft) and/or permanent teeth (DMFT). The World Health Organization (WHO 1988) had as its goal for the year 2000 that 50% of 5- to 6-year-olds would be free from caries and that 50% of 12-year-olds would have a DMFT of no greater than 3. However, despite earlier indications that the WHO targets might be achieved (Downer 1991), subsequent surveys have shown that, particularly in areas of social deprivation, dental caries seems to be increasing (Jones et al 1997).

There are wide regional variations in dental health in the UK; in 1988, the prevalence of caries among 5-year-olds in Scotland was 58%, compared with 44% in England, and in 12-year-olds the figures were 61% and 50%, respectively (O'Brien 1994).

The Consumers' Association (1997) found great variations in provision of NHS dental treatment and also in charges for private treatment. Thomas et al (1997) reported a 56% increase since 1989 in attendance at a free hospital dental emergency clinic, with many inappropriate self-referrals.

15.2 Consider why regional variations might exist.

Promoting oral health

Nurses in all spheres of practice (see Box 15.1) can help with early education in the simple preventive measures that are the key to oral health, and to identify orodental problems early and thus minimise some of their distressing consequences (Oral Health Group 1996, Levine 1996a).

See Wray & Gibson (1997) for illustrations of oral soft tissue disease and Sweeney & Bagg (1997) for an interactive programme on the mouth.

Oral hygiene. Parents should introduce a dental hygiene routine as soon as their child's first teeth appear, using a soft, baby toothbrush. Most children will require supervision until they are 7 or 8 years old.
The teeth should be brushed last thing at night and, ideally, after every meal. The toothbrush should be held at an angle of 45° and the teeth brushed horizontally to avoid damage to the gums. All exposed surfaces of the teeth should be cleaned and the mouth rinsed well during and after brushing.
Toothbrushes should be renewed every 3 months, and hard brushes should be avoided as they can damage tooth enamel and gums.
Toothpaste with added fluoride is recommended, except in areas with fluoridated water. Toothpaste with sugar added to improve flavour should be avoided. Sensitivities to certain toothpaste ingredients (e.g. cinnamon-aldehyde, menthol and peppermint) occur occasionally and will resolve spontaneously when use is discontinued (Lamey et al 1990, Morton et al 1995).
Dental floss with or without added fluoride may be used to clean between the teeth. Overzealous use can damage the gums and it is best not used by children. Similar care should be taken in the use of toothpicks.
Disclosing tablets can be useful to demonstrate how plaque is left after inadequate brushing. Chewed after cleansing, the tablet produces a stain on any teeth still covered with plaque. Correct brushing should then remove the plaque.

Box 15.1 Contribution of nurses to orodental health

Health visitors
Encourage oral hygiene in childhood and visits to dentist and orthodontist. This is a primary preventive function of the health visitor. Educate on oral cancer prevention (smoking, alcohol and other substance abuse)

School nurses
Demonstrate dental hygiene. Alert parents to the need for children's visits to the dentist. Encourage healthy eating principles

Occupational health nurses and practice nurses
Educate on adverse effects of smoking and excessive alcohol. Raise awareness of symptoms of intraoral cancer. Advise on good handwashing practices and healthy eating

District nurses
Identify potential problems in elderly people. Advise on continued dental examination. Raise awareness of oral cancer

Nurses caring for elderly people
As above. Increase mouth comfort and self-esteem

Nurses working with those with learning disability
Supervise early and continued dental care and thus minimise need for restorative dentistry

Midwives
Give dental care advice in pregnancy

All nurses
Encourage and/or assist with oral hygiene for patients' comfort and health. Have dental/oral health literature available

An assessment of oral care products can be found in Consumers' Association (1997).

Common misconceptions. Chewing gum after meals to increase saliva is of limited value in reducing decay. To be of any benefit, sugar-free gum must be chewed for 20 min and be backed up by other forms of dental care.

Chewing an apple after a meal does not clean the teeth. Rather, it leaves an acidic deposit which encourages development of plaque.

15.3 How good an example do you set in the practice of oral hygiene?

Diet. Research by System Three Scotland (1994) found that although there was awareness among parents and grandparents of the harmful effects of sugar on children's teeth, and some changes in attitude regarding its consumption, there were areas of confusion and misinformation about hidden sugar content of various foods and doubts about control over its intake by children. The 1990 Diet and Nutritional Survey of British Adults (Gregory 1990) found the daily consumption of sugar to be approximately 95 g (19 teaspoons), which is over 50% more than the recommended maximum intake of 60 g, or 10% of dietary energy (12 teaspoons). Nurses could contribute to health education in this area, and emphasise the cariogenic action of non-milk sugars, which include fruit juices, honey and table sugar (Department of Health 1989).

See Rugg-Gunn (1993) for information on diet and oral health, and Oral Health Group (1996) for an oral health programme and list of resources.

15.4 Examine the contents labels of the prepared foods you normally buy. Do any of these products contain more sugar than you had realised?

Access to dental care. Often, the dental surgery is the first remembered clinical setting for health care. If these first visits are reasonably pleasant, then a positive attitude may be created towards future regular dental check-ups, and subsequent serious disease can then be diagnosed early. However, it seems possible that changing factors in delivery of dental care may affect the future dental health of the nation. These factors include regional variation in accessibility of NHS dentistry, increased treatment charges and changes in funding of dental services (Curzon & Pollard 1997, Pitts 1997).

Early access to orthodontic services, particularly for those with congenital abnormalities, will help to minimise problems in later life.

15.5 Consider that those who were children when the WHO set its targets in 1988 are now adults. Is their attitude to dental treatment likely to have changed? If so, why?

Fluoride is a substance naturally present in some areas in water. It is taken up by growing teeth and makes enamel harder and more resistant to the development of caries. The incidence of caries has been shown to be high in areas with low levels of fluoride, particularly in areas of deprivation (Jones et al 1997). Despite well documented evidence of the benefits of fluoride, controversy still continues over the practice of adding it to the water supply.

Fluoride supplements can be given to children from the age of 6 months. Dentists, chemists and health visitors should be able to advise on the correct amount required locally. Overdosing causes fluorosis, which can cause 'mottling' of teeth (brown spots with white opacities).

See Levine (1996a,b) for further information on dental health education.

Dental and periodontal disease

PATHOPHYSIOLOGY

Plaque is a firmly adherent, non-calcified deposit of bacteria, mucus, food particles and cellular debris which accumulates on the surface of a tooth, particularly at the base. It forms rapidly in the absence of good oral hygiene and reacts immediately with sugar to form an acid which can attack and erode tooth enamel, leading, if unchecked by adequate saliva combined with good dental hygiene, to gum disease and dental caries.

Calculus is hard mineralised plaque which requires removal by a dental surgeon or dental hygienist.

Caries is progressive, localised decay of teeth caused by bacterial action. It is characterised by demineralisation of the inorganic portion and destruction of the organic substance of the tooth.

Gingivitis (inflammation of the gums). Normal gums are pink (e.g. in Caucasians) or brown (e.g. in Asian or African people) and are firm. In gingivitis, the gums are purple-red, soft and puffy, tender, and may bleed easily. Regular oral hygiene and dental care reduce this reversible stage of gum disease.

Untreated, gingivitis can lead to gum recession and the formation of pockets (found in 75% of dentate adults) around the base of teeth, in which plaque and calculus can collect. Further infection from bacteria in plaque may lead to periodontitis.

Periodontitis is characterised by gradual loss of the supporting membrane of the teeth and erosion of supporting bone. Membrane and bone, once destroyed, cannot be replaced and subsequent loosening of teeth occurs. In 1988, 69–75% of dentate adults had periodontal disease (Todd & Lader 1991).

Acute ulcerative gingivitis is an uncommon condition caused by a mixed infection of a bacillus and spirochaetes. Poor oral hygiene, smoking, throat infections and stress can contribute. This condition is also seen in HIV infection. The gums are sore and bleed easily and ulcers develop which may spread more deeply. A characteristic foul smell is associated with this condition. Cervical or neck lymph glands may be enlarged.

Common presenting symptoms. The patient commonly presents to his general medical practitioner (GMP) or general dental practitioner (GDP) with a combination of symptoms which may include toothache, bleeding gums and emission of pus from the gums (pyorrhoea). If oral hygiene has habitually been poor, the patient is more likely to wait until pain is severe before presenting. Many people fear going to the dentist and delay for as long as possible.

MEDICAL MANAGEMENT

Investigations include X-rays, sialograms (see Appendix 1) and relevant blood tests.

Dental surgery or outpatient procedures. Most orodental problems are treated in dental surgeries (NHS or private practice). Treatments such as extractions, fillings, root treatment for dental abscess, and restorative work such as fitting crowns and dentures are carried out with the patient under a local anaesthetic administered by the dentist. Some procedures necessitate general anaesthesia, which is administered by an anaesthetist. Treatment of gingivitis is with mouthwashes and metronidazole or penicillin. Scaling, i.e. removal of plaque and calculus, is carried out when swelling has subsided.

In-patient or day-case procedures. Procedures which can be classed as minor oral surgery but which may require hospital treatment include:

- removal of impacted wisdom teeth
- removal of dental cysts
- removal of salivary glands or ducts
- apicectomy (excision of apex of tooth root)
- preprosthetic surgery
- placement of implants.

Patients may be referred to a dental hospital/school or to an oral/maxillofacial unit.

Patients with certain conditions or who are taking certain types of drugs will require hospital admission and special monitoring as follows:

- diabetes mellitus — insulin dosage must be monitored; there is a risk of delayed healing
- heart valve disease — monitoring is very important as infection can lead to bacterial endocarditis (see Ch. 2)
- steroid drugs — must be monitored; healing may be delayed
- anticoagulants — must be monitored; there is increased risk of haemorrhage.

NURSING PRIORITIES AND MANAGEMENT: ORODENTAL DISEASE

Nursing considerations

Outpatient care. Individuals treated in dental surgeries or as hospital outpatients will require reassurance and advice on aftercare at home. The nurse should make available written information such as that presented in Box 15.2 and ensure that the patient understands and can carry out instructions for self-care and knows where to call for advice should problems arise.

In-patient care. Admission is usually on the day preceding or the actual day of surgery and discharge is on the day after. The patient's stay may be longer, however, if any of the special considerations listed above apply.

The preparation of patients for anaesthesia is described in Chapter 26. Because of 'dentist phobia', patients undergoing dental surgery often experience anxiety which may seem disproportionate to the size of the procedure, and need much reassurance.

Postoperatively, the patient may experience considerable pain, swelling and bruising. Nursing Care Plan 15.1 gives an example of the care that is required following a wisdom tooth extraction.

On discharge, the patient should be given clear, adequate information on self-care and a number to call should further advice be needed.

Promoting oral health and comfort in special client groups

Most people are able to maintain good oral hygiene independently throughout much of their lives. Others, for reasons of physical or cognitive disability, or infirmity due to illness or advanced age, will need supervision and assistance in carrying out dental and periodontal care routines. The importance of this aspect of daily care must not be minimised, as poor orodental health can seriously compromise the individual's well-being, both functionally and socially.

Physically disadvantaged and those with learning difficulties

Individuals with limited motor control or manual dexterity may require help with brushing teeth. Toothbrushes with adapted handles are available to aid gripping and the nurse should be aware of how these can be obtained (often from an occupational therapist). Many people with limited movement depend on the mouth and teeth to hold or control equipment; it is thus especially important that their teeth are kept in good condition. Occasionally, it is difficult to gain the cooperation of a disadvantaged person who needs dental treatment; in such cases, general anaesthesia may be required even for a simple procedure. The practice of good oral hygiene is obviously preferable to repeated general anaesthesia.

Elderly people

Adequate dental care for elderly people can greatly enhance quality of life with regard to comfort, self-image and social interaction (Fiske et al 1990). However, Holmes (1996) commented that 'much of the care is not supported by research, and oral-care practices have remained unchanged for many years'.

Box 15.2 Information for patients having minor oral surgery

Following surgery to your mouth, you can expect some swelling and discomfort. This may last for some days. The following information will help you in the postoperative period.

On the day of treatment

1. Rest for a few hours. You do not necessarily have to lie down, however
2. Avoid strenuous exercise for 24 h
3. Avoid rinsing your mouth for 24 h, even if it tastes unpleasant. Rinsing may disturb any blood clots and start up bleeding
4. Your lips and/or tongue may be numb. Be careful not to bite or burn them inadvertently
5. Avoid hot fluids, alcohol, hard foods and cigarettes
6. Pain or soreness can be relieved with a mild painkiller, e.g. Co-codamol or paracetamol (no more than eight tablets in 24 h for an adult)
7. Should the wound begin to bleed, apply a compress (a clean cotton handkerchief rolled up is ideal). Place this on the bleeding point and bite firmly on it for 10 min, or longer if necessary
8. If you are at all worried, or if anything untoward occurs such as prolonged bleeding, excessive pain or swelling, please telephone the oral surgery department where you received treatment.

On the day after treatment

A mouthwash can now be used to cleanse the mouth. It is not necessary to purchase a proprietary mouthwash, although you can if you wish. It is the mechanical action of washing out the mouth which is of importance, rather than the substance used.

Warm salty water is very effective to cleanse and freshen the mouth. Dissolve half a teaspoon of salt in a tumbler of warm water. Hold a mouthful of the solution in the mouth for a minute or two and then spit it out. Finish the tumbler in the same way. Repeat the procedure several times a day for 5 days.

Follow-up

You will have been given another appointment if further treatment is necessary. If you have any problems please contact the oral surgery department for advice.

Nursing Care Plan 15.1 Care of a patient following removal of impacted wisdom teeth

Nursing considerations	***Action/intervention***	***Expected outcome***
1. Pain due to manipulation of jaw	❒ Administer adequate analgesia and monitor its effect	Patient is free of pain
2. Risk of haemorrhage	❒ Withhold mouthwashing overnight	Blood clot left undisturbed; bleeding minimised
3. Vomiting because of swallowed blood from tooth socket	❒ Give constant reassurance; stay with the patient or allow him privacy according to his wishes	Patient is comforted; dignity and self-esteem respected
4. Personal hygiene	❒ Provide frequent sponging, especially of face and hands	Comfort maintained
5. Oral hygiene	❒ Provide gentle, warm saline mouthwashes the morning after; gentle brushing, avoiding socket	Mouth is freshened; debris removed; haemorrhage avoided
6. Risk of infection	❒ Administer antibiotics if prescribed ❒ Implement special precautions for patients at risk	Infection avoided; normal healing takes place
7. Discharge	❒ Evaluate outcome of treatment and postoperative care ❒ If the patient is fit for discharge: give after-care information; refer to community nurse and hygienist; arrange return appointment	Patient is confident that he can perform self-care; professional supervision is continued

Many elderly people now retain their natural teeth and regular dental check-ups should be encouraged by community nurses. Good oral hygiene and regular assessment of oral/dental health for elderly people in hospital should form part of any nursing care plan. However, Samaranayake et al (1995) found considerable unmet dental need among a group of 147 elderly people in five long-stay wards.

Elderly people in general have specific problems relating to oral health as follows (the figures in parentheses are from Samaranayake et al 1995):

- Gum retraction/resorption — this occurs naturally, causing root surfaces to be exposed, and with natural wear of the teeth can necessitate repair work.
- Dry mouth (35%) — this can lead to a coated tongue (56%) and increases the risk of decay.
- Ill-fitting dentures (45%) — as a result of the natural resorption of the alveoli when teeth are lost. Continuous wearing of dentures can lead to the development of *Candida*-associated denture stomatitis (19%) (refer to the section on infections). Dentures should therefore be removed at night, cleaned and kept in water or a weak solution of Milton or other proprietary cleanser. Dentures left dry for any length of time can shrink.
- Angular cheilitis (25%).
- Loss of appetite — elderly people who have lost interest in meals should be examined for any of the above and for early indications of intraoral cancer. Specialist opinion should always be sought for any ulcer which does not heal within 2–3 weeks (Williams 1990).
- Reduced manual dexterity and general weakness.

Q **15.6** Consider your nursing care of elderly patients. Do you always give the same quality of care to teeth as to washing face and hands and combing hair?

Acutely ill people

During the acute phase of any illness, the patient may require assistance or supervision in carrying out oral hygiene, but the objective should be to encourage optimum independence as far as possible.

Jamieson et al (1997) describe mouth care in detail and the student is referred to that text for general procedures. See Wray & Gibson (1997) and Sweeney & Bagg (1997) for illustrations of oral disease which the nurse might encounter during routine oral inspection and which would warrant seeking specialist advice.

Many acutely ill people suffer from stomatitis and/or candidiasis and will require special measures. These are further discussed in the following section.

INFECTIONS AND INFLAMMATORY CONDITIONS OF THE MOUTH

These can give rise to considerable pain and discomfort, and the individual, already often ill, debilitated and poorly nourished, can become more so if the oral condition is not reversed. The mouth may be affected by the following:

- local and systemic infections (see Table 15.3)

- oral manifestations of a generalised systemic disease:
  —gastrointestinal and nutritional disorders (see Chs 4, 20 and 21, and Table 15.4)
  —blood (haemopoietic) and endocrine disorders (see Chs 5 and 11)
  —dermatological disorders (see Ch. 12).

Stomatitis

PATHOPHYSIOLOGY

Stomatitis, or inflammation of the mouth (stoma), is sometimes referred to as mucositis and can be caused by:

- vitamin deficiency (B_{12}; folic acid)
- viral infection, including HIV
- radiotherapy to head and neck
- chemotherapy
- bone marrow transplantation (BMT) and graft-versus-host disease (GVHD)
- liver failure
- renal failure.

Common presenting symptoms. In this condition, cell regeneration in the epithelium of the mucous membrane cannot keep pace with the rate of destruction which occurs as a result of any of the above. The mucosa becomes thin and there is erythema and some loss of taste. Later, oedema develops and the mucosa breaks down at the slightest trauma, giving rise to haemorrhage and ulceration.

The pain caused by stomatitis can be excruciating. One patient described drinking water as being 'like swallowing broken glass'.

Table 15.3 Common local and systemic infections affecting the mouth. (Adapted from Lamey & Lewis 1988)

Infection/organism	*Oral presentation*	*Cause/effect*
Candidiasis (moniliasis), *Candida albicans*	Different presentations are recognised and may be found at the same time, especially in terminal illness, and when associated with HIV and AIDS. Anorexia is common (Challacome 1991, Ventafridda et al 1995). Different presentations of candidiasis are described below (Challacombe 1991)	Destruction of normal oral flora due to immunosuppression caused by, e.g., antibiotics, cytotoxic drugs, radiotherapy to head and neck, HIV, severe debilitation post-surgery, anaemia and other blood disorders, diabetes mellitus; terminal illness (identified in 75–89% of patients; Ventafridda et al 1995)
Acute pseudomembranous candidiasis (thrush)	White-yellow plaques like milk curds, easily wiped off, leaving painful, bleeding surface	May also occur in oropharynx (?cause of anorexia); in infants (poor hygiene) highly infectious; advanced HIV (Palmer et al 1996)
Acute atrophic (or acute erythematous) candidiasis	Minimal white plaques, painful erosion of dorsum of tongue	Often related to use of broad-spectrum antibiotics
Chronic atrophic (or chronic erythematous) candidiasis	Erythema, oedema, often with clear demarcation from normal tissue (areas in contact with dentures — denture stomatitis)	Poor oral hygiene, xerostomia, smoking. Occurs in 65% of denture-wearing elderly people
Chronic hyperplastic candidiasis	Firm adherent white patches or tiny nodules on erythematous base; can resemble leukoplakia (a pre-cancerous condition)	Usually associated with HIV
Candidal cheilosis (often found with chronic atrophic candidiasis)	Soreness, redness and cracks at corner of mouth	Habitual licking
Chickenpox (varicella)	Occasionally vesicles develop on oral mucosa	Similar to characteristic vesicles on skin
Herpes labialis (cold sore), herpes simplex virus type I	Vesicular eruption on lip; patient is not always aware of infective nature — virus present in saliva	Often follows primary herpetic infection; stress, fever, local irritation. Exposure to sunlight may reactivate the virus
Herpes zoster (shingles), varicella zoster virus	Affects one or more branches of trigeminal (CN V) nerve, usually unilaterally	As above
Herpangina, Coxsackie virus group A	Multiple ulcers and erythema affecting palate and fauces	Mild, short-lasting
HIV infections/AIDS (see also candidiasis particularly pseudomembranous)	Oral disease present in 80% of patients with AIDS and 50% of patients with HIV (Palmer et al 1996) Oral manifestation may be first clinical sign; may present as hairy leukoplakia (Epstein–Barr virus has been isolated)	Early management advised to avoid serious complications when immune system is further suppressed (Scully et al 1991)
Kaposi's sarcoma (KS)	Red-blue or purple patches on skin of cheek or oral mucosa	50% of patients with KS have oral lesions (Scully et al 1991)
Bell's palsy — viral infection of facial nerve (CN VII)	Drooping of mouth, unable to close eye or wrinkle forehead	Very disfiguring; patient feels stigmatised

Table 15.4 Gastrointestinal and nutritional disorders affecting the mouth. (Adapted from Lamey & Lewis 1988)

Disorder	*Oral presentation*	*Cause/effect*
Gastro-oesophageal reflux (bulimia)	Erosion of teeth due to exposure to gastric acid from self-induced vomiting	Tooth erosion may be first indication of disorder
Crohn's disease	Irregular swelling of lower lip, angular cheilitis and folded thickening of oral mucosa	Mainly due to lymphoedema Sensitivity to foods, flavouring, dyes and preservatives
Coeliac disease	Recurrent oral ulceration	Caused by folic acid deficiency
Pernicious anaemia	Generalised papillary loss with mucosal atrophy	Caused by vitamin B_{12} deficiency
Iron deficiency anaemia	Atrophic glossitis	Less severe than that due to folic acid or vitamin B_{12} deficiency

A sore mouth is one of the side-effects that makes chemotherapy, radiotherapy to the head and neck area or preparation for BMT an unhappy experience for many people (see Ch. 31). In health, saliva normally helps to clear the mouth of harmful pathogens, but in these patients saliva becomes increasingly viscoid and xerostomia (dry mouth) develops which upsets the normal pH balance (Holmes 1997), creating an ideal environment for invasion by *Candida albicans*.

Candidiasis (thrush)

PATHOPHYSIOLOGY

Candidiasis, candidosis or moniliasis is caused by infection with *Candida* (*Monilia*) *albicans*, a yeast-like fungus normally found in the respiratory, alimentary and (in females) genital tracts of healthy people. Oral candidiasis is very common in people who are ill, debilitated, elderly or terminally ill. Presentation and predisposing factors are summarised in Table 15.3.

Systemic diseases showing oral manifestations

These include blood disorders such as leukaemia (bleeding gums), polycythaemia vera (bright red oral mucosa) and thrombocytopenic purpura (petechiae on tongue). For greater detail on these conditions, see Chapter 11. In dermatological conditions (see Ch. 12), examples of oral symptoms are Koplick's spots in measles and oral vesicles in chickenpox (varicella).

Burning mouth syndrome

Although this condition is neither inflammatory nor infective, it is relatively common, particularly among elderly women. The oral mucosa appears entirely normal, but the sufferer complains of continuous or intermittent burning sensation on tongue, palate, lips and lower alveolus.

Aetiological factors include vitamin deficiency, allergies, haematological disorders, undiagnosed diabetes, xerostomia and cancerphobia, the latter, in particular, causing much anxiety. Patients should be advised to seek specialist advice when the problem can usually be readily managed (Lamey 1996).

MEDICAL MANAGEMENT OF INFECTIONS AND INFLAMMATORY CONDITIONS

Treatment begins with the identification of the pathogen by culture swab or saliva washings. An appropriate antibiotic or antifungal agent is prescribed. Finlay et al (1996) found daily fluconazole more efficacious than amphotericin lozenges in the treatment of oral candidiasis during radiotherapy and it is also recommended for prophylaxis in recurrent candidiasis in patients with AIDS (Regnard et al 1997). To achieve maximum effect, topical drugs should be applied after oral hygiene procedures have been carried out. All patients having radiotherapy, chemotherapy or preparation for BMT should be referred for dental assessment before treatment starts (Maximiw & Wood 1989).

If the patient is being treated for a systemic disease, his medication should be reviewed with appropriate consideration of drug interactions. Only if the symptoms become severe will causative treatments such as radiotherapy be withdrawn temporarily.

Appropriate mouthwashes may be prescribed; again, drug interactions should be avoided (Barkvoll & Attramadal 1989).

NURSING PRIORITIES AND MANAGEMENT: INFECTIONS AND INFLAMMATORY CONDITIONS OF THE MOUTH

Many patients with these conditions are already ill people; to have to cope with an excruciatingly painful mouth can often overwhelm them completely and lead to total demoralisation. Nurses write frequently about oral care, but despite that, Ventafridda et al (1995) comment that 'many aspects of oral care need to be better defined'. Much of the ritual of oral care is unsuited to a sick person with acute stomatitis and/or candidiasis. However, there is evidence that protocols are being developed for oral care for seriously ill patients, e.g. in BMT (Porter 1992, Armstrong 1994, Coleman 1995), head and neck radiotherapy (Feber 1995, Little 1996, McIlroy 1996), intensive care (Kite 1995) and advanced cancer (Krishnasamay 1995).

Nursing responsibilities for oral care

It is difficult to encompass the many aspects of oral care in a limited text, but the student is invited to consider the following when caring for individuals and to challenge inappropriate practice.

Self-care should be encouraged whenever possible as patients know what their own mouths will tolerate (Little 1996) and are more likely to comply.

Assessment. The condition of the oral cavity may change from day to day; frequent assessment is vital, using a tool and chart to record changes. On the one hand, the patient may find it intrusive, but on the other, if the patient is self-caring, it can be used as an opportunity to supervise and offer encouragement. Holmes & Mountain (1993) and Coleman (1995) evaluate oral assessment tools which have benefits in different care settings.

Frequency. There is general agreement that care should be regular, but opinions vary as to frequency. Four times daily may be adequate for some patients, but those able to tolerate only rinsing or even just moistening may benefit from half-hourly care.

This may be an opportunity for relatives to contribute to care (Watson 1989). Cleaning before meals may improve appetite (Roberts 1990).

Regimen. A simple regimen is recommended. For dentate patients, a soft toothbrush and dentifrice are familiar. If there is fragile mucosa, foam sticks may remove debris but will not remove plaque. Gauze swabs held in forceps or wrapped around a finger are too rough and may remove a layer of regenerating epithelium. Irrigation with a syringe may be appropriate in some circumstances, but forceful use may damage mucosa. Following intraoral surgery, a patient may find it difficult to adapt to the changes inside his mouth because of alteration to contour and presence of insensate flaps (Little 1996), so supervision may be necessary to ensure removal of debris.

Cleansing agents. A mouth with acute stomatitis can be regarded as an open wound. Discussing painful wound dressings, Hollinworth (1997) reiterates that 'gentle irrigation with normal saline or tap water is usually effective for cleaning wounds'. Gooch (1985), Miller (1987) and Jenkins (1989) all recommend using tap water as an oral cleansing agent, and one must consider if water is not more appropriate for a patient with a painful mouth than some other traditionally recommended preparations.

Advantages and disadvantages of some oral care preparations described over two decades are summarised in Table 15.5.

Other more esoteric recommendations for oral care in a palliative care setting include pineapple chunks, cider and soda mouthwash for a 'dirty' mouth; and semi-frozen tonic water and gin, or fruit juice for a dry mouth (Regnard et al 1997).

From the information contained in Table 15.5, it can be seen that there is considerable variation in the opinions of practitioners from different care settings, and no one agent has been proven to be completely beneficial and harmless. In the absence of research evidence, it seems prudent to use only tap water or saline for patients with severe mucositis.

Temperature is important. Ice cubes may seem soothing if a mouth feels inflamed, but may delay the healing process. Warm solution is recommended for wound irrigation (Hollinworth 1997); it should assist in healing a damaged mouth and is often preferred by patients.

Analgesia must always be adequate and timed appropriately, e.g. to give maximum benefit at mealtimes and to cover periods away from the ward or home when receiving treatment. Opioids may be appropriate; topical anaesthesia including benzydamine mouthwash, mucaine or lozenges containing local anaesthetic may be used (Regnard et al 1997).

Dignity and self-esteem. Consideration should be given at all times to the importance to the patient of maintaining dignity and self-esteem. A sore mouth can be a further demoralising factor for a patient already under stress. All nursing care plans for oral care must form part of holistic care and must consider any therapeutic measures being implemented by other members of the multidisciplinary team.

Reference should also be made to oral hygiene as described earlier in this chapter, in Chapters 26–33 and in Jamieson et al (1997) considering each individual's needs.

OROFACIAL TRAUMA

Traumatic injury to the mouth or face typically gives rise to much anxiety concerning disfigurement. Moreover, because of the high vascularity of this area, blood loss at the time of injury may be considerable and the patient and his companions or relatives are likely to be very alarmed.

Soft tissue injuries to the face range from simple lacerations, knife wounds and bites to multiple injuries resulting in tissue loss. Bone injuries include fracture of the mandible and fracture of the maxillae, malar (zygomatic) and nasal bones (middle third fracture). The signs and symptoms of different types of fracture are summarised in Table 15.6.

Causes

Violence

During the period 1973–90, recorded woundings and assaults at one centre showed a sixfold increase (Shepherd et al 1993). Football hooliganism and attacks on public transport personnel are increasing. Shepherd (1989) argued that reasons for increases in violent crime include drug abuse, unemployment, inner-city deprivation and racism. Interpersonal violence is now the leading cause of facial fractures in many centres (Asadi & Asadi 1997).

Injury is usually caused by a direct blow from a fist or weapon. Many injuries occur in the course of unprovoked muggings and the victim may be in a state of shock (see Ch. 18). Many incidents are associated with excessive consumption of alcohol (Pernanen 1991). In a large study, Pernanen found that 73% of female assaults took place in the home, and 58% knew their assailant very well (37%) or fairly well (21%). In contrast, only 26% of male assaults happened at home, the remainder being at work, in the drinking place or on the street. Many researchers suspect that a significant percentage of assault cases go unreported, particularly among younger women. Lydon (1996) suggests the following reasons for this: fear due to repeated psychological abuse; fear of reprisals; fear for their children's safety or that they will be taken into care; and financial dependence on the assailant. Lydon comments that domestic violence is often trivialised and challenges nurses to be proactive in trying to bring to the fore this serious issue in our society. The Zero Tolerance campaign (theme: 'violence against women and children is a crime'), which started in Edinburgh and spread country-wide, is a very successful example of raising awareness of this issue (see Women's Aid, 'Useful addresses', p. 579).

Q **15.7** Discuss how you would react if you suspected that someone presenting to the A&E outpatient department had been assaulted by someone they know well.

Road traffic accidents (RTAs)

Facial injuries following RTAs (much reduced since seat belt legislation — Department of Health 1978) may involve lacerations, fractures and eye damage and may be compounded by other injuries.

Industrial injuries

Accidents in the workplace involving machinery or equipment are often followed by claims for compensation. Nurses should therefore not comment on the circumstances of any incident, either in person or by telephone, other than by using standard statements agreed by hospital policy (UKCC 1992).

Sports injuries

These are usually the result of a collision, fall or blow from a ball, bat or other piece of equipment. Facial injury is estimated to occur in 4–18% of sports injuries (Bayliss & Bedi 1996). Wearing helmets or gum shields may reduce injury.

Table 15.5 Advantages and disadvantages of mouth care preparations, 1977–97

Preparation	*Advantages/recommended by*	*Disadvantages/not favoured by*
Hydrogen peroxide	Topical germicidal, mechanical cleansing properties (Maurer 1977) Useful for loosening necrotic ulcers, crusting and debris (Crosby 1989) Weak solution may help dry crusted mucosa (Roberts 1990)	Forms medium for candidiasis (Segelman & Doku 1977) Causes burning if incorrectly diluted (Howarth 1977, Crosby 1989) No scientific or clinical basis for use (Daeffler 1980, Tombes & Gallucci 1993) May act as irritant to tongue when stomatitis is present; potentially dangerous if cough reflex is absent (Thurgood 1994)
Sodium bicarbonate	Alkaline component, has cleansing properties (Campbell 1987, Dudjak 1987) Useful for dry crusted mucosa (Roberts 1990) Use only if tenacious mucus present	Causes burning if incorrectly diluted (Howarth 1977, Crosby 1989) Will not remove thick tongue coating (Hallett 1984) Negates bacteriostatic, acidic properties of saliva (Gooch 1985) Use not advised, should be subject to investigation (Tombes & Gallucci 1993)
Lemon and glycerine		Lemon is acidic and glycerine is hypertonic, exhausts salivation process (Roth & Creason 1986, Crosby 1989) Has no place in oral cancer care (Roberts 1990)
Glycothymoline		Only transiently refreshing (Howarth 1977) No place in oral cancer care (Roberts 1990)
Chlorhexidine	Reduces plaque, effective for 2 h (Gibbons 1983, Crosby 1989) Prophylactic against *Candida* in BMT patients (Ferretti et al 1987) Use only after presence of infection is established (Dudjak 1987) Twice daily use advised to control bacteria (Roberts 1990)	Avoid use with nystatin, reduces efficacy (Barkvoll & Atramadal 1989) No significant improvement for leukaemia patients; rather, causes stinging of mucosa (Wahlin 1989) If dilution too strong, causes mucosal burning, stains teeth (Roberts 1990) Unpleasant taste (Thurgood 1994)
Fluoride rinse	Eliminated caries after radiotherapy (Roth & Creason 1986, Crosby 1989)	
Saliva substitutes	Increases comfort before eating or speaking, e.g. to relatives Recommended by several authors	Excessive use may cause discomfort (Holmes 1997)
Saline	Palliative treatment for leukaemia gingivitis; post-radiotherapy problems (Segelman & Doku 1977) Promotes healing and granulation tissue (Daeffler 1980) Alternative to hydrogen peroxide (Tombes & Gallucci 1993) Patients having oral radiation (Feber 1995) Recommended for wound healing (Hollinworth 1997)	
Prostaglandin E_2	Used topically — reduced mucositis in radiotherapy and chemotherapy (Matejka et al 1990) Protects GI tract mucosa (Calman & Langdon 1991)	
Tap water	Recommended by Gooch (1985), Miller (1987), Jenkins (1989)	
Effervescent ascorbic acid	Dislodges debris (Watson 1989) Part of hospice oral care protocol (Accord Hospice, Paisley 1998)	
Dentifrice and toothbrush	Recommended by several authors since Howarth (1977)	

Table 15.6 Characteristics and management of maxillofacial fractures (Note — there will be considerable variation in presentation and in the timing of manipulative procedures, in accordance with the exact site and combination of fractures)

Fracture	*Signs and symptoms*	*Management*
Fractured nasal bones	Nasal deviation or flattening; bruising	Manipulation of nasal bones and septum; nasal pack and plaster of Paris for 1–2 weeks
	Septal haematoma causing obstructed breathing	Drainage of haematoma
		Complicated fracture may need open reduction and internal fixation (ORIF)
Fractured malar bone	Black eye; swelling over cheek, sometimes flattening; anaesthesia of areas supplied by injured nerves (infraorbital and superior dental); inability to open mouth; diplopia	Elevation of malar bone through incision in temporal region Fixation by wiring of bone and packing of maxillary antrum is sometimes required
'Blow-out' fracture of malar	Periorbital haematoma; diplopia	Insertion of implant to orbital floor to stop eye dropping
Fractured maxilla/middle third fracture	Grossly swollen face; failure of teeth to occlude properly; bilateral periorbital haematoma; fractured nasal bones; teeth may be loosened; CSF rhinorrhoea	Reduction and fixation of fractures by eyelet wires, cap splints, etc., plaster of Paris head cap or halo frame (see Figs 15.3–15.6) Antibiotics
Fractured mandible with/without other fractured facial bones	Displaced or undisplaced; local pain and swelling; severe pain on opening mouth; sublingual haematoma	Undisplaced: usually no treatment Displaced: reduction with wires or splints depending on site of fracture

Accidents

Accidental falls are common among elderly people, often resulting in facial injury. The underlying cause of the fall may require investigation (Chew & Edmondson 1996).

Burns

The treatment of burn injuries is discussed in detail in Chapter 30. It can be emphasised here, however, that to assist in the prevention of contractures of the mouth and subsequent difficulty in function or administration of a general anaesthetic, burns patients should be encouraged to drink from a cup as early as possible and avoid the use of straws.

Q **15.8** Take a few sips of a drink directly from a cup and then with a straw. What do you observe about the maxillofacial movement required for these two actions?

MEDICAL MANAGEMENT

Immediate intervention. Emergency treatment of all traumatic injuries will involve whatever resuscitative measures are required to maintain the patient's airway, breathing and circulation and to circumvent the development of clinical shock (see Chs 18 and 27). Priorities for intervention will have to be set if multiple injuries exist. A full physical examination will involve neurological observations and X-rays as appropriate, and will be followed by referral to the appropriate specialists, e.g. maxillofacial, orthopaedic or ophthalmic surgeons. Cannell et al (1996) state that, in using an injury assessment tool (Ali & Shepherd 1994) when assessing multiply injured patients, maxillofacial injuries often tend to be underscored and that a maxillofacial surgeon should be involved as soon as possible to minimise facial deformity. However, the person with a maxillofacial injury with minimal displacement of bone and no symptoms of head injury may delay attending for treatment until, eventually, swelling and bruising make the injury appear more alarming.

Treatment of maxillofacial injuries. The signs and symptoms of maxillofacial injuries, together with appropriate treatments, are summarised in Table 15.6.

Soft-tissue injuries require thorough cleansing (this may entail scrubbing of the wound under general anaesthesia) to remove glass, debris, gravel, dirt and so on. Failure to adequately clean the injury will lead to 'tattoo scarring', i.e. a permanent blue-grey scar. Facial suturing should adhere to plastic surgical techniques (McGregor & McGregor 1995).

Bone injuries. The objectives of treatment are to restore pre-existing anatomy, functional occlusion of teeth and facial appearance. The commonest method of immobilisation now employed is open reduction and internal fixation (ORIF) of the fracture using either a rigid plate or mini-plates. However, other methods may still be successfully used and are also briefly described:

- *Interosseous plating*. The fracture is exposed, reduced (i.e. repositioned) and fixed with a rigid plate or mini-plates. This may be left in situ permanently or removed after 3 months (see Fig. 15.3).
- *Eyelet wiring*. Wires are twisted around the upper and lower teeth, leaving a loop (eyelet). The teeth are then brought into proper occlusion and wired together (see Fig. 15.4).
- *Arch bar wiring*. This technique is similar to eyelet wiring but is used when fewer teeth exist. A malleable bar is fitted over the gum and wired as above.
- *Gunning splint*. This is used if dentures are absent or ill-fitting. 'Dentures' without teeth are fitted and wired to each other (see Fig. 15.5).
- *Cast cap splinting*. Metal alloy splints are made from dental impressions and cemented onto the teeth. The jaws are then wired together or fixed with rubber bands.

Undisplaced fractures of the mandible generally require no surgical treatment.

A fractured maxilla can be immobilised internally or externally, depending on the precise nature of the injury. Internal fixation can be achieved by means of metal plates or with internal suspension

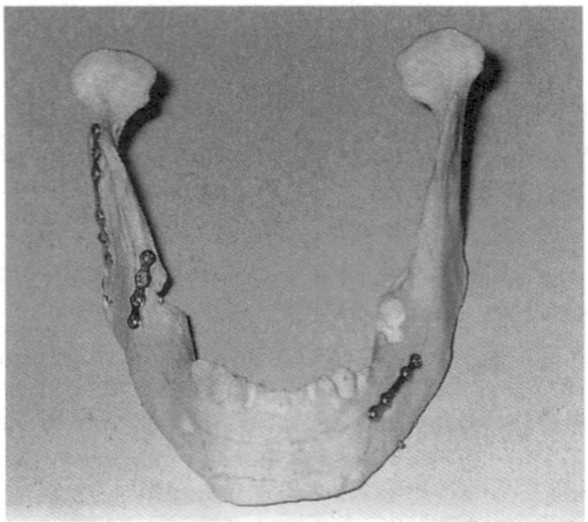

Fig. 15.3 Interosseous plating.

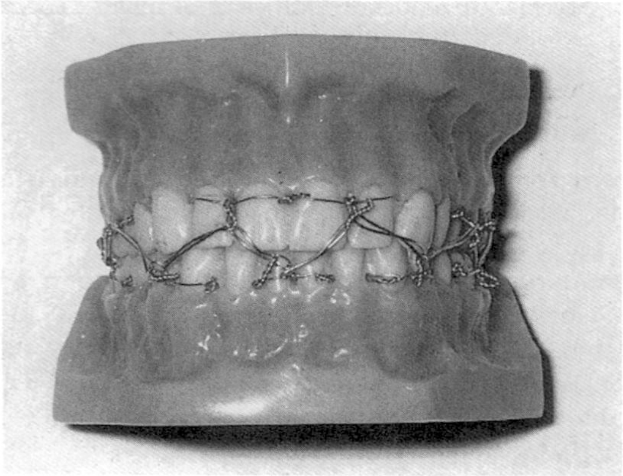

Fig. 15.4 Eyelet wiring.

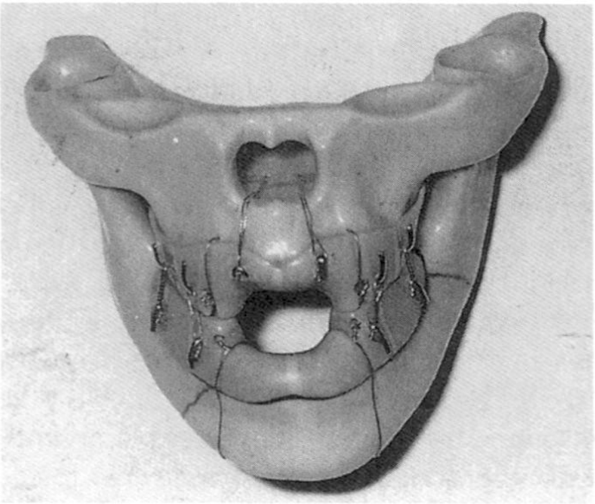

Fig. 15.5 Gunning splint.

wires. The latter hold the maxilla and mandible in occlusion and are fixed to the malar or frontal bone.

External fixation is now less commonly seen but may be achieved by the following means:

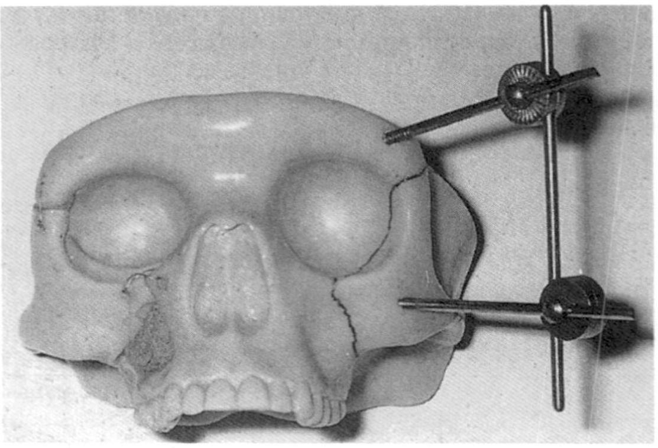

Fig. 15.6 Model showing fractures of malar or zygomatic bones and maxillae. The right bones have been wired, an implant placed in the floor of the orbit, and packing inserted in the maxillary antrum. On the left side, fractures are stabilised by means of a form of external fixation.

- Le Vant or box frame — a metal frame is screwed to the skull through the supraorbital ridge. Rods are then attached to dental splints and secured to the frame
- plaster of Paris head cap firmly fitted to the skull
- halo frame — a metal frame fixed to the skull.

The latter two are much less commonly used methods.

Treatment of a fractured malar (zygoma) may take the following forms:

- elevation through incision in the temporal region
- wiring of the fracture and packing of the maxillary antrum to maintain stability (see Fig. 15.6)
- K-wires (rigid wires) in one or more directions; the ends are cut just clear of the skin
- an implant may be necessary to repair a shattered orbital floor (see Fig. 15.6).

Fractured nasal bones may also form part of a compound facial injury. Here, the fracture is reduced by manipulation of the nasal bones and immobilised by a plaster of Paris splint.

For further information on the treatment of maxillofacial injuries, see Williams (1994).

NURSING PRIORITIES AND MANAGEMENT: OROFACIAL TRAUMA

Orofacial injuries vary widely both in presentation and in their impact upon the individual's lifestyle and psychological well-being. Case Histories 15.1 and 15.2 outline the experiences of two patients admitted to hospital after receiving blows to the face. Each has different needs, priorities and concerns, and hence different requirements for nursing care. While the treatment of individuals who have suffered orofacial trauma must take into account a range of physical and emotional considerations, only that care which is specific to the mouth and face will be described here. General pre- and postoperative care is discussed in Chapter 26; reference to other chapters will be made as appropriate.

Case History 15.1 Ms Y

Ms Y, aged 23, was brought to the A&E department by a neighbour who heard a disturbance and found her dazed. She was found to be suffering from concussion, a fractured malar bone and facial lacerations, and was admitted to the ward. Ms Y explained that she received these injuries when she tripped and fell against a door.

Ms Y was told that she would have to have the fractured malar reduced and stabilised under anaesthetic. She was assured that the operation was not a major procedure, but that the fracture would simply be fixed by means of wires. She was also given general information on preoperative procedures and postoperative care.

As well as wiring the fractured malar bone, the surgeon inserted a gauze pack soaked in Whitehead's varnish into the maxillary antrum to support the orbital floor. A small portion was left protruding into the mouth through an incision in the upper gum. The nurse explained to Ms Y that it was important for her not to disturb this, and that she should take care not to use mouthwash too vigorously.

She was able to take a soft diet, however, and was advised to continue with soft foods for 7–10 days and to take as much protein as possible to promote healing.

After the incident, Ms Y was also suffering from diplopia (double vision) as a result of a slight displacement of one eye. This persisted and she was later referred for orthoptic exercises.

While she was on the ward, Ms Y began to disclose some of her domestic problems, first to her primary nurse and then to the medical social worker who, with Ms Y's agreement, had become involved. Ms Y indicated that she would consider accepting assistance from a women's support group. The social worker arranged for Ms Y's children to be cared for until she was ready for discharge.

Ms Y's discharge was planned well in advance. Through liaison with women's support agencies, she was assisted in reviewing her home circumstances and was offered alternative accommodation with her children.

Case History 15.2 Mr J

Mr J, aged 30, was assaulted while returning from an evening out with friends. He was unconscious for a short time after the incident. He was brought to the A&E department in the recovery position to prevent blood from inside his mouth trickling down the pharynx (and potentially the trachea) and causing respiratory distress. (Fortunately, he had not suffered pneumothorax, in which case he might not have been able to lie in this position.) It was difficult to restrain him as he was restless from the combined effects of blows to the head and the alcohol he had taken. He was found to be suffering from a middle third fracture, a fractured mandible, fractured ribs and facial lacerations.

Mr J was advised that his jaws would have to be wired together and external fixation applied, but he had difficulty concentrating and absorbing information. His wife was present during the discussion. She was very anxious and mentioned that she had been concerned by the fact that her husband had been drinking more lately.

When he awoke from the anaesthetic, Mr J was quite frightened, as he did not remember much of what had been explained to him preoperatively. The nurse in the recovery ward told Mr J to breathe deeply and encouraged him to relax. She then explained again what had happened and what was preventing him from opening his mouth. She explained why it was important for him not to disturb the fixation, but also assured him that if it ever became urgent for him to release his jaw, the necessary equipment was at hand. She then stayed with Mr J until the feeling of the wires became more familiar to him, and ensured that adequate analgesics and sedation were being administered (see Ch. 19).

Mr J had some problems in the first few postoperative days when he accidentally turned in bed and knocked his frame. He was somewhat apprehensive about having a visit from his active 2-year-old daughter.

He was able to take only a liquid diet, and so liquidised meals were provided with supplementary drinks. He was advised that he could obtain a prescription from his GP for high-calorie drinks during the time when the wiring was in place.

Mr J was surprised at how quickly the appearance of his injury improved. His facial wounds healed quite rapidly and he was encouraged that within a few months the scars would fade and become less noticeable.

While he was still in hospital, he was encouraged to review his alcohol intake and was given information on the effects of alcohol abuse and on local self-help groups from whom he and his family could obtain support as he addressed his dependency problem (see Ch. 36).

Life-threatening concerns

For patients who have suffered maxillofacial injury, the immediate priority of intervention is likely to be to maintain the airway. Respiratory difficulty and haemorrhage will require immediate care.

Respiratory difficulty

This problem can vary in severity and may be due to swelling of the tongue caused by oedema or haematoma, or to the patient's inability to control the tongue because of disturbance of the muscle attachments. If the patient is conscious, he should be sat up and propped forward as soon as possible, if other injuries allow. The airway must be kept clear. If the maxilla is fractured, it may be necessary to insert two fingers into the patient's mouth and hook behind the hard palate to re-establish the airway. In severe cases, early intubation or tracheostomy may be necessary.

Haemorrhage

There may be significant haemorrhage from middle third fractures resulting in cheek swelling, and nasal packing may be required. Bleeding may also be profuse when soft tissue injury has occurred, and immediate measures may be necessary, e.g. applying pressure on a bleeding point or pressure point, until ligation of the damaged vessel can be performed. Bleeding can also be controlled by holding the skin edges together with Steristrips until suturing can be carried out.

Shock

Nursing and medical staff must be alert to the warning signs of shock and should be prepared to take urgent action (see Ch. 18).

Major nursing considerations

Observation and monitoring

Vital signs (temperature, pulse, respiration and blood pressure) should be recorded at regular intervals. Neurological observations may be appropriate (see Ch. 9).

Rhinorrhoea. The nurse should also watch for the presence of rhinorrhoea (nasal discharge) caused by leakage of cerebrospinal fluid (CSF). This can occur in fracture of the maxilla if the cribriform plate of the ethmoid bone is disturbed. CSF gives a positive reaction to Dextrostix.

Eye integrity/vision (see also Ch. 13). The nurse should check for abnormal pupil reactions, proptosis and acute pain. Vision should be checked hourly at first, especially if the patient cannot open his eyes because of oedema. The nurse should gently open the eyes and check pupil reaction. Any rapid decrease in visual acuity can indicate retrobulbar haemorrhage, which can lead to blindness and requires urgent action. Double vision can indicate a fracture of the orbital floor.

Major patient problems

Pain

Pain must be assessed (see Ch. 19) but is not normally a major early problem. It is important, however, not to underestimate the patient's pain and to explain why analgesics may have to be withheld initially while investigations are carried out (see Ch. 27).

Anxiety

Anxiety caused by fear of disfigurement and scarring may be the first concern of many patients and relatives. An injury to the eye will be a source of further anxiety.

Patients and relatives should be given the opportunity to talk about their fears, particularly in the early stages when profuse bleeding may make the injury look horrific. Nurses should offer the reassurance that healing is usually rapid and that as much as possible will be done to minimise scarring. However, it is equally important not to raise expectations unduly. Some people have unrealistic ideas about the results that surgery can produce, and it is unfair to allow them to imagine that what existed before can always be fully restored. Scars can fade and may be camouflaged, but it is not always possible to disguise the disfigurement caused by major tissue loss or bone displacement and it may be appropriate to introduce psychological support at an early stage (Partridge 1993).

Nurses should also bear in mind that post-traumatic amnesia, in which the patient has no recall of events immediately preceding the incident (see Ch. 17), may give rise to psychological distress later should the memory of the event return (see Box 15.3).

Other considerations

Every effort should be made to clean blood and debris from the patient before his relatives see him, in order to avoid unnecessary distress. Dirty clothing should be removed, observing local policy for the care of patients' property.

Box 15.3 Post-traumatic amnesia

A well publicised example of post-traumatic amnesia is the case of Trevor Rees-Jones, the sole survivor of the crash which killed Diana, Princess of Wales, in 1997. Despite wearing a seat belt, Mr Rees-Jones sustained multiple head and facial injuries, which required many reconstructive operations. Although he made a good physical recovery and was able to work, after a year he still had no memory of the events leading up to the crash (*The Times*, 4 August 1998).

Oral hygiene should be carried out within the limitations of the patient's condition. For example, a blood clot should be left undisturbed as far as possible to minimise further bleeding, but broken teeth, debris and so on should be removed if this has not already been done. Gentle irrigation with warm saline may be helpful.

Nursing care in surgical interventions

Patients who have soft tissue injury without bone damage will have suturing and/or reconstruction carried out as soon as possible.

Many patients with maxillofacial fractures will require surgical intervention to reduce and stabilise the fracture. The timing of this surgery will vary according to the patient's overall condition and the amount of localised swelling which may make assessment of the fracture difficult. In many cases, fixation is best left for a few days; if his general condition permits, the patient may be discharged home for the interim. Alternatively, direct transfer to a specialised unit may be arranged.

Postoperative management

The overall aim of postoperative management is to assist the patient as necessary with the activities of daily living and to help him to achieve independence in these activities as soon as possible.

Monitoring vital signs. In the initial postoperative period, the patient's vital signs should be recorded every 15 min. As his condition stabilises, the patient can gradually be raised to a sitting position to aid respiration, help drainage and minimise oedema. The patient should be encouraged to maintain an upright position even at night. Individuals who find it very difficult to sleep sitting up may find that resting against pillows placed in armchair fashion helps. A reclining armchair, if available, can be useful later if other injuries permit this.

Respiration. The patient may have a nasal airway in situ to assist breathing and this will need occasional suction to be kept clear. The mouth may also need gentle suction if the patient is afraid to swallow saliva for fear of choking. The patient should be encouraged to relax and to practise gentle swallowing movements.

Oral hygiene. It will be very important to help the patient maintain good oral hygiene. If the jaws have been wired, a soft toothbrush or Q-tips can be used to keep the anterior surface of the teeth and splints clean. The inside of the mouth can be cleansed with mouthwash taken through a straw (or a feeding cup with a spout) and squeezed out between the teeth. An alternative method is to irrigate the mouth through gaps between the teeth, using a rubber ball (chip) syringe, letting the fluid run out.

Preventing wound infection. The skin entry points of external fixation should be kept free of crusting by cleaning with normal saline. An ointment such as sterile petroleum jelly may be applied.

Sutures to facial lacerations can be kept clean with normal saline and removed in 3–4 days to minimise scarring. Supporting Steristrips may then be applied over the wound for a further 3–4 days. Any intraoral lacerations are usually repaired using catgut, which will be absorbed, but the mouth should be checked in case any non-absorbent sutures have been used, e.g. inside the lip.

Maintenance of fixation. The guiding principle of the treatment of maxillofacial fractures is, as for any other types of fracture, to obtain healing in the optimal position (e.g. that which maintains proper occlusion). In order for callus to form, and thus for healing to take place, the bone must remain immobile. Many patients will have fractures fixed with internal metal plates. However, if the jaw is immobilised by other means, appropriate instruments for releasing the fixation (i.e. wire cutters, or scissors for elastic bands) must always be available at the patient's bedside for immediate use should any danger of airway obstruction arise.

Instruments for tightening screws should also be at hand, and the fixation checked at regular intervals. Most patients will be aware if it becomes loose, but elderly people or those with head injury may not be. To avoid confusion, only those instruments appropriate for loosening or tightening the individual's particular type of fixation should be available at the bedside.

Nutrition (see also Ch. 21). A nasogastric tube may be inserted to allow for postoperative aspiration and/or drainage of old blood. Oral feeding should be encouraged as soon as possible, and there are particular problems if the jaws must be kept wired for several weeks. A liquid diet must be taken, which may make it difficult for the patient to consume sufficient calories to maintain body weight. All food must be liquidised and supplemented with 'sip feeds', of which a wide variety is now available. Frequent, small meals should be taken throughout the day.

The dietician should be consulted, ideally before the surgery takes place, to assess the patient's dietary requirements. Elderly patients with a low body mass index (BMI) will require special monitoring and encouragement. This is especially important if food is served by non-nursing personnel who may not appreciate the significance of unfinished meals.

Q **15.9** How can a calorie intake adequate to promote healing be provided within the constraints of a hospital setting for Ms Y (Case History 15.1), who has no interest in food, and Mr J (Case History 15.2), whose injuries prevent him from eating solid food?

Allaying fears. Nursing staff should bear in mind that the patient is likely to be very alarmed when he recovers from anaesthesia to find that interdental or external fixation is in place, even if he had been informed that this would be necessary. It is important that the patient is given some means of expressing his feelings and concerns and is briefed fully on how he will be able to manage basic functions such as eating and how he will be able to avoid choking should he need to cough up phlegm or to vomit.

Communication will be frustrating for the patient initially if his jaws have been fixed, but most difficulties will be overcome by otherwise healthy people, given sufficient encouragement and reassurance in the early stages. Writing pads, 'magic' slates, picture cards and other aids may be used to facilitate communication. Special care will be needed for patients with learning difficulties.

Mobility. When and how well the patient will be able to mobilise will depend on the nature of any other injuries incurred. Patients with facial injuries can be up on the day following surgery, but there are obvious restrictions if a maxillocranial frame is in place.

Q **15.10** Stop and reflect on how your own activities would be affected if you had metal rods protruding from your head.

Body image. Disfigurement caused by facial injuries is of great concern to most patients, and for the majority scarring will be a source of continuing anxiety.

Many people will be reluctant to look at themselves in a mirror following surgery and should not be forced to do so. It might help for the nurse to ask the patient if he would like her to describe how his face looks to her; if her account is matter-of-fact and accepting, he may be more willing to look at himself. Unfortunately, for many people, disfigurement will give rise to deep feelings of grief and loss which may never be completely resolved, and specialist help may be needed (Robinson et al 1996).

Discharge planning

Patients who are fit and who can maintain adequate self-care can be discharged when postoperative swelling has subsided. They should be provided with written instructions on diet and oral hygiene, and given a telephone number to call in case of emergency. Referral to the community nurse should be made for care of wounds, checking of fixation and assessment of diet. A follow-up appointment should be made for the patient to return after 4–6 weeks to have the fixation removed.

Elderly patients who are frail may never recover fully from maxillofacial injury and surgery. Some who are fit to go home may well be too afraid or self-conscious to go out again. The community nurse is in an ideal position to encourage such individuals to venture into the outside world again. Some may require long-term care, whether within the family, in sheltered housing or in an appropriate home.

TUMOURS OF THE MOUTH

Oral cancer is more common than is often realised, the mortality rates being comparable with malignant melanoma and cervical cancer, which are subject to more publicity and screening programmes (Brown & Langdon 1995). Much of it could be prevented, as early diagnosis leads to cure, and nurses in their role as health educators can make a significant contribution to its reduction (see Box 15.1, p. 559).

Treatment of intraoral tumours is frequently carried out in specialised units. However, as the use of advanced reconstructive techniques becomes more widespread and patients are discharged into the community at an earlier stage, often to continue treatment as outpatients, nurses in more general areas of practice are likely to encounter these patients. To help to ensure continuity of care from hospital to the community, it is important for general nurses to have an understanding of the long-term problems faced by these patients (Espie et al 1989, Freedlander et al 1989, Kelly 1994).

Treatment plans vary from centre to centre and there are different schools of thought within the medical profession as to which treatment schedule best promotes survival and, also important, a good quality of life (McAndrew 1990). However treated, it is likely that many patients will suffer some disruption of several basic mechanisms which control the functions of eating and speaking. Patients may be left with short-term, long-term or permanent malfunction, which will vary greatly from patient to patient and is dependent on many factors. Table 15.7 indicates some of the malfunctions following surgery and/or radiotherapy.

It must be stressed that each patient is very much an individual whose needs and priorities will differ significantly from those of another patient with a seemingly similar problem. There can therefore be no set plan of care, and nurses must be ready and equipped to modify their ideas (working in conjunction with the other members of the multidisciplinary team and with the patient) to meet the individual's needs. As rehabilitation may take many months or years, it is often necessary for this multidisciplinary liaison to continue for some considerable time to ensure the best possible quality of care.

The pathophysiology and common presenting symptoms of tumours of the mouth are described under the following headings:

- tumours of the lips
- tumours of the floor of the mouth and tongue

Table 15.7 The effects of intraoral disease and treatment on the mechanisms of eating

Normal mechanism and cranial nerves involved	*Disruption caused by intervention*	*Effects*
Teeth bite and chew food, powered by muscles of jaw and supplied by trigeminal (5th cranial) nerve	Teeth may be extracted due to caries or to give access to tumour	Soft food only can be taken until fitting of dentures, if this is possible
Saliva secreted by parotid gland (9th cranial nerve), submandibular and sublingual glands mixes with food	Glands may be excised during surgery or damaged by radiotherapy	Dry mouth (xerostomia) Stomatitis Thrush
Tongue and teeth powered by muscles of jaw break down food and form it into bolus	Muscles damaged or weakened by surgery and trauma	Re-education of eating skills will be needed
Mouth kept closed by superficial facial muscles (supplied by CN V and CN VII) Buccinator prevents food gathering in cheek pouches	Internal contours of mouth are altered; lack of control, temporomandibular joint malfunction	Drooling Food gathers in mouth Trismus — mouth cannot open
Tongue helps propel food to back of mouth and into contact with oral part of pharynx	Excision of part or whole tongue. Tongue becomes fixed or insensate	Patient needs to push food to oropharynx
Simultaneously with above, muscles of soft palate elevate and tighten, straightening out to close off nasal cavity and preventing food from entering it	Damage to palate and nerves allows food to enter nasal space	Food, liquids come down nose unless obturator (see Box 15.4) can be fitted
Larynx rises under shelter of epiglottis to close off airway, preventing entry of food	CN IX damage causes paralysis of pharyngeal muscles	Aspiration of fluid to lungs necessitates permanent tracheostomy and gastrostomy

- tumours of the palate
- tumours of the salivary glands.

However, because the separate functions of the mouth, e.g. speaking, chewing and swallowing, are frequently interdependent, medical and nursing management will be discussed with reference to the whole mouth.

Tumours of the lips

PATHOPHYSIOLOGY

Benign tumours, including granulomata, are treated by simple excision.

Malignant disease may take the form of basal cell carcinoma (BCC, often called 'rodent ulcer' because of its pattern of 'eating' or 'gnawing into' tissue) or squamous cell carcinoma (SCC). Malignant melanomas may also rarely occur on the lips (see Ch. 12).

Predisposing factors include prolonged, unprotected exposure to sunlight (e.g. among outdoor workers), fair skin and pipe smoking. The lower incidence of lip cancers among women may possibly be due to the barrier effect of cosmetics.

Common presenting symptoms. Basal cell carcinoma may appear as a nodule or as a small, unstable ulcerating area with persistent crusting. It may also be diffuse and invasive. The patient often reports: 'I thought it had healed up, but I kept knocking the top off it'. The ulcer may have 'pearlised' rolled edges. These tumours are generally slow-growing and do not metastasise, although occasionally a tendency to multiple BCCs is seen.

Squamous cell carcinoma is more aggressive and, if untreated, may assume the 'cauliflower' look of a malignant ulcer and will eventually fungate and cause severe pain.

Tumours of the floor of the mouth and tongue

PATHOPHYSIOLOGY

Tumours of the tongue account for about one-third of all intraoral tumours in the UK. Others included in the category of the floor of the mouth are found on the lower alveolus, tonsillar fossae and retromolar trigones, and about 90% are of the SCC type (Smith 1989). The incidence is twice as common in men as in women, and although there was a dramatic fall from the start of this century until the 1970s, both incidence and mortality rates now appear to be rising, especially in younger men in almost all EC countries. In the UK, a north–south divide is noted, with a higher incidence in Scotland and northern England (Cancer Research Campaign 1993).

Spread usually involves the local lymph nodes (e.g. cervical, submandibular, submental). Distant metastases occur rarely in the lung.

Predisposing factors. Heavy smoking combined with excessive alcohol consumption is associated with these cancers. In countries where tobacco-chewing is common (e.g. India) the incidence of oral cancer is relatively high (Smith 1989). Chewing tobacco teabags or the use of nicotine chewing gum is also thought to contribute. However, tumours do occur in patients who have never smoked and who seldom or never take alcohol. There is thought to be a relationship with chronic oral infections, e.g. syphilis, herpes simplex virus, human papilloma virus and HIV (Smith 1989). Poor oral hygiene and nutritional deficiencies are often present and may be causative factors (Cancer Research Campaign 1993). Diets high in fruit (Winn 1995) and antioxidants (Garewal 1995) are thought to be preventive factors.

Common presenting symptoms. These cancers may become apparent in a variety of ways. In the early stages, intraoral SCC is easily mistaken for infection, irritation from dentures or a simple aphthous ulcer. Dysplasia, abnormal mucosa, which presents as white patches (leukoplakia) or red patches (erythroplakia), is a precancerous condition which can revert to normal if the individual stops smoking. Unchecked, this condition will usually become malignant (Williams 1990). More advanced tumours are usually unmistakable, but many patients present late for various reasons, including fear, misdiagnosis and self-neglect.

Tumours of the hard and soft palate

PATHOPHYSIOLOGY

These tumours may arise from the epithelium of the mucous membrane (SCC), in the maxillary sinuses, in the maxilla or in the minor salivary glands in the palate. They are less common than tumours of the floor of the mouth, but are potentially more disfiguring, as spread may occur locally to the floor of the orbit or to the eye.

Common presenting symptoms. Onset may be insidious. The patient may notice a dull ache for some time and may complain of 'sinusitis'. The pain will eventually increase and swelling may develop over the cheek. There may be some displacement of the eye (proptosis) in advanced cases. Rarely, a malignant melanoma appears as a pigmented lesion of the palate and goes unnoticed until the individual presents with a secondary tumour of the cheek or neck.

Tumours of the salivary glands

PATHOPHYSIOLOGY

The most common cause of swelling of the parotid gland is mumps (acute parotitis), an infectious, inflammatory condition that usually resolves without treatment. Mumps may, however, be relatively severe in adults and lead to pancreatitis or orchitis.

Benign (pleomorphic salivary adenomas, PSAs) or malignant tumours may develop in the parotid, submandibular, sublingual and other minor salivary glands. Salivary gland ducts may become blocked by small accretions (see 'Orodental disease', p. 559).

Common presenting symptoms. The patient presents with a swelling, which is often asymptomatic and therefore sometimes long-standing, in the area of the affected gland. If left untreated, a parotid gland tumour may involve the facial nerve (cranial nerve VII), resulting in facial palsy, a severe disfigurement.

MEDICAL MANAGEMENT OF TUMOURS OF THE MOUTH

Tests and investigations. A treatment plan for malignant tumours will be devised on the basis of careful staging of the cancer (see Table 15.8 and Ch. 31). Investigation may include the following:

- history
- physical examination — visual and by palpation
- blood tests
- diagnostic X-rays — face and jaw; chest and spine as appropriate
- orthopantomogram (OPT; see Appendix 1)
- sialogram (see Appendix 1)
- CT (computed tomogram) scan
- MRI (magnetic resonance imaging; see Ch. 31)
- EUA (examination under anaesthetic)
- videofluoroscopy (see Appendix 1)
- fine needle aspiration (see Appendix 1)
- biopsy — results are essential for staging disease and planning treatment.

The patient's age, general physical condition and mental outlook will also be taken into consideration.

Treatment. Patients are often seen at a combined clinic, which can be very stressful (Telfer & Shepherd 1993). Different specialist consultants can plan treatment, which may be radical, i.e. intended to effect a cure, or conservative, i.e. intended to alleviate pain, prevent fungating tumours and subsequent haemorrhage. Radical treatment may involve extremely difficult adjustments for patients and, for some, a significant reduction in the quality of life (Espie et al 1989, Freedlander et al 1989).

The treatment options for oral tumours are radiotherapy, surgery and, less commonly as first-line treatment, chemotherapy. These treatment modes may be used singly or in combination; sequence and timing vary from one centre to another.

Chemotherapy is usually given concurrently with other treatment. It may be used to reduce the bulk of some tumours prior to surgery or in cases of recurrent tumours (see also Ch. 31).

Radiotherapy can be given as the sole treatment, or pre- or postoperatively. It may take either of the following forms:

- teletherapy (external radiation) by means of megavoltage machines or supervoltage machines
- brachytherapy, in which a radioactive source is placed in or near the tumour, e.g. interstitial needles to tumours of the lip or oral cavity. This treatment is being used increasingly in tongue cancer to try to maximise quality of life (Harrison 1997).

Many tumours (e.g. SCC) are highly curable by radiotherapy. Sarcoma and malignant melanoma, on the other hand, are less radiosensitive (see also Ch. 31, Snape & Robinson 1996, Holmes 1997).

Surgical excision. Treatment by this method ranges from small local excisions with direct closure, to major operations with full reconstruction. Benign tumours are usually excised.

Some centres carry out excision of tumours initially with secondary reconstruction later; others carry out immediate reconstruction. Table 15.9 summarises current surgical procedures.

Both radiotherapy and surgery treat squamous cell carcinoma successfully, either independently or in combination, but there is lack of agreement among medical practitioners as to the best timing of each.

See McGregor & McGregor (1986) for detailed information on surgical and other therapies for cancers of the mouth.

Table 15.8 TNM classification for lip and oral cavity. (Adapted from Sobin & Wittekind 1997)

T: Primary tumour	
T1	Tumour <2 cm
T2	Tumour >2–4 cm
T3	Tumour >4 cm
T4	Tumour invading adjacent structures
N: lymph nodes (neck)	
N1	Ipsilateral single node <3 cm
N2	Ipsilateral single node >3–6 cm
	Ipsilateral, multiple nodes <6 cm
	Bilateral, contralateral nodes <6 cm
N3	Node >6 cm
M: distant metastases	
M0	No distant metastases
M1	Distant metastases

Table 15.9 Surgery for tumours of the mouth

Site	*Excision*	*Reconstruction*
Superficial lesion of lip, leukoplakia	Shaving	None
Lip, parotid gland, T1 tumour of mouth	Simple excision	None: direct (primary) closure
Lip	Wedge excision	Direct closure
Tongue	Local excision	Split-skin graft
Lip, alveolus, tongue	Local excision	Local flap (many varieties: Abbe, tongue, buccal, nasolabial, etc. See Soutar & Tiwari 1996)
Mouth/pharynx (all sites), cheek, neck	Local/wide excision ± neck dissection	Free flap common in many centres (Webster & Soutar 1986)
As above (especially for recurrent tumour as palliative procedure)	As above	Pedicled flap (deltopectoral, pectoralis major)

Nurses should be aware of the effect of radiation on the epithelium (see Ch. 31, Little 1996, Snape & Robinson 1996, Holmes 1997). Following radical radiotherapy, healing after surgery may be delayed; occasionally, orocutaneous (between mouth and skin) fistulae may develop. A late effect may be bone necrosis (osteoradionecrosis).

Follow-up and after-care will require outpatient appointments at regular intervals for at least 5 years. Dental and/or prosthetic provision may include dentures, obturators (see Box 15.4) and other prostheses provided by members of the multidisciplinary team as and when necessary. Referral to other consultants (e.g. ENT, ophthalmic, thoracic and neurological specialists) will be made as appropriate. Speech therapy and dietary advice will be essential for many patients.

NURSING PRIORITIES AND MANAGEMENT: TUMOURS OF THE MOUTH

The presence of an oral tumour may not give rise to immediate life-threatening concerns, except where a long-neglected tumour causes respiratory distress or haemorrhage.

Patients will vary widely in the symptoms with which they present, and usually require much reassurance when a biopsy confirms the diagnosis. They will be admitted as soon as appropriate treatment has been arranged, or immediately if disease is advanced. A gastrostomy (see Ch. 21) may be planned if swallowing difficulties are anticipated. The nurse may require to be the patient's advocate, to ensure that he has adequate understanding before he consents to treatment. Referral to the primary care team and/or Macmillan or Marie Curie home care nurses will be beneficial to many patients for support before definitive treatment starts.

Immediate nursing priorities

Nursing intervention in the early stages of treatment will focus on controlling pain (see Ch. 19), relieving anxiety, encouraging self-care in oral hygiene, and nutritional assessment (see Ch. 21). Supplementary feeding may be necessary, as weight loss is common among this group of patients. Existing physical conditions must of course be taken into account in any nursing plan. An additional concern may be the assessment and control of alcoholism. Excessive consumption of alcohol is a causative factor in many cases of oral cancer, and advice and information on limiting the intake of alcohol may be given by nurses (see Ch. 36).

Box 15.4 Obturators

Obturators are prostheses which are designed to fill a defect in the palate after maxillectomy. They are fitted in three stages:

1. *Surgical splint*. Fitted during surgery to hold a skin graft in place and/or avoid collapse of the cheek and upper lip. After about 2 weeks, it is replaced by a temporary obturator.
2. *Temporary obturator*. Used throughout radiotherapy. This allows the patient to become accustomed to wearing and handling an obturator.
3. *Definitive obturator*. Fitted after shrinkage of defect. It may be composed of a soft malleable 'bung' which fills the defect, and a denture which fits over the bung.

Without the obturator, the patient will be unable to speak or eat properly, and fluid will run into the nasal cavity. With a well-fitting obturator, the patient can eat and speak normally.

The obturator must be removed after meals and cleaned by brushing or by immersion in a proprietary cleaning solution (if the obturator has been 'built up', cleanser should not be used). The mouth must be rinsed after all food to prevent accumulation of plaque, debris, etc.

Preoperative preparation

Giving information

All patients will require adequate and honest information about the proposed treatment and its implications (see Ch. 31). In view of the many variations in procedures, and the diverse presentations and responses to treatment that are possible, nurses should be wary of giving information based on limited knowledge of apparently similar cases. What is feasible for one person may not be possible for another, and expectations (or anxieties) should not be raised unduly.

The patient should, however, be allowed to voice his concerns about the disease and its implications for normal functioning (e.g. speaking and eating) and for appearance. Many patients also have a deep fear of cancer and may have misconceptions about prognosis and the likely course of the disease. It is important for their needs to be recognised and any unfounded anxiety relieved.

Strategies for sensitive listening are described in Porritt (1990).

A multidisciplinary approach

A successful outcome will depend in part on the continuity of care provided by the multidisciplinary team. Along with medical staff, the nursing team will include ward, theatre and HDU nurses, specialist nurses, community nurses and possibly Macmillan and Marie Curie nurses. The following professionals also contribute to care, and the nurse must be aware of each team member's role and facilitate liaison wherever appropriate:

- Dietician — assesses dietary intake and advises staff and patient on maintaining adequate nutrition; liaises with pharmacy, the nutritional support person in the commercial companies and the community dietician for provision of enteral feeding equipment
- Speech and language therapist — advises patient on pre- and postoperative exercises to assist with speech and swallowing difficulties; advises on alternative means of communicating if loss of voice is permanent (see Ch. 14)
- Physiotherapist — gives instruction and assistance with pre- and postoperative exercises to assist breathing, expectoration, limb and shoulder movements
- Dentist (associate specialist) or prosthodontist — assesses need for dental care (especially when radiotherapy is part of treatment) and fits obturator and/or dentures
- Dental hygienist — advises patient on care of teeth and oral hygiene, especially during radiotherapy and/or chemotherapy
- Maxillofacial technician — advises on whether provision of a prosthesis is realistically possible; designs, constructs and fits when appropriate for each individual patient
- Medical social worker — gives information and advice on availability of grants for special needs; arranges home help, day care
- Hospital chaplain or other religious counsellor — gives spiritual comfort and practical help
- Voluntary support agencies — provide emotional and practical support for patient and family.

Case History 15.3 Mrs C

Mrs C, a 45-year-old housewife with two teenage children, was referred to an oncology unit from a dental hospital after she reported that she had had a lump in her mouth for some weeks. No lymphatic nodes were palpable in her neck and Mrs C was not too concerned that she might have cancer because she had never smoked and rarely took alcohol. She and her husband were consequently very shocked when they were given the result of a biopsy which showed squamous cell carcinoma.

She was assured that the disease was treatable and was advised to have surgical excision in the first instance, possibly followed by radiotherapy. Liaison was immediately set up with a Macmillan nurse, who visited her at home and discussed with Mrs C and her family their fears about cancer.

Mrs C felt that she did not want her husband to visit her until 3 or 4 days after the surgery. Her husband, however, felt anxious at not seeing her and came to visit of his own accord on the first postoperative day. The nurse prepared him for how his wife would look, and although he was initially shocked by her appearance, he felt that the result was not as bad as he had anticipated. He was also able to appreciate the rapid improvement which had taken place by the second day.

For herself, Mrs C was glad that he had visited. She felt more alert than she had believed possible. She also noticed the relief on her husband's face on his second visit and was able to believe him when he said she looked much better. On the third day, having prepared them, he brought their two children.

Three years later, Mrs C is attending the outpatient clinic for regular follow-up appointments. She has upper and lower dentures, which she wears all day, and is able to chew, swallow and speak well. She is socially very active and has adjusted well to the effects of her surgery, although she feels anxious every time she visits the clinic. Even after 3 years, she admits, 'I worry in case they find anything'.

15.11 In what ways would each member of the team be able to contribute to the care of the patient described in Case History 15.3 while in hospital and in the community?

Postoperative care

The postoperative nursing care of individuals who have undergone major surgery for intraoral cancer is highly specialised and combines the skills of many specialities. There will be variations in procedures and approaches among centres, and each patient will require a highly individualised plan for care.

Many centres reconstruct facial defects using free tissue transfer. Figure 15.7 outlines nursing procedures for the monitoring of free flaps.

Webster & Soutar (1986) describe 20 free flaps. See also Coull & Wylie (1990) and Coull (1992) for a discussion of nursing responsibility for monitoring free flaps.

Participation of relatives

Oral tumours and the effects of treatment may have far-reaching consequences not only for the patients concerned but also for their families (Espie et al 1989, Freedlander et al 1989, Kelly 1994). Relatives must often provide care for the patient after discharge. They are likely to experience much anxiety and to need maximum support. Nurses must help them through this very stressful time.

Relatives will need constant reassurance, especially during the early postoperative days, and should be counselled before the first postoperative visit, which is usually very stressful (see Case History 15.3).

It is advisable to reinforce and supplement verbal advice with written information, particularly with regard to oral hygiene, diet, radiotherapy, chemotherapy and local support groups. Local written information is now often available and general information booklets are also available, e.g. BACUP, Cancerlink.

Altered body image

The impact of surgery to the face and mouth upon day-to-day function is visible to everyone. Basic activities such as breathing, eating and drinking may have to be performed with some loss of dignity. This, together with the disfiguring effects of the surgery, will require the patient to accept an altered body image, which can be a very difficult adjustment to make. Below, a patient describes, in a diary shared with the author (Kelly 1987), how she feels about her swollen face:

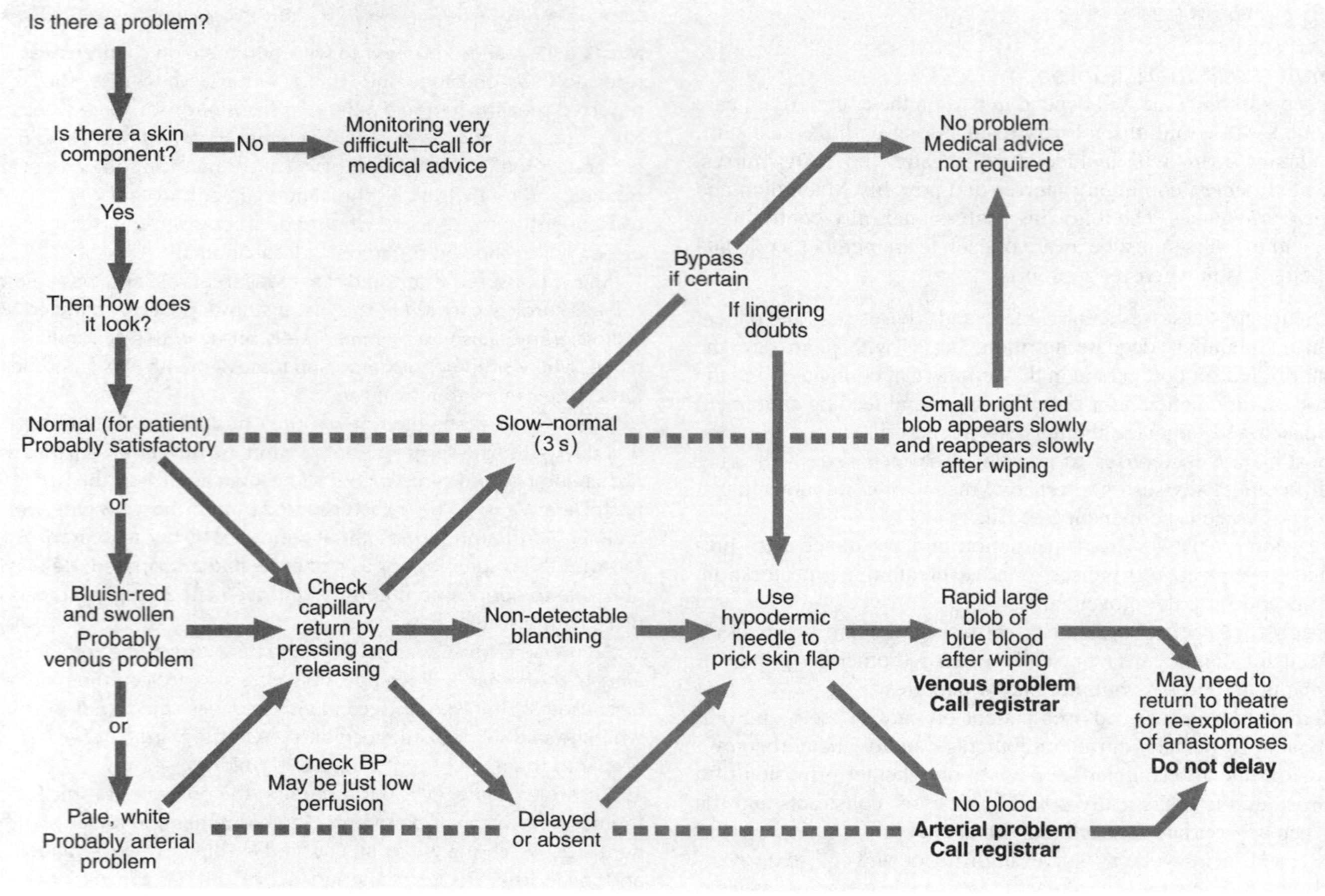

Fig. 15.7 An algorithm for monitoring free flaps.

He said I was 'round the corner'— but I don't really feel like it. He said the swelling would come down when I start moving around.
I asked about my face which is freakish and he said when I start walking about, gravity would reduce it. So I have now started, every time I go to the toilet, walking two laps of the ward — or when I am unleashed!

The patient now refers to being disconnected from drainage and feeding tubes —another assault on body image:

I feel a bit shy about it. I feel a freak especially when I see in a mirror — avoid mirrors meantime!

Another patient who had undergone several operations, commented: 'Each time, I feel I am a little less of the person I once was'. Remarks such as 'Of course, until I get my teeth, I can't go anywhere' are also frequently heard. It is worth noting that for many patients, after this type of surgery, dentures (if they can be worn) may be purely cosmetic rather than functional. Many patients, e.g. those who have had a tracheostomy, will be temporarily unable to speak following their surgery. It is important for nurses to bear in mind that it may be difficult for these individuals to convey their emotions in writing and that it may be necessary to 'read between the lines' in order to fully appreciate the extent of their emotional pain. The effects of a permanent tracheostomy are discussed in Chapter 14.

Q

15.12 Consider how Mrs C in Case History 15.3 is likely to feel about her condition and the consequences of treatment. How is her body image likely to be affected?

Discharge planning

Prior to the patient's discharge, liaison should be established with the GP and community nurse and appropriate appointments and home visits arranged. In many cases a Macmillan nurse will have visited the patient in the ward and will continue to give support at home. Each of these professionals will coordinate subsequent visits through the local health centre according to her assessment of the patient's needs and should be encouraged to contact any member of the hospital team for help and support at any time.

Particular advance planning will be required if the patient's social circumstances are less than optimum; for example, many patients live alone or in hostel accommodation, and early liaison with social workers will ensure that the best possible social support is provided.

Rehabilitation

Following discharge after major oral surgery and radiotherapy, the process of rehabilitation may not be complete for a period of some months or even years. Patients will need ongoing support as they learn to cope with changes in lifestyle and in the activities of daily living (see Ch. 34). Planning for rehabilitation should start from the day of admission and must take into account the following considerations:

- *Living arrangements*. The patient may need to live with relatives temporarily or permanently, or may need rehousing if he is to live alone. Long-term nursing support (e.g. from Macmillan and Marie Curie nurses) and community-based services (e.g. Meals-on-Wheels) may need to be arranged.
- *Breathing*. Patients with a tracheal stoma will need to be instructed in its management and will need support in adjusting to their altered appearance.
- *Oral hygiene; eating and drinking*. The patient or his carer will need to be proficient in maintaining oral hygiene and using special equipment for delivering enteral feeds if necessary.
- *Communication*. Training in alternative forms of communication will be needed to compensate for a loss in speech.
- *Psychological support*. The patient should receive pre-discharge counselling to help him adjust to an altered body image. Ongoing professional support may be needed for some time after discharge as the patient readjusts to life in the community (Robinson et al 1996), and patients and family should be able to contact members of the hospital team for support and advice.
- *Work*. The patient will need help in adjusting to new employment circumstances, whether he changes his job, stops working or returns to his previous job and learns to cope with his changed appearance and function and with the reactions of colleagues.
- *Education*. The patient may need information on such matters as nutrition, giving up smoking and reducing alcohol intake. He and his family should be informed about local self-help groups where they can obtain practical and psychological support.

Collyer (1984) provides many examples of how disfigured people have been rehabilitated and of the difficulties they overcame during that process.

15.13 Consider how you might go about planning the long-term rehabilitation of Mrs C in Case History 15.3.

Nursing and stress

Caring for patients with intraoral tumours can give rise to considerable stress. Nurses may find this area of care quite harrowing: unfortunately, ward nurses frequently see patients return with a recurrence of the cancer, and some may question whether radical treatment has in fact been justified.

Liaison with outpatient clinics will make it apparent, however, that many patients do in fact survive to lead fulfilling lives for many years after treatment.

Staff support in cancer nursing is discussed by Tschudin (1996) (see also Chs 17 and 31 of this book).

See Rhys-Evans (1996) for further information on tumours of the head and neck.

REFERENCES

Accord Hospice 1996 A protocol for oral care. Accord Hospice, Paisley

Ali T, Shepherd J P 1994 The measurement of injury severity. British Journal of Oral and Maxillofacial Surgery 32(1): 13–18

Armstrong T S 1994 Stomatitis in the bone marrow transplant patient: an overview and proposed oral care protocol. Cancer Nursing 17(5): 403–410

Asadi S G, Asadi Z 1997 The aetiology of mandibular fractures at an urban centre. Journal of the Royal Society of Health 117(3): 164–167

Barkvoll P, Attramadal A 1989 Effect of nystatin and chlorhexidine digluconate on candida albicans. Oral Surgery 67: 279–281

Bayliss T, Bedi R 1996 Oral, maxillofacial and general injuries in gymnasts. Injury 27(5): 353–354

Brown A E, Langdon J D 1995 Management of oral cancer. Annals of the Royal College of Surgeons of England 77: 404–408

Calman F M B, Langdon J 1991 Oral complications of cancer. British Medical Journal 302: 485–486

Campbell S 1987 Mouth care in cancer patients. Nursing Times 22(83): 59–60

Cancer Research Campaign 1993 Oral cancer: factsheet 14.1–5. CRC, London

Cannell H, Paterson A, Loukota 1996 Maxillofacial injuries in multiply injured patients. British Journal of Oral and Maxillofacial Surgery 34: 303–308

Challacombe S 1991 Revised classification of HIV-associated oral lesions. British Dental Journal 170: 305–306

Chew D J, Edmondson H D 1996 A study of maxillofacial injuries in the elderly resulting from falls. Journal of Oral Rehabilitation 23(7): 505–509

Coleman S 1995 An overview of the oral complications of adult patients with malignant haematological conditions who have undergone radiotherapy or chemotherapy. Journal of Advanced Nursing 22(6): 1085–1091

Consumers' Association 1997 Looking after your teeth. Which (August): 8–15. CA, Hertford

Crosby C 1989 Method in mouth care. Nursing Times 85(35): 38–41

Curzon M E J, Pollard M A 1997 Do we still care about children's teeth? British Dental Journal 182(7): 242–244

Daeffler R 1980 Oral hygiene measures for patients with cancer, Part 1. Cancer Nursing 3(6): 427–431

Department of Health (Committee on Medical Aspects of Food Policy) 1989 Report on health and social subjects, No 37. Dietary sugars and human disease. Report of the panel on dietary sugars. HMSO, London

Department of Health and Social Security 1978 Road accident statistics. HMSO, London

Downer M C 1991 The improving dental health of United Kingdom adults and prospects for the future. British Dental Journal 170: 154–158

Dudjak L 1987 Mouth care for mucositis due to radiation therapy. Cancer Nursing 10(3): 131–133

Espie C A, Freedlander E, Campsie L M, Soutar D S, Robertson A G 1989 Psychological distress at follow-up after major surgery for intraoral cancer. Journal of Psychosomatic Research 33(4): 441–448

Feber T 1995 Mouthcare for patients receiving oral irradiation. Professional Nurse 10(10): 666–670

Ferretti G A, Hansen I A, Whittenburg K, Brown A T, Lillich T T, Ash R C 1987 Therapeutic use of chlorhexidine in bone marrow transplant patients: case studies. Oral Surgery 63(6): 683–687

Finlay P M, Richardson M D, Robertson A G 1996 A comparative study of the efficacy of fluconazole and amphotericin B in the treatment of oropharyngeal candidiasis in patients undergoing radiotherapy for head and neck tumours. British Journal of Oral and Maxillofacial Surgery 34(1): 23–25

Fiske J, Gelbier S, Watson R M 1990 The benefit of dental care to an elderly population assessed using a sociodental measure of oral handicap. British Dental Journal 168: 153–156

Freedlander E, Espie C A, Campsie L M, Soutar D S, Robertson A G 1989 Functional implications of major surgery for intraoral cancer. British Journal of Plastic Surgery 42: 266–269

Garewal H 1995 Antioxidants in oral cancer prevention. American Journal of Clinical Nutrition 62(6): 1410–1416S

Gibbons D E 1983 Mouthcare procedures. Nursing Times 79(7): 30

Gooch J 1985 Mouth care. Professional Nurse 1(3): 77–78

Gregory J 1990 The dietary and nutritional survey of British adults. HMSO, London

Hallett N 1984 Mouth care. Nursing Times 159(21): 31–33

Harrison L B 1997 Applications of brachytherapy in head and neck cancer. Seminars in Surgical Oncology 13(3): 177–184

Hollinworth H 1997 Less pain, more gain. Nursing Times 93(46): 89–91

Holmes S 1996 Nursing management of oral care in older patients. Nursing Times 92(9): 37–39

Holmes S 1997 Radiotherapy, 2nd edn. Lisa Sainsbury Foundation Series. Austin Cornish, London

Holmes S, Mountain E 1993 Assessment of oral status: evaluation of three oral assessment guides. Journal of Clinical Nursing 2(1): 35–40

Howarth H 1977 Mouth care procedures for the very ill. Nursing Times 73(10): 354–355

Jamieson E M, McCall J M, Blythe R, Whyte L A 1997 Clinical nursing practices, 3rd edn. Churchill Livingstone, Edinburgh

Jenkins D 1989 Oral care in the ICU: an important nursing role. Nursing Standard 7: 24–28

Jones C M, Taylor G O, Whittle J G, Evans D, Trotter D P 1997 Water fluoridation, tooth decay in 5 year olds and social deprivation measured by the Jarman score: analysis of data from British dental studies. British Medical Journal 3: 514–517

Kelly R 1987 A study of patients who have undergone surgery for cancer in the head and neck region. Unpublished paper (accessible from author)

Kelly R 1994 Nursing patients with oral cancer. Nursing Standard 8(32): 25–29

Kite K 1995 Changing mouthcare practice in intensive care: implications of the clinical setting context. Intensive & Critical Care Nursing 11(4): 203–209

Krishnasamay M 1995 Oral problems in advanced cancer. European Journal of Cancer Care 4: 173–177

Lamey P-J 1996 Burning mouth syndrome. Dermatological Clinics 14(2): 339–354

Lamey P-J, Lewis M A O 1988 Oral medicine. Pocket picture guides series. Lippincott, Philadelphia, PA

Lamey P-J, Rees T D, Forsyth A 1990 Sensitivity reaction to the cinnamonaldehyde component of toothpaste. British Dental Journal 168: 115–118

Langley J 1989 Working with swallowing disorders. Winslow Press, Bicester

Levine R S (ed) 1996a A handbook of dental health for health visitors, midwives and nurses. Health Education Authority, London

Levine R S (ed) 1996b The scientific basis of dental health education, 4th edn. Health Education Authority, London

Little J 1996 Head and neck cancer: oral care during radiotherapy. Nursing Standard 10(22): 39–42

Lydon C 1996 Too slap happy. Nursing Times 92(45): 48–49

McAndrew P G 1990 Oral cancer and precancer: treatment. British Dental Journal 168: 191–198

McGregor I A, McGregor A D 1995 Fundamental techniques of plastic surgery and their surgical applications, 9th edn. Churchill Livingstone, Edinburgh

McIlroy P 1996 Radiation mucositis: a new approach to prevention and treatment. European Journal of Cancer Care 5(3): 153–158

Martin V 1995 Helping parents cope: cleft lip, cleft palate. Nursing Times 29(31): 38–40

Matejka M, Nell A, Kment G, Schein A, Leukauf M, Portender H, Mailath G, Sinzinger H 1990 Local benefit of prostaglandin E2 in radiochemotherapy-induced oral mucositis. British Journal of Oral Maxillofacial Surgery 28: 89–91

Maurer J 1977 Providing optimum oral health. Nursing Clinics of North America 12: 671–685

Maximiw W G, Wood R E 1989 The role of dentistry in patients undergoing bone marrow transplantation. British Dental Journal 167: 229–234

Miller R 1987 Oral health care for the hospitalised patient: the nurse's role. Journal of Health Education 26(9): 362–366

Morton C A, Garioch J, Todd P, Lamey P J, Forsyth A 1995 Contact sensitivity to menthol and peppermint in patients with intra-oral symptoms. Contact Dermatitis 32(5): 281–284

O'Brien M 1994 Children's dental health in the United Kingdom 1993. Office of Population Censuses and Surveys. HMSO, London

Oral Health Group 1996 Promoting oral health. Health Education Group for Scotland, Edinburgh

Palmer G D, Robinson P G, Challacombe S J et al 1996 Aetiological factors for oral manifestations of HIV. Oral Diseases 2(3): 193–197

Partridge J 1993 The psychological effects of facial disfigurement. Journal of Wound Care 2(3): 168–171

Pernanen K 1991 Alcohol in human violence. Guilford Press, New York

Pitts N B, 1997 Do we understand which children need and get appropriate dental care? British Dental Journal 182(7): 273–278

Porter H 1992 Oral care for BMT patients. Nursing Standard 7(6): 54–55

Regnard C, Allport S, Stephenson L 1997 ABC of palliative care: mouth care, skin care and lymphoedema. British Journal of Medicine 315: 1002–1005

Roberts H 1990 Mouthcare in oral cavity cancer. Nursing Standard 4(19): 26–29

Robinson E, Rumsey N, Partridge J 1996 An evaluation of the impact of social interaction skills for facially disfigured people. British Journal of Plastic Surgery 49(5): 281–289

Roper N, Logan W W, Tierney A J 1996 The elements of nursing: a model for nursing based on a model of living, 4th edn. Churchill Livingstone, Edinburgh

Roth P T, Creason J 1986 Nurse administered oral hygiene: is there a scientific basis? Journal of Advanced Nursing 11(3): 323–331

Samaranayake L P, Wilkieson C A, Lamey P J, MacFarlane T W 1995 Oral disease in the elderly in long-term hospital care. Oral Diseases 1(3): 147–151

Scottish Office Department of Health 1995 The oral health strategy for Scotland. Scottish Office Department of Health, Edinburgh

Scully C, Porter S R, Luker J 1991 An ABC of oral health care in patients with HIV infection. British Dental Journal 170: 149–150

Segelman A, Doku H 1977 Treatment of oral complications of leukaemia. Oral Surgery 45: 469–477

Shepherd J P 1989 Surgical, socio-economic and forensic aspects of assault: a review. British Journal of Oral and Maxillofacial Surgery 27: 89–98

Shepherd J P, Ali M A, Hughes A O, Levers B G 1993 Trends in urban violence: a comparison of accident department and police records. Journal of the Royal Society of Medicine 82(2): 87–88

Smith C J 1989 Oral cancer and precancer: background, epidemiology and aetiology. British Dental Journal 167: 377–383

Snape D, Robinson A 1996 Radiotherapy In: Tschudin V (ed) Nursing the patient with cancer, 2nd edn. Prentice-Hall, London, ch 4

Sobin L H, Wittekind C 1997 (eds) UICC TNM classification of malignant tumours, 5th edn. Wiley-Liss, New York

Soutar D S, Tiwari R (eds) 1996 Excision and reconstruction in head and neck cancer. Churchill Livingstone, Edinburgh

System Three Scotland 1994 Scottish health survey 1994. Report prepared for the Health Education Board for Scotland, Edinburgh

Telfer M R, Shepherd J P 1993 Psychological distress in patients attending an oncology clinic after definitive treatment for maxillofacial malignant neoplasia. International Journal of Oral and Maxillofacial Surgery 22(6): 3347–3349

The Times 1998 Tuesday August 4, p 1

Thomas D W, Satterthwaite J, Shepherd J P 1997 Trends in the referral and treatment of new patients at a free emergency dental clinic since 1989. British Dental Journal 182(1): 11–14

Thurgood G 1994 Nurse maintenance of oral hygiene. British Journal of Nursing 3(7): 332–334, 351–353

Todd J E, Lader D 1991 Adult dental health 1988, United Kingdom. HMSO, London

Tombes M B, Gallucci B 1993 The effects of hydrogen peroxide rinses on the normal oral mucosa. Nursing Research 42(6): 332–337

Tschudin V 1996 Staff support. In: Tschudin V (ed) Nursing the patient with cancer, 2nd edn. Prentice-Hall, London, ch 27

United Kingdom Central Council for Nursing, Midwifery and Health Visiting (UKCC) 1992 Code of professional conduct for the nurse, midwife and health visitor. UKCC, London

Ventafridda V, Ripamonti C, Sbanotto A, de Conno F 1995 Mouth care. In: Doyle D, Hanks G W C, MacDonald N (eds) Oxford textbook of palliative medicine. Oxford University Press, Oxford, ch 4.10

Wahlin Y B 1989 Effects of chlorhexidine mouthrinse on oral health in patients with acute leukaemia. Oral Surgery 68: 279–287
Watson R 1989 Care of the mouth. Nursing 3(11): 20–24
Webster M H C, Soutar D S 1986 Practical guide to free tissue transfer. Butterworth, London
Williams J L 1990 Oral cancer: clinical features. British Dental Journal 168: 13–16
Wilson K J W, Waugh A 1996 Ross & Wilson: anatomy and physiology in health and illness, 8th edn. Churchill Livingstone, Edinburgh
Winn D M 1995 Diet and nutrition in the aetiology of oral cancer. American Journal of Clinical Nutrition 61(2): 437– 445S
World Health Organization 1988 Oral health global indicator for 2000. WHO, Geneva

FURTHER READING

Collyer H 1984 Facial disfigurement: successful rehabilitation. Macmillan, London
Consumers' Association 1997 Looking after your teeth. Which August: 8–15. CA, Hertford
Coull A 1992 Making sense of surgical flaps. Nursing Times 88(1): 32–34
Coull A, Wylie K 1990 Regular monitoring: the way to ensure flap healing. Nursing priorities following flap repair and reconstruction surgery. The Professional Nurse 6(1): 18–21
Henderson D 1985 A colour atlas and text book of orthognathic surgery. The surgery of facial skeletal deformity. Wolfe, London
Holmes S 1997 Radiotherapy, 2nd edn. Lisa Sainsbury Foundation Series. Austin Cornish, London
Jamieson E M, McCall J M, Blythe R, Whyte L A 1997 Clinical nursing practices, 3rd edn. Churchill Livingstone, Edinburgh
Johnson D R, Moore W J 1997 Anatomy for dental students, 3rd edn. Oxford University Press, Oxford
Kemble J V H, Lamb B E 1984 Plastic surgical and burns nursing. Baillière Tindall, London
Langley J 1989 Working with swallowing disorders. Winslow Press, Bicester
Levine R S (ed) 1996a A handbook of dental health for health visitors, midwives and nurses. Health Education Authority, London
Levine R S (ed) 1996b The scientific basis of dental health education, 4th edn. Health Education Authority, London
McGregor I A, McGregor F M 1986 Cancer of the face and mouth. Churchill Livingstone, Edinburgh
Oral Health Group 1996 Promoting oral health. Health Education Group for Scotland, Edinburgh
Porritt L 1990 Interaction strategies, 2nd edn. Churchill Livingstone, Edinburgh
Rhys-Evans F 1996 Tumours of the head and neck. In: Tschudin V (ed) Nursing the patient with cancer, 2nd edn. Prentice-Hall, London, ch 11
Rugg-Gunn A J 1993 Nutrition and dental health. Oxford University Press, Oxford
Snape D, Robinson A 1996 Radiotherapy. In: Tschudin V (ed) Nursing the patient with cancer, 2nd edn. Prentice-Hall, London, ch 4
Sweeney M P, Bagg J 1997 Making sense of the mouth (video and CD-ROM). Partnership in Oral Care, Glasgow
Webster M H C, Soutar D S 1986 Practical guide to free tissue transfer. Butterworth, London
Williams J L 1994 (ed) Rowe and Williams maxillofacial injuries, 2nd edn. Churchill Livingstone, Edinburgh
Wilson K J W, Waugh A 1996 Ross & Wilson: anatomy and physiology in health and illness, 8th edn. Churchill Livingstone, Edinburgh
Wray D, Gibson J 1997 Oral medicine. Churchill Livingstone, Edinburgh

USEFUL ADDRESSES

CancerBACUP
3 Bath Place
London EC2A 3DR
also:
30 Bell Street
Glasgow G1

British Dental Health Foundation
Eastlands Court
St Peter's Road
Rugby CV21 3QP

Cancerlink
11–21 Northdown Street
London N1 9BN
also:
Unit 1
West Upper Level
25 Johnston Terrace
Edinburgh EH1 2NH

Changing Faces
1–2 Junction Mews
Paddington
London W2 1PN

CLAPA (Cleft Lip and Palate Association)
134 Buckingham Palace Road
London SW1 9SA

Cranio-Facial Support Group
44 Helmsdale Road
Leamington Spa
Warks CV32 7DW

Disfigurement Guidance Centre
52 Crossgate
Cupar
Fife KY5 5HS

Health Education Board for Scotland (HEBS)
Woodburn House
Canaan Lane
Edinburgh EH10 4SG

Let's Face It
62 Fortescue Road
Edgeware
Middlesex HA8 0HN

PINNT (Patients on Intravenous and Nasogastric Nutrition Therapy)
258 Wennington Road
Rainham
Essex RM13 9UU

Smoke line
Tel (freephone): 0800 84 84 84

The Centre for Women's Health
6 Sandyford Place
Sauchiehall Street
Glasgow G3 7NB

Women's Aid
Norton Park
57 Albion Road
Edinburgh EH7 5QY
(see also local telephone directory for nearest centre)

THE IMMUNE SYSTEM AND INFECTIOUS DISEASE

16

Marion C. Stewart

INTRODUCTION

The immune system is a complex and fascinating network of cells and proteins which is programmed to respond to the many challenges presented to it by foreign particles, microorganisms (such as bacteria, viruses, fungi and protozoa) and tumour cells. Its function is to protect the body from anything that could be harmful. In order to carry out this function, it has to be able to recognise 'self', which is tolerated, and 'non-self', which it attacks and attempts to eliminate or destroy.

Human beings and animals have a number of non-specific barriers to foreign substances; for example, the intact skin protects the body from invasion and substances in some body fluids help to kill microorganisms (see Fig. 16.1). It is when these barriers fail or are compromised that the specific immune responses come into play.

Healthy individuals can fight off infection by immune mechanisms, and in many cases immunity to a disease occurs after a single encounter with the infectious organism. Sometimes, the system is unable to function normally because of an immune deficiency or a functional disorder. When a large number of microorganisms enter the body, the immune system may function normally but still be too slow to prevent the person from developing the infectious disease. Immune suppression can occur as a result of other disease; it can also be iatrogenic, resulting from drug treatment or radiotherapy.

Epidemiology

Methods of reporting the diseases of the immune system vary and in some instances yield only an estimate of their occurrence. Statistics about infectious diseases, however, are more readily available because of the statutory requirement for notification of certain infections (Bannister et al 1996).

So important is the immune system that few people, if any, can survive with a severe immune defect. Nonetheless, nurses are likely to encounter a range of immune disorders in their work. Hyperactive disorders such as asthma (see Ch. 3) are thought to affect around 5% of adults and 10% of children in the UK (Crockett 1993), while up to 15% of the population suffer from allergies to common substances such as grass pollens, animal danders and food allergens (Brostoff et al 1991). Genetic factors are important in these diseases, but it is thought that environmental pollution is also

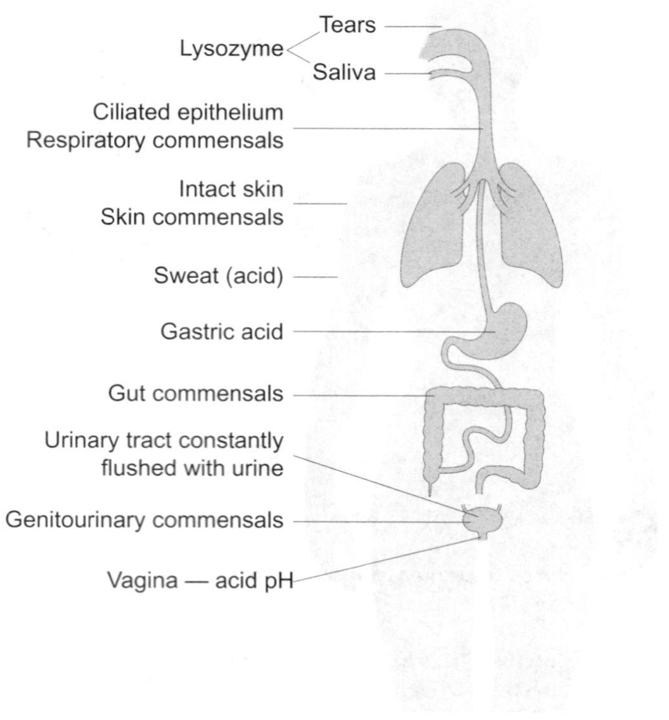

Fig. 16.1 Barriers to infection.

Box 16.1 ***Escherichia coli*** **0157 (Chief Medical Officer 1996, Public Health Laboratory Service 1997)**

- This is a strain of *E. coli* which produces potent toxins called verocytotoxins. These can cause severe disease in humans
- The organism is found in the intestines of healthy cattle, and human infection occurs through eating inadequately cooked minced beef, or other contaminated foods such as milk, cooked meat or meat pies and raw vegetables
- The infectious dose is low, i.e. consumption of a very small number of organisms can result in infection
- The toxin helps the organism to adhere to the lining of the intestine, causing diarrhoea, abdominal cramps and, in severe cases (approximately half of those affected), haemorrhagic colitis with bloody diarrhoea
- It can also affect other organs by damaging the vascular endothelium, causing, for example, haemolytic uraemic syndrome (particularly in children and the elderly) or thrombotic thrombocytopenic purpura
- The incubation period can be from 1 to 14 days, and is typically 3 days
- There is no specific treatment for the infection. Clinical management depends on symptoms
- Infected patients are barrier-nursed, in 'source' isolation, if they are in hospital
- Food hygiene, in particular adequate cooking/reheating of meat products and careful handling of all cooked foods, is critical in preventing infection

a contributing factor. Advances in medical treatment have meant that organs can now be transplanted with a degree of success, and malignancies controlled if not eliminated. Unfortunately, organ transplantation and cancer therapy involve the destruction or suppression of vital components of the immune system, thus predisposing the patient to overwhelming infection. The autoimmune diseases, in which the body attacks its own cells, are comparatively rare and their cause is not completely understood at present.

Infectious diseases have been around for centuries, but many factors have influenced the pattern of their occurrence in recent years. Smallpox has virtually been eradicated from the world by the widespread use of vaccination, and vaccination has also had a significant effect in reducing the incidence of many other diseases such as polio, whooping cough, measles and rubella. The decline in tuberculosis has probably been due more to improved sanitation, hygiene, nutrition and housing than to vaccination, although anti-tubercular drugs have had a significant effect. However, tuberculosis is on the rise again and is seen in some patients with human immunodeficiency virus (HIV) infection and the acquired immune deficiency syndrome (AIDS) (see Ch. 37). Of particular concern are the strains of the tubercle bacillus which are antibiotic-resistant, known as multi-drug resistant or MDR-TB.

Some infections have been recognised only in the last 20–25 years, e.g. Legionnaire's disease in 1976, and AIDS in the 1980s. Others, such as *Campylobacter* and toxoplasmosis, are identified more frequently than in the past.

Some hazards arise from behaviour and lifestyle. Around 16 000 new cases of sexually transmitted disease are reported in Scotland each year (I & SD 1996). Intravenous drug misuse leads to the risk of blood-borne disease such as hepatitis B or HIV infection through the sharing of contaminated injection equipment. (These diseases are also transmitted sexually.)

Changes in cooking and eating habits (e.g. a reliance on microwave ovens and fast foods) have emphasised the necessity for thorough and adequate cooking of all foods which are known to be frequently contaminated with organisms such as the *Salmonella* species. Processed foods can also be a problem; for example, soft cheeses, paté and yoghurt have on occasion been found to be contaminated with *Listeria monocytogenes*. The verocytotoxic strains of *Escherichia coli*, such as *E. coli* 0157 are an increasing concern, because of the associated morbidity and mortality (Box 16.1).

Increased foreign travel has meant that diseases can cross borders as easily as their hosts or victims. Malaria, for example, is often contracted abroad, but becomes apparent only after the traveller returns home.

Food poisoning is one of the most common notifiable infectious diseases in the UK. Measles is still extremely common in spite of the reduction in cases by large-scale vaccination programmes. It is likely that the increase in HIV infection and AIDS throughout the world will influence the future incidence of other infectious diseases.

The problem of antibiotic resistance makes treatment of infections caused by organisms such as methicillin-resistant *Staphylococcus aureus* (MRSA; see Box 16.7, p. 593) and vancomycin-resistant enterococci (VRE) very difficult.

The nurse's role

The nurse is in an ideal position to educate people about the avoidance and management of infectious diseases. A home visit to any patient is an ideal opportunity to assess and give advice on food safety and on the prevention of infection through good hygiene. A patient recovering from salmonellosis or hepatitis B may be anxious about transmitting the infection to others and require practical advice; such advice should emphasise what can, as well as what cannot, be done.

For infectious patients who are unable or unwilling to act upon such advice, special arrangements may have to be made to ensure that others are not put at unnecessary risk. The assessment of the patient as an individual is particularly important in these circumstances.

ANATOMY AND PHYSIOLOGY

The lymphoid system

The lymphoid (or lymphatic) system consists of organs and tissues made up of cells which are involved in the immune response. These structures may be described as being either primary or secondary, as follows.

Primary lymphoid organs

The thymus gland and the bone marrow are known as primary lymphoid organs. Lymphocytes develop in the bone marrow (see Ch. 11). T lymphocytes differentiate in the thymus gland, and B lymphocytes differentiate in the bone marrow. It is in the organ where they differentiate that lymphocytes acquire the surface receptors which enable them to recognise antigens.

Secondary lymphoid organs

The spleen and lymph nodes are known as secondary lymphoid organs, as are other areas of lymphoid tissue which are associated with mucosal surfaces in the body, such as in the respiratory, gastrointestinal and genitourinary systems. The spleen contains white blood cells, or leucocytes (see Ch. 11), and is involved in the breakdown of erythrocytes, leucocytes and platelets. The lymph nodes are small collections of lymphoid tissue (1–25 mm in diameter) which are found all over the body, often where lymphatic vessels branch. Lymph nodes act as filters, trapping any foreign materials or antigens so that they can be attacked and destroyed by specialised white blood cells which accumulate there in large numbers.

For further information, see Wilson & Waugh (1996).

Types of immune response

Two types of immune response are involved in recognising and eliminating any 'foreign' material which enters the body. These are:

- *Non-specific or innate immunity*, by which any foreign cell or particle is identified as such and attacked. Even tumour cells which arise in the body's own tissues can be recognised as foreign and may be destroyed. This response is non-specific in that it is the same whether the foreign particle or antigen is a bacterium, a particle of asbestos or anything else. The response occurs as soon as the antigen is encountered. No 'memory' is involved and a second contact with the same antigen will produce the same response at the same rate.
- *Specific or adaptive immunity*, in which special cells (B and T lymphocytes) are programmed to respond to recognised antigens. This response is highly specific: each lymphocyte is equipped to recognise only one antigen. Once contact has been made with that antigen and it has been destroyed, some 'memory' cells (see p. 584) remain in the body. If the same antigen is encountered again, these cells are stimulated to reproduce, and the response is both faster and greater.

Box 16.2 Components of the immune system

Cells
Leucocytes (white blood cells)
- Granular (granulocytes or polymorphonuclear leucocytes)
  —neutrophils
  —basophils and mast cells
  —eosinophils
- ***Non-granular (agranulocytes)***
  —Mononuclear phagocytes (monocytes and macrophages)
  —Lymphocytes
  B lymphocytes
  T lymphocytes

Chemicals
Complement
Cytokines, e.g. interferons
Inflammatory mediators, e.g. histamine
Antibodies (immunoglobulins)

Cells and chemicals involved

Box 16.2 summarises the components of the immune system.

Cells

The cells involved in the immune response are white blood cells (leucocytes). These may be granular (also called granulocytes or polymorphonuclear leucocytes) — the neutrophils, basophils and eosinophils — or non-granular (also called agranulocytes) — the mononuclear phagocytes (monocytes and macrophages) and lymphocytes. In this section these cells will be described according to their function.

Phagocytes have the ability to recognise foreign material and to engulf and digest microorganisms by a process called phagocytosis. Three different cells are classed as phagocytes, namely neutrophils, monocytes and macrophages.

Neutrophils are small cells and live only for a few days. They originate in the bone marrow and circulate in the blood.

Monocytes are roughly the same size as neutrophils. They also originate in the bone marrow and circulate in the blood, but they may enter the tissues, where they become macrophages.

Macrophages are larger than neutrophils and monocytes. They are long-lived and are found in the tissues, principally in the liver, spleen, lymph nodes and lungs. Mainly involved in non-specific immunity, they are also activated by lymphokines, which are produced by some T cells in the cell-mediated immune response (see p. 586). Phagocytosis can take place only if the invading cell becomes adherent to the surface of the phagocyte. This occurs by a chemical attraction between the surface of the phagocyte and antigen. The process can be assisted by complement (see p. 584) and by antibodies.

Accessory cells. These cells function by releasing chemicals which are harmful to invading organisms. This group of cells comprises eosinophils, basophils and mast cells.

Eosinophils are capable of phagocytosis, but their main function is to attach themselves to larger parasites such as helminths (worms) and kill them by releasing harmful substances. They may also help to control the inflammatory response by breaking down histamine. There is an increase in the number of eosinophils in people suffering from allergic conditions or from parasitic infections.

Basophils and mast cells contain histamine and other chemicals which give rise to an inflammatory response when released. They are important in some allergies, e.g. hay fever (see p. 596). Basophils circulate in the bloodstream. Mast cells, although similar in function, are located in connective tissues and mucous membranes.

Lymphocytes originate in the bone marrow as stem cells and subsequently differentiate into the following types:

B cells are the lymphocytes which produce antibodies. They differentiate in the bone marrow and then mature in the secondary lymphoid tissues. The antigen receptor on their surface is specific for one antigen only. B lymphocytes are capable of 'memory' and are specialised to deal with microorganisms which do not, of their own accord, enter host cells (e.g. circulating bacteria).

T cells have various functions. They originate in the bone marrow and then mature and differentiate in the thymus gland. They are also antigen-specific and have an antigen receptor which is similar in structure and function to that of the B cells. T lymphocytes are capable of 'memory' and are specialised to deal mainly with microorganisms which invade host cells (e.g. viruses).

T cells can be broadly divided into two groups:

- T-helper cells
- T-cytotoxic cells.

T-helper cells are subdivided into the cells which interact with B cells, helping them to produce antibody, and the cells which assist the mononuclear phagocytes, helping them to destroy intracellular pathogens.

T-cytotoxic cells destroy host cells which are infected by viruses or other intracellular pathogens.

Chemicals

Complement is the collective name for a group of proteins which induce chemical reactions and are involved in the control of inflammation. Their three main functions are:

- To coat microorganisms with a substance which phagocytic cells can recognise. This ensures that the microorganism adheres to the surface of the phagocytic cell.
- To activate the destruction of the microorganism inside the phagocyte once ingestion has taken place. Complement also participates in the acute inflammatory response by inducing vasodilation and increasing the permeability of the capillary endothelium.
- To assist in the lysis of invading cells.

Cytokines are molecules (mainly proteins), of which there are several types, whose function is to signal between cells during the immune response. Interferons are one example. There are many different interferons and they protect cells of the same species from viral attack. They are synthesised by virally infected cells and secreted into the extracellular fluid. Here they bind to specific receptors on other, non-infected cells, which 'surround' the infected cell and prevent the spread of virus.

Histamine is released by mast cells when they degranulate after adhering to a microorganism. It gives rise to increased vascular permeability, arteriolar dilatation, smooth muscle contraction in the respiratory and alimentary tracts, and increased secretion of respiratory mucus.

Antibodies are the principal substances involved in the adaptive or specific immune response. Collectively known as immunoglobulins, they are proteins capable of recognising and binding to their own specific antigen (usually a microorganism).

Antibodies are produced by B lymphocytes and, once formed, circulate in the plasma. They have three functions:

- to bind to antigens
- to bind to phagocytes
- to activate the complement pathway.

There are five classes of antibody: immunoglobulin G (IgG), IgA, IgM, IgD and IgE. Each of the five classes may be produced with specificity for a single antigen. Their structure varies according to function and they are present in different amounts in the bloodstream (see Box 16.3).

Box 16.3 Immunoglobulins

Immunoglobulins are proteins with known antibody activity. They form the central component of the immune system and are synthesised by lymphocytes and plasma cells. The five classes of immunoglobulins are as follows:

- IgM — the first immunoglobulin to appear in the bloodstream in the primary response to infection. Since it disappears fairly quickly after the antigen disappears, it is an indicator of current or very recent infection.
- IgG — produced in large quantities in both the primary and secondary responses to infection. It is also important as a defence against infection in the first few weeks of life, being the only immunoglobulin which crosses the placenta to the fetus.
- IgA — secreted onto the luminal surface of the respiratory, alimentary and genitourinary tracts and present in saliva, tracheobronchial and genitourinary secretions as well as in the serum. It is important in preventing the entry of microorganisms from the external orifices of the body.
- IgE — normally found on the surface membrane of basophils and mast cells. It is associated with allergic reactions such as hay fever.
- IgD — present in small quantities bound to B cells where it aids in the 'memory' function.

Immunoglobulins can be taken from a donor by plasmapheresis and given:

- to someone who has been exposed to a pathogen and is not immune, e.g. antitetanus immunoglobulin (Humotet)
- as short-term prophylaxis, when exposure is anticipated and there is not time for vaccine to take effect, e.g. tick-borne encephalitis
- to someone who is heavily immunosuppressed, following exposure to a pathogen which could cause serious infection because of an inadequate immune response.

Passive immunisation with immunoglobulins does not confer long-term protection: this requires vaccination (see p. 585).

The immune response

The non-specific immune response

When a foreign substance enters the body, the first line of defence is the non-specific immune response, which comprises the following components:

- mechanical barriers (e.g. cilia in the upper respiratory tract)
- phagocytes
- chemicals (complement, the interferons)
- substances found in body secretions (e.g. lysozyme, gastric acid).

These defences can be effective on their own, but help is sometimes needed from adaptive or specific immune response mechanisms.

Disadvantages of the non-specific response are as follows:

- The cells can differentiate between 'self' and 'non-self' but cannot recognise specific antigens.
- It does not adapt after exposure, i.e. the same level of response is produced for each exposure to an antigen.
- It does not have a 'memory' and so cannot prevent the individual from developing the same infection a second time.

The specific immune response: natural immunity

The specific immune response involves the lymphocytes and comprises the humoral or antibody-mediated response (initiated by B lymphocytes) and the cell-mediated response (initiated by T lymphocytes). These responses are described separately here, but they interact with each other as well as with non-specific factors. The humoral response deals mainly with extracellular organisms, and the antibodies which it produces are present in the serum. The cell-mediated response is important for dealing with intracellular organisms.

Specificity. When it is first exposed to an antigen, the circulating lymphocyte differentiates to recognise and bind to that one particular antigen. This recognition and binding is like a lock and key mechanism on a door. Many different keys may go into the same lock, but only one will fit closely enough to turn in the lock and open the door (the primary response).

On re-exposure to the antigen, perhaps many years later, the remaining progeny of that cell (memory cells) will be stimulated to replicate (the secondary response).

Antibody-mediated immune response. This response may be described in terms of its primary and secondary phases.

Primary response. The first time an antigen is encountered in the body it takes about 2 weeks for a corresponding antibody to be detectable in the blood. The production of this antibody is called the primary response. Although the immune system reacts immediately to antigens, the synthesis of antibodies takes some time. An antigen binds to its specific receptor on the surface of the B lymphocyte, triggering the following sequence of events:

1. The B lymphocyte is stimulated to develop into a plasma cell and to undergo multiple divisions so that identical plasma cells are formed.
2. The plasma cells synthesise antibodies.
3. Some B cells differentiate to become memory cells, which persist and replicate in the body long after the invading antigen has been dealt with (see Fig. 16.2).
4. Once sufficient quantities of an antibody have been produced to destroy all the antigen, the plasma cells die, leaving memory cells ready to respond to a future attack by that antigen.
5. Antibodies bind to the antigen, activating the complement system.
6. When several antibodies bind to one antigen, the complex thus formed is chemically attracted to the surface of phagocytic cells, resulting in the formation of an antigen–antibody–phagocyte complex.
7. The presence of antibodies seems to trigger the phagocyte into action, resulting in ingestion and digestion of the bacterium.

The time interval between contact with the antigen and the production of antibodies (IgM) may allow disease to develop in the individual due to the effects of the antigen (e.g. infection from microorganisms).

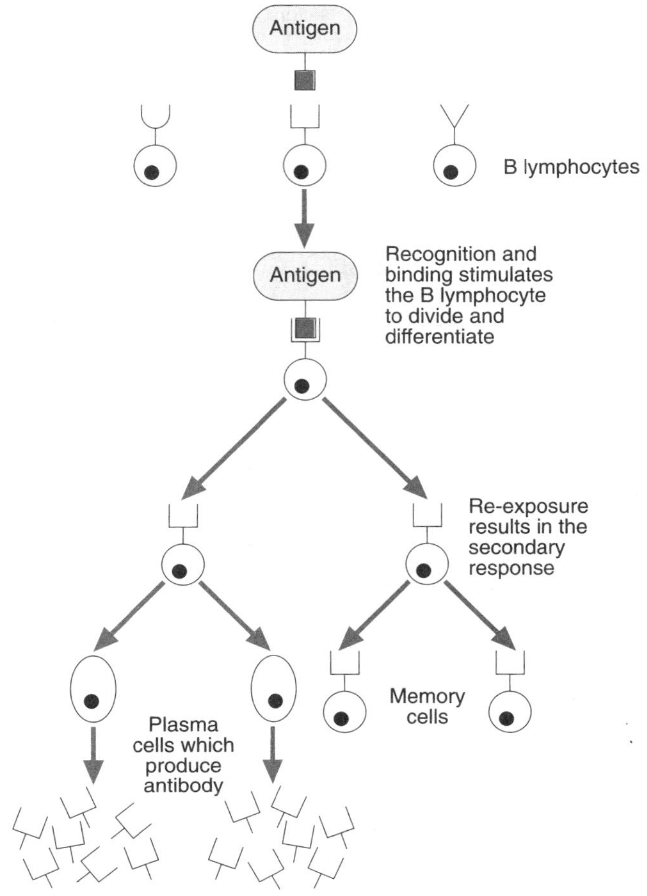

Fig. 16.2 The primary immune response.

Secondary response. When the body encounters an antigen for the second time (or subsequently), the memory cells respond rapidly by producing plasma cells, which then produce antibodies. This response occurs within a few days and, together with any residual antibody from the primary response, usually prevents disease from developing. In other words, the individual is immune.

Immunisation: artificial immunity

Vaccination or immunisation is a means of artificially invoking a primary immune response to a particular microorganism (antigen) so that when the antigen is subsequently encountered, the individual will be immune to it. The principle of immunisation is to introduce altered microorganisms or toxins into the body so that the individual does not develop the disease, but does mount an immune response. In other words, it mimics the natural response to infectious disease. Booster doses may be required months or years after the first dose of a vaccine in order to maintain an adequate level of memory cells. There are three types of vaccine:

- *Live attenuated vaccines*. Laboratory culturing of virulent strains of some organisms causes them to lose their virulence. These are then capable of inducing immunity without causing disease. The bacille Calmette - Guérin (BCG: tuberculosis) and rubella vaccines are of this type. It can be dangerous to administer a live vaccine to someone who is immunosuppressed.

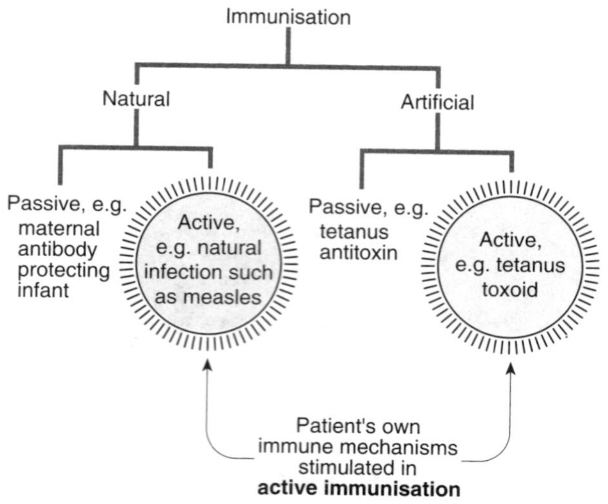

Fig. 16.3 Natural and artificial immunity. (Reproduced with kind permission from Kirkwood E, Lewis C 1989 Understanding medical immunology, 2nd edn. Copyright John Wiley & Sons Ltd.)

- *Toxoids*. The toxin produced by the bacterium is chemically modified by formalin treatment so that its toxicity is lost but it retains its antigenicity and is therefore still capable of inducing an immune response. The tetanus toxoid is an example of this type.
- *Killed vaccines*. These are preparations in which the organisms have been killed by heat or chemicals; the whooping cough vaccine is one example.

Immunity can therefore be natural (acquired in utero or after infectious disease) or artificial (acquired after immunisation). Figure 16.3 illustrates the processes involved in natural and artificial immunity.

Cell-mediated immune response. As it is not possible for antibody to reach microorganisms which live inside host cells, e.g. viruses, a different system, known as the cell-mediated immune response, carries out this function. There has to be a way for the T lymphocyte to recognise an infected cell and this involves the major histocompatibility complex (MHC). The MHC is a group of molecules which are important in interactions between cells in the immune system, in particular in the recognition of infected cells. One of these molecules is present on the surface of the cell in association with antigen, and this is what the T cells recognise and bind to. T-helper cells recognise and bind to the antigen and MHC molecule on the surface of macrophages, producing cytokines (see p. 584) which activate the macrophage and kill the intracellular microorganism. Cytotoxic T cells are also antigen-specific, having acquired a specific antigen receptor during their maturation in the thymus gland. They recognise antigen in association with the MHC on virally infected cells, which they destroy.

Once all the antigen has been destroyed, the immune response is 'switched off' until the next time. The involvement of other cells (e.g. mast cells) in the immune response has been discussed on page 583.

CONTROL OF INFECTION

Considering their disparity in size, the relationship between humans and the microorganisms with which they share the world is a paradoxical one. Some of these organisms can cause severe disease and even death in their host if the conditions are favourable for them to do so. On the other hand, some microorganisms are normal inhabitants of the human body (e.g. on the skin and in the gut), and without them we should be in grave danger of invasion by pathogenic (disease-producing) organisms. This situation can arise when people are treated unnecessarily with antibiotics which kill the useful microorganisms that normally compete with invading bacteria.

Disease-producing organisms

Why are some organisms pathogenic and others not? The extent to which an organism is capable of producing disease will depend on the nature of the organism, its location, the numbers present and the state of the host's defences. It is not possible to classify all organisms as either pathogens or commensals (commensals are those which normally live harmlessly on or in the body), for some commensals can be pathogenic if they are transferred to a more susceptible site. For example, *E. coli* is a normal commensal in the gastrointestinal tract, but it can cause urinary tract infection if it gets into the bladder (Duerden et al 1993) (see Ch. 8). Urinary tract infection is commoner in females than in males because of the close proximity of the anus to the urethra. The female urethra is also shorter.

The first microorganisms a healthy newborn baby encounters are those in the birth canal of its mother and on the hands of its attendants. The baby's skin very quickly becomes colonised, and once feeding is established the gut is also colonised. These organisms are usually those which constitute the normal flora (or commensals) of the body (Table 16.1), but can also include disease-producing organisms.

There are other organisms which are always considered to be pathogenic, as they inevitably produce disease if they are introduced into the body in large enough numbers; one such example is *Salmonella typhimurium*.

Table 16.1 Normal commensal microorganisms

Site	*Organism*
Skin	*Staphylococcus epidermidis* Diphtheroids *Corynebacterium* sp.
Mouth and throat	Staphylococci Streptococci Anaerobes *Neisseria* sp.
Nose	Staphylococci Diphtheroids
Gut	*Escherichia coli* *Klebsiella* sp. *Proteus* sp. *Streptococcus faecalis* *Clostridium perfringens* Yeasts (*Candida*)
Kidneys and bladder	Normally sterile
Vagina	Lactobacilli Streptococci Staphylococci Anaerobes

Control of infection in patient care

Nurses have a responsibility not only to assist individuals to return to good health, but also to prevent further illness while the healing process is taking place. Patients should also be given the information they need in order to stay healthy. For example, a patient at home with a urinary catheter should be taught how to keep the urethral meatus clean and to prevent the introduction of bowel or other organisms; also, an elderly patient with a venous ulcer (see Ch. 2) should be reminded that by scratching the affected area, infection is likely to be caused by the introduction of organisms into a site where they will readily grow and multiply. Nurses also have a responsibility to prevent the spread of infection from one person to another (cross-infection or exogenous infection), whether from patient to nurse, nurse to patient, nurse to nurse, or patient to patient. Nurses must all do what they can to ensure the safety of patients and of other health care staff.

Q **16.1** How might infection spread within a hospital setting?

The patient with an infection may not know the importance of even the simplest measures (e.g. thorough handwashing) to prevent it spreading. Many people have misconceptions about how infections are acquired, and it may be helpful if the nurse asks the patient what she understands about her illness so that appropriate information can be given. At times, the nurse may have to use a great deal of subtlety to persuade the patient to change her behaviour.

Infections acquired in hospital are called 'nosocomial' or hospital-acquired infections. The problem of infection is much greater in hospital than at home, for a number of reasons, including the following:

- Sick people are gathered together.
- Each has a large number of attendants — nurses, doctors, physiotherapists, domestics and many more.
- Normal skin barriers are broken by surgery and invasive procedures.
- Many patients are given antibiotic therapy.
- Equipment and instruments may be used for a number of patients.
- Food is cooked and stored in bulk.
- Stress, which is thought to lower resistance to infection, is caused by being in hospital.

Nevertheless, the principles of controlling infection should be applied in the home as well as the hospital setting; at all times, the nurse must do everything he can to prevent the spread of infection. Indeed, this is part of the nurse's professional responsibility (UKCC 1992). Most health boards/authorities and NHS Trusts have a control of infection nurse who gives advice and provides information to all health care staff (Hospital Infection Working Group 1995).

Q **16.2** How would you protect yourself from getting an infection at work?

Microorganisms cannot walk, jump, or fly: they have to be transferred, usually in body fluids or on the surface of articles or hands. It follows, therefore, that any body fluid is capable of transmitting infection and that the hands of doctors and nurses, as well as instruments and other equipment used on patients, are potential means of transfer.

Policies

Many arrangements and procedures in health care are governed by legislation or by guidelines issued from time to time by the UK Health Departments: the Department of Health (DoH) in England, formerly the Department of Health and Social Security (DHSS); the Scottish Office Department of Health, formerly the Scottish Office Home and Health Department (SOHHD) in Scotland; the Welsh Office in Wales; and the Department of Health and Social Services (DHSS) in Northern Ireland. Documents governing infection control are numerous and are updated from time to time. Health boards/authorities and Trusts are expected to have up-to-date local policies based on national guidelines.

Policies that cover every eventuality are so lengthy and cumbersome that they are unlikely to be read or used. In addition, individualised care precludes the writing of very detailed guidelines, because the assessment of the patient as an individual determines the care required. Policies that are easy to understand and apply are more likely to be followed, but in order to achieve simplicity without compromising safety, it may be necessary to set general rules which are more than may be required in each individual case.

In this chapter, examples are given of policy requirements as well as of additional measures that can be taken. It is important that nurses become familiar with existing control of infection policies in their place of work.

Safe working practice

Safe working practice entails making sure that one does not put oneself or others at unnecessary risk of acquiring an infection (see Box 16.4). It is not always possible to identify people who have transmissible infections; indeed, many (such as symptomless hepatitis B carriers) will be unaware of the fact themselves. By relying solely on identification, the nurse may unknowingly expose himself to pathogens. Safe practice involves:

- good hand hygiene
- universal blood and body fluid precautions
- cleaning, disinfection or sterilisation of equipment, instruments and surfaces
- correct use of disinfectants
- aseptic technique
- safe disposal of waste, sharps and linen
- isolation precautions when patients have a known or suspected infection.

Each of these elements of safe practice will now be considered in turn.

Hand hygiene

Hands should ideally be washed after each patient contact. This is not always possible, however, and an alcohol wipe or hand-rub (if approved by the Control of Infection Committee) may be used instead.

Box 16.4 Safe practice: preventing infection

- Wash hands thoroughly and frequently
- Cover all cuts and broken skin with a waterproof plaster
- Wear the appropriate protective clothing for contact with all body fluids and substances
- Keep immunisations up to date
- Be familiar with procedures for needlestick injury and accidental contamination with body fluid

Liquid antibacterial soaps (e.g. those containing chlorhexidine or povidone-iodine) have been shown to kill a higher percentage of microorganisms than soap and water (Ehrenkranz 1992). Some authorities advocate the use of an antibacterial cleanser after the hands have been contaminated with a body fluid (including contact with contaminated equipment) and before an aseptic procedure is carried out (e.g. wound dressing or emptying a urinary catheter drainage bag). Others believe that a soap and water wash is adequate, as it has not been proved that the reduction in number of microorganisms achieved by using an antibacterial soap actually reduces the incidence of infection in patients, although this has been demonstrated in intensive care units (Bryan et al 1995).

It is important that all surfaces of both hands are washed thoroughly, taking particular care with the areas likely to be missed (Taylor 1978a,b), i.e. the fingertips, finger webs and the backs of the thumbs. The hands should first of all be wetted, the soap applied and used to wash them, and then they should be rinsed and thoroughly dried, preferably with paper towels. A study which investigated the change in bacterial counts on the hands after drying found that the number of bacteria on the hands was considerably reduced after using paper towels, but greatly increased after using hot air hand dryers (Knights et al 1993). The taps should be turned off with the elbow or wrist.

Q **16.3** Why should you not turn the taps off with your hands?

If elbow or wrist-action taps are not available, a paper towel should be used to turn off the tap. Handwashing is essentially simple, easily forgotten, but nonetheless crucial to safe patient care (see Box 16.5) — just think of all the things one does with one's hands!

Universal blood and body fluid precautions

The UK Health Departments (1998) consider that blood, body fluids likely to contain blood, and certain other body fluids such as cerebrospinal fluid are capable of transmitting infection, and recommend that precautions are taken in the handling of these body fluids. Some authorities believe that all body fluids should be treated as if they were infectious, given the difficulty in identifying people who have transmissible infections, e.g. *Salmonella* excretors or hepatitis B carriers. If the nurse assumes that all body fluids might be infectious, then unnecessary risks will be avoided.

Box 16.5 Hand hygiene

Hands should be washed:

AFTER
- Examining or caring for a patient
- Going to the toilet
- They have been contaminated with body fluids
- Leaving an isolation room

BEFORE
- Leaving a patient or work area
- Eating or serving food
- Carrying out an aseptic procedure
- Entering a protective isolation room

Box 16.6 Universal blood and body fluid precautions

- Cover cuts and broken skin with a waterproof plaster
- Wear disposable gloves if you are going to be handling blood or body fluids
- Wear a disposable apron (and perhaps a gown) if your uniform or clothing is likely to be contaminated
- Wear a facemask and protective visor or spectacles if you think your eyes or mouth might be splashed

In this chapter, the term 'universal precautions' refers to measures taken to protect health workers when they have contact with blood or other body fluids from anyone, regardless of whether that individual is known to have an infection or not. All patients are thus treated in the same way, except when additional isolation precautions are required (see p. 592; Box 16.6; Research Abstract 16.1).

Q **16.4** Critically review the article in Research Abstract 16.1 (Courington et al 1991) and then discuss the implications of the research findings.

Cleaning, disinfecting and sterilising equipment, instruments and surfaces

Instruments, equipment and surfaces used in patient care may be 'sterile', 'disinfected' or 'clean', depending upon the standard of cleanliness demanded by the patient's condition and by the nature of the procedure being carried out.

Sterilisation. A sterile object is one which is free from all microorganisms, including spores. Sterilisation in hospitals can be reliably done only by heat, using an autoclave.

Spores are formed by some bacteria such as *Clostridium tetani* or *C. perfringens* when they encounter adverse conditions. The bacterium encases itself in a tough, resistant shell which allows it to survive for weeks or months in dust or soil. When conditions

Research Abstract 16.1

Observational studies carried out by Courington et al (1991) measured adherence to universal precautions by doctors, medical students and nurses in three surgical patient care areas (operating theatre, surgical ICU and surgical wards), before and after a specific educational programme aimed at improving compliance.

Common infractions were:

- theatre — failure to wear eye protection
- surgical ICU — failure to wear gloves and eye protection
- surgical ward — failure to wear gloves.

Percentage infractions before and after the educational programmes to improve compliance were:

	Before	After
Theatre	75%	81%
Surgical ICU	75%	40%
Surgical ward	30%	32%

Courington K R, Patterson S L, Howard R J 1991 Universal precautions are not universally followed. Archives of Surgery 126: 93–96 become favourable (i.e. in the presence of warmth, moisture and a food source), the spores germinate and regain all the properties of bacteria. Spores are difficult to kill, requiring a sterilisation process to ensure their destruction.

16.5 When could spores germinate in a patient in hospital?

Surgery and traumatic injury present the greatest risk for infection caused by spores. This is because deep tissues or body cavities may be penetrated and inadvertently implanted with spores. Sterilisation is required for all instruments which are used subcutaneously (under the skin) or submucosally (across mucous membrane into a sterile cavity); this includes surgical instruments, injection needles, urinary catheters and instruments being passed into the uterus. Ideally, it is carried out in a hospital sterilisation and disinfection unit (HSDU).

Once instruments have been sterilised, they must be kept sterile until they are used. This is done by packing the instrument (before autoclaving but after thorough cleaning and drying) in a special autoclave bag made of paper which is permeable to steam but impermeable when dry. The autoclave uses steam under pressure (usually at 134°C for 3 min) which penetrates the bag. The packs are then dried before the cycle is complete. As long as the packaging remains undamaged and dry, the contents of the bag should be sterile. The pack should therefore be checked for damage and signs of dampness before it is used. Dentists, general practitioners and some hospital departments may use a small autoclave suitable only for naked (i.e. unpackaged) instruments. These autoclaves are useful in situations where sterile instruments are required for immediate use only, as sterility cannot be maintained.

Special autoclave tape, or a small coloured panel on the bag, is used to indicate if a pack has been sterilised. The appearance of dark stripes on the tape, or a colour change in the panel, indicates that the pack has been through a sterilisation process.

Instruments that have been used on patients at risk from Creutzfeldt–Jakob disease are treated differently from all other surgical instruments. Creutzfeldt–Jakob disease, which affects the central nervous system, causing senile dementia and psychosis, is caused by an agent which is resistant to the normal sterilisation and disinfection procedures (i.e. autoclaving at 134°C for 3 min or immersion in glutaraldehyde). Contaminated instruments from someone at risk of developing this disease may have to be destroyed (SEHD 1993a).

Contaminated instruments from people with tuberculosis, HIV or hepatitis are sometimes autoclaved before they are handled in the HSDU. This may not be necessary if an automatic wash process at 98°C for 5 min is performed.

Disinfection ensures freedom from harmful microorganisms, but not from spores, and is recommended for all instruments and surfaces which have been:

- in contact with body fluids, tissues, broken skin or mucosal surfaces, pathological specimens or cultures
- used by, or on, patients with known or suspected infection
- about to be used by, or on, severely immunosuppressed patients.

Disinfection is necessary to prevent cross-infection. It can be achieved using heat or chemicals; for small items, heat is the best method. Most microorganisms are destroyed by a temperature of 80°C held for 1 min, but a higher temperature is required to kill the hepatitis B virus (Kobayashi et al 1984). Equipment that is used in such close proximity to the patient that trauma to mucosal surfaces or contact with broken skin is likely (e.g. ENT instruments, sigmoidoscopes and breast pumps) may provide a vehicle for blood-borne viruses, such as hepatitis B, and should be cleaned and disinfected at a higher temperature, such as 93°C for 10 min in a washer disinfector.

Vaginal instruments, which may provide a vehicle for heat-resistant papillomaviruses, should be autoclaved at 134°C. Body fluid containers, e.g. bedpans, urinals, suction jars and washbowls, are unlikely to be traumatic or to provide a vehicle for blood-borne transmission, and should be cleaned and disinfected at 80°C for 1 min in a washer disinfector designed for that purpose (see Research Abstract 16.2).

An autoclave can be used for disinfection where a washer/disinfector is not available, in which case the items must be thoroughly cleaned and dried first. They do not need to be individually wrapped, as sterility does not need to be maintained. The disinfection process is used simply to kill any microorganisms which have been deposited on an instrument before it is used for another patient. Figure 16.4 gives an example of a policy for the disinfection of small items.

Chemical disinfectants can be used to disinfect heat-sensitive instruments (e.g. flexible endoscopes), but the process is fraught with difficulties. Some of the problems with the use of chemicals are as follows:

- They are not all effective against commonly encountered microorganisms.
- They tend to be inactivated by body fluids, and so the surfaces of the item must be clean before it is immersed.
- The correct strength must be used.
- Steps must be taken to ensure that all surfaces of the instrument are in contact with the disinfectant and that all air is removed.
- Ample time is required.

Research Abstract 16.2

A study by Greaves (1985) examined infection control practices relating to bedbaths and washbowls. Part of the study looked at the use and misuse of washbowls. One bowl in each of three wards was marked, and then observed twice daily for 5 days. In addition, 11 random bowls were sampled for microbiology by being rinsed out with normal saline and the resulting fluid sent for culture.

Articles of clothing (e.g. pants, nightdresses, scrotal supports) were found soaking in some of the bowls. Bowls were mostly communal, were frequently left wet and were stacked upright, one on top of the other.

Questioning on other wards revealed that nine out of 13 used some sort of disinfectant for cleaning the bowls, but most used Hibiscrub (a liquid antibacterial soap for handwashing). Of the 11 bowls randomly sampled, only two showed 'no growth'. Others showed the presence of microorganisms which could potentially cause infection if they reached a susceptible site.

Greave's recommendations were as follows:

- Hospital patients should be supplied with their own bowls.
- These bowls should be washed with detergents and hot water after use, and dried and stored inverted, preferably in the patient's locker.
- Before a bowl is used for another patient, it should be disinfected; stericol, a phenolic, is recommended.

Greaves A 1985 We'll just freshen you up, dear. Nursing Times Journal of Infection Control Nursing 81(10) Suppl: 3–8

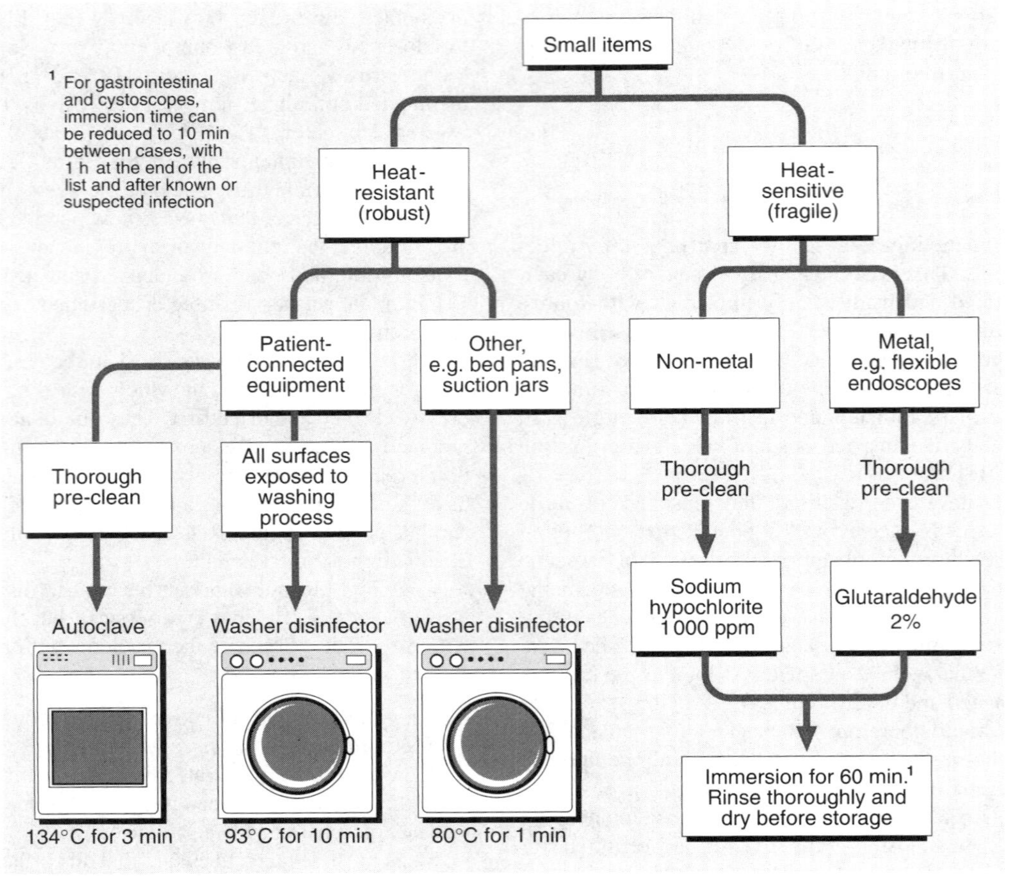

Fig. 16.4 An example of a policy for disinfection of small items. (Reproduced with kind permission from Dr A B White.)

- Thorough rinsing after immersion is essential.
- Once diluted, most disinfectants quickly deteriorate.
- It is necessary to check that the material from which the instrument is made is compatible with the disinfectant to be used. For example, soft porous rubber as well as plastic may absorb phenolics and glutaraldehyde, and hypochlorite will damage metal and some fabrics.
- Disinfectants are toxic and can cause skin reactions.

Heat-sensitive instruments may be chemically disinfected, using either sodium hypochlorite 1000 ppm (for non-metallic items) or glutaraldehyde 2% (for instruments which are incompatible with hypochlorite). A Control of Substances Hazardous to Health Regulations (COSHH) assessment is required (see below).

Flexible endoscopes are heat-sensitive and are usually disinfected chemically, although new methods using low temperatures, such as gas plasma, are now being developed and tested for efficacy and suitability. These instruments are expensive, and because of the speed with which endoscopy is performed, a large number of instruments would be required if each instrument was to be immersed for 1 h. As a compromise, endoscopes which are considered unlikely to be contaminated with mycobacteria are generally immersed for a shorter time (see Fig. 16.4). On the basis that all bronchoscopes could be contaminated with mycobacteria, and that this is more likely than with gastrointestinal or cystoscopes, some authorities recommend that all bronchoscopes be immersed for 1 h if they cannot be heat-disinfected. Scopes entering a sterile cavity, such as arthroscopes and laparoscopes, should of course be sterile. This is possible chemically with immersion for 3–10 h (Medical Devices Agency 1996), but autoclavable arthroscopes and laparoscopes are now available.

COSHH (1988) requires users of chemicals such as glutaraldehyde to take steps to minimise the hazards to staff in the use of such substances if there is not an acceptable alternative chemical or process. Totally closed machines to prevent the escape of vapour are being developed, and air extraction systems may also be required to keep the amount of aldehyde vapour below the minimum acceptable level. If glutaraldehyde must be used, staff exposure to it should be minimised, and gloves, masks and visors or goggles worn. New disinfectants are being developed, such as peracetic acid and chlorine dioxide, but they are expensive, and safety precautions are still required for their use. The problems of chemical disinfection and the COSHH regulations are discussed by Babb (1990).

Instruments should not be stored in disinfectants, but removed after the required immersion time, rinsed thoroughly and stored dry. Disinfection is carried out preferably in an HSDU, but may be done on the ward; if the process is carried out correctly there should be no risk to patients or staff.

When dealing with patient-connected equipment, it is important to establish whether items are reusable (i.e. they can be processed and used again), for single use or for single patient use, so that they can be treated accordingly.

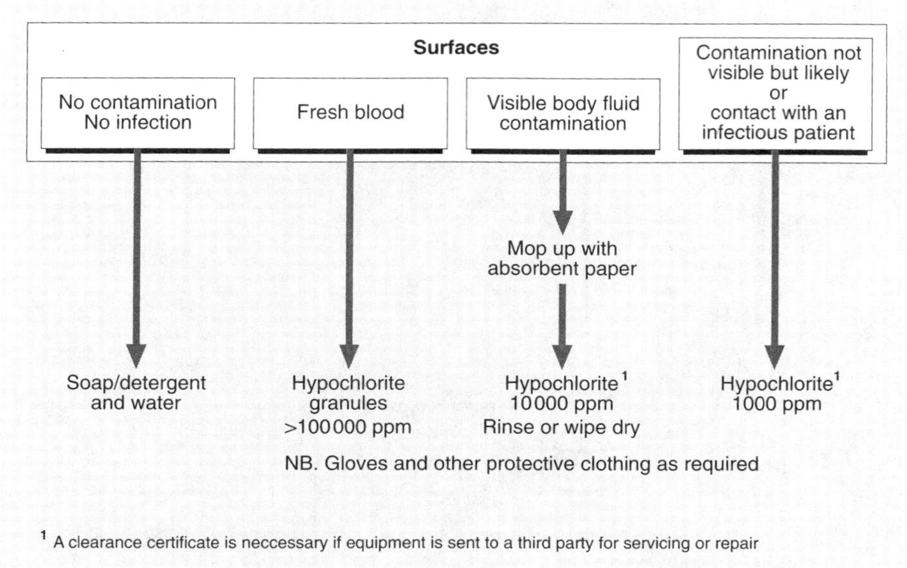

Fig. 16.5 An example of a policy for spillage: surfaces and equipment. (Reproduced with kind permission from Dr A B White.)

Spillage. The management of spillage must adhere to locally prescribed policy. Normally, spillage of body fluid on a floor or other surface should first of all be mopped up using disposable paper, cloth or a mop with a detachable head which is sent to the laundry after use. Gloves must be worn. The spillage area should then be wiped with a disinfectant, e.g. sodium hypochlorite 10 000 ppm. The disinfectant should be rinsed off and the surface dried afterwards; this is especially important if the surface will come into contact with the skin, e.g. a toilet seat. Disinfectants are also used for wiping down surfaces which have been in contact with patients with known or suspected infection. All surfaces should be left dry after cleaning or disinfection.

Strong chlorine-releasing granules (>100 000 ppm) can be poured over fresh blood spills; these will absorb the blood and disinfect it before it is cleared up. They are, however, extremely pungent and care is necessary in their use. With other body fluid spillages, it is probably more effective and less messy to clear up the spillage first (using disposable paper) and then to disinfect the area.

Hypochlorite 1000 ppm may be used where body fluid contamination is probable even though the surface looks clean, and for well-sponged fabrics and thoroughly pre-cleaned metal surfaces.

Alcohol is a useful cleaning agent for clean, hard surfaces such as glass, but is not suitable for disinfecting dirty surfaces, e.g. commodes, because of its poor penetration when organic material is present (Rutala 1996).

Figure 16.5 provides an example of a policy for the disinfection of surfaces. The certificate referred to in the figure is required for all medical equipment and devices sent to a third party for investigation, inspection, repair or servicing (MAC 1996). It serves as a warning to the receiving department that, where dismantling of the item is required, a hazard may still exist and precautions will be necessary.

Cleaning. Ordinary cleaning with soap or detergent and water is adequate when there is no contamination with blood or body fluid, and no contact with patients with known or suspected infection.

Aseptic technique

An aseptic technique is carried out in a clean environment using sterile equipment. The procedure is carried out in such a way as to minimise the likelihood of infection being introduced to the site. It is used for wound dressings, urinary catheterisation, manipulation of intravenous infusions and other situations where the skin is broken. Hands should be thoroughly washed (see p. 588) and only sterile materials (e.g. gloves, instruments, etc.) should be used.

Safe disposal

Waste. Procedures in the safe disposal of clinical and household waste are as follows.

Clinical waste consists of human tissue, blood or other body fluids; excretions; drugs, swabs or dressings; and syringes, needles or other sharp instruments. It includes all waste arising from medical, nursing, dental or similar practice, investigation, treatment, care, teaching and research (HSAC 1992).

Household or domestic waste consists of all non-hazardous waste generated in the course of normal life.

Waste identification. Colour-coded bags make it easy to distinguish between clinical and household waste. Health workers should check which colours are used in their area of work. Most health boards or authorities have adopted the national colour code (HSAC 1992), which is as follows:

- human tissue, dialysis waste and waste from the isolation nursing of patients with infectious disease should be placed in thick yellow plastic bags
- sharps should be placed in the designated yellow sharps box immediately after use, by the person using them, and not left for someone else to clear up
- other clinical waste should be discarded in thin yellow plastic bags. See end note on page 609.

Incineration is mandatory for most clinical waste, and is the preferred option for all clinical waste. There are some exceptions

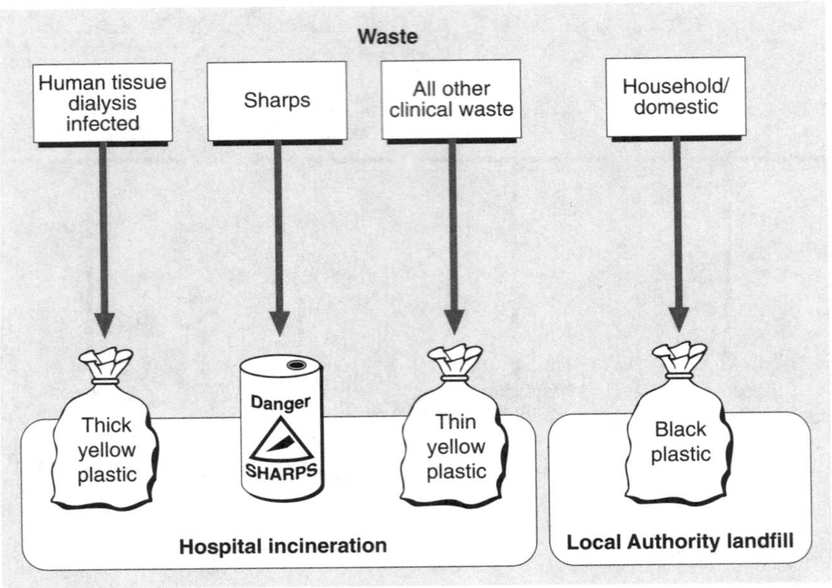

Fig. 16.6 An example of a waste disposal policy. (Reproduced with kind permission from Dr A B White.)

to this rule. Certain items of waste can be placed in striped black-and-yellow bags and disposed of by licensed landfill. New technologies for heat disinfection prior to landfill offer an alternative method for some categories of clinical waste.

Clinical waste arising from home treatment must not enter the domestic waste system (HSAC 1992). Some health boards/authorities in urban areas may make special arrangements for the uplift of clinical waste through the environmental health or cleansing department, but this can be difficult in rural areas.

Figure 16.6 gives an example of a waste disposal policy.

Linen. Procedures for the safe laundering of hospital and domestic linen are as follows.

Hospital laundry. All hospital linen is disinfected using either heat or chemicals. Heat is the method of choice, and temperatures and holding times are laid down by the NHS Executive (1995) and SOHHD (1993). Chemicals, e.g. sodium hypochlorite, may be used for fabrics which are likely to be heat-labile, such as personal clothing, so that they can be washed at a lower temperature (40°C), although if fouling is likely to be frequent, it is advisable for the patient to buy clothing that will withstand the disinfection temperatures.

It is a national requirement that linen is sorted in the ward into used (soiled and fouled) linen and infected linen. What follows in this section is an example of a local laundry policy.

Figure 16.7 outlines a laundry policy in which linen is sorted into the following categories:

- used (no longer fresh)
- fouled (contaminated with body fluid)
- infected (used for a patient with known or suspected infection)
- heat-labile (unable to withstand thermal disinfection temperatures).

White outer bags identify all used linen. Red outer bags are used for potentially infected linen. Blue outer bags are used for personal clothing.

In addition, alginate stitch or soluble panel bags are used for all fouled or infected linen before it is placed in the outer laundry bags (totally water-soluble bags may also be used). This prevents seepage through the outer bag during transit and protects laundry staff as the bag should be placed straight into the laundry machine without being opened. When the washing process has started, the soluble panel dissolves to allow the contents to be washed and heat-disinfected. The remains of the bags must be removed before the linen is placed in the dryer.

It is important that no extraneous items are inadvertently sent to the laundry, as sharp items can damage linen and cause injury to the laundry staff.

In this policy, used and fouled linen is thermally disinfected at 71°C for 3 min. A higher temperature (93°C for 10 min) is recommended for all infected linen in order to inactivate the hepatitis B virus and make the linen safe to handle.

Laundry in the home. Most linen and clothing can be washed in the usual way at home. Fouled linen is washed at 60°C, and infected linen at 90–95°C (in an automatic washing machine). In some areas, it may be possible for contaminated linen to be collected and laundered by the hospital laundry and then returned clean.

Barrier nursing or isolation precautions for patients with known or suspected infection

Patients who suffer from an infectious disease or who are colonised or infected with organisms such as MRSA (see Box 16.7) are a potential source of infection to others. Particularly in hospital, where patients are especially vulnerable, it is important to take precautions to prevent the spread of infection. These precautions are known as barrier nursing, source isolation, or simply isolation precautions, meaning that attempts are made to stop the microorganisms from spreading to other patients and staff. The implied 'barrier' or 'isolation' simply means keeping someone who may be an infection risk away from others who might be susceptible, i.e. in a single room if possible, and wearing appropriate protective clothing when caring for them and when touching contaminated surfaces or equipment.

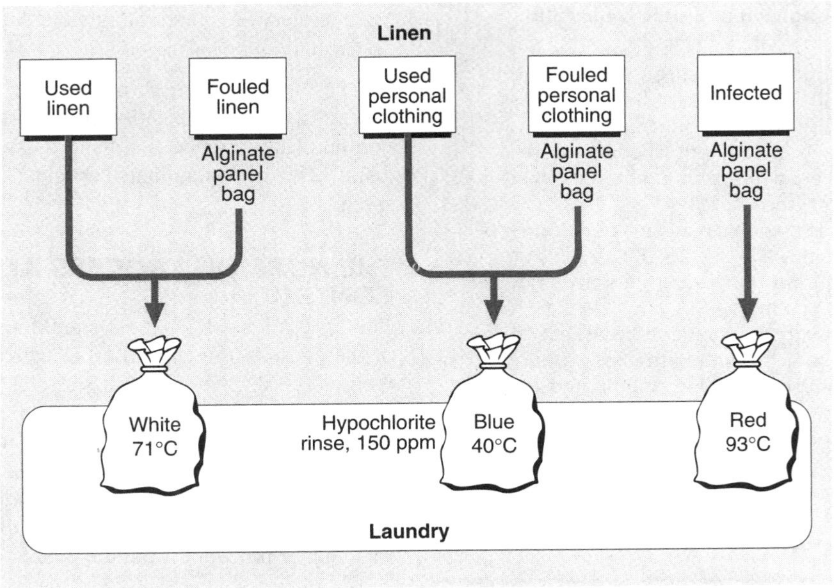

Fig. 16.7 An example of a linen laundering policy. (Reproduced with kind permission from Dr A B White.)

Box 16.7 Methicillin-resistant *Staphylococcus aureus* (MRSA)

- *Staphylococcus aureus* is a bacterium which is present in the nose and/or skin of approximately 50% of the population
- There are many strains of *S. aureus*. Some are resistant to many antibiotics; these are known as MRSA
- Most people with MRSA are colonised only (see p. 592), but sometimes MRSA cause infection
- MRSA are a problem in hospital because of the danger of spread, particularly to vulnerable patients, e.g. those in ICUs, people undergoing orthopaedic or vascular surgery and the immunosuppressed
- MRSA are not a risk to healthy people, including pregnant women, young children and babies
- Management of people with MRSA depends on where the organism is, where the person is (e.g. orthopaedic ward, long-stay hospital or at home) and the vulnerability of other people in that person's environment
- Patients in hospital with MRSA are usually barrier-nursed (source isolation) in single rooms, or 'cohorted' together in a larger area
- MRSA are mainly spread by hands (hence the importance of handwashing) but can also be spread by skin scales, dust and contaminated equipment or fabrics
- The management of MRSA varies both between and within hospitals, depending on local circumstances, and is based on risk assessment
- Antiseptics are used for staff handwashing and may be used for body and hair washing in colonised patients, in order to try to eliminate carriage

Some people believe that if universal precautions are carried out, there is no need to take further isolation precautions with patients who have a known or suspected infection. However, certain things are required when a patient is known to have a transmissible infection, namely a thick yellow waste bag (HSAC 1992), a red linen bag (SOHHD 1993b, NHS Executive 1995) and an appropriate warning to other departments so that the same precautions can be taken there. In addition, we know that universal precautions are not always carried out properly (see Research Abstract 16.1) and that universal precautions do not encompass the unseen contamination which can result from patient rather than staff behaviour — e.g. when a person suffering from salmonellosis has diarrhoea, does not wash her hands properly and touches door handles and the furniture around her or even hands sweets or food to other people.

Patients suffering from an infectious disease and their families at home will need advice about how to prevent the spread of infection. In the case of home helps, the diagnosis need not be disclosed, but precautions that are needed when handling body fluids and contaminated surfaces or furniture should be carefully explained. Handwashing is the most important precaution in these circumstances.

The hazard in nursing people with infection is the infectious body fluid(s), and the aim of protective clothing is to prevent contact with the infectious fluid(s) and with any surface that may have been contaminated, by touch, splash or with airborne particles, e.g. dust containing the infectious agent.

Another kind of barrier nursing, often known as reverse barrier nursing or protective isolation, is used when an individual is particularly susceptible to infection, e.g. neutropenic patients (see Box 16.8 and Ch. 11).

One way of determining the precautions required is to ascertain which body fluids or substances are infectious and how far those infectious fluids are spreading into the environment, and to use the following categories:

- *exudate precautions* — for infection confined to an internal body fluid or discharge capable of occlusion
- *standard isolation* — when infectious fluid contaminates the patient's skin and immediate environment by direct contact
- *strict isolation* — when infectious fluid (including airborne particles) contaminates the entire room.

Box 16.8 Reverse barrier nursing or protective isolation

- Some authorities recommend or practise this type of isolation, although there is little evidence for its effectiveness
- The aim is to minimise the introduction of harmful microorganisms into the environment of someone whose immune system is severely depressed, e.g. patients with a very low white cell count (see Ch. 11)
- Some immunosuppressed patients may also be a source of infection, e.g. people with AIDS (see Ch. 37).
- The emphasis is on ensuring that everything entering the room is as germ-free as possible
- Protective clothing is worn to prevent the nurse from infecting the patient, rather than the other way around
- Good handwashing and properly decontaminated equipment are essential
- Some specialist units have sophisticated facilities which include filtered ventilation
- A 'clean diet' may be advised, i.e. avoiding foods like raw fruit and vegetables which could be contaminated and therefore hazardous in these circumstances

An explanation of how these precautions work in practice is given in the section on 'Infectious diseases' (see pp. 600–608).

Most books on infection control have a section on barrier nursing, and a recent guideline produced by the Hospital Infection Control Practices Advisory Committee (HICPAC 1996) gives a comprehensive account of current thinking as well as references to previous work.

Isolation can be a very stressful experience (Knowles 1993), but this is not in itself a reason for failing to isolate someone if her condition warrants this precaution for the safety of others. Criticism of isolation often relates to the way it is done rather than to the requirement for isolation itself. It is important, therefore, to do everything possible to lessen the patient's anxiety, loneliness and boredom.

Improving the quality of life for patients in isolation. A patient in isolation requires skilled and sensitive care, as she is in effect cut off from the outside world and from normal human contact. It is important, therefore, that the patient's needs are discussed, agreed and recorded in the care plan. Loneliness is often a major problem: allocating one nurse on each shift to be responsible for the patient will help, as long as that nurse spends time with the patient at frequent intervals. Extra staff may be required. Encouraging relatives to visit at different times of the day can help, as can the offer of a television, telephone, radio or cassette player. Favourite leisure activities such as card games, sewing or knitting will help to pass the time.

The patient needs to have some privacy and should not feel that she is constantly being watched. Patients suffering from diarrhoea are often acutely aware of smells and may welcome the offer of a deodorising room spray or a few drops of an essential plant oil such as lavender placed on a tissue in the room.

Patients with infections not requiring isolation. Some infections are caused by organisms which are normally found in the environment but have caused disease because:

- they have infected a susceptible site, e.g. *E. coli* in the urinary tract
- they have gained access due to impaired host defences, e.g. candidiasis (thrush) in an immunosuppressed patient
- their spores have been implanted deep in the tissues as a result of surgery or a penetrating wound, e.g. gas gangrene caused by *Clostridium perfringens*.

These patients can be nursed in a multi-bed ward and do not necessarily require isolation precautions. Treatment of the infection and safe practice (i.e. hand hygiene, safe disposal, adequate disinfection of contaminated articles) should be enough to prevent spread.

THE NURSING PROCESS AND INFECTION CONTROL

The assessment of a patient should always include consideration of the possible infection risks to which she might be exposed, as well as the degree to which she presents a risk to other people. This will be reflected in the care plan. All individuals are at risk of acquiring an infection while in hospital, but the very young, the very old and those who are immunosuppressed, debilitated or undergoing surgery or invasive procedures are especially vulnerable. Urinary catheters, intravenous therapy, enteral feeding and many other procedures put the patient in danger of infection.

Q **16.6** What would be the dangers of bacterial contamination of nasogastric feeding solutions?

Enteral feeds should be prepared using hygienic practices (Anderton 1995). Equipment used in preparation must be adequately disinfected and correctly stored. (Feeds prepared locally are refrigerated immediately and administered as soon as possible after preparation. Commercially prepared feeds carry instructions about shelf-life and storage.) Feeding solutions are an ideal breeding ground for bacteria, particularly at room temperature. It is therefore essential to give the feed within the specified time in order to prevent bacterial multiplication and possible gastrointestinal upset (see Nursing Care Plan 16.1).

The Bowell–Webster risk guide (Bowell 1990) is a helpful reminder in assessing a patient's risk of infection (see Table 16.2).

Anticipation of potential problems is essential in patient care. For example, the passage of a urinary catheter should remind the nurse of the infection risks involved and lead him to assess how much the patient needs to be taught about subsequent self-care. In the case of immunosuppressed patients (see Ch. 11), the greatest risk is endogenous infection (self-infection), caused by the patient's own microorganisms entering a susceptible site or by reactivation of latent infection, e.g. cytomegalovirus. Although endogenous infection is more difficult to prevent than cross-infection, the nurse can still teach the patient how to minimise the risk. This not only helps the individual to stay free from infection, but also encourages a positive attitude, allowing her to feel that she can contribute to her own well-being.

Health and safety

Nurses have a duty of care to others, as stated in the Health and Safety at Work etc Act (1974). This duty can be expressed in health care situations in a number of ways, which include:

- Implementing measures in accordance with safe working practice (see p. 587) to ensure that no harm results from actions or omissions.
- Notifying other departments that precautions need to be taken with the body fluids of an infectious patient being transferred there.

Nursing Care Plan 16.1 Preventing bacterial contamination during nasogastric feeding
Mr W is a 46-year-old bachelor who works as a travelling salesman. He suffers from an inflammatory bowel disease which has recently become unmanageable. He has been admitted to hospital for enteral nutrition to improve his nutritional state prior to surgery.

Nursing considerations	***Action***	***Rationale***	***Evaluation***
1. Nasogastric tube may have caused trauma to mucosal surfaces, resulting in mild immunosuppression/ potential risk of infection	❒ Keep mouth clean and comfortable by giving mouthwashes every 2 h ❒ Encourage Mr W to clean his teeth regularly	The patient is not able to drink much fluid and his mouth may become very dry. Salivary flow may be diminished	Patient's mouth is clean and moist, and salivary flow is adequate
2. Danger of bacterial multiplication in hospital/ prepared feed unless refrigerated, and administered within given time	❒ Administer 500 ml feeds within 4 h at a consistent rate and record on fluid balance chart	If the feed is left at room temperature for longer than this, bacterial counts will rise rapidly	Feed administered to time except 12.00–14.00 h when detached while patient at X-ray. Remaining feed discarded and fresh feed commenced at 14.00 h
	❒ Use a fresh reservoir and giving set for each 500 ml feed	Even after the feed has been given, a fine film remains on the inside of the reservoir and giving set: bacteria will have begun to replicate	Reservoir and giving set changed after each 4-hourly feed
	❒ Observe patient for nausea, vomiting, abdominal pain, diarrhoea	Any signs of gastroenteritis should be reported	No signs of gastroenteritis. Feed appears to be tolerated well

Table 16.2 The Bowell–Webster risk assessment guide for identifying patients at risk of infection. (Reproduced with kind permission from Bowell 1990)

General factors	*Local factors*	*Invasive procedures*	*Drugs*	*Disease*
Age	*Oedema*	*Cannulation*	Cytotoxics	Carcinoma
Very young	Pulmonary	Peripheral		
Very old	Ascites	Central	Antibiotics	Leukaemia
	Effusion	Parenteral		
Nutrition			Steroids	Aplastic anaemia
Emaciated	*Ischaemia*	*Catheterisation*		
Thin	Thrombus	Intermittent		Diabetes mellitus
Obese	Embolus	Closed drainage		
Dehydrated	Necrosis	Irrigation		
				Liver disease
Mobility	*Skin lesions*	*Surgery*		Renal disease
Limited	Trauma	Anaesthesia		
Immobile	Burns	Wound		AIDS
Temporary	Ulceration	Wound drainage		
Permanent		Wound/colostomy		
	Foreign body	Implant		
Mental state	Accidental			
Confused	Planned	*Intubation*		
Depressed		Endobronchial suction		
Senile		Humidification		
		Ventilation		
Incontinence				
Urine				
Faeces				
Temporary				
Permanent				
General health				
Weak				
Debilitated				
General hygiene				
Dependence				
Mouth/teeth				
Skin				

- Staying home from work if one is unwell, particularly if the illness could be communicated to others, e.g. diarrhoea.
- Being aware of one's immune status regarding infectious diseases such as rubella, chickenpox, measles, tuberculosis, tetanus, hepatitis B, poliomyelitis, etc. Nurses can obtain advice from their general practitioner (GP) or from their employer's occupational health department.

Further information about immunisation can be found in DoH (1996).

Confidentiality

People suffering from infection are often embarrassed and sometimes depressed because of isolation precautions and the feeling that they are in some way 'dirty'. Nurses are legally responsible for keeping confidential any information given to them by patients and may divulge such information only when it is necessary to do so for the benefit of the patient or the safety of others (UKCC 1992). Nurses should reassure the patient that this is the case, in order to minimise any embarrassment or unease she may feel. It is also helpful to inform the patient about infection control procedures and the reasons for having them.

DISORDERS OF IMMUNITY

Four types of immunity disorder can be identified:

- immunodeficiency
- hypersensitivity
- autoimmune disease
- graft rejection after transplantation.

In this chapter, only the first three are addressed.

IMMUNODEFICIENCY

Immunodeficiency can be primary or secondary in nature, as outlined in the following.

Primary immunodeficiency

Primary immunodeficiency states are very rare, but may arise under either of the following two conditions:

- there are not enough cells available
- the number of cells is adequate but they have a functional defect.

These problems will be discussed in relation to the cells and proteins involved, i.e. impairment of phagocytes, B lymphocytes or of T lymphocytes.

16.7 Recall the cells and proteins that are involved in the immune response.

Impairment of phagocytes

Phagocyte impairment may occur in the following forms:

- *Neutropenia* — a low number of neutrophils (see p. 583). This condition can be congenital (very rare), secondary to drug or radiation therapy (see Ch. 31) or overwhelming infection, or associated with the autoimmune diseases (see p. 598).
- *Functional defects* — abnormalities in phagocyte structure or function. These can result in the inability of phagocytes to localise in an inflammatory site, or in their inability to ingest and digest microorganisms.
- *Failure of complement activation*. There are many steps in the complement pathway, and many components are involved or created during complement activation. Some appear to be more important than others (Roitt 1994). Absence of one of the complement components can make phagocytosis difficult, as it is easier for the granular leucocytes to ingest microorganisms if their outer surface is coated with complement.

16.8 Recall the function of B lymphocytes and try to work out what will happen if they are deficient.

Impairment of B lymphocytes

Occasionally B lymphocytes fail to mature properly in the bone marrow, resulting in B-cell deficiency and therefore diminished antibody production. People with B-cell deficiency are particularly prone to bacterial infections, e.g. *Staphylococcus aureus* (Roitt 1994).

Impairment of T lymphocytes

T-cell deficiency occasionally occurs in children in whom absence of the thymus gland means that the cells cannot differentiate to become T lymphocytes. People with T-cell deficiency are particularly prone to some viral infections, e.g. varicella (Roitt 1994).

Secondary immunodeficiency

This occurs as a result of some other condition, and an individual suffering from secondary immunodeficiency is sometimes called a 'compromised host'. This term simply means that the person's immune defences are in some way reduced or compromised, making her particularly susceptible to infection (Weir & Stewart 1993).

The commonest clinical situations in which this happens are lymphoma, malnutrition, chemotherapy, AIDS (see Ch. 37), and in people who are post-transplant.

HYPERSENSITIVITY

An excessive immune response (hypersensitivity) can result in damage to normal tissue. This response may be immediate or delayed. Four types of hypersensitivity reaction have been described: types I, II and III are antibody-mediated; and type IV is mediated mainly by T cells and macrophages (Roitt et al 1996).

Type 1: anaphylactic or immediate hypersensitivity. In this type of immune response, excessive IgE production results in IgE binding to mast cells which, when the antigen is encountered, release histamine, giving rise to an acute inflammatory reaction. This response develops within minutes of exposure to the antigen and will recur on subsequent encounters.

The reaction can be local, as in asthma (see Ch 3), hay fever and eczema, or systemic, as in anaphylactic shock. Typical antigens are the house dust mite, pollen and foodstuffs such as shellfish, eggs and nuts (an increasing problem with allergy to nuts has resulted in many food labels indicating whether the product contains nuts). The nature of the symptoms will depend on whether the antigen is encountered locally or systemically, or absorbed via the intestine.

Atopy is a term used to describe the tendency of 10–15% of the population to suffer from allergic diseases such as asthma, eczema, hay fever, urticaria and food allergy (Brostoff et al 1991). There is often a familial (genetic) disposition to this condition.

Type II: antibody-dependent cytotoxic hypersensitivity. In this type of response, antibodies react to normal tissue cells, which then bind to complement or to phagocytes, resulting in lysis or phagocytosis of the cell. This can occur as a result of 'foreign' antigens entering the body, e.g. a mismatched blood transfusion (see Ch. 11) or a transplant, or can be induced by drugs or infections which appear to alter cell surface antigens such that an attack by native antibodies ensues.

Type III: immune-complex-mediated hypersensitivity. In this form of hypersensitivity, large immune complexes (i.e. antigens bound to antibodies; see p. 585) form in excess and are deposited in the capillary endothelium of the kidney, joints, skin and other sites. They may activate complement and attract phagocytes, resulting in mast cell degranulation and local or general inflammation. The inflammation may be acute, as in serum sickness; chronic, as in glomerulonephritis; or both, as in farmer's lung (see p. 598). This type of hypersensitivity resembles an anaphylactic reaction, but takes longer (several hours or longer) to develop.

Type IV: cell-mediated or delayed hypersensitivity. In this type of immune reaction, sensitised T cells, on repeat contact with an allergen (antigen), release cytokines (soluble chemicals) which attract phagocytes and function without the presence of antibodies. These reactions cause chronic and sometimes extensive inflammation and are apparent a few hours after exposure to the antigen.

This type of immune response is the basis of the Mantoux test (see p. 605), which is given to find out whether a person has tuberculosis, has developed immunity to tuberculosis or is not immune. It also gives rise to contact dermatitis (see Ch. 12) and sarcoidosis (see p. 598), and contributes to graft rejection.

Anaphylactic shock (type I)

Anaphylactic shock is a sudden and severe form of type I hypersensitivity reaction, where there is an inappropriate or excessive response to some foreign material such as an antibiotic or other drug, a vaccine or a bee sting.

PATHOPHYSIOLOGY

IgE antibodies are the mediators of this reaction. The mechanism is similar to that of hay fever, except that the response is systemic rather than localised.

Common presenting symptoms. The characteristic feature of anaphylactic shock is collapse within seconds or minutes after exposure to the offending allergen. Usually this follows an injection, or less commonly ingestion, of the offending antigen. Laryngeal oedema manifests as swelling in the throat, hoarseness or stridor. Examination of the patient shows an urticarial skin rash which may be localised or widespread. The rash is itchy and can coalesce to form giant hives. In anaphylaxis, urticaria is part of a life-threatening condition. However, urticaria can present independently as a mild type I hypersensitivity and can be alleviated by the application of antihistamine creams.

Angioedema resulting from a sudden increase in vascular permeability can lead to oedema of the skin, respiratory obstruction and severe hypotension, the result of which may be fatal.

MEDICAL MANAGEMENT

There is not usually time for investigations in patients with anaphylactic shock. The diagnosis must be made rapidly. Treatment in mild cases is with subcutaneous adrenaline to restore blood pressure and relax the airways. This can be repeated at 3-min intervals. Severe cases require intensive cardiovascular and respiratory support with adrenaline given intravenously. Antihistamines may also be given to counter the harmful effects of the histamine released by mast cells. Corticosteroids are sometimes given but have a delayed effect, as they act on the immune system and do not counter the chemicals already released.

NURSING PRIORITIES AND MANAGEMENT: ANAPHYLACTIC SHOCK

Life-threatening concerns

Anaphylactic shock may occur suddenly and unexpectedly and is life-threatening, especially in circumstances where emergency facilities are not available. Death may ensue if prompt action is not taken. Maintenance of airway, breathing and circulation are paramount. Emergency procedures are as follows (see also Ch. 18):

1. Place the patient flat (to help restore blood pressure) in the left lateral position and insert an airway to prevent respiratory obstruction.
2. Give adrenaline intramuscularly (unless the patient's condition is good and there is a strong central pulse).
3. Give oxygen by face mask if it is available.
4. Send for medical aid (GP or hospital doctor) or ambulance (dial 999); ask a relative, if present, to stay with the patient while you do this.
5. Be prepared to institute cardiopulmonary resuscitation.
6. Check pulse and blood pressure regularly and after any drug treatment.

Major patient problems

Should the patient survive, she is likely to experience severe anxiety after the event. The question of how to prevent a similar occurrence will need to be explored and the cause of the reaction investigated. People with frequent unpreventable attacks should have a Medic-Alert card or bracelet, and relatives should be supplied with, and taught how to administer, adrenaline.

Transfusion reaction (type II)

This is a type II antibody-dependent cytotoxic hypersensitivity. An adverse reaction to a blood transfusion can occur when the immune system mounts an antibody response to the transfused blood. For details of this kind of reaction and the associated medical and nursing care, see Chapter 11.

Serum sickness (type III)

This condition is a type III immune-complex-mediated hypersensitivity reaction to foreign serum, i.e. that of another species. It occurs when the immune system recognises the proteins in an introduced serum as foreign and produces antibodies against them. Antigen–antibody complexes (known as immune complexes) form and may be deposited in the skin, joints, heart and kidneys, resulting in a temperature rise, urticarial skin rash, swollen lymph glands/nodes and swollen and painful joints. Serum sickness was common in the days when horse serum was used as a source of immunoglobulin (Roitt 1994). Its occurrence led to the development of blood transfusion-derived products such as Humotet (human antitetanus immunoglobulin). Insulins used in diabetes are now produced by genetic engineering to avoid allergic reactions to non-human insulin components (see Ch. 5).

Farmer's lung (type III)

PATHOPHYSIOLOGY

Also known as extrinsic allergic alveolitis, this is a type III hypersensitivity reaction in which inhalation of fungal spores in dust from mouldy hay causes an allergic reaction and deposition of immune complexes in the alveoli and bronchioles. The spores act as an antigen. As the name suggests, this disease is common in farm workers.

Common presenting symptoms. Within 6–8 h of exposure, the sensitised person will develop symptoms, i.e. dry cough, dyspnoea without wheeze, headache and chest tightness accompanied by fever and malaise. The symptoms usually subside when exposure to the antigen ceases. However, prolonged exposure can lead to permanent disability due to interstitial fibrosis.

MEDICAL MANAGEMENT

Diagnosis is usually made on the history. Diagnostic investigation is seldom required or done. The patient is advised to avoid inhalation of the spores.

Treatment. In severe cases, corticosteroids such as prednisolone may be given to suppress the inflammatory response. Patients with hypoxia may require high-concentration oxygen therapy (see Ch. 3).

NURSING PRIORITIES AND MANAGEMENT: FARMER'S LUNG

Depending on the severity of symptoms, respiratory support may be required (see Ch. 3).

Prevention

Farm workers are advised to take the following precautions:

- avoid creating dust when working
- wear a suitable dust respirator if contact is unavoidable
- make sure indoor working areas are well ventilated
- use an industrial vacuum cleaner to remove dust from the inside of buildings
- wear protective clothing at work; do not take work clothing home.

Employers have a duty under the Health and Safety at Work etc Act (1974) and the COSHH regulations (1988) to provide a safe working environment and to inform and instruct employees about health risks and the precautions to be taken. Employees have a duty to follow such advice. A leaflet entitled 'Farmer's lungs' is produced by the Health and Safety Executive (1990) and gives helpful information to both farmers and their employees.

Sarcoidosis (type IV)

This is a type IV hypersensitivity reaction, the cause of which is as yet unknown.

PATHOPHYSIOLOGY

This disease may take a subacute or chronic form and is characterised by disturbances in cell-mediated immunity in which the balance between the different types of T lymphocyte is altered. Lesions or granulomas develop in the lungs, liver, spleen, parotid glands, joints, skin, eyes, mediastinal and superficial lymph nodes, and phalangeal bones. In the subacute form, often discovered incidentally on routine chest X-rays, the lesions usually resolve spontaneously without treatment, but in chronic sarcoidosis they may lead to the production of fibrous tissue, causing permanent damage, e.g. interstitial fibrosis in the lungs; myocardial damage leading to cardiac arrhythmias; skin rashes; and damage to the iris possibly leading to blindness. Although the disease may involve other organs, the severity of their involvement is variable. The disease is primarily pulmonary.

Common presenting symptoms. Most patients have pulmonary symptoms, i.e. dyspnoea on exertion and unproductive cough in addition to general malaise, weakness, loss of appetite, fever and weight loss. Lymph node enlargement may also be detected on examination.

MEDICAL MANAGEMENT

Investigations. Diagnostic investigation includes chest X-ray and lung function tests (see Ch. 3). Biopsy of the lung or other tissue can confirm the diagnosis. In some cases, a Kveim test is used to confirm the diagnosis. Intradermal infection of sarcoid tissue produces a characteristic microscopic appearance on biopsy 4–6 weeks later (typical of type IV).

Treatment of chronic sarcoidosis occasionally involves the administration of corticosteroids, to suppress the immune (type IV) reaction, often for several years. Oxygen is given in acute or severe cases.

NURSING PRIORITIES AND MANAGEMENT: SARCOIDOSIS

The priorities in nursing care will depend on the level of impairment caused by the granulomatous lesions. Commonly, there is respiratory impairment and occasionally a potential for cardiac arrhythmias. Vision may be affected and liver function disturbed. Sarcoidosis may not be the prime reason for admission to hospital but must not be neglected in setting priorities for care. The British Lung Foundation publishes a factual leaflet about sarcoidosis, available from their offices.

AUTOIMMUNE DISEASES

These disorders occur when the body's tolerance to 'self' breaks down, and autoantibodies (antibodies against 'self' antigens) are formed. Autoimmune disorders may be:

- organ-specific (focusing on one tissue)
  —Hashimoto's thyroiditis
  —pernicious anaemia (see Ch. 11)
- generalised
  —rheumatoid arthritis (see Ch. 10)
  —systemic lupus erythematosus (SLE)
  —sarcoidosis.

It is not properly understood why autoantibodies sometimes cause disease. Their production may be initiated by minor changes in cells or by the exposure of previously 'hidden' cells as a result of damage, infection or genetic mutation, resulting in 'new' surface antigens being presented to the immune system. Autoimmune diseases may also involve a hypersensitivity reaction, whether immediate or delayed.

Goodpasture's syndrome (anti-GBM disease)

PATHOPHYSIOLOGY

People with this rare disorder develop antibodies to their ow kidney glomerular basement membrane (GBM). These antibodies bind to the glomerular membrane, fix complement and cause

glomerulonephritis. They may also be deposited in the basement membranes of the lung alveoli. The cause of this disease is not known. It is potentially fatal and is commoner in young men than in others. Fortunately, it is rare.
Common presenting symptoms, which may be acute and severe, include:

- haematuria, mild or severe
- haemoptysis, dyspnoea, cough.

MEDICAL MANAGEMENT

History and examination. The onset can be rapid, with symptoms of nephritis and pulmonary haemorrhage.
Investigations. Urinalysis will confirm haematuria and proteinuria, and a chest X-ray will determine the degree of lung involvement. The diagnosis is confirmed if serology or kidney or lung biopsy reveals the presence of anti-GBM antibodies. Blood chemistry shows raised serum creatinine and blood urea nitrogen. Urine collection would demonstrate reduced creatinine clearance, indicating some degree of kidney failure.
Treatment. This disease must be treated urgently, as renal and respiratory failure can occur. High-dose parenteral corticosteroids (e.g. prednisolone) are given, sometimes in conjunction with a cytotoxic drug such as azathioprine or cyclophosphamide. Plasmapheresis may be carried out to remove circulating anti-GBM antibodies. If renal failure develops, dialysis will be undertaken. Kidney transplant may be required but can be attempted only after intensive plasmapheresis to ensure that no circulating anti-GBM antibodies remain. Oxygen therapy and assisted ventilation (see Ch. 29) may be required if respiratory failure develops.

NURSING PRIORITIES AND MANAGEMENT: GOODPASTURE'S SYNDROME

Patients with Goodpasture's syndrome will present with both respiratory and renal failure which may require intensive nursing support.

Myasthenia gravis

This rare autoimmune disease is thought to be caused by a disorder of the thymus gland, whereby it produces defective T lymphocytes. It usually occurs in individuals aged between 15 and 50 years, and is more common in females than in males.

PATHOPHYSIOLOGY

The defective T cells stimulate B cells to produce antibodies to the acetylcholine receptors in the neuromuscular junction. Acetylcholine allows the normal transmission of impulses from the motor nerves to voluntary muscle (see Ch. 10).

The autoantibodies react with the acetylcholine receptor, blocking the attachment of the neurotransmitter and thus preventing normal muscular activity.

Complement fixation may also result in destruction of the receptors.
Common presenting symptoms. The classic symptom of myasthenia gravis is that some muscle groups tire quickly. Movement may be strong at first but rapidly weakens. Localised symptoms include diplopia or ptosis (see Ch. 13) due to weakness of the extraocular muscles, as well as weakness in chewing, swallowing, talking and moving the limbs. The muscles around the shoulder girdle are those most commonly affected.

Symptoms are often worse at the end of the day or after exercising. Double vision or progressively quieter speech may be early symptoms. Respiratory muscles may be affected, resulting in a weakened cough. Relapses sometimes occur after infections or following emotional disturbance.

MEDICAL MANAGEMENT

History and examination. The patient presents with a history of muscle weakness and inability to sustain muscle power, e.g. difficulty in brushing hair. Anti-acetylcholine receptor antibodies can be detected in the serum.
Investigations. Diagnosis is assisted by giving an intravenous injection of a short-acting anticholinesterase. Muscle power improves within 30 s of the injection and often persists for 2–3 min as a result of the temporary increase in acetylcholine at the damaged neuromuscular junction.
Treatment. Anticholinesterase drugs such as pyridostigmine or neostigmine are used. Pyridostigmine is the drug of choice: 60–120 mg orally 2–8 hourly are given, depending on the duration of the effect, which can be measured during a supervised trial of the drug. Thymectomy or plasmapheresis can be done, or corticosteroids given, to influence the autoimmune process more directly.
'Cholinergic crisis' may occur as a consequence of drug therapy. The patient becomes paralysed, pale and sweaty, salivates excessively and has persistently small pupils. This occurs as a result of excessive acetylcholine, which causes hyperstimulation of the acetylcholine receptors. It requires urgent medical attention.

NURSING PRIORITIES AND MANAGEMENT: MYASTHENIA GRAVIS

Life-threatening concerns

The consequences of cholinergic (or myasthenic) crisis are life-threatening. Paralysis of the respiratory muscles can rapidly lead to severe hypoxia; consequently, the patient may require resuscitation and ventilation (see Ch. 29). Baseline and repeat peak flow monitoring may be necessary. Some drugs, including common antibiotics, can cause deterioration.

Major patient problems

These include fatigue and muscle weakness. Patients may need help with eating, drinking, washing and dressing. Difficulty with swallowing can lead to choking, and reduced mobility may lead to pressure sores (see Ch. 23).

Further considerations

Most people suffering from myasthenia gravis continue to live independently at home for as long as possible. Their nursing care, when required, will depend on the severity of symptoms. The potential seriousness of their condition may not be obvious. The educational aspect of community care for family and friends will be a priority. Advice on a nutritious diet is particularly important where chewing and swallowing are impaired. Small mouthfuls of food should be chewed slowly before swallowing. Soft, moist food is usually easiest to manage. Choking is a danger, but can often be avoided by helping the patient to concentrate on chewing and then swallowing. Eye care may be required if blinking is impaired; this may include the use of eye drops to prevent dryness of the cornea (see Ch. 13). If breathing is made difficult by respiratory muscle fatigue, the patient may be more comfortable sitting up, or propped up in bed.

Useful advice is available in leaflets from the Myasthenia Gravis Association (See p. 610).

Systemic lupus erythematosus

Systemic lupus erythematosus (SLE) is an uncommon multisystem disorder in which autoantibodies against a variety of cellular antigens are produced. Thus any cell or tissue can be affected. Women are more often affected than men, and onset usually occurs in young adulthood. It is commoner in people of Afro-Asian and Chinese origin than in others.

PATHOPHYSIOLOGY

The cause of this disease is not known, although both genetic and environmental factors (e.g. the effect of sunlight, drugs, hormone levels or viral infections) have been suggested. Damage is caused by the deposition of immune complexes in the tissues (a type III hypersensitivity reaction) and by the autoantibodies reacting directly with normal tissue cells (a type II hypersensitivity reaction).

Common presenting symptoms are often vague and non-specific, so that other illnesses or psychological problems may be considered responsible. Joint symptoms (arthritis, polyarthralgia), fever, rashes and Raynaud's disease are common features. Fatigue is a common non-specific symptom, and skin rash, usually on areas which are exposed to sunlight such as the face, neck and scalp, may occur; characteristically, this is a 'butterfly rash' across the nose and cheeks. Nephritis is common, along with decreased urine output.

Vasculitis, especially in the smaller blood vessels, can give rise to skin rash or ulceration, nephritis, neuropathy or stroke. There may be poor peripheral perfusion, due to inflammation and consequent occlusion of small blood vessels. There may also be cardiopulmonary symptoms, including decreased cardiac output due to pericarditis, myocarditis, endocarditis and pulmonary infarction.

Occasionally there is cerebral inflammation leading to confusion, epilepsy or psychiatric symptoms.

MEDICAL MANAGEMENT

History and examination. As the symptoms of SLE are diverse, and their severity highly variable, a thorough history will be required. There may be external signs of tissue damage (such as skin rash) which will assist the doctor in making a diagnosis. Some patients will have lymphadenopathy and an enlarged spleen. Other features will depend on the specific organs involved.

Investigations. In the course of diagnostic investigation, the erythrocyte sedimentation rate (ESR; see Appendix 1) will usually be found to be raised. Antinuclear antibodies will be found in the serum of most patients with this disease. Some patients will have detectable anti-DNA antibodies and circulating immune complexes. Anaemia, leucopenia and thrombocytopenia (see Ch. 11) may be present on haematological examination. Depending on the organs involved, renal, cardiac or respiratory function may be altered.

Treatment is aimed at relieving symptoms and preventing organ damage. Non-steroidal anti-inflammatory drugs (NSAIDs) such as ibuprofen may help to alleviate joint pain and other symptoms. Antimalarial drugs are sometimes used, as they can reduce the frequency of exacerbations of skin and joint lesions. Corticosteroids, e.g. prednisolone, are given when major organs (heart, lung, kidney, brain) are involved.

NURSING PRIORITIES AND MANAGEMENT: SYSTEMIC LUPUS ERYTHEMATOSUS (SLE)

The specific care of patients with SLE depends very much on the stage of the disease and on the organs involved. In any event, the aim is to alleviate symptoms as they present.

Life-threatening concerns

Depending on the nature and severity of organ involvement, myocardial infarction, respiratory failure and renal failure may ensue. Appropriate resuscitative measures are described in Chapters 2, 3 and 8.

Major patient problems

As fatigue is common, the patient should be encouraged to have adequate rest. For patients who have experienced alteration in bowel habit, dietary advice may help. Patients may experience confusion, depression due to CNS involvement, or fears about prognosis. Epilepsy may also occur.

Poor peripheral circulation leading to cold hands and feet may develop. Patients are also likely to become susceptible to infection due to the debilitating effects of the disease process and the immunosuppressive effects of treatment.

Further considerations

Both pregnancy and the contraceptive pill have exacerbating effects on this disease. Patients suffering from photosensitivity should be encouraged to minimise exposure to sunlight and to protect the skin when exposure is unavoidable. Emotional support will be needed as this is a chronic disease of uncertain progression. Patient literature is available from the Lupus Erythematosus Society.

INFECTIOUS DISEASES

'Infectious' (or 'communicable') diseases are illnesses caused by microorganisms which are not normally present in or on the body, such as salmonellosis, hepatitis B and tuberculosis. Such infections contrast markedly with those which are acquired as a result of poor asepsis in invasive techniques or as a consequence of antibiotic therapy, immunosuppressive drugs or inadequate handwashing. Infectious diseases can be caught by anyone, at any time, in any place, and do not usually result from a particular nursing or medical procedure. This does not mean, however, that they cannot be spread from person to person; this presents a particular danger when patients with infectious disease are nursed in hospital.

Causes

Infectious diseases are generally caused by:

- bacteria, e.g. salmonellosis, meningococcal meningitis
- viruses, e.g. hepatitis, chickenpox
- protozoa, e.g. malaria, toxoplasmosis, amoebic dysentery.

Knowledge of the organism that is causing the disease is important in the planning of care.

Transmission

Most infectious diseases are ingested (e.g. hepatitis A), inhaled (e.g. tuberculosis) or inoculated (e.g. hepatitis B). Inoculation in this context refers to blood or body fluid entering a cut or skin abrasion or being splashed onto mucous membranes; it can also occur following needlestick injury. The organisms can be transmitted directly (i.e. straight from one person to another through direct contact with the infectious body substance) or indirectly (i.e. deposited on hands or surfaces where they can be picked up by touch).

Some infectious diseases are so common in the population that only general care is needed. Many people suffer from cold sores (herpes simplex), but the common-sense precautions of avoiding mucous membrane contact until the sores have healed, careful handwashing and washing of cutlery and cups, and not sharing toothbrushes, razors or face cloths are usually enough to prevent transmission.

Diseases like chickenpox are so common and so easily transmitted that special precautions to prevent their spread in the community are rarely necessary, although these may need to be enforced in settings such as hospitals and schools where there are particularly susceptible individuals. Other common diseases are preventable by an active immunisation programme; for example, immunisation against diphtheria, pertussis (whooping cough), tetanus; poliomyelitis; measles, mumps and rubella and *Haemophilus influenzae* type B is now offered for all infants. It is still advisable, however, for pregnant women (because of the risk of damage to and/or infection in the fetus during pregnancy) and people who are immunosuppressed to keep away from anyone known to have an infectious disease.

Immunity to infectious diseases

Q **16.9** Review your knowledge of how immunity comes about (see p. 583).

Immunisation against many diseases is carried out during childhood, with booster doses being required only in later life (DoH 1996). A booster dose is a smaller dose of a vaccine which boosts the level of memory cells (specific to the given antigen) circulating in the bloodstream (see Fig. 16.2).

Nurses and health visitors have an important role to play in encouraging parents to have their children vaccinated. Vaccination should be carried out by staff who are aware of the risks and the benefits. Some parents are afraid that their child might develop an adverse reaction to a vaccine; this is an uncommon occurrence, however, and few of the children so affected have developed serious complications (DoH 1996). In the late 1970s in England and Wales, the percentage of infants vaccinated against whooping cough fell dramatically due to public concern about vaccine-damaged children (although such cases were very rare). There was a concurrent rise in the number of whooping cough cases reported (Wilks et al 1995), a proportion of which had serious systemic complications.

MEASURES TO PREVENT SPREAD OF INFECTIOUS DISEASE

Planning the care of patients with an infectious disease requires the following preliminary steps:

- finding out the diagnosis or provisional diagnosis
- ascertaining which body fluid/substance is infectious
- assessing how far that body fluid is likely to travel from the patient into the environment
- finding out the period of communicability.

At this point, the details of care planned for a patient in her own home and those for a patient in hospital will diverge. At home, the patient will have been in contact only with family and friends; in hospital she will be among other sick people who may be particularly susceptible to infection. In hospital, there is also the problem of the large number of people who will be in contact with the patient. Directly involved are nurses, doctors, physiotherapists, radiographers, domestics and porters; indirectly involved are laundry workers and staff working in sterilising and disinfecting units handling contaminated equipment.

Q **16.10** Consider how measures to prevent the spread of infection would apply to a patient with urinary incontinence who is practising clean intermittent self-catheterisation at home (see Ch. 24).

Hospital care: barrier nursing/isolation precautions

Barrier nursing may be carried out in hospital when a patient is suffering from an infectious disease which could be passed on to other patients or staff. The precautions required will vary according to which body fluid is infectious and how far that body fluid is likely to spread into the environment. Three things are required for the spread of infection:

- a source of infection
- a means of transfer
- a susceptible host.

As discussed earlier, it is advised that universal blood and body fluid precautions are adopted as safe working practice. This is important because, for every person who is known to be infectious, there may be many more who have not been identified. Moreover, additional precautions may be required in the care of a patient known to be infectious, e.g. red laundry bags, thick yellow waste bags, the disinfection of surfaces that may have been contaminated and warnings to other departments (see p. 588). There are different types of isolation precautions, but some arrangements are standard for all types, as follows:

- Accommodation — single room with washbasin is advisable, preferably with own toilet and shower/bath.
- Protective clothing — worn as appropriate.
- Crockery — heat-disinfected or disposable.
- Linen — laundered as infected.
- Refuse — disposed of in a thick yellow plastic sack (refer to local policy).
- Laboratory specimens — may need a 'danger of infection' sticker on container and request form.
- Body fluids — must be disposed of carefully, without splash, and any spillage dealt with using the correct strength of disinfectant.
- Room cleaning — should be done using the appropriate disinfectant, and cloths and mop-heads either disposed of or laundered as infected.
- Hands — washed and dried thoroughly before and after leaving an isolation room.
- Visitors — restricted if the nature of the disease and the state of the patient warrant.
- Repairs — external surfaces of all equipment should be disinfected before removal from the ward, and the service department should be notified in advance, in writing, if an infection hazard still exists (MAC 1996).
- Transport — if it is essential that a patient is moved to another department, the nurse must inform that department of the precautions being taken in the ward, without divulging the diagnosis. Porters and ambulance staff may also need to be informed.
- Accidents involving blood or body fluid should be reported immediately to the nurse in charge, who will initiate the local accident procedure. Always encourage a fresh injury (e.g. needlestick injury) to bleed, and wash off any contamination.
- Death of a patient with an established transmissible disease — it is sometimes recommended that the body is placed in a

sealed cadaver bag after the last offices have been carried out (Healing et al 1995), for the protection of anyone subsequently handling the body. Undertakers must be informed that a risk of infection exists (DHSS 1988).

Three categories of isolation precautions will now be described:

Exudate precautions. This category is appropriate for patients with a known infection in which the infectious body fluid (exudate) is normally contained (i.e. not contaminating the environment). Protective clothing is required only at times when there is contact with the exudate. Examples of this are changing a wound dressing for a hepatitis B carrier, and toileting a patient with salmonellosis who no longer has diarrhoea, is continent and cooperative, and practises good hand hygiene.

Standard isolation. This category is appropriate when the infectious body fluid is contaminating everything used by or touched by the patient, and the contamination is restricted to the patient's immediate surroundings because she is confined to bed. Staff should wear protective clothing for direct nursing care and when touching any items that may have been contaminated. Disposable crockery and cutlery are advisable. Surfaces touched by the patient must be disinfected. Examples of this are the patient with salmonellosis who has diarrhoea and is bedridden, and a hepatitis B carrier with a discharging wound where the discharge cannot reliably be contained by an occlusive dressing.

Strict isolation. In this type of isolation, everything within the patient's room may be contaminated, for one of the following reasons:

- The patient has infectious diarrhoea, is ambulant and mobile, practises poor hand hygiene and may touch anything in the room.
- The patient has an infection which is spread by upper respiratory tract secretions or saliva and is highly productive of those secretions.
- The disease is a skin infection and there is desquamation.

Protective clothing is required on entry to the room for any purpose. Negative ventilation (i.e. extract) should be used if available for patients with respiratory or skin infections. All horizontal surfaces and equipment in the room must be disinfected.

It will be apparent from the above descriptions that it is not the infectious agent itself which determines what type of isolation precautions will be required, but the mode of transmission, the stage of the disease and the state of the patient. It is essential, therefore, that each patient is individually assessed and that care is reviewed on a daily basis. Care should be planned and discussed with the patient, where possible, and the reasons for any precautions carefully explained to her and to her relatives.

Home care

In the case of patients being nursed at home, the risk of cross-infection is confined to family members and anyone visiting the household, e.g. the community nurse, health visitor, GP, home help or friends. Isolation precautions may consist of wearing the appropriate protective clothing (gloves and apron) when contact with body fluid or contaminated surfaces is likely, and careful handwashing after removing the gloves and apron and before leaving the house. Nurses should remember that taps, towels and door handles may be contaminated if the patient's hygiene is poor; it is useful to carry some paper towels in addition to a small container of antibacterial handwashing solution. The use of an alcohol hand-rub after leaving the house may also be advisable.

The patient and/or her relatives may need advice on washing clothes or dishes. Generally, hot soapy water is adequate for dishes, which are best left to drip-dry, and a 'hot' wash (60°C, or 90–95°C if available on the machine) is satisfactory for linen (see p. 592). A laundry service may be available through the local health board/authority. Clinical waste should be disposed of in the appropriately coloured bag designated for clinical waste in the community (see p. 592), and special collection arrangements may have to be made.

Other isolation precautions are rarely necessary at home, and many are not practicable.

Choosing a disinfectant

Most health boards/authorities have a disinfectant policy which states the disinfectants that have been tested and approved for use.

Q **16.11** Check the disinfectant policy for your health board to find out which agents are recommended.

Despite the disadvantages of chemical disinfectants, chemicals are still necessary for dealing with large surfaces after spillage or infection (see p. 591). It must be remembered that some materials are incompatible with certain disinfectants and that disinfectants will not work in some situations, e.g. on carpets. Carpets are almost impossible to disinfect adequately and it is not advisable in hospital to carpet areas where body fluid spillage is likely to occur.

SALMONELLOSIS

PATHOPHYSIOLOGY

Salmonellosis is caused by one of about 200 serotypes of the genus *Salmonella* which cause disease in humans and animals (Grist et al 1993). Only a few of these are encountered in the UK. The organism is ingested; common sources are contaminated meat and poultry products (Benenson 1995) and untreated milk (Department of Health Working Group 1994). The incubation period is 12–72 h.

Some salmonelli, e.g. *S. typhi* and *S. paratyphi*, can cause enteric fever.

Common presenting symptoms are highly variable, ranging from mild symptoms to life-threatening septicaemia. Normally, the effects of infection are acute enterocolitis with diarrhoea, abdominal pain and nausea; less frequently, they include vomiting, fever, headache and toxaemia. Rarely, arthritis, cholecystitis, endocarditis, pyelonephritis, meningitis or pneumonia occur.

MEDICAL MANAGEMENT

Investigations. Diagnostic investigation includes stool bacterial culture while diarrhoea persists. If enteric fever, septicaemia or a focal infection is suspected, blood cultures during the acute stage of the illness are done. Serological tests are of little value except in the detection of a 'carrier'.

Treatment. Rehydration and electrolyte replacement may be necessary in the treatment of severe enterocolitis. Antibiotics are not generally given in uncomplicated intestinal infection as they tend to prolong the excretion of the organism. Antibiotics are given if the disease is severe with evidence of systemic spread and/or a vulnerable patient, e.g. frail or elderly. Antibiotics are absolutely indicated in enteric fever caused by *S. typhi* and *S. paratyphi* (Farthing et al 1996). Ciprofloxacin is exceedingly active and is the drug of choice in all cases of salmonellosis and enteric fever. It is not licensed, however, for use in pregnancy or in those under 18 years of age. Chloramphenicol is a useful alternative, although it can be associated with side-effects such as severe haematological disorders. Other drugs such as ampicillin, trimethoprim/sulphamethoxazole and third-generation cephalosporins (e.g. cefotaxime) have also been used.

NURSING PRIORITIES AND MANAGEMENT: SALMONELLOSIS

Many people with salmonellosis become ill at home, often after a cold buffet or an undercooked meal or after eating poultry. Eggs may also be contaminated (Hobbs & Roberts 1993). Most people will wait to see if the symptoms subside before contacting their GP, but if a particular item of food is suspect they may seek help earlier.

Institutional outbreaks can and do occur (Wall et al 1996) and are usually a result of defects in food hygiene, either at kitchen or at ward level. Cross-infection in the ward can occur, either directly from a patient with salmonellosis to another person, or via nurses' hands if hygiene is poor. However, the cause of such outbreaks is not always identified.

The nurse is unlikely to be involved in caring for a patient at home with acute salmonellosis, unless there are concurrent problems. The community nurse or health visitor may be involved in helping to obtain faecal specimens from other members of the family and in trying to trace the source of infection, in conjunction with the environmental health officer and the consultant in public health medicine (Communicable Diseases and Environmental Health; variously termed medical officer for environmental health, consultant in communicable disease control). Such visits are an excellent opportunity for health education in general and food hygiene as part of a planned programme which takes into account family needs.

Life-threatening concerns

Those that may arise are septicaemia, focal sepsis, severe fluid and electrolyte imbalance, and dehydration.

Major patient problems

These include skin excoriation from severe diarrhoea, fever, abdominal pain, nausea, loss of appetite and weakness because of constant diarrhoea (see Nursing Care Plan 16.2).

Further considerations

Specific ongoing nursing care

Ongoing care comprises the following aspects:

- preventing the spread of infection and teaching handwashing
- ensuring that fluid intake is adequate (see Ch. 20)
- ensuring that nutrition is adequate (see Ch. 21), while trying to accommodate the patient's wishes (this can be difficult in hospital, where there is central catering and where meals are delivered at specific times)
- keeping the anal region clean and dry and applying a barrier cream to prevent excoriation
- ensuring that the patient can manage to get to the toilet or has a commode at the bedside and has the opportunity to wash her hands afterwards
- designating one nurse on each shift (in hospital) to look after the patient. It is important for nurses to spend time with the patient to give reassurance and counteract the loneliness of isolation
- encouraging visitors to visit at different times of the day
- identifying a carer at home
- encouraging self-care and independence
- trying to ensure privacy as far as possible
- being sensitive to any odour problem; discussing this with the patient might help.

Nursing Care Plan 16.2 Managing problems of a patient with salmonellosis
Mr G is 67 years old and has been admitted to hospital from a local nursing home because he has salmonellosis. He is confined to bed and has frequent diarrhoea.

Nursing considerations	*Action*	*Rationale*	*Evaluation*
1. Isolation precautions required because: **• Mr G has salmonellosis** **• He is bedridden** **• He has diarrhoea and experiences difficulty in using bedpans**	❐ Standard isolation ❐ Wear disposable gloves when handling faeces or any items touched or used by Mr G ❐ Wear plastic apron and mask if there is danger of splash ❐ Wear gown if uniform is likely to be contaminated, e.g. during lifting	Mr G is bedridden, has diarrhoea and finds it difficult to use bedpans and so his immediate environment (bed linen, items touched by him) might be contaminated Protective clothing is necessary only when there is contact with faeces, or when items touched or used by the patient are being handled. The type of protective clothing worn will depend on the procedure being carried out	No spread of salmonellosis to any other patients or staff in the ward
2. Mr G will need company and distraction while in the single room	❐ Allocate one nurse to look after him on each shift. Try to ensure frequent visits and company. Put a TV in his room	Loneliness is common when patients are isolated; aim to do the same for Mr G as you would if he were in a multi-bed ward	
3. Mr G is embarrassed by constant diarrhoea and occasional accidents	❐ Try to ensure privacy		

Box 16.9 Patient education: prevention and management of salmonellosis

In discussing with the patient and her relatives the management of *Salmonella* poisoning in a home care setting and in giving instruction on how to prevent its recurrence, the nurse should:

- stress the need for fluids and for nourishing and tempting meals
- teach and demonstrate good hand hygiene
- teach skin care and its importance
- explain the need to keep surfaces clean, e.g. toilets, door handles, taps
- offer reassurance that efforts will be made to trace the cause
- explain the importance of food hygiene, stressing the following points:
  - —defrost frozen foods thoroughly before cooking
  - —do not store raw foods above cooked foods in the fridge (to prevent contamination through dripping)
  - —do not use the same utensils or surfaces for cooked and raw foods
  - —cook food at the recommended temperature for the required time; if the food is to be stored, chill it as quickly as possible
  - —keep foods hot or cold, not warm
- reassure the patient that recovery is the usual outcome
- ask if the patient's work involves food handling; if it does, check with the doctor about the need for clearance specimens.

In hospital, the nurse should follow the above outline but in addition:

- Explain treatment and give information and reassurance about isolation procedures and why they are needed
- Assure the patient that by the time she is discharged home, isolation precautions should be minimal, i.e. care with faeces and exudate precautions.

Excretion of the organism may persist long after the symptoms have disappeared — sometimes for months or years. This is only significant in people whose work involves food handling.

Care with faeces will be needed in the home, with particular attention to surfaces which may be contaminated. In hospital, isolation precautions will be required (see Box 16.9). The degree of isolation will depend on the state of the patient and on how far faecal matter is likely to be spread into the environment.

HEPATITIS B

Hepatitis B is a viral infection which is transmitted from mother to child (mostly at birth), sexually, by blood contact (especially needle-sharing by intravenous drug abusers) and needlestick injury. It is endemic in some parts of the world. The virus, HBV, has been found in most body secretions and excretions, but only blood, saliva, semen and vaginal secretions have been shown to be infectious (Benenson 1995). Hepatitis B was formerly seen in people who had received blood and blood products and in people who had been given injections with contaminated needles. These risks have largely been eliminated in the developed countries by the screening of blood donors, the testing of donor blood and the single use of sterile syringes and needles. The main risk to health care workers is that of inoculation with infected blood, either through needlestick injury with a contaminated needle or by being splashed with infected blood on skin abrasions or mucous membranes.

PATHOPHYSIOLOGY

The virus is made up of several particles, each of which is capable of inducing an immune response. HBsAg (hepatitis B surface antigen) is the first antigen to appear in the blood after infection. The presence of anti-HBs in the blood is the best measure of immunity to the virus.

Acute hepatitis B may have one of four outcomes:

- complete recovery
- fulminant hepatitis — rare but frequently fatal
- carrier state — HbsAg-positive
- chronic hepatitis — may lead to cirrhosis of the liver and to hepatocellular carcinoma (see Ch. 4).

Some people become infected with the hepatitis B virus without developing the acute disease (this is known as subclinical infection) and may develop the carrier state. These individuals may be unaware of the infection and of their potential for transmitting the virus to others.

The incubation period for hepatitis B is 45–180 days (Benenson 1995). Onset is insidious.

Common presenting symptoms are highly variable, ranging from unapparent infection or malaise with abnormal liver function tests to cases of fatal acute hepatic necrosis. Normally, anorexia, nausea, vomiting, abdominal discomfort and fever occur, followed perhaps by arthralgia, urticaria or glomerulonephritis (caused by antigen–antibody complexes) progressing to jaundice.

MEDICAL MANAGEMENT

Investigations are serological. HBsAg is indicative of infection and infectivity and occurs both before and during the acute illness. This finding must be interpreted with caution, however, as HBsAg may still be present in carriers and the chronically infected who have become jaundiced from some other cause. Carriers are of high infectivity when HBeAg is present (a marker of replication in the liver), and low infectivity when anti-HBeAg is present. HBV DNA is a more sophisticated measure of replication, infectivity and the progression to chronic liver disease. IgM anti-HBc is an antibody to the 'c' or 'core' antigen which may be present during the diagnostically difficult 'window' when HBsAg and anti-HBs are in equivalence and neither is detectable in the serum. Serial estimation of these, other antigens/antibodies, other viruses such as hepatitis D and the liver enzymes may be necessary to establish the stage and progression of the disease.

Treatment. There is no effective treatment for the acute disease. Bed rest is not of proven value but it would seem wise to avoid strenuous exercise during the acute phase. Effective vaccines are available and are recommended for health care personnel working with patients, particularly high-risk patients, and those in contact with blood, particularly when handling sharp instruments. Prophylaxis (vaccination and/or specific immunoglobulin) is also given after inoculation accidents and to sexual contacts of HbsAg-positive persons as well as to infants born to HbsAg-positive mothers. Chronic hepatitis B may be treated by immunosuppression with a tapering course of corticosteroids such as prednisone for 6 weeks, but now recombinant interferon or interleukin-2 is favoured. Liver transplantation, however, may still be the last recourse for a patient with advancing chronic disease.

Some health care staff (e.g. surgeons, midwives) are required to demonstrate their immunity to hepatitis B virus before they are allowed to perform procedures (known as 'exposure-prone procedures', EPP) where their gloved hands may be in contact with sharp objects (e.g. needles, instruments, spicules of bone) inside a body cavity or wound and where their hands are not always completely visible (UK Health Departments 1993).

NURSING PRIORITIES AND MANAGEMENT: HEPATITIS B

Since there is no treatment for acute hepatitis B, nursing priorities are to alleviate symptoms and to support the patient until the disease has run its course. People with acute hepatitis B may stay at home, requiring admission to hospital only when they are too ill to be looked after at home or when they require specific medical intervention.

Life-threatening concerns

Fulminant hepatitis will lead to gross liver failure and all of the associated problems (see Ch. 4).

Major patient problems

These include lethargy, weakness, nausea, vomiting and anxiety about transmission.

Further considerations

Specific ongoing care

This includes the following interventions:

- preventing the spread of infection
- encouraging the patient to rest; lethargy and weakness are often the first symptoms to arise and the last to go away
- ensuring that fluid intake is adequate (see Ch. 20).
- accurate recording of fluid balance
- ensuring that nutrition is adequate (see Ch. 21)
- providing skin care and change of position
- ensuring that the patient can manage to get to the toilet or has a commode at the bedside
- designating one nurse per shift to look after the patient in hospital; loneliness and dejection can be minimised by talking with the patient and discussing her needs — access to a telephone, television and other diversions may be important
- encouraging relatives and friends to stagger visiting times
- encouraging self-care and independence (see Box 16.10)
- exercising care with blood if the nurse is caring for the patient at home.

In hospital, isolation precautions will be required during the acute illness. The patient must not share razors and toothbrushes with others.

Box 16.10 Patient education: management of hepatitis B

In discussing with the patient and her relatives the management of hepatitis B infection at home, the nurse should:

- stress the need for rest and for adequate fluids and nourishment
- explain the importance of position changes and how to care for the skin
- explain about how the virus can be passed on to others
- teach and demonstrate hand hygiene
- discuss the possibility of hepatitis B vaccination for the patient's partner
- offer emotional support and include the family in the assessment of the patient and care planning
- provide written information if available.

In a hospital setting, the nurse should also explain about isolation precautions and why they are necessary.

Some patients may be concerned about their employment outlook because they have had hepatitis B or are carriers. In general, this is not a barrier to future employment; the patient should be encouraged to discuss the matter with her own doctor, and possibly with her employer's occupational health physician.

Depending on how the infection was contracted, the patient may need advice about the possibility of HIV infection. It could also be helpful to the patient to discuss the sharing of information about her illness with others; the patient's wishes in this regard should be documented in the care plan.

PULMONARY TUBERCULOSIS

Pulmonary tuberculosis is now the most common form of tuberculosis infection, although other systems are sometimes affected, e.g. the genitourinary or skeletal systems. It is more common in immigrants from countries which have a higher prevalence of tuberculosis than the UK (Mandal et al 1996). This disease is notifiable in the UK.

PATHOPHYSIOLOGY

Pulmonary tuberculosis is a bacterial infection caused by *Mycobacterium tuberculosis* (also known as the tubercle bacillus). The bacteria enter the body by being inhaled; once they reach the epithelial surface of the alveolus, they cause swelling of the epithelial cells and local capillary dilatation. Although some organisms will be engulfed by alveolar macrophages (see p. 583), they will not be destroyed and will continue to multiply; some will escape and may enter the bloodstream, with the potential to infect any other organ in the body (miliary TB). Lymph nodes are often infected.

Invasion of the lung tissue gives rise to an inflammatory reaction in which the infected alveoli fill up with fluid, macrophages and bacteria. The resultant lung damage eventually leads to fibrosis, which will be visible on a chest X-ray. The primary lesion in the lung is often asymptomatic and confined to one area. Healing of the lung tissue occurs, sometimes leaving an area of calcification.

The patient becomes Mantoux-positive 4–6 weeks after primary infection, i.e. she will develop a hypersensitivity reaction to an injection of tuberculin (see Appendix 1). A chronic cough with mucopurulent sputum develops as the disease becomes more advanced.

Dormant bacilli may be reactivated by an alteration in immunity resulting from age, malnutrition or other diseases. People with AIDS (see Ch. 37) are prone to developing tuberculosis. People with pulmonary tuberculosis are considered to be infectious until they have had 2 weeks of appropriate chemotherapy (Joint Tuberculosis Committee 1994).

Common presenting symptoms. Normally the initial infection is unapparent. Pulmonary disease is characterised by cough, fever, fatigue and weight loss, and less frequently by haemoptysis, chest pain or erythema nodosum. Extrapulmonary disease is less common but can involve most organs of the body, causing, for example, meningitis, lymphadenitis, pericarditis, pleurisy, nephritis, cystitis, osteomyelitis, arthritis, laryngitis or peritonitis.

MEDICAL MANAGEMENT

Investigations. Diagnostic investigation includes chest X-ray, often with tomograms. Microscopy and culture of sputum, gastric washings, urine, CSF, aspirate or biopsy material are performed as appropriate. Histology of biopsy material is done. Skin testing with tuberculin may be performed, especially in the young.

Treatment. Normally, pulmonary tuberculosis is initially treated with a combination of isoniazid, rifampicin, ethambutol and pyrazinamide to avoid emergence of bacterial resistance. (If the isolate is shown to be sensitive, one or two of the drugs may be discontinued after 2 months.) Other antibiotics may be used when resistance is present or likely to be a problem, and particularly in patients from abroad. Ethambutol is not normally given to patients under 5 years of age or to very elderly individuals. Therapy continues for at least 6 months.

NURSING PRIORITIES AND MANAGEMENT: PULMONARY TUBERCULOSIS

The main aims in nursing patients with pulmonary tuberculosis are to establish drug therapy and to encourage compliance. The underlying health of these patients may not be good and their nutritional status is often poor. The prospect of having to take a large number of tablets regularly over a long period of time is daunting, and the side-effects of some drugs may make some people stop taking them. A great deal of support and encouragement will be needed (Sarafino 1990).

Once a person is diagnosed as having pulmonary tuberculosis, it is important that she is kept away from anyone who is immunosuppressed. Contacts may require follow-up; in the case of staff, this is done by the occupational health department. Non-staff contacts such as family members can be referred to a chest physician.

A sputum specimen sent to bacteriology will be examined directly under the microscope for the presence of tubercle bacilli. If these bacilli are seen, the report will state 'AAFB (acid alcohol fast bacilli) seen on direct film', 'film positive', 'smear positive' or 'ZN (Ziehl–Neelsen) positive', and the patient will be considered to have 'open' pulmonary tuberculosis. This simply means that there are enough bacilli in the sputum for them to be easily seen in a small sample, and therefore that the sputum is infectious to others. Culture of the organism may take 3–6 weeks and is necessary to make a firm diagnosis (there are mycobacteria other than *M. tuberculosis*). Infectivity also depends on whether or not the person is 'productive' — a person who is highly productive of sputum and is film-positive is much more likely to infect others than someone who is film-positive and not coughing up any sputum at all.

Life-threatening concerns

Respiratory failure may develop if the patient is too weak to cough. Tuberculosis in people who are immunosuppressed, such as AIDS patients, can result in serious illness.

Major patient problems

These include difficulty in maintaining the drug regimen and in learning to cough in a safe way.

Further considerations

Specific ongoing care

Nursing care and physiotherapy for people with pulmonary tuberculosis are similar to those for patients with any other respiratory infection (see Ch. 3). The dietician may be asked to advise on appropriate diet.

The risk of spreading the infection to others is greatly reduced when the person remains at home, in which case care with sputum is usually all that is necessary. There is some debate as to whether isolation precautions are required for patients with pulmonary tuberculosis in hospital. Recent advice (Joint Tuberculosis Committee 1994) recommends that the patient who is smear-positive should be segregated in a single room for 2 weeks, but that other isolation precautions (gowns, masks, special crockery, etc.) are unnecessary. This document, however, also states that people who are smear-positive are infectious. Because of this, some isolation precautions may still be taken, e.g. wearing a mask when one is within 3 feet of the patient when she is coughing. Masks should be untied, carefully removed and discarded, and the hands washed afterwards.

Staff who have been in close respiratory contact with patients with open pulmonary tuberculosis may be screened by Mantoux tests and, if necessary, by chest X-ray. Other staff contacts may receive TB contact cards.

Patients are sometimes found to have tuberculosis when they are being investigated in hospital for chest disease. Other patients in the same room may be notified through their GP. If these contacts are likely to have a prolonged stay in hospital, their consultant may also be notified.

There may be difficulties in explaining the importance of drug therapy, particularly if English is not the patient's native language. Tracing and follow-up of contacts of people with pulmonary tuberculosis is important. Those relatives and friends of the patient who have been in close respiratory contact are generally referred to an infectious diseases physician for examination and follow-up. The British Thoracic Society recommends that there should be trained tuberculosis health visitors or nurses to provide support in implementing policies for screening, follow-up and contact tracing (Joint Tuberculosis Committee 1994).

Q

16.12 Miss A is a 78-year-old woman who has lived alone since her sister's death a year ago. Recently, she lost her appetite and developed a persistent cough. A sputum specimen was taken and open pulmonary tuberculosis diagnosed. Normally a pleasant, cooperative person, Miss A was grumpy and resentful when the nurse visited her at home, and there were soiled tissues strewn all over the bed and floor. Devise a care plan to prevent the spread of infection from sputum and saliva.

MENINGOCOCCAL INFECTION

Infections caused by a Gram-negative bacterium, *Neisseria meningitidis*, are commonly known as meningococcal infections.

PATHOPHYSIOLOGY

The organism is inhaled and may enter the bloodstream via the nasopharynx, giving rise to bacteraemia and, frequently, pyogenic meningitis. It is the most common cause of bacterial meningitis in the UK (Haslett et al 1999). The disease usually starts with signs of upper respiratory infection, followed after a day or two by headache, vomiting, fever and a petechial rash.

Common presenting symptoms are highly variable. They may be inapparent or consist of local symptoms if there is nasopharyngeal infection only. The disease may be invasive, with fever, septicaemia, a petechial or macular rash and, rarely, pneumonia or joint involvement. It may be meningeal, with fever, intense headache, stiff neck, nausea and vomiting. Delirium and coma may supervene. Fulminating cases may present with sudden shock, extensive purpura and disseminated intravascular coagulation (see Ch. 18).

MEDICAL MANAGEMENT

Investigations. Diagnostic investigation consists of microscopy and culture of CSF as well as CSF cellular and chemical analysis. Detection of antigens in the CSF is usually carried out by immunocoagglutination techniques. Blood and throat swab or skin lesion culture is done. Molecular techniques such as polymerase chain reaction (PCR; see Appendix 1) on blood and CSF are performed in specialist centres.

Treatment. The drug of choice in the treatment of meningococcal infections in the UK is benzyl penicillin, given in high dosage parenterally, commenced as soon as the diagnosis is suspected. If the bacteriological diagnosis cannot be established with certainty (or when there is allergy to penicillin) then broad-spectrum treatment is often given to cover other bacterial pathogens; this usually consists of a high-dose injectable cephalosporin such as cefotaxime. Chloramphenicol is a suitable alternative. Close household and respiratory secretions/salivary contacts are given a short course of rifampicin or ciprofloxacin to eradicate nasopharyngeal carriage. This is also given to the index case, as penicillin does not eradicate carriage.

NURSING PRIORITIES AND MANAGEMENT: MENINGOCOCCAL INFECTION

Life-threatening concerns

This disease is life-threatening. Death may occur due to fulminating septic shock (see Ch. 18), which has a high mortality rate if not detected in its early stages.

Major patient problems

Meningeal irritation may result in neck stiffness. Vomiting and sweating may lead to dehydration and electrolyte imbalance (see Ch. 20).

Further considerations

The patient with meningococcal meningitis is infectious, and isolation precautions, especially taking care with upper respiratory tract secretions and saliva, will be required until antibiotics have been administered.

Informative leaflets are available from the National Meningitis Trust (See p. 610).

16.13 Create a care plan for a young woman admitted to hospital with all of the typical features of meningococcal meningitis.

CHICKENPOX AND SHINGLES

Chickenpox and shingles are caused by the same virus, known as the varicella zoster virus (VZV). Primary infection causes chickenpox (varicella), and most people have chickenpox only once, since infection usually confers lifelong immunity. The virus remains latent, however, and recurrence in a different form — shingles (herpes zoster) — can occur months or many years after the initial infection and on more than one occasion.

Chickenpox is highly infectious, from both respiratory droplets and skin lesions. Although common in children, it also affects adults, sometimes causing severe disease. Shingles is usually seen in older people (50–80 years of age) and only the skin lesions are infectious. People can develop chickenpox after contact with someone suffering from shingles; but shingles cannot be contracted from a person suffering from chickenpox. This is because shingles occurs as a result of reactivation of the VZV, whereas primary infection results in chickenpox (which may be subclinical). Contact with chickenpox or shingles, in someone who is not already immune, can result in primary infection.

Nursing staff should be aware of their immune status (see Box 16.11). (The nurse's immune status is normally determined from his personal history. Only in the event of a unit being unable to provide sufficient immune staff would it be necessary to resort to an IgG test (see Box 16.3 p. 584) for the presence of antibodies.) A nurse who is not known to be immune should not nurse someone with chickenpox or shingles. This is because people who are incubating the disease are infectious for several days before they develop symptoms, and they may inadvertently infect others before they are aware they have caught the disease themselves. It is also advisable for pregnant staff to keep away from patients with chickenpox or shingles.

Chickenpox

PATHOPHYSIOLOGY

The incubation period of chickenpox is 2–3 weeks, commonly 13–17 days. The disease is communicable from 5 days before the onset of the rash until 6 days after the first crop of vesicles has appeared.

Common presenting symptoms. Initial symptoms are usually a slight fever and the development of a skin rash which is maculopapular at first, becomes vesicular and then forms a scab. The lesions do not all occur at the same time but in succession, so that

Box 16.11 Staff contacts with infectious diseases of childhood

The following questions should be posed in determining which staff members should provide nursing care for patients with diseases such as measles, mumps, rubella and chickenpox:

1. Are the staff members known to be immune (e.g. rubella antibody-positive) or have they been immunised? In the case of a disease that produces lasting immunity, have they had the disease themselves?
2. Are they working with susceptible patients, e.g. neonates, young children, the seriously ill or the immunosuppressed?

If the answer to '1' is 'yes', it is usually all right for the staff members to work as usual.

If the answer to '1' is 'no' and to '2' is 'yes', the staff members should be reassigned to a non-susceptible area until the incubation period is over.

In circumstances where there is any doubt, the control of infection or occupational health department should be consulted.

on different parts of the body they may be at different stages. Areas of the body that are normally covered by clothing often have more lesions than exposed parts.

MEDICAL MANAGEMENT

Treatment. There is specific treatment for chickenpox with acyclovir but this is usually not recommended for uncomplicated disease. Antibiotics may be given for secondary infection of vesicles. Zoster immunoglobulin can be given to those at special risk (e.g. the immunosuppressed) who have been in contact with the disease and have not had it themselves.

NURSING PRIORITIES AND MANAGEMENT: CHICKENPOX

Life-threatening concerns

Rarely, chickenpox can cause severe illness. The most common cause of death in adults with the disease is primary viral pneumonia, which is treated with parenteral antiviral agents. Children may develop septic complications or encephalitis. The disease can be severe in the immunosuppressed.

Major patient problems

The rash may cause irritation and discomfort, and secondary bacterial infection of lesions can occur.

Further considerations

Chickenpox is highly infectious, both from respiratory secretions and from skin discharges. Strict isolation will be required until the period of communicability is over. (Protective clothing must be worn for every entry to the room; the door must be kept closed, and negative ventilation used if available. All items in the room will be contaminated and will therefore require disinfection.)

Shingles

PATHOPHYSIOLOGY

Common presenting symptoms. The first symptoms the person notices are often pain and paraesthesia in the affected area; this is usually the trunk but can be the face or a limb. A rash appears, starting with a macule on which vesicles develop over several days. The vesicles, which are a grey colour, dry up and crust over, usually in a week or so. The rash is characteristically restricted to the area supplied by the sensory nerves of one or an associated group of dorsal root ganglia. Subsequent healing may take several weeks, and residual or prolonged pain occurs in about 10% of cases.

MEDICAL MANAGEMENT

Treatment involves administering analgesics, acyclovir and sometimes applying idoxuridine paint to the vesicles in the early stages. Early acyclovir treatment may prevent development of severe disease.

NURSING PRIORITIES AND MANAGEMENT: SHINGLES

Shingles can flare up spontaneously or may follow treatment for another disease, e.g. radiotherapy, where the patient is immunocompromised.

Major patient problems

Pain and discomfort may result from the lesions, which may persist for a long time. The patient may experience anxiety and depression if the condition fails to improve; this is especially common among elderly patients. A sympathetic and optimistic attitude can do a lot to make the symptoms more bearable.

Further considerations

Care of the skin condition is similar to that for other skin disorders (see Ch. 12); it should be borne in mind that the lesions will be susceptible to secondary bacterial infection.

If the person is in hospital, she should be kept apart from other vulnerable patients. Isolation precautions may be necessary until the lesions have crusted over. The type of isolation will be determined by the extent and location of the lesions and whether they can be adequately covered to prevent contamination of outer clothing or bed linen. Only immune staff should nurse patients with shingles (see Box 16.11).

CONCLUSION

This chapter has outlined the function of the immune system and explained how the components of the immune response come together to protect the body from foreign material, whether microorganisms, allergens or tumour cells. Unfortunately, things can go wrong. Deficiencies, whether of cells or of proteins, can impair the immune system in its response.

Immune deficiency can be acquired, either through infection, e.g. HIV/AIDS (see Ch. 37), or as a result of medical treatment, e.g. immunosuppression during and after cytotoxic drug administration or radiotherapy (see Ch. 31). Hypersensitivity gives rise to a whole range of 'allergic' conditions, and the autoimmune diseases cause considerable morbidity and mortality. Infectious diseases have been with us for centuries and although some have become less common, others have stepped in to take their place.

Nursing care, in whatever context, involves a thorough assessment of each patient as an individual. Potential problems include the risk of the spread of infection, either through people (other patients, staff) or through inanimate objects (equipment, instruments). Some of the issues surrounding hospital-acquired infection (also called nosocomial infection) are discussed in Chapter 23. The safety of our patients is, to a large extent, in our own hands. It is up to us to do everything we can to make sure that the environment in which we care for people is, indeed, a safe one.

Q

16.14 A 70-year-old woman is at home suffering from *Campylobacter jejuni* enteritis. She is fully mobile and has profuse diarrhoea but seems to make it to the toilet in time. Although she tells you she has understood what you told her about the disease, during your visit she went to the toilet and did not wash her hands afterwards. Her grandchildren (aged 3 and 7 years) visit her regularly and she always has a supply of fruit and sweets for them.

- Devise a nursing plan for this patient for home care.
- Devise a nursing plan for hospital care.
- What advice would you give to this patient and her family about hygiene?
- Think about how you might try to ensure that your advice was followed.

16.15 Arrange to spend some time with the infection control nurse in your health board/authority/Trust. Find out what he does and how his work relates to patient care.

Q **16.16** Ask if you can visit the microbiology laboratory in your hospital. Find out what information is required on the specimen request form and why it is important. Ask to see what happens to the various specimens and which tests are carried out.

Q **16.17** Arrange to visit your HSDU. Watch how instruments are received, unwrapped, washed, dried, packed and autoclaved, or disinfected.

16.18 Discuss with a community nurse how the control of infection can be achieved in the patient's home, e.g. hand hygiene, use of protective clothing, aseptic techniques and disinfection of equipment.

ENDNOTE

National guidelines related to infection control are reviewed and updated regularly. As this book goes to print in 2000, UK health authorities/boards and Trusts are interpreting recent documents (HSAC 1999). New guidelines will be issued to registered nurses, and it is therefore important to check local policy for waste disposal. If necessary, consult local infection control specialists for advice.

ACKNOWLEDGEMENTS

The author wishes to extend her thanks to Dr A B White (formerly Consultant Microbiologist and Control of Infection Officer), Dr A J Hay (Consultant Microbiologist and Infection Control Doctor), Dr D O Ho-Yen (Consultant Microbiologist) and Dr M M Steven (Consultant Physician), all of Raigmore Hospital, NHS Trust, Inverness, for their generous assistance in the preparation of this chapter.

REFERENCES

Anderton A 1995 Reducing bacterial contamination in enteral tube feeds. British Journal of Nursing 4(7): 368–376
Babb J R 1990 Chemical disinfection and COSHH: safe and effective work practices. Institute of Sterile Services Managers Journal 1(10): 9–12
Bannister B A, Begg N T, Gillespie S H 1996 Infectious disease. Blackwell Science, Oxford
Benenson A S (ed) 1995 Control of communicable diseases manual, 16th edn. American Public Health Association, Washington
Bowell B 1990 Assessing infection risks. Nursing 4(12): 19–23
Brostoff J, Scadding G K, Male D, Roitt I M 1991 Clinical immunology. Gower Medical Publishing, London
Bryan J L, Cohran J, Larson E L 1995 Hand washing. A ritual revisited. Critical Care Nursing Clinics of North America 7(4): 617–625
Chief Medical Officer 1996 *E. coli* 0157 (SODH/CMO (96)22). Scottish Office Department of Health, Edinburgh
Control of Substances Hazardous to Health Regulations (COSHH) 1988 HMSO, London
Courington K R, Patterson S L, Howard R J 1991 Universal precautions are not universally followed. Archives of Surgery 126: 93–96
Crockett A 1993 Managing asthma in primary care. Blackwell Scientific, Oxford
Department of Health Working Group 1994 Management of outbreaks of foodborne illness. Department of Health, Wetherby
DHSS 1988 Information to undertakers: infectious diseases. PL/CMO (88) 7. DHSS, London
DoH 1996 Immunisation against infectious disease (Edward Jenner bicentenary edition). HMSO, London
Duerden B I, Reid T M S, Jewsbury J M 1993 Microbial and parasitic infection, 7th edn. Edward Arnold, London
Ehrenkranz N J 1992 Bland soap handwash or hand antisepsis? The pressing need for clarity. Infection Control and Hospital Epidemiology 13: 299–301
Farthing H, Feldman R, Finch R et al 1996 The management of infective gastroenteritis in adults. A consensus statement by an expert panel convened by the British Society for the Study of Infection. Journal of Infection 33: 143–152
Greaves A 1985 We'll just freshen you up, dear…. Nursing Times Journal of Infection Control Nursing 81(10) (suppl): 3–8
Grist N R, Ho-Yen D O, Walker E, Williams G R 1993 Diseases of infection: an illustrated textbook, 2nd edn. Oxford University Press, Oxford
Haslett C, Chilvers E R, Hunter J A, Boon N A (eds) 1999 Davidson's principles and practice of medicine, 18th edn. Churchill Livingstone, Edinburgh
Healing T D, Hoffman P N, Young S E J 1995 The infection hazards of human cadavers. Communicable Diseases Report (CDR) Review 5(5): R61–68
Health and Safety Executive 1990 Farmer's lungs. Health and Safety Executive, London
Health and Safety at Work etc Act 1974 HMSO, London
Health Services Advisory Committee (HSAC) 1992 The safe disposal of clinical waste. HMSO, London
Hobbs B C, Roberts D 1993 Food poisoning and food hygiene, 6th edn. Edward Arnold, London
Hospital Infection Control Practices Advisory Committee (HICPAC) 1996 Guideline for isolation precautions in hospitals, Part 2. Recommendations for isolation precautions in hospitals. American Journal of Infection Control 24(1): 32–45
Hospital Infection Working Group 1995 Hospital infection control. Department of Health, London
Information and Statistics Division (I & SD), NHS in Scotland 1996 Scottish health statistics. I & SD, NHS in Scotland, Edinburgh
Joint Tuberculosis Committee of the British Thoracic Society 1994 Control and prevention of tuberculosis in the United Kingdom: code of practice. Thorax 49: 1193–1200
Kirkwood E, Lewis C 1989 Understanding medical immunology, 2nd edn. Wiley, Chichester
Knights B, Evans C, Barrass S, McHardy B 1993 Hand drying: a survey of efficiency and hygiene. University of Westminster, London
Knowles H 1993 The experience of infectious patients in isolation. Nursing Times 89(30): 53–56.
Kobayashi H, Tsuzuki M, Koshimizu K et al 1984 Susceptibility of hepatitis B virus to disinfectants or heat. Journal of Clinical Microbiology 20(2): 214–216
Mandal B K, Wilkins E G L, Dunbar E M, Mayon-White R T 1996 Lecture notes on infectious diseases, 5th edn. Blackwell Science, Oxford
Medical Devices Agency (MDA) 1996 Decontamination of endoscopes. MDA 9607. Medical Devices Agency, London
Microbiology Advisory Committee (MAC) 1996 Sterilisation disinfection and cleaning of medical equipment, Part 2. Medical Devices Agency, Department of Health, London

NHS Executive 1995 Hospital laundry arrangements for used and infected linen (HSG(95)18). NHS Executive, London
Public Health Laboratory Service (PHLS) 1997 PHLS vero cytotoxin – producing *Escherichia coli* 0157. Factsheet. PHLS, London
Roitt I 1994 Essential immunology, 8th edn. Blackwell Scientific, Oxford
Roitt I, Brostoff J, Male D 1996 Immunology, 4th edn. Mosby, London
Rutala W A 1996 APIC guideline for selection and use of disinfectants. American Journal of Infection Control 24(4): 313–342
Sarafino E P 1990 Health psychology: biopsychosocial interactions. John Wiley, New York
Scottish Executive Health Department (SEHD) 1999 Variant Creutzfeldt-Jakob Disease (vCJD): minimising the risk of transmission. Scottish Executive, Edinburgh
Scottish Office Home and Health Department (SOHHD) 1993 Hospital laundry arrangements for used and infected linen. MEL (1993)7. SOHHD, Edinburgh
Taylor L J 1978a An evaluation of hand-washing techniques — I. Nursing Times 74(2): 54–55
Taylor L J 1978b An evaluation of hand-washing techniques — II. Nursing Times 74(3): 108–110
United Kingdom Central Council (UKCC) 1992 Code of professional conduct for the nurse, midwife and health visitor, 3rd edn. UKCC, London
UK Health Departments 1998 Guidance for clinical health care workers: protection against infection with blood-borne viruses. HMSO, London
UK Health Departments 1993 Protecting Health Care Workers and Patients from Hepatitis B. HMSO, London
Wall P G, Ryan M J, Ward L R, Rowe B 1996 Outbreaks of salmonellosis in hospitals in England and Wales: 1992–1994. Journal of Hospital Infection 33(3): 181–190
Weir D M, Stewart J 1993 Immunology, 7th edn. Churchill Livingstone, Edinburgh
Wilks O, Farrington M, Rubenstein D 1995 The infectious diseases manual. Blackwell Science, Oxford

FURTHER READING

Advisory Group on Infection 1998 Scottish Infection Manual. Scottish Office Department of Health, Edinburgh
Akerman V, Dunk-Richards G 1991 Microbiology: an introduction for the health sciences. Harcourt Brace Jovanovich, Sydney
British Lung Foundation 1996 Sarcoidosis. British Lung Foundation, London
British Medical Association 1989 A code of practice for sterilisation of instruments and control of cross-infection. British Medical Association, London
Burton G R W 1992 Microbiology for the health sciences, 4th edn. Lippincott, Philadelphia
DoH 1996 Immunisation against infectious disease (Edward Jenner bicentenary edition). HMSO, London
Fenelon L E 1995 Protective isolation: who needs it? Journal of Hospital Infection 30(suppl): 218–222
Health Services Advisory Committee 1999 Safe disposal of clinical waste. HMSO, London
Horton R, Parker L 1997 Informed infection control nursing. Churchill Livingstone, Edinburgh
Larson E, Kretzer E K 1995 Compliance with handwashing and barrier precautions. Journal of Hospital Infection 30(suppl): 88–106
Levy J 1989 Listeria and food poisoning: a growing concern. Maternal and Child Health 14: 380–383
Mallett J, Bailey C (eds) 1996 The Royal Marsden NHS Trust manual of clinical nursing procedures, 4th edn. Blackwell Science, Oxford
Microbiology Advisory Committee (MAC) 1991 Health Circular HC(91) 33. Decontamination of equipment, linen or other surfaces contaminated with hepatitis B and/or human immunodeficiency viruses. Department of Health, London
Mooney B R, Reeves S A, Larson E 1993 Infection control and bone marrow transplantation. American Journal of Infection Control 21: 131–138
MRSA Working Party of the Royal College of Nursing 1992 Introduction to methicillin resistant *Staphylococcus aureus*. Scutari Projects, Harrow
Philpott-Howard J, Casewell M 1994 Hospital infection control policies and practical procedures. WB Saunders, London
Rubin R H, Tolkoff-Rubin N E 1989 Infection: the new problems. Transplantation Proceedings 21(1): 1440–1445
Stewart M 1993 Skills for caring: hygiene for care. Churchill Livingstone, Edinburgh
Wilson K J W, Waugh A 1996 Ross and Wilson's anatomy and physiology in health and illness, 8th edn. Churchill Livingstone, New York
Working Party of the British Society for Antimicrobial Chemotherapy and the Hospital Infection Society 1995 Guidelines on the control of methicillin-resistant *Staphylococcus aureus* in the community. Journal of Hospital Infection 31: 1–12
Working Party Report 1988 Cleaning and disinfection of equipment for gastrointestinal flexible endoscopy. Gut 42: 585–593
Working Party Report 1998 Revised guidelines for the control of methicillin-resistant *Staphylococcus aureus* infection in hospitals. Journal of Hospital Infection 39: 253–290

USEFUL ADDRESSES

British Lung Foundation
78 Hatton Garden
London EC1N 8JR

Health and Safety Executive Information Centre
Baynards House
1 Chepstow Place
Westbourne Grove
London W2 4TF

Lupus UK
1 Eastern Road
Romford
Essex RM1 3NH

Myasthenia Gravis Association
Chester Park
Alfreton Road
Derby DE1 4AS

British Liver Trust
Ransomes Europark
Ipswich
Suffolk IP3 9QG

National Meningitis Trust
Fern House
Bath Road
Stroud
Glos. GL5 3TJ

COMMON PATIENT PROBLEMS AND RELATED NURSING CARE

SECTION 2

SECTION CONTENTS

STRESS

Vivian Leefarr

17

INTRODUCTION

'Stress' is a word that frequently enters into everyday conversation as people remark on the difficulties and challenges of life. Most people would probably describe themselves as being 'stressed' from time to time, but what does this really mean? Is stress something that resides within the environment, in situations that are threatening, harmful or unpleasant, or is it essentially an internal state, an effect of the individual's perception of what is happening to him? Benner & Wrubel (1989) define stress as 'the disruption of meanings, understanding and smooth functioning so that harm, loss or challenge is experienced and sorrow, interpretation, or new skill acquisition is required'.

Stress research is a highly complex field involving a number of sciences, including biology, physiology, psychology and sociology. These disciplines take different approaches to the definition, observation and measurement of stress. When biologists and physiologists talk of sources of stress, they are referring to empirical phenomena. Their interest is in examining identifiable events and their measurable effects upon the organism or system being stressed. Anything which affects the equilibrium of the organism may be described as a stressor; this would include bacterial or viral infections, dehydration, excessive cold or heat, inadequate food, and so on.

Social scientists view stress in terms of the pressures upon the individual to conform (or not) to societal norms. The inherent values expressed in a society's organisation and functioning may themselves be a source of stress to the individual. Modern industrial society, for example, provides food, safety and shelter for its members in return for a commitment to work, often at some sacrifice to personal interests, leisure and family life.

Psychologists view stress from the perspective of the interaction of individuals and groups with the environment, describing the effects of stress on cognition, emotional well-being and behaviour.

It is important for nurses to have a clear understanding of the concept of stress as they endeavour to provide the best possible care for their patients. It is essential to appreciate why patients might be feeling stressed and how their anxiety might be alleviated. In relation to the nurse's own well-being, an understanding of stress and its effects is equally important. Nursing is physically and emotionally strenuous work, and it is vital for nurses to be able to recognise the signs of stress in themselves and to know how to go about managing stress in their daily work.

This chapter begins by outlining some of the more influential models for describing stress. These include definitions of stress as a type of stimulus, as a response, or as an interaction between an individual and his environment. The second section of the chapter describes in some detail the effects of stress upon physiological systems. This provides a basis for the third section, which examines the relationship between stress and disease.

The discussion then turns to the concept of coping, and various cognitive and behavioural mechanisms by which people commonly attempt to deal with stress are outlined. This is followed by a description of the therapeutic strategies that are available to assist the individual in managing stress. The chapter ends with a discussion of stress in nursing, identifying some of the most significant sources of stress in this very demanding profession and suggesting ways in which vital support can be given to nurses to enable them to meet the emotional demands of patient-centred care.

MODELS OF STRESS

The physicist Robert Hooke (1635–1703) used the word 'stress' in the 17th century to refer to the ratio of an external force (created by a load) to the area over which that force was exerted. The resultant strain created a deformation or distortion of the object by what became known as Hooke's law (Cox 1989).

There is an interesting similarity between this use of the word stress and its modern application in the realm of human emotion and behaviour; indeed, people frequently use words such as 'weight' and 'strain' when describing their feelings of anxiety and stress.

In the 20th century, the adoption of the concept of stress by the biological and behavioural sciences has resulted in the formulation of a number of models to describe stress and its effects:

- stimulus-based model
- response-based model
- the transactional model
- the phenomenological approach.

Each of these models and its implications for nursing practice will be described in the following sections.

The stimulus-based model

In this model the person is viewed as being constantly exposed to external or environmental 'stressors' in his daily life, e.g. the demands of work, family responsibilities, bereavement or disablement, or more specific stressors such as smells or poor lighting. Stress arises from the environment and is external to the individual. It has the potential, however, to cause distressing feelings and/or physical symptoms and to undermine well-being.

In the stimulus-based model, stress is a state that can generally be empirically observed, measured and evaluated, and which can potentially be removed or altered to reduce the individual's stress: it is possible, in theory, to make noisy neighbours quieter, a cold working environment warmer, or poor lighting conditions more satisfactory. As an approach to identifying areas that might be improved to increase productivity, this model has some appeal for industrial planners and managers (Sutherland & Cooper 1990).

Limitations of the model. In many situations, such as a bereavement or disablement, the original stressor cannot be changed or adapted to reduce distressing feelings. Even in relatively simple situations such as that illustrated in Case History 17.1, removing the stressor is not necessarily a straightforward matter. It quickly becomes apparent that the stimulus-based model has substantial shortcomings when considered in relation to the breadth of human experience (Sutherland & Cooper 1990). Whilst it has some application in limited contexts, such as certain working environments, it does not explain why some people experience stress in certain situations while others, in similar circumstances, do not. Nor does it explain why a given situation may be stressful for a person at one time but not at another. Moreover, this model offers no explanation as to why a person may be stressed in response to apparently neutral stimuli such as birds, spiders or aeroplanes. Lazarus (1966) argued that it is not possible to evaluate the human experience of stress objectively; only a personal account of feelings and experiences can adequately convey the nature of an individual's stress.

The response-based model

In this model, the word 'stress' is used to describe the experience of a person who feels himself to be in a threatening or difficult situation. Stress is thus a person's response to threat and, unlike in the stimulus-based model, is not inherent in the environment or situation. By using this approach, it is possible to make sense of an individual's unique stress responses and even of responses that might seem, within the stimulus-based model, to be irrational, such as a fear of birds, spiders or flying.

The systems model of the human stress response

A response-based model that considers the human stress response as 'a multi-factorial, interactive, dynamic, phenomenon' is the systems model described by Everly & Sobelman (1987). In this model the stress response is defined as consisting of six components:

1. Environmental stimuli. Some environmental stimuli, or stressors, activate the stress response as a direct consequence of their physical or biochemical properties, i.e. their effects are not mediated by cognitive–affective evaluation. Examples of such stressors are caffeine, nicotine and extremes of heat and cold. Many environmental stimuli are not, however, intrinsically harmful but are perceived as such by the individual and, in this way, set the stage for activation of the stress response.

2. Cognitive–affective domain. Everly & Sobelman (1987) describe this as 'the critical "causal" phase in most stress responses', in that it is the individual's interpretation of the environment that gives rise to most stress reactions. The perspective that the individual takes towards his environment will be determined by 'biological predispositions', 'personality patterns', 'learning history' and 'available resources'. Everly & Sobelman argue that cognitive appraisal precedes emotional response.

Case History 17.1 J

A health visitor could not understand initially why her client, J, an unsupported mother of two, appeared to be tense and unhappy when they met at the child surveillance clinic. She asked how J was feeling, and J described how she had new neighbours in the flat above her who played loud music until early in the morning, preventing her and her two children from getting enough sleep. She had tried to talk with them but they had been hostile towards her and made her feel apprehensive. She didn't dare complain to them again. The lack of sleep was affecting J and her children. J had difficulty concentrating at work and felt like crying frequently during the day; the children were overtired and generally irritable, making it even more difficult for her to cope.

The health visitor asked J if she could intervene by contacting the housing department on her behalf, but J said that she was afraid that this would make matters worse.

Note: The author wishes to state that all case histories used in this chapter are fictional.

3. Neurological triggering mechanisms. The locus coeruleus, limbic system and hypothalamic nuclei are the anatomical sites for 'the integration of sensory, cognitive, affective, and visceral activity' (Everly & Sobelman 1987). In response to cognitive–affective appraisal, these structures trigger neurological and endocrine reactions. They also seem to be involved in a feedback system in which visceral and somatic efferent messages are relayed in response to emotional arousal. Everly & Sobelman suggest that 'these centers seem capable of establishing an endogenously-determined neurological tone that is potentially self perpetuating' and which 'may, over time, serve as the basis for a host of psychiatric and psychophysiologic disorders'.

4. The physiological stress response axis. The stress response itself occurs sequentially along the neurological, neuroendocrine and endocrine axes and results in neural and hormonal activity directed at target organs.

Neurological axis. Neurological activity is especially evident in reactions to sudden acute stress and results in direct activation of the sympathetic nervous system (seen as raised heart rate and blood pressure, etc.) and the parasympathetic nervous system (seen as constricted pupils, increased salivation, urinary bladder contraction, etc.) and in the transmission of messages to skeletal muscle (resulting in contraction).

Neuroendocrine axis. This is based in the adrenal medullae and plays an important role in longer-term arousal. Release of the catecholamines noradrenaline and adrenaline by the adrenal medullae results in such sympathetic responses as increased cardiac output and diminished blood flow to the skin and gastrointestinal system (see p. 619).

Endocrine axis. This axis also plays an important role in chronic arousal. Here the hypothalamus, pituitary gland, adrenal cortex and thyroid gland are stimulated serially to release into the circulatory system the range of hormones described on page 619.

5. Coping. In this final phase of the stress response, the individual attempts to reduce his level of arousal by manipulating the environment or making cognitive adjustments.

6. Target-organ effects. If coping is unsuccessful and arousal is either excessive or prolonged, the physiological processes of the stress response are likely to lead to target organ dysfunction or disease.

Limitations of the model. One of the problems in viewing stress as a response only is that this can lead to the assumption that the occurrence of stress in the life of the individual is solely his own responsibility. The descriptive term 'coping' used in a technical sense by stress researchers to describe physiological and psychological ways of adapting to stress can also be used in an emotive way in everyday discourse to describe an individual's lack of mastery in stressful circumstances. Thus someone who 'copes' with stress masters a situation in a positive way, whilst someone who does not 'cope' is lacking in this ability. Such judgements on self or others can have a harmful emotional effect on the individual.

Q **17.1** Is shedding tears of sadness in such a circumstance a sign of one's inability to cope?

Hans Selye's general adaptation syndrome

Hans Selye's extensive physiological research as an endocrinologist (Selye 1936, 1946a,b, 1976) was largely based upon the response-based model of stress. His hypothesis was that all organisms placed under stress behaved in a particular way physiologically, regardless of the nature of the stress. Given the presence of a stressor such as severe heat or cold, the response of the organism would be of a uniform nature. Selye concentrated mainly upon a set of physiological responses to stress, which he called the general adaptation syndrome. This syndrome is divisible into three phases: alarm reaction, resistance and exhaustion (see p. 618).

Limitations of the model. Whilst Selye's work was highly influential in early stress research, it is now felt that his model does not take full account of the individuality of psychological and physiological responses. Nor does it consider the role of the appraisal of stressful situations, which is now considered to precede each response. Lazarus (1966) argued that there is a circularity about Selye's model in so far as something about the stimulus elicits a particular stress response while something about the response indicates the presence of a stressor.

Q **17.2** Physical stressors such as disease or injury may well result in death, but how might the individual respond to psychological or social stressors such as bereavement or unemployment?

The transactional model

A behavioural model of stress that incorporates a dynamic view of the individual and his interaction with the stress in his environment is called a transactional model. The person appraises, or seeks meaning in, what is perceived to be a potentially threatening situation in an attempt to respond in a way that minimises the distress. The process of appraisal is highly individual; each person will perceive a threatening situation differently and attach his own meanings to it (Lazarus & Folkman 1984, Cox 1989). Moreover, the relationship between the individual and his environment is a dynamic one which constantly changes as the process of appraisal continues.

Nursing application. Case History 17.2 highlights how the transactional model of stress has clear advantages for the clinical nurse. Although Mr P's feeling of terror was related to the stressor of being in hospital and the prospect of surgery, these circumstances in themselves did not fully account for his state of mind. His feeling of stress derived from his appraisal of the situation, and this appraisal reflected his childhood experience. The transactional model of stress recognises that a person such as Mr P, rather than being a passive recipient of stress, interacts actively with a situation.

Cox's man–environment model

Cox (1989) defines five stages within his man–environment model:

1. Source of demand — a situation is perceived as threatening
2. Individual's perception of demand, and coping based upon personality and early experiences
3. Psychophysiological changes in response to the perceived threat
4. Coping responses and consequences — how the individual sets about dealing with the threat
5. Feedback — both physiological and psychological.

Cox describes the 'demand' as arising from the individual's psychological and physiological needs. The individual attempts to understand the demand and his ability to do this determines the way he sets about coping. Stress may occur at a time of hopelessness, when the person understands the nature of the threat but is unable to respond in a way that diminishes or removes it. At this time, physiological responses also become active as methods of

Case History 17.2 Mr P

Nurse T was asked to interview Mr P on his admission to the ward for minor dental surgery the following day. Mr P, a 32-year-old engineer, was married and had two children, a girl and a boy. He lived with his family near the hospital and worked in a factory in a nearby town. During the interview, Nurse T noticed that while Mr P appeared to be in good health and to have a clear understanding of the surgery he was about to undergo, he seemed uneasy. Knowing that many patients feel apprehensive before having surgery, she asked him how he was feeling. Mr P replied: 'I feel silly, stupid and embarrassed about it but I am very scared — have been since I got the appointment in the post — can't understand why! I haven't been able to sleep for the past week and when I do I have awful dreams.'

The nurse talked further with Mr P about his feeling of fear. She asked him if he had ever been in hospital before and he recalled with some difficulty how as a small child he had been admitted as an emergency for a circumcision. As he talked he realised how frightened he had been at that time and that when he had been readmitted for an inflamed wound, his fear had become even greater. He remembered that his mother had been unable to stay with him.

The following day Mr P had his surgery. Before leaving the ward he said to Nurse T that he had felt better after talking with her. He had still felt afraid but the powerful feeling of terror had gone.

coping with stress. At each stage of the model, the individual receives evaluative feedback.

Limitations of the model. Given the complexity of individual experiences and coping stategies, it is extremely difficult to subject transactional models of stress such as Cox's man–environment model to empirical evaluation.

17.3 Discuss how the terms 'stress' and 'stressor' are used differently within various models of stress.

The role of appraisal

How individuals appraise, or find meaning in, adversity is crucial to how they withstand it. As we will see with the concept of resilience (p. 617; see also 'hardiness', p. 623), some people (e.g. patients with cancer or AIDS — Polk 1997) can withstand and survive the adversity whilst others cannot. So appraisal is crucial to the individual's ability to continue a healthy life after catastrophe or illness, and of course, as with resilience, the personal traits of the person will influence his ability to find meaning in what is happening to him.

Appraisal then becomes an interpretative process involving perception, intuition and reason by which the person feeling stressed distinguishes between safe and threatening situations. While not all situations involving feelings of stress are severe, it is worth remembering here that people experiencing stress may be 'in extremis' or very seriously ill. The cognitive process of appraisal as described here may, in fact, be a spontaneous emotional reaction rather than a well thought-out process.

People are unique in their experiences and personalities, and because no two people, and no two situations, are exactly the same, the appraisal will be about the meaning that the person finds within the circumstances.

The phenomenological approach

Phenomenological approaches to knowledge emphasise the importance of the object as it appears within a context rather than the object in itself. Thus a phenomenological approach to stress rests largely upon the description given by the individual of his own experience of stress. The writings of phenomenological philosophers such as Merleau-Ponty and Heidegger describe human experience as 'being-in-the-world' whereby each person is defined by his own thoughts, feelings, memories, relationships and social settings. Mind and body are not described as separate but as one integral whole (Dreyfus 1987, Benner & Wrubel 1989). The body is the physical means of knowing and sensing the world, and with disablement or disease the experience of the person will be impaired (Benner & Wrubel 1989). Whether the impairment is of the mind or the body, the whole experience of the person will be affected.

This view of human experience invites the clinician to use an intuitive approach when working with people who are distressed, because it acknowledges the complexity of individual responses, and recognises that providing the right kind of help is, similarly, a complex and subtle task.

Case History 17.3 underlines the fact that a solution to a problem which may seem reasonable to one person may present insuperable difficulties to another. In order to understand his colleague's rejection of his suggestion, L would need to know more about why C overeats. If it were possible to ask her about her feelings, she might offer one or more reasons for her behaviour. For instance:

- she may feel anxious and unhappy as a student and feel reassured when she eats sweet foods
- she may have started overeating as a child at a time of family distress
- she may have been abused as a child
- she may feel sexually unattractive and find eating a means of gaining consolation
- she may feel constantly hungry.

Nursing application. The description of human experience from a phenomenological viewpoint attributes to the person a wisdom about himself and his problems that cannot easily be gained from an 'objective' position (Benner & Wrubel 1989). But does this mean that the clinical nurse is merely a passive observer when working with distressed people? If suggestions and advice cannot be offered in any but the most uncomplicated situations, then what help *can* be offered?

The most effective help that can be given by the clinical nurse is support in enabling the person to identify what is causing his stress and to deal with it in his own way. This does not entail the nurse, however subtly, suggesting what she thinks the patient should do. Rather, it involves being aware and respectful of the patient's right to choose what is appropriate for himself. This is not a passive position for the clinical nurse to take but, in fact, a highly interactive and enabling one (Rogers 1974, Kennedy 1990, Egan 1997).

Case History 17.3 L and C

L, a student nurse, notices at mealtimes that her colleague C often mentions her distressed feelings about her weight. Knowing that she frequently eats sweets and cakes, L suggests to her that all she would need to do to lose weight would be to stop eating between meals. C, however, rejects this option as being too difficult to carry through.

Case History 17.4 Miss H

J had been an experienced health visitor for a number of years, working with a general practice in a rural area. She had been visiting Miss H for a year or two and had been alerted by the home help to the possibility that she was not eating as regularly as she ought. Miss H was 86 years old and had lived alone for 20 years since her father had died. She had always been fiercely independent, but her home help telephoned on Thursday morning to ask if Miss H could be visited urgently.

When J visited she found Miss H sitting in her kitchen with her elderly cat on her lap. It was apparent that the cat had died. Miss H's home help thought that she had been sitting with her cat throughout the night and was worried that she had not eaten or moved. J did not know what to do and so sat quietly beside Miss H for some time. She felt it would somehow be wrong to try to separate her from her lifelong friend.

After a while Miss H and J talked quietly about her cat and how he had become ill and died during the night. Miss H said that she did not know whether she would be able to live without him. Much later, however, she agreed to put the cat out in the garden and allowed a neighbour to come and bury him. When the village heard what had occurred, many people came forward to give Miss H sympathetic support and to keep her company.

In Case History 17.4, J, a health visitor, does not attempt to deal with the situation by taking action or giving suggestions, even though her concern that Miss H had not eaten or moved for some time might have prompted her to do so. J's support and concern do, however, enable Miss H to talk about how she feels and then to accept help in dealing with the body of her cat.

This example also underlines a further facet of stress, i.e. that people often experience stress when they are not themselves being threatened. Stress can arise as an empathic response through the perception of the stress experienced by another. When J perceives the intense distress of her client, she too may experience that distress.

Phenomenology, appraisal and the role of stress

In a sense, all appraisal is phenomenological because it rests upon the individual's own attribution of meaning to a situation (Lazarus & Folkman 1984). Personality can, however, play a large part in determining what features of his environment an individual attends to, and what he attends to is a feature of the meaning that a situation has for him (Lazarus & Folkman 1984, Benner & Wrubel 1989). Rather than describing the individual as 'appraising' a situation, however, Benner & Wrubel (1989) prefer to speak of him 'being in' a situation. They emphasise that the attribution of meaning to a situation is unique for every individual, even though many people's interpretations appear to coincide. Taking this even further, they argue that there are no situations with an objective reality beyond the highly individual interpretations that are put upon them.

For Benner & Wrubel (1989), stress is woven into the fabric of our 'being in the world' and is not 'out there' to be dealt with. From this point of view, it would be harmful to suppress painful emotions, as these assist us in our interpretations of the world. Emotions such as anger or guilt give guidance to people about what is happening to them in the world. To teach people to relax may give them some short respite from painful tension until they are ready to confront their problems again and may be useful for this reason, but to teach relaxation as a way of dealing with problems is surely misguided. Stress is part of the person's self, his concerns, thoughts, feelings about the past and future, memories and relationships to others and to objects.

The concept of resilience

An interesting and developing concept for nurses is that of resilience in individuals, which enables them to 'spring back' following distressing events (Jacelon 1997). The research indicates that people who can spring back have a constellation of personality traits such as above-average intelligence, interest in life, a positive outlook and flexibility. Those who can visualise their own future are also more likely to be resilient.

The notion of resilience as a process is less well researched, although nurses will recognise the individual learning and change described by Polk (1997) as 'survival, recovery and rehabilitation'. Those able to undergo this process are more likely to be members of social groups, to have friends and family, hope and the ability to find meaning and purpose in their experience of life.

Of course, the important thing to be learned from this research for nurses working clinically is how to identify ways to enable those without the personality traits or social systems in place (Dewar & Morse 1995) to be helped towards rehabilitation, education and consolation. Why is it that some people have these abilities whilst others do not? As nurses, we must also ask ourselves what are the developmental aspects of a person's life that create a more resilient personality?

PHYSIOLOGICAL RESPONSES TO STRESS

The role of hormones in responses to stress

In 1935, Cannon summarised the response to external threat as a 'flight, fight or fright' reaction; this has often been called the 'acute stress response'. There are, in fact, many stress-provoking events in life. Real and imagined psychosocial stressors are an essential component of living and, when present to a moderate degree, have been described as 'eustress' since they optimise performance and improve learning. It is when a threat is perceived to be greater, endangering either a person's reputation or even life itself, that one sees the full manifestations of the acute stress response. After events such as a car crash, bomb explosion or unexpected physical attack, alarm occurs, activating the rapid physiological adaptations of the acute stress response (see below). This can, in some circumstances, be life-saving. Consider, for example, the situation in which smoke suddenly appears in a room and, all too soon, the first flames begin to spread — a person will often find a sudden unexpected ability for rapid action to deal with such an emergency. Along with a surge of physical strength, there will be an increased ability to tackle the flames and a marked enhancement in the ability to run and thereby escape the danger. Such a response is enabled by a release of hormones brought about by activation of the adrenal medulla.

An alarm reaction of lesser magnitude is a common occurrence in the more ordinary trials of life. This occurs, for example, in such circumstances as running out of petrol on the motorway en route to an important engagement, losing one's front door keys, or being with someone who unexpectedly becomes acutely ill. The severity of the alarm reaction varies considerably between different individuals and also between different occurrences of a similar situation. Thus, when a person breaks down on the motorway for a second time, he may feel even more distressed than on the first occasion; alternatively, he may be more confident in his ability to deal with the event and consequently less 'stressed'.

Psychosocial stress derives not merely from external problems or dangers but from the way in which people attempt to manage these problems. Ostell (1991) describes stress as the state of affairs that exists when the way in which people attempt to manage problems taxes or exceeds their coping resources. When the response to a stressor is severe, normal social relationships can be affected as aspects of the 'flight, fight or fright' response impinge upon rational behaviour.

Stress provoking events additional to psychosocial stressors include aversive physical stimuli such as excessive noise, cold or heat, and physiological imbalances such as those associated with sleep deprivation, lack of food or chronic pain. Each of these stressors not only acts to bring about hormonal changes associated with the acute stress response, but also has its own selective effects on physiological functioning.

An example of such a selective effect can be seen in the body's response to cold. In cold conditions, the body seeks to maintain homeostasis by redistributing the blood supply to less exposed areas and by increasing body temperature via the mechanical act of shivering and the increased secretion of thyrotrophin-releasing hormone from the hypothalamus. Thyrotrophin-releasing hormone stimulates the pituitary gland to secrete thyroid-stimulating hormone (TSH); this causes enhanced release of the thyroid hormones thyroxine and tri-iodothyronine, which raise basal metabolic rate and hence increase heat production and core temperature.

Thus, in seeking to maintain constancy of the internal environment when this is threatened by a stressor, the body employs a range of physiological mechanisms. Some stressors are short-lived, in which case the body may be able to react to the situation and quickly resolve the disturbance evoked by the stressor. Other stressors may last for days, months or even years. There are many circumstances of chronic stress, as when people must live with circumstances such as chronic disease or social disharmony. Where there has been repeated exposure to a particularly stressful or aversive event, there can be a further reaction characterised by a conditioned fear response to any neutral stimulus experienced at the same time as the previous stress. This effect is responsible for many of the anxiety reactions or acts of avoidance some people show in response to specific harmless objects.

The general adaptation syndrome

As discussed, on page 615, Selye, in his response-based model of stress noted that diverse noxious stimuli, which challenged the ability of the body to maintain homeostasis, induced a common pattern of effects (Selye 1936, 1976). He found, initially, that the injection of an extract of cattle ovary into rats appeared to stimulate a triad of responses: hypertrophy of the adrenal glands, atrophy of the lymphoid tissue and ulceration of the stomach. He subsequently noted the same effects when the animals were subjected to other stressors such as extremes of temperatures or the injection of modestly noxious chemicals. Selye deduced that, whatever the nature of the stressor, it resulted in a pattern of non-specific responses that formed part of what he described as a general adaptation syndrome (GAS). These responses, providing they where not overwhelming, enabled a physiological adaptation to take place (Selye 1976).

The syndrome is divisible into three phases. In the first of these, 'the alarm reaction', the adrenal glands are activated. The adrenal medulla, together with the sympathetic nervous system, prepares the body for flight or fight following cognitive appraisal of the threat. If the stress continues, the triggering of neural and endocrine responses in the alarm reaction is followed by the second phase of the stress response, 'resistance'. Stimulation of the hypothalamo-pituitary–adrenal axis results in increased secretion of corticosteroids. In this phase, the internal responses of the body stimulate tissue defences and achieve the maximum adaptation possible. The final phase of the general adaptation syndrome is 'exhaustion', in which the body may succumb to the stressor.

The general adaptation syndrome provides a somewhat simplistic model of the actual responses of the body and fails to take full account of the individual nature of psychological and physiological responses.

The acute stress response

During the alarm reaction to stress, a series of physiological responses involving limbic and brain stem structures is triggered (Gray 1987, Fox 1990). Neural pathways from the amygdaloid nuclei in the limbic system mediate responses to emotional stress, and pathways from the reticular formation in the brain stem mediate responses to traumatic stressors such as pain and injury. This activates the hypothalamopituitary–adrenal axis and results in the secretion of a range of hormones, as illustrated in Figure 17.1.

An immediate response to threat or stress involves the neural connections from the hypothalamus to the sympathetic outflow, activating both postganglionic sympathetic nerves and preganglionic sympathetic nerves passing to the adrenal medulla. This is

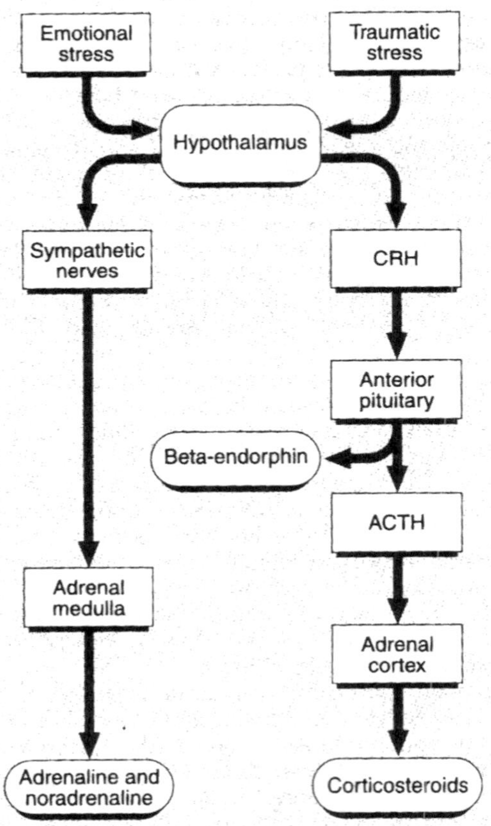

Fig. 17.1 Hormone secretion in response to stress.

the emergency reaction described by Cannon (1935). In the adrenal medulla, acetylcholine released at preganglionic sympathetic nerve terminals activates the chromaffin cells to secrete adrenaline and noradrenaline. In humans, adrenaline is secreted in greater amounts than noradrenaline. The release of these hormones takes place in a matter of seconds or minutes.

The hormones liberated from the adrenal medulla have many effects which facilitate emergency reactions. For example, adrenaline and noradrenaline improve cardiac and respiratory function. Heart rate and force of contraction are increased. Bronchioles are dilated and the depth and rate of respiration are increased. Blood flow is redistributed to areas of need, i.e. the heart and skeletal muscles. Blood glucose and basal metabolism are raised and blood clotting facilitated. The increase of blood glucose is due mainly to the actions of adrenaline on the liver to promote glycogen breakdown and enhance gluconeogenesis from fatty acids and proteins. Adrenaline also acts on the pancreas to inhibit insulin secretion. The piloerection and pupillary dilatation so characteristic of the behaviour of fighting cats represent yet another physiological consequence of hormone release from the adrenal medulla. Sweating by the eccrine glands is increased. In the meantime, functioning of the digestive tract is reduced and urinary sphincters are closed. The physiological effects of noradrenaline and adrenaline are explained in Chapter 5. Adrenaline acts on α- and β-adrenoceptors, whereas noradrenaline acts predominantly on α-adrenoceptors.

In the more long-term responses to stress described by Selye, the centre of activity passes from the adrenal medulla to the adrenal cortex, and to the hypothalamus and pituitary, which are responsible for activating the adrenal cortex. Corticotrophin-releasing hormone (CRH) is secreted by the hypothalamus as well as by extrahypothalamic sites in the brain. CRH acts on the anterior pituitary gland, stimulating the secretion of adrenocorticotrophic hormone (ACTH) and beta-endorphin. Beta-endorphin reduces susceptibility to pain and is probably one of the means by which stress and the stimuli of conditioned fear give rise to endogenous analgesia. Other factors influence the release of ACTH, including antidiuretic hormone (ADH) and hypothalamic vasoactive intestinal peptide (VIP). The ACTH liberated by the anterior pituitary acts to stimulate cells in the adrenal cortex to secrete corticosteroids.

Glucocorticoids secreted by the adrenal cortex play a key role in adaptation to stress (Bowman & Rand 1980). Cortisol (hydrocortisone) accounts for about 95% of the glucocorticoid activity of the adrenal cortex. Glucocorticoids modify metabolism so as to increase blood glucose concentrations. They do this by mobilising tissue protein and amino acids and by these actions may induce a negative nitrogen balance. Glucocorticoids are needed to enable other hormones to bring about mobilisation and metabolism of fat. These metabolic effects of glucocorticoids ensure the supply of adequate fuel to the cells when the body is under stress, and in this respect the adrenal cortex provides an important back-up system for the adrenal medulla. In addition, glucocorticoids play important roles in the proper functioning of many organ systems and tissues in the body, including lymphoid tissue, the cardiovascular system, skeletal muscle and the nervous system.

Glucocorticoids such as cortisol and corticosteroid possess appreciable mineralocorticoid activity, retaining sodium chloride and indirectly increasing extracellular fluid volume, although they are much less potent in this respect than aldosterone. The secretion of aldosterone is not regulated by ACTH, and so its release is independent of the stress response. Mineralocorticoid activity by hormones such as cortisol may in part underlie important, though poorly understood, actions on the cardiovascular system. An increase of extracellular fluid volume can be of great importance under circumstances when stressors induce shock or when there is loss of body fluids after haemorrhage or burn injury.

Additionally, glucocorticoids can decrease the number of circulating lymphocytes, eosinophils and basophils and, at pharmacological concentrations, suppress the immune response. Finally, in addition to their direct effects, the corticosteroids exert an enabling influence on the actions of several other hormones and are, in fact, necessary for the body to show a full response to the adrenaline and noradrenaline released from the adrenal medulla. As a result of its wide-ranging functions, especially in the maintenance of fluid and electrolyte balance, the adrenal cortex is essential to life.

The chronic stress response

Clearly, as Selye (1976) found, there are limits to the body's ability to maintain its stage of resistance and adaptation in the face of continuing stress; environmental stressors can be toxic and physiologically overwhelming. Where the person is physiologically challenged but not overwhelmed, in conditions of prolonged stress, enlargement of the adrenal glands and thymicolymphatic atrophy will occur. When stress persists beyond a certain period of time, disturbances occur in the homeostatic balance of the body and there is an ever-increasing danger that disease processes will be precipitated.

An important part of the body's defence mechanism in the stage of resistance is the pituitary secretion of ACTH, which in turn stimulates the adrenal cortex to release corticosteroids. One of the early signs of the body's inability to meet the demands of unremitting stress is a blunting of the amounts of ACTH released by the anterior pituitary in response to that stress (Schatzberg & Nemeroff 1988). Under these circumstances, the adrenal cortex frequently shows hyperplasia, which persists despite the reduced secretion of ACTH. This blunting of the ACTH response to stress also occurs in long-standing timidity, which is possibly due to high arousal together with slow habituation to the stressors. This is coupled with an associated enlargement of the adrenal glands and hypersecretion of adrenal steroids under comparatively non-threatening circumstances. Likewise, blunting of the ACTH responses to stressors is seen in depressive illness and in many forms of anxiety. In depressed individuals, there is frequently a high corticosteroid excretion associated with enlargement of the adrenal glands and an increase in the concentrations of CRH in cerebrospinal fluid.

Emotional as well as hormonal changes characterise chronic stress. These include a decreased sensitivity to rewards and a withdrawal from decision-making characteristic of fatigue. This can progress to the condition known as 'burnout', a complex phenomenon involving extreme physical and emotional distress which, for the individual, is linked to organisational factors (Melchior et al 1996, Farrington 1997). In burnout the person feels physical fatigue along with a lack of involvement, sympathy or respect for colleagues and clients. At its final stage, chronic stress is followed by exhaustion and collapse. Long-lasting stress in which there is a poor coping strategy is correlated with increased occurrence of a variety of diseases (Levi 1971). These may be described as diseases of adaptation and are related to deranged secretion of adaptive hormones in the stage of resistance. These conditions include digestive disturbances, hypertension, myocardial infarction, allergies and sleep disturbances. Such chronic stress may also lead to anxiety, depression or behavioural disturbances, such as appetite disorders or increased usage of alcohol, tobacco, caffeine and drugs.

Due to the prevalence of cardiovascular disease in Western society, particular attention has been paid in recent years to the relationship of stress to hypertension, myocardial dysfunction leading to unexpected sudden death, and to coronary atherosclerosis and myocardial infarctions (Matthews et al 1986). It has been noted that vascular responses to a series of acute stresses in normotensive people living under permanent emotional stress sometimes become protracted and exaggerated. The excess of mineralocorticoid secretion in response to the stress in these persons raises peripheral resistance, and many later develop permanent hypertension.

Unexpected sudden death arising from cardiac failure has been found frequently to follow emotional upheaval or shock. It may be caused either by adrenosympathetically induced ventricular fibrillation or by apparent vagal stimulation and cardiac standstill. The increase in blood concentrations of glucocorticoids, mineralocorticoids and catecholamines as a result of stress can derange the vital myocardial electrolyte equilibrium. In a series of unexpected sudden deaths, the postmortem catecholamine concentrations in the blood were found to be excessively high, almost as high as in fatal adrenaline poisoning.

Finally, increase in the blood concentrations of adrenaline, by its enhancement of platelet aggregation, can promote thrombus formation in atherosclerotic coronary arteries and thus lead to myocardial infarction. Statistical data show a close correlation between the high incidence of ischaemic heart disease in professional persons exposed to demanding occupational stress and in the 'Type A' individual, characterised by time consciousness, irritability and driving ambition (see p. 623).

In view of the serious consequences of excessive or prolonged stress in combination with poor coping strategies, it can be seen that improvements to the working environment and social milieu, together with 'stress education' to lessen reactivity to adverse circumstances, might have as profound an impact on the health of a community as did the improvements to diet and sanitation in the mid-19th century.

STRESS AND DISEASE

Migraine

Migraine headaches have been known about for well over 2000 years and it is estimated that they are experienced by 10% of the population (Blau 1987). It is recognised that they are not caused solely by stress but have a number of precipitating factors such as menstrual cycle, diet, sounds and smells which, in conjunction with a feeling of stress, may trigger an attack. Many people report that the attack, paradoxically, occurs after the cessation of the stressful event.

For many people, migraine is a very debilitating and distressing condition. An analogy is of a storm building up and causing, instead of lightning, wind and rain, intense pain, nausea and vomiting, often lasting for several hours. The person is often prevented from continuing with normal activities. The phases of an attack are outlined in Box 17.1.

Box 17.1 Migraine phases (Blau 1987)

Migraine attacks follow a pattern consisting of the five phases described below. The third and fourth phases are prerequisites of a diagnosis of classical migraine.

1. Prodrome
- Subtle symptoms; may not be noticed
- Craving to eat sweet food
- Mood variations
- Tiredness
- Mild photophobia
- Heightened visual perception

2. Aura
- Multicoloured visual disturbances
- Scotoma with flickering, scintillating edge
- Tingling of face, sometimes one sided
- Numbness of face

3. Headache
- Slowly developing throbbing pain
- Lasts 2–72 h

4. Resolution
- Sleep is major resolving mechanism
- Vomiting

5. Postdromal phase
- 'Washed-out' or drained feeling
- Euphoria
- Impaired concentration
- Irritability
- Cerebral flow observations indicate that anomalies can outlast headache by 24 h

Physiologically, the hypothesis put forward to explain migraine (Blau 1987) is that stress causes cerebral hypoxia through increased activity in catecholamine pathways. This suggestion is supported by the observation that cerebral oxygen consumption rises when the individual is stressed. The role of the catecholamines, adrenaline, noradrenaline and dopamine is to activate the cerebral metabolism. If the nerve fibres penetrate deeply enough into the brain, the sympathetic nervous system could release noradrenaline and increase neuronal metabolism in the surrounding tissue. In this hypothesis stress increases cerebral metabolism thereby increasing the risk of migraine.

Treatment

The person should, if possible, identify the precipitating factors of his migraine attacks and avoid them. The pain can be treated with analgesics in conjunction with metoclopramide for the nausea; the latter will also improve the uptake of the analgesic from the intestine (Blau 1987).

Depression

It is not the case that everyone who feels stressed also has depression or anxiety, but the illness of depression can be the outcome of feelings of stress; conversely, people experiencing depression can also become stressed (Box 17.2).

It is difficult to formulate an exact definition of depression and its relationship to stress. The experience of depression seems to range from unpleasant but normal feelings of being 'fed up' to severe states of mental ill-health requiring psychiatric intervention. It is important to recognise that depression, which is a serious mental illness, can be life-threatening, as suicide and self-harm are frequent outcomes in severe depression. It is vital for health professionals to be alert to this possibility. According to Hawton (1989):

> *Among people who kill themselves, or who attempt suicide, approximately two-thirds have visited doctors, usually their general practitioners, within the month beforehand.*

Box 17.2 Depression: the facts (Paykel & Herbst 1989)

- 1 in 1000 of the general population are admitted to psychiatric hospitals annually with depression
- 3 in 1000 are referred by their GP to psychiatrists
- 2 in 1000 are treated for depression as outpatients
- General practitioners treat 3% of patients with depression, although it is estimated that a further 3% go unrecognised following a consultation with their doctor
- Prevalence of depression in the population is estimated at about 5%

Symptoms of depression

The presence of depression is often not obvious to the clinician, as observable signs do not always indicate the unpleasantness of the feelings that the individual is experiencing. Some symptoms, however, particularly when they occur in combination, strongly indicate the presence of depression. Symptoms often associated with depressed states include early morning wakening, a feeling of grinding tiredness, loss of energy, loss of interest in sexual relationships, loss of appetite, feeling 'down' and a feeling of bad temper. The link between anxiety and depression is debatable, but if we dispense with this division, the list of potential symptoms of depression might be expanded to include panic or anxiety attacks.

Feelings associated with depression

The relationship between stress and depression is an extremely close one. Some people experiencing depression feel stressed by, amongst other things, their inability to continue with day-to-day concerns. Others, who are burdened by overwhelming demands, respond by becoming depressed. What is not understood is why some people respond to stress by becoming depressed whilst others show other emotions such as anger.

People experiencing depression often describe their circumstances in terms that denote an ongoing feeling of oppression, as of being under a cloud, of everything looking black or grey, or of being in a tunnel without an end. Feelings of hope diminish, to be replaced by feelings of hopelessness. Depressed people often feel uncared for and alone even when this is not the case. Undertaking tasks or projects often becomes impossible as inertia takes the place of activity. Depressed individuals often blame themselves for problems in their relationships or daily lives where others who are not depressed might show anger. This leads to the hypothesis that depression is anger turned in on itself when for some reason it cannot be expressed openly (Freud 1917, Worden 1991).

People experiencing feelings of depression may have additional problems such as sleeplessness, anxiety and eating disorders. They may also be prey to overwhelming and terrifying urges to commit suicide as a way of freeing themselves from a seemingly hopeless situation.

Causes of depression

Depression can occur at any time in life and may follow on from any painful event or loss, such as the death of a loved one or the loss of a job. Depression which does not have an obvious cause when it occurs in adulthood may be the result of early childhood loss or distress. Individuals who have been the victims of sexual, physical or emotional abuse as children may suffer depression as adults in a delayed response to the loss associated with abuse, which is triggered by a more recent experience of distress. Early unresolved loss has been suggested as a possible explanation for the distressing symptoms of depression following childbirth. The depression of a parent witnessed in childhood may, for some, be at the root of depression experienced in adulthood (Miller 1987).

Q **17.4** Identify five stressors in each of the following categories:

(a) emotional
(b) physical
(c) environmental
(d) societal.

Anxiety attacks

Anxiety or panic attacks are characterised by severe sympathetic arousal, often in the absence of any obvious or immediate stressor. Panic attacks are a common presenting problem in those visiting their general practitioner (GP) with feelings of stress. During an attack, the person often experiences intense fear accompanied by physiological signs such as palpitations, sweating, trembling, rapid respiration and pallor. The fear may be associated with a fear of collapse, death or a need to escape. Sufferers often explain that they feel that their heart might burst.

By explaining the nature of these attacks, the nurse can sometimes bring an element of relief to the sufferer. It is true that the circularity of being afraid of the fear often intensifies the symptoms. Practical advice on the management of attacks is also helpful (see Case History 17.5).

Anxiety attacks are symptomatic of underlying distress. They can be acute and of rapid onset, occurring perhaps only once or twice, or can develop into a chronic symptom. Attacks may occur at any time, causing intense feelings of fear where there is no obvious cause, such as fear or discomfort in a centre seat at the cinema or on a bus. The stressor causing the attack may only become apparent (if at all) upon later introspection or therapy.

Post-traumatic stress disorder

This condition, which has been recognised for a number of years, can affect people who have experienced any serious accident or trauma outside the range of their normal experience, such as a severe road traffic accident, rape, physical attack, plane crash, bomb blast or war. The disorder can follow one or more of such events and can occur not only in those directly involved but also in those called to assist, such as emergency workers or onlookers. The greater the scale of the accident, the more likely it is for post-traumatic stress disorder to arise.

The person having escaped adversity and perhaps having a sense of relief at having escaped unharmed can be very perplexed at the occurrence, sometimes a considerable time after the event, of distressing symptoms. There may be a loss of memory and total amnesia and sufferers often report feeling psychically numbed (McKinley & Brooks 1991). Symptoms may include:

- mood swings and feelings of aggression
- feelings of alarm, anxiety and irritability
- feeling jumpy
- flashbacks to the original trauma — these leave the person feeling as though he were back in the situation of the trauma
- lack of interest in pleasurable events
- panic, phobic and depressed feelings
- sleep disturbances, e.g.
  —waking in alarm and not being able to get back to sleep
  —difficulty in getting off to sleep
  —early morning waking
  —distressing nightmares
  —night sweats.

Case History 17.5 Midwifery Sister D

Midwifery Sister D had been working very hard in her new post in the labour suite and she discussed with her colleagues her feeling of apprehension that she might make a mistake or be unable to deal with the management responsibility that her new post entailed. The suite was often understaffed, and although she realised that this was not her responsibility, she felt guilty about the demands it placed upon her colleagues. On her night off she went with one or two friends to a pub and although she had not drunk a great deal she knew that she had exceeded her usual limit.

The following morning she awoke with a feeling of unease that she found difficult to describe. She experienced something like a feeling of agitation but her skin also felt as if it were 'crawling'. She had planned to go for a walk with her friends but when she reached the park where she was to meet them the feeling she had experienced throughout the morning became much more intense. She became sweaty, had great difficulty in breathing and felt very afraid. Feeling her pulse, she realised that her heart was beating very fast. Sister D later described her fear that she might collapse and die during this attack. This feeling lasted for 10 minutes. Her friends took her home, and later she contacted her family doctor.

This episode was described by the doctor, following some routine investigations, as an anxiety attack. He explained what had happened physiologically and was able to offer reassurance. He suggested that she either attend a stress reduction workshop or talk to a counsellor, and reduce her coffee and alcohol consumption. After Sister D had taken the opportunity to talk about her fears and problems with a counsellor, she felt more able to deal with her new job. She noticed, however, that when she began to feel tired and worried, the physical signs of sweating and palpitation would re-emerge. She used this as an indication that she needed a rest. Sister D also noticed that alcohol exacerbated the problem, as it had during her first attack.

Postviral fatigue syndrome (myalgic encephalomyelitis)

The symptoms of this puzzling illness, which is also referred to as chronic fatigue syndrome and which seems to have close links with depression, include extreme muscle fatigue, poor memory and concentration and slips of the tongue (Wessley 1990). This condition can cause considerable distress and disability over a period of months and sometimes years. The individual may, with devastating consequences, be unable to continue full- or even part-time work or may be forced to take frequent periods of sick leave. This and other implications of the illness can cause stress to loved ones and adversely affect the well-being of the family as a whole.

Fatigue and depression as sequelae to infection have long been recognised, particularly in relation to Epstein–Barr, Coxsackie and other enteroviruses. It is important, however, that postviral fatigue syndrome not be mistaken for psychiatric illness (Calder et al 1987). Indeed, even today, not all GPs recognise postviral fatigue as a condition (Ho-Yen & Macnamara 1991).

Some commentators advise rest, while others, recognising the adverse effects of long-term inactivity, advise exercise. Good emotional support is vital, and it is most important that depression, where present, is treated (Lynch et al 1991). Other treatments are aimed at the detection of possible allergies and/or candidiasis and at maintaining a good diet. There is an extremely active ME association which often has local branches (see 'Useful addresses', p. 633).

THE CONCEPT OF COPING

Used in a neutral sense, the term 'coping' refers to the way in which the individual responds to a stressful situation or to the perception of threat, by attempting consciously and unconsciously to maintain an equilibrium. It can be revealing, however, to reflect upon everyday usage of the word, as it can be a value-laden term used in intrinsically judgemental descriptions of an individual's degree of mastery over a situation or environment. Consider the degree of approval or disapproval that might be implied in the following statements:

- 'She cannot cope.'
- 'He finds it difficult to cope with exams.'
- 'He couldn't cope with the patient's relatives.'
- 'She coped well in her first managerial position.'

The association of 'coping' with mastery and of 'failure to cope' with weakness should not be automatic. It may be the case that the individual who succumbs to feelings of stress is more able to sense tension in a situation than the person who gives the appearance of coping well. The person who removes himself from a situation may in fact be 'coping' with it, by acknowledging that distancing or disengagement is the best way in the circumstances to preserve emotional health or physical safety. In some situations, the determination to persevere or to achieve mastery can be a damaging choice, ending in disease.

Different situations demand different strategies for coping. In some cases the individual may need to confront a difficulty or overcome an obstacle. In other circumstances, he must learn how to carry on with his life in the face of an ongoing situation such as bereavement, disability or unemployment. What 'coping' entails will depend upon the individual's unique circumstances and needs, and various models such as resilience and hardiness have been put forward in an attempt to identify the factors that contribute to an individual's style of coping.

Models of coping

An understanding of the models of coping can enhance the ability of the nurse to care compassionately for patients who are experiencing stress.

One of the most well-known approaches to the concept of coping focuses on the role of personality in the individual's response to stressful events and identifies 'Type A' behaviours (see below) which characterise the individual as being particularly susceptible to the health risks associated with stress. In an alternative and influential approach which discusses coping within the context of stress, burnout, support and hardiness, Kobasa (1979) attempts to identify those who are particularly resilient, i.e. who exhibit hardiness under stress (Duquette et al 1995). Those with hardiness are less likely to have physical or psychological symptoms, are less likely to become emotionally exhausted and have a sense of personal achievement (Dillard 1990). This concept has many similarities with that of resilience (see p. 617).

Some models describe coping in terms of the palliation strategies; for example, strategies that may be sought by those experiencing the early stages of burnout are exercise, relaxation, prescribed medication, drug abuse, smoking and alcohol consumption. Other models describe coping in terms of problem-solving, or, as in

Lazarus' (1966) approach, in terms of a dynamic process by which the individual engages himself with the source of stress. It is also possible to discuss coping in terms of defence mechanisms that the individual employs to preserve himself from a perceived threat (see p. 624).

Coping and personality

Some people appear to be relatively unaffected by traumatic events, while others seem to be quite unable to withstand what might appear to the onlooker as minor upheavals. Researchers have attempted to identify personality 'types' which are more likely than others to cope effectively with stress, by isolating relatively stable and highly consistent inborn personality dispositions or traits which enable the individual to function well in difficult situations. Such traits may be related to, for example, conformity or non-conformity, conscientiousness, compulsive behaviour, or the ability to suppress, repress or sublimate feelings.

Type A behaviour. Extensive research into the question of whether there are certain people who experience stress more acutely than most others, and who are more likely to succumb to cardiac or circulatory disease as a result, has identified a 'Type A' individual who is at particular risk from the effects of stress. Type A behaviour is not, strictly speaking, a trait; traits are by definition inborn, whereas Type A behaviour appears to be learned by social modelling. Type A people both wish to achieve and are high achievers (Westra & Kuiper 1997) and are more likely to have a job-centred lifestyle than one based upon interpersonal contacts with others (Fukunishi & Hattori 1997). Type A behaviour seems to have very positive short-term consequences; for example, in business or other organisations, people who show involvement, drive and initiative are often highly valued, although this behaviour may be linked to suppressed feelings of hostility and anger, which confer different cardiovascular disease risks (O'Connor et al 1995, Miller et al 1996). The long-term consequences of Type A behaviour, however, are often negative. The Type A person is typically observed engaged in polyphasic activity, concurrently undertaking a number of tasks; characteristics associated with this personality type include time urgency, hostility, difficulty in expressing anger, impatience, desire for control and aggression. The following interrelated elements are present in the personality:

- a set of beliefs about oneself in relation to the world
- a set of values which merge with motivation and commitment
- a set of beliefs about lifestyle that are focused upon achievement and control.

Type A individuals invest a great deal of themselves in their lifestyle and expend a great deal of energy in maintaining control. When challenged, their response is often highly emotional; this is likely to stimulate frequent surges of catecholamine secretion, which is likely to induce, in the physically unhealthy person, coronary heart disease. These people often show signs of raised serum cholesterol levels, raised serum fats and diabetic-like traits; at the same time they are frequently smokers who do not have time for regular exercise. Understandably, Type A behaviour is often highly destructive to relationships with family members, friends or colleagues.

It is important to bear in mind that people can change their learned behaviours and improve their ability to cope with certain experiences. In addition, there can be some degree of habituation to stressors such that they seem less stressful over time.

Personality and health. Kobasa (1979) examined the mediating effects of personality, not in relation to stress and disease, but in relation to stress and health. Whilst much research effort had been directed towards understanding the role of mediators such as early childhood influences, physiological predisposition and social resources in relation to the onset of disease, Kobasa asked why some people can be under considerable stress but not become ill. Using the social readjustment rating scale (Holmes & Rahe 1967), she tested the following hypotheses:

- People who have a greater sense of control over their own lives will remain healthier than those with a sense of powerlessness.
- People who have a sense of commitment to various areas of their lives will be healthier than those who have a sense of alienation.
- People who view change as a challenge will remain healthier than those who view change as a threat.

Kobasa postulated a state of hardiness in the personalities of those who can be stressed without becoming ill. The hardy person has certain characteristics, including:

- a clear sense of self and of personal meaning
- an understanding of values, goals and capabilities and a belief in their importance
- a vigorous involvement in and commitment to his own environment
- an internal locus of control
- active involvement in change.

The process model of coping

Lazarus & Folkman (1984) described coping in terms of a dynamic process involving movement, force and energy within the individual and his relationship with the source of stress. An important feature of the process approach is that it reflects the fact often observed in clinical settings that an individual's response to his situation changes and evolves over time. This response is highly complex and unique to each individual and might be described as occurring in stages, although these stages are not sequential or predictable.

Worden (1991), for example, described four tasks of mourning that the individual must complete in order to emerge from a state of grief:

- accepting the reality of the loss
- experiencing the pain of grief
- adjusting to an environment from which the deceased is missing
- withdrawing emotional energy and reinvesting it in another relationship.

For the individual, these tasks of mourning may not be sequential, but may be experienced instead as an 'ebb and flow' of feelings. For the nurse, Worden's definition of the tasks of grieving will give an indication of the direction that a person might take in his mourning. For the individual concerned, the stages passed through might be recognised only in hindsight.

The process approach emphasises that the individual copes with stress in a unique way that is governed by both childhood and adult experience. The ability to cope is shaped by the developmental processes that the individual undergoes from birth to death. The individual's perspective will change continually, and situations that may be stressful at one time may be viewed differently at another stage of life.

PSYCHOLOGICAL DEFENCES

While it is possible to think of defence mechanisms as both conscious and unconscious strategies of self-protection against perceived threat, these mechanisms may seriously compromise the effective functioning of the individual. Defence mechanisms operate essentially by restricting situations which are seen as threatening, narrowing down the individual's field of action to one that is manageable. They enable the individual, often against overwhelming odds, to maintain an equilibrium of feelings, thoughts and actions in daily life.

Problems arise when they feature inappropriately, as when a defence mechanism first acquired to combat severe or terrifying feelings in one domain becomes active without cause in another, perpetuating the emotional disturbance that gave rise to the mechanism in the first place. This may occur some time after the original experience, and the content of that experience may not be accessible to the person even after therapy. While it is useful for the clinician to bear in mind that unresolved conflict may exist, the detailed and often long-term task of helping the person to understand the extent of his defences is best left to therapists and counsellors.

Defences may be compared to a sea wall in that the magnitude of the original intense fear and distress will determine the height, breadth and depth of the defence. These defences are not always infallible, however; they can be breached during sleep, under the influence of alcohol and other drugs, and in conditions of stress.

A number of defence mechanisms have been identified, the most common of which are listed in Box 17.3.

MANAGEMENT OF STRESS

The management of stress can be approached in a number of ways. One of these is to offer the individual the opportunity to examine the sources of his stress in present or childhood experience and to consider ways of modifying his responses to that stress. This kind of therapy can be provided by a psychotherapist, clinical psychologist or qualified counsellor. The nurse should be familiar with the basic approaches available within psychological therapy; two significant models, patient-centred therapy and cognitive therapy, are described on page 625.

Some individuals suffering from acute anxiety or depression may find it impossible to confront the source of their difficulty and to make constructive changes without first being given some relief from their distressing feelings. Here, carefully monitored drug therapy can facilitate recovery and change. Again, the nurse should be familiar with the most common pharmaceutical agents used in this type of treatment; these are briefly described on pages 626–627.

The individual suffering from stress can also learn a number of techniques that will assist him to reduce or manage his stress in day-to-day life. Techniques such as relaxation, yoga, biofeedback, visualisation and meditation have all gained in credibility and popularity in recent years. When taught well and followed up with continuing support, courses in such techniques can help people to adopt a new approach to the problem of stress. Moreover, learning a new skill such as deep relaxation can impart to the individual a feeling of well-being which may facilitate positive change in various areas of his life. We should remind ourselves, however, that if stress lies in the interaction between the person and his environment, or in the meaning he attributes to his situation, then clearly a short workshop on relaxation (for example) cannot hope to seriously address the source of his stress. Indeed, it should be borne in mind that there is a potential for courses in stress reduction to exacerbate the problem if the individual is made to feel that any stress that is not helped by the techniques offered is intractable or somehow abnormal.

Box 17.3 Defence mechanisms

Repression
Unconsciously keeping unacceptable feelings out of awareness. Not acknowledging angry or jealous feelings towards others.

Disavowal or denial
This defence blocks out a perception from memory. Someone whose father left the family at birth may unconsciously think of him as having died rather than confront the feelings of loss and anger.

Projection
In projection, people unconsciously attribute to others their own aggressive or angry feelings. The feeling that one is being 'got at' by a colleague may be a projection of one's own angry negative feelings towards the colleague.

Introjection
The acceptance of another's values and opinions as one's own. A young person living with a domineering parent may unconsciously accept the attitudes of the parent rather than risk confrontation.

Reversal
This is the process of detaching a feeling from the person or object to whom it should be directed and directing it to oneself instead. A wish to physically harm another may instead become a process of self-harm.

Displacement
Strong feelings towards another person may be directed towards someone less dangerous than the original source of the feeling. A child experiencing powerful and angry feelings towards a mother may punish a favourite doll instead.

Isolation
In isolation, a feeling is detached from a thought in order to deprive the thought of emotional significance. Nurses sometimes describe helping at the scene of an accident without being in touch with the experience of the associated feelings.

Reaction formation
Unacceptable feelings disguised by repression of the real feeling and the reinforcement of the opposite feeling. A husband caring for a disabled wife may feel angry at her dependence, but instead shower her with loving attention.

Rationalisation
In rationalisation, false reasons are found to justify unacceptable attitudes. Following the termination of an employment contract, a person might claim to be pleased to be no longer employed, rather than acknowledge painful feelings of worthlessness.

Conversion
This is the process of converting a psychological disturbance into a physical disorder. A feeling of panic or fear accompanied by physical symptoms may be regarded as physical symptoms alone by the person, to unconsciously avoid confronting the cause.

Therapy

Psychodynamic therapy

Although Freud, as a psychoanalyst, was working mainly with people who were seriously mentally ill, many of the theoretical concepts he used can be applied to the contemporary experience of individual stress (Freud 1914). He did not, however, use the term 'stress' in his work with his patients, but used instead the diagnosis of neurosis, melancholia and hysteria to designate particular types of symptoms.

Since Freud began writing his important works, from 1896 onwards, psychoanalysis has developed many schools and approaches (Bateman & Holmes 1996). Psychoanalytical and psychodynamic therapies are predicated upon the belief that a large part of the person's psychic life is unconscious. The analogy of an iceberg is helpful here — the person is unaware of the influences that may be affecting his conscious life (Stafford-Clark 1987). Within the unconscious are wishes, uncomfortable memories, hurts or traumas that have been pushed out of consciousness and kept repressed, but which have an important effect upon the person's conscious life and especially upon relationships with others.

In psychoanalytic or psychodynamic therapy, the person seeking help is encouraged to work with the therapist in a way that enables the features of the unconscious relationships that are so destructive to emerge. For instance, a person who as a small child experienced the depression of a parent, and who unconsciously blamed himself for what was happening to that parent, might in adult life treat those with whom he has a close relationship as if they were psychically fragile. In so doing, the person is transferring his unconscious relationship with the parent — which might also, for example, be full of frustration and anger — onto adult conscious relationships. This is called transference, and the therapist then works with the patient to explore consciously the meanings of the transference, to enable the person to change his way of being. To be able to help the patient through the transference, the therapist must herself have undergone personal therapy.

Person-centred therapy

Person-centred therapy was first described by the psychologist Carl Rogers (1974). In the therapeutic setting, the counsellor works with the client in a way that enables him to explore his own feelings. Rogers' core conditions of unconditional acceptance, warmth, genuineness and empathy are used by the counsellor to enable the client to begin to develop trust and then to move on to greater understanding of his own feelings. Thorne (1990) emphasised that to be able to help the client achieve this, the counsellor must be congruent. The counsellor's own behaviour must closely match her own feelings.

Cognitive therapy

In 1963–64 the psychologist A T Beck identified certain manifestations of 'thought disorder' (Dryden 1990) by which people entertain thoughts that, in a number of ways, harm them. According to Beck's theory, people ordinarily function effectively in their day-to-day lives as problem-solvers. For example, the nurse who considers applying for promotion may try to consider objectively whether she has the relevant experience, training and personality for the job. If, however, she is feeling depressed, her thoughts might be negative or destructive, as in 'Why apply for this? I wouldn't get it anyway. I'm no good at anything'.

Cognitive therapists work closely with people to help them identify negative or dysfunctional thoughts and to replace them with positive, enabling thoughts which will help them to cope with difficult situations. This approach attempts to relieve disabling psychological symptoms while reinforcing the person's own psychological responses. At the same time, it offers detailed analysis of interpersonal or other situations that cause problems. This type of therapy does not seek first and foremost to find the causes of distress by, for instance, re-examining childhood trauma; nor is it centred on the person's own feelings to the same degree as client-centred therapy. It is, rather, directed towards the alleviation of distressing symptoms with a view to enabling the person to have positive experiences in his day-to-day life and thus enhance his ability to deal with other new challenges. The underpinning theory is that if the person can change the way that he reacts to situations and relationships, by dealing with them differently, then his experiences and relationships will improve, thus creating a positive cycle. Cognitive therapists work with people experiencing anxiety and phobias as well as other psychological problems.

Finding and choosing therapeutic help

There are a number of ways to find therapeutic help with feelings of stress, although the availability of some types of psychotherapy will depend upon where in the UK the person seeking help lives. Whilst many people travel long distances to see a counsellor or psychotherapist, the regular nature of the consultations, which may be weekly, may indeed cause an added burden if extensive travel is required.

If psychotherapeutic help is sought through the NHS, a referral can be made by the GP. Many departments of clinical psychology will accept self-referrals, but will ask to contact the person's GP.

Where the therapy being sought is private, the person pays a fee for each consultation, in contrast to help through the NHS which is free. There are a number of ways to contact a therapist, and various professional bodies for counselling and psychotherapy will give suggestions (see 'Useful addresses', p. 633).

For therapy to be effective it must respond to the person within his own frame of reference and be relevant to his own life from his own unique perspective. Finding an appropriate form of therapy can be very difficult for the individual, and many people are reluctant to approach a professional agency or voluntary organisation for assistance with personal problems. Many people think about it and wait for long periods before plucking up the courage to seek help, and often their first point of contact is with a member of the primary care team at their local surgery; this may be the GP, the practice nurse or another member of the primary care team, such as the health visitor or community psychiatric nurse. The practice nurse, or nurse practitioner (Martin & Starling 1989) undertaking screening programmes, is in a uniquely placed position to be able to listen to patients who are distressed (Cunningham 1996).

Often, merely discussing the problem with a member of the practice team can provide great relief. However, when further help is required, the patient can be referred to other mental health specialists, such as:

- the practice counsellor
- community psychiatric nurse
- a clinical psychologist
- community psychiatrist
- community mental health team.

The GP may also wish to discuss with the patient the possibility of prescribing antidepressants, and will be able to ensure that the patient is not suffering from an organic illness such as hyper- or hypothyroidism or anaemia which can cause symptoms similar to depression. Reassurance can be given that panic attacks are not life-threatening and advice can be given on how to deal with them. The GP can also authorise official sick leave to enable the patient to rest.

The therapist–client relationship

People are highly individual in their feelings, experiences, backgrounds and personalities. A model of therapy which is helpful to one person may not suit another, and a therapist who is helpful to one person may fail to establish a good rapport with another. For this reason it is important for therapists to be clear with their clients about the way they work, what the work involves, its likely duration and, if private consultation is sought, its cost. It is possible for the client to change therapists if the therapy does not seem to be helpful, although there is one major proviso to this. For personal change to take place, therapist and client must work closely in a relationship of trust. This will enable the therapist to reflect back and challenge the behaviour that is causing the client distress. The fact that this can be an unsettling experience for the client may not be the right reason for him to leave therapy. Nevertheless, the therapist should be willing to discuss any feeling on the client's part that the therapy is detrimental or unhelpful and, if appropriate, to give guidance on finding an alternative therapist.

The person wishing to become a therapist must undertake extensive training, which involves the study of theory as well as undertaking supervised work with clients. Nurses working in clinical settings can undertake shortened courses which will help them to develop the necessary skills to listen in a therapeutic way to people in their daily work. An example of therapeutic listening is given in Case History 17.6.

Case History 17.6 Mrs A

Mrs A cares for her mentally and physically handicapped son, J, at home with the help of the community nursing service and the local social work department. She is 68 years old and a widow; her son is 29. He is visually impaired and unable to communicate easily by speaking. He is always incontinent. Although he can walk, Mrs A always has to guide him. Getting him out of bed and dressed in the morning is very heavy work for her.

Mrs A has known her community nurse, B, for a number of years. B feels a sense of despair that Mrs A never has any freedom from J and has rarely had any time to herself in the years she has known her. B has tried repeatedly, both by herself and in conjunction with social work colleagues, to plan some respite care for J. This planning has taken the form of a provision for day care at a local day centre and periods of respite care at a local residential unit. But somehow when the time came for J to attend, Mrs A managed to avoid sending him. The only assistance she will accept is from the local care attendant team; one helper, who has become a friend, sits with J for 2 hours while Mrs A does her shopping.

One day B was able to sit and talk with Mrs A whilst J was asleep. By listening carefully to her, B realised that Mrs A felt extremely guilty about J's handicap. She felt that she had caused J's condition by not taking sufficient rest during her pregnancy, and she relieved her feelings of guilt by caring for him all the time. She was also extremely fearful of what would happen to J after she died.

B listened to Mrs A carefully as she talked about her painful feelings, and was aware that she had not been able to share these feelings with anyone before. She did not try to make Mrs A feel better by taking away her feelings of guilt, nor did she try to reassure her. Instead, she simply listened carefully and attentively.

They did not talk again about this problem although B was ready to listen if Mrs A wished to raise the subject again. Some time later, however, Mrs A asked B if she could help her organise some day care for J, as it would help him to get used to other people. B was then able to arrange respite care for J, which also enabled B to get some rest.

Drug therapy

The personal experience of stress can be so severe and overwhelming that the individual finds himself unable to take any action to alleviate his feelings. Severe anxiety or depression, perhaps in combination with an overpowering feeling that a serious physical illness is lurking, can have an immobilising effect on the person so that even the prospect of action to alleviate symptoms is daunting. When people feel as severely distressed as this, they may begin to entertain thoughts of suicide.

Drug therapy can help to alleviate severe distress by relieving its most acute symptoms and thus enabling emotional rest to take place. Some drugs are intended to help with sleeplessness, while others which do not have a tranquillising effect will permit those taking them to continue to work, to problem-solve, to drive, and so on. Drug therapy should always be supplemented by continuing monitoring and support by the medical practitioner. The following provides a brief overview of the main types of drugs used in the treatment of stress-related conditions.

For more detailed information on drug therapy the reader is referred to Lacey (1996).

Tricyclic and related antidepressants

The most common antidepressant drugs used in severe stress and depression are the tricyclic and related groups. These are usually prescribed to people suffering from moderate to severe depression, although it is important to realise that they work by alleviating symptoms. This can be useful; for instance, the person who is debilitated by anxiety might be able to find ways of living that are more constructive once his feelings of anxiety are lifted. These drugs may not be helpful, however, when the depression is related to bereavement, an unhappy working environment, overwhelming family responsibilities or disturbing memories of abuse or neglect, for it is only when the underlying cause of depression can be understood that the person is likely to obtain any lasting benefit.

Management. The person prescribed tricyclic antidepressants must be seen frequently following prescription. These drugs can take 2–4 weeks to begin to have an effect; during this time the patient may feel isolated and helpless. Side-effects include the following:

- constipation
- sleepiness
- dry mouth
- blurred vision
- urinary retention
- sweating.

Tolerance seems to develop over time and some of the side-effects become less unpleasant.

If the individual's depression is severe, he may feel like killing himself. Careful support and perhaps hospitalisation may be essential at this time. Treatment with this group of drugs should be continued for at least 1 month (BMA 1998). Reduction or withdrawal of the drug should be carried out very slowly to avoid severe symptoms such as strange, fragmented dreams, headaches, recurrence of anxiety, depression or restlessness.

Selective serotonin reuptake inhibitors

This group of drugs block the reuptake of 5-hydroxytryptamine (5-HT), producing an increase in the amount of the neurotransmitter at central synapses.

Monoamine oxidase inhibitors (MAOIs)

This group of drugs prevents the breakdown of monoamine neurotransmitters, thereby prolonging their action. They are recommended for people with depression, anxiety and somatic complaints, for patients who do not respond to tricyclics and patients with agoraphobia.

Lithium

Lithium possibly decreases noradrenaline release and enhances its reuptake. Lithium salts are used to treat mania and hypomania, and to prevent mania and depression.

Trazodone Hydrochloride

This drug exhibits antiserotonin and α-receptor antagonist properties. Its sedative properties are useful in the treatment of anxiety.

Benzodiazepine tranquillisers

The benzodiazepine group of drugs fell into disrepute when people who had been taking them for long periods found that their original symptoms were often intensified and that the drugs were addictive. It is recommended that these drugs are prescribed for periods not exceeding 2 or 3 weeks and that careful supervision is provided by the GP (BMA 1998).

Other means of stress reduction

Exercise

Although there is strong anecdotal and research evidence that regular vigorous exercise has a positive effect upon the individual's ability to deal with feelings of depression and stress, the palliative effects of exercise are not generally accepted or understood; for instance, those taking physical exercise may have considerable light exposure and this may have a therapeutic effect upon feelings of depression (Groom & O'Connor 1996). There is evidence that aerobic exercise may trigger panic attacks in those already experiencing them (Reif & Hermanutz 1996). Proponents of exercise as a means of stress reduction argue that exercise is generally essential for psychological, physiological and social development, having a direct effect upon feelings of self-esteem. (Segar et al 1998). However, in the treatment of depression, aerobic exercise in particular is efficacious (Beesley & Mutrie 1997, Moore & Blumenthal 1998). Physical fitness is seen as a positive aid towards emotional stability. Guidelines for exercise as a means towards stress reduction are given in Box 17.4.

Box 17.4 Guidelines for exercise

- Any exercise is good
- Set aside a specific time for exercise. Treat that time as sacrosanct, but do not feel worried if it is necessary for some reason to miss a session
- Exercise at least three times a week if possible, for at least half an hour
- Exercise should be gentle but vigorous; build up slowly to a good exercise level
- If in doubt, have a health check and talk over your exercise programme with your general practitioner prior to starting

Exercise works in a paradoxical manner in reducing stress; it is, itself, a physical stressor causing an acute stress response but nonetheless functions as a relaxant. The physiological effects of exercise include increased blood flow and oxygen consumption as well as changes in blood pressure, heart rate, respiration and metabolic rate.

Physical exercise can act as a relaxant for a number of reasons:

- Most exercise involves effort and concentration and it can be difficult to sustain anxious thought whilst engaged in physical exercise.
- Meeting a physical challenge can give the individual a sense of achievement.
- During strenuous exercise the body produces noradrenaline and endorphins; these substances help to alleviate depression and bring about feelings of happiness and tranquillity.
- Exercise can be taken alongside other people and so can diminish feelings of social isolation.

Relaxation

Relaxation along with other alternative therapies, such as aromatherapy, guided imagery and massage (Vines 1994), has long been known to help alleviate feelings of stress and to enhance health-seeking behaviours. Relaxation may take various forms, including relieving muscle tension (e.g. through exercise), taking time off, either on a daily or weekly basis or as a scheduled holiday, and meditation. Everly & Benson (1989) discuss the response elicited physiologically and psychologically by certain types of meditative relaxation. They identify two components of these meditation techniques (Knight 1995) which cause the relaxation response and a reduction in feelings of stress:

- the repetition of a word, sound, phrase, liturgical prayer
- the positive disregard of everyday thoughts when they come to mind.

There are six types of activity which specifically foster this type of relaxation:

- meditation
- autogenic training
- pre-suggestion hypnosis
- prayer (repetitive or liturgical)
- yoga exercises
- *t'ai chi chu'an.*

For many people these techniques produce a sense of well-being as well as an increase in concentration and energy. They also produce the following physiological changes (Everly & Benson 1989):

- decreased oxygen consumption and carbon dioxide elimination with no change in the respiratory quotient
- reduced heart and respiratory rates and lowered blood lactate
- reduced blood pressure (during exercise).

Everly & Benson (1989) show that during relaxation there are physiological alterations consistent with a decrease in central and peripheral adrenergic excitation, and that people who undertake regular meditative relaxation (see Box 17.5) recover faster from stressful events than those who do not relax in this way.

Paradoxically, for some people experiencing anxiety, the effort of trying to relax can intensify their feelings of panic (Heide & Borkovec 1983). Feelings of not being in control intensify and the experience of relaxing, by not being achievable, becomes a negative one.

Box 17.5 Guidelines for meditative relaxation

Setting the scene
- Find a quiet, warm, comfortable room where you are unlikely to be disturbed (try to exclude children, pets, ticking clocks or telephones)
- Meditate sitting upright and well supported in a comfortable chair. Rest the feet flat on the floor and the hands loosely in your lap
- Have a watch or clock in clear view. The session lasts 20 minutes. If you feel that you are likely to fall asleep, set an alarm
- Loosen any tight clothing; slip off your shoes if this makes you more comfortable
- Meditate whilst neither too hungry nor too full
- Try to meditate twice each day for 20 minutes. Because you may feel deeply relaxed, it is better not to meditate close to bedtime, as this might interfere with your sleep patterns

The process
- During the process of meditation you will remain completely conscious
- You may prefer to meditate with your eyes closed. Begin the process by taking one or two deep, relaxing breaths
- Gently begin to count, either on each inhalation or exhalation, with the number one, then two, then three... Every time you become aware of a thought, any thought, calmly return to number one. It is unlikely, though, that after a number of years of regular meditating you will go beyond the number one; indeed, the principle of this sort of meditation is not one of mastery, but of the gentle pushing aside of thoughts to enable the body and the mind to achieve complete rest
- You may find that you have spent the whole session thinking over a problem. If so, do not worry; before you finish the session gently return to the counting, for 1 or 2 minutes
- If you find that you have fallen asleep, do not worry about this. It may be that you are very tired and your body needs sleep. Before finishing the relaxation, gently return to the counting for 1 or 2 minutes. If you find that during the meditation, you have solved a major problem, written a poem or worked out a solution, before finishing the session, gently return to your counting
- At the end of the session, before moving, stretch gently and sit with the eyes closed for a few moments

STRESS IN NURSING

Sources of stress

Nursing can be an extremely exciting and satisfying profession. The rewards of seeing patients move from ill-health to health and from disability to independence are great. To nurse a dying person in a way that enables him to die without pain and with dignity can also be very fulfilling. When nurses have the benefit of comprehensive managerial and educational support plus clinical supervision, there is a general enhancement of all aspects of work (Hallberg 1994). When formal support does not exist, nursing is by its very nature likely to cause some degree of stress. In certain cases the nurse may find that she is unable to help the patient recover and is only able to offer support as he comes to accept permanent disablement or chronic disease. The nurse may feel that her role is a passive and unhelpful one and she may feel frustrated and distressed by her inability to help. As Menzies (1960) wrote:

> *Nurses are in constant contact with people who are physically ill or injured, often seriously. The recovery of patients is not certain and will not always be complete. Nursing patients who have incurable diseases is one of the nurse's most distressing tasks. Nurses are confronted by the threat and the reality of suffering and death as few lay people are. Their work involves carrying out tasks which, by ordinary standards, are distasteful, disgusting and frightening... The work situation arouses very strong and mixed feelings in the nurse: pity, compassion and love; guilt and anxiety; hatred and resentment of the patients who aroused these strong feelings; envy of the care given to patients.*

Patient-centred care

In 1960, Menzies described nurses as working in a task-oriented way with patients. This way of working allowed nurses only minimal contact with each patient and, Menzies hypothesised, enabled them to be emotionally defended against feelings of anxiety caused by contact with patients. Because they were always moving on to the next task, they did not have time to listen to their patients. This defence, Menzies argued, while offering protection against anxiety, was a source of dissatisfaction for the nurse and impeded personal growth and maturation.

Soon after this, the curriculum in nurse education began to change. The earlier emphasis on 'training' and the learning of nursing tasks was replaced, albeit gradually, with a more balanced curriculum. Nurses are now being educated to use a more holistic and individualised approach to patient care with more emphasis upon the psychological and interpersonal underpinnings to clinical work, where the nurse is encouraged to enter into a cooperative contract with the patient in the planning of care. Nurses are being asked to work in this way in the face of budgetary constraints and sometimes inadequate staffing levels. The difficulties of putting this approach into practice may contribute to increased stress, anxiety and disenchantment. After all, it is inherent in this approach that nurses no longer have the benefit of the defences previously offered by task-oriented care (Menzies 1960), which protected them from the rigours associated with close interpersonal contact with patients. If nursing education is to give students and qualified nurses the ability to interact more closely with patients then, as a comcomitant to this, it must also teach methods of giving and getting support.

Stress can be described as 'sticky', and nurses who care on a daily basis for those who are ill and distressed, afraid or dying may find that some of the distress adheres to them. Over a period of time the distress can accumulate, particularly if the nurse also has personal problems. Thus, it is important that nurses themselves have peace of mind and good mental health, so as to be able to identify the sources of their own stress, and good support and supervision of nurses at all stages of their career is axiomatic.

Working with dying patients

The nurse caring for terminal patients may experience strong feelings during the period before the patient dies and may also grieve following the death. When the nurse is working in a clinical setting such as oncology, the grief may become compounded by factors such as a personal relationship with the family or a decision not to continue with treatment. Other factors, such as the nurse's personal experience of death, e.g. in her own family, may further compound the grief (Feldstein & Gemma 1995) (Case History 17.7). A sense of relief may be felt that the person who has been cared for over a long period has died, particularly if the patient has been severely ill. Some nurses, however, work in clinical settings where death may be sudden rather than timely, such as operating

Case History 17.7 Community Nurse E

E is a community nursing sister in a small town. She is attached to a busy general practice where other team members work together sharing patient care. They also spend some social time together and are generally able to give support to one another when it is needed.

E had been closely involved with the care of Mrs M, a 45-year-old woman suffering from multiple sclerosis. E had shared Mrs M's care with a colleague, but during the last year she had visited the family on almost a daily basis on her working days, as the nursing care required increased in complexity. Throughout the year Mrs M's condition deteriorated considerably. She died before Christmas, shortly after being admitted to the local general hospital.

E had got to know Mrs M's family well and following her death she tried on a number of occasions to visit them. This became increasingly difficult as time went on and E found herself driving longer distances than necessary to avoid passing their house. She began to feel extremely distressed by this and suffered from overwhelming feelings of guilt. She also found that she was short-tempered with her own family and began taking some sick leave just to give herself a break. She could not understand why she was feeling as she did and felt ashamed.

Later she was able to talk over her feelings with a colleague. This woman, who had also been a bereavement counsellor, working for Cruse (see 'Useful addresses', p. 633), gently suggested that perhaps E had also 'lost' Mrs M and was also grieving. E soon found herself talking about the feelings she had experienced following the death of her own mother a number of years before and her strong feelings of guilt at not being with her when she died.

E later felt able to visit the family. She was able to talk openly and with affection of Mrs M and she was able to return to them on later occasions. E also took the opportunity offered by her colleague to informally talk over the experience of visiting Mrs M's family and of her own feelings. She felt as if a weight had been lifted from her shoulders.

theatres (Edwards 1997). Psychiatric nurses also experience sudden death when patients tragically commit suicide (Midence et al 1996). Within the busy clinical context of a hospital or general practice, it can be difficult to share feelings arising from these experiences in a way that can bring relief (Kushnir et al 1997).

Fear of dying

Many studies looking at stress in nursing draw attention to the distressing aspects of working with people who are dying and the emotional strain of caring for them and their families through this extremely difficult time, while at the same time offering skilled compassionate care (Spencer 1994). It would be misleading, however, to say that working with terminally ill people is always distressing or stressful in predictable ways, for, as has been discussed (see p. 616), the experience of stress is related both to the person and to the situation. A philosophy of palliative care that offers nurses a model encompassing the concepts of control, challenge and commitment may enable them to develop and retain hardiness (Hutchings 1997).

Unlike many people in society, nurses regularly care for people who are dying and their families, and in this way they are confronted with the reality that others may have the opportunity to repress: the fear of dying and the concomitant anxiety, which may be expressed in somatisation and isolation (Feldstein & Gemma 1995).

The feeling of fear and anxiety that can surround the process of death may be non-specific and, as such, difficult to understand. As with physiological responses to stress, the symptoms may seem far removed from the causes, e.g. the development of painful headaches or anxiety that might follow a bereavement.

Lazarus & Folkman (1984) describe a type of coping that is not related to mastery of a situation but is an experiential learning process. This model is particularly relevant to the situation of professionals working clinically with dying people. For example, in Case History 17.7, E is not looking for help in problem-solving when she shares her feelings with her colleague. Rather, she is working through a process of grief and self-understanding which started at the time of her mother's death and which she finally comes to recognise through her relationship with Mrs M's family.

Grief and bereavement are generally not pathological states. They are normal, if often very painful, aspects of human experience. Coming to terms with loss can present the person with an opportunity for personal growth, although this may not be realised for a considerable period; if the process of mourning is suppressed, however, grief can become a source of depression or chronic stress (Worden 1991).

When in the presence of a dying patient, who is perhaps frightened or experiencing pain, the nurse may, as well as feeling distressed by her patient's suffering, be acutely aware of the possibility of the same thing happening to herself or her family. It is hardly surprising that this area of care can be one that causes distressing feelings for nurses, especially in a society such as ours that does not give great recognition to the reality of death and dying.

Support and clinical supervision for nurses

There is a long tradition in the UK of supervision amongst counsellors and psychotherapists. This practice has become enshrined in the accreditation of counsellors currently offered by the British Association for Counselling and is a requirement of other bona fide qualifying bodies for counselling and psychotherapy (see 'Useful addresses', p. 633). The principle is that the person who is undertaking counselling work meets regularly with a supervisor, i.e. someone who is doing similar work and has skills of giving support, to discuss confidentially her feelings about her work. Nurses who listen carefully to their patients are doing work that is intense, exacting and difficult, and supervision can offer them invaluable support (Ayer at al 1997, Begat et al 1997).

The clinical supervisor's work is not just to reassure the nurse, but also to allow the emotional disturbance to be felt within the safer setting of the supervisory relationship, where it can be survived and reflected upon. The development of a reflective approach to both educational needs and professional support in the context of a therapeutic relationship with the patient is the positive outcome of clinical supervision (Scanlon & Weir 1997).

Supervision is essential for those who call upon their inner resources in an effort to listen empathically to others (Palsson et al 1994). Supervision can enable nurses to develop an awareness of the full extent of their therapeutic role in working with patients. Good regular supervision can also prevent the nurse from succumbing to emotional fatigue, disillusionment and apathy (see Box 17.6).

Box 17.6 Guidelines for using clinical supervision and support

For the patient
When support or clinical supervision is sought by the clinical nurse in her work with a patient, it is essential that the strictest confidentiality is maintained. The patient is never mentioned by name and any identifying characteristics are carefully removed from the presentation. If the patient is known to the supervisor or if in a group setting the patient is recognised by another person in the group, then in the interests of the patient's privacy, the person who knows the patient should withdraw from the group or the discussion should not take place.

For the nurse
The focus of supervision is upon the feelings and thoughts of the nurse seeking support. Although the problems she encounters in working with the patient are important, the nurse's reaction to these problems is of more importance and should be the focus of supervision (British Association for Counselling 1996).

The nurse seeking supervision, however, should be aware of the special demands that this implies (Hawkins & Shohet 1989):

> *Before entering this relationship, however, we believe that supervision begins with self-supervision; and this begins with appraising one's motives and facing parts of ourselves we would normally keep hidden (even from our own awareness) as honestly as possible.*

The search for support must be a voluntary step taken by the clinician, who recognises the value to herself of this help.

Every health worker whose job involves some aspect of counselling should be aware of the kinds of supervision that are available. Support may take the following forms:

Individual supervision. The nurse and supervisor meet regularly (e.g. 1 or 2 h each month) to discuss areas of work and the nurse's feelings. A contract for working together is agreed at the outset.

Group supervision. Groups can be both creative and therapeutic as supervisory tools. They can be 'open', with people joining and leaving them during the life of the group, or 'closed', with not more than eight members and a coordinator meeting regularly (Corey & Corey 1992).

Team supervision. Many nurses work in teams, either with colleagues from the same discipline or in multidisciplinary groups. Informal or formal sharing can take place when support is needed from a group of people who are experiencing similar stressful situations. The disadvantage of this arrangement is that the individual will have to share feelings with others who will continue to be colleagues; this may compromise the degree of openness that can be achieved.

Peer supervision. In this model the clinical nurse talks with someone who is working, as she is, with patients and so understands the type of work that is being undertaken.

Ad hoc sharing. The value of sharing problems with a trusted friend, relative or colleague on an ad hoc basis should not be underestimated as a means of relieving intense feelings of stress. While this outlet for stress has the advantage of immediacy and informality, the confidante may not feel as bound to confidentiality as she might in a more formal arrangement.

Q **17.5** Imagine that following a time spent nursing a particular patient you feel unhappy and troubled and that your sleep is disturbed by nightmares. You recognise that you would like to talk about your feelings with someone.

Write a few lines about the advantages and the disadvantages as you see them, of talking to:

(a) your line manager
(b) your tutor or lecturer
(c) a friend or relative
(d) a colleague
(e) a professional helper such as a counsellor, general practitioner or psychotherapist.

Triads. The triad model (see Box 17.7) created by the Tavistock Institute of Human Relations as a support and training model is especially suitable for people working in shifts, as it requires a group of only three people working together. This model is appealing in that the small number of people taking part makes it relatively easy to implement. If a working agreement is carefully formulated at the outset, this model does not lose any of the formal constraints that are essential in any system of professional support.

Box 17.7 The triads model of supervision

Triads provide an opportunity for three persons to 'tune in' to each other on an emotional and cognitive level in a process that is non-threatening. The purpose of a triad is to create an association of the three people involved which allows them to explore issues in a positive manner with a view to facilitating insight and resolution. Everything that takes place in a triad is confidential to its three members.

There are three roles in the triad:

- presenter
- listener
- observer.

The presenter takes no longer than 5 minutes to talk about something that concerns her.

The listener does not interrupt the presenter, but listens until she is finished. The listener may then ask questions, make observations, obtain clarification, refresh her memory on what was said, and enable the presenter to amplify her remarks if she wishes to do so. The listener will try to be aware of whether or not a particular interpretation or conclusion was helpful.

The observer simply observes the interaction between the presenter and the listener. Her role is to be alert to the feeling level of the interchange, the non-verbal messages given by both participants and the quality of the listening and responding. She then conveys her observations to the others.

The three persons in the triad then reflect on the value of the exercise. They are then encouraged to work together with parity. They will each have the opportunity, in turn, to exercise each of the roles, completing the exercise within an hour.

17.6 Take a few moments to think about your clinical working environment. Would you like more support in the work that you do?

Write a few lines under the following headings to describe how you feel you might be better supported:

(a) emotional
(b) educational
(c) organisational
(d) managerial.

17.7 Set aside 10–15 min for this exercise. Think back over your last working day and think of the patients with whom you worked. Try to answer in as straightforward a manner as possible the following questions:

Can you think of one person who has 'stayed with' you since you stopped work? Perhaps you have been thinking of this person whilst doing other activities.

Ask yourself:

(a) How did I feel whilst speaking with my patient?
(b) What were we talking about?
(c) How did we end our discussion? How did I feel about this?
(d) What will happen next? How do I feel about this?

CONCLUSION

Stress is not in itself a pathological or abnormal phenomenon. Indeed, it is hard to imagine how any individual might go through life without being faced with stressful situations. For some individuals, stress can, to a significant degree, be treated as a challenge and as a spur to personal growth and maturation. Why it is that certain people seem better able than others to withstand stressful conditions has been the subject of a great deal of debate as researchers have attempted to identify the physiological, psychological and social factors that mediate the experience of stress.

The fact that the word 'stress' can be used freely in daily conversation without invoking the negative connotations of 'mental illness' perhaps indicates how the potentially grave effects of stress can be underestimated or obscured. As this chapter has shown, stress can be closely associated with serious physical, emotional or psychiatric illness, including heart disease, depression and compulsive behaviours. Stress can also give rise to detrimental coping behaviours such as drug, alcohol and other forms of substance abuse (see Ch. 37). For this reason it is vital that stress is taken seriously by health professionals and that its mechanisms and effects are clearly understood.

From the nurse's perspective, perhaps the most important aspect of the experience of stress is its uniqueness for each individual. The experience of stress, like the experience of pain, must be assessed in each patient, and approaches to stress management must be congruent with the individual's personality, experiences and values. It is hoped that this chapter has assisted the nurse in formulating a practical understanding of stress and its effects, and will enable her to make a positive contribution to the treatment and management of stress and stress-related disorders in her patients. It is also hoped that the reader will be able to meet with greater confidence the challenge of recognising and coming to terms with the effects of stress in her own professional and personal life.

REFERENCES

Ayer S, Knight S, Joyce L, Nightingale V 1997 Network. Practice-led education and development project: developing styles in clinical supervision. Nurse Education Today 17(5): 347–358

Bateman A, Holmes J 1996 Introduction to psychoanalysis. Routledge, London

Begat I B E, Severinsson E I, Berggren I B 1997 Implementation of clinical supervision in a medical department: nurses' views of the effects. Journal of Clinical Nursing 6(5): 389–394

Beesley S, Mutrie N 1997 Exercise is beneficial adjunctive treatment in depression [letter; comment]. British Medical Journal 315(7121): 1542–1543

Benner P, Wrubel J 1989 The primacy of caring. Addison Wesley, London

Blau J N (ed) 1987 Migraine: clinical, therapeutic, conceptual and research aspects. Chapman and Hall, London, ch 11, pp 185–204

Bowman W C, Rand M J 1980 Textbook of pharmacology, 3rd edn. Blackwell, Oxford, pp 19.30–19.39

British Association for Counsellors 1996 Code of ethics and practice for counsellors. BAC, Rugby

British Medical Association and Royal Pharmaceutical Society of Great Britain 1998 British National Formulary. BMA, London

Calder B D, Warnock P J, McCartney R A, Bell E J 1987 Cocksackie B viruses and the post viral fatigue syndrome: a prospective study in general practice. The Journal of the Royal College of General Practitioners 294(37): 11–15

Cannon W B 1935 Stresses and strains of homeostasis. American Journal of Medical Science 189: 1

Corey M S, Corey G 1992 Groups: process and practice. Brooks/Cole, California

Constantini A, Solano L, Di Napoli R, Bosco A 1997 Relationship between hardiness and risk of burnout in a sample of 92 nurses working in oncology and AIDS wards. Psychotherapy and Psychosomatics 66(2): 78–82

Cox T 1989 Stress. Macmillan Educational, London

Cunningham J 1996 For better or for worse. Practice Nurse 12(10): 624–627

Dewar A L, Morse J M 1995 Unbearable incidents: failure to endure the experience of illness. Journal of Advanced Nursing 22: 957–964

Dillard N L 1990 Hardiness and academic achievement. Indiana University School of Nursing D.N.S.

Dreyfus H L 1987 From depth psychology to breadth psychology: a phenomenological approach to psychopathology. In: Messer S B, Sass L A, Woolfolk R L (eds) Hermeneutics and psychological theory. Rutgers University Press, New Brunswick, NJ

Dryden W 1990 Individual therapy. Open University Press, Milton Keynes

Duquette A, Kerouac S, Sandhu B K, Ducharme F, Saulnier P 1995 Psychosocial determinants of burnout in geriatric nursing. International Journal of Nursing Studies 32(5): 443–456

Edwards J 1997 Sudden death and the theatre nurse. British Journal of Theatre Nursing 6(12): 11, 13–14

Egan G 1997 The skilled helper: a systematic approach to effective helping. Brooks/Cole, California

Everly G S, Benson H 1989 Disorders of arousal and the relaxation response: speculations on the nature and treatment of stress related diseases. International Journal of Psychosomatics 36(1–4): 15–21

Everly G S, Sobelman S H 1987 The assessment of the human stress response: neurological, biochemical and psychological foundations. AMS Press, New York

Farrington A 1997 Strategies for reducing stress and burnout in nursing. British Journal of Nursing 6(1): 44–50
Feldstein M A, Gemma P B 1995 Oncology nurses and chronic compounded grief. Cancer Nursing 18(3): 228–236
Fox S I 1990 Human physiology, 3rd edn. W C Brown, Dubuque, pp 293–303
Freud S 1914 The psychopathology of everyday life. Penguin, London
Freud S 1917 Mourning and melancholia. Standard edition, vol X1V. Hogarth Press, London
Fukunishi I, Hattori M 1997 Mood states and type A behaviour in Japanese male patients with myocardial infarction. Psychotherapy & Psychosomatics 66(6): 314–318
Gray J A 1987 The physiology of fear and stress. Cambridge University Press, Cambridge
Groom K N, O'Connor M E 1996 Relation of light and exercise to seasonal depressive symptoms: preliminary development of a scale. Perceptual and Motor Skills 83(2): 379–383
Hallberg I R 1994 Systematic clinical supervision in a child psychiatric ward: satisfaction with nursing care, tedium, burnout, and the nurse's own report on the effects of it. Archives of Psychiatric Nursing 8(1): 44–52
Hawkins P, Shohet R 1989 Supervision in the helping professions. Open University Press, Milton Keynes
Hawton K 1989 Suicide and the management of attempted suicide. In: Herbst K R, Paykel E S (eds) Depression: an integrated approach. Heinemann Medical/The Mental Health Foundation, Oxford
Heide F, Borkovec T 1983 Relaxation-induced anxiety. Journal of Consulting and Clinical Psychology 51: 171–182
Holmes T H, Rahe R H 1967 The social readjustment rating scale. Journal of Psychosomatic Research 11: 213–218
Ho-Yen D O, Macnamara I 1991 General practitioners' experience of the chronic fatigue syndrome. The British Journal of General Practice 41: 349
Hutchings D 1997 The hardiness of hospice nurses. The American Journal of Hospice & Palliative Care 14(3): 110–113
Jacelon C S 1997 The trait and process of resilience. Journal of Advanced Nursing 25(1): 123–129
Kennedy E 1990 On becoming a counsellor: a basic guide for non-professional counsellors. Gill and Macmillan, Dublin
Knight S 1995 Use of transcendental meditation to relieve stress and promote health. British Journal of Nursing 4(6): 315–318
Kobasa S C 1979 Stressful life events, personality and health: an inquiry into hardiness. Journal of Personality and Social Psychology 37(1): 1–11
Kushnir T, Rabin S, Azulai S 1997 A descriptive study of stress management in a group of paediatric oncology nurses. Cancer Nursing 20(6): 414–421
Lazarus R S 1966 Psychological stress and the coping process. McGraw-Hill, New York
Lazarus R S, Folkman S 1984 Stress, appraisal, and coping. Springer, New York
Levi L (ed) 1971 Society, stress and disease, vol 1. Oxford University Press, Oxford, pp 280–366
Lynch S, Seth R, Montgomery S 1991 Antidepressant therapy in the chronic fatigue syndrome. The British Journal of General Practice 41(349): 121–127
Martin A C, Starling B P 1989 Managing common marital stresses. Nurse Practitioner: American Journal Of Primary Care 14(10): 11–12, 14–16, 18
Matthews K A (ed) 1986 Handbook of stress, reactivity and cardiovascular disease. Wiley, New York
Mckinley B, Brooks N 1991 Post traumatic stress disorder explained. Nursing Standard 5(19): 35–38
Melchior M E W, Philipsen H, Abu-Saad H H, Halfens R J G, van de Berg A A, Gassman P 1996 The effectiveness of primary nursing on burnout among psychiatric nurses in long stay settings. Journal of Advanced Nursing 24(4): 694–702
Menzies I E P 1960 A case study of the functioning of social systems as a defence against anxiety. Human Relations 13(2): 95–123
Midence K, Gregory S, Stanley R 1996 The effects of patient suicide on nursing staff. Journal of Clinical Nursing 5(2): 115–120
Miller A 1987 The drama of being a child. Virago, London.
Miller S B, Dolgoy L, Friese M, Sita A 1996 Dimensions of hostility and cardiovascular response to interpersonal stress. Journal of Psychosomatic Research 41(1): 81–95
Moore K A, Blumenthal J A 1998 Exercise training as an alternative treatment for depression among older adults. Alternative Therapies in Health and Medicine 4(1): 48–56
O'Connor N J, Manson J E, O'Connor G T, Buring J E 1995 Psychosocial risk factors and nonfatal myocardial infarction. Circulation 92(6): 1458–1464
Ostell A 1991 Coping, problem solving and stress: a framework for intervention strategies. British Journal of Medical Psychology 64: 11–24
Palsson M E, Hallberg I R, Norberg A1994 Systematic clinical supervision and its effects for nurses handling demanding care situations. Cancer Nursing 17(5): 385–394
Paykel E S, Herbst K R (eds) 1989 Depression: an integrated approach. Heinemann Medical/The Mental Health Foundation, Oxford
Polk L V 1997 Toward a middle-range theory of resilience. Advanced Nursing Science 19(3): 1–13
Reif W, Hermanutz M 1996 Responses to activation and rest in patients with panic disorder and major depression. British Journal of Clinical Psychology 35(pt4): 605–16, Nov.
Rogers C R 1974 On becoming a person. Constable, London
Schatzberg A E, Nemeroff C B (eds) 1988 The hypothalamic–pituitary–adrenal axis: physiology, pathophysiology and psychiatric implications. Raven Press, New York, pp 55–66
Selye H 1936 Syndrome produced by diverse nocuous agents. Nature (London) 138: 32
Selye H 1946a The general adaptation syndrome and the diseases of adaptation. Journal of Clinical Endocrinology 6: 117
Selye H 1946b What is stress? Metabolism 5: 525
Selye H 1976 The stress of life. McGraw-Hill, New York
Spencer L 1994 How do nurses deal with their own grief when a patient dies in an intensive care unit, and what help can be given to enable them to overcome their grief effectively? Journal of Advanced Nursing 19: 1141–1150
Stafford-Clark 1987 What Freud really said. Pelican Books, London
Thorne B 1990 Person-centred therapy. In: Dryden W (ed) Individual therapy psychotherapy handbooks. Open University Press, Milton Keynes
Vines S W 1994 Relaxation with guided imagery: effects on employees' psychological distress and health seeking behaviours. American Association of Occupational Health Nursing Journal 42(5): 206–213
Wessley S 1990 Postviral fatigue syndrome. Update 41(12): 10–13
Westra H A, Kuiper N A 1997 Cognitive content specificity in selective attention across four domains of maladjustment. Behaviour Research & Therapy 35(4): 349–365
Worden J W 1991 Grief counselling and grief therapy: a handbook for the mental health practitioner. Routledge, London

FURTHER READING

Alexander D A 1990 Psychological intervention for victims and helpers after disasters. British Journal of General Practice 40: 345–348
Asterita M 1985 The physiology of stress. Human Sciences Press, New York
Bailey R, Clarke M 1989 Stress and coping in nursing. Chapman and Hall, London
Beck A T 1976 Cognitive therapy and the emotional disorders. International Universities Press, New York
Beck A T 1989 Love is never enough. Viking Penguin, London
Bowlby J 1980 Attachment and loss, vol 3: loss, sadness and depression. Tavistock, London
Burnard P 1989 Existentialism as a theoretical basis for counselling in psychiatric nursing. Archives of Psychiatric Nursing 3(3): 142–147
Everly G S, Smith K 1987 Occupational stress and its management. In: Humphrey J (ed) Human stress: current selected research, vol 2. AMS Press, New York, pp 235–246
Hawkins P, Shohet R 1989 Supervision in the helping professions. Open University Press, Milton Keynes
Kobasa S, Maddi S, Kahn S 1982 Hardiness and health: a prospective study. Journal of Personality and Social Psychology 42: 168–177

Kobasa S, Puccetti M 1983 Personality and social resources in stress resistance. Journal of Personality and Social Psychology 37: 1–11
Kubler-Ross E 1982 Living with death and dying. Souvenir Press, London
Lacey R 1996 Mind. Complete guide to psychiatric drugs: a layman's guide to antidepressants, tranquilisers and other prescription drugs. Vermillion, London
Oatley K 1989 The importance of being emotional. New Scientist (Aug): 33–36
Palmer J A, Palmer L K, Michiels K, Thigpen B 1995 Effects of type of exercise on depression in recovering substance abusers. Perceptual & Motor Skills 80(2): 523–530
Parkes C M 1972 Bereavement. Tavistock, London
Parkes C M 1972 Determinants of outcome following bereavement. Omega 6: 303–323
Payne R, Firth-Cozens J 1988 Stress in health professionals. Wiley, Chichester
Price V A 1982 Type A behaviour pattern. Academic Press, London
Schatzberg A E, Nemeroff C B (eds) 1988 The hypothalamic–pituitary–adrenal axis: physiology, pathophysiology and psychiatric implications. Raven Press, New York, pp 55–66
Sedgwick A W, Paul B, Plooij D, Davies M 1989 Follow-up of stress management courses. Medical Journal of Australia (May): 485–486, 488–489
Segar M L, Katch V L, Roth R S et al 1998 The effect of aerobic exercise on self-esteem and depressive and anxiety symptoms among breast cancer survivors. Oncology Nursing Forum 25(1): 107–113
Selley C 1991 Post-traumatic stress disorder. The Practitioner, 235(1506): 635–641
Smith D L 1990 Psychodynamic therapy. In: Dryden (ed) Individual therapy. Open University Press, Milton Keynes
Stoltenberg C D, Delworth U 1988 Supervising counsellors and therapists. Jossey-Bass, San Francisco
Sutherland V J, Cooper C L 1990 Understanding stress. Chapman and Hall, London
Yalom I D 1968 Existential psychotherapy. Basic Books, New York

USEFUL ADDRESSES

British Association for Counsellors
1 Regent Place
Rugby
Warwickshire CV21 2PJ

British Migraine Association
178a High Road
Byfleet
Surrey KT14 7ED

CRUSE Bereavement Care
Scottish Headquarters
18 South Trinity Road
Edinburgh EH5 3PN

Depressives Anonymous
36 Chestnut Avenue
Beverly
North Humberside HU17 9OU

Keep Fit Association
16 Upper Woburn Place
London WC1H 0QG

Manic Depression Fellowship
21 St George's Rd
London SE1 6ES
0171 793 2600

Mental Health Foundation
24 George Square
Glasgow G2 1EG

Migraine Trust
45 Great Ormond Street
London WC1N 3HD

MIND (National Association for Mental Health)
22 Harley Street
London W1N 2ED

Myalgic Encephalomyelitis (ME) Association
PO Box 8
Stamford-le-Hope
Essex SS17 8EX

RELATE (National Marriage Guidance Council)
Herbert Gray College
Little Church Street
Rugby
Warwickshire CV21 3AP

The Samaritans
17 Uxbridge Road
Slough
Berkshire SL1 1SN

The Scottish Institute of Human Relations
56 Albany Street
Edinburgh EH1 3QR

Tavistock Institute
Tavistock Centre
120 Belsize Lane
London NW3 5BA

United Kingdom Council for Psychotherapy
167 Great Portland Street
London W1N 5FB

Westminster Pastoral Foundation
23 Kensington Square
London W8 5HN

SHOCK

Dorothy J. Armstrong

18

INTRODUCTION

Despite advances in diagnosis, treatment and management, shock remains one of the leading causes of death in the critically ill patient. It is important that nurses from all areas of clinical practice have the knowledge required to identify patients at risk and ensure timely and appropriate intervention is carried out.

The aim of this chapter is to facilitate the understanding of the pathophysiology of shock and the nursing care required.

In any environment, awareness of the predisposing factors which may lead to shock, early detection and prompt action are vital to a good prognosis. Caring for patients who are suffering from shock requires not only an understanding of the pathophysiology of shock and the principles of its treatment and management, but also an awareness of the devastating psychological and social impact such a sudden change from health to illness can have on patients and their families.

THE PATHOPHYSIOLOGY OF SHOCK

Circulatory haemostasis exists when the circulating blood volume and the vascular tone of blood vessels are in dynamic equilibrium. Shock is a state in which tissue perfusion is inadequate to maintain the supply of oxygen and nutrients necessary for normal cellular function and disequilibrium ensues. The cells may also be unable to extract and utilise normally the reduced supply of substrates and oxygen which is delivered.

Shock syndromes have traditionally been categorised according to the underlying cause, namely:

- *Hypovolaemic* — due to reduction of blood volume
- *Cardiogenic* — due to myocardial damage
- *Distributive* — due to altered vascular resistance. This category includes septic shock, neurogenic shock, spinal shock and anaphylactic shock.

The stages of shock

Before considering specific types of shock it is necessary to understand the basic pathophysiological processes which produce the clinical picture typically observed in shock. These processes can be divided into four stages (Quaal 1992):

1. *Initial stage.* There are no signs and symptoms but cellular changes begin to occur in response to a disturbance in cell perfusion and oxygenation. This disturbance progresses to a change from aerobic to anaerobic cellular metabolism, in which production of lactic acid and pyruvic acid leads to metabolic acidosis.
2. *Compensatory stage.* Physiological adaptations occur in an attempt to overcome the original problem, e.g. hypovolaemia.

3. *Progressive stage*. Compensatory mechanisms begin to fail and produce adverse effects.
4. *Refractory stage*. Pathophysiological processes set in motion cannot be arrested or reversed. Death is imminent.

It is important to understand that the stages of shock comprise continuous and complex processes and that there is usually no sudden transition from one stage to the next. It should also be noted that in septic shock the early clinical picture is altered. For example, the presence of endotoxins produces a hyperdynamic state with depressed left ventricular function. This occurs even when the endotoxin is experimentally injected into healthy people (Suffredini et al 1989).

The compensatory stage

When circulation becomes inadequate due to the reduction of circulating fluid, pump failure or massive vasodilatation, various mechanisms are activated in response to hypotension, hypoxaemia or acidosis, or a combination of these. These mechanisms may be neural, hormonal or chemical, but since the body functions as a whole system they are closely interlinked.

Neural mechanisms. Hypotension leads to decreased stimulation of the aortic and carotid sinus baroreceptors, which in turn reduces impulses to the vasomotor centre and thus reduces inhibition of the vasoconstrictor centre. This stimulates the sympathetic nervous system, resulting in the activation of the stress response (see Fig. 17.1, p. 618). This response includes the discharge of the catecholamines, namely adrenaline and noradrenaline, resulting in vasoconstriction in the skin, kidneys, gastrointestinal tract and other organs while blood supply to the heart and brain is preserved. Vasoconstriction and increased heart rate may initially restore the arterial blood pressure to normal, but peripheral resistance will be raised, making the myocardium work harder to maintain cardiac output. Urinary output and peristalsis will decrease, and the individual's skin will become pale and cool. Sympathetic nervous system stimulation will also result in increased respiratory rate and depth, dilated pupils and increased sweat gland activity, causing the 'clammy' skin typically found in all forms of shock other than early septic shock.

Hormonal mechanisms. Adrenaline secreted by the adrenal medulla stimulates the anterior pituitary gland to release adrenocorticotrophic hormone (ACTH), which causes the adrenal cortex to release glucocorticoids such as hydrocortisone and mineralocorticoids such as aldosterone.

Glucocorticoids raise blood sugar by increasing gluconeogenesis and thereby the availability of glucose for energy. In addition, the glucocorticoids mobilise amino acids from the tissues and decrease protein synthesis. They also reduce glucose uptake by the cells and mobilise fatty acids from the adipose tissue into the plasma. Cortisol shifts cell metabolism from glucose to fatty acids for energy, enhancing fatty acid oxidation, and also reduces tissue destruction by stabilising lysosomal membranes (Quaal 1992).

Aldosterone decreases excretion by increased reabsorption of sodium and chloride by the kidney, and increases excretion of potassium and hydrogen ions. Thus metabolic acidosis and hypokalaemia can occur. The high serum osmolality resulting from a high concentration of sodium chloride stimulates the hypothalamic osmoreceptors to release antidiuretic hormone (ADH) from the posterior pituitary gland.

ADH stimulates an increase in renal water reabsorption, in an attempt to restore normal serum osmolality and thus increase circulating fluid and blood pressure.

Noradrenaline secretion by the adrenal medulla results in renal artery vasoconstriction, which in turn stimulates secretion of renin by the kidney. In the circulation, renin reacts with angiotensinogen, producing angiotensin I. This is converted by an enzyme in the lungs to angiotensin II, which causes venous constriction and increases aldosterone release, thus leading to increased fluid and sodium retention, increased blood volume and therefore increased venous return, blood pressure and renal perfusion.

Thyroxine secreted by the thyroid gland sensitises the beta-receptors in the heart to noradrenaline and so increases heart rate, systolic pressure, stroke volume and cardiac output.

Chemical mechanisms. Poor lung perfusion leads to ventilation–perfusion mismatch and decreased oxygen tension in the circulating blood. This is detected by chemoreceptors in the aorta and carotid bodies. The carbon dioxide concentration falls as the respiratory rate increases and the amount of carbon dioxide is 'blown off' thus producing a respiratory alkalosis. Cerebral blood vessels constrict in response to decreased carbon dioxide tension leading to cerebral hypoxia. Subsequently, the acid–base balance is further complicated by a metabolic acidosis resulting from the anaerobic metabolism of glucose to lactic acid.

These mechanisms may initially combine to compensate for the initial problem, but unless the latter is promptly and successfully overcome, more clinical signs will become evident. The typical clinical picture at this stage of shock is of a patient with cool, pale, clammy skin, decreased urinary output, increased heart rate and decreased bowel sounds. The patient may be anxious, restless or confused due to the cerebral effects of hypoxia, hypocapnia and sympathetic nervous system stimulation.

Anxiety will intensify the physiological responses to stress and thus it is very important for the nurse to provide much needed reassurance to both the patient and her relatives during a major life crisis.

The progressive stage

Although the compensatory mechanisms may at first appear to reverse the effects of shock, if the cause is not treated appropriately then the next stage of shock becomes evident.

With decreased perfusion, the supply of oxygen and nutrients to the cells will be inadequate to produce sufficient adenosine triphosphate (ATP) (see Fig. 18.1). The sodium pump will fail and sodium will increase inside the cells while potassium leaks out (see Fig. 18.2). This can result in hyperkalaemia, which may in turn cause cardiac arrest. The anaerobic metabolism which results from an inadequate oxygen supply will increase the production of lactic acid, resulting in a metabolic acidosis. The consequences of the increasing acidosis and hypoxia are that the precapillary sphincters become fatigued, causing collapse of the microcirculation and increasing hydrostatic pressure and capillary leakage. Haemoconcentration and viscosity will increase. Sludging in the microcirculation may lead to disseminated intravascular coagulation (DIC, see p. 651), one of the complications of shock. Figure 18.3 illustrates the vicious cycle of shock.

Prolonged vasoconstriction and its impact on cell function will soon compromise the functioning of the vital organs, as follows:

- The kidneys will be unable to filter, excrete and reabsorb fluid normally. Urinary osmolality will fall, and output will be reduced to below 20 mL/h. Acute tubular necrosis may occur, causing a marked rise in blood urea and creatinine.

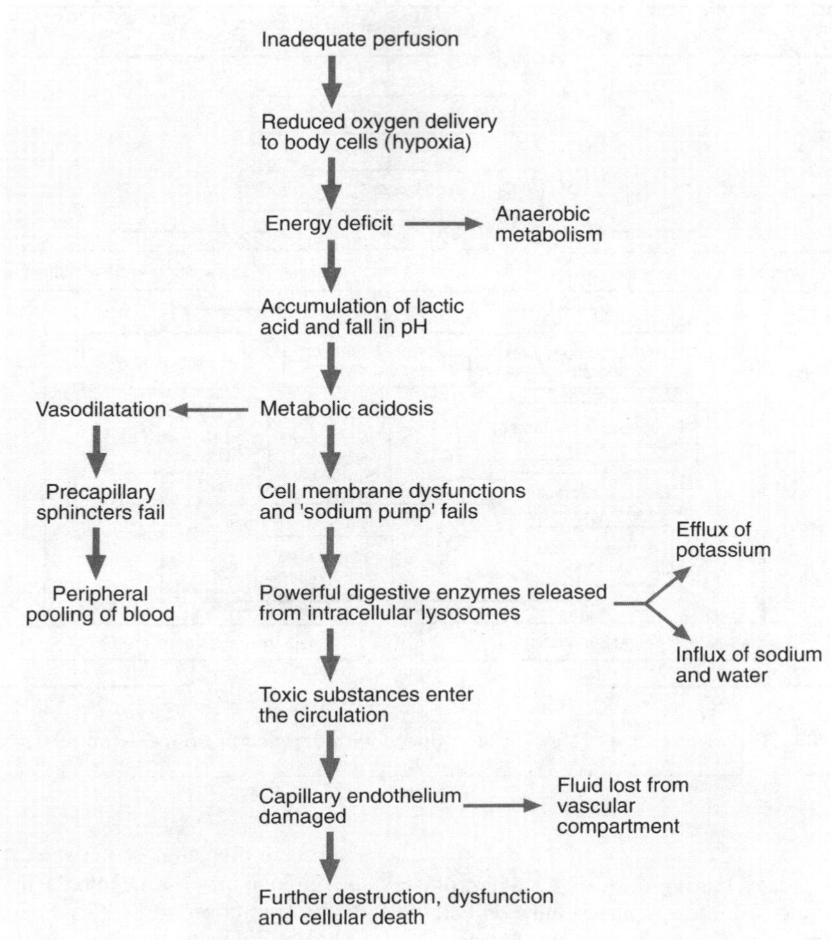

Fig. 18.1 Effects of inadequate perfusion on cell function.

- Pancreatic cells will release the enzymes amylase and lipase into the circulation, contributing to the formation of myocardial depressant factor (MDF), which decreases myocardial contractility.
- The lungs will become less compliant as fluid and plasma proteins leak into the interstitium, altering osmotic pressure and leading to pulmonary oedema. This in turn reduces gaseous exchange and may result in adult respiratory distress syndrome (ARDS, see p. 650). Hydrostatic or cardiac pulmonary oedema may occur as the heart fails. All of these changes will increase hypoxia and acidosis.
- The heart will eventually fail as coronary perfusion and oxygen supply become inadequate to meet the demands of the myocardium, which will be working hard to maintain blood flow by pumping rapidly against high resistance and disadvantaged by the effect of MDF.
- Ischaemic damage to the intestinal mucosa will release bacteria and toxins from the gut into the circulation.
- Alteration in cerebral function may have a number of effects, ranging from a dulling of responses to major behavioural changes.

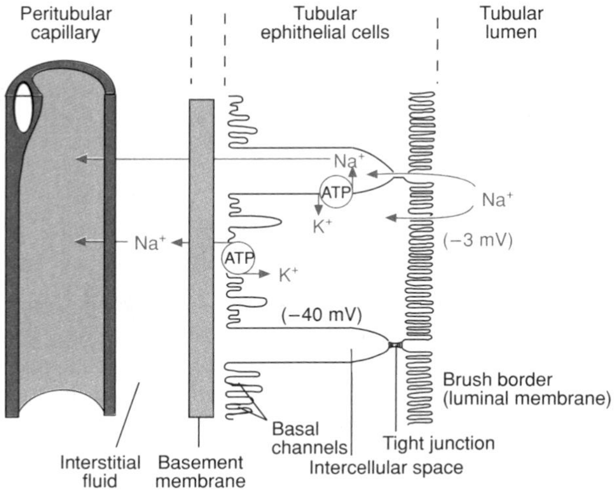

Fig. 18.2 The sodium–potassium pump. (Reproduced with permission from Guyton & Hall 1996.)

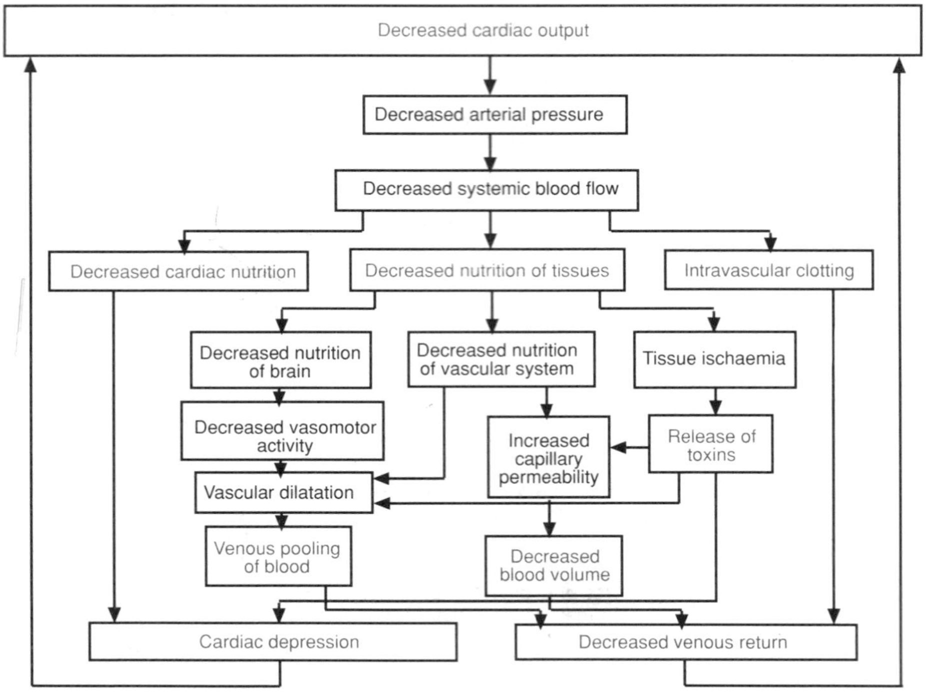

Fig. 18.3 The vicious cycle of shock. (Reproduced with permission from Guyton & Hall 1996.)

The refractory stage

Continuing circulatory collapse, increasing acidosis, sludging of red cells and platelets and decreased intravascular volume will all contribute to decreasing perfusion of tissues. Massive bleeding due to DIC may also exacerbate this effect. Inadequate ventilation will lead to increasingly inadequate oxygenation. Renal failure will contribute to increasing metabolic abnormalities, and vital centres in the brain will eventually cease to function due to ischaemia and hypoxia. If the refractory stage is reached, the shock is irreversible and death will occur.

TYPES OF SHOCK

Specific aspects of the pathophysiological processes of shock will be evident according to the type of shock which is occurring. The following sections will therefore describe the distinguishing features of hypovolaemic shock, cardiogenic shock and the different forms of distributive shock.

Hypovolaemic shock

This is the most common type of shock. Its primary cause is loss of fluid from the circulation, which may be described as:

- *external fluid loss* — due to superficial bleeding, vomiting, diarrhoea, overuse of diuretics, burns or diabetes insipidus
- *internal fluid loss* — due to internal bleeding such as haemothorax or bleeding into tissues at fracture sites after injuries; to paralytic ileus, intestinal obstruction or acute dilatation of the stomach; or to gross ascites.

While internal conditions may not be an obvious cause of fluid loss, their effect can be very serious. For example, 1 L (around 20% of the blood volume of an average man) or more of fluid may be sequestered in the gastrointestinal tract during paralytic ileus and/or acute dilatation of the stomach, and the same volume or more of blood may escape into the tissues and/or thorax as a result of multiple injuries.

The physiological implications of hypovolaemia are:

reduced blood volume
↓
decreased venous return
↓
decreased cardiac output
↓
reduced tissue perfusion.

In early hypovolaemic shock, the compensatory mechanisms already described (see p. 636) are activated when the blood pressure starts to fall. These mechanisms will compensate for up to 10% reduction of the circulating volume of a healthy person without the development of marked symptoms. However, if a greater volume of fluid is lost and is not replaced quickly, the compensatory mechanisms may fail quite suddenly, in which case the patient's condition will deteriorate rapidly. It should be recognised that in older people the cardiovascular system is often less able to cope with haemodynamic changes, and the heart may be less able to pump faster and harder in order to maintain cardiac output against high peripheral resistance.

Recognising hypovolaemic shock

The following signs and symptoms of hypovolaemic shock are reliable only if they are considered in relation to one another and to the patient's previous, stable, condition. Nevertheless, whenever several of these indicators occur together, the possibility of shock should be considered, as a successful outcome depends upon early intervention. The nurse should therefore be alert to the following:

- narrowing of the pulse pressure, i.e. a reduced difference between systolic and arterial pressures due to decreased stroke volume and increased peripheral resistance indicating vasoconstriction of the skin and viscera (see Daily 1992 for more information)
- anxiety, restlessness and confusion, which may indicate decreased cerebral perfusion and oxygenation
- a rapid, weak, thready pulse, due to low blood flow despite a rapid heart rate
- cool, clammy skin due to vasoconstriction and sympathetic stimulation of sweat glands
- decreased urinary output, due to renal artery vasoconstriction and endocrine compensatory mechanisms
- rapid and deep respirations in response to sympathetic nervous system stimulation, hypoxia and acidosis
- lowered body temperature, which may be related to altered metabolism, perfusion and oxygenation and, possibly, heat loss from evaporation of sweat from the skin
- thirst and a dry mouth related to fluid depletion and possibly to sympathetic nervous system stimulation
- fatigue, probably related to inadequate perfusion and oxygenation of the tissue and vital organs.

As stated earlier, it is relatively easy to diagnose hypovolaemic shock when a patient is bleeding externally. Diagnosis is more difficult when hypovolaemia is developing as a consequence of an internal crisis. Nurses must be alert to recognise the above signs and context of the crisis and to ensure that prompt action is taken and/or help is sought.

Cardiogenic shock

This type of shock is caused by abnormalities in the functioning of the heart, and is particularly problematic in patients who have suffered an acute myocardial infarction. Cardiogenic shock can perhaps best be understood with reference to the physiological processes that contribute to the normal circulation of blood.

Q

18.1 Refresh your knowledge of cardiac function by reviewing Chapter 2.
18.2 Review the terms listed in Box 18.1 to ensure that you understand how they would be applied in the course of treatment and monitoring for cardiogenic shock.

Haemodynamic changes leading to the development of cardiogenic shock

When myocardial ischaemia and infarction occur, the contractility of the ventricles may be impaired. Ischaemic muscle is deprived of adequate oxygen and substrates for effective contraction, and infarcted muscle or scar tissue is unable to contract. When there is a rapid reduction in the amount of functional myocardium (e.g. when 40–50% is damaged), cardiac output will fall to a level insufficient to maintain adequate arterial pressure and tissue perfusion. In addition, since the left ventricle is not being effectively emptied, pressure will rise in the left atrium, the pulmonary circulation and the right side of the heart. As the pulmonary artery wedge pressure (PAWP) rises above 18 mmHg, pulmonary oedema will eventually ensue, reducing oxygenation. Thus, not only will the tissues be poorly perfused, but also the blood which does reach them will carry less oxygen.

Pump failure (i.e. reduced contractility of the damaged myocardium) and ensuing hypoxia and acidosis activate the compensatory mechanisms of shock. The resulting tachycardia and vasoconstriction will increase the workload of the impaired myocardial muscle. As shock progresses, without effective intervention the vicious circle of effects shown in Figure 18.3 will result in progressive deterioration and eventual release of MDF (see p. 637) which will depress myocardial contractility even further.

Box 18.1 Key terms relating to cardiac status

Cardiac output
This is the product of the heart rate multiplied by the stroke volume and represents the amount of blood ejected from the heart each minute. In the adult, cardiac output is normally 5–8 L/min.

Cardiac index
This is patient's cardiac output divided by her body surface area. It indicates how many litres per minute per square metre of body surface the heart ejects. The normal range of an adult is 2.7–4.3 L/min per m^2.

Stroke volume
This is the amount of blood delivered to the aorta during a left ventricular contraction (normally 80–120 mL in an adult). Three factors influence stroke volume: preload, afterload and contractility.

Preload
Indicators are central venous pressure (CVP) and pulmonary artery wedge pressure (PAWP). By means of a CVP transducer, right atrial pressure can be measured. CVP reflects the pressure in the right atrium and systemic veins but does not reliably reflect left ventricular pressures. PAWP gives an indication of the compliance of the left ventricular myocardium during diastole and the left atrial filling pressure necessary to fill the left ventricle with blood prior to systole.

Afterload
This is the resistance to systolic ejection of blood from the ventricle and can be assessed by measuring pulmonary vascular resistance and systemic vascular resistance. The pulmonary vascular resistance is the ratio of the pressure drop across the pulmonary vascular system to the total flow passing through the pulmonary circulation. Systemic or peripheral vascular resistance is a measurement of the vascular resistance to blood flow.

Contractility
This refers to the ability of the myocardium to contract effectively and act as a pump to maintain the circulation of blood.

Signs of cardiogenic shock

The signs of cardiogenic shock include:

- systolic pressure <80 mmHg
- tachycardia and a weak, thready pulse
- cold, clammy skin
- oliguria — urine output <20 mL/h
- confusion
- mottling of the extremities, particularly the legs
- if measured pulmonary artery wedge pressure is >18 mmHg, cardiac index is <1.8 L/min per m^2 (see Box 18.1).

Despite modern advances in haemodynamic monitoring and therapy, the mortality rate of patients with cardiogenic shock remains over 80% (Jowett & Thompson 1989, Quaal 1992).

Distributive shock

Septic shock

Despite progression in the treatment of sepsis and septic shock, the incidence over the past 30 years has continued to rise, with the mortality rate remaining at 40–70% (Jackson 1994). Septic shock is commonly seen as a complication of bacterial infection and is characterised by a wide range of metabolic and haemodynamic abnormalities (Bone 1991).

Gram-negative and Gram-positive organisms. Septic shock may be caused by any invading microorganism. However, this condition is commonly associated with Gram-negative bacteria such as *Escherichia coli, Klebsiella, Pseudomonas, Bacteroides* and *Proteus*. Gram-negative bacteria contain a lipopolysaccharide in their cell walls called endotoxin. When released into the bloodstream, endotoxin produces a variety of adverse biochemical changes and activates immune and other biological mediators that contribute to the development of septic shock (Hudak & Gallo 1994).

Gram-positive organisms such as *Staphylococcus, Streptococcus* and *Pneumococcus* are also implicated in the development of sepsis. The British tabloid newspapers have recently coined the term 'flesh-eating bug' to describe the invasive necrotising fasciitis caused by group A *Streptococcus*. This virulent bacterium is associated with septic shock and organ failure. Necrotising fasciitis can present suddenly and must be treated with radical surgery and supportive therapy in an intensive care unit (Ward & Walsh 1991).

Phases of septic shock. The clinical effects of septic shock occur in two distinct phases. Ferguson (1991) describes these as the warm hyperdynamic stage and the cold hypodynamic stage.

The hyperdynamic phase. This first stage is characterised by the following:

- high cardiac output
- low systemic vascular resistance
- vasodilatation
- volume depletion and hypotension
- fever and chills
- low urine output
- tachycardia
- tachypnoea
- restlessness, agitation and confusion.

Edwards (1993) describes the haemodynamic changes in septic shock as primarily reduced left ventricular preload, myocardial depression and vasodilatation. He suggests the resulting hypovolaemia may be due to absolute volume depletion as a result of vomiting, diarrhoea, sweating, hyperventilation and generalised fluid loss due to increased tissue permeability.

The hypodynamic phase. Following the hyperdynamic phase, the hypodynamic stage occurs. This is characterised by:

- high systemic vascular resistance
- vasoconstriction
- hypotension
- hypoperfusion
- cold, clammy skin
- subnormal or elevated temperature
- depressed conscious level.

At this stage, clinical findings begin to resemble more closely those typically associated with shock. Catecholamine release results in vasoconstriction and the patient's skin becomes cold, moist and possibly mottled at the peripheries. The pulse becomes rapid, thready and weak, and ECG changes suggest an inadequate coronary blood flow. Patients who reach this clinical state are particularly at risk of developing multisystem failure.

During this phase it is common for haematological problems to become evident. The released endotoxins damage the endothelium and cause adhesion of platelets and subsequent destruction of the microcirculation. These effects, together with the activation of the coagulation and fibrinolytic systems, may give rise to DIC (see p. 651). Hyperventilation persists but fails to overcome hypoxia. Lactic acid builds up and there is increasing metabolic acidosis, further compromising cell function.

Edwards (1993) states that other important clues to the gravity of the condition are the presence of septic encephalopathy (which presents as confusion or drowsiness) and bradycardia. Whatever the clinical impression, a patient presenting with these signs would be near to death (see Case History 18.1 and Nursing Care Plan 18.1).

Q **18.3** Which stage of shock do the clinical findings in Case History 18.1 represent: hyperdynamic or hypodynamic?

Neurogenic shock

This type of distributive shock is associated with the central nervous system. It can occur when a disease process, drug or traumatic injury blocks sympathetic nerve impulses from the brain's vasomotor centre and thus increases parasympathetic activity. Neurogenic shock produces a picture of vasodilatation with loss of vascular tone. Venous return is reduced, cardiac output falls and hypotension rapidly follows.

There are a number of preconditions which may, over the course of several hours, or even a few weeks or months, lead to the development of neurogenic shock. One of the most common causes is spinal anaesthesia, especially that which extends up the length of the spinal cord and results in a blockage of sympathetic impulses. Cerebral trauma such as contusions or concussion (particularly to the brain stem or medulla oblongata) may also produce severe neurogenic shock. Another potential cause is spinal cord trauma in which all reflex activity below the level of the lesion is lost.

Case History 18.1 **Mr R (see also Nursing Care Plan 18.1)**

Mr R, a 50-year-old bank manager, was admitted to the surgical unit for a hemicolectomy for diverticular disease. The surgery went according to plan and Mr R appeared to be progressing well. On the fifth postoperative day, however, the staff nurse noticed that he looked ill, and Mr R admitted that he was 'not so well today'. Physical findings included:

- tachycardia
- tachypnoea
- warm, pink skin
- restlessness
- pyrexia
- polyuria.

The doctor concluded that Mr R was in the early stages of septic shock. Nursing staff then implemented the interventions summarised in Nursing Care Plan 18.1.

Nursing Care Plan 18.1 Mr R — care of a patient with septic shock (see Case History 18.1)

Nursing considerations	***Goal***	***Action***	***Rationale***
1. Potential risk of fluid volume depletion due to peripheral vasodilation and capillary leakage	To restore and maintain circulating blood volume	❒ Assess vital signs, skin colour and capillary refill time	Depending on the shock phase, Mr R may present with an increased cardiac output, which causes a flushed, pink appearance. As the hypodynamic phase develops, the cardinal signs of shock become evident (see p. 639)
		❒ Ensure i.v. access with a minimum of two large-bore catheters	Fluid volume loss due to redistribution requires blood, colloid and crystalloid replacement
		❒ Monitor and record vital signs and core body temperature	Alterations in vital signs determine stability, improvement or deterioration and indicate whether changes need to be made to therapy
		❒ Insert a urinary catheter	Renal function is a good indicator of overall tissue perfusion. A urine output of 0.5–1.0 mL/kg per h is desirable. In the early stages of septic shock, an inappropriately large volume of urine may be passed due to renal vasodilation caused by bacterial toxins. In such circumstances, urine output can be more than 100 mL/h
		❒ Assist with the insertion of a pulmonary artery catheter	Ideally the left ventricular function should be monitored by means of a PA catheter. If this is not possible then a central line will monitor the CVP and serve as a guide to fluid replacement
		❒ Administer and evaluate the effectiveness of inotropic agents: • dobutamine • dopamine • dopexamine	Inotropic agents increase cardiac output and therefore improve renal, coronary, mesenteric and cerebral blood flow
2. Potential for impaired gas exchange due to interstitial fluid overload	Restore and maintain optimal pulmonary function	❒ Assess Mr R's respiratory status, rate and rhythm: • Is he distressed? • Does he have any bronchospasm? • Monitor arterial blood gases • Monitor O_2 saturation via pulse oximetry	Escalating demands on the cardiovascular system increase oxygen consumption. In the early hyperdynamic stage, the ABGs may be relatively normal and it is not until the hypodynamic stage is reached that they reflect hypoxia or metabolic acidosis
		❒ Encourage Mr R's cooperation in optimising respiratory function by means of: • breathing exercises • chest physiotherapy • incentive spirometry (see Ch. 3) • progressive O_2 therapy	Mr R may eventually need intubation and ventilation to maintain acceptable ABGs. To try to avoid this the nurse can employ these interventions
		❒ Administer bronchodilators as prescribed by the physician	Bronchodilators cause airway dilatation by acting directly on β_2 receptors
3. Potential for further systemic infection	Reduce or eliminate the systemic risk of further infection	❒ Administer appropriate antibiotic therapy via i.v. route	Antibiotics are given i.v. to ensure a high level of the drug in the blood, body cavity fluids and tissues
		❒ Minimise the introduction of further infection by: • careful and frequent handwashing • maintaining aseptic techniques for all invasive procedures	Shock states alter the immune response and these patients are even more susceptible to infection. The increased use of invasive monitoring techniques offers more opportunities for invading pathogens
		❒ Perform frequent bacteriological screening	The use of antibiotic 'cocktails' to treat one organism may allow others to proliferate

Spinal shock

Trauma to the head, neck, back or shoulders resulting from an accident may cause injury to the vertebral column and/or spinal cord. Spinal injuries are most prevalent among young men who have been previously healthy and for whom the injury is a catastrophic event necessitating major changes in lifestyle.

The degree and type of force exerted on the spine at the time of injury will determine the nature and severity of the injury. The most frequently seen and, unfortunately, the most damaging type of spinal injury as a result of a road traffic accident (RTA) is a sudden hyperflexion and rotation with fracture-dislocation of the vertebral column at C5 and C6, and T12 to L1. Within 30–60 min of the trauma, autonomic and motor reflexes below the level of the injury are suppressed. This state is known as spinal shock and it may last hours or even weeks. It is probably a result of the sudden cessation of efferent impulses from the supraspinal centres.

Anaphylactic shock

This type of shock is life-threatening if it is not dealt with immediately. It arises when the individual develops a hypersensitivity response to an antigen, drug or foreign protein in which the release of histamine causes widespread vasodilatation resulting in hypotension and increased capillary permeability with loss of fluid into the interstitium.

The main causes of systemic anaphylaxis are insect bites and stings (particularly from bees and wasps) and drugs (notably penicillin). Occasionally, diagnostic contrast media may also precipitate anaphylactic reactions.

Q **18.4** What precautions might be observed before a patient undergoes a diagnostic test involving a contrast medium?

The individual developing anaphylactic shock presents with a combination of the following symptoms:

- skin eruptions, large weals
- local oedema, particularly around the face
- a weak and rapid pulse
- laryngeal stridor, dyspnoea, cough and, occasionally, cyanosis.

Treatment will be urgently needed because of the respiratory problems caused by local tissue swelling, laryngeal oedema and/or bronchospasm in addition to circulatory insufficiency (see Ch. 16. p. 597).

Box 18.2 provides a summary of interventions used in the treatment of shock.

FIRST AID TREATMENT FOR SHOCK

Nurses may occasionally be called upon to help people on the street or in other public places who have gone into shock as the result of an accident, heart attack or severe allergic reaction, and so should be aware of the appropriate first aid to give in the absence of clinical facilities.

The main objectives of intervention in such an emergency should be:

- to maintain an adequate supply of blood to the heart, lungs and brain
- to ascertain the cause of the shock
- to limit haemorrhaging and prevent further injury
- to arrange for transfer to hospital.

Box 18.2 Definitive and supportive therapy in clinical shock. (Adapted from Rice 1991)

Definitive therapy

Hypovolaemic shock
- Maintain or increase intravascular volume
- Decrease any future fluid/blood loss via i.v. fluid regimen
- Give supplementary O_2 therapy

Cardiogenic shock
- Reduce cardiac muscle damage by O_2 supply and reduce cardiac demand by O_2 therapy and cardiac medication to dilate the coronary vessels and by decreasing pain and activity
- Increase effectiveness of heart as a pump via inotropic medication

Septic shock
- Restore adequate intravascular volume via i.v. fluids
- Give supplemental O_2 therapy
- Identify and control source of infection via bacterial screening
- Administer appropriate antibiotics
- Remove nidus of infection if possible

Anaphylactic shock
- Identify and remove causative antigen
- Reduce effects of mediator substances that have caused massive vasodilatation, e.g. give adrenaline to restore vascular tone, antihistamines to reverse histamine effects, bronchiolators to oppose bronchial constriction
- Give O_2 therapy and i.v. fluid replacement

Supportive therapy
- Give adequate ventilation and oxygenation via optimal airway maintenance, optimal breathing technique and supplemental O_2
- Maintain or restore adequate perfusion of tissues to ensure oxygen delivery, via maintenance of cardiac pump to effectively circulate the blood and medication to improve contractility and reduce cardiac workload
- Maintain or restore metabolic equilibrium
- Reverse metabolic acidosis via hyperventilation and, if severe, by i.v. sodium bicarbonate administration

Box 18.3 lists the steps to take in the event of an emergency, especially where hypovolaemic shock is suspected or imminent.

MANAGEMENT AND TREATMENT OF SHOCK

In its early stages, shock demands immediate intervention. Treatment must begin even before a primary diagnosis is confirmed; otherwise the pathophysiological process of the shock reaction may quickly become irreversible. Re-establishing perfusion of the vital organs is essential. The nurse should be confident in the 'ABC' of resuscitation (see Ch. 2, p. 232, and Ch 27, p. 836). The patient may require immediate intubation in the accident and emergency (A&E) department or protection of her airway by the insertion of an artificial airway. Immediate oxygen therapy will be required, possibly with assisted ventilation. In the obviously hypovolaemic patient, rapid fluid replacement will be required. The nurse's role in carrying out or assisting with these measures will be crucial from the outset.

The nurse must know what actions will be necessary for the particular type of shock that has developed. She must understand

Box 18.3 Emergency interventions at the scene of an accident

1. Immediately reassure and comfort the person.
2. Check the airway for patency. If breathing is laboured or difficult, lie the individual in the recovery position if it is safe to do so. This will reduce the risk of aspiration of stomach contents. The jaw may need to be lifted, without hyperextension of the neck, to aid in the maintenance of the airway. Loosen any tight clothing, especially around the neck. *NB — do not attempt to move the person if there is any likelihood of cervical or other spinal injury.*
3. If haemorrhaging is obvious, try to control it by applying pressure.
4. Ask someone reliable to call 999. Give clear instructions, i.e. what kind of help is needed and the correct location of the accident. People tend to panic when a crisis occurs and someone needs to assume the position of leader and maintain an air of calm efficiency. Discourage onlookers from gathering as this only distresses the individual even further.
5. If relatives or friends are at the scene, ask them for a quick history. This may help to ascertain the cause of the shock.
6. Someone may be able to provide a blanket or coat to cover the person. However, do not accept the offer of a hot water bottle, as the application of heat would only increase peripheral vasodilatation and draw some of the blood supply away from the vital organs.
7. If the person complains of thirst, moisten the lips with water but do not allow drinking.
8. If a cardiac or respiratory arrest develops, commence artificial resuscitation immediately.
9. Transfer the person to hospital as soon as possible.
10. Try to ensure safety, considering the cause of the problem. For example, in the case of an RTA, ask someone to warn and divert traffic, taking care for his or her own safety.

Box 18.4 Identifying patients at risk of experiencing shock

- Has the patient experienced multiple trauma?
- Has the patient had surgery recently?
- Has the patient suffered severe burns?
- Is the patient postpartum?
- Does the patient have a history of oesophageal varices or peptic ulceration?
- Is the patient taking anticoagulant therapy?

The above factors put the patient at risk of ***hypovolaemic*** *shock.*

- Has the patient experienced chest pain recently or suffered a myocardial infarction — especially in vessels supplying the anterior wall of the left ventricle?
- Does the patient have a history of cardiac failure or cardiac dysrhythmias?

The above factors put the patient at risk of ***cardiogenic*** *shock.*

- Does the patient have impaired immunity, e.g. is she suffering from AIDS or cancer or undergoing chemotherapy?
- Does the patient have a resistant deep-seated infection?
- Is the patient seriously ill and requiring multiple invasive catheters and devices?

The above factors put the patient at risk of ***septic*** *shock.*

- Does the patient suffer from any disordered state resulting in impaired nervous stimuli to vascular shock muscle?
- Has the patient experienced recent spinal anaesthesia?
- Has the patient experienced trauma to the brain and/or spinal cord?

The above factors put the patient at risk of experiencing ***neurogenic*** *or* ***spinal*** *shock.*

- Does the patient have significant allergies or sensitivities?
- Is the patient undergoing tests requiring contrast media?

The above factors put the patient at risk of experiencing ***anaphylactic*** *shock.*

the rationale behind all interventions, bearing firmly in mind the overall aims of treatment, which are:

- to restore and maintain the circulating blood volume, ensuring that oxygenation and plasma osmotic pressure are adequate
- to achieve and maintain effective cardiac function
- to prevent complications.

As well as being able to recognise the warning signs of shock (see p. 638), the nurse should be able to identify those patients who are most at risk of developing shock. When obtaining a patient's initial history the nurse should take note of the risk factors listed in Box 18.4.

18.5 (a) Read Case History 18.2. In your opinion, is Mr A suffering from shock? If so, which type?
(b) Why might his abdomen be rigid?
(c) What initial steps should medical and nursing staff take?

Management and treatment of hypovolaemic shock

Regardless of what may have triggered the patient's hypovolaemia, the restoration of circulating fluid volume is the key to management. As soon as the patient's airway has been secured and oxygen therapy instituted, the next priority is to assess circulatory status and commence replacement i.v. fluids via two large-bore cannulae. The nurse needs to ask:

- What kind of fluid is required?
- How much fluid does the patient need?

Clinical opinion varies with regard to resuscitative fluids. Fluid therapy should be guided clinically, by changes in respiratory rate, heart rate and blood pressure. Edwards (1993) describes central venous pressure monitoring as being misleading, as the readings may be high even in the presence of profound hypovolaemia due to the homeostatic mechanisms of maintaining the blood pressure.

Crystalloids

Normal saline solution (sodium chloride 0.9%) is often the first replacement fluid administered to the shocked patient, although its large concentration of chloride ions could be disadvantageous to the patient whose renal function is already impaired. It may also cause hypernatraemia, hypokalaemia or a hyperchloraemic metabolic acidosis.

Case History 18.2 Mr A

Mr A, aged 35, is married and has two young children. While travelling to work one morning he was involved in an RTA. Within 30 minutes he was admitted to the nearest A&E department, where initial assessment showed the following:

Vital signs
- Blood pressure — systolic = 70 mmHg but diastolic difficult to hear
- Heart rate — 150/min; pulse weak, thready and rapid
- Respirations — 40/min; breathing shallow
- Temperature — 35.5°C

Neurological signs
- Little response to painful stimuli
- Poor gag and cough reflex
- Right pupil unresponsive to light
- Left pupil reacting sluggishly
- Glasgow Coma Scale score = 4

General examination
- Large swelling in right occiput
- Rigid abdomen; bowel sounds absent
- Obvious fracture to right femur with large gaping wound
- Possible fractured pelvis
- Skin moist and clammy; mouth dry

Dextrose 5% is not considered a suitable fluid for the patient in shock, although it may maintain water balance and supply the calories necessary for cell metabolism.

Hartmann's solution is one of the most common resuscitative fluids used in haemorrhagic shock. Essentially it is an electrolyte solution consisting of sodium chloride, potassium chloride, calcium chloride and sodium lactate in water. Since it closely resembles blood plasma, but without the formed elements, it can be used as an emergency plasma expander until blood has been grouped and cross-matched. It rarely causes any adverse reactions and is inexpensive and readily available.

Colloids
When crystalloid fluids do not reverse the hypovolaemia, a colloid solution may be administered. A colloid is a solution containing large particles, such as protein, which help to restore the interstitial osmotic pressure. Examples of colloids are albumin and fresh frozen plasma. However, increasingly, synthetic solutions are being used due to the expense of human products.

Dextran is a synthetic colloidal solution that simulates the effects of albumin. It provides rapid plasma volume expansion when compatible blood or blood products are unavailable. Advantages of dextran include its long shelf-life, its reasonable cost and the fact that it presents no risk of hepatitis or AIDS transmission. It may, however, interfere with blood typing and cross-matching, as it tends to coat the cells. It has also been known to cause allergic reactions.

Other colloids include polygeline (Haemaccel), succinylated gelatin (Gelofusine) and hetastarch (Hespan).

Combined solutions
Despite their advantages, it is argued that the crystalloid group of solutions dilute the plasma proteins and reduce the plasma oncotic pressure. This leads to changes in cell wall permeability, resulting in increased fluid leakage across the capillaries into the interstitial space and hence oedema, particularly in the lungs. Ledingham & Ramsay (1986) suggest that the best results are achieved by using a combination of crystalloid and colloid solutions, citing evidence that the cell's oxygen consumption is higher with a combination of both solutions.

Blood
The rapid replacement of blood and blood products is essential in the haemorrhagically shocked patient. It is often necessary to use a pressure infuser to increase the rate of delivery and a blood warmer to bring the blood up to body temperature in order to avoid excessive cooling of the patient (see Ch. 27).

Autotransfusion. This procedure involves collecting the lost blood from the patient, treating the blood with an anticoagulant and reinfusing the patient (Tortora & Grabowski 1996). Autotransfusion is a popular practice in large trauma centres.

Management and treatment of cardiogenic shock
The main goals of therapy in cardiogenic shock are:

- to re-establish circulation to the myocardium
- to minimise heart muscle damage
- to improve the effectiveness of the heart as a pump.

Damage to cardiac muscle can be minimised by improving the heart's oxygen supply and, at the same time, reducing its own oxygen demand. Oxygen supply can be increased by the administration of a high percentage of O_2 via a non-rebreathing face mask. Jowett & Thompson (1996) state that 'high oxygen concentrations (100%) are required and toxicity rarely occurs because of arteriovenous shrinking in the lungs'. Oxygen demand can be reduced by placing the patient in a comfortable position (Boore et al 1987) and keeping her at rest. Analgesics to control pain will also aid in the reduction of O_2 demand.

The effectiveness of the heart's pumping action can be enhanced by the use of inotropic agents, which increase the force of contraction and improve systolic ejection of blood (Rice 1991).

The catecholamines such as adrenaline and noradrenaline are commonly used to improve contractility and correct hypotension, and since the patient with myocardial ischaemia and impaired myocardial contractility will also be at risk of arrhythmias, antiarrhythmic agents may also be administered.

Drugs commonly used
Catecholamines function by stimulating the smooth muscle receptors of the myocardium. This leads to an increase in the contractility of the myocardium and thereby increases cardiac output, raises arterial pressure and improves tissue perfusion.

Dopamine is one such agent frequently used in cardiogenic shock; it does have the disadvantage, however, of producing an atrial tachycardia. Dobutamine is another catecholamine which acts directly on the beta-adrenergic receptors in the myocardium and has an inotropic and chronotropic effect.

Dopexamine hydrochloride is a more recent catecholamine which increases cardiac output and improves peripheral circulation. Its dopaminergic properties, with resulting effects on splanchnic and renal blood flow, may help to prevent development of renal failure in septic shock (Kaukinen et al 1991). Enoximone and milrinone are phosphodiesterase inhibitors marketed for intravenous use in patients with cardiac failure. Both drugs strengthen cardiac contraction and dilate peripheral vessels, reducing ventricular preload and afterload. In some cases, drugs may be prescribed to decrease afterload. Here, the goal of therapy is to decrease vascular resistance, improve the ventricles' emptying capacity and, in so doing, to lower the filling pressure of the heart. Nitroprusside is probably the drug most frequently used for this purpose in short-term applications.

The intra-aortic balloon pump (IABP)

The IABP is often used in conjunction with drugs to improve afterload. It assists a weakened or damaged left ventricle by aiding left ventricle ejection and thus improving coronary artery and peripheral tissue perfusion.

There are various types of IABPs, all of which work on the same principle. The catheter is inserted via the femoral artery and the balloon is advanced into the aorta just distal to the left subclavian junction. The catheter is then attached to a pump which inflates the balloon with carbon dioxide or helium during diastole and in so doing increases intra-aortic blood pressure, thereby improving coronary artery perfusion.

Ventricular assist device

For some patients, the above therapies are not sufficient and ventricular assist may be needed. This device is basically a pump to bypass a failing ventricle, which physically removes blood from the circulation allowing the ventricle to rest and recover. A large-bore cannula is inserted from the atria to drain blood to the pump and back via another inflow cannula from the pulmonary artery or aorta. The decision to use a ventricular assist device should not be taken lightly, due to the possibility of life-threatening complications such as arterial occlusion or pulmonary embolism, and in addition requires highly skilled nursing expertise.

For further information, see Coombs (1993a).

Management and treatment of septic shock

The first stage in treatment of septic shock is directed at restoring the patient's circulating volume, which may initially correct hypotension and the cardiac index (see Box 18.1).

Cultures should be taken from all possible sites of infection and sensitivities determined. It may in some cases be necessary to treat the septic focus surgically, e.g. by drainage of abscesses or debridement of infected or necrotic tissue.

The critically ill patient is likely to have a number of invasive monitoring devices, all of which provide an opportunity for pathogens to invade the body. In view of this risk, antibiotics are usually commenced before any definitive results arrive from the bacteriology laboratory.

Blood gases

Blood gases should be monitored regularly. Access can be gained by arterial cannulation and increasingly nurses are taking responsibility for arterial line sampling in the light of the *Scope of Professional Practice* document (UKCC 1992). Many patients with septic shock present with a mixed acidosis due to a respiratory and metabolic element. Treating the cause is obviously vital and most patients will require artificial ventilation in a critical care unit.

Nitric oxide and nitric oxide inhibitors

Although still in the experimental stages, treatment of septic shock with nitric oxide and/or nitric oxide inhibitors is having noteworthy results (Kalweit 1997). The action of nitric oxide was first discovered by Furchgott as early as 1980. Many studies have been carried out to determine the benefits of treatment and successful applications have been made in North America, Europe and Australia (Cuthbertson & Webster 1995).

Vasoactive substances essential in the physiological regulation of blood vessel tone are produced within the endothelial layer of the pulmonary vasculature. One of these substances is endothelium-derived relaxing factor (EDRF). Nitric oxide is the gaseous form of this potent vasodilator.

The physiological effects of nitric oxide. The release of nitric oxide is responsible for many physiological effects, including control of vessel tone and tissue perfusion, platelet aggregation, white cell function and neuronal activity. Nitric oxide is produced by the enzyme nitric oxide synthase from the substrate amino acid L-arginine. The nitric oxide produced then diffuses to the vascular smooth muscle layer, stimulating the enzyme guanylate cyclase. Guanosine triphosphate is formed, which then catalyses the production of guanosine monophosphate. This chemical cascade is responsible for smooth muscle relaxation and vasodilatation.

In septic shock, endotoxin stimulates the formation of excessive amounts of endogenous nitric oxide, resulting in profound vasodilatation and hypotension.

Nitric oxide inhibitors. Nitric oxide inhibitors administered by i.v. infusion are currently being investigated for the treatment of severe hypotension associated with septic shock (Crowley 1996).

Inhalational nitric oxide. Nitric oxide in the form of inhalation therapy is currently being used successfully for the treatment of adult respiratory distress syndrome (ARDS, see p. 650) and pulmonary hypertension in many critical care units. One of the most useful features of nitric oxide is its lack of effect on the systemic circulation. Controlled administration of nitric oxide optimises gas exchange by opening up the pulmonary blood vessels to extract the maximum amount of oxygen as the blood flows through the lungs. The result is an improvement in overall gas exchange and the elimination of carbon dioxide. Because nitric oxide selectively ventilates areas of the lungs, lower oxygen concentrations and decreased ventilator pressures can be used on critically ill patients requiring ventilator support. Cardiac function is also enhanced because the nitric oxide-induced vasodilatation reduces pulmonary artery pressure and thus the stress on the right ventricle.

Microcirculatory changes

The patient suffering from septic shock needs particular nursing attention to the condition of her skin. The administration of inotropic agents increases peripheral vasoconstriction and the resulting decrease in tissue perfusion puts the patient at risk of pressure sores. Moreover, the patient may not be sufficiently haemodynamically stable to allow frequent repositioning or assessment of pressure areas. Such critically ill patients often require the expertise of a tissue viability nurse or specialist nurse to assess and implement a strategy for the prevention of pressure sores (see Ch. 29). A number of therapeutic beds are now available for purchase or rent which will provide appropriate therapy, and in addition some beds rotate the patient, providing a useful adjunct to postural drainage and physiotherapy (James 1997).

Management and treatment of anaphylactic shock

Swift recognition of anaphylactic shock, which results from a severe allergic reaction to a specific antigen, is vital to the individual's survival. Intervention should aim first at identifying and removing the cause. If this is not possible, the effects of the reaction must be reversed.

In extreme circumstances, intubation and artificial ventilation may be needed to overcome respiratory complications. The drug of choice is i.v. adrenaline to restore vascular tone. Aminophylline may be given to counteract bronchoconstriction and antihistamines may be administered to reverse the adverse effect of the mediator histamine involved in the reaction. As with other forms of shock, oxygen therapy and i.v. fluid replacement will usually be required (see also Ch. 16, p. 597).

Definitive and supportive therapy

From the above it can be seen that the interventions used in the treatment and management of shock may be described as either 'definitive' or 'supportive'(Rice 1991). The goal of definitive therapy is to locate and correct the cause of the shock and to restore and maintain adequate perfusion and oxygenation of the tissues, while the goal of supportive therapy is to improve oxygen delivery to the tissues, to restore and maintain tissue perfusion, and to restore cellular function.

For further reading on the management of fractures and burns, see Chapters 10 and 30, respectively.

MONITORING THE PATIENT IN SHOCK

Monitoring and observation of the patient's ever-changing condition will allow for the prompt correction of deficits. The following are the most important indicators of tissue perfusion and will be discussed in the following sections:

- cardiac status
- respiratory status
- haemodynamic status
- level of consciousness
- renal function
- body temperature
- skin condition.

Monitoring cardiac status

Electrocardiography

An electrocardiogram (ECG) is a recording of the electrical activity of the myocardium and indicates the changes which occur as a result of contraction. The contraction of any heart muscle is associated with electrical changes called depolarisation and these can be detected by electrodes attached to the surface of the body (see Ch. 2). An ECG can be obtained quickly in an A&E department or with a portable electrocardiograph at the site of an accident and can give useful information about the rate and rhythm of the heart. Thus, if arrhythmias arise they can be detected and treated immediately. All patients who are likely to be suffering from shock should be monitored by electrocardiograph. In addition, heart sounds should be assessed, as should major arterial pulses for rate, rhythm and pressure.

Q **18.6** What might cause a shocked patient to experience: A

(a) tachycardia — heart rate ≥100 beats/min

(b) bradycardia — heart rate ≤60 beats/min?

Monitoring respiratory status

The shocked patient's respiratory status may change rapidly and therefore should be monitored at frequent intervals, allowing for the early detection of potential deterioration. In the early stages, the nurse should be alert to hyperventilation, resulting in respiratory alkalosis followed by fatigue of the respiratory muscles. This may lead to shallow breathing and the risk of respiratory distress, necessitating mechanical ventilation.

Monitoring oxygen saturation

The level of O_2 saturation in the patient's blood (S_aO_2) will give some indication of respiratory status. Continuous monitoring will give valuable information on the individual's response to interventions and can provide early warning of hypoxaemia. Both invasive and non-invasive techniques are available for S_aO_2 measurement.

Pulse oximetry. Arterial O_2 saturation along with pulse rate can be monitored continuously by means of a non-invasive electronic device called a pulse oximeter. This functions by measuring the absorption of red and infrared light passed through living tissue (usually a finger, toe or ear lobe). Since results correspond closely to arterial blood gas values, this instrument reduces the need for blood samples. Readings are not affected by skin colour but can be distorted by high blood bilirubin levels (as in jaundice) and in cases of carbon monoxide poisoning and smoke inhalation. Results for very heavy smokers may also be difficult to interpret. Coull (1992) gives further details on the operation of the pulse oximeter.

The fibreoptic catheter. The fibreoptic catheter can be used to measure the patient's venous oxygen saturation. This pulmonary artery catheter contains two optical fibres: one transmits light from the optical module to the catheter tip, and the second collects reflected light at the catheter tip and transmits it back to the optical module. These signals are transmitted to a computer which calculates oxygen saturation percentage values. These values are continuously displayed in numerical form and recorded as a graph. Acceptable oxygen saturation levels are considered to be above 90%, although observing for changes in trends should be the nursing priority.

Monitoring haemodynamic status

In the shocked patient, blood pressure may initially be kept within normal limits by the compensatory mechanisms described earlier (see p. 636). However, as shock progresses and cardiac output decreases, blood pressure will fall. In progressive decompensating shock, the use of a sphygmomanometer to estimate blood pressure is inaccurate and inadequate, and more sophisticated investigation will be required.

Central venous pressure (CVP) monitoring

CVP is the blood pressure within the right atrium and vena cava. Its measurement can give information about blood volume or venous system capacity. It can also give an indication of vascular tone and pulmonary vascular resistance, as well as of the effectiveness of the right heart pump. However, it does not measure left ventricular function and it can be unreliable in the critically ill patient with chronic lung disease, right and left heart failure and valve disease.

CVP monitoring reflects the rate of blood return to the right side of the heart and can be an accurate guide for fluid replacement. A CVP of about 0.5 cmH_2O in the presence of a low arterial blood pressure usually indicates hypovolaemia, while a CVP above 14 cmH_2O in the presence of a low arterial blood pressure indicates cardiac failure (see Fig. 18.4).

Technique. A large-bore catheter should be inserted under aseptic conditions into the internal or external jugular, subclavian or femoral veins either using the percutaneous technique via a large-bore needle or by means of a venous cutdown by a member of the medical staff. The site of the central line is checked radiologically prior to the commencement of fluid therapy.

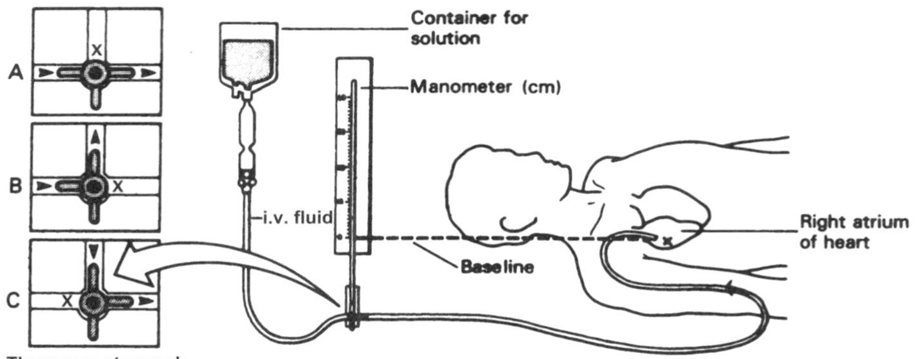

Fig. 18.4 Diagram of a CVP water manometer. A: Before measuring central venous pressure (CVP), the infusion flow is to the patient and the three-way stopcock is closed to the manometer. B: To measure CVP, the stopcock is turned so that it is closed to the patient. This allows the manometer to be refilled with fluid. C: The stopcock is turned so that it is closed to the infusion fluid. This allows a free flow of fluid from the manometer to the intravenous catheter. The fluid level will fall until the level corresponds with the pressure in the right atrium or superior vena cava. (Adapted from Jamieson et al 1997.)

In the intensive therapy or high-dependency unit, a transducer can be attached to the central line in order to obtain a waveform and digital display of the CVP reading in mmHg. Continuous monitoring will indicate the effectiveness of treatment.

Central venous lines, although extremely important for a critically ill patient, present a danger of bacterial infection. Nurses can make an important contribution to care by ensuring that aseptic techniques are adhered to when the line is inserted initially and that the insertion site is kept clean and dry. Once it is no longer needed, the line should be removed as quickly as possible to reduce the risk of infection.

Arterial pressure monitoring

An accurate assessment of blood pressure can be made by measuring the arterial pressure directly. This is performed by medical staff by the insertion of a flexible catheter into an easily accessible artery. The most commonly used site is the radial artery, as the line can be readily secured and observed at this point, and the hand has a good collateral circulation. Other frequently used sites include the brachial, femoral and dorsal arteries.

Once the catheter is inserted, it is attached to a bag of normal saline, which is normally pressurised to around 300 mmHg (see Fig. 18.5). Approximately 2–3 mL/h of the solution is delivered into the artery to maintain patency. By means of a transducer the arterial waveform is displayed on a monitor along with arterial pressure readings.

Patients with an arterial catheter in place require constant nursing supervision, in order to ensure that the catheter does not become disconnected, as the patient could exsanguinate in a matter of minutes. The nurse should ensure that the catheter is securely positioned and covered with a sterile dressing. In addition, the catheter should be clearly labelled to prevent the line being used as an injection port.

For further information see Allan (1989).

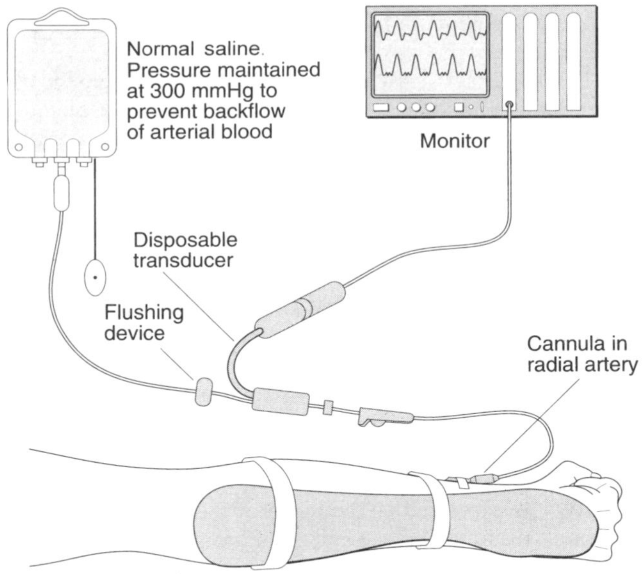

Fig. 18.5 Arterial pressure monitoring equipment.

The normal waveform will indicate that the arterial catheter is functioning and that the digital blood pressure display is accurate. The nurse must be able to recognise its distinct pattern, which is composed of a systolic upstroke and a dicrotic notch on the downstroke (see Fig. 18.6). The dicrotic notch occurs as a result of the aortic valve closing and a simultaneous increase in aortic pressure. If this pattern becomes dampened, the nurse must be aware that it may indicate a clot in the catheter, air in the line or pressure from the tip of the catheter against the vessel wall itself.

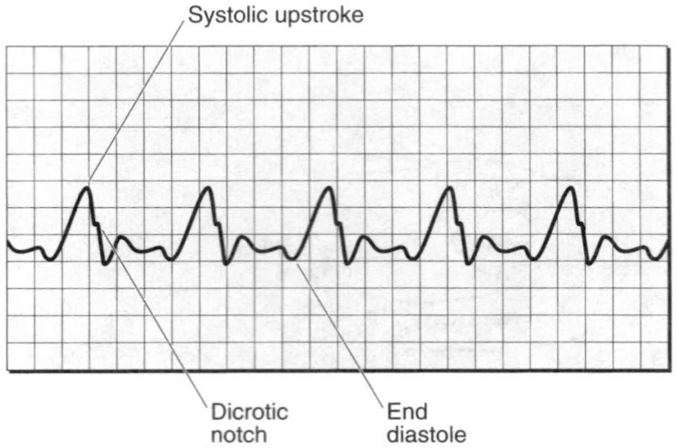

Fig. 18.6 Normal arterial waveform.

Pulmonary artery pressure monitoring

The pulmonary artery, flow-directed, balloon-tipped catheter has made possible the safe and easy assessment of left ventricular function (Fig. 18.7). Cardiac output, right and left ventricular pressures, and pulmonary capillary wedge pressures can all be measured using this catheter. The readings obtained allow the clinician to determine the intervention and therapies required (see Fig. 18.8).

Pulmonary artery catheter insertion. The catheter must be inserted by experienced medical staff under sterile conditions, using an appropriate introducer and catheter.

The catheter is usually inserted at the bedside where the patient is constantly monitored. An image intensifier is not required, as the characteristic pressure changes which take place in each chamber can be viewed on the cardiac monitor. The catheter can be inserted via either a peripheral or a central vein. Possible sites include the internal jugular, subclavian, basilic and cephalic veins.

Monitoring pulmonary wedge pressure. By measuring the pulmonary artery wedge pressure (PAWP) the clinician gains an accurate picture of the patient's left-sided cardiac function (see Fig. 18.8). In order to measure PAWP, the balloon is inflated with approximately 1.0 mL of air. This will enable the catheter tip to be wedged in a smaller branch of the pulmonary artery. When the vessel has been totally occluded, the catheter's distal port will detect the pressure within the occluded vessel and will display the resulting waveform and pressure reading on the monitor.

PAWP is expressed as the mean of the diastolic and systolic pressures, the normal range being 8–12 mmHg.

18.7 If the patient has a PAWP of <8 mmHg what does that indicate?
18.8 If the PAWP is >25 mmHg, what might be the medical diagnosis?

Monitoring cardiac output. By means of the pulmonary catheter with a thermistor (temperature probe) in place, the patient's cardiac output (see Box 18.1 p. 639) can be calculated using the thermodilution technique (see Fig. 18.9). This involves injecting a 10 mL bolus of dextrose 5% or normal saline through the proximal port into the right atrium. This fluid must be cooler than the patient's blood so that the temperature change which occurs as the blood mixes with the fluid can be detected by the thermistor in the pulmonary artery. The results are relayed to a cardiac output computer

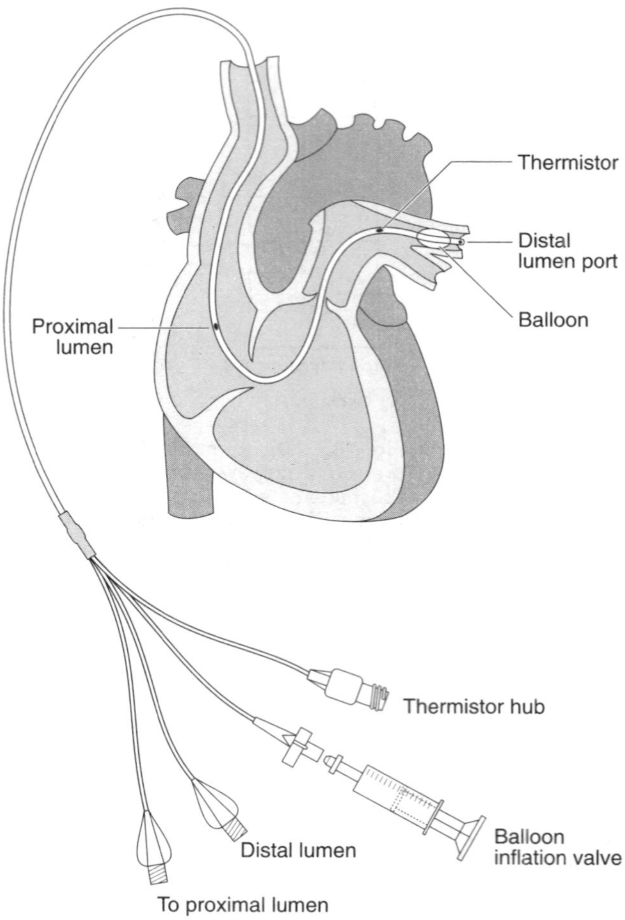

Fig. 18.7 A pulmonary artery catheter. *Distal lumen*: located at the tip of the catheter in the pulmonary artery. Pulmonary artery pressure (PAP), pulmonary artery wedge pressure (PAWP) and mixed venous gas pressures are obtained at this port. *Proximal lumen*: used for central venous pressure (CVP) monitoring or main fluid infusion lumen. It is situated in the right atrium and can also be utilised to measure the right atrial pressure. *Balloon inflation valve*: the balloon situated at the end of the catheter may be inflated to read the PAWP. *Thermistor hub*: situated 4 cm from the tip of the catheter and used to measure cardiac output by thermodilution methods (see Fig. 18.9).

and displayed in L/min. This procedure is usually carried out at least three or four times and the mean value taken as the cardiac output.

For further reading, see Coombs (1993b).

The nurse's responsibilities. As soon as the PAWP reading is obtained, the balloon must be deflated, as prolonged occlusion of the pulmonary artery will cause pulmonary infarction. The nurse must observe the catheter waveform carefully and ensure that the catheter does not migrate up into a branch of the pulmonary artery and occlude it. A flat or dampened trace will indicate that this has occurred and that the balloon needs to be checked. Sometimes, if the patient is asked to cough, the tip of the catheter may be freed. However, this method is not always effective and the doctor should be notified if a dampened waveform persists.

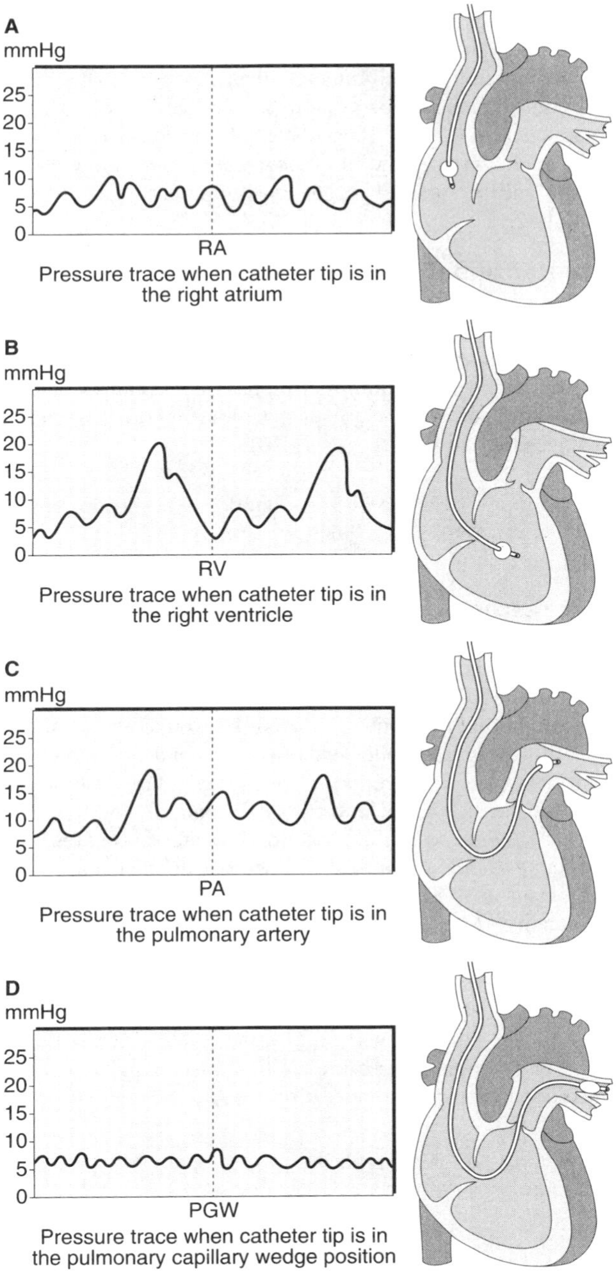

Fig. 18.8 Waveform changes during monitoring by pulmonary artery catheter. (A) The catheter is advanced by the doctor until it is in the right atrium. The balloon is then inflated. (B) The balloon carries the catheter through the tricuspid valve and into the right ventricle. (C) The pressure of blood flow carries the catheter through the pulmonary valve into the pulmonary artery. (D) When the catheter has become wedged in a branch of the pulmonary artery, the balloon is deflated and falls back into the pulmonary artery, where it can be used to monitor continuously the pulmonary artery pressure.

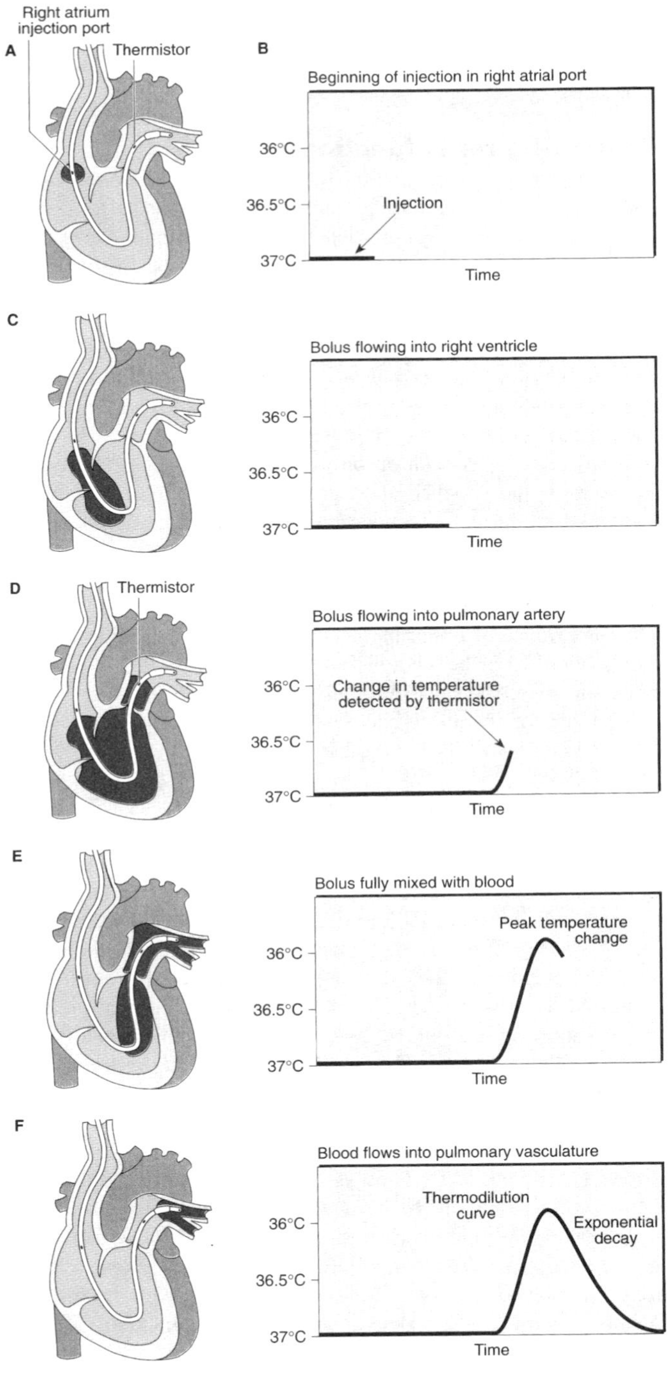

Fig. 18.9 The thermodilution technique for assessing cardiac output.

Monitoring level of consciousness

In the early stages of shock, the patient may still be quite alert and anxious. She may complain of pain and may be able to give a history which will help the clinician to establish a diagnosis. However, if her cerebral perfusion pressure falls, with resulting cerebral hypoxia, she will gradually become less coherent and may eventually become comatose. The nurse should observe the patient carefully at this stage and ensure an airway is maintained. It may be advisable to place her in the lateral position. In a clinical setting, medical staff may elect to intubate and artificially ventilate the patient. The Glasgow Coma Scale (see Fig. 28.4, p. 857) is a useful tool with which to assess the patient's cerebral function. For a detailed discussion of consciousness levels, see Chapter 28, page 853.

Monitoring renal function

Renal function is a very good indicator of tissue perfusion and should therefore be monitored carefully in patients suffering from shock. Since the kidneys are dependent on adequate tissue perfusion, a drop in urinary output will indicate poor perfusion. Unless the patient is dehydrated, urinary output should be 0.5–1.0 mL/kg per hour.

Urinary catheterisation and hourly urine volumes can assist in early detection of decreasing renal perfusion.

Measurement of specific gravity and osmolality will reflect the concentration of the urine. In the early stages of shock, when urine volume falls, the concentration of excreted waste products rises. However, if the shocked state progresses, urine volumes remain low but the ability to concentrate the urine and blood and the osmolality are fixed or low (Rice 1991).

Monitoring body temperature

The importance of obtaining accurate body temperature measurements should not be underestimated, as many clinical interventions are based on these readings. These factors, as well as procedures for obtaining accurate core temperature readings, are described in detail in Chapter 22.

Observing skin condition

Direct observation of the skin colour, temperature and condition will reflect the stage of shock that the patient is in. Intense activation of the sympathetic nervous system will result in pale, clammy skin and a dry mouth. Failure of capillary refill will indicate sustained and prolonged vasoconstriction. If oxygen delivery is severely impaired, the skin will become cold, mottled and cyanosed. However, it should be noted that the clinical picture in septic shock is different. In the early stages of this type of shock, the skin becomes warm, dry and flushed as bacterial toxins cause vasodilatation.

Laboratory and diagnostic tests

Arterial blood gas (ABG) analysis can give some indication of circulatory efficiency. In the early stages of shock, it is not uncommon to find a fall in the partial pressure of oxygen ($P\text{O}_2$) and a rise in the partial pressure of carbon dioxide ($P\text{CO}_2$). However, $P\text{CO}_2$ may fall due to hyperventilation. With an increase in anaerobic metabolism and in the production of lactic acid, metabolic acidosis is frequently seen in the severely shocked patient.

Information on a range of diagnostic tests is given in Appendix 1.

COMPLICATIONS OF SHOCK

Renal failure

When the crisis of shock occurs, blood flow to the kidneys is reduced both by the original hypovolaemic or other circulatory problem and by the vasoconstriction which occurs as part of the body's compensatory mechanisms (see p. 636).

Q **18.9** What are the functions of noradrenaline?

In addition to the reduction of blood flow to the kidneys, there is also a change in the flow within the kidneys. Blood flow is directed away from the renal cortex to the renal medulla to preserve the function of the juxtamedullary nephrons. This is essential if the countercurrent system of concentrating the urine is to function (see Ch. 8). If, however, the shock persists without prompt treatment, then the countercurrent mechanism will fail and the urine will become dilute, leading to the early stages of acute renal failure.

Haemofiltration

Many patients with acute renal failure will require renal replacement therapy as part of their treatment. Haemofiltration is the removal of excess fluid and waste products from the blood by a filter in conjunction with fluid replacement. Increasingly, haemofiltration is being used in the critical care area and offers a number of advantages to dialysis (see Fig. 18.10).

For further reading see Woodrow (1993) and Kirby & Davenport (1996).

Adult respiratory distress syndrome (ARDS)

ARDS is characterised by acute, severe and progressive respiratory distress, increased stiffness of the lungs and diffuse lung opacification. At cellular level, a number of substances are activated, including macrophages, platelets, proteases, lysosomes, endotoxins, polymorphonuclear lysosomes and free oxygen radicals, which cause damage to the alveolar capillary membrane and lead to the classic sign of pulmonary oedema. In addition, surfactant production is decreased, secondary to atelectasis, resulting in dyspnoea. Although treatment has become sophisticated, there is still no drug or procedure which will cure ARDS. The mortality rate remains about 60% and has shown little reduction despite increased technology and intervention. Appropriate supportive nursing care is of paramount importance (Hamner 1995). Generally patients presenting with ARDS will be nursed in an intensive care unit and will require mechanical ventilation with positive end expiratory pressure (PEEP). Increasingly, inhalational nitric oxide is being used to treat severe ARDS (see p. 645).

Q **18.10** What is PEEP?

Positioning of patients

The body position of critically ill patients may have a profound effect on arterial oxygenation (Richardson 1997). A number of studies have examined the effects of nursing the patient supine, lateral or prone. A review of the literature suggests that the common practice of supine positioning may be erroneous. Nursing critically ill patients prone is challenging to nurses but may prove to be beneficial to those patients who do not respond to conventional therapies and high inspired oxygen concentrations (Lasater-Erhard 1995). Although the efficacy of the prone position remains controversial, Thomas (1997) suggests that reversal of the gravitational forces increases perfusion to ventilated regions with resolution of ventilation–perfusion mismatch (see Ch. 29).

Newer treatments also include pressure-controlled inverse ratio ventilation.

See Ahrens et al (1996) for further reading.

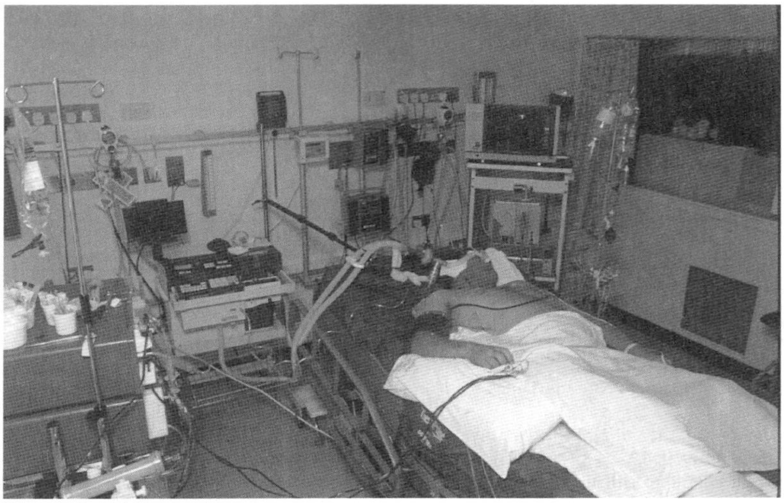

Fig. 18.10 Patient on haemofiltration therapy. (Reproduced with kind permission from West Lothian NHS Trust.)

Disseminated intravascular coagulation (DIC)

Some of the pathophysiological processes leading to DIC have already been described in relation to septic shock (see p. 640). In DIC the patient's normal clotting mechanisms do not function correctly. Clots may be produced in capillaries where they are not required, and sites where clotting factors could be utilised are deprived of them. Fibrinolytic (clot-dissolving) factors then go into action where they are not needed, and the end result is uncontrolled haemorrhage.

Early clinical signs usually include bleeding from venepuncture sites, the mucous membranes, wounds or drain sites. Treatment is aimed at replacing the clotting factors by administering blood and blood components, platelets, fresh frozen plasma and possibly cryoprecipitates. Sometimes it is advisable to administer some heparin to slow or stop the clotting process before the clotting factors are replaced.

CONCLUSION

Although there have been important advances in the resuscitation and treatment of patients in shock in recent years, survival can still be improved by early recognition and supportive therapy (Edwards 1993).

Assisting individuals suffering from shock, whether in a hospital or a community setting, presents the nurse with a major challenge to her clinical skills. Intervention will require not only a sound understanding of the pathophysiological process of shock but also the ability to act swiftly on the basis of that understanding and to assist with a range of resuscitative and investigative procedures. Above all, the nurse is in a unique position to ensure that patients and their loved ones are supported and informed throughout this life-threatening experience.

REFERENCES

Bone R C 1991 Sepsis, the sepsis syndrome, multiorgan failure: a plea for comparative definitions. Annals of Internal Medicine 114: 332–333

Boore J R P, Champion R, Ferguson M C 1987 Nursing the physically ill adult. Churchill Livingstone, Edinburgh

Coull A 1992 Making sense of pulse oximetry. Nursing Times 88(32): 42–43

Crowley S R 1996 The pathogenesis of septic shock. Heart and Lung 25(2): 124–133

Cuthbertson B H, Webster N R 1995 Nitric oxide in critical care medicine. British Journal of Hospital Medicine 54(11): 579–582

Daily E K 1992 Haemodynamic monitoring. In: Guzzetta C E, Dossey B M (eds) Cardiovascular nursing: holistic practice. Mosby, St Louis, MO, pp 183–184

Edwards J D 1993 Management of septic shock. British Medical Journal 306: 1661–1664

Ferguson J 1991 Septic shock in the critically ill patient. Surgical Nurse 4(2): 22–24

Guyton A C, Hall J E 1996 Textbook of medical physiology. WB Saunders, London

Hamner J 1995 Challenging diagnosis: adult respiratory distress syndrome. Critical Care Nurse 15(5): 46–51

Hudak C M, Gallo B M 1994 Critical care nursing: a holistic approach. J B Lippincott, Philadelphia

Jackson J 1994 Endotoxin and the sepsis syndrome: do we cause more harm than good? British Journal of Intensive Care (suppl): 14–19

James H 1997 Pressure sore prevention in acutely ill patients. Professional Nurse 12(suppl 6): S8–10

Jamieson E M, McCall J M, Blythe R, White L A 1997 Guidelines for clinical nursing practices. 3rd edn. Churchill Livingstone, Edinburgh

Jowett N I, Thompson D R 1996 Comprehensive coronary care. Scutari, Harrow

Kalweit S 1997 Inhaled nitric oxide in the ICU. Critical Care Nurse 17(4): 26–32

Kaukinen S, Schavikin L, Kaukinen L 1991 Dopeximine hydrochloride in sepsis. Clinical Intensive Care 2(suppl 3): 47–49

Lasater-Erhard M 1995 The effect of patient position on arterial oxygen saturation. Critical Care Nurse 15(5): 31–36

Ledingham I M, Ramsey G 1986 Hypovolaemic shock. British Journal of Anaesthesia 58: 169–189

Quaal S J 1992 The person with heart failure and cardiogenic shock. In: Guzzetta C E, Dossey B M (eds) Cardiovascular nursing: holistic practice. Mosby, St Louis, MO, pp 329–332

Rice V 1991 Shock: a clinical syndrome. Parts 1–4. Critical Care Nurse 11(4–7): 20–27, 74–82, 34–39, 28–39

Richardson A 1997 Turning a patient prone with ARDS. Nursing in Critical Care 2(4): 197–199
Suffredini A F, Fromm R E, Parker M M et al 1989 The cardiovascular response of normal humans to the administration of endotoxin. New England Journal of Medicine 321: 280–287
Thomas C 1997 Use of the prone position: the ventilation/perfusion relationship in ARDS. Care of the Critically Ill 13(3): 96–99
Tortora G J, Grabowski S R 1996 Principles of anatomy and physiology. HarperCollins College, New York
United Kingdom Central Council of Nursing, Midwifery and Health Visiting 1992 Scope of professional practice. UKCC, London
Ward R G, Walsh M S 1991 Necrotising fasciitis: 10 years' experience in a district general hospital. Surgery 78: 488

FURTHER READING

Ahrens T S, Beattie S, Nienhaus T 1996 Experimental therapies to support the failing lung. AACN Clinical Issues: Advanced Practice in Acute and Critical Care 7(4): 507–518
Allan D 1989 Making sense of arterial catheterisation. Nursing Times 85(40): 45–47
Coombs M 1993a Ventricular assist devices for the failing heart: a nursing focus. Intensive and Critical Care Nursing 9: 17–23
Coombs M 1993b Haemodynamic profiles and the critical care nurse. Intensive and Critical Care Nurse 9: 11–16
Hagland M R 1996 Septic shock: a case study. Intensive and Critical Care Nursing 12: 55–59
Hayes E E 1990 Needs of family members of the critically ill patient: a Northern Ireland perspective. Care of the Critically Ill 6(1): 27–28
Kirby S, Davenport A (1996) Haemofiltration/dialysis treatment in patients with acute renal failure. Care of the Critically Ill 12(2): 54–58
Manifold S L 1995 Case history: traumatic adult respiratory distress syndrome – a multisystem approach. International Journal of Trauma Nursing 1(3): 74–81
McLuckie A, Bihari D 1994 Sepsis in the intensive care unit. Care of the Critically Ill Patient 10(6): 276–279
Moxham J, Goldstone J 1994 Assisted ventilation. BMJ Publishing Group, London
Roberts S L 1988 Cardiogenic shock: decreased coronary artery tissue perfusion. Dimensions of Critical Care Nursing 7(4): 196–208
Sandrock J 1997 Managing hypovolaemia. Nursing 27(12): 32aa–32ee
Vonfrolio L G, Noone J 1995 Self test: recognising signs of shock. Nursing 25(7): 18–21
Woodrow P 1993 Resource package: haemofiltration. Intensive and Critical Care Nursing 9: 95–107

PAIN

Sue Duke

19

INTRODUCTION

Melzack & Wall (1988) describe pain as a complex experience encompassing sensory, emotional, cognitive and behavioural components. Interaction between these components is influenced by physiological, psychological and sociocultural factors. These factors make pain unique for each individual, every time it is experienced. This means that although pain is a common experience, it is difficult to understand what pain is like for another person. This understanding is hampered by the lack of research addressing the lived experience of pain, in contrast to a vast body of research into the pathophysiology of pain and treatment modalities. Nevertheless, some recent research addresses this deficit and offers nurses ways of caring and supporting people in pain. Here is how one person described the pain she experienced: 'Bodily feelings were shrieking agony at the top of their voices, mental feelings were fury and total frustration' (Seers & Friedli 1996).

Another quote from the same study describes the overwhelming nature of pain:

> Pain is now beyond coping with…it has stopped me leading my whole life. I'm petrified they'll say I have to learn to live with this level of pain…I would rather die. I'd like to be unconscious. Deep inside I feel suicidal…Can't see through the pain when there is so much and I know I do not want to live with it.

Q **19.1** Think about a time when you were in pain. Write down your description of this experience. Compare your description with the discussion below.

Pain has been described and defined by a number of authors. Many definitions emphasise the physiological dimension of pain. For example, the International Association for the Study of Pain (IASP) (1986) define pain as the sensation caused by noxious (i.e. tissue damaging) or potentially tissue-damaging stimuli. However, this definition has been challenged by Wall (1989a) who argues that it is too simplistic and does not account for other peripheral stimuli, for central nervous system (CNS) activity and the variable way in which the nervous system responds to stimuli, especially after injury.

The conception of pain as a sensation has also been criticised by Bendelow & Williams (1995) from a sociological perspective. They argue that such emphasis elevates sensation over emotion and ignores social and cultural perspectives. They cite Morris (1991) who suggests that pain emerges at the intersection of bodies, minds and cultures. Some definitions have tried to encompass this interaction, e.g. National Institutes of Health (1987):

> Pain is a subjective experience that can be perceived directly only by the sufferer. It is a multidimensional phenomenon that can be described by pain location, intensity, temporal aspects, quality, impact and meaning. Pain does not occur in isolation but in a specific human being in psychosocial, economic, and cultural contexts that influence the meaning, experience and verbal and non-verbal expression of pain.

However, some argue that pain is very difficult to define. Scarry (1985) proposes that this is due to the essential qualities of pain being its invisibility and its inexplicability. As Madjar (1997) points out, these qualities make it possible to be physically near someone in pain and not be aware of it. McCaffery (1972) comes closer to addressing the invisibility of pain with her succinct definition: 'Pain is whatever the experiencing person says it is, existing whenever he says it does'. This definition has been criticised for encouraging practitioners to take the patient's report of pain at face value. For example, Price & Cheek (1996) argue that it does not take into account that a patient's verbal description of his pain may be swayed by the context of care. Patients may minimise their pain for a variety of environmental reasons such as perceived peer pressure from other patients and nurses not to be a nuisance and superficial communication with health care professionals. In addition, encouraging practitioners to accept the patient's report does not enable patient or practitioner to understand the pain being experienced. Thus Price & Cheek argue that pain must be framed within the context of patients' experience and the depth of interaction between practitioner and patient.

The importance of understanding the experience of pain is similarly stressed by sociologists who describe the embodiment of pain, where the body becomes a central aspect of the experience of pain (Bendelow & Williams 1995). Such a perspective recognises that pain takes over lived space and time, and relations with others and one's self.

In addition, McCaffery's (1972) definition may not be helpful if, as Scarry (1985) suggests, pain is difficult to describe. Indeed, the public expression of pain is dependent on language (Waddie 1996) and on an individual's ability to put his experience into words. This perhaps explains why, as yet, no definition adequately describes the feelings of being trapped in a body where pain has become a master and tormentor, 'calling attention to itself and robbing the person of sleep and rest' (Madjar 1997).

From the discussion of the definitions of pain, it can be seen that it is a very complex experience to interpret. This chapter tries to outline key features of this experience, to demonstrate the interaction between the physiological sensation of pain and its perception, and to discuss the nursing implications. The chapter begins by describing the physiology of pain. This may seem contradictory in light of the above discussion, but it gives a framework for the discussion of theories of pain, factors influencing pain perception and the nursing assessment and management of pain.

ANATOMY AND PHYSIOLOGY: THE EXPERIENCE OF PAIN

Q **19.2** Before reading the next section, try to describe the pathway of pain from being kicked on the shin to becoming aware of what has happened.

Nociceptors

Like all sensations, pain is recognised by specific receptors. These are called nociceptors — free sensory nerve endings that detect physical and chemical damage to the tissues and form a widespread and overlapping network in almost all tissues of the body. Like other neurones, nociceptors are classified according to their speed of conduction and their diameter. Most nociceptors fall into the A and C group of sensory neurones. Nociceptors are structurally similar to other sensory neurones but differ in respect of their thresholds (the minimum stimulus that activates them) and their specificity (Francis 1987). Some nociceptors, such as the fast conducting myelinated A-delta (A-δ) neurones, are unimodal and respond to high threshold mechanical stimulus. Other A-δ neurones are bimodal, responding to both chemical and mechanical or thermal stimuli. Most of the slower conducting non-myelinated C fibres are polymodal and respond to chemical, thermal, mechanical and light touch. The differentiation between A and C nociceptors is a fundamental principle of the gate control theory of pain, which is discussed below. However, it is important to appreciate that this differentiation is simplistic since there is a dynamic interaction between all nociceptors.

Chemical stimulation is usually a result of tissue damage and the subsequent release of chemicals around the free nerve endings. These chemicals are released by damaged cells and by the action of neurotransmitters released by nociceptors. For example, damaged cells synthesise prostaglandins and leucotrienes from membrane phospholipids. The neurotransmitter substance P and other peptides are released from C fibres, causing sensitisation, vasodilatation and leaking of blood vessels. In addition, substance P induces histamine release from mast cells and 5-hydroxytryptamine (5-HT or serotonin) from platelets. Chemicals are also released from the sympathetic fibres and contribute to pain and aspects of the inflammatory process (Melzack & Wall 1988; see also Ch. 23, p. 739).

Such chemicals either directly initiate a response in the nociceptor or sensitise it to further stimulation, i.e. lower the threshold. Inhibiting these chemicals can reduce pain. For example, corticosteroids, such as prednisolone and dexamethasone, can reduce inflammation and inhibit the enzyme phospholipase A_2 that initiates prostaglandin and leucotriene synthesis. Similarly, aspirin and other non-steroidal anti-inflammatory drugs (NSAIDs) inhibit the enzyme cyclooxygenase, responsible for the synthesis of prostaglandins from arachidonic acid (usually a membrane-bound fatty acid).

Peripheral nerve pathways

Once a nociceptor has been activated, an electrical impulse is conducted along afferent (i.e. sensory) neurones to the CNS. This is achieved through the exchange of sodium and potassium across the neurone membrane through the sodium pump; a specialised membrane-bound protein. In some kinds of nerve pain, this exchange of ions across the membrane can be disrupted, causing haphazard 'firing' along the length of the neurone. This can sometimes be rectified by local anaesthetic drugs such as the anticonvulsant or antiarrhythmic drug groups which act by blocking sodium channels and thus prevent firing (Colvin & McClure 1997).

Spinal cord pathways

Nociceptors communicate with the CNS at the dorsal horn of the spinal cord (see Fig. 19.1). The dorsal horn is the posterior part of the grey, butterfly-shaped area seen on cross-section of the spinal cord. This is surrounded by white matter — myelinated axons stretching the length of the spinal cord. These fibres are either ascending or descending pathways connecting the brain with the dorsal horn.

The grey matter comprises the cell bodies of interneurones, small neurones that link the peripheral nervous system with the CNS via specialised nerve pathways. Cross-section of the spinal cord shows a loose structural organisation of these cells in 10 layers called lamina. Six of these laminae are in the dorsal horn and roughly correspond to the cells responsible for nociception. The outer two, laminae I and II, comprise the substantia gelatinosa, identified by Melzack & Wall (1988) as a key area in nociception, central to the gate control theory. However, recent research has shown that most noxious stimuli are assessed by nociceptive-specific (NS) cells in lamina I (Lima 1997). Other stimuli, such as those caused by heat, pressure and touch, are assessed by wide dynamic range (WDR) neurones predominately found in laminae IV, V and VI (Lima 1997). Thus peripheral fibres interact with NS and WDR fibres depending on the stimulus they are conveying. The role of the NS and WDR neurones in assessing impulses from the peripheral nervous system is an important one and determines whether the impulse will be transmitted to the brain (Wall 1989b). For example, recent research has shown that brief stimuli are sufficient to activate NS neurones, whereas prolonged stimulation is required to activate WDR neurones (Lima 1997). Lima (1997) suggests that the evidence now available points to NS and WDR neurones being part of two distinct but complementary nociceptive systems.

Ascending pathways

Ascending pathways consist of neurones that link the dorsal horn with centres in the brain. There has been an explosive growth of knowledge about these pathways during the last few years. Perhaps the most important information to come to light is the number of pathways identified in nociception and their role in a compound processing system activated by any kind of sensory input.

From a review of research using chemical and electrophysiological tracing techniques, Lima (1997) has identified the following ascending tracts as nociceptive pathways: lateral spinothalamic, medial spinothalamic, spinomesencephalic, spinoreticular medial, spinocaudal ventrolateral medullary reticular, spinodorsomedullary reticular, spinosolitary, spinohypothalamic, spinoamygdalian and spino-orbital cortex. However, although all of these pathways are capable of transmitting pain, they are not, in most cases, pain-specific. Each of these tracts connects a particular area of the dorsal horn with a specific area in the brain. While much remains to be discovered about the operation of these tracts, their apparently overlapping functions may include (Melzack & Casey 1968, Willis 1989):

- signalling the 'sensory–discriminative' aspects of pain (e.g. location, identification)
- signalling its 'motivational–affective' aspects (e.g. unpleasantness of the sensation, desire to escape, anxiety)

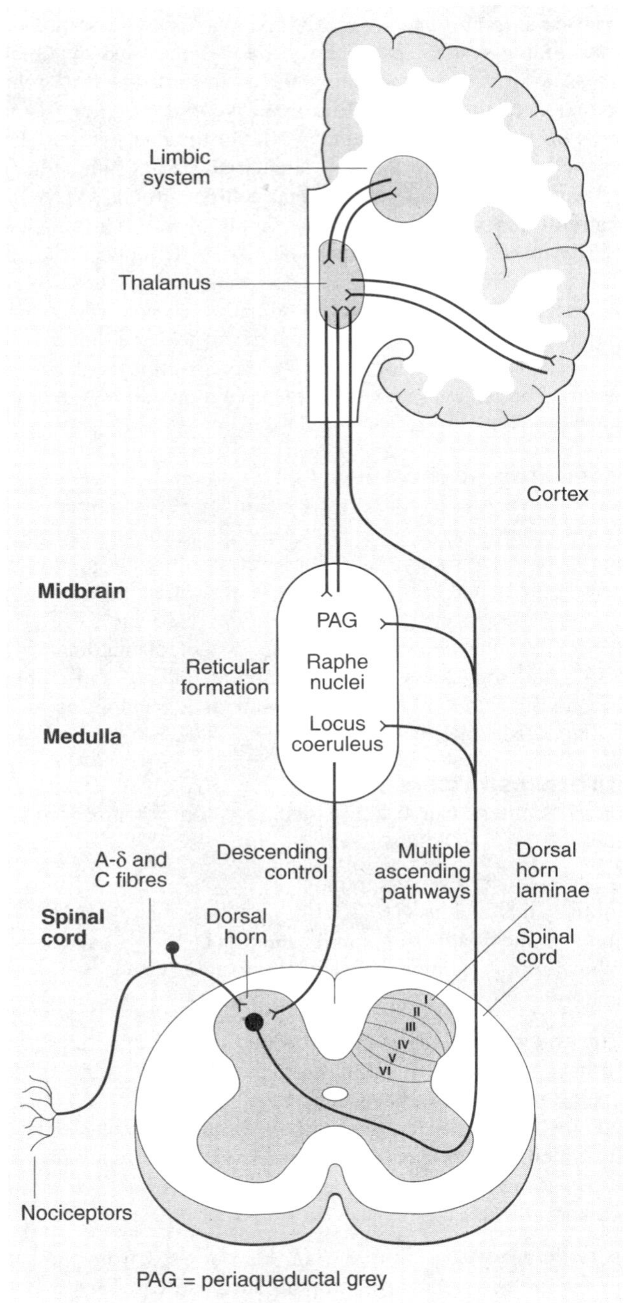

Fig. 19.1 Diagrammatic representation of some neural pathways involved in pain transmission.

- triggering motor and autonomic responses
- activating descending analgesia systems.

Brain mechanisms

From the number of ascending tracts described above, it can be seen that many areas of the brain are involved in pain transmission. Each of these centres interacts to receive and integrate sensory inputs, relate them to past experiences and thus bring about behaviour to promote survival. Central to these centres is the reticular formation in the central core of the medulla, pons and midbrain. The reticular formation contains the periaqueductal grey

(PAG), the locus coeruleus and the raphe nuclei. Of these, the PAG has particular importance for receiving inputs from the frontal cortex, the limbic system (particularly the thalamus and hypothalamus), as well as some ascending tracts. In turn, the PAG relays information to the nuclei of the rostal ventral medulla (RVM), such as the nucleus raphe magnus (NRM), the nucleus reticularis magnocellularis (Rmc), the reticularis paragigantocellularis (Rpgl) and the medullary adrenergic cellular groups (MA). The neurotransmitters involved in this relaying of information appear primarily to be 5-HT and neurotensin (NT). Through these connections the PAG has a monitoring as well as a response role in pain sensation and perception, coordinating a negative feedback loop between the ascending tracts and the cortex, and the descending tracts and the dorsal horn. It is proposed that this feedback loop modulates the responses of convergent (multireceptive) neurones (Bouhassira et al 1995).

Descending pathways

Descending pathways connect the brain centres described above with the dorsal horn. They have a key role in the modulation of pain, primarily through the release of specialised neurotransmitters at the dorsal horn. The principal neurotransmitters associated with these pathways are noradrenaline (NA) and 5-HT. They coexist with other neuropeptides such as the encephalins. There is also some suggestion that the inhibitory amino acid gamma-aminobutyric acid (GABA) is involved at a local level in the dorsal horn (Melzack & Wall 1988).

Neurotransmitters

Neurotransmitters can be classified into four groups (Kruk & Pycock 1991):

- cholines such as acetylcholine
- amino acids such as GABA
- monoamines such as dopamine and 5-HT
- neuropeptides (endogenous opioids) such as encephalins and endorphins.

The following discussion will focus on neuropeptides since these have a key role in inhibiting pain, and understanding how they act can inform clinical practice.

Neuropeptides are morphine-like substances produced by the body, which bind to specific receptor sites on neurones involved in pain pathways. Neuropeptides are derived from three distinct precursor molecules:

- *beta-lipotrophin*, a pituitary hormone derived from the same precursor as adrenocorticotrophic hormone (ACTH); it is the precursor for beta-endorphin, a stable peptide chain of 30 amino acids
- *encephalin*, which contains methoimine encephalin and leucine encephalin, two very short peptides, each having five amino acids which alone are very short-acting (less than a minute) and unstable
- *dynorphine*.

Neuropeptides tend to bind with specific receptors and are found throughout the CNS. The opioid group of analgesics works by mimicking the effect of endogenous neuropeptides, binding to opioid receptors and thus inhibiting pain transmission.

Summary

Pain transmission is a complex process involving peripheral and central mechanisms that interact dynamically to receive, monitor and modulate stimuli. Whether the stimuli are perceived as painful or not depends on a variety of factors which interplay with the central mechanisms at the cortex and limbic system.

THEORIES OF PAIN

Many theories of pain have been put forward, all of which contribute to our understanding of the phenomenon and lead to a more comprehensive understanding of the interaction between the sensation and experience of pain. Four of the most influential theories of pain are briefly described here. A more comprehensive overview of these theories is given in Melzack & Wall (1988).

The specificity theory

This theory has been very influential and continues to influence practice today. The philosopher Descartes (1596–1650) proposed that there was a direct channel for pain from the periphery of the body to the brain. This concept was developed in the 19th century to include the existence of a specific pain system that carried messages from pain receptors to a pain centre in the brain. Eventually the spinothalamic tract was postulated to be the pain pathway, and the pain centre was thought by some to be located in the thalamus (Melzack & Wall 1988).

However, research and clinical evidence suggest that this theory is too simplistic. For example, Melzack & Wall (1988) describe how surgical lesions of the peripheral and central nervous systems, which one might expect to abolish pain in a direct pathway system, are often unsuccessful. Conversely, in phantom limb pain an individual will experience pain from a part of a limb that is no longer present. Moreover, there are many examples of people being hurt in accidents or sporting events and not experiencing pain at the time of the injury.

The pattern theory

The pattern theory develops the concept that any stimulus is capable of producing pain if it reaches sufficient intensity. However, the pattern theory differs from the specificity theory in that it proposes that all fibre endings are alike (except innervate hair cells) and that the pattern for pain is produced by intense stimulation of non-specific receptors (Melzack & Wall 1988). The pattern theory also suggests that successive impulses which, alone, would not be of sufficient intensity to produce pain can collectively 'summate' to reach a critical firing level. This is known as temporal (over time) summation. Furthermore, the theory suggests that summation can be prevented by a specialised input-controlling system, consisting of rapidly conducting fibres. Melzack & Wall (1988) later developed this notion of a two-fibre system — a slow pain system and a fast modulating system — in the gate control theory.

The affect theory

This older theory dates back to Aristotle, who developed Plato's theory about extremes and opposites. Aristotle argued that pain was the opposite of pleasure and that both pain and pleasure were 'quales' — emotional qualities of the soul. An important part of Aristotle's differentiation between pleasure and pain was his belief that pleasure is good whereas pain is bad. Thus Aristotle viewed both pain and pleasure as having moral value and, indeed, he argued that these quales were fundamental moral drives directing human action. Furthermore, he suggested that pain could be overcome by reason.

Although this theory originated in the third century BC, it was still influential at the turn of the century. Melzack & Wall (1988) suggest that the development of knowledge about neurophysiology during the 20th century overshadowed this theory and the importance of the emotional component of pain. However, it is likely that this theory still influences many people, who see pain as a form of punishment for wrong-doing of some kind. Indeed, the word pain derives from the Greek word for punishment (*poine*) and this interpretation of pain may not be far from that intended by Aristotle.

The gate control theory

The gate control theory of pain, developed by Melzack & Wall (1965), combines pertinent aspects of older theories with an account of what happens in clinical practice. According to this theory, the transmission of information from a potentially painful stimulus can be modified by a gating mechanism situated in the substantia gelatinosa in the dorsal horn of the spinal cord (see Fig. 19.2). This mechanism can increase or decrease the flow of nerve impulses from the periphery to the CNS. If the gate is open, impulses pass through; if it is partially open some pass through; and if shut no impulses get through and pain is not experienced.

Melzack & Wall (1965) argued that whether the gate is open or closed is determined by:

- activity in small diameter fibres (A-δ and C fibres, which transmit pain)
- activity in large diameter fibres (A-β fibres, which transmit touch)
- descending influences from higher centres, including those concerned with motivational and cognitive processes.

Melzack & Wall (1965) proposed that the substantia gelatinosa is activated by large A-β fibres (shut the gate) and, conversely, inhibited by small A-δ and C fibres (open the gate). This activity then influences the information sent to the brain, which in turn initiates descending inhibitory controls depending on the information from other areas such as the cortex.

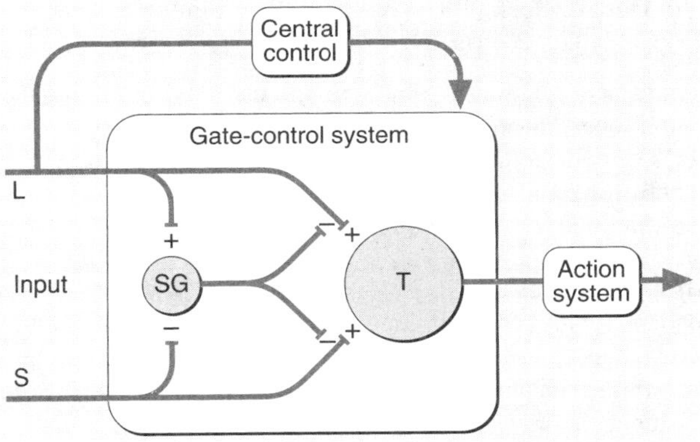

Fig. 19.2 The gate control theory of pain. +, excitation; –, inhibition; L, large diameter fibres; S, small diameter fibres. The fibres project to the substantia gelatinosa (SG) and the first central transmission (T) cells. The inhibitory effect exerted by the SG on the afferent fibre terminals is increased by activity in the L fibres and decreased by activity in the S fibres. The central control trigger is represented by a line running from the large fibre system to the central control mechanisms; these mechanisms, in turn, project back to the gate control system. The T cells project to the action system. (Reproduced with kind permission of Penguin Books Ltd, Harmondsworth from R Melzack and P D Wall, The Challenge of Pain, 2nd edn, 1988, copyright © Ronald Melzack and Patrick D Wall 1982, 1988.)

Implications of the gate control theory

The physiology of pain has developed since the gate control theory was first proposed. However, the inherent fundamental principles have stood the test of time and influenced pain management. Clinically the gate control theory has been applied to nursing care by McCaffery & Beebe (1994), who advocate that it provides a framework for understanding pain and on which various pain relief measures can be developed. For example, the use of touch and massage can stimulate the skin, increasing large fibre (A-β) activity and thereby closing the gate at the spinal cord level and relieving pain. This rationale also explains the benefit of the advice: 'rub it better'.

Closing the gate at the brain stem level can sometimes be achieved by ensuring sufficient sensory input, e.g. by using distraction and imagery (see p. 671). Similarly, at the level of the cortex/thalamus the gate can be closed by reducing anxiety, e.g. by providing accurate information about the cause, likely course and relief of pain and thereby increasing the patient's confidence and sense of control.

Developments since the gate control theory

The pain control system described by the gate control theory is one that acts rapidly. Research has demonstrated the existence of 'plasticity' or adaptability in the nervous system, which allows for both rapidly transmitted impulses and slow-onset, long-duration changes. It is thought that C fibres, especially those originating in deep tissues, trigger these slower messages (Wall 1989a). This prolonged mechanism, referred to as 'wind up', results in a sustained experience of pain (Wall 1989a) which may account for some cases of chronic pain. In addition, there is some evidence that chronic pain can be explained by changes in central neural function (Coderre et al 1993).

Q

19.3 Think back to the experience of pain that you described in question 19.1 and to your experiences of caring for people in pain. From these experiences, make a list of factors that might influence someone's pain. Organise your thoughts under the following headings: factors related to individual differences; factors related to small systems such as families and care teams; and factors related to organisations, society and cultures. Compare your thoughts with the following discussion.

FACTORS INFLUENCING THE EXPERIENCE OF PAIN

Individual differences

Past learning

Learning about pain takes place throughout life, through the process of socialisation. If a child falls over and hurts his knee, he learns that this feeling is called pain and he also learns how he is expected to react by the response that he elicits — e.g. sympathy and a cuddle may reinforce crying when in pain, whereas ignoring the complaint and subsequent praise may reinforce the minimisation of pain.

Gender

The evidence surrounding the effect of gender on pain and its expression is inconclusive. It has been suggested that men are able to tolerate more pain than are women. However, this may be due to the different ways in which men and women are socialised

(Bendelow 1993). For example, in some societies men are expected to be 'brave', whereas women are expected to be expressive or 'emotional'. These expectations may explain why Davitz & Davitz (1981) found that the nurses in their study tended to see female patients as suffering more physical pain and psychological distress than male patients.

Age

The evidence with respect to the influence of age on the experience of pain is conflicting (Harkins et al 1984). It has been suggested that age diminishes the experience of pain. However, this is in contrast to evidence that many elderly people live in the community with pain that severely reduces their quality of life and do not seek help because they feel their pain is to be expected and tolerated (Walker et al 1990, Yates et al 1995):

> Well, I just realised that I've got to live with it you know...it's always there...it's no good. I've just got to learn to live with it, I know fully well that nothing will help me now (Yates et al 1995).

Personality

An individual's personality will influence the way in which he expresses and copes with pain. For example, drawing on Eysenck's theory of the personality, several studies have demonstrated that an internal locus of control in combination with active coping strategies leads to less depression and pain compared with an external locus of control and passive coping strategies (Rosenteil & Keefe 1983, Brown & Nicassio 1987, Crisson & Keefe 1988, Hakapaa et al 1991). Snow-Turek et al (1996) and Reitsma & Meijler (1997) suggest that a person's ability to cope with and accommodate pain in his life influences his disability and quality of life. Walker et al (1990) found that the elderly were less likely to be able to do this if they were lonely or coping with other problems such as financial difficulties or the illness or death of a friend.

Meaning of pain

Pain will have different meanings for different people. Some patients may view pain as a punishment, while others may see it as having some value for self-testing or personal growth; yet others may see it as something that must be cured. Pain from a recurrence of cancer is likely to have a different significance for the patient than pain following routine elective surgery. For example, people with cancer often fear that pain means they are getting worse or that pain will increase as death approaches (Ferrell et al 1991a,b). Pain following surgery is more expected, although patients often underestimate the intensity of the pain to be experienced (Carr 1990, Carr & Thomas 1997) and this may lead them to worry that the pain signifies complications. Chronic pain may also have implications for the individual's self-image by necessitating a change in or loss of role. The meaning of pain will also be influenced by individual pain beliefs (Kotorba 1988, Williams & Thorn 1989). For example, Williams & Thorn (1989) described three dimensions encompassing such beliefs: whether an individual blames himself for the pain; whether he sees pain as mysterious; and whether he sees pain as something that has to be endured. They argued that any of these beliefs can negatively influence the intensity of the pain, compliance with medication and self-esteem, and be indicative of psychological distress and external locus of control.

Body part affected

The part of the body involved may influence the expression of pain (Meinhart & McCaffery 1983). Some areas of the body, such as the rectum or genitals, may be difficult to refer to for some people, and thus pain in these areas may go unreported. The assessment and relief of pain in these areas therefore need very skilled management.

Factors related to systems such as families and care teams

Interaction between the person in pain and their partner

Pain rarely has an isolated influence. The experience of pain interacts with relationships. Witnessing pain is distressing (Taylor et al 1990) and can affect the physical and psychological health of a partner (Turk et al 1987). Family carers in Ferrell et al's (1991a) study described feelings of fear, suffering, helplessness, heartbreak and denial. They quote one spouse who said: 'It is the saddest thing in the world. I share her pain. If she hurts, I hurt. What else can I say?'. These feelings concur with those reported elsewhere (Dura & Beck 1988). Sometimes, such feelings can influence the way in which couples communicate and cope with the experience. In chronic pain, this can lead to coping which reinforces an individual's disability. For example, Romano et al (1995) and Schwartz et al (1996) have found that, in cases of chronic pain, physical and psychosocial disabilities are more likely in those whose spouses respond in a concerned way and less likely in those whose spouses respond in a negative way.

Family dynamics

Families play an important role in the health of individuals (Snelling 1991) and in their care (Ferrell et al 1991b). Thus pain will be influenced by family members and how they cope; this will depend on the resources available to them and whether or not pain is seen as a crisis (Turk et al 1987). Families who can cope with pain can positively influence an individual's experience of pain through support. However, families who have ineffective coping responses may aggravate an individual's pain and, in turn, the family dynamics (Dura & Beck 1988, Snelling 1991, Schwartz et al 1996). Dura & Beck (1988) observed that families unable to cope are typically characterised by:

- enmeshed relationships where interactions are polarised — either overprotective or detached
- lack of cohesion within the family group
- controlling and manipulative behaviour
- conflict and a lack of expression of their feelings.

Team dynamics

A patient's pain can be influenced by the response of health care professionals to it. Edgar (1993) argues that if a nurse can be with someone in pain without becoming unduly distressed, then nurse and patient are likely to interact in a way that encourages discussion and communication. However, if a nurse feels overwhelmed by such situations then she is likely to use distancing strategies such as depersonalising the pain and playing down its severity (Harrison 1991). Such strategies will not only result in poor assessment of pain, but also exacerbate distress. An individual's experience of pain will also be influenced by the way in which the health care team functions. Nursing is a predominantly team endeavour, irrespective of where it is taking place. May (1990) suggests that this limits the action of individual carers. For example, effective pain relief post-operatively is dependent on a congruent plan between anaesthetists, ward-based nursing and medical personnel, general practitioners and district nurses. Where there is disagreement about a care plan, tension may arise and this can be displaced onto the patient (Nievaard 1987), negatively affecting the experience of pain.

Social and environmental factors

Culture

Each cultural group has its own behaviours, beliefs and values which it regards as normal and correct, and these expectations appear to influence responses to pain. For example, most British people traditionally value control over the display of emotions — maintaining a 'stiff upper lip' — which has the effect of discouraging people from complaining about pain.

A classical study by Zborowski (1952) illustrates this link between behaviours, beliefs and values. Men from three groups were compared: 'old Americans' (i.e. their grandparents or earlier forebears were born in America and they did not identify with a particular cultural group), Italian Americans and Jewish Americans. The 'old Americans' attempted to avoid showing any pain, tended to withdraw and preferred to be alone when in severe pain. The Italian and Jewish Americans, however, openly expressed their pain and did not want to be alone. The Italian Americans were concerned with relief of their pain, while the Jewish Americans were concerned about the implications of their pain for the future. This study has been criticised for selecting people whose cultures may have been 'diluted' by their residence in America.

Other cultural differences have been demonstrated by Moore (1990), who found that whilst Anglo-American patients preferred pills and injections, Chinese patients preferred external agents such as oils, salves and massage to help them cope with pain. Differences between American and Japanese patients with low back pain were evaluated by Brena et al (1990), who found that the Americans in their study had greater dysfunction than the Japanese patients, despite similar medical findings. However, the sample size was small and such findings need to be interpreted with caution.

Social conditioning/group pressure

The reactions of others may affect an individual's expression of pain. In a seminal study, Craig & Weiss (1971) set up an experiment in which the research assistants were led to believe that three actors were experiencing pain as a result of receiving electric shocks. In fact, these individuals were not experiencing electric shocks, but they nevertheless acted out three different types of behaviour in response to the pain they were supposed to be experiencing — passive behaviour, neither tolerant nor intolerant of the pain; intolerant behaviour, indicating they were intolerant of or could not bear the pain; and tolerant or 'brave' behaviour in the face of the pain. The research participants were then exposed to one of these actors, depicting one type of pain response behaviour, and electric shocks of increasing strength were administered to the participants. It was found that those who were exposed to a passive model were able to tolerate a shock of 6.3 milliamps (mA) before describing it as painful; those exposed to an intolerant model described the shock as painful at 2.5 mA; and those exposed to a tolerant model described it as painful at 8.65 mA. These results suggest that peer pressure or social modelling may influence the report of pain. The results do not, however, suggest that the threshold for pain is different between individuals, because similar studies using electric shocks without models of pain behaviour have found pain to be reported at similar levels (Melzack & Wall 1988). (It is interesting to note that, nowadays, such an experiment would be most unlikely to go ahead as it would not gain ethical approval.)

Organisational factors

The reactions of others can operate within hospital settings. Thus, a patient may respond according to how he feels he should respond rather than according to the level of his pain. Davidson (1988) suggests that organisations utilise a variety of strategies to manage difficult situations such as pain. He describes these strategies as the 'institutional denial of pain'. The most powerful of these strategies is to render the patient a passive receiver of care. Carr & Thomas (1997) described how some patients can be reluctant to tell nurses that they are in pain because they feel dehumanised and helpless while in hospital.

KEY CONCEPTS IN PAIN

Acute and chronic pain

Acute and chronic pain are terms often used in pain management to categorise types of pain experience with a view to selecting the correct approach to management. In the following discussion it should be remembered, however, that these two types of pain are interrelated and that their management will have similarities as well as important differences (see also Ch. 32).

Q **19.4** Before reading the following section, discuss with a colleague the differences between acute and chronic pain. How might these differences influence a patient's experience and management?

Acute pain

Acute pain is usually a warning against injury. For example, the pain experienced after touching something hot acts as a disincentive to return the hand to the hot surface, thus averting additional injury. It may also result in rest, which promotes healing. In addition, acute pain promotes survival. In rare cases of congenital insensitivity to pain, life expectancy is considerably shortened due to unrecognised trauma and subsequent infections (Sternbach 1989). Acute pain usually has a well-defined course and disappears once the injury is healed. It can, however, be intermittent. Examples of acute pain are pain after surgery and pain from a fractured bone.

Effects of acute pain on physiological mechanisms. Pain can elicit a variety of physiological mechanisms that are similar to those evoked by other stressors. This can make interpretation of responses difficult and should not be relied upon. Typical responses include the 'fight or flight' reaction, with sympathetic dominance and vagal inhibition resulting in inhibition of gastric mobility, nausea and vomiting, and glycogen liberation from the liver into the blood as an energy source. This increases oxygen consumption, blood pressure, pulse and vasoconstriction. On the other hand, pain can occasionally evoke parasympathetic stimulation, which results in a decrease in pulse and blood pressure. These responses have important implications for patient care. For example, nausea and vomiting will make an adequate intake of fluids unlikely. Pain will result in immobility and an increased risk of stasis complications such as chest infection, deep vein thrombosis and pressure sores.

Psychosocial effects of acute pain. Anxiety is often part of the experience of acute pain. This may be due to the unexpectedness of injury or the stress of surgery. The experience of anxiety is associated with a response from the sympathetic nervous system that interacts with the transmission of pain, with the effect that the sensation of pain is heightened. The increase in pain may be interpreted as indicating complications, and this in turn may heighten anxiety. Thus a vicious cycle is set up between anxiety and pain (Peck 1986). This cycle can be broken by strategies such as information, explanation and adequate pain management.

Chronic pain

In contrast to acute pain, chronic pain usually has no clear function as a warning system and persists after healing. Rather than promoting survival, it is usually destructive physically, psychologically and socially (Sternbach 1989). Chronic pain is often defined in terms of arbitrary time periods, such as duration greater than 3 or 6 months, but many authors see this as unhelpful. Chronic pain is frequently divided into two categories: chronic non-malignant pain and cancer pain.

Chronic non-malignant pain. This sort of pain is sometimes referred to as 'benign' pain, but since it can affect the patient and family in many negative ways, 'non-malignant' seems a more appropriate term. Many different types and intensities of pain fall into this category, e.g. chronic low back pain and phantom limb pain. Sometimes a physical cause for the pain may be identified, but this is not always the case and this is frequently a cause of distress (Seers & Friedli 1996). Patients with non-malignant pain often have long histories of pain and have typically tried various treatments without lasting success. Such pain is poorly understood and there is much controversy as to how it should be treated. In many cases it must be agreed that the aim of treatment cannot be to stop the pain, but to help the patient cope with it.

The most effective relief for patients with chronic non-malignant pain is often obtained through multidisciplinary pain clinics (Flor et al 1992) (see p. 670) in which the whole pain experience is considered and treatments such as graded exercise and activity, medication reduction, and cognitive and behavioural therapy are explored. Portenoy (1996) argues that long-term opioid therapy may be appropriate for a selected subgroup of patients with chronic non-malignant pain and may be pursued without the development of significant toxicity or side-effects. Whatever the approach, pain management will need to be incorporated into everyday life. McCaffery & Beebe (1994) outline some useful guidelines for nursing people with chronic pain.

Cancer pain. Stjernsward & Teoh (1990) have estimated that 3.5 million people worldwide suffer from cancer pain daily. However, not all people with cancer have pain. When it is present, it may be due to tumour growth in soft tissues, bone and hollow viscera, which activates nociceptors. Tumours may also compress and infiltrate nerves, causing neuropathic pain (Scott 1989). Pain may also be associated with cancer therapy, i.e. surgery, chemotherapy and radiotherapy (see Ch. 31). The management of cancer pain has developed from Saunders' (1976) pioneering work in the hospice movement which emphasised the need to give regular analgesics and to titrate dosages in accordance with need.

Effects of chronic pain on physiological mechanisms. Chronic pain differs from acute pain physiologically in that the 'fight or flight' reaction ceases over time and therefore the physiological indicators that may be associated with acute pain will not be present. Nevertheless, people with chronic pain will have physiological changes such as sleep disturbance, irritability, fatigue, reduced motor activity and reduced pain tolerances (McMillan 1996). These changes share many characteristics with depression (Sternbach 1989) and stress (Walker et al 1989). It can be argued that these physiological responses also have behavioural components.

Psychosocial effects of chronic pain. Coping with pain over long periods of time is psychologically draining and can give rise to a range of emotional responses. Anxiety is a significant feature of cancer pain (Velikova et al 1995) and depression, anger and frustration are common. In addition, an individual's life can be utterly altered and devastated by this experience: work, home and social relationships can all be affected (Snelling 1991). Kopp et al (1995) found that chronic pain reduced family activity. This can lead to a lowered self-esteem and be compounded if interactions with others centre on the pain, so reinforcing a 'sick role'. This may lead the individual to regard himself as chronically disabled and thus lead to further disability.

Chronic pain also has economic consequences for the community as a whole by virtue of the work days lost and the increased use of health care facilities.

Pain tolerance and pain threshold

These are important concepts that must be carefully distinguished from one another. Pain threshold is 'the least experience of pain which a subject can recognise' (IASP 1986). Laboratory studies of pain have demonstrated that pain thresholds are fairly constant across the population. In other words, the vast majority of people agree on the point at which a sensation becomes painful.

Pain tolerance is 'the greatest level of pain which a subject is prepared to tolerate' (IASP 1986). Pain tolerance has also been described as 'the duration or intensity of pain that a person is willing to endure' (McCaffery & Beebe 1994). The concept of pain tolerance is problematic since it implies that some degree of endurance can be expected.

Referred pain

Normally, if one stubs a toe or cuts a finger, it is apparent exactly where the injury has occurred. However, this localisation of pain is limited to the skin. Pain from the viscera and from deep somatic tissue can be felt in apparently unrelated but predictable locations. For example, the pain of a heart attack is often referred to the left arm, and pain in the early stages of appendicitis may appear to originate from above the umbilicus. Pain is usually referred to a structure developed from the same embryonic structure or sclerotome.

Another type of referred pain is associated with trigger points. These are small hypersensitive regions in muscle or connective tissue that can be located in the area of pain or some distance from it. This referred pain does not follow any known dermatomes, but stimulation produces pain in a relatively constant and predictable location (Meinhart & McCaffery 1983).

BARRIERS TO PAIN MANAGEMENT

Q **19.5** Before reading this section, consider your own feelings about pain and pain relief. If you were in pain, what sorts of things would be important to you to help you cope? Would this be different if you were at home rather than in hospital? Would different things be important for different types/causes of pain?

Theory–practice gap

There is a gap between theory and practice in current pain management. Despite significant developments in research-based knowledge, people still experience pain that could be adequately relieved. A recent study by Carr & Thomas (1997) found that over three-quarters of patients experienced pain postoperatively which they described as severe: 'tearing', 'harsh' or 'excruciating'. These results are very similar to those reported by Seers (1989) 8 years previously and to those reported by McQuay et al (1997) in a literature review of acute pain. This lack of progress reflects the comments in a report by the Royal College of Surgeons and College of

Anaesthetists (1990) that: 'treatment of pain after surgery...has been inadequate and has not advanced significantly for many years'.

The picture is no better with respect to chronic pain, particularly chronic malignant pain, which on the whole is easier to relieve. The World Health Organization (WHO) has published guidelines for the treatment of cancer pain (see Box 19.1), which a number of studies have found to be effective (e.g. Walker et al 1989). However, these guidelines are frequently not utilised in practice. For example, in a sample of 401 people referred to a pain unit with difficult to manage cancer pain, in most cases the treatment previously prescribed was inadequate: 10% of the sample were receiving no analgesics; 66% were prescribed analgesics irregularly or at intervals that were too far apart; 27% were prescribed inadequate doses of non-opioids; and 42% were prescribed inadequate doses of opioids. When these inaccuracies were rectified, most of the patients experienced adequate pain relief (Grond et al 1991).

19.6 Why do you think that the gap between theory and practice exists in respect of pain management? What would influence your ability to provide adequate pain relief for someone you were looking after?

Inadequate professional education and training

A number of researchers have demonstrated that there is insufficient education in pain management throughout the world (McCaffery & Ferrell 1994, 1995, Brunier et al 1995, Clarke et al 1996, Kubecka et al 1996). This can lead to attitudinal barriers and inappropriate behaviours in pain management (Edwards 1990). For example, most nurses in these studies did not understand the fundamental principles of pain relief or take responsibility for pain assessment, and they misunderstood the extent to which opioids induce respiratory depression and addiction. However, such attitudes have been shown to respond positively to education when this is provided (Brunier et al 1995, McCaffery & Ferrell 1995, Dalton et al 1996).

Box 19.1 WHO guidelines on treating cancer pain. (Reproduced with kind permission from WHO 1986)

1. Cancer pain can, and must, be treated.
2. A thorough history should first be obtained and the patient examined carefully. Acute conditions that require specific treatment should be excluded.
3. Drugs usually give good relief, provided the right drug is administered in the right dose at the right intervals.
4. For persistent pain, the drugs should be taken regularly 'by the clock' and not 'as required'.
5. For mild to moderate pain, the patient should be prescribed a non-opioid drug and the dose adjusted to the optimum level. If necessary, an adjuvant drug should also be used.
6. If or when this treatment no longer relieves pain, a weak opioid drug should be prescribed in addition to the non-opioid drug, together with an adjuvant, if appropriate.
7. If and when these no longer relieve pain, the patient should be prescribed a strong opioid, together with a non-opioid adjuvant drug, if appropriate.
8. The patient must be supervised as often as possible to ensure that treatment continues to match the pain and to minimise side-effects.

Professional and cultural biases in inferences of pain

At the beginning of the chapter, it was argued that it is very difficult to know what anyone's experience of pain is like. However, many studies have shown that nurses make assumptions and judgements about the amount or type of pain their patients are suffering which significantly influence the quality of care provided.

There is a significant body of evidence that supports the view that nurses and other health care professionals view pain as 'normal' or to be expected and thus underestimate the severity of the patient's experience (Carr 1990, Walker et al 1990, Carr & Thomas 1997). Harrison (1991) suggests that nurses become desensitised to people's distress over time. This might explain the findings from a study by Perry & Heidrich (1982) in which nurses working in a burns unit for fewer than 5 years rated pain as more severe than those who had been on staff for more than 5 years. This is supported by Mason (1981) who found that nurses with less than 1 year's experience inferred more pain than those with 6–10 years' experience. However, Dudley & Holm (1984) found that the number of years that had elapsed since qualification did not affect nurses' inferences of pain. Similarly, Davitz & Davitz (1981) found that some nurses consistently inferred a relatively high and some a relatively low degree of suffering. This may be influenced by personal experience. For example, Holm et al (1989) found that nurses were generally more sympathetic if they had themselves experienced intense pain.

There is also a body of evidence that suggests that factors influencing the patient's experience of pain also influence a nurse's judgement of pain. For example, Davitz & Davitz (1981) found that patients' religious or ethnic backgrounds influenced nurses' inferences of pain and psychological distress, with Jewish and Spanish patients being thought to have most pain and Oriental and Anglo-Saxon patients as suffering least.

Furthermore, there is evidence that nurses make judgements about pain based on whether or not they believe it has a cause. Wakefield (1995) found that nurses believe that pain can, and should, only be manifest in the presence of an identifiable cause. Similarly, Taylor et al (1984) found that nurses rated pain as less intense when no physical cause could be found and this was supported by Halfens et al (1990) who replicated Taylor et al's study with a Dutch population.

The belief that pain should only be manifest in the presence of an identifiable cause has a profound effect on patients, as illustrated by another example from the study by Seers & Friedli (1996):

> I had something that was medically unacceptable. The GP labelled me as neurotic because they couldn't find anything wrong. Their dismissive 'unlistening' attitude to my mysterious pain almost amounts, in my opinion, to mental cruelty.

This persistence in a reductionist approach influences pain relief. Wakefield (1995) reported that if no cause was identified, nurses were likely to believe that patients were trying to get analgesics by immoral means. Similarly, nurses were more likely to label patients as complainers if they felt that they were exaggerating their report of pain (Davitz & Davitz 1981) or that they were not coping adequately with their pain (Salmon & Manyande 1996). Likewise, Lander (1990a) suggested that unpopular or difficult patients are often labelled as not having 'real' pain.

Inadequate assessment and evaluation

Assessment is fundamental to pain management but is inhibited by many factors (see Allcock 1996). For example, nurses continue to rely on their ability to judge a patient's pain rather than asking the patient himself about it (McCaffery & Ferrell 1997). Few nurses accurately document their pain assessment or their evaluation of the effectiveness of any drug or comfort measure given to relieve pain (Albrecht et al 1992, Clarke et al 1996, Dalton et al 1996). Many nurses assume that a patient who does not appear to be in pain is in no discomfort when the opposite might be true. Moreover, they assume that analgesics have been effective because the patient does not say anything to the contrary (Bourbonnais & Mackay 1981, Choiniere et al 1990). Ten misconceptions that commonly compromise pain assessment are listed in Box 19.2.

Inadequate pain relief

Both nurse and patient may view pain as something to be tolerated and the patient may feel that an uncomplaining attitude is expected of him (Yates et al 1995). As one patient explained: 'I keep quiet even if the pain is severe, I don't want to get into the nurses' bad books' (Seers 1987). Carr & Thomas (1997) suggest that the depersonalisation, helplessness and passiveness that are inherent in being a patient may explain this attitude. In addition, research has shown that both patients and nurses often have low expectations of analgesics, and accordingly are satisfied with pain 'relief' that allows significant levels of pain to remain (Cohen 1980, Weis et al 1983, Cartwright 1985, Yates et al 1995, Carr & Thomas 1997).

Low expectations regarding pain relief may also derive from certain beliefs about the risks of analgesics, as described in the following.

Fear of the effects of opioids

Fear of addiction. Adequate pain relief is frequently influenced by the fear that pain-relieving drugs may cause addiction — a fear held by nurses (Lander 1990b, Brunier et al 1995, Closs 1996, McCaffery & Ferrell 1997), patients (Walker et al 1990) and their carers (Ferrell et al 1991a,b, Berry & Ward 1995). However, this fear is groundless, as the two following studies demonstrate. Porter & Jick (1980) reviewed nearly 12 000 records of patients taking at least one opioid and found only four cases of addiction in patients with no previous history of addiction; only one of these cases required treatment. Correspondingly, Perry & Heidrich (1982) reviewed 10 000 hospitalised burn patients, among whom the prolonged use of opioids was common, and found no cases of iatrogenic addiction.

Nevertheless, despite evidence to the contrary, fears of addiction are often expressed. For example, Seers (1987) found that over 75% of the patients in her study disliked taking 'pain killers' or would take them only if the pain was severe. One said: 'Once you get used to them you've had it'; and another: 'I'd rather suffer in silence than rely on them'. Some patients do not want to take an analgesic as they feel it will not work later when they 'really need it'.

Box 19.2 Ten myths and misconceptions surrounding pain assessment. (After McCaffery & Beebe 1994)

Misconception 1. *The health care team is the authority on the existence and nature of pain.*
In fact, the professional does not necessarily see the situation as the person in pain does. He or she must accept the patient as an authority on his own pain.

Misconception 2. *We can rely on our personal values and intuitions to judge whether a person is lying about his pain.*
This is not a professional approach. The professional response is to believe the person in pain or to give him the benefit of the doubt.

Misconception 3. *Pain is largely an emotional or psychological problem, especially in a person who is anxious or depressed or whose pain is unclear.*
Reacting to pain with emotion does not mean that the pain is caused by an emotional problem.

Misconception 4. *Lying about pain is common.*
In fact, this would seem to be rare. It is important to avoid the inaccurate labelling of patients as malingerers.

Misconception 5. *A person who obtains benefits because of pain is exaggerating his pain.*
Using pain to one's advantage is not the same as malingering and it is not easy to assess what constitutes using pain for advantage.

Misconception 6. *If there is no obvious physical cause for pain, its existence may be doubted.*
All pain is a result of physical and mental events and, whatever its cause, is real to the person in pain.

Misconception 7. *Pain is accompanied by physiological and/or behavioural changes which can be used to confirm the existence and severity of pain.*
Physiological signs such as an increase in blood pressure and pulse do adapt over time. Behavioural cues such as guarding, bracing, moaning and grimacing can be unreliable, and a lack of pain expression does not necessarily mean a person is not in pain. People in pain may choose to hide it, taking pride in their self-control. Fatigue can also reduce expressions of pain.

Misconception 8. *Similar physical stimuli produce similar pain in different people.*
There is no direct relationship between the pain stimulus and the perception of pain. Two people who have had an identical operation may experience very different levels of postoperative pain, and the duration and intensity of their pain cannot be predicted with any certainty.

Misconception 9. *People with pain should have a high tolerance for pain.*
Pain tolerance varies from one person to another and in the same person in different situations. What may be tolerable during
the day may become intolerable at night when there are fewer distractions from the pain. If health professionals reward a high pain tolerance, this may encourage patients not to express pain. This may control pain expression, but it does not control pain.

Misconception 10. *People who obtain pain relief from placebos are malingering or their pain is not real.*
There is no evidence for this. Placebos may increase patients' expectations for relief, which in turn may reduce anxiety and pain. There is some evidence, moreover, that placebos activate endogenous pain relief mechanisms such as the endorphins (see p. 656).

Seers' findings demonstrate that some fears of addiction are influenced by confusion surrounding the terms 'addiction', 'tolerance' and 'dependence'. McCaffery & Beebe (1994) define addiction as the behaviour of 'obtaining and using a drug for its psychic effects, not for approved medical reasons'. Tolerance is the term used to describe when the repeated administration of a given dose of an opioid becomes less effective and larger doses are needed. Dependence is the term given to the physiological changes that occur when an opioid is given over time and where withdrawal symptoms occur if it is abruptly stopped. McCaffery & Beebe (1994) point out that such symptoms rarely appear in a clinical setting because analgesics are usually titrated to pain. For example, postoperative pain subsides gradually and the dosage of analgesic opioids is accordingly reduced. The overwhelming majority of patients stop taking opioids when the pain stops. If a patient is reluctant to take analgesics, McCaffery & Beebe (1994) suggest asking the following question: 'Would you want to take medication if you were not in pain?'.

Fear of respiratory depression. Adequate pain relief is also influenced by fears of respiratory depression (Brunier et al 1995, Closs 1996). However, this is an unlikely complication when the dose of the opioid is gradually increased and titrated to the degree of pain experienced. Respiratory depression is more likely to occur following surgery when this titration is not possible and when an anaesthetic has been given. It is wise to monitor respiration and level of arousal following the first dose of an opioid, but fears of respiratory depression should never prevent an opioid from being given to someone in pain.

Other fears. The fear of losing control or of experiencing strange feelings causes some patients to avoid analgesics. As one patient in Seers' (1987) study remarked: 'It's a funny feeling — I hate it not being yourself'.

Fear of sedation may be a worry for patients; however, McCaffery & Beebe (1994) argue that the sedative effect of an analgesic usually subsides after several days.

Fear of injections may pose a problem for some patients (Seers 1987, Berry & Ward 1995); in such cases an alternative route of administration could be considered.

Inadequate prescription

Pain relief will be ineffective if analgesics are not prescribed frequently enough or in large enough doses. Although it may be difficult to predict an adequate dose for an individual, drugs and doses should be titrated to the pain report rather than giving a standard amount.

Inadequate administration

Many analgesics are prescribed, especially after surgery, 'as needed' or *pro re nata* (PRN). If they are given 'as needed', titrated to effect, the flexibility that this mode of prescribing allows could help the patient to obtain optimum relief, particularly if analgesics are given as soon as the pain begins (McCaffery & Beebe 1994). Thus, the success of this approach depends upon adequate assessment and on judicious timing of each dose.

However, as Mather & Mackie (1983) discuss, PRN is sometimes wrongly interpreted as 'as little as possible'. This is supported by Closs (1990), who found that only 30–35% of the maximum doses of analgesics prescribed were actually given in the immediate postoperative period. Carr & Thomas (1987) found that nurses frequently gave the minimum dose prescribed irrespective of the severity of the pain. Similarly, PRN prescriptions have disadvantages for people with chronic pain, as in these cases pain is very unlikely to diminish but remains a constant feature of that person's life. However, PRN doses may have a role in chronic pain when used for breakthrough pain, i.e. pain that breaks through an analgesic regimen that is given at regular intervals throughout the day and that normally reduces an individual's pain to an acceptable level (Portenoy & Hagen 1990).

In view of the disadvantages and misuse of PRN prescriptions, many authors advocate giving analgesics 'around the clock' at set times depending on the drug used. This method has been shown to maintain constant plasma blood levels of the drug (Fig. 19.3) and thus prevent the peaks and troughs associated with PRN prescription (Hanks et al 1996). This method of administration breaks the pain–anxiety cycle and decreases the patient's anticipation of pain worsening or returning. In addition, Keefe (1989) suggests that this method has advantages for patients with chronic non-malignant pain by dissociating their pain from the positive reinforcement of obtaining analgesics. Lutz & Lamer (1990), on the other hand, argue that, in the case of postoperative care, around-the-clock administration may result in patients being overmedicated. However, if this occurs, it is likely to be due to an inappropriate analgesic dose being prescribed.

If around-the-clock administration is used, it is important to continue this throughout the 24-h period, to maintain a constant blood plasma level so that pain does not return. Depending on the drug used, this may mean that it will be necessary to wake the patient. This may not seem ideal, but pain may wake the patient later anyway and prove to be much more difficult to control than if it were treated before becoming severe. In cancer pain which is being managed with oral morphine or diamorphine, it is possible, without ill effect, to double the dose at bedtime to avoid having to wake the patient (Hanks et al 1996).

Constant blood plasma levels of drugs can also be attained by using continuous infusion pumps. These are typically used in cancer

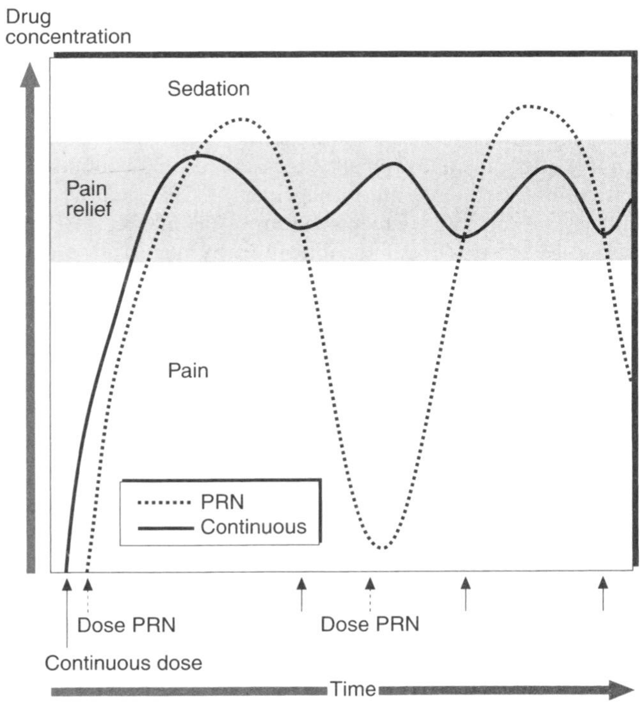

Fig. 19.3 PRN versus around-the-clock administration of analgesics.

pain subcutaneously, in chronic non-malignant pain epidurally, and in postoperative pain intravenously or epidurally. These pumps frequently incorporate a boost facility, enabling the patient or carer to give a small additional dose when required. This will be discussed below in more detail under patient-controlled analgesia (PCA).

PAIN MANAGEMENT

The role of the nurse

Q **19.7** What do you think your role is in pain management? What do you think you do as a nurse that will influence the patient's experience of pain?

Nurses have a very significant role to play in pain management. They are responsible for assessing, delivering and monitoring the effectiveness of any treatment prescribed. However, it must be appreciated that the success of treatment is likely to depend upon the relationship developed between the nurse and the patient. In turn, this is influenced by the quality of communication between the nurse and other members of the multiprofessional team. While communication will not be discussed in depth here, it is important to reinforce that, if communication between the nurse and other professionals is compromised, this will negatively influence the care received by patients (Nievaard 1987). Similarly, if the nurse does not understand the concerns of patients she will not be able to anticipate them and patients may go without support and treatment that might otherwise alter their experience and enable them to cope more effectively.

An important aspect of understanding patients' concerns is to ask about them and to listen carefully to the patients' replies. In a study with cancer patients at home, Ferrell et al (1991a,b) asked patients' carers what nurses and doctors could do to help to relieve pain. They identified that nurses and doctors needed to: be there and offer hope; explain; be honest and listen; address addiction concerns; and help with giving medications. Many of these themes are addressed by other authors and affirmed in other research studies. For example, roughly 50% of a sample of 190 older people in the community emphasised the importance of nurses' attributes, such as understanding, sympathy, reassurance and confidence, in contributing to their pain management (Walker et al 1990). Similarly, postoperative patients in Carr & Thomas's (1997) study emphasised the emotional support given by nurses. One patient said:

> If she (the acute pain nurse) had just walked away I don't know what I would have done. Her being with me enabled her to understand what I was going through. I didn't feel alone. I felt that I had someone who was helping...you know. She was sort of experiencing it with me. Really, it was a wonderful feeling in that way...that she was with me.

Information and explanation are important aspects of support and therefore crucial to the nurse's role. The purpose of these activities is to ensure the patient has realistic expectations and that the nurse works towards achieving these. The aim is to achieve congruence between patients' expectations and their experience, since this has been shown by studies to reduce distress (Suls & Wan 1989, Carr & Thomas 1997). In their review of this area, Suls & Wan (1989) found that patients who are briefed on the procedures they are to undergo and the sensations they are likely to experience show the most consistent reductions in pain reports, negative affect and other related distress.

Congruence between expectation and experience will also depend on the type of pain. In non-malignant pain it may not be possible to achieve much of a reduction in pain, although much can be done to help people cope. On the other hand, in acute and cancer pain it might be realistic to work towards considerable pain relief. However, despite advances in pain management, few doctors and nurses work towards this goal and this may influence patient experience. For example, Weis et al (1983) found only 21% of the doctors and nurses in their study had this aim. Likewise, in a sample of 117 nurses, Cohen (1980) found that during the first two postoperative days, 1% of nurses aimed for complete pain relief, 59% aimed to relieve as much pain as possible, 39% aimed to relieve pain just enough for the patient to function, and 1% aimed to relieve pain to a level where the patient could just tolerate it.

The findings are compounded by research identifying that patients do not realise that they can ask for pain relief (Seers 1990, Carr 1990, Carr & Thomas 1997). One postoperative patient in Seers' (1990) study, said:

> It would be useful if you were told you should ask for a painkiller. You drift in and out of sleep and pain. I presumed I'd had one and they would come with another. You don't realise you can ask between when they come round. One nurse on a shift mentioned it but that was way after the op. She said 'If you don't need it now you can always ask in half an hour.' If I'd known that initially it would have been helpful.

Similarly, Owen et al (1990) found that over two-thirds of the patients in their study would wait until they were in severe pain before requesting an analgesic or would not ask at all. Carr & Thomas (1997) suggest that this is due both to the lack of information and to the fact that patients can see that nurses are busy: 'Well you could see the bells ringing here, there and everywhere and I wasn't that bad, so why worry them'. On the other hand, research by Salmon & Manyande (1996) suggests that this is due to nurses' underestimation of patients' ability to cope with pain and they therefore do not offer enough analgesia.

The nurse's role in chronic pain extends to the family. Stiles (1990) identified pain management as an important aspect of the nurse–family relationship in cancer pain. Similarly, Rowat & Jeans (1989) urged a collaborative approach to the management of chronic non-malignant pain, to enable adaptation, enhanced quality of life, improved pain control and coping. This approach avoids the pitfall of treating pain as an isolated symptom.

Part of the nurse–family relationship is to recognise that family members have information needs of their own, particularly if they are the key carers. The carers in Ferrell et al's (1991b) study of cancer pain identified the need to have the following concerns addressed: fears of the future — whether the pain would get worse; understanding why their loved one had pain; concerns about medication; fears about how to give medication and how to manage pain at home.

The role of the person in pain

The role of patients in the management of their own pain has been largely ignored. In part, this can be explained by the way in which health care professionals have encouraged a passive patient role, as discussed above. In addition, patients have not been given sufficient information about pain relief (Owen et al 1990, Carr & Thomas 1997), with the result that they have low expectations about what level of relief can be achieved.

Health care professionals can encourage patients to play a role in their pain management by adopting a partnership approach to care, involving patients in the assessment of their pain and its relief. This approach can foster a sense of control and reduce reliance on health care professionals. Control can be enhanced by giving adequate information about pain and pain relief prior to surgery (Carr & Thomas 1997) and by the self-administration of drugs, e.g. by the use of PCA, postoperatively. In addition, with appropriate instruction and support, patients may contribute to their pain management by using complementary methods of pain relief (see p. 670). Patients can also be helped to have a sense of control in their pain management if their coping strategies are built on rather than ignored (Arathuzik 1991). Thus, finding out how people cope with pain becomes a crucial part of assessment.

The role of family members and carers

Family members have a key role in pain management. Ferrell et al (1991a) noted that family carers contribute to pain assessment by identifying the nature of pain through descriptors such as those used by patients — e.g. 'aching', 'horrendous', 'excruciating' — and by referring to anatomical locations of pain. Carers are also perceptive as to the degree to which pain is hidden by patients or minimised: 'a lot of the time I can sense what she is going through, but she doesn't want to burden others, so she minimizes'. However, the degree to which family carers' assessment of pain is congruent with that of the patient is dependent on the severity of the pain. McMillan (1996) found that congruence was more likely when pain was at its least rather than when it was at its worst, which is likely to be due to the distress experienced by family members when the patient's pain is severe.

Family members also play a very significant role in pain relief at home. With respect to people with cancer pain, Ferrell et al (1991b) found that carers often had a 24-h responsibility for deciding which analgesic to give and when. In addition, they were involved in reminding and encouraging the patient to take the analgesic and in keeping a record of what was taken and when. They were also involved in non-pharmacological pain management such as positioning, massage, the use of heat, cold and touch, and the use of talk and other distraction techniques.

Pain assessment

Pain assessment is an important and crucial nursing activity that must be carried out as part of the initial nursing assessment and at regular intervals thereafter in order to obtain a complete and evolving picture of the patient's pain.

Pain assessment is complex and dependent upon the interaction between patient and nurse. It includes observing the patient's behaviours, taking account of relevant physiological measurements, interviewing the patient and understanding his concerns. Assessment may incorporate a framework such as a pain assessment tool, but it should be remembered that a pain tool is only one facet of an adequate assessment.

Observation

> **19.8** Discuss with your colleagues what sorts of verbal and non-verbal clues might indicate that a patient is in pain.

Observation of pain is difficult and unreliable but is usually based on verbal clues such as direct statements, as well as moaning, crying or sighing and grimacing, and non-verbal clues such as guarding, bracing and lying perfectly still. However, these clues do not have to be present for someone to be in pain. Indeed, such clues are frequently absent in chronic pain and may also be absent when someone is distracted, e.g. by a television programme or visitors. Thus, caution should be exercised in the interpretation of non-verbal signals and they should not replace other pain measurements (Keefe 1989). However, they remain an important source of assessment for people who cannot respond verbally, such as those who are unconscious or disorientated and confused. Where this is the case, observational assessment needs to be systematic and may be enhanced by the use of an observational tool such as that reported by Simons & Malabar (1995).

Measuring physiological responses

Pain assessment may include measurement of blood pressure, pulse and respiration. However, these responses are not reliable indicators of pain, as discussed above.

Asking the patient

In pain assessment, the observation of behaviour and measurement of physiological responses should be subsidiary to direct consultation with the patient. However, as discussed above, nurses undervalue this facet of assessment, resulting in few patients ever being asked about their pain (Donovan et al 1987, Carr & Thomas 1997). This results in a discrepancy between patients' experience of pain and nurses' judgement of it (Seers 1989, Choiniere et al 1990, David & Musgrave 1996).

> **19.9** Compare your perception of a patient's pain with his own description. Do the two versions match?

The expression of pain is dependent on language (Waddie 1996) and the adjectives that patients use to describe it. Common descriptors include: throbbing, shooting, stabbing, sharp, cramping, gnawing, hot/burning, aching, heavy, tender, splitting, tiring/exhausting, sickening, fearful and punishing/cruel (Melzack & Torgerson 1971). The words that people use to describe their pain can be dependent upon their culture. Nevertheless, studies have shown a fairly consistent usage. For example, Gaston-Johansson et al (1990) found that different cultural groups rated 'pain' as the most intense sensation, followed by 'hurt' and lastly 'ache' as the least intense. However, it is important to be aware that some people may not actually use the word 'pain' when asked about their discomfort and may even deny having pain. Therefore it can be helpful to incorporate words such as 'ache', 'hurt', 'sore' and 'discomfort' into an assessment.

> **19.10** Try to describe a recent pain, such as a headache or toothache, to your group. What was the sensation like? How did it make you feel, think and behave? Look at the differences and similarities between pain descriptions within the group.

Assessment content

The general points that pain assessment must cover include:

- location of the pain
- intensity of the pain
- patterns of the pain
- effects of the pain.

Location. Nurses need to know where a patient is experiencing pain in order to take account of this in their care. For example, they need to know where to avoid touching when giving care. In

The London Hospital
PAIN OBSERVATION CHART

This chart records where a patient's pain is and how bad it is, by the nurse asking the patient at regular intervals. If analgesics are being given regularly, make an observation with *each* dose and another *half-way between* each dose. If analgesics are given only 'as required', observe two-hourly. When the observations are stable and the patient is comfortable, any regular time interval between observations may be chosen.

To use this chart, ask the patient to mark all his or her pains on the body diagram. Label each site of pain with a letter (i.e. A, B, C, etc).

Then at each observation time ask the patient to assess:

1. The *pain in each separate site* since the last observation. Use the scale above the body diagram, and enter the number or letter in the appropriate column.
2. The *pain overall* since the last observation. Use the same scale and enter in column marked *overall.*

Next, record what has been done to relieve pain. In particular:

3. Note any *analgesic* given since the last observation, stating name, dose, route and time given.
4. Tick any other *nursing care* or *action taken* to ease pain.

Finally note any *comment on pain* from patient or nurse (use the back of the chart as well, if necessary) and initial the record.

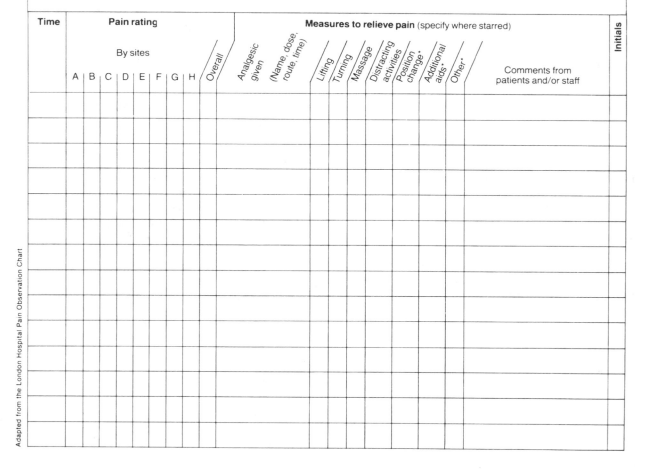

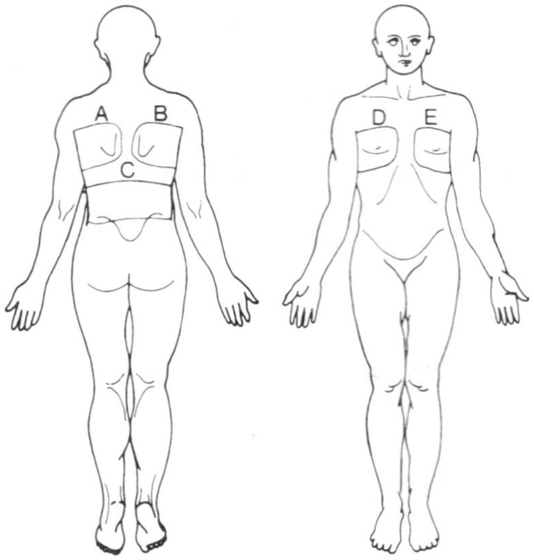

Date ______________ **Sheet number** ______________ **Patient identification label**

Time	Pain rating: By sites A	B	C	D	E	F	G	H	Overall	Measures to relieve pain (specify where starred): Analgesic given (Name, dose, route, time)	Lifting	Turning	Massage	Distracting activities	Position change*	Additional aids*	Other*	Comments from patients and/or staff	Initials

Adapted from the London Hospital Pain Observation Chart

Fig. 19.4 The London Hospital Pain Chart. (Reproduced with kind permission from Raiman 1987.)

addition, location can give information about the possible mechanisms of the pain and whether treatment is being effective. The location of pain is frequently recorded on a body chart such as that illustrated in The London Hospital Pain Observation Chart (see Fig. 19.4). Body outline charts are particularly helpful when the patient has more than one pain, e.g. following trauma, or is in chronic pain, as they enable the nature of each pain to be depicted. In addition, they enable a patient to pinpoint precisely where pain is felt, which can help in gaining a picture of the patient's experience.

Intensity. It is important to assess the intensity of an individual's pain, since this will often determine the analgesic administered. Typically, intensity is determined using a scale designed to enable the patient to rate the degree of pain felt. These scales can also be used to note any change in pain levels following an intervention or to indicate when the 'worst pain' or 'least pain' was felt, thus giving a profile of the pain experience over time. Scales can also be used to help the patient quantify the distress caused by the pain or to determine at what level of intensity the patient would like to be given analgesics. It should be remembered, however, that this level is not necessarily constant and that the patient's pain tolerance may fluctuate from day to day or within a 24-h period. Three pain scales in current use are described below.

Patterns. Pain often follows a pattern that gives a clue about its nature and what can be done to relieve it. For example, the pain in arthritis is often worse in the morning and knowing this can influence the medication that is given at night in an attempt to alleviate it. Similarly, chronic pain is sometimes worse when the individual is tired; knowing this can help the individual to plan his day. Questions that enable such patterns to be identified include:

- When did the pain start?
- How long does it last?
- Is it intermittent or continuous?
- What makes it better?
- What makes it worse?
- Do you have your own methods of relieving and coping with the pain?

In addition, it is important to ask: 'Is there anything else that you can tell me that may help us work with you to get the best possible control of your pain?' (McCaffery & Beebe 1994).

Effects. The nurse should also determine how the individual's pain affects daily activities such as sleeping and socialising. Patients with chronic pain, for example, may find that they are prevented from working and that they have difficulty getting adequate sleep. This is important because disruption of these things will affect an individual's quality of life and can lead to depression.

Using pain assessment scales

It can be very difficult to convey the precise quality of such a complex and subjective experience as pain. The nurse may find that the use of one or more of the assessment tools described here will help the patient to communicate his needs. The three discussed below have been demonstrated to be both reliable and valid.

Visual analogue scale (VAS). This is usually a 10 cm line with the words 'no pain at all' at one end and a phrase such as 'agonising pain' or 'worst pain possible' at the other end (see Fig. 19.5). The line is usually horizontal but can be vertical. The patient is asked to mark this line at whatever point he feels corresponds to the degree of pain he is experiencing at that moment. The assessor then measures in cm from the left-hand side of the pain scale to the mark in order to obtain the pain 'score'.

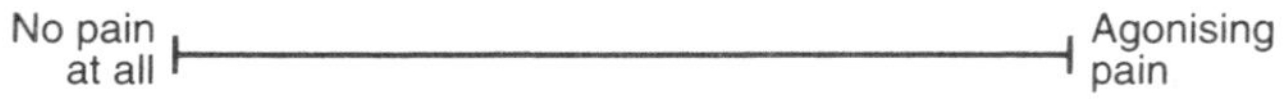

Fig. 19.5 The visual analogue scale.

The advantages of this scale include the absence of numbers or words along it; the person in pain is not forced to assign a precise numerical value to the pain or to choose a word that does not exactly represent it. Some patients, however, will find this scale too abstract and will be unable to think about their pain in reference to a line. Sriwatanakul et al (1982) found that 4% of the patients in their study were unable to understand the scale; Kremer et al (1981) found that 11% of their sample were unable to complete it and that it was especially difficult for elderly people. However, Choiniere & Amsel (1996) have addressed these problems through the development of a visual analogue thermometer (VAT). This consists of a red opaque band that slides across a card marked between the anchor descriptors to the place that depicts the patient's pain. The patient is told to think of the tool as a thermometer that measures pain rather than temperature. This tool has the advantage that the patient does not have to put a mark on a line and there are millimetre markings on the back of the tool that saves the assessor from measuring the line. Choiniere & Amsel's research found that patients preferred the VAT to a VAS and concluded that the VAT was a valid and accurate tool for clinical use.

Numerical rating scale (NRS). This scale is like the VAS but is calibrated with the numbers 0–10 (see Fig. 19.6). The patient is asked to make a mark at a point that indicates the intensity of his pain. Even with the added numerical guideline, not all patients find this scale easy to use. Jensen et al (1986, 1989) found that a 0–10 scale was a useful clinical index of pain intensity with post-operative patients, but that a 0–100 scale appeared to be the most effective for patients with chronic pain. Paice & Cohen (1997) demonstrated that numerical scales can be administered verbally without jeopardising the validity of the tool. They suggest this can be helpful, for example, when assessing pain over the telephone or when the patient is acutely ill.

Verbal rating scale (VRS). This scale provides graded categories, e.g. 'no pain at all', 'slight pain', 'moderate pain', 'very bad pain' and 'agonising pain' (see Fig. 19.7). The patient marks whichever category is most like his pain and is assigned a score from 0 to 4. The advantage of this scale is that many patients find it easy to use (Kremer et al 1981). Its disadvantages include the

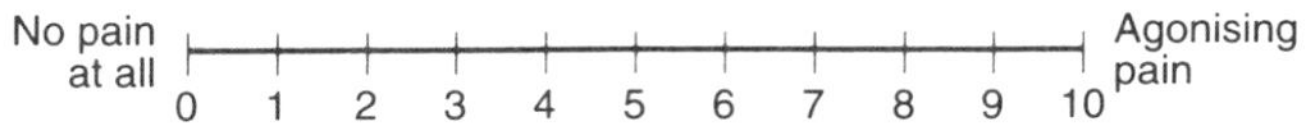

Fig. 19.6 The numerical rating scale.

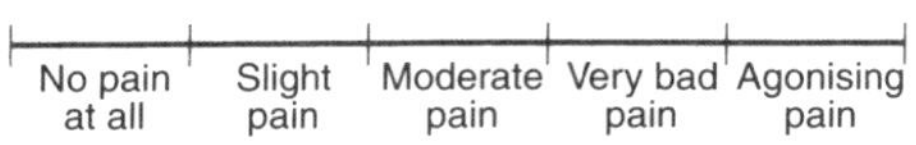

Fig. 19.7 The verbal rating scale.

fact that there are fewer points than on a 0–10 scale and so it is not as sensitive. For example, a patient may rate himself as being in 'moderate' pain before and after an intervention, although he has noticed some worsening, or easing, of his pain.

The visual, numerical and verbal pain scales rate intensity, which is only one aspect of pain. They can also be used to rate how distressing the pain is, e.g. from 'not at all distressing' to 'extremely distressing'. Turk (1989) points out that pain intensity may not be seen by the person in pain in a linear fashion, and that forcing a judgement onto a linear scale may constrain and distort the results. Furthermore, the effectiveness of any of the above assessment tools may be distorted by inadvertent and deliberate denial or minimisation of pain (McCaffery & Beebe 1994).

> **19.11** How would you feel if a patient told you he had pain, but told the doctor he had no pain? How would you feel if a patient told you he had no pain, but reported pain to the doctor? Can you explain this from the patient's perspective?

The scales described above are simple forms of pain assessment tools. Many tools are more comprehensive and incorporate a body outline and words that can be used to describe the pain, e.g. the McGill Pain Questionnaire (MPQ) and The London Hospital Pain Chart (Fig 19.4). The latter has been adapted for use with postoperative patients by Sofaer (1984) and for use with orthopaedic patients by Davis (1988). Some charts, such as that designed by McCaffery & Beebe (1994), enable respiration, blood pressure, pulse and level of arousal to be recorded and include a 'plan and comments' column for strategies to improve or maintain pain control. For people being cared for at home, pain diaries are useful assessment tools and are usually kept by the patient to record intensity of pain, effect of medication, other pain-relieving measures used and major activities (e.g. lying, sitting, walking) over a period of a week or so. This can give nurses and doctors an overall picture of the person's pain, which can be more useful than a description of the pain at the time of the appointment.

The type of pain chart used should be appropriate to the care setting (e.g. hospital or home) and should be one to which the patient can respond. The frequency of recording will depend on the patient's situation and the nature of his pain, but must be adequate for continuous evaluation of interventions. Pain charts can provide an invaluable basis for discussion with other members of the health care team and can help the nurse present objective information about the pain.

Pain relief

This section provides an overview of a variety of strategies employed to provide relief from pain. It is not a detailed review of opioid and non-opioid drugs and adjuvant medications. The reader can gain in-depth information from pharmacology texts such as Rogers & Spector (1989) and from pharmacists.

Analgesics

The most common pain-relieving measure is the administration of drugs to achieve analgesia, which may be defined as the 'absence of pain in response to stimulation which would normally be painful' (IASP 1986). Analgesics are commonly divided into three groups: non-opioids, weak opioids and strong opioids. Opioid analgesics such as morphine predominantly act centrally, whereas non-opioids such as aspirin predominantly act peripherally. The principles of analgesic pain management are summarised in points 5, 6 and 7 in Box 19.1 (See p. 661). These principles can be applied to acute pain in reverse (McQuay et al 1997). Underpinning these principles is the importance of titrating the drug and the dose given to the severity of pain. The tendency is for physicians to underprescribe them, for nurses to underadminister them, and for patients not to ask for them (McCaffery & Beebe 1994).

However, whilst many pains respond to non-, weak or strong opioids, adjuvant medication may be needed to enhance their effects or to treat non-opioid-responsive pain such as neuropathic pain. For example, anticonvulsants and antiarrhythmics can stabilise firing across neurone membranes (Colvin & McClure 1997); antidepressants can modulate pain transmission at the dorsal horn (McQuay et al 1996); and corticosteroids can decrease swelling surrounding nerves and inhibit prostaglandin synthesis.

Careful documentation of the effects of analgesics is important for evaluation of the drug and dose given. This important aspect of pain management is frequently overlooked (Albrecht et al 1992, Dalton et al 1996) and can negatively affect patient care.

Placebos

The word 'placebo' comes from the Latin 'I shall please'. It refers to 'any medical treatment...or nursing care that produces an effect in a patient because of its implicit or explicit intent and not because of its specific nature or therapeutic properties' (McCaffery & Beebe 1994).

> **19.12** What would your reaction be if a patient reported that an analgesic worked within seconds of it being given?

It is a common misconception that people who are helped by placebos were exaggerating their pain in the first place. However, placebos may relieve pain because they cause an expectation of pain relief that may trigger the release of the body's natural opioids, endorphins (Levine et al 1978). It is therefore important not to make judgements about pain based on the perceived analgesic effect alone and to recognise that patients may gain a therapeutic effect from having had their pain taken seriously. Occasionally, placebos will be given to patients as part of a 'blind' clinical trial, but only if they have given consent.

Drugs and legislation

It is important to be familiar with a number of Acts of Parliament, and health and professional guidelines which control the prescription, supply and administration of many drugs used to relieve pain. These include the Misuse of Drugs Act (1971) and the Department of Health (1989) guidelines on the Act and on the Misuse of Drugs Regulations (1985). In addition, the administration of medication by nurses is subject to professional standards published by the UKCC (1992a).

Much interest has been shown over the last few years about nurse prescription of a limited range of drugs. Analgesics that are part of these arrangements are generally available 'over the counter' and this legislation has therefore made little impact on pain management.

Routes of administration

Analgesics are administered via a number of routes — oral, intramuscular, intravenous, rectal, sublingual, buccal, transdermal, subcutaneous, by inhalation, intrapleural, respiratory and spinal — depending on such factors as efficacy, convenience, desired onset of analgesia, acceptability to the patient, side-effects and cost. The choice of route should be made after a careful consideration of the comparative risks and benefits of the various routes possible for a given drug. The following discussion provides only a brief introduction to the routes of analgesic administration in common use.

For more detailed information, the reader is referred to McCaffery & Beebe (1994).

Oral. Tablets or liquids are usually easy to administer and place no restrictions on patient mobility. However, their effectiveness is dependent on patient compliance. Sustained-release preparations can enhance compliance by limiting the number of tablets needed each day and they have the advantage of attaining consistent blood plasma levels. However, absorption of drugs given by the oral route will be compromised if the patient has nausea and vomiting. In addition, this route has the disadvantage that it is susceptible to the first-pass effect in the liver and intestine, by which some of the drug is metabolised and thus inactivated before it enters the circulation. The oral route is often thought to be appropriate only for mild to moderate pain, but there is much research to show that oral opioids such as morphine can be effective against severe pain if they are given regularly and the dose titrated to the pain (Hanks et al 1996).
Intramuscular. This route is often used in the treatment of post-operative pain. It has the advantage that it enables the rapid absorption of drugs, although oily solutions may be more slowly and erratically absorbed. The injection of the solution can be painful, particularly if the volume of drug exceeds 4 mL. It also has the disadvantage that it takes time to prepare the injection and have it checked, which can delay analgesia for the patient.
Intravenous. The action of analgesics administered by this route is rapid in onset but of short duration, and therefore a continuous infusion rather than bolus injection may be more effective in maintaining analgesia. Giving drugs by the i.v. route is an extended role for the nurse that requires training following registration as outlined in the *Scope of Professional Practice* (UKCC 1992b).
Rectal. Drugs given by the rectal route are absorbed across the mucous membrane and generally the bioavailability of opioids given via this route is similar to that obtained via the oral route (Hanks et al 1996). Indeed, there is some indication that this route may be better, because the first-pass effect might be avoided as a result of the venous drainage (McQuay 1990). However, absorption can be incomplete or erratic, particularly if the patient is constipated. This is a useful route for people unable to take drugs by the oral route, e.g. if they have nausea and vomiting or difficulty in swallowing. Examples of analgesic drugs given in this way include the NSAID diclofenac (Voltoral) and the opioids oxycodone and morphine. Most drugs come as a suppository preparation. These preparations have the advantage that they can be given at home and are useful in the management of terminally ill people. However, some people find drug administration by this route unacceptable.
Sublingual and buccal. In sublingual administration, the medication is placed under the tongue; in buccal administration it is placed between the upper lip and gum or between the cheek and gum. These routes may avoid the first-pass effect and are rapid in onset of action. However, they have the disadvantage that the patient may inadvertently swallow the drug, and buccal administration may be difficult if the patient has upper dentures. Examples of analgesic drugs given in this way are the opioids buprenorphine and dextromoramide.
Transdermal. This is a relatively new method of pain relief which involves placing a drug-containing patch directly onto the skin, where absorption occurs. The opioid drug fentanyl has been shown to give effective pain relief by this route and is currently licensed for people with cancer pain. Patches need to be changed, usually every 3 days, and therefore the number of tablets taken is reduced and compliance increased. Research has shown that once the correct dose is achieved to manage the pain, this route of providing analgesia is effective and improves the person's quality of life (Ahmedzai & Brooks 1997). Successful management of cancer pain by this route is dependent on the patch being in contact with the skin and the availability of oral morphine for 'breakthrough' pain. In addition, absorption can be speeded up by warmth, so care is needed when bathing or sunbathing.
Subcutaneous infusions may be very useful for people who need continuous pain control. Storey et al (1990) concluded that this method offers a simple, safe and effective alternative to i.v. or i.m. injections when oral medications cannot be used, and can be safely used in the patient's home. Examples of analgesic drugs given by this route include opioids (see Portenoy 1996) and NSAIDs (see Myers & Trotman 1994). Irritation can occur with some drugs given by this route.
Inhalation. This route enables rapid absorption of gaseous, volatile and atomised substances. For example, nitrous oxide (Entonox) administered with a mask or inhaler can help the patient to deal with bursts of pain, as in childbirth, or during dressing changes or other painful minor procedures. However, this route has the disadvantage that it can be difficult to give an exact dose and it may cause irritation to the airway.
Spinal. This route enables drugs to be given directly into the epidural or subarachnoid space of the spinal column. This gives rapid onset of effect and can offer effective pain relief for a wide variety of acute and chronic pains (see Boys et al 1993, Van Dongen et al 1993, McQuay et al 1997). Drugs typically given by this route include opioids and anaesthetic agents which, if given together, can have a synergistic effect. Because of the direct access to the central nervous system afforded by this route, much smaller doses are required. Whilst this route has many advantages, it has important and potentially serious complications such as respiratory depression and dramatic lowering of blood pressure. Giving drugs by this route is an extended role for the nurse and subject to the same requirements as discussed under the i.v. route. Despite the need for caution, many people with chronic pain are managed at home for long periods of time, with spinal analgesia administered via a small portable syringe pump.
Changing the route of administration. A number of studies have shown that patients are likely to experience an increase of pain postoperatively when the route of administration is changed, e.g. from continuous infusion to an oral route. This may be due to lack of knowledge in respect of equianalgesic conversion from one route to another (McQuay 1990, Du Pen & Williams 1994), although conversion charts are available to help in this process (see McCaffery & Beebe 1994). However, Carr & Thomas (1997) found that it was due to nurses giving too low a dose of analgesics within the range prescribed, which may be part of nurses' underestimation of pain.

Patient controlled analgesia (PCA)

PCA refers to the administration of analgesics by any appropriate and safe route over which the patient has control. It usually refers to the self-administration of i.v. boluses of an opioid analgesic via a specifically designed pump. The pump is set with 'lock-out' intervals and doses to regulate the dose of drug received. This method is typically used postoperatively, but some interest has been shown in using it for people with cancer pain (Walsh et al 1992). Nevertheless this method is dependent on the patient being able and willing to use it, although satisfaction is generally high (Sidebotham et al 1997, Snell et al 1997). PCA has been found to be a safe method of analgesic administration although side-effects such as nausea and sedation have been reported from the opioids used (Sidebotham et al 1997). There is some evidence that PCA offers improved pain relief and quicker recovery following surgery, resulting in earlier discharge (Clark et al 1989, Thomas 1989, Thomas & Rose 1993). However, these results were not demonstrated in a random control study undertaken by Snell et al (1997) in which no significant difference was found. Thomas & Rose (1993) pointed out that the efficacy of PCA will be influenced by the opioid chosen, the setting chosen for the demand dose and the lock-out interval, and patient psychological variables.

The evidence is also contradictory in terms of whether PCA influences the amount of analgesic required during hospital admission when compared with nurse-administered systems such as drug rounds. Some suggest that PCA can result in a lower total dose of opioids during the patient's time in hospital (Hunter 1993, Thomas & Rose 1993), whereas others have found the opposite (Clark et al 1989) and a few have found no difference (Estok et al 1987, Snell et al 1997). It is likely that the differences in study results can be explained by the regularity with which the comparison groups were given analgesics (Williams 1996), confirming the importance of giving analgesics in a way which achieves a constant plasma level (p. 669).

The reader is referred to Williams (1996) for a more comprehensive review of PCA and Mather & Woodhouse (1997) for a review of the pharmacokinetic perspective of PCA.

Other medical interventions

Local anaesthesia and regional nerve blocks. These interventions work by injecting local anaesthetic (sometimes together with a steroid) near to or in a peripheral nerve or major nerve plexus or into the spine. There can be adverse reactions and complications, however the pain-relieving effects often outlast the duration of the local anaesthetic. A review of the use of peripheral nerve blockade in chronic pain is given by Lamacraft et al (1997), and King & Jacob (1993) review the nursing care related to such procedures.

Surgery. Nerves can be transected in an attempt to reduce or eliminate intractable pain. Although this measure may work initially, because there are so many pain pathways, the pain often returns and may be worse. Examples of surgical methods of pain relief include sympathectomy and cordotomy. The reader is referred to Melzack and Wall (1988) for details.

Radiotherapy, chemotherapy and hormone therapy may relieve pain by reducing invasive tumours. These therapies are reviewed in detail by Hoy (1989). Radiopharmaceuticals such as strontium chloride-89 have also been shown to be effective for pain due to bone metastases (Robinson et al 1995). There is also growing evidence that bisphosphonates such as pamidronate are effective in relieving bone pain (Body et al 1996). The reader is also referred to Chapter 31.

Specialised pain services

Acute pain services. In response to continuing documentation of inadequate postoperative pain relief and the introduction of techniques such as PCA, some centres have set up a multidisciplinary acute pain service (see, e.g., Ready et al 1988, Ready 1989). These services are responsible for the day-to-day management of acute pain after surgery. They ensure that the level of pain relief and monitoring is appropriate and provide in-service training for medical and nursing staff. They may also be involved in auditing outcomes and undertaking clinical research. Evidence of the effectiveness of such services is sparse, but there is some indication that they can improve patient outcome (Mackintosh & Bowles 1997).

Hospice/palliative care teams working in hospitals and in the community have a wealth of expertise in pain and symptom control and can be a valuable resource. A study by Bruera et al (1989) on the influence of a pain and symptom control team (PSCT) on the management of pain in patients not under the direct care of the PSCT found that higher doses of opioids were prescribed 3 years after the PSCT was set up. However, two-thirds of medication was still prescribed PRN, despite the recommendation that opioids be administered regularly. Bruera et al concluded that while the presence of the PSCT had resulted in some changes, more instruction or discussion was needed in many areas.

Pain clinics. Chronic pain is recognised as a syndrome in its own right and pain clinics often, although not exclusively, treat patients with chronic non-malignant pain. Clinics are often multidisciplinary and may be staffed by anaesthetists, nurses, psychologists, physiotherapists, occupational therapists and pharmacists. The aim of pain clinics is to increase the person's ability to function and lead a more fulfilled life. People with chronic non-malignant pain have been successfully treated on an in-patient basis (Gottlieb et al 1977), on an outpatient basis (Skinner et al 1990), and using 'field management', whereby behavioural assessment and treatment strategies are implemented in the patient's own home and work environments (Cott et al 1990).

Complementary methods of pain relief

'Complementary' methods of pain relief have gained in popularity and include distraction, relaxation imagery, transcutaneous electrical nerve stimulation (TENS), massage, the application of heat or cold, hypnosis, biofeedback and acupuncture. There is some overlap between certain of these techniques; for example, imagery contains elements of distraction and relaxation.

As with all aspects of pain management, the success of the therapy will be dependent on the quality of the relationship between the therapist and the patient. Indeed, Stacey (1988) suggests that many people seek complementary therapies in order to have the opportunity to talk about their concerns. In addition, many nurses have incorporated complementary therapies into nursing practice in order to develop their caring relationship with patients (Tutton 1991, Closs 1996). However, before incorporating complementary therapies into nursing practice the Royal College of Nursing (RCN) advocates that four factors must be taken into account (Stevenson 1992):

- the likely response to therapy
- adequate preparation of the practitioner
- the relationship between current treatment and the proposed complementary therapy
- agreement on acceptable therapies.

It is important to remember that many nurses may use such complementary techniques without valuing them as such. For example, a nurse may distract a patient during a dressing change by asking him about a holiday or his family. Furthermore, many patients incorporate complementary techniques into their lives without realising it — they might, for example, use distraction such as watching television or listening to music to help their pain.

Nevertheless, it is important to remember that whilst many people find complementary therapies helpful, some are sceptical. In part, this is due to the lack of sound research demonstrating their effectiveness, but it may also be due to pharmacological methods being seen as the only legitimate treatment for pain. In addition, it is important to appreciate that some people, when offered complementary therapies, might feel there is an implication that their pain is 'all in the mind'. Some people may also refuse complementary therapies because they believe that their pain is too bad. If complementary therapies are offered, explanation about them is best given when pain is either not present (i.e. before surgery) or not at its worst.

Distraction

Distraction involves diverting attention away from the distressing stimulus so that it is no longer the main focus. This can be achieved by encouraging patients to participate in activities that they find absorbing, e.g. conversation, watching television, listening to music or undertaking planned activities, or by focusing on everyday stimuli in the immediate environment. For example, Copp (1974) found that patients resorted to counting bricks on a wall or repeating words or phrases to cope with pain. Distraction can give patients a sense of control over their pain and can improve mood (McCaffery & Beebe 1994). However, it also has the following potential disadvantages:

- the validity of the individual's pain may be doubted if distraction is successful
- distraction does not reduce the need for analgesics
- no lasting effect follows a period of distraction; indeed, an individual may be more aware of the pain afterwards
- distraction needs energy and therefore a person might feel fatigued and irritable afterwards.

Relaxation

McCaffery & Beebe (1994) define relaxation as 'a state of relative freedom from both anxiety and skeletal muscle tension'. Relaxation may help to reduce the distress associated with having pain, rather than the pain itself. Relaxation needs to be taught; face to face teaching has been found to be more effective than using taped instructions (Sears & Friedli 1996), although once the patient has been given personal instruction, he could be given a tape to refresh his memory.

Various methods may be used to promote relaxation; some of these highlight breathing techniques and others attempt to focus the attention sequentially on various parts of the body and then 'letting go' of the tension in those areas. Relaxation can be used to help people cope with specific painful procedures or events or to help people live with chronic pain. Relaxation has been found to reduce postoperative pain (Clum et al 1982), tension headache (Cox et al 1975), chronic low back pain (Philips 1988), chronic non-malignant pain (Seers & Friedli 1996) and cancer pain (Sims 1987). In contrast, Levin et al (1987) found no significant effect of relaxation on postoperative patients; this was confirmed in a review by Good (1996).

For more detailed information, see McCaffery & Beebe (1994).

Guided imagery

This technique involves using the imagination to help control pain. Typically it involves a variety of senses in conjuring up an image. For example, an image about the seaside might include 'seeing' the sand and waves at a beach, 'hearing' the waves and the wind, 'feeling' the sand and the warmth of the sun, 'smelling' the sea air and 'tasting' the salty sea spray.

Evidence for the effectiveness of imagery is weak. In a review, Wallace (1997) found few controlled studies, lack of control groups, small sample sizes, weak theoretical frameworks and few complete descriptions of the nature of the pain being treated. However, notwithstanding methodological problems, some studies suggest benefit, particularly when a person chooses his own image and controls when to use it. Swinford (1987) found that relaxation and imagery decreased pain on the first and second days after surgery. Horan et al (1976) found that dental patients given pleasant images to dwell on had less discomfort than a control group, and Kearney (1992) described the positive effect of imagery in cancer pain. However, it should be noted that imagery should not be used in people who are psychotic (McCaffery & Beebe 1994).

Cutaneous stimulation

Transcutaneous electrical nerve stimulation (TENS). In this intervention low-voltage electrical stimulation is delivered via electrodes placed on the skin near to or on the site of pain. This usually causes a sensation of vibration or tingling and can be used in an intermittent or continuous mode. The device is powered by a battery pack and can be operated by the patient. In a review of clinical pain conditions successfully and unsuccessfully treated with TENS, Woolf (1989) concluded that while TENS could be useful in a wide variety of acute and chronic conditions, reducing or eliminating mild to moderate pain, it appeared to be less effective against severe pain. However, Librach & Rapson (1988) suggested that this may be due to the intensity of frequency used. TENS is not suitable for people with cardiac pacemakers or people suffering from senility and should not be placed over a pregnant uterus or the carotid sinus (McCaffery & Beebe 1994).

Massage. The laying on of hands is described by Haldeman (1989) as 'unquestionably the oldest, most universally utilised and probably the most appreciated means of relieving pain and suffering'. The reader is referred to this source for a description of different massage and manipulation techniques. Massage should not be confused with therapeutic touch, a technique designed to realign energy fields through the transfer of energy from a healer or therapist.

For further reading on therapeutic touch see Wright (1987) and Wyatt & Dimmer (1988).

Heat and cold. The application of heat or cold may relieve pain through a 'counter-irritant' effect as well as by direct effects on peripheral and free nerve endings (Lehmann & de Lateur 1989). Care should be taken with patients with impaired sensation or reduced level of consciousness who could damage their skin without realising it while using these methods.

Hypnosis

The nature of hypnosis and the mechanism of its effects are unclear. However, it seems to be an altered state of consciousness in which concentration is focused and distractions are minimised. Success appears to be determined by the individual's ability to respond to suggestion (Orne & Dinges 1989), although the person may choose to inhibit this responsiveness. In addition, it seems to be dependent on the type of pain being treated, the context and goals of treatment, the skill of the therapist and the expectations and motivations of the patient. This technique is not one that should be attempted without special training.

Biofeedback

Biofeedback is a method used to encourage and develop relaxation skills. An individual is encouraged to use relaxation to alter specific body functions, such as muscle tension, blood pressure, pulse and/or temperature. Information about these functions is fed back to the individual as he relaxes. This enables him to learn how to positively influence tension and anxiety. However, from a literature review, Jessup (1989) concluded that biofeedback has no advantage over relaxation, both being equally effective.

Acupuncture

Acupuncture originated in China thousands of years ago. It involves inserting needles into the skin at specific acupuncture or Hoku points that are located in a series of channels or meridians. These needles may be manipulated to maximise the effect. The mechanism of action has been the subject of many debates, and activation of endorphins has been implicated. From a review of 14 studies, Patel et al (1989) concluded that, whilst most results favoured acupuncture for chronic pain, there were various potential sources of bias that precluded a conclusive finding.

In acupressure, the acupuncture points are stimulated by pressing and/or rubbing rather than by the insertion of needles.

Behaviour therapy

The development of behaviour therapy programmes for pain management owes much to Fordyce (1978), who first drew attention to the rewards a person in chronic pain may receive for 'pain behaviour', such as sympathy, attention and exemption from certain tasks. Since behavioural psychologists believe that all behaviour is governed by its consequences, they feel that by discouraging pain behaviours (such as moaning or grimacing) and encouraging 'well behaviours', the professional can help the person adopt a more normal pattern of behaviour. This has been described as operant conditioning. A cognitive–behavioural approach (e.g. Turk & Meichenbaum 1989) includes the modification of the patient's thoughts and feelings as well as his behaviours; it also includes a commitment to behaviour therapy procedures in promoting change, such as graded practice and homework assignments. This type of approach can also be achieved as group therapy (Weir et al 1988). Pain clinic programmes usually contain some element of behaviour therapy.

Chiropractic and osteopathy

There is much overlap between the methods and techniques of chiropractic and osteopathy, with what Tanner (1987) describes as 'subtle' differences. He argues that chiropractors are more likely to emphasise the structure of the spine, whereas osteopaths emphasise abnormal movement of the spine. Research supporting these practices is sparse. However, Meade et al (1990) found that patients with chronic low back pain benefited more from consulting a chiropractor than from a traditional hospital outpatient treatment and argued for chiropractic to be offered under the National Health Service. However, several authors (Graham et al 1990, Greenough 1990) have disputed this conclusion.

Other therapies

Space precludes discussion of other therapies such as faith healing, herbal remedies, music therapy, art therapy, aromatherapy and reflexology. However, much of what has already been said above is equally applicable to these therapies in that they promote well-being and relaxation and may decrease anxiety and thus pain. Art and music therapy may also enable active expression of feelings, which can contribute towards pain relief.

19.13 Discuss with your colleagues whether anyone has had any experience of these therapies used in pain relief.

Support and self-help groups

People suffering from pain often seek help from relatives and friends before approaching a professional such as their GP within the health care system. Zola (1973), who argued that only a small number of people present to a doctor, confirmed this. Examining the 'trigger' that converts a 'person' into a 'patient' can help to determine how best to help those who do seek help. Examining this in people with chronic pain, Reitsma & Meijler (1997) found that those employing effective coping strategies were less likely to be consumers of health care. In contrast, those people without effective coping strategies were more likely to see themselves as patients and have a greater degree of disability. This suggests that if individual coping skills are developed then disability and distress might be reduced. Emotional coping skills may be developed through self-help groups and organisations such as The National Back Pain Association and The British Migraine Association. Problem-solving skills may be developed using information obtained from the many books now available, a selection of which include Sternbach (1987), Broome & Jellicoe (1987), Gingell (1988), Hewitt (1982), Benson & Klipper (1975) and Tanner (1987).

CONCLUSION

Pain and its relief form a central part of nursing in almost all care settings. Ongoing education for health professionals and an understanding of the complexities of pain and its management are crucial in forming a sound basis for practice. Lander (1990b) describes education as probably 'the single most important tool for improving pain management'. The person in pain should be believed, his pain should be systematically assessed, treated and reassessed, and he should be involved in pain management whenever possible. Pain and its relief need to be given a high priority in care, and health professionals should be accountable for the pain relief of people in their care. Indeed, 'failure to treat pain is inhumane and constitutes professional negligence' (Meinhart & McCaffery 1983). Nurses are in the fortunate position of being able to make an important contribution towards the comfort and well-being of people in pain.

REFERENCES

Ahmedzai S, Brooks D 1997 Transdermal fentanyl versus sustained release morphine in cancer pain: preference, efficacy and quality of life. Journal of Pain and Symptom Management 13(5): 254–261

Albrecht M N, Cook J E, Riley M J, Andreoni V 1992 Factors influencing staff nurses' decisions for non-documentation of patient response to analgesia administration. Journal of Clinical Nursing 1(5): 243–251

Allcock N 1996 Factors affecting the assessment of postoperative pain: a literature review. Journal of Advanced Nursing 24(6): 1144–1151

Arathuzik D 1991 Pain experience for metastatic breast cancer patients. Cancer Nursing 14(1): 41–48

Bendelow G A 1993 Pain perceptions, emotions and gender. Sociology of Health and Illness 15(3): 273–294

Bendelow G A, Williams S J 1995 Sociological approaches to pain. Progress in Palliative Care 3(5): 169–174

Berry P E, Ward S E 1995 Barriers to pain management in hospice: a study of family caregivers. The Hospice Journal 10(4): 19–33

Body J J, Coleman R E, Piccart M 1996 Use of bisphosphonates in cancer patients. Cancer Treatment Reviews 22: 265–287

Bouhassira D, Gall O, Chitour D, Le Bars D 1995 Dorsal horn convergent neurone: negative feedback triggered by spatial summation of nociceptive afferents. Pain 62(2): 195–200

Bourbonnais F E, Mackay R C 1981 The influence of nursing intervention on chest pain. Nursing Papers 13(3): 38–48

Boys L, Peat S J, Hanna M K, Burn K 1993 Audit of neural blockade for palliative care patients in an acute unit. Palliative Medicine 7: 63–65

Brena S F, Sanders S H, Motoyama H 1990 American and Japanese chronic low back pain patients: cross-cultural similarities and differences. Clinical Journal of Pain 6(2): 118–124

Brown G K, Nicassio P M 1987 Development of a questionnaire for the assessment of active and passive coping strategies in chronic pain patients. Pain 31(1): 53–64

Bruera E, MacMillan K, Hanson J, MacDonald R N 1989 Palliative care in a cancer centre: results in 1984 versus 1987. Journal of Pain and Symptom Management 5(1): 1–5

Brunier G, Carson M G, Harrison D E 1995 What do nurses know and believe about patients' pain? Results of a hospital survey. Journal of Pain and Symptom Management 10(6): 436–445

Carr E C J 1990 Postoperative pain: patients' expectations and experiences. Journal of Advanced Nursing 15(1): 89–100

Carr E C J, Thomas V J 1997 Anticipating and experiencing post-operative pain: the patient's perspective. Journal of Clinical Nursing 6(3): 191–201

Cartwright P D 1985 Pain control after surgery: a survey of current practice. Annals of the Royal College of Surgeons 67: 13–16

Choiniere M, Melzack R, Girard N, Rondeau J, Paquin M J 1990 Comparisons between patients' and nurses' assessment of pain and medication efficacy in severe burn injuries. Pain 40(2): 143–152

Choiniere M, Amsel R 1996 A visual analogue pain thermometer for measuring pain intensity. Journal of Pain and Symptom Management 11(5): 299–311

Clark E, Hodsman N, Kenny G 1989 Improved postoperative recovery with patient-controlled analgesia. Nursing Times 85(9): 54–55

Clarke E B, French B, Bilodeau M L, Capasso V C, Edwards A, Empoliti J 1996 Pain management knowledge, attitudes and clinical practice: the impact of nurses' characteristics and education. Journal of Pain and Symptom Management 11(1): 18–31

Closs S J 1990 An exploratory analysis of nurses' provision of postoperative analgesic drugs. Journal of Advanced Nursing 15(1): 42–49

Closs S J 1996 Pain and elderly patients: a survey of nurses' knowledge and experiences. Journal of Advanced Nursing 23(2): 237–242

Clum G A, Luscomb R L, Scott L 1982 Relaxation training and cognitive strategies in the treatment of acute pain. Pain 12(2): 175–183

Coderre T J, Katz J, Vaccarino A L, Melzack R 1993 Contribution of central neuroplasticity to pathological pain: review of clinical and experimental evidence. Pain 52(3): 259–285

Cohen F 1980 Postsurgical pain relief: patients' status and nurses' medication choices. Pain 9(2): 265–274

Colvin L A, McClure J H 1997 Local anaesthetics: structure-activity relationships and their role in pain treatment. Pain Reviews 4: 59–77

Copp L A 1974 The spectrum of suffering. American Journal of Nursing 74(3): 491–495

Cott A, Anchel H, Goldberg W M, Fabich M, Parkinson W 1990 Non-institutional treatment of chronic pain by field management: an outcome study with comparison group. Pain 40(2): 183–194

Cox D J, Freundlich A, Meyer R G 1975 Differential effectiveness of electromyograph feedback, verbal relaxation instructions, and medication placebo with tension headache. Journal of Consulting and Clinical Psychology 43(6): 892–898

Craig K D, Weiss S M 1971 Vicarious influences on pain threshold determinations. Journal of Personality and Social Psychology 19(1): 53–59

Crisson J E, Keefe F J 1988 The relationship of locus of control to pain coping strategies and psychological distress in chronic pain patients. Pain 35(1): 147–154

Dalton J A, Blau W, Carson J et al 1996 Changing the relationship among nurses' knowledge, self-reported behaviour and documented behaviour in pain management: does education make a difference? Journal of Pain and Symptom Management 12(5): 308–319

David Y B, Musgrave C J 1996 Pain assessment: a pilot study in an Israeli bone marrow transplant unit. Cancer Nursing 19(2): 93–97

Davidson P 1988 Facilitating coping with cancer pain. Palliative Medicine 2: 107–114

Davis P S 1988 Changing nursing practice for more effective control of postoperative pain through a staff initiated programme. Nurse Education Today 8(6): 325–331

Davitz J R, Davitz L J 1981 Inferences of patients' pain and psychological distress: studies of nursing behaviors. Springer, New York

Department of Health 1989 Guide to The Misuse of Drugs Act 1971 and The Misuse of Drugs Regulations 1985. DoH, Welsh Office, Scottish Office, London

Donovan M, Dillon P, McGuire L 1987 Incidence and characteristics of pain in a sample of medical surgical inpatients. Pain 30(1): 69–78

Dudley S R, Holm R 1984 Assessment of the pain experience in relation to selected nurse characteristics. Pain 18(2): 179–186

Du Pen S L, Williams A R 1994 The dilemma of conversion from systemic to epidural morphine: a proposed conversion tool for treatment of cancer pain. Pain 56(1): 113–118

Dura J R, Beck S J 1988 A comparison of family functioning when mothers have chronic pain. Pain 35(1): 79–89

Edgar L 1993 The psychological aspects of pain. In: Carroll D, Bowsher D (eds) Pain management and nursing care. Butterworth Press, Oxford

Edwards W T 1990 Optimizing opioid treatment of postoperative pain. Journal of Pain and Symptom Management 5(suppl 1): S24–36

Estok P M, Glass P S A, Goldbert J S, Freibergen J J, Sladen R N 1987 Use of PCA to compare intravenous with epidural administration of fentanyl in the postoperative patient. Anesthesiology 67: A230

Ferrell B, Rhiner M, Cohen M Z, Grant M 1991a Pain as a metaphor for illness. Part 1: impact of cancer pain on family caregivers. Oncology Nurse Forum 18(8): 1303–1308

Ferrell B, Cohne M Z, Rhiner M, Rozek A 1991b Pain as a metaphor for illness. Part 2: family and caregiver's management of pain. Oncology Nurse Forum 18(8): 1313–1322

Flor H, Fydrich T, Turk D C 1992 Efficacy of multidisciplinary pain treatment centers: a meta-analytic review. Pain 49(2): 221–230

Fordyce W E 1978 Learning processes in pain. In: Sternbach R A (ed) The psychology of pain. Raven Press, New York, pp 49–72

Francis I W 1987 The physiology of pain. In: Boore J R P, Champion R, Ferguson M C (eds) Nursing the physically ill adult. Churchill Livingstone, London

Gaston-Johansson F, Albert M, Fagan E, Zimmerman L 1990 Similarities in pain descriptors of four different ethnic-cultural groups. Journal of Pain and Symptom Management 5(2): 94–100

Good M 1996 Effects of relaxation and music on post-operative pain: a review. Journal of Advanced Nursing 24(5): 905–914

Gottlieb H, Strite L C, Koller R, Mardorsky A, Hockersmith V, Kleeman M, Wagner J 1977 Comprehensive rehabilitation of patients having chronic low back pain. Archives of Physical Rehabilitation 58: 101–108

Graham G P, Dent C M, Fairclough J A 1990 Low back pain: comparison of chiropractic and hospital outpatient treatment. British Medical Journal 300: 1647

Greenough C G 1990 Low back pain: comparison of chiropractic and hospital outpatient treatment. British Medical Journal 300: 1648

Grond S, Zech D, Schug S A, Lynch J, Lehmann K A 1991 Validation of World Health Organization guidelines for cancer pain relief during the last days and hours of life. Journal of Pain and Symptom Management 6(7): 411–422

Hakapaa K, Jarvikoski A, Mellin G, Hurri H, Luoma J 1991 Health locus of control beliefs and psychological distress as predictors for treatment outcome in low back pain patients: results of a 3 month follow up of a controlled intervention study. Pain 46(1): 35–41

Haldeman S 1989 Manipulation and massage for the relief of pain. In: Wall P D, Melzack R (eds) Textbook of pain, 2nd edn. Churchill Livingstone, Edinburgh, ch 69, pp 942–951

Halferns R, Evers G, Abu-Saad H 1990 Determinants of pain assessment by nurses. International Journal of Nursing Studies 27(1): 43–49

Hanks G, de Conno F, Ripamonti C et al 1996 Morphine in cancer pain: modes of administration. British Medical Journal 312: 823–826

Harkins S W, Kwentus J, Price D D 1984 Pain and the elderly. In: Benedetti C, Chapman C R, Moricca G (eds) Advances in pain research and therapy, vol 7. Recent advances in the management of pain. Raven Press, New York, pp 103–121

Harrison A 1991 Assessing patients' pain: identifying reasons for error. Journal of Advanced Nursing 16(9): 1018–1025

Holm K, Cohen F, Dudas S, Medema P G, Allen B L 1989 Effect of personal pain experience on pain assessment. Image. Journal of Nursing Scholarship 21(2): 72–75

Horan J J, Layng F C, Pursell C H 1976 Preliminary study of effects of 'in vivo' emotive imagery on dental discomfort. Perceptual and Motor Skills 42: 105–106

Hoy A M 1989 Radiotherapy, chemotherapy and hormone therapy: treatment for pain. In: Wall P D, Melzack R (eds) Textbook of pain, 2nd edn. Churchill Livingstone, Edinburgh, ch 71, pp 966–978

Hunter D 1993 Acute pain. In: Carroll D, Bowsher D (eds) Pain management and nursing care. Butterworth Press, Oxford, ch 5

International Association for the Study of Pain (IASP) 1986 Pain terms: a current list with definitions and notes on usage. Pain 27: S215–221

Jensen M P, Karoly P, Braver S 1986 The measurement of clinical pain intensity: a comparison of six methods. Pain 27(1): 117–126

Jensen M P, Karoly P O, Riordan E F, Bland F, Burns R S 1989 The subjective experience of acute pain: an assessment of the utility of 10 indices. Clinical Journal of Pain 5(2): 153–159

Jessup B A 1989 Relaxation and biofeedback. In: Wall P D, Melzack R (eds) Textbook of pain, 2nd edn. Churchill Livingstone, Edinburgh, ch 73, pp 989–1000

Kearney M 1992 Imagework in a case of intractable pain. Palliative Medicine 6: 152–157

Keefe F J 1989 Behavioral measurement of pain. In: Chapman C R, Loeser J D (eds) Issues in pain measurement. Advances in pain research and therapy, vol 12. Raven Press, New York, ch 32, pp 405–424

King V M F, Jacob P A 1993 Special procedures. In: Carroll D, Bowsher D (eds) Pain management and nursing care. Butterworth Press, Oxford, ch 15

Kopp M, Richter R, Rainer J, Kopp-Wilfing P, Rumpold G, Walter M H 1995 Differences in family functioning between patients with chronic headache and patients with low back pain. Pain 63(2): 219–224

Kotorba J A 1988 Perceptions of death, belief systems and the process of coping with chronic pain. Social Science and Medicine 17(10): 681–689

Kremer E, Atkinson J H, Ignelzi R J 1981 Measurement of pain: patient preference does not confound pain measurement. Pain 10(2): 241–248

Kruk Z L, Pycock C J 1991 Neurotransmitters and drugs, 3rd edn. Chapman and Hall, London

Kubecka K E, Simon J M, Boettcher J H 1996 Pain management of hospital-based nurses in rural Appalachian area. Journal of Advanced Nursing 23(5): 861–867

Lamacraft G, Molley A R, Cousins M J 1997 Peripheral nerve blockade and chronic pain management. Pain Reviews 4: 122–147

Lander J 1990a Clinical judgements in pain management. Pain 42(4): 15–22

Lander J 1990b Fallacies and phobias about addiction and pain. British Journal of Addiction 85(6): 803–809

Lehmann J F, de Lateur B J 1989 Ultrasound, shortwave, microwave, superficial heat and cold in the treatment of pain. In: Wall P D, Melzack R (eds) Textbook of pain, 2nd edn. Churchill Livingstone, Edinburgh, ch 68, pp 932–941

Levin R F, Malloy G B, Hyman R B 1987 Nursing management of postoperative pain: use of relaxation techniques with female cholecystectomy patients. Journal of Advanced Nursing 12(4): 463–472

Levine J D, Gordon N C, Jones R T, Fields H L 1978 The mechanism of placebo analgesia. Lancet 2: 654–657

Librach S L, Rapson L M 1988 The use of transcutaneous electrical nerve stimulation (TENS) for the relief of pain in palliative care. Palliative Medicine 2: 15–20

Lima D 1997 Functional anatomy of spinofugal nociceptive pathways. Pain Reviews 4: 1–19

Lutz L J, Lamer T J 1990 Management of postoperative pain: review of current techniques and methods. Mayo Clinic Proceedings 65(4): 584–596

McCaffery M 1972 Nursing management of the patient in pain. Lippincott, Philadelphia, PA

McCaffery M, Beebe A 1994 Pain: clinical manual for nursing practice. Mosby, Aylesbury

McCaffery M, Ferrell B R 1994 Nurses' assessment of pain intensity and choice of analgesic dose. Contemporary Nurse 3(2): 68–74

McCaffery M, Ferrell B R 1995 Nurses' knowledge about cancer pain: a survey of five countries. Journal of Pain and Symptom Management 10(5): 356–369

McCaffery M, Ferrell B R 1997 Nurses' knowledge of pain assessment and management: how much progress have we made? Journal of Pain and Symptom Management 14(3): 175–188

Mackintosh C, Bowles S 1997 Evaluation of a nurse-led acute pain service. Can clinical nurse specialists make a difference? Journal of Advanced Nursing 25(1): 30–37

McMillan S C 1996 Pain and pain relief experienced by hospice patients with cancer. Cancer Nursing 19(4): 289–307

McQuay H 1990 The logic of alternative routes. Pain and Symptom Management 5(2): 75–77

McQuay H, Moore A, Justins D 1997 Treating acute pain in hospital. British Medical Journal 314: 1431–1535

McQuay H, Tramer M, Nye B A, Carroll D, Wiffen P J, Moore R A 1996 A systematic review of antidepressants in neuropathic pain. Pain 68(2): 217–227

Madjar I 1997 The body in health, illness and pain. In: Lawler J (ed) The body in nursing. Churchill Livingstone, London, ch 5, p 62

Mason D J 1981 An investigation of the influence of selected factors on nurses' inferences of patients' suffering. International Journal of Nursing Studies 18(4): 251–259

Mather L, Mackie J 1983 The incidence of postoperative pain in children. Pain 15(3): 271–282

Mather L E, Woodhouse E 1997 Pharmacokinetics of opioids in the context of patient controlled analgesia. Pain Reviews 4: 20–32

May C 1990 Research on nurse-patient relationships: problems of theory, problems of practice. Journal of Advanced Nursing 15(4): 307–315

Meade T W, Dyer S, Browne W, Townsend J, Frank A O 1990 Low back pain of mechanical origin: randomised comparison of chiropractic and hospital outpatient treatment. British Medical Journal 300: 1431–1437

Meinhart N T, McCaffery M 1983 Pain: a nursing approach to assessment and analysis. Appleton-Century-Crofts, Norwalk

Melzack R, Casey K L 1968 Sensory, motivational, and central control determinants of pain: a new conceptual model. In: Kenshalo D R (ed) The skin senses. Thomas Springfield, Illinois

Melzack R, Torgerson W S 1971 On the language of pain. Anesthesiology 34(1): 50–59

Melzack R, Wall P D 1965 Pain mechanisms: a new theory. Science 150: 971–979

Melzack R, Wall P D 1988 The challenge of pain, 2nd edn. Penguin, Harmondsworth

Misuse of Drugs Act 1971 HMSO, London

Moore R 1990 Ethnographic assessment of pain coping perceptions. Psychosomatic Medicine 52: 156–170

Morris D 1991 The culture of pain. University of California Press, Berkeley

Myers K G, Trotman I F 1994 Use of ketolorac by continuous subcutaneous infusion for the control of cancer-related pain. Post Graduate Medical Journal 70: 359–362

National Institutes of Health Consensus Development Conference 1987 The integrated approach to the management of pain. Journal of Pain and Symptom Management 2(1): 35–44

Nievaard A C 1987 Communication climate and patient care: causes and effects of nurses' attitudes to patients. Social Science and Medicine 24(9): 777–784

Orne M T, Dinges D F 1989 Hypnosis. In: Wall P D, Melzack R (eds) Textbook of pain, 2nd edn. Churchill Livingstone, Edinburgh, ch 77, pp 1021–1031

Owen H, McMillan V, Rogowski D 1990 Postoperative pain therapy: a survey of patients' expectations and their experiences. Pain 41(3): 303–307

Paice J A, Cohen 1997 Validity of a verbally administered numeric rating scale to measure cancer pain intensity. Cancer Nursing 20(2): 88–93
Patel M, Gutzwiller F, Marazzi A 1989 A meta-analysis of acupuncture for chronic pain. International Journal of Epidemiology 18(4): 900–906
Peck C L 1986 Psychological factors in acute pain management. In: Cousins M J, Phillips G D (eds) Acute pain management. Churchill Livingstone, Edinburgh, ch 10, pp 251–274
Perry S, Heidrich G 1982 Management of pain during debridement: a survey of US burn units. Pain 13(3): 267–280
Philips H C 1988 Changing chronic pain experience. Pain 32(2): 165–172
Portenoy R K 1996 Opioid therapy for chronic non-malignant pain: a review of the critical issues. Journal of Pain and Symptom Management 11(4): 203–217
Portenoy R K, Hagen N A 1990 Breakthrough pain: definition, prevalence and characteristics. Pain 41(2): 273–281
Porter J, Jick H 1980 Addiction rare in patients treated with opioids. New England Journal of Medicine 302(2): 123
Price K, Cheek J 1996 Exploring the nursing role in pain management from a post-structuralist perspective. Journal of Advanced Nursing 24(5): 899–904
Raiman J 1987 Pain. In: Collins S, Parker E (eds) Essentials of nursing, 2nd edn. Macmillan, London, ch 5, pp 70–90
Ready L B 1989 Acute pain services: an academic asset. Clinical Journal of Pain 5(suppl 1): S28–33
Ready L B, Oden R, Chadwick H S, Benedetti C, Rooke G A, Caplan R, Wild L M 1988 Development of an anesthesiology-based postoperative pain management service. Anesthesiology 68(1): 100–106
Reitsma B, Meijler W J 1997 Pain and patienthood. The Clinical Journal of Pain 13: 9–21
Robinson R G, Preston D F, Schiefelbein M, Baxter K G 1995 Stontium 89 therapy for the palliation of pain due to osseous metastases. Journal of American Medical Association 4(5): 420–424
Rogers R C, Spector H J 1989 Aids to clinical pharmacology, 2nd edn. Churchill Livingstone, Edingburgh
Romano J M, Turner J A, Jenson M P, Friedman L S, Bulcroft R A, Hops H, Wright S F 1995 Chronic pain patient-spouse behavioural interactions predict patient disability. Pain 63(3): 353–360
Rosenteil A K, Keefe F J 1983 The use of coping strategies in chronic low back pain patients: relationships to patient characteristics and current adjustment. Pain 17(1): 33–44
Rowat K M, Jeans M E 1989 A collaborative model of care: patient, family and health care professionals. In: Wall P D, Melzack R (eds) Textbook of pain, 2nd edn. Churchill Livingstone, Edinburgh, ch 75, pp 1010–1014
Royal College of Surgeons and College of Anaesthetists 1990 Commission on the provision of surgical services. Report of the working party on pain after surgery. Royal College of Surgeons, London
Salmon P, Manyande A 1996 Good patients cope with their pain: postoperative analgesia and nurses' perceptions of their patients' pain. Pain 68(1): 63–68
Saunders C 1976 Care of the dying, 2nd edn. Macmillan/Nursing Times, London
Scarry E 1985 The body in pain. Oxford University Press, New York
Schwartz L, Slater M A, Birchler G R 1996 The role of pain behaviours in the modulation of marital conflict in chronic pain couples. Pain 65(2/3): 227–233
Scott J F 1989 Carcinoma invading nerve. In: Wall P D, Melzack R (eds) Textbook of pain, 2nd edn. Churchill Livingstone, Edinburgh, ch 42, pp 598–609
Seers C J 1987 Pain, anxiety and recovery in patients undergoing surgery. PhD thesis, University of London (unpublished)
Seers K 1989 Patients' perceptions of acute pain. In: Wilson-Barnett J, Robinson S (eds) Directions in nursing research: ten years of progress at London University. Scutari, London, ch 12, pp 107–116
Seers K 1990 Early discharge after surgery: its effects on patients, their informal carers and on the workload of health professionals. Daphne Heald Research Unit Report, Royal College of Nursing, London
Seers K, Friedli K 1996 The patients' experience of their chronic non-malignant pain. Journal of Advanced Nursing 24(6): 1160–1168
Sidebotham D, Dijkhuizen M R J, Schug S A 1997 The safety and utilization of patient controlled analgesia. Journal of Pain and Symptom Management 14(4): 202–209
Simons W, Malabar R 1995 Assessing pain in elderly patients who cannot respond verbally. Journal of Advanced Nursing 22(1): 663–669
Sims S E 1987 Relaxation training as a technique for helping patients cope with the experience of cancer: a selective review of the literature. Journal of Advanced Nursing 12(5): 583–591
Skinner J B, Erskine A, Pearce S, Rubenstein I, Taylor M, Foster C 1990 The evaluation of a cognitive behavioural treatment programme in outpatients with chronic pain. Journal of Psychosomatic Research 34(1): 13–19
Snell C C, Fothergill-Bourbonnais F, Durocher-Hendrikis S 1997 Patient controlled analgesia and intramuscular injections: a comparison of patient pain experiences and post operative outcomes. Journal of Advanced Nursing 25(4): 681–690
Snelling J 1991 The effects of chronic pain on the family unit. Journal of Advanced Nursing 19: 543–551
Snow-Turek A L, Norris M P, Tan G 1996 Active and passive coping strategies in chronic pain patients. Pain 64(3): 455–462
Sofaer B 1984 Pain: a handbook for nurses. Harper and Row, London
Sriwatanakul K, Kelvie W, Lasagna L 1982 The quantification of pain: an analysis of words used to describe pain and analgesia in clinical trials. Clinical Pharmacology and Therapeutics 32(2): 143–148
Stacey M 1988 The sociology of health and healing. Unwin Hyman, London
Sternbach R A 1989 Acute versus chronic pain. In: Wall P D, Melzack R (eds) Textbook of pain, 2nd edn. Churchill Livingstone, Edinburgh, ch 14, pp 242–246
Stevenson C 1992 Appropriate therapies for nurses to practise. Nursing Standard 6(50): 51–52
Stiles M 1990 The shining stranger: Nurse-family spiritual relationship. Cancer Nursing 13: 235–245
Stjernsward J, Teoh N 1990 The scope of the cancer pain problem. In: Foley K M, Bonica J J, Ventafridda V (eds) Advances in pain research and therapy, vol 16. Raven Press, New York, pp 7–12
Storey P, Hill H H, St Louis R H, Tarver E E 1990 Subcutaneous infusions for control of cancer symptoms. Journal of Pain and Symptom Management 5(1): 33–41
Suls J, Wan C K 1989 Effects of sensory and procedural information on coping with stressful medical procedures and pain: a meta-analysis. Journal of Consulting and Clinical Psychology 57(3): 372–379
Swinford P 1987 Relaxation and positive imagery for the surgical patient: a research study. Perioperative Nursing Quarterly 3(3): 9–16
Tanner J 1987 Beating back pain: a practical self-help guide to prevention and treatment. Dorling Kindersley, London
Taylor A G, Lorentzen L J, Blank M B 1990 Psychological distress of chronic pain sufferers and their spouses. Journal of Pain and Symptom Management 5(1): 6–10
Taylor A G, Skelton J A, Butcher J 1984 Duration of pain condition and physical pathology as determinants of nurses' assessments of patients in pain. Nursing Research 33(1): 4–8
Thomas V 1989 Predicting PCA. Nursing Standard 3(18): 34–35
Thomas V, Rose F D 1993 Patient controlled analgesia: a new method for old. Journal of Advanced Nursing 11(1): 1719–1726
Turk D C 1989 Assessment of pain: the elusiveness of latent constructs. In: Chapman C R, Loeser J D (eds) Issues in pain measurement. Advances in pain research and therapy, vol 12. Raven Press, New York, ch 22, pp 267–279
Turk D C, Meichenbaum D H 1989 A cognitive-behavioural approach to pain. In: Wall P D, Melzack R (eds) Textbook of pain, 2nd edn. Churchill Livingstone, Edinburgh, ch 74, pp 1001–1009
Turk D C, Flor H, Rudy T E 1987 Pain and families I: etiology, maintenance and psychological impact. Pain 30(1): 2–27
Tutton L 1991 An exploration of touch and its use in nursing. In: McMahon R, Pearson A (eds) Nursing as therapy. Chapman and Hall, London, ch 7
UKCC 1992a Scope of professional practice. UKCC, London
UKCC 1992b Standards for the administration of medicines. UKCC, London
Van Dongen R T, Cruel B J, De Bock 1993 Long term intrathecal infusion of morphine and morphine-bupivacaine mixtures in the treatment of cancer pain: a retrospective analysis of 51 cases. Pain 55(1): 119–123
Velikova G, Selby P J, Snaith P R, Kirby 1995 The relationship of cancer pain to anxiety. Psychotherapy and Psychosomatics 63: 181–184
Waddie N A 1996 Language and pain expression. Journal of Advanced Nursing 23(5): 868–872
Wakefield A B 1995 Pain: an account of nurses' talk. Journal of Advanced Nursing 21(5): 905–910
Walker J M, Akinsanya J A, Davies B D, Marcer D 1989 The nursing management of pain in the community: a theoretical framework. Journal of Advanced Nursing 14(1): 240–247
Walker J M, Akinsanya J A, Davies B D, Marcer D 1990 The nursing management of elderly patients with pain in the community: study and recommendations. Journal of Advanced Nursing 15(4): 1154–1161
Walker V A, Hoskin P J, Hanks G W, White I D 1988 Evaluation of WHO analgesic guidelines for cancer pain in an acute-based palliative care unit. Journal of Pain and Symptom Management 3(3): 145–149

Wall P D 1979 On the relation of injury to pain. Pain 6(3): 253–264
Wall P D 1989a Introduction. In: Wall P D, Melzack R (eds) Textbook of pain, 2nd edn. Churchill Livingstone, Edinburgh, pp 1–18
Wall P D 1989b The dorsal horn. In: Wall P D, Melzack R (eds) Textbook of pain, 2nd edn. Churchill Livingstone, Edinburgh, ch 5, pp 102–111
Wallace K G 1997 Analysis of recent literature concerning relaxation and imagery interventions for cancer pain. Cancer Nursing 20(2): 79–87
Walsh T D, Smyth E M, Currie K, Glare P A, Schneider J 1992 Pilot study, review of the literature, and dosing guidelines for patient controlled analgesia using subcutaneous morphine sulphate for chronic cancer pain. Palliative Medicine 6: 217–226
Weis O F, Sriwatanakul K, Alloza J L, Weintraub M, Lasagna L 1983 Attitudes of patients, housestaff, and nurses toward postoperative analgesic care. Anaesthesia and Analgesia 62: 70–74
Weir R, Woodside R, Crook J 1988 Group therapy for chronic pain patients: a review of complexity. The Pain Clinic 2(2): 109–120
Williams C 1996 Patient-controlled analgesia: a review of the literature. Journal of Clinical Nursing 5(3): 139–147
Williams D A, Thorn B E 1989 An empirical assessment of pain beliefs. Pain 36(3): 351–358
Willis W D 1989 The origin and destination of pathways involved in pain transmission. In: Wall P D, Melzack R (eds) Textbook of pain, 2nd edn. Churchill Livingstone, Edinburgh, ch 6, pp 112–127
Woolf C J 1989 Segmental afferent fibre-induced analgesia: transcutaneous electrical nerve stimulation (TENS) and vibration. In: Wall P D, Melzack R (eds) Textbook of pain, 2nd edn. Churchill Livingstone, Edinburgh, ch 63, pp 884–896
World Health Organization 1986 Cancer pain relief. WHO, Geneva
Yates P, Dewar A, Fentiman B 1995 Pain: the views of elderly people living in long term residential care settings. Journal of Advanced Nursing 21(4): 667–674
Zborowski M 1952 Cultural components in response to pain. Journal of Social Issues 8(4): 16–30
Zola I K 1973 Pathways to the doctor: from person to patient. Social Science and Medicine 7: 677–689

FURTHER READING

Benson H, Klipper M Z 1975 The relaxation response. Collins, London
Broome A, Jellicoe H 1987 Living with your pain. British Psychological Society/Methuen, Leicester
Gingell J 1988 A safety net when experts fail. Action Group for the Relief of Pain and Distress, Bristol
Hewitt J 1982 The complete relaxation book. Rider, London
McCaffery M, Beebe A 1994 Pain: clinical manual for nursing practice. Mosby, Aylesbury
Mather L E, Woodhouse E 1997 Pharmacokinetics of opioids in the context of patient controlled analgesia. Pain Reviews 4
Melzack R, Casey K L 1968 Sensory, motivational and central control determinants of pain: a new conceptual model. In: Kenshalo D R (ed) The skin senses. Thomas, Springfield, Illinois
Melzack R, Wall P D 1988 The challenge of pain, 2nd edn. Penguin, Harmondsworth
Sternbach R A 1987 Mastering pain. A twelve-step regimen for coping with chronic pain. Arlington, London
Tanner J 1987 Beating back pain: a practical self-help guide to prevention and treatment. Dorling Kindersley, London
Williams C 1996 Patient-controlled analgesia: a review of the literature. Journal of Clinical Nursing 5(3): 139–147
Wright S M 1987 The use of therapeutic touch in the management of pain. Nursing Clinics of North America 22(3): 705–714
Wyatt G, Dimmer S 1988 The balancing touch. Nursing Times 84(21): 41–42

USEFUL ADDRESSES

The British Migraine Association
178a High Road
Byfleet
Weybridge
Surrey KT14 7ED

The National Back Pain Association
31–33 Park Road
Teddington
Middlesex TW11 0AB
http://www.backpain.org/intr.htm

Self-help in pain groups (SHIP)
c/o Room 27
Walton Hospital
Liverpool L9 1AE

Migraine Sufferers Support Group
http://www.migraine.co.nz/mssginfo.htm

FLUID AND ELECTROLYTE BALANCE

20

Mary Gobbi

INTRODUCTION

Monitoring and manipulating body fluid and electrolytes form a crucial aspect of nursing care. For the average male, only about 18% of the body weight is protein (with 15% fat and 7% minerals); 60% is water. For health, body water and electrolytes must be maintained within a limited range of tolerances. Homeostatic mechanisms regulate parameters such as body fluid volume, pH and electrolyte concentrations, maintaining a delicate, dynamic balance which can be destabilised during illness. In extreme cases, the fluid or electrolyte deficit can lead to death. Consequently, nurses must have a clear understanding of fluid and electrolyte homeostasis so that they can assess fluid and electrolyte status, anticipate/recognise deterioration and implement corrective interventions.

Nursing interventions in relation to fluid therapy may range from encouraging the patient to drink her afternoon cup of tea to managing a complicated intravenous fluid regimen. Ill-defined terms such as 'restrict fluids' or 'push fluids' and instructions to record fluid intake/output or daily weight are commonly encountered, but without a knowledgeable appreciation of the physiology and pathophysiology of fluid and electrolyte balance there is a real risk that these tasks will be performed in a somewhat mechanistic fashion, without sufficient thought.

This chapter reviews the normal mechanisms which regulate body fluid and outlines some of the basic adaptive responses to stress. The regulation of acid–base balance is also considered, along with basic principles in the management of fluid and electrolyte disorders. Throughout the chapter, typical clinical situations where fluid and electrolyte control may be embarrassed are reviewed. Reference is made to the ethical dilemmas which may be associated with the administration/withdrawal of hydration measures.

Students who are unfamiliar with the physiology of fluid, electrolyte and acid–base balance are advised to read this chapter in conjunction with their physiology textbook. It is important for the reader to be familiar with units and terms such as 'moles', 'molality', 'equivalents', 'diffusion', 'osmosis', 'osmoles', 'osmolality', 'tonicity' and 'filtration'.

For more detailed information, see Timberlake (1988) and Smith & Kinsey (1991).

Nursing goals in the care of patients with existing or potential fluid and electrolyte problems include:

- the promotion and maintenance of a healthy pattern of fluid intake/output appropriate to the patient's lifestyle and wishes
- the detection of existing or potential fluid and electrolyte imbalances
- the re-establishment of fluid and electrolyte balance when homeostasis is disturbed
- the development of educational programmes on the maintenance of fluid and electrolyte balance.

It is hoped that this chapter will provide some of the essential background knowledge necessary to achieving these aims.

BODY WATER

Water has a range of functions within the body which are essential to sustaining life and maintaining health. These include:

- giving form to body structures and cushioning the body from shock
- acting as a transport medium for nutrients, electrolytes, blood gases, metabolic wastes, heat and electrical currents
- providing insulation
- aiding in the hydrolysis of food
- acting as a medium and reactant in chemical processes
- acting as a lubricant.

Body tissues contain varying proportions of water, ranging from 10% for fat to 83% for blood. A young 70 kg man of average build has a total body water (TBW) of about 63% of body weight, or 45 L. The percentage of body weight represented by the TBW varies from one individual to another, depending on factors such as age, sex and build. Fat contributes little towards TBW and is the main source of this variation. A 70 kg woman of average build would have a TBW of about 52% (36 L) due to the greater proportion of adipose tissue. In both sexes, the percentage of body water tends to decrease with age. Lean tissue has a fairly constant water content of 71–72 mL/100 g, and if adipose tissue is disregarded as a non-functional storage tissue, then the TBW of the lean body mass is about 73%. As water makes up nearly three-quarters of the body's active tissues, homeostatic regulation of body fluids is essential to normal function and health.

Fluid compartments

Body water is distributed between two major compartments: the intracellular fluid (ICF) and the extracellular fluid (ECF). The distinction between the two compartments is maintained by the selective permeability of cell membranes. The intracellular environment is not homogeneous but varies greatly between cell types. However, all cells can tolerate only a limited variation in the volume and composition of their ICF before function is disrupted.

Large proteins which are synthesised by the cell remain trapped inside as they are too big to pass through the membrane. However, the membrane is freely permeable to water. Selective membrane transport processes regulate the distribution of electrolytes, and hence water, across the cell membrane. The ICF has been estimated to be approximately 40% of TBW, or about 28 L in a 70 kg male.

The ECF bathes and surrounds the cells, forming a relatively constant environment. It has a smaller volume than the ICF, accounting for about 20% of TBW (or 14 L), and can be divided into four subcompartments:

- the extravascular fluid (interstitial or tissue fluid)
- inaccessible bone water (skeletal water)
- the intravascular fluid compartment (blood plasma)
- transcellular fluids.

Interstitial fluid includes lymph and accounts for about 15% (10.5 L) of TBW. Interstitial fluid is defined by two membranes: the cell membrane separates it from the ICF, and the capillary endothelium separates it from plasma. Interstitial fluid forms the interface and exchange route between the ICF and plasma. Plasma represents about 4% of body weight (3 L).

Transcellular fluids are specialised fluids which are separated from the ECF by an additional epithelial cell layer. They include:

- cerebrospinal fluid (CSF)
- aqueous and vitreous humour of the eye
- glandular secretions
- synovial fluid
- pleural fluid
- peritoneal fluid
- glandular secretions
- saliva and other gastrointestinal secretions
- respiratory tract fluid
- fluid within the urinary system.

Transcellular fluid volume is highly variable, and some transcellular fluids have a very high turnover (in the gastrointestinal tract alone it can be greater than 20 L/day). Some water is trapped in the deeper layers of bone; this is inaccessible and, because it does not readily exchange with the rest of the ECF, is difficult to measure. The relative contribution of each compartment is summarised in Box 20.1. In infants and children, although the actual ECF volume is much smaller than in adults, the ECF:ICF ratio is larger, i.e. the ECF represents a greater percentage of the TBW, and fluid loss can rapidly lead to dehydration. The consequences of ECF losses from, for example, vomiting, sweating or diarrhoea are potentially more serious in the infant than in the adult.

Solutes and electrolytes

Body fluids cannot be equated simply with water, as they also contain dissolved substances or solutes as well as larger particles in

Box 20.1 Distribution of body water in the average young adult male. (After Edelman & Liebman 1959)

Fluid compartment	Percentage of TBW	
Intracellular fluid	55	
Extracellular fluid	45	
Extravascular fluid		(20.0)
Inaccessible bone water		(15.0)
Intravascular fluid		(7.5)
Transcellular fluid		(2.5)
	100	

Assuming that the individual's body contained 40 L of fluid, the average distribution would be as follows:

Fluid compartment	Volume (L)	
Intracellular fluid	22	
Extracellular fluid	18	
Extravascular fluid		(9)
Inaccessible bone water		(6)
Intravascular fluid		(3)
Transcellular fluid		(1)
	40	

suspension (colloids). Solutes may be complete molecules (non-electrolytes) or parts of molecules (electrolytes). Measures of body fluid volume such as the litre refer to the volume of water and its dissolved solutes. Glucose is a good example of a non-electrolyte. It dissolves in body water but does not dissociate into component parts. An electrolyte, however, will dissociate in solution into its constituent ions. Sodium chloride is the most important example of this. In solution, a molecule of sodium chloride dissociates into a positively charged sodium ion (cation) and a negatively charged chloride ion (anion). Sodium is the dominant cation in the ECF but smaller concentrations of potassium, magnesium and calcium ions are present. Chloride and bicarbonate are the major extracellular anions.

Inside the cell, potassium is the dominant cation. Lower concentrations of magnesium, calcium and sodium are also present. Intracellular anions include phosphate, sulphate and intracellular proteins which also behave as anions. The cell regulates the movement of ions across its membrane, and maintenance of an appropriate distribution of ions between the ECF and ICF is essential for cell function, particularly in excitable tissues such as nerve and muscle.

Fluid exchange

Fluid exchange between ICF and ECF

The movement of body fluids and their constituents between the different compartments involves both active and passive transport processes. The main mechanisms which enable body fluids to enter the cell membrane are (Guyton & Hall 1996):

- diffusion
- facilitated diffusion
- voltage-gated channels
- ligand-gated channels
- active transport.

Lipid-soluble substances diffuse directly through the cell membrane, while water and electrolytes utilise channels formed by membrane proteins. The membrane is freely permeable to water but is only selectively permeable to electrolytes. Permeability is affected by the size and charge of the hydrated ion; for example, the membrane is 50–100 times more permeable to K^+ than to Na^+. Movement into the cell via membrane proteins may be by simple diffusion, facilitated diffusion (carrier-mediated transport) and active transport. Glucose, for example, enters the muscle cell by facilitated diffusion under the influence of insulin. The most important example of active transport is the sodium–potassium pump. This pump is a membrane protein that couples the active transport of Na^+ out of the cell with the active transport of K^+ inwards. It requires energy derived from the hydrolysis of ATP (adenosine 5-triphosphate) to function.

Tissue–capillary fluid exchange

Just as the cell membrane separates the ICF from the ECF, the capillary wall represents the boundary between the intravascular and interstitial compartments of the ECF. The capillary wall is selectively permeable to substances of a molecular weight less than 69 000 g and to lipid-soluble molecules. The exchange of water, electrolytes, metabolites and waste products between the plasma and interstitial fluid occurs at the capillary. Fluid movement is determined by three forces: diffusion, osmosis and filtration. The capillary endothelium is freely permeable to water and solutes but the larger plasma proteins are retained. At the arterial end, fluid is forced out of the capillary by hydrostatic pressure. As water is lost from the capillary, the plasma proteins become more concentrated and the colloid osmotic or oncotic pressure exerted by the plasma proteins increases. (Oncotic pressure means osmotic pressure caused by the presence of colloids, i.e. colloid osmotic pressure.) At the venous end, the hydrostatic pressure is lower and the osmotic pressure draws fluid back into the capillary.

Because the capillary endothelium is a very imperfect barrier, plasma proteins may leak into the interstitial fluid, complicating the situation described above. If these proteins were not removed, the oncotic pressure of the interstitial fluid would rise, disrupting capillary fluid exchange and favouring retention of water in the interstitial spaces. The lymphatic system is central to maintaining interstitial fluid volume. Blind-ended lymphatic capillaries in the interstitium are more permeable than the capillaries and easily take up and remove plasma proteins and fluid from the interstitial space. The fluid formed in these vessels — lymph — is carried through the lymphatic system, eventually returning to the circulation via the central lymphatic and the thoracic duct.

As approximately 20% of body fluid is found in the interstitial or tissue spaces, the maintenance of fluid volume in this compartment plays a key role in homeostasis. Normally, a dynamic equilibrium exists which maintains the extracellular fluid content of both the plasma and the tissue spaces. However, this delicate balance can easily be disturbed by the following factors:

- *Alterations in capillary pressure*. Changes in pressure at either end of the capillary will alter net movement of fluid. Increased arterial pressure or venous congestion will both tend to favour the loss of fluid to the interstitial space. Examples include hypertension, hypotension, heart failure, and arterial or venous obstruction.
- *Alterations in the plasma proteins*. A reduction in plasma proteins due to malnutrition, liver or renal disease, loss of circulating plasma or leakage of proteins into the tissue fluids will alter the osmotic pressure gradient and prevent fluid being reclaimed from the tissue spaces. Failure of the lymphatics to remove this fluid will increase the osmotic pressure of the interstitial fluid and favour fluid retention.
- *Changes in the integrity of the capillary membranes*. Factors which alter the normal mechanisms regulating the permeability/pore size of the capillary membranes also change the osmotic or hydrostatic pressures. These effects may be local or systemic. Examples include membrane damage from burns, anoxia, pressure, septicaemia and the presence of inflammatory mediators such as bradykinin or histamine.
- *Accumulation of metabolites*. An accumulation of metabolites within the tissue fluid can alter the hydrostatic and colloidal osmotic pressures with consequent changes in fluid movement. For example, in some states of shock or tissue hypoxia, the cumulative effects of lactic acid and carbon dioxide when combined with vasoactive substances may result in oedema.

Oedema

Oedema is an accumulation of fluid in the interstitial spaces or other sites such as the pericardial sac, between the pleura, in the peritoneal cavity or within the joint capsule. Oedema alters the natural turgor of the tissue spaces and may be noticed by swelling or distension. If the swollen tissue is indented by slight pressure, it is called pitting oedema. In the case of blocked lymphatics, protein leakage from the capillaries is not reclaimed from the tissue fluid and the oedema so caused is firm due to the presence of the proteins and does not tend to pit — a characteristic sign of lymphoedema. Oedema may be localised (as in the case of inflammation and tissue damage) or generalised (as seen in heart failure).

General features

Oedema presents several problems to the patient. Its characteristic features may be described as follows:

- it accumulates in dependent areas, especially soft tissues
- it presents as swelling and distension which sometimes 'pits' under pressure
- it hinders the diffusion of gases and transport of nutrients and waste products
- the oedematous tissues lose integrity and are easily traumatised
- tissues adjacent to the oedema may be damaged by the pressure.

Management

It is important to ascertain the cause(s) of the oedema before initiating any nursing actions.

Q **20.1** Why are the following situations managed differently? A
(a) Oedema caused by a deep vein thrombosis
(b) Oedema caused by a soft tissue injury
(c) Oedema due to arterial insufficiency and the accumulation of metabolites liberated from hypoxic cells
(d) Oedema due to protein loss
(e) Oedema due to cardiac failure.

Consideration of the points listed below may enable a safe, effective plan of care to be initiated which is specific to the person concerned.

1. Identify the cause of the oedema and ascertain the appropriate management by liaising with medical staff and other health professionals (e.g. physiotherapists may advise in the case of sports or orthopaedic problems).
2. Consider the use and effects of gravity, which may alter fluid drainage or blood flow.
3. Monitor and record the extent and nature of the oedema. Communication between day and night staff may identify oedema due to the effects of gravity/position. For example, oedematous feet in the evening may appear to be resolved by a night in bed, only to be replaced in the morning by sacral or orbital oedema (recognised by puffy eyes).
4. Assess the effects of the oedema on local tissues and take appropriate action. For example, sacral oedema increases the risk of a pressure sore, and severe oedema of the fascia may restrict blood flow and lead to tissue hypoxia.
5. Implement medical therapies with appropriate interventions, e.g. administration of diuretics.
6. Consider the potential implications and complications of specific types of oedema (e.g. pulmonary or cerebral) and initiate appropriate nursing assessment.
7. Consider how oedema may restrict movement, alter a person's self-image and cause practical difficulties in daily life. Ankle oedema may be exacerbated by tight-fitting shoes, whilst ascites may cause respiratory embarrassment and affect the body image. Attention to small details may greatly enhance the comfort of a person with oedema.

Q **20.2** Why should one try to avoid giving injections in oedematous areas? A

Q **20.3** What advice could you give to an elderly person who suffers from persistent ankle oedema and who wishes to buy a new pair of shoes? A

WATER AND ELECTROLYTE HOMEOSTASIS

Constancy of the internal environment is essential for efficient cell function. In health, the volume and composition of the different fluid compartments is finely regulated, with daily fluctuations in TBW of less than 0.2%. Water and electrolytes are ingested and absorbed through the gastrointestinal (GI) tract, although a small volume of water is produced through the oxidation of hydrogen in food. Excess water, electrolytes and waste products are excreted via the kidneys and in faeces. Additional water and salt loss occurs via the skin and respiratory tract.

Since losses from the GI and respiratory tracts are not subject to fine regulation, the kidney is the main regulator of fluid and electrolyte balance. Plasma represents about 4% of the body weight, or only 3 L, but the glomerular filtration rate is 125 mL/min, or about 180 L a day. This means that the 3 L of plasma contained within the body is filtered and reabsorbed about 60 times a day! With such a large turnover, the kidney can exert a major influence on plasma composition and, through plasma, on the composition of interstitial and, ultimately, intracellular fluid. Basal urine production in the absence of fluid ingestion is about 300 mL/day. The maximum rate seen in some disease states is 23 L/day, and a normal volume might be around about 2–2.5 L/day. The kidney regulates not only fluid volume, but also electrolyte composition, osmolality and pH. Central to the renal regulation of body fluid, osmolality and volume is the kidney's role in the handling of sodium and water.

Q **20.4** How much daily water is required by a 26-year-old woman who weighs 62 kg? How much extra water might she need if she had a pyrexia of 39°C? A

Regulation of ECF volume, osmolality* and sodium

Volume and osmolality regulation involves a series of homeostatic mechanisms which regulate the constancy of the ECF. Although the plasma compartment is small, it is dynamic, with shifts in volume and pressure occurring in response to internal and external stimuli. The rapid turnover of the plasma makes it the ideal target for regulatory mechanisms. Although plasma volume and osmolality are monitored, sodium is also a major factor in the regulation of ECF. Changes will also occur in the interstitial and intracellular fluid volumes, but these are usually slower than changes in plasma volume and the body can adapt to them with less functional disruption. The kidney regulates sodium and water ingestion/excretion under the influence of two hormones, aldosterone and vasopressin (also known as antidiuretic hormone, ADH), with additional input from the renin–angiotensin system and other factors.

Osmolality and ADH

Within the hypothalamus are specialised cells called osmoreceptors which monitor and respond to changes in plasma osmolality.

*The concentration of a solution defined in terms of the number of osmoles per kg of solvent; this is a measure of a solution's osmotic property.

They are very sensitive and respond to changes of as little as ±3 milliosmoles (mosmol). Plasma osmolality is normally in the range of 280–290 mosmol/kg water. The osmoreceptors respond to variations in plasma osmolality by stimulating two mechanisms: ADH release and thirst.

ADH acts on the epithelial cells of the nephron collecting ducts to increase tubular permeability to water and therefore water reabsorption. If a large volume of water is ingested, the plasma sodium is diluted, causing a fall in the plasma osmolality. This fall is registered by the osmoreceptors, with a resultant decrease in ADH release. Lowered plasma ADH then results in decreased tubular permeability, less water is reabsorbed and water is excreted in the form of a more dilute urine. Conversely, if plasma osmolality is increased, e.g. after fluid loss or after the ingestion of excess salt, a higher plasma ADH results with an increased permeability of the collecting ducts, and water is absorbed to dilute the hypertonic plasma.

The presence of a non-absorbable solute in the tubular lumen will increase water loss. For example, when plasma glucose levels are raised (as in diabetes mellitus) and filtered glucose exceeds the ability of the nephrons to reabsorb it, urine production is increased. The glucose exerts an osmotic force, keeping water in the tubule. Osmotic diuresis can also be induced therapeutically by the i.v. administration of a non-absorbable molecule such as mannitol.

Other factors affecting ADH regulation of osmolality. ADH release may be altered by some drugs, including nicotine and alcohol. Alcohol inhibits the release of ADH, with a resulting diuresis. Nicotine, morphine and barbiturates are drugs which increase ADH release. Adrenal insufficiency alters the renal response to water loading. Deficiency in adrenal glucocorticoids causes an increase in distal tubular permeability to water. Water reabsorption is increased and dilute urine cannot be produced. Tubular response to ADH is decreased and, even in the absence of ADH, permeability to water remains high.

Regulation of ECF volume and sodium

ECF volume is principally determined by sodium, and body sodium is regulated by the kidney mainly under the influence of aldosterone. Aldosterone is a mineralocorticoid essential for sodium (with associated water) reabsorption. It has a complex effect: it stimulates Na^+ reabsorption but is not the main regulator of Na^+ reabsorption (excess aldosterone production does not usually lead to excess sodium retention). When aldosterone is lacking, Na^+ reabsorption does not occur; this can rapidly lead to death from sodium and water depletion. Aldosterone is also important in hydrogen/potassium ion exchange in the kidney, and in the reabsorption of sodium in the gut and from sweat and the salivary glands. Aldosterone release is stimulated by plasma potassium concentration, plasma sodium concentration and changes in ECF volume. Increases in serum potassium levels of as little as 0.1 mmol can cause a marked increase in aldosterone release.

However, hypovolaemia, which reflects a fall in sodium content (as opposed to concentration), will increase aldosterone secretion via the renin–angiotensin system. Changes in the effective circulating volume (i.e. the blood volume actually perfusing the tissues, which may be less than the total blood volume) stimulate renin release.

Renin is a proteolytic enzyme released when sodium loss causes a drop in the effective circulating volume. Renin acts on a plasma protein called angiotensinogen, causing it to release angiotensin I. Angiotensin I is in turn split by a converting enzyme into angiotensin II. Angiotensin II has several actions:

- it is a potent vasoconstrictor
- it stimulates the release of aldosterone
- it increases the reabsorption of sodium by the proximal convoluted tubule
- it acts upon the hypothalamus, which then stimulates the thirst centre and increases ADH secretion.

DISORDERS OF WATER AND SODIUM BALANCE

Water volume and sodium imbalances frequently occur in combination with other electrolyte problems, although occasionally they occur alone. Principal causes of disturbance can be related to insufficient or excessive intake or output, problems in the regulation of intake and output, or problems related to fluid shifts within the body. Let us begin by considering the effects of water deprivation (dehydration) and excessive intake (water overload).

Fluid volume deficit (see Boxes 20.2 and 20.3)

An ECF volume deficit will arise when water loss exceeds water intake. Insufficiency of intake may be related to a number of factors. For example, a patient may be reluctant to swallow because of oral or pharyngeal pain and so may take in less fluid and food. Depressed, anorexic, nauseous or fatigued patients may also fail to take in adequate fluid. Patients suffering from neuromuscular impairment or who are unconscious will have an impaired ability to swallow and thus will also be prone to fluid volume deficit.

Dehydration

Strictly speaking, dehydration refers only to water losses from the body which exceed intake, leaving the person with a corresponding accumulation of sodium (hypernatraemic dehydration). However, 'free water' losses are unusual and it is more common for water to be lost in conjunction with sodium and/or in its role as the biological solvent. Dehydration may thus be isotonic, hypernatraemic or hyponatraemic with respect to the ECF. Isotonic dehydration occurs when the fluid lost is isotonic with the ECF in respect to the water and sodium content, whilst in hyponatraemic dehydration the sodium losses exceed the water losses.

Water-only depletion causes a volume deficit in the ECF. Sodium concentration is increased (hypernatraemic dehydration) with a consequent rise in osmolality and haematocrit (PCV, see Appendix 2). If the dehydration is not resolved, the cells will ultimately become dehydrated. Compensatory mechanisms initially maintain blood pressure, heart rate and haematocrit, but as the dehydration continues, blood pressure falls, pulse volume weakens, and heart rate and haematocrit rise. Haemoconcentration also causes apparent rises in haemoglobin and albumin levels. Eventually the person will be unable to meet the obligatory volume necessary to excrete waste products in the urine. The sequelae of this — metabolite accumulation, acidosis, renal failure and toxaemia — may lead to death.

Dehydration can be assessed according to the approximate percentage of body water that is lost; in the adult this may be defined as follows:

- mild: 4% (3 L)
- moderate: 5–8% (4–6 L)
- severe: 8–10% (7 L).

Management of dehydration is often complex, especially in severe states where there is gross derangement of body chemistry. In mild to moderate dehydration, fluid losses should be replaced slowly to prevent sudden shifts of water and/or electrolytes

Box 20.2 Causes of fluid volume deficit and excess. (Adapted with kind permission from Lippincott Williams & Wilkins, from Porth C M 1998 Pathophysiology: concepts of altered health state, 5th edn.)

Fluid deficit

Inadequate fluid intake
- Unconsciousness, inability to express thirst, inability to gain access to fluids
- Oral trauma or dysphasia
- Impaired thirst mechanism
- Withholding of fluids for therapeutic reasons
- Anorexia
- Nausea
- Depression

Excessive fluid losses
- Gastrointestinal losses
  —vomiting
  —diarrhoea
  —laxative abuse
  —gastrointestinal suction
  —fistula drainage
- Urine losses
  —diuretic therapy
  —osmotic diuresis (hyperglycaemia)
  —adrenal insufficiency
  —salt wasting renal disease
  —polyuria due to diabetes insipidus
- Skin losses
  —fever
  —exposure to hot environments
  —burns and wounds that remove skin

Third space losses (Na^+ and H_2O)
- Intestinal obstruction
- Oedema
- Ascites
- Burns (especially in first few days)

Fluid excess

Excessive sodium and water intake
- Excessive dietary intake
- Excessive administration of sodium-containing i.v. fluids
- Excessive ingestion of sodium-containing foods or medications

Inadequate renal losses
- Renal disease
- Congestive heart failure
- Cirrhosis of the liver
- Increased corticosteroid levels
  —glucocorticoids (Cushing's syndrome)
  —hyperaldosteronism

between fluid compartments which would aggravate ionic balance. However, as severe dehydration (as seen in diabetes insipidus) may lead to fatal hypovolaemia, aggressive therapy is required. The effects of hyponatraemia and hypernatraemia which may accompany dehydration will be discussed later (see p. 683).

Gastrointestinal losses

Within the gastrointestinal tract there is a continuous exchange of fluids, with most of the fluid produced being absorbed. Illnesses which present with diarrhoea or vomiting, or conditions in which fistulae, drainage tubes or GI suction are involved, can result in excessive fluid volume losses (potentially up to about 8–9 L/day).

Box 20.3 Signs and symptoms of fluid volume deficit and excess. (Adapted with kind permission from Lippincott Williams & Wilkins, from Porth C M 1998 Pathophysiology: concepts of altered health state, 5th edn.)

Fluid deficit
- Thirst
- Acute weight loss
  —mild extracellular deficit: 2% loss
  —moderate extracellular deficit: 2–5% loss
  —severe extracellular deficit: 6% or more
- Alteration in renal function
  —decreased urine output
  —increased urine osmolality in specific gravity
- Alteration in cardiovascular function
  —increased serum osmolality
  —increased haematocrit
  —increased BUN (blood urea nitrogen)
  —decreased vascular volume
  —tachycardia
  —weak and thready pulse
  —postural hypotension
  —decreased vein filling and increased vein refill time
  —hypertension and shock
- Other
  —loss of intercellular fluid
  —dry skin and mucous membrane
  —cracked and fissured tongue
  —decreased salivation and lacrimation
  —neuromuscular weakness
  —fatigue
  —increased body temperature

Fluid excess
- Acute weight gain — in excess of 5% body weight
- Alteration in cardiovascular function
  —full and bounding pulse
  —venous distension
  —increased ECF
  —pitting oedema
  —puffy eyelids
- Alteration in respiratory function
  —pulmonary oedema
  —shortness of breath
  —râles
  —dyspnoea
  —cough

Continuous GI or fistula drainage will have the same consequences for a patient as severe diarrhoea and vomiting.

Urinary loss

Patients who have incurred head injury, who have undergone hypophysectomy or who have a primary diagnosis of diabetes insipidus may excrete excessive volumes of water and electrolytes due to a disruption in the hypothalamopituitary release of ADH. Diabetes insipidus occurs when there is either a deficiency in the manufacture and release of ADH, or an inability of the kidney to respond to ADH. ADH deficiency and its consequences are discussed in Chapter 5.

Osmotic diuresis

In osmotic diuresis, polyuria results from the presence of large quantities of solutes in the blood which enter the glomerular filtrate and are not reabsorbed. The high osmolality produced in the renal tubules inhibits the action of ADH and prevents reabsorption of water. This principle can be used to produce an osmotic diuresis therapeutically, e.g. mannitol can be administered to reduce intracranial pressure.

Osmotic diuresis will occur in the following circumstances:

- when the production of large particles exceeds the body's ability to reabsorb or excrete them — classic examples are glucose excess in diabetes and urea excess in renal failure
- when solutes which can be filtered by the kidney are not reabsorbed (e.g. when mannitol and polysaccharides are administered)
- when substances are infused beyond the capacity of the nephron to reabsorb them (e.g. sodium chloride and urea).

Skin losses

The loss of sodium and water from the skin increases dramatically during excessive sweating or if large areas of the skin have been damaged. For example, in extreme hot weather as much as 1.5–2.0 L/h can be lost through sweat. In the patient with fever, water loss may be up to 3 L/24 h. Burns patients suffer excessive fluid losses; evaporation losses may be from 0.8 to 2.6 mL/kg for each percentage point of burn area (Porth 1998). Total loss from burns can be as much as 6–8 L/24 h.

Third space losses

The concept of the 'third space' is used to describe the presence of fluids in areas of the body where they are usually absent or present only in small quantities, e.g. the peritoneal cavity. Although not lost from the body, the fluid is physiologically unavailable and thus many of the effects of fluid loss may be produced. Whilst the total body weight may remain constant with no net change in body water, the distribution of fluid within the body may be altered. The difficulty in ascertaining the actual problem experienced by a patient is illustrated in the self-assessment question below.

Q **20.5** Mrs Jones, aged 26, is receiving a continuous infusion of opiates to relieve postoperative pain, and she has a urinary catheter in situ. Mrs. Jones' urinary output has been measured at under 25 mL/h for the past 3 h. A
(a) Identify at least five potential causes of this reduced urinary output.
(b) How might you ascertain which was the most likely cause?

While diagnosis is the physician's role, astute nursing assessment and implementation of a sound plan of care for such a patient may prevent or anticipate likely problems in relation to the patient's fluid and electrolyte balance.

Q **20.6** What might be the significance of a patient complaining of being very thirsty? A

Fluid volume excess (see Boxes 20.2 and 20.3)

The retention of fluid results in a fluid volume excess. Such an imbalance can be caused by overloading with fluids or by reduced functioning of the body's homeostatic mechanisms responsible for maintaining fluid and electrolyte balance. Circulatory overload is a condition associated with an increase in the intravascular blood volume. It is most often observed during the administration of i.v. fluids or in blood transfusion, especially if the amount or rate of the administration is excessive. Isotonic fluids such as 0.9% sodium chloride (normal saline) or Ringer's lactate contain large amounts of sodium, e.g. in Ringer's lactate the sodium content is 131 mmol/L. With some patients, e.g. those who are elderly or who have a history of heart disease, careful attention needs to be paid to i.v. fluid therapy. Other sources of sodium gain include some proprietary drugs (e.g. Alka Seltzer) or the frequent use of hypertonic enemas.

Effects of drinking large amounts of hypotonic fluid, e.g. water. When a large volume of water is ingested, it begins to be absorbed within about 15 min, in consequence of which the osmolality of the blood decreases. This causes an inhibition of the production and secretion of ADH. Absence of ADH makes the distal convoluted tubule and collecting duct impermeable to water and so more urine is excreted in the kidney, thus producing a more dilute urine and a water diuresis. Following a single large intake of oral fluid, the maximum effect upon diuresis will be noticed about 40 min later. A similar effect is achieved if a bolus or fluid challenge of i.v. fluid is administered.

Water intoxication. The kidney has a maximum rate at which it can excrete fluid. If water (or hypotonic i.v. fluid) ingestion exceeds this capacity, then the ECF remains hypotonic. The hypotonic ECF results in fluid moving into the ICF, with a subsequent swelling and bursting of cells. In the brain, this is most serious, causing raised intracranial pressure, convulsions and death.

Fluid volume adjustments

Chapter 2 described how the circulatory system comprises the arterial system of high pressure and low volume and the venous system which operates with a lower pressure and higher volume. Approximately 55% of the plasma volume is in the venous system, 10% in the arterial system and the remaining 35% distributed in the heart, lungs and capillaries. Thus changes in volume are usually accommodated by the venous system. The effect of gravity upon fluid in the circulatory system is marked, causing pooling of blood in the venous system with a consequent reduction in the arterial blood volume. If an individual stands for a prolonged period, particularly in a warm environment, there is a reduction in arterial flow to the cells; inadequate venous return then leads to a fall in end-diastolic volume and hence cardiac output. Inadequate perfusion of the brain can then lead to fainting.

The tissue spaces can accommodate large volumes of fluid, but the process is slow and causes less disturbances to the ICF or plasma. Adults can usually tolerate changes of about 2 L in the tissue spaces before there are noticeable signs of a volume shift. This 'hidden' accumulation of fluid may, however, be noticed by changes in body weight, 1 L of water being equivalent to 1 kg.

THE ELECTROLYTES

Sodium

Sodium is a major cation found in the ECF, and its concentration is maintained within the range 135–145 mmol/L. Its importance for a number of body functions is related to its role in maintaining the osmolality of extracellular fluids, normal muscular functioning, acid–base balance and a number of other chemical reactions. While hyper- or hyponatraemia usually indicates changes in body water content rather than in the intake of sodium, it is not unknown for individuals to have bizarre eating habits and thus become hypernatraemic. Furthermore, as sodium is the main extracellular cation, addition of substances to the plasma may cause a dilution effect rather than an actual loss of sodium. For example, serum sodium may appear to have fallen when glucose levels suddenly rise either due to hyperalimentation or in diabetes mellitus. Sodium losses may occur from the GI tract, kidney, skin or traumatised limbs.

Normally, the kidneys are extremely efficient in controlling sodium when the intake is reduced. Hyponatraemia, i.e. sodium depletion in the extracellular fluids, is defined as a sodium concentration in the blood of less than 135 mmol/L. The loss of sodium from the ECF is usually as a result of excessive fluid loss and not a deficit in intake. Signs, symptoms and causes of sodium imbalance are listed in Boxes 20.4 and 20.5.

Chloride

Chloride is ingested either with sodium or as potassium chloride. Normal daily intake is about 70–120 mmol, and the minimum requirement is 75 mmol. Chloride output is via sweat (15 mmol/L), gastric juice (90–150 mmol/L) and other intestinal secretions (50–100 mmol/L). Renal excretion is in conjunction with ammonia (NH_4Cl) and occurs mainly in the proximal tubule. Reabsorption occurs in the ascending limb and is passively linked with Na reabsorption. Cl^- reabsorption is inversely linked to bicarbonate. As Cl^- is linked to Na^+ reabsorption, aldosterone is an indirect regulator.

Potassium

Potassium (K) is the major intracellular cation. The body contains 2900–3500 mmol of potassium, of which 98% is intracellular and 2% is in the ECF. The intracellular potassium level is approximately 150 mmol/L, as compared with a plasma concentration of 3.5–4.8 mmol/L. Of the body's potassium, 90% is exchangeable while the remaining 10% is bound (mainly in the red blood cells). Men have about 45 mmol/kg body weight and women about 37 mmol/kg body weight of exchangeable K. The total body K declines significantly with increasing age in both sexes. Potassium continually leaks out of the cells, but a high intracellular level is maintained by the sodium–potassium pump. Although extracellular K is low, both intracellular and extracellular K are essential for normal physiological function.

As the muscle cell membrane potential is largely a function of the ratio of intracellular K^+ to extracellular K^+, any alteration of this ratio can adversely affect neuromuscular function. The low ECF potassium means that large changes can occur in total body potassium without a significant effect on plasma K^+.

Potassium is acquired through the diet. Although the potassium content of food varies widely, any diet providing sufficient energy will invariably supply more than enough K, and a normal intake would be 40–200 mmol a day. Potassium is not as well conserved by the kidney as sodium and the minimum daily K loss is about

Box 20.4 Signs and symptoms of sodium imbalance. (Adapted with kind permission from Lippincott Williams & Wilkins, from Porth C M 1998 Pathophysiology: concepts of altered health state, 5th edn.)

Hyponatraemia
- Serum sodium <135 mmol/L
- Decreased serum osmolality
- Dilution of other blood components, e.g. haematocrit, BUN (blood urea nitrogen)
- Increased water content of brain and nerve cells
- Headache
- Mental depression
- Personality changes
- Confusion
- Apprehension and feeling of impending doom
- Lethargy, weakness
- Stupor
- Coma
- Convulsions
- Gastrointestinal disturbances
- Anorexia, nausea and vomiting
- Abdominal cramps
- Increased ICF
- Fingerprinting over the sternum

Hypernatraemia
- Serum Na^+ >148 mmol/L
- Increased serum osmolality
- Thirst
- Oliguria or anuria
- High specific gravity of urine
- Intracellular dehydration
- Skin dry and flushed
- Mucous membranes dry and sticky
- Tongue rough and dry
- Subcutaneous tissue firm and rubbery
- Agitation and restlessness
- Decreased reflexes
- Manic behaviour
- Convulsions and coma
- Change in body temperature
- Decreased vascular volume
- Tachycardia, decreased blood pressure
- Weak and thready pulse

Box 20.5 Causes of sodium imbalance (Adapted with kind permission from Lippincott Williams & Wilkins, from Porth C M 1998 Pathophysiology: concepts of altered health state, 5th edn.)

Hyponatraemia
- Excess sodium loss
  - —sweating
  - —gastrointestinal losses
  - —diuresis
- Sodium dilution
  - —overinfusion of sodium-free i.v. solutions
  - —psychogenic polydipsia
  - —ingestion of tap water during periods of sodium restriction
  - —repeated use of tap water enemas
- Hormone-induced water gains
  - —SIADH (syndrome of inappropriate ADH secretion)
  - —ADH agonists (e.g. oxytocin)

Hypernatraemia
- Excessive sodium intake
  - —rapid or excessive parenteral infusion of sodium chloride or sodium bicarbonate
  - —excessive oral intake
- Decreased extracellular water
  - —increased insensible water loss, e.g. burns, diaphoresis, hyperventilation
  - —water diarrhoea
  - —hypertonic tube feeds
- Water deprivation — unconscious, debilitated patient (thirst excess)
- Diabetes insipidus — tracheobronchitis
- Decreased water intake
  - —unconsciousness or inability to express thirst
  - —oral trauma or inability to swallow
  - —the withholding of water for therapeutic reasons

40 mmol: obligatory losses are approximately 15–20 mmol from the gastrointestinal tract and skin and 10–20 mmol in urine. Dietary K is usually sufficient to cover the individual's needs but additional potassium may be required during trauma and stress. Potassium excretion is regulated mainly by the kidney, and plasma K^+ levels are regulated by both renal mechanisms and shifts between the intracellular and extracellular compartments. Although only small amounts are normally lost through the GI tract, diarrhoea and vomiting can quickly lead to potassium imbalances.

Box 20.6 outlines some other factors influencing potassium levels. Signs and symptoms of potassium imbalance are listed in Box 20.7. Potassium cannot be conserved by the body, and so a daily intake is required. In the proximal tubule, 80–90% of filtered potassium is reabsorbed; this is essentially an obligatory process little influenced by regulatory factors. Renal regulation of potassium excretion occurs in the distal tubule and collecting duct. Aldosterone is the regulatory hormone for potassium ions. A rise in plasma K^+ concentration increases aldosterone secretion, resulting in increased potassium excretion; a fall in plasma K^+ decreases aldosterone secretion.

Box 20.6 Factors associated with potassium imbalance. (Adapted with kind permission from Lippincott Williams & Wilkins, from Porth C M 1998 Pathophysiology: concepts of altered health state, 5th edn.)

Hypokalaemia

Inadequate intake
- Inability to eat/debilitation
- Potassium-deficient diet
- Administration of potassium-free massive parenteral solutions
- Anorexia
- Alcoholism

Excessive gastrointestinal losses
- Vomiting
- Diarrhoea
- Prolonged gastric suction
- Fistula drainage
- Laxative abuse

Excessive renal losses
- Diuretic phase of renal failure
- Diuretic therapy
- Increased mineralocorticoid levels
- Cushing's syndrome
- Primary aldosteronism
- Treatment with glucocorticoid hormones

Intercellular shift
- Treatment for diabetic acidosis/alkalosis, either metabolic or respiratory

Hyperkalaemia

Excessive intake or gain
- Excessive oral intake
- Excessive or rapid parenteral infusion
- Tissue trauma, burns and crushing injuries

Inadequate renal losses
- Renal failure
- Adrenal insufficiency
- Addison's disease
- Potassium-sparing diuretics

Hyperkalaemia

Body regulation of potassium is geared mainly towards management of hyperkalaemic states, with general excretion occurring via the colon and kidney, whilst serum levels are also influenced by the catecholamines, the pancreatic hormones (insulin and glucagon) and by acid–base states. Due to the cation exchange mechanism which operates in the regulation of acid–base balance, potassium secretion is increased by the nephron in alkalotic states and decreased in acidosis. For example, in metabolic alkalosis the potassium levels rise in the ICF to compensate for hydrogen ion loss. Potassium levels are thus high in the nephron and so excretion takes place with a resultant total body loss of potassium.

Changes in serum potassium levels tend to reflect either total body changes of potassium or movement of potassium from one fluid compartment to another. Potassium levels are interrelated with sodium and body water levels. This relationship is disturbed by illness, especially if cell membrane function is disrupted. Cell membrane function is itself very susceptible to changes in potassium concentrations; even small alterations affect membrane excitation, with potentially dire consequences for cardiac tissue. In diabetes mellitus, the administration of insulin causes potassium to enter the cells with glucose in a cotransporter system, leading to a fall in serum potassium. Thus potassium depletion decreases insulin secretion, with the cells having a lower tolerance to glucose. This action of insulin can be utilised in the management of patients with hyperkalaemia: insulin and glucose can be administered to reduce serum potassium.

Hyperkalaemia may also be managed by creating GI losses through the induction of diarrhoea or by using an ion exchange (i.e. a sodium or calcium resin which exchanges with the potassium). Intravenous calcium may temporarily reverse the toxic effect of potassium upon cardiac tissue.

Box 20.7 Signs and symptoms of potassium imbalance. (Adapted with kind permission from Lippincott Williams & Wilkins, from Porth C M 1998 Pathophysiology: concepts of altered health state, 5th edn.)

Hypokalaemia
- Serum K^+ <3.5 mmol/L
- Muscle tenderness, paraesthesia or cramps
- Weakness, muscle flabbiness
- Paralysis
- Postural hypotension
- Increased sensitivity to digoxin
- Arrhythmias
- Anorexia, vomiting, abdominal distension, paralytic ileus
- Shortness of breath, shallow breathing
- Low osmolality and specific gravity of urine
- Nocturia
- Thirst
- Confusion, depression
- Metabolic alkalosis

Hyperkalaemia
- Serum K^+ >5.5 mmol/L
- Paraesthesia
- Weakness and dizziness
- Muscle cramps
- Nausea, diarrhoea, intestinal colic, gastrointestinal distress
- Peaked T waves
- Depressed ST segments
- Depressed P wave and widening of QRS segment
- Cardiac arrest

Hypokalaemia

Management of hypokalaemia involves the treatment of any accompanying alkalosis or potassium losses. Potassium supplements may be given orally or intravenously. However, i.v. potassium can cause peripheral vein phlebitis and overly rapid infusion may cause cardiac dysrhythmias and death. Intravenous potassium should not be added to blood products, where it may cause erythrocyte lysis, nor should it be added to solutions of mannitol, amino acids or lipids, as precipitation may occur. Nursing considerations in the administration of potassium are summarised in Boxes 20.8 and 20.9.

Calcium

Calcium is the fifth most abundant element in the body, constituting 2% of body weight. Of the total body calcium, 99% is found in bone, 0.5% in teeth and the remaining 0.5% in soft tissues. Total plasma content is low (8 mmol) and over half of this is bound to albumin. Binding to plasma proteins is pH-sensitive, so that acidosis can cause an increase in plasma Ca^{2+} without changes in the total Ca^{2+}. Spuriously high Ca^{2+} levels will be measured if a tourniquet is used to obtain blood for calcium levels. This is due to venous constriction increasing fluid loss with an apparent concentration of the Ca-binding plasma proteins. Normal plasma levels are 2.2–2.6 mmol/L and urinary excretion is 2.5–7.5 mmol/day.

Calcium is required for a range of physiological functions, including:

- calcification of bones and teeth
- regulation of cell metabolism
- excitability of nerve and muscle, synaptic neurotransmitter release, muscle contraction
- cardiac conduction
- haemostasis
- complement activation.

Calcium is an important intracellular cation, with free calcium ion levels of 10^{-7} mol/L. Within the cell, calcium may be contained within organelles or bound to proteins. A calcium/magnesium ATPase may maintain the concentration gradient of calcium across the cell membrane.

Bone calcium, found in the hydroxyapatite form, provides a large reserve of calcium. The continual formation and destruction of bone, together with soft tissue calcium and calcium in the ECF, provides a small, exchangeable pool which can compensate for decreases in plasma Ca.

Calcium is ingested through the diet. Its absorption from the gut varies according to the presence of vitamin D, parathyroid hormone, growth hormone, corticosteroids and lactose (see Ch. 5). Calcium exists in two major forms within the ECF: as plasma, namely as freely ionised calcium ions; and as a complex bound to proteins (usually albumin). It is the freely ionised calcium which is important for nerve and muscle function. In the plasma, the ratio of the two forms of calcium is usually 50:50, although in the tissue fluid there is only freely ionised calcium.

The location of plasma calcium varies according to pH. The more acidic the plasma, the less protein is available for binding with calcium, and thus the free calcium ion level rises. In a patient with alkalosis there may be signs of hypocalcaemia because the free ions are reduced, yet total plasma levels remain unchanged. Any sudden change in pH will change the free calcium levels and cause clinical effects. This is one reason why in the treatment of metabolic acidosis (e.g. after a cardiac arrest) any infused sodium bicarbonate should be given slowly and with caution. Where there is a low serum albumin, the free calcium ion level will be normal, although the total plasma calcium will be low. Calcium should not be added to blood, lipid, bicarbonate or amino acid preparations, as precipitation may occur.

Box 20.8 Oral potassium supplements: nursing implications. (Adapted from Metheny 1996)

Common side-effects of oral potassium are nausea, vomiting, GI discomfort and diarrhoea. These are due to GI irritation and can be reduced by the steps listed below. Because of these side-effects, patient compliance may be poor, limiting the effectiveness of the supplements. Liquid preparations are preferred to slow-release tablets. Potassium-sparing diuretics are used where possible as they do not require potassium to be supplemented, unlike other diuretics. Potassium supplements can be a cause of hyperkalaemia.

To prevent gastrointestinal irritation/ulceration:

- Always dilute potassium preparations according to the manufacturer's instructions
- Advise patients to sip the diluted solution slowly, over a 5–10 min period
- Effervescent products must be fully dissolved and should not be swallowed until they have stopped fizzing
- Advise the patient to drink a full glass of water with slow-release tablets to help them dissolve in the GI tract
- Give potassium supplements after meals
- Observe patients on slow-release potassium tablets for signs of GI bleeding
- Check manufacturer's information before crushing potassium tablets. Some types must not be crushed.

Box 20.9 Critical precautions to observe when administering i.v. potassium. (Adapted from Metheny 1996)

- Never give a rapid bolus of potassium, as this may cause cardiac arrest
- Always dilute potassium ampoules before administration. Usual concentration is 40 mmol/L (range 40–60 mmol/L); do not exceed 80 mmol/L
- 10 mmol/h via a peripheral line and 20 mmol/h via a central line are maximum recommended infusion rates
- Maximum adult dose is 100–200 mmol/24 h
- Avoid giving higher concentrations of i.v. potassium via a peripheral vein, as this causes venous pain and sclerosis
- Use an infusion pump to control rate when giving higher concentrations intravenously. Observe closely for signs of extravasation
- Observe for signs of thrombophlebitis
- Use ready-prepared solutions when possible
- Ensure thorough mixing of the infusate when potassium is added to infusion solutions. Never add potassium to an infusion bag which is hanging in the upright position because the patient may receive a bolus of undiluted potassium due to inadequate mixing
- Avoid i.v. potassium if the patient is dehydrated or has seriously impaired renal function. Adequate urine flow is required before i.v. potassium can be administered
- Monitor the patient carefully, noting urine flow, cardiovascular parameters, infusion rate and infusion site. Potassium is highly irritating if it leaks into subcutaneous tissues and may lead to serious tissue damage

It is known that cardiac muscle contraction is dependent not only upon the concentration of calcium ions but also upon the acidity of the extracellular environment. Myocardial depression may occur when there is a rapid drop in calcium levels, as for example following massive blood transfusion when the calcium may have been chelated by the citrates and the bone reservoir cannot release calcium quickly enough to compensate.

The myocardial depression will be aggravated in states of shock where there is poor coronary perfusion. The normal ionic regulation of the cardiac cells is disturbed when there is myocardial necrosis; in this circumstance calcium ions can pour into the cells and overactivate the ATPases, which in turn aggravate and worsen the cardiac necrosis. Thus, where the cell becomes overloaded with calcium ions, uncoordinated and disturbed waves of contraction spread through the muscle, inhibiting effective contraction. Unfortunately, following myocardial ischaemia, immediate reperfusion of the cells with oxygen and nutrients does not necessarily reverse the problem.

Calcium-blocking drugs such as verapamil, nifedipine and beta-blockers can slow the entry of calcium into the cells, thus reducing the effects of the necrosis. Calcium blockers may be used for their two major effects, namely to relax muscle and cause vasodilatation, and to alter cardiac rhythm.

Digoxin is known to ultimately change intracellular calcium levels through its action upon the sodium–potassium pump. It is this action which enables digoxin to improve the contractility of cardiac muscle.

The causes and symptoms of calcium deficit and excess are listed in Boxes 20.10 and 20.11.

Tetany

If there is a decrease in extracellular freely ionised calcium ions then a condition known as hypocalcaemic tetany may be observed. In the absence of sufficient calcium ions in the ECF, neurotransmission is inhibited, but the deficit of calcium ions in the cell leads to an excitatory effect on nerve and muscle cells, giving rise to increased motor activity. The outcome of this neuromuscular activity is marked spasms of skeletal muscle, particularly affecting the larynx and extremities. If laryngospasm becomes severe, then the person may suffer respiratory obstruction and arrest. Early signs of hypocalcaemia are described in Box 5.4 (p. 149).

ACID–BASE BALANCE

Body fluids are normally slightly alkaline, within a pH range of 7.36–7.44 (H^+ concentration ($[H^+]$) 35–45 nmol/L). Blood has a H^+ concentration of 40 nmol/L, or a pH of 7.4. Acidaemia occurs when the arterial blood pH is less than 7.36 (greater than 44 nmol/L H^+). An arterial pH greater than 7.44 (or less than 36 nmol/L H^+) is alkalaemia. The body enzymes which control most physiological processes are optimally active within the normal pH range, and variations from this range can rapidly result in severe disability or death. It is therefore essential to understand the basis of acid–base balance in health and the effects of disease on this balance. A pH outside the range 6.9–7.7 is incompatible with life and variations outside 7.36–7.44 are serious and may be difficult to rectify. Whilst the blood pH is maintained at a slightly alkaline level, the pH of urine is frequently acidic as the body seeks to excrete surplus acids which have been produced by both metabolic and respiratory processes.

How the body attempts to maintain its internal environment at an optimal pH will now be outlined and a few situations in which acid–base balance is disrupted will be reviewed. The long-term regulation of pH occurs through the lungs and kidneys, whilst

Box 20.10 Causes of calcium deficit and excess. (Adapted with kind permission from Lippincott Williams & Wilkins, from Porth C M 1998 Pathophysiology: concepts of altered health state, 5th edn.)

Hypocalcaemia

- Impaired ability to mobilise calcium from bone — hypoparathyroidism
- Abnormal calcium binding
  —decreased serum albumin
  —decreased pH
  —increased free fatty acids
  —rapid transfusion of citrated blood
- Abnormal losses — cardiovascular, inadequate vitamin D
- Impaired absorption
- Renal failure
- Liver disease

Hypercalcaemia

- Excessive gains
  —increased intestinal absorption
  —excessive vitamin D
  —excessive dietary intake
  —milk alkali syndrome
- Increased bone resorption
- Increased levels of parathyroid hormone
- Inadequate losses
- Renal insufficiency

Box 20.11 Signs and symptoms of calcium deficit and excess. (Adapted with kind permission from Lippincott Williams & Wilkins, from Porth C M 1998 Pathophysiology: concepts of altered health state, 5th edn.)

Hypocalcaemia

- Serum calcium <8.5 mg/dL
- Increased nerve excitability
  —paraesthesia
  —skeletal muscle cramps
  —abdominal spasms and cramps
  —hyperactive reflexes
  —carpopedal spasm
  —laryngeal spasm
  —positive Chvostek's sign
  —positive Trousseau's sign
- Renal failure
- Hypotension
- Cardiac insufficiency
- Failure to respond to drugs that act via calcium-mediated mechanisms

Hypercalcaemia

- Serum calcium >10.5 mg/dL
- Altered neural and muscular activity
- Muscle weakness and atrophy
- Ataxia, loss of muscle tone, lethargy
- Stupor and coma
- Cardiovascular alterations
  —hypertension
  —shortening of the QT interval
  —AV block
- Anorexia, nausea, vomiting, constipation

buffers in the blood provide an immediate response to changes in pH. With adjustments in respiratory rate, carbon dioxide levels (and hence pH) can also change. The response involving the kidney is slower and sometimes referred to as the 'renal lag'. The kidney's ability to regenerate bicarbonate ions whilst excreting hydrogen ions enables it to aid the regulation of pH.

Acidosis and alkalosis

The terms acidosis and alkalosis refer to abnormal situations which lead to acidaemia and alkalaemia, respectively, if there are no secondary compensatory mechanisms to reverse the situation. Both situations can be equally disruptive.

Acidosis occurs when there is a high hydrogen ion concentration and thus a low pH (below 7.36). It can arise through:

- metabolism of proteins producing sulphuric and phosphoric acids
- anaerobic metabolism producing lactic acid
- metabolism of fats producing acetoacetic acid and ketone bodies
- excessive intake of acidic products orally or intravenously
- excessive loss of bicarbonate from the body
- hypoventilation with resulting retention of carbon dioxide.

Alkalosis occurs when there is a loss of hydrogen ions or a gain in bicarbonate ions and hence a correspondingly high pH (greater than 7.44). Alkalosis can occur through:

- excessive loss of gastric juices, e.g. vomiting, gastric aspiration
- excessive intake of alkaline products, e.g. overdose of antacids
- hyperventilation with resulting removal of carbon dioxide.

Changes in carbon dioxide tension with a respiratory origin result in respiratory acidosis or alkalosis. Changes in bicarbonate levels reflect metabolic causes: metabolic acidosis or alkalosis. Whilst the primary causes may be metabolic or respiratory, the adaptive responses involve both systems and lead to compensatory states. Occasionally both metabolic and respiratory problems occur simultaneously and a confused picture presents, as in respiratory failure in a patient with renal failure.

Buffers

Q **20.7** Refer to your physiology textbook to review the Henderson–Hasselbalch equation.

Regulation of blood pH at all levels involves complex chemical reactions in which buffers play a critical role. Buffers are substances which prevent major changes in the pH of a solution by removing or releasing hydrogen ions. In humans there are three main buffer systems:

- carbonic acid bicarbonate
- phosphate and sulphate compounds
- proteins and haemoglobin (main ICF system).

Buffers are found in both the ICF and the ECF and enable products to be safely transported to the site of excretion.

Carbonic acid bicarbonate

This is the main buffer in humans and will serve as an illustration of the role of buffers in the body. This mechanism operates through the following reversible reaction:

$$H_2O + CO_2 \rightleftharpoons H_2CO_3 \rightleftharpoons H^+ + HCO_3^- \text{ (bicarbonate ion)}$$

In situations where hydrogen ions are added to body fluids, they combine with the bicarbonate ion:

$$H^+ + HCO_3^- \rightleftharpoons H_2CO_3$$

In situations where the hydrogen ion levels become low or there is an excess of hydroxyl ions, carbonic acid dissociates, releasing hydrogen ions into solution:

$$H_2CO_3 \rightleftharpoons H^+ + HCO_3^-$$

In alkalotic states, the level of bicarbonate ions rises (metabolic alkalosis) or the amount of carbon dioxide in solution falls (respiratory alkalosis). In acidic states the level of bicarbonate decreases (metabolic acidosis) or the amount of carbon dioxide in solution rises (respiratory acidosis). There is thus a reciprocal relationship between the levels of carbon dioxide and the bicarbonate ions. This dynamic relationship, which enables pH to be regulated, is utilised in several ways within the respiratory system and the renal tubule. The enzyme carbonic anhydrase catalyses the formation of carbonic acid from water and carbon dioxide. Acetazolamide is an example of a drug which blocks carbonic anhydrase and thus inhibits both the regeneration of bicarbonate ions and the production of hydrogen ions in the renal tubule.

Alterations in the pH of the body may be indicated by clinical signs and laboratory results. The acidity of plasma is determined using arterial blood gas samples, but changes in other body fluids may be detected by testing urine, intestinal fluids, CSF and other exudates.

Handling blood gases

Obtaining a sample for the analysis of blood gases can be effected by direct arterial puncture or the withdrawal of blood from an arterial line. The nurse responsible for the patient will need to ensure that several precautions are taken to prevent a false result. The specimen form should include details such as the following:

- temperature
- respiratory pattern
- concentration of oxygen in the inspired gases
- any relevant recent therapies (e.g. physiotherapy, administration of bicarbonate or blood)
- time the sample was taken.

The sample should be collected in a small syringe (1 or 2 mL), to which a small quantity of dilute heparin (100 units/mL) has been added to prevent coagulation. The amount of heparinised saline added should be just enough to fill the dead space of the syringe. In the case of collecting a blood sample from an arterial line, it will be necessary first to withdraw and discard the heparinised saline in the arterial line tubing (excess heparin itself reduces the measured pH). A second syringe may then be used to withdraw the arterial blood itself. As soon as the sample has been collected, a bung or stopper is attached to the end to prevent air contamination. The syringe should be labelled and sent to the laboratory as soon as possible. If the ambient temperature is warm then the sample can be transported in ice. The arterial line will need to be flushed and reset in order to remove the blood which has been drawn back into the line. With direct puncture, firm digital pressure will be required over the puncture site for at least 5 min to prevent arterial haemorrhage or subsequent aneurysm formation. The circulation of the limb distal to the puncture should be checked later. Normal blood gas results are listed in Box 20.12.

The acidotic/alkalotic states

Q

20.8 Disorders of acid–base balance are primarily respiratory or metabolic in origin. From the information given so far, you should be able to draw up a chart to indicate how the respective acid/base states may influence the pH, the bicarbonate ion levels (HCO_3^-) and the partial pressure of carbon dioxide in the plasma ($P\text{CO}_2$) in:
(a) metabolic acidosis
(b) respiratory acidosis
(c) metabolic alkalosis
(d) respiratory alkalosis.

Box 20.12 Normal blood gas results (slight variations according to local laboratory)

pH	7.36–7.44
[H+]	35–45 nmol/L
$P_a\text{CO}_2$	4.6–5.6 kPa (35–42 mmHg)
$P_a\text{O}_2$	11.3–14 kPa (90–105 mmHg)
HCO_3	23–31 mmol/L
Standard HCO_3^-	22–26 mmol/L
Base excess	−2 to 2 mmol/L
Saturation O_2	97%

Recognition and management of metabolic alkalosis

Metabolic alkalosis is caused by a loss of hydrogen ions (e.g. through vomiting) or a gain of alkali, as seen in the excess intake of sodium bicarbonate. It is characterised by high pH and a high concentration of bicarbonate ions. This rise in pH decreases the ionisation of calcium, thus giving signs of hypocalcaemia. Indicators of hypokalaemia may also arise. The respiratory response seeks to compensate for the alkalosis by raising the $P\text{CO}_2$ through a decreased respiratory effort: thus a respiratory acidosis may accompany the metabolic alkalosis. The increasing numbers of bicarbonate ions utilise free sodium ions, thus decreasing the ratio of free sodium ions to chloride ions. There is a slight renal compensation which attempts to conserve hydrogen ions. Usually, a metabolic alkalosis is successfully treated by management of the cause with appropriate monitoring of any hypokalaemia and/or by restoration of fluid volume. Occasionally, acidification of the plasma may be required, or the administration of acetazolamide to inhibit carbonic anhydrase.

Antacid use. Antacids are bases used to neutralise the acidity of gastric juices. Injudicious use can lead to metabolic alkalosis and problems associated with other side-effects of the substances used. Most antacids comprise a combination of aluminium or magnesium hydroxides, or derivatives of carbonates. It is important that patients who take antacids are aware of the necessity to keep within the prescribed doses and to report side-effects or failure of the therapy to their physician or community pharmacist; some antacids, for example, are contraindicated with peptic ulcers.

Recognition and management of metabolic acidosis

Metabolic acidosis is characterised by a low pH and low levels of bicarbonate ions. The lowered pH leads to a compensatory respiratory drive to hyperventilate, thus causing a transitory fall in the $P\text{CO}_2$. If this is successful, the pH will return towards normal. However, if the acidosis is severe, cardiac output may drop with accompanying bradycardia (because acidosis impairs cardiac contractility). Renal compensation is made through the excretion of extra hydrogen ions. Hyperkalaemia may also be present, depending upon the cause of the acidosis. The features of the underlying acidotic state (e.g. peripheral vasodilatation) will also be present. Treatment may involve the administration of bicarbonates, but it is important to recall that each mmol of sodium bicarbonate given contains 1 mmol of sodium ions. The three most common causes of metabolic acidosis are renal failure, diabetic ketoacidosis and hypoxia.

Recognition and management of respiratory alkalosis

The most common cause of respiratory alkalosis is an anxiety attack which has led to the person noticeably hyperventilating. The subsequent removal of carbon dioxide leads to a raised pH and eventually a fall in the bicarbonate level when renal compensation has occurred. The aim in managing the anxiety attack is to enable the person to breathe more slowly, to calm her (with a sedative if necessary) and, if it is safe, to enable her to rebreathe her expired air, thus raising the carbon dioxide level. (This can be achieved by having the person breathe in and out of a paper bag. While this technique is effective, it must be supervised to ensure that the person does not suffocate or do it to excess.) Other instances of alkalosis will require management of their specific causes.

Recognition and management of respiratory acidosis

Respiratory acidosis is caused by an excess of carbon dioxide. It is most frequently caused by primary disorders of the respiratory tract or by conditions which affect the respiratory centre (e.g. drug overdose and central nervous system problems). Faults in the management of mechanical ventilation may also lead to respiratory acidosis.

Respiratory acidosis may be detected when the underlying respiratory problem is recognised (e.g. asthma or bronchitis) and/or when the signs of acidosis become apparent. People with chronic respiratory problems may of course already have well-established compensatory mechanisms; for example, in chronic obstructive airways disease (COAD) there may be a renal compensation which retains bicarbonate ions to counter the respiratory acidosis generated by a chronic high level of $P\text{CO}_2$. In these situations, biochemical results may have a different significance from those associated with acute respiratory acidosis.

NURSING CONSIDERATIONS IN MAINTAINING FLUID AND ELECTROLYTE BALANCE

Assessment

Assessing hydration

The effects of a fluid loss or gain depend to a large extent on the volume of the loss or gain and the rate at which it occurs. Effects are more acute when they develop rapidly, when the person is elderly and when the person is debilitated. Signs and symptoms observed by the nurse will depend upon the effects of the fluid loss or gain on the serum osmolality. A major problem in the assessment of fluid and electrolyte imbalance is that significant changes occur before they can be detected by clinical measurements such as blood pressure or central venous pressure.

Changes in tissue fluid volume are noticed mainly through observation of mucous membranes and skin elasticity (the latter is more easily observed over bony prominences). With an infant, the anterior fontanelle provides a good indication of hydration status. In an elderly person it is difficult to detect changes in skin turgor due to the gradual loss of skin elasticity with age. However, changes in the presence or absence of oedema may be a useful indicator. Alterations in the ICF volume are very difficult to detect — except in the brain, where changes in intracranial pressure may be manifest.

The nurse should remember, when assessing hydration status, that the mucous membranes in the mouth may become dry for a variety of reasons, e.g. the use of anticholinergic drugs, mouth breathing, oxygen administration or dehydration itself. In a patient who is mouth breathing or on oxygen therapy, hydration status may be checked by inspecting the membrane between the cheek and gum wall, which should stay moist if the patient is sufficiently hydrated. Examination of the veins in the hand can also give a useful indication of a person's state of hydration — normally, elevation or dependency of the hand causes the veins to empty or fill within 3–5 s.

Q

20.9 What are the other indicators of a person's state of hydration? (see Box 20.3 p. 682).

Assessing fluid and electrolyte status

The nurse's frequent contact with the patient should enable him to detect any disturbances or features which may be related to fluid and electrolyte status. Unfortunately, nursing management of patients' needs for food and fluid is often neglected and notoriously full of errors and confusion (see Research Abstract 20.1, p. 692). In illness, certain groups of patients, such as the elderly, children and pregnant women, are particularly susceptible to fluid and electrolyte problems. Others are at risk by virtue of an underlying pathological problem and/or as a result of nursing or medical interventions.

Q

20.10 Make a list of any reasons which may cause a person to have a problem in managing her fluid and electrolyte balance. A

A number of parameters may indicate changes in fluid or electrolyte status, but minor changes are often recognised only by those familiar with the person. This emphasises the importance of communication between nurses (e.g. at handover reports) and with carers (e.g. relatives may notice changes). The rapid detection of patterns and trends can be important in identifying deterioration or improvement in the patient's condition.

A structured approach to nursing assessment should facilitate the identification of actual and potential patient problems. Indeed, the initial assessment may not be completed until a 24-h observation of the patient has been undertaken. Assessment of the patient's fluid and electrolyte status frequently involves the use of a fluid balance chart.

Jones (1975) published the results of a study into the nutritional care of unconscious patients being fed by a nasogastric tube. Amongst the many findings of this study were several points pertinent to the fluid status of the patient. We suggest that you consult this study which discusses some of the errors commonly made in fluid measurement and administration, problems which are still valid today. Metheny (1996, Ch. 2) identifies other potential sources of error when recording fluid input and output.

Q

20.11 Carry out the activities listed below. What are the implications of your findings in respect to a patient's hydration status?

(a) Measure out 100 mL quantities of liquid using a syringe or i.v. burette and inject them into the following utensils, observing the water levels:
- urinal
- catheter bag
- usual measuring jugs
- standard hospital glass, cup and cereal bowl.

(b) Determine how much liquid is contained by the standard hospital glass, cup and bowl when:
- full to the brim
- half full
- filled to the level usually served by the catering staff.

20.12 Select a suitable person on your next clinical allocation and make an assessment.

(a) What is the state of the person's hydration?
(b) What is the person's ability to regulate fluid and electrolyte intake and to excrete necessary fluids?
(c) Give reasons for your conclusions.

Monitoring

The two most important components of monitoring a patient's fluid balance are measurements (or estimations) of fluid intake/output and weight. Insensible fluid losses are estimated according to standard norms, with adjustments made for factors such as the following:

- body temperature
- ambient temperature
- basal metabolic rate
- respiratory rate
- respiratory assistance (e.g. use of oxygen, humidification)
- other pathologies
- fluid content in stools
- internal losses due to fluid movement
- losses through skin trauma.

Whilst some losses and gains have to be estimated, in appropriate circumstances others can be measured:

- content of food and fluids
- i.v. fluids
- GI gains through enteral sources
- GI losses
- losses from fistulae and drains
- urine.

Unfortunately, the fluid content of food and fluid intake is usually estimated rather than measured. Indeed, some 'fluid foods' such as soups and custards are not necessarily included in fluid recording. This is particularly important in patients who are restricted to a liquefied diet or volume control and who seek strategies to avoid the restriction!

Fluid balance charting: possible sources of error

Nurses should be aware of the many ways in which the accuracy of fluid intake/output calculations may be compromised. Examples include:

- duplication or omission of items
- use of estimations rather than measurements

- arithmetical errors
- fluids counted in theatre transferred to ward chart
- shift change errors, i.e. in carrying forward from the previous shift
- mixing colloidal and crystalloid calculations
- recording wrong i.v. bag — confusion between treatment chart and fluid chart
- failure to observe patterns in consecutive daily balance
- the patient is unable to accurately recall events.

Measurement errors also arise when inappropriate utensils are used. To reduce the margin of error, low volumes of urine should be measured in containers with graduations designed for low volumes. Large volumes measured from catheter bags may prove to be different if the bag is emptied and then measured from a rigid jug. Similarly, i.v. fluid bags may contain more than the actual amount specified. Understanding the relative acceptable margins of error is an essential but neglected aspect of fluid monitoring. In a fit, healthy person, small errors may not be significant, but in a vulnerable person they can lead to inappropriate treatment regimens with consequent problems.

Managing fluid and electrolyte therapy

Aims

The aims of all fluid and electrolyte therapy are:

- to regulate, where possible, the patient's fluid and electrolyte balance by controlling the content and volume of the oral/enteral route; when oral/enteral routes are inadequate, venous access is used
- to control excessive losses and gains, e.g. by means of surgical intervention to prevent blood loss or by the use of diuretics to regulate fluid balance.

Both the medical and nursing management of the patient's fluid and electrolyte status will be derived from the initial assessment. The patient may require one or more of the following interventions:

- assistance with the maintenance of normal fluid and electrolyte requirements; this usually occurs for a short period of time in a previously well-nourished person, e.g. following surgery or during a brief period of coma
- correction of fluid/electrolyte imbalances
- parenteral nutrition (PN).

Occasionally, a person will require all three measures simultaneously; for example, someone with a major injury to the abdomen may need immediate correction of blood losses and electrolyte disturbances. There would then be a need to ensure that normal fluid and electrolyte requirements are met, with consideration being given to changes in demand due to the injury. If oral/enteral feeding is unlikely to be resumed within a couple of days then immediate plans should be made to commence parenteral feeding.

In deciding on the most appropriate plan for a patient, consideration is given not only to the content of the therapy, but also to the resources available, the patient's coexisting problems (e.g. cardiac failure or diabetes) and the particular hazards associated with the respective methods of administration. The timing, rate and duration of the therapy can also determine which route is most sensible.

Determining the volume and content of the therapy

The regimen prescribed for the patient will be based upon the following essential considerations:

- what needs to be replaced — measured and insensible or hidden losses from the body
- what needs to be removed — where there is excess production or excretory failure
- what needs to be adjusted — where there is translocation of fluids or electrolytes
- what needs to be halted — the cause of the problem, e.g. vomiting, haemorrhage.

The identification of these requirements will be based on nursing observation, medical assessment and laboratory analysis of specimens. However, the method of administration will influence the nature of the fluid regimen. Fluids can be administered through the rectum and through ostomies, although these routes are not always efficient. When the oral route is inadequate, arteriovenous (AV) access may be used for i.v. therapy, or AV shunts for dialysis. Fluid and electrolyte regulation may also involve the use of human or artificial membranes in the case of peritoneal dialysis or haemodialysis. Subcutaneous infusions (hypodermoclysis) are infrequently used for fluid or electrolyte therapy, although they may be used in the absence of facilities or personnel to administer i.v. therapy. Subcutaneous infusates need to match ECF, with absorption dependent upon the vascular condition of the area concerned. Eventually the tissues will no longer be able to absorb fluid and will become swollen and hard. In complex situations a variety of routes for therapy may be employed.

Routes for fluid and electrolyte therapy

The oral route. Replacing fluids via the oral route is without doubt the safest method. In a healthy adult who has no circulatory or renal insufficiency, the need for fluid is 1500–3000 mL/24 h. Replacing fluids orally will involve identifying the person's preferred drinks and then making these available (where reasonable) in the desirable quantity.

In some situations the patient may be prescribed 'restricted fluids', the amount usually being stated. For example, a person with renal failure may have a restricted fluid intake of 1000 mL/24 h. In other circumstances the nurse may be instructed to 'encourage fluids', especially when the goal is to prevent urinary stasis in the catheterised patient.

Two key points for the nurse to bear in mind when caring for persons requiring replacement of fluid and electrolytes by the oral route are as follows:

- Always ascertain the exact meaning of any vague verbal or written orders concerning fluid replacement, e.g. 'push fluids', 'encourage fluids', 'taking sips'. Remember that fluid and electrolyte balance is important and that the nurse has a key role to play in preventing further problems.
- If at all possible, know exactly how much fluid a person is required to have over a 24-h period. Medical orders can easily be written to identify appropriate daily fluid intake targets, e.g. 2000–2500 mL/24 h.

Sometimes patients on fluid replacement therapy still complain of thirst. Whilst the thirst reflex will be permanently relieved if the thirst sensors in the hypothalamus are no longer stimulated, a temporary depression of the thirst mechanism has been associated with interventions related to the oropharyngeal region (Anderson & Rundgren 1982). The patient troubled by thirst may be comforted by the following nursing actions (Woodtli 1990):

- carrying out frequent oral hygiene
- applying lubricant on lips

- giving mouth rinses
- choosing carefully the type and temperature of fluids
- offering ice chips for the patient to suck.

The parenteral route. For a number of patients, fluid and electrolyte therapy must be administered via the parenteral (i.v.) route. Parenteral fluid administration enables solutions to enter into the extracellular compartment directly, enabling a rapid and controlled method of delivery. Managing an i.v. therapy regimen has become a common nursing responsibility, although in most health authorities it is clearly seen as part of an extended nursing role (Speechley & Toovey 1987).

Before commencing an i.v. therapy regimen, assessment should consider the adequacy of the person's renal/cardiac function and her current fluid/electrolyte status, referring to such objective measures as laboratory studies, body surface area and intake/output.

Major complications of i.v. therapy

While, due to advances in technology, i.v. therapy is now relatively safe, it is still possible for serious complications to arise. Unfortunately, as Speechley & Toovey (1987) remarked, these complications are sometimes regarded as routine occurrences or a mere 'nuisance', but to overlook or underestimate the potential risks of i.v. therapy is to lose sight of the aim of therapy, which is to effectively replace fluid and electrolytes without causing the patient discomfort or further injury (see Research Abstract 20.1).

Phlebitis and extravasation are the two most commonly encountered problems. In their review of the literature, Adams et al (1986) found several factors associated with an increased incidence of phlebitis:

- cannula location — insertion in the lower extremities or movable joints gave an increased risk
- duration of therapy — increasing length of time raised the incidence, especially over 24 h
- blood flow problems in the region
- inadequate sterilisation of the cannula site
- pre-existent infection within the body
- pH and osmolality of the fluid — acidic infusates in particular
- particulate matter which contaminated the delivery system.

Research Abstract 20.1

Nystrom et al (1983) published the findings of a European multicentre trial whose purpose was to survey the incidence of bacteraemia and the use of intravenous devices in surgical patients. The study sample comprised 1016 patients in 42 hospitals across eight countries. The survey demonstrated that 62.9% of the patients received an i.v. device at some point in their hospital stay (in the UK this figure was 39.9% in those with a peripheral device and 2.5% in those with a central line). The incidence of thrombophlebitis was 10.3% (UK 15.1%), with the incidence of bacteraemia as follows:

- patients without an i.v. — 1.5 in 1000, of which 0.5 per 1000 was a nosocomial infection
- patients with peripheral device only — 6.9 in 1000, of which 3.7 per 1000 were nosocomial
- patients with a central device — 59 per 1000, of which 44.8 per 1000 were nosocomial.

Nystrom B, Larsen S O, Dankert J et al 1983 Bacteraemia in surgical patients with intravenous devices: a European multicentre incidence study. Journal of Hospital Infection 4: 338–349

Selecting the site

Patients who are particularly vulnerable to complications are those with existing infections or immune suppression and those whose restlessness or mental state may lead them to traumatise the cannula site. As Maki et al (1973) have pointed out, the cannula site is similar to an open surgical wound containing a foreign body and should be treated as such.

See Peters (1984) for a summary of the potential complications associated with i.v. devices.

Some practical considerations are involved in site selection, namely:

- the nature and anticipated duration of the therapy
- situational and environmental factors
- patient and safety factors
- availability of products
- staff expertise.

Insertion of the i.v. cannula is an extended role of the nurse and is usually undertaken by medical staff (see Davies 1988). However, communication between patient, nurse and doctor may enable a more effective and safe selection of site, materials and insertion technique.

In life-threatening circumstances, the selection of the i.v. site is largely dependent upon the expertise of the staff available, the products to hand and the purpose of the line. Whilst infection control measures are important, at the scene of a disaster or accident, environmental contaminants may be inevitable and speed may take priority. The more invasive the procedure, the greater is the importance of environmental control. Where possible, central lines (especially those involving a cutdown procedure) should be inserted in an operating theatre. Local factors which may be controlled during the time of insertion include the elimination of airborne contaminants and the avoidance of debris or bacteria entering via the insertion site.

Patient factors. Patient mobility and comfort may be enhanced or hindered by site selection. It is wiser and causes less discomfort to site the i.v. cannula away from movable joints or sites where clothes may rub. Skin areas which are vulnerable to breakdown should also be avoided, including areas which are burned, oedematous, traumatised, inflamed or affected by dermatological conditions such as eczema or psoriasis. The integrity and state of the veins themselves should influence selection.

The safety of lines in patients who are restless often poses a practical problem for nursing staff. Stability of the line may be enhanced by the method of attachment to the patient, and applying principles of counter-traction through the use of loops may prevent unnecessary trauma. Personal and environmental hygiene factors may necessitate that the insertion site be covered.

Central lines

Chapter 18 discusses the management of central lines used for the measurement of central venous pressure (CVP). Rainbow (1989) summarises the potential problems associated with the insertion, maintenance and removal of CVP lines. Similar principles apply when the central line is used for the long-term administration of infusates (e.g. patients requiring PN, cytotoxic and antibiotic therapy). However, the greatly increased incidence of complications associated with the use of central lines necessitates a very cautious and competent approach to their management. Mennim et al (1992) remind us of the danger of venous embolism associated with central line removal, although this is also a potential problem during insertion.

Types of parenteral fluids

The nature of the products to be infused determines both the number and location of the lines. Some infusates cannot be mixed, and if concurrent administration is required, two or more lines may be needed. Infusates which increase the likelihood of microbial contamination include those used in PN, especially those containing high concentrations of glucose. Each infusate carries with it particular risks, and nurses should familiarise themselves with the specific potential side-effects associated with different infusates.

Broadly speaking, the infusates commonly used in i.v. therapy as opposed to PN may be categorised as follows:

- colloidal solutions:
  —blood and blood products
  —plasma and plasma substitutes
- crystalloids — water, electrolytes and isotonic solutions.

Infusates can also be categorised in respect to their tonicity, as described below.

Isotonic solutions have the same osmolarity (tonicity) as serum or other body fluids and expand the intravascular compartment without affecting the intracellular and interstitial compartments.

Hypotonic solutions have a lower serum osmolarity and cause body fluids to shift away from the blood vessels and into the intracellular and interstitial spaces to areas of higher osmolarity. Hypotonic solutions may be used in the case of cellular dehydration due to diabetic ketoacidosis.

Hypertonic solutions cause fluid to move from the interstitial and intracellular compartments towards the intravascular compartments. For example, hypertonic saline will increase plasma and interstitial fluid osmolality.

Q

20.13 This résumé of the numerous issues involved in the safe management of a person with an i.v. device illustrates the complexity and importance of skilful and knowledgeable nursing practice. The professional accountability of the nurse practitioner is outlined in the UKCC's *Scope of Professional Practice* (UKCC 1992) which includes reference to the *Code of Professional Conduct* (UKCC 1992a), the *Standards for the Administration of Medicines* (UKCC 1992b) and *Records and Record Keeping* (UKCC 1993). In the light of these standards, why not evaluate the 'customs and practices' in your own clinical areas? It would be a useful management exercise to attempt to devise some criteria/standards which could be employed to evaluate the effectiveness of local policies.

20.14 How might you recognise signs of a problem associated with the maintenance of i.v. therapy? A

20.15 What specific problems may be encountered by a person with an infusion device who is being cared for at home? A

The subcutaneous route In patients who are older with impaired venous access, confusion, or non compliance with an alternative route, or in the terminally ill individual, the use of subcutaneous fluid administration (SFA) can be both appropriate and preferred (Mansfield et al 1998). The sites of choice for this administration include the anterior or lateral aspects of the chest wall, the abdominal wall, the anterolateral aspects of the thigh and the scapula. The site of the subcutaneous administration should be regularly inspected and changed every 24 h.

Dehydration and hydration in the terminally ill individual

The ethical debate continues as to whether to withhold or withdraw intravenous, subcutaneous, or naso-gastric hydration in the terminally ill patient. Nurses may well be presented with situations where a decision regarding hydration of their patients must be made. Nurses need to be knowledgeable of the benefits and disadvantages of both terminal dehydration and the rationale for hydration. Decisions made must be individualised and based on careful assessment that considers the problems related to dehydration, the potential risks and benefits of fluid replacement and the patient's and family's wishes.

For further discussion of this important issue in nursing care see Craig (1996), Smith (1997) and Jackonen (1997). The reader may also refer to Chapter 33.

PROBLEMS ASSOCIATED WITH DISORDERS OF FLUID AND ELECTROLYTE BALANCE

This section will outline some areas in which patients commonly experience difficulties with fluid and electrolyte control. Nurses in many areas of practice will encounter patients whose fluid and electrolyte balance has been challenged with potentially dire consequences, e.g. patients with burns, cardiac failure or respiratory problems. The reader is referred to the relevant chapter of this book for information on fluid and electrolyte management in these more specialised contexts.

Gastrointestinal disorders

Disorders of the GI system are very likely to lead to derangements in the normal balance of fluid and electrolytes, with subsequent problems in acid–base control. Fundamental problems can arise in circumstances such as the following:

- fluids are lost from the body by vomiting, diarrhoea or stomas
- the body is unable to absorb ingested fluids and foods
- the usual GI fluids are produced either normally or in excess but the body is unable to reabsorb them; thus the gut acts as a third space, as seen in paralytic ileus
- body fluids leak into the gut or GI fluids leak into adjacent organs or cavities (which again act as a third space) — examples include GI bleeding from oesophageal varices or GI ulcers, fistulae and peritonitis.

It is possible for several of these conditions to occur simultaneously, e.g. in a person with intestinal obstruction who is vomiting, has abdominal distension from the obstruction and may develop paralytic ileus. Two common problems of the GI tract which can be fatal if left untreated are vomiting and diarrhoea.

Vomiting

Losses of fluid through vomiting can rapidly cause dehydration and, if prolonged or severe, may lead to metabolic alkalosis and malnutrition. Following surgery to the thoracic and abdominal regions, vomiting can exacerbate the pain experience and delay healing due to the strain imposed upon the abdominal muscles. In the case of a person's inability to protect her airway (e.g. through coma), inhalation of vomitus may lead to inhalation pneumonia and possibly death.

Vomiting causes fluid loss through the ejection of recently ingested foods and fluids, the loss of gastric or upper intestinal juices, the loss of blood from GI lesions and the prevention of oral fluid and nutritional replacement. Thus prolonged or severe vomiting requires not only the prevention and/or control of the vomiting itself, but also adequate fluid replacement.

The loss of gastric juices, which contain hydrochloric acid and potassium ions, initially leads to metabolic alkalosis due to a surplus of bicarbonate ions. In severe, prolonged vomiting without adequate nutritional replacement, the body begins to metabolise fats as an energy source, producing ketone bodies and further exacerbating the metabolic acidosis.

Thus fluid and electrolyte losses caused by vomiting may be summarised as follows:

- depletion of the ECF volume
- hypochloraemia (Cl^- loss)
- alkalosis
- hypokalaemia
- possible acidosis
- anaemia due to any blood losses.

Nursing management. The actual control and the prevention of further episodes of vomiting will depend upon the cause of the vomiting and on available resources. However, whilst the person is vomiting some practical measures can help to alleviate some of her distress. These include providing a receptacle to vomit into, ensuring privacy if possible, and providing something to wipe away the vomit and mucus. The controlled use of breathing and swallowing techniques can sometimes enable the person to regain control of the waves of contraction that accompany the vomiting episode.

The nurse's ability to enable a person to adopt such techniques often rests on his interpersonal skills and confidence. The use of touch can also help the person to relax and thus avoid unnecessary muscular contractions which may aggravate any wound pains. (In the presence of a wound, it is important for the patient or nurse to support this.) When the immediate episode is over, a method of refreshing the mouth is essential. Judicious use of pharmacological agents may prevent vomiting episodes, especially if their timing is sequenced for maximum benefit, e.g. taken before anticipated triggers. With very severe vomiting episodes there is a risk that inhalation may occur; in such cases observation of the person's breathing pattern is essential (indeed, occasionally gastric contents may be emitted via the nose).

If a person vomits whilst a nasogastric tube is in place, the nurse should investigate the following possibilities:

- Is the tube blocked, kinked, in the wrong place or spigoted?
- Is the tube too fine for the aspirate?
- Does the frequency of gastric aspiration need to be altered?
- Is there a deterioration in the patient's condition, e.g. haemorrhage?
- Should the tube be removed?

The best action is to leave the tube on free drainage and aspirate unless this is contraindicated. At a suitable juncture, the effectiveness of the tube should be re-evaluated.

Q

20.16 What actions could be taken when the following patients seem likely to vomit? A

(a) A person with a spinal injury.
(b) A person with a wired jaw.

20.17 What is the significance of the information that may be obtained through observation of vomitus and the accompanying episodes of vomiting? A

Diarrhoea

Diarrhoea occurs when the body is unable to reclaim/absorb the fluids in the intestinal tract and the peristaltic contractions of the gut expel the intestinal contents. Generally, intestinal fluids are isotonic with the ECF until the colon is reached, at which point the contents gradually become hypotonic due to the colon's role in water reabsorption. Severe and prolonged diarrhoea as seen in cholera or in some forms of infant enteritis can lead to severe electrolyte imbalance, dehydration and ultimately death if treatment is unsuccessful or delayed. The fluid losses may cause:

- depletion of ECF volume
- hyponatraemia
- hypokalaemia
- metabolic acidosis due to loss of HCO_3^- in the digestive juices
- severe water dehydration (if the problem is located in the colon).

The causes of diarrhoea are identified and its nursing and medical management discussed in Chapter 4. Fluid and electrolyte replacement is an essential component in the management of the effects of diarrhoea, with accompanying management of the causative agent. Oral rehydration therapy is frequently employed in cases of enteritis and dehydration, providing the gut is able to absorb ingested fluids (see Box 20.13).

Q

20.18 Why do oral preparations to rehydrate a person suffering from diarrhoea/dehydration contain salts and glucose? A

Box 20.13 Contents of a solution to use in oral rehydration therapy (to be reconstituted with water to make a total volume of 1 L) (British National Formulary 1998)

Substance	WHO formulation
Sodium chloride	3.5 g
Potassium chloride	1.5 g
Sodium citrate	2.9 g
Anhydrous glucose	20.0 g

This combination gives (mmol/L):

- sodium: 90
- potassium: 20
- chloride: 80
- citrate: 10
- glucose: 111.

In UK practice, where less severe forms of dehydration are found than in developing countries, the sodium content is slightly less and the glucose higher. It is important to ensure that the water additive is safe and free from contaminants.

Special needs of the person undergoing surgery

The person undergoing surgery, whether elective or emergency, is particularly vulnerable to several disturbances of fluid and electrolyte balance. Disturbances in the composition and placement of the body fluids and electrolytes accompany many procedures and include blood loss, dehydration from preoperative fasting, bowel preparation (e.g. mannitol administration to clear the gut) and surgical exposure. Problems due to the underlying pathology and the patient's general health status exacerbate the situation. Surgery/trauma causes a defensive metabolic response which conserves water and sodium and changes the plasma levels of sodium, potassium, nitrogen and albumin. The basis of the response is vasoconstriction of the renal artery and the release of ADH, whilst any changes in blood pressure which affect the juxtaglomerular apparatus will stimulate the renin/aldosterone systems. This response enables conservation of plasma volume and the retention of sodium, whilst an increase in catecholamines raises the cardiac output and heart rate.

The renal response to trauma usually takes 24–72 h to recover and during this time the patient is unable to cope normally with electrolyte control and cannot produce hypotonic urine. The risks of fluid overload and water intoxication are thus high; yet, conversely, inadequate replacement therapy may lead to dehydration and shock. Thus, in a vulnerable person it is important not only to measure daily fluid balance but also to keep a record of the consecutive daily balances over the first 72 h. Oedema may occur due to changes in vascular permeability, with translocation of fluids into the third space. The fundamental nursing activities of patient assessment and effective implementation of treatment regimens are often critical to the patient's recovery.

By convention, it is normally assumed that intraoperative fluid losses are replaced in theatre and that fluid balance recording commences postoperatively from a state of 'zero' balance. It is important to note the losses during surgery in order to anticipate any potential problems, which should be indicated in the theatre notes and postoperative guidelines from the anaesthetist. However, the picture is occasionally confused by poor record-keeping and inadequate communication, which may cause the postoperative fluid balance data to be misleading. Insensible losses may also pass unnoticed, e.g. loss from sweating (as in shock or pyrexia).

Q

20.19 Select a person who is to undergo surgery and whom you can follow up postoperatively. Assess your chosen patient and identify his or her actual and potential needs with particular reference to:

(a) comfort needs in respect of hydration and elimination
(b) potential fluid and electrolyte losses or gains
(c) other factors influencing fluid and electrolyte balance
(d) the changing needs of the patient from the preoperative assessment through surgery to the postoperative phase.

Critically evaluate the planned and implemented nursing care of your selected patient in respect of the identified problems derived from items (a)–(d).

REFERENCES

Adam S D, Killien M, Larson E 1986 In line filtration and infusion phlebitis. Heart & Lung 15(2): 134–140
Anderson B, Rundgren M 1982 Thirst and its disorders. Annual Review of Medicine 33: 231–239
British National Formulary 1998 No. 35 (March). Pharmaceutical Press, London
Davies S 1988 The role of nurses in intravenous cannulation. Nursing Standard 12(17): 43–46
Edelman I S, Leibman J 1959 Anatomy of body water electrolytes. American Journal of Medicine 27: 256–278
Guyton A C, Hall J E 1996 Textbook of medical physiology, 9th edn. WB Saunders, Philadelphia
Jackonen S 1997 Dehydration and hydration in the terminally ill: care considerations. Nursing Forum 32(3): 5–13
Maki D G, Goldman D, Rhame S 1973 Infection control in IV therapy. Annals of Internal Medicine 79(6): 867–887
Mansfield S, Monaghan Hall J 1998 Subcutaneous administration and site maintenance. Nursing Standard 13(12): 56–62
Mennim P, Coyle C F, Taylor J D 1992 Venous air embolism associated with the removal of CV catheter. British Medical Journal 305(6846): 171–172
Metheny N 1996 Fluid and electrolyte balance: nursing considerations, 3rd edn. Lippincott, Philadelphia
Nystrom B, Larsen S O, Dankert J et al 1983 Bacteraemia in surgical patients with intravenous devices: a European multicentre incidence study. Journal of Hospital Infection 4: 338–349
Porth C M 1998 Pathophysiology: concepts of altered health state, 5th edn. Lippincott, Philadelphia
Rainbow C 1989 Monitoring the critically ill patient. Heinemann, Oxford
Smith S A 1997 Controversies in hydrating the terminally ill patient. Journal of Intravenous Nursing 20(4): 193–200
Speechley V, Toovey J 1987 Problems in i.v. therapy. Professional Nurse 2(8): 240–242
UKCC 1992a Code of professional conduct. UKCC, London
UKCC 1992b Standards for the administration of medicines. UKCC, London
UKCC 1993 Records and record keeping. UKCC, London
UKCC 1994 The scope of professional practice. UKCC, London
Woodtli A O 1990 Thirst: a critical care nursing challenge. Dimensions of Critical Care Nursing 9(1): 6–15

FURTHER READING

Barta M 1987 Correcting electrolyte imbalance. Registered Nurse 50(2): 30–34
Bland J H 1963 Clinical metabolism of body water and electrolytes. Saunders, London
Craig G M 1996 On withholding artificial hydration and nutrition from terminally ill sedated patients. The debate continues. Journal of Medical Ethics 22: 147–153
Dougherty L 1992 Intravenous therapy. Surgical Nurse 5(2): 10–13
Fan S T, Teoh-Chan C H, Lau K F, Chu K W, Kwan A K, Wong K K 1988 Predictive value of surveillance skin and hub cultures in central venous catheters sepsis. Journal of Hospital Infection 12(3):191–198
Feluer L 1980 Understanding the electrolyte maze. American Journal of Nursing 80(9): 1591–1595
Gamble J L 1954 Chemical anatomy, physiology and pathology of ECF, 6th edn. Harvard University Press, Harvard

Ganong W F 1997 Review of medical physiology, 18th edn. Appleton & Lange, New York

Green J H 1976 An introduction to human physiology, 4th edn. Oxford University Press, Oxford

Green J H 1978 Basic clinical physiology, 3rd edn. Oxford University Press, Oxford

Haynes S 1989 Infusion phlebitis and extravasation. Professional Nurse 5(3): 160–161

Haynes S 1991 CVP monitoring. Professional Nurse 6(12): 727–729

Hecker J, Swartz M (eds) 1982 Current topics in infectious diseases. McGraw-Hill, New York

Hinchliff S M, Montague S E, Watson R (eds) 1996 Physiology for nursing practice, 2nd edn. Baillière Tindall, London

Holmes O 1993 Human acid-base physiology: a student text. Chapman and Hall, London

Jones D C 1975 Food for thought. Royal College of Nursing, London

Lamb J F, Ingram C G, Johnston I A, Pitman R M 1992 Essentials of physiology, 3rd edn. Blackwell Scientific Publications, Oxford

McVicar A, Clancy J 1992 Which infusate do I need? Professional Nurse 7(9): 586–591

Maki D G 1977 Preventing infection in IV therapy. Current Research Anaesthesia and Analgesics 56(1): 141–153

Maki D G, Goldmann D, Rhame S 1993 Infection control in IV therapy. Annals of Internal Medicine 79(6): 867–887

Maki D G, Ringer M 1987 Evaluation of dressing regimens for prevention of infection with peripheral IV catheters. Journal of American Nursing 258(17): 2396–2403

Manley K M 1992 Flow control devices in intravenous therapy. Surgical Nurse 5(3): 11–15

Marieb E N 1998 Human anatomy and physiology, 4th edn. Benjamin Cummings, California

Metheny N 1996 Fluid and electrolyte balance: nursing considerations, 3rd edn. Lippincott, Philadelphia

Millam D 1988 Managing complications of IV therapy. Nursing 88 18(3): 34–42

Miller J 1988 Recording the CVP. Professional Nurse 3(6): 188–189

Miller J 1989 Intravenous therapy in fluid and electrolyte balance. Professional Nurse 4(5): 237–240

Morling S 1998 Infusion devices: risks and user responsibilities. British Journal of Nursing 7(1): 13–20

Neeser M, Ruedin P, Restellini J P 1992 Thirst strike: hypernatraemia and acute prerenal failure in a prisoner who refused to drink. British Medical Journal 304(6838): 1352

Peters J L 1984 Peripheral venous cannulation: reducing the risks. British Journal of Parenteral Therapy March: 56–68

Rochon P A, Gill S S, Litner J et al 1997 A systematic review of the evidence for hypodermoclysis to treat dehydration in older people. Journal of Gerontology: Medical Sciences 52A(3): M169–176

Smith E, Kinsey M 1991 Fluids and electrolytes: a conceptual approach, 2nd edn. Churchill Livingstone, Edinburgh

Stonehouse J, Butcher J 1996 Phlebitis associated with peripheral cannulae. Professional Nurse 12(1): 51–54

Timberlake K 1988 Chemistry, 4th edn. Harper Collins, New York

NUTRITION

21

Mary Gobbi Colin Torrance

INTRODUCTION

Eating and drinking are an integral part of human existence. An adequate intake of food and water is required to maintain physiological function, to allow for growth and maintenance of tissues, and to provide energy to meet the demands of daily living. Eating and drinking have been identified as forming one of the 12 essential activities of living (ALs) in Roper et al's (1996) model of living. Although a biological necessity, eating and drinking have a significance beyond the merely physiological, forming an important part of social and psychological well-being. In any society, food production and preparation are central activities; even in developed countries where food is abundant, the preparation and consumption of food may take up several hours a day. Meals are used as a time for families to come together; food or drink may be offered to make a guest feel welcome; and formal meals may be a feature of family, religious or national ceremonies. Illness or hospitalisation can alter eating habits with important psychological as well as nutritional effects. The AL of eating and drinking is influenced by a range of factors, including physical, psychological, social, cultural, religious, environmental and economic factors. Nursing interventions should be based on both a physiological and psychosocial assessment of the nutritional needs of the individual. Presenting a well-balanced meal is of little value if the patient is unable or unwilling to eat. Discharging a patient home with a diet sheet that includes items that are economically or culturally unacceptable is equally futile.

The importance of nutritional care within nursing has been well recognised. Henderson (1960) stated that 'there is no more important an element in the preparation for nursing than the study of nutrition', and Florence Nightingale was as influential in the development of dietetics as in nursing. However, it has been well demonstrated that the provision of food and fluids has largely been relegated to ancillary staff and that there is still a need to raise nurses' awareness of the importance of nutrition in patient well-being (see Research Abstract 21.1). The nurse's role in nutritional care spans the wellness–illness continuum from involvement in health education, such as giving advice on a 'healthy' diet, to the management of parenteral nutrition (PN) regimens. Helping an

Research Abstract 21.1

Kowanko et al (1999) conducted a small survey of nurses' attitudes and knowledge about nutrition and the provision of food to patients in an Australian hospital. Their findings were consistent with the work of Perry (1997) in the UK, namely that nurses' knowledge about nutritional care was 'not well developed' with few nurses being able to accurately define a 'healthy diet'. Nurses seemed unaware of the likelihood of malnutrition in their clinical areas and articulated a lack of knowledge and skill. Nurses reported problems with the catering services, expressing uncertainties about their role and responsibilities in relation to the catering staff. Some nurses commented that time pressure and other activities meant that feeding patients became a 'low priority' task in practice.

The study demonstrated that in the absence of accurate nutritional knowledge, good catering services and a positive attitude towards nutritional care, patients are likely to receive inadequate advice, be inappropriately assessed and receive insufficient food, of the wrong sort, or none at all.

Kowanko I, Simon S, Wood J 1999 Nutritional care of the patient: nurses' knowledge and attitudes in an acute care setting. Journal of Clinical Nursing 8(2): 217–224.

individual to meet his basic need for food is as critical a component of nursing care as ensuring adequate oxygenation. In this chapter we will consider normal nutrition and the basic need for food, the role of food in health and disease, non-nutritional aspects of eating and drinking, assessment of nutritional status and the nurse's role in planning and implementing nutritional care.

Normal nutrition

To maintain healthy function, an adequate supply of the essential nutrients is required. The exact composition of the diet can vary enormously — foods common in one culture may be unacceptable in another — but the constituents will belong to one of the six main macro- and micronutrient groups: protein, carbohydrate, fat, vitamins, minerals and, of course, water. In addition, many non-nutrient compounds or unavailable carbohydrates are included in the diet and have their own importance, e.g. fibre, whilst other non-nutrients like food colourings, flavourings and preservatives, which are useful in the cooking and commercial production of food. Some may be associated with disease in susceptible individuals. Contamination of food is common. Improperly prepared or stored food may harbour organisms causing food poisoning; typical culprits found in undercooked chicken are bacteria belonging to the genus *Salmonella*. *Clostridium botulinum* is an anaerobic bacterium which may multiply in inadequately preserved (often home-canned) foods and produces a powerful toxin that interferes with synaptic transmission. Outbreaks of food poisoning due to *Escherichia coli* are now increasingly common. Elderly people and children are particularly susceptible and severe outbreaks in Lanarkshire and Cumbria have attracted national attention and resulted in several deaths. Box 21.1 lists some major food contaminants of possible toxicological importance.

Q **21.1** What safety precautions are taken in the hospital environment to reduce the likelihood of food poisoning? Check your local policies.

Box 21.1 Sources of food contamination. (Adapted from Kilgore & Li 1980)

During food production
- Animal and insect filth, whole or parts of insects
- Parasites
- Microorganisms
- Agrochemical residues (pesticides, fungicides, etc.)
- Drugs (antibiotic, growth hormones)
- Toxic metals (especially mercury and the heavy metals)

During processing
- Animal and insect filth, whole or parts of insects
- Microorganisms and microbial toxins
- Foreign bodies and processing residues

During packing and storage
- Animal and insect filth
- Labelling materials
- Microorganisms and microbial toxins
- Chemical migrants from the packaging materials

Although synthetic foods containing all the known nutrients can be formulated, no single naturally occurring food can meet all the daily nutritional demands. Many foods contain the essential six nutrients, but the proportion of each varies and a range of different foods is necessary to provide the daily requirement of individual nutrients. In general, plant products are richer in carbohydrate but lower in protein and fats than are animal products. Plants are the major source of fibre. Some foods are particularly rich in a single nutrient, although they may contain other nutrients; thus meat should be classed as protein-rich rather than as a protein, as it also contains a lot of fat and other nutrients. Cereals are rich in carbohydrate; wheat flour, for example, is over 70% carbohydrate, but it also has more than 10% protein and 12% fat. Very few foods, such as sugar (almost pure carbohydrate) or cooking oils (almost pure fat), fall predominantly into one nutrient group.

Nutrients have a complex role in physiological function and most nutrients are involved in several processes. Iron is required for oxygen transport within the red blood cell but is also important in several enzyme systems, e.g. as part of prolyl hydroxylase, an essential enzyme in collagen formation. Nutrients may form the structural material of the body, provide energy for metabolism or help in the regulation of physiological processes. A single nutrient may be necessary for one or all these functions, e.g. carbohydrate, fat and protein are all sources of energy. Although carbohydrate and fat are the diet's predominate energy source, protein has the same energy value as carbohydrate (Box 21.2). Water, protein, fat, minerals and carbohydrate form the structural elements of the body. Minerals and vitamins are important in regulatory processes, but protein and fats, as hormones and enzymes, also contribute to metabolic regulation. Non-nutrients such as fibre are important for physiological function, and others such as caffeine and food additives may fulfil other lifestyle functions and possibly

Box 21.2 Energy value of major nutrients

Carbohydrate	16 kJ/g (~4 kcal/g)
Protein	17 kJ/g (~4 kcal/g)
Fat	38 kJ/g (~9 kcal/g)
Alcohol	29 kJ/g (~7 kcal/g)

contribute to disease. Alcohol is calorie-rich and has a complex role in many societies but is damaging if it contributes a major proportion of dietary energy.

The healthy diet

Normally, the diet provides an adequate supply of all the nutrients (and important non-nutrients such as fibre) that are necessary to satisfy the needs of body cells. Whilst the healthy person can tolerate short-term fluctuations in nutrient intake, a persistent deficiency of any of the nutrients will impair function (see Table 21.1). There must be enough:

- water
- protein for tissue repair, maintenance and growth
- carbohydrate and fat for energy
- vitamins and minerals for the regulation of physiological processes.

The diet must supply the essential nutrients, i.e. those which are necessary for survival but cannot be synthesised by the body from other sources. Some amino acids, for example, are required for health but are not dietarily essential as they can be synthesised by the body in sufficient quantities to meet metabolic needs. The diet should supply all these necessary components in the correct quantities and proportions, whilst avoiding excessive intake. For optimal health, nutrient intake must balance nutrient usage; an excess intake may be nearly as damaging as a deficiency. Western society has demonstrated that the adverse effects of overeating may be as serious as chronic undernutrition. Recently, health problems have been identified due to excessive intake of a single nutrient taken in the form of vitamin supplements — a typical example is vitamin A which is toxic in high doses.

Actual requirements will vary depending on the person's size, age, gender, activity level and state of health. The reference nutrient intakes (RNI) of some major nutrients for different groups within the British population are listed in Table 21.2. However, recently the Scientific Committee for Food has decided to give, not just one, but three reference values for a nutrient. In addition to the RNI, there is the lower reference nutrient intake (LRNI), the intake below which most individuals would be unable to meet metabolic requirements, and the estimated average requirement (EAR).

Table 21.1 A summary of clinical signs of nutritional significance (Miller & Torrance 1991)

Area	*Signs*	*Deficiencies*
Hair	Dull/dry Thin/sparse Easily falls out Loss of colour Alopecia	PEM Essential fatty acids
Face	Moon-face Enlarged thyroid Nasolabial seborrhoea Seborrhoeic dermatitis	PEM Iodine Riboflavin, niacin, zinc
Eyes	Dryness, softening/ inflammation of cornea Pale conjunctiva Conjunctivitis Keratomalacia Loss of vision, night blindness	Vitamin A, B complex, iron, folate
Lips	Angular stomatitis, cheilosis	Riboflavin, niacin, iron
Tongue	Glossitis, red, swollen	Folate, B complex iron
Gums	Reddened, spongy, receding, bleeding	Vitamin C
Nails	Spoon-shaped	Iron
Skin	Dryness, petechiae, ecchymoses, oedema, colour changes, texture changes Follicular hyperkeratosis Pellagrous dermatosis	Vitamins A, C and K, niacin
Musculo- skeletal	Fat and muscle wasting Fatigue, stiffness, pain	PEM, vitamin D
Neurological	Paraesthesia, sensory loss Irritability, confusion, depression Motor weakness, hypoflexia	B complex, thiamine PEM

For further information on dietary requirements, see Department of Health (1991) and Scientific Committee for Food for the European Community (1993).

To remain healthy, individuals may need to modify their diet to meet changes in metabolic demand, e.g. during pregnancy, lactation (Box 21.3) and disease. Effective nutritional nursing depends on assessing the patient to identify current needs and helping him to identify ways of meeting these nutritional requirements that fit in as much as possible with his usual food habits and preferences. In addition, an RNI has not been fully established for all the essential nutrients. A varied diet remains the best way to ensure an adequate intake of all the essential nutrients.

21.2 Apart from pregnancy and lactation, when else during their lifespan may a person have sudden changes in their nutrient demand?

Food groups

For patients needing special diets, detailed assessment, food analysis and dietary planning are important, but for many patients it may be more appropriate to adopt a more general approach to nutritional education. The food group approach aims to inform and encourage the patient to eat a balanced diet, one in which major food groupings are all represented, providing a sufficient variety of foods to meet all nutrient requirements. One of the most widely used of these divides foods into five basic groups: cereals/bread/potatoes; fruit and vegetables; milk and diary products; meat, fish and alternatives and foods containing fats and sugar. Box 21.4 demonstrates a four-group plan based on an adult's daily needs. Such a plan needs modification for groups with special nutritional needs, such as children, teenagers, pregnant women and nursing mothers. A more complex food exchange system is required for those with a known metabolic condition such as diabetes mellitus. One group meriting special mention are vegetarians, for whom the normal four-food group plan with a reliance on meat as a protein source is obviously unacceptable. Vegetarians

Table 21.2 Reference nutrient intakes for vitamins (Reproduced with permission from Department of Health 1991 Dietary reference values for food energy and nutrients for the United Kingdom. Report of the Panel on Dietary Reference Values of the Committee on Medical Aspects of Food Policy (COMA). (Report on Health and Social Subjects 41) HMSO, London)

Age	*Thiamin mg/day*	*Riboflavin mg/day*	*Niacin (nicotinic acid equivalent) mg/day*	*Vitamin B_6 mg/day*[a]	*Vitamin B_{12} µg/day*	*Folate µg/day*	*Vitamin C mg/day*	*Vitamin A µg/day*	*Vitamin D µg/day*
0–3 months	0.2	0.4	3	0.2	0.3	50	25	350	8.5
4–6 months	0.2	0.4	3	0.2	0.3	50	25	350	8.5
7–9 months	0.2	0.4	4	0.3	0.4	50	25	350	7
10–12 months	0.3	0.4	5	0.4	0.4	50	25	350	7
1–3 years	0.5	0.6	8	0.7	0.5	70	30	400	7
4–6 years	0.7	0.8	11	0.9	0.8	100	30	400	—
7–10 years	0.7	1.0	12	1.0	1.0	150	30	500	—
Males									
11–14 years	0.9	1.2	15	1.2	1.2	200	35	600	—
15–18 years	1.1	1.3	18	1.5	1.5	200	40	700	—
19–50 years	1.0	1.3	17	1.4	1.5	200	40	700	—
50+ years	0.9	1.3	16	1.4	1.5	200	40	700	[b]
Females									
11–14 years	0.7	1.1	12	1.0	1.2	200	35	600	—
15–18 years	0.8	1.1	14	1.2	1.5	200	40	600	—
19–50 years	0.8	1.1	13	1.2	1.5	200	40	600	—
50+ years	0.8	1.1	12	1.2	1.5	200	40	600	[b]
Pregnancy	+0.1[c]	+0.3	[d]	[d]	[d]	+100	+10	+100	10
Lactation									
0–4 months	+0.2	+0.5	+2	[d]	+0.5	+60	+30	+350	10
4+ months	+0.2	+0.5	+2	[d]	+0.5	+60	+30	+350	10

[a] Based on protein providing 14.7% of EAr for energy.
[b] After age 65 the RNI is 10 µg/day for men and women.
[c] For last trimester only.
[d] No increment.

Box 21.3 Calcium requirements during lactation

The calcium requirement of lactating women provides a striking example of how requirements for a nutrient can vary in health. A non-pregnant woman has a calcium RNI of 500 mg, whereas the RNI during lactation is 1200 mg; therefore the woman's normal diet would need modification to meet her increased requirements for calcium during lactation.

can be classed as lacto-ovo-vegetarians, i.e. those who use animal products such as milk and eggs but exclude animal flesh (meat, fish and poultry), and vegans who avoid all animal products and eat only plant foods. Box 21.5 illustrates a modified five-group plan for vegetarians.

Food plans of this type provide an easily understandable guide for balanced eating, but an individual following such a plan can still become deficient in some nutrients. Vitamins B_6 and E, and minerals such as iron, magnesium and zinc are sometimes deficient. The quality of the foods consumed can also be an important factor, as economic or ethnic factors may influence food choices within the groups. However, the simplicity of the approach with the division of foods into easily recognised groups can make it an effective way of providing patients with nutritional education.

Box 21.4 Five-food group plan for adult's daily requirements

- *Cereals/bread/potatoes* — Make these the main part of every meal. Whole grain products are preferred. This group provides carbohydrates (starch) fibre, (non-starch polysaccharide), some calcium, iron and B vitamins.
- *Fruit and vegetables* — Aim to eat at least five portions a day. Eat a wide variety of fresh, frozen, canned or juiced fruit and vegetables. This group provides Vitamin C and A, folates, fibre and some carbohydrate.
- *Milk and diary products* — Eat moderate amounts of these foods. Lower fat alternatives are preferred. This group provides protein, calcium and Vitamins A B_{12} and D.
- *Meat, fish and alternatives* — Eat moderate amounts of these foods. Lower fat alternatives preferred. Include two portions of fish each week, one of which should be oily fish. This group provides protein, iron, zinc, magnesium and B vitamins.
- *Fats and sugars* — Eat fatty foods sparingly and choose low-fat alternatives if possible. Fats contain Vitamins A, D and E and essential fatty acids. Eat sugary foods infrequently and in small amounts as sugar contributes to tooth decay and contains no other nutrients.

THE MAJOR NUTRIENTS

The essential nutrients are water, carbohydrate, protein, fat, vitamins and minerals. Water is the major component of the body and the diet must include a sufficient quantity to meet daily needs. Energy supply is the primary function of carbohydrate but it also has a protein-sparing action, an antiketogenic effect, a protective

Box 21.5 Five-food group plan for vegetarian adults' daily requirements

- *Cereals/bread/potatoes* — Make these the main part of every meal. Whole grain products are preferred. This group provides carbohydrates (starch) fibre, (non-starch polysaccharide), some calcium, iron and B vitamins.
- *Fruit and vegetables* — Aim to eat at least five portions a day. Eat a wide variety of fresh, frozen, canned or juiced fruit and vegetables. This group provides Vitamin C and A, folates, fibre and some carbohydrate.
- *Milk and milk alternatives* — Eat moderate amounts of these foods. Lower fat alternatives are preferred. This group provides protein, calcium and Vitamins A B_{12} and D. Alternatives include Vitamin B_{12} soya milk and vegetarian cheese.
- *Alternatives to meat and fish* — In vegetarian diets, it is not sufficient just to avoid meat. Such food must be replaced by other foods from the same food group. Choose protein-rich plant foods such as pulses, soya bean, quorn, nuts and seeds. Eat moderate amounts of these foods. Lower fat alternatives preferred. This group provides protein, iron, zinc, magnesium and B vitamins.
- *Fats and sugars* — Eat fatty foods sparingly and choose low-fat alternatives if possible. Fats contain Vitamins A, D and E and essential fatty acids. Eat sugary foods infrequently and in small amounts as sugar contributes to tooth decay and contains no other nutrients.

NB
Vitamin B_{12} is an essential vitamin in animal foods. Strict vegetarians (vegans) must rely on Vitamin B_{12} fortified soya or cereals. Regular supplements may be required.
Vegetarian diets are high in fibre, which absorbs water. It is important to drink plenty of fluid (2–3 litres a day).

function and a role in the synthesis of many body materials. Proteins are required for a range of functions. Some are key components in structure, some are hormones and enzymes, yet others have a role in immunity, blood clotting and transport of body substances, and others in the regulation and the maintenance of osmotic pressure. Fats (oils and waxes) are necessary for a number of physiological functions, and fat is the richest source of energy available to the body. Vitamins are required for the regulation of metabolic processes. They act as cofactors, coenzymes or as components of coenzymes and enzymes. The final group of essential nutrients is the minerals. More than 24 minerals may be required for physiological functioning and these can be divided into the major minerals, trace elements and putative trace elements.

Only a brief review of the major nutrients is possible here — for further details the reader is directed to Garrow & James (1993).

Carbohydrates

Carbohydrate is the main energy source for the body, and in its simplest form, glucose, it is the preferred fuel for the brain. Although fat has a higher calorific value, it is less efficiently used by the brain, and a high-fat diet increases the risk from some diseases. The three major carbohydrate groups in food are sugars, starches and the complex polysaccharides. The fruits, flowers, roots, leaves and stalks of plants provide carbohydrate, but leaves and stalks tend to have the more indigestible polysaccharide, cellulose, and so provide dietary fibre. Berries and fruits are rich in sugars while roots and seeds are usually excellent sources of the digestible polysaccharide starch. Foods rich in starch and fibre are recommended as the main energy source in a healthy diet. However, it is necessary to distinguish between useful carbohydrate sources, those which supply starch and fibre, and sources of questionable nutritional value which supply mainly processed sugars or 'empty calories'.

Proteins

The DoH (1991) recommendation for protein intake is calculated on the basis of 0.75 kg protein/kg body weight per day. Some amino acids are synthesised by the body; others, the dietarily essential amino acids, cannot be synthesised and must be obtained from food. Dietary protein is required primarily for the growth and maintenance of body tissue, but proteins fulfil many roles and protein function can be summarised into three broad categories: structural maintenance, physiological regulation and, in extremis, as an energy supply. Proteins are required to build new tissue during growth or replace tissue lost through injury, e.g. new blood cells after haemorrhage. Less obviously, protein is required to replace tissues lost on a daily basis — hair, nail, skin cells and blood cells need constant replacement. In fact, nearly all cells need replacing on a regular basis and, in addition, cell proteins are regularly replaced and renewed. Almost all enzymes and many hormones are proteins, so the regulatory role of proteins is profound.

Proteins are found in most foods, including meat, fish, cereals, legumes, fruit and vegetables, but the amount and quality of protein varies. A high-quality protein with a high biological value would be one that contains all the essential amino acids and is easily digested and absorbed. In general, the amino acids from animal products such as eggs, meat, milk and fish are well absorbed (over 90%), amino acids from legumes (e.g. beans, peas, lentils, etc.) are about 80% absorbed, and those from grains and other plant sources are between 60 and 90% absorbed. Animal products represent the best sources of quality protein but tend also to increase fat intake. Legumes come close in protein quality, avoid the problem of fat and contain many additional minerals and vitamins. If plant foods are to provide the major source of protein, it usually requires a wider mix to ensure an adequate supply of all the essential amino acids. For health, it is probably better to reduce the current level of animal protein in the Western diet and increase the use of legumes and cereals. However, no nutrient can be considered in isolation, and animal products are good sources of other nutrients, e.g. vitamin B_{12}, vitamin D and bioavailable iron.

Fats

Fats provide a concentrated energy source and are the body's largest energy store. Fat provides an important insulating layer beneath the skin and surrounds some body organs, giving support and cushioning the organs from mechanical trauma. Fat is a structural element forming, for example, the major component of the cell membrane. It is also required for effective neural function — myelin is a form of fat. Fats are used in the formation of substances such as lipoproteins, cholesterol and phospholipids and the steroid hormones. Adequate dietary fat is important, as the essential fatty acids and the fat-soluble vitamins are found mainly in fatty foods. Dietary fat provides energy and cholesterol to supplement the body's endogenous cholesterol supply. Fats are also important in foods for giving aroma and flavour, and they contribute to the feeling of satiety. Fat greatly increases the palatability of food and so has gained a prominent place in the Western diet. In some countries, 40–45% of food energy may be derived from fat. While sufficient fat is vital for health, excess intake is associated with a number of health problems, including obesity, cardiovascular disease and perhaps cancer. Excess of animal fats may be the particular problem.

Vitamins

Apart from vitamin D, which can be synthesised through the action of sunlight on the skin, and vitamin K which can be synthesised by intestinal bacteria, all the vitamins must be obtained from the diet. Since they are not consumed by the reactions they regulate, only small amounts are needed and a varied diet will normally supply all the vitamins required. The two main groupings are the fat-soluble and the water-soluble vitamins. The fat-soluble vitamins are absorbed from the small intestine along with dietary fat. They are found in foods such as fish, meat, butter, milk and plant oils. The fat-soluble vitamins can be stored in the liver and adipose tissues; therefore excessive intake (hypervitaminosis) can lead to toxic levels. Water-soluble vitamins are easily lost from foods and the body; little storage occurs and hypervitaminosis for these vitamins is rare. Vitamin deficiency often results from a more widespread nutritional disruption but some specific deficiencies and disease states are important. Vitamin deficiency usually affects the water-soluble vitamins, but in severe trauma or illness the fat-soluble vitamins may also be involved.

Minerals

The major minerals — calcium, phosphorus, sodium, potassium, chlorine, magnesium and sulphur — are essential for health and are required in amounts over 100 mg/day. Trace elements are required in much smaller amounts (under 100 mg/day) and play an essential role in human nutrition. A balanced diet featuring a range of different foods is likely to meet daily requirements for the major minerals and trace elements. A mineral is established as essential when deficiency can be shown to produce an impairment which can only be reversed or prevented by supplementation with that particular element. Trace elements are important as enzyme components or as structural components. Of particular nutritional significance are iron, iodine and zinc. Iodine deficiency in the form of endemic goitre is characterised by marked enlargement of the thyroid gland. It occurs in areas where water and soil are deficient in iodine. Zinc is present in body tissues in larger amounts than all of the other trace elements. It is involved in a number of enzyme reactions and is particularly important in periods of growth and during wound healing. Animal products are the main sources of zinc. Cereals and legumes are poorer sources. Marginal deficiency may occur in the elderly and the hospitalised patient with poor appetite.

The major function of iron is as a component of haemoglobin, but it may also be important in many enzyme processes and in the immune response. Iron is not excreted by the body but small amounts are lost mainly through the gastrointestinal (GI) tract in blood, desquamated cells and bile. Basal losses in the female are negligible, but menstruation adds an additional variable loss, and pregnancy and lactation increase requirements. Although most foods are rich in iron, iron deficiency is one of the major nutritional diseases in the world. This is due not so much to a lack of iron but to a lack of bioavailable iron. Iron in the form of haem as found in meats is 20–40% available, whereas iron in most plant foods is often less than 5% available. In addition, a number of dietary factors may influence iron absorption (see Torrance 1992).

NUTRITIONAL INTERVENTION

Dietary manipulation is a useful adjunct to the treatment of many diseases; for example, special diets may help in renal disease, GI disease and cardiovascular disease, and are essential in the management of diabetes mellitus and conditions such as phenylketonuria (PKU). Diets may be used to increase or decrease intake of specific nutrients, to help control body weight or to improve nutrition in the undernourished. A detailed consideration of diet therapy is beyond our remit, but before discussing the nurse's role in helping a patient meet his nutritional needs, a brief discussion of obesity and its management is presented. Obesity is the major nutritional disorder of our society and provides a good example of an overall approach to diet management. Paradoxically, severe malnutrition is a major problem worldwide and a degree of malnutrition may be relatively common in the hospitalised patient.

Obesity

Obesity is the condition of excessive accumulation of fat in the body, leading to an increase in weight beyond that considered desirable with regard to the individual's height, bone structure and age. It has a complex aetiology related to food habits and intake, exercise and activity patterns and individual metabolic rate (Mela & Rogers 1998). Obesity is considered a major health problem of the Western world. Fat people tend to die younger than comparable lean people and obesity is linked with many common disorders (Simopoulos 1985). The extra strain placed on the musculoskeletal system may contribute to arthritic disease, particularly of the lower spine, hips and knees. Abdominal muscle may fail, resulting in abdominal hernias. Fatty leg muscle may be inefficient, reducing the effectiveness of the muscle pump and predisposing to varicose veins. Excess fat in the thoracic cavity may impair breathing (Pickwickian syndrome). Obesity is linked with cardiovascular disease, including atherosclerosis and hypertension, which may progress to angina pectoris and heart failure. Other diseases associated with obesity are gall bladder disease and non-insulin-dependent diabetes mellitus. Figure 21.1 summarises some of the complications of obesity. The psychological and social effects of obesity can also be profound. Thinness is the current, perceived norm for Western societies and fat people may suffer social and employment discrimination, insurance rates will be higher, and current fashions may not be available in larger sizes. Obesity may engender a negative body image and this may be reinforced by the way society views and treats fat people.

In general, obesity results from an increased food intake or a reduced level of activity, i.e. over a significant period of time energy intake exceeds energy expenditure. Overeating is the major cause, but this does not mean that all fat people simply overeat. Currently, much research is focused on the role of leptin, a potent anorectic agent found in adipose tissue (Zhanget 1994, Elmquist et al 1998). Studies on twins suggest that genetic factors may be involved in obesity. Newman et al (1937) found that fraternal twins had a greater weight difference than identical twins. However, they also showed a greater difference in weight between twins raised apart compared with twins raised together, suggesting that environmental factors (family environment) may have the greater influence. The importance of the family environment is confirmed by studies of adopted children where there is little evidence of weight differences between the adopted and biological siblings (Garn & Bailey 1976). In a later report, Garn & Clark (1976) recorded a high correlation between the skinfold measurements of parents and child. Although this research is now somewhat dated, the view is still held that the family's attitude to food and food habits are major factors in obesity.

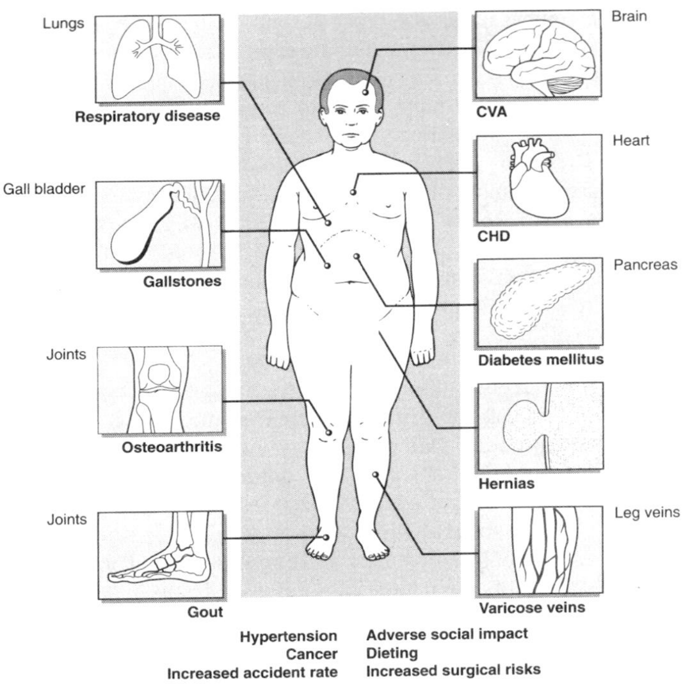

Fig. 21.1 Adverse effects of obesity.

The importance of socioeconomic factors is clear and, although its exact nature is uncertain, the relationship between socioeconomic status and obesity is particularly strong in women. In a major American study, an inverse relationship between obesity and socioeconomic status was demonstrated: 5% of upper status women; 16% of middle status women; and 30% of lower status women were obese (Goldblatt et al 1965). The situation is complicated, however, by the findings that racial, ethnic and religious factors also have an influence.

Popular opinion suggests a glandular basis for obesity, but there is little evidence for an endocrine origin in most cases. Individual differences in metabolic rate and handling of nutrients have also been suggested, but there is no clear evidence that fat people metabolise fuel foods more efficiently than lean people.

For a detailed review of obesity, see Mela & Rogers (1998).

A number of approaches are available to deal with excess weight, ranging from severe diets to surgical gastric partitioning and liposuction, from diuretics to appetite suppressors, and from fad diets to counselling and self-help groups. As the problem is in most cases due to overeating, diet therapy and counselling/support comprise perhaps the major approach. A balanced approach to eating and increased exercise are the mainstays of weight reduction. Reducing diets are perhaps the main area of popular interest, with exponents recommending high-fibre diets, low-calorie diets, tropical fruit diets, banana and milk diet, and a number of specialised powder and food-bar diets. Some of these diets may restrict calories and other nutrients to such a degree that they can only be used under medical supervision. Behavioural changes, peer support and a sensible diet as typified by the Weight Watchers programme are to be recommended. Going on a diet is not enough — one must stay on a diet to lose weight and then adopt healthy eating patterns to maintain an ideal body weight. Episodic dieting where the individual swings from overeating to very low calorie intake and back to overeating may be more injurious than obesity itself.

A reducing diet should be planned after nutritional assessment and should take into account the patient's lifestyle and food habits. It must supply sufficient energy for resting energy expenditure (REE) and normal activity but exclude excess energy intake. Restriction of fat and an increase in the use of complex carbohydrate (including fibre) are usually recommended. Choices should still be made from the usual food groups to ensure enough vitamins and minerals. Defining the exact amount of energy required depends on the individual, but most women will need at least 5 MJ (1200 kcal) per day, and bigger or more active women and men may need 6–7.5 MJ (1500–1800 kcal) daily. Diets providing less than this should probably only be undertaken on medical advice. It is important to establish a realistic level of energy intake.

Undernutrition

Undernutrition is an endemic problem; protein-energy malnutrition (PEM) affects large numbers of the world's population and contributes significantly to human mortality and morbidity. However, in developed countries, outright starvation is unlikely but levels of undernutrition do exist. Certain groups may be at particular risk, including the homeless, the elderly, alcoholics, those with behavioural disturbances of eating such as anorexia nervosa, and the hospitalised patient.

Metabolically active disease can alter or increase the need for nutrients. Disease processes may reduce food intake or absorption of nutrients; pyrexia and infection may increase metabolic rate and nutritional demands; surgery and trauma have a profound impact on metabolism, initiating a complex neuroendocrine response which shares some of the characteristics of the body's response to starvation (Torrance 1991). Undernutrition is often associated with chronic disease and is a risk whether the patient is nursed at home or in hospital, but there is also evidence of significant undernutrition in medical and surgical wards. Tierney (1996) has reviewed the literature on malnutrition in hospital patients and the elderly in particular. Surveys have suggested that between 22 and 50% of hospitalised patients could suffer from malnutrition. Bistrian et al (1974, 1976) found that protein-energy malnutrition (PEM) was common in both surgical and medical patients. Medical patients were more energy-depleted than surgical patients but had better protein status. In a UK study of 105 surgical patients, only 22 of them had any comments in their records about their nutritional status and less than one-fifth had been weighed during their period of hospitalisation (Hill et al 1977). A small study by Todd et al (1984) on medical, surgical and orthopaedic wards indicated that 24% of patients had a food intake below the level predicted for REE and 16% had less than the recommended daily amount of protein.

In surgical patients, undernutrition is associated with increased postoperative morbidity and mortality and studies have demonstrated that preoperative nutritional support can reduce these rates (Delmi et al 1990). Postoperative infection is particularly linked to undernutrition. Infection can induce a stress-related, catabolic response similar to that seen in surgical trauma and it is also often associated with anorexia. The link between nutrition and immunodepression is complex, but it is clear that a wide range of immunological functions may be affected. Nearly all dietary elements can be important in resistance to infection, but adequate levels of protein, carbohydrate, types of fat, iron and zinc may be of particular significance.

A study of nursing nutritional care is reported in Coates (1985).

21.3 Coates considered the issue of nutritional care in relation to the nutritional needs of patients, record-keeping and organisation of nursing care. What ward-based factors do you think influence a patient's nutritional needs and nursing management?

Hospitalisation may predispose to undernutrition due to a number of factors. The patient may find that the anxiety and unfamiliarity of the environment reduce his appetite. Food may not be to his taste and the presentation of meals and environment for eating less than ideal. Investigations may require periods of fasting and missed meals may not be replaced. Of particular interest is the practice of preoperative fasting, reviewed by Torrance (1991). Routine practice is to fast patients for a minimum of 4 h before surgery, in order to empty the stomach and avoid perioperative or postoperative vomiting and the risk of aspiration into the lungs. However, actual fasting times for elective surgery ranging from 5 to 22 h have been reported, and in one study only 16% of patients on an afternoon list were fasted for 6 h or less (Smith 1972, Thomas 1987, Chapman 1996); 33% had been deprived of food for more than 13 h. For patients on the morning list, 10 h was the minimum length of fast. The theoretical 4–6 h preoperative fast appears to result in practice in periods of abstinence that might be better termed preoperative starvation, which could lead to a state of catabolism which may be detrimental to a patient undergoing major surgery (Short 1983). Jester & Williams (1999) discuss strategies to reduce unnecessary preoperative fasting.

21.4 Patients attending as outpatients for procedures on a day basis may have been advised to fast before or after the procedure. In respect of the patient's nutritional needs, review your hospital's practices in relation to the information given to patients attending day care and the advice given to them on discharge.

The remainder of this chapter will explore the nurse's role in nutritional assessment and ensuring an adequate intake of food — encouraging oral intake and managing artificial feeding by enteral and parenteral routes.

NUTRITIONAL ASSESSMENT

The first stage in nutritional intervention is assessment, identifying the individual's current nutritional status, normal eating habits and risk of developing nutritional imbalances, and establishing a baseline for monitoring changes in status. Important aspects of nutritional assessment are clinical and dietary history, physical examination, biochemical tests and immunological tests. Tables of normal values, expected weight for height, etc., are useful, but it must be remembered that nutritional care, like other aspects of nursing care, must be individualised and patient-centred. Obtaining the patient's confidence is as important as mastering technical procedures and measurement tools. Assessment and analysis should allow needs and goals to be set with the patient, and nursing interventions can be planned to meet these needs (see McLaren & Green 1998, Pedder 1998). As always, interventions should be recorded and regularly evaluated and modified as the patient's condition progresses.

Increasingly, nutritional factors are being recognised as influencing a number of disease processes, and in developed societies, diseases linked to lifestyle, including eating habits, are particularly important. Modern nursing requires an advanced understanding of nutritional issues and nurses need to be able to assess nutritional needs rapidly and accurately in both the hospital and community setting. Dietary assessment is a key skill for any nurse today. Bond (1997) uses a number of case studies to illustrate the importance of nutrition in a range of different settings. Bond's comprehensive resource pack *Eating Matters* should be essential reading for all health care professionals. The importance of a multidisciplinary approach is discussed by Steele (1998) and Lancaster (1998).

The dietary and clinical history

The dietary and clinical history provides a range of information on food intake, eating habits, food preferences, medications, medical conditions and other factors that may influence the individual's intake, digestion and absorption of nutrients. It is important to establish normal weight and any recent losses or gains. The nurse should also ask about changes in appetite, taste or smell, dental problems or problem dentures, food restrictions (allergies, cultural/ethnic factors, individual choices), food habits and meal pattern, economic/social factors (e.g. cooking facilities), medical conditions restricting intake or influencing GI function, medications (laxatives, antibiotics, etc.) and use of alcohol or drugs. The patient's usual activity level and exercise interests are also relevant. Box 21.6 provides a more complete summary of the type of data required.

If necessary, a 24-h recall using a questionnaire and interview is useful to determine the patient's consumption over the last 24 h. However, it is very subjective and care must be taken to ensure that the previous 24-h intake was typical for the patient. If poor nutrition is suspected, a daily food record might be useful and this is especially important if the patient is subjected to extensive investigations which might require fasting or risk missing mealtimes.

Physical examination

The patient's general appearance and fit of clothes should be noted, as should the condition of the hair, skin, eyes, mouth, neurological and musculoskeletal systems. Table 21.1 gives a brief summary of changes to look out for in the physical assessment.

Anthropometric evaluation

Anthropometric measurements provide an objective assessment of nutritional status — height, weight, skinfold thickness and muscle mass are the commonly used parameters. Although not routinely used by nurses, the skills could be easily taught and provide a useful addition to the physical examination. Non-invasive, low-cost approaches to nutritional screening are preferable (Bond 1997) and nurses are well placed to carry out this type of assessment. More shared learning between nurses and dieticians would help to strengthen these skills and improve nutritional care for patients. Regular checks of accuracy and, if necessary, recalibration are essential for all anthropometric equipment including scales.

Height and weight. Body weight is a useful indicator of nutritional status; it should be recorded on admission and monitored regularly. To ensure accuracy, the patient should, if possible, be weighed on the same scales at the same time each day, and preferably in the same clothes, and after emptying bladder and bowels. Single measurements of weight are of limited value, but serial measurements permit trends in weight loss to be identified; a rapid loss of 10% suggests mild undernutrition. A weight loss of 20%

Box 21.6 Data required from a dietary and clinical history (Miller & Torrance 1991)

Activity levels
- Occupation
- Exercise pattern

Appetite
- Good, poor, recent changes
- Changes and/or problems with the sense of taste or smell
- Effects of stress

Factors influencing food habits
- Cultural/ethnic influences
- Religion
- Educational level
- Nutritional knowledge/insight
- Eating patterns/family meal patterns

Gastrointestinal status
- Indigestion, 'heartburn'
- Flatulence, constipation
- Diarrhoea

Medical conditions/special diets
- Chronic diseases, e.g. diabetes, ulcerative colitis, coeliac disease
- Special diets, e.g. diabetic diet, low-salt diet, lactose-free, etc.

Social drug use
- Alcohol consumption, amount and frequency
- Smoking
- Other recreational drugs

Economic/social
- Income, spending on food
- Social benefits/services
- Cooking facilities and other services, e.g. meals on wheels

Foods
- Likes/dislikes
- Type/amount
- Food restrictions — allergies, intolerance
- Fluid intake — type, amount, frequency

Medications
- Type, dose, frequency
- Length of treatment
- Use of laxatives, emetics
- Vitamins or other supplements

Other problems
- Dental problems, dentures
- Problems with chewing/swallowing
- Physical or mental handicaps

indicates moderate and 30% severe malnutrition. However, caution is required when interpreting rapid weight losses; factors such as dehydration or oedema can complicate the clinical picture. Height is another useful indicator of under- or overnutrition, most often combined with weight for comparison with ideal values of weight for height and sex as obtained from standard weight/height tables.

Body mass index. Another, more recent, way of classifying weight is to use the body mass index (BMI). This is simply the body weight in kilograms (kg) divided by the height in metres squared (m^2). For example, someone with a body weight of 57 kg and a height of 1.62 m has a BMI of $57/1.62^2 = 22.3$ kg/m^2. The BMI tends to vary between 20 and 30. The ideal range is 20–25; 25–30 indicates overweight and a ratio of over 30 indicates obesity.

Triceps skinfold thickness (TSF). Skinfold measurements provide a good estimate of endogenous body fat. A number of sites can be used but the triceps is the most accessible and reproducible. Skinfold callipers such as the Holtain calliper are used, the measurement being made on the posterior aspect of the upper, non-dominant arm, midway between the olecranon and acromial process. A fold of skin is grasped between the thumb and forefinger and the callipers applied while the arm is relaxed and an average of three readings is recorded. Readings will not be accurate if oedema is present. The TSF can be compared with values from standard tables: less than 60% of standard will indicate severe malnutrition; less than 90% moderate malnutrition. Training is required for accurate measurement using skinfold callipers and other measures such as arm circumference are recommended for routine use.

Mid-arm circumference (MAC). Estimates of skeletal muscle mass can be obtained by measuring mid-arm circumference. The non-dominant arm is bent at right angles to the body and the mid-point between the acromial process of the scapula and the olecranon process of the ulna marked. Using indelible ink will help to ensure that later measurements can be made at exactly the same place. MAC is measured at this point with the arm relaxed. The undernutrition can be recognised by comparing the measured MAC with standard tables. It is important to use a high-quality, non-stretch anthropometric tape measure.

Mid-arm muscle circumference (MAMC). MAMC is calculated by the following equation using both triceps skinfold thickness (TSF) and mid-upper arm circumference (MUAC); it provides an index of skeletal muscle mass alone:

$$\text{MAMC (cm)} = \text{MUAC (cm)} - \pi \times \text{TSF (mm)}$$

where π is 3.14. MAMC is a useful indicator of PEM; less than 90% of standard indicates moderate and less than 60% severe PEM.

Laboratory investigations

Laboratory measurements are another useful source of objective data. A number of parameters, obtained from investigation of plasma, blood cells, urine and tissues (e.g. hair, liver, bone), can be measured to assess protein, fat, vitamin and mineral status.

Nitrogen balance. Nitrogen balance studies provide an index of protein status. Nitrogen balance is determined by estimating protein intake and subtracting urinary nitrogen excretion with an allowance for nitrogen loss via hair, skin and faeces. Additionally, losses from wound drainage or GI fistulae must be considered. A positive nitrogen balance indicates that the patient is in an anabolic state, while a negative balance indicates catabolism. A loss of 5–10 g/day would be defined as a mild negative balance, 10–15 g/day as moderate and over 15 g/day as severe.

Serum proteins. Total serum protein provides an estimate of nutritional status but is a relatively insensitive measure. Measurement of individual plasma proteins is sensitive. Albumin, transferrin, prealbumin and retinol binding protein, the major plasma proteins, are synthesised in the liver. Serum albumin levels reflect the protein status of the blood and internal organs. However, serum albumin is slow to reflect changes in nutritional status, and therefore low albumin levels represent long-standing PEM. Many disease states result in depressed albumin levels,

Table 21.3 Serum proteins of nutritional significance (Miller & Torrance 1991)

Protein	*Half-life*	*Other factors influencing levels*
Albumin	20 days	Extravascular pool, stress, trauma, infection
Prealbumin	2 days	Trauma, sepsis, cancer
Transferrin	7–8 days	Iron deficiency
Retinol binding protein	12 h	Vitamin A status

including liver disease, advanced kidney disease, sepsis and cancer. However, albumin has a long half-life (20 days) and there is a large reserve, so serum albumin levels will only fall after sustained protein loss. Accepted standards for serum albumin vary, but less than 3 g/dL suggests significant PEM. Other serum proteins, e.g. transferrin, have a shorter half-life and are more responsive to nutritional changes, providing an earlier indication of nutritional depletion than albumin (Table 21.3). However, as a large number of disease conditions, including trauma and sepsis, can alter serum protein levels, these parameters (like all biochemical data) need to be used with caution and in conjunction with other nutritional indicators and the clinical data.

Other parameters. Laboratory investigation can also assess more specific nutritional components. Fat status can be evaluated by measuring serum cholesterol, triglycerides or lipoproteins. Specific vitamins (e.g. vitamins C, D, B_1) or minerals (e.g. iron, zinc) can be assayed. Tests of immune function such as total lymphocyte count or skin testing are also useful indicators of nutritional depletion.

Accurate nutritional assessment relies on utilisation of data from a number of sources. Data from only one source can be open to misinterpretation due to the many factors, such as disease processes, that can influence individual parameters. A combination of dietary history, clinical examination, anthropometric measurements and laboratory studies is required to gain an accurate picture of the patient's nutritional status and to diagnose malnutrition.

ENCOURAGING THE PATIENT TO EAT

Nurses are ideally placed to help patients, whether at home or in hospital, to manage their nutritional needs. However, dieticians and occupational therapists are invaluable as the members of the health care team with special expertise in dietary and functional aspects of nutritional care. Nutritional assessment identifies dietary needs but a full nursing assessment will help in identifying the patient's ability to meet those needs and the level of intervention required. Nursing interventions may include the provision of nutritional education, assisting and encouraging an oral intake or managing an artificial (either enteral or parenteral) feeding regimen.

It is important to acknowledge that food has a number of non-nutritional roles, fulfilling a range of psychosocial needs. Eating will have very different expectations and associations for different people. Loss of menu choice, unfamiliar foods, food presentation, ethnic or cultural preferences, eating alone, eating in company, timing of meals, and even the eating utensils, can all influence the patient's motivation to eat. The patient's psychological state, e.g. stress due to the hospital environment or illness, may modify eating behaviour. Physical factors such as ability to manipulate cutlery, ability to chew and swallow, to taste food, even to reach food independently, will also be important. Assessment of all aspects of the patient and his environment that might influence food intake and enjoyment is critical. A carefully planned, nutritionally correct diet is of no value if the patient cannot or chooses not to eat the food. In managing an artificial feeding regimen, ensuring the provision of the essential nutrients is critical, but an understanding of the equipment and feeds used, essential monitoring, infection risks, psychological impact, and metabolic or mechanical complications is also required.

Oral intake

A number of individual factors (physical and psychological) and environmental or organisational factors will influence the patient's ability or willingness to eat an adequate diet. For an individual to successfully ingest an adequate oral diet, a number of activities are required and have to be assessed:

- Is the patient able to go shopping and to choose and purchase appropriate foods?
- Is his nutritional knowledge adequate for informed choice and has he the financial resources to purchase the required foods?
- Once purchased, can he easily transport food home or is a delivery service available?
- Are there adequate facilities for storing food at home (e.g. refrigerator)?
- Are adequate cooking facilities available and can the patient use them safely?
- Can the patient feed himself or does he need help?

If a deficit occurs in any of these areas, the nurse may need to look at alternative strategies; the occupational therapist may have a major role in assessing the home environment.

Shopping for food can be difficult for disabled people, the ill elderly and some patients with behavioural disturbances. Mobile shops and delivery services may overcome these problems, if they are available and the individual can cope with ordering the food. However, where these services are unavailable or psychiatric or communication difficulties limit their use, the patient will require outside assistance. The family or informal carers may be involved, as can social services (e.g. home helps) or voluntary agencies.

Food preparation can also be a problem. The home environment should be assessed for access to the kitchen, and access to worktops, cupboards, fridges and cookers. For example, a patient who is dependent on a wheelchair may need substantial alteration to the kitchen to enable independent food preparation. Patients with chronic illness such as multiple sclerosis or rheumatoid arthritis may have limited mobility or may find food preparation tiring and need adapted equipment and lightweight cooking utensils. Perceptual problems and confusion may also interfere with independent food preparation. Again, if the patient cannot cope, or he can only cope with assistance, family or community services may need to be involved.

Physical factors influencing eating

To eat and drink normally requires the ability to transfer food to the mouth, the ability to chew and the ability to swallow. It is important to realise that while manual dexterity with eating implements such as knives and forks is usually assessed, in some cultures the norm is to eat with the fingers or to use alternative

Box 21.7 Physical factors influencing eating

Oral cavity
- Congenital abnormalities, e.g. cleft lip and palate
- Dentition — natural teeth, dentures, edentulous
- Oral health — xerostomia, gingivitis, stomatitis, mouth ulcers, pain
- Sensory — temperature sensation, taste, smell

Chewing and swallowing
- Age
- Dentition
- Dysphagia
- Achalasia

Dexterity/mobility
- Perceptual problems
- Upper limb function
- Mobility
- Positioning

Others
- Dyspnoea
- Pain

implements such as chopsticks. Sensory function is also important; appetite is improved and eating is easier if we can see, smell and taste the food. Digestion and absorption of the nutrients are dependent on effective GI function, and utilisation is dependent on metabolism. Box 21.7 lists physical factors that influence eating. The state of the teeth and mouth is important. Cleft lip and cleft palate are examples of congenital abnormalities that reduce a baby's ability to suck. Teeth are needed for effective chewing; edentulous patients may require food of a softer texture or cut into smaller pieces but seldom a diet of only mashed or minced foods. Edentulous patients can suffer from malnutrition. In one study of 130 healthy individuals carried out as long ago as the 1960s, it was found that protein intake was inversely correlated with chewing ability (Davidson et al 1962). If the oral tissues are dry, inflamed or painful, the patient may be reluctant to eat. In xerostomia, artificial saliva can be used to help lubricate food. Oral health may also contribute to improving the taste/enjoyment of a meal; poor oral hygiene can mask taste and reduce appetite. The number of taste buds per papilla of the tongue decreases with age and taste changes can occur in some conditions such as cancer. Strohl (1983) has suggested the use of mouthwashes prior to food for cancer patients with taste alterations. In the elderly, the sensations of sweet and salty tend to deteriorate, while sour and bitter tastes are better detected. They may therefore prefer more highly seasoned food.

The odour of food is an important aspect of taste and enjoyment. Conditions such as upper respiratory tract infections can cause a temporary reduction in the sense of smell. Rare conditions causing anosmia may alter the patient's perception of food. Ageing may also be associated with alterations in the sensation of smell. Reduced oral sensitivity or confusion may cause the temperature of food to be misjudged, resulting in a greater risk of scalds and burns. The visual appearance of food is also important; meals that look unappetising or are poorly presented may reduce interest in eating. The visually impaired will appreciate knowing where different foods are positioned on the plate.

The texture of food and the patient's perception of his ability to chew it are also important. Problems with mastication appear to increase with age and may often be related to poorly fitting dentures. In some conditions there may be difficulty in coordinating chewing, and the movements of the mouth may be uneven with a tendency for food to dribble out of one side.

Dysphagia is defined as difficulty in swallowing and has a number of causes. It may be due to neurological injury, as in stroke, mechanical or motor obstruction of the oesophagus, oesophagitis and oesophageal cancer. Odynophagia — pain associated with swallowing — is often due to reflux of gastric acid. Achalasia is a condition in which the smooth muscle of the lower oesophagus and cardiac sphincter of the stomach fail to relax leading to dysphagia, vomiting and odynophagia. The degree of dysphagia must be assessed. It may be that only soft foods or liquids can be tolerated. If oral intake is problematic, supplementary artificial feeding can be instigated. If oral intake is not possible, parenteral or tube feeding is required.

Reduced mobility may cause problems in access to foods, choice of place for eating and attaining a comfortable eating position. Care and perhaps some dietary alterations may be required if supine or prone positions have to be adopted for eating. Any impediment of arm or hand movement or hand–eye coordination may diminish the ability to eat. The patient may need assessment for eating aids such as cutlery with special grips or shapes. If the patient has to eat one-handed, stabilisation of plates and the provision of plate guards may help. Drinking may also be a problem and special cups and glasses are available. If the patient suffers from muscle weakness, special lightweight utensils can be ordered. A number of diseases may result in problems with feeding, but stroke is an example of a disease which can markedly alter many aspects of feeding behaviour. The nurse can assess eating skills, and an occupational therapy consultation will help in the identification of suitable eating aids.

Organising effective mealtimes

Ensuring a supply of nutritious food, at the right temperature and in an attractive and hygienic manner, is the responsibility of both nursing and catering services. Although nurses remain responsible for ensuring adequate nutrition, their role in the preparation and distribution of food has tended to be reduced. Food preparation is not usually a nursing task, but the nurse is responsible for ensuring that food is ordered and may have to act as a buffer between the patient and the centralised catering services. Meals are often delivered to the wards preplated in heated trolleys at times dictated by catering service needs. With the withdrawal of Crown Immunity, reheating of meals or preparation of small snacks in the ward kitchen is discouraged. However, some patients may need or prefer more frequent, smaller meals. Patients may miss meals due to investigations, treatments, etc., and obtaining meals in these cases can be difficult if catering services are inflexible. In one study it was found that for some patients, food had to be ordered 2 days in advance, which is not always possible in the acute areas (DHSS & Welsh Office 1976).

Mealtimes

Ideally, mealtimes should be a planned part of nutritional care; used appropriately they can be an effective therapeutic event. Meals are often the focal point of the day, providing landmarks that break up the day and lend a familiar pattern to the ward routine. For the elderly person at home, the arrival of a midday meal may be an important social event; in a busy ward sharing a table may help patients to break down barriers. Mealtimes must not be considered as an inconvenience, disrupting ward activities three times a day. Rather they should be orchestrated to be, where possible, a pleasurable social activity. Properly managed they can provide a useful focus for the social activities of the ward. To make the most of meals, they should be planned in relation to timing, environment and, of course, menu and nutritional value. A King's Fund study (1986) indicated that 'food should be given priority over other work when it appears on the ward'.

Ideally the timing of meals would be flexible, allowing individual patients to continue with their normal pattern of mealtimes. Unfortunately the necessities of catering for large numbers preclude this. Mealtimes should not coincide with other structured ward activities such as drug rounds, shift handovers or staff breaks, since there is a risk that they will then be hurried and unsatisfactory for both nurse and patient. Some patients may like to take their time over meals and others may require assistance in eating. Hovering staff, in a hurry to clear away dishes, will not encourage appetite. Even when meals are preplated and the trays distributed by domestic staff, it is essential for the nurse to be involved.

Timing of meals may have to be a compromise, reflecting the needs of the individual, the ward and the catering service. Breakfast need not be inflexible, especially if cold cereals or a continental style breakfast have been chosen. Midday is probably an appropriate time for lunch for most people but it may not be the main meal of the day for some. The evening meal is often the main meal for working people but in hospital it may occur too early, at around 17.00 h. It also tends to leave a long gap before breakfast. A snack and hot drink later in the evening may be essential. In the hospital surveyed by Simon (1991), breakfast was delivered at 09.30 h, lunch at 11.30 h and tea at 17.30 h. This resulted in a gap of only 2 h between breakfast and lunch. Not surprisingly, the late breakfast was eaten well but lunch poorly! Kirk (1990) also found that timing of meals influenced how much was eaten. Some flexibility over mealtimes is preferable in the acute setting but it is essential that an effort is made to meet residents' needs and norms in long-term care.

Ideally the patient will have a choice of where he eats. While some may prefer to eat by their bed or in their own room, a separate dining area, distinct from the bed spaces and treatment area of the ward, is required. The nature of the open ward, with inevitable sights, sounds and smells of illness, is not conducive to appetite. The dining area should be decorated to provide a social atmosphere and provided with small tables to allow patients to eat in their natural groupings. Provision for those who wish to eat alone or who need assistance is also necessary. Forcing relative strangers to eat together or to have to watch a person with eating difficulties will not aid appetite. Even if the eating area also has to double as the day room, it can be specifically set up at mealtimes. Tables should be bright and clean, and tablecloths, large napkins and other civilised accoutrements will help. Having large numbers of visitors in the ward while patients are eating may be a disadvantage. If a patient has visitors during meals, a phenomenon described by Holmes (1987) as 'feeding time at the zoo' might occur, with the patient having to eat surrounded by his visitors. If possible, it might be better for the patient and visitors to go to the cafeteria and eat together.

Food presentation

Although nurses do not always serve meals, it is important for them to make sure that each of their patients receives the right food in sufficient quantities. It is then easier to ensure adherence to dietary regimens and, after a meal, to estimate the patient's intake. The patient needs to be active in food selection. Helping him to fill in a menu card or offering him a choice from a bulk trolley is an important nursing function. Foods should be attractively served, with small inviting portions (usually they are too large) placed separately on the plate. Presenting a heaped plate of food to an ill person with a poor appetite will be counterproductive. For some, large portions of food can be daunting (see Research Abstract 21.2). In a study of anorexia nervosa sufferers, it was found that they exaggerated the size of food portions and might find smaller portions more tempting (Yellowlees et al 1988). The temperature of food is another factor that affects appetite; cold food was one problem noted in the DHSS & Welsh Office (1976) study. It is also important that food is served using a no-touch technique. Chipped or cracked crockery will not clean properly and can become a source of cross-infection.

Research Abstract 21.2
Improving presentation of food to the terminally ill patient

Williams & Copp (1990) carried out a study of food presentation to terminally ill cancer patients. They identified problems with ordering food 24 h in advance. Patients often could not remember what they had ordered; 85% found portions too large and off-putting. They also felt embarrassed about leaving food. Food was often too dry; more sauces and gravy were recommended. Food was often cold, meals too early or late, and food presentation poor.

The plated meals were replaced with a bulk trolley system. This allowed the primary nurses to serve their own patients. Patients made their choices from the food available, and portion size, order and timing of courses could be individualised. Other changes made included the use of smaller, decorated plates and bowls (to reduce portions), serviettes and individual salt and pepper pots on each tray. These changes improved enjoyment of meals and avoided complaints about the temperature, portion size and dryness of food.

Williams J, Copp G 1990 Food presentation and the terminally ill. Nursing Standard 4(5): 29–32.

For further information, see Patients' Association (1993).

21.5 Discuss the management issues that might arise from adjusting food presentation, timing and service.

Assisting patients to eat

When someone has difficulty eating, it becomes the nurse's privilege to help him with this basic activity of living. Feeding a patient requires considerable care and sensitivity. Having to be fed is a threat to the individual's integrity and self-esteem. This should be recognised and every effort made to minimise the negative aspects. Before preparing for the meal, the dependent patient should be offered a bedpan or urinal, followed by handwashing facilities. Eating is easier and more normal sitting out of bed, but the bedfast patient can be sat upright and made comfortable. An appropriate table is required so the patient can have his food set before him, allowing him to see the food and indicate preferences. The patient can be offered the opportunity to clean his teeth or use a mouthwash before (and after) the meal.

The nurse should sit level with the patient and encourage a relaxed social atmosphere. The patient's food habits must be identified and the rate and manner of feeding should be at the patient's normal pace and pattern. Plenty of time is essential to allow the patient to chew, to pause between mouthfuls and to have a drink when desired. If protection for the clothing is required, a normal serviette can be used. Plastic bibs or rolls of paper towel will damage self-esteem. Normal crockery should be used if the nurse is feeding the patient; if the patient is able to participate, then feeding aids may improve his independence. Spoons have their place but knife and fork should be used for the main course. The nurse should check that plates and food are at an appropriate temperature and ensure that any bones or fruit pips are removed.

Feeding a patient or assisting him in feeding himself is an essential nursing function. The patient should be closely observed and assessed for developing independence in eating. What he can do for himself he must be given the time and encouragement to attempt. Food and drink can be positioned on the dominant side, well within reach. If the patient cannot manage to pour a drink, a glass can be left ready filled. If he cannot manage to cut up his food, the nurse can do this but encourage him to do the rest. By giving the patient her full attention and allowing the patient to control the process of feeding as much as possible, the negative effects of having to be fed can be alleviated. As with any nursing activity, assisting with eating necessitates assessment of the individual, identification of problems and the required interventions, and evaluation and reassessment as the activity proceeds or the patient progresses.

Patients with poor appetite or dysphagia may not be able to ingest enough solid food to meet nutritional needs, and supplements of liquid foods between meals may be required. A number of supplementary oral or sip feeds are available. These may be powdered feeds added to milk or complete formulas. Many sip feeds can also be used as tube feeds. Although providing a range of nutrients, they are particularly useful for providing a supplementary energy intake. Patients may need some persuasion to take supplementary feeds and they may reduce food intake at meals. Barnes (1989) has suggested adding supplementary calories in the form of glucose powder to foods such as porridge and soups to overcome this problem. If a patient has a poor intake or requires assistance with feeding, it is useful to chart daily intakes of food and fluid and to note any successful feeding strategies in the nursing records.

ENTERAL FEEDING

Enteral or tube feeding involves delivering nutrients directly to the stomach or small intestine. Its success depends on normal absorption, but it provides a way of avoiding the oral route. The major enteral route is via a nasogastric tube, but longer tubes can be passed directly to the small intestine (nasoduodenal and nasojejunal). Less commonly a tube can be passed via the mouth — the orogastric route. Another form of enteral feeding is via tubes surgically inserted through the body wall into the oesophagus (oesophagostomy), the stomach (gastrostomy) and jejunum (jejunostomy). Gastrostomy is the most commonly used of the enterostomies.

For further information, see White (1998).

Nasal insertion is often preferred for short-term alimentation; it is well tolerated if a small-bore, flexible tube is used. Enterostomies are more likely to be used for long-term feeding or if transnasal passage is difficult. If feeding is likely to last for longer than 6 weeks or there is a risk of aspiration, enterostomy feeding is preferable. If the expected duration is less than 6 weeks and aspiration is not a major risk then the nasoenteral route can be used (Cataldo & Smith 1980).

Tube feeding represents a more 'normal' mode of feeding than the intravenous (i.v.) route. It has many benefits and is based on the maxim 'if the gut works, use it', although this is not an infallible guide. With appropriate patient selection, tube feeding can be used to meet all the daily demands for nutrients and water. It has been shown to be cost-effective and, because digestion and absorption follow a more physiological pattern, it helps to maintain normal structure and function in the small intestine (Rombeau & Jacobs 1984). In general, tube feeding can be considered as more cost-effective and less hazardous than intravenous alimentation. It remains an invasive treatment with complications as well as benefits. The relative simplicity of the method may result in the nursing skills and responsibilities involved being underestimated; as reported by Jones (1975), the management of enteral feeding may often be delegated to very junior nurses. In common with many 'basic' nursing skills, the management of tube feeding requires a considerable level of knowledge and expertise to ensure a satisfactory outcome for the patient.

Indications for enteral feeding

The enteral route can be considered for any patients unable to meet all their nutritional needs by oral ingestion. A voluntary oral intake of less than 80% of normal daily requirements indicates the need for supplementary feeding. Enteral feeding can be used as the sole form of nutrition or as a supplement to oral intake. The two major requirements for enteral feeding are:

- a sufficient area of functioning small intestine for absorption of nutrients
- convenient access for introduction of nutrients.

Provided that access, absorption and the availability of a suitable feed can be ensured, the majority of medical and surgical patients can tolerate enteral feeding (Moghissi & Boore 1983). Indeed, relatively few conditions preclude enteral feeding, but those that do include malfunctioning of the GI tract and major upper alimentary tract surgery. Tube feeding is contraindicated in adynamic ileus, total intestinal obstruction, some types of malabsorption and intractable vomiting, when parenteral nutrition should be considered. The unconscious patient can tolerate enteral feeding but the danger of aspiration must be recognised. If the comatose patient has serious pulmonary disease, vomiting or hiccuping and lacks a gag response then parenteral feeding is recommended; if a gag response is present and pulmonary dysfunction minimal then nasojejunal feeding can be considered (Shils 1988). High-output fistulae, particularly upper alimentary fistulae which cannot be bypassed by the feeding tube, are a contraindication (Moghissi & Boore 1983, Shils 1988). Tube feeding is indicated in a wide range of clinical situations; major indications are listed in Box 21.8. As transnasal tubes represent the commonest approach to tube feeding, they will be the focus of the rest of this section.

Nasoenteral feeding

Nasoenteral feeding is indicated when short-term nutritional support is required. Nasoenteric tubes include nasogastric, nasoduodenal or nasojejunal tubes. As the transnasal route does not interfere with oral function, nasoenteric feeding can be used to supplement oral intake. The traditional nasoenteral tube was a wide-bore rubber

Box 21.8 Indications for enteral feeding

Increased nutritional needs
- Protein-energy malnutrition
- Persistent anorexia
- Hypercatabolic states — burns, major sepsis, severe trauma

Compromised oral access to GI tract
- Facial/oral surgery
- Head and neck surgery
- Oesophageal stricture, surgery, fistula
- Carcinoma of the mouth or upper alimentary structures
- Functional or mechanical obstructions

Inability to eat
- Unconscious
- Confused/uncooperative

Unwillingness to eat
- Odynophagia — mucositis, pharyngitis, oesophagitis
- Persistent anorexia, e.g. related to chemotherapy or radiotherapy
- Psychiatric disorders resulting in a refusal to eat (anorexia nervosa)
- Cancer cachexia/anorexia
- Persistent nausea and vomiting

Danger of aspiration
- Dysphagia
- Neurological disorders with loss of cough reflex

Gastrointestinal disorders
- Fistula
- Short bowel syndrome
- Malabsorption syndromes
- Inflammatory bowel disease

or PVC tube such as the Ryle's tube. Although still used they are poorly tolerated and can cause pressure necrosis of the nares and oropharynx (Rombeau & Jacobs 1984). The wide bore may encourage cardiac sphincter incompetence and increase the risk of gastric reflux and aspiration (Cataldo & Smith 1980, Silk 1980, Janes 1982). Fine-bore feeding tubes of silicone or polyurethane are now available. These are softer, more pliable tubes that are better tolerated by the patient and less likely to cause pressure ulceration or sphincter problems. However, they are more difficult to insert (a wire introducer may be required) and, due to the narrow lumen, are prone to blockage. The tube can pass into the trachea without causing laryngeal spasm or respiratory distress and the position of the tube has to be checked by X-ray (the tubes usually have a weighted, radio-opaque tip). A tendency to collapse on aspiration makes it difficult to check for gastric acid. Choice of tube depends on the patient and the intended feed. In general a tube with the smallest bore compatible with the viscosity of the enteral formula should be used. Ports and connections on enteral feeding tubes and equipment must not be compatible with i.v. infusion sets.

The patient should be in an upright position while the tube is being inserted to avoid the risk of intracranial insertion. The length of tube required can be estimated by measuring the distance from the bridge of the nose to the ear lobe plus the distance from the tip of the nose to the xiphisternum (Delaney 1991). In general, a 36-inch tube is used for nasogastric intubation, and a 43-inch tube for the nasoduodenal/jejunal route. If radiography is not used, another method of checking placement must be adopted. Two main methods are aspiration with pH testing and air injection. Injecting 2–5 mL of air while listening over the stomach with a stethoscope for the whoosh or gurgling of the injected air is a common practice. Research by Metheny et al (1990) indicate that this is not a reliable method. Problems associated with this method listed by Delaney (1991) include:

- small-bore tubes do not always allow the entry of sufficient air for diagnosis
- vigorous peristalsis may mimic the sound of injected air
- there is a danger of pneumothorax if the tube is in the lungs
- an inexperienced nurse may misinterpret the sounds heard.

Kennedy (1997) summarises the issues associated with enteral feeding and the critically ill patient.

Selection of enteral feeds

The range of enteral feeds, oral or tube, is large. In general, hospitals tend to use commercially prepared feeds as these are of known nutritional content, sterile and designed for ease of nasoenteral administration. These feeds may be whole protein (polymeric) feeds or specialised partially digested (peptide) or fully digested (elemental) feeds. Specialised feeds are of importance where absorption is impaired as in inflammatory bowel disease.

Prescription of a tube feed depends on a complete assessment of the patient's nutritional needs. Protein content varies between 1.2 and 10 g/100 mL, energy content between 188 and 837 J/100 mL (45–200 kcal). The osmolality of feeds ranges from 184 to over 900 mosmol/kg. As most feeds are hyperosmolar, they can cause GI disturbances when feeding is being initiated or if they are infused too rapidly. Nutrient content will vary according to assessed need and disease state.

Methods of administration

Nasoenteral feeds can be delivered by intermittent bolus or continuous feeding (see Kennedy 1997). Bolus feeding was the traditional approach when large-bore nasogastric tubes were used. Gravity- or pump-controlled drip infusion can be intermittent or, more usually, continuous. Bolus feeding can be organised to reflect more closely the normal eating pattern, it permits free movement between feeds and is particularly convenient for home enteral nutrition. Its disadvantages are that it is more likely to result in feelings of nausea, vomiting, intestinal distension, cramps and diarrhoea. There is an increased risk of reflux and aspiration. Hanson et al (1975) reported that problems with tachycardia, nausea, gagging and regurgitation increased in normal subjects due to rapid feeding. To avoid overloading the stomach, the bolus should be limited to a maximum of 300 mL (Janes 1982) and sufficient time, 10–15 min, allowed to deliver the bolus. The risk of aspiration can be reduced by feeding the patient in an upright position and maintaining this position for an hour after the feed. As discussed, the position of the tube should be checked and if the gastric residue exceeds 75–100 mL the feed should be withheld (Holmes 1987). Flushing of the tube with water after the feed will help to reduce blockage and additionally may help by reducing the osmolality of the feed. For bolus feeding, it is probably better if the feed is approximately at body temperature.

Intermittent feeding by gravity or peristaltic pumps over a period of 30–40 min may be better tolerated than a bolus feed. However, for many patients continuous feeding is adopted. The feeding regimen may extend from 16 to 24 h. The advantages of continuous feeding are that it delivers a lower volume per hour, resulting in a smaller residual volume, reduces the risk of aspiration and increases patient tolerance. The major disadvantages are cost and the reduction in patient mobility, although the patient can move around with the enteral feeding set supported on a wheeled drip stand. The initial delivery should be at a rate of 25–50 mL/h and then it should be slowly increased until the desired rate is attained. It is also desirable to start with dilute feeds until the bowel has adapted (Chernoff 1983). The temperature of the feed is probably less important during continuous administration. Gormican (1970) and Kagarva-Busby et al (1980) have reported an association between cold feeds and diarrhoea, but other authors have found no adverse effects from administering cold tube feeds (Holt 1962, Fason 1967, Williams & Walike 1975).

The equipment for continuous feeding consists of the nasoenteral tube, a reservoir, a giving set and possibly a peristaltic pump. The reservoir may be a rigid plastic or glass bottle or a PVC bag. In addition there is a proliferation of products designed for use with particular tubes, or combining reservoir and giving set. PVC bag-type reservoirs can be difficult to fill and calibration is less reliable. Bottles require an airway but are easier to fill and allow more accurate monitoring of the volume administered. Reservoirs should not be used for more than 24 h. A number of peristaltic pumps are available for ensuring accurate delivery of feeds and these may be required for more viscous formulas. Use of a pump is convenient but does not remove the nurse's responsibility for monitoring the delivery of the nasoenteric feed.

Complications of enteral feeding

If patient selection and monitoring has been appropriate then the complications of enteral feeding can be prevented or identified and rectified at an early stage. Complications are rarely serious enough to discontinue feeding, but care is necessary to minimise their impact. Complications can be classed into three broad groups: mechanical, metabolic and gastrointestinal (see Tables 21.4–21.6).

Table 21.4 Mechanical and infectious complications of enteral feeding

Complication	*Prevention*	*Treatment*
Tube blockage	Flush tube with water when feed stopped/interrupted Maintain continuous flow Use correct feeding tube/nutrient solutions combinations	Flush tube Replace tube
Knotted tubes	Use acid-resistant tubes Use unweighted tubes Replace regularly Remove tubes with care	Note any pain on tube withdrawal If knotted end can be seen through the mouth, grip with forceps, pull out of mouth and cut; remove rest of tube as normal. If not seen, further investigation required
Misplacement	Insert tube with patient in an upright position Use correct type, length of tube Check position by aspiration and pH or by X-ray Particular care needed if the patient lacks a gag reflex, is unconscious or has severe facial injuries	Withdraw and replace
Displacement	Secure firmly; explain need for tube to patient Check position at least daily Marking the tube at the nares will facilitate monitoring of position	Replace tube
Aspiration	Elevate head of bed during continuous feeding, 30 min after intermittent feeding Correct placement of tube Check position before starting feed Use nasojejunal feeding Avoid use of large-bore tubes	Discontinue tube feeding
Discomfort	Ensure hydration Encourage nose breathing Lubricate lips Provide regular oral care Secure tube firmly Use smallest appropriate bore of tube	Give water by mouth if possible
Acute otitis media	Use small-bore, soft feeding tube	Change to other nostril Antibiotic therapy
Mucosal erosion (nares, nasal septum, nasopharynx, gastrointestinal mucosa)	Secure tube firmly to avoid Keep mucosa moist (see discomfort above) Avoid Ryle's or other wide-bore tubes Inspect nares daily	
Aspiration pneumonia	Avoid aspiration as above Risk greater if patient supine, unconscious, when cardiac sphincter is incompetent or if a Ryle's tube is used	
Contamination	Avoid non-sterile feeds Take care when handling feeds or equipment Change giving sets regularly Change bags/bottles after 24 h	

Table 21.5 Metabolic complications of enteral feeding. (Adapted from Forlaw & Williamson 1986)

Complication	*Monitoring*	*Intervention*
Hyperkalaemia	Routine electrolytes	Use lower potassium feed
Hyponatraemia	Routine electrolytes	Restrict water
Hypophosphataemia	Routine electrolytes	Phosphate supplements
Hyperglycaemia	Blood glucose testing Serum glucose level Urinalysis — glycosuria, ketones	Reduce infusion rate Administer insulin
Uraemia	Check blood and urine urea regularly Assess hydration Assess protein intake	Deal with dehydration Correct any protein/energy imbalance
Overhydration	Accurate daily intake/ output recording Weight regularly	Reduce flow rate
Dehydration	Accurate daily intake/ output recording Weight regularly	Additional water

Table 21.6 Gastrointestinal complications of enteral feeding. (Adapted from Taylor 1989, and Forlaw & Williamson 1986)

Complication	*Prevention*	*Treatment*
Nausea and vomiting	Avoid high fat or hyperosmolar feeds Avoid rapid infusion rates Use low lactose or lactose-free formulas Elevate head or bed during feeds Initiate feeding with low volume or dilute feeds Increase concentration and rate slowly Use enteral pump	Reduce infusion rate Dilute feed Change to lower fat formula Change to lower lactose or lactose-free feeds
Diarrhoea	Monitor antibiotic therapy Avoid hyperosmolar feeds If patient has not been eating or has been on PN, introduce enteral feeding slowly (gut atrophy) Use isotonic formula if appropriate Use lactose-free feeds Monitor hydration	Dilute feed Change to lactose-free feed Consider i.v. antibiotics or changing to better absorbed antibiotics Oral rehydration solutions might be required Check feeds for contamination
Constipation/overflow	Use fibre-containing feed Encourage mobility Monitor frequency and consistency of stool Ensure adequate water intake	Extra fluid and bulking agents Enemas or laxatives as appropriate
Distension/cramps	Commence feeding with slow rate and dilute feeds Use lactose-free formula	Reduce infusion rate Dilute formula Change to lactose-free feed

Careful monitoring of the patient is essential. Monitoring is required to prevent complications developing and to ensure that nutritional goals are being met. Daily recording of intake and output is essential, including calculation of nutritional content. Nutritional monitoring using anthropometric and biochemical parameters is also required. General monitoring of the patient and equipment is necessary to identify any technical problems. Monitoring of the patient receiving tube feeding has been extensively discussed by Moghissi & Boore (1983).

The psychological effects of tube feeding should also be considered, since food has a profound influence on psychosocial well-being. For a patient with facial injuries who is unable to chew, the enteral tube may represent control and relief from his anxieties over nutrition, but for others it may be yet another assault on their self-image and feelings of loss of control over their own lives. Enteral feeding can lead to a marked change in a patient's attitude to food. The nurse should try to:

- understand what tube feeding means to the patient and family
- encourage the patient to express his feelings about the feeding regimen
- ensure that nursing management recognises and meets the patient's needs
- discuss the duration and management of the regimen with the patient.

If tube feeding is likely to be a long-term intervention or is to be continued at home, then patient and family education becomes a priority. Padilla et al (1979) addressed some of the psychological aspects of tube feeding.

PARENTERAL NUTRITION

In parenteral feeding, nutrients in solution are infused directly into the venous system, usually via a large, central vein into the right atrium (Finlay 1997). Parenteral nutrition (PN) may be used as a supplement to oral or nasogastric feeding or it can be the sole form of feeding. This invasive technique is associated with several hazards and problems and should only be used when other methods have been excluded. The function of parenteral feeding is to provide the patient with adequate nutrients and water during a period of stress/illness when other methods of feeding are either impractical or inadequate. The need for parenteral feeding can be identified by accurate clinical and nutritional assessment and by anticipating the patient's nutritional needs as his condition or treatment progresses. Parenteral feeding is best initiated before the patient deteriorates. Early intervention can prevent or reduce the likelihood of other complications arising. Nurses have a major role in the management of PN and the important aspects to consider include:

- indications for PN
- assessment of needs and selection of nutrient solutions
- infusion systems for PN
- monitoring and management of PN
- complications of PN
- evaluation of PN.

Indications for PN

The risks and expense associated with PN are significant and three general factors should be considered when deciding to use this form of feeding:

- the availability of the GI system
- the degree of malnutrition
- the metabolic status of the patient.

PN will be the method of choice if the GI system is unavailable for use. Major abdominal surgery or injury, GI obstruction, fistula or malignancy, inflammatory disease of the bowel or malabsorption syndromes can all rule out the use of enteral feeding. Psychiatric disturbances, severe anorexia or coma may also indicate a need for PN. As discussed earlier, undernutrition may be common in some groups of hospitalised patients. Severely malnourished patients may not be able to tolerate the oral or enteral intake required to rectify their nutrition deficits, and supplementary parenteral feeding should be considered. In some cases of GI disease, the patient may be severely malnourished and require preoperative PN to prepare for the increased metabolic demands after surgery. Severe trauma, including extensive surgery, some malignancies and major sepsis, can induce a state of hypercatabolism which imposes an enormous demand on nutritional resources. If exogenous nutrients are not available, the catabolic demands can result in a marked loss of body tissues.

PN should be considered if a patient is severely malnourished before surgery or if he has not eaten for 5 days and is not expected to eat for another 7 days. PN may also be required in patients who are likely to be starved for over 5 days and have a history of a 7–10% loss of body weight in the preceding 2 months. With these basic considerations in mind, appropriate use of PN would include:

- Nutritional preparation of severely malnourished patients prior to surgery, e.g. those with mechanical obstruction of the oesophagus due to stricture or cancer, swallowing difficulties, gastric obstruction, severe gastric ulceration, cancer of the stomach or congenital abnormalities.
- Trauma to the GI system which may result in an inability to ingest or absorb foods. This trauma may be due to incidents or surgery or be secondary to other disease processes, e.g. fistula, perforated bowel, facial injuries, oesophageal injuries or intestinal tumours.
- Postoperative complications delaying enteral feeding, e.g. paralytic ileus, obstruction, short bowel syndrome, fistulas, peritoneal sepsis.
- Patients suffering from acute or chronic GI inflammation which is not responding to treatment, e.g. Crohn's disease, ulcerative colitis, severe gastroenteritis.
- Insufficient oral intake or malabsorption, e.g. in cancer and cancer chemotherapy or radiotherapy, severe trauma, burns, sepsis and other conditions resulting in a hypermetabolic state, major hepatic disease, pancreatitis, coma, nausea and vomiting secondary to CNS disease, anorexia nervosa, severe or chronic malnutrition.

Whilst there may be 'typical' indications for PN, each patient will have individual needs and pose a challenge to the staff. In order to successfully support and maintain a patient with PN, a team approach is needed, involving not only the nursing and medical staff but also the nutritionist, pharmacist and community nurses if the patient is to receive therapy at home. Specialist nutrition teams assist patients and carers to manage PN successfully at home, giving advice on such things as storage of PN bags, management of the regimen and equipment use.

Nutritional assessment and monitoring

Nutritional assessment for PN is carried out using the standard methods discussed earlier — dietary history, anthropometric measurements, laboratory and immune function data and clinical evaluation to identify requirements and deficits. Baseline measurements must be established; monitoring is critical during the stabilisation period and regular checks are still required once PN has been established. Local protocols for monitoring the progress of PN should be consulted. In addition, the patient's psychological status should be sensitively evaluated.

Venous access

Parenteral nutrition can be administered through a peripheral or central vein. Peripheral cannulation is not usually suitable for parenteral feeding as the solutions infused are often hypertonic and chemical irritation will result in thrombophlebitis. If peripheral cannulation is used, it should only be for 24–48 h before resiting the cannula, and the leg veins should be avoided.

Central venous catheterisation is currently the route of choice, although Colagiovanni (1997) advocates the use of peripheral vein access for short-term use, i.e. less than 14 days. The superior vena cava is the preferred vessel, as the inferior vena cava is more difficult to reach. Infusion into the vena cava promotes rapid dilution of the hyperosmolar infusates. The vena cava can be accessed by direct cannulation via the subclavian, external jugular, internal jugular or brachiocephalic veins. Catheters can be inserted by percutaneous puncture, a cutdown procedure or sometimes using a tunnelling technique. With tunnelling, there is some distance between where the catheter enters the skin and the point at which it enters the vein, which may facilitate better positioning of the catheter and reduce the risk of infection. Central venous catheterisation can also be carried out through a peripheral vein using a long catheter that is threaded up to the vena cava. Regardless of the approach adopted, an aseptic insertion technique and careful insertion site management are essential (see Ch. 20). The central venous line should ideally be inserted in the operating theatre where maximum control of the environment is possible. After insertion of the cannula, an X-ray should be performed to ensure that extravasation has not occurred.

Administration equipment

A large variety of i.v. cannulae and catheters are available for parenteral feeding. A rigid cannula is more likely to damage the internal lining of the vein and cause phlebitis. A flexible, strong catheter made from an inert, soft material is ideal. It should also be detectable by X-ray. Polyurethane catheters are often used although other materials are common. Infusion sets with Luer locks should be used. Flow control is important, and if infusion pumps are not available a burette can be used to limit the volume infused. In-line filters can be used to reduce phlebitis due to particulate and bacterial contamination.

Solutions for PN

Parenteral nutrition must meet all of the patient's requirements for water, energy, amino acids, vitamins, major minerals and trace elements. The fluid intake should cover loss via urine, faeces (especially if diarrhoea occurs), respiration, perspiration and any abnormal losses via wounds or drains. An estimate of fluid loss for an average adult would be 2.5–3.0 L/day. Energy and protein requirements should be determined after nutritional assessment and additional demands due to the medical condition taken into account. The need for water-soluble and fat-soluble vitamins, minerals and trace elements may be increased by the disease process. To meet all these needs, a variety of i.v. solutions are required. Table 21.7 lists nutrient solutions. Energy can be obtained from carbohydrate, fat or alcohol preparations. Carbohydrate and alcohol may be provided in amino acid solutions or supplied as separate sugar (dextrose, fructose or sorbitol) solutions.

Alcohol can be infused directly as ethanol but is commonly given with amino acids. A number of different amino acid solutions are available with varying proportions of essential and non-essential amino acids. They may contain additional energy sources. Fat is provided by soya bean oil emulsions with added glycerol and triglycerides. Vitamins, minerals and trace elements can be provided by a number of additive preparations (Table 21.8). Nutrients may be infused separately, but it is now common for pharmacy departments to prepare, under aseptic conditions, 3 L bags containing all the nutrients (except possibly fat) prescribed for the individual patient. These large bags reduce the frequency at which bags have to be changed, reduce the risk of infection and are much easier to manage for the patient receiving home PN.

Complications of PN

A number of complications are associated with PN, some of which have been dealt with by the use of the 3 L bag system, which provides most of the nutrients required over 24 h in a sterile, stable and more compatible format. When fluids had to be administered singly or in tandem, the sudden changes in the nature of the fluid meant marked fluctuations in body chemistry. Fat solutions are usually given separately, but some centres practise TNA (total nutrient admixture of triple mix) with some success. Possible problems with TNA include the following:

- a shorter shelf-life
- support for more bacterial growth
- more expensive plasticiser-free bags may be needed
- possible incompatibility with infusion pumps
- 0.22 mm bacterial filters cannot be used.

In addition, the 3 L system may lead to waste if the patient's nutrient needs change rapidly and bags in progress have to be abandoned.

Table 21.7 Some examples of nutrient solutions for PN

Product (manufacturer)	*Nitrogen (g/L)*	*Energy (kJ/L)*	*K^+ (mmol/L)*	*Na^+ (mmol/L)*	*Mg^{2+} (mmol/L)*	*Cl^- (mmol/L)*	*Acet⁻ (mmol/L)*	*Others (per L)*
Amino acids								
Aminoplasmal L5 (Braun)	8.03	850	25	48	2.5	31	59	Acid phosphate 9 mmol Malate 7.5 mmol
Aminoplex 5 (Geistlich)	5.00	4200	28	35	4.0	43	28	Ethanol 5% Sorbitol 125 g Malic acid 1.85 g
FreAmine III 8.5% (Kendall)	13.00	1400	—	10	—	<3	72	Phosphate 10 mmol
Perfusin (Kabi)	5.00	500	30	40	5.0	9	10	Malate 22.5 mmol
Synthamin 9 (Clintec)	9.10	1000	60	70	5.0	70	100	Acid phosphate 30 mmol
Vamin 9 (Kabi)	9.40	1000	20	50	1.5	55	—	Ca^{2+} 2.5 mmol
Lipid								
Intralipid 10% (Kabi)	—	4600	—	—	—	—	—	Fractionated soya oil 100 g Glycerol 22.5 g
Lipofundin S 10% (Braun)	—	4470	—	—	—	—	—	Soya oil 100g
Carbohydrate–electrolytes								
Glucoplex 1000	—	4200	30	50	2.5	67	—	Acid phosphate 18 mmol Anhydrous glucose 240 g Zn^{2+} 0.046 mmol
Plasma-Lyte 148 (Baxter) (water)	—	80	5	140	1.5	98	27	Gluconate 23 mmol
Plasma-Lyte 148 (Baxter) (dextrose 5%)	—	880	5	140	1.5	98	27	Gluconate 23 mmol Anhydrous glucose 50 g

Table 21.8 Nutrient additives for PN (adults)

Product (manufacturer)	*Purpose*	*Composition*	*Comments*
Addamel (Kabi)	Electrolytes and trace elements	Ca^{2+} 5 mmol, Mg^{2+} 1.5 mmol, Cl^- 13.3 mmol Traces: Fe^{3+}, Zn^{2+}, Mn^{2+}, Cu^{2+}, F^-, I^- (per 10 mL ampoule)	Addition to Vamin range (except Vamin 18)
Addiphos (Kabi)	Electrolytes	Phosphate 40 mmol, K^+ 30 mmol, Na^+ 30 mmol (per 20 mL ampoule)	Addition to Vamin range and glucose solutions
Additrace (Kabi)	Trace elements	Traces: Fe^{3+}, Zn^{2+}, Mn^{2+}, Cu^{2+}, Cr^{3+}, Se^{4+}, $Mb6^+$, F^-, I^- (per 10 mL ampoule)	Addition to Vamin range
Multibiona (Merck)	Vitamins	Ascorbic acid 500 mg Dexpanthenol 25 mg Nicotinamide 100 mg Pyridoxine 15 mg Riboflavin 10 mg Thiamine 50 mg Tocopheryl acetate 5 mg Vitamin A 10 000 units (per 10 mL ampoule)	Addition to infusion solutions
Solvito N (Kabi)	Vitamins	Biotin 60 μg Cyanocobalamin 5 μg Folic acid 400 μg Glycine 100 mg Nicotinamide 100 mg Pyridoxine 15 mg Riboflavin 10 mg Sodium ascorbate 113 mg Sodium pantothenate 16.5 mg Thiamine 3.1 mg	Addition to glucose infusions Intralipid (powder for reconstitution)
Vitalipid N (Kabi)	Vitamins	Vitamin A 330 units Ergocalciferol 20 units Tocopherol 1 unit Phytomenadione 15 μg (per mL)	Addition to Intralipid (10 mL ampoule)

NB: Amino acid and fat solutions are available in many different strengths and formulations, e.g. Intralipid 20%, Vamin 18 (18 g/L nitrogen), Synthamin 14 (14 g/L nitrogen). Paediatric and other special formulations are also available.

General complications associated with PN can be classed as:

- complications associated with the i.v. route, especially with central venous access
- complications associated with the nature of the feeding regimen
- difficulties arising from coexisting medical problems
- the psychosocial impact of artificial feeding upon the patient.

Colagiovanni (1997) discusses the nursing monitoring strategies for patients receiving PN in hospital.

Complications of the intravenous route

Chapter 20 considers the general problems of i.v. therapy. In PN, particular risks are those related to the long-term use of a central venous catheter and the administration of large quantities of viscous and hypertonic fluid. Mechanical problems of PN are listed in Box 21.9. Many of the complications associated with catheter insertion can be reduced by restricting insertion to experienced personnel.

Air embolism can occur during insertion when the syringe is removed; a head-down tilt will reduce the likelihood of this, because venous pressure is raised, preventing air aspiration. Intravenous administration sets must have a safety valve to prevent air entry if the fluid container is allowed to run empty. Pneumothorax is a common complication, although the incidence is reduced by using experienced personnel; haemothorax, brachial plexus injury and subclavian artery damage can also occur. Catheter displacement usually occurs during insertion and can be ascertained by radiography. Catheters may also become displaced during dressing changes, especially when adhesive transparent dressing are used (Moghissi & Boore 1983). Displacement can result in hydropneumothorax. Displacement of a peripheral PN cannula can result in serious extravasation and tissue necrosis. Catheters should be well secured when initially inserted. Catheter fracture and embolus are very rare with modern equipment.

Box 21.9 Mechanical complications of PN

- Air embolism
- Catheter displacement/accidental withdrawal
- Catheter infection and sepsis
- Catheter fracture and catheter embolus
- Catheter blockage

Catheter blockage can be due to blood or fat emulsions clotting within the lumen of the catheter. Blockage due to fats may also form at two-way taps and connections which are encouraged by interruption of flow. The need to change fluid bags should be foreseen and changeover accomplished with minimum delay. Slow infusion of hyperosmolar dextrose may also increase the risk of clotting at the catheter tip. Heparinisation may be useful when a catheter is not in use. Catheters should only be irrigated with caution and never if there is no blood return. As with general i.v.

therapy, local and systemic infections are a serious risk. It is a particular risk for the patient with a long-term cannula who may be immunocompromised and is receiving fat and hypertonic glucose solutions. These form an ideal growth medium if there is a breach of sterility. The sources of infection in PN are essentially the same as those discussed in Chapter 20 for peripheral i.v. lines. Stopcocks should be avoided and giving sets and infusion bags changed every 24 h.

These complications can be avoided or reduced if attention is paid to the management of the line. Poor management increases the risk of infection, and Finnegan & Oldfield (1989) consider catheter infection to be almost totally preventable. Scrupulous attention to the care of the insertion site, infusion lines and bag changes is essential, and hospital protocols should be observed. It is also important to reduce the number of 'breaks' in the infusion system and feeding lines should not be used for the administration of medications or the withdrawal of blood.

Complications associated with the infusion fluid

Satisfying the nutritional requirements of an individual through the i.v. route poses complex administration problems. Calorific intake, nitrogen balance and amino acids for protein synthesis need to be regulated together with the normal and specific constituents of the diet. An understanding of the processes involved in the absorption and metabolism of the i.v. products used in PN enables the nurse to appreciate the potential complications that may arise during therapy. On the whole, these complications are metabolic or are associated with the nature of the fluid being administered or the speed of administration, e.g. over- or under-infusion. The biochemical problems arise because the body's attempts to utilise different energy sources have metabolic effects; for example, high-carbohydrate infusions produce raised levels of carbon dioxide which in turn influence the respiratory pattern, particularly of patients with concurrent respiratory problems. Metabolic complications are identified in Table 21.9.

Table 21.9 Metabolic complications associated with parenteral nutrition

Nutrient	*Associated complications*
Carbohydrate	Hypoglycaemia Hyperglycaemia Hyperosmolar coma Respiratory distress Fatty liver
Amino acids	Raised blood urea Acid–base abnormalities Hepatic encephalopathy Raised ammonia levels, especially in the newborn
Fats	Overinfusion Acute reactions Immunosuppression Poor utilisation of fats, e.g. liver disease Reduced pulmonary function
Deficiencies	Fatty acids: linoleic acid Minerals: pH Vitamins, both fat- and water-soluble Trace elements, e.g. Fe, Se, Zn, Cu
Toxicity	Vitamin A
Others	Acid–base disturbances Hepatic toxicities

In order to detect and prevent these complications, accurate and continuous monitoring of the patient's condition is necessary, e.g. the routine monitoring of blood glucose levels with the prescription of appropriate insulin regimens. Nursing assessment of the patient is essential to monitor the patient's progress and response to therapy. Effective management of the patient with PN involves all members of the health care team. Body biochemistry will be monitored by both the nurse and the physician so that estimations of the patient's nutritional requirements may be made in conjunction with the nutritionist. The clinical pharmacist will then be responsible for preparing the prescribed i.v. regimen and advising on any potential administration problems.

Coexisting medical problems

The complexity of managing the patient receiving PN is often related to underlying medical problems, e.g. patients with hypertension, arthritis, diabetes, and renal, hepatic or respiratory diseases. Whatever the coexisting medical problems, they will influence the patient's need for, or response to, nutritional support and must be considered in the patient's nursing and medical management.

Psychosocial effects

Most patients on PN receive nothing by mouth and may rapidly lose the normal sensations and drives associated with both the physical and social aspects of eating. It is important to support the patient and family during this period, and they may require appropriate counselling related to the underlying illness. Hopefully, for those for whom parenteral feeding is not a lifetime necessity, PN will be gradually supplemented with oral or enteral feeding and the patient weaned gradually from therapy. During this adaptation period the patient may experience difficulties in ingesting food and suffer from diarrhoea, constipation, nausea, vomiting and the sensation of fullness. Loss of weight or absence of chewing may also have led some to experience problems with ill-fitting dentures. Some patients find it difficult to resume normal eating habits. At this stage, liaison with the family, the nutritionist and sometimes the occupational or speech therapist may prove of great value in restoring both eating habits and a pleasure in food.

For further information, see Henry (1997) and Reilly (1998).

FUTURE DIRECTIONS

In 1994, the British Association for Parenteral and Enteral Nutrition issued two reports (BAPEN 1994a,b) which highlight some of the issues for the future. The first report, *The Organisation of Nutritional Support in Hospital*, stated that over two-thirds of UK hospitals lacked a formal nutritional team and made four key recommendations:

- All patients in UK hospitals diagnosed as malnourished or at risk of developing malnutrition should have access to a nutritional support team.
- All patients at risk of developing malnutrition should be routinely screened prior to or on admission to hospital.
- A nutrition steering committee should be set up in all major hospitals or hospital groups to set standards and take responsibility for catering services, dietary supplementation and nutritional support.
- The nutrition steering committee should appoint nutritional support teams to implement the agreed standards.

The second report, *Enteral and Parenteral Nutrition in the Community*, recognised the growing need for nutritional support within community care. At any one time there are about 4000 patients receiving tube feeding at home and another 300 receiving home PN. The report recommends setting up local and national audit systems to monitor the cost and effectiveness of home nutrition services. It also recommends the establishment of expert, multidisciplinary nutrition teams to provide for administration, education and support of home nutrition services. Nurses clearly have an opportunity within these developments to reclaim nutrition as a key element of effective nursing care.

ACKNOWLEDGEMENTS

The author wishes to express her gratitude to Pamela A. Jackson, Lecturer in Nursing, Head of Acute Care Nursing Dept, Southampton General Hospital, Southampton, and Rosemary Richardson, Senior Lecturer-Dietetics, Queen Margaret University College, Edinburgh, for their advice and assistance with this chapter.

REFERENCES

Barnes E 1989 Increasing energy intake in hospital food. Nursing Standard 4(5): 30–31
Bistrian B R, Blackburn G L, Hallowell E et al 1974 Protein status of general surgical patients. Journal of the American Medical Association 230: 856–860
Bistrian B R, Blackburn G L, Vitale J et al 1976 Prevalence of malnutrition in general medical patients. Journal of the American Medical Association 235: 1567–1570
Bond S 1997 Eating matters. Centre for Health Services Research, University of Newcastle, Newcastle-upon-Tyne
British Association for Parenteral and Enteral Nutrition (BAPEN) 1994a The organisation of nutritional support in hospital. British Association for Parenteral and Enteral Nutrition, Maidenhead
British Association for Parenteral and Enteral Nutrition (BAPEN) 1994b Enteral and parenteral nutrition in the Community. British Association for Parenteral and Enteral Nutrition, Maidenhead
Cataldo D B, Smith L 1980 Tube feedings: clinical application. Ross Laboratories, Columbus
Chapman A 1996 Current theory and practice: a study of pre-operative fasting. Nursing Standard 10(18): 33–36
Chernoff R 1983 Enteral support: introduction to nutritional support. 7th Clinical Congress of American Society for Parenteral and Enteral Nutrition, Washington, DC
Colagiovanni L 1997 Parenteral nutrition. Nursing Standard 12(9): 39–43
Davidson C S, Livermore J, Anderson P, Kaufman S 1962 The nutrition of a group of apparently healthy aging persons. American Journal of Clinical Nutrition 10: 181–199
Delaney C J 1991 Nasogastric intubation: use and abuse. Surgical Nurse 4(3): 4–9
Delmi M, Rapin C H, Bengoa J M, Delmas P D, Vasey H, Bonjar J P 1990 Dietary supplementation in elderly patients with fracture of neck of femur. Lancet 335(8696): 1013–1016
Department of Health 1991 Dietary reference values for food energy and nutrients for the United Kingdom. Report of the Panel on Dietary Reference Values of the Committee on Medical Aspects of Food Policy (COMA). Report on health and social subjects 41. HMSO, London
Department of Health and Social Security and Welsh Office Central Health Services Council 1976 The organisation of the in-patient's day. HMSO, London
Elmquist J K, Maratos-Flier E, Saper C B, Flier J S 1998 Unraveling the central nervous system pathways underlying responses to leptin. Natural Neuroscience 1(6): 445–450
Fason M F 1967 Controlling bacterial growth in tube feeding. American Journal of Nursing 67: 1246–1247
Finlay T 1997 Making sense of parenteral nutrition in adult patients. Nursing Times 93(2): 35–36
Finnegan S, Oldfield K 1989 When eating is impossible: TPN in maintaining nutritional status. Professional Nurse 4: 271–275
Forlaw L, Williamson I J 1986 Advances in nutritional support. In: Tierney A J (ed) Clinical nursing practice. Churchill Livingstone, Edinburgh
Garn S M, Bailey S M 1976 Fatness similarities in adopted pairs. (Letter.) American Journal of Clinical Nutrition 29: 1067–1068
Garn S M, Clark D C 1976 Trends in fatness and the origins of obesity. Pediatrics 57: 443–455
Goldblatt P B, Moore M E, Stunkard A J 1965 Social factors in obesity. Journal of the American Medical Association 192: 1039–1044
Gormican A 1970 Prepackaged tube feedings. Hospital 44: 58–60
Hanson R L, Walike B C, Grant M, Kubo W, Bergstrom N, Padilla G, Wong H L 1975 Patient responses and problems associated with tube feeding. Washington State Journal of Nursing 47(1): 9–13
Henderson V 1960 Basic principles of nursing care. International Council of Nurses, Geneva
Hill G L, Pickford G A, Young C J et al 1977 Malnutrition in surgical patients. An unrecognised problem. Lancet 1: 689–692
Holmes S 1987 Artificial feeding. Nursing Times 83(31): 4958
Holt E 1962 A study of premature infants fed cold formulas. Journal of Paediatrics 61: 556–561
Janes E M H 1982 Nursing aspects of tube feeding. Nursing 2(4): 101–104
Jester R, Williams S 1999 Pre-operative fasting: putting research into practice. Nursing Standard 13(3): 33–35
Jones D 1975 Food for thought. Royal College of Nursing, London
Kagarva-Busby K, Heitkemper M M, Hansen B et al 1980 Effects of diet temperature on tolerance of enteral feedings. Nursing Research 29: 276–280
Kennedy J 1997 Enteral feeding for the critically ill patient. Nursing Standard 11(33): 34–43
Kilgore W W, Li M-Y 1980 Food additives and contaminants. In: Doull J, Klassen C D, Amdur M O (eds) Toxicology. Macmillan, New York, pp 593–607
King's Fund 1986 A review of hospital catering. King's Fund, London
Kirk S L 1990 Adequacy of meals served and consumed at a long-stay hospital for the elderly. Care of the Elderly 2(2): 77–80
Kowanko I, Simon S, Wood J 1999 Nutritional care of the patient: nurses' knowledge and attitudes in an acute care setting. Journal of Clinical Nursing 8(2): 217–224
Lancaster R 1998 Lifting the lid. Nursing Standard 12(46): 20–22
McLaren S, Green S 1998 Nutritional screening and assessment. Nursing Standard 12(48): 26–29
Mela D J, Rogers P J 1998 Food, eating and obesity: the psychological basis of appetite and weight control. Chapman and Hall, London
Methaney N, McSweeney M, Wehrle M A et al 1990 Effectiveness of the auscultatory method in predicting feeding tube location. Nursing Research 39: 262–267
Miller B, Torrance C 1991 Nutritional assessment. Surgical Nurse 4(5): 21–25
Moghissi K, Boore J R P 1983 Parenteral and enteral nutrition for nurses. William Heinemann Medical Books, London
Newman H H, Freeman F N, Holzinger K J 1937 Twins: a study of heredity and environment. University of Chicago Press, Chicago
Padilla G V, Grant M, Wong H et al 1979 Subjective distresses of nasogastric tube feeding. Journal of Parenteral and Enteral Nutrition 13: 53–57
Pedder L 1998 Nursing's nutritional responsibilities. Nursing Standard 13(9): 49–55
Perry L 1997 Nutrition: a hard nut to crack: an exploration of the knowledge, attitudes and activities of qualified nurses in relation to nutritional nursing care. Journal of Clinical Nursing 6(3): 315–324

Rombeau J L, Jacobs D O 1984 Nasogastric tube feeding. In: Rombeau J L, Caldwell M D (eds) Clinical nutrition, vol I. Enteral and tube feedings. WB Saunders, Philadelphia, pp 261–274
Roper N, Logan W W, Tierney A J 1996 The elements of nursing, 4th edn. Churchill Livingstone, Edinburgh
Shils M E 1999 Modern nutrition in health and disease, 9th edn. Williams & Wilkins, London
Short E A 1983 Perioperative starvation – an often underrecognised condition. The Australian Nurses Journal 13: 47–52
Silk D B A 1980 Enteral nutrition. Hospital Update 8: 761
Simon S 1991 A survey of the nutritional adequacy of meals served and eaten by patients. Nursing Practice 4(2): 7–11
Simopoulos A P 1985 The health implications of overweight and obesity. Nutrition Reviews 43(2): 33–40
Smith S H 1972 Nil by mouth? Royal College of Nursing, London
Steele C 1998 The links in the food chain. Nursing Standard 12(49): 25–27
Strohl R A 1983 Nursing management of the patient with cancer experiencing taste changes. Cancer Nursing 6(5): 353–359
Taylor S J 1989 Preventing complications in enteral feeding. Professional Nurse 4(5): 247–249
Thomas E A 1987 Preoperative fasting – a question of routine? Nursing Times 83: 46–47
Tierney A J 1996 Undernutrition and elderly hospital patients: a review. Journal of Advanced Nursing 23(2): 228–236
Todd E A, Hunt P, Crowe P J et al 1984 What do patients eat in hospital? Human Nutrition: Applied Nutrition 38A: 294–297
Torrance C 1991 Preoperative nutrition, fasting and the surgical patient. Surgical Nurse 4(4): 4–9
Torrance C 1992 Absorption and function of iron. Nursing Standard 6(19): 25–28
Williams J, Copp G 1990 Food presentation and the terminally ill. Nursing Standard 4(5): 29–32
Williams K R, Walike B C 1975 Effect of temperature of tube feeding on gastric motility of monkeys. Nursing Research 24: 4–9
Yellowlees P M, Roe M, Walker M K, Ben-Tovim D I 1988 Abnormal perception of food size in anorexia nervosa. British Medical Journal 296(6638): 1689–1690
Zhang Y, Proenca R, Maffei M, Barone M, Leopold L, Friedman J M 1994 Positional cloning of the mouse obese gene and its human analogue. Nature 372: 425–432

FURTHER READING

Association of Community Health Councils 1997 Hungry in hospital? Association of Community Health Councils for England and Wales
Bond S 1997 Eating matters. Centre for Health Services Research, University of Newcastle, Newcastle-upon-Tyne
Colagiovanni L 1997 Parenteral nutrition. Nursing Standard 12(9): 39–43
Coates V 1985 Are they being served? Royal College of Nursing, London
Cole K D, Jones F A 1995 Interdisciplinary teams for the solution of nutritional problems. In: Morley J E, Glick Z, Rubenstein L Z (eds) Geriatric nutrition: a comprehensive review, 2nd edn. Raven Press, New York, pp 367–375
Department of Health 1991 Dietary reference values for food energy and nutrients for the United Kingdom. Report of the Panel on Dietary Reference Values of the Committee on Medical Aspects of Food Policy (COMA). Report on health and social subjects 41. HMSO, London
Department of Health 1992 The nutrition of elderly people. Report 43 on health and social subjects. HMSO, London
Finnegan S 1989 Mechanical complications of parenteral nutrition. Professional Nurse 4: 325–327
Garrow J S, James W P T 1993 Human nutrition and dietetics, 9th edn. Churchill Livingstone, Edinburgh
Hasan M, Meara R J, Bhownick B K et al 1995 Percutaneous endoscopic gastrostomy in geriatric patients: attitudes of health care professionals. Gerontology 41(6): 326–331
Henry L 1997 Parenteral nutrition. Professional Nurse 13(1): 39–42
Holmes S 1998 Food for thought. Nursing Standard 12(46): 23–27
Kennedy J 1997 Enteral feeding for the critically ill patient. Nursing Standard 11(33): 34–43
Lennard-Jones J E 1992 A positive approach to nutrition as treatment. Report of a working party on the role of enteral and parenteral feeding in hospital and a home. King's Fund, London
McWhirter J P, Pennington C R 1996 A comparison between oral and nasogastric nutritional supplements in malnourished patients. Nutrition 12(7–8): 5502–5506
Mela D J, Rogers P J 1998 Food, eating and obesity: the psychological basis of appetite and weight control. Chapman and Hall, London
Nutrition in practice 1997 Nursing Times 93–94 (parts 1–11) (occasional series)
Patients' Association 1993 Catering for patients in hospital: guidelines on hospital food. Patients' Association, London
Pi-Sunyer F X 1988 Obesity. In: Shils M E, Young V R (eds) Modern nutrition in health and disease, 7th edn. Lea & Febiger, Philadelphia, pp 795–816
Reilly H 1998 Parenteral nutrition: an overview of current practice. British Journal of Nursing 7(8): 461–467
Scientific Committee for Food for the European Community 1993 Report on proposed nutrient and energy intakes for the European Community. (Editorial.) Nutrition Reviews 51(7): 209–212
Shils M E (ed) 1999 Modern nutrition in health and disease, 9th edn. Williams & Wilkins, London
Starkey J F, Jefferson P A, Kirby D F 1988 Taking care of percutaneous endoscopic gastrostomy. American Journal of Nursing 1(42): 42–45
Taylor S, Goodinson-McLaren S M 1992 Nutritional support: a team approach. Wolfe, London
White S 1998 Percutaneous endoscopic gastrostomy. Nursing Standard 12(28): 41–45
Wykes R 1997 The nutritional and nursing benefits of social mealtimes. Nursing Times 93(4): 32–34

TEMPERATURE CONTROL

Charmaine Childs

22

INTRODUCTION

The aim of this chapter is to give the student nurse a basic understanding of the factors and processes which are involved in thermoregulation, i.e. the maintenance of body temperature at a near-constant level. Only when the nurse has a clear understanding of these physical, physiological and biological mechanisms will he be able to provide rational treatment for patients whose thermoregulatory system is disturbed (Edwards 1998). There are a number of reasons why body temperature might rise or fall out of the 'normal' range, and it is essential that the treatment the patient receives for an alteration in body temperature does not cause the problem to worsen. Unfortunately, it often happens that a patient's condition is exacerbated by attempts to correct a rise or fall in deep body (core) temperature. Excellence in clinical practice cannot be achieved without a proper understanding of the patterns of normal body temperature and of the pathological processes which give rise to problems.

Taking a person's temperature with a clinical thermometer is one of the most commonly used methods for detecting disturbances in health (Cutter 1994). It is therefore an extremely important clinical measurement but one which in practice is often done rather badly. The responsibility of the nurse, whether practising in the home or hospital, is to record an accurate measurement which can be used with confidence to guide decisions about treatment. Simply recording a temperature measurement without appreciating what it reflects about the person's condition is not good nursing practice. The nurse needs to understand the factors which contribute to the production of body heat, why normal body temperature is 'set' at about 37°C, and how much this can be expected to vary in health and illness. He must also understand in what circumstances treatment should be given for alterations in body temperature.

NORMAL BODY TEMPERATURE

'Body temperature' is a general term frequently used to refer to a person's temperature, without regard to the site at which that temperature was taken. However, since temperature varies so much across the skin surface and within the tissues of the body, it is good practice to avoid the use of this rather vague term and to report the temperature of the site used, e.g.: 'Axilla temperature of Mr A on admission to hospital was 36.9°C', or 'Oral temperature of Mrs B was 37.1°C'.

The temperature of the tissues of the body

Surface temperature

The body is not at a uniform temperature at all sites or in all tissues. Under most circumstances, the skin surface is the coolest area. The skin is often referred to as the 'shell' and the organs, blood and deeper tissues as the 'core' of the body (Tortora & Grabowski 1996). Skin temperature varies very much in accordance with air temperature (see Fig. 22.1) and will be considerably lower than oral, axillary or rectal temperature.

Q

22.1 After examining the temperature data given in Figure 22.1, answer the following questions:

(a) What is the reason for the change in the size of the shell between A and C?

(b) What is the explanation for the higher skin temperatures at the extremities in A compared with C?

(c) What do you notice about the skin temperatures measured over the thigh, leg, foot and toe in A? Why is the pattern of skin temperature in A different from those in B and C?

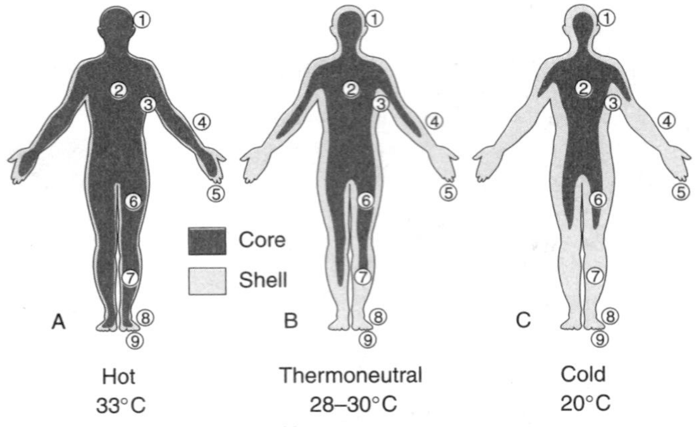

	Site	A (°C)	B (°C)	C (°C)
1	Scalp	36.0	34.8	32.8
2	Chest	35.8	34.5	31.3
3	Axilla	36.5	36.4	36.4
4	Arm	35.9	33.5	27.6
5	Finger	35.9	33.2	21.0
6	Thigh	35.2	33.4	27.8
7	Leg	35.3	30.1	25.2
8	Foot	35.5	29.7	22.7
9	Toe	36.2	29.1	21.4

Fig. 22.1 Core temperature and temperature of the skin surface at various sites in a hot, thermoneutral and cold environment. (Based on an original figure by Aschoff & Wever, cited in Stainer et al 1984, with additional data from Childs C.)

Deep body (core) temperature

The body core is well protected from the environment but not all of the organs contained within it are at the same temperature. The liver, kidney, brain and myocardium, for example, have a high metabolic rate and consequently a higher temperature than tissues with a lower rate of metabolic activity such as smooth muscle (Houdas & Ring 1982). Whilst there are slight differences in the temperature of different organs, for the purpose of patient measurement there are only a few sites where deep body temperature can be measured reliably without causing pain or distress. A recent study in children has shown that deep body temperatures measured with a thermistor inserted into the rectum and a thermistor incorporated into a urinary bladder catheter are almost identical (Childs et al 1999). Rectal temperature is an accurate method for measuring deep body temperature (Jensen et al 1994) and one can probably dispense with the notion that rectal temperature is slow to change, lagging behind temperature measurements made at other sites.

It is important to be precise when taking a patient's temperature. This means that the same site and the same method should be used each time the nurse takes a patient's temperature. If this is not possible and the site must be changed, then the temperature chart should be marked to show the change of site. It is also important to be consistent in the way in which a temperature measurement is taken, e.g. by leaving the thermometer in situ for the same duration each time. For these reasons, the taking of temperatures should always be done by qualified nurses or students under supervision and should not be delegated to health care assistants. The advantages and disadvantages of the oral, axillary and rectal sites for temperature measurement are listed in Table 22.1.

REGULATION OF BODY TEMPERATURE

Current understanding is that mammalian thermoregulation is controlled by the brain. Observations made in the early 19th century found that the body cooled down after severe damage to the spinal cord. This finding led people to believe that the nervous system was important in thermoregulation. Over a century later, Bazett and Penfield (see Bligh 1972) showed just how important the brain was (particularly the hypothalamus) in the control of body temperature.

Even though a hypothalamic nerve cell or group of cells has still not been identified as the precise location for the control of body temperature, the pre-optic region within the anterior portion of the hypothalamus has been shown to be vital for an intact thermoregulatory system.

Information from thermoreceptors in the skin and in the deeper organs is integrated within the hypothalamus. Outgoing, or efferent signals stimulate changes in either heat gain or heat-losing processes if the temperature of the blood bathing the cells of the hypothalamus starts to change from that of the body's own thermostat or 'set-point' temperature. An intact nervous system is essential, not only to permit the transmission and reception of afferent signals but also to allow the transmission of signals to effector organs such as muscles (for shivering) and sweat glands.

If incoming information indicates that the body is above or below its normal thermostat temperature (Fulbrook 1993), often referred to as the temperature 'set-point', an 'error signal' is received. The error signal is a useful concept borrowed from engineering theory to describe incoming sensory signals which differ from the brain's thermostat reference temperature. When an error signal is received, the nervous system stimulates activities which protect the person from overheating or from becoming too cold. If the former situation occurs, mechanisms will be stimulated to

Table 22.1 Sites for body temperature measurement: advantages and disadvantages

Site	*Nursing practice*	*Advantages*	*Disadvantages*
Mouth (posterior sublingual pocket)	Leave mercury-in-glass thermometer in situ for 8 min	Safe and accessible, particularly in adults and older children. Reliable indication of 'core' temperature	Inaccurate results after recent hot or cold drinks, food or smoking Wait 20–30 min before taking measurement in these circumstances
Axilla	Place in centre of armpit, hold arm against chest. Leave in position for 9 min	Ideal for temperature measurement in babies and toddlers	Less accurate than oral or rectal measurements but can be a reasonable indicator of core temperature if thermometer is left in situ for the required length of time. Since it is a measurement which is not taken in a body cavity, there is more chance of external influences affecting the result
Rectum	Insert rectal thermometer 4 cm into the anus (adults) or 2–3 cm in an infant. Leave in situ for 4 min	Suitable site for babies or for unconscious patients who need continuous temperature monitoring	Unacceptable for routine monitoring in some conscious patients, although seriously ill patients with fluctuating conscious levels may require rectal temperature monitoring. Rectal temperature may be higher than at other sites. There is a lag phase between the true 'core' temperature and the rectal temperature
Ear (e.g. using the Core Check™ thermometer; model 2090, Ivac, Basingstoke, UK)	Gently pull the pinna of the ear backwards. Insert the ear piece into the auditory canal. The thermometer emits a 'buzz' when the measurement is complete	Simple and quick. The measurement takes only 1–2 s. Plastic disposable probe cover limits cross-contamination	The ear piece can be difficult to place correctly in babies. Measurements may be inaccurate if not placed correctly. False low readings occur when ears are cold. There can be temperature differences between ears. Nurses should take an average of two ear temperatures (right and left) whenever possible

promote heat loss; in the latter case, mechanisms to conserve or produce heat will be activated. In this way, deep body temperature is prevented from fluctuating greatly from its biological set-point.

Mechanisms of heat conservation and heat production

There are many circumstances which could cause the temperature of the blood bathing the cells of the hypothalamus to rise above or fall below the set-point temperature of 37°C. These include exposure to modest or extremely high air temperatures as well as disturbances in the rate of heat produced or lost from the skin surface. When conditions such as these alter the hypothalamic temperature, even if only very slightly, homeostatic mechanisms are brought into operation to restore core temperature to 37°C.

Heat conservation (see Fig. 22.2A)

If a person becomes cold and core temperature falls slightly, signals from peripheral thermoreceptors in the skin are interpreted at the pre-optic region of the hypothalamus to stimulate the heat-promoting centre to begin actions to retain heat and/or to increase the amount of heat produced within the body, the aim being to restore body temperature to 'normal'.

Behavioural thermoregulation. The ability of humans to conserve heat by putting on more clothes or seeking shelter is often overlooked as a most important aspect of thermoregulation, but these are, in fact, the first protective thermoregulatory responses to feeling cold. Very young and very old people, as well as those who are immobile due to illness or sedation, are unable to protect themselves from cold and are therefore more vulnerable to changes in environmental temperature. It then becomes the responsibility of the nurse to place his patient in a warm and comfortable situation so that body temperature does not fall.

Peripheral vasoconstriction. At about the same time that a person begins to recognise feelings of cold, changes in the flow of blood to peripheral tissues also occur. Nerve impulses from the area of the hypothalamus concerned with heat conservation cause blood vessels, particularly in the hands, feet, ears and nose, to constrict. Sympathetic stimulation to nerves supplying the blood vessels in these regions (described as acral regions) results in peripheral vasoconstriction and a reduced flow of warm blood from internal organs to the skin. This means that heat is retained or stored in the body, where it maintains the core tissues at or close to 37°C.

In situations where body temperature continues to fall, despite the above measures, additional mechanisms that involve heat production come into play (see non-shivering and shivering thermogenesis below) in order to restore body temperature to normal.

Q **22.2** What steps should be taken by a nurse to help a patient with a low core temperature to retain body heat? What are the harmful or adverse effects of allowing a patient to shiver continuously?

Heat production

In a healthy 20-year-old adult, the metabolic rate is between about 35 and 39 kcal/m^2 body surface per h. In an infant the metabolic rate is 53 kcal/m^2 per h. This difference can be explained by the fact that the rapid synthesis of cells in the growing body of a child contributes to an increased metabolic heat production. Metabolic rate can be increased well above the normal limit for a given age in sick or injured patients, particularly those who are febrile and/or have an infection (Childs & Little 1994, Jenney et al 1995). Patients suffering from serious burns (see Ch. 30) have been shown to undergo a large increase in metabolic rate (Wilmore 1977), but more recent studies have indicated that the increase in metabolic activity is not as great as was once thought and that the most likely explanation for this is the change in the management of burn wounds, i.e. by the early surgical removal of dead and necrotic tissue and its replacement with healthy skin grafts (Childs 1994).

Any situation or series of events which increases the rate of chemical reactions in cells (and thus the rate of oxygen uptake by the cells) increases metabolic rate and the amount of metabolically produced heat (Frayn 1997). If deep body temperature is within the normal range, the additional heat generated must be matched by an increase in the rate of heat loss from the body surface; otherwise, deep body temperature will rise.

Non-shivering thermogenesis. Although peripheral vasoconstriction is very effective in helping to conserve heat, heat production itself may need to increase in order to restore body temperature to

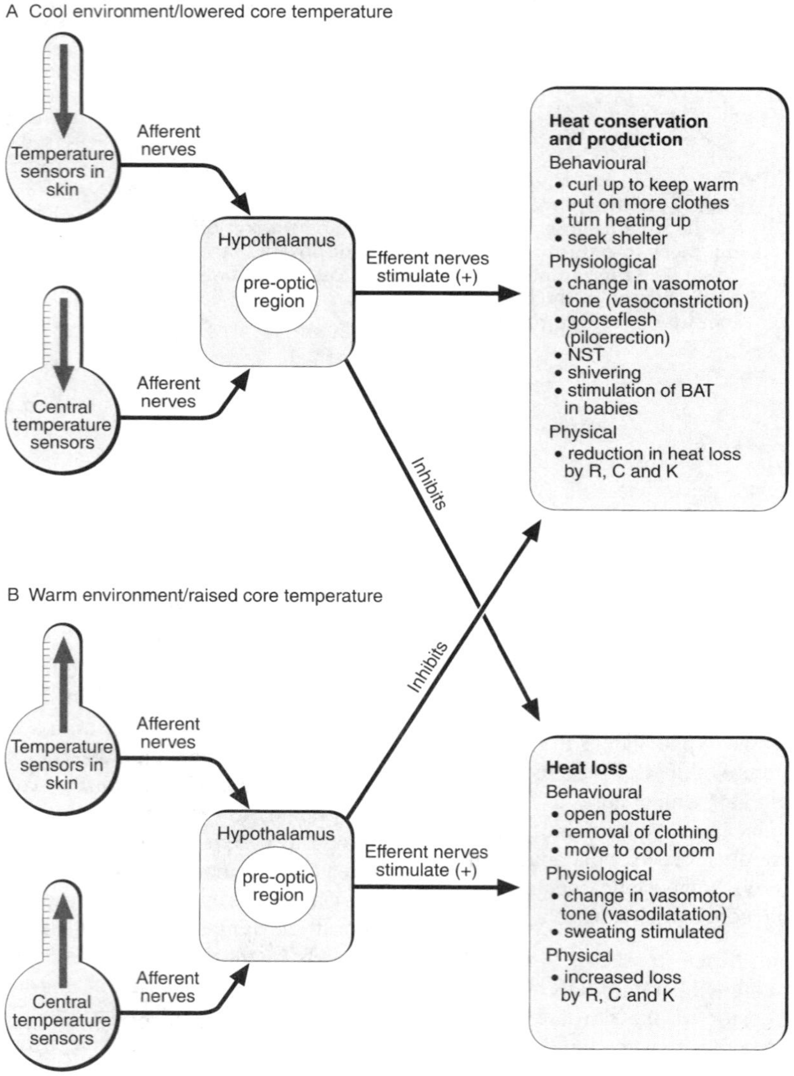

Fig. 22.2 Control of body temperature. A: Responses to a cool environment or lowered core temperature. B: Responses to a warm environment or raised core temperature.

normal. Initially, this is achieved by non-shivering thermogenesis (NST). As its name implies, NST does not involve muscular contraction to produce heat, although muscle tissue is the most important source of chemically produced heat (Jansky 1979). Other important heat-producing organs are the brain and liver. NST is controlled by the sympathetic nervous system and is stimulated by the release of the hormone noradrenaline.

Shivering thermogenesis. Shivering is an easily recognisable feature of a person who feels cold or whose body temperature has fallen. The heat conservation area of the brain stimulates an increase in muscle tone (i.e. shivering) which can increase heat production by five times the basal rate (Morgan 1990). Shivering occurs in most skeletal muscles but is of greatest intensity in the neck and of least intensity in the legs. The repetitive contraction of muscle is not, however, a very economical process, for only 40% of the heat generated in shivering is retained by the body.

Mechanisms of heat loss (see Fig. 22.2B)

High air temperatures and strenuous exercise can raise the temperature of the blood so that heat-losing mechanisms are initiated and heat-conserving mechanisms are inhibited. The series of events which protect the brain (and core tissues) from reaching dangerously high temperatures are as follows:

1. A higher air temperature heats the skin and the resultant change in skin temperature is detected by skin thermoreceptors, which signal the thermoregulatory centre.
2. The first reaction of the person is to reduce the amount of body insulation by removing some clothing.
3. At about the same time, blood vessels in acral regions dilate so that more blood is brought to the surface of the skin.
4. Providing the air temperature is lower than the skin temperature, heat will be lost by radiation and convection (see Table 22.2). If the air temperature is higher than skin temperature, the person will gain heat from the environment. This is why evaporative heat loss becomes so important when the temperature gradient between skin and air temperature is narrow.
5. Stimulation of sweat glands in hot conditions is controlled by the sympathetic nervous system. Production of a fluid consisting mostly of water (but also containing salt, urea, lactic acid and potassium ions) onto the skin causes cooling when the thermal energy needed to transfer the fluid to a gas is absorbed by the surrounding air from the skin surface. This transfer of energy from a fluid to a gaseous state is called vaporisational heat loss.

Q

22.3 What is the most important route for heat loss in a warm environment?

22.4 What is the collective term used to describe heat loss by radiation and convection?

22.5 Find out which areas of the body are described as 'acral regions'. What is their specific function in thermoregulation?

22.6 After a bath, patients often feel cold and uncomfortable if the nurse is slow in helping them to dry themselves. What is the cause of this feeling of discomfort when the body is wet and the room temperature low? Why would leaving the door of the bathroom open make the patient feel cold? How can the nurse improve the patient's comfort when preparing her for a bath?

FLUCTUATIONS IN A HEALTHY PERSON'S TEMPERATURE

Humans are capable of surviving in a range of climates. This is because they are able to make both physiological and behavioural adjustments which prevent deep body temperature from rising above or falling below approximately 37°C. Like many mammals, humans have the ability to increase the amount of heat in the body as air temperature falls or to increase heat loss when conditions become uncomfortably hot.

Normal temperature range

Although central or hypothalamic temperature is set at a relatively constant level, fluctuations do occur in healthy people, e.g. following exercise. No harm is done to the cells of the body by a change in temperature, providing core temperature does not rise above or fall below certain limits. Indeed, the ability of the thermoregulatory system to stimulate changes in heat production or heat loss indicates that the system is operating efficiently.

DuBois's now classic monograph (1948) illustrates the range of 'normal' temperature in health. In the early morning or during cold weather, body temperature may fall to 35–36°C. After moderate exercise (and also, for example in crying babies), core temperature may rise to about 38°C. Following hard exercise, body temperature may rise to 40°C. An increase of about 5°C above 37°C indicates a serious disruption of thermoregulation and a person's life may be at risk if deep body temperature rises above 43°C or falls below 24°C.

Q

22.7 During one shift of duty, find out how many patients have a high temperature and then answer the following questions:

(a) Give the highest and lowest measured temperatures for each of the patients you have identified as having a pyrexia.
(b) State the site used to measure deep body temperature for each patient.
(c) Has the pyrexia been reported?
(d) What are the possible reasons for the pyrexia?
(e) Has the cause been identified and treated?
(f) How frequently is the temperature being monitored?

Circadian rhythm

Body temperature fluctuates in a characteristic pattern over a 24-h period. It is thought that this pattern derives from regular alterations in the set-point of the hypothalamic thermostat. Thus, like many other physiological functions, thermoregulation displays a circadian rhythm or diurnal variation (Davis & Lentz 1989). This rhythm persists in health and even during short periods of night work. Eventually, however, regular night work will reverse the pattern so that lower temperatures occur during the day and higher temperatures at night.

In general, the lowest temperatures recorded over a 24-h cycle will be approximately 0.5°C lower than the plateau temperature. The highest temperature during the evening may be as much as 1.0°C above the early morning temperature.

The circadian rhythm of deep body temperature does not occur in babies (Lorin 1982, Peterson et al 1991) but develops during early childhood, when fluctuations may be more marked than in the adult.

An awareness of the normal changes in deep body temperature in health is necessary if nurses are to interpret temperature

Table 22.2 Principles of heat transfer

Route for heat loss	*Principle*	*Relevance to clinical practice*
Radiation (R)	Transfer of energy in the form of electromagnetic waves. The human body emits heat as infrared radiation. At the same time all dense objects (furniture, buildings, other people) are also radiating heat. The rate at which heat is emitted from the human body is dependent upon the temperature difference (gradient) between the skin and other objects and surfaces in the room. If the skin is hotter than the average temperature of objects in the room, heat will be lost. If the objects in the room are hotter, the body will gain heat	A person, naked, sitting quietly in a room at 25°C loses between 50 and 70% of heat by R, the major route for heat loss under such conditions. As air temperature increases, the temperature gradient between skin and air falls such that less heat is lost by this route. As air temperature rises towards skin temperature (35°C), the gradient will be so small that very little heat loss can take place by this route. Evaporative heat loss then becomes an important route for heat loss
Convection (C)	Air (or water) next to the body warms and moves slowly away because warm air is less dense and rises. As it moves away from the body, cooler air replaces it. This process can be speeded up if a strong draught (e.g. electric fan) is used to force the air away and cause a rapid replacement of warmed air with cool air	Nurses frequently increase the rate of heat loss by convection by placing electric fans close to their patients. This can be a very efficient way to lower skin temperature, but frequently the cool stimulus results in an inappropriate response, i.e. peripheral vasoconstriction. Heat retention within core tissues then causes core temperature to rise rather than fall. In febrile patients who have an elevated set-point, the use of electric fans is likely to exacerbate the problem of pyrexia
Conduction (K)	Heat loss by K involves transfer of thermal energy from atom to atom. The skin must be in contact with cooler or hotter objects for heat exchange to take place by K	Critically ill patients are often nursed on special beds designed to reduce the incidence of pressure sores. These beds are often maintained at a constant temperature to help prevent heat loss from the body. Sometimes the thermostat can fail and patients have been known to overheat or to cool because the temperature of the bed is too high or too low. This is an example of heat loss or heat gain by conduction. Patients must be protected from body temperature disturbances of an iatrogenic nature such as this
Evaporation (E)	Evaporation of water from the skin and respiratory passages is the most important route for heat loss in hot conditions. The evaporation of water occurs when energy transforms water and sweat droplets to a gas. The heat (or thermal energy) needed to drive this process is taken from the body. Thus the more water there is on the skin, the more heat is taken from the body to turn it into a gas (vaporisation). The more heat removed from the body in the process of E, the more the body cools. The function of sweat (produced under the control of the sympathetic nervous system) as an agent for vaporisational heat loss can be enhanced by spraying the body with a fine mist of warm water	Patients with a high core temperature may not always sweat. During a rise in rectal temperature the body responds as though it were too cold and if patients are observed carefully it will be seen that their skin is dry. At this stage the hypothalamic set-point is above normal but the body continues to activate heat-conserving mechanisms to achieve the new set-point temperature. Only when the patient has reached the new central temperature set-point will heat loss by all routes (E included) be activated. Thus when nurses notice that patients with a high core temperature are sweating, it is more likely to indicate that core temperature has reached the new set-point. A fall in body temperature may then follow

measurements correctly. A moderately elevated oral temperature recorded during the afternoon should be monitored closely before treatment is started. If the cyclical nature of oral temperature is not appreciated, treatment for pyrexia could be instigated for what is essentially a normal temperature.

Q

22.8 For this project you will need to measure the temperature of a healthy person every 2–4 h. You will need to ask for help from your partner, parents,

Q

22.8 (*cont'd*)
siblings or friends — someone who will not mind being woken at night for the sake of this exercise. Plot your subject's oral temperature every 2–4 h for 24 h onto graph paper. From the data you collect, try to identify a circadian rhythm in your subject. State the highest and lowest temperatures recorded over the 24-h period. You should now be able to state the overall variation in body temperature of a healthy subject.

Other factors which affect a healthy person's temperature

Age. The age of a patient must be taken into account in the interpretation of body temperature.

Babies and young children. Early studies (e.g. Bayley & Stolz 1937) showed that rectal temperature begins to rise during the first 7 months of life, remaining fairly constant until the age of 2 years, after which it begins to fall. Average rectal temperature at 1 month of age was 37.1–37.2°C, at 8 months 37.6–37.7°C, and at 18 months 37.7°C. By the time the children in their study approached their third birthday, rectal temperature had settled to values around 37.1°C.

Healthy children tend to have a higher deep body temperature than adults and therefore their 'normal' range differs slightly. Higher temperatures in early childhood are thought to be a result of increased cellular and metabolic activity. The newborn baby and the young of most mammals are particularly well adapted to generating body heat. This adaptation is vital for survival; human infants have a large body surface area in proportion to their weight and are therefore vulnerable to the effects of cold. They are unable to shiver and cannot increase body insulation by adding extra layers of clothes by themselves. However, they do have an important source of body heat in the form of brown adipose tissue (BAT), a specialised fat which can be found around the kidneys, between the shoulder blades, around the great vessels and deep within the axillae (Rothwell 1989, Frayn 1997).

A large amount of heat is produced by this unique tissue, which requires a large supply of blood and oxygen in order to fulfil this function (the dense vascular supply is responsible for the brown colour of this tissue). Brown fat becomes much less important in maintaining the temperature of the body as a baby gets older.

Adults and elderly people. The importance of BAT for heat production in an adult is not clear but is probably minimal. Unlike small infants, who rely principally on 'switching on' heat production to maintain a stable deep body temperature, adults are more efficient at conserving body heat. In other words, they rely on preventing body heat from being lost, either by putting on more clothes (behavioural thermoregulation) or by vasoconstriction at the extremities (physiological thermoregulation).

Older people, however, often have lower body temperatures than children or younger adults. There are a number of reasons for this. After the age of about 50 years, metabolic rate starts to fall. This results in a lower rate of heat production within the body, and consequently, deep body temperature tends to be lower. In addition, social and economic factors contribute to the inability of some elderly people to keep warm, particularly in winter. As people grow older, it is more difficult for them to detect extremes in temperature; this puts them at risk of hypothermia and hyperthermia (see Box 22.1). In warm conditions, for example, deep body temperature in the older person may rise slightly because the ability to sweat is reduced. Evaporative heat loss is therefore less efficient at a time when increased heat loss is needed to keep the temperature within the normal range.

Exercise. Hard exercise can raise oral and rectal temperature by several degrees. Temperatures above 40°C have been recorded in marathon runners, and after a game of rugby rectal temperatures over 39°C can occur (Mitchell & Laburn 1985). This rise in temperature can persist for many hours and represents an imbalance between heat production and heat loss (see pp. 721–723).

The menstrual cycle. It is now well recognised that 80% of healthy ovulating women have higher oral temperatures at the time of ovulation. A record of early morning oral temperature can be used to predict the time of ovulation in healthy women. On waking, oral temperature should be recorded before doing any work or exercise. These measurements should be made on a daily basis throughout the cycle. A slight drop in temperature occurs 24–36 h after ovulation. Temperature then rises abruptly by 0.3–0.4°C and continues at this slightly higher level for the rest of the cycle. Three days after the onset of the higher temperature is generally thought to coincide with the end of the fertile phase.

The occurrence of 'hot flushes' in the menopause is discussed in Box 22.2.

Box 22.1 Helping the elderly to keep warm in winter

There will always be cold spells during the winter months and some will be much worse than others. Weathermen frequently refer to the more extreme conditions as a 'cold snap' and their advice, particularly to elderly television viewers, is to make sure that they keep warm. The problem is that keeping warm usually means keeping the heating on for longer than usual with a consequent rise in heating bills. In recognition of this, the Government has recently provided a small annual winter fuel payment to all pensioners. However, elderly people become cold for many reasons and at times other than during extremely cold spells.

The older housing stock in which many elderly people live becomes damp and cold if maintenance and repairs are not kept up to date. It is expensive to keep old houses warm at any time of year, but particularly in winter. If elderly people cannot be persuaded to keep their heating on during the winter, it can be helpful for family, friends and neighbours to offer good advice about keeping warm.

The obvious suggestion for someone on a low pension would be to heat just one room, i.e. the room in which she spends most of her time. An alternative is to conserve body heat by wearing extra layers of clothes. These should be comfortable but effective in retaining body heat. The most important principle to remember is that there is no particular merit in one kind of material as compared with another except in its capacity to trap air. Clothes made of cotton are as good as down feathers in this respect. The problem is that feathers can be easily compressed, and when this happens the insulating properties are reduced. It is worth advising people who use a down quilt and their covers to keep it 'fluffed' for maximum insulation.

Covering the parts of the body which are exposed to draughts (i.e. hands, feet and head) should be done in much the same way as for a person in a cold climate. Although the head is generally heated by a plume of warm air rising upwards from the body (Clarke & Edholm 1985), this band of warm air can be blown away if the person is in a draught. People who spend a lot of time relatively immobile in a draughty house should be advised to wear something on their head like a hat, cap or even a Balaclava. The reasons for taking so much care to keep warm are obvious: lives can be saved by these simple yet effective actions.

Q **22.9** When you have the opportunity, either at work or at home, record the temperatures of three or four people before and after they take a hot drink and before and after they smoke a cigarette. What differences do you observe?

Box 22.2 Hot flushes

The exact cause of 'hot flushes' in menopausal women is not known, but there is evidence that a defect in thermoregulatory function may be responsible for the discomfort and distress associated with the hot flush. The two physiological changes which characterise hot flushes are sweating and cutaneous vasodilatation. During a hot flush, central temperature falls in response to heat lost from the skin surface after peripheral vasodilatation and sweating. Sufferers feel very warm and uncomfortable and want to cool themselves. Since the flushes frequently occur at night (night sweats), they can cause great distress and make it difficult to get a good night's sleep.

It is thought that hot flushes are the result of a sudden fall in the central hypothalamic thermostat. This would result in the body being too hot and stimulating heat loss mechanisms such as sweating and vasodilatation. In a recent study, 29% of women who had between 3 and 12 months' amenorrhoea and 37% of postmenopausal women experienced hot flushes several times a day (Guthrie et al 1996). Because hot flushes occur during the climacteric and are associated with cessation of ovarian function, their underlying cause is thought to lie in changes in the endocrine system. Reporting of hot flushes is greatest 3 months or more after the final menstrual period. The frequency of hot flushes is associated with increasing follicle-stimulating hormone (FSH), a reduction in oestradiol, and a history of menstrual complaints (Guthrie et al 1996).

Eating a meal. The process of breaking down and metabolising food produces body heat. This effect was originally described as the specific dynamic action (SDA) of food. Metabolism of protein was found to have a greater effect in generating heat than the metabolism of carbohydrate or fat (Ashworth 1969). However, the SDA or 'diet-induced thermogenesis' (DIT, the term more often used today) is used to describe the heat generated from the gastrointestinal activity of absorbing and digesting the nutrients in a meal (Frayn 1997). DIT will be responsible for the increased metabolic rate after a meal and some authors believe that DIT can produce a slight rise in core temperature.

The source of body heat (chemical thermogenesis)

Heat is expressed in 'energy units' called calories (cal), or more usually in the larger units, kilocalories (1 kcal = 1000 cal). The SI unit for energy is the kilojoule (1 kJ = 4.18 kcal).

Since nurses are involved in measuring the temperature of the tissues of the body, it is important for them to understand how body heat is generated. Most of our energy for growth and repair of tissues, for work and for body warmth comes from the food we eat. Different foods provide different amounts of energy. Most packaged foods have a label which gives the amount of energy (kcal or kJ) contained in an average serving (or per 100 g) when oxidised or burned by the body. Heat is a by-product of oxidation and the process by which it is produced is called chemical thermogenesis. The rate at which heat is produced is called the metabolic rate.

Metabolic rate

If a semi-nude man fasts overnight for 12 h, resting quietly (awake) in a warm (28–30°C) room, his metabolic rate, or energy expenditure, will be at a minimum or basal level (basal metabolic rate, BMR). If the man increased his activity, by walking, exercising or even shivering, his demand for energy and thus his metabolic rate would increase. When this happens, some of his energy would be used to do external work (between 2 and 25%, depending on the activity), but most would be lost as heat.

A business person spending most of his day at the office and doing little exercise can expect to increase his energy requirements by 25–40% above the basal rate during the course of a day. Assuming that all his energy requirements were provided from the food he ate on that day (100%), approximately 10% would be lost as heat as a by-product of the work involved in processing his food, 50% would be lost as heat in the conversion of potential energy in food to high-energy biochemical bonds and 20% would be lost as heat as a result of internal work (respiration, cell pumps, glandular activity). In this example, only 20% of the individual's energy intake would be used for external work (e.g. muscular contraction) and the rest (80%) would be lost as heat (Wilmore 1977).

It is clear that our utilisation of food energy is a very inefficient process. Most of our energy intake is lost as heat. However, the rate at which heat is produced does not necessarily reflect the rate at which it is lost from the body: heat can be retained and stored. One of the most important stimuli for body heat storage is a slight fall in core temperature, particularly if the person is in a cool environment.

THE MEASUREMENT OF BODY TEMPERATURE

Thermometers

The clinical thermometer

The development of a reliable thermometer was made possible only after scientists came to an agreement about the meaning of temperature and devised a scale to measure it. The scale we are most familiar with in clinical practice is the Celsius or centigrade scale determined by Anders Celsius (1701–1744). The mercury-in-glass thermometer has been the standard temperature-taking instrument for the last century. For many years it has been the most practical way of measuring oral, axilla and even rectal temperature, but some hospital trusts are encouraging the use of new and more sophisticated instruments which are quicker and easier to use (see Table 22.1, p. 721). Ear thermometers, for example, are becoming very popular as a method for measuring 'core' temperature in children's hospitals and can even be bought 'off the shelf' for use at home (Childs et al 1999).

Electronic thermometers

Electronic thermometers like the 'IVAC' are very accurate instruments and are often more suitable for measuring a patient's temperature than clinical thermometers, because a measurement only takes about 1 min. Electronic thermometers are usually used for 'spot' measurements of oral and axilla temperature, but they can be inserted into the rectum if necessary. This is a great advantage when one considers the time needed to obtain an accurate oral or axilla temperature measurement (Haddock et al 1996) with a mercury-in-glass thermometer (see Table 22.1, p. 721) and how difficult it can be to take a baby's or toddler's temperature if she is upset or uncooperative.

Infrared radiation thermometers

A new type of thermometer is now available which measures temperature in the ear, more precisely at the tympanic membrane (Fraden 1991, Fraden & Lackey 1991, Edge & Morgan 1993) (see Table 22.1, p. 721). This thermometer determines temperature by detecting infrared radiation emitted from the tympanic membrane.

It was recognised for some time that because of the very good blood supply to the tympanic membrane, measurement of its temperature would provide a very useful indication of deep body temperature. However, it has taken many years to develop a thermometer which is safe to use, even in children, and which does not present any risk of perforation to the ear drum. The new tympanic membrane thermometers are simple to use; the probe is placed in the external auditory canal (it does not have to touch the tympanic membrane itself) and a recording is available in 1–2 s. Studies using a Thermoscan™ tympanic membrane thermometer (Talo et al 1991) compared the temperature at three different sites: the ear, mouth and rectum. The difference between average ear and rectal temperatures was found to be 1.1°C (rectal temperature 37.7°C, mean ear temperature 36.6°C). Mean oral temperature was 36.8°C. Recent studies have shown that ear thermometers are not always reliable (Brogan et al 1993, Childs et al 1999) and there can be quite large differences in the temperature of a patient's ears. This finding should alert nurses to make sure that the patient's measurement is made in the same ear. A second or even third measurement should be made to check the reliability. It is best to record an average of about three readings.

Small infrared thermometers have also been developed to measure the skin surface temperature. The great benefit of these instruments is that they can be held in the hand; the thermometer does not need to touch the skin, just be held a few cm from the surface and a measurement can be made in a few seconds. This is a useful way to measure skin temperature, e.g. after vascular surgery or after trauma, since the temperature of the skin surface gives a reasonable indication of skin blood flow (Stoner et al 1991). In plastic surgery, surface temperature measurements are a useful and often important way of diagnosing burn depth (Cole et al 1990, 1991, Wyllie & Sutherland 1991), the deeper burn being colder than surrounding tissue (see Ch. 30). After transplantation of skin flaps, a change in temperature of a flap could indicate poor vascular supply (if lowered) or infection (if raised).

Liquid crystal thermometers

Some liquids have special properties which resemble certain characteristics of crystals. When these substances are placed under a form of stress, e.g. a change in temperature, their optical properties cause them to change colour. These 'liquid crystals' can be used to indicate temperature by being mounted in a flexible plastic sheet which can then be placed directly onto the surface of the body. Obviously, this sort of thermometer cannot be used for temperature measurement in body cavities. Changes in colour at different temperatures are easily detected and provide a simple (albeit imprecise) means of taking temperatures.

Taking temperatures

Recording accurate temperatures depends not only on having a reliable instrument but also on clinical skill. Even the most accurate of instruments will give an incorrect reading if the nurse has a poor temperature-taking technique. Table 22.1 gives some useful tips to help the nurse improve clinical practice.

Q

22.10 Ask a qualified nurse to help you with this exercise. With a patient's consent and cooperation, measure oral and axilla temperature at intervals of 1, 3, 5 and 9 min. Compare the results. Are there differences in the values recorded at the two sites?

Q

22.11 If you have some experience of using an electronic thermometer, comment on the advantages (if any) of this technique of measuring deep body temperature compared with the mercury-in-glass thermometer.

22.12 Ask the ward sister or charge nurse on the ward where you are working to tell you about the cost of temperature-taking and how much of the ward/unit budget is allocated to temperature measurement.

DISTURBANCES IN TEMPERATURE REGULATION

The aim of this section is to supplement the nurse's understanding of thermal physiology with examples of abnormal responses which disturb the thermoregulatory system, causing illness, discomfort or even death.

Table 22.3 gives examples of clinical conditions associated with a rise in body temperature. The causes of increased body temperature can be divided into two categories:

- a rise due to fever
- an increase as a result of heat illness.

It is very important to recognise the fundamental differences between the two main causes of raised body temperature as well as to appreciate their implications for treatment.

Fever

The high 'core' or deep body temperature associated with fever is due to an upward movement in the central set-point temperature in the hypothalamus (see p. 720). If the set-point is shifted from 37°C to, say, 39°C by the action of pyrogens (cytokines) released, for example, during infection, the thermoreceptors in the brain will detect a discrepancy between the set-point temperature and the temperature of the blood circulating (at 37°C) through the hypothalamus (this is the error signal described on p. 720). Since the blood temperature is lower than the new, raised set-point temperature, heat gain mechanisms will be stimulated to achieve an increase in the temperature of the 'core'. This can be detected in a person's behaviour as she pulls on more bedclothes or turns the heating up. Patients do this even when their core temperature has started to rise. Their hands and feet feel cold as skin blood flow is diverted away from the 'shell' to the central 'core'. The patient may also start to shiver (very vigorous shivering is called a rigor). The occurrence of febrile convulsions in young children is discussed in Box 22.3.

Despite the gradual development of fever and higher core temperature, the heat loss mechanisms are inhibited or 'switched off'. These thermoregulatory changes help the temperature to reach the new set-point level. At this stage, the nurse should not try to lower the patient's temperature by cooling her either by tepid sponging or with electric fans, because in so doing he will counteract the heat conservation mechanisms already in operation (Bruce & Grove 1992). However, once the temperature of the blood and core tissues is at the new 'set-point' level and sufficient heat has been stored within the body to sustain the new set-point temperature, the patient will become more comfortable despite her high temperature.

The set-point will not remain at the higher level. Eventually, the biological effects of the pyrogen will wear off and the thermoregulatory 'set-point' abruptly returns to normal. When this

Table 22.3 Changes in body temperature

	Cause	*Clinical examples*	*Appropriate treatment*
Fever	Elevation of hypothalamic set-point by endogenous pyrogens such as cytokines, interleukin-1 (IL-1) and interleukin-6 (IL-6). Both are released from the patient's own white cells in response to bacterial or viral infection or to damage to skin and tissues	Infection: bronchitis, malaria, sepsis, meningitis Trauma: burn injury, minor and major surgery, myocardial infarction, thrombophlebitis	Antipyretic drugs like aspirin or paracetamol return altered set-point temperature to a lower level. Avoid external cooling as this may exacerbate the rising core temperature
Heat illness	Increased metabolic heat production, *or* Reduction in the rate of heat loss (by R, C and E) from the body surface (see Table 22.2)	Heat stroke resulting from high air temperature, overwrapping (children/elderly) and excessive clothing, or due to increased exercise or work in hot conditions where dehydration and reduced sweating are common associated factors	External cooling: 1. Increase radiant and convective heat loss by removing clothing and helping 'stir' the air around the subject. Avoid cold draughts. Do not use ice packs, as these can increase vasoconstriction 2. Increase evaporative heat loss by applying a fine mist of warm water (40°C) over the body and exposing as much of the skin surface as possible to the air
Malignant hyperpyrexia	Largely unknown. Patients found to have an underlying inborn error of muscle metabolism (Britt 1979) usually triggered by general anaesthesia	Hyperthermia occurs shortly, or immediately, after general anaesthetic, in apparently normal patients. Once body temperature starts to go up, it does so very rapidly, and by as much as 1°C every 5 min. Temperatures as high as 46°C may be reached, with tachycardia, cyanosis and loss of consciousness (Lorin 1982)	Active cooling, maintenance of cardiac output, correction of metabolic disturbances, e.g. hyperkalaemia, acidosis. Administration of dantrolene sodium

happens the patient will feel uncomfortable and hot. Hands, face and feet will become red as peripheral vasodilatation replaces vasoconstriction. Vasodilatation allows skin blood flow to reach the most superficial layers of skin so that heat exchange from core tissues to the surface can take place. The patient should be put in the best position to allow dissipation of body heat naturally. Forcing heat loss by causing excessive draughts or allowing the temperature of the room to fall so low that the patient quickly becomes cold will make her uncomfortable and possibly induce peripheral vasoconstriction again. If this happens, heat loss by radiation and convection will be reduced. Patients often have a drenching sweat when their set-point returns to normal. It is, however, possible to encourage heat loss by evaporation by spraying the patient with a fine mist of warm water. The use of non-steroidal anti-inflammatory drugs (NSAIDs) in the treatment of fever is discussed in Box 22.4.

How fever develops

A rapidly expanding area of biology is the study of cytokines, which are peptide molecules released from a variety of cells, including those of the immune system (see Ch. 16). They allow communication to occur between cells so that the internal environment is regulated following inflammation, injury or sepsis and during healing. For many years, the substances thought to be responsible for the fever associated with infection, tissue breakdown and necrosis (e.g. after traumatic injury or myocardial infarction) were a group of peptides called endogenous pyrogens (EPs). The endogenous pyrogens have recently been shown to include specific molecules and are now collectively called interleukins.

Interleukin-1 (IL-1) is generally believed to be the pyrogen which acts in the brain to raise the set-point temperature to a higher level (Stainer et al 1984). IL-1 is not easily detected in plasma (Childs et al 1990) and its role as a circulating pyrogen is unclear. Its release in the brain is probably stimulated by other interleukins produced outside the brain. Interleukin-6 (IL-6) is a cytokine produced by a number of different cells (activated macrophages, monocytes, keratinocytes, fibroblasts and endothelial cells, to name a few). It is thought that IL-6 released at the site of inflammation or injury triggers the production of IL-1 in the brain. In the brain, IL-1 probably stimulates production of a group of substances called prostaglandins. These substances are thought ultimately to be responsible for elevating the thermoregulatory set-point.

Chills and rigors

A sudden onset of fever with a 'chill' or 'rigor' is characteristic of some diseases. The chills associated with malaria are well known and are often portrayed in novels and films as a serious symptom of tropical disease. Repeated rigors are typical of pyrogenic infections and bacteraemia but are now also recognised as a symptom of viral as well as bacterial infections and even of non-infectious disease. Rigors and chills were once taken to confirm diagnosis of certain illnesses, but because they are now known to be associated

Box 22.3 What to do in the event of a febrile convulsion

Febrile convulsions occur in 40 out of 1000 children and it has been estimated that 30% of all convulsions in children occur during a febrile episode. About 2–5% of all children have at least one convulsion in association with fever by the time they are 5–7 years of age.

Febrile convulsions generally occur in normal children between the ages of 6 months and 5 years. Simple febrile convulsions are probably not harmful. They are brief, lasting only seconds or a few minutes. They occur soon after the onset of fever and it is the height of the fever rather than the speed of the rise in temperature that is thought to be an important contributing factor. However, there are some situations in which a rapidly developing high fever (of 39–40°C) in infants and young children is not associated with convulsions (Childs 1988) and this raises questions about the precise contribution of level of fever and rapidity of onset to the development of a convulsion.

Certain infections, particularly those of the central nervous system, have a particularly high incidence of associated seizures. Bacterial and viral meningitis have been associated with a high incidence of convulsions, but these conditions may well precipitate convulsions by virtue of the nature of the underlying disease rather than because of the fever *per se*.

Nurses play an important role in the acute management of the child with a febrile convulsion. Convulsions can cause fear and misunderstanding and, since they generally occur in very young children, the parents may feel particularly helpless. Health visitors are often in a good position to explore these fears and misconceptions with parents and to provide them with information about what to do if their child experiences a febrile convulsion; this information will help to reduce anxiety and feelings of helplessness.

When a convulsion starts, the child needs to be protected from falling on the floor or against furniture. If she is in a cot or bed, care should be taken to prevent her from falling out or hitting herself against sharp corners which may be within reach. The airway should be cleared but nothing should be inserted into the mouth. A common misconception is that the use of spoons or gags is necessary to prevent the tongue from blocking the airway. This practice is dangerous and can harm the child. As long as the nurse puts the child in the recovery position (see Ch. 26), observes the airway and takes the necessary actions to maintain a clear airway by, for example, wiping away accumulated secretions, little more can be done. However, if the convulsion does not resolve after a period of 10–20 min, drugs may be needed to control it. In such a case, medical help will be needed.

In addition to protecting the child from injury during the convulsion, the nurse should document its characteristics. Notes should be made relating to the child's temperature at the time of the convulsion or the last measurement made before it started, the type of movements made during the convulsion, where they started, how they developed and for how long they lasted. The clinical condition of the child should also be described.

with a variety of diseases, their diagnostic importance has been diminished.

A chill or rigor is accompanied by intense feelings of cold. The patient's skin will be white and cold and she will probably pull her bedclothes tightly around her body and curl up into a ball. Her teeth may chatter and she will be very uncomfortable. Intense shivering and violent jerking movements will be uncontrollable.

Box 22.4 Non-steroidal anti-inflammatory drugs (NSAIDs)

In addition to their anti-inflammatory effects, NSAIDs are antipyretics. They act by inhibiting the production of prostaglandins from arachidonic acid in the cyclo-oxygenase pathway.

Since 1986, the NSAID aspirin (acetylsalicylic acid) has been withdrawn from general use in children under the age of 12 years because of the association between this drug and a serious condition called Reye's syndrome.[a] Paracetamol (acetaminophen) is now the most commonly used antipyretic in children. Although not an NSAID, its antipyretic properties are thought to lie in its ability to prevent the synthesis of prostaglandins, which are thought to affect the temperature set-point when released into the brain (see p. 720).

Antipyretic drugs are not effective in conditions where high core temperatures are caused by heat illness; neither are they effective in lowering normal body temperature.

[a] Reye's syndrome is a rare illness that occurs typically in children and teenagers. The onset is usually during a viral illness like influenza or chickenpox. This is then followed by protracted vomiting and neurological changes at just about the time when the child is beginning to recover from the original illness (Ward 1997). The use of aspirin during the illness has been identified as a factor contributing to the very serious metabolic disorders associated with it (encephalopathy and fatty degeneration of organs). Unexpected vomiting and disturbed brain function after a viral illness are symptoms of Reye's syndrome in children and teenagers, but in infants the symptoms may be slightly different and include diarrhoea, breathing difficulties and fits. The number of cases reported has fallen in countries where aspirin has been withdrawn from use in children (Larsen 1997).

Fever in myocardial infarction

Myocardial infarction is an example of a condition in which there is an acute rise in deep body temperature. Typically, body temperature rises after the first 24 h to 37.8–39.9°C and remains elevated for 2–3 days. Temperatures may be even higher. By day 5, however, deep body temperature returns to normal. It is thought that the pattern of elevated body temperature reflects necrosis of myocardial tissue (see Ch. 2).

If fever persists after the fifth day, the nurse should consider infection (e.g. pneumonia, thrombophlebitis or a systemic infection) as a possible cause.

Q

22.13 Each of the following illnesses and conditions may result in fever:

- otitis media
- meningitis
- blood transfusion
- acquired immune deficiency syndrome (AIDS).

Construct a table to give the cause of the fever and its appropriate nursing care. You will need to refer to Nursing Care Plan 22.1 as well as to other chapters in this book to complete the table. When you have done so, answer the following questions:

(a) What is the common cause of the raised deep body temperature in the above examples?
(b) Why would you expect your chosen methods of treatment to be effective in lowering deep body temperature in each case?

Fever or heat illness?

It is important at this point to clear up some of the confusion which sometimes surrounds the use of the word 'fever' to describe an elevated body temperature. 'Fever' is often used as a general term to describe a rise in body temperature, but in fact it has specific characteristics. To add to the confusion, the words 'hyperthermia' (wrongly) and 'hyperpyrexia' (correctly) are also used to describe 'fever'. In caring for patients with an elevated deep body temperature, it is important to appreciate the distinction between the mechanisms of fever on the one hand, and of heat illness on the other. The nurse should ask himself when planning to treat the patient: 'Does this patient have a high temperature because she has an altered set-point (if this is the case the patient is febrile) or is she hot because she has a problem dissipating her body heat (if this is the case the patient is not febrile but has hyperthermia)?'. The problem is that, in many cases, it is difficult to be sure of the cause of high body temperature.

How heat illness develops. Heat illness is a term which includes these three clinical conditions:

- heat cramps
- heat exhaustion
- heat stroke.

An elevated body temperature is not a diagnostic criterion for heat illness, but it may occur in association with clinical symptoms secondary to environmental heat stress or to a disturbance in the body's ability to dissipate body heat.

The aetiology of heat illness is quite different from that of fever. Fever and the concept of an upward resetting of the hypothalamic set-point have already been discussed. Heat illness can be a minor medical problem or so severe that it poses a threat to life. It is caused not by the production of endogenous pyrogens but by a variety of other factors (e.g. drugs, extremely hot and humid conditions, overwrapping, excessive work in a hot environment) which cause an excess amount of heat to build up which cannot then be dissipated quickly enough from the body surface. The mildest form of heat illness is heat cramp, and the most severe is heat stroke (see Case History 22.1).

Table 22.4 presents some of the signs which may alert the nurse to the fact that a patient is becoming overheated.

Nursing care of a febrile patient

Fever may start abruptly with a shaking chill or it can develop without the patient even being aware that her temperature has gone up. When measured, core temperature may remain high or it may fluctuate (Edwards 1998). A fluctuating temperature with peaks and troughs can occur naturally, as discussed on page 723, but often in hospital it is a consequence of giving antipyretic drugs such as aspirin or paracetamol. A peak and then a trough in temperature can be produced by giving an antipyretic. This pattern should not be considered a natural fluctuation in temperature, but one caused by the treatment given to the patient. The nurse must be able to differentiate between fluctuating fevers brought about by repeated administration of antipyretic drugs and fevers which fluctuate independently of external factors.

Case History 22.1 Mr G

While making her weekly call to the home of Mr G, an 81-year-old widower, the community nurse finds her patient in the garden sitting in his wheelchair in a state of collapse. A relative arrives shortly afterwards and explains that since it was a nice day she thought Mr G would benefit from some fresh air and sunshine whilst she did his shopping.

Mr G feels hot and his hands and feet are red and sunburned. His skin is dry (he is not sweating) and his lips are slightly cracked. His axilla temperature (measured when taken indoors) is 39.2°C.

After being taken indoors, Mr G is sponged with warm water and his clothing removed or loosened. Cool drinks are given and his temperature gradually returns to normal over the next 4 h.

Table 22.4 Clinical appearance and observations of an apyrexial patient who complains of feeling hot: evidence for behavioural and physiological thermoregulation

Observation	*Response*
The bedclothes have been pushed to the bottom of the bed by the patient	This is a behavioural response to the sensation of feeling too warm. Removal of bedclothes/clothing exposes a larger area of the body surface for heat exchange by radiation and convection. If bedclothes/clothing are removed then sweat can freely evaporate to the room and so facilitate evaporative heat loss
Close inspection of the patient shows that the skin of the hands and feet is red and the veins in these areas dilated	Under control of the sympathetic nervous system, veins of the feet and hands vasodilate due to a reduction in vasomotor tone. Blood is therefore directed to the skin surface and the result is that the core tissues extend to the shell (see p. 720). This is why the skin appears to be flushed. The skin is now at a higher temperature, thus creating a wider temperature gradient between the body and the environment. The greater the temperature difference between the body surface and its surroundings, the greater the heat loss by dry routes
Small droplets of sweat appear on the forehead and trunk	Sweating is stimulated in response to either an increase in skin temperature or a rise in core temperature. (Note the exception to this described in Table 22.2.) Sweating occurs first on the forehead, followed by the upper arms, hands, thighs, feet and, finally, the abdomen. Sweating has been shown to start when the average skin temperature is 34°C; as skin temperature increases so does the sweat rate.

Nursing Care Plan 22.1 Care of a febrile patient

Time scale	*Problem*	*Action*	*Rationale*
08.00	When measured, the patient's oral temperature has risen to 37.5°C	❐ Measure patient's temperature every 10 min	During a chill, frequent measurements should be made to determine the pattern of temperature and the maximum values reached
09.00	Oral temperature continues to rise, and now does so rapidly and is accompanied by shivering. The trunk is hot but the limbs are cold	❐ Cover the patient's body with blankets and raise the air temperature slightly. Avoid exposing the patient to cold draughts	At this stage the temperature regulating system is disturbed. Mechanisms are initiated to raise body heat to meet the new, raised set-point temperature. Any attempt at this stage to cool the patient will worsen her chill and delay the time in which the new set-point temperature is reached
11.00	Oral temperature has reached a plateau of 39.5°C	❐ Once deep body temperature has settled and is no longer rising, temperature measurements can be made every 30 min	A person's temperature can be considered to be stable when there are at least two consecutive readings of the same value over a period of 1 h. Once the temperature is stable, measurements can be made every 2–4 h but observations of the patient's general condition should continue
11.30	Pulse rate has increased to 100 beats/min and respiratory rate to 20/min	❐ Frequent observations of pulse and respiratory rate should be part of the overall assessment of the febrile patient	As body temperature goes up so does cellular activity; in other words, there is a rise in metabolic activity. There are direct effects upon the cardiovascular and pulmonary systems as a consequence of a rise in temperature and metabolic activity. Metabolic activity increases by 13% for every 1°C rise in core temperature. Because of the increased energy demands brought about by fever, a persistent pyrexia represents a drain on energy stores. In addition, febrile patients become anorexic and are reluctant to eat and so their energy intake falls. A poor energy intake in conjunction with increased energy expenditure results in negative energy balance or weight loss
11.45	An antipyretic has been prescribed to lower core temperature	❐ Administer aspirin/paracetamol as indicated. Note the patient's temperature at the time of giving the drug. Monitor the patient's temperature regularly (every 15 min) and record the changes on the patient's temperature chart. This will allow the nurse to be able to describe for himself the efficacy of the treatment given	Antipyretics such as aspirin return the upwardly reset temperature to the original set-point level of approximately 37°C. Once this happens the excess heat stored within the body represents an excessive heat load which must be dissipated. In addition to heat loss by the dry routes, radiation, convection and evaporative heat losses are switched on and patients may sweat profusely. Body temperature subsequently falls
		❐ Remove blankets and switch off any form of external heating	During the phase of heat dissipation the surface of the body needs to be exposed so that heat loss by all routes can be encouraged
13.00	The patient's mouth is dry. She is drenched in sweat and feels uncomfortable	❐ Frequent mouth care should be given if the patient cannot eat or drink, but whenever possible clear fluids should be encouraged. These can be refreshing and can provide glucose for energy	Some authors claim that as much as 3 L water can be lost each day in a febrile sweating person. An inadequate fluid intake is accompanied by excretion of a small amount of concentrated urine. An inadequate urine output indicates poor hydration and this is often accompanied by the development of sordes. Drenching sweats are uncomfortable, particularly if nightwear and sheets are wet. The patient can be made more comfortable by giving her a bedbath and by sponging her with warm water. Cold water should be avoided as this causes external cooling and worsens the feeling of discomfort

Nursing the patient with fever is a skill. It demands knowledge of the mechanisms of thermoregulatory disturbance as well as good clinical practice. The care that might be given to a febrile patient in the course of a few hours is described in Nursing Care Plan 22.1.

Hypothermia

The physiological mechanisms that lead to the development of hypothermia can be explained with reference to the hillwalker described in Case History 22.2. With nightfall, a drop in air temperature will stimulate a number of physiological responses to limit the rate of heat loss from the surface of Mr E's body. First of all, a fall in skin temperature, detected by skin thermoreceptors, will cause a reduction in blood flow to the skin of the extremities. Whilst peripheral vasoconstriction is extremely effective in maintaining body temperature with a moderate fall in air temperature, the conditions on the hillside will be more severe and eventually peripheral vasoconstriction will become maximal. When the vessels cannot constrict further, other mechanisms will be stimulated to prevent a further fall in deep body temperature. This will involve activation of the thermoregulatory mechanisms of heat production.

The first response to a modest reduction in air temperature which causes mild sensations of discomfort is an increase in non-shivering thermogenesis (NST; see p. 722). Shivering quickly follows NST as the major thermoregulatory mechanism to raise heat production as air temperature and deep body temperature fall. The main stimulus to shivering thermogenesis is a fall in skin temperature, but the intensity of shivering increases when core temperature falls as well. Shivering starts first in the muscles of the jaw and progresses to all muscles. Although shivering increases heat production by about five times the basal rate, only about 48% of the heat produced is retained within the body (Glickman et al 1967). The rest is lost as wasted heat from the body surface. Although shivering is not a very economical process, it is very important in humans to increase heat production and so prevent an excessive fall in core tissue temperatures.

Shivering is maximal when core temperature is about 35°C. It does not go on indefinitely in response to continued cold exposure but stops when deep body temperature falls to about 32°C. By this time the energy stores in skeletal muscle will be exhausted (the muscular contractions of shivering rapidly utilise these stores). The cold also prevents optimum contraction of muscle tissue.

As the protective thermoregulatory mechanisms fail, core temperature falls further and body systems begin to fail. Although the hillwalker in Case History 22.2 initially took sensible steps to protect himself from the cold and exposure, his loss of body heat continued. Under less severe conditions, his normal thermoregulatory mechanisms would have been adequate to prevent a serious fall in deep body temperature. The duration of exposure in Mr E's case was obviously of major importance in the development of hypothermia.

Case History 22.2 — Mr E

Mr E, a novice hillwalker, becomes separated from his fellow hikers and is lost for many hours in the mountains of the Lake District. As evening approaches, the air temperature falls and Mr E begins to feel tired, hungry and cold. After putting on an extra woollen jumper he sets off to find shelter. He is found early the next morning huddled under an outcropping of rock. The rescue team recognise that he is suffering from hypothermia and take him to hospital.

On his admission to hospital, his rectal temperature is found to be 33.8°C. Although mortality accompanying this degree of cold exposure is approximately 50% (Houdas & Ring 1982) and Mr E is confused and unable to speak clearly when found, he does in fact recover after successful rewarming and emergency treatment.

Q **22.14** Why is it so important for Mr E (Case History 22.2) to find shelter on the hillside? Why would rain have made the hillwalker's problem of becoming cold worse?

Causes of accidental hypothermia

Although accidental hypothermia does occur in fit young people, it is more often seen in neonates shortly after birth or in the elderly living at home. These people are vulnerable to the effects of cold, particularly during the winter months. Resistance to cold in the fit and healthy person depends upon an efficient thermoregulatory system (see Fig. 22.2). Some impairment of thermoregulation may play a role in the predisposition of elderly people to the adverse effects of cold. Perception of cold, for example, may be impaired and the individual may therefore not behave appropriately (such as not putting on more clothes when cold). Many elderly people become chair- or bed-bound, so it is impossible for them to get extra clothes even when they do feel the cold. Those caring for elderly patients at home can help by leaving extra clothes close at hand so that they can be used when needed. A hat may be useful to reduce heat loss from the head. Warm drinks will help to warm the body (see Box 22.1, p. 725).

Although the young of most mammalian species have additional protection from the cold in the form of brown fat (BAT) (p. 725), the elderly do not have the same resource for generating heat within the body, and NST and shivering thermogenesis may not be as efficient as in the younger adult. In addition, malnutrition and hypothyroidism, if present, can all reduce the ability of the body to produce heat when needed (see Box 22.5). Hypoglycaemia may also be a problem in the elderly diabetic patient, as it inhibits shivering (Gale et al 1981).

Intoxication with alcohol can be an important cause of hypothermia. Alcohol inhibits the availability of glucose. As a consequence, the hypoglycaemia which follows excessive alcohol ingestion then leads to an inhibition of shivering thermogenesis in response to cold.

In the UK, accidental hypothermia in the elderly is considered to be common, but the true incidence of hypothermia is difficult to define (Hislop et al 1995). In a Scottish survey, the rate of presentation of hypothermia was 1 in 14 000 people (Office of Population Census and Surveys 1991). Mortality rate from hypothermia is considered to be about 40% (Stoner & Randall 1990).

Accidental hypothermia is preventable. A recent study (Donaldson et al 1998) has shown that even in the coldest regions of the earth, Eastern Siberia, people took action to prevent excessive cold. They wore very warm clothing, stayed indoors in warm houses and this prevented the increases in mortality from hypothermia seen in winter in milder regions of the world. These are simple actions, but yet in the UK each year we read and hear of deaths in the elderly which we all know are preventable given that elderly people could be encouraged and helped to keep warm.

The importance of temperature measurements in elderly people at home

When the community nurse visits elderly patients during the winter months, some assessment of their thermoregulatory system

Box 22.5 Hypothermia in malnourished elderly people

During the winter months we often hear of elderly people becoming hypothermic after an injury, usually a fall. Why do some injured elderly people have such a problem in maintaining their body temperature at or around 37°C?

Do the elderly become hypothermic because they get cold as a result of the fall (e.g. outside in the snow) or is there another reason? Studies have shown that very thin elderly women are more prone to fracture of the femur. They do not, as popularly believed, fall outside the home — 80% of falls in one study occurred indoors (Allison 1997). On admission to hospital with a fractured femur, thin elderly women had the lowest core temperatures, i.e. less than 35°C (Bastow et al 1983), and failed to generate body heat when body temperature dropped. However, if body weight was restored, the expected response (i.e. thermogenesis) to a cold stimulus returned (Mansell et al 1988).

It seems that in thin, underweight patients the central thermoregulatory 'thermostat' does not respond in the usual way to the cold, and if the patient is injured the problem is worsened. Injury *per se* has its own effects on thermoregulation, resulting in an inability to produce heat by shivering when body temperature falls. Body temperature of injured patients can fall well below 35°C (at which shivering is maximal in healthy subjects exposed to cold) before shivering heat production begins.

In summary, very thin, undernourished elderly people have a problem maintaining their body temperature because they do not produce heat when they need it most, i.e. when core temperature falls. When people get cold, they become confused and muscles get stiff, so it is not surprising that frail and elderly people are most at risk of a fall, especially in winter. Whether in the community or in hospital, nursing care should be directed towards ensuring that elderly people maintain their body weight and are protected from the cold. By doing this, injury and hypothermia may be prevented.

should be made. If the nurse thinks that the patient's house is too cold, he should assess whether there is a risk of hypothermia. The nurse should carry a low reading thermometer. Cold patients are often reported to have deep body temperatures exactly equal to the lowest value on a clinical thermometer (35°C). In fact, the body may be much colder than 35°C, but the nurse has overlooked using a low reading thermometer. The true temperature of the patient is therefore not recorded.

Rewarming the hypothermic patient

Safe rewarming of an individual who has developed hypothermia is a difficult task which must be undertaken with care, as death can occur, often some hours later, even after an apparently successful rescue. In one tragic incident, 16 people fell into the sea off the coast of Greenland. A rescue ship arrived quickly and brought all 16 people on board. The survivors were given hot drinks and wrapped in warm covers and, although they were alive at rescue, all died a short while later (Marcus 1979). The reason for this may have been the occurrence of 'after-drop', first described during the Second World War as a late effect of prolonged immersion in cold water. Although after-drop has not yet been fully explained, it is thought that, as the patient is warmed, skin blood flow increases, bringing a large volume of very cold blood from the extremities to the heart. This results in ventricular fibrillation and death follows.

The most appropriate way to rewarm a hypothermic patient after immersion in cold water also applies to the person subjected to cold exposure. The first step is to stop any further heat loss from the body. Once this is done, the body will gradually warm up. This is called 'passive' rewarming. Next a shock blanket is used to retain body heat. When the patient is warmed passively, a rise in core temperature occurs by a gradual build-up of body heat as a natural consequence of the metabolic activity of the body. Providing most of this heat is conserved, the temperature of the body will gradually rise (Stoner & Randall 1990). If core temperature is above 32°C, passive rewarming is the method of choice.

If core temperature is below 32°C and the patient is a young adult who has become hypothermic through immersion in cold water or from exposure, active rewarming of the core tissues is required. There are a number of methods available (King & Hayward 1989), namely:

- gastric lavage with warmed saline
- the introduction of warmed humidified gases via a ventilator
- the administration of warmed intravenous fluids
- peritoneal lavage.

Rewarming the elderly hypothermic patient by active rewarming is a safer method to use, but some external heating will probably be necessary as well (Stoner & Randall 1990). If this is done, the patient's cardiovascular system should be monitored carefully.

In all patients it is important to remember that if the skin surface is warmed first, blood flow to the extremities will be increased. For elderly people with pre-existing cardiovascular disease, this could precipitate a fall in blood pressure. With active rewarming, core temperature can rise from 0.6 to 1.9°C/h (Stoner & Randall 1990). As core temperature rises, shivering may start and will become maximal at about 35°C.

Local cold injuries (see also Box 22.6)

Frostbite

When tissue freezes, ice crystals form and the substances in tissue fluid become concentrated. The ice crystals can be many times the size of the cell itself. The degree of cell death after freezing depends on the concentration of the solute. Tissue damage resulting from freezing very much resembles a burn injury.

The milder form of freezing injury is called 'frost nip'. The extremities (nose, ear lobes, cheek, fingertips, hands and feet) can be affected, but treatment is by simple rewarming of the affected area. A more serious form of cold injury is frostbite. In this condition, blood vessels are damaged and blood circulation stops. The congested blood causes agglutination of cells, resulting in thrombus formation. The severe conditions which result in frostbite can mean that the person is so cold that she neglects to care for the frostbitten tissues and that, if rewarming does occur because of improvements in weather conditions, the frostbitten areas become macerated.

Treatment for frostbitten limbs should be aimed at warming the core tissues first before treating the local damage. The affected limb can then be immersed in water at 10–15°C. The water temperature should then be raised every 5 min by 5°C to a maximum of 40°C.

Once the core and the affected extremities have been rewarmed, the patient should remain on bed rest. The affected limbs should be elevated and tetanus toxoid administered. Antibiotics may be necessary if there is any evidence of infection. Local treatment should consist of care of the wound with early physiotherapy.

Box 22.6 The metabolic 'cost' of a polar expedition

In 1992, two explorers, Mike Stroud and Sir Ranulph Fiennes, completed the first unaided crossing of Antarctica. The 1700 km journey took 95 days.

Throughout the journey the men conducted a series of medical experiments to assess the effect of the extreme climate and hard work on their bodies. In air temperatures of between −10 and −50°C and strong winds, the men dragged their sleighs for 10–12 h each day. The journey took these men to the limits of human endurance. Despite a high food intake, each man lost an extreme amount of weight (26% and 29%), all of their body fat as well as a proportion of lean tissue (muscle). As body fat (and therefore insulation) was lost, the men felt even colder and weaker and they became extremely malnourished. The hard work, the extreme cold over such a long time, together with a number of injuries, resulted in an enormous demand for energy. The food they ate was not enough to stop them from breaking down their energy stores of fat, and as time went on they also began to break down their muscle to provide a source of energy. The results of the tests and measurements on their body composition illustrate how the human body adapts to the most extreme conditions and climate (see Stroud 1993, 1997, 1998).

Raynaud's phenomenon

Raynaud's phenomenon occurs most often in young women and is due to abnormal stimulation of vasoconstrictor nerves (see Ch. 2). The cause of this abnormal vasoconstriction is thought to be emotional upset and, often, cold weather. The fingers are mainly affected; spasm of the digital arteries causes sluggish circulation in the fingers, which then become cyanosed. The intense vasoconstriction causes the arteries to empty of blood and this leads to the typical 'dead', white appearance of the fingers. When the vasoconstrictor spasm has passed the circulation starts to flow. At this stage the individual experiences intense pain, throbbing and tingling. In some patients, vasoconstriction can be so severe and prolonged that the skin of the fingertips becomes ulcerated and necrosed, a condition known as 'Raynaud's disease'. Raynaud's phenomenon generally worsens in winter.

Nursing care of individuals with Raynaud's phenomenon should be directed towards helping them to avoid the stimuli which they know cause their fingers (and toes) to go 'dead'. For some people, simply wearing gloves may be sufficient precaution. Pocket handwarmers are very useful in preventing attacks but they should be used before the person goes out into the cold, as once the hands have become cold a pocket handwarmer is unlikely to be sufficient to prevent vasoconstriction. In severe cases, vasodilator drugs or sympathectomy may be necessary.

Q

22.15 Now try to apply the knowledge you have gained in reading this chapter to the following situations. In formulating your answers, refer to the relevant sections of this chapter as well as to the books and articles listed in the references and further reading.

22.16 An elderly patient (Mrs K) was being cared for by her husband until his recent death. Now alone, Mrs K is visited daily by her daughter and the community nurse. Mrs K has become very depressed, her appetite is poor and she has lost weight. On one of your morning visits, you find Mrs K collapsed in the cold hallway of her home. You suspect she may have been on the floor for some hours. You notice that her skin is very cold. Her axilla temperature is 34°C.

(a) What is the rationale for the immediate management of this patient?
(b) What steps would you take to rewarm the patient at home and once admitted to hospital?
(c) What method of temperature measurement would be needed to record deep body temperature?
(d) What would you expect the method of rewarming to be in the A&E department?
(e) What advice would you give to the patient's family so that further episodes of hypothermia could be avoided?

Q

22.17 In the following situations, what decisions would you consider appropriate in the management of a patient with a disturbance in body temperature? (Note: you may decide that no action is necessary in some cases; if so, give your reasons.)

(a) A patient admitted to hospital with abdominal pain has had a fluctuating oral temperature (between 36.5 and 37.5°C) for 2 days. When you last took her temperature it was 39°C and she was complaining of feeling cold. Her hands and feet were cold and she looked 'mottled' blue. The patient then starts to shiver.
(b) A patient on his second postoperative day has had a raised axilla temperature for 6 h. Treatment with aspirin was given 30 min previously. The patient is flushed and droplets of sweat are present on his forehead.

REFERENCES

Allison S P 1997 Impaired thermoregulation in malnitrition. In: Kinney J M, Tucker H N (eds) Physiology, stress, and malnutrition – functional correlates, nutritional intervention. Lippincott-Raven, Philadelphia, pp 571–593

Aschoff J, Wever R 1958 cited in Stainer M W, Mount L E, Bligh J 1984 Energy balance and temperature regulation. Cambridge University Press, Cambridge

Ashworth A 1969 Metabolic rates during recovery from protein–calorie malnutrition: the need for a new concept of specific dynamic action. Nature 223: 407–409

Bastow M D, Rawlings J, Allison S P 1983 Undernutrition, hypothermia and injury in elderly women with fractured femur: an injury response to altered metabolism. The Lancet 1: 143–146

Bayley N, Stolz H R 1937 Maturational changes in rectal temperature of 61 infants from 1–36 months. Child Development 8(3): 195–206

Bligh J 1972 Neuronal models of mammalian temperature regulation. In: Bligh J, Moore R E (eds) Essays on temperature regulation. North-Holland, Amsterdam

Britt B A 1979 Etiology and pathophysiology of malignant hyperpyrexia. Federation Proceedings 38: 44

Brogan P, Childs C, Phillips B M, Moulton C 1993 Evaluation of a tympanic thermometer in children. The Lancet 342: 1364–1365
Bruce J, Grove S 1992 Fever: pathology and treatment. Critical Care Nurse 12(1): 40–49
Childs C 1988 Fever in burned children. Burns 14(1): 1–6
Childs C 1994 Studies in children provide a model to re-examine the metabolic response to burn injury in children treated by contemporary burn protocols. Burns 20: 291–300
Childs C, Little R A 1994 Acute changes in oxygen consumption and body temperature after burn injury. Archives of Disease in Childhood 71: 31–34
Childs C, Harrison R, Hodkinson C 1999 Tympanic membrane temperature as a measure of core temperature. Archives of Disease in Childhood 80(3): 262–266
Childs C, Ratcliffe R J, Holt I, Hopkins S J 1990 The relationship between interleukin-1, interleukin-6 and pyrexia in burned children. In: The physiological and psychological effects of cytokines. Wiley, New York
Clarke R P, Edholm O G 1985 Man and his thermal environment. Edward Arnold, London
Cole R P, Jones S G, Shakespeare P G 1990 Thermographic assessment of hand burns. Burns 16: 60–63
Cole R P, Shakespeare P G, Chissell H G, Jones S G 1991 Thermographic assessment of burns using a non permeable wound covering. Burns 17: 117–122
Cutter J 1994 Recording patient temperature – are we getting it right? Professional Nurse 9(9): 608–612
Davis C, Lentz M J 1989 Charting oral temperature: circadian rhythms to spot abnormalities. Journal of Gerontological Nursing 15: 34–39
Donaldson G C, Ermakov S P, Komarov Y M, McDonald C P, Keatinge W R 1998 Cold related mortalities and protection against cold in Yukutsk, Eastern Siberia: observation and interview study. British Medical Journal 317: 978
DuBois E F 1948 Fever and the regulation of body temperature. Thomas, Springfield, IL
Edge G, Morgan M 1993 The Genius infrared tympanic thermometer. Anaesthesia 48: 604–607
Edwards S L 1998 High temperature. Professional Nurse 13(8): 521–526
Fraden J 1991 The development of the Thermoscan® instant thermometer. Clinical Paediatrics 30(4): S11–12
Fraden J, Lackey R P 1991 Estimation of body temperature from tympanic measurements. Clinical Paediatrics 30(4): S65–70
Frayn K N 1997 Metabolic regulation – a human perspective. Portland Press, Oxford
Fulbrook P 1993 Core temperature measurements in adults: a literature review. Journal of Advanced Nursing 18(9): 1451–1460
Gale E A M, Bennett T, Green H, Macdonald I A 1981 Hypoglycaemia, hypothermia and shivering in man. Clinical Science 61: 463–469
Glickman N, Mitchel H H, Keeton R W, Lambert E H 1967 Shivering and heat production in men exposed to intense cold. Journal of Applied Physiology 22: 1–8
Guthrie J R, Dennerstein L, Hopper J L, Burger H G 1996 Hot flushes, menstrual status, and hormone levels in a population-based sample of midlife women. Obstetrics and Gynecology 88: 437–442
Haddock B J, Merrow D L, Swanson M S 1996 The falling grace of axillary temperature. Pediatric Nurse 22(2): 121–125
Hislop L J, Wyatt J P, McNaughton G W, Ireland A J, Rainer T H, Olverman G, Laughton L M 1995 Urban hypothermia in the west of Scotland. British Medical Journal 311: 725
Houdas Y, Ring E F J 1982 Human body temperature. Plenum Press, New York
Jansky L 1979 Heat production. In: Lomax P, Schonbaum E (eds) Body temperature regulation, drug effects and therapeutic implications. Marcel Dekker, New York
Jenney M E M, Childs C, Mabin D, Beswick M V, David T J 1995 Oxygen consumption during sleep in atopic dermatitis. Archives of Disease in Childhood 72: 144–146
Jensen B N, Jeppesen L J, Mortensen B B, Kjaergaard B K, Andreasen H, Glavind K 1994 The superiority of rectal thermometry to oral thermometry with regard to accuracy. Journal of Advanced Nursing 20(4): 660–665
King G, Hayward J S 1989 Hypothermia and drowning. Medicine International 2964–2967
Larsen S U 1997 Reye's syndrome. Medicine, Science and the Law 37: 235–241
Lorin M I 1982 The febrile child. Wiley, New York
Mansell P I, Fellows I W, Macdonald I A, Allison S P 1988 The syndrome of undernutrition and hypothermia – its physiology and clinical importance. Quarterly Journal of Medicine 69: 842--843
Marcus P 1979 The treatment of acute accidental hypothermia: proceedings of a symposium held at the institute of Aviation Medicine. Aviation Space Environmental Medicine 50: 834–843
Mitchell D, Laburn H P 1985 Pathophysiology of temperature regulation. The Physiologist 28(6): 507–517
Morgan S 1990 A comparison of three methods of managing fever in the neurological patient. Journal of Neuroscience Nursing 22(1): 19–24
Office of Population Census and Surveys 1991 Population census 1991. HMSO, London
Peterson S A, Anderson E S, Lodemore M, Rawson D, Wailoo M P 1991 Sleeping position and rectal temperature. Archives of Disease in Childhood 66: 976–979
Rothwell N J 1989 Brown fat: a biological furnace. Biological Sciences Review (March): 11–14
Stainer M W, Mount L E, Bligh J 1984 Energy balance and temperature regulation. Cambridge University Press, Cambridge
Stoner H B, Barker P, Riding G S G, Hazelhurst D E, Taylor L, Marcuson R W 1991 Relationships between skin temperature and perfusion in the arm and leg. Clinical Physiology 11: 27–40
Stoner H B, Randall P E 1990 The metabolic aspects of hypothermia. In: Cohen R D, Lewis B, Alberti K G M M, Denman A M (eds) The metabolic and molecular basis of acquired disease. Baillière Tindall, London
Stroud M A 1993 Shadows on the wasteland. Jonathan Cape, London
Stroud M A 1997 Thermoregulation, exercise and nutrition in the cold: investigations on a polar expedition. In: Kinney J M, Tucker H N (eds) Physiology, stress and malnutrition: functional correlates, nutritional intervention. Lippincott-Raven, Philadelphia, pp 571–593
Stroud M A 1998 Survival of the fittest? Jonathan Cape, London
Talo H, Macknin M L, Medendorp S V 1991 Tympanic membrane temperatures compared to rectal and oral temperatures. Clinical Pediatrics (suppl): 30–35
Tortora G J, Grabowski S R 1996 Principles of anatomy and physiology, 8th edn. Harper Collins, London
Ward M R 1997 Reye's syndrome: an update. Nurse Practitioner 12: 45–53
Wilmore D W 1977 The metabolic management of the critically ill. Plenum, London
Wyllie F J, Sutherland A B 1991 Measurement of surface temperature as an aid to the diagnosis of burn depth. Burns 17: 123–128

FURTHER READING

Campbell K 1983 Taking temperatures. Nursing Times (Aug 10): 63–65
Childs, C. 1994 Temperature regulation in the burned patient. British Journal of Intensive Care 4: 129–134
Litsky B Y 1976 A study of temperature taking systems. Supervisor Nurse 7: 48–53
Stoner H B 1971 The effect of injury on shivering thermogenesis in the rat. Journal of Physiology 63(3): 427–429
Stroud M A 1993 Shadows on the wasteland. Jonathan Cape, London
Stroud M A 1997 Thermoregulation, exercise and nutrition in the cold: investigations on a polar expedition. In: Kinney J M, Tucker H N (eds) Physiology, stress and malnutrition: functional correlates, nutritional intervention. Lippincott-Raven, Philadelphia, pp 571–593
Stroud M A 1998 Survival of the fittest? Jonathan Cape, London

WOUND HEALING

Sue Bale

23

INTRODUCTION

For most healthy individuals, the term 'wound' conjures up thoughts of a cut, a graze or even a surgical incision which heals rapidly without difficulty. For nurses, however, the management of wounds is a complex aspect of patient care, requiring much skill and expertise. A nurse may care for a patient with a wound in a variety of settings; ranging, for example, from patients with surgical incisions nursed in hospital, to patients with chronic leg ulcers nursed in their own homes, to patients with industrial injury or trauma treated in their workplace.

We might be tempted to forget the impact that wounds have on an individual. Pain, fear and scarring are the most obvious, but individuals vary in their response to having a wound. For some, restriction in social activity, or the financial implications of not being able to work, should also be considered alongside the psychological effects of altered body image.

Tissue injury and the resulting wound problems have existed for as long as humans have walked the earth (Leaper 1998). For many centuries, trauma and war injury caused most wounds. A variety of readily available materials were used as wound coverings, the forefathers of today's dressing materials. Prehistoric humans had a wide range of salves, which were used to achieve haemostasis, and plant extracts, herbs, cold water, snow and clay were used to ease pain. Surprisingly, throughout human history, wound management has been well documented. One of the first ever records of wounds was found in cave paintings.

Archaeologists have found skulls dating back to the New Stone Age that show evidence of healing following skull trephining. This demonstrates not only that this surgical procedure was performed then, but also that people survived it long enough to heal. Injuries which did not result in death were likely to have been lacerations, contusions (bruises) and fractures. First-aid priorities in these situations would have been to arrest bleeding, bring the tissue edges together, hold them in place and protect the damaged tissues with a covering.

Scandinavian folklore (Forrest 1982) suggests that for thousands of years plant extracts have been applied to wounds for a variety of reasons. Of these 2500 agents, some were antimicrobial, others astringent and others used to effect healing. Towards the end of the Roman era, Galen (the famous Greek physician and anatomist, AD 129–200) developed his theory of laudable pus — *pus bonum et laudabile*. The basis of this theory was that, should a wound become infected, its temperature would increase and this localisation of infection should be allowed to continue. Galen wrote that, when infection localised and then discharged itself, the wound would go on to heal without problems. In the years that followed, medical practitioners became so keen on this idea that they believed not only that pus was acceptable, but also that it was essential and desirable for good wound healing. Clean, uninfected wounds were inoculated with various noxious substances in order to stimulate pus formation. These practices continued from the 7th to the 14th century. It was not until the 19th century that Pasteur and Lister managed to persuade their medical colleagues that mortality rates could be reduced by using antiseptics and aseptic principles.

Throughout time, individual species have varied in the way in which their tissues are renewed. Primitive vertebrates such as reptiles and amphibians have retained the ability to regenerate lost tissue. However, in humans, only liver and epidermal tissue can regenerate. Where tissue loss in humans occurs, healing is achieved by tissue repair.

The healing process depends on a number of factors, and in order for it to proceed at its optimal rate the individual concerned should be in good health. The nurse who cares for a patient with wounds has an important role in promoting health. Her skills as a health promoter and health educator will be called upon to minimise the healing time.

As in other aspects of nursing, the issue of clinical effectiveness and the delivery of evidence-based care are being debated within wound management. As wound healing is a relatively new speciality, there are considerable gaps in our knowledge, although research strategies are being developed (Cullum & Roe 1995).

Definition of a wound

A wound can be defined as a defect or breach in the continuity of the skin. This is an injury to the skin or underlying tissues/organs caused by surgery, a blow, a cut, chemicals, heat/cold, friction/shear force, pressure or as a result of disease, such as in leg ulcers and carcinomas.

Box 23.1 lists the terms that are used in wound healing.

Wound types and the classification of wounds

The ability to deal with injury quickly and effectively has been important throughout human evolution for survival of the species.

There is no clear-cut method of classifying wounds. Some practitioners refer to wounds by anatomical site, e.g. abdominal wall wounds, axillary wounds. Others classify wounds by their depth, e.g. epidermal loss, subcutaneous wounds. Another possible classification is by degree of tissue loss. In the first group, there are wounds with little or no tissue loss where the skin edges can be brought together and sutured. In the second, there has been substantial tissue loss and the skin edges cannot be brought together.

Box 23.1 Terms used in wound healing

Aseptic technique. A precautionary method, using sterile equipment and a 'no-touch' technique to prevent infection.
Autolysis. The disintegration or breakdown of cells or tissues by endogenous enzymes.
Autolytic debridement. The natural process by which the body's own enzymes degrade devitalised tissue on a wound bed.
Chemotaxis. The process by which chemical attractants (kinins) stimulate polymorphs to move towards damaged cells.
Collagen. Fibrous protein strands which provide the strength and structure of granulation tissue.
Collagenase. An enzyme which breaks down collagen during remodelling.
Debridement. The removal of devitalised tissues from a wound.
Dehiscence. Bursting open of a wound.
Elastin. Fibres in connective tissue which provide elasticity.
Epithelium. The cells which form the epidermis.
Exudate. The extracellular fluid which bathes a wound and is rich in nutrients, phagocytes and antibodies.
Granulation. The process of healing by secondary intention.
Ground substance. A gel-like material in which connective tissue cells and fibres are embedded.
Necrotic tissue. Dead tissue, often black in colour.
Pus. A protein-rich liquid consisting of exudate, dead macrophages and bacteria.
Slough. Devitalised white/yellow tissue — dead tissue that separates (and is 'sloughed' off) from healthy tissue after inflammation and infection.
Tensile. The ability to be stretched.
Wound abscess. A localised collection of pus, caused by invading microorganisms, which forms as a result of liquefaction of disintegrated tissue and an accumulation of polymorphs — the process of abscess development is in response to the defences of the body attempting to 'wall off' the damage.

Epidemiology

The epidemiology of wounds is not clearly documented. Because patients with wounds can be found in almost every speciality, information relating specifically to wounds is not collected. However, although there are currently no centrally collected data on wounds, information is available for some wound types.

Leg ulcers

Leg ulcers have been described as 'loss of skin below the knee on the leg or foot which takes more than 6 weeks to heal'(Dale et al 1983). Leg ulceration has affected humans over the centuries (Louden 1982) and is associated with venous disease of the lower limb in approximately 80% of cases (Cullum et al 1997).

The largest survey of patients with leg ulcers was carried out in the Lothian and Forth Valley Leg Ulcer Study in 1985 (Callam et al 1987) (see Table 23.1).

The social and economic burden of managing these patients is great. Estimates vary; Lees & Lombert (1992) estimate the costs to be up to £600m annually, Morison & Moffatt (1994) between £150 and £600m annually, and Cullum et al (1997) £230–£400m annually for the UK alone. Around 100 000 patients in the UK have an open leg ulcer requiring treatment at any one time (Lees & Lombert 1992). The cost of home care has been estimated at a

Table 23.1 Leg ulcers — prevalence

Prevalence 10 per 1000 in adult population
36 per 1000 in over-65s

Age (years)	*Sex ratio (male:female)*
Under 65	1:1
65–74	1:2.6
75–84	1:4.8
85+	1:10.3

Table 23.2 Leg ulcers — healing time and recurrence (Dale & Gibson 1986)

Time to heal	*%*	*Recurrence*	*%*
<3 months	21	1 episode	33
3 months–1 year	29	2–5 episodes	46
1–5 years	40	Over 6 episodes	21
Over 5 years	10		

minimum of £400m and this figure is likely to increase with the rising numbers of elderly in the population (Moffatt 1995). For the most part these patients are cared for by their GP and community-based nurses within the community setting. However, there is an increasing trend towards referral to a specialist leg ulcer service or centre.

The individual's lifestyle can be greatly affected by the presence of a leg ulcer. These are wounds which are difficult to manage, traditionally slow to heal and, even once healed, likely to recur (Table 23.2).

Pressure sores

Throughout the history of nursing, the issue of patients developing pressure sores has been associated with guilt and failure (Dealey 1997). Indeed, it has been suggested that 95% of pressure sores are preventable (Waterlow 1988). In long-term facilities as well as in the acute hospital setting, incidence and/or prevalence of pressure sores are being used as key quality indicators in patient care. This has been supported by the Department of Health in the document *Pressure Sores: a Key Quality Indicator* (Department of Health 1993b). There is a growing awareness that the problem of pressure sores in patient care is not only a nursing issue but also involves medical staff, management and government. Improvement in patient care needs a number of approaches, including the development of local (Trust-wide) prevention strategies and educational programmes for all health care professionals (Dealey 1997).

Pressure sores are among the most difficult wound types to manage. UK surveys have documented the prevalence rate as being between 10.3 and 18.6% (Clark & Cullum 1992, O'Dea 1993).

The incidence of pressure sores within hospital ranges from 4.3 to 43% (Gebhardt 1992, Clark & Watts 1994). The variation in rates depends on the speciality in which the patients are being nursed; orthopaedic units and wards where patients are elderly, immobile, chronically ill and disabled have the higher rates.

In the community, the costs have been estimated to be a minimum of £250 000 a year in one community unit (Preston 1991). The cost implications of a patient developing a pressure sore are high. Such patients need to spend longer in hospital and, even when discharged home, frequently require a district nurse to continue treatment. This financial cost is thought to be rising, although no data have been collected. In 1973, the estimate was around £60m (*The Lancet*, Editorial 1973), in 1982 it was £150m (Scales et al 1982), and it subsequently increased to £300m in 1988 (Waterlow 1988) and £755m in 1993 (Department of Health 1993c). If one takes into consideration the rising numbers of elderly and debilitated people, the figure could be much higher today.

The personal costs to the individual of developing a pressure sore also need to be taken into account. Apart from the disappointment of having discharge postponed and return to normal function delayed, there is the pain and distress, all of which are difficult to measure (Dealey 1997).

Given the suggestion that 95% of pressure sores can be prevented (Waterlow 1988), highlighting the extent of the challenge for practising nurses is clear (p. 752).

Q **23.1** Review the structure and function of the skin (see Cameron 1997).

THE PHYSIOLOGY OF WOUND HEALING

A number of cell types are involved in the process of healing (Table 23.3).

Tissue repair

The wound healing process is one whereby the continuity and strength of damaged tissues are restored by the formation of connective tissue and regrowth of epithelium. The process can be divided into four phases (Fig. 23.1) but, since wound healing is a continuous biological process, there is some overlap between them (Table 23.4).

Phase I — inflammation

As soon as wounding occurs, the wound bleeds, platelets stimulate coagulation and a fibrin clot quickly forms.

An inflammatory reaction takes place at the wound site, and histamine, prostaglandins and activated complement proteins are released. This causes the surrounding blood vessels to dilate and become more permeable. Inflammatory exudate, containing plasma proteins, antibodies, some erythrocytes and white blood cells (neutrophils and monocytes), flows into the damaged area.

Phase II — destructive phase

Polymorphonuclear leucocytes (polymorphs) begin the process of clearing the wound area of debris. Polymorphs ingest damaged cells and are attracted to the site of the wound by chemotaxis. During this time the numbers of monocytes (which later become

Table 23.3 Important cells in wound healing

Cell	*Function*
Endothelial cells	Help to achieve haemostasis
Polymorphs	Take part in the initial inflammatory response
Macrophages	Digest debris and stimulate other cells to function
Fibroblasts	Produce collagen
Myofibroblasts	Aid wound contraction by producing mature collagen

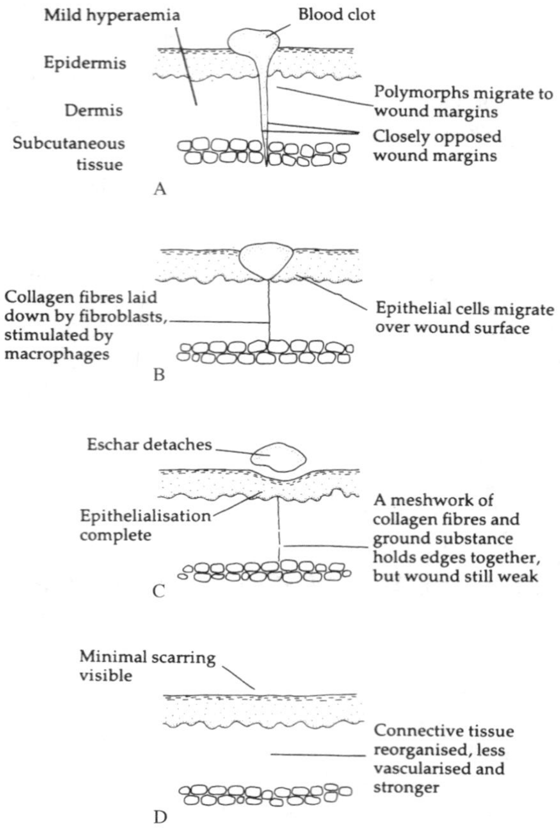

Fig. 23.1 Wound healing by primary intention. A: Inflammation/destructive phases. B, C: Proliferation/reconstruction phase. D: Maturation phase. (Adapted from Morison et al 1997.)

macrophages) present increase. It is the macrophages which, through phagocytic activity, clear debris from the wound site. This phase can be looked on as one of biological cleansing. It does, however, make a considerable metabolic demand on the body. Much heat and fluid can also be lost where a cavity wound exists. The shorter the duration of this phase, the better, because as it nears completion, proliferation or formation of new tissue can begin. Following the destructive phase, the wound site is prepared for the repair process to begin.

Phase III — proliferation/reconstruction

During this phase, tissue repair takes place. The increasing numbers of macrophages present play an important role. They:

- have a phagocytic action on cell debris and bacteria
- are able to break down numerous complex molecules into simple sugars and amino acids which can then provide nutrition to the wounded area
- attract fibroblasts to the wounded area and also enhance their multiplication (through monocyte-derived growth factor, MDGF)
- stimulate fibroblasts to produce collagen, fibronectin and ground substance, which form the mass of connective tissue
- produce a variety of proteins (e.g. interferon and enzymes such as lysozyme) and lipids.

A comprehensive understanding of the full role of the macrophage does not as yet exist. However, its importance in coordinating tissue repair is without doubt.

Table 23.4 Phases of wound healing

Phase	*Time after sustaining wound*
Inflammation	0–3 days
Destructive phase	2–5 days
Proliferation	4–28 days or until defect is filled
Maturation	15 days–1 year

The role of fibroblasts. Fibroblasts greatly increase in numbers during this phase of healing and produce the basic materials which form granulation tissue. Fibroblasts will multiply rapidly in the well-nourished individual and, to be most effective, need adequate amounts of vitamin C, ferrous iron, oxygen and nutrients.

Fibroblasts produce:

- fibronectin, which forms the framework for tissue by holding collagen and cells together whilst attaching them to the ground substance
- elastin, a protein which gives elasticity to tissue, although production is limited in scar tissue
- ground substance, which forms the mass of connective tissue and is made up of proteoglycans (glycoproteins formed of subunits of polysaccharide chains with amino acids).

As the wound defect is filled with newly formed tissue, fibroblast and macrophage numbers and activity decrease.

Re-epithelialisation. Following complete filling of the wound defect with granulation tissue, the open wound surface is ready to be covered by epithelium. Epithelialisation of the relatively large area is achieved by migration into it of epithelium from two sources. At the wound edges, epithelial cells divide and, gradually, epithelium migrates from the edges towards the middle of the wound. At the same time, any epithelial cells near hair follicles, which might be present deep in the dermis, divide rapidly. Islands of epithelium appear wherever a follicle is present. Cells migrate from these islands to meet each other, while cells from the edges of the wound grow inwards to cover the raw surface.

Phase IV — maturation

Vascularisation of the wounded area decreases during this phase. Although the wound appears closed or healed to the naked eye, much activity continues. The immature collagen laid down in phase II is gradually replaced by a mature collagen. The formation of new collagen and the lysis of immature collagen are balanced so that the amount of collagen present at any one time remains constant. The immature collagen is laid down in a random, haphazard fashion, its function being to fill the wound defect as quickly as possible. Mature collagen is laid down following lines of tension within the wound, and at the same time it is cross-linked to give strength. Tensile strength at 14 days in sutured wounds is only about 10% of the original strength of the skin. Tensile strength is gained over a period of months, and a year after wounding will have reached only about 70% of its original value.

Healing by primary/first intention

When injury occurs, whether through accident or as a surgical necessity, the aim of treatment is to effect complete healing as quickly as possible with minimal scarring.

To achieve this, the method of choice is healing by primary intention, which occurs when wound edges are in apposition (Fig. 23.1). This is only possible where there is adequate, mobile tissue and no complicating bacterial contamination. In situations where contamination is suspected, closure of the wound is accompanied by the use of prophylactic systemic antibiotics. For healing to take place by primary intention, the wound edges need to be closely approximated and held together until the wound has healed sufficiently. The skin may be closed by using adhesive tapes, clips, or continuous or interrupted sutures. The skill of the surgeon ensures that the sutures are not inserted too tightly and that the skin edges are closely apposed. The choice of suture material depends on the type of tissue being closed and on the particular function of the tissue.

Healing by secondary intention

Where there is significant tissue loss and/or bacterial contamination, wounds are usually left open to heal by secondary intention through the formation of granulation tissue and, later, wound contraction (Fig. 23.2). Due to the amount of tissue excised or lost during injury, wound healing is a longer process, taking weeks or even months to complete. The healing process itself proceeds in much the same way as for healing by primary intention. The proliferative phase is much extended, as this is when granulation tissue forms and fills the wound defect. It is generally accepted that the length of time a wound takes to heal depends on its original size, i.e. small wounds heal more quickly than larger ones, and it is therefore possible in some wound types (pilonidal sinus, abdominal and axillary wounds) to predict when wounds of a given size that are free from infection will heal (Marks et al 1983).

For methods of wound closure and types of suture material, see Morison et al (1997) and Bale & Jones (1997).

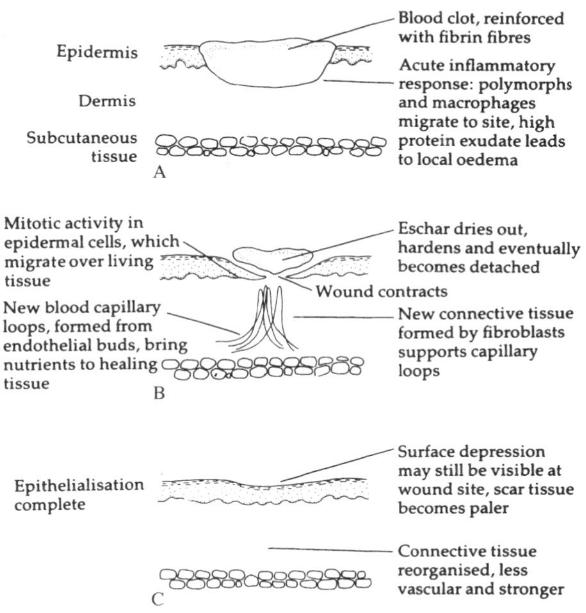
Blood clot, reinforced with fibrin fibres
Epidermis
Acute inflammatory response: polymorphs and macrophages migrate to site, high protein exudate leads to local oedema
Dermis
Subcutaneous tissue
A
Mitotic activity in epidermal cells, which migrate over living tissue
Eschar dries out, hardens and eventually becomes detached
Wound contracts
New blood capillary loops, formed from endothelial buds, bring nutrients to healing tissue
New connective tissue formed by fibroblasts supports capillary loops
B
Surface depression may still be visible at wound site, scar tissue becomes paler
Epithelialisation complete
Connective tissue reorganised, less vascular and stronger
C

Fig. 23.2 Wound healing by secondary intention. A: Inflammation/destructive phase. B: Proliferation/reconstruction phase. C: Maturation phase. (Adapted from Morison et al 1997.)

Scar tissue

A scar is the mark that may remain after a wound has healed. A scar consists of relatively avascular collagen fibres covered by a thin layer of epithelium.

Most scars fade with time (see Table 23.5) and the resultant cosmetic effect is generally acceptable, but abnormal scarring can lead to problems, as follows:

- stretching of scar tissue — this can occur where sutures have been removed prematurely, especially over areas that are under tension, e.g. the skin over the scapula and back are common sites where stretching occurs
- hypertrophic scar tissue — here collagen lysis and collagen production are out of synchrony and excessive tissue lies within the boundaries of the scar
- keloid — this is a protuberant, prominent scar which results from excessive collagen formation in the dermis during connective tissue repair.

Hypertrophic and keloidal scarring are examples of excessive scar formation. Such scarring is more common in young people, especially during pregnancy and puberty, and also in deeply pigmented skins, the peristernal area being particularly susceptible.

A number of factors influence scarring (see Table 23.6).

Why some wounds are sutured and others are left open

Wound closure (enabling wounds to heal by primary intention) is considered to be the method of choice whenever possible, as healing by primary intention is much quicker than healing by secondary intention.

Wound closure is undertaken where:

- the procedure will result in cosmetically acceptable scars (adhesive tapes and clips can be used to avoid undesirable suture marks)
- sufficient mobile tissue exists to allow the edges of the wound to be brought together easily without tension or without causing trauma (which could lead to subsequent wound breakdown)
- the wound site is clean, e.g. when an operation is considered to be a clean procedure as in excision of lipoma (a benign tumour containing fatty tissue).

Secondary intention is chosen as the method of healing where:

- the final cosmetic effect is likely to be an improvement over either skin grafting or suturing
- there is insufficient tissue to allow the wound edges to be approximated, e.g. in some chronic open wounds such as pressure sores (see p. 752) and leg ulcers (see p. 755)
- the wound area is heavily contaminated or infected, i.e. in a dirty injury or a dirty surgical procedure such as excision of an infected pilonidal sinus.

Table 23.5 The maturation of scar tissue

Time after sustaining wound	*Characteristics of scar*
0–28 days	The scar is fragile and soft
28 days–3 months	The scar becomes denser, stronger and is red or purplish in colour
3 months onwards	Over time the colour fades to white and the tissues become softer and more elastic

Table 23.6 Factors influencing scarring

Cause of injury		*Race*	*Age*	*Wound site*
Burn/trauma	*Surgery*			
1. Over joints contractures can occur 2. Dirty injuries caused by gravel can cause pigmentation	1. The skill of the surgeon 2. The type of suture material used, i.e. non-absorbable sutures cause extra scars alongside the wound	1. Extreme hypertrophic scarring is common in deeply pigmented races and rare in Caucasian races	1. In infancy and childhood, scars resolve quickly 2. In pregnant women, hypertrophic scarring is more common	1. Scars which follow the body's natural lines of skin tension do best 2. Scars which cross skin folds do less well 3. Scars on the shoulders, sternum and back produce unsightly scarring

FACTORS THAT ADVERSELY AFFECT HEALING

Q **23.2** Before considering factors that adversely affect wound healing, identify the requirements for optimal wound healing.

A number of factors can adversely affect the normal rate of healing, slowing it down and, in severe cases, impairing it altogether. These factors can be intrinsic or extrinsic.

Intrinsic factors

Advanced age. The metabolic rate of individuals gradually slows down with advancing years. This is reflected in wound healing, the rate of which is relatively slow in the elderly. This is in marked contrast to the rate of healing in young children and in pregnancy when the metabolic rate is increased.

Impaired nutritional status. Well-nourished individuals have a plentiful supply of the proteins, carbohydrates, fats, vitamins and minerals that are essential for normal healing. Good nutrition should be encouraged throughout the healing period. Those patients undergoing surgery should be carefully assessed, as their nutrition may be poor in the perioperative period as a result of preoperative fasting or postoperative dietary restrictions (see Ch. 21). For some patients it is not always easy to maintain adequate nutrition, e.g. an elderly person living alone or a terminally ill patient who is unable to eat. The importance of diet cannot be overstressed, and wherever possible the nurse should ensure that the patient receives all the nutrients required for healing. The advice of a dietician may be sought in an attempt to improve the nutritional status of vulnerable individuals.

Dehydration. The metabolic processes of an individual require about 2500 mL of water every 24 h (see Ch. 20). A dehydrated individual will not be able to metabolise efficiently and this will adversely affect the healing process.

Disease processes. The generalised metabolic effects of a number of disease processes can delay healing. Diabetes, cancer, inflammatory disease and jaundice are included in this group, as is any disease that impairs the body's immune response.

Impaired blood supply to the area. Where the blood supply to the wounded area is impaired, insufficient nutrients and oxygen are supplied and the healing period is prolonged. This happens in patients with peripheral vascular disease and lower limb ulcers.

Smoking adversely affects the healing process in a number of ways:

- Smoking (and the absorption of nicotine) has a vasoconstricting effect. After smoking one cigarette, peripheral blood flow has been shown to be depressed by 50% and to remain so for more than an hour.
- Nicotine was first shown to have an adverse effect on the immune response by reducing IgG concentrations (Corre et al 1971).
- It was found, when looking at the healing of abdominal wounds, that the overall cosmetic effect of a scar was poorer in patients who were smokers (Siana et al 1992). The main influences of nicotine and carbon dioxide relate to the effects on peripheral tissues, with a reduction in oxygen tension in these tissues and the formation of thrombi.

Extrinsic factors

Poor surgical technique. Where tissues are handled roughly during surgery, they can be damaged, resulting in haematoma formation. This can lead to the development of wound infection as the haematoma is broken down. A dead space may also occur if tissues are not correctly approximated during surgery; again this encourages the development of wound infection. Where sutures are inserted too tightly, the tissue becomes damaged and tissue death can occur.

Drug treatments. A whole range of drug therapies can affect the healing rate. The cytotoxic drugs given during chemotherapy can destroy healthy cells as well as malignant cells. Ideally, their use is withheld until any wound healing is complete. Steroids can also slow down, or prevent, healing taking place and their use is closely monitored in individuals with wounds.

Inappropriate wound management. The healing process may be adversely affected by the use of poor dressing technique, the wrong dressing material or antiseptics where they are not needed (see p. 748).

Adverse psychosocial factors. A wide variety of psychosocial factors can have an adverse effect on wound healing, e.g. lack of understanding and acceptance of the treatment regimen, or anxiety associated with changes in work, income, personal relationships and self-image (Morison et al 1997).

Infection. Of all the factors which can delay or prevent healing, infection is the most important.

WOUND INFECTION

A wound is a breach in the skin which, until complete healing is achieved, presents a risk of infection to the individual. However, infection in a healing wound delays healing and may even cause wound breakdown, herniation of the wound and complete wound dehiscence. The clinical signs and symptoms of a wound infection are summarised in Box 23.2. Despite all the technological advances that have been made in surgery and wound management, the problem of wound infection persists. This happens because the causes of wound infection are very varied and are often linked to the individual's general condition; both nutritional status and immune status are important factors in resistance to infection (Bale & Jones 1997).

The wound environment can itself encourage bacterial growth. Some organisms (anaerobes) thrive in wounds with a poor oxygen supply. A wound bed or area which is free from haematomas and dead tissue and is clean reduces the risk of infection.

The way in which the wound is managed can also affect infection. Contamination by bacteria, through poor technique on the part of the nurse, poor hygiene or incontinence on the part of the patient, can all increase the risk of wound infection.

The consequences of wound infection vary depending upon the environment in which the individual is being nursed.

In a hospital, a patient with a surgical wound infection poses a considerable risk to other patients with wounds on that ward. At home, that patient is less of a risk to his family and community, who are unlikely to be vulnerable.

Factors that predispose to wound infection

Factors associated with the patient

There are several factors which, in addition to delaying the healing process, can predispose a patient to wound infection. These can be identified on first assessment:

- Poor nutritional status — McLaren (1997) has described in detail the effects of deficiencies in nutrition on wound healing. Protein-energy malnutrition (PEM) has been linked to hospitalisation and impacts on all aspects of patient care, including developing pressure sores and influencing postoperative wound infection.
- Immunosuppression — suppression of the immune system (e.g. in diabetes mellitus or after steroid therapy) can lead to an increased rate of infection (Kindlen & Morison 1997).
- Excessive body weight.
- Advanced age.

Box 23.2 Clinical signs and symptoms of wound infection

The local effects of wound infection are:

- Pain — throbbing
- Redness
- Swelling — of the area surrounding the wound
- Discharge — haemoserous and/or purulent
- Loss of function — to protect the area
- Unhealthy appearance of the wound bed (p. 745)

Wound infection prolongs the inflammatory healing phase and delays healing by secondary intention. Systemic effects on the patient are:

- Raised temperature
- Increased metabolic rate
- General malaise
- Anorexia

Factors specifically related to the hospital environment

- Adverse spatial arrangements — when too many patients are nursed in close proximity to each other, especially in an open ward, the wound infection rate increases. An increase occurs when there are more than 25 patients being nursed in an open ward (Bibby et al 1986).
- Length of preoperative stay — the wound infection rate is linked to the length of time a patient spends in hospital prior to operation. The longer this period, the more likelihood there is of the individual being colonised by the pathogenic bacteria that are found in hospitals.
- Inappropriate preoperative care — patients who are not shaved preoperatively have the lowest clean wound infection rate, at 0.9%. This increases to 2.5% when patients are shaved (Spencer & Bale 1990).
- Prolonged operative procedure — the longer the operation, the greater is the risk of infection in clean wounds (Cruse & Foord 1980).
- Surgical contamination — in clean elective surgery (e.g. excision of a benign breast lump), the rate of infection is between 1 and 2%. In emergency operations where the area is contaminated (e.g. for perforated bowel), the rate soars up to 40% (Westaby 1985).
- Use of drains — the presence of a drain increases the risk of wound infection. It is lowest with closed drainage systems (Redivac) and highest with open drainage systems (e.g. corrugated drains) (Cruse & Foord 1980).

As a wound infection develops, localisation of the infection leads to the formation of a wound abscess. This may drain through the suture line or into the wound in the case of cavities. Occasionally, if deep-seated, the abscess will need a surgical incision to drain it properly. Where partial wound breakdown occurs, extra caution is needed to carefully explore and assess the wound as being suitable for healing by secondary intention (Bale & Jones 1997).

Sources of wound infection

Endogenous. Organisms found on the patient's own skin are endogenous sources of wound infection. These organisms (usually *Staphylococcus aureus* or gut commensals) are either present under normal circumstances or are hospital pathogens that colonise the body after the patient is admitted to hospital. *Staph. aureus* is found on the skin and sometimes in the upper respiratory tract. This organism does not normally affect the patient adversely, but when a wound has been created, *Staph. aureus* can invade the wound from adjacent skin or be breathed into the wound from the nose.

Exogenous. Infections from exogenous sources are those that occur following contamination of the wound from outside of the patient. This may happen in theatre or later in the ward when pathogens are allowed to fall onto the wound and penetrate it. Bacteria such as *Pseudomonas aeruginosa* can be found in wet areas or where moisture is present, i.e. in water, other fluids or ventilators. *Ps. aeruginosa* is also found in flower vases, sinks and drains.

Accidental injuries are highly likely to have been contaminated by bacteria. *Clostridium tetani* and *Clostridium welchii* are present in the soil and can be hazardous to the individual. People who garden or receive minor injuries in their gardens are at risk and should be immunised.

Bacteria

Bacteria consist of a variety of single-celled organisms which have a primitive nucleus with no nuclear membrane. Bacteria do vary in size, but are larger than viruses and can be seen under a light microscope. Bacteria reproduce by simple binary fission, i.e. each bacterial cell divides into two, both of which can divide again. The rate of division of bacteria, and so multiplication, depends on their environment, and in suitable conditions they divide rapidly.

Many of the harmful effects of bacteria on humans are caused by products of the bacteria, namely toxins, when these are released into the bloodstream. Endotoxins are released when a bacterial cell dies and breaks up, whereas exotoxins are continually released by thriving bacteria.

Bacterial cell walls. The cell wall of a bacterium can have a number of characteristics. These ultimately influence how capable a host will be at destroying that bacterium (Box 23.3). It is the cell wall that the body's immune system penetrates in order to destroy it.

Q **23.3** Identify the major microorganisms that cause wound infection. Can you identify their sources?

WOUND MANAGEMENT — A HOLISTIC APPROACH

In the past, many aspects of nursing care have been administered in a disjointed way using a task-oriented approach. Wound management has been no exception, all wounds being managed in much the same way, regardless of the needs of the individual or the environment in which he is being cared for.

Ideally, management of a patient with a wound uses an organised approach (Bale & Jones 1997). This begins with an initial assessment (Box 23.4) of both the patient and the wound so that the management can be planned. Following implementation, evaluation of that management is required to ensure that the needs of the patient have been met.

This approach can be adapted to suit the environment in which the patient is being cared for, whether this be in the patient's own home or in the hospital setting.

Nursing developments in wound management are undergoing rapid change, so it is important that nurses keep pace with current research findings. Journals, study days and conferences provide access to much of the research-based data and to cost-effectiveness studies. A whole range of written material, workbooks, videos, the internet and CD-ROMs on individual products is available from pharmaceutical companies and, while these may be biased, they can contain useful information on handling and application techniques, and on product range and sizes.

Box 23.3 Gram-positive versus Gram-negative bacteria

The differing characteristics of the bacterial cell wall can be determined by the staining reaction first used by Professor Hans Gram in the late 19th century. Gram, who developed the procedure quite accidentally, found that due to the properties of the cell wall, certain bacteria retain staining with crystal violet and resist any attempt to decolorise with ethanol. Other bacteria lose the stain, or respond to decolorisation and then respond to a pink counterstain. The former are described as Gram-positive bacteria and include such organisms as the cocci and clostridia. The latter are described as Gram-negative and include such organisms as *Escherichia coli* and *Pseudomonas aeruginosa*. This staining reaction is now considered a major classification distinction between bacteria.

Box 23.4 Assessment in wound care

1. Assess the patient:
- Identify factors that might impede healing, such as intercurrent disease processes or certain medications (see p. 742)
- Where disease processes are identified, attempt to ensure that they are corrected
- Where they cannot be corrected, build an expected delay in healing into the nursing care plan

2. Assess the wound:
- Consider whether the wound is healthy for the stage of healing and free from infection
- Assess the wound's physical characteristics
- Where appropriate, measure and record wound size

3. Assess the environment in which the patient is being nursed

4. Assess the appropriateness of wound agents and wound dressing materials

Assessment of the patient

When managing patients with wounds, it is easy to get carried away solely by assessment of the wound. Do not forget that the whole patient needs to be cared for, not just the wound. Whether the patient is being managed in the hospital or in the home, or is young or old, assessment of the patient's general condition should be undertaken. This is done to identify any of the factors which might impair the wound-healing process (p. 742). For those factors discovered which are reversible, treatment should be sought. For those factors uncovered for which no treatment is possible, some degree of delay should be anticipated and allowed for in the nursing care plan.

For further reading, see Bannon (1993). In this article, the author explains the importance of the holistic approach to wound care in the setting of an intensive care unit.

Assessment of the wound

Once the patient has been assessed in order to identify any factors that might affect healing, the next logical step is assessment of the wound being managed. A little time and thought taken at this stage can save much work later, ensure treatment is straightforward and avoid many pitfalls (Bale & Jones 1997).

Assessment of wounds that are healing by primary intention

Three questions need to be answered when assessing wounds that are healing by primary intention:

What has caused this wound? The answer may be surgical incision to perform an operation, or surgical excision of an abscess. Once the cause of the wound has been established, the expected prognosis for complete healing can be estimated. For example, a surgical incision in a fit, 20-year-old woman to remove a benign breast lump should result in a wound which will heal quickly and without complications. Compare this situation to an elderly lady who has had emergency bowel surgery for removal of a cancer. The expected healing potential here is not as good as in the first case (Spencer & Bale 1990).

Is the wound healthy for the stage of healing? During the first 3 days of healing by primary intention, the area surrounding the wound will be swollen, indurated and often painful. This is normal during the inflammatory phase of healing. This can be illustrated by looking at a wound 2 days postoperatively. The patient experiences some difficulty in moving around and the incision area appears red, sore, swollen and inflamed. Whereas this is normal at this stage of the healing process, it would not be considered normal if the patient presented with the same symptoms 7–10 days postoperatively, and would indicate the presence of infection. Recognising what is normal throughout the healing process is essential. Only when this has been achieved can the abnormal be identified.

What needs to be done in the days before the sutures or clips are removed? Nothing; if the wound remains healthy during the early days, the original dressing (if unstained and intact) can be left in place until the wound closure material is removed.

Box 23.5 Taking a wound swab

Points to remember:

- Use an aseptic technique
- Use a sterile, microbiological cotton wool swab
- This swab should be moistened in a transport medium before use
- If the wound is flat or shallow, gently rotate the swab across the middle of the wound bed. Care needs to be taken not to contaminate the swab with skin flora from the edges of the wound
- If the wound is deep, or has a recess, insert the swab into the depths of the wound. Bacteria present in the depths of a wound are different and more likely to be pathogenic than bacteria on the surface of a wound
- Carefully replace the swab directly into its storage tube containing culture medium
- Deliver to the laboratory as soon as possible, but at the latest within 24 h
- Record antibiotic drugs being given, the site of the wound, together with any other information likely to be of help to the laboratory

Assessment of cavity wounds

If wound management materials are to be used effectively, the appropriate product must be applied to the wound throughout the stages of healing. It is essential that the nurse is aware of what she requires from a dressing material in order to ensure that each product is used cost-effectively. During the assessment the following factors should be taken into consideration (Bale 1993).

Appearance of the wound bed. In the pre-granulation stage, cavity wounds often appear red and raw, and have a very uneven surface of adipose tissue. It is important to recognise that this is normal for this early stage of healing. Within 10–13 days, however, the appearance of the wound will change as granulation tissue is formed. A healthy wound should be pale pink in colour (sometimes covered with a pale yellow membrane), pain-free and should not bleed easily if touched. If infection is present, the appearance of the wound will alter. The colour of the tissue may change to a dark red and the wound will show a tendency to bleed easily on light contact and become uncomfortable or painful. Superficial bridging of tissue can also be seen within the cavity. As the presence of infection can delay healing, prompt treatment is needed in these situations. For deep-seated infection, a wound swab (Box 23.5) followed by the appropriate course of antibiotics is generally indicated, but more superficial infections can sometimes be treated topically. Until the infection is cleared no dressing material will be fully effective.

Wound size. In general, the larger a wound, the longer it will take to heal; therefore the size of a wound provides a useful indication of the probable healing time. The healing rates of some wound types, such as pilonidal sinus excisions, axillary wounds and abdominal wall wounds, have been carefully measured, and so it is possible with these wound types to predict with some accuracy how long they will take to heal (Marks et al 1983).

The size of a wound may also influence the choice of dressing. Whilst small cavities may be dressed with one of a number of products, it may not be practical to use some products on larger wounds where multiple pieces or packs would be required. In these situations, the choice of dressing material may be limited to products which provide the bulk with just one or two packs. This is an especially important consideration in the community where the available size range of modern dressing materials is limited.

Wound measurement. In order to assess the effectiveness of a particular treatment, it is necessary to monitor changes in the size of the wound. For the majority of wound situations this should be the way a wound progresses towards complete healing. Surgically created cavities are usually of even contour and depth; the length and breadth of such a wound can generally be determined fairly easily. Weekly measurement is sufficient and steady progress should be evident (Bale 1992).

Wound volume is more difficult to assess and does not really offer any advantages over the measurement of linear dimensions.

Chronic wounds, such as pressure sores, are often more difficult to measure as these wounds can extend under the skin edge. The simplest way of assessing the extent of these wounds is to measure by using a probe in the wound, under the edge of the cavity, and marking the boundary on the skin with an ink marker. This outline of the extent of the wound can then be traced onto paper and stored as a permanent record of wound progress.

For leg ulcers, the circumference of the wound can be traced onto clean acetate or plastic sheets and, again, can be stored as a permanent record.

Re-measurement of chronic wounds may only be necessary every 2–3 weeks, as healing is generally slower in these situations. Accurate measurement and keeping of these records avoid the need to depend upon clinical impression. More sophisticated and expensive methods of wound measurement are available, including structured light which assesses wound area and volume using parallel beams of light (Plassman & Jones 1992). The use of photography, especially instant Polaroid, is valuable in providing a permanent record of the appearance of the wound.

Q **23.4** How are wounds measured in the areas in which you have worked? Devise a way of recording the wound dimensions in the care plan of one of your patients.

Wound shape. When managing cavity wounds, it is necessary to recognise the importance of wound shape. Ideally, cavities created surgically should be boat- or saucer-shaped, with evenly sloping sides. Where pockets, tracts or sinuses occur within a cavity, drainage of exudate may be inadequate, and this in turn may greatly delay healing. Poor wound shape also restricts the range of dressing materials that can be used. For example, a long narrow cavity will require a dressing material that is conformable enough to be inserted into the restricted space but which can be easily removed from the depth of the wound without leaving behind fibres and particles which could then become a focus for infection.

In a wound where the shape is so poor that progress towards healing is unacceptably slow, surgical revision may be required in order to create a wound with more regular contours. This is occasionally necessary when wounds which have undergone primary closure subsequently break down. Pressure sores are particularly prone to develop into poorly shaped wounds and, as surgical revision here is not always possible or advisable due to the poor health of the individual, careful choice of an appropriate dressing material is essential (Bale 1992).

Exudate production. Cavities vary enormously in the amount of exudate they produce. New, surgically created wounds can exude heavily, whereas some deep pressure sores produce very little exudate. This variation will affect management, especially the choice of dressing material. Some products are highly absorbent and able to deal with copious discharges, whereas others have a limited capacity for absorption. The inappropriate use of a dressing material can sometimes have serious consequences. If, for example, a dressing material is chosen that is unable to cope with heavy exudate production, the surrounding skin can quickly become macerated. Alternatively, a very hydrophilic dressing material applied to a lightly exuding wound may cause excessive drying of the wound surface, delaying healing and sometimes even causing pain.

Presence of slough or necrotic tissue. When slough or necrotic tissue is present on the wound surface, healing will be delayed or, in some cases, prevented altogether. This material needs to be loosened and removed to allow wound healing to progress. This procedure is known as debridement and is a difficult task which requires intensive and skilled nursing intervention (see p. 747) (Bale 1996).

Assessment of the physical environment

The place where patients are nursed can have an effect on their progress. Patients being nursed in a hospital are in a controlled environment. Their dietary intake and fluid balance can be monitored and their general well-being assured. For 24 h each day, nursing care is available and, to a great extent, the nurse 'controls' the environment in which the patient is being nursed. In the community, when patients are being cared for in their own homes, the nurse has far less control over what happens in the environment of the patient. As a guest, the district nurse is able to advise and recommend an adequate food and fluid intake but is unable to monitor this accurately, as she is only available for a comparatively short period once or twice a day.

Creating an environment for healing

Principles of moist wound healing

Healing proceeds at its optimal rate when the wound is enclosed in a warm, moist environment (Fig. 23.3). Under these conditions, cellular activity is maximised; the benefits of such an environment have been recognised since the early 1960s (Winter 1962, Turner 1985). This is true for the whole spectrum of wounds encountered, from superficial cuts and grazes to large, extensive granulating wounds. Exposure of a wound to the air precipitates drying out of the wound surface and scab formation (Thomas 1990a).

Nurses should be mindful of the importance of providing a suitable environment for wound healing when choosing a wound management material. The term 'dressing' is a misnomer in the 1990s. The concept of a dressing 20 years ago was one of some form of absorbent cotton/gauze-type material that was used to soak up excess wound secretions and protect the wound from trauma. By the 1990s a whole range of sophisticated materials had been developed to cater for the diversity of individual wound situations. Many of these materials interact with the wound surface (so-called interactive materials) and are designed to optimise the local conditions for wound healing (Thomas 1990a). Box 23.6 summarises the characteristics of an ideal wound dressing material.

As new therapies continue to be developed, the use of growth factors, cultured human skin and synthetic substitutes are being introduced into patient care (Gentzknow et al 1996). Although such therapies are not appropriate for many patients whose

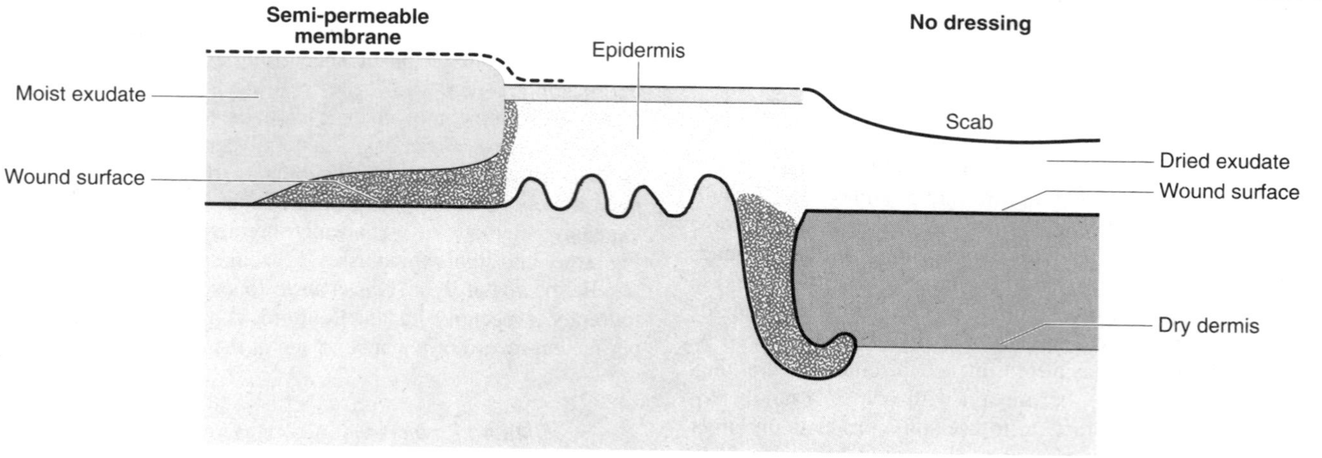

Fig. 23.3 Healing of skin wounds with and without a semi-permeable membrane dressing (Adapted from Winter 1962).

Box 23.6 Characteristics of an ideal dressing (Morison et al 1997)

- Non-adherent
- Impermeable to bacteria
- Capable of maintaining a high humidity at the wound site while removing excess exudate
- Thermally insulating
- Non-toxic and non-allergenic
- Comfortable and conformable
- Capable of protecting the wound from further trauma
- Requires infrequent dressing changes
- Cost-effective
- Long shelf-life
- Available both in hospital and in the community

wounds are healing rapidly, their use can be invaluable for wounds in life-threatening and other difficult situations such as burns and chronic and indolent ulcers.

Principles of cleansing

Why cleanse a wound? Sutured wounds rarely need cleansing unless leakage has occurred. In this situation the suture line can be gently, aseptically cleansed with sterile normal saline. With open wounds, strict asepsis is not always required. The patient can use the bath or preferably the shower to irrigate the wound with warm water (Harding 1992). For patient comfort, fluids used for wound cleansing should be warmed to body temperature. The main reason for cleansing open cavity wounds is to remove any loose debris and excess wound secretions. A shower is particularly useful in achieving this. The gently flushing action of the spray will remove any particles which are loose, and flushing for 10–15 s is usually sufficient. If bathing, the wound should be flushed by splashing water into it. Wounds of the lower limb can be bathed in a bucket or bowl, gently splashing the wound to remove loose debris. A bucket can be lined with a commercial bin liner. This protects the bucket from contamination and makes cleaning of the bucket much easier and so reduces the potential risk of cross-infection.

The role of antiseptics and topical agents. The actions of the whole range of antiseptics and cleansing agents are generally poorly understood. These lotions are widely used to mechanically cleanse wounds at dressing changes, and also as topical applications which stay in contact with the surface of the wound. In the past, nurses have been taught that all bacteria are bad for a wound and that wounds should be kept bacteria-free and sterile. Along with this went teaching that antiseptics which eradicate bacteria are therefore good and should be used routinely to keep the bacterial count at the wound surface as low as possible. There are a few situations where this is the case, i.e. in the treatment of burns and some immunocompromised patients and in some wounds which have undergone primary closure. For open wounds, the role of bacteria is somewhat different. All wounds become colonised by bacteria from the surrounding skin which are particular to that individual. Their presence does not affect the healing rate in many cases and these bacteria are extremely difficult to get rid of completely (Leaper 1986).

Bacterial studies on pilonidal sinus excisions, axillary wounds and abdominal wall wounds have shown that the vast majority of bacteria present in these wound types do not cause problems to the patient or, in fact, delay healing (Marks et al 1983). In a similar study looking at the bacteriology of leg ulcers, the presence of bacteria on the wound surface again did not delay healing (Eriksson 1984). Patients with leg ulcers appeared to keep their initial bacterial flora irrespective of the type of treatment and its eventual outcome. The organisms here included *Staphylococcus aureus*, *Escherichia coli* and *Pseudomonas aeruginosa*.

Nurses should use a realistic approach when cleansing wounds. Many antiseptics have a short-lived action and so bacteria will quickly re-colonise the wound surface. If these organisms are not harmful then why seek to eradicate them? Since the mid-1980s there has been debate within the nursing, medical and pharmaceutical professions as to the effectiveness of antiseptics, especially chlorinated solutions. Thomas (1990b) has made recommendations based on the available research that hypochlorite solutions should not be used routinely. There are, however, many clinicians who have successfully used these solutions over a number of years and advocate their use (Langridge 1990). The problem is yet to be resolved due to the lack of in vivo studies demonstrating their effects on healthy human tissue. The general guidelines issued by Thomas (1990b) should be followed if chlorinated solutions are to be used. Their use should be restricted to infected, sloughy and necrotic wounds and then only for short periods of time (maximum 7 days). These solutions are best not used on healthy tissues due to their potentially cytotoxic effects.

Removal of devitalised tissue

Chemical debridement. Before the advent of modern dressing materials, a range of chemicals was applied to sloughy and necrotic tissue in an attempt to soften and remove it (Bale 1996), but with varying degrees of success. In their use with harder necrotic tissue, which forms an eschar, these agents have difficulty in penetrating the surface and so are ineffective. About 100 mL of a solution which contains 0.25% w/v chlorine is needed to dissolve 1 g of sloughy tissue (Thomas 1990b), making this an apparently ineffective debriding treatment. Further work with Eusol on necrotic tissue showed that, after immersion for 24 h, the tissue remained unchanged (Thomas 1990b). Where granulation tissue is present, damage can occur due to the toxicity of the chemicals. However, it must be said that many nurses, both in the hospital and in the community, have successfully used these products for many years (Table 23.7). In these cases, the chemicals are generally used in the short term, for around 5–7 days, and the surrounding skin is well protected with a barrier cream. The experience and expertise of the user are the key to their success.

Enzymatic agents. These are designed to remove slough and necrotic tissue. A mixture of streptokinase and streptodornase is thought to act on slough and necrotic tissue without affecting viable tissue. It can be applied directly to the area or injected into an eschar. The latter procedure should only be carried out by experienced practitioners (Thomas 1990a). Alternatively, an eschar can be scored with a scalpel prior to application of the enzymes. A range of bacterial, plant-derived and fish-derived enzymes has been developed. Preliminary studies demonstrate a high potency of some of these (Glyantsev et al 1997).

Surgical debridement. It is sometimes possible for a surgeon to excise devitalised tissue with or without anaesthesia depending on the site and depth of the problem. The advantages of this method are that debridement is instant and a healthy cavity results. Where patients are being cared for in the community, access to the surgeon may be limited and this is not always a practical alternative for many patients. Less radical sharp debridement can be undertaken at the patient's bedside (Bale 1996).

Modern wound dressing materials. A number of these materials will effectively remove devitalised and necrotic tissue without damaging either the skin surrounding the wound or healthy tissue within the wound. Included in these are the hydrogels, hydrocolloids and the polysaccharides (Table 23.8).

Hydrogels and hydrocolloids quickly rehydrate devitalised tissue which has become dehydrated. Under moist conditions, the normal autolytic processes facilitate separation of viable from non-viable tissue. As the sloughy and necrotic tissue loosens, it can be wiped away or carefully pared off (Thomas 1990b).

Table 23.7 Topical cleansing agents

Agent	*Action*
Cetrimide	Bacteriostatic (against Gram-negative bacteria)
Chlorhexidine	Bacteriostatic (against both Gram-positive and Gram-negative bacteria)
Hydrogen peroxide 1000	Oxidising agent
Hypochlorites Eusol Eusol and paraffin Chloramin T Milton Dakin's solution Chlorasol	Oxidise and hydrolyse nitrogenous materials
Iodine preparations Aqueous solutions Alcoholic lotions	Powerful antimicrobial action
Proflavin cream	Mild bacteriostatic (against Gram-positive bacteria)

Table 23.8 Dressing materials

Material	*Presentation*	*Action*	*Advantages*	*Disadvantages*	*Suitable for*
Absorbent cotton and gauze	Variety of pads, rolls, squares and ribbon gauze	Absorbent material	Absorbent and cheap	Allows strike-through Adheres to granulation tissue and can become embedded in it Needs frequent dressing changes	As an outer layer for extra absorbency Should not be a primary contact material
Low-adherence dressing	Flat sheets in a variety of sizes	Absorbent for lightly exuding wounds	When used correctly has low adherence with wound surface	Allows strike-through when used in moderately to heavily exuding wounds and in these situations can stick	As a primary wound contact material for lightly exuding wounds, i.e. suture lines, superficial injuries, some superficial leg ulcers and pressure sores and at the end stage of healing
Tulle	Sheets of various sizes have paraffin and other substances impregnated in them	Non-adherent when used for lightly exuding wounds	Cheap When sufficient is applied correctly, will not adhere to wound surface	When used in moderately or heavily exuding wounds or when the exudate is particularly sticky, can adhere to the wound surface and be difficult to remove Impregnates can be allergenic especially with leg ulcer patients	Superficial open wounds which are lightly exuding
Semi-permeable film	Sheets of various sizes	Moisture-retaining adhesive film Allows gaseous exchange	Maintains moisture and fulfils a number of the criteria of a good dressing	Can peel off Can leak if wound exuding (although this can be prevented by aspiration of excess fluid)	Shallow superficial open wounds, suture lines, prophylaxis on pressure sores

Table 23.8 (*cont'd*)

Material	*Presentation*	*Action*	*Advantages*	*Disadvantages*	*Suitable for*
Paste bandage	7.5 cm × 4 m impregnated bandages used in conjunction with a compression bandage	Depends on the substance impregnated	Cheap, low-adherent Usually only needs changing weekly	Some patients develop allergies Does need skill to apply correctly, can cause damage if applied too tightly or with poor technique	Leg ulcer of venous origin, can be cut into strips for use on fungating lesions
Impregnated textile (Inadine, Poviderm)	Sheets of various sizes	Bactericidal	Low-adherence Delivers iodine to wound	Reaction if patient allergic to iodine When used inappropriately in lightly exuding wounds, can stick	Superficial leg ulcers and pressure sores and infected (especially pseudomonal) superficial open wounds
Dextranomers (Iodoflex, Iodosorb)	Paste, ointment	Cleansing and debriding by osmotic action at the wound surface and bactericidal	Will debride sloughy and necrotic matter	Possible allergic reaction to iodine	Sloughy, dirty and necrotic wounds, also for leg ulcers and pressure sores
Foam (Lyofoam, Allevyn, Lyofoam E, Tielle, Cavicare)	Sheets of various sizes, liquid base and catalyst but also need disinfectant to clean foam stent	Absorbent foams When poured, forms an exact cast of the wound	Infrequent dressing changes by the nurse, patient manageable	Not for use in irregularly shaped cavities	Superficial open wounds and cavity wounds
Hydrocolloid Hydrofibre	Wafers, beads, powder and paste	Dissolves into a gel on contact with wound secretions and this provides a healing environment, may stimulate formation of granulation tissue	Infrequent dressing changes Improved healing in chronic wounds	Offensive smell may be produced by the dressing as it degrades Not for infected wounds Occasionally, maceration of surrounding skin	Granulating wounds, especially chronic wounds
Hydrogel	Sheets and sachets	Provides a healing environment	Rehydrates dry areas Soothes painful areas Quickly removes necrotic tissue and slough from a wound surface Infrequent dressing changes	Can cause maceration of the surrounding skin Can be difficult to keep in place and may leak	Painful flat areas, burns, fungating lesions, cavity wounds, leg ulcers, pressure sores, sloughy and necrotic wounds
Alginate	Sheets, ribbon gauze	Provides a healing environment when dissolved into a gel	Absorbent material Infrequent dressing changes Can be used in sinuses and irregularly shaped wounds	Can build up on the wound edge Can be difficult to keep in place	Open wounds, chronic wounds, both regularly and irregularly shaped wounds

Excessive granulation

From time to time, re-epithelialisation fails to take place due to the presence of excessive granulation tissue or 'proud flesh'. Treatment is needed to flatten the granulation tissue so that it is level with the epithelial edge, as new epithelium cannot migrate up over this 'proud flesh'. An application of 75% silver nitrate sticks will cauterise the tissue, but a less traumatic method is the use of a cream containing a corticosteroid, although this should be used under medical supervision. The need for careful assessment is paramount in the successful treatment of cavity wounds. When planning a wound care programme, consideration of these factors should provide the nurse with an accurate picture of the needs of each patient and also provide some assistance with the dressing selection process.

Therapies of the future

Unlike traditional cotton absorbent materials, some of the modern dressings available interact with the wound (e.g. hydrocolloids, hydrogels, alginates). The trend to develop interactive products continues. Outside the UK, other countries are using agents to stimulate the healing process. These include the use of growth factors such as bFGF (basic fibroblasts growth factor), TGFb (transforming growth factor, b family), the interleukin family of proteins, and PDGF (platelet-derived growth factor) (Hopkinson 1992). Research continues to determine which wounds are likely to benefit most from the application of such agents.

A range of cultured skin and living skin equivalents has been developed. These are expensive to produce and are recommended for indolent wounds, burns and diabetic foot ulceration (Gentzknow et al 1996). This technology is unlikely to be widely available in the community but could enhance the care and improve outcomes for patients with the most difficult wound healing problems.

Dressing change techniques

Throughout the UK there are many different policies, procedures and protocols for dressing changes. However, the general principles remain the same.

A dressing needs changing when:

- there is a specific purpose, e.g. to remove sutures
- clinical signs of infection are present
- wound discharge has leaked through the dressing
- cleansing of an open wound is necessary — this may be as frequently as twice a day or as infrequently as once a week (see Table 23.8 for different dressings)
- special treatments are needed, e.g. burns dressings.

Aseptic technique

In hospital. When dressing changes are being performed within a hospital, the nurse must always take into consideration the possibility of transferring bacteria from one patient to another, due to the close proximity in which patients are cared for. This is more of a risk when several patients with wounds are being nursed in the same ward and by the same nurses. Once a wound has become contaminated, clinical infection can quickly develop. Aseptic technique aims to prevent pathogenic organisms from contaminating a wound (Box 23.7).

In hospital, dressings are generally changed using an aseptic technique. There may, however, be occasions when dressing changes require a technique that is socially clean without being fully aseptic.

Box 23.7 Principles of aseptic technique

- Perform the procedure in an area which is closed, clean and well ventilated at least 1 h after periods of activity — bedmaking and ward cleaning, for example, increase the circulation of dust particles and airborne bacteria
- Use a clean trolley — this should be thoroughly cleaned daily and wiped with an alcoholic solution before and after use
- Wash hands (p. 588) before, after and at any point during the procedure should they become contaminated. The use of an alcoholic hand-rub can sometimes be substituted
- Wear a clean plastic apron to protect the patient from bacteria on the nurse's uniform
- Use sterile equipment for the procedure — be aware of how your health authority/board identifies equipment which is sterile and therefore safe to use
- Discard equipment which has broken or damaged packaging
- Use sterile fluids and dressing materials
- Prepare equipment before dressings are removed
- Use gloves to remove any dressings and dispose of both immediately
- Carry out the procedure using forceps or sterile gloves, discarding equipment as it becomes contaminated
- Dispose of used equipment in the appropriate bin

It is an individual nurse's responsibility to understand the principles of asepsis and adapt her knowledge to the situation being managed.

In the community. In the hospital, equipment is provided which allows the nurse to manage safely all the wound management situations she may encounter. Maintaining asepsis may pose different problems in the patient's own home. The district nurse may have little control over the cleanliness of the area and needs to take extra care when changing dressings. It is just as important in the community to avoid cross-infection between households and contamination of wounds. The district nurse in these situations has many opportunities for health education.

The place for a clean technique

For many dressing changes, the use of a clean technique (Table 23.9) is safe and acceptable. The types of wound suitable for this method include the majority of granulating wounds.

Involving the patient in wound care

Whether the patient is being cared for at home or in hospital, there are many opportunities for the nurse to involve the patient in his wound management. This is important in giving the patient a sense of independence and will help the individual to return to normality. Patients with sutured wounds can be taught to monitor themselves for clinical signs of infection and to give good self-care in terms of nutrition, fluid intake, rest and avoidance of excessive movement of the affected area. Patients with open wounds can become much more involved. In addition to the self-care elements outlined above, they can be taught about the appearance of the wound surface and what can be expected to happen during the healing phase. In the community, patients and their relatives can be taught the basic dressing-change technique where asepsis is not necessary and the district nurse can assume a supervisory role. This obviously depends on individual circumstances and the patient's level of understanding, but certainly many patients with open wounds are able to play a major role in wound management. This is important as the patient begins to resume a more normal lifestyle and it also avoids the need for routine daily visits by the district nurse.

Table 23.9 Clean technique

Procedure	*Rationale*
1. Use non-sterile gloves to remove dressing. Change gloves	Protects both nurse and patient from cross-infection
2. Shower or bathe patient's wound	Mechanically removes loose wound debris (NB — ensure thorough cleansing of shower/bath whether at home or in hospital)
3. Use clean bowl/bucket with bin liner for patients with small wounds or foot/leg wounds in the home	Prevents contamination of equipment
4. Use clean paper or a clean towel to dry area surrounding wound	Prior to application of dressing, area needs to be dry
5. Encourage patient involvement in treatment	Increases patient compliance and encourages return to normal activity

Patients with chronic wounds, such as leg ulcers and pressure sores, need special help, but it is very important to gain their cooperation. Patients with venous leg ulcers (see p. 756) need to be taught leg elevation techniques and calf pump muscle exercises to stimulate the circulation and aid drainage of the lower limb. Carers of patients with pressure sores (see p. 752) need to be taught how to correctly lift, turn and position, and handle the patient. They also need to know how the pressure-relieving aids work, so that these are used correctly all the time and not just when the district nurse is in the home.

Nurse prescribing

Nurses working in the community play an integral part in the management of patients with wounds. The need for patients to receive a high standard of wound care in the community is of paramount importance as more and more patients are being cared for outside of hospital (Bale 1991).

For district nurses, the vast majority of their wound management workload concerns chronic wounds. Only 1% of patients with leg ulcers, for example, are managed in hospital. It is the district nurse who is faced with the long-term management of such wounds. Difficulties arose in the community when, following patient assessment, district nurses had to have the necessary dressing prescribed by the general practitioner. This 'rubber stamping' was both time-wasting and frustrating for the nurse. In response to a directive from the 1987 Primary Health Care White Paper 'Promoting better health', an Advisory Group was set up to investigate the professional and ethical issues surrounding nurse prescribing and make recommendations. In 1991, the Advisory Group recommended that 'suitably qualified nurses in the community should be able, in clearly defined circumstances, to prescribe from a limited list of items' (O'Dowd 1998). Pilot sites have successfully evaluated nurse prescribing and it has now been introduced.

As far as wound management is concerned, this list includes an extensive range of primary wound contact materials, bandages and dressing-retention materials (Bale 1991).

Auditing care

The use of audit consists of systematically looking at nursing practice, the peer reviewing of the results of specific interventions, the identification of problems and solutions followed by the implementation of change. The undertaking of clinical audit has been recognised by the Department of Health (1993a) as a useful method of evaluating and reassessing the quality of care given to patients. With regard to wound care, the incidence of pressure sores can be used as a key quality indicator (Department of Health 1993b).

Standard-setting

The setting of standards is another method of improving quality of care for patients. The standard-setting cycle is used to achieve a standard which individuals, teams and organisations can agree upon. Standards must to be relevant to care, understandable, measurable, behavioural and achievable (Marr & Geibing 1994). As with the audit cycle, the process includes peer review, problem identification and change management. Both audit and standard-setting are dynamic, practical processes.

Wound management policies and guidelines

There has been an increasing trend towards standardising wound management in health Trusts throughout the UK, by providing written policies, protocols and guidelines. The best of these are produced from systematic reviews of the literature covering randomised, controlled trials (Cullum et al 1997). Given the rapid development of wound dressings and associated devices (such as bandages and pressure-relieving equipment) and the wide range of therapies available to patients, such protocols and guidelines can promote enhanced quality of care for patients by ensuring they receive treatment which is research-based.

The transition from hospital to home

The transition from hospital to home for patients with wounds usually happens without any problems. Liaison nurses are often available to organise the discharge home and to arrange for any visits needed by the district nurse for the newly discharged patient. In accident and emergency departments, a liaison service may also be available. It is important, though, that wherever patients receive treatment they have a point of contact so that they are well supported when discharged home (Bale & Jones 1997).

Provision of materials in hospitals and in the community

Nurses may be unaware of the vast differences which exist in the provision of wound management materials to patients cared for in the hospital compared with those managed in the community. Although most hospitals impose some form of restriction on which materials are provided, generally all the main groups of manufactured materials are available for use in the hospital. These are supplied not only to in-patients but also to outpatients who are under the care of a hospital consultant. All materials needed for in-patient treatment are provided without direct cost to the individual patient. It is the norm, then, for patients treated in hospital to have access to a comprehensive range of wound management materials for their wound care, and supplies of these continue as long as the patient remains in hospital. Patients managed in the community are in a different position. Materials needed for their treatment are generally obtained from the general practitioner, who writes a prescription for those items required. Unless the patient is exempt from paying, a charge is made for each item dispensed. Provision is made to enable patients to purchase a 'season ticket' lasting 4 months or 1 year.

Apart from direct costs which may be incurred, the range of materials available on FP10 prescription is less comprehensive than that available within hospitals. The products that can be prescribed are listed in the Drug Tariff which is controlled by the Department of Health.

Q **23.5** Ask the pharmacist what products are available on FP10 to patients in the community. Look also at the sizes of prescribable products.

The Drug Tariff shows the current list of modern products. Although at first sight it would appear that it includes materials from all groups, the range of sizes is very restricted. In turn, this restricts the sizes of wounds that can be managed or increases the number of smaller packets required for each dressing change.

Expectations of outcome and effectiveness of treatment

Following individual patient and wound assessment, the nurse should have reasonable expectations regarding the prospects of achieving complete healing. In some wounds, complete healing is expected rapidly, as in primary wound closure following excision of a lipoma in a healthy young person. For others, the prognosis for healing is not so good, e.g. an elderly lady with arthritis and a venous leg ulcer. The expected outcome affects the choice of treatment for individual patients. For patients with a poor prognosis for healing, treatment is often directed towards minimising symptoms and preventing further wound breakdown. This situation can arise in terminally ill patients with superficial pressure sores where the aim is to prevent deterioration of the sore into deeper tissues. Patient comfort and convenience become the priorities and provide some measure of the effectiveness of the treatment. Where healing is expected, effectiveness means complete healing is achieved in the minimal number of days.

Cost-effectiveness

Efficacy is also measured in terms of the cost of treatments. Hospital doctors, general practitioners and the pharmacists who supply materials for wound management can be misled into believing that, because the initial cost of a material is high then it follows that the total treatment costs will also be high. The modern wound dressing materials are very much more expensive to buy per unit than traditional materials. However, the modern materials can often be left on the wound for several days and, in some cases, for a full week. Traditional, cheaper materials need daily or twice-daily dressing changes and the equipment needed during these frequent dressing changes increases the total treatment costs dramatically. If nursing time is also taken into consideration, then the cost of using traditional, cheap materials increases again (Bale 1989a,b).

It is important, when comparing the costs of modern and traditional materials, to look at:

- how long the product can be left on the wound
- how much nursing time is needed to change and apply dressings
- the benefits of using a material which is interactive and so stimulates tissue growth to achieve rapid healing or stimulate healing in a chronic wound.

Clinical evidence for improvement in healing or other outcome measures

It is in the area of materials that there has been most benefit, especially in the community, where much of the chronic wound care is undertaken. Modern materials are helping to achieve healing in these difficult wounds and enabling more efficient use of nurses' time.

Discharging such patients after many months, if not years, of treatment also improves their quality of life.

SPECIFIC WOUND TYPES

Pressure sores

Definition. A pressure sore is an area of localised damage to the skin and may involve underlying structures. Tissue damage can be restricted to superficial epidermal loss or extend to involve muscle and bone (Banks 1992).

The prevention and management of pressure sores present major challenges for nurses. The pressure sore problem is widespread and persistent, affecting patients from all walks of life and with a range of illnesses. It causes diminished quality of life and distress to patients and carers and it makes major financial demands on the health service. As a result, in many hospital and community trusts, nurses are now supported by a 'tissue viability service' (Dealey 1997). For nurses, the difficulties arise in trying to identify patients who might develop a pressure sore, and when they are at risk of doing so.

It is a basic responsibility of nurses to:

- accurately assess the patients in their care for being 'at risk' of developing a pressure sore
- ensure that any predisposing factors are reduced
- ensure that patients are nursed on the most suitable surface, depending on their individual needs
- ensure that established pressure sores are efficiently managed
- undertake regular and ongoing reassessments of individual patients; a patient's needs vary from one day to the next, and in the very ill from one hour to the next.

Aetiology

Pressure sores result from areas of previously healthy tissue becoming devitalised, resulting in localised tissue death. Pressure sores develop in a number of ways:

- as a result of direct, unrelieved pressure of soft tissues against bone
- where friction occurs between the patient and the surface of a bed or chair; this can happen if the patient is moved and the skin is dragged over a sheet
- as a result of the shear force which frequently accompanies both direct pressure and friction; shear forces develop in tissues that are distorted and pulled, so that the blood supply is disrupted.

Classification

In order to assess the extent or degree of damage, several gradings have been developed for the classification of pressure sores (Torrence 1983, Hibbs 1988, AHCPR 1992, Department of Health 1993b, Reid & Morison 1994).

There are four- and five-stage systems which classify by the extent and depth of the tissues damaged. One such, the National Pressure Ulcer Advisory Panel (NPUAP) Classification (AHCPR 1992), is as follows:

- *Stage I* — non-blanchable erythema of intact skin: the heralding lesion of skin ulceration.
- *Stage II* — partial-thickness skin loss involving epidermis and possibly also the dermis. The ulcer is superficial and presents clinically as an abrasion, blister or shallow crater.
- *Stage III* — full-thickness skin loss involving damage or necrosis of subcutaneous tissue that may extend down to, but not through, underlying fascia. The ulcer presents clinically as a deep crater with or without undermining of adjacent tissue.
- *Stage IV* — full-thickness skin loss with extensive destruction, tissue necrosis or damage to muscle, bone or supporting structures (e.g. tendon or joint capsule). Undermining and sinus tracts may also be associated with stage IV pressure ulcers.

Assessment of risk

In an acute illness, even the most unlikely individual may become 'at risk' of developing a pressure sore; therefore, all patients should be assessed on admission either to a hospital ward or unit or onto a district nurse's caseload — 'The importance of assessing all patients (except perhaps some short-stay cases) cannot be over emphasised' (Waterlow 1992). A combination of disease processes and/or drug therapies or surgery, for example, can quite suddenly put an individual into an 'at risk' category.

The following types of patients are at risk of developing pressure sores:

- the elderly
- the immobile, e.g. paraplegic, following orthopaedic surgery

Table 23.10 Norton risk scale (Norton et al 1962)

A *Physical condition*		*B* *Mental condition*		*C* *Activity*		*D* *Mobility*		*E* *Incontinent*	
Good	4	Alert	4	Ambulant	4	Full	4	Not	4
Fair	3	Apathetic	3	Walk/help	3	Slightly limited	3	Occasional	3
Poor	2	Confused	2	Chairbound	2	Very limited	2	Usually/urine	2
Very bad	1	Stuporous	1	Bedfast	1	Immobile	1	Double	1

Scoring system: total score of 14 and below = at risk of developing a pressure sore.

- those with sensory loss, e.g. comatose, diabetic
- those with a range of systemic diseases, e.g. anaemia, peripheral vascular disease, carcinoma
- those having a range of drug therapies, e.g. anti-inflammatories, cytotoxics, steroids
- the incontinent
- poorly nourished individuals
- the obese and those with below-average body weight.

Several scales and scoring systems have been devised for assessing risk, the most widely used being the Norton scale (Table 23.10) and the Waterlow score (Fig. 23.4). Traditionally, the Waterlow scoring system has been widely used in the UK because it takes many factors into consideration. It is comprehensive and yet easy to use (Morison et al 1997). There are many other risk assessment scores available, including those of Douglas (Pritchard 1986), Lowthian (1987) for orthopaedic patients (Fig. 23.5) and Bradon (Flanagan 1993) and the Walshall Community Pressure Sore Risk Calculator (Milward 1993).

With so many risk assessment systems available, it is inevitable that criticism has arisen. Because the Norton scale was devised using elderly patients, it has been suggested that its use is limited for younger people. It has also been criticised for not being sufficiently comprehensive to cover other risk factors such as nutrition. Bridel (1993) reviewed three scoring systems and came to the conclusion that there were problems with validity in these systems.

The reasons for the widespread use of the Waterlow and Norton scoring systems, and for their popularity, are probably that both are easy to use and take a matter of minutes to complete. Both reasons are important if all patients are to be regularly reassessed. Some health authorities and health boards have adapted these scoring systems to suit their own patients' needs and as part of a pressure sore prevention policy. However, all health care professionals have a duty towards their patients, the responsibility for taking action being crucial once risk is identified (Dealey 1997).

A risk assessment scoring system is only useful, however, if it is used regularly — on admission and again each time the patient's condition changes. The scores need to be accurately documented and then used to determine the most appropriate pressure-relieving devices on which to nurse the patient.

23.6 What scoring system does your ward/area use? Where is the score documented and how often are patients reassessed?

For further information, see Bridel (1993) and Dealey (1997).

Prevention of pressure sores

Once patients have been identified as being 'at risk', they should be nursed on the most appropriate surface (Box 23.8). This includes not only the mattress on the bed but also any chairs in which they may sit during the day (Dealey 1992). Other areas worth considering are theatre operating tables and trolleys on which patients are transported around the hospital.

For further reading, see Hibbs (1991).

Liaison with other professionals may be indicated, for example with the physiotherapist to assess the degree of mobility an individual has and where help and treatment can be given.

Attempts to reduce friction and shearing when nursing patients are essential. At home this is easier than in hospital where sheets are often starched. Where possible, patients should be nursed on soft sheets or covered with a duvet, as hard rigid surfaces increase friction.

Friction also increases with moisture. As increased skin moisture can result from incontinence and sweating, these should be avoided where possible.

Nutrition and fluid balance also need attention. It has been estimated that dehydrated patients and patients in a negative nitrogen balance are more likely to experience tissue breakdown.

Pressure sore prevention policies. These are designed to rationalise and standardise patient care so that all patients receive a reasonable level of care. They also help to ensure that the available pressure-relieving equipment is used most efficiently.

Management of patients with established pressure sores

In addition to providing a suitable surface for the patient to be nursed on, ensuring adequate nutrition and using good handling techniques when moving a patient, local care of the pressure sore needs to be considered (Morison et al 1997).

Stage 1. Although no ulcer is present, tissues will rapidly deteriorate if pressure is not relieved as a matter of urgency.

Stage 2. These superficial wounds usually need a dressing to assist tissue recovery and to protect the area. A common cause of such sores is either friction or, more usually, a combination of friction and shear force.

Elimination of the cause is needed to avoid further and more extensive damage. Several materials can be chosen as dressings which will provide a healing environment: semi-permeable films, occlusive alginates, foam sheeting and hydrocolloids are all good examples (Table 23.8). Where incontinence is a problem, occlusive or semi-occlusive materials are invaluable.

A

WATERLOW PRESSURE SORE PREVENTION/TREATMENT POLICY
Ring scores in table, add total, several scores per category can be used

Build/weight for height	★	Skin type Visual risk areas	★	Sex Age	★	Special risks	★
Average	0	Healthy	0	Male	1	**Tissue malnutrition**	★
Above average	1	Tissue paper	1	Female	2		
Obese	2	Dry	1	14 – 49	1		
Below average	3	Oedematous	1	50 – 64	2	e.g. Terminal cachexia	8
		Clammy (temp.↑)	1	65 – 74	3	Cardiac failure	5
Continence	★	Discoloured	2	75 – 80	4	Peripheral vascular disease	5
		Broken/spot	3	81 +	5	Anaemia	2
Complete/ catheterised	0					Smoking	1
Occasion. incont.	1	**Mobility**	★	**Appetite**	★	**Neurological deficit**	★
Cath./incontinent of faeces	2	Fully	0	Average	0	e.g. Diabetes, M.S., CVA	
Doubly incontinent	3	Restless/fidgety	1	Poor	1	Motor/sensory paraplegia	4–6
		Apathetic	2	N.G. tube/		**Major surgery/trauma**	★
		Restricted	3	fluids only	2		
		Inert/traction	4	NBM/anorexic	3	Orthopaedic – below waist, spinal	5
		Chairbound	5			On table >2 hours	5
						Medication	★
						Cytotoxics, High dose steroids Anti-inflammatory	4

Score	10+ at risk	15+ high risk	20+ very high risk

© J Waterlow 1991 Obtainable from Newtons, Curland, Taunton TA3 5SG

B

REMEMBER: TISSUE DAMAGE OFTEN STARTS PRIOR TO ADMISSION, IN CASUALTY.

ASSESSMENT : (see over) If the patient falls into any of the risk categories then preventive nursing is required.
PREVENTION : A combination of good nursing techniques and preventive aids will definitely be necessary.

Preventive aids:

Special mattress/bed:	10+ Water mattresses, e.g. Dyson, Spenco, Vaperm, Topper. 15+ Large cell ripple, e.g. Huntleigh, Water beds. 20+ Pegasus Airwave, Clinitron, Mediscus.	Mechanical aids:	Real sheepskins – sacral, heel/ elbow pads, e.g. Pegasus Lamb Pads, Gel protection Bed Cradle
Chair:	Correct for patient protection – side/seats, movement, e.g. Nestor, Roho, Jay.	Patient aids:	Monkey Pole Hand Lifts
Bed clothing:	i) Cotton cellular blanket ii) Duvet iii) Vapour permeable mattress cover. iv) Pillows	Operating table/ Theatre trolley	e.g. 'Moulding Top' e.g. Topper, Waffle
Nursing care:	Pain control Turning / 30° tilt Passive movements Nutrition – high protein, minerals, vitamins	Skin care	General hygiene, NO rubbing. Prevent shearing force damage e.g. correct lifting & positioning Dress with inert covering e.g. Opsite

IF TREATMENT IS REQUIRED, FIRST REMOVE PRESSURE

WOUND CLASSIFICATION :

Blanching hyperaemia	STAGE I	Is wound RED?	YES Semi-occlusive dressing Bioclusive, Tayederm.
Non-blanching hyperaemia	STAGE II	Is wound RED, clean but not healed?	YES Granuflex, Lyofoam, Scherisorb, Sorbsan, Silastic Foam (deep)
Ulceration progresses	STAGE III	Is wound YELLOW/ infected/inflamed?	YES Sorbsan, Scherisorb, Debrisan Granuflex
Ulceration extends	STAGE IV	Infected?	YES Sorbsan packing, Isosorb, Actisorb, Flamazine (for pseudomonas), Debrisan.
Infective necrosis	STAGE V	Is wound BLACK/ necrotic?	YES Debride – surgical excision Granuflex, Scherisorb, Varidase

Fig. 23.4 The Waterlow pressure sore prevention/treatment policy. (With kind permission from Waterlow 1991.)

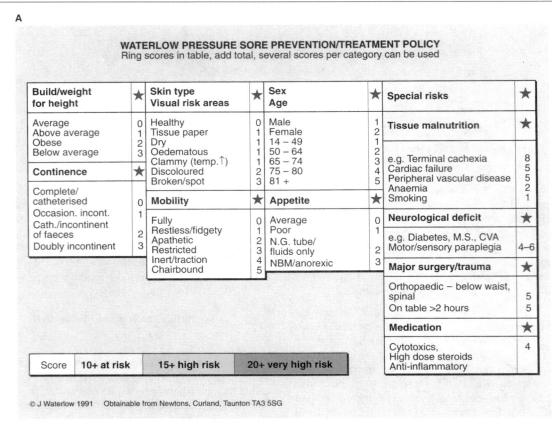

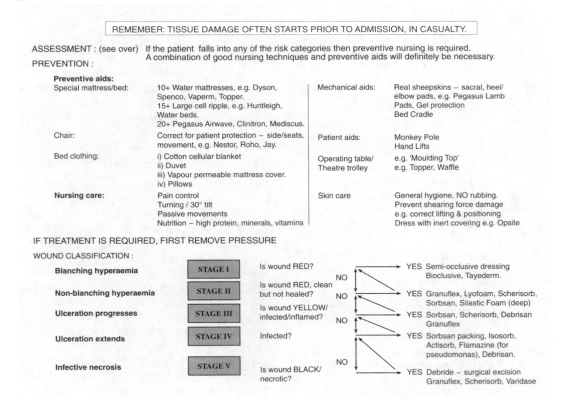

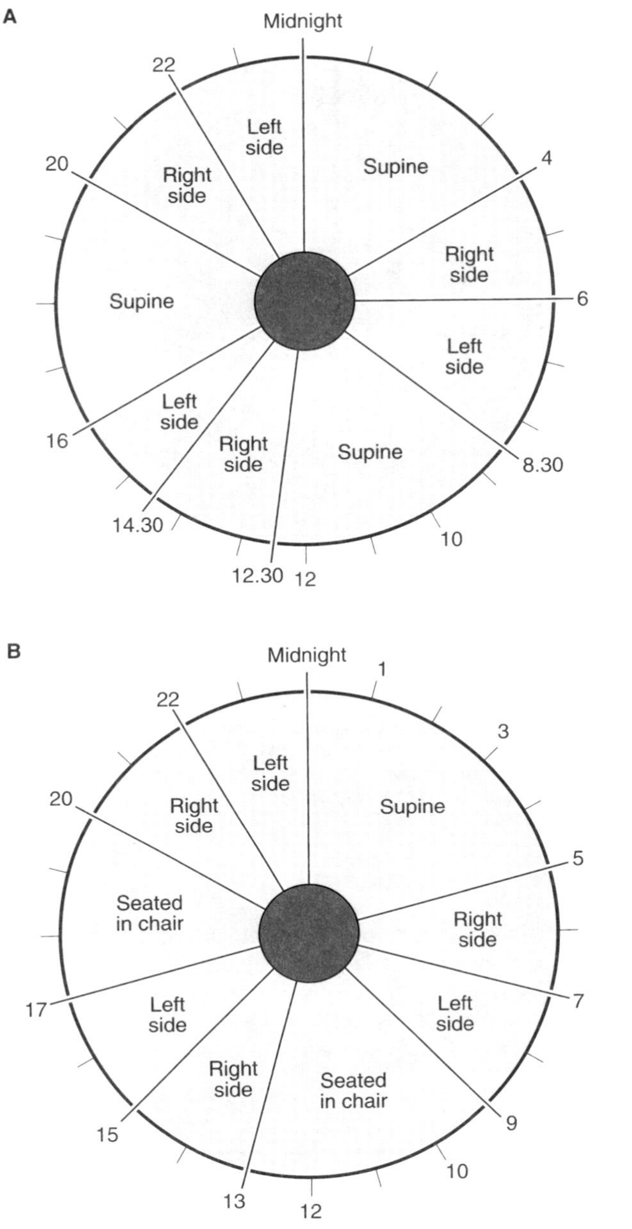

Fig. 23.5 Lowthian's 24 h turning clocks. Turning schedules for (A) bed-bound patients and (B) chair-fast patients. (Adapted from Lowthian 1987.)

Stages 3 and 4. These deeper wounds are much more difficult to manage. They often have an irregular contour with the wound extending under the skin edge. Assessment is needed of the full extent of the wound (see p. 745). Other problems related to wound shape are sinus formation, which requires careful management, and packing and/or irrigation. This is a situation where surgical intervention may be needed.

Necrotic tissue and slough deep within these extensive wounds must be removed if healing is to proceed, and there are several ways of achieving this (Bale 1996) (see p. 747). One important point to remember is that, until all the devitalised tissue has been removed, the full extent of the pressure sore cannot be realised. The development of severe tissue damage is a serious and potentially hazardous situation for a patient. Ninety per cent of patients with necrotic pressure sores of the trunk die within 4 months (Bliss 1990).

Box 23.8 The range of pressure-relieving devices (Dealey 1992)

Low-risk patients
- Sheepskins
- Hollow-core fibre pads
- Bead overlays
- Foam overlays
- Gel pads

Medium-risk patients
- Foam overlays
- Foam replacement mattresses
- Combination foam/water mattresses
- Combination foam/gel mattresses
- Alternating air pads
- Water beds
- Double-layer alternating air pads

High-risk patients
- Double-layer alternating air pads
- Air-flotation pads
- Dynamic air-flotation mattresses
- Air-wave mattresses
- Air-fluidised beds

Other nursing considerations

The management of an established pressure sore is costly in both economic and personal terms. Prevention of pressure sores is often far cheaper than management (Dealey 1997). Health service managers are able to cost the treatment of pressure sores more accurately and with the call for pressure sores to become a notifiable condition (Dealey 1992) more emphasis is being put on prevention.

Patient education

In the prevention and management of pressure sores, patients have an important role to play. Young, chronically disabled patients can be taught various methods of regularly relieving pressure by changing position (Thomas et al 1990). Patients who are not able to take such an active part in their own management can be taught the value of and need for the changes of position that nurses and other carers carry out for them. Compliance increases when patients understand why intervention is necessary.

Education leaflets can also be useful. An extract from a typical patient information leaflet demonstrates how the nurse and the patient share in the prevention of pressure sores (Box 23.9).

In the USA the NPUAP has issued guidelines for the prevention and treatment of pressure sores for professionals, carers and patients (AHCPR 1992).

Leg ulcers

Leg ulceration is essentially a community-based problem and a difficult problem to treat, with only about 1% of these patients admitted to and treated in hospital (Callam et al 1985). The day-to-day care of patients with these wounds is undertaken in the community by the district nurse and general practitioner. The major cause of leg ulceration in the UK is chronic venous insufficiency associated with venous hypertension (70–75%). Between 20 and 30% of patients with a leg ulcer have some degree of ischaemia.

Box 23.9 Extract from an education leaflet: preventing pressure sores (Morison et al 1997)

As most pressure sores are the result of staying in one position for too long, the answer is to:

Relieve the pressure by changing position

Ideally, you should get up out of bed or your chair at least once every 2 h during the day and take a short walk. This activity also helps your blood circulation and stops your muscles getting lax.

If you are confined to a chair, you should lift your bottom off the seat for a few moments every half hour by pushing up on the arms of the chair.

If you have to stay in bed, then your bed may be fitted with a 'monkey pole' or rope ladder — the nurse will show you how to use this to lift yourself off the bed.

If your pressure sore is extensive or deep, or your movement is very restricted, a special movement chart will be devised for you by the nursing staff to keep you off the sore as much as possible, and you may be given a special bed or mattress.

Diabetes, vasculitis and trauma are other causes of leg ulceration. It follows that one of the most important stages in the assessment of these patients is to diagnose the aetiology of the ulcer, as that dictates the most appropriate method of management. Such diagnosis is achieved by conducting a lower limb assessment in conjunction with the use of a hand-held Doppler (Morison & Moffatt 1994) (see Box 23.10).

Venous stasis leg ulcers

This is the most commonly encountered group of leg ulcers, occurring frequently in elderly female patients. Damage to the veins deep in the calf causes incompetence of the perforators (the veins which link the deep and superficial veins in the calf) (Fig. 23.6).

Drainage of the skin in the lower leg is affected, leading to oedema, induration and pigmentation. Fibrin is laid down around the capillaries in this area, which interferes with oxygen diffusion into the tissues. Following this, any knock or minor injury to the lower leg leads rapidly to breakdown of the skin and ulceration. Most commonly, ulceration occurs around the medial malleolus; the ulcers are shallow and pain is not usually a factor.

A typical past history reveals previous phlebitis, deep vein thrombosis (DVT), leg fracture or severe leg injury, or varicose veins.

It can take months and even years for these wounds to heal. Because of the poor condition of the tissues, ulceration can recur and these patients need to wear compression stockings even after healing, to help maintain drainage of the affected limb.

For further reading, see Morison & Moffatt (1994) and Cullum & Roe (1995).

Assessment. One of the primary aims of assessment in a patient with an ulcer is to determine the cause of that ulcer. This is frequently undertaken by both the nurse and doctor working together as part of the primary health care team. This assessment includes:

- taking a comprehensive medical history which might indicate the presence of venous disease, e.g. history of previous DVT, venous claudication, previous vein surgery or pelvic trauma
- undertaking a thorough clinical examination to support the medical history

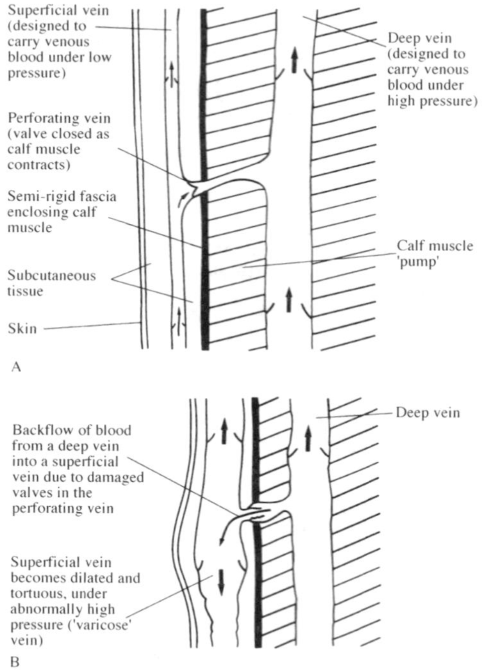

Fig. 23.6 A: Healthy, intact valves prevent back-flow of blood from the deep to the superficial veins. B: An incompetent valve in a perforating vein allows back-flow of blood from the deep to the superficial venous system. (Reproduced with kind permission from Morison & Moffatt 1994).

- undertaking the appropriate investigations: a Doppler assessment will give the ankle pressure index (Box 23.10) but other investigations may include haemoglobin to exclude anaemia, ESR to indicate the presence of infection, glucose levels to exclude diabetes mellitus, and wound swab where infection is suspected.

Box 23.10 How to take the ankle pressure index

- Lay the patient flat and allow the patient to rest quietly for 20 min. This is necessary to eliminate the effects of gravity on the legs
- Place sphygmomanometer cuff on the upper arm, apply gel over the brachial artery. Hold Doppler probe at a 45° angle and measure the systolic pressure
- Place the sphygmomanometer cuff around the malleolus (should the ulcer be sited here, place the cuff above the ulcer). Apply gel around either the dorsalis pedis or posterior tibial pulse
- Locate the pulse and inflate the cuff until Doppler sound disappears. Gradually deflate the cuff and, when sound returns, record this as the ankle systolic pressure. The ankle pressure index is calculated by dividing the ankle pressure reading by the brachial pressure reading

Normal ankle pressure index ≥1
Abnormal ankle pressure index ≤1
If ankle pressure index ≤0.8, the arterial impairment is significant

Management

Bandaging. The most important component in the treatment of venous stasis ulcers is the control of oedema by compression bandages or support stockings (Morison & Moffatt 1994). Compression bandages are designed to give a graduated compression that provides more support at the ankle and less at the knee, to compensate for the failure of the perforators in the leg. The bandages need to be worn constantly during the day when the patient is walking and upright, to reduce oedema. It may be necessary to prescribe diuretics to assist drainage of oedema.

The principles of compression bandaging are to:

- bandage from toes to below the knee (see Fig. 23.7)
- apply graduated compression by applying even tension to a compression bandage; more pressure is applied to the ankle and less as the circumference of the leg increases to the knee — 30–40 mmHg of pressure may be required at the ankle, graduating to 15–20 mmHg below the knee (Morison & Moffatt 1994)
- maintain the level of compression
- ensure that the bandage/stocking does not slip, causing constriction of the limb (Morison & Moffatt 1994).

The pressure exerted by a bandaging system can be calculated using Laplace's law (Box 23.11).

Selection of a bandage depends on the amount of compression required. Three grades of compression bandage are available:

- grade I provides very light compression or support for mild oedema
- grade II provides moderate compression at the ankle of between 18 and 24 mmHg
- grade III provides strong compression, giving between 25 and 35 mmHg at the ankle.

Control of infection. Where pain, cellulitis, erythema, enlarging of the ulcer and purulent discharge occur, antibiotics may be necessary to control the infection. These should be administered systemically. Superficial infection can sometimes be controlled by the topical application of an antiseptic.

Physiotherapy. Exercises to stimulate the calf muscle pump (which assists venous return) can be taught to each patient, and these are encouraged regularly throughout the day to stimulate circulation and aid drainage of the lower legs. Some period of leg elevation should also be encouraged around the middle of the day, again to allow drainage of the lower legs.

Dressings. Dressing management should be carefully considered once the factors outlined above have been successfully tackled. The ulcer should be assessed (as for wounds, p. 744) and the appropriate material then selected (p. 748). Caution should be exercised with dressings and lotions as these patients quickly develop sensitivities to many of the commonly used products. The simplest treatments should be used first. Paste bandages with elastic compression bandages, hydrocolloid wafers, alginate sheets, impregnated textile dressings and polysaccharide dressings, all used with a good compression bandage, are suitable for these wounds.

A complete treatment package of a suitable wound contact dressing combined with adequate compression therapy, physiotherapy and education are likely to produce the best patient outcomes.

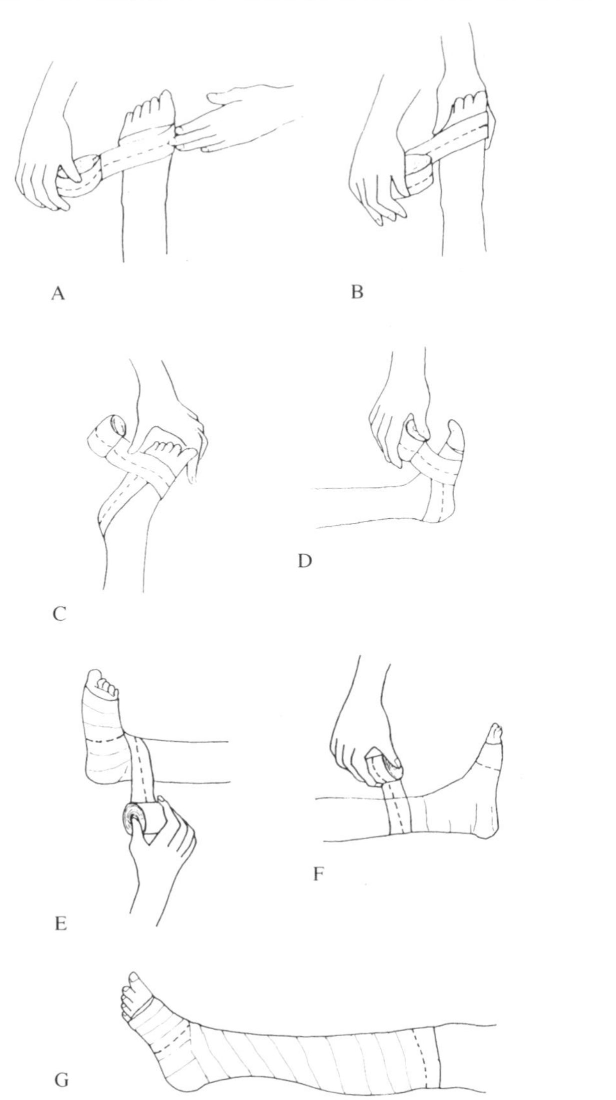

Fig. 23.7 Elastic web bandage. A: Start bandage on the inner side of the sole of the foot, with the lower edge of bandage at the root of the toes. Turn $1\frac{1}{2}$ times round the foot. B**:** The thumb fixes the bandage for the start of the turn around the heel. C: View from the outer side of the foot. Thumb and finger hold bandage in place prior to completing turn around base of toes. D: View from the inner side of the foot. E: View from the outer side of the foot. Continuation of the bandaging, keeping lower edge of the bandage along red or blue line of the previous turn. F: View from the outer side of the foot. Tension used is about half the full stretch of the bandage. G: View from the outer side of the leg. Note the position of the final turn of bandage immediately below the knee. (Reproduced with kind permission from Ryan 1991.)

Arterial ulcers

These are a result of arteriosclerosis obliterans and thromboangiitis obliterans (Cullum 1994) of the lower leg and so are a very different problem from ulcers arising from venous disease (see Table 23.11). Arteriosclerosis may occur anywhere throughout the arterial circulation, so causing narrowing and occlusion due to calcification of the artery wall. Damage to the arteries supplying the leg can be caused by vascular disease and this gradually occludes and blocks them. Additionally, infarction of smaller arteries is caused by embolus formation, which causes ischaemia in the area of skin normally supplied by that artery. What follows is a very rapid breakdown of the skin. The characteristics of these ulcers are

Box 23.11 Formula for calculating the pressure exerted by a bandaging system (Morison & Moffatt 1994)

$$P = \frac{T \times N \times \text{constant}}{C \times W}$$

P = sub-bandage pressure
T = tension
N = number of layers
C = limb circumference
W = width of bandage

a history of intermittent claudication and rapid onset of a deep ulcer which is often extremely painful. Relief is gained by lowering the affected limb and hanging it over the edge of the bed or chair. These patients rarely go to bed to sleep, or if they do, they have to get up in the night because of the pain. They tend to sleep in a chair, which allows the affected limb to hang down. These ulcers can occur anywhere on the lower leg, but usually present on the foot and lateral aspect of the lower leg. Foot pulses are often absent or very difficult to palpate. Doppler assessment reveals a pressure index of below 0.8. The patient may also have a history of cardiovascular disease, typically hypertension, myocardial infarction, strokes or transient ischaemic attacks.

Management. Surgical intervention may be necessary to improve the circulation or to debride dead tissue within the ulcer, and skin grafting may be considered. Light bandaging only is applied to keep a dressing in place; compression is to be avoided at all costs as this would further impede an already poor blood supply to the area.

Healing of these wounds is slow and the prognosis for eventual healing often poor. Treatment aims to keep the patient as comfortable as possible and to achieve debridement and cleansing where necessary. Useful dressings include alginate sheets, medicated dressings and hydrogel sheets.

Mixed aetiology ulcers

Around 20% of venous ulcers also have a significant arterial blood supply deficiency (Morison & Moffatt 1994). This further complicates management, as control of oedema is needed but without restricting the already poor blood supply.

Diagnosis. Accurate diagnosis is fundamental to successful treatment. Those giving care should be absolutely certain of exactly what the aetiology of the ulcer is before any type of treatment begins. Lower limb assessment together with Doppler assessment (p. 756) will assist diagnosis. Clearly, if arterial problems are allowed to go unrecognised and strong compression bandaging applied, treatment will not only be ineffective but could also cause the patient harm. Information on other types of leg ulcer is summarised in Box 23.12.

Patient education

Individual education regarding wound management can have a dramatic effect on progress.

This aspect of care is particularly appropriate in patients with leg ulcers, especially venous leg ulcers, as unless these patients know the cause of their ulcer, they may not comply with treatment. Leg exercises, leg elevation and the need for adequate compression are the key factors to success. Without this education the patient is not fully equipped to participate in management of the ulcer. Patient education can be helped by providing leaflets which can be read at home (Box 23.13).

Sutured wounds

Although the vast majority of sutured wounds heal without complication, there is a need for careful observation of both the patient and the wound site:

- Observe the patient for changes in vital signs, pulse, temperature, or malaise which could indicate the presence of infection, especially wound infection.
- Observe the wounded area for signs of infection after the initial inflammatory response has taken place, i.e. redness, swelling, pain, discharge, heat.

When are the sutures removed? The best time for removal of suture material depends upon a number of factors:

- The site of the wound — wounds on the head and neck usually heal within 2 days due to the rich blood supply to the area, whereas wounds on the back may take 10–14 days to heal. The skin here is thicker and less well supplied with blood.
- Patient variation — if, during suture removal, the wound begins to gape then the nurse should stop and refer to the

Table 23.11 Characteristics of venous and arterial disease of the lower limb

Characteristic	*Venous disease*	*Arterial disease*
Site of ulcer	Around the 'garter' area, commonly above the medial malleolus	Anywhere on the lower limb including the foot, but commonly affecting the toes
Depth of ulcer	Shallow and spreading	Deep, with a punched-out appearance
Presence of oedema	Common, due to poor venous return	Often not detected
Onset	Gradual, unless precipitated by trauma	Rapid
Pain	Often uncomfortable, nagging in character	Pain on elevation of limb relieved by lowering it (the blood flow is increased when the limb is in the dependent position). The pain of ischaemia can be unremitting
Temperature of foot	Warm and well perfused	Cool or cold and poorly perfused
Condition of the skin surrounding the ulcer	Lipodermatosclerosis present Varicose eczema	
Ankle pressure index	>0.8	<0.8

Box 23.12 Other types of leg ulcers (Browse & Burnard 1982)

- *Vasculitic ulcers* (2.5%) — these are due to connective tissue disease (e.g. rheumatoid arthritis, scleroderma), and also occur on the lower leg. They are unusual and extremely difficult to manage due to the underlying disease process and the drug therapies that these patients require.
- *Diabetic ulcers* (5.0%) — these occur most commonly on the foot. Again, due to the general condition of the patient, they heal slowly. It is worth noting that diabetics may give a falsely high reading on Doppler assessment due to peripheral hypertension. The management of rheumatoid and diabetic ulcers is generally under specialist care and treatment is prescribed by the individual consultant.
- *Traumatic ulcers* (2%).
- *Miscellaneous causes* (1%) — neoplastic and tropical ulcers are examples in this category.

surgeon for advice. The skin edges can be pulled back together and held for a few more days with paper sutures.

- Cosmetic considerations — it should also be noted that leaving sutures in for too long can cause excessive scarring.

In general, the principles for managing sutured wounds are to leave the wound undisturbed and the theatre dressing intact unless either the patient or the wounded area begins to develop signs which indicate the presence of infection (Bale & Jones 1997). Disturbing dressings unnecessarily can lead to the entry of bacteria into the wound itself or disturb the newly forming epithelium. Local wound infection can slow down the rate of healing and also increase the amount of scar tissue produced. Careful postoperative observation is important. Ultimately a severe wound infection can spread into the tissues and also the bloodstream, causing septicaemia which could be life-threatening (Spencer & Bale 1990).

Traumatic wounds

Patients who present to the accident and emergency department with traumatic wounds need special consideration. These patients may be shocked or have other injuries and their wounds are often contaminated due to the nature of the trauma (see Ch. 27).

These wounds are frequently an irregular shape, with varying degrees of tissue loss. Due to contamination, wound closure is often not attempted. Mechanical cleansing of the wound is undertaken to remove debris such as glass, wood or tarmac. Where wound closure is attempted, antibiotic cover is given to prevent infection.

Patients with extensive injuries are admitted for in-patient treatment. However, the majority of patients with wounds are discharged home to be cared for in the community. They may be instructed to care for the wound themselves or told to return to the accident and emergency department for any dressing changes, or the community nurse may be asked to take over the wound management.

For further information, see Bale & Jones (1997), part 2: intervention.

Box 23.13 An education leaflet for patients with venous ulcers and their carers: how to care for your legs (Morison & Moffatt 1994)

How long must I keep the dressing and bandage (or stocking) in place?
Wear the support bandages or elastic support stockings as advised by the doctor and nurse. They will make arrangements for your next dressing change.

Do not be tempted to look under the bandage or disturb the dressing in the meantime, as this may delay healing. It is particularly important not to scratch the skin around the ulcer as this skin is easily damaged.

Ask for help AT ONCE if:

- Your leg itches excessively, is hot, or more painful than usual
- You feel that the bandage is too tight anywhere
- You lose sensation in your toes, or they turn cold or blue
- You need any other advice.

Contact person:

Contact telephone number:

Can I exercise?
Yes. Exercise is good for your circulation and your general health. If possible, take a gentle walk every day. Even indoors, you can bend and stretch your toes while sitting, and bend, flex and circle your ankles to prevent them from becoming stiff. It is important not to stand still for too long. It is a good idea to do the dishes and the ironing sitting down, if you can obtain a chair of the correct height.

Should I sit with my legs up?
Yes. Sitting with your legs hanging down is almost as bad as standing in one place for too long. You should sit with your legs supported on a stool, on a cushion or pillow, i.e. above the level of your hips. It is also helpful to raise the foot of your bed 9 inches (23 cm), as this aids return of blood from the legs to the heart overnight.

Do I need a special diet?
You do not need a special diet, but try to eat a balanced one that includes protein (meat, fish, eggs), fresh fruit and vegetables. Being overweight does not help the circulation in your legs. Ask the doctor for advice on weight loss if this is a problem for you.

Are there any other ways I can help my legs?
Yes.

- Avoid knocks to your legs, as this could lead to another ulcer.
- Keep your legs warm, but do not sit too close to the fire as this can damage the skin.
- Do not wear anything tight around the tops of your legs, such as garters or girdles, as your circulation will be hindered.
- Stop smoking.

Malignant wounds

This is one group of wounds where healing is not always the expected outcome of wound management. These wounds include fungating carcinoma of the breast, fungating lesions of malignant melanoma and a variety of other non-healing, extending or fungating wounds. Mortimer (1993) has defined the term 'fungating' as describing a malignancy which has ulcerated and infiltrated through the epithelium. Fungating wounds can result either in a protruding growth or in an ulcerating cavity (Carville 1994). These patients are generally managed by a combination of hospital and home care and over a period of time become well known to both agencies.

The growth of tumours is a complex process which controls blood flow and tissue oxygenation (Grocott 1995). Hypoxia of the tissues causes tissue breakdown and encourages anaerobic and aerobic bacterial growth, producing malodour.

Problems encountered with malignant wounds (see Ch. 31) are as follows:

- *Wound site*. Often these wounds are present in an area which is extremely difficult to dress in terms of keeping the dressing in place, e.g. on the chest wall, in the groin and on the lower limb.
- *Exudate production.* The exudate tends to be thick and sticky. Many dressings which do not adhere to other wound types will do so in the presence of this particularly viscous exudate. The hydrogel sheets and gel are very useful dressings for these wounds.
- *Pain*. Where nerve endings are exposed, changing dressings and rubbing of dressings can be problems. Keeping the wound covered reduces the irritation to the nerve endings, and using gel dressings reduces pain at dressing changes.

Where healing is not the ultimate aim, wound management should maximise convenience and minimise distress.

For further reading, see Morison et al (1997), Chapter 11.

Burns

The management of burns is a specialised area (see Ch. 30). The treatment given depends on the individual burns unit. However, all follow the same basic principles for management. Treatment will depend on the physical well-being and age of the individual, the area burnt and the depth and extent of the burn.

Psychosocial factors

The presence of a wound will inevitably have some effect on well-being. There may be no difficulty when a wound is small and heals rapidly, but for many patients some degree of anxiety is felt relating to the wound. This can disrupt sleep patterns, increase the perception of pain and even suppress the immune system. In more serious wounds, a disturbance of body image may also cause lasting distress, particularly if the patient is unprepared for this (Lacey & Birchnell 1986).

23.7 How would you help the following patients to overcome their fears and worries?

- An elderly lady living alone has a chronic venous ulcer requiring frequent dressing by the community nurse. She is increasingly confined to the house.
- A small girl recovering from a hernia repair fears that when the sutures are removed her wound will break open.
- A young woman has been mugged on her way home from work. The knife wound to her face required suturing in the accident and emergency department. She has had no opportuniy to see the wound and is fearing the worst.

CONCLUSION

The effective management of patients with wounds requires an understanding of the healing process in conjunction with an organised approach to both assessment and management, and includes:

- assessment of the individual's overall health, taking into account factors which might impair healing
- assessment of the wound
- planning the management of the individual, taking into account the social and physical environment, and using the most appropriate dressing materials available
- involving the patient, where possible, in wound care
- evaluation and reassessment of the individual until the wound heals or the needs of the patient change.

23.8 Which types of dressing materials are available in your hospital/community?

Estimate the cost of dressings needed to manage four different patients for 1 week. Include dressing packs, surgical tapes and lotions as well as the dressing materials themselves.

How much variation is there between the four? Which patient is the most expensive to manage?

23.9 Go to the operating theatre and find out how pressure sores are prevented in theatre.

23.10 Go to the hospital pharmacy/chemist's shop to find out how dressing materials are ordered and dispensed. Who decides which products are made available in the hospital?

REFERENCES

Agency for Healthcare Policy and Research 1992 Pressure ulcers in adults: prediction and prevention. Clinical practice guideline No 3. AHCPR Publication No 92. 0047. AHCPR, Rockville, USA

Bale S 1989a Cost effective wound management in the community. Professional Nurse 4(12): 598–601

Bale S 1989b Research in the community. Nursing Times 84(38): 73–75

Bale S 1991 Nurse prescribing wound management in the community. Nursing Standard 5(8): 29–31

Bale S 1992 A holistic approach and the ideal dressing: cavity wound management in the 1990s. In: Horne E M, Cowan T (eds) Staff nurse's survival guide, 2nd edn. Wolfe, London, pp 261–268

Bale S 1993 Wound assessment. Surgical Nurse 6(1): 641–645

Bale S 1996 A guide to wound debridement. Journal of Wound Care 6(4): 179–182

Bale S, Jones V 1997 Wound care nursing: a patient centred approach. Baillière Tindall, London

Banks V 1992 Pressure sores: a community problem. Journal of Wound Care 1(2): 42–44

Bibby B A, Collins B J, Ayliffe G 1986 A mathematical model for assessing the risk of post-operative wound infection. Journal of Hospital Infection 8: 31–38

Bliss M 1990 Geriatric medicine. In: Bader D L (ed) Pressure sores. Clinical practice and scientific approach. Macmillan, London

Bridel J 1993 Assessing the risks of pressure sores. Nursing Standard 7(25): 32–35

Browse N L, Burnard K G 1982 The cause of venous ulceration. Lancet ii: 243–245
Callam M J, Harper D R, Dale J J, Ruckley C V 1987 Chronic ulceration of the leg: clinical history. Lothian and Forth Valley Leg Ulcer Study. British Medical Journal Clinical Research 294(6577): 929–931
Callam M J, Ruckley C, Harper D, Dale J J 1985 Chronic ulceration of the leg – extent of the problem and provision of care. British Medical Journal 290: 1855–1856
Cameron J 1997 Dermatological aspects of wound healing. In: Morison M, Moffatt C, Bridel-Nixon J, Bale S (eds) Chronic wounds. Mosby, London
Carville K 1994 Assessment and management of cancerous wounds. Primary Intention 2(1): 20–26
Clark M, Cullum N 1992 Matching patients' needs to pressure sore prevention with the supply of pressure redistributing mattresses. Journal of Advanced Nursing 17: 310–316
Clark M, Watts S 1994 The incidence of pressure sores within a National Health Service trust hospital during 1991. Journal of Advanced Nursing 20: 30–36
Corre F, Lellouch J, Schwartz D 1971 Smoking and leucocyte counts. Lancet 2: 632–634
Cruse P J E, Foord R 1980 The epidemiology of wound infection: a 10 year prospective study of 62,939 wounds. Surgical Clinics of North America 60(1): 27–40
Cullum N 1994 The nursing management of leg ulcers in the community: a critical review of the research. HMSO, London
Cullum N, Roe B 1995 Leg ulcer research and practice: the way forward. In: Cullum N, Roe B (eds) Leg ulcers: nursing management. Scutari Press, London
Cullum N, Sheldon T A, Fletcher A, Semlyen A, Glanville J, Sharp F 1997 Compression therapy for venous leg ulcers. Effective Health Care 3(4): 1–12
Dale J, Callam M J, Ruckley C, Harper D R, Berry P N 1983 Chronic ulcers of the leg: a study of prevalence in a Scottish community. Health Bulletin (Edin) 41: 310–314
Dale J, Gibson B 1986 The epidemiology of leg ulcers. Professional Nurse 1(8): 215–216
Dealey C 1992 How are you supporting your patients? A review of pressure relieving equipment. In: Horne E M, Cowan T (eds) Staff nurse's survival guide, 2nd edn. Wolfe Publishing, London
Dealey C 1997 The politicisation of pressure sores. In: Managing pressure sore prevention. Mark Allen, Guildford
Department of Health 1993a Clinical audit. Department of Health, London
Department of Health 1993b Pressure sores. A key quality indicator. Department of Health, London
Department of Health 1993c The costs of pressure sores. Department of Health, London
Eriksson G 1984 Bacterial growth in venous leg ulcers – its clinical significance in the healing process. An environment for healing: the role of occlusion. The Royal Society of Medicine, London
Flanagan M 1993 Pressure sore risk assessment scales. Journal of Wound Care 2(3): 162–167
Forrest R O 1982 Early history of wound treatment. Journal of the Royal Society of Medicine 75: 198–205
Gebhardt K 1992 Preventing pressure sores in orthopaedics. Nursing Standard 6(23): 3–5
Gentzknow G D, Iwasaki S D, Hershon S 1996 Use of dermagraft, a cultured dermis, to treat diabetic foot ulceration. Diabetes Care 19(4): 350–354
Glyantsev S P, Adamyan A A, Sakharvoc I Yu 1997 Collagenase in wound debridement. Journal of Wound Care 6(1): 13–16
Grocott P 1995 The palliative management of fungating malignant wounds. Journal of Wound Care 4(5): 240–242
Harding K G 1992 The wound programme. Centre for Medical Education, University of Dundee, Dundee
Hibbs P J 1988 Pressure area care for the City and Hackney Health Authority. Prevention plan for patients at risk from developing pressure sores. Policy for the management of pressure sores. City and Hackney Health Authority, London
Hopkinson I 1992 Growth factors and extracellular matrix biosynthesis. Journal of Wound Care 1(2): 42–50
Kindlen S, Morison M 1997 The physiology of wound healing. In: Morison M, Moffatt C, Bridel-Nixon J, Bale S (eds) Nursing management of chronic wounds, 2nd edn. Mosby, London
Lacey J H, Birchnell S A 1986 Body image and its disturbance. Journal of Psychosomatic Research 30(6): 623–631
Langridge C J 1990 Ban on hypochlorites is stupid. Hospital Doctor 10(32): 10
Leaper D J 1986 Antiseptics and their effect on healing tissue. Nursing Times 82(23): 45–47
Leaper D J 1998 History of wound healing. In: Leaper D J, Harding K G (eds) Wounds: biology and management. Oxford University Press, Oxford
Lees T A, Lombert D 1992 Prevalence of lower limb ulceration in an urban health district. British Journal of Surgery 92: 1032–1034
Louden I S L 1982 Leg ulcers in the 18th and early 19th centuries. Journal of the Royal College of General Practitioners 32: 301–309
Lowthian P 1987 The practical assessment of pressure sore risk. Care, Science and Practice 5(4): 3–7
McLaren S 1997 Nutritional factors in wound healing In: Morison M, Moffat C, Bridel-Nixon J, Bale S (eds) Nursing management of chronic wounds, 2nd edn. Mosby, London
Marks J, Hughes L E, Harding K G, Campbell H, Ribero C D 1983 Prediction of healing time as an aid to the management of open granulating wounds. World Journal of Surgery 7: 641–645
Marr H, Geibing H 1994 Quality assurance in nursing: concepts, methods and case studies. Campion, Edinburgh
Milward P 1993 Scoring pressure sore risk in the community. Nursing Standard 3(8): 50–55
Moffatt C 1995 The organisation and delivery of leg ulcer care. In: Cullum N, Roe B (eds) Leg ulcers. Scutari Press, London
Morison M, Moffatt C, Bridel-Nixon J, Bale S 1997 A colour guide to the nursing management of chronic wounds, 2nd edn. Mosby, London
Morison M, Moffatt C J 1994 A colour guide to the assessment and management of leg ulcers, 2nd edn. Mosby, London
Mortimer P 1993 Skin problems in palliative care: medical aspects. In: Doyle D, Hanks G, MacDonald N (eds) Oxford textbook of palliative medicine. Oxford Medical Publications, Oxford
Norton D, McLaren R, Exton-Smith A N 1962 Investigation of geriatric nursing problems in hospital. National Corporation for the Care of Old People, London (reissued 1975, Churchill Livingstone, Edinburgh)
O'Dea K 1993 Prevalence of pressure damage in hospital patients in the UK. Journal of Wound Care 2(4): 221–225
O'Dowd A 1998 Back bench driver. Nursing Times 94(35): 16
Plassman P, Jones B F 1992 Measuring leg ulcers by colour-coded structured light. Journal of Wound Care 1(3): 35–38
Preston K 1991 Counting the costs of pressure sores. Community Outlook 1(9): 19–24
Pritchard V 1986 Calculating the risk. Nursing Times 82(8): 59–61
Reid J, Morison M 1994 Towards a consensus: classification of pressure sores. Journal of Wound Care 3(3): 157–160
Ryan T 1991 The management of leg ulcers. Oxford University Press, Oxford
Scales J T, Lowthian P T, Poole A G et al 1982 'Vaperm' patient support system: a new general purpose hospital mattress. Lancet 2: 1150–1152
Siana J E, Frankild S, Gottrup F 1992 The effect of smoking on tissue function. Journal of Wound Care 1(2): 37–41
Spencer K, Bale S 1990 A logical approach: management of surgical wounds. Professional Nurse 5(6): 303–306
The Lancet 1973 The costs of pressure on the patient (editorial). Lancet 2: 309
Thomas A, Krowskop S L, Noble G, Noble P 1990 Pressure sore management and the recumbent person. In: Bader D L (ed) Pressure sores: clinical practice and scientific approach. Macmillan Press, London
Thomas S 1990a Wound management and dressings. The Pharmaceutical Press, London
Thomas S 1990b Eusol revisited. Dressing Times 3: 1
Torrence C 1983 Pressure sores: aetiology, treatment and prevention. Croom Helm, Beckenham
Turner T D 1985 Semiocclusive and occlusive dressings. In: Ryan T (ed) An environment for healing: the role of occlusion. Royal Society of Medicine Congress and Symposium, Series 8
Waterlow J 1988 Prevention is cheaper than cure. Nursing Times 84(25): 69–70
Waterlow J 1991 A policy that protects: the Waterlow pressure sore prevention/treatment policy. In: Horne E M, Cowan T (eds) Staff nurse's survival guide, 2nd edn. Wolfe, London
Westaby S (ed) 1985 Wound care. William Heinemann Medical Books, London
Winter G D 1962 Formation of the scab and rate of epithelialization of superficial wounds in the skin of the young domestic pig. Nature 193: 293–294

FURTHER READING

Barbenel J C, Jordan M M, Nichol S M, Clark M O 1977 Incidence of pressure sores in the Greater Glasgow Health Board Area. Lancet 2: 548–550

Bader D L (ed) 1990 Pressure sores: clinical practice and scientific approach. Macmillan Press, London

Bale S, Jones V 1997 Wound care nursing: a patient centred approach. Baillière Tindall, London

Bannon M 1993 Healing the whole person. Nursing Times 89(13) (Wound Care Supplement): 62–68

Bridel J 1993 Assessing the risks of pressure sores. Nursing Standard 7(25): 32–35

Cullum N, Roe B 1995 Leg ulcers. nursing management: a research-based guide. Scutari Press, London

Dealey C 1991 The size of the pressure sore problem in a teaching hospital. Journal of Advanced Nursing 16: 663–670

Dealey C 1997 Managing pressure sore prevention. Mark Allen, Guildford

Dealey C 1999 The care of wounds. Blackwell Scientific Publications, Oxford

Goldstone L A, Goldstone J 1982 The Norton score: an early warning of pressure sores. Journal of Advanced Nursing 7: 419–426

Hibbs P J 1991 The economics of pressure sore prevention. In: Bader D (ed) Pressure sores: clinical practice and scientific approach. Macmillan Press, London

Krasner D, Kane D 1997 Chronic wound care: a clinical source book for healthcare professionals, 2nd edn. Health Management Publications, USA

Morison M, Moffatt C J 1994 A colour guide to the assessment and management of leg ulcers, 2nd edn. Mosby, London

Morison M, Moffatt C J, Bridel-Nixon J, Bale S 1997 A colour guide to the nursing management of chronic wounds, 2nd edn. Mosby, London

Roberts B V, Goldstone L A 1979 A survey of pressure sores in the over-sixties on two orthopaedic wards. International Journal of Nursing Studies 16: 355–364

Video cassettes

Harding K G, Bale S, Banks V, Jones V 1992 Nursing chronic wounds in the community. Medical Television Productions, London

Harding K G, Bale S, Lewis B, Banks V 1992 Nutrition and wound healing. Purvis-Wickes Video Projects, London

USEFUL ADDRESSES

The Wound Care Society
PO Box 263
Northampton NN3 4UJ

The European Pressure Ulcer Advisory Panel
Wound Healing Institute
Churchills Hospital
Headington
Oxford OX3 7LJ

The Tissue Viability Society
Wessex Rehabilitation Unit
Odstock Hospital
Salisbury

Venous Forum of the Royal Society of Medicine
The Ashdown Hospital
Burrell Road
Haywards Heath
West Sussex RH16 1UD

European Wound Management Association
88 White Hart Lane
Tottenham N17 8HP

CONTINENCE

24

Jean Swaffield

INTRODUCTION

Having control over urinary and faecal elimination is an expected norm within every society. In all but the very young, incontinence is generally not viewed with sympathy, and the real suffering it causes to the individual and her carers has not received the attention it deserves. Epidemiological research has shown that the number of people suffering from incontinence in some form or other far exceeds the number of cases reported to health professionals. An underlying theme of this chapter is the need to acknowledge the extent of the problem and to promote continence by improving screening practices and raising public and professional awareness of preventive measures against incontinence and of the range of treatments available.

Incontinence is a symptom that is often wrongly labelled as a disease. This chapter describes the underlying conditions that can prevent the acquisition of continence or provoke its loss. It is argued that a sound understanding of the causes and types of incontinence is essential for its proper investigation, treatment and management and that diagnostic assessment must recognise the individuality of each patient. Similarly, where incontinence is intractable, assessment for aids and equipment must be sensitive to the values, needs and priorities of each patient in order to ensure that an optimum quality of life is achieved.

Throughout the chapter the nurse is encouraged to take a positive, problem-solving approach towards this often hidden problem, to assess his own attitudes towards the subject of incontinence, and to base his nursing decisions and actions on up-to-date, research-based knowledge.

URINARY CONTINENCE

The acquisition of continence in early childhood is a much valued developmental milestone. In the adult, the ability to control urinary and faecal elimination is largely taken for granted, and a loss of continence will have profound implications for the individual's ability to participate fully within society. While it may be deemed acceptable for a child to have an occasional 'accident', this is not generally the case for adults. The subject of incontinence is one which many people find difficult to discuss openly, and one which is poorly understood. Clear definitions and sound knowledge have been lacking, and certain mistaken beliefs in the recent past — such as the assumption that incontinence is untreatable — which were once entrenched, are now being challenged.

The onus is on health professionals to foster a change in social attitudes by acquiring a clear understanding of how continence is attained and how incontinence can develop. In the role as health educator, the nurse can make an important contribution to the promotion of continence among those groups who are particularly vulnerable.

Defining continence

Continence may be defined in terms of the actions and abilities necessary for the appropriate management of urinary and faecal elimination. These include:

- recognising the need to pass urine or faeces
- identifying the correct place to pass urine or faeces
- delaying elimination until the appropriate place is reached
- reaching the correct place
- passing urine or faeces appropriately once a suitable place is reached.

Acquiring continence

Urinary continence cannot be acquired until the physiological systems necessary for micturition have matured. Once the prerequisite physical development has taken place, becoming continent is a matter of imitation, skill attainment and social conditioning.

The anatomy of the bladder is detailed in Chapter 8. The bladder is a simple organ which has a dual function: it acts as a reservoir for urine and it expels urine at the volition of the individual. Urine remains in the bladder as long as the intravesical pressure does not exceed the urethral resistance.

In normal micturition, the contraction of the detrusor muscle of the bladder induces the bladder neck to open while the pelvic floor muscles and the external sphincter relax. For a child to obtain continence, she must acquire control of the mechanisms for preventing the bladder from automatically emptying when it is full; this is usually achieved by the age of 3 years.

The neurological control of the bladder at birth involves a simple sacral reflex arc whereby automatic filling and emptying of the bladder are under the control of sacral segments 3 and 4 of the spinal cord. Stretch receptors in the bladder wall are activated by urine accumulation. These relay impulses with increasing frequency through the parasympathetic nerves to the spinal cord until the motor parasympathetic nerves react by causing the bladder muscles to contract and the urethra sphincter to open, whereupon reflex emptying occurs.

In order to achieve continence, a child needs to become aware of the sensation of the bladder becoming full and through trial and error attempt to overcome the reflex emptying mechanism by using the pelvic floor to keep the urethral sphincter closed. The sensory tracts of the spinal cord involve the cerebral cortex in the brain to overcome or inhibit the contractions; this requires practice as well as maturation of the central nervous system (see Fig. 24.1).

Continence thus involves the active inhibition of nerve impulses. When micturition is initiated, the brain ceases to send out inhibitory impulses, allowing the spinal reflex arc to be completed. Figure 24.2 illustrates the innervation of the bladder.

'Normal' patterns of micturition can vary markedly from one individual to another. Most people empty their bladders four to six times a day and have a bladder capacity of up to 600 mL; this may be altered, however, by age, fluid intake, perspiration, body temperature, activity and stress. People in a state of anxiety generally feel the need to empty their bladders more often; in the event of acute emotional distress or sudden shock, it is possible for incontinence to occur.

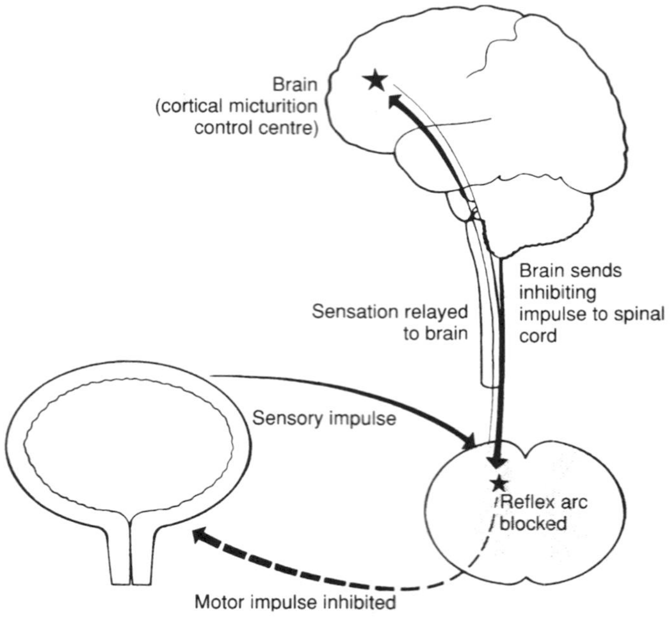

Fig. 24.1 Bladder-filling phase. The brain inhibits the spinal reflex arc. (Reproduced with kind permission from Coloplast Foundation 1987.)

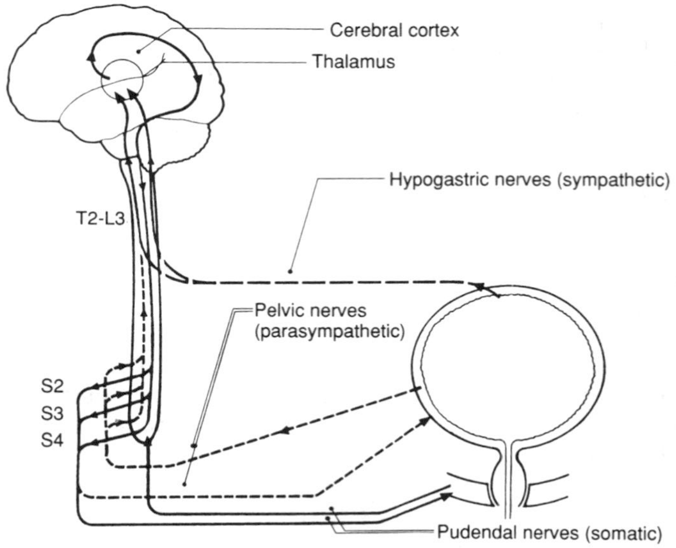

Fig. 24.2 Nerve pathways between the bladder, spine and micturition control centre. NB — nerves supplying the urethra have been omitted for clarity. (Reproduced with kind permission from Coloplast Foundation 1987.)

ATTITUDES TOWARDS INCONTINENCE

In modern British society, attitudes towards many previously taboo subjects are rapidly changing. This is particularly evident in the topics that are now permissible within 'polite' conversation, e.g. sex, AIDS and homosexuality. Incontinence is also gradually becoming an acceptable subject for open discussion and began to be addressed in newspaper and magazine articles, radio and television programmes openly from 1985 onwards (Glew 1985, Horsfield 1986, Walker 1987), as well as in medical journals. Nevertheless, certain myths still persist, such as the notion that incontinence is an inevitable consequence of old age. Such mistaken ideas must be dispelled in favour of seeking the real cause of incontinence in any given case.

For the nurse, perhaps the best starting point in this process of re-education is an examination of her own preconceptions of incontinence, since it has been demonstrated that nurses to a large degree reflect the views of the society that they serve (Fielding 1986, Ewles & Simnett 1992). Self-appraisal of one's own attitude to the subject of incontinence may be a necessary prerequisite to the effective nursing of incontinent patients.

Types of incontinence

The International Continence Society (ICS), which has tried to regulate the terminology associated with the lower urinary tract, has defined urinary incontinence as 'a condition in which involuntary loss of urine is a social or hygienic problem and is objectively demonstrable' (ICS 1984, Anderson et al 1988).

Urinary incontinence may take a variety of forms:

- stress incontinence
- urge incontinence
- overflow incontinence
- reflex incontinence
- enuresis
- immobility incontinence.

It is only when the specific type and cause of an individual's incontinence are known that appropriate treatment can be offered.

Stress incontinence results from a failure of the urethral sphincter to remain closed when sudden abdominal pressure on the bladder occurs, e.g. during coughing, sneezing or laughing. The weak pelvic floor allows the urethra to descend and the sphincter to open, releasing urine.

Urge incontinence results from the contraction of the detrusor muscle of the bladder as if to void, when only small amounts of urine have accumulated in the bladder. This may be caused by overactive detrusor function (motor urgency) or by hypersensitivity (sensory urgency).

Overflow incontinence occurs as a consequence of urinary retention, which may in turn result from:

- an obstruction, e.g. that caused by a tumour, faecal impaction, or an enlarged prostate gland
- an underactive detrusor muscle, producing a flaccid bladder and thus failing to generate enough pressure to open the urethra
- failure of the urethra to open.

Reflex incontinence may occur as a result of damage to the spinal cord and loss of sensation associated with the desire to micturate, leading to failure to inhibit the simple reflex arc.

Enuresis refers to any involuntary loss of urine. Nocturnal enuresis is the term for urinary incontinence which occurs during sleep in the absence of any organic disease or infection. Nocturia refers to being woken at night by the urge to pass urine.

Immobility incontinence. The individual with this type of incontinence would in favourable circumstances be able to remain continent but is prevented by pre-existing disease or disability from gaining access to an appropriate place at an appropriate time to pass urine. Diseases which may affect mobility and dexterity, and therefore continence, are multiple sclerosis, spina bifida, arthritis and spinal cord injury. In addition, conditions associated with ageing, such as slowness of movement, pain, stiffness, inability to climb stairs or difficulty in manipulating fastenings, may all contribute to incontinence.

EPIDEMIOLOGY

In conducting their seminal research into the prevalence of incontinence, Thomas et al (1980) used the following definition to identify all those in two London health districts over the age of 5 years who were incontinent: 'involuntary excretion or leakage of urine and/or faeces in inappropriate places or at inappropriate times and production of two or more "accidents" a month or continuous leakage of urine'. This categorisation included individuals with 'long term catheters and urinary diversions'.

In the early stages of the study, this definition was applied to known patients who were already in touch with health and social services agencies. These individuals were monitored over a 1-year period, and the following information was obtained:

Age (years)	*Percentage of incontinence in this sample*
15–64	0.2% in women
	0.1% in men
65+	2.5% in women
	1.3% in men

In an extension of the study, a postal questionnaire was sent to all individuals over the age of 15 on the lists of 12 general practitioners (a total of 22 430 patients). An 89% return was obtained. The results, when compared with those of the first study, were illuminating, as they revealed a markedly higher incidence of incontinence, as follows:

Age (years)	*Percentage of incontinence in this sample*
15–64	8.5% in women
	1.6% in men
65+	11.6% in women
	6.9% in men

While incontinence was the most prevalent among elderly women, its occurrence was significant across all age groups. Stress incontinence was reported less commonly by nulliparous than by parous women of all ages, and was especially prevalent among those who had borne four or more children. Urge incontinence also occurred more commonly among parous than nulliparous women. No significant class differences were found among men or women, but individuals of Afro-Caribbean or part Afro-Caribbean descent were more likely to have some form of incontinence than those with an Asian background. However, differences have been found among groups of Asiatic women working in the east end of London (Haggar 1995).

The most important finding of the study, however, was the 1:10 ratio of known to unknown cases of incontinence. This means that for every incontinent person who is known to medical or social services professionals, there are 10 others who are unidentified and require help. As further in-depth interviews revealed, many people try to 'cope' with moderate to severe problems of incontinence without professional support. These findings identify the need for health care workers to take advantage of all appropriate opportunities in hospital or community care settings to identify those who require assessment and treatment for incontinence.

Brocklehurst (1993), in an analysis of a MORI poll, suggests that there is now some improvement in the number of people coming forward for help. Recent national awareness campaigns coordinated by the Department of Health and the Continence Foundation, starting in 1994, as well as a Continence Foundation Help Line, all help to direct people to the professional services that they need, by helping to remove the stigma in talking about the problem (Willis 1996).

The most recent figures presented by the Royal College of Physicians (1995) show an increase in the number of people with incontinence, but this may in fact be evidence of more people coming forward for help or admitting the problem.

Surveys of health care institutions and social services homes between 1964 and 1986 showed a high prevalence of incontinence and suggested that this was to some extent a consequence of the quality of care given. A high failure rate in addressing the problems of incontinence was apparent and this was attributed to insufficient knowledge (Egan et al 1983), a factor also noted over 30 years ago by Townsend (1964) and confirmed by Edginton et al (1986).

The implication of these research findings is that there is a need not only to identify patients who are incontinent, but also to improve public and professional understanding of incontinence, to evaluate services available for those requiring assessment and to improve methods of treatment and management.

Q

24.1 Determine how many patients in your ward or on your community list are incontinent.
24.2 What percentage of your caseload does this represent?
24.3 To the best of your knowledge, how many of those who are incontinent have been fully investigated?
24.4 From what you have been told, try to identify the type of incontinence suffered by each person.
24.5 Compare your findings with the work of Edginton et al (1986), Gilleard (1981) and McLaren et al (1981) or, if you are working in the community, with Thomas et al (1980).
24.6 Discuss your findings with a senior member of staff in your working area.

Sociological factors in underreporting of incontinence

The fact that incontinence remains to such a large extent a hidden problem among the general population can be attributed in part to the reluctance of many people to admit to their incontinence and seek treatment. The failure to report symptoms is of course not limited to individuals who are incontinent; indeed, it has been estimated that only 20% of people needing treatment for illness of any kind attend for medical advice (Patrick & Scambler 1986).

Sociologists have investigated the factors that may prompt an individual to seek a medical opinion. Their findings suggest that such decisions are rarely made in isolation. Scambler (1986), assessing the work of Zola (1973), suggests that people present with illness not only when there is a distressing symptom such as pain, but also in response to 'triggers' that arise out of social and personal interaction, including:

- interpersonal crises
- perceived interference of the health problem with social or personal relations
- sanctioning pressures from others to consult a doctor
- perceived interference of the problem with vocational or physical activity
- reaching a personal deadline for the resolution of symptoms.

Scambler (1986) also cites cultural variations as a partial determinant of who will consult a doctor and who will try to self-treat.

The fact that it is 'comparatively rare for someone to decide in favour of or against a visit to the surgery without discussing his or her symptoms with others' — Freidson (1970) refers to this as 'a lay referral system' — may go some way towards explaining why incontinence is underreported. Many people prefer not to mention their incontinence to others, and so the opportunity for friends to encourage them to seek advice does not arise. Moreover, it may also be true that in the case of women, the private and, to some degree, secretive management of menstruation gives an easily transferable model of management to follow should incontinence develop. Many women conceal the leakage of urine as they have concealed menstruation previously, and some also accidentally discover that the use of a tampon will temporarily lessen the problem of stress incontinence. The bulk of the tampon in the vagina pushes against the urethra and thus helps to keep the urethral sphincter closed.

For many people, incontinence is a source of embarrassment or shame rather than a signal to them that they should seek medical help. The dysfunction is seen mainly in terms of its social consequences rather than as a symptom of a possible underlying illness or disease process.

Personal and social attitudes towards incontinence are not, however, the only factors that account for the underreporting of this widespread health problem. The way that particular health services are marketed or presented can also influence an individual's decision whether to seek help or cope on her own (Armstrong 1980).

It is therefore important that services available through the National Health Service (NHS) reflect positive approaches to the promotion of continence, and progress on this is demonstrated in the setting of standards by nurses and monitoring of services and treatment by quality assurance audits (ACA 1993, National Institute for Nursing 1995, Swaffield 1995). In line with patient charter initiatives, a 'charter for continence' has been developed by a group of professional organisations (Box 24.1).

Box 24.1 Charter for Continence*

The Charter for Continence presents the specific needs and rights of people with bladder or bowel problems. It outlines the resources available and the standards of care that can be expected.

As a person with bladder or bowel problems you have the right to:

- Be treated with sensitivity and understanding
- Become continent if achievable
- Receive a thorough individual assessment of your condition by a doctor or nurse knowledgeable in this aspect of care
- Request specialist advice about continence care
- Be provided with a clear explanation of your diagnosis
- Participate in a full discussion of treatment options, their advantages and disadvantages
- Be provided with full, impartial information on the range of products which are available and how to obtain them
- Expect products to have clear instructions for use
- Receive regular reviews of treatment and be given the opportunity to change treatments if your condition has changed
- Be made aware of any treatments or products as they become available
- Be provided with a personal contact point able to give you ongoing advice and support

*Developed by The Continence Foundation, InconTact, Association for Continence Advice (ACA), the RCN Continence Care Forum, the Enuresis Resource and Information Centre (ERIC), the Spinal Injuries Association and the Multiple Sclerosis Society. (Produced by an educational grant from Bard Ltd, March 1995.) (Reproduced with kind permission from Coloplast Ltd)

A Cochrane Urinary and Faecal Incontinence Review Group (CURE), based at the University of Aberdeen, has been set up to prepare, maintain and disseminate systematic reviews of the effectiveness of the interventions for incontinence, including prevention, treatment and rehabilitation, concentrating on randomised controlled trials.

Care pathways, a process approach to managing integrated patient-focused care, are being designed to improve quality and standards of care for all incontinent people (Bayliss et al 1998).

An audit package 'Promoting continence' has now been developed which can be used on a single patient, multiple patients or for a faculty audit. It covers urinary incontinence, faecal incontinence and faecal incontinence and urethral catheter management (Royal College of Physicians 1998). It is intended to encourage staff to reflect on their management of incontinence and to consider areas where action needs to be taken to achieve high standards of care.

Identifying patients

Most people who are incontinent do not regard themselves as ill. It is therefore incumbent upon nurses and other professionals working in hospitals and the community to take advantage of every opportunity to identify those who are suffering in silence. Table 24.1 outlines potential opportunities for professionals to identify patients with incontinence problems and demonstrates that it is not always medical professionals who have the greatest opportunity to help people with problems of incontinence. This supports the view that non-medical professionals and others should become better informed about this aspect of health. Chemists and home carers, to choose two very different examples, are well placed to provide information and foster positive attitudes towards treatment and should be included in educational initiatives to promote continence.

PRIMARY REASONS FOR INCONTINENCE

Delay in achieving continence

In childhood, the acquisition of the skills needed to become continent may be delayed. Nocturnal enuresis may be a particular problem, especially among boys (Thomas et al 1980). Nocturnal enuresis may present as a primary or secondary feature; its cause is not known. Although it often spontaneously resolves itself, it is sometimes not resolved during childhood. In such cases it may remain a problem throughout life if it is not treated (Feneley 1987, Walker 1987, Shapiro 1989, Butler 1994). In 1997, the National Health Service Centre for Reviews and Dissemination published a systematic review of the effectiveness of interventions for managing childhood enuresis. Its impact on the family has been researched by Morison (1996).

Sometimes mental or physical handicap will prevent a person from attaining continence. Professionals working with individuals with mental handicap, however, should base their interventions on

Table 24.1 Lifespan opportunities for helping people who are incontinent (Reproduced with kind permission from the Continence Foundation)

		Sources of help	
Lifespan stage	*Potential problem areas*	*Nurses*	*Others*
Childhood	'Potty' training Enuresis Urinary control Learning disability Ureteric reflux	Health visitor, clinic nurse, school nurse, practice nurse, community learning disability nurse, nursery nurse, paediatric nurse	Doctor, consultant, portage staff, social worker, dietician, teachers
Teenager	Body function Sex education Cystitis	Health visitor, school nurse/matron, family planning nurse	Teachers, health educator, product reps, youth club leader
Pregnancy, childbirth	Antenatal frequency Difficult birth — tissue/nerve injuries, postnatal stress incontinence	Health visitor, midwife, district nurse	GP, gynaecologist, obstetrician, self-help groups, chemist
Adulthood and hormone changes	Symptoms of incontinence from urological, gynaecological, neurological, psychological conditions	Well-women's nurse, practice nurse, clinic nurse, district nurse, health visitor, outpatients/ occupational health nurse, specialist ward or urodynamics nurse	Urologist, neurologist, psychologist, physiotherapist, occupational therapist, dietician, keep-fit teacher, GP
Old age	As above, combined with the ageing process, prostatic enlargement and disability	District nurse, health visitor, practice nurse, day/ward nurse, geriatric nurse	Home help, home carers, social workers and aides, old age club leaders, senior citizens organisers, GP, geriatrician

the assumption that although the process of toilet training will be slow, continence will eventually be achieved (Maleham 1993). Some children are incapable of acquiring continence because of spinal lesions, as in spina bifida. Others are prevented by other congenital malformations. A baby who is continuously wet or shows signs of leaking should always be investigated for either congenital fistula or failure to empty the bladder. Such symptoms should be taken seriously, for ureteric reflux caused by failure of the bladder to empty will put pressure on the kidney and may cause infection and life-threatening damage.

Problems in maintaining continence

Childbirth. Giving birth can cause damage to the mother's pudendal nerve, preventing the tone of the pelvic floor muscles from returning to normal. This has been shown to be particularly significant in the development of stress incontinence in women who have had four or more children (Thomas et al 1980). Henry et al (1982) suggest that prolonged second-stage labour, the delivery of large babies and the use of forceps put mothers at particular risk of damage to the pudendal nerve.

Chronic disorders. Cerebral, nerve or muscle damage can have varying effects on continence, as can trauma and damage resulting from injury or accident (see Fig. 24.3). Tumours or growths in the area of the bladder or cauda equina are also contributory factors, as is constipation. The process of ageing may itself have an effect on the lower urinary tract system and its control.

Drugs. Many drugs, especially diuretics, can have an effect on the bladder and its function. They may cause incontinence because of the sheer volume of output that they induce, and because of the demands they place on elderly or handicapped individuals in reaching a place to pass urine in time.

The sedative and diuretic effects of alcohol can also contribute to incontinence. Sedatives and hypnotics make people less responsive to signals from the bladder. Anticholinergic drugs and others with some anticholinergic action, such as phenothiazines and antidepressants, can cause retention in people with previously normal bladder function. Beta-blockers also generate a variety of urinary dysfunctions. Keister (1989) has shown that numerous drugs taken by the elderly have the potential to cause incontinence.

For further information see Trounce (1997).

The effects of ageing. Age can also affect an individual's ability to maintain continence. It should be emphasised, however, that while incontinence is more prevalent among elderly people (especially women), it is not an inevitable consequence of ageing. Nonetheless, research suggests that around 20% of admissions to long-term care for the elderly may be a direct result of incontinence (Shuttleworth 1970).

With age comes an increasing degeneration of the glomeruli in the kidneys; their function is reduced by up to 50% by the age of 80, thus impairing the ability of the kidney to concentrate urine. This consequence of ageing occurs alongside a decrease in the bladder's urine-storing capacity (Wysocki 1983).

The failure of the kidneys to dispose of sufficient waste products from the body means that at night they remain very active. An increased nocturnal output of urine results, leading to a change in the individual's rhythms of micturition.

Ageing may also have some effect on the cerebral control of micturition, through the diminishing of cell function. Ageing of the cerebral cortical neurones diminishes their effectiveness in inhibiting the sacral reflex arc, so that involuntary emptying of the bladder occurs.

In elderly women, vaginal dryness, soreness and atrophic changes may give a number of clues as to why incontinence has developed. Glycosuria or atrophic changes in the vulva may lead to vaginitis and urethritis (note that the lining of the vagina is continuous with that of the urethra). After the menopause, hormonal changes resulting in a decrease of oestrogen can cause dryness in the vagina and urethra. This may interfere with functioning of the moist seal at the urethral sphincter in the urethra, producing incompetency and thus allowing urine to leak through (Ritch 1988).

Constipation is one of the main causes of urinary incontinence. Because of the anatomical proximity of the rectum to the urethra, it is possible for the urethra to be closed off by a faecal mass (see Fig. 24.4). This can lead to failure of complete voiding and thus stasis of urine, which in turn can lead to an infection in the bladder. A full rectum, patulous anus and distended rectal walls are all signs of constipation.

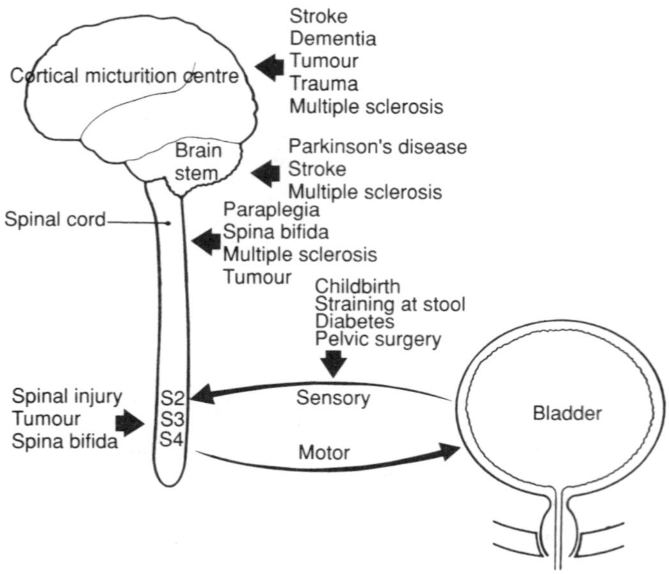

Fig. 24.3 Possible neurogenic causes of incontinence. (Reproduced with kind permission from Coloplast Foundation 1987.)

PROMOTING CONTINENCE: A PROBLEM-SOLVING APPROACH

The problem-solving approach to nursing intervention consists of four stages:

1. Identifying the problem through assessment
2. Setting goals
3. Implementing care or treatment
4. Evaluating outcome to ascertain that the goals have been achieved.

The involvement of the patient in all aspects of the nursing process will help to improve motivation and willingness to agree to treatment and will enhance the patient's feeling of independence and self-esteem.

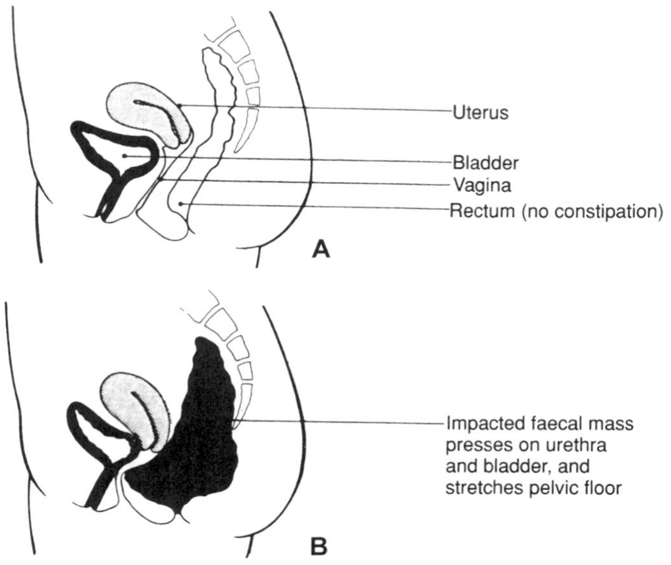

Fig. 24.4 How constipation can cause incontinence. Female, side view. (A) Normal. (B) Impacted. (Reproduced with kind permission from Coloplast Foundation 1987.)

Assessment

Assessment should be carried out with reference to a professionally agreed protocol and be individualised. It is vital that this assessment is conducted with a view to ascertaining the cause of any incontinence, for only then can the correct type of treatment be instigated. In collecting information from patients, the nurse must have a clear understanding of the rationale behind his questions and of the implications for diagnosis and treatment of the patient's responses (see Table 24.2).

A full assessment should include:

- the patient's own account of the problem
- a detailed history, using closed and open-ended questions
- recording of micturition and incontinence over a few days
- physical examination by medical staff
- urine testing
- further investigations as required.

Assessment should take place in a private setting and allow adequate time for the patient to air concerns and ask questions.

Questioning the patient

In order to establish a good rapport with the patient, it is important to meet her own agenda when discussing the potentially embarrassing topic of incontinence. Open-ended questions such as 'Tell me about the problems with wetting that you have been having' or 'Could you describe what happens when wetting occurs' will give the patient a greater opportunity to relate her problem in detail than questions that require a simple 'yes' or 'no' response, and will allow her to set out her own agenda for the interview. However, yes/no questions are useful with patients who are acutely embarrassed and have trouble finding a comfortable vocabulary to describe their problems.

The nurse's choice of language and sensitivity to the patient's preferred terminology will be important to the patient's comfort during the assessment interview. Patients generally use terms such as 'passing water', 'peeing' or 'making water' rather than medical terms such as 'micturition' or 'voiding' and many find words such as 'accidents', 'wetting' or 'leaking' more acceptable than the term 'incontinence'. Where the patient uses a euphemism or is vague, the nurse should seek clarification if there is any danger of misunderstanding, e.g. by asking 'When you said "at it" did you mean "having intercourse"?' or 'What do you mean by "a little"?'.

Other specific questions may be indicated when the assessment is of a patient with a pre-existing illness, e.g. multiple sclerosis, or where bleeding, pain or discharge has occurred. Obviously, some questions (such as those concerning childbirth or prostate problems) will be gender-specific. Supplementary questions can be asked by means of a written assessment form.

Table 24.2 provides a checklist of questions that can be used during the assessment interview, together with a rationale for each item of information requested. These questions should be posed only after the patient has described her symptoms and has been given the opportunity to articulate her own agenda of concerns.

Charting information

The patient's history may yield enough information to determine the type and cause of her incontinence. A baseline chart recorded over a few days can confirm the accuracy of the history by supplying information indicating frequency of micturition and incontinence and, where required, the volume of urine passed. Charting such information again at intervals of a few weeks or at the end of treatment will produce a means of evaluating the treatment implemented. Any chart provided should be straightforward and easily understood so that patients will not be discouraged from using it, for the success of any future treatment will depend upon the patient's motivation.

After careful explanation, the patient should be given the chart to fill in for a few days. Suggestions that the chart is hung with a pen on the back of the bathroom door at home, or kept available in the bedside locker in hospital, are useful in reminding the patient to fill them in. The times of voiding and times of wetting are the most important pieces of information. While amounts lost may be too subjective to be useful, complicated before and after testing of pads is possible if objective testing is required (Sutherst et al 1986). Ticking or a collection of ++++ may be sufficient. A full fluid chart is rarely required, although issuing a jug and persuading the patient to measure output for a day may be useful in some cases.

The above approach is advocated for most patients, whether in the hospital or the community, and many specialists in the field of incontinence suggest that complicated investigations and admission to hospital to discover the type of incontinence among the majority of patients seen are not required (McGrother et al 1987).

For many patients this assessment will indicate the likely type, or cause, of the incontinence and the problem can be identified.

Physical examination

Women. In women, a physical examination can determine whether atrophic vaginal changes, vaginitis or soreness from excoriation are features, and whether prolapse(s) or constipation is present. In the case of genuine stress incontinence, provocative testing such as asking the patient to cough while she is in a semi-recumbent position may demonstrate leakage. Assessing the ability of the pelvic floor to contract may be achieved by placing two gloved fingers in the vagina and asking the patient to tighten the pelvic floor muscles.

Men should be examined for prostate enlargement and to determine whether the bladder is palpable. If a bladder is palpable or

Table 24.2 Incontinence assessment questions

Question	*Rationale*
How long have these symptoms been present?	The symptoms may have begun at a life crisis or on taking a new drug, or they may have been a long-standing problem, but some new development has prompted the patient to ask for help
Are you wet every time?	It is important to establish the degree and frequency of wetting
How many times do you pass water each day?	A baseline needs to be established in order for progress to be charted
Are you wet at night as well as by day?	This gives an indication of the degree of the problem as well as the type of incontinence
Are you aware of the need to go to the toilet before you are wet?	This will determine whether signals are normal or absent
Do you have feelings of urgency to go to the toilet?	This indicates whether signals are present and their degree of urgency
Do you lose urine if you laugh, jump or run?	A positive response often indicates genuine stress incontinence
Do you pass small amounts of urine?	Passing small amounts of urine may be due to urge, stress or overflow incontinence. It may also be indicative of reduced fluid intake
Do you pass a full stream?	Passing a full stream suggests the bladder capacity is normal
Is the stream of urine poor?	The flow rate may indicate a degree of obstruction or the bladder's inability to contract
Does passing urine sting?	Stinging urine usually indicates infection or a sore or broken area
Does the urine have a strong smell?	Urine invaded with bacteria or concentrated often has a strong smell
Do you have difficulty in starting to pass urine?	Hesitancy may be caused by an obstruction, e.g. prostatic enlargement
Do you dribble urine before or after going to the toilet?	Dribbling before suggests overflow; dribbling after suggests a failure to completely empty the bladder or an incompetent sphincter
Do you need to use pads or other aids, and if so how many and how often?	The answer may indicate the degree of urine loss
Are you constipated?	Constipation is the most common cause of urinary incontinence
Have you had any operations 'down below' (lower abdomen)?	Surgical trauma may be significant
Have you difficulty in getting to the toilet, problems with undoing clothes or any sight problems?	If the patient has problems with mobility or dexterity, clothes may need to be adapted and toilet seats raised. Supports to steady patients and aids to help them locate the toilet may be required
Are you taking any medication?	Many drugs can affect the functioning of the urinary tract
Is the patient mentally aware?	Senile dementia may be the cause of incontinence due to a failure to remember the routines of the day

the history suggests inability to empty the bladder completely, it may be necessary to ask the patient to pass urine, after which a catheter can be introduced so that the residual volume of urine can be assessed.

Urine testing. A urine sample may be obtained and examined for signs of infection, blood or glycosuria, and a midstream sample sent for culture and sensitivity analysis. Routine testing of urine can identify problems which may contribute to incontinence; haematuria, for example, may be an indication of infection, stones in the bladder or tumours. The neuropathy that may accompany diabetes mellitus may eventually result in damage to the receptors in the bladder demonstrated by proteinuria. However, protein in urine, together with a cloudy appearance and a strong smell, is a sign of a urinary tract infection.

Further investigations

Once the type of incontinence in question has been diagnosed, goals can be set for the patient's achievement or recovery of continence. If the incontinence is of an intractable nature, requiring long-term management rather than cure, further assessment for aids or equipment will be required. It may also be the case that further investigation into the cause of the incontinence is needed and that referral is indicated.

Urodynamics. Where the information given suggests urge incontinence or mixed symptoms, patients are often referred for urodynamic testing and further investigation. Patients will want to know what this involves and it is an important part of the nurse's role as advocate to explain these procedures to them.

Urodynamic testing measures the pressure and flow relationships in the bladder and urethra. It can aid diagnosis of the type of incontinence by showing sphincter incompetence, bladder instability, overflow incontinence, urethral instability and problems with voiding due to obstruction or an underactive detrusor. The procedure is invasive, unpleasant, potentially very embarrassing, but not painful. Clear explanations and psychological support must be given to the patient throughout.

For the test, the patient usually attends with a full bladder, in itself a potentially distressing requirement. Urine is passed while sitting on an adapted commode with a flow meter attached. Flow rates are recorded, as are volumes and time taken, using a transducer which relays to the urodynamic printer. On catheterisation the residual volumes can then be accurately measured.

Following the patient's emptying of the bladder, the patient lies on the couch. Two catheters are passed into the bladder — a filling catheter (Jacques) and a fine epidural cannula — and a special balloon catheter is placed in the rectum. The patient is then transferred to the commode and the tubes joined up to the urodynamic equipment. Care in taping the catheters and holding them in place while transferring the patient is essential.

The bladder is then gently filled with saline via the Jacques catheter and the other catheter records the pressures. The balloon catheter in the rectum is used to record the abdominal resting pressure and the increase when coughing, talking, straining, etc. This is subtracted from the bladder pressure reading to record the actual bladder pressure.

During the filling phase, patients need to report their first need to pass urine and subsequently the onset of a strong desire to pass urine. During the test or at the close of the procedure, provocative testing can then be undertaken, such as coughing, standing or jumping. Any leakage is recorded by the flow meter or by observation, possibly by listening. Urethral pressure profiles may also be recorded as the catheters are removed from the bladder.

In the case of urine flow, it is possible to time the speed and flow of urine and to contrast this with normal outputs (Dove 1987).

Radiography. Radiographs can reveal signs of stones or large tumours in the bladder and may be required to assess the extent of faecal impaction in the colon and to show any narrowing or obstruction.

Videocystourethrography affords the opportunity to observe the bladder and the urethra on a video screen during filling and emptying.

Cystoscopy. A cystoscope is an instrument fitted with a fine telescope which is introduced via the urethra into the bladder. Modern types of cystoscope are quite flexible and allow the procedure to be carried out with only a local anaesthetic. It allows the urologist the opportunity to inspect the bladder and urethra, observing for tumours, stones, strictures and the condition of the mucosa. Further information on this procedure is given in Chapter 8.

Planning and implementing care

Effective treatment can be implemented only when the type of incontinence has been correctly diagnosed. This may seem obvious, but research has shown that doctors have often prescribed the wrong treatment for incontinence because of a lack of understanding of its causes, that drugs have therefore been used wrongly and that women who have had children have been advised that incontinence is inevitable (Horsfield 1986, Walker 1987).

Treatments for incontinence include pelvic floor exercises, bladder training, the administration of anticholinergic drugs, clean intermittent self-catheterisation, advice on diet, relieving underlying medical conditions and surgical intervention. These forms of treatment, together with their application in different forms of incontinence, are described below.

Pelvic floor exercises

These exercises are primarily intended to increase the strength of the levator ani muscles and to evoke their contraction without simultaneously increasing intra-abdominal pressure. In women, assessment of the ability to 'squeeze' the muscles around the vagina and teaching them to continue these exercises to improve their tone can counteract any descent of the pelvic floor and help

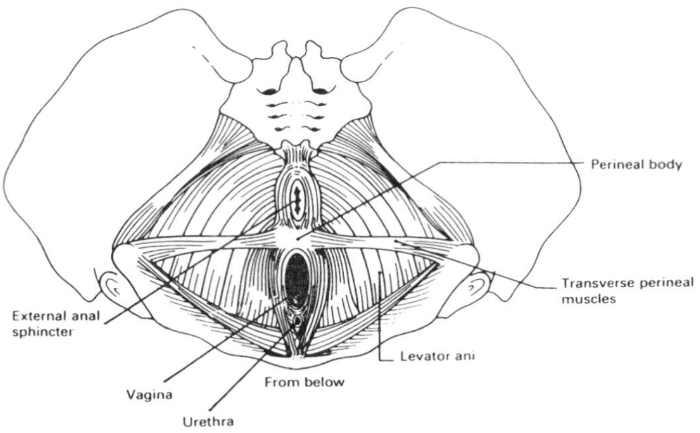

Fig. 24.5 The female pelvic floor muscles viewed from below. (Reproduced with kind permission from Farrer 1986.)

restore the normal anatomical relationships and sphincter function. Figure 24.5 illustrates the position of the muscles of the pelvic floor in women.

Genuine stress incontinence in men or women (see p. 765) is the main problem for which pelvic floor exercises may be used. This type of incontinence occurs when the pelvic floor is unable to absorb a sudden abdominal pressure and allows the urethral sphincter to open, i.e. the intravesical pressure overcomes the intraurethral pressure.

Pelvic floor exercises can also be useful for patients with urge incontinence. Sitting down when strong 'signals' occur and carrying out pelvic floor exercises can help the patient to overcome urgency signals and encourage the bladder to fill a little more before needing to be emptied.

Pelvic floor exercises are also useful following prostatectomy to stop postmicturition dribble and should be taught preoperatively.

Identifying the pelvic floor muscles. Before patients can perform pelvic floor exercises they must be able to identify two specific muscles:

- *the levator ani* — patients can locate this by imagining that they have diarrhoea and need to tighten their back passage muscle in order to get to the toilet without an accident
- *the pubococcygeus* (the anterior portion of the levator ani; see Fig 24.5) — this can be located when passing urine: while in full stream, patients should try to stop, or at least slow, the flow and then try to remember which muscle was used in order to do this.

It is essential that patients identify the correct muscles; crossing the legs and pulling in 'tummy' or buttock muscles will not be correct.

Motivation and practice. In order to encourage compliance, the nurse must ensure that the patient has understood the instructions on performing the exercises and is motivated to practise them over a 3-month period (Montgomery 1986, Laycock 1987). In carrying out the exercise, the patient should tighten the two muscles of the pelvic floor to the count of 5, five times; this should be repeated hourly through the day.

Supplementary techniques. Physiotherapists employ a range of equipment and techniques to help patients to overcome stress incontinence. Electrical stimulation and interferential treatment are the main therapies in use (Laycock & Green 1988).

The use of cones of various weights, which are carried in the vagina, has gained popularity (Peattie et al 1988) and can supplement pelvic floor exercises (Laycock 1992). A disposable type has been introduced which is 5 cm long and plastic-coated with a string attached to the narrow end to aid removal. Motivation and support of patients appear to be important elements in achieving success with this treatment.

A perineometer can also be used in therapy for stress incontinence. This instrument is a probe which is placed in the vagina or rectum to measure the strength of the pelvic floor contraction. This procedure used in conjunction with biofeedback (see Ch. 17) has been shown to be beneficial for stress and urge incontinence (Taylor & Henderson 1986, Holmes 1990). In this treatment the patient watches a gauge which shows intravesical pressure in the bladder; she then experiments with relaxing muscles or holding contractions to reduce the rise in pressure or to contract the urethra in order to prevent urine escaping. With practice, the patient will then be able to apply this technique to retaining urine when necessary in everyday life.

Evaluation. The success of these conservative approaches to achieving continence may be measured objectively by recording the weight of pads for urine loss, and subjectively by the patient's reports on the number of pad changes required per day. Female patients can check their ability to tighten the pelvic floor muscles by placing two fingers in the vagina and squeezing. The long-term effectiveness of simple interventions such as pelvic floor exercises or bladder training was demonstrated by O'Brien & Long (1995) and that of devices by Nygaard (1995).

Q **24.7** While discussing the rehabilitation of her mother following a mild stroke, Mrs M confides to you that she is occasionally wet after lifting her mother. What is your role here and what advice may be given as to treatment?

Bladder retraining

For the patient with urge incontinence, bladder retraining in conjunction with anticholinergic drugs is the main treatment.

The aim of this form of treatment is for the bladder to 'learn' to increase its capacity and for the urethral sphincter to maintain its ability to remain sealed as the bladder fills, thereby lengthening the intervals between voiding.

Method. The treatment begins with a baseline measurement of bladder capacity (i.e. the amount of urine passed) at the time of assessment. In stages the patient then learns to hold on for a few minutes more between the bladder signal and going to the toilet. As each lengthened interval is achieved and maintained, new objectives are set for the next few days.

Anticholinergic drugs are a useful adjunct to bladder retraining, as they reduce the initial urge to void and thereby help to increase bladder capacity. When the patient achieves an acceptable social interval between toilet visits, the drugs are then reduced and eventually discontinued; attempts by the patient to maintain the same regimen as when taking the medication are instigated. If the same interval between passing urine is maintained, the treatment is seen as successful.

Anticholinergic drugs are contraindicated in patients with glaucoma (see Ch. 13). The normal side-effect of a dry mouth should be explained to patients using this medication.

Evaluation. Whatever the degree of success of the treatment, toileting regimens will remain individual to each patient. In order to evaluate progress, a further continence chart should be completed after a few weeks' treatment and again towards the end of treatment. Comparison of the charts, showing both voiding intervals and quantities, will allow an objective evaluation to be made as to the success of the treatment.

Q **24.8** Mrs C needs to pass urine frequently. She tells you that she has had a 'poor' bladder for about 10 years which often wakes her at night, as well as 'keeping her on the run' during the day. After referral for urodynamics and further investigations, it is confirmed that she has urge incontinence. You are requested to instigate her treatment of a course of anticholinergic drugs and bladder training. What plan of action would you implement?

Clean intermittent self-catheterisation

This technique is employed by patients with voiding difficulties caused by conditions such as an atonic bladder or dysynergia (in which bladder contraction does not synchronise with opening of the urethral sphincter). It has also been used in conjunction with the passing of 'sounds' for urethral adhesion or prostate enlargement (adhesions are often due to healing from infections and prostate enlargements may restrict the diameter of the urethra). Clean intermittent self-catheterisation has also been of particular benefit to individuals with multiple sclerosis (Sibley 1988), spina bifida (White 1990), paraplegia and prostate obstruction.

Intermittent self-catheterisation is a relatively simple treatment for incontinence which is known to have been used in ancient times. The ancient Egyptians used reeds, and the ancient Chinese onion stems. The Roman encyclopaedist, Celsus, mentions the use of catheters in his writings (c. 30 BC) and in 11th century Europe, silver catheters are known to have been in use (Bard 1987, Seth 1987).

Assessment of the suitability of intermittent self-catheterisation for a particular patient must include identification of the specific type of incontinence and an evaluation of the manual dexterity, mental alertness and motivation of the individual. Children as well as adults have been successful in learning the technique. In some cases it may be appropriate for partners or family members to be taught to carry out the catheterisation.

The procedure of self-catheterisation simulates normal voiding; the bladder is allowed to fill, the clean catheter is introduced and the bladder is then completely emptied. This prevents the build-up of residual urine in the bladder, which otherwise may cause:

- damage to the stretch receptors
- overflow incontinence
- urine reflux into the ureters and kidneys leading to pressure which may cause renal damage and give rise to infection.

Unlike long-term catheterisation, in which aseptic technique and good management are of paramount importance, self-catheterisation may seem unhygienic. However, the clean technique is not associated with bladder infection, as the bladder is completely emptied each time a catheter is passed (Murray et al 1984).

The clean intermittent self-catheterisation technique requires the patient to be able to identify the urethra. A small catheter (a Jacques catheter) is introduced several times a day. The same catheter is used repeatedly; after use it is rinsed under the tap, dried and placed in a polythene bag, ready for use again. It is replaced weekly.

Evaluation. Most patients find that inserting the catheter becomes easier with each attempt. The success of the treatment can be measured in terms of the improved quality of life it offers to patients who were continually wet or who previously had to visit hospital emergency departments to seek relief from pain caused by failure to empty their bladder.

Q **24.9** Mrs F, who is 42 years old, has multiple sclerosis. Although she has had symptoms of urge incontinence and frequent bouts of infection, she has now passed into a dysynergia phase in which large residuals of urine occur and clean self-catheterisation is required. She has fairly good manual dexterity. Outline a plan for teaching her self-catheterisation.

Managing symptoms related to underlying medical disorders

Some types of incontinence can be reduced by treating the underlying medical disorder such as constipation, anal fissure and vaginitis.

Relieving constipation. Constipation as a causative factor in urinary retention and subsequent incontinence is described on page 768. In the treatment of constipation, the faecal mass can be cleared by such means as arachis oil retention enemas followed by a course of evacuation enemas over a period of a few days. When the main mass of faeces has been cleared, laxatives may be prescribed to clear any residual material.

An investigation of the cause of the constipation must be undertaken to establish that it is not caused by medication or by any underlying pathology. Dietary factors should also be assessed.

Preventing constipation. Patients who are prone to constipation should be encouraged to be as active as possible. Requests by elderly patients to go to the toilet should always be responded to as quickly as possible, in order to ensure that the gastrocolic reflex is never ignored. In the patient's home, this may necessitate structural adaptations to make the toilet more accessible or the installation of a chemical or macerating toilet or commode in the patient's bedroom or sitting room.

A lack of privacy, time or comfort in an institutional care setting can easily interfere with the maintenance of good bowel habits. Where patients share facilities, nurses and carers must apply standards that allow patients to retain dignity and privacy.

Constipation can be prevented by the introduction of adequate fibre or roughage into the diet, in conjunction with an intake of approximately 8 cups of fluid a day. A dental check-up may be necessary to ensure that patients will be able to manage the raw or chewy food typical of a high-fibre diet. Individuals who are forced by dental problems to eat only soft foods will be susceptible to constipation.

Confusional states. For patients with senile dementia or other confusional states, adherence to a regular routine will help to reinforce the need to go to the toilet at particular times during the day. If a high-roughage diet is encouraged and usual patterns of defaecation maintained (usually a half hour after breakfast or other meals), it may be possible to prevent constipation. Subsequent 'spurious' diarrhoea which occurs when the mass of faeces breaks down and mucus and faeces flow away — causing faecal incontinence associated with a characteristic, penetrating smell — can then be avoided. It is probably preferable for patients with senile dementia to be taken to the toilet at normal intervals rather than to be asked to adapt to new regimens such as using a commode in the sitting room.

Problems related to bowel evacuation. Anal fissures and haemorrhoids need to be healed and soothed in order that constipation caused through pain and avoidance can be prevented. Analgesic medication taken over a long period should always be accompanied by a regular laxative to prevent constipation from developing.

Vaginal dryness or vaginitis may be treated with oestrogen creams or oral supplements. Patients should be referred to a doctor if vaginal prolapse or procidentia is evident. For women who are not sexually active and prefer not to have surgery, ring pessaries may be used to correct the uterine displacement. This appliance will need to be changed at intervals of 3–6 months.

Q **24.10** Mr G has been drawn to your attention because of increasing agitation, exacerbated by what appears as diarrhoea and incontinence of faeces. What aspects of his regimen would be considered in his assessment and what therapies would you implement with his carer to promote continence?

Referring patients

It is the responsibility of the nurse to investigate the causes of a patient's incontinence by careful history-taking. The findings of the history can then be supplemented with a baseline chart (see p. 769) which records the times that the patient passes urine and/or faeces. Patients should not be referred without this data as this will delay treatment.

In a busy surgery or hospital situation, the significance of a patient's wetness may not be fully appreciated. In his role as patient advocate, the nurse should make a case for further investigation, as quite often the individual feels embarrassed by her problem and is unable to convince the doctor of its impact on her social life.

For the nurse who is inexperienced in dealing with the problems of incontinence, a continence advisor or a trained nurse with a specialist interest in continence may be able to act as a resource person and help the nurse gain confidence in his own ability to interpret the data obtained from the patient history and the baseline incontinence chart.

Where the incontinence is not understood, or appears to be outside the scope of the treatments available to the nurse, the patient should be referred to the appropriate professional. This may be a gynaecologist, urologist, geriatrician, physiotherapist, neurologist or psychiatrist.

Surgical intervention

Surgery for stress incontinence. Although conservative measures are generally tried initially, some cases of stress incontinence in women can only be treated by means of surgical intervention. Operations for genuine stress incontinence may be carried out by a vaginal or a suprapubic route. The operation of choice for stress incontinence is suprapubic, whereby the bladder neck is hitched up or supported with sutures or with the patient's own connective tissue. The sling passes around the bladder neck and is usually attached to the ileopectineal ligaments or the rectus sheath. The most common operation is the colposuspension, in which the paravaginal fascia is sutured to the ileopectinal ligament.

Intervention for prostatic enlargement. Where the prostate partially or completely obstructs the urethra, failure to empty the bladder may occur as well as overflow incontinence. Failure to assess the patient accurately may lead to failure in treatment (Neal et al 1987). Transurethral resection of the prostate (TURP) is the most common surgical intervention performed for an enlarged prostate. This operation is fully described in Chapter 8, but a recent prostatectomy audit showed that only 70% of operations were successful (Rouse 1996).

While patients may have experienced overflow incontinence previously, if damage occurs to the sphincter during the operation, dribbling incontinence may develop postoperatively and in some cases may be permanent. Gentle pressure behind the scrotum on the perineum or bulbospongiosum can help to prevent postmicturition dribbling. Incontinence aids such as dribble pouches or Y-front marsupial pants with pads for those with a retracted penis should be available in hospitals and in the community. Also available are Y-front pants with a plastic-backed gusset to prevent leakage.

Pelvic floor exercises (see p. 771) should be learned preoperatively and practised diligently following surgery.

Incontinence within the institutional setting

The health problems generated by the institutionalisation of patients were graphically described by Townsend (1964) and Robb (1967) in their seminal research. In some care settings, especially long-stay wards, nurses may still find that the care they give actually causes such problems as incontinence. This is often due to a task-oriented style of nursing and a failure to individualise care, causing patients to become overdependent on the institutional regimen. Studies of hospitalised patients by Miller (1984, 1985) and Donaldson (1983) showed that a number of functions of daily living tended to decline even in patients whose physical state remained steady. They concluded that increased dependency and decline in function were induced by ward routines. The loss of continence was one area in which this tendency was apparent. Miller (1984) also showed that in one ward where a systematic and individualised 'nursing process' approach was used, the incidence of incontinence fell. The introduction of the 'named nurse' (Scottish Office 1992) with the emphasis on individual assessment may help accurate patient assessment.

However, research by Cheater & Hawthorn (1987) into problems of urinary incontinence among elderly patients in hospital wards still reflected some confusion in nursing approaches to incontinent patients. That study indicated that the term 'urinary incontinence' was subject to individual interpretation and that there was a low level of agreement among qualified nurses in identifying and characterising instances of incontinence.

Cheater & Hawthorn's study found that assessment was lacking in detail and that possible causes of incontinence were identified in less than 12% of cases. Incontinence charts were highly subjective; it could be inferred from the recorded periods of continence, the researchers pointed out, which nurse was on duty at a given time. They suggested that if rehabilitation is to take place then 'there has to be a more consistent and systematic means of identifying, articulating and communicating the problem of incontinence'.

The King's Fund (1983) report *Action on Incontinence* revealed that in the pre-registration education and training of doctors and nurses, as little as 10 minutes may be devoted specifically to incontinence, and that some textbooks fail to refer to it at all.

Clegg (1980) argued that the ward sister is the key figure in health education and that she should be re-educated in the area of incontinence therapy. Copperwheat (1985) showed, from her experience of caring for elderly people on a ward, that it is important to start with a good basic knowledge of incontinence in order to have continual communication with colleagues and work as part of a team, and to start the therapy programme with one or two patients, building up the numbers of successful cases gradually.

Some nurses have made a start by introducing into their ward philosophy the intention 'to reduce the level of incontinence in elderly people who are resident in hospital'; Southern & Henderson (1990) reported a reduction of incontinence episodes by 40% when this standard was implemented in their units.

Evaluation

The last stage of the problem-solving approach to nursing is to evaluate the care given and assess whether the goals set have been achieved. At this point new problems may come to light, in which case the nursing process will begin again with an assessment for this new problem.

Q **24.11** Fully assess the next patient suffering from incontinence who is admitted to your ward or whom you meet in the community. Outline your strategy for care resulting from this assessment.

Continence advisory services

Health authority board services

Nurses may find that, within their own health area, there is a well-established continence advisory service which offers support in the promotion of continence in the community and hospital setting. These services were established during the 1980s from very small but significant beginnings.

In 1977 Dame Phyllis Friend suggested that health authorities should direct attention to the problems of incontinence by taking the following measures (DHSS 1977):

- making local arrangements for the assessment and provision of aids and equipment
- holding seminars to discuss and disseminate information and research findings on matters related, in particular, to the promotion of continence
- making simple local arrangements (in nursing libraries or other suitable areas) for the exhibition of literature and examples of aids and equipment
- identifying the subject of incontinence in the workload of an appropriate nursing officer, who will then act as a resource person for nurses and health visitors in all fields of the service.

The King's Fund Group (1983) made further recommendations, which included:

- the appointment of continence advisors to all health authorities
- the inclusion of the subject of incontinence in all nursing curricula
- activation of a major campaign of public awareness through the media, chemists' shops and public information posters, indicating where to obtain help
- the introduction of a special course for nurses and other professionals on continence promotion and incontinence management.

A review of continence services by the Department of Health resulted in a report which recommended models of good continence services across a district (DoH 1991).

The Association for Continence Advice (ACA)

From a small group of interested people, an Association of Continence Advisors was formed in 1980. The association, which changed its name in 1990 to The Association for Continence Advice, is multidisciplinary and now has over 700 members, including international members and representatives from appropriate manufacturers.

Continence advisors

The instigation of the post of continence advisor originally within the health authorities, but now within Trusts, has been of key importance in the struggle to improve care for individuals suffering from incontinence. In addition to carrying a small caseload of their own, continence advisors attempt to alter public opinion through education and discussion in the media, set up services, and work to improve the knowledge base of nurses and medical professionals. Within the Trusts, networks have been set up to facilitate communication among, and to give support to, professionals working in the area of incontinence therapy. In order to expand the knowledge base of continence advisors and to provide peer support, the ACA organises branch meetings, holds annual conferences and issues four newsletters a year. The ACA has always maintained that the role of the continence advisor is primarily that of educator or resource person (ACA 1985). The setting up of linkage schemes in some regions has helped continence advisors to disseminate information to nurses at all levels, to encourage uniformity of care across authorities and to motivate and support nurses who are trying to put improved assessment techniques into practice.

MANAGING INTRACTABLE INCONTINENCE

In some patients, incontinence will unfortunately be intractable. The key to successful assessment of these patients for aids and equipment is, as always, to determine individual needs and priorities with a view to improving quality of life. The problem-solving approach should again be applied, taking into account:

- financial considerations
- lifestyle
- home conditions
- the degree and frequency of micturition or defaecation.

Aids and equipment

Aids and equipment are now being formally submitted to evaluation by product trials (Medical Devices Agency 1996a,b, 1997, 1998a,b). Early trials and reports included Fader et al (1987) and Ryan-Woolley (1987).

The type of aid that should be recommended for an individual will depend upon the specific type of incontinence from which she suffers. The assessment of a patient for aids or equipment must be informed by an understanding of the cause of her incontinence.

Aids to enhance mobility and stability, raised toilet seats, portable bidets or commodes and clothes that have been chosen or adapted for ease of access may be helpful to many individuals. Aids to personal cleansing can also be made available to help the patient maintain independence and dignity.

Urinals for women

For women confined to a wheelchair, incontinence may derive from an inability to transfer. Here a 'turtle cone' with attached tubing may be the answer, or, if the individual is confined to bed, a 'Femina bedpan' with tubing. These are fully described in the Continence Products Directory (Continence Foundation 1996).

For some women with arthritis who are taking diuretics and find that they cannot get to the toilet in time, a small slimline jug may be the solution. The patient stands and passes urine into this container and then, when able, takes it to the toilet for emptying or waits until assistance is available.

Pads and pants

For men and women who cannot achieve urinary control, a wide range of appliances, pads and pants is available. For up-to-date details on these, the reader is again directed to the *Continence Products Directory* (Continence Foundation 1996) or PromoCon in Manchester or to the nearest continence service, which will be able to provide information on the availability of particular pads in the local hospital and community.

Many pads can be obtained by mail order. The availability of aids and the process of collection or delivery vary for each area (Devlin 1985, Egan et al 1985). The type of pad and bed protection that an individual will be able to use will depend on the laundry facilities available and the role and time available of any carer involved with the patient. During assessment for such aids, patients should be asked if they have a washing machine, whether they will need to use a launderette or if a laundry service is provided by their local area health authority. It should be also established whether there are local facilities for collecting large amounts of incontinence aids refuse.

The pads available fall into the following categories:

Light incontinence. To collect small amounts of urine, and in cases where frequent changes are required, adhesive sanitary towels, marsupial pants and pads, small pads with stretch net pants, disposable pants and washable pants with protective waterproof gussets can all be used satisfactorily.

Medium and heavy incontinence. For medium and heavy incontinence, larger plastic-backed pads can be used with stretch net pants. Where hygiene is a concern or where large amounts of reflux emptying occurs, all-in-one adult diapers or nappy-style pads are available. A thin liner inside the pad may be useful where faecal incontinence also occurs. The liner can easily be separated from the pad and flushed with its contents down the toilet.

Bed pads are used as an extra protection for furniture and should not be sat or lain upon directly by the patient unless there are clear indications for using them in this way, e.g. where skin care of terminal patients presents a problem. Plastic mattress covers are also available to prevent soiling. Reusable bed pads can be purchased by those who have the necessary laundry facilities to cope with them and the finances to purchase at least three (one on the bed, one in the wash and one available for replacement). These particular aids are sometimes provided through local health services.

Products for men

Most urinary equipment designed to enable men to combat incontinence is available on prescription. New equipment is being developed and introduced quite rapidly and is frequently being tested in field trials (Pomfret 1990). Dribble pouches are available to accommodate small amounts of urine loss while sheaths (urodomes) with varying types of adhesive fixings and attachments are continually being refined.

Urethral occlusive devices are available but should be used with caution. Cautious introduction of surgical radio receiver implants have been used to aid continence and micturition (Schreiter 1985).

Pad and pants systems with Y-front marsupial pouches are particularly useful for men with a retracted penis and dribbling problems.

Obtaining further information

Many other aids are available in addition to those mentioned above which may prove helpful to particular patients. During assessment for aids and equipment, it may be advisable to consult an occupational therapist, physiotherapist or continence advisor on the range of supplies available in a particular health area. The patient may wish to investigate aids to daily living on view in regional aids centres or in specialist outlets.

Financial support and advisory service

Individuals who are incontinent or who care for an incontinent person may be eligible for a number of benefits such as Disability Living Allowance, Attendance Allowance and other loans: claim packs for these are now available. Further information can be obtained from local social security offices and post offices. Information is also available on the web site at 'http://www.dss.gov.uk'.

A number of voluntary agencies may also be able to offer practical support. For children, the Family Fund can give help with washing machines, tumble driers and bedding. Services such as 'Crossroads' may be available to provide respite care so that carers can have a break from their responsibilities, and in some areas day centres are available for patients to attend.

Advisory services

Nurses should be aware of the free advice on benefits that is available to patients, e.g. through freephone services. In some local authorities, welfare rights officers are also available to advise patients.

Q **24.12** When you are in your local post office or library, take note of any free literature or available benefits. Jot down the reference numbers of leaflets that may be relevant to your patients or build up a collection to refer to as particular questions on benefits arise.

Long-term catheter care

Long-term catheterisation is used in the management of incontinence only after all other treatment possibilities have been eliminated. It should not be undertaken without due consideration of the patient's lifestyle, preferences and likely level of compliance. The potential effect of long-term catheterisation on sexual relationships should also be considered (Webb 1985). The patient should be made aware of what catheter management will entail before the procedure is carried out (Heenan 1990). Catheter care is an important part of the nurse's role in the hospital and the community; an understanding of the principles of catheter selection and drainage system management together with skill in patient education are, of course, prerequisites for this. The anatomy and physiology of the lower urinary tract system and the selection and management of catheters are outlined in Chapter 8. The following exercise will help readers to review their knowledge.

Q **24.13** Mr A, who is 69 years old, has been sent home from hospital with a Foley catheter in place. He will need advice and information. Ascertain whether your knowledge base will be adequate to give good management care of his catheter and drainage system by considering the following questions.

Q **24.13** *(cont'd)*
(a) State four situations in which catheterisation would be justified. (A)
(b) Define what is meant by a Foley catheter.
(c) When is a large balloon catheter (30 ml) used?
(d) When is a small balloon catheter (5–10 ml) used?
(e) State four other features which should be considered in the selection of a catheter.
(f) What materials can be used to make catheters?
(g) What is a catheter with a hole below the balloon called?
(h) Can air, saline or other substances be used to fill balloons? Justify your answer.
(i) How many mL of fluid are used to fill a 5 ml balloon?
(j) What conditions are correct for the storage of catheters? What conditions should be avoided?

Preventing urinary tract infection

Urinary tract infection is the most common of all infections acquired in hospital, accounting for about 30% of the total (Meers et al 1980, Mulhall et al 1988). However, infection in the catheterised patient is not inevitable and can be prevented when the potential entry points of infection are properly managed.

Q **24.14** In Figure 24.6, can you identify the potential entry points for infection? What techniques can be used to prevent infection at each of these entry points? (A)

Considerable and ongoing research is being carried out on catheter management and, in keeping with the UKCC *Code of Professional Conduct* (UKCC 1994), all nurses involved in catheter care should keep abreast of new research findings in this area.

Bladder lavage

Catheter and bladder lavages or washouts have enjoyed a vogue in recent years as a means of reducing urinary infection, catheter encrustation and debris and are often cited as preventive measures in the nursing of catheterised patients. Nurses should be clear that

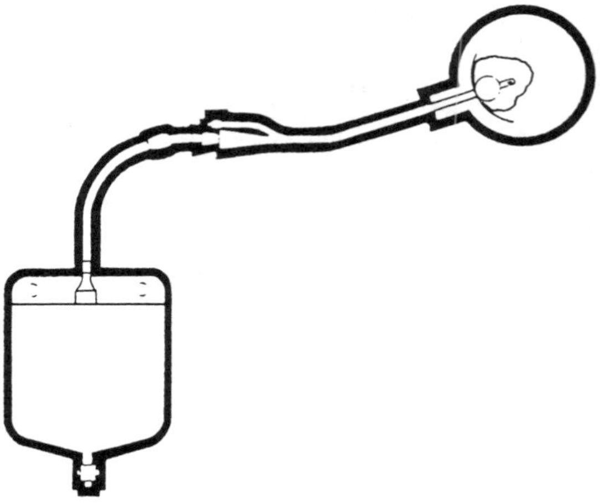

Fig. 24.6 Schematic of urethal catheter (see Self-assessment Question 24.14).

there is a difference between bladder irrigation and bladder lavage or washout. Strictly speaking, irrigation refers to the continuous washing out of the bladder (see Ch. 8). There is also disagreement as to whether these procedures should be carried out at all, as they disrupt the 'closed system' approach to management. Research findings suggest that bladder lavage is harmful (Elliott et al 1989, Bailey 1991) and should be carried out only where it is particularly indicated, never routinely (Roe 1990).

The use of prophylactic antibiotic therapy is not recommended (Slade & Gillespie 1985); instead, the ingestion of extra fluid to wash through the system is seen as the appropriate means of preventing infection and the accumulation of debris.

Nursing Care Plan 24.1 demonstrates the use of a problem-solving approach in identifying a patient's problems in caring for his catheter. It proceeds from identification of problems to setting goals with the patient and his relatives and then breaking down nursing interventions into their smallest components so that they can be carefully monitored and evaluated.

Supplying catheter equipment

Following the introduction of nurse prescribing, certain qualified nurses working within the community can now order the supplies required by catheterised patients. Patients should be given a list of all of their equipment, including sizes, types and capacity, as well as the name of a reliable chemist, retailer or mail order supplier. Appropriate details may be obtained by referring to the *Continence Products Directory* (Continence Foundation 1996) and the *Nurses' National Formulary*, which is to be updated biannually. Assessment of products is now being undertaken by the Medical Devices Agency (1996a,b, 1997, 1998a,b).

Emergency help and contact numbers. All catheterised patients in the community should be given a 24-hour contact number from which to gain help in an emergency. Practical advice on what to do in certain emergencies and on what constitutes a real problem should be given in writing to patients and carers. Roe (1987) suggests that the patient should be advised to notify her district nurse or doctor if any of the following occurs:

- catheter falls out
- urine is not being drained
- persistent pain
- fever
- blood in the urine.

Sexuality

Incontinence does not suddenly remove sexual desire (Broomhead 1986), even if it often causes people to refrain from sexual activity. Although many professionals may not see this aspect of their patient's well-being as a priority, patients who have been sexually active and are suddenly faced with incontinence caused by injury, childbirth or disease, as well as those who are facing progressive incontinence as a result of chronic disease, will have to make a difficult adjustment to changes in their sexual lives.

Problems of sexuality and incontinence affect both the young and the old. An unmet need was clearly identified when various readers of *Woman* magazine voluntarily replied to a questionnaire on incontinence (Glew 1986). One in three of the respondents had never mentioned their problem to their husbands and 25% of those aged 25–34 had told no one at all, including their own doctor. Thirty-eight per cent found the subject of incontinence too difficult to discuss with family and friends — 1 in 5 because they were embarrassed, and 1 in 5 because they worried about what others would think.

Of the respondents, 65% had suffered from incontinence for more than 2 years; 57% said their problem started with childbirth while 17% reported that intercourse produced leakage. The respondents identified anxiety in their sexual relationships as the main effect of incontinence; this included the difficulty of explaining the problem to a partner and the embarrassment of accidents that occurred during intercourse. These problems were severe enough to cause marriages to break up, yet a quarter of the women accepted their situation as 'a woman's lot'.

Glover et al (1986) conducted a study in four London boroughs to determine how many patients with urinary symptoms due to bladder neuropathy experienced difficulties with sexual intercourse; this formed part of a larger study of the management of urinary symptoms in neurological disease. Of the 252 patients interviewed, 216 (86%) were questioned about sexual intercourse, 86% of whom answered the complete questionnaire. Difficulties with intercourse were reported by 48% of those with multiple sclerosis and 63% of those with other neurological diseases. Difficulties were more commonly reported by men (71%) than by women (40%). A further 12% were refraining from sexual intercourse.

The nurse's attitude

Following a review of the nursing literature on human sexuality, as early as 1979 Brower & Tanner concluded that most nursing authors were not concerned with the sexuality of their patients and its implications for nursing care. More recently, Booth (1990) confirmed that this is especially the case with respect to older people.

These findings serve to remind us that nurses involved in counselling must examine their own attitudes and feelings relating to the subject of sexuality. Counselling with regard to the implications of incontinence for the individual's sexuality should be initiated only when the patient signals that she is ready to address the issue. However, the nurse may need to introduce the subject and thereby give the patient 'permission' to voice her concerns. Nurses may be prevented by inexperience and embarrassment from discussing questions of sexuality comfortably with their patient. Nelson (1977) argued that this difficulty is related to the fact that it can take individuals, including nurses, many years to form personal values regarding sex.

Practical problems and solutions

Certain issues concerning sexuality and incontinence may be dealt with in a practical manner, as outlined in the following.

Nocturnal enuresis is likely to inhibit both social and sexual intercourse and should be treated. The numbers of adults who are afflicted with this problem is uncertain; one indicator of its prevalence in the UK is the finding that it may affect in the region of 1% of entrants to the armed forces (de Jonge 1973), although problems with methodology and epidemiology are reported (Krantz et al 1994, Morison 1996).

It is important to chart the patient's pattern of enuresis before treatment is commenced. Often a form of bladder training is tried initially whereby the patient learns to hold onto urine longer during the day. The main treatment for nocturnal enuresis in the teenager and adult is to introduce the use of a personal alarm system. A small electrode attached to a battery alarm system about the size of a matchbox is pinned to the patient's nightgown or pyjamas. When the first drop of urine touches the electrode, a signal is activated and wakes the patient.

The prescription of desmopressin is helpful but does not cure the problem. This drug is available as a spray and consists of a

Nursing Care Plan 24.1 Management of an indwelling catheter

Problem	***Goal***	***Nursing Action***	***Evaluation***
2/7/2000 Unable to manage catheter and urine bag due to lack of knowledge and lack of manual dexterity	2/7/2000 To successfully and confidently manage care of his catheter and urine bags in as safe a manner as possible, by the time of his discharge: 9/7/2000	2/7/2000 Assess patient's ability to cope with buttons and zips	2/7/2000 While dressing himself today, patient was able to manage zip, but was slow with buttons
		3/7/2000 Change leg bag today and explain equipment and procedure	3/7/2000 Took a great deal of interest in the management and asked how the catheter stayed in
		4/7/2000 Discuss with patient and daughter the general management of the catheter	4/7/2000 Married daughter visited, says she can visit him every day at home and phone him. She thinks he could cope if instruction was given
		4/7/2000 Arrange a plan of teaching with patient and carer	4/7/2000 Married daughter coming on 5/7/2000 at 10.00 h for a teaching session
		5/7/2000 Display of equipment and information session Provide written information	5/7/2000 Patient and daughter took interest and a number of queries were raised
		5/7/2000 Extra leg bag change Patient to change leg bag and put on night 'add-on' bag with supervision	5/7/2000 Managed leg bag Night-time bag put on correctly but forgot to open valve
		6/7/2000 Night nurse to supervise night-time add-on bag application	6/7/2000 With prompting, remembered to open valve
		7/7/2000 Night nurse to supervise removal of night-time bag	7/7/2000 Remembered to close valve Successful in removal, drainage and disposal
		7/7/2000 Liaison with district nurse for supervision at home	7/7/2000 Contacted Sr G. Discussed patient's progress. Will visit 8/7/2000 p.m.
		7/7/2000 Supply patient with all equipment, written instructions and phone numbers for emergencies	7/7/2000 Patient read all the information and was able to identify each piece of equipment and how used. Given DN's number and info on visit
		8/7/2000 Discussion with patient and daughter on diet, emergencies, care and storage of equipment	8/7/2000 Daughter and patient happy about discharge on 9/7/2000 Able to change add-on bag successfully this morning
		9/7/2000 Discharge 10.00 h	9/7/2000 Patient discharged, confident about catheter management. Has 2 weeks' supply. Daughter thanked staff for teaching session

form of the antidiuretic hormone vasopressin. A single intranasal dose taken at night lasts for 10–12 h; this affords control of enuresis without affecting daytime urine production. Prolonged use is not recommended as adverse effects on the nose have been reported as well as water intoxication (NHS Centre for Reviews and Dissemination 1997).

An excellent resource centre dealing with all aspects of enuresis is the Enuresis Resource and Information Centre (ERIC; see 'Useful addresses', p. 782). Many helpful pamphlets are available from the centre for adults as well as children.

Cystitis involves either an infection or an inflammation of the bladder. The causal bacteria is usually *Escherichia coli*. It occurs most commonly in women, because of the anatomical closeness of the urethra, vagina and anus, and in some women may be linked to sexual intercourse. Incontinence rarely develops, but frequency and pain are present. When this occurs, many couples curtail their sexual activity, which may lead to tension in the relationship.

Careful hygiene, wiping the vulval area from front to back and avoiding contact by the penis or fingers with the anus during intercourse may prevent problems. Passing urine before and after intercourse has been found to be effective. Drinking copious amounts of water to flush the bladder can help when an attack occurs. Its management can also involve antibiotic therapy or self-help techniques (Shreeve 1986).

Preparation for intercourse

For many women who are incontinent, orgasm produces further episodes of urine loss. Passing urine before sexual intercourse may help. Protecting the bed and discussing the problem with one's partner can help to make the wetting less of an issue.

Catheterised patients need not avoid intercourse. For men, the catheter may be strapped to the underside of the penis, and may in some individuals with a degree of impotence also help rigidity. In women the catheter may be strapped to the inner thigh (Broomhead 1986).

Counselling. Open and reflective counselling will help to reveal the extent of any sexual problems experienced by the incontinent patient. If the patient's difficulties are not easily resolved, she should be referred to experts in sexual counselling who are available either in the hospital or in the community, or to other appropriate agencies such as the Association to Aid the Sexual and Personal Relationships of People with a Disability (SPOD). The nurse should be prepared to furnish information on these organisations and details of how to obtain an appointment.

The reader is referred to Fairburn et al (1983) and Webb (1985) for discussion of the issues surrounding the management of sexual problems.

FAECAL INCONTINENCE

While urinary incontinence is more prevalent in the population than faecal incontinence, the latter is the more distressing problem. Faecal incontinence is socially even more unacceptable than urinary incontinence and raises strong emotions among carers who have to deal with it. It is a source of discomfort and acute embarrassment for the sufferer, and contributes to feelings of helplessness and a loss of self-esteem.

Thomas et al (1984) found that 1 in 200 adults (0.5%) experience regular faecal incontinence. It is especially prevalent among elderly people (Johansen & Lafferty 1996) and those requiring long-term care. However, cohort research studies are discovering a number of women with damaged levator ani function following vaginal delivery (MacArthur et al 1997). Most cases, however, can be cured and the remainder can be made more manageable with proper care (Henry 1983).

Normal defaecation

Defaecation is the expulsion of faecal matter from the rectum with the aid of peristaltic movements of the muscular walls of the intestine (see Ch. 4). The rectum is stimulated to empty from impulses received from mass peristalsis, often starting from the gastrocolic reflex. The need for defaecation is felt as a response to distension of the sigmoid colon and the stimulation of the receptors. Further information on normal bowel function can be found in Chapter 4.

Anxiety can produce an urge to defaecate more often and in situations of extreme crisis faecal control can be temporarily lost.

The causes of faecal incontinence must be determined before treatment is instigated. Other than simple constipation and impaction, the cause of faecal incontinence is usually damage to the pelvic floor and anal sphincters, resulting in an inability to recognise that the rectum is full or to distinguish between flatus and faeces. The resulting incontinence may be due to constipation, faecal impaction, diarrhoea or spurious diarrhoea. The causes of faecal incontinence vary from an episode of diarrhoea or severe constipation, which is within normal limits, to underlying pathological disease or injury.

Constipation

The constipated patient may complain of headache, general malaise and lack of appetite. Abdominal discomfort, rectal fullness and cramps may also be reported. During examination, the abdomen can be measured for signs of increasing distension (Bishop 1982).

In people with a normal bowel, constipation may be caused by any of the following:

- a low-fibre diet
- low fluid intake
- ignoring the signals to defaecate
- pain in the anorectal region from haemorrhoids or fissures, or inability to position oneself comfortably in the necessary position, leading to avoidance of defaecation
- mouth pain leading to intake of soft foods only
- dental problems leading to inability to cope with foods that need to be chewed
- intake of narcotic analgesics, sedatives or hypnotic drugs.
- unacceptable toilet conditions
- unfamiliar surroundings or circumstances leading to loss of habit
- inability to recognise social expectations, as in some cases of mental handicap, senile dementia or excessive consumption of alcohol.

Where constipation is not relieved by the regimen described earlier in the chapter (see p. 773), or where no obvious cause is found, the problem may be due to damage to the pelvic floor and anal sphincter or to some other pathology, such as loss of rectal sensation as a result of surgery, injury or tumour. Other contributory problems include endocrine and metabolic reasons for dehydration and neurological damage.

Diarrhoea can also occur within normal limits; common causes are infection, inflammation in the bowel or rectum, excessive use of laxatives and the ingestion of certain foods or drugs. Parasitic infection can also cause diarrhoea.

Abnormalities resulting in faecal incontinence

The most common cause of faecal incontinence is damage to the puborectalis muscle and nerves, resulting in a failure of the valve at the anorectal flap or angle and associated lack of control and sensation. This may have been caused by straining at stool (Snooks et al 1985), trauma in childbirth (Swash 1988, MacArthur et al 1997, Sultan & Kamm 1997), congenital abnormalities or damage sustained during surgery. Atonic muscles may also preclude adequate pushing to expel the faeces.

In the assessment of faecal incontinence, a history of the complaint and an explanation of what previously constituted a normal habit should be obtained in order to establish the specific type of incontinence. Bleeding, loss of sensation and the presence of mucus are all symptoms that should be investigated. A full description of the incontinence and its frequency are also important to the diagnosis. Liquid leakage is quite different from true diarrhoea.

Following a rectal examination, referral for a plain X-ray, proctoscopy, barium enema and stool culture may be necessary (see Ch. 4).

Interventions may be quite conservative, involving such measures as changing the diet and making toilets more accessible. In some cases, however, surgery will be indicated. Recently some pioneering treatment using electrical stimulation has been reported (Matzel et al 1995). Gastrointestinal management of diarrhoea is fully described in Chapters 4, 20 and 21.

For a full account of the operations currently used to correct problems with the anorectal flap, see Parks (1986, pp. 88–90).

REFERENCES

Anderson J, Abrams P, Blaivas J G, Stanton S L 1998 The standardisation of terminology of lower urinary tract function. Scandinavian Journal of Urology and Nephrology 114(suppl): 5–9

Armstrong D 1980 An outline of sociology as applied to medicine. John Wright, Bristol

Association for Continence Advice 1985 Guidelines on the role of the continence advisor. ACA, London

Association for Continence Advice 1990 Directory of continence and toileting aids. ACA, London

Association for Continence Advice 1993 Guidelines for continence care. ACA, London

Bailey S 1991 Using bladder washouts. Nursing Times 87(24): 75–76

Bard 1987 You, your patients and urinary catheters. Bard, Crawley

Bayliss V K A, Cheery M, Salter E A 1998 Proposal for the development of care pathways. Continence ACA 18(2): 17–18

Bishop F K 1982 Notes from a district nurse. Community Outlook Nursing Times July 14: 195–196

Booth B 1990 Does it really matter at that age? Nursing Times 86(3): 50–52

Brocklehurst J C 1993 Urinary incontinence in the community: analysis of a MORI poll. British Medical Journal 306: 832–834

Broomhead L 1986 Incontinence: a personal account. Nursing 3(10): 11

Brower H T, Tanner L A 1979 A study of older adults attending a programme on human sexuality: a pilot study. Nursing Research 28(1): 36–39

Butler R 1994 Nocturnal enuresis – the child's experience. Butterworth Heinemann, Oxford

Cheater F, Hawthorn P 1987 Incontinence: a nursing perspective. Short report. Nursing Times 83(46): 46

Clegg 1980 Report on the standing commission on pay comparability. HMSO, London

Coloplast Foundation 1987 Objective: continence. Coloplast, Huntingdon, Cambs

Continence Foundation 1996 Continence products directory. Continence Foundation, London

Copperwheat M 1985 Putting continence into practice. Geriatric Nursing 5(3): 4–8

de Jonge G A 1973 Epidemiology of enuresis. In: Kolvin I, Mackeith R C, Meadows S R (eds) Bladder control and enuresis. Heinemann, London

Department of Health 1991 Agenda for action on continence services. DoH, London

Devlin R 1985 Are they being served? Community Outlook Nursing Times 81: 25–26

DHSS 1977 CNO (SNC) (77)1. HMSO, London

Donaldson L J 1983 Survival and functional capacity. Journal of Epidemiology and Community Health 37: 176–179

Dove D 1987 The five second flow test in urinary assessment. The Professional Nurse 2: 171

Edginton A, Shepherd A, Bainton D 1986 'D' is for dignity. Health and Social Services Journal 96: 50–51

Egan M, Playmet K, Thomas T, Meade T 1983 Incontinence in patients in two district general hospitals. Nursing Times 79(5): 22–24

Egan M, Thomas T, Meade T 1985 Mix and match. Community Outlook Nursing Times 81: 32–37

Elliott T J J, Gopal Rao G, Rigby R C et al 1989 Bladder irrigation or irritation? British Journal of Urology 64(4): 391–394

Ewles L, Simnett I 1985 Promoting health. Wiley, Chichester

Fader M J, Barnes K E, Malone-Leed et al 1986 Incontinence garments: results of a DHSS study. Health Equipment Information 159. DHSS/King's Fund, London

Farrer H 1986 Gynaecological care. Churchill Livingstone, Edinburgh

Feneley R C L 1987 Enuresis at twenty-five. British Medical Journal 294: 391–392

Fielding P 1986 Attitudes revisited: an examination of student nurses' attitudes towards older people in hospital. Royal College of Nursing, London

Freidson E 1970 Profession of medicine. Dodd Mead, New York

Gilleard C J 1981 Incontinence in the hospitalized elderly. Health Bulletin 391: 58–61

Glew J 1985 Incontinence: what every woman should know. Woman magazine, 9 March, pp 30–32

Glew J 1986 A woman's lot. Nursing Times 82(15): 69–71

Glover D, Thomas T, North W et al 1986 Urinary symptoms and sexual difficulties. Nursing Times 85(15): 72–75

Haggar V 1995 Strong developments. Nursing Times 91(33) (continence supplement)

Heenan A 1990 Indications for long term catheterization. Nursing Times 86(14): 70–71

Henry M 1983 Faecal incontinence. Nursing Times 79(33): 61–62

Henry M M, Parks A G, Swash M 1982 The pelvic floor musculature in the descending perineum syndrome. British Journal of Surgery 69: 470–472

Holmes P 1990 Mind over bladder. Nursing Times 86(4): 16–17

Horsfield M 1986 Incontinence: a young woman's problem. She magazine, October, pp 86–87

International Continence Society (ICS) 1984 The standardisation of terminology of the lower urinary tract function. ICS, London

Johanson J F, Lafferty J 1996 Epidemiology of faecal incontinence. The silent affliction. Americal Journal of Gastroenterology 91(1): 33–36

Keister K J 1989 Medication of elderly institutionalized incontinent females. Journal of Advanced Nursing 14(11): 980–985

King's Fund 1983 Action on incontinence. Report of a working group No 43. King's Fund, London

Krantz I, Jykas E, Ahlberg B M, Wedel H 1994 On the epidemiology of nocturnal enuresis – a critical review of methods used in descriptive epidemiological studies on nocturnal enuresis. Scandinavian Journal of Urology and Nephrology (suppl) 163: 75–82

Laycock J 1987 Graded exercises for the pelvic floor muscles in the treatment of urinary incontinence. Journal of Physiotherapy 73(7): 371–373

Laycock J 1992 Pelvic floor re-education for the promotion of continence. In: Roe B H (ed) Clinical nursing practice. Prentice Hall, Englewood Cliffs, NJ, p 102

Laycock J, Green R J 1988 Interferential therapy in the treatment of incontinence. Physiotherapy 74(4): 161–168

MacArthur C, Bick D E, Keighley M R B 1997 Faecal incontinence after childbirth. British Journal of Obstetrics and Gynaecology 104: 46–50
McGrother C W, Castleden C M, Duffin H, Clarke M 1987 Provision of services for incontinent elderly people at home. Journal of Epidemiology and Community Health 40(2): 134–138
McLaren S M, McPherson F M, Sinclair F et al 1981 Prevalence and severity of incontinence among hospitalised female psycho-geriatric patients. Health Bulletin 38: 62–64
Maleham T 1993 A dry run. Nursing Times 89(30): 66–68
Matzel K E, Stadelmaier U, Hohenfellner M et al 1995 Electrical stimulation for the treatment of faecal incontinence. The Lancet 346: 1124
Medical Devices Agency 1996a Disability equipment assessment – catheters for intermittent self-catheterisation. No. A18. MDA, Surbiton
Medical Devices Agency 1996b Disability equipment assessment – sterile leg bags. No. A20. MDA, Surbiton
Medical Devices Agency 1997 Disability equipment assessment – catheter valves. No. No. A22. MDA, Surbiton
Medical Devices Agency 1998a Disability equipment assessment – enuresis alarms – an evaluation. No. A22. MDA, Surbiton
Medical Devices Agency 1998b Disposable, shaped bodyworn pads with pants for heavy incontinence. An evaluation. No. IN.1. MDA, Surbiton
Meers P C, Ayliffe G A, Emmerson A M et al 1980 Report on the national survey of infection in hospital. Journal of Hospital Infection 2(suppl): 1–11
Miller A 1984 Nurse-patient dependency. Journal of Advanced Nursing 9: 479–486
Miller A 1985 Nurse-patient dependency: is it iatrogenic? Journal of Advanced Nursing 10: 63–69
Montgomery E 1986 Pelvic power. Community Outlook Nursing Times 82: 33–34
Morison M 1996 Family perspectives on bed wetting in young people. Avebury, London
Mulhall A B, Chapman R G, Crow R A 1988 Bacteriuria during indwelling urethral catheterization. Journal of Hospital Infection 11: 253–262
Murray K, Lewis P, Blannin J et al 1984 Clean intermittent self-catheterization in the management of adult lower urinary tract infection. British Journal of Urology 56: 379–380
National Institute for Nursing 1995 An evaluation of nursing developments in incontinence care. Report no. 10. NIN, Oxford
Neal D E, Styles R A, Ng T, Powell P H, Thong J, Ramsden P D 1987 The relationship between voiding pressures, symptoms and urodynamic findings in 253 men undergoing prostatectomy. British Journal of Urology 60: 554–559
Nelson S E 1977 All about sex for students. American Journal of Nursing 77(4): 611–612
NHS and Community Care Act 1990 HMSO, London
NHS Centre for Reviews and Dissemination 1997 A systematic review of the effectiveness of interventions for managing childhood nocturnal enuresis. CRD report 11. The University of York, York
Nygaard I 1995 Prevention of exercise incontinence with mechanical devices. Journal of Reproductive Medicine 40(2) 89–94
O'Brien J, Long H 1995 Urinary incontinence: long term effectiveness of nursing interventions in primary care. British Medical Journal 311: 1208
Patrick D S, Scambler G (eds) 1986 Sociology as applied to medicine. Baillière Tindall, London
Peattie A B, Plevnik S, Stanton S L 1988 Vaginal cones: a conservative method of treating genuine stress incontinence. British Journal of Obstetrics and Gynaecology 95: 1049–1053
Pomfret I 1990 All shapes and sizes. Journal of District Nursing 8(12): 9–10
Ritch A E S 1988 The use of oestrogen in incontinence in the elderly. Measuring and managing incontinence. Geriatric Medicine and Kabivitrium Ltd
Robb B 1967 Sans everything: a case to answer. Nelson, London
Roe B 1987 Catheter care. A guide for users and their carers. Wallace, Colchester
Roe B 1990 Catheter prescribing and the use of antimicrobials. Nursing Times 86(14): 65–68
Rowse A 1996 A voiding problem. Nursing Times 92(suppl): 41
Royal College of Physicians 1995 Incontinence: causes, management and provision. A report from the Royal College of Physicians. RCP, London
Royal College of Physicians 1998 Promoting continence – clinical audit scheme for urinary and faecal incontinence. RCP, London
Ryan-Woolley B 1987 Aids for the management of incontinence. King's Fund, London
Scambler G 1986 Illness behaviour. In: Patrick D L, Scambler G (eds) Sociology as applied to medicine. Baillière Tindall, London
Schreiter F 1985 Bulbar artificial sphincter. European Urology 11: 294–299
Scottish Office NHS in Scotland 1992 The named nurse national guidelines. SO, Edinburgh
Seth C 1987 Incontinence: doing it yourself. Nursing Times Community Outlook 83: 11–12
Shapiro R 1989 A shameful secret. Community Outlook Nursing Times 85: 21–23
Shreeve C 1986 Cystitis: the new approach. Thorsons, Northamptonshire
Shuttleworth K E D 1970 Urinary tract diseases: incontinence. British Medical Journal 4: 727–729
Sibley L 1988 Confidence with incontinence. Nursing Times 84(46): 42–43
Slade N, Gillespie W A 1985 The urinary tract and the catheter: infection and other problems. Wiley, Chichester
Snooks S J, Barnes P R H, Swash M et al 1985 Damage to the innervation of the pelvic floor musculature in chronic constipation. Gastroenterology 89: 971–981
Southern D, Henderson P 1990 Tackling incontinence. Nursing Times 86(10): 36–38
Sutan A H, Kamm M A 1997 Faecal incontinence after childbirth. Commentary. British Journal of Obstetrics and Gynaecology 104: 979–982
Sutherst J R, Brown M C, Richmond D 1986 Analysis of the pattern of urine loss in women with incontinence as measured by weighing perineal pads. British Journal of Urology 58: 273–278
Swaffield J 1995 Quality audit – a review of the literature concerning delivery of continence care. Journal of Clinical Nursing 4: 277–282
Swash M 1988 Childbirth and incontinence. Midwifery 4: 13–18
Taylor K, Henderson J 1986 Effects of biofeedback and urinary stress incontinence in women. Journal of Gerontological Nursing 12(9): 25–30
The Continence Foundation, Incon Tact, Association for Continence Advice (ACA), the RCN Continence Care forum, the Enuresis Resource & Information Centre (ERIC), the Spinal Injuries Association, the Multiple Sclerosis Society 1995 Charter for Continence. The Continence Foundation, London
Thomas T M, Egan M, Walgrove A et al 1984 The prevalence of faecal incontinence. Community Medicine 6: 216–220
Thomas T M, Plymet K R, Blannin J et al 1980 Prevalence of urinary incontinence. British Medical Journal 281: 1243–1245
Townsend P 1964 The last refuge: a survey of residential institutions and homes for the aged in England and Wales. Routledge and Kegan Paul, London
UKCC 1994 Code of professional conduct for the nurse, midwife and health visitor, 2nd edn. UKCC, London
Walker I 1987 The one problem we still can't talk about. Living magazine, May, pp 102–104
Webb C 1985 Sexuality, nursing and health. HM and M, Chichester
White M 1990 Independence for the handicapped child. Nursing Times 86(7): 69–72
Willis J 1996 Outreach for prevention. Nursing Times 92(suppl): 15
Wysocki R 1983 Urinary incontinence and the older adult. Australian Nurses' Journal 12(11): 49–50, 52
Zola I 1973 Pathways to the doctor: from person to patient. Society of Scientific Medicine 7: 677–689

FURTHER READING

Badger F J, Drummond M F, Isaacs B 1983 Some issues in the clinical, social and economic evaluation of new nursing services. Journal of Advanced Nursing 8(6): 478–494
Bard 1984 Guidelines for the management of catheterized patients. Bard, Crawley
Dobson P 1990 Update on ERIC. Nursing Times 86(7): 75
Fairburn C G, Dickerson M G, Greenwood J 1983 Sexual problems and their management. Churchill Livingstone, Edinburgh
Parks A G 1986 Faecal incontinence. In: Mandelstam D (ed) Incontinence and its management. Croom Helm, Beckenham

Syred M E J 1981 The abdication of the role of health education by hospital nurses. Journal of Advanced Nursing 6: 27–33

Trounce J 1997 Clinical pharmacology for nurses, 15th edn. Churchill Livingstone, Edinburgh

Webb C 1985 Sexuality, nursing and health. HM and M, Chichester

World Health Organization 1975 Education and training in human sexuality: the training of health professionals. WHO, Geneva

USEFUL ADDRESSES

ACA (Association for Continence Advice)
Winchester House
Kennington Park
Cranmer Road
The Oval
London SW9 6EJ

Continence Foundation
307 Hatton Square
16 Baldwins Gardens
London EC1N 7RJ

ERIC (Enuresis Resource and Information Centre)
34 Old School House
Britannia Road
Kingswood
Bristol BS15 2DB

PromoCon Disabled Living
4 Chad's Street
Manchester M8 8QA

SPOD (Association to Aid the Sexual and Personal Relationships of People with a Disability)
286 Camden Road
London N7 0BJ

SLEEP

S. José Closs

25

INTRODUCTION

The intriguing subject of sleep has been much written about. What happens when we fall asleep? Despite hundreds of years of observations of sleep and, more recently, extensive and systematic research, the mechanisms and functions of sleep are still poorly understood. Many theories, both physiological and behavioural, have been postulated, but there is still much to discover. Nevertheless, sleep is something that everyone does, and from which 'beggars in their beds take as much pleasure as kings' (Thomas Dekker 1604)*. Although there have been individuals who maintain that they never sleep, so far such claims have always been discredited after careful monitoring. Everyone sleeps.

Ageing both exacerbates existing sleep disorders and introduces new ones. Given that the numbers of elderly people are rapidly rising, this is an area of increasing concern in nursing practice. An understanding of the structure and probable functions of sleep should allow nurses in all fields of care to help patients to get the best possible sleep, both at home and under the rather more difficult conditions in hospital. This chapter aims to provide both theoretical and practical information about sleep which is relevant to nurses working in hospital and in home care settings.

*Thomas Dekker (c. 1572 – c. 1632), English playwright

THE IMPORTANCE OF THE SLEEP–WAKE CYCLE

Primarily, it is our circadian rhythms that dictate when it is time to sleep. The word circadian is derived from the Latin *circa* ('about') and *diem* ('a day') and refers to the physiological and behavioural patterns that repeat every 24 h. Under normal circumstances, these rhythms are synchronised by external time cues, such as the light–dark cycle, and by social time cues, such as mealtimes. These synchronising cues are known as Zeitgebers ('time-givers'). It seems, however, that there are internal as well as external synchronisers. Many studies have confirmed that endogenous 'clocks' govern the function of every living tissue. These clocks are coordinated directly or indirectly by the brain. It is probable that the 'pacemaker' controlling the sleep–wake cycle is situated in the suprachiasmatic area of the hypothalamus, since bilateral lesions in this area abolish the normal circadian pattern of rest and activity. When humans are placed in an environment free of time cues, their circadian rhythms usually take on a 'natural period', which occasionally lasts fewer than 24 h but is usually about 25 h or sometimes more. This natural periodicity is known as free-running.

The sleep–wake cycle coincides with other circadian rhythms, such as 24-h fluctuations in body temperature, heart rate and plasma levels of anabolic and catabolic hormones. Catecholamines and cortisol potentiate stress responses (see Ch. 17), which are likely to be high among patients in intensive care units (see Ch. 8). If subjects are allowed to free-run, i.e. they are isolated from all cues signalling the time of day, then their various circadian rhythms tend to become dissociated from one another. For example, it has been shown that in the absence of time cues the rest–activity cycle may have a period of, say, 33 h, whereas body temperature might have a 24.5-h cycle.

Desynchronisation of circadian rhythms has been shown to disrupt not only temperature and sleep–wake patterns, but also pulse rate, respiration, arterial pressure, diuresis and excretion of electrolytes. This acute desynchronisation can produce symptoms such as fever, alcohol hangover, migraine and some mental disorders. Weitzman et al (1970) showed that EEG recordings of subjects following a phase shift of the sleep–wake cycle revealed changes in sleep structure similar to those found in endogenously depressed individuals. These included an increased time before the onset of rapid eye movement (REM) sleep (see p. 785) and more night-time awakenings. It has been suggested that endogenous depression might result from a long-term mismatch between metabolic rhythms and the sleep–wake cycle.

People have highly individual 24-h routines. Many rise in response to an alarm clock at a specific time that allows them to arrive at work punctually. Patterns of activity tend to be dictated by work, family and social commitments, as well as by the individual's particular requirements for sleep. For most people, the propensity to fall asleep peaks twice during the day. The first peak is at the usual bedtime and the second is after lunch (whether or not lunch has actually been eaten), when people in some countries customarily take a siesta.

Normal sleep–wake cycles may be disrupted by many different events. For example, new parents may find that 'night is turned into day' for the first 3 months or so of their baby's life.

It is not only the young whose sleep patterns differ from those of the normal adult. The circadian rhythms of older people tend to weaken as they age. This results in less night-time sleep, more awakenings at night and sometimes more daytime napping. This has implications for those who care for elderly people, both in hospital and at home (see Ch. 5). In hospital, routines should be relaxed in order to accommodate the relatively irregular sleeping habits of elderly patients. At home, carers who have to get up several times throughout the night in order to attend to the needs of an elderly relative often find that fatigue reduces their ability to cope effectively, particularly if they also have to work during the day.

Shiftwork is another common cause of disruption to the sleep–wake cycle. Student nurses working night shifts for the first time may be surprised at their difficulty in adjusting to a new pattern of rest and activity. The degree of difficulty is highly individual, some nurses finding it relatively easy to adjust while others find it virtually impossible to get enough sleep during the day, when there is usually more noise and when Zeitgebers which normally prompt night-time sleep are absent. Those nurses who do not sleep adequately may not be able to function efficiently throughout the night, resulting in a reduction in the quality of care that they give. The possibility of dangerous errors, such as in the administration of drugs, also becomes more likely.

Since the average free-running day is about 25 h, people tend to adjust to changes in the rest–activity cycle more easily when the cycle is being lengthened. Travelling west rather than east and changing one's work shift to a later rather than an earlier period in the day are easier adjustments to make.

The circadian disruptions which occur upon the patient's admission to hospital may result from the absence or adjustment of the Zeitgebers normally responsible for synchronisation, as well as from stresses such as pain and anxiety. Of necessity, hospitals impose unfamiliar lighting conditions and altered times for meals (or their absence) and awakening. Floyd (1984) found that psychiatric hospital in-patients slept less than a matched group of outpatients and that their normal times of sleeping and activity appeared to be altered by the hospital's rest–activity schedule. However, psychiatric pathology itself may interfere with sleep patterns, a point which is discussed later (see p. 789).

Although much of the experimentation on desynchronisation has been conducted under tightly controlled circumstances, some of its findings may be applicable to daily life. It appears that the disruption of normal circadian rhythms (and, in particular, of the sleep–wake cycle) leads to numerous adverse physiological and psychological consequences. These are detrimental to patients in the community and particularly undesirable for hospital patients, who are subject to many additional stresses. Since the two major synchronising rhythms appear to be those of sleep and body temperature, nurses should try to maintain an awareness of these and attempt, where appropriate, to help patients to synchronise them with their normal patterns.

Q **25.1** Discuss with your colleagues how nurses can use the notion of circadian rhythmicity to help patients to sleep better, both in hospital and in the community.

DESCRIBING SLEEP

For the most part, modern researchers have tended to use objective criteria to describe sleep, usually in terms of physiological events occurring during specific stages of sleep. These include changes in the electrical activity of the brain and fluctuations in the secretion of various hormones. It is important to bear in mind, however, that it is the individual's subjective experience of sleep which is of greatest importance in an assessment of the quality of that sleep. Even when an EEG indicates that sleep has been long and continuous, if the individual feels that he has slept badly, he cannot be contradicted. Conversely, if a patient habitually sleeps for only 2 h a night, but claims that this amount is adequate, leaving him rested and refreshed, then there is nothing wrong with his sleep.

In addition to recognising the importance of sleep as a subjective experience, it is also useful to have some basic knowledge about the structure and function of sleep. This may be put to good use in attempting to understand patients' sleep difficulties and their implications and in planning interventions.

The structure of sleep

Electroencephalography is a relatively new technology which has enabled researchers to describe the structure of sleep in terms of types of gross electrical activity which take place in the brain. This is achieved by attaching electrodes to the scalp, which then conduct the electrical current generated by various areas of the brain to a device which allows them to be viewed. Usually this is either a TV monitor or an electroencephalograph, which inscribes a permanent trace of brainwaves on paper (i.e. an electroencephalogram, or EEG), in a manner similar to the recording of the electrical activity of the heart by an electrocardiograph (see Ch. 2). EEGs and other recordings have shown that there are two distinct types of sleep.

NREM sleep

NREM (non-rapid eye movement, or orthodox, sleep) comprises four stages, as described by Rechtschaffen & Kales (1968). In each stage, electrical activity of the brain progressively slows and increases in amplitude (see Fig. 25.1).

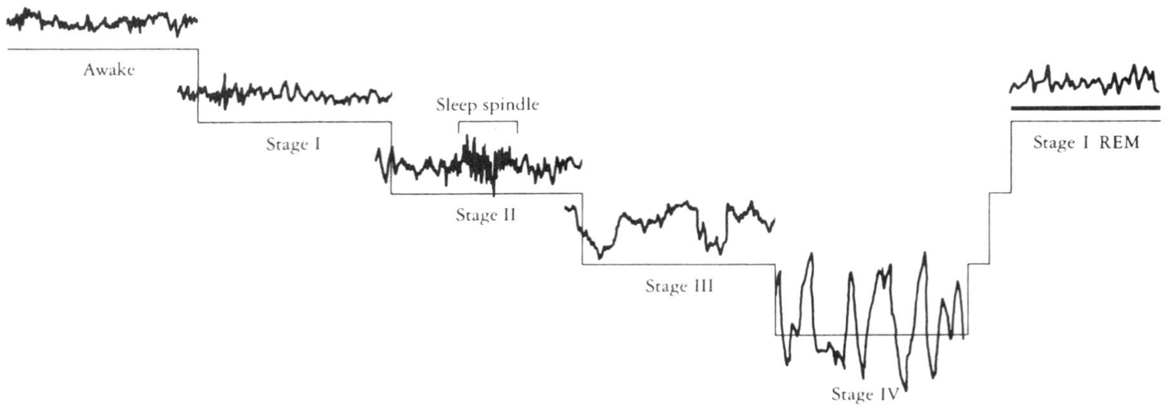

Fig. 25.1 Progressive changes in the EEG following the onset of sleep. (From SLEEP, by J. Allan Hobson. Copyright © 1995 by J. Allan Hobson. Reprinted by permission of W.H. Freeman and Company.)

Stage 0 or W (wakefulness). During wakefulness, the EEG is characterised by generally low-voltage activity at 4–25 Hz. Sinusoidal alpha waves are present when the subject is awake with his eyes closed.

Stage I (drowsing). The alpha rhythm (8–12 Hz) begins to fluctuate and slow, rolling eye movements appear on the electro-oculogram (EOG), which records electrical activity associated with eye movements. During stage 1, the pupils constrict and dilate at intervals of roughly 1–3 s. The EEG shows mostly low-voltage, mixed-frequency activity at 2–7 Hz. This is the lightest stage of sleep. If asked, the subject may report that he felt drowsy but was awake. Even though the subject may feel fully alert, it is likely that observers will note his reduced attentiveness. Some simple perceptual distortions (i.e. daydreams) may occur during stage 1 sleep.

Stage II (light sleep). The alpha rhythm disappears and 'sleep spindles' of 12–14 Hz, lasting at least 0.5 s, appear. These spindles are the most consistent characteristic of stage 2 sleep. This phase of altered consciousness is such that, if awakened, most people recognise that they have been asleep. It is in stage 2 that body movements begin to diminish and dreams involving a storyline first appear. Dream recall on waking, however, is far less vivid than for REM sleep.

Stage III (slow wave sleep). The amplitude of the EEG increases, and 20–49% of the trace records delta activity (i.e. less than 2 Hz with amplitudes greater than 75 mV from peak to peak). Spindles are rarely seen. Body movements continue to diminish. The distinction between stages 3 and 4 is somewhat arbitrary, since the increase in the proportion of delta waves occurs gradually.

Stage IV (slow wave sleep). Over 50% of the EEG shows delta activity. High-amplitude slow waves are indicative of this stage. There is a high degree of immobility and intense external stimuli are required to arouse the subject. Large increases in the secretion of growth hormone occur.

By convention, and throughout this chapter, stages 3 and 4 are considered together and termed slow wave sleep (SWS). The distinctions between wakefulness, stage 1, stage 2, SWS and REM are qualitative, involving clearly observable physiological differences, while the distinction between stages 3 and 4 seems arbitrary.

REM sleep

The second type of sleep is known as rapid eye movement (REM) or paradoxical sleep and is characterised by dreaming, muscular relaxation and high levels of physiological arousal. In order to identify this phase of sleep, extra electrodes can be applied to the face to detect electrical activity due to eye movement, and below the chin to detect muscle tone. These may then be recorded as an EOG and EMG (electromyogram) to augment the information gained from the EEG. If all these electrical signals are recorded overnight, the result is a complex series of parallel traces known as a polysomnogram. From this, the most reliable indicator of REM, i.e. the disappearance of skeletal muscle tone, can be visualised. The EEG recorded during REM sleep is virtually indistinguishable from that taken during wakefulness, showing low-amplitude, mixed frequency activity. During REM sleep, muscle tone is lower than in any other sleep stage. Blood pressure fluctuates, pulse and respiration rates increase and may become irregular, oxygen consumption increases, premature ventricular contractions may occur and there is penile tumescence in men and increased vaginal secretion in women. The eye movement which occurs in REM sleep usually consists of rapid darting movements of the eyes under closed lids, occurring in bursts of 3–10 s at intervals of 30–40 s. These do not always occur, and if they are absent this is most likely to be during the first REM period of the night. If subjects are woken up they frequently report that they have been dreaming; consequently, REM sleep is frequently referred to as dreaming sleep.

During a night's sleep, both REM sleep and all four NREM stages may occur many times, usually in a cyclical fashion (see Fig. 25.2). Sleep usually begins with stage 1 (drowsing) and progresses through stage 2 to SWS. This 'deep' sleep is frequently followed by a brief return to stage 2 before an episode of REM. The pattern then repeats, usually starting from stage 2. The duration of this cycle may vary considerably according to age and other factors, but in young healthy adults it lasts approximately 100 min.

The first part of the night tends to contain more SWS, while the latter part of the night contains a higher proportion of REM. Interestingly, even during the day, people undergo 100 min cycles of alertness and drowsiness, although they are usually unaware of these. During sleep, shifts from stage to stage tend to accompany body movements. Shifts to light sleep tend to occur suddenly, whereas shifts to deep sleep tend to be gradual.

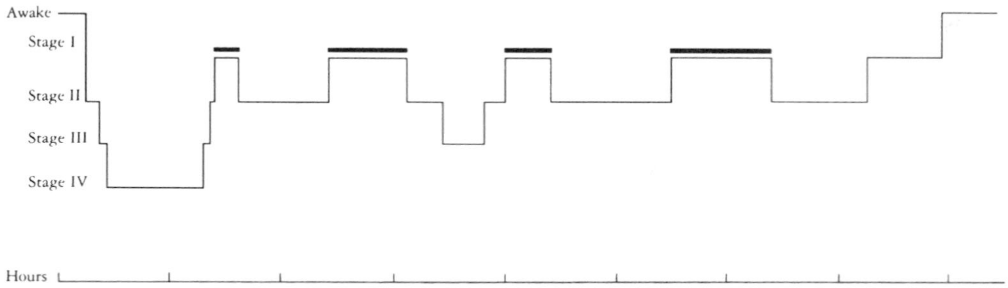

Fig. 25.2 Sleep architecture showing one night's progression of sleep cycles. (From SLEEP, by J. Allan Hobson. Copyright © 1995 by J. Allan Hobson. Reprinted by permission of W.H. Freeman and Company.)

Normally, sleep in healthy young adults comprises approximately 4% stage 1, 50% stage 2, 23% SWS and 23% REM sleep (Johns 1984).

PHYSIOLOGICAL CONTROL OF SLEEP

Precisely how and why people sleep remains the subject of much research. At present it appears that the brain has several interlinked sleep centres. Some relate to the onset and timing of sleep, some to REM sleep, others to NREM sleep and others to wakefulness. In addition, there are several putative, naturally occurring sleep substances which seem to be diffused throughout the brain.

Neurological control

The neurological control of sleep is complex and is not yet completely understood. The medulla, pons and midbrain comprise the brain stem (see Ch. 9) and accommodate many of the anatomical structures which govern sleep and wakefulness. The cell network known as the reticular formation is located within the brain stem and contributes to several aspects of brain function. Implicated in the regulation of sleep and wakefulness is the reticular activating system (part of the reticular formation), which describes collectively specific structures within the brain stem and the thalamus.

NREM sleep mechanisms in the basal forebrain interact with reticular systems, producing characteristic slow wave electrical activity in the cerebral cortex. The REM sleep generator in the pons interrupts this process periodically, reactivating the brain.

Neurotransmitters

Three different neurotransmitters are implicated in the regulation of sleep and wakefulness. These are noradrenaline, acetylcholine and 5-hydroxytryptamine (5-HT, also called serotonin), each produced by different sets of cells within the pons. Noradrenergic neurones are responsible for the arousal of the cortex observed during wakefulness and REM sleep. Cholinergic cells facilitate REM sleep, while cells producing 5-HT appear to be responsible for the maintenance of NREM sleep and to play an important role in the regulation of REM sleep.

Sleep substances

Theories claiming the existence of sleep substances have gained popularity from the beginning of this century. These are claimed to be naturally occurring substances which accumulate in the central nervous system (CNS) and cause sleep. Several sleep substances have been isolated, but it is not known whether they are central to the regulation of sleep or part of a larger and more complex system.

FUNCTIONS OF SLEEP

Despite enormous research efforts, the only universally agreed reason for sleeping is to avoid being sleepy. Interpretations of research findings vary, but it is generally considered that sleep is a restorative process (Adam & Oswald 1983). It has also been suggested, however, that sleep is merely an instinctual behaviour, a genetic remnant of earlier days when immobility at night aided survival. Horne (1988) proposed that some sleep is obligatory (SWS and about two-thirds of REM) and some optional (stages 1 and 2 and one-third of REM). He argued that the obligatory portion of sleep is essential only for the functioning of the brain and that other organs may require only physical rest and feeding for restitution.

Although these are the most widely accepted theories, there are many others concerning the purpose of sleep. A symposium in 1995 proposed many possibilities, including the resetting of physiological systems, growth, energy conservation, modulation of immune functions, homeostatic restoration of brain function, maintenance of inherited behaviours, creativity and others (Moorcroft 1995). Overall, however, sleep appears to have a major role in the maintenance and/or restoration of physical and cerebral functioning.

SWS and restorative processes

The direct study of sleep and tissue restitution in human subjects presents practical and ethical difficulties. Obviously it would be unacceptable to deprive people who have sustained injury of sleep in order to study the effects of sleep on healing. A rather less direct way of investigating body restoration is to study circadian variations in the levels of anabolic and catabolic hormones. These regular fluctuations suggest that anabolic processes occur during the sleep period. In humans, protein synthesis is inhibited by hormones such as cortisol, glucagon and catecholamines, which reach their highest levels during the day. During sleep, energy expenditure in the tissues falls and the energy stored within the cells as adenosine triphosphate (ATP) rises to levels which become sufficiently high for protein synthesis to occur. The first episode of night-time SWS coincides with peak levels of secretion of human growth hormone (HGH), which stimulates protein and RNA synthesis and amino acid uptake. Consequently, as a recent overview of research into the functions of sleep suggested, peak tissue-building processes are associated with SWS (Shapiro & Flanigan 1993). The onset of SWS is also associated with increased immunological activity. Further, SWS is the sleep state which has the highest positive correlation with the length of prior wakefulness and therefore appears to be associated with restorative properties. All this evidence supports the assertion that sleep, and in particular SWS, is essential for tissue restoration.

REM sleep

The function of REM sleep is more difficult to explain. Babies have large amounts of REM sleep, whereas elderly sufferers of chronic brain degeneration have a reduced duration of REM sleep. This implies that REM sleep has a possible role in brain metabolism. Human studies of REM sleep deprivation have not yet produced a clear picture of its effects. There have been tentative suggestions that REM sleep is involved in the integration of emotional experiences and entirely new material, but does not affect tasks such as learning word lists or the assimilation of familiar sorts of experience. It seems possible that REM sleep is involved in learning and memory, but research has so far failed to provide convincing evidence to support these ideas.

Effects of sleep deprivation

Total sleep deprivation has been shown to result in clear signs of CNS impairment and there is evidence of physiological damage as well. Rechtschaffen & Bergmann (1995) reported a series of experiments which deprived rats of sleep and found that they suffered 'severe pathology and death' whereas control rats did not. The major pathology caused was impaired thermoregulation, together with ulcerative and hyperkeratotic skin lesions, but they were unable to identify a specific link between sleep deprivation and the resulting pathology. Human research is also somewhat inconclusive (Horne 1983). Total sleep deprivation for 48 h in humans results in changes in CNS function, such as behavioural irritability, suspiciousness, speech slurring and minor visual misperceptions. These may be accompanied by increased suggestibility and/or a reduction in motivation and willingness to perform tasks. In hospital, this could impede mobilisation and other aspects of self-care. For patients in the community, this could reduce efficiency at work and affect social and family relationships. Detrimental psychological effects of sleep deprivation observed in hospital patients include lethargy, irritability, confusion and, in more extreme cases, delusions and paranoia.

A meta-analysis of 19 research studies which addressed the effects of sleep loss suggested that the effects of such deprivation may well be underestimated (Pilcher & Huffcutt 1996). From a total sample of almost 2000 people, they concluded that mood was the aspect of human functioning which suffered most. They also found that partial sleep deprivation produced a greater impairment of cognitive and motor functioning than either short-term or long-term sleep deprivation.

Both acute and prolonged sleep disturbances, including delirium, have been observed in acute care settings (Cronin-Stubbs 1996). Hartmann (1973) assessed sleep requirements by interview and questionnaire and found that stress and illness were virtually always accompanied by an increased subjective sleep need. Taken together, these observations support the hypothesis that sleep aids healing, suggesting that conditions favourable to sleep should be encouraged in all areas where patients are suffering from infection or trauma or are recovering following surgery.

Q **25.2** Given that postoperative patients require frequent observation and attention, how can nurses help to ensure that these patients get adequate sleep in the period immediately following surgery?

NORMAL SLEEP

No matter what objective recordings of sleep might indicate about its duration, continuity or 'architecture', if the sleeper is satisfied with his sleep, then it may be considered to be normal. A good, restful night's sleep and a good day's refreshed and efficient wakefulness are, of course, interrelated. Even though their relationship is not one of simple cause and effect, each depends on the quality of the other.

Individual requirements for sleep vary enormously. A range of 3–12 h of sleep per night has been cited as normal by Johns (1984). The average is about 7.5 h, although the duration of sleep has a normal distribution (see Fig. 25.3).

Some people habitually take a nap during the day, while many do not. In addition, some people are early risers while others are more active in the evening and tend to go to bed late. The tendency of individuals to 'morningness' or 'eveningness' was first reported by Horne & Ostberg (1976) who described such people as 'larks' and 'owls'. Hospital routines tend to override these individual variations in behaviour, with a possible outcome of disturbed sleep patterns for some.

Factors affecting normal sleep

There are many factors which may affect normal sleep, including age, gender, diet and ambient temperature. These influences should be taken into account in nursing assessments of patients' sleep, since the normal habits and needs of individuals may bear little resemblance to one another.

Age

Over half of those aged 65 or more tend to have problems sleeping (Ancoli-Israel 1997). These changes in sleep patterns associated with ageing have been well documented (see Fig. 25.4). While

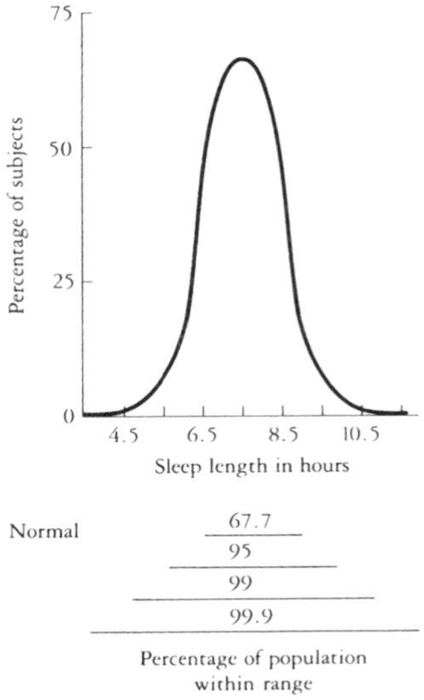

Fig. 25.3 Normal frequency curve of sleep durations. (From SLEEP, by J. Allan Hobson. Copyright © 1995 by J. Allan Hobson. Reprinted by permission of W.H. Freeman and Company.)

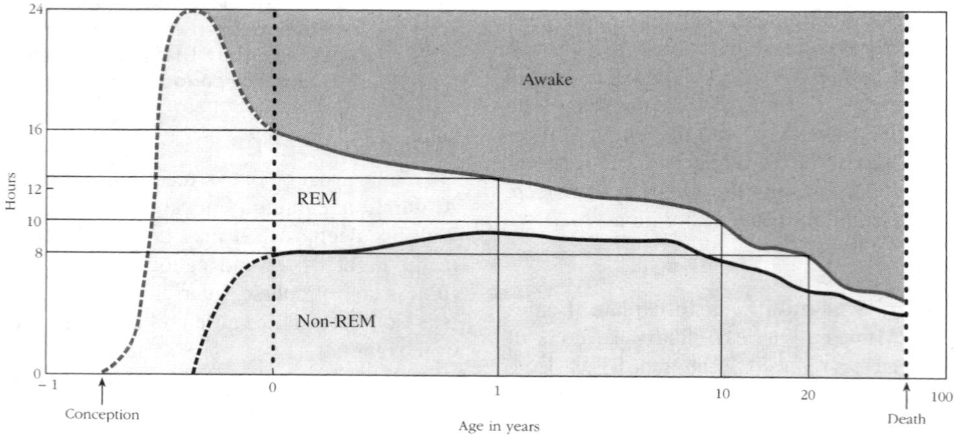

Fig. 25.4 Relative proportions of each 24-h day spent awake, in REM sleep and in NREM sleep over a lifetime. (From SLEEP, by J. Allan Hobson. Copyright © 1995 by J. Allan Hobson. Reprinted by permission of W.H. Freeman and Company.)

neonates may spend 18 out of 24 h asleep, young adults may sleep for 8 h, while elderly individuals might sleep for 6. Elderly people tend to sleep less, to spend more time in bed, to have comparatively less stage 4 and REM sleep and to have more shifts between sleep stages than younger people.

These changes have been attributed to age-related loss of neurones and progressive fragmentation of circadian rhythmicity. Elderly people have increased amounts of wakefulness after sleep onset. Ancoli-Israel et al (1989) found that 41% of a sample of patients in a nursing home woke frequently due to apnoeic disturbances and leg jerks (see Research Abstract 25.1). Webb & Swinburne (1971) attributed 38% of night-time awakenings among elderly people to pain and physical discomforts such as bladder distension and urinary urgency. Awareness of such problems should prompt nurses to alleviate discomfort as far as possible and to encourage regular bowel and bladder habits (see Ch. 35).

Elderly people sustain an absolute and a relative reduction in time spent in stage 4 sleep, which may even disappear in a quarter of those in their sixth decade of life. Concurrently, they have an increased total duration of stage 1 sleep and an increase in the number of shifts into stage 1. The total sleep time (TST) is either reduced or unchanged in elderly people as compared with younger groups, although the time in bed tends to increase. This appears to be because older people spend more time lying in bed at night without attempting to sleep or while unsuccessfully trying to sleep, and lying in bed resting or napping during the day. Obviously, these sleep patterns would be considered abnormal in a younger age group, but should cause no concern amongst the elderly; wards with large proportions of elderly patients should consequently adjust their routines in order to accommodate such sleep habits.

Zepelin et al (1984) studied subjects aged 18–71 years and found a correlation between a decline in the intensity of noise required to arouse individuals from sleep and increasing age. This reduction was present in all sleep stages but was greatest in stage 4. Since noise disturbs normal sleep stage progression and increases frequency of awakening, it may be that noise reduction in hospital is of particular importance in optimising the sleep of the elderly.

Research Abstract 25.1
Sleep fragmentation in patients from a nursing home

It is well known that many elderly people sleep poorly. Many try to lengthen their sleep by spending more time in bed. This then has a detrimental effect on sleep: increased time in bed makes sleep more fragmented and chronic bed rest interferes with the circadian sleep–wake rhythm.

The sleep of a group of institutionalised patients was monitored in order to compare it with that of similar elderly people in the community. Sleeping EEGs, respiratory movements and general body movements were recorded for 200 institutionalised elderly people. Recordings were made over two nights for 62% of the patients, and over one night for the remainder. These began at about 16.30 h and finished the following morning.

Findings showed a remarkable amount of sleep disturbance and related daytime sleepiness. The average duration of time in bed was 15.5 h, in which patients were asleep for about 8 h and awake for 7.5 h. In order to obtain that amount of sleep, the patients spent an extended amount of time in bed during the day, since they averaged no more than 39.5 min of sleep per hour in any hour of the night. Of the group studied, 50% woke up at least two or three times each hour, and 41% had frequent disturbances due to sleep apnoea.

Although nursing home residents slept on average only 1 h longer than elderly patients living independently, they had to spend substantially more time in bed to obtain the same amount of sleep.

Recommendations were made by the authors of the study to improve the sleep of elderly people by restricting time in bed, encouraging activity during the day and reducing daytime napping.

Ancoli-Israel S, Parker L, Sinaee R, Fell R L, Kripke D F 1989 Sleep fragmentation in patients from a nursing home. Journal of Gerontology 44(1): pp. 18–21

For an elderly person, the knowledge that degenerative changes in sleep patterns are commonly experienced and are therefore not necessarily pathological might be quite reassuring. Although some caution should be exercised lest treatable problems relating to sleep are overlooked, nurses have an important role to play in educating their patients about the predictable changes that occur in sleep habits with advancing age.

Gender
Research has shown that there are some interesting differences between the sexes in terms of their satisfaction with sleep. Men have more disturbances in sleep than women from early adulthood onward (Webb 1982), frequently due to nocturnal penile tumescence occurring during REM sleep. Wever (1984) found that women sleep significantly longer than men, although it is well recognised that women complain of problems with sleeping more than men do and that they consume far more sleep-inducing drugs. While this difference is evident from early adulthood, it becomes clearly marked in middle age.

Body weight
Weight gain is associated with an increased duration of sleep, while weight loss is associated with shorter sleep. This has been confirmed by several studies of anorexic individuals. As body weight falls, so does total sleep, which also becomes more broken and is interrupted by earlier waking. A small-scale study by Adam (1977) found a significant positive correlation between body weight and REM whereby the greater an individual's weight, the more REM sleep he has. A larger study of 36 subjects by the same author (Adam 1987) confirmed that both total and percentage REM correlated with body weight, although the reasons for this were not clear.

Exercise
The effect of exercise on normal sleep is not straightforward. Research studies have produced conflicting evidence: some have shown that exercise increases the duration of SWS, while some have found no effect and others a negative effect on sleep. A recent meta-analysis of 38 studies showed that exercise had different effects on different stages of sleep (Youngstedt et al 1997). The changes were somewhat modest, the greatest one being an increase of 10 min on SWS. However, most of this research has focused on good sleepers. A randomised controlled trial of depressed elderly people showed that exercise had a more profound effect on poor than on good sleepers (Singh et al 1997). It appears that, overall, exercise has a small sleep-promoting effect for many people, provided that it is not taken late in the evening.

Heredity
Finally, sleep quality and length appear to be influenced by genetic factors. This was demonstrated by Partinen et al (1983), who studied the sleep of 2238 monozygotic and 4545 dizygotic twin pairs. Familial clustering of narcolepsy (see p. 790) and idiopathic insomnia has also been observed. It may be worth noting a family history of sleep difficulties when assessing a patient, since it may not always be possible to remedy inherited sleep problems by means of nursing interventions.

Q **25.3** Discuss with your colleagues any changes in sleep patterns that have been experienced by elderly patients in your care. Consider which may be due to inevitable age-related physiological changes and whether any adverse consequences are likely.

COMMON SLEEP DISORDERS
Although the existence of sleep disorders has long been recognised, it is only in the past few decades that the seriousness of these has been acknowledged and a greater understanding of them has developed. Epidemiological studies in Europe and the USA have indicated that 14–40% of the population of Europe and the USA report difficulties in sleeping, with about 17% considering the problem to be serious. Insomnia is the most common complaint and may be defined as 'a subjective problem of insufficient or nonrestorative sleep despite an adequate opportunity to sleep' (Gillin & Byerley 1990). General practitioners have reported that one-third of the subjective complaints made by their patients are of difficulties in sleeping.

Researchers have investigated sleep difficulties for patients at home and in hospital. A large multinational study of about 8000 patients in the community who had attended sleep clinics showed that 25% suffered from various insomnias, while 39% suffered from excessive daytime sleepiness (Coleman 1983). Smirne et al (1983) investigated sleep disorders of patients in general hospital wards, asking them about their sleep prior to admission. Of 2518 people, 25% reported some kind of sleep disturbance. These figures indicate that sleep presents difficulties for about a quarter of the population, posing a challenge to nurses in all fields of care.

There are different ways of grouping sleep disorders, but the revised International Classification of Sleep Disorders (Diagnostic Classification Steering Committee 1990) is probably the most widely accepted system. It recognises four broad diagnostic classes which collectively subsume some 88 distinct sleep/wake irregularities. These four classes are the dyssomnias, parasomnias, sleep disorders associated with medical/psychiatric disorders and proposed sleep disorders. By far the most frequently reported and treated complaints, however, are the disorders of initiating or maintaining sleep, or the insomnias. Some of the more common factors which disturb sleep are discussed below.

Factors disrupting normal sleep
Anxiety and depression
Anxiety and depression frequently interfere with sleep, and each of these is relatively common among the general population. Most people suffer at some time from occupational stress, family tension, bereavement, divorce, illness and so on. Admission to hospital may be a major cause of anxiety, with all the accompanying worries with regard to illness, investigations, surgery and so forth.

The increased activity of the sympathetic nervous system due to anxiety results in an increase in plasma noradrenaline levels. This in turn results in sleep changes similar to those seen in normal elderly adults (less stage 4 and REM sleep, and more stage shifts and awakenings), who also undergo elevations of daytime and night-time plasma noradrenaline.

Insomnia due to depression has been associated with raised levels of monoamine oxidase, which catabolises the neurotransmitters noradrenaline and 5-HT, each of which is involved in sleep onset and maintenance. Depressed patients therefore tend to experience difficulty falling asleep, an increased number of awakenings during the night and early morning waking. Nursing staff should encourage depressed and anxious patients to discuss their feelings and, if possible, assist them to deal with underlying difficulties (see Ch. 17). Alerting medical staff to the apparent existence of anxiety and depression should ensure that the patient receives appropriate medical or psychological treatment.

Physical illness

Cardiac and pulmonary diseases often worsen during the night. The incidence of asthma attacks increases during the latter half of the night, while angina, cardiac dysrhythmias and nocturnal dyspnoea are all likely to worsen during sleep (see Chs 2 and 3).

Metabolic disorders such as Cushing's disease, Addison's disease and diabetes mellitus may disrupt normal sleep patterns. Hyperthyroidism may reduce sleep time and hypothyroidism increase it (see Ch. 5). Diseases which mobilise the immune system, whether viral, bacterial or fungal, may be associated with increased sleepiness (see Ch. 16).

Since many areas of the brain are implicated in sleep regulation, any pathology impinging on these sites can cause problems. A rise in intracranial pressure from whatever cause increases sleepiness, which in some cases leads to coma and death. Interference with the brain stem or hypothalamus may affect the onset and maintenance of sleep (see Chs 9 and 28).

Sleep-induced nocturnal myoclonus

This condition is characterised by repetitive twitching of the legs occurring at regular intervals of 20–60 s. These episodes may last from a few minutes to several hours, and either or both legs may twitch. This does not always disturb the individual, unless he is a light sleeper or the twitching is severe enough to arouse him from 'deep' sleep. Associated with this condition is restless legs syndrome, where an unpleasant, crawling sensation is experienced in the calves or thighs. Nocturnal myoclonus has been associated with the use of tricyclic antidepressant drugs (see Ch. 17) and chronic uraemia (see Ch. 8).

Narcolepsy

This disorder occurs in about 4 in 10 000 people and can be described as an imbalance between wakefulness, REM sleep and NREM sleep. Sleep frequently intrudes into wakefulness and this change in conscious state is often triggered by strong emotions such as anger or laughter. It is REM sleep which intrudes, either partially or totally, producing the possibility of four different symptoms, as follows:

- excessive daytime sleepiness
- cataplexy, when only the muscular paralysis of REM occurs: the sufferer may be awake but is paralysed
- sleep paralysis, a type of cataplexy which occurs at sleep onset (paralysis which occurs on waking from REM is benign)
- REM dreaming during wakefulness: hypnagogic hallucinations.

Pain

Sleep problems are commonly experienced by people who live with chronic pain. Such pain may be due to arthritis, cancer and low back injury and is often described as intractable. Some types of chronic pain, such as that from gastric ulcers or dyspepsia, have a circadian rhythm of increasing intensity at night. GPs tend to manage such pain pharmacologically, sometimes by aiming to relieve the cause, but more often providing symptomatic relief by means of analgesics. Sometimes the use of antidepressant drugs is successful, since some chronic pain syndromes can be associated with depression.

Nurses are closely involved in the delivery of pain relief in hospital because of their 24-h contact with patients. Jones et al (1979) studied intensive care patients and found that pain was ranked second to discomfort as contributing to sleep loss. Pain has been shown to be a major cause of sleep loss in the postoperative period (see Research Abstract 25.2) (Seers 1987, Southwell & Wistow 1995, Closs & Briggs 1997). Postoperative patients have strong views about sleep and pain (Closs 1991; see Box 25.1, p.788). If nurses are to be able to help patients cope with pain, they must perform an accurate nursing assessment of quality of sleep (see p. 793).

Research Abstract 25.2
A study of patients' and nurses' assessments of sleep in hospital

In this study, 454 hospital patients completed questionnaires about their sleep. This included patients on medical, surgical, care of elderly people and acute psychiatric wards. Questionnaires were also distributed to 129 nurses working on those wards. Patients and nurses then answered questions concerning the same nights in hospital.

Half of the patients reported that they could not sleep through the night and were consequently sleep-deprived. The main factors which patients reported as disturbing their sleep were discomfort (including beds and pillows and particularly the use of plastic covers on them), pain, noise, being too warm and worries. Half were dissatisfied with both settling and waking times.

There were differences in emphasis between patients' and nurses' views of environmental factors disruptive to sleep. More patients than nurses reported noise outwith the ward, emergencies, patients making a noise, nurses' shoes and nurses talking to one another. More nurses than patients reported treatments, commodes/bedpans, toilets flushing and nurses talking with patients. Nurses were more aware of noise generated by their own work and were largely unaware of the noise they caused by chatting to each other and from their shoes.

In view of the mismatch between nurses' and patients' perceptions, the authors emphasised the need to elicit patients' perspectives on care. However, the two groups were in agreement that patients did not get as much sleep as they needed. It was recommended that nurses, managers and others should take action to ensure that patients' sleep should be disrupted as little as possible. Nurses need to be aware when patients are awake, and take steps to ease pain, discomfort and worries. It is also important to minimise the wide range of possible disturbances during the night.

Southwell M T, Wistow G 1995 Sleep in hospitals at night: are patients' needs being met? Journal of Advanced Nursing 21 (6): 1101–1109

Diet

There has been much research into the effects of diet on sleep. Brezinova & Oswald (1972) investigated the reasons why Horlicks malted beverage seems to enhance sleep. A link was noted between habitual bedtime practices and sleep: those who normally ate little or nothing before bedtime had no improvement in sleep after having Horlicks, while those who usually did have a bedtime drink slept better after Horlicks. Hot milky drinks are provided in many hospitals in the late evening, but these may not suit everyone. It should be remembered that many people take an alcoholic 'nightcap' at home, and if they are normally heavy drinkers they will suffer from withdrawal symptoms in hospital if they are not permitted to drink alcohol.

Withdrawal from alcohol will result in disturbed sleep, as will withdrawal of hypnotics (sleep-inducing drugs). It should be noted that alcohol is not a good hypnotic, since although it accelerates

Box 25.1 What patients say about postoperative sleep and pain (From Closs 1991)

Effects of tiredness on postoperative pain
- 'The pain is more nagging and it's harder to put up with if you're tired.'
- 'If you're tired, the pain's more draining, more severe, a down-puller. It can actually make you feel depressed.'
- 'If you're tired and in pain, you want to give up quicker. You could have shot me yesterday for all I cared.'

Effects of sleep on pain intensity
- 'If you've slept well, the pain isn't as bad a blow when you waken. If you don't sleep you wonder when it'll ever end. It's a vicious circle.'
- 'If you're tired you're narky, if you're narky it hurts worse.'
- 'Sleep makes you relax and takes away some of the pain.'

Effects of sleep on coping with pain
- 'It's essential — you can't cope with anything unless you've slept, especially pain.'
- 'You're not so well able to cope if you're tired, you have a good attitude if you're rested.'
- 'It's impossible to cope properly if you haven't slept well.'

Effects of sleep on recovery
- 'Sleep is the best healer in the world. You know it's going to take longer to get better if you can't get your sleep.'
- 'You've got to get a good sleep before you get anything else. You feel fresh and don't get crabby, you can deal with the pain and everything else and it speeds up your recovery.'
- 'Sleep is a great healer — that's why I don't understand why they wake you up early in the morning. I think, why, what is it for? Certainly not for the patient. It makes you agitated. It's all done to their rules.'

sleep onset it disturbs sleep patterns later on in the night (Williams et al 1983) and can cause early waking due to a full bladder. Drinks such as tea, coffee and cola contain caffeine and therefore act as stimulants, disturbing normal sleep patterns. Karacan et al (1976) showed that coffee disturbed sleep even in those who felt unaffected by it.

The biochemical effects of diet on sleep are unclear, but avoiding stimulants and adhering to routines appear to enhance sleep. Although research in this area has so far been inconclusive, community nurses might be able to help poor sleepers simply by giving them dietary advice, while hospital nurses should allow patients to eat or drink as they would at home prior to bedtime, as far as that is feasible.

Drugs

There are many drugs which affect sleep, hypnotics being perhaps the best known. In addition, there are many others which have side-effects on sleep, including antidepressants, antihistamines, anticonvulsants and alcohol. L-dopa and beta-blockers may produce vivid dreams and nightmares, while diuretics increase urine production leading to bladder distension and therefore nocturia. Other drugs such as amphetamines and caffeine stimulate the CNS, delaying sleep onset and reducing total sleep time.

Sleep position and snoring

Sleep positions have been associated with objective and subjective sleep quality. Poor sleepers appear to spend a greater proportion of their time on their backs with their heads straight and to change position more frequently than better sleepers (Koninck et al 1983). Snoring and sleep apnoea have been associated with subjects who sleep flat on their backs. Since these symptoms are undesirable for the sleeper himself, and snoring may disturb others sleeping within earshot, nurses could perhaps encourage and assist poor sleepers to adopt alternative positions for sleeping. Many snorers may have problems such as sleep apnoea which are amenable to some kinds of treatment, as discussed later.

Often married couples, of whom one is an intractable snorer, may find this to be a real problem. It is by no means unknown for a chronically sleep-deprived spouse to request, at best, to sleep in a different room, or at worst to begin divorce proceedings. As Anthony Burgess said: 'Laugh and the world laughs with you, snore and you sleep alone'. There are devices available which dilate the nostrils during sleep, and some that are worn like wristwatches which are noise-sensitive and deliver mild electric shocks when snoring begins. The efficacy of such devices is variable.

Respiration

Hypoventilation and breathing irregularities are common during normal sleep but may sometimes be clinically important. Normal changes include the hypoxaemia and hypercapnia due to the slight reduction in metabolic rate which occurs during NREM sleep; in REM sleep irregular breathing is the norm.

Patients at home who have respiratory difficulties might benefit from advice regarding sleep position and the use of pillows to prop themselves up in order to maximise lung expansion. In hospital, nurses should ensure that any patients with respiratory difficulties (such as postoperative patients or those with respiratory tract infections) receive adequate support and assistance, particularly regarding oxygen administration, posture, deep breathing and coughing.

Sleep apnoea syndrome

This problem was first recognised about 25 years ago. The literal meaning of sleep apnoea is cessation of breathing during sleep. Often these episodes are repetitive and each may last up to a minute or even longer. Such apnoeas frequently cause the sleeper to wake, in some cases many times during the night. The main symptom resulting from this disorder is usually daytime sleepiness, although some sufferers complain of insomnia.

There are two main types of sleep apnoea: central sleep apnoea is caused by impaired neurological control of breathing, so that the intercostal muscles fail to contract; obstructive apnoea is the result of obstruction of the airway, e.g. by large tonsils, a large or oedematous soft palate, fat deposits around the airway, retrognathia or micrognathia (see Ch. 15). The cause may be treated if the problem becomes severe. Obesity is common among these patients, in which case weight loss is usually the first approach to relieving the problem. For the more severe cases, continuous positive airway pressure (CPAP) during the night may help, while corrective surgery may be required for others.

Temperature

Even slight changes in ambient (room) temperature may affect an individual's normal sleep–wake cycle. Kendel & Schmidt-Kessen (1973) pointed out that unclothed and uncovered subjects awoke from cold at 26°C and below. Total sleep deprivation has been shown to decrease the mean daily body temperature and to increase subjective feelings of cold (Horne 1985). Fever is associated with a greater number of awakenings, increased total waking time and reduced amounts of SWS and REM sleep. Elevated ambient temperature produces similar results. The duration of the REM phase is shortened in artificially induced fever as well as at high ambient temperature. Zulley (1980) found that the higher the body temperature at sleep onset, the longer the duration of sleep, while REM sleep was negatively correlated with body temperature. These findings suggest that active management of pyrexial patients, perhaps by giving antipyretic drugs such as aspirin (or paracetamol for children), might improve their sleep.

Room temperature should be carefully monitored on general wards so that it may be maintained at a comfortable level, and patients should be encouraged to request more or fewer bedclothes as required. Elderly people are particularly vulnerable, especially at home, since their ability to perceive temperature changes is often diminished. Community nurses are well placed to identify at least some of those individuals susceptible to hypothermia, and have a useful role in advising them about adequate clothing, bedding and heating in their home (see Ch. 22, p. 733).

Noise

Noise can disturb sleep under all sorts of circumstances. In the home, mothers may wake at the slightest whimper from their children, while others successfully adjust to the difficulties of living under noisy flight paths near airports. Although noise is often detrimental to sleep, there are occasions when the opposite is the case. People often become used to noise at night. For example, those who live near a busy main road may have great difficulty sleeping in a quiet environment. Similarly, town dwellers might have problems sleeping for the first few nights of a quiet country holiday, or a patient who has a long stay in a noisy hospital ward might have some difficulty readjusting to the quietness of his home environment. Individuals become habituated to the normal circumstances surrounding their sleep.

In hospital, noise poses a considerable problem, particularly in acute areas (Soutar & Wilson 1986, Aaron et al 1996). Patients' sleep may be disturbed by a wide variety of sounds, including noise made by other patients, nurses talking, footsteps, telephones, traffic, equipment alarms, squeaky doors, trolleys, rattling windows and many others (Closs 1988a, Southwell & Wistow 1995, Simpson et al 1996). If possible, nurses should acquaint their more long-term patients with the unfamiliar sounds on the ward. This may help them to become accustomed to these noises and develop the ability to sleep through them. While some noise is unavoidable at night, careful maintenance of equipment and precautions such as wearing soft-soled shoes can considerably improve the night-time hospital environment (see Research Abstract 25.2).

Q **25.4** Mr B is a 47-year-old man who had an appendicectomy 3 days ago. His physical recovery has been straightforward, but he is feeling very tired and has been finding it difficult to sleep at night. Consequently, he has been reluctant to get up and walk and has been taking short naps throughout the day. (A)

Q **25.4** *(cont'd)*
Construct a care plan, giving possible reasons for Mr B's inadequate sleep, suggesting possible nursing interventions and stating the expected outcome of these.

Parasomnias

Sleepwalking

This behaviour, when it occurs, commences during SWS, although the somnambulist appears to be in a part-sleeping, part-waking state. It can be very dangerous: sufferers have been known to walk out of windows and to attack family members. During an episode of sleepwalking, the individual is usually uncommunicative and returns to bed spontaneously, rarely remembering the event the next morning. Sleepwalking is difficult to treat, so it is advisable to take precautions such as locking windows at night.

Night terrors and nightmares

Night terrors also arise during SWS and occur mostly in children. The sufferer often screams and shows signs of panic, such as a dramatic rise in heart rate, respiratory distress and sweating. He may be very difficult to arouse, but usually calms down within a few minutes, usually without waking up. Most people remember nothing about the incident. Nightmares occur during REM sleep and are often remembered very vividly on waking.

METHODS OF ASSESSING SLEEP

While sleep assessment in clinical settings has been attempted by many researchers, the methods used have not always been suitable for general use by nurses (Closs 1988b). In general, these methods of assessing sleep can be classified into groups: those which rely on patients' subjective reports of their sleep and those which obtain objective measurements of either physiological events which coincide with sleep or psychological attributes reflecting the effects of sleep (see Box 25.2).

Many of the objective methods of sleep assessment available involve the use of expensive and sometimes unwieldy equipment. In most cases, nurses would have neither access to such equipment nor the expertise to use it. In addition, although these methods may be suitable for relatively healthy, stress-free individuals, most hospital patients would probably find such monitoring anxiety-provoking, restrictive or uncomfortable.

Box 25.2 Approaches to the assessment of sleep (Closs 1988b)

Subjective assessment of sleep
- Visual analogue scales
- Subjective rating scales
- Questionnaires
- Interviews
- Daily sleep charting (sleep diary)

Objective assessment of associated physiological/psychological events
- Polysomnography
- Observation of sleeper
- Arousal thresholds
- Body movements
- Vigilance and sleepiness
- Electrodermal activity

Nursing assessment of sleep

The assessment of sleep is an important part of the general assessment of patients. While it is appropriate for researchers and clinicians in other disciplines to use sophisticated monitoring equipment, nurses must rely on their communication skills, by both questioning patients carefully and listening to what they tell them. Although people are unable to give accurate reports of the actual time it takes them to fall asleep, or how long they lie awake in the small hours, they can give reliable accounts of changes in their sleep patterns. For example, people suffering from insomnia will generally overestimate how long it takes them to fall asleep, and underestimate how long they spend asleep, but will nonetheless give realistic reports of changes in their sleep habits.

Although in hospital it is possible for nurses to observe patients during the night, this is a notoriously inaccurate way to determine the quality or quantity of someone's sleep (Aurell & Elmqvist 1985). In a home care setting, patients' reports of sleep are all the nurse has to go on. Consequently, the ability of nurses to make useful assessments of sleep depends on the acquisition of good communication skills. As Morgan (1987) points out, the only realistic method of assessing the quality of patients' sleep is to ask them about it. Not all patients, of course, will be able to give their own account. In such cases, information might be gained from non-verbal clues, the descriptions provided by relatives and carers, and from nursing and medical records.

Communication skills in the assessment of sleep

Communication between patients and nurses in hospital wards has been studied by researchers including Macleod Clark (1983) and Hewison (1995). They found that patients' queries were frequently blocked by nurses, that communications were often discouraged and that patients were typically asked questions which were closed or leading. If patients are to communicate their concerns, they must be given clear opportunities and encouragement to do so. This applies to community nurses as much as to hospital nurses, although the former are more likely to identify chronic rather than acute problems. Encouraging patients, where possible, to talk about themselves, their feelings and their needs is vital. The use of open-ended questions and prompts can facilitate disclosure. For example, a closed question such as 'Did you sleep well last night?' is more likely to produce a polite and possibly meaningless 'Yes, thank you' than asking, 'How did you sleep last night? Did you have any problems?'. The latter query provides a clearer invitation for the patient to inform the nurse of any difficulties. If the patient appears reluctant to complain, it could be helpful to follow up such a question with gentle prompting.

Body language is also important here: patients are less likely to be forthcoming if the nurse speaks from an uncomfortable distance, looking as if she is about to leave for some more important task. Planned nurse–patient interactions can provide ample opportunities for discussion and nursing assessment. In addition to general questioning about sleep, nurses might ask some specific questions. These could include details such as time of settling down to sleep, time of morning waking, duration of sleep, night-time disturbances, diet, medication, pain, anxieties and so on. The patient's disclosures should be recorded in nursing notes so that each nurse participating in his care is aware of his needs.

Once an assessment of the patient's sleep has been made, nursing care relevant to sleeping habits may be planned. Nurses can help by providing information about sleep that enables patients to have realistic expectations. In addition, they can give basic guidelines for improving sleep through attention to sleep hygiene, i.e. behaviour and attitudes conducive to healthy sleep patterns. Among the factors concerned are attitudes towards sleep, the sleep environment, attention to diet, sleep scheduling, pre-sleep activities and daytime behaviours. If the patient requires specialised help, the nurse should alert the appropriate professionals. In the community, this may be the GP or clinical psychologist, while in hospital it is usually the house officer.

HELPING PATIENTS TO SLEEP

The points listed in Box 25.3 should be borne in mind by nurses as they assist patients to cultivate healthy sleep patterns.

Q

25.5 A middle-aged woman complains to a community nurse that she is having great difficulty in getting to sleep at night. She says that, as a result, she needs to take naps during the day. In addition, she has found no help from taking drinking chocolate immediately before going to bed. What advice could the nurse give?

PHARMACOLOGICAL TREATMENTS FOR INSOMNIA

Hypnotic drugs

The major treatments available for insomnia are pharmacological. The majority of hypnotics which are currently prescribed belong to the benzodiazepine group, and include temazepam, triazolam, nitrazepam and others. These provide temporary symptomatic relief and are not a cure. The sleep produced by these drugs does not resemble natural sleep: the duration of stage 2 sleep is increased at the expense of REM sleep and SWS. However, even though the structure of sleep is changed by these drugs, most physiological processes associated with SWS continue as usual. It is difficult, therefore, to comment on the difference between the quality of sleep induced by hypnotics and that of normal sleep.

The effects of benzodiazepines vary, particularly with regard to their duration of action. Nitrazepam has quite long-lasting effects and is used less commonly than other forms, particularly among the elderly, in whom the drug's 'hangover effect' may cause loss of balance and result in falls. Triazolam has effects of very short duration, while those of temazepam last for a moderate period.

There are other types of hypnotic now coming onto the market. Cyclopyrrolones such as zopiclone and the newer imidazopyridines such as zolpidem are both fast-acting with a short half-life (Reite et al 1997). They appear to be as effective as the benzodiazepines, but with fewer side-effects. Short-acting hypnotics tend to be favoured, since they are less likely to produce hangover effects during the day.

While these drugs are initially effective in inducing sleep, their regular use produces 'tolerance'. As time goes on, the body requires increasingly large doses of the drug to achieve the same effect. The effectiveness of most hypnotic drugs is diminished after 3–14 days of use.

Although hypnotics can provide short-term improvement in sleep, long-term use can result in more problems with sleep. After an initial improvement, hypnotics may actually cause tiredness because of the reduction in SWS and REM sleep. When hypnotics are withdrawn, the patient may suffer from rebound insomnia. This involves extreme feelings of edginess, greater difficulty in falling asleep and more intense dreams and nightmares. These symptoms gradually diminish over time. In spite of these drawbacks, the short-term use of hypnotics can be highly beneficial.

Box 25.3 Basic information and advice for poor sleepers

- Patients' expectations of sleep should be realistic. Many people think that there is something wrong with their sleep if they do not get 8 h every night. Such incorrect assumptions may in themselves cause anxiety and sleep disturbance. The great individual differences in sleep requirements and the normal effects of ageing should be clearly explained in order to instil realistic attitudes towards sleep.
- Most people experience short episodes of poor sleep for which no particular treatment is needed. There is no evidence that transient insomnia has a detrimental effect on health. Chronic insomnia (lasting for at least 3 weeks) may require detailed assessment and treatment. If it is clear that the insomnia is transient, nurses may be able to reassure their patients on this point, and in so doing help them to overcome insomnia by reducing their anxiety about sleep loss.
- People suffering from insomnia tend to stay in bed even when they are unable to sleep. This interferes with their sleep by reducing the psychological association between bed and sleep. They should, if possible, avoid going to bed until they are sleepy, and if they cannot sleep, they should then get up and do something else. For example, they might read, watch television or engage in any other activity they enjoy, preferably something relaxing.
- It helps to establish a regular time of waking up in the morning, even if the previous night's sleep was unsatisfactory. This strengthens the circadian rhythm and should be adhered to at weekends as well as weekdays. A reliable alarm clock or perhaps the assistance of a relative or friend can help to ensure a regular waking time.
- Patients who have difficulty sleeping at night may reduce their night-time sleep drive if they take daytime naps. Avoiding daytime naps also helps to reinforce circadian rhythmicity. Naps may be avoided by planning activities that can coincide with the times that naps are desired, so that there is always an alternative to napping available. If a post-lunch nap is to be missed, for example, the individual could plan to walk the dog or fetch a newspaper at that particular time.
- Poor sleepers should try to reserve the evening hours for relaxation and leisure activities. They should avoid strenuous mental or physical exertion immediately preceding bedtime, with the exception of sexual activity, which may increase relaxation and encourage sleep. The development of calming pre-sleep rituals such as reading can help patients drift off to sleep.
- Hunger and thirst can disturb sleep. If this is a problem, a light snack should be taken at bedtime. This may be anything, provided that it does not contain stimulants. A milky drink and a biscuit or a piece of fruit may be appropriate. There is no evidence to suggest that eating cheese before going to sleep has any adverse effects. Some may wish to keep a drink beside the bed in case they wake up during the night feeling thirsty.
- Many poor sleepers are sensitive to the stimulants found in some foods. It takes at least 8 h to metabolise caffeine, so caffeine-containing beverages and foods should be omitted from the diet after midday. This includes tea, coffee, cola and chocolate. It is possible to buy caffeine-free tea and cola as well as coffee, for those who wish to take such drinks in the evening.
- Sleep is disturbed by the use of nicotine as well as by withdrawal from nicotine. Thus the prevention of disturbed sleep is yet another good reason for not smoking. The role of the nurse as health educator is important here since many people are unaware of any connection between smoking and poor sleep.
- Although small amounts of alcohol hasten sleep onset, larger amounts disturb sleep later on in the night. The detrimental effects of alcohol on sleep can therefore outweigh any benefits. Again, the nurse may have an opportunity to provide health education in this regard, as it is a common misconception that alcohol enhances sleep.
- The sleep-disturbing side-effects of drugs such as antihypertensives and anti-asthmatics should be understood. It might be that the patient has not linked his sleep difficulty with his medication. An explanation of such a connection could provide valuable reassurance. If disturbed sleep is accounted for in a rational manner in this way, the patient may perceive it as less of a problem.
- Sudden noises are more disturbing than constant ones. If occasional loud noise is inevitable, using earplugs or masking the disturbing noise with a monotonous background sound such as that made by an electric fan can help.
- Nurses should endeavour to create conditions favourable for sleep. Most people sleep best in a quiet, darkened room on a firm mattress which is large enough to allow movement and stretching. Individual preferences, however, should be respected as far as is feasible.
- Being too hot or too cold can disturb sleep. Ambient temperature should be comfortable, and the amount and type of bedding adjusted to suit the individual.

For example, an anxious patient due to have surgery may greatly benefit from the limited use of hypnotics over, perhaps, 3 or 4 perioperative nights.

Herbal remedies

Although several herbs are claimed to have sleep-inducing properties, valerian is the only one whose use has been scientifically evaluated. Valerian taken orally has been shown to reduce significantly the time taken to fall asleep (Lindahl & Lindwall 1989). However, other unproven herbal remedies may be effective, not least by virtue of a placebo effect.

PSYCHOLOGICAL AND BEHAVIOURAL TREATMENTS FOR INSOMNIA

While pharmacological treatments of insomnia are palliative, psychological treatments aim to deal with the cause of the sleeplessness. In some cases, insomnia may be attributed to physiological or psychological overactivity. Stress is a common cause of sleep disturbance and can be dealt with by a variety of techniques (see Ch. 17, pp. 624–628). However, some individuals who suffer from insomnia are constitutionally poor sleepers who are unlikely to respond to any treatment. These people usually have difficulties sleeping throughout their lives, and the process of ageing is likely to further reduce the quality of their sleep. For those whose sleeplessness is associated with physiological or psychological hyperactivity, many non-pharmacological methods of treating insomnia have been attempted, with varying degrees of success. Four of the most widely known — relaxation therapy, paradoxical intention, associative learning technique and cognitive therapy — are discussed below. The choice of strategy depends on the cause of the sleeplessness, individual temperament and personal preference.

Relaxation techniques

Emotional problems such as anxiety can be modified using various types of relaxation therapy, which aims to reduce physical and mental tension. Autogenic training teaches people to concentrate on sensations of warmth and heaviness in their limbs by repeated suggestion. Progressive muscular relaxation achieves a similar effect by the alternate tensing and relaxing of a series of muscles. These methods have been successful in helping people to fall asleep and in increasing their satisfaction with sleep (Borkovec 1982, Lacks 1987).

Paradoxical intention

Paradoxical intention has been used with success in the treatment of patients who are particularly anxious about their difficulty in falling asleep. This anxiety produces the opposite of the desired effect, making patients too tense to fall asleep. When such individuals are instructed to stay awake all night, their anxiety about falling asleep is reduced, paradoxically allowing them to relax and fall asleep (Ascher 1980).

Associative learning technique

This is a useful technique where the bed and the bedroom have become associated in the patient's mind with sleeplessness. For such people, going to bed is an aversive stimulus which produces an aroused state. Bootzin (1972) devised a method of avoiding all behaviours in the bedroom not associated with sleep, such as reading, eating, watching television or just lying awake. Individuals are instructed to go to bed only when they are sleepy and to get up if they lie awake for more than 10 min. Eventually this re-establishes the psychological association between bed and sleep.

Cognitive therapy

Cognitive refocusing can be used by an individual who is plagued by intrusive and repetitive thoughts which keep him awake. Usually these are problems and worries which the individual can learn to control, first by recognising that he cannot solve his problems by turning them over and over in his mind at night, and second, by learning to suppress the troubling thoughts, often by concentrating on alternative, benign thoughts. Other techniques employed by cognitive therapists include meditation and guided imagery (see Ch. 17).

For the most part, therapies for helping individuals to overcome sleeping difficulties are currently provided by clinical psychologists. While in some areas of the UK it may be possible for community patients to be referred to such specialists for help, clinical psychologists are a rare commodity in most general hospitals. If nurses could learn some of the simpler techniques (such as relaxation therapy) they might well be able to make a significant contribution to helping patients to sleep. Health visitors are already becoming involved in successful schemes designed to help adults with insomnia (Eaton 1996) and others may also develop such skills. Since sleep is such a fundamental activity of life and is essential to good health, this extension of the nurse's role would seem perfectly legitimate.

CONCLUSION

Sleep is a complex and universal behaviour which is prone to disruption by numerous internal and external influences. Since everyone needs sleep, every nurse needs to understand it and to know how patients may be helped when problems arise. This chapter has offered basic information on the structure and function of sleep, the importance of the sleep–wake cycle, normal and abnormal causes of sleep disturbance and strategies for treating patients' problems. The most crucial point to remember is that everyone is different: behaviours, attitudes and problems are highly individual. Consequently, nursing care both in hospital and in the patient's home should include careful assessment of sleep, since many difficulties can be overcome by simple changes in lifestyle and by adjustments to the individual's expectations of sleep. Where more serious problems occur, help from other health care professionals may be needed.

REFERENCES

Aaron J N, Carlisle C C, Carskadon M A, Meyer T J, Hill N S, Millman R P 1996 Environmental noise as a cause of sleep disruption in an intermediate respiratory care unit. Sleep 19(9): 707–710

Adam K 1977 Body weight correlates with REM sleep. British Medical Journal 1: 813–814

Adam K 1987 Total and percentage REM sleep correlate with body weight in 36 middle-aged people. Sleep 10(1): 69–77

Adam K, Oswald I 1983 Protein synthesis, bodily renewal and the sleep-wake cycle. Clinical Science 65(6): 561–567

Ancoli-Israel S 1997 Sleep problems in older adults: putting myths to bed. Geriatrics 52(1): 20–30

Ancoli-Israel S, Parker L, Sinaee R, Fell R L, Kripke D F 1989 Sleep fragmentation in patients from a nursing home. Journal of Gerontology 44(1): pp18–21

Ascher L M 1980 Paradoxical intention. In: Goldstein A, Foa E B (eds) Handbook of behavioural interventions: a clinical guide. Wiley, New York, pp 266–321

Aurell J, Elmqvist D 1985 Sleep in the surgical intensive care unit: continuous polygraphic recording of sleep in nine patients receiving post-operative care. British Medical Journal 290: 1029–1032

Bootzin R R 1972 Stimulus control treatment for insomnia (summary). Proceedings of the 80th annual convention of the American Psychological Association 7: 395–396

Borkovec T D 1982 Insomnia. Journal of Consulting and Clinical Psychology 50(6): 880–895

Brezinova V, Oswald I 1972 Sleep after a night-time beverage. British Medical Journal 2(5811): 431–433

Closs S J 1988a A nursing study of sleep on surgical wards. Nursing Research Unit report. Department of Nursing Studies, University of Edinburgh

Closs S J 1988b Assessment of sleep in hospital patients: a review of methods. Journal of Advanced Nursing 13(4): 501–510

Closs S J 1991 A nursing study of patients' night-time sleep, pain and analgesic provision following abdominal surgery. Nursing Research Unit report. Department of Nursing Studies, University of Edinburgh

Closs S J, Briggs M 1997 Evaluation of an intervention to improve post-operative sleep and pain control in orthopaedic patients at night. Report for the NHS Executive Northern & Yorkshire, University of Hull, Hull

Coleman R M 1983 Diagnosis, treatment and follow-up of about 8000 sleep/wake disorder patients. In: Guilleminault C, Lugaresi E (eds) Sleep/wake disorders: natural history, epidemiology and long term evolution. Raven Press, New York, pp 87–97

Cronin-Stubbs D 1996 Delirium intervention research in acute care settings. In: Annual Review of Nursing Research, vol. 14. Springer, New York, ch 3

Diagnostic Classification Steering Committee (Thorpy M J, Chairman) 1990 The international classification of sleep disorders: diagnostic and coding manual. American Sleep Disorders Association, Rochester, MN

Eaton L 1996 Health visitors tackle adult insomnia. Health Visitor 69(8): 312

Floyd J A 1984 Interaction between personal sleep–wake rhythms and psychiatric hospital rest–activity schedule. Nursing Research 33(5): 255–259

Gillin J C, Byerley W F 1990 The diagnosis and management of insomnia. The New England Journal of Medicine 322(4): 239–248

Hartmann E L 1973 The functions of sleep. Yale University Press, New Haven

Hewison A 1995 Nurses' power in interactions with patients. Journal of Advanced Nursing 21(1): 75–82

Hobson J A 1995 Sleep. Scientific American Library, New York

Horne J A 1983 Human sleep and tissue restitution: some qualifications and doubts. Clinical Science 65: 569–578

Horne J A 1985 Sleep function with particular reference to sleep deprivation. Annals of Clinical Research 17(5): 199–208

Horne J A 1988 Why we sleep: the functions of sleep in humans and other mammals. Oxford University Press, Oxford

Horne J A, Ostberg O 1976 A self-assessment questionnaire to determine morningness – eveningness in human circadian rhythm. International Journal of Chronobiology 4: 97–110

Johns M W 1984 Normal sleep. In: Priest R G (ed) Sleep: an international monograph. Update Books, ch 1

Jones J, Hoggart B, Withey J, Donaghue K, Ellis B W 1979 What the patients say: a study of reactions to an intensive care unit. Intensive Care Medicine 5: 89–92

Karacan I, Thornby J I, Anch M, Booth G H, Williams R L, Sallis P J 1976 Dose-related sleep disturbances induced by coffee and caffeine. Clinical Pharmacology and Therapeutics 20: 682–689

Kendel J, Schmidt-Kessen W 1973 The influence of room temperature on night-time sleep in man (polygraphic night-sleep recordings in the climate chamber). In: Koella W P, Levin P (eds) Sleep. Karger, Basel, pp 423–425

Koninck J, De Gagnon P, Lallier S 1983 Sleep positions in the young adult and their relationship with the subjective quality of sleep. Sleep 6(1): 52–59

Lacks P 1987 Behavioural treatment for persistent insomnia. Pergamon Press, New York

Lindahl O, Lindwall L 1989 Double blind study of a valerian preparation. Pharmacology Biochemistry and Behavior 32(4): 1065–1066

MacLeod Clark J 1983 Nurse–patient communication in surgical wards. In: Wilson-Barnett J (ed) Nursing research: ten studies in patient care. Wiley, Chichester

Moorcroft W H 1995 The function of sleep. Comments on the symposium and an attempt at synthesis. Behavioural Brain Research 69(1–2): 207–210

Morgan K 1987 Sleep and ageing. Croom Helm, London

Partinen M, Kaprio J, Koskenvuo M, Langinvainio H 1983 Genetic and environmental determination of human sleep. Sleep 6(3): 179–185

Pilcher J J, Huffcutt A I 1996 Effects of sleep deprivation on performance: a meta-analysis. Sleep 19(4): 318–326

Rechtschaffen A, Bergmann B M 1995 Sleep deprivation in the rat by the disk-over-water method. Behavioural Brain Research 69(1–2): 55–63

Rechtschaffen A, Kales A 1968 A manual of standardised terminology, techniques and scoring system for sleep stages of human subjects. US Dept. of Health, Education and Welfare, Bethesda, MD

Reite M, Ruddy J, Nagel K 1997 Evaluation and management of sleep disorders. American Psychiatric Press, Washington

Seers C J 1987 Pain, anxiety and recovery in patients undergoing surgery. Unpublished PhD thesis, University of London

Shapiro C M, Flanigan M J 1993 ABC of sleep disorders. Function of sleep. British Medical Journal 306: 383–385

Simpson T, Lee E R, Cameron C 1996 Relationships among sleep dimensions and factors that impair sleep after cardiac surgery. Research in Nursing & Health 19(3): 213–223

Singh N A, Clements K M, Fiatarone M A 1997 A randomized controlled trial of the effect of exercise on sleep. Sleep 20(2): 95–101

Smirne S, Franceschi M, Zamproni P, Crippa D, Ferini-Strambi L 1983 Prevalence of sleep disorders in an unselected in-patient population. In: Guilleminault C, Lugaresi E (eds) Sleep/wake disorders: natural history, epidemiology, and long term evolution. Raven Press, New York, pp 61–71

Soutar R L, Wilson J A 1986 Does hospital noise disturb patients? British Medical Journal 292: 305

Southwell M T, Wistow G 1995 Sleep in hospitals at night: are patients' needs being met? Journal of Advanced Nursing 21(6): 1101–1109

Webb W B 1982 Sleep in older persons: sleep structures of 50 to 60 year old men and women. Journal of Gerontology 37: 581–586

Webb W B, Swinburne H 1971 An observational study of sleep of the aged. Perception and Motor Skills 32: 895–898

Weitzman E D, Kripke D F, Golmacher D, McGregor P, Nogire C 1970 Acute reversal of the sleep–waking cycle in man. Archives of Neurology 22: 483–489

Wever R A 1984 Properties of human sleep–wake cycles: parameters of internally synchronised free-running rhythms. Sleep 7: 27–51

Williams D L, McLean A W, Cairns J 1983 Dose-response effects of ethanol on the sleep of young women. Journal of Studies on Alcohol 44: 515–523

Youngstedt S D, O'Connor P J, Dishman R K 1997 The effects of acute exercise on sleep: a quantitative synthesis. Sleep 20(3): 203–214

Zepelin H, McDonald C S, Zammit G K 1984 Effects of age on auditory awakening thresholds. Journal of Gerontology 39(3): 294–300

Zulley J 1980 Timing of sleep within the circadian temperature cycle. Sleep Research 9: 282

NURSING PATIENTS WITH SPECIAL NEEDS

SECTION 3

SECTION CONTENTS

THE PATIENT FACING SURGERY

26

Sheila E. Rodgers

INTRODUCTION

This chapter aims to give an overview of the nursing care required by patients facing surgery. Discussion will include not only those interventions relevant to the period of hospitalisation, but also the support needed by patients during the diagnostic process and during their eventual rehabilitation at home. Patients undergo many types of surgery for a wide range of reasons, but the principles of care can to a large degree be generalised with reference to particular types of procedure. It should be stressed, however, that individuals often react quite differently to a given disease or treatment. What one person may regard as a 'minor' procedure may cause extreme anxiety in another. Nursing staff must be sensitive to each patient's individuality and try to appreciate the significance of the experience of surgery from the patient's own perspective.

Q **26.1** Think of an intervention or form of treatment you have experienced, such as removal of wisdom teeth, a cervical smear or suturing of a cut. What sort of fears did you have, however irrational they might seem now?

No attempt has been made to apply any one model of nursing throughout the chapter, although it might be suggested that appropriate models can be selected according to the nature of the patient's illness and the care required. The present chapter does, however, highlight advances in care that are made possible by the use of primary nursing (see Manthey 1981, Allsopp 1991, Ersser & Tutton 1991) and through care pathways (see Wigfield & Boon 1996).

Changing patterns of surgical care

Advances in surgical technology have had a dramatic effect in recent years on the experience of patients undergoing surgery. Interventions now available range from laser treatment to shatter (ablate) renal stones (lithotripsy) to stapling and suturing of the bowel to restore continuity. Laparoscopic angiographic catheterisation, endoscopy and laser techniques can now incorporate treatment often at the time of investigation, and as treatments in their own right are replacing many standard invasive surgical techniques (Frost 1993). Arthroscopy is now the method of choice in managing tears of the menisci in the knee. Many gynaecological procedures can be carried out laparoscopically, e.g. excision of ovarian cysts and tubal ligation.

There have been recent developments in laparoscopic cholecystectomy, which for some patients can now be carried out as day surgery (Prasad & Foley 1996). The procedure takes only 40–90 minutes in experienced hands, leaving the patient with very little scarring or pain, and requiring only a 1- or 2-day stay in hospital (McGinn et al 1995). Many patients return to work within 1 week (Dubois et al 1990). In comparison, the standard treatment for gallstones — cholecystectomy — involves scarring, a 7–10 day stay in hospital and 6 weeks off work (Cheslyn-Curtis & Russell 1991).

Day surgery has become possible for many general surgical patients. In Scotland, the proportion of elective patients treated as day cases rose from 38% in 1991–92 to 52% in 1994–95 (Scottish Office Department of Health 1996). In 1995, throughout the UK, some 20% of all cases were day-case patients (Office of Health Economics 1995). The trend seems set to continue and will lead to a further decrease in morbidity, shorter length of stay and increased patient turnover. This in turn has increased the responsibilities of informal carers and community nurses.

There are increasing numbers of elderly people in our society. It is estimated that, in 2001, 16% of the UK population will be aged 65 and over, with a continued increase in the proportion of those aged 75 and over (Office of Health Economics 1995). With advances in medical and nursing care, the elderly are more likely to survive and achieve a good quality of life following surgery. Surgeons are now able to offer procedures to people who in previous years would not have been considered fit for surgery.

The nature of surgical services is changing rapidly to keep pace with technology and with advances in knowledge and skills. Not least among the factors affecting surgical care are changes in the overall approach to nursing practice. A study of one surgical ward demonstrated that many improvements in nursing practice, including the introduction of primary nursing, could be made without any need for increased staffing levels. During this time there were no obvious changes in medical practice, but a significant fall in postoperative complications, reduced length of stay and an increase in patient satisfaction were noted. These effects were attributed to changes in nursing practice (Malby 1991).

The nurse's role in surgical care will continue to evolve rapidly in response to the shift toward day-case and short-stay surgery, which will intensify the needs of patients during their time in hospital and put increased emphasis on pre- and postoperative care in the community. Developments in nurse-led initiatives such as gynaecology assessment units (Bell 1996) and nurses carrying out endoscopies (Hughes 1996) will further expand the role of nurses in perioperative care.

PRE-SURGICAL CARE

Classification of surgery

Some patients experience a long period of ill-health or disability before undergoing an operation; others experience a sudden illness or injury that necessitates immediate surgery. The degree of urgency of a surgical intervention is a useful criterion for its classification and prioritisation. An elderly patient with osteoarthritis of the hip who requires a total hip replacement operation would normally not be classified as an urgent case, but would be put on a waiting list and admitted 'electively'. However, if the same patient had fallen and fractured the neck of the femur, repair or (more commonly) total replacement of the hip to prevent further deterioration and ensure a speedy recovery would be regarded as 'essential'.

A given operation may be performed for different classifications of surgery. Surgery for a strangulated hernia will be handled as an emergency, whereas surgery for an irreducible hernia will be considered as essential, and for a reducible one as elective. Patients requiring essential surgery will be admitted to hospital within a week or two, but elective patients may have to wait for some considerable time. In 1994, there were 608 000 patients waiting for general surgery in the UK (Office of Health Economics 1995).

Within the *Patient's Charter* (DoH 1991), patients are guaranteed a maximum waiting time for elective surgery of 18 months in England. There has been some debate as to the usefulness of this focus on waiting times. To say that all patients receive surgery within 18 months may meet a standard, but for an individual who requires surgery within several weeks the standard cannot apply. For those waiting for some types of surgery, such as hip replacement, a 1 year wait may be intolerable. However, within the guarantees of the *Charter*, medical staff can no longer delay non-urgent surgery beyond 18 months in order to treat more urgent, but not immediately life-threatening, cases.

Presenting for surgery

Q **26.2** Ask a patient who has recently experienced surgery what signs and symptoms first brought her attention to her illness. What was it that made her seek out treatment? How does she define ill-health?

Personal definitions of health and ill-health and the decision to seek treatment are influenced by a range of factors, such as previous experience, social context, perceived severity of the illness and judgements as to whether treatment would be beneficial.

In Case History 26.1(A), Mr W was reluctant to take time off work to seek treatment but eventually came to a point where pain and discomfort made it impossible for him to carry on. In Case History 26.2, Mrs B was very reluctant to seek help, partly due to her fear of having cancer and partly due to what she felt was an embarrassing symptom. She had also convinced herself that she merely had haemorrhoids and could treat the condition herself.

In Case History 26.3(A), Mr L's community nurse had been alerted to problems developing and had contacted his general practitioner (GP) to initiate treatment. However, she remained worried about Mr L as, although the abscess was small, it was not reducing. She knew Mr L well and was sensitive to the deterioration in his general condition. She pursued her reassessment of Mr L and liaised with the GP, the consultant, the patient's wife and the surgical ward nurse in providing care.

Pathways and progress

Patients may be referred for surgery by different paths. Figure 26.1 represents the progress of Mr W and Mr L through the health care system, and Figure 26.2 that of Mrs B. Patients might enter these pathways at various points; Mrs B, for example, was taken straight to accident and emergency (A&E) by ambulance without seeing her GP about the illness. Patients may also be transferred from other wards. For example, a patient on a medical ward may undergo investigations which lead to a diagnosis that necessitates surgical treatment and therefore transfer to a surgical ward. A few patients admitted as emergencies may go straight to theatre from A&E and be admitted to the surgical ward following the operation. Some patients may need to go back to theatre or the intensive

Case History 26.1(A) Mr W

Mr W was a 42-year-old man who worked for a large construction company. He was married and had three young children. They enjoyed a comfortable lifestyle and had bought their own home that year. Mr W had been able to get some overtime work and this helped considerably with the mortgage repayments.

Mr W had been having some pain and swelling in his groin for some time, but it usually resolved on its own over time. However, over the past few weeks the swelling had got worse and was limiting the range of work he could do. One day when he was in obvious discomfort he was told by the foreman to see the occupational health nurse.

The nurse quickly assessed the extent of his inguinal hernia and rang Mr W's GP to make an urgent appointment. Before leaving the treatment room, she fitted him with a scrotal support and gave him some simple analgesia.

Mr W returned to light duties after a couple of days' sick leave. He thanked the nurse and returned the support she had given him. She was pleased to see Mr W looking relaxed and comfortable. She instructed him to continue to wear the support and gave him an extra one to help with laundering. He told her that his GP was referring him for surgery, but he was worried about taking time off work and being able to carry on with his job. The nurse reassured him that he would eventually be able to return to a full range of duties once he had completely recovered. She also suggested that if he were able to give up smoking he would have less of the cough that was partly exacerbating his hernia, and that he would have a better chance of a quick recovery after the anaesthetic. Mr W had always found he put on weight when he stopped smoking and was already moderately overweight. They discussed a plan of how he might give up smoking, including the use of chewing gum and nicotine patches. He knew his wife would be very supportive but was less sure of his mates, whom he met in the pub on Friday nights. The nurse also gave him a booklet on healthy eating to take home and look at with his wife. He quickly identified that his fried breakfasts and love of chips and beer were major sources of imbalance in his diet.

Several weeks later, the nurse spotted Mr W as she was touring the shop floor. He called her over to tell her that he had not had a cigarette for 3 weeks. He had saved the money he would have spent on cigarettes, which he felt would go some way towards keeping the family solvent during his sick leave. He also told her that he had a date for his operation at the end of the month. They talked about what sort of work he would be able to do after the operation. Mr W felt he knew the nurse well enough now to ask her about the effect of the operation on his ability to have sex and whether it would make him sterile. She reassured him on these points and explained that the operation would tighten a track through to his scrotum and would not affect his genitals. She did warn him, however, that he might be a little tender in the groin for the first week.

therapy unit (ITU) if their condition deteriorates or requires further intervention. Occasionally, a lengthy convalescence or rehabilitation may be required in another ward or hospital.

There are a number of patients, such as M (see Case History 26.4(A)), whose illness is of a chronic nature, and who will be readmitted to the surgical ward on one or more occasions. Patients

Case History 26.2 Mrs B

Mrs B was a 78-year-old woman who had lost her husband several years ago. Her eldest daughter lived nearby and was very supportive. Mrs B now lived in sheltered housing, which was a relief to her daughter, as she had previously lived in an isolated country cottage. Her sight had gradually deteriorated in recent years and the arthritis in her fingers and knees limited what she could do. At the time Mrs B became ill, she was pleased that she still had her own home, and enjoyed going to the local day centre twice a week.

One of the care assistants at the day centre was a little concerned that Mrs B did not seem to be enjoying the singing quite so much as before and spent much of the afternoon dozing. Mrs B, being an independent and spirited lady, thanked the young girl for her concern and joked that she wasn't getting any younger and that there was no need to worry about her.

Mrs B thought long and hard that evening. She had been constipated for some time but had put it down to old age. Now she was also passing blood, and although she was frightened that it might be 'something nasty', she had decided that it must be piles. She had bought some ointment and laxatives from the chemist, but was reluctant to go to her GP, who had visited her when she just moved into the area. He was a nice young man, but she did not want him to examine her.

Several weeks later, the driver of the day centre minibus got no reply at Mrs B's door when he called to collect her. Worried that she might have fallen, he called the warden, who had a key to the flat. Mrs B was found still in her bed, in obvious pain and sweating profusely. The warden called an ambulance immediately and then phoned Mrs B's daughter. Mrs B was then taken to the A&E department of the local hospital.

Case History 26.3(A) Mr L

Mr L was a 56-year-old man who had suffered from multiple sclerosis for many years. He lived at home with his wife and, with the help of the community nurses, normally coped well with his disability. He now had no sensation or power in his legs, but was able to transfer to and from and get about in his wheelchair. He was extremely knowledgeable about his illness and had a very positive approach to living with his disability.

The community nursing sister had worked out a plan of care with Mr and Mrs L to ensure that they received appropriate help and care and that the necessary equipment and aids were provided. She would visit every second day to give bowel care, as Mr L had no voluntary control over his bowels. Recently, she noticed a small red area developing on Mr L's buttock. She checked the inflation pressure in his Rohoe cushion and with Mr L decided to increase the frequency of pressure relief (i.e. raising himself off the seat of his chair).

The next time the nurse visited, a small abscess had begun to form with some obvious pus, and she phoned Mr L's GP, who then arranged to visit him at home the following day. The GP lanced the abscess with a scalpel and took a specimen of pus to send to the laboratory for culture and sensitivity. As the result could take several days to come back, Mr L was started on a course of antibiotics which would be appropriate for common skin infections.

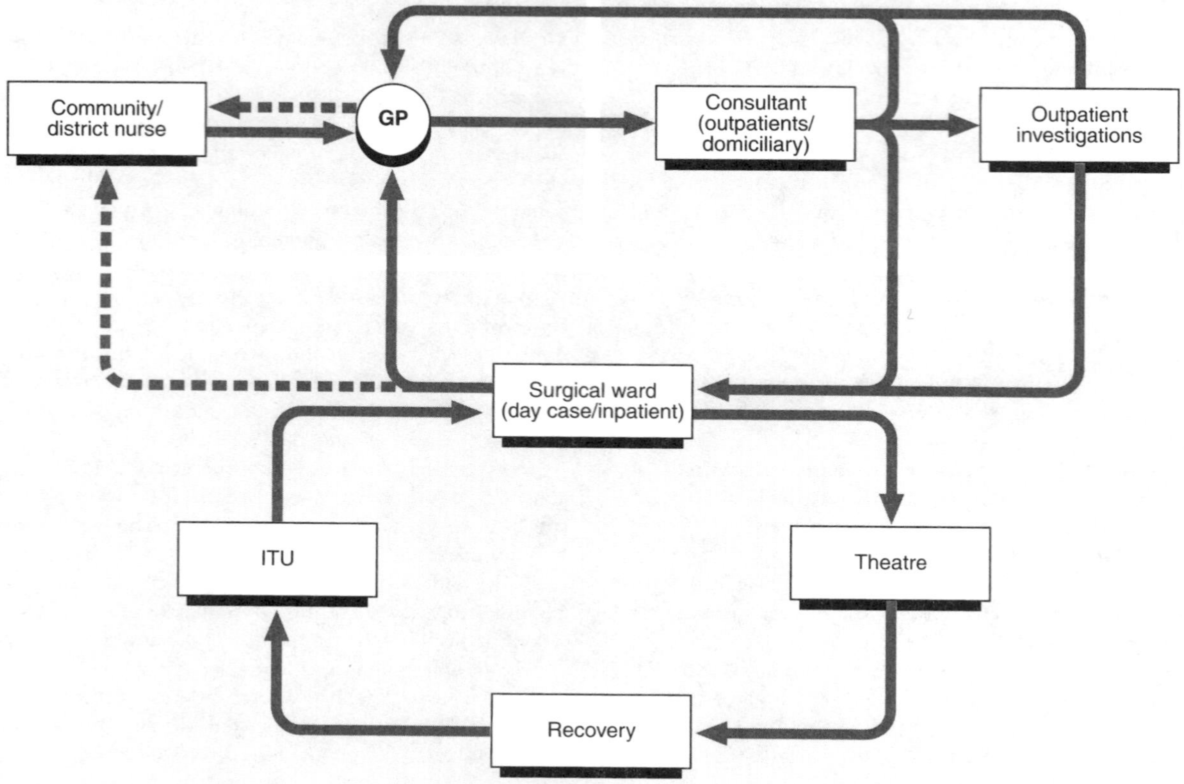

Fig. 26.1 Pathways to essential and elective surgery.

with Crohn's disease can present at an early age and may require repeated interventions and admissions to hospital throughout their lives. In a busy surgical ward these patients require a sensitive approach. One must not assume that because a patient has been through a procedure before, she will need less support or information than she did the first time.

The vast majority of patients are admitted to hospital from home and return to their own homes. The GP can be seen as the gatekeeper to services, as unless the illness is a sudden emergency or an accident, he is the one who will refer the patient for further care under the hospital consultant. However, as with Mr L and Mr W, community nurses can be the first point of contact for the patient, referring the patient to the GP or seeking the GP's advice for further treatment. Community nurses have established lines of communication with the wards but these tend to be unidirectional, moving from ward to community nurse.

A substantial morbidity exists among patients on waiting lists for surgery. Those waiting for hip surgery, for example, may suffer restricted activity and constant pain. Those awaiting gallstone surgery may suffer recurrent bouts of severe abdominal pain. Mr W is fortunately supported by his occupational health nurse, who institutes measures to reduce discomfort and prevent further injury while he waits for treatment.

26.3 What actions might a community nurse take to improve the health of these patients awaiting surgery?

INFORMED DECISION-MAKING

The aim of this section is to introduce the issue of informed consent for surgery by discussing nursing responsibilities and highlighting some areas for ethical debate.

For a wider discussion on the ethical aspects of consent, see Thompson et al (1994) and Tingle & Cribb (1995).

The decision to operate

Once the outcome of investigations are known and have been considered in the light of the patient's presenting signs and symptoms, the surgeon can make a definite or provisional diagnosis and recommend a course of action. This may involve diagnostic, curative or palliative surgery, a combination of these, or no surgical intervention at all. If the patient can be treated as successfully without surgical intervention, then the relevant alternatives will be pursued. Consider the following examples:

- A middle-aged woman is found to have Stage 2A cervical cancer (see Ch. 31) with infiltrating lymph nodes when she undergoes examination under anaesthesia (EUA). It is decided that surgery is not appropriate. She is referred to an oncologist, who prescribes a course of radical radiotherapy.
- Another patient has been referred to hospital for an oesophagoscopy and gastroscopy after complaining of heartburn. He is found to have a hiatus hernia and is prescribed an

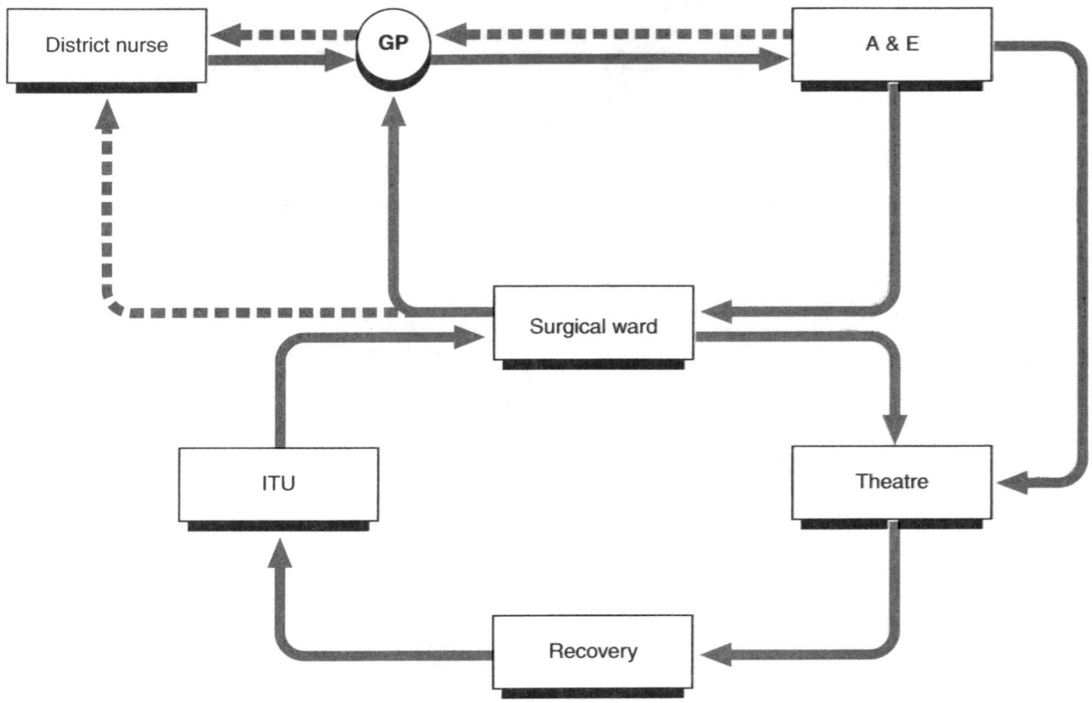

Fig. 26.2 Pathways to emergency surgery.

Case History 26.4(A) M

M was a 23-year-old hotel receptionist who had suffered from Crohn's disease for as long as she could remember. She had been in and out of hospital on account of her condition on many occasions. This time she was sent straight up to the ward after her appointment in the outpatients' department. The primary nurse who had looked after her on two earlier occasions felt a real friendship with her. When the nurse greeted her on the ward, M burst into tears. M told her how she had developed a horrible faecal discharge from her vagina and that she had been admitted for more investigations. She was pyrexial, looked pale, and with her small frame appeared extremely fragile. The primary nurse offered her a single room as she was obviously distressed by her uncontrolled diarrhoea.

Once M had telephoned her boyfriend, with whom she had been living for the past year, and had taken time to collect her thoughts, she was visited by the consultant. He suggested that a fistula was the cause of the current problem and that the best plan of action would be to close it surgically. M was informed that there was a chance that she would need a defunctioning stoma and spent some time talking to the primary nurse and the night staff about it.

The next day M started her bowel preparation. This consisted of 4 L of Go-lytely to be taken over the next 24 h. She was not allowed to eat that day but could take extra drinks of clear fluids if she wanted. She discussed with the primary nurse the use of large pads to absorb leakage from her vagina. She was also given some soft wipes and a tube of barrier cream to avoid excoriation of the perianal area by the diarrhoea.

antacid and gelling agent (Gaviscon). The nurse in outpatients gives him advice on sleeping propped up at night, avoiding certain foods and on how to take his medication.

- M (see Case History 26.4(A)) has been making frequent visits over the last few months to see her medical consultant about her vaginal fistula. Despite enteral diets, anti-inflammatory agents and antibiotics, the fistula does not resolve. She is referred to the surgeon and subsequently admitted to the surgical ward.

It might appear from these brief descriptions that it is the medical staff who take the decision on the course of treatment to be given. However, whereas the doctor decides what treatment appears to be the most appropriate, it is the informed patient who must make the final decision as to what treatment is accepted (UKCC 1996). Thus the woman with cervical cancer is offered either radiotherapy or surgery, but is advised by her doctor that radiotherapy would be more suitable in her particular case. The doctor considers that the extent of surgery that would be necessary and the risks and morbidity associated with surgery outweigh the benefits. After being informed of and discussing the survival rates and adverse effects of both forms of treatment, the patient opts for radiotherapy.

Informed consent

When patients undergo any type of intervention or procedure, they must give their consent. Touching someone without their consent and without lawful justification could be construed as trespass, civil assault or battery (Dimond 1990).

In practice, it is preferable to obtain verbal rather than written consent from the patient for low-risk procedures, such as having a chest X-ray or being given suppositories. However, when a patient is to undergo surgery or any invasive procedure (and when a general or local anaesthetic is required), it is advisable and standard practice to obtain her written consent. As it is the medical team who are in charge of these procedures, they are ultimately responsible for obtaining the written consent from the patient. The doctor signing the consent form with the patient has to ensure that:

- the patient understands the information, and not just that it has been given and received
- the extent of the information is sufficient for that patient to make the decision.

The role of the nurse

The nurse has an important role to play in obtaining consent prior to surgery. For a patient to give a valid consent, she must comprehend fully what she is consenting to, i.e. her consent must be informed. The nurse can provide the team with a knowledge of the patient's individual need for information and her comprehension of the information given.

The nurse will also provide the patient with information about the procedure and the recovery period and may be able to clarify points previously discussed between patient and doctor. However, the nurse cannot and must not be the provider of information in order for the doctor to obtain informed consent for surgery. This is a medical staff responsibility.

There may be occasions when the nurse considers he needs to obtain written consent from the patient for a particular procedure or treatment. In this instance, providing the information for consent is the nurse's responsibility, as he is in charge of the procedure.

The need for informed consent raises several legal and ethical issues for nurses and patients. The current social climate emphasises consumerism and patients' rights. Patients have an increased desire to be 'partners in care', i.e. to be well informed and to take responsibility for their own health. Patients have the right to be given an adequate explanation of proposed treatment, including any risks and alternative treatments. Nurses have a vital role to play in ensuring a patient's needs for information are met and that a full discussion takes place (Alderson & Helms 1995).

However, there may be occasions when the patient is less than fully informed. The depth and complexity of information held by medical staff may be overwhelming for a lay person. This consideration must be balanced against individual needs and consumer demands. There have been some instances where patients have attempted to sue health authorities for lack of information about potential risks or side-effects of treatment (*Sidway v. Bethlem Royal Hospital* 1985). There is now a heightened awareness of the need to explain potential adverse as well as beneficial effects of treatment. With some procedures, the risks are now clearly stated on the consent form itself. Both the chance of occurrence and the severity of potential adverse effects of the procedure must be addressed in considering whether to inform the patient of them. For example, a myelogram carries only a small risk of seizures and loss of power in the limbs, but as the effect on the patient would be severe, it is important to inform her of these risks.

There may be occasions when medical staff deliberately withhold certain information in the belief that it would be detrimental to the patient to have this information. This is perfectly legal if the doctor is deemed to be acting in the patient's best interests. Our moral principles tell us that one should always tell the truth. However, if knowledge of the truth would have a negative effect upon the patient then a difficult decision has to be made. If the individual has expressed a desire for full information about her diagnosis, the decision becomes clearer. It would not be legal or ethical to withhold information on the grounds that the patient might refuse treatment if she were given the full facts.

Q

26.4 A young woman is told she has ovarian 'cysts' and, although distressed at requiring an oophorectomy and possibly a hysterectomy and so losing the ability to have children, she consents to the operation. Her husband and the surgeon have agreed that she would not cope well with knowing her true diagnosis of ovarian cancer at this time, and so withhold this information from her. She then questions the ward nurses, at first indirectly and then directly with questions such as 'It's cancer, isn't it?' and 'This is going to be the end of me, isn't it?'.

What might you do or say if faced with such a situation in the ward? How might the patient react if you told her you were not able to answer her questions? Discuss the example with your nursing and medical colleagues.

In theory, a nurse could face disciplinary action or even dismissal if he were to go against the surgeon's expressed wish to withhold information. This is highly unlikely if the nurse was clearly acting in the patient's best interests. Gillan (1994) suggests that nurses lack the confidence, knowledge and debating skills to challenge medical staff when information is withheld. However, it is more usual for nursing and medical staff to be sensitive to the individual needs of the patient and to work collaboratively with the patient and her family to resolve any such moral dilemmas.

In some cases, the patient may be too ill to comprehend what is proposed sufficiently well to give informed consent. When an adult patient is unable to give informed consent, e.g. when she is unconscious or mentally unfit, her relatives have no legal right to give or, perhaps more importantly, to refuse consent. Good practice would dictate that relatives are consulted and a decision made in the patient's best interest. However, the ultimate decision in this case is the doctor's.

For further reading, see Brennan (1989).

Similarly, relatives have no legal rights in determining whether information should be given to or withheld from the patient. In fact, the doctor or nurse would be in breach of confidentiality if he were to tell the relatives first, or to tell them at all, without the patient's expressed consent. However, if the information is withheld from the patient, how can the patient consent to it being divulged (UKCC 1996)?

Resolving dilemmas

When a patient is too ill to be told or cannot give informed consent, then medical and nursing staff must carry out their professional duty to act in the patient's best interests, whilst considering the wishes of the relatives.

The UKCC *Code of Professional Conduct* (UKCC 1992) provides nurses with guidelines on professional practice (see UKCC 1996 for more detailed discussion on truthfulness and consent). Nurses are required to follow the code in terms of acting to safeguard the patients' interests and to work in a collaborative and cooperative manner with other health care professionals.

It is essential that nurses are familiar with the code and apply it in everyday practice. Guidelines on informed consent have also been produced for doctors and nurses (DoH 1990, Medical Defence Union 1997).

PREOPERATIVE PREPARATION

Preoperative preparation might begin long before the patient is admitted to a hospital ward. Mr W's occupational health nurse and Mr L's district nurse were both involved in preparing their patients for surgery. As this aspect of care has already been considered, this section refers to the immediate preoperative period following admission to hospital.

Patients arrive for admission having experienced very different types of preparation. Mrs B had no preparation at all, being taken to A&E as an emergency. Mr L had already seen his consultant surgeon at home the day prior to admission and had discussed the need for hospital admission and possible surgery with him and the district nurse. Mr W had visited the ward 1 week earlier and met his primary nurse. She had talked to him along with a small group of patients coming in for day-case and short-stay surgery over the next couple of weeks. He had received a booklet about the ward and had some blood tests, a chest X-ray and an ECG. He arrived on the ward on the morning of admission having had nothing to eat or drink since going to bed the night before. The primary nurse showed him to a chair where he could wait for a bed to become available. She had also received a phone call to say that Mrs B was to be admitted from A&E as an emergency, and was also aware that Mr L would be arriving in time for the consultant's round later that morning.

All of these patients, whether emergency, essential or elective admissions, would require appropriate preoperative assessment, information about their care, and safe preparation for anaesthetic and surgery.

Assessment

Assessment of the patient is required in order to identify any special needs, to highlight potential problems and to provide a baseline against which to measure postoperative progress. Ideally, the primary nurse would admit the patient himself in order to establish a relationship and to enable him to directly observe and question the patient. He may also use other sources of information, such as existing medical or nursing records, the patient's relatives and other health care professionals to form a complete picture. The way a nurse assesses a patient will vary according to the model used. This might be one developed by the ward nurses or an established model such as Roper et al's (1996) activities of daily living model or Johnson's (1980) behavioural system model. But while each nurse's approach to, and description of, the delivery of care may be different, the needs of the patient remain essentially the same. Care pathways have been developed to outline these needs for some types of surgery. They detail the care that a particular group of patients will receive and at what point in their stay. Deviations from this pathway are recorded for quality assurance purposes and to enable individual variation in care. This approach to care has led to a reduction in length of hospital stay for some patients and has facilitated a continuance of care in the community for others (Calligaro et al 1996, Schaldach 1997).

Giving information

Reducing preoperative anxiety and stress is not only desirable on humanitarian grounds, but also promotes recovery. Giving the patient information and emotional support preoperatively is known to substantially reduce pre- and postoperative anxiety (Martin 1996, Gammon & Mulholland 1996) and also has a direct effect on reducing postoperative complications, partly by increasing compliance. Patients who have received structured preoperative information or teaching have been found to mobilise earlier postoperatively, to have a shorter postoperative hospital stay (Gammon & Mulholland 1996) and to have a reduced need for analgesia postoperatively (Hayward 1975, Shade 1992, Teasdale 1993, Martin 1996) as compared with patients who receive standard ward or unstructured preparation. However, preoperative information-giving remains a neglected aspect of care in a wide number of hospitals (Dale 1993). Lack of information has also been found to be a major source of dissatisfaction among day-case patients (Edmondson 1995).

It is important that patients receive information at an appropriate level and on matters that do in fact concern them — not simply on what the nurse assumes they will be anxious about. Mitchell (1997) argues that giving every patient volumes of information will not lead to a reduction in anxiety for all. Information given should be dependent on the patient's individual preference and need, and be of high quality. Watts & Brooks (1997) studied patients admitted to an intensive care unit following surgery. They found that information about the management of pain and nausea and mouth care was important for patients. This information was thought to give reassurance in terms of bodily comfort and also that they would be closely monitored by a nurse postoperatively. Potential anxiety about using a bedpan or a bottle could also be reduced by giving information about the use of urinary catheters.

Q **26.5** How will this knowledge change the way you would approach giving information to your preoperative patient?

Skilled, systematic and sensitive assessment is essential in determining what is important for the individual. Sensitive, open questioning can determine what the patient already understands and what she would like to know more about. Simply giving a factual account of what will occur is insufficient. Patients want to know what to expect and how it will feel. They also need the opportunity to discuss their fears and worries. Factual and sensory information, coping strategies and counselling are then the essential components of preoperative education. During the admission procedure Mr W told his primary nurse that he was afraid of feeling pain during the operation, as he knew he could be awake throughout the procedure. The nurse then described to him what kind of sensations he might expect:

> Once all the checks and preparations have been completed in the ward, you will be given a tablet that will make you feel a little drowsy and more relaxed. The checks will take place again when you get to theatre and a nurse will stay with you at all times. When you go into theatre, the doctors will put up a screen using green cloth so you won't have to watch what is happening. They will also give you an injection around the top of your leg to begin to numb the area. It feels like a scratch under the skin as they make sure the skin is numb before giving you a deeper dose of anaesthetic. You will probably feel quite sleepy during the procedure, but you may feel the doctor pressing around the area, although there should be no pain or discomfort. You will never lose consciousness and would always be able to tell the doctor if you felt anything. If you would like to listen to some music on the headphones when you are in theatre, let me know before you go up and I can show you what tapes we have. A lot of people find it takes their mind off things and helps them relax. Remember there is always a nurse with you whom you can talk to or ask about things whilst you are in theatre. How do you feel about things now?

Q **26.6** Can you identify the information given here in terms of knowledge, sensory information and coping strategies?

When and how information is given will influence its effectiveness. Many patients have difficulty in remembering verbal information; while a personal, verbal explanation is invaluable in that it allows for feedback from the patient, it has a poor recall over time. Moran & Kent (1995) found that short-stay patients were most often dissatisfied with the extent of information given after the outpatient appointment prior to surgery. They advocate the wider use of pre-assessment clinics (Burns 1993) where nurses can address this problem, and the development of information leaflets and patient-held shared care records to enable full information exchange between hospital and community staff and the patient. Nelson (1996) found that patients had a strong preference for information to be given in a pre-admission programme prior to cardiac surgery. Pre-admission information allows for emotional adjustment over a longer period and enables patients to share information with and seek support from their families. Recall of information is also improved when information is given in a more relaxed setting. Beddows (1997) found that patients who were given information in their own homes prior to admission and again on admission were less anxious than those who were given information on admission only.

Pre-admission booklets for surgical patients can be beneficial in reducing patient anxiety and improving outcomes. Law (1997) found that preoperative information needed to be written down as a back-up to verbal advice given. Information leaflets are not, therefore, a substitute for personalised explanation but do provide a constant reference source and can prepare patients to use their contact time with nurses more effectively. This allows the nurse to focus on areas of concern and to devote more time to counselling than to information-giving, as in reality it is often difficult to complete both tasks well in the busy preoperative period. Thus, in the example given above (Mr W), the primary nurse was able to spend some time providing more detailed information and coping strategies as Mr W had already read about his operation and visited the ward to familiarise himself with the environment.

Preoperative information booklets should be easy to read without being patronising. Print size, reading ease and vocabulary should all be considered and the use of jargon avoided. A booklet must also be comprehensive, as this improves recall and compliance with instructions (Bradshaw et al 1975). Many wards produce their own booklets about the ward and general information about surgery. Some also have leaflets about specific operations which can be sent or given to the patient with the ward and/or hospital booklet prior to admission.

Preoperative education aims to produce a well-informed consumer, to promote healthy choices and to reduce anxiety. The informed patient is better equipped to make good decisions about her care and to discuss her treatment fully and openly with staff. In this sense, information also serves to produce a more autonomous patient (Ewles & Simnet 1992). One must then respect the view that the well-informed patient has the right to reject advice or treatment against professional judgement for personal reasons (Fahrenfort 1987). What the professional advocates may conflict with what the patient wants. Simply informing someone of an objective fact that appears rational (e.g. smoking causes lung cancer) will be insufficient in some cases to promote healthy behaviour or coping mechanisms (Galvin 1992).

For further reading on patient education, see Kiger (1995).

Safe preparation for anaesthesia and surgery

In the admission assessment, the patient's specific needs and potential problems may be identified. The general risks associated with anaesthesia and surgical intervention will also be taken into account in any related medical or nursing procedure. Patients undergoing surgery require medical assessment, the nature of which will depend on the extent of surgery, the age of the patient and on any pre-existing medical conditions. Mr W was given a chest X-ray to screen for any abnormalities of the lungs, a blood test for urea and electrolytes and a full blood count. An ECG was performed to rule out cardiac dysfunction, as it is important to ensure that a patient has no gross abnormalities of the cardiovascular and respiratory systems prior to the administration of an anaesthetic. The anaesthetist was pleased that Mr W had managed to stop smoking, and relieved that he no longer had a productive cough. Smoking considerably increases the risk of chest infection and atelectasis postoperatively.

Risk of chest infection

All patients receiving a general anaesthetic are at risk of developing a chest infection; this is one of the most common complications after surgery (Dilworth & Pounsford 1991). Drugs and gases used in anaesthesia are drying to the respiratory tract and inhibit the action of the cilia. Secretions of mucus become thick and tenacious, causing partial obstruction of the lower airways. Cigarette smoking also damages and paralyses the cilia and leads to excess mucus production. The secretions eventually pool in the base of the lungs and plug the bronchioles. The retained secretions obstruct the lower airways, inhibiting gaseous exchange and providing a source of bacterial infection.

Artificial ventilation during the operation is at tidal volume and does not fully inflate the lung (see Ch. 3). Normally, a person will sigh intermittently or increase demands for oxygen by activity, so fully inflating the lungs and preventing stagnation and atelectasis. Changes of position, movement and coughing all serve to dislodge excess mucus or fluid, which is then expelled from the lungs as sputum. The patient will be lying still and unable to cough or sigh throughout the operation when under a general anaesthetic. There will also be a period of inactivity postoperatively and perhaps a reluctance to breathe deeply or cough if there is abdominal or thoracic pain.

Patients should be advised to stop smoking, at least for 2 weeks prior to surgery, if not for good. Haddock & Burrows (1997) found that nurses could have a significant impact on helping smokers to quit before surgery by giving constructive advice and information in the pre-admission stage. All patients, regardless of whether they are smokers or not, must be taught deep breathing exercises and coughing. It can be difficult to teach a patient to contract the diaphragm in order to breathe deeply preoperatively, let alone postoperatively. The tendency is to use intercostal and accessory muscles to lift the rib cage and draw the abdomen in. Although instruction may be the responsibility of the physiotherapist in some wards, it will still require reinforcement from the nursing staff. In this context, the need for early mobilisation can be described to the patient.

For further reading on deep breathing exercises see Webber & Pryor (1994).

26.7 Try some deep breathing exercises yourself. Did you draw your abdomen in and lift the rib cage? Try to breathe using the diaphragm. Place one hand on your abdomen. Breathe in through your nose while you try to feel your abdomen pushing your hand out (as the diaphragm moves downwards and displaces the stomach).

Risk of deep vein thrombosis (DVT) and pulmonary embolism (PE)

An intravascular clot or thrombus is most likely to occur when the following three conditions (known as Virchow's triad) exist:

- trauma — damaged endothelium
- stasis — slow blood flow
- hypercoagulable blood.

Thrombus formation is initiated by the activation of factor XII in reaction to exposure to collagen filaments in the damaged endothelium. This results in platelet aggregation, formation of thrombin from circulating prothrombin, and stimulation of the production of insoluble fibrin from fibrinogen (see Ch. 11, p. 432).

It has been found that during surgery, the veins of the lower leg distend by up to 48% (Coleridge Smith et al 1991). This distension leads to subluminal endothelial damage, which can provide a site for clot formation. In the soleal and gastrocnemius veins, the blood flow is highly dependent on exercise, and so these are often the site of initial thrombus formation following prolonged periods of inactivity and lack of calf muscle pressure to assist venous return. The general adaptation reaction to the stress of surgery (see Ch. 17, p. 615) results in reduced levels of the coagulation inhibitors protein C, protein S and antithrombin III. Fibrin clots may be gradually broken down by the enzyme plasmin in a process called fibrinolysis. However, the thrombus may persist, causing some degree of venous obstruction. In a small proportion of cases, a fragment of the clot breaks away, forming an embolus. The embolus may travel through the venous system, through the right side of the heart and into the pulmonary arteries. Here it becomes lodged at a point where the arteries become too small to allow the embolus to pass through. The extent of the resultant pulmonary infarct depends on the size of the vessel occluded. Some patients may have no signs or symptoms of either DVT or PE if thrombi are small and infrequent (see Ch. 2, p. 54 for signs and symptoms). However, large thrombi can be devastating, causing sudden death in 50% of patients with pulmonary embolism.

All surgical patients are exposed to a number of risk factors for DVT. The incidence of DVT in patients undergoing various types of vascular surgery was found to be between 9 and 14% despite standard prophylaxis with anticoagulants (Fletcher & Batiste 1997). The incidence in patients undergoing abdominal surgery and neurosurgery has been reported as lower than this at around 5%, again with anticoagulant prophylaxis (Flinn et al 1996, Kakkar et al 1997). During the preoperative assessment, the nurse should assess the patient for the presence of known risk factors. Caprini et al (1988) have categorised risk of thrombosis into low-, moderate- and high-risk categories (see Fig. 26.3). A similar scale

Risk factors

Age 40–60 yrs = 1 point	☐	Trauma	☐
61–70 yrs = 2 points	☐	Theatre time = 2 hours +	☐
70+ yrs = 3 points	☐	Total joint replacement	☐
History of DVT/PE = 3 points	☐	Pelvic long bone fracture	☐
Immobilisation	☐	Leg: oedema, ulcer, stasis	☐
Varicose veins	☐	Malignant disease	☐
Obesity	☐	Pregnancy	☐
Myocardial infarction	☐	Inflammatory bowel disease	☐
Congestive heart failure	☐	Sepsis	☐
Stroke	☐	Oestrogen therapy (including contraceptive pill)	☐
Hypercoagulable states	☐		

Score one point for each risk factor except where noted. Calculate degree of risk as follows:

1 point = low risk
2–4 points = moderate risk
4+ points = high risk

Fig. 26.3 Assessing the risk of deep vein thrombosis in surgical patients. (Adapted from Caprini et al 1988.)

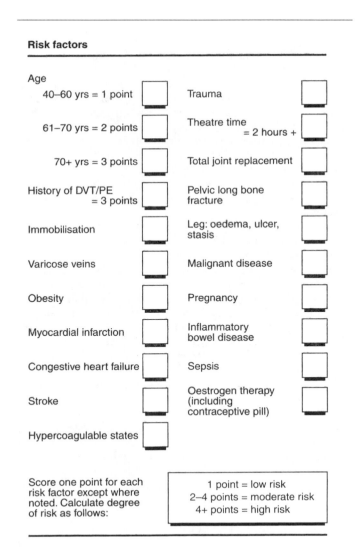

was developed by Autar (1996) but it has only been tested on a small population of orthopaedic surgery patients and so has limited generalisability.

The preventive measures taken by medical and nursing staff will depend on the level of risk for DVT and potential bleeding complications in individual patients. It is now generally accepted that patients in all risk categories should use graduated compression stockings (Caprini et al 1988, Jeffery & Nicolaides 1990). These stockings create a decreasing pressure gradient in the leg from around 18 mmHg at the ankle to 8 mmHg at the thigh (full length) or to 14 mmHg at the calf (below-knee length). The gradient increases blood flow in the femoral vein and prevents the venous distension that causes endothelial damage (Coleridge Smith et al 1991). Graduated compression stockings reduce the incidence of postoperative DVT by approximately 60% (from 30 to 11%) in general surgical patients. Reductions in incidence among orthopaedic and gynaecological patients have also been demonstrated (Turner et al 1984).

The nurse should ensure that a well-designed and well-fitting stocking is applied. Stockings are fitted according to calf size and leg length and are available in a wide variety of sizes. If stockings roll down, a constricting band is created which may cause higher pressures, leading to an inverse gradient and delayed venous emptying. For this reason, below-knee stockings have been found to be more comfortable for low-risk patients who are ambulant. Knee-length stockings have been shown to be as effective as full-length ones in increasing blood flow in the deep veins (Lawrence & Kakkar 1980), resulting in no significant difference in the incidence of DVT in patients wearing above- or below-knee stockings (Porteous et al 1989). It is, however, recommended that full-length stockings are used for patients in moderate- and high-risk categories. The patient should wear the stockings from admission to discharge unless she is in a low-risk category and fully ambulant in the preoperative period, when the stockings can be applied prior to theatre.

Other measures that should be encouraged where possible are early activity and hourly leg exercises. The patient should be taught to dorsiflex the foot preoperatively. This will assist venous return by the action of the calf muscle compressing blood in the deep veins. Deep breathing exercises will also aid the respiratory pump as deep inspiration reduces intrathoracic pressure and hence increases venous return. In addition, of course, ensuring adequate hydration will reduce hypercoagulability.

For high-risk patients, sequential pneumatic compression of the legs has been shown to be effective (Caprini et al 1988). This can be achieved by two plastic sleeves fitted over graduated compression stockings. The sleeves have small separate pockets at different levels up the leg. A pump inflates the pockets in order from ankle to thigh so that a wave-like action passes up the leg, 'milking' the blood up towards the heart (see Fig. 26.4). Teaching leg exercises and applying graduated compression stockings and/or sequential pneumatic compression devices (SCD) prevent DVT by their action on two aspects of Virchow's triad, namely stasis and endothelial damage. Hypercoagulability can be avoided to some extent by adequate hydration but will be stimulated in any event by the general adaptation to stress response and by the effects of surgery initiating clotting mechanisms. Medical staff will seek to minimise hypercoagulability with the administration of anticoagulants (with all but low-risk patients). The value of prophylactic low-dose heparin to prevent DVT and PE in general surgical patients is well known. To be effective it must be given at least 2 h prior to surgery (Collins et al 1988). The risk of bleeding complications is minimal unless the patient has a clotting disorder; in such a case, administration of anticoagulants would have to be monitored closely and its value judged carefully against the risk of DVT. Small wound haematomas may be more likely to occur in the patient receiving low-dose heparin, but when cared for correctly do not usually pose a threat.

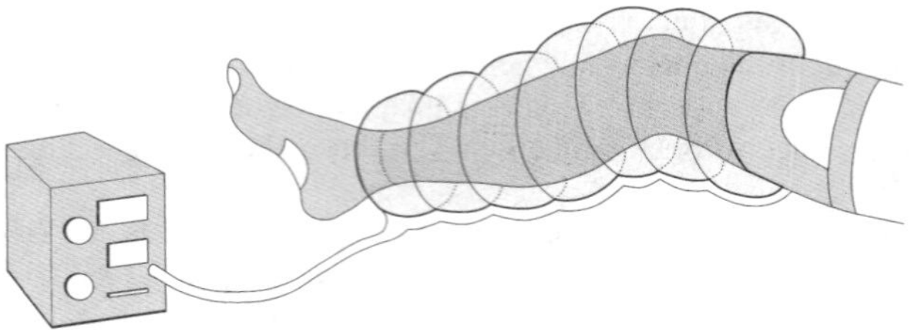

Fig. 26.4 Sequential pneumatic compression.

26.8 Work out the risk of DVT in the four patients below. Plan care appropriate to each individual in order to prevent DVT.

- Mr W is going to theatre later that morning to have a hernia repair under a local anaesthetic.
- Mrs B is to go straight from A&E to the operating theatre as her abdominal X-rays and clinical findings show that she has peritonitis due to perforation of the bowel.
- Mr L is scheduled for theatre the following day to excise and debride his perianal abscess.
- M is due to go to theatre for repair of her vaginal fistula in 2 days when she has completed her bowel preparation.

Preoperative fasting

Patients who are to receive a general anaesthetic, heavy sedation or a local anaesthetic with the possibility of proceeding to a general anaesthetic are all at risk of aspiration pneumonia (sometimes termed Mendelson's syndrome). When a patient is anaesthetised or unconscious, the swallowing reflex is absent. From the point of induction of the anaesthetic, there is a risk that stomach contents may reflux and be inhaled through the open larynx into the lungs. This inevitably causes respiratory embarrassment and leads to the development of a diffuse chest infection. The risks are minimised partly through the administration of certain drugs (see p. 809) but also by fasting the patient of both diet and fluids.

Different foodstuffs pass through the stomach at different rates. Gastric emptying is usually complete for most meals in 4–5 h. Even fasting patients may have up to 200 mL in the stomach (Pritchard & Walker 1984). Taking this into account, the minimum preoperative fasting period is usually 4 h for fluids and 6 h for food. However, a study by Phillips et al (1993) found there was little difference in residual volume when patients were allowed to drink clear fluids up until the time of the premedication (approximately 2 h preoperatively). The patients had no problems with aspiration or regurgitation and they were less thirsty and more comfortable.

A classic study by Hamilton Smith (1972) found that patients were often fasted preoperatively for much longer than necessary.

A small replication study by Thomas (1987) found that little had changed, with patients on the morning list for theatre being fasted for 10–18 h whilst those on the afternoon list were fasted for 5–22 h. Chapman (1996) found that patients continue to be fasted for prolonged periods, with those on a morning list fasted for an average of 12 h and those on the afternoon list for 8 h.

The undesirable results of prolonged fasting are mainly dehydration and electrolyte imbalance (the liver has glycogen stores sufficient to maintain blood sugar levels for about 18 h). In elderly patients this occurs more rapidly and can lead to confusion. All patients experience, to some extent, feelings of starvation and a dry mouth. Some might not understand the reasons for fasting and eat or drink against advice.

Doctors and nurses are not unaware of proper fasting times, but tend to set a wide margin of safety and fast patients for at least 6 h. Theatre times are always approximate, apart from that of the first person on the list, as one cannot be entirely sure how long each operation will take. Surgeons may decide to alter the order of patients on the list, but this should not form part of everyday practice. Nurses work to the earliest likely time for theatre, but this often proves to be much later. A lack of individualised care leads to the imposition of one fasting time for all patients on the theatre list. A patient on the morning list is then fasted from midnight, but if she is last on the morning list she may not go to theatre until 14.00 h and thus will have fasted for at least 14 h. Individual fasting times and close liaison with the anaesthetist can resolve such problems.

Patients must be given adequate information in order to understand what they cannot eat or drink, for how long, and how to care for a dry mouth in the meantime. If the patient has oral medication prescribed during the fasting time, it should not be routinely withheld; rather, medical staff should be consulted as to whether the drug should be given or not. Tablets can be taken with 30–60 mL of water.

To return to our case histories, Mrs B was to go to theatre as an emergency, so it was not possible to ensure she had fasted for at least 4 h. In this case, her stomach was emptied by aspirating the contents through a nasogastric tube. Mr W had come into hospital on the morning of theatre but had received instructions about fasting in his booklet from the ward the week before. He was not sure whether he could have an early morning cup of tea and had asked his primary nurse about this during his visit. As theatre would not start until 09.30 h she advised him he might have a drink at 06.00 h but nothing after that. In fact, Mr W was third on the list and did not go up to theatre until 11.30 h.

Q **26.9** Observe how long patients are fasted preoperatively in your ward experience. How would you explain to a patient the necessity of fasting prior to theatre?

Skin preparation

Preparation of the skin before theatre can help to reduce the incidence of postoperative infections. Another important factor is the exposure to nosocomial pathogens. The risk of infection can be reduced by shortening the length of preoperative stay. It has already been proposed that by reducing preoperative anxiety, psychological and physiological stress can be reduced and the incidence of postoperative infection lowered (Boore 1978).

Preparation of the skin formerly included shaving the site of the operation. However, shaving leaves small cuts and abrasions that can give rise to infection. Research has demonstrated that shaving delays discharge on average from 7.3 to 9.1 days (Editorial, *The Lancet*, 1983). However, if sticking plaster is to be used, hair removal may be justified on humanitarian grounds. Hair removal may also be necessary if the hair occludes the surgeon's vision of the operation site or if adhesive leads are to be applied, requiring a good skin contact. For example, a patient undergoing angiographic surgery may have the cannula inserted via the femoral artery in the groin. A pressure dressing is essential postoperatively, which necessitates the use of strong adhesive tape in the groin.

If hair removal is necessary then hair clippers or depilatory cream can be used. A patch test for sensitivity to creams must be carried out before use. Application of depilatories must also be avoided around sensitive mucous membranes in the genital area. When creams cannot be used and clippers are not available, a well-lubricated shave with a sharp razor immediately prior to theatre may be sufficient. This does, however, carry a higher risk of infection than the use of creams or clippers (McIntyre & McCloy 1994). In some centres the shave may be carried out by the theatre orderly once the patient is anaesthetised.

The bacterial count on the skin can be actively reduced by having the patient shower prior to theatre with a skin antiseptic such as Hibiscrub, which is chlorhexidine-based (Brandberg & Anderson 1980). Bathing should be avoided where possible, as bacteria may multiply in the warm water and there is a risk of cross-infection from organisms already present in hospital baths. The patient should be asked to shower several hours prior to theatre and to dress in a fresh theatre gown (Freshwater 1992). It is unnecessary to change bed linen that is clean.

Specific measures

Premedication (premed) is the term used for drugs given to the patient before leaving the ward for theatre. These drugs constitute part of the anaesthetic and are used to prepare the patient to receive a general or local anaesthetic. They are often also used to relax the patient and relieve anxiety (see Table 26.1). The 'premed' is prescribed by the anaesthetist after he has assessed the patient for the administration of the anaesthetic. The prescription may be made at a set time or 'on call', i.e. the anaesthetist will phone the ward to ask the nurse to administer the prescribed drug when he is sure how long it will take for the patient to be called to theatre.

The nurse must ensure that the consent form has been signed and that all other preoperative checks are complete before giving the premed. The patient should then be advised to rest and asked not to get out of bed unsupervised if the premed contains a strong sedative or narcotic agent.

Some patients will require very specific types of preoperative preparation as ordered by medical staff. That most commonly seen is bowel preparation prior to surgery on the gastrointestinal tract or pelvic organs. If a paralytic ileus is anticipated, or the bowel is to be opened (resulting in risk of infection), then some form of bowel preparation is usually necessary. This generally consists of oral laxatives and purgatives, or suppositories and enemas to clear the bowel, with oral antibiotics to reduce bacterial flora.

Again returning to our case histories, Mr W's anaesthetist prescribed him a sedative (diazepam 5 mg) as a premedication as he was aware that Mr W was particularly anxious. Mr W had also borrowed one of the personal stereos from the ward and was enjoying listening to a Simon and Garfunkel tape. While research into the effects of music on anxiety and postoperative pain remain inconclusive, predominantly due to a lack of studies in the area, many patients do find listening to music a helpful distracter at this stage (Good 1996).

Table 26.1 Common premedications

Drug	*Usual adult dose*	*Route*	*Effects*
Diazepam (Valium)	2–10 mg	Oral	Sedative: reduces tension and anxiety. Decreases muscle tone and potentiates non-depolarising muscle relaxants. Induces mental detachment and amnesia
Temazepam	10–20 mg	Oral	Sedative: reduces tension and anxiety. Induces drowsiness
Morphine sulphate, papaveretum[a] (Omnopon)	5–15 mg 10–20 mg	i.m. i.m.	Narcotic analgesic: induces drowsiness, reduces anxiety, induces mental detachment, respiratory depression[b], nausea[b]
Atropine	0.6 mg	i.m.	Anticholinergic: reduces smooth muscle tone, reduces bronchial and salivary secretions; blocks vagus nerve, preventing bradycardia due to vasovagal stimulation (from passage of endotracheal tube)
Hyoscine (scopolamine)	0.2–0.4 mg	i.m.	Anticholinergic: reduces smooth muscle tone, reduces bronchial and salivary secretions and blocks vasovagal stimulation (as atropine). Depresses CNS. Antiemetic. Causes restlessness and delirium in elderly patients[b]

[a]Papaveretum must not be used in women of child-bearing potential (Committee on Safety of Medicines 1991).
[b]Unwanted/undesirable effect.

Table 26.2 Preoperative checks

Criteria	*Action*	*Rationale*
Identification	Prepare two name bands with patient's full name, hospital unit number, date of birth, home address (as a minimum), plus ward and consultant Clearly note allergies on the anaesthetic sheet and on wrist bands as well as the drug Kardex Ensure site is correctly marked with indelible ink	Correct identification of patient Avoidance of all allergens Correct identification of site
Documentation	Ensure that medical notes, nursing notes, signed consent form, X-rays and anaesthetic sheet accompany patient to theatre	Ready availability of all necessary information
Fasting	Check with patient when she last had anything to eat or drink	Prevention of aspiration pneumonia
Empty bladder	Ask patient to pass urine prior to administering premed	To prevent damage to full bladder during surgery To enable complete bed rest after premed To prevent postoperative discomfort due to a full bladder
Risk of diathermy burns	Ask patient to remove all jewellery, hair pins and other items containing metal (wedding rings may be covered with tape)	To remove all metal that may concentrate the diathermy current
Prostheses	Ask patient to remove all prostheses, e.g. dentures, hearing aids, contact lenses, false eyes, glasses, etc.	To prevent harm caused by prostheses To prevent loss
Care of valuables	Offer to receive valuables into safekeeping for the patient	Patient will be away from the ward and unfit to be responsible for her valuables
Circulatory assessment	Ask patient to remove all make-up, lipstick and nail varnish	To facilitate observation of colour of skin, lips and nail beds

Theatre safety

The nurse must ensure that certain preoperative checks are carried out before the patient receives the premed and leaves the ward to go to theatre. Preoperative checks should be completed prior to administration of the premed as the results of the checks may necessitate a delay in going to theatre. Moreover, the patient should not have received sedative or narcotic agents before signing the consent form. Many hospitals have created their own checklists to complete. Examples of criteria for checklists are given in Table 26.2.

In order for patients to understand and cooperate with preoperative procedures, adequate explanation and reassurance must be given. However, the nurse should also be aware that some information might cause unnecessary distress. For example, Mrs B did not want to remove her wedding ring. The nurse offered to tape this for her, but Mrs B said that she had never taken if off and that it would be secure. The nurse did not want to frighten her by telling her that it was to protect her from being burnt by the use of electric current to seal blood vessels during the operation. Many patients would have visions of being electrocuted. Instead the nurse said that if she didn't lock all the patients' valuables away, she had to secure them with tape for security and to protect items from any antiseptics that might be spilt. Mrs B happily agreed to this and was relieved that she could continue to wear her ring.

There are some patients who greatly rely on their hearing aids and/or glasses. In such cases, glasses or hearing aids can be labelled with adhesive tape and worn by the patient until he is anaesthetised. A note should be made to this effect on the checklist or anaesthetic form.

During the immediate preoperative period, the patient may feel extremely vulnerable and afraid. She will be wearing a flimsy gown with nothing underneath; she may have removed her dentures and be unable to see well without her glasses; and she will feel drowsy from the premed. Anxiety about the impending operation can be high. It is during the immediate preoperative period that patients often feel most vulnerable and anxious, yet tend to receive minimal care (Thompson 1990). Reassurance by the nurse at this time and sometimes distraction can be helpful. Also, the patient should be encouraged to rest. Nursing Care Plan 26.1 summarises the preoperative care given to Mr W.

PERIOPERATIVE SAFETY

Caring for the patient in theatre

The patient arrives in the operating theatre accompanied by a nurse from the ward and a porter or operating department assistant (ODA). Patients may be brought to the theatre on a trolley or, in some cases, on the bed from the ward. Once the patient transfers to the theatre table the bed is taken to a holding area. The patient is

Nursing Care Plan 26.1 Preoperative care for Mr W (see Case Histories 26.1A and B)

Nursing considerations	***Action***	***Rationale***	***Evaluation***
Anxiety due to: • hospital environment • diagnosis/prognosis • anaesthesia and surgery	❐ Ensure Mr W is informed of and understands diagnosis, procedure, likely postoperative progress ❐ Provide opportunity to discuss fears and anxieties ❐ Enhance or supplement coping mechanisms (e.g. use of personal stereo)	To reduce anxiety and promote recovery	Anxiety is reduced to an acceptable level
Haemorrhage and shock*	❐ Record vital signs as baseline ❐ Encourage intake of fluids until 4 h before theatre ❐ Ensure blood tests and blood grouping completed	To make data available for postoperative comparison To maintain good fluid balance To ensure availability of blood products in case transfusion is necessary To ensure good haemoglobin status	Staff are prepared to deal with bleeding and shock is prevented
Wound infection*	❐ Have Mr W shower with Hibiscrub ❐ Provide clean theatre gown ❐ Remove hair in the groin area with depilatory (patch test should be done at preoperative visit)	To reduce skin flora To prevent obstruction of surgeon's view and prevent pain on removal of adhesive dressing	No infection occurs
Chest infection*	❐ Teach deep breathing and coughing exercises ❐ Continue to support Mr W in not smoking	To fully inflate lungs and clear stagnating secretions Patient is under stress and may return to inappropriate coping mechanisms	No infection occurs
Deep vein thrombosis*; pulmonary embolism*	❐ Teach leg exercises and stress importance of early mobilisation ❐ Fit and apply graduated compression stockings ❐ Teach deep breathing exercises (see above)	Contraction of calf muscle and graduated external compression; increase blood flow in the femoral vein and promote venous return	Thrombosis and embolism are prevented
Aspiration pneumonia*	❐ Have Mr W fast 4 h (fluids) and 6 h (food) preoperatively from 06.00 h	Stomach must be empty prior to anaesthesia; Mr W may need general anaesthetic	Vomiting is prevented
Theatre safety	❐ Complete checklist prior to administration of premed (see Table 26.2)	See Table 26.2	Patient is safely prepared for anaesthetic and surgery

* Potential problem

then transferred straight back onto her bed at the end of the operation. This reduces the discomfort of transferring from a trolley to the bed in the ward, and reduces the amount of patient lifting by nurses, porters and ODAs.

The anaesthetic or theatre nurse receiving the patient goes through the preoperative check (as in Table 26.2) again. Once this is complete, the ward nurse will usually return to the ward. If the patient is especially nervous or a little confused, it can be comforting if a nurse who knows her well can stay with her until the induction of anaesthesia. All patients must be supervised by a nurse in this pre-induction time, as the patient may have received premedication and is in an extremely stressful and unfamiliar environment. It is now common practice for theatre nurses to visit their patients preoperatively to carry out a nursing assessment and to introduce themselves and give any information required about patient care in theatre (Roberts 1991).

In emergency cases, the theatre nurse may continue the preoperative preparation. For example, Mrs B's daughter arrived at the hospital just as these preparations were being carried out. She was escorted to theatre by the A&E nurse and saw her mother for a few minutes in the anaesthetic room before she was anaesthetised. The theatre nurse briefly explained what was happening, and once her mother was asleep made a cup of tea for her daughter and let her make a phone call from the Sister's office. She then phoned the primary nurse, who sent a nursing auxiliary to bring Mrs B's daughter up to the ward where she was waiting to meet her.

The roles of the theatre staff are summarised in Box 26.1. The anaesthetist will visit the patient preoperatively in the ward, not only to assess the patient's ability to tolerate the anaesthetic, but also to introduce himself to the patient and give information and reassurance. He will also prescribe a premedication if one is to be given.

If the patient has minimally invasive surgery or investigations, e.g. colonoscopy, endoscopic retrograde cholangiopancreatography (ERCP) or cardiac catheterisation, a general anaesthetic may not be used. Instead, the patient may be sedated by drugs such as diazepam or midazolam, which also have amnesic properties — this helps the patient to be less aware of what is happening and to remember less about the procedure. In this situation, an anaesthetist may not necessarily be present but would be available should the need arise to proceed to a general anaesthetic or should other supportive treatment be required. The nurse may act as the surgeon's assistant and take part of the responsibility for monitoring the patient's condition, or some specialist nurses may conduct endoscopies independently.

In main theatres, at least two nurses as well as the anaesthetist and surgeon will be present. One nurse acts as the circulating nurse and the other is the scrub nurse. The scrub nurse wears sterile gloves and will provide instruments for the surgeons, assist where necessary and ensure safety with equipment during the operation (see Box 26.1).

The emphasis of the nursing role in theatre is on patient safety and teamwork. Each professional has an important part to play in the patient's passage through theatre. As the team members develop trust and understanding amongst themselves, it may be difficult initially for the student to appreciate the communication links in place, especially when staff have half their faces covered with a mask!

Box 26.1 The roles of the theatre staff

The anaesthetic nurse

- Receives the patient in the reception area of the anaesthetic room
- Checks patient in, deals with any irregularities
- Helps to relieve patient anxiety
- Assists in the induction (and maintenance) of anaesthesia
- Performs emergency preparation of patients for theatre
- Uses and checks anaesthetic equipment
- Maintains patient safety and comfort

The anaesthetist

- Visits the patient preoperatively:
  - — to assess fitness for anaesthesia
  - — to provide information and reassurance
  - — to prescribe a premedication
- Induces and maintains anaesthesia
- Monitors patient's condition during surgery
- Provides supportive treatment, e.g. fluid replacement, Po_2 level maintenance, correction of arrhythmias
- Initiates postoperative analgesia

The circulating nurse

- Assists with the provision of equipment
- Maintains nursing records
- Positions the patient
- Ensures safety with regard to instruments and swabs
- Cleans and sterilises equipment
- Observes, measures and records vital signs

The scrub nurse

- Positions the patient
- Provides appropriate sterile equipment
- Assists the surgeon
- Protects the patient's dignity
- Prevents diathermy and pressure injuries
- Ensures safety with regard to instruments and swabs
- Manages the high-risk patient

The recovery room nurse

- Maintains patency of the airway
- Observes patient for level of consciousness and safety
- Observes vital signs: colour, respiration, temperature (core and peripheral), pulse, blood pressure, fluid intake and output, wounds and drainage, specific checks as required
- Assesses pain and nausea and administers analgesics and antiemetics
- Reassures the patient and provides a quiet environment
- Provides total patient care
- Provides documentation and facilitates communication

Environmental safety

The environment in the operating theatre is designed to minimise the risk of exogenous infection to the patient. Some of the measures used to ensure safety are as follows:

- Clean filtered air is pumped into clean areas. Air pressure is higher inside the theatre than outside, in order to maintain an air flow from the theatre to the outside. This prevents potentially contaminated air from the rest of the hospital moving into the theatres.
- Humidity is also controlled through the ventilation system to prevent static electricity build-up and the risk of sparks, as flammable gases may be in use. Staff are required to wear antistatic shoes (clogs or boots are usually worn). All equipment must have antistatic rubber wheels or covers.

- Clean and dirty areas are delineated by doors or a line on the floor. All personnel moving into clean areas must be clean and appropriately dressed (see below). All items brought into clean areas must be clean. All dirty items leaving theatre should do so via dirty areas. It is essential that staff are aware which are the dirty and the clean areas and corridors. The use of sticky mats at the main entrance to theatre was thought to reduce contamination from the feet of staff entering theatre. This has now been shown to be ineffective and the practice should be discontinued. Similarly, the use of overshoes has been questioned, as there is a risk of contaminating the hands by handling the overshoes to take them off, which may outweigh the benefits of wearing them (Carter 1990).
- The numbers and movement of staff inside theatres are kept to an absolute minimum to reduce the number of skin scales shed and mixing of air.
- All staff entering clean areas are appropriately dressed. Clean theatre dresses or trouser suits are worn. Hair is completely covered by a bonnet-style cap and all jewellery, especially on the hands, is removed. Masks are worn inside the theatre itself to reduce airborne organisms. (Masks should be handled only by the tapes once applied, as the main fabric of the mask becomes contaminated with moisture and microorganisms which can then be transmitted on the hands.)
- Staff do not leave the theatre area when dressed in theatre clothing as the clothing can become contaminated.
- A sterile field is created around the patient. The patient and trolleys in this area are all covered with sterile drapes. The surgeon and scrub nurse wear sterile gloves and gowns to work within the sterile field.

Safety of the patient

The patient's safety in theatre is further ensured by the following precautions:

- Transfer to operating table and positioning is carried out with extreme care. The preoperative visit by the theatre nurse enables her to assess for any potential problems, especially in relation to joint mobility and the risk of developing pressure sores. Special types of pressure-relieving mattresses can be used with high-risk patients. Once patients are anaesthetised, they may lose muscle tone. Care should be taken with all limbs; for example, if the arm is left to hang over the edge of the table, irreparable damage to the brachial plexus may result. The nurse must also be aware of the risk of back pain to the patient, which may require special supports to the lower back (Rafferty 1988).
- The diathermy pad is carefully positioned. A self-adhesive pad may be used and the pad is usually placed under the buttocks or strapped to the thigh to ensure good contact over the entire surface. A poor contact by only part of the surface may concentrate the current, causing it to leave a burn.
- Swabs, needles and instruments used during theatre are counted and checked throughout and at the end of the operation by the scrub and circulating nurses. This ensures that all items used are accounted for and none left inside the patient.
- Allergies to drugs, skin antiseptics and dressings are assessed preoperatively by the theatre nurse and anaesthetist, so the use of any allergens can be avoided.
- The patient's skin is cleaned at the start of the procedure with an antiseptic solution to reduce skin flora and the risk of endogenous infection. Some surgeons also use a sterile plastic adhesive drape over the skin (Incisa-drape) through which to make the incision. This prevents the surgeons' and nurses' sterile gloves being contaminated with the patient's skin flora.
- Prophylactic antibiotics may be given (usually intravenously) during the operation, or the site of the surgery may be irrigated with an antibiotic solution. These measures are usually taken only if there is a specific risk of contamination, or if contamination from an abscess or the gastrointestinal tract is already present.
- During surgery the patient is at risk of primary haemorrhage. When an incision is made, the patient will bleed until a clot is formed or until the pressures within the vessel and the cavity into which it is bleeding have equalised. Bleeding during surgery is minimised by the use of clamps and ligatures, local pressure or diathermy to seal small vessels. Topical haemostatic agents such as cellulose and collagen may also be used. To facilitate the surgeon's vision, the site of operation is kept free of blood by swabs or suctioning. The circulating nurse may weigh the swabs to estimate blood loss and note the volume of blood in the suction bottle to estimate 'total blood loss'.
- Special procedures must be followed for the care of the patient identified as a carrier of certain infectious diseases — commonly blood-borne diseases with a high morbidity and mortality (see Ch. 11). To prevent cross-infection and to reduce risks involved with cleaning and spillages, disposable equipment may be used where possible (see Ch. 16). In many hospitals, such procedures are now followed for all patients as it is often not known whether a patient is a carrier of an infectious disease. The surgeon and scrub nurse may wear two pairs of gloves, and the patient might not be taken into the recovery room after the operation, in case of further blood loss, but recovered in theatre instead. The patient should be at the end of a theatre list to enable recovery in theatre and to allow thorough cleaning and disinfection of the theatre before it is used again.

In summary, the safety of the patient in theatre is the prime responsibility of all members of the theatre team. The Royal College of Nursing and the Medical Defence Union both have codes of practice for operating department safety; these might be consulted as further reading (National Association of Theatre Nurses 1988).

Anaesthesia

An anaesthetic is used to block any sensations of pain during surgery. It may be applied locally or regionally to the area of surgery or generally throughout the body. A brief introduction to the use of anaesthetics is given here.

For further information on anaesthesia, please consult Trounce (1997).

Local anaesthesia

Local anaesthesia blocks transmission of pain from the region operated upon. In some cases, only the sensory receptors may be blocked; this is more correctly termed local analgesia. A local anaesthetic is often combined with adrenaline to constrict blood vessels and delay absorption of the anaesthetic into the bloodstream. This reduces the amount of local anaesthetic required and prolongs its action. Types and common uses of local anaesthetics are summarised in Table 26.3. Epidural or spinal anaesthetics may be used when a general anaesthetic could be harmful or is undesirable, e.g. in elderly patients with arteriosclerosis or diabetes, in patients with respiratory disorders and in patients with

Table 26.3 Local anaesthetics

Method of administration	*Effect*	*Example of drugs and their uses*
Topical: solution or cream applied to skin or mucous membranes	Blocks local sensory nerve receptors	Lignocaine, benzocaine Minor ENT procedures Insertion of cannulae
Infiltration: injection into surgical site	Blocks local sensory nerve receptors	Lignocaine, procaine Removal of skin moles Insertion of Hickman line Drainage of abscess
Nerve block: injection close to relevant nerve trunk	Blocks conduction of sensory impulses to central nervous system	Lignocaine with adrenaline Brachial plexus procedures on the arm (Bier's block) Intercostal blocks for pain relief
Epidural: injection into space outside the dura	Blocks nerves as they enter the spinal cord	Lignocaine, bupivacaine Rectal or pelvic surgery Caesarean section
Spinal: injection into the subarachnoid space below the 2nd lumbar vertebra	Blocks preganglionic fibres (motor and sensory) Position of patient determines distribution of drug and spinal nerves affected	Bupivacaine, lignocaine Amputation Abdominal surgery

hypertension. The procedure causes hypotension and so should be avoided in patients with this condition. Care must be taken to prepare the patient psychologically in order to reduce anxiety and ensure cooperation. Psychological support continues throughout the operation and the nurse should ensure that the patient's vision of the procedure is adequately screened.

Both Mr W and Mr L were conscious during their operations. Mr W had his operation under a local anaesthetic, but Mr L had such extensive demyelinisation that he had no motor or sensory function below the waist. The anaesthetist had fully assessed the sensation around Mr L's sacrum and was satisfied that the area was already anaesthetised and Mr L would feel no pain. He did prescribe a sedative for both patients and the nursing staff ensured that their vision was screened. Both patients were reassured and informed of progress throughout the operation by the surgeon and the nurse.

General anaesthesia

General anaesthesia is characterised by loss of consciousness, analgesia and muscle relaxation. These effects occur according to the stage of anaesthesia, as follows:

Stage 1. The pain is reduced or relieved, but the patient is still conscious. Heavy sedation can produce 'dissociative anaesthesia' and some muscle relaxation, while local analgesics supplement pain control as necessary. The patient may remain drowsy but conscious throughout the procedure.

Entonox (50% oxygen with 50% nitrous oxide) can be self-administered during childbirth or painful procedures to achieve stage 1 anaesthesia for pain control. This application is discussed with other methods of pain relief in Chapter 19.

Stage 2. Consciousness is lost, but the patient may exhibit wild movements and irrational behaviour. With intravenous induction of anaesthesia, this stage is passed through very quickly and may be more in evidence when the patient is recovering from anaesthesia.

Stage 3. Breathing becomes regular and there is relaxation of the muscles along with loss of reflexes. This is the level of surgical anaesthesia. The degree of muscle relaxation required to facilitate surgery can be achieved by deepening this stage but this has undesirable side-effects such as fall in cardiac output, respiratory depression and liver damage. To overcome this problem, muscle relaxants can be administered to enable a relatively light anaesthetic to be used and so reduce the risks of anaesthesia in the elderly and those with cardiovascular and respiratory complications. This has also aided the development of day-case surgery.

Premedication can be used to relieve anxiety, induce a state of analgesia, reduce bronchial and salivary secretions, prevent vasovagal stimulation (mainly bradycardia) and make the patient less aware and somewhat drowsy. Usually, a sedative or anxiolytic is given orally, or a narcotic analgesic with an anticholinergic agent is given as an intramuscular injection (see Table 26.1).

The induction of anaesthesia is usually achieved with a short-acting intravenous agent administered with a short-acting muscle relaxant (see Tables 26.4 and 26.5). This rapidly produces surgical anaesthesia, in which the patient is unable to maintain her own airway (due to lack of reflexes) and the muscles of breathing are paralysed. An endotracheal tube is passed through the relaxed larynx and artificial ventilation is maintained throughout the operation. Anaesthesia can be maintained during surgery, usually by means of inhaled anaesthetics and a longer-acting muscle relaxant. At the end of the operation, the anaesthetic gas is discontinued and the effects of the muscle relaxant are reversed with the appropriate drug. The patient gradually regains consciousness, passing through stages 2 and 1 of anaesthesia and regaining muscle tone, which enables her to breathe independently. During this time, the patient is transferred to the recovery room.

Recovery from anaesthesia

Once surgery is completed, the patient will normally be kept in the recovery room until the immediate effects of the anaesthetic have worn off. The patient should be able to maintain her own airway and be considered stable before transfer back to the ward. In some cases the patient will be transferred directly to the intensive therapy unit while she continues to be intubated and her respiration is maintained by artificial ventilation.

Whilst the patient is still unconscious, the nurse must ensure that the airway is kept open. This can be achieved by placing the

Table 26.4 General anaesthetics

Method of administration	*Effect*	*Example of drugs and their uses*
Intravenous: for induction	Sedation, surgical anaesthesia Respiratory depression Some cause hypotension	Thiopentone, methohexitone, ketamine, propofol Induction of anaesthesia Short surgical procedures, EUA, dental extraction
Inhalation: for maintenance of anaesthesia	Surgical anaesthesia Some cause hypotension, nausea and vomiting	Halothane, nitrous oxide, isoflurane Maintenance of anaesthesia Wide range of surgical prodedures

Table 26.5 Muscle relaxants

Name of drug	*Effect*	*Use*
Suxamethonium (depolarising): binds and blocks acetylcholine receptors	Skeletal flaccid paralysis Increased K^+ release Rarely: prolonged apnoea and malignant hyperpyrexia	Short-acting (15 min) Induction, manipulations, ECT No drug available to reverse effects
Tubocurarine and pancuronium (non-depolarising) Prevents acetylcholine gaining access to receptor site	Skeletal flaccid paralysis Can cause hypotension	Longer-acting (30–45 min) Maintenance of relaxation during anaesthesia or controlled ventilation Reversed by neostigmine (anticholinesterase — raises levels of acetylcholine)

patient in a lateral or semi-prone position, tilting the head backwards and pulling the mandible forwards, or inserting a Guedal airway. If a Guedal airway is used, it can be left in position until the patient expels it spontaneously as reflexes return. There is a risk of aspiration pneumonia should the patient vomit while regaining consciousness; therefore, suction equipment must be available. Anaesthetics, muscle relaxants, narcotics and severe pain itself can cause nausea and vomiting. Pain must be adequately controlled and antiemetics may be required.

The nurse should observe the patient's level of consciousness and be aware that a stage of excitement (stage 2) may occur. Close observation and the use of side rails may be required. Many patients will be prescribed oxygen until fully awake, in order to maintain Po_2 while there is still some respiratory depression due to anaesthesia. The patient should be encouraged to commence deep breathing and leg exercises as soon as she regains consciousness.

As the patient regains consciousness, the nurse should bear in mind that hearing is usually one of the first senses to return. Verbal reassurance that the operation is over should be given. It may be appropriate to return hearing aids and spectacles at this point. The patient should be allowed to rest as quietly as possible during this period and will usually fall asleep after regaining consciousness. Close and frequent observation of vital signs is required for the early detection of changes in the patient's condition. During the recovery period the patient is especially at risk of reactionary haemorrhage as her blood pressure rises (hypotension is often induced during surgery due to anaesthetic agents). A ligature or clot may become dislodged, leading to signs of haemorrhage and hypovolaemic shock (see p. 638). Observation of wound dressings and wound drainage will also aid assessment of the patient in the recovery period.

In surgery, the patient may have had a large surface area exposed, leading to loss of body heat. Shivering will have been suppressed, due to the use of skeletal muscle relaxants. The environmental temperature in theatres is therefore kept fairly high, but patients may still have a low body temperature. As well as feeling uncomfortable, the patient may also suffer adverse effects on postoperative recovery. A drop of 2°C during colorectal surgery has been shown to triple wound infection rates and to lead to an increased length of stay (Kurz et al 1996). Extra blankets and 'space blankets' can be used, but the nurse must be wary of warming the patient too quickly, as this can lead to peripheral vasodilation and a fall in blood pressure.

Pain control begins before, or as, the patient regains consciousness. A patient such as Mr W may have the operation site infiltrated with more lignocaine at the end of surgery to provide local anaesthesia. Adrenaline may be given with the lignocaine to cause vasoconstriction and so localise the effects of the lignocaine. This type of analgesia for herniorrhaphy has been found to provide good pain control and reduce recovery time to around 3 h for day-case surgery patients (Morris 1995). The anaesthetist may also prescribe some narcotic analgesia and some simple oral analgesia for the patient's return to the ward.

Some patients may have an epidural infusion commenced at the end of the operation or, as with Mrs B, be commenced on an i.v. infusion of morphine. Some patients may be able to administer a type of i.v. infusion of a narcotic drug (patient-controlled analgesia, PCA) themselves (see p. 669). Many patients will receive their first dose of intramuscular analgesia in the recovery room. The patient's pain should be controlled before she leaves the recovery room. In a partly conscious patient, a sudden rise in blood pressure and restlessness may indicate the presence of pain. The nurse must also be aware that narcotic analgesia may cause a fall in blood pressure and respiratory depression, and that severe pain in itself can lead to shock and shallow breathing.

The patient may spend several hours in the recovery room and will, in many regards, require the same care as an unconscious patient (see Ch. 28). Most patients will require attention at least to the mouth (mucous membranes will be dry due to anticholinergic drugs, fasting and perhaps dehydration) as well as pressure area care. The recovery room nurse will document the care given and provide a summary to the ward nurse who collects the patient. In this way, continuity of care can be achieved. The role of the recovery room nurse is summarised in Box 26.1.

Nursing Care Plan 26.2 Care for Mrs B on sixth postoperative day (see Case History 26.2)

Nursing considerations	***Action***	***Rationale***	***Evaluation***
Abdominal pain	❒ Administer i.v. analgesic pump as prescribed ❒ Increase rate 30 min prior to activity as prescribed ❒ Record respiratory rate hourly ❒ Ensure that Mrs B is positioned comfortably ❒ Encourage her to support wound on moving ❒ Apply heating pad to abdomen for 'wind' pains	To prevent pain and foster recovery by enabling Mrs B to cough, exercise, rest and sleep comfortably	Mrs B is sufficiently pain-free to cooperate with therapy
Fluid and electrolyte imbalance*	❒ Administer i.v. infusion as per chart (change giving set at 24 h) ❒ Observe pulse and BP 6-hourly ❒ Observe for dyspnoea ❒ Record all fluid intake and output ❒ Observe for nausea, vomiting and diarrhoea	To detect any signs of dehydration and electrolyte imbalance early	Fluid and electrolytes maintained at satisfactory levels
Paralytic ileus	❒ Observe for passage of flatus/ faeces in stoma bag ❒ Administer antiemetics as prescribed ❒ Give oral fluids: water 60 mL/h	To detect return of normal peristalsis To prevent nausea and dehydration	Mrs B is comfortable until normal peristalsis returns
Retention of urine*	❒ Remove urinary catheter ❒ Take catheter specimen of urine for culture and sensitivity ❒ Observe urine outpu	To prevent retention of urine and related infection	Diuresis is adequate
Wound infection*	❒ Check wound daily for colour, exudate and temperature ❒ Record axillary temperature 6-hourly ❒ Observe exudate from wound drain; shorten drain according to medical staff's instructions	To detect early signs of infection and promote healing	Wound is kept free of infection
Pressure sores*	❒ Nurse Mrs B on low air loss mattress ❒ Change her position $\frac{1}{2}$-hourly in bed; do not have her lie on left shoulder ❒ When Mrs B is sitting, have her stand hourly to relieve pressure ❒ Parental nutrition as prescribed (see Ch. 21)	To prevent loss of skin integrity	Mrs B does not develop pressure sores

POSTOPERATIVE CARE

All patients require close observation during the immediate postoperative period in order to detect any complications early on. This close observation may be continued for hours or days for the patient requiring intensive nursing care, or perhaps for an hour or two if a local infiltration of anaesthetic or a very light general anaesthetic has been used. The next stage of postoperative care focuses on recovery and repair along with the active prevention of complications. Rehabilitation will be achieved at a different pace and to differing levels by each patient. The patient with a hip replacement may find that her joint pain is almost immediately reduced postoperatively and that her functional ability is far better than before the operation. Some patients may not be able to achieve the desired level of recovery and others may be aiming for palliation rather than cure.

For purposes of clarity, this section will focus on the postoperative recovery, repair and rehabilitation most commonly experienced during the hospital stay, while the next section ('Rehabilitation') focuses on continued care after discharge from hospital. It is recognised, however, that many patients will still be recovering from the effects of the anaesthetic, which can take up to 24 h to be eliminated from the body, after discharge following day surgery. Examples of postoperative care are given in Nursing Care Plans 26.2 and 26.3.

Shock and haemostasis

Shock is discussed here with specific application to the care of surgical patients. For a wider discussion of the types and mechanisms of shock and their signs and symptoms, see Chapter 18.

When the patient returns from theatre to the ward, she requires frequent observations for signs of impending shock or haemorrhage.

Nursing Care Plan 26.2 (*cont'd*)

Nursing considerations	***Action***	***Rationale***	***Evaluation***
Chest infection*	❒ Administer antibiotics as prescribed ❒ Keep Mrs B as upright as possible in bed ❒ Assist her with hourly deep breathing exercises with Triflo ❒ Assist with chest physiotherapy twice daily ❒ Encourage coughing and expectoration ❒ Observe temperature and respiration	To provide prophylaxis against infection and to prevent the build-up of secretions	No shortness of breath; sputum is clear
Deep vein thrombosis and pulmonary embolism*	❒ Assess daily for calf tenderness and inflammation ❒ Use TED stockings, full length ❒ Encourage hourly leg exercises ❒ Administer Minihep as prescribed ❒ Encourage early mobilisation, e.g. walking to toilet and back twice daily with nurse; sit out 1–2 h as able	To detect early signs of thrombus or embolus and encourage good circulation	No detection of DVT
Pain in knees and left shoulder	❒ Ensure Mrs B's position is comfortable ❒ Administer analgesia as prescribed ❒ Apply heating pad ❒ Assist with passive exercise and gentle massage	To alleviate pain and prevent stiffness	Mrs B's comfort is maintained at acceptable level
Inability to maintain own hygiene	❒ Encourage Mrs B in self-care tasks ❒ Assist with washing only for areas she cannot reach, i.e. back and lower half ❒ Assist with oral hygiene as required ❒ Encourage use of talcs and perfumes as desired ❒ Change and wash TED stockings daily ❒ Give psychological support when Mrs B changes nightclothes in view of stoma's effect on body image (see Nursing Care Plan 26.3)	To promote return to independence To help Mrs B maintain dignity	Mrs B is able to resume self-care and to cope with changed body image

* Potential problem

As blood pressure continues to rise, there is a continued risk of reactionary haemorrhage for the first 24 h. Hypovolaemic shock may also occur due to a slow, continuous loss of fluid; this might be a slowly bleeding vessel or the pooling of fluid in the gastrointestinal tract during the paralytic ileus that occurs as a consequence of surgery. The loss of fluid may be detected as soakage on the dressing or blood in the wound drains, but if the patient is bleeding into a body cavity or losing fluid into the gut it may be less obvious. Distinction should also be made between hypovolaemic and other forms of shock, i.e. cardiogenic, septic, anaphylactic and neurogenic.

Cardiogenic shock is caused essentially by failure of the heart to pump and maintain adequate cardiac output. Possible causes following surgery may be pulmonary embolus causing massive resistance to the output from the right side of the heart, fluid overload and concomitant heart failure, anaesthetic depression of cardiac output, or myocardial infarction. Patient signs and symptoms and measurement of central venous or pulmonary wedge pressures along with other vital signs can help the nurse to distinguish between hypovolaemic and cardiogenic shock.

Secondary haemorrhage can occur 1–7 days postoperatively due to vessel erosion by infection or from a long, slow bleed. The patient may collapse suddenly and will usually need to return to theatre. Fortunately, this is not a common problem.

The patient may also be at risk of neurogenic shock (usually due to severe pain), anaphylactic shock (usually due to drug reactions) and septic shock (from infections occurring following surgery).

Nursing Care Plan 26.3 Stoma care plan for Mrs B (see Case History 26.2)

Nursing considerations	***Action***	***Rationale***	***Evaluation***
Patient's lack of knowledge about her colostomy	❒ Explain the reasons for the colostomy, liaising with medical staff ❒ Assess Mrs B's level of understanding and her wish for knowledge ❒ Include Mrs B's daughter in teaching ❒ Provide a colostomy booklet for Mrs B to read and to use as a guide for teaching ❒ Give basic information about appliances ❒ Discuss the effects of colostomy on lifestyle ❒ Check Mrs B's retention of information from previous sessions	To provide a sound basis for good stoma care	Mrs B acquires an understanding of the rationale of stoma care
Anxiety about stoma formation and change in body image	❒ Encourage Mrs B to voice fears; provide reassurance in the form of accurate information ❒ Introduce Mrs B to a suitable visitor with a colostomy ❒ Support Mrs B in her grief, provide privacy, passive listening, counselling, touch ❒ Provide support for daughter	To provide an outlet for anxiety	Mrs B is better able to adjust to her new situation
Lack of skill and confidence to care for the colostomy	❒ Implement the following stages: • encourage Mrs B to look at stoma; give reassurance • show her how to check and clean stoma, then supervise as she does this • discuss the range of appliances available, and guide her in making a suitable choice • show Mrs B how to fit appliance and teach skin care • encourage her to fit appliance under supervision and to check and clean stoma independently • encourage her to care for stoma independently	To build confidence by helping Mrs B to succeed at each stage	Mrs B achieves independence in colostomy care
Inability to cope with the stoma at home*	❒ Refer Mrs B to a community stoma nurse at least 1 week prior to discharge ❒ Give advice and information on the following as appropriate: diet; fluid and electrolyte balance; alcohol consumption; clothing; prescriptions; flatus control; disposal of appliances; travel; pursuing hobbies and interests; intimate relationships; local colostomy association; attitudes of loved ones ❒ Provide on discharge: supply of equipment; prescription care; prescription exemption form	To prepare Mrs B for her discharge home	The transition from hospital to home care is smooth; Mrs B feels that she is able to cope

* Potential problem

The aim of nursing observations in the first 24 h following surgery is to detect changes that might indicate the initial stages of compensation to hypovolaemic shock. As the circulating volume falls, the nurse may see increased loss of blood on dressings or in wound drainage bags or bottles. There will be a slight rise in heart rate to maintain cardiac output but no change or a slight rise in systolic blood pressure. Peripheral vasoconstriction to conserve blood supply to vital organs (brain, heart, lungs, liver, kidneys) may lead to a clammy, sweaty appearance. The vasoconstriction of the veins maintains diastolic (end) volume and therefore increases stroke volume. This, along with increased cardiac contractility, maintains blood pressure to at least pre-shock levels. As the brain is extremely sensitive to hypoxia, the patient may also appear restless.

If the blood or fluid loss continues, then these mechanisms may eventually fail to compensate effectively. There may then be further vasoconstriction of the arterioles to increase peripheral resistance. There is also reduced parasympathetic activity to increase heart rate and stroke volume, resulting in increased cardiac output. At this point the heart rate increases further and blood pressure begins to fall. Urine output decreases rapidly (due to decreased renal perfusion over and above the effects of increased antidiuretic hormone (ADH) and aldosterone; see p. 636) as blood flow is conserved to maintain the brain, heart and lungs as a priority. The patient appears breathless, centrally cyanosed and may be quite confused due to hypoxia. The signs and symptoms of the initial compensation and failing compensation are summarised in Box 26.2.

Shock must be detected at the first level of compensation and not when the classic picture of the falling blood pressure and rising pulse occurs and a crisis ensues. If a patient is allowed to continue at the first level of compensation, all but the vital organs will be deprived of oxygen and newly anastomosed tissue will have an increased tendency to breakdown and infection due to prolonged vasoconstriction and hypoxia.

The nurse should report any significant changes to the nurse in charge of the patient's care, who may then decide to call in the medical staff. Actions to correct shock must be taken swiftly and must be appropriate to the type of shock diagnosed. Raising the foot of the bed to aid venous return could have disastrous effects in patients undergoing gastrointestinal surgery. If there is bleeding or large volumes of fluid due to paralytic ileus or obstruction in the abdomen, these contents would fall against the diaphragm, impeding respiratory and cardiac function.

Aggressive fluid replacement in elderly patients can lead to heart failure, arrhythmias and cardiogenic shock. Needless to say, increasing the i.v. infusion rate would not help to maintain circulating volume.

Once the doctor has assessed the patient, oxygen therapy may well be started or increased to reduce hypoxia. In hypovolaemic shock the lost fluid must be replaced or returned to the circulation. Some patients may have large amounts of fluid available in the body — as in paralytic ileus or peripheral oedema — but in the wrong body compartment. This fluid can be drawn back into the circulation by treating the cause and by raising the osmotic pressure of the circulation.

Crystalline fluids can be given intravenously but are soon lost from the circulation. Plasma protein substitutes (PPS, Gelofusine or Haemaccel) can be given as plasma expanders. These raise the osmotic pressure and draw extracellular fluid into the circulation. Interstitial fluid also moves into the capillaries as hydrostatic pressure falls in response to lowered blood pressure and arteriolar constriction. In haemodynamic shock, rapid transfusion of blood may be required and should be given through a blood warmer. Central venous pressure measurements are of great value in assessing the volume of blood returning to the heart and the heart's ability to pump (see Ch 18). A central venous line may be inserted as an emergency in a patient whose shock proves difficult to manage. Nursing Care Plan 26.4 illustrates the type of nursing care required to detect the early signs of shock.

Box 26.2 Signs and symptoms of shock, by stages

Initial compensation

- Appears sweaty, clammy, pale
- Peripheral cyanosis
- Appears restless; may complain of feeling generally unwell
- Falling urine output but may remain above 30 mL/h
- Increase in pulse rate
- Slight rise in systolic blood pressure
- Increased soakage of blood on wound dressings and in wound drains

Failing compensation

- Appears cold, sweaty
- Central cyanosis
- Appears confused, often agitated, and then increasingly drowsy
- Urine output falls below 30 mL/h
- Tachycardia
- Fall in blood pressure
- Large volumes of blood may be lost

Fluid balance

Most patients experience some loss of fluid during surgery which may be compounded by electrolyte disturbances resulting from the illness itself or trauma during surgery. Preoperative dehydration due to excessive fasting should be avoided (see p. 808). Patients having a general anaesthetic will be fasted postoperatively until they are fully conscious and the cough and swallowing reflexes have returned. Some may be required to fast for longer than this when there is a paralytic ileus or after facial or laryngeal surgery. These patients require fluid and electrolyte replacement via the i.v. route to meet normal demands (some require over and above this volume to replace fluid lost at theatre).

Fluid balance can be significantly affected by the physiological response of the body to the stress of surgery. Glucocorticoid secretion increases reabsorption of sodium and water in the renal nephrons with a reciprocal loss of potassium and hydrogen ions. Elevated levels of antidiuretic hormone (ADH) also increase water reabsorption and high aldosterone levels increase sodium reabsorption further. The net effect is to increase the extracellular fluid volume and reduce urine output. Consequently, it would not be unusual for a well-hydrated patient to retain fluid and have a high positive fluid balance for the immediate postoperative period (Bove 1994).

As a result of trauma to the tissues during surgery, the intracellular electrolyte potassium is released. This is excreted in part exchange for retained sodium. Potassium levels will be closely monitored by medical staff in patients who have undergone major surgery and appropriate replacement with i.v. fluids given.

Many surgical patients complain of thirst and a dry mouth postoperatively. This is due partly to dehydration and partly to the anticholinergic drugs given during the operation to reduce salivary

Nursing Care Plan 26.4 Immediate postoperative care plan for M (see Case History 26.4(A) and 26.3(B))

Nursing considerations	***Action***	***Rationale***	***Expected outcome***
Shock due to haemorrhage and pain*	❒ Observe TPR and BP $\frac{1}{2}$-hourly ❒ Observe for pallor, sweating and confusion ❒ Record urine output hourly ❒ Give O_2 therapy at 4 L /min as prescribed ❒ Implement pain control (see below) ❒ Check wound and drains $\frac{1}{2}$-hourly ❒ Maintain circulatory volume as prescribed	To ensure pulse is maintained at 65–90, BP at 100/65 to 140/95, urine output at ≥30 mL/h	Shock does not develop
Abdominal pain	❒ Provide patient-controlled analgesia as prescribed ❒ Record respiratory rate hourly ❒ Assess effectiveness of analgesia using appropriate assessment tool ❒ Ensure comfortable positioning ❒ Encourage M to support wound while moving	To control pain and enable deep breathing exercises to be performed	Pain is kept at an acceptable level
Fluid and electrolyte imbalance*	❒ Provide i.v. infusion as per chart; change giving set after 24 h ❒ Observe for dyspnoea, irregularities in CVS ❒ Record all fluid intake and output ❒ Observe for nausea, vomiting and diarrhoea	To maintain circulatory volume	Fluid and electrolytes maintained at satisfactory levels
Paralytic ileus	❒ Allow nil by mouth, provide oral hygiene hourly ❒ NG tube, free drainage: aspirate hourly ❒ Observe for flatus ❒ Administer antiemetics as prescribed	To accommodate loss of normal peristalsis To detect return of peristalsis	M is comfortable until peristalsis returns
Loss of bladder tone	❒ Observe and record urine output; urinary catheter with 10 mL balloon inserted in theatre ❒ Perform catheter care morning and evening ❒ Maintain asepsis of closed drainage system	To prevent urinary retention and infection	Diuresis satisfactory Urinary tract does not develop infection

secretions. Until the effects of the anaesthetic have worn off fully, thirst is therefore an unreliable measure of hydration.

Metabolic and stress responses

Surgery and general anaesthesia are major stressors which result in the 'general adaptation syndrome' (Selye 1976). The psychological effects of stress are often seen as anxiety and withdrawal in surgical patients and are addressed in detail in Chapter 17. The importance of adequate preoperative education and counselling in minimising stress is discussed on page 805.

The physiological effects of stress can be reduced by controlling anxiety preoperatively and continuing this postoperatively.

In the immediate postoperative period (and up to 4 days after a major operation) the patient utilises protein as a source of energy along with fats and carbohydrates. The amino acids act as a source of glucose for the brain. Blood glucose levels can be elevated, resulting in glycosuria. This will be a cause for concern and careful monitoring in diabetic patients and in those receiving parenteral nutrition. It is important that patients are in a nutritional state sufficient to withstand this period of catabolism and negative nitrogen balance. The loss of nitrogen can also be reduced by administration of an amino acid solution (e.g. Vamin) but requires administration of glucose as an energy source to allow amino acids to be used for protein synthesis. This solution is similar to that used in parenteral nutrition but omits lipids. It contains less glucose and can be administered peripherally. If the patient has a poor nutritional status, and/or is undergoing major surgery with or without prolonged fasting, parenteral nutrition is generally indicated.

Most patients can tolerate catabolism and some starvation for approximately 1 week after major surgery (Canizaro 1981). Many become anabolic after a couple of days and begin to rebuild proteins, while hormones released in stress decrease. A large diuresis and negative fluid balance may be seen at this point. Chapter 21 describes nursing interventions to improve the nutritional status of the patient and provides a complete discussion of parenteral nutrition.

Nursing Care Plan 26.4 (*cont'd*)

Nursing considerations	***Action***	***Rationale***	***Expected outcome***
Wound infection*	❒ Check wound and drains ½-hourly ❒ Do not disturb dressing until 48 h postoperatively ❒ Observe vaginal loss twice daily	To promote healing and prevent infection	Wound begins to heal normally
Pressure sores*	❒ Change M's position according to comfort needs and prior to hyperaemia of skin ❒ Observe for reddening of pressure areas ❒ Ensure skin is clean and dry ❒ Use Spenco mattress	To safeguard skin integrity	M does not develop pressure sores
Deep vein thrombosis and pulmonary embolism*	❒ Administer Minihep as prescribed ❒ Use TED stockings below knee ❒ Assist with leg exercises hourly ❒ Have patient sit out for bed-making on first morning postop	To encourage good circulation, especially venous return	No thrombosis or embolism
Chest infection*	❒ Nurse M as upright as possible ❒ Assist with deep breathing exercises hourly ❒ Encourage coughing and expectoration ❒ Assist with chest physiotherapy	To prevent build-up of secretions and resulting infection	Chest remains clear
Inability to maintain own hygiene	❒ Assist M to wash and change into own nightclothes when appropriate ❒ Provide bed bath with complete assistance on first day postop ❒ Provide oral hygiene as required ❒ Change and wash TED stockings daily	To assist M in maintaining dignity and regaining independence	M's comfort and hygiene maintained
Anxiety about outcome of surgery	❒ Reassure M about the outcome of the operation ❒ Repeat information as required if she is drowsy post-anaesthetic	To reduce anxiety	M is encouraged about prospects for the future

* Potential problem

Pain

In 1990 a study reported that 75% of surgical patients suffered severe pain (Royal College of Surgeons 1990). Six years later, Field (1996) found that nurses consistently underrated patients' postoperative pain and made little use of pain assessment tools. Despite advances in pain management technology, it would appear that progress has been slow, as acute pain services remain underdeveloped and underfunded (Davies 1996). While thoracic and abdominal operations tend to cause the most pain, minor procedures can also cause severe pain. Firth (1991) found that 53% of patients having day surgery suffered moderate to excruciating pain. Being in pain was rated as the most anxiety-provoking issue for surgical patients (Biley 1989). Clearly, postoperative pain deserves close attention in nursing practice, research and education. The issues relating to pain specifically in the postoperative period are discussed here. The reader is also referred to Chapter 19, where broader but equally pertinent issues are addressed.

Pain control after surgery is a prime concern on humanitarian grounds alone. It also has significant effects on other aspects of the patient's recovery. Good pain control also allows for early activity, so minimising problems of immobility such as chest infections, urinary tract infections, deep vein thrombosis, pressure sores and muscle wasting. Pain after surgery has also been cited as one of the main reasons for poor sleep (Closs 1992). Elderly patients are at an increased risk of the complications described above. It should not be assumed that they have higher pain thresholds, but they may receive slightly lower doses of analgesics as their clearance and metabolism of analgesics are slower. Accurate and systematic assessment of pain is essential. Seers (1987) found that nurses in her study consistently underestimated the intensity of patients' postoperative pain, stating: 'Patients' ratings of pain cannot be predicted by the type of operation or time since surgery'.

One source of controversy in pain management concerns the assessment of pain as part of the diagnostic process. The nature of the pain (especially in abdominal pain) is an important diagnostic sign, which often results in medical staff withholding analgesics until a full assessment and provisional diagnosis have been arrived at. The nurse then has to deal with the complaints or signs of obvious and sometimes severe pain from the patient while the doctor refuses to prescribe analgesics. The need for urgent examination of the patient followed by administration of a short-acting analgesic such as pethidine or Entonox should be stressed.

Meanwhile, the nurse will require all his skills to comfort and reassure the patient physically and emotionally and will need to be assertive in ensuring that medical staff are kept fully informed of the patient's condition.

Postoperative pain can vary according to the site of the incision, being greater with midline, subcostal and intercostal incisions (see Fig. 26.5). The small incisions made by laparoscopes usually cause the least discomfort.

Controlling pain in the immediate postoperative period is the responsibility of the anaesthetist. The anaesthetist visits the patient preoperatively and will usually discuss pain control with her. This not only reduces one of the patient's main anxieties, but also allows the anaesthetist to make a full assessment of that individual's needs. Narcotic analgesics are the mainstay of postoperative pain control. Some commonly used analgesics are given in Table 26.6. Intramuscular injection is the most commonly used method of administration, but is not always the most effective. The patient must understand that the drug is not absorbed to therapeutic levels immediately, so she will need to be informed to ask for analgesia as the pain starts to build up. Otherwise, she may wait until the pain is unbearable (suffering the ill-effects of this pain) and continue to suffer for a further 15–20 minutes until the injection takes effect. Prompt administration is essential with this method to prevent long periods of severe pain. Plasma drug levels can vary enormously and drugs are often short-lived, requiring administration every 4 h or so. Nurses should bear in mind that patients may fear the discomfort of the injection itself.

Some newer methods of pain control aim to prevent such large fluctuations in plasma levels. Continuous infusions of narcotic agents can be given through the intravenous, subcutaneous or epidural routes. Intravenous infusion can be advantageous as it enables the rate of infusion to be altered immediately, according to the patient's respiratory rate, as narcotic drugs may depress respirations if too large a dose is given. Patient-controlled analgesia (PCA) allows the patient to control the administration of small boluses of intravenous narcotic. A special infusion pump is set to give a specific volume of solution (and therefore a set dosage according to the dilution of the drug) when the patient presses a hand-held button. The machine is programmed to provide a bolus only after a certain length of time has elapsed (lockout) and a maximum total number of boluses over a time period. PCA can be very effective with a cooperative patient. Mackintosh & Bowles (1997) found that patients using PCA postoperatively gained significantly greater relief of pain than those receiving intramuscular injections.

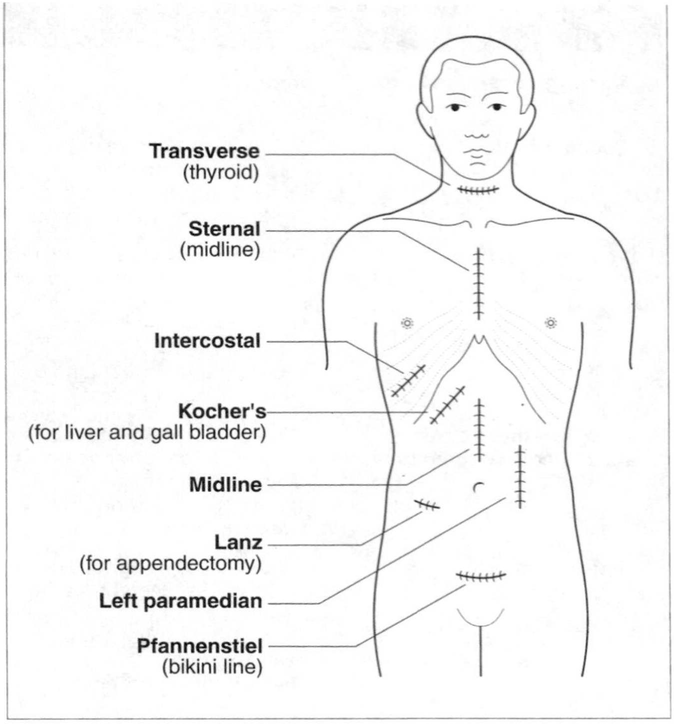

Fig. 26.5 Some incision lines used in surgery.

All narcotic agents have similar side-effects, i.e. central nervous system and cardiovascular depression, and can lead to addiction. Some may induce nausea and vomiting (see Trounce 1997 for further detail). Fear of respiratory depression and of causing

Table 26.6 Analgesics commonly used in postoperative pain control[a]

Method of administration	*Example of dug used*	*Example of types of surgery*
Epidural infusion	Bupivacaine and lignocaine	Major pelvic or lower abdominal, e.g. colectomy
Intravenous or subcutaneous infusion	Diamorphine, papaveretum[b] (Omnopon)	Major pelvic or abdominal, e.g. gastrectomy
Intramuscular injection	Morphine sulphate, pethidine, papaveretum[b], codeine	Many types, e.g. total hip replacement Specifically used in neurosurgery
Nerve blocks and local anaesthetic	Lignocaine with adrenaline	Thoracic surgery, wound areas can be infiltrated after surgery
Sublingual	Buprenorphine	Many types of major and minor surgery
Oral	Meptazinol, diclofenac sodium (Voltarol), co-proxamol, co-dydramol, paracetamol	Many products are available Used in continued recovery and rehabilitation or alone after minor surgery

[a]For further reading see Trounce (1990).
[b]Papaveretum must not be used in women of child-bearing potential (Committee on Safety of Medicines 1991).

Table 26.7 Some specific causes of postoperative pain and discomfort

Cause	*Suggested nursing action*
Joint, neck and back pain and stiffness	Prevent overextension of the neck at intubation point. Exert care in assessment and positioning of patients with rheumatoid arthritis and osteoarthritis. Assist with frequent change of position and passive exercises. Administer analgesics (NSAIDs can be given as suppositories as well as orally). Provide massage, heat pads.
Anastomatic leak (in GI surgery)	Observe for signs and symptoms of peritonitis, gradual or sudden onset of abdominal pain and shock, pyrexia, shallow breathing, abdominal distension, obvious change in drain output. Alert nurse in charge of the patient and/or medical staff immediately.
Nasogastric (NG) tube	Keep nasal passages clean, lubricate with petroleum jelly. Ensure tape is secure, clean and does not obscure view. Support the weight of the tube and/or bag by taping or pinning it to nightclothes (this also helps to prevent the tube being pulled out by sudden movement). Pass NG tubes while the patient is under anaesthetic where possible.
Wound drains	Wound drains with softer tubes cause less pain. Sudden or severe pain at a drain site should be reported. (In case of anastomatic leak or haemorrhage, relieve weight of drainage bags by regular emptying, if appropriate). Secure drains well with tape to prevent pulling on the securing suture. Label tubes if there is more than one. (The exit may become obscured from view by securing tape.) Provide analgesia cover prior to drain removal. Encourage patient to use relaxation techniques to reduce muscle tension.
Sutures, clips, staples	Sutures should not normally be a cause of pain. Deep tension sutures, wounds under tension (e.g. perianal) or clips catching on nightclothes can cause discomfort. Check wounds daily for signs of infection. Teach patient to support wound when coughing and moving. Cover clips with a light dressing to prevent catching. Provide reassurance and encourage use of relaxation techniques on suture removal.
Dressing changes	These should not be painful for the vast majority of patients, provided good practice is followed. Irrigate wounds with warm saline to clean and use non-adherent wound care products. Wounds tend to become painful when granulating, as nerve endings are exposed. Any adherent dressings should be soaked to aid removal. Excess hair should be removed at operation site prior to surgery (see p. 809). Analgesics ranging from paracetamol to a general anaesthetic may be required for some dressings. Entonox can be extremely useful in providing short-acting pain relief during dressing changes.
Urinary retention	Observe urine output in uncatheterised patients having pelvic or abdominal surgery, or reduced mobility postoperatively. (Urinary catheters should be inserted in theatre if their need can be predicted.) Observe for a palpable bladder and rising blood pressure. (These signs may also be present in a catheterised patient if the catheter blocks up; measurement of specific gravity of the urine indicates if urine output is truly falling as urine becomes more concentrated.) Ensure privacy and comfortable positioning of patient when bedpans or bottles are being used. Discuss continued retention with medical staff and perform residual catheterisation if necessary, leaving the catheter in situ. Blocked catheters should be irrigated or changed. (See Ch. 24 for care of patients with urinary catheters.)
Colic and wind	When the patient's paralytic ileus is resolving strong pains and spasmodic muscle contractions may be experienced. Pockets of gas may also have collected in the GI tract and may cause distension. Early and frequent mobilisation can reduce these pains. With approval of medical staff, peppermint water can be given, or, if appropriate, peppermint oil can be used in aromatherapy. Antispasmodic drugs are not usually prescribed, as they can cause a return of the ileus and constipation. Heat pads and gentle massage (by experienced hands) can be helpful.

addiction often leads to doctors underprescribing and nurses underadministering. Seers (1987) found that 85% of nurses in her study overestimated the risk of addiction to narcotic analgesics. The major narcotic agents (except buprenorphine) can be reversed with naloxone should respiratory depression occur. It should also be remembered that respiration will in fact be hindered by inadequate pain control (see p. 821). Addiction is unlikely when narcotics are administered only in the postoperative period.

The variety of causes of postoperative pain and discomfort and the wide range of nursing interventions available (see Table 26.7 and Case Histories 26.1(B), 26.3(B) and 26.4(B)) clearly demonstrate that the nurse has a key role to play in alleviating postoperative pain. Primary nursing may also improve the quality of care in postoperative pain, as one experienced nurse and his team of associates can get to know the patient well. Detailed knowledge of the patient and her reaction to pain assists in planning and evaluating care, while the close relationship between nurse and patient instils trust and confidence. This not only reassures the patient, but also has a placebo effect that supplements the analgesia administered.

The therapeutic contribution of the nurse in relation to pain control is fully addressed in Chapter 19. The nurse's knowledge base with regard to pain assessment, measurement and relief, his assertiveness and communication skills, his knowledge of the psychological impact of surgery and pain, and his use of complementary therapies such as relaxation and massage are all vital elements of his ability to provide effective postoperative pain control.

Case History 26.1(B) **Mr W (cont'd from Case History 26.1(A), p. 000)**

Mr W had had his incision site for inguinal hernia repair infiltrated with lignocaine at the end of the operation. He did not experience any pain on return to the ward and was up and about that evening. He had some difficulty with lower back stiffness and pain, but found some relief from a gentle back massage by an associate of the primary nurse who had taken a course in this technique. She also used some aromatherapy oils to help him relax and get to sleep that evening. Mr W did not require any analgesia until the following morning, when he took some co-proxamol before getting up. After being seen by medical staff he got ready to go home. He had already bought some paracetamol to take at home as instructed in his preadmission booklet.

Case History 26.3(B) **Mr L (cont'd from Case History 26.3(A), p. 000)**

Mr L had no sensory perception in his lower back or perianal area, and therefore experienced no pain from the wound. He did, however, experience some considerable discomfort from the removal of the Elastoplast securing his i.v. cannula. A large piece of tape had been stuck onto his very hairy arm. Fortunately, the tape was not waterproof and could be soaked with plaster remover to dissolve the adhesive. The primary nurse shaved his arm around the new cannula and applied a sterile dressing film. She also made a mental note to mention the incident to the house officer responsible for the previous cannula dressing.

Case History 26.4(B) **M (cont'd from Case History 26.4(A), p. 000)**

M had had a couple of operations over the last few years for her Crohn's disease. She did not like having injections to control the pain and had become more frightened and anxious about pain with each operation. The anaesthetist decided she would be a good candidate for patient-controlled analgesia (PCA) and spent some time teaching her about this preoperatively. M kept her infusion until she was able to manage her pain control with a simple compound analgesic. She made a quick postoperative recovery and said she had experienced far less pain than with her previous operations. She had also felt reassured that pain relief would be there as soon as she needed it.

Nausea and vomiting

These problems are now less common, as modern-day anaesthetics have fewer side-effects than drugs used formerly. However, some patients will experience nausea and vomiting due to inadequate pain relief, as a side-effect of narcotic analgesia or due to the collection of secretions in the stomach. The premedication atropine (see Table 26.1, p. 802) reduces gastric motility and can slow stomach emptying. Paralytic ileus can lead to the accumulation of a large quantity of gastrointestinal secretions. Some patients may have some bleeding into the stomach postoperatively which can induce nausea (e.g. in partial gastrectomy). Patients who have a history of travel sickness or migraine are also more likely to suffer postoperative nausea and vomiting (Blinkthorne 1995).

Phillips & Gill (1993) found that postoperative nausea and vomiting can be reduced by the use of acupressure bands on the wrist. Patients who wore the bands not only reported less sickness, but also required significantly fewer doses of antiemetics.

Sleep

Research has demonstrated that surgical patients have greatly disrupted sleep patterns (Closs 1992). In addition to the factors affecting the sleep of all hospital patients, surgical patients are exposed to many others. Pain, general discomfort and restricted positioning can cause disturbed sleep. Postoperative patients may experience hypoxia and hypercapnia due to anaesthetic sedation or shock severely compromising CNS control of sleep (see Ch. 25).

In the postoperative period, frequent observations and recordings are necessary, often into the first postoperative night. These disturbances, along with the general noise generated by procedures, new admissions and emergency action necessary at night, all add to the disruption of patients' sleep. Sleep is especially important for the postoperative patient as protein synthesis takes place predominantly during sleep and rest. Growth hormone is secreted during periods of REM sleep. Sleep and rest are essential not only for a feeling of well-being but also for anabolism and tissue repair.

Pain control and general comfort measures are paramount in promoting a good night's sleep. Pulse oximeters can be useful to indicate hypoxia at night in vulnerable patients; however, they require careful use to prevent undue disturbance. Nursing observations should be minimised to safe levels and noise reduced where possible.

Elimination

Constipation is a common problem which arises as a consequence of immobility, the use of narcotic analgesics and dehydration. Conversely, diarrhoea can occur as postoperative paralytic ileus resolves. Patients may experience colicky pain due to flatus and muscle spasm; this can be reduced by increasing mobility and administering peppermint water (see Table 26.7). Ensuring adequate hydration and early mobilisation help prevent constipation before it becomes necessary to resort to oral laxatives. Diarrhoea following paralytic ileus will resolve spontaneously in a couple of days. Oral fluids and diet may be introduced gradually to prevent nausea and vomiting.

Urinary retention may occur due to immobility or the relaxation of bladder muscle tone by anaesthesia, or as the result of paralytic ileus following abdominal or pelvic surgery. When urinary retention is anticipated, the patient should be catheterised in theatre to minimise discomfort. Otherwise, patients should be given the opportunity for privacy and assistance to assume a normal position to pass urine where possible. If retention leads to distension of the bladder and discomfort, or is a cause for concern, a residual catheterisation may be done. The catheter can then be left in situ should the residual exceed approximately 300 mL.

Once the paralytic ileus resolves (as detected by return of bowel sounds or passage of flatus or faeces), the urinary catheter is usually removed. If the catheter is used for monitoring in haemodynamic shock, or in retention due to immobility, it can be removed when monitoring is no longer required or the patient is mobile enough to pass urine successfully.

Use of urinary catheters should be avoided where possible due to the associated risk of infection (Winn 1996). The postoperative patient may also be at risk of urinary infection without catheterisation, as a result of immobility. A small volume of concentrated urine will remain in the bladder for prolonged periods, providing a medium for the growth of bacteria.

Following some surgical procedures on the bladder, continued blood loss and clot formation may obstruct the urethra. To prevent this, patients are catheterised with a three-way catheter (sometimes called a 'triple lumen') and continuous irrigation given to the bladder to wash out potentially obstructing clots or debris.

Wound care

Wound care is given with the aim of promoting healing and minimising the risk of infection (see Nursing Care Plan 26.4). Methods of promoting healing depend very much on the individual patient's circumstances. Factors that need to be considered, especially with the surgical patient, are prolonged hypoxia due to shock, dehydration or local pressure; protein calorie malnutrition; and the local wound dressing. Factors to be considered in all patients with regard to wound healing are discussed in Chapter 23. Prevention of infection begins in the preoperative period with reduction of anxiety and skin and bowel preparation (see p. 809). Asepsis in theatre reduces the threat of exogenous infection (see p. 812). The use of wound drains, prophylactic antibiotics and aseptic technique, along with precautions against haematomas, will help to reduce wound infections postoperatively. However, some patients will be more at risk of infection than others, depending on the type of surgery and on exposure to endogenous bacteria (see Table 26.8).

In the immediate postoperative period, the wound and any drains to the operation site must be checked frequently for signs of bleeding. To assess the degree of soakage on a wound dressing, a ballpoint or felt-tipped pen can be used to mark the margin of the soakage. Any advancing margin of soakage can then be easily detected. Volume markings on drainage bottles and bags give a clear indication of the amount of blood or fluid lost (large volumes of bloodstained fluid may be due to the fluid used to wash out a cavity but this should still be reported). Wound dressings should not be changed as they become soaked with blood; instead, fresh pads should be added on top to promote clot formation under both dressings. To disturb dressings on the first or second postoperative day also increases the risk of infection.

The aim of wound drains is to drain blood and inflammatory exudate, to prevent haematoma formation and to give an indication of blood loss. Some drains may have suction applied to collapse the space left in the tissues after an operation. Drains can also indicate when an anastomosis has broken down (discharging blood, digestive or faeculent fluid) and when an abscess has resolved (cessation of discharge of pus). Some examples of the more common types of wound drain are given in Figure 26.6.

To prevent infection, the entry site should be dressed aseptically and a closed drainage system maintained. If bags or bottles need to be changed (when the vacuum is lost or the receptacle is full or heavy) then asepsis should be maintained and sterile equipment used. The decision to remove the drain is made by the doctor when there is minimal or no further drainage. Non-vacuum drains may be shortened before removal to encourage the space left behind to collapse and granulate. Otherwise a cavity might be left that could fill with fluid and give rise to an abscess. Before a drain is removed, the patient will require an explanation and reassurance, and often analgesic cover. Vacuum drains should have their suction released and securing sutures will need to be removed. Relaxation exercises can help to reduce the patient's anxiety and muscle tension. Drains that do not move smoothly may be eased by rotating the tube slightly. Traction should not be applied to drains if they are stuck. Such cases must be referred to the medical staff.

Drains that are shortened require securing to prevent them falling back into the patient as the securing suture has been removed. A large, sterile safety pin can be passed through the tube to prevent this from occurring. As the weight of a Penrose drain may pull out the entire length of the tube, these are usually cut and a pin inserted through the end of the tube, which is then sealed inside a drainage bag applied over the drain site (see Fig. 26.6D). This also enables the patient to be more mobile, as a long drainage bag is not needed. Furthermore, it is often more comfortable as the extra weight of the long tube is removed.

After the first 24 h, the wound and drains should be checked for signs of infection. As stated previously, wound dressings should not be disturbed for the first 48 h to reduce the risk of infection. However, most infections typically do not appear until at least 3 days postoperatively. Regular temperature monitoring may also detect signs of infection. Patients discharged home within the first 2 days after an operation should be taught how to recognise a wound infection and know whom to report it to. Community and practice nurses may continue checks on patients with wounds who have been discharged home early.

After 48 h, wounds healing by 'primary intention' have laid down a top layer of epithelium across the top of the wound. The wound is effectively sealed from exogenous infection and may be exposed to air, which also allows for easy observation. Dressings are not necessary unless the patient has clips or staples that may

Table 26.8 Risk of infection in different types of surgery[a]

Type of surgery	*Percentage of patients with infected wounds (% risk)*	*Example of types of operation*
Clean: hollow organs not opened, no preoperative inflammation or infection	2–5%	Inguinal hernia repair, mastectomy, total hip replacement
Clean contaminated: hollow organs (not bacteriologically clean, e.g. respiratory and urinary tract) opened	5–10%	Transurethral resection of prostate, pneumonectomy, elective cholecystectomy
Contaminated: in areas known to be heavily contaminated, e.g. lower GI tract or in the presence of infection	10–50%	Large bowel surgery, traumatic wounds, abscesses

[a]For further reading see Hare & Cooke (1991), Ayliffe et al (1993) and Richold (1990).

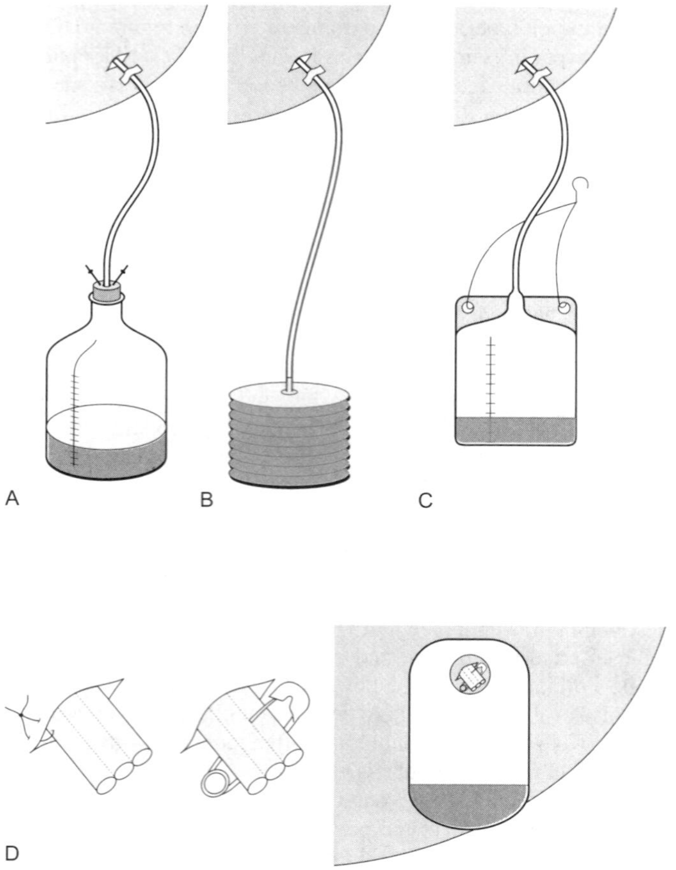

Fig. 26.6 Some types of wound drain. A: Redivac drain (prongs come together as vacuum is lost). B: Concertina-type drain. C: Simple tube/Penrose drain. D: Corrugated drain: secured by a suture and then a safety pin as the drain is shortened to prevent it from falling back into the patient. Fluid drains down the channels and into a bag.

catch on clothing or there is continued discharge from the wound. Some wounds may be left to heal by 'secondary intention' due to lack of tissue to close the wound or to the presence of infection in the tissues where closure may well lead to abscess formation. Care of these types of wounds is discussed in Chapter 23.

Wounds heal at different rates according to growth rate and blood supply of the local tissues and the patient's general physical condition (see Box 26.3). Clips would be removed from a thyroidectomy incision line at 2–3 days postoperatively, whereas Mrs B's abdominal sutures were not removed until 12 days postoperatively. There is an increasing trend towards the use of absorbable continuous sutures where good healing is expected. This is especially useful when the patient is to be discharged home in the first few days. Most patients are also relieved to hear that they do not have sutures to be removed. Some types of sutures and their removal are shown in Fig. 26.7. Patients discharged home with non-absorbable sutures in situ may be referred to the community or practice nurse for their removal.

Potential complications

Virtually all surgical patients will be at some risk of developing deep vein thrombosis (DVT), pulmonary embolism (PE), chest infection and atelectasis. Prevention is the mainstay of care and is described on pages 807–808. Preventive measures such as leg and breathing exercises, thromboembolic deterrent (TED) stockings and subcutaneous heparin are all continued throughout the postoperative recovery. Early mobilisation contributes significantly to the prevention of not only the complications just mentioned, but also the risks of immobility to which many patients are exposed. Mrs B's care exemplifies the type of proactive preventive measures required (see Nursing Care Plan 26.3).

Box 26.3 Examples of factors that may predispose patients to delayed wound healing

Mrs B (see Case History 26.2)

- High risk of wound infection due to:
  —perforated bowel
  —unprepared bowel
- Anaemia (preoperative)
- Malnutrition (preoperative) and fasting (postoperative)
- Prolonged shock (postoperative)
- Immunosuppression (due to cancer and prolonged stress)
- Lack of preoperative skin preparation
- Age

M (See Case History 26.4(A) and 26.4(B))

- Steroid therapy (pre- and postoperative)
- Contamination of wound (bowel opened and infection present)
- Low body fat/protein reserves
- Pre-existing inflammatory condition

Communication

When the patient recovers from a general anaesthetic, the first sense to return is that of hearing. Care of the patient in the recovery room can be enhanced by having aids to communication, e.g. hearing aids and glasses, available. A number of patients, especially the elderly or the very ill, become and remain confused postoperatively (Carter 1989). This may be due to the effects of

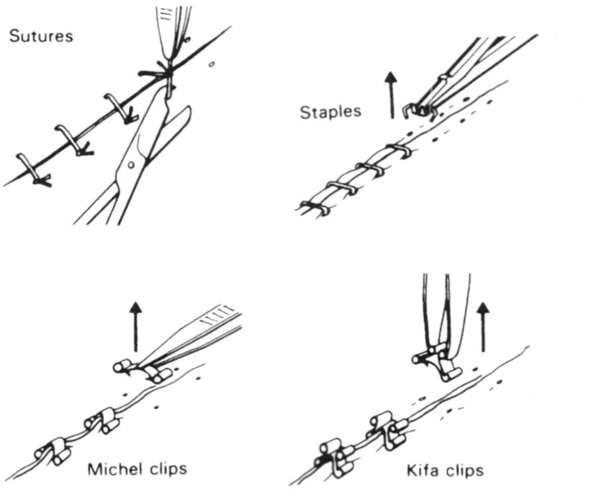

Fig. 26.7 Some common types of sutures and their removal. (Reproduced with kind permission from Jamieson et al 1998.)

the anaesthetic or to systemic illness. Efforts must be made to treat the cause, and nursing measures to reorientate and minimise confusion should be taken. The use of anticholinergic drugs that cross the blood–brain barrier, such as atropine and hyoscine, should be avoided in the elderly as they may cause confusion. Narcotic analgesics are undoubtedly the cause of delirium in some patients. Alternative non-narcotic analgesics such as diclofenac sodium (Voltarol) might be employed.

Patients with provisional diagnoses are often anxious to speak to the doctor about findings in theatre and their prognosis. When information is withheld, a moral dilemma may exist for nursing staff (see p. 805). Patients are often reluctant to raise all their concerns with the consultant or registrar surrounded by his entourage of juniors on ward rounds. The nurse has an important role to play in clarifying the patient's understanding and answering questions where possible or referring the patient's queries to others to be dealt with. The patient can experience an anxious time waiting to learn of her diagnosis if samples have been sent to the pathology laboratories for examination. Support for the patient will be required from the nurse and the patient's family (who themselves may require support) and is often gained informally from other patients.

Good communication among professionals in the postoperative period is essential. Medical and nursing staff must rely on one another for information and advice in order to provide a coordinated plan of care. In primary nursing, one nurse can become extremely knowledgeable about his patients and is the central focus for channelling information among health care professionals. This is equally true in the case of short-stay patients, who require intensive discharge planning and a highly coordinated plan of care (Sutherland 1991).

Body image

Our body image is our perception of our own appearance, which might be quite different from our actual physical appearance. This mental picture of ourselves is influenced not only by physical appearance but also by our attitude towards ourselves. Fawcett & Fry (1980) describe this as 'body attitude'. Body image forms part of our total self-concept and, as such, can have enormous impact on psychological, sociocultural and physical concepts of self (Blackmore 1989).

Body image can be altered by a change in physical appearance or body attitude, or both. If this alteration leads to a negative self-concept, educational and psychological support will be necessary to help the patient regain a positive self-concept. Mr W's body image became very positive after his operation as his appearance was restored in line with cultural values such as youth, health, beauty, intactness and vigour. His ability to provide for his family was restored and he would be seen by his workmates as able to cope with all aspects of his job again. Fortunately, the occupational health nurse had already provided education to correct his misconception about the operation's effect on his sex life and fertility.

M needed much psychological support from her primary nurse. She understood how a vaginal fistula had formed and how it could be treated, but felt that her sexual relationships and ability to have children might be affected. She could not come to terms with the continuous loss of fluid through her vagina and having to wear large incontinence pads. She associated wearing the pads with babies and the debilitated elderly patients she had seen in the wards previously. She felt everyone could see the pads and could detect an unpleasant odour from her.

For further reading on women with Crohn's disease and sexual problems, see McHenry (1991) or in relation to cancer see Burt (1996).

The primary nurse provided a listening ear for M so that she could talk about her fears and her new relationship with her boyfriend. The nurse also comforted and reassured her.

Mrs B recovered from the anaesthetic to find herself attached to tubes, loosely draped in a hospital gown and, worst of all, wearing a colostomy bag. As Mrs B went to theatre as an emergency, there was no time to prepare her for this. At first, she was totally disgusted by the stoma and refused to look at it. She was only able to begin to accept it and learn about it once she learned that it could be reversed in several months' time. Her attitude towards her body was also influenced by knowing that she had had cancer. Mrs B saw cancer as stigmatising and she felt that everyone would know she had a bag and why. Her self-esteem was severely threatened. Mrs B's stoma care plan (see Nursing Care Plan 26.3, p.818) outlines the care planned by the primary nurse to help her cope with this threat.

See Black (1994) for further reading on the management of patients undergoing stoma surgery.

Mrs B had a considerable need for education but required support — often given non-verbally through touch or by simply having someone with her before she was able to usefully receive any information. Her body image and self-esteem were helped enormously by a visitor from the colostomy association. Mrs B was surprised to see someone with a colostomy looking so well and normal. Her primary nurse also asked the stoma nurse to visit Mrs B in hospital to offer expert advice, to begin to establish a relationship and to plan her home care for after discharge. The therapeutic role of the nurse in offering psychological support should not be underestimated (Jenkinson 1996).

It is not only the patient with obvious outward structural changes in appearance who experiences a change in body image. Perceived or actual alterations in function can change body attitude and thus body image and self-concept. Some may be positive, others negative, but it is certain that all surgical patients are affected to some extent.

DISCHARGE PLANNING

Discharge plans aim to provide a smooth transition from hospital to home for continued patient care. Research has highlighted problems in discharge planning, including the lack of adequately documented plans and poor communication (Tierney et al 1994). Anderson & Helms (1995) found that information passed to the community carers on discharge was of poor quality and often late. It can be helpful if the care and discharge planning of a patient are coordinated by one nurse (Sutherland 1991). Victor et al (1993) suggest that the named nurse should take responsibility for coordinating discharge plans. Continuous responsibility is a feature of primary nursing that facilitates this approach. Ersser & Tutton (1991) state:

> the primary nurse is in a position to develop a greater knowledge of a smaller number of patients and...to engage in direct communication with all those involved in a patient's care. This would also suggest that practices which rely on careful co-ordination, such as discharge planning, may improve under this system.

In a busy surgical ward there is often an urgent need for beds, which can lead to a hasty and poorly planned discharge. All patients are referred to their GP on discharge from hospital by the surgeon (see Figs 26.1 and 26.2). The primary nurse will decide whether the patient needs to be referred to the community nurse as well. Referrals can be made for nursing interventions ranging from wound care — checking for signs of infection, changing dressings or removing sutures — to providing psychological support for the patient and her family, especially where cancer has been diagnosed with a poor prognosis. If patients are able to attend the health centre or clinic for wound dressing procedures, then arrangements for an appointment can be made before discharge. It should be remembered when starting a patient on a course of treatment that not all wound dressing materials are available in the community.

However, information for community nurses should not be solely procedural or task-centred — mental state, mobility, social circumstances and what the patient has been told must also be included. Raiwet et al (1997) argue that care maps covering the whole patient care episode, including community care, can facilitate continuity of care.

Worth et al (1994) argue that community nurses can have a vital role to play in discharge planning. A personal phone call, a copy of the care plan on discharge or a visit by the community nurse to the ward can all be useful. Mrs B's stoma nurse had visited her in hospital on several occasions prior to discharge and had liaised closely with her primary nurse to ensure she was well prepared to go home. Mr L's community nurse called in to the ward to see him and the primary nurse, who was able to discuss the discharge arrangements and to ensure that the community nurse had a copy of Mr L's care plan and was familiar with the low air loss mattress. She also provided enough dressing material for Mr L's wound for the first week at home.

Careful discharge planning is essential as the decreasing length of in-patient stay means that less time is available for planning. Forward planning and continuous responsibility as an element of primary nursing may help nurses to achieve the goal of effective discharge preparation.

Discharge teaching

Patient teaching for discharge begins on or before the day of admission to hospital. Mr W had received a booklet at his preoperative visit to the hospital which helped him plan for convalescence at home. He also had learned about healthy diet, interventions to help him stop smoking and expected function and return to work from his occupational health nurse.

Patients require specific information to continue their recovery from surgery, but the opportunity for more general health education can also be taken.

For further reading on patient education see Kiger (1995).

The opportunity to teach patients about their care on discharge may be limited, as with day-case patients, or more prolonged, as during an in-patient stay after major surgery. Information can also be given to relatives (when acceptable to the patient) to enable them to continue to support their loved one at home.

Some patients may be quite unsure or have misconceptions about how they should progress during their recovery at home. In day-case surgery it is essential that patients understand that the anaesthetic may take a full 24 h to be eliminated from the body. Therefore they must not drive home, should be continuously accompanied for the first 24 h after surgery and should not drive to work the following morning. Some individuals expect to feel fully fit and to be able to care for themselves as normal immediately they are discharged. Many will feel a little insecure without the presence of the nurse and feel anxious about their health.

The type of information required in discharge after surgery has been summarised in a patient booklet by Vaughan (1988). Carapeti et al (1998) describe how patients were treated as a day case for haemorrhoidectomy, but the success of this was dependent on detailed discharge planning. This involved not only information-giving but also a 24 h contact number and a kit with drugs and dressings.

Mrs B was to return home for several months before the surgeon would consider reversing her colostomy. She had to be independent in caring for her stoma and so required staged teaching and much support (see Nursing Care Plan 26.3). She had a booklet to reinforce the teaching given by the nurses, which also acted as a focus for discussions of the stoma with her daughter. Mr and Mrs L were shown how to use the low air loss mattress they had hired for Mr L to use at home. The primary nurse also explained to Mr L how to use a urinary sheath and pointed out how to avoid common problems with it. Mr L quickly became independent and proficient in using the sheath.

All patients should be clear about seeking advice or treatment from the most appropriate source on discharge. Referral to community nurses and GPs, when possible, establishes continued support and may be preferable to telling patients just to ring the ward.

REHABILITATION

Rehabilitation of the patient does not take place exclusively in either hospital or home, but is nonetheless an increasing focus of care in the community setting. The needs of patients in terms of recovery from surgery do not differ dramatically from the time they leave hospital to their arrival at home. Discharge from hospital is therefore a stage in patient care, involving transfer of care from one setting to another. The plan of care for the discharged patient may thus address similar problems to that of the patient who continues her recovery in hospital. Many interventions described in the sections on postoperative care will be equally relevant to the patient in hospital or at home.

Rehabilitation can be a lengthy process, requiring continued support by community nurses, or a short event with minimal professional intervention. Mrs B was visited by the community nurse at home to assess her self-care deficits using Orem's model (Orem 1995). She was also visited regularly by the stoma care nurse whom she had first met in hospital. Mr L's district nurse continued to care for his wound on discharge, following a very similar pattern of care to that given in hospital. M saw her practice nurse once to make sure that her abdominal wound was healing well, and Mr W talked to his occupational health nurse about resuming a full range of duties.

The demands made by postoperative patients in the community have increased enormously in recent years. This is partly due to an ageing population making greater demands on the service. The elderly are known to be vulnerable on discharge and are more likely to have contact with community nurses (Dash et al 1996). The trend towards day-case surgery and early discharge (see p. 800) places more responsibility for postoperative care in the hands of community health care workers.

Jester & Turner (1998) describe a hospital at home scheme which enables early discharge home into the care of a multiprofessional care team. These trends have also been driven partly by public demand. In 1991, the Audit Commission reported that 80% of day-case patients preferred to be treated as a day case. A small qualitative study by Otte (1996) found that patients who had previous experience as an in-patient preferred to have surgery as a day case. An increasing number of patients are therefore recovering from surgery at home.

Patients undergoing surgery demand a range of care from nurses in both the hospital and community settings, in both the pre- and postoperative periods. Whilst care can often appear to be focused on performing tasks in a standardised manner, it has been proposed here that patients enter the surgical experience for a wide variety of reasons with quite differing health care needs. The nurse is ideally placed to not only coordinate and humanise the surgical experience, but also to facilitate a safe and speedy recovery in an individualised manner.

REFERENCES

Alderson P 1995 Consent to surgery: the role of the nurse. Nursing Standard 9(35): 38–40

Allsop C 1991 Primary nursing in a surgical unit. In: Ersser S, Tutton E (eds) Primary nursing in perspective. Scutari, London

Anderson M, Helms L 1995 Communication between continuing care organisations. Research in Nursing and Health 18: 49–57

Audit Commission and the National Health Service in England and Wales 1991 Measuring quality: the patient's view of day surgery. HMSO, London

Autar R 1996 Nursing assessment of clients at risk of deep vein thrombosis (DVT): the Autar DVT scale. Journal of Advanced Nursing 23(4): 763–770

Beddows J 1997 Alleviating preoperative anxiety in patients: a study. Nursing Standard 11(37): 35–38

Bell K 1996 The establishment of a gynaecology assessment unit. Nursing Times 92(10): 27–29

Biley F C 1989 Perceptions of stress in pre-operative patients. Journal of Advanced Nursing 14(7): 575–581

Blackmore C 1989 Altered images. Nursing Times 85(12): 36–39

Blinkthorne K 1995 Prepared for a smooth recovery? Nursing Times 91(28): 42–44

Boore J R P 1978 Prescription for recovery. Royal College of Nursing, London

Bove L A 1994 How fluids and electrolytes shift after surgery. Nursing 94: 34–39

Bradshaw P W, Ley P, Kinnay J 1975 Recall of medical advice, comprehensibility and specificity. British Journal of Sociology and Clinical Psychology 14: 55–62

Brandberg A, Anderson I 1980 Whole body disinfection. Royal Society of Medicine International Congress and Symposium, Series 23. Royal Society of Medicine, London Academic Press

Burns S 1993 Surgical nurses in outpatient clinics. Surgical Nurse 6(5): 6

Calligaro K D, Miller P, Dougherty M J, Raviola C A, Delaurentis D A 1996 Role of nursing personnel in implementing clinical pathways and decreasing hospital costs for major vascular surgery. Journal of Vascular Nursing 14(3): 57–61

Canizaro P C 1981 Methods of nutritional support in the surgical patients. In: Yarborough M F, Curreri P W (eds) Surgical nutrition. Churchill Livingstone, Edinburgh

Caprini J A, Scurr J H, Hasty J M 1988 Role of compression modalities in a prophylactic program for deep vein thrombosis. Seminars in Thrombosis and Haemostasis 14(suppl): 77–87

Carapeti E A, Kamm M A, McDonald P J, Phillips K S 1998 Double blind randomised controlled trial of effect of metronidazole after day case haemorrhoidectomy. The Lancet 351(9097): 169–172

Carter C 1990 Ritual and risk. Nursing Times 86(13): 63–64

Carter M 1989 Effects of anaesthesia on mental performance in the elderly. Nursing Times 84(4): 40–42

Chapman A 1996 Current theory and practice: a study of pre-operative fasting. Nursing Standard 10(18): 33–36

Cheslyn-Curtis S, Russell R C G 1991 New trends in gallstone management. British Journal of Surgery 78: 143–149

Closs S J 1992 Patients' night-time pain, analgesic provision and sleep after surgery. International Journal of Nursing Studies 29(4): 381–392

Coleridge Smith P D, Hasty J H, Scurr J H 1991 Deep vein thrombosis: effects of graduated compression stockings on distension of the deep veins of the calf. British Journal of Surgery 78: 724–726

Collins R, Scrimgeour A, Yusuf S, Peto K 1988 Reduction in fatal pulmonary embolism and venous thrombosis by perioperative administration of subcutaneous heparin. New England Journal of Medicine 318: 162–173

Committee on Safety of Medicines 1991 Genotoxicity of papaveretum and noscapine. Current Problems 31 (June)

Dale F 1993 Post operative pain in the elective surgical patient. British Journal of Nursing 2(17): 842–849

Dash K, Zarle N C, O'Donnell L, Vince-Whitman C 1996 Discharge planning for the elderly. A guide for nurses. Springer, New York

Davies K 1996 Findings of a national survey of acute pain services. Nursing Times 92(17): 31–33

Department of Health (NHS Management Executive) 1990 A guide to consent for examination or treatment. DHSS Health Publications Unit, London

Department of Health 1991 The patient's charter. HMSO, London

Dilworth J P, Pounsford J C 1991 Cough following general anaesthesia and abdominal surgery. Respiratory Medicine 85(suppl): 13–16

Dimond B 1990 Legal aspects of nursing. Prentice-Hall, Hemel Hempstead

Dubois F, Icard P, Berthelot G, Levard H 1990 Coelioscope cholecystectomy: preliminary report of 36 cases. Annals of Surgery January 211: 60–62

Editorial (Lancet) 1983 Preoperative depilation. Lancet I: 311

Edmondson M 1995 Day surgery: handling patients' complaints. Nursing Standard 9(47): 25–28

Ersser S, Tutton E 1991 Primary nursing in perspective. Scutari, London

Ewles L, Simnett I 1992 Promoting health: a practical guide. Scutari, London

Fahrenfort M 1987 Patient emancipation by health education: an impossible goal? Patient Education and Counselling 10(1): 25–37

Fawcett J, Fry S 1980 An exploratory study of body image dimensionality. Nursing Research 29(15): 324–327

Field L 1996 Factors influencing nurses' analgesia decisions. British Journal of Nursing 5(14): 838–844

Firth F 1991 Pain after day surgery. Nursing Times 87(40): 72–76

Fletcher J P, Batiste P 1997 Incidence of deep vein thrombosis following vascular surgery. International Angiology 16(1): 65–68

Flinn W R, Sandager G P, Silva M B, Benjamin M E, Cerullo L J, Taylor M 1996 Prospective surveillance for perioperative venous thrombosis. Archives of Surgery 131(5): 472–480

Freshwater D 1992 Preoperative preparation of the skin – a review of the literature. Surgical Nurse 5(5): 6–10

Frost J 1993 Clinical application of lasers. Professional Nurse 8(5): 298–303

Galvin K T 1992 A critical review of the health belief model in relation to cigarette smoking behaviour. Journal of Clinical Nursing 1: 13–18

Gammon J, Mulholland C W 1996 Effect of preparatory information prior to elective total hip replacement on post-operative physical coping outcomes. International Journal of Nursing Studies 33(6): 589–604

Gillan I 1994 The right to know: the nurse's role in informing patients. Nursing Times 90(35): 46–47

Good M 1996 Effects of relaxation and music on post operative pain: a review. Journal of Advanced Nursing 24: 905–914

Haddock J, Burrows C 1997 The role of the nurse in health promotion: an evaluation of a smoking cessation programme in surgical pre-admission clinics. Journal of Advanced Nursing 26(6): 1098–1110

Hamilton Smith S 1972 Nil by mouth. Royal College of Nursing, London

Hayward J 1975 Information: a prescription against pain. Royal College of Nursing, London

Hughes M 1996 Key issues in the introduction of nurse endoscopy. Nursing Times 92(8): 38–39

Jamieson E M, McCall J M, Blythe R, Whyte L A 1997 Guidelines for clinical nursing practice, 3rd edn. Churchill Livingstone, Edinburgh
Jeffery P C, Nicolades A N 1990 Graduated compression stockings in the prevention of deep vein thrombosis. British Journal of Surgery 77(4): 380–383
Jenkinson T P 1996 The nurse as significant other for surgical patients. Professional Nurse 11(10): 651–652
Jester R, Turner D 1998 Hospital at home: the Bromsgrove experience. Nursing Standard 12(20): 40–42
Kakkar V V, Boeckl O, Boneu B et al 1997 Efficacy and safety of a low-molecular-weight heparin and standard unfractionated heparin for prophylaxis of postoperative venous thromboembolism: European Multicenter Trial. World Journal of Surgery 21(1): 2–9
Kurz A, Sessler D, Lenhardt R 1996 Perioperative normothermia to reduce the incidence of surgical-wound infection and shorten hospitalization. New England Journal of Medicine 334(19): 1209–1215
Law M 1997 A telephone survey of day surgery eye patients. Journal of Advanced Nursing 25: 355–363
Lawrence D, Kakkar W 1980 Graduated static external compression of the lower limb: a physiological assessment. British Journal of Surgery 67: 119–121
Mackintosh C, Bowles S 1997 Evaluation of a nurse led acute pain service. Can cinical nurse specialists make a difference? Journal of Advanced Nursing 25(1): 30–37
Malby R 1991 Audit audibility in a nursing development unit. Nursing Times 87(19): 35–37
Manthey M 1981 The practice of primary nursing. Blackwell Scientific, Boston
Martin D 1996 Pre-operative visits to reduce patient anxiety: a study. Nursing Standard 10(23): 33–38
McGinn F P, Miles A J, Uglow M, Ozmen M, Terzi C, Humby M 1995 Randomized trial of laparoscopic cholecystectomy and mini-cholecystectomy. British Journal of Surgery 82(10): 1374–1377
McIntyre F J, McCloy R 1994 Shaving patients before operation: a dangerous myth? Annals of The Royal College of Surgeons of England 76: 3–4
Medical Defence Union 1997 Consent to treatment. Medical Defence Union, London
Mitchell M 1997 Patients' perceptions of pre-operative preparation for day surgery. Journal of Advanced Nursing 26(2): 356–363
Moran S, Kent G 1995 Quality indicators for patients' information in short stay units. Nursing Times 91(4): 37–40
Morris J 1995 Monitoring post operative effects in day surgery patients. Nursing Times 91(10): 32–34
Nelson S 1996 Pre-admission education for patients undergoing cardiac surgery. British Journal of Nursing 5(6): 335–340
Office of Health Economics 1995 Compendium of health statistics, 9th edn. Office of Health Economics, London
Orem D 1995 Nursing: concepts of practice, 5th edn. Mosby, St Louis
Otte D I 1996 Patients' perspectives and experiences of day case surgery. Journal of Advanced Nursing 23(6): 1228–1237
Phillips K, Gill L 1993 A point of pressure. Nursing Times 89(45): 44–45
Phillips S, Hutchinson S, Davidson T 1993 Preoperative drinking does not affect gastric contents. British Journal of Anaesthetics 70: 6–9
Porteous M J, Nicholson E A, Morris L T, James R, Negus D 1989 Thigh length versus knee length stockings in the prevention of deep vein thrombosis. British Journal of Surgery 76: 296–297
Prasad A, Foley R J 1996 Day case laparoscopic cholecystectomy: a safe and cost effective procedure. European Journal of Surgery 162(1): 43–46
Pritchard A P, Walker V A 1984 The Royal Marsden Hospital manual of clinical nursing policies and procedures. Harper & Row, London
Rafferty A 1988 Postoperative backache. Nursing Times 84(46): 32–35
Raiwet C, Halliwell G, Andruski L, Wilson D 1997 Care maps across the continuum. Canadian Nurse 93(1): 26–30
Roberts S 1991 Operation reassurance. Nursing Times 87(40): 70–71
Roper N, Logan W, Tierney A 1996 The elements of nursing, 4th edn. Churchill Livingstone, Edinburgh
Royal College of Surgeons of England and the College of Anaesthetists 1990 Pain after surgery. Royal College of Surgeons, London
Schaldach D E 1997 Measuring quality and cost of care: evaluation of an amputation clinical pathway. Journal of Vascular Nursing 15(1): 13–20
Scottish Office Department of Health 1996 Health in Scotland. The Stationery Office, Edinburgh
Seers K 1987 Perceptions of pain. Nursing Times 83(48): 37–39
Selye H 1976 The stress of life, 2nd edn. McGraw-Hill, New York
Shade P 1992 PCA: can client education improve outcomes? Journal of Advanced Nursing 17: 408–413
Sidway versus Bethlem Royal Hospital Governors and others 1985 1, ALL, ER 643
Sutherland E 1991 All in a day's work. Nursing Times 87(11): 26–30
Teasdale K 1993 Information and anxiety: a critical reappraisal. Journal of Advanced Nursing 18: 1125–1132
Thomas E A 1987 Preoperative fasting: a question of routine. Nursing Times 83(49): 46–47
Thompson E 1990 Preoperative visiting. British Journal of Theatre Nursing 27: 4
Tierney A, Worth A, Closs S J, King C, Macmillan M 1994 Older patients' experiences of discharge from hospital. Nursing Times 90(21): 36–39
Turner G M, Cole S E, Brooks J H 1984 The efficacy of graduated compression stockings in the prevention of deep vein thrombosis after major gynaecological surgery. British Journal of Obstetrics and Gynaecology 91: 588–591
UKCC 1992 Code of professional conduct for the nurse, midwife and health visitor, 3rd edn. UKCC, London
UKCC 1996 Guidelines for professional practice. UKCC, London
Vaughan B 1988 Discharge procedures: discharge following surgery. Nursing Times 84(15): 28–33
Victor C, Young E, Hudson M, Wallace P 1993 Whose responsibility is it anyway? Hospital admission and discharge of older people in an inner London district health authority. Journal of Advanced Nursing 18: 1297–1304
Watts S, Brooks A 1997 Patients' perceptions of the pre-operative information they need about events they may experience in the intensive care unit. Journal of Advanced Nursing 26(1): 85–92
Wigfield A, Boone E 1996 Critical care pathway development: the way forward. British Journal of Nursing 5(12): 732–735
Winn C 1996 Basing catheter care on research principles. Nursing Standard 10(18): 38–40
Worth A, Tierney A, Lockerbie L 1994 Community nurses and discharge planning. Nursing Standard 8(21): 25–30

FURTHER READING

Ayliffe G A J, Collins B M, Taylor L J 1993 Hospital-acquired infection: principles and prevention, 2nd edn. Wright, Bristol
Black P K 1994 Management of patients undergoing stoma surgery. British Journal of Nursing 3(5): 211–212, 214–216
Brennan A 1989 Clinical conundrum. Nursing Times 87(20): 48–49
Burt K 1995 The effects of cancer on body image and sexuality. Nursing Times 91(7): 36–37
Clarke P, Jones J 1998 Brigdens operating department practice. Churchill Livingstone, Edinburgh
Devine E C 1992 Effects of psychoeducational care for adult surgical patients – a meta analysis of 191 studies. Patient Education and Counselling 19(2): 129–142
Dykes P C, Wheeler K (eds) 1998 Planning, implementing and evaluating critical pathways. Churchill Livingstone, Edinburgh
Feber T 1996 Promoting self-esteem after laryngectomy. Nursing Times 92(30): 37–39
Hare R, Cooke M 1991 Bacteriology and immunology for nurses, 7th edn. Churchill Livingstone, Edinburgh
Hughes A 1991 Life with a stoma. Nursing Times 87(25): 67–68
Johnston M, Vogele C 1993 Benefits of psychological preparation for surgery, a meta analysis. Annals of Behavioural Medicine 15(4): 245–256
Kiger A 1995 Teaching for health: the nurse as health educator. Churchill Livingstone, Edinburgh
McHenry C 1991 Silent suffering. Nursing Times 87(46): 21
Markanday L (ed) 1997 Day surgery for nurses. Whurr, London
Myers C 1997 Stoma care nursing: a patient centred approach. Arnold, London

National Association of Theatre Nurses 1988 Code of practice: guidelines to total patient care and safety in practice in operating theatres. National Association of Theatre Nurses, Harrogate
Richold J C 1990 Postoperative surgical wound infection. Nursing Times 86(17): 56
Salter M (ed) 1997 Altered body image: the nurse's role. Wiley, Chichester
Smith S 1996 Discharge planning: the need for effective communication. Nursing Standard 10(38): 39–41
Sutherland E 1996 Day surgery – a handbook for nurses. Baillière Tindall, London
Thompson I, Melia K, Boyd K M 1994 Nursing ethics, 3rd edn. Churchill Livingstone, Edinburgh
Tingle J, Cribb A 1995 Nursing law and ethics. Blackwell Science, Oxford
Trounce J 1997 Clinical pharmacology for nurses, 15th edn. Churchill Livingstone, Edinburgh
Vaughan B, Hanford L 1997 Time of transition. Nursing Times 93(47): 36–38
Webber B A, Pryor J A 1994 Physiotherapy for respiratory and cardiac problems. Churchill Livingstone, Edinburgh

THE PATIENT WHO EXPERIENCES TRAUMA

27

Marie-Noelle Orzel

INTRODUCTION

Every year, 15 million patients attend accident and emergency (A&E) departments in England and Wales (Audit Commission 1996). They present with a wide variety of injuries or conditions, some that may be considered as life-threatening and others which are relatively minor. This means that nurses working within an A&E environment are required to have a broad knowledge base and a wide range of skills to enable them to meet the needs of all patients. This chapter considers this diverse nature of A&E nursing. As many of the medical and surgical conditions have been discussed in other areas of this book, this chapter will focus on the concept of trauma. It will outline the process of triage which is used to assess and prioritise patients and how this incorporates the SOAP model (Hnott & Davis 1984) for planning and implementing care.

Two case studies will be used to highlight the principles of emergency nursing care and will examine what is meant by trauma, by exploring the range of injuries that may be encountered by an A&E nurse, whilst highlighting key principles of care. The case studies will focus on:

- the care of a patient who is multiply injured and who therefore requires immediate resuscitation
- the care of a patient who attends with a minor injury and who is assessed, diagnosed, treated and discharged independently by a nurse.

Whilst trauma accounts for a large proportion of A&E work, it is important to consider other distinct areas of practice that require specific skills to enable the nurse to meet both the patient's and the family's physical and psychosocial needs. Bereavement is an extremely sensitive and emotional area of A&E nursing, as relatives and friends have had no opportunity to anticipate or prepare themselves for their sudden loss. Principles of caring for families during their crises will be explored with specific reference to the loss of a baby as a result of sudden infant death syndrome (SIDS). It is also important to acknowledge the A&E staff's personal needs during these difficult periods, and the concept of critical incident stress debriefing (CISD) will be outlined.

A&E departments provide an interface between the community and the hospital setting. Operating an 'open door' philosophy confronts the A&E nurse with many practical and ethical challenges which are often linked to wider sociological and political issues. Strategies that may be adopted to prevent incidents of violence and aggression will be discussed and the A&E nurse's responsibility to the law highlighted. The dynamic nature of the A&E environment means that the workload is often unpredictable and A&E nurses have to be prepared for the unexpected. For this reason, a section of this chapter is devoted to the key aspects of an A&E department's response to disasters which involve large numbers of casualties. It will also consider the subsequent psychological impact this may have on the survivors, their families, the witnesses and the rescuers and health care workers involved both at the scene of the disaster and within the hospital environment.

Throughout the chapter, the importance of patient and family involvement in the planning and delivery of nursing care will be emphasised.

What is trauma?

Trauma may be defined as any physical wound or injury. It can be caused by a variety of accidents but may also be self-inflicted or result from acts of violence. The impact of traumatic events on victims, witnesses and staff may also cause psychological problems long past the event itself (Chandler 1993) and this is discussed later in this chapter under post-traumatic stress disorder. The severity of the wound or injury may be as minor as a simple graze which can be self-treated within the home environment or one which requires more specialised treatment in a hospital A&E department. Conversely, the trauma victim may present with life-threatening multiple injuries, such that he is vulnerable to imminent death within the initial hours following the causative event. In England alone, 630 000 people are admitted to hospital each year via A&E units, following an injury or poisoning (Department of Health 1994). Trauma is the main cause of death in young people. Annually in the UK, 14 500–18 000 deaths occur as a result of trauma, with 60 000 patients being admitted to hospital each year as a result of a road traffic accident (RTA) (Driscoll et al 1993). Whilst there has been legislation to reduce the number of accidents, e.g. the wearing of seat belts for car users, helmets for motorcyclists, drink driving laws (Hill 1990) and the Health and Safety at Work Act (Health & Safety Commission 1974), society can still view risk-taking behaviour as a positive characteristic so that these measures are not always adhered to (Fiest & Brannon 1988). Despite this, statistically there has been a reduction in the incidence of trauma, but still the cost to the health service of caring for injured people is £300 million/year (Central Statistics Office 1994). It is for this reason that A&E nurses must be able to meet the immediate needs of patients who attend with both life-threatening and less serious conditions.

Reception in A&E

A&E departments are designed to accommodate patients who arrive by a variety of means and who present with a diversity of problems. Within the NHS it is generally accepted that the general practitioner (GP) is the primary source of medical care through whom patients are referred to hospital facilities and specialist practitioners. Those who require acute specialist care will more often than not be admitted through the A&E department and will be seen and assessed by the relevant medical or surgical team. However, patients present to A&E departments via other channels. With the knowledge that they can gain immediate access to hospital facilities without GP referral, many individuals self-present to A&E units. Other patients are referred via occupational health services and schools. Generally, more seriously ill or injured patients will arrive via the local ambulance service either by road transport or, in more extreme cases, by helicopter. Usually these patients arrive singly, but on occasion, as in the case of RTAs that involve several vehicles, there will be several patients arriving at one time, often with injuries of differing severity.

For this reason the A&E environment must be flexible. The physical division of any department facilitates this. There are usually two points of access to the clinical area, one for ambulance patients which provides direct access into the clinical area, and one for other patients which leads into a reception and waiting area. In most units there are separate areas allocated to treat patients with minor injuries and areas that contain individual examination cubicles for those who require a more thorough examination. All departments have a designated resuscitation area for those patients who present with life-threatening conditions. Larger departments may have separate plaster areas, theatres for minor operations and specially equipped cubicles for eye and dental problems. In departments where children are seen, it is recommended that there are separate waiting areas and cubicles which are suitably decorated and equipped to meet the needs of children (RCN 1994).

A&E departments cannot follow a 'first come, first served' policy. As has already been discussed, a large number of patients attend A&E departments each day. There is also only a finite number of health care workers available to care for them. For this reason priorities have to be set by assessing each patient's needs. This is supported by the government's initiative *The Patient's Charter*, which states that all patients should be seen immediately and their need for treatment assessed (DoH 1991). A nationally recognised system to ensure that patients are seen in order of priority, based on their physical and psychosocial needs, is the 'triage' system (Manchester Triage Group 1997).

Triage

Triage is the first point of contact a patient has with a health care professional in an A&E department and the triage process is integral to the clinical management of any A&E department. It is usually performed by nursing staff and in practical terms involves a nursing assessment of the patient's illness or injury to determine a priority of care. Priority setting is an important aspect of the triage concept and follows logically from a comprehensive assessment that allows the nurse to prioritise the patient's condition in relation to the severity of the illness or injury. This in turn ensures that the patient receives the most appropriate care based on the seriousness of his condition, whilst considering both the resources that are available and the demands being made on the service. The assessment technique must be comprehensive enough to allow for accurate decision-making but brief enough to ensure the smooth continuous functioning of the triage system. Although the purpose of triage is not to diagnose, the nurse has to be able to recognise clinical signs and symptoms and use this knowledge when deciding a priority of care. Nurses who practise triage have to be able to collect pertinent information whilst discriminating between the relevant and irrelevant factors in a short period of time. For this reason they need to be experienced and have competent interpersonal skills which allow them to complete the process rapidly (Manchester Triage Group 1997). Often the nurse practising this role is working under stress. She has to be able to react to both verbal and non-verbal responses, as well as being aware of her own verbal and non-verbal techniques, to ensure that an accurate assessment is made and all the relevant data are gathered. One way of ensuring that the correct information is collected is to use a nursing model. By using a model, all nurses working within its framework use the same guidelines (Sbaih 1992). The framework that has been used extensively in the A&E setting is that of the

Box 27.1 SOAP assessment model

S Subjective information refers to the information that is obtained by listening to the patient and recording the history obtained — it is what the patient says

O Objective information is obtained from observing the patient, including the clinical observations completed during the physical examination of the patient — it is what the nurse finds

A Assessment refers to what the nurse identifies as the patient's problem and is based on both the subjective and objective information. It should also include any relevant social factors

P Plan refers to what the nurse plans to do with the patient. This includes any immediate first aid and the priority awarded in relation to the assessment of the patient's condition

problem-oriented nursing record, known as the SOAP model (Hnott & Davis 1984, Blythin 1988). Box 27.1 demonstrates an application of this model which includes the collecting of subjective and objective information.

Using this information, the triage nurse must make an accurate prioritisation in relation to the patient's needs. In smaller departments, the triage nurse will see all patients. In larger units there may be separate triage nurses — one who assesses those patients with minor injuries who walk into the department, and one who assesses patients who have sustained major injuries. However, there has to be close liaison between the two to ensure that patients are prioritised appropriately. Priorities can be described as either colours or numbers, but they usually correlate to a patient's condition, e.g. requiring immediate treatment such as in a resuscitation scenario, urgent treatment, semi-urgent attention, the condition is non-urgent or, if the injury is particularly minor, that no harm would come to the patient if treatment were delayed. Table 27.1 demonstrates a priority rating guide in relation to ankle injuries.

IMMEDIATE TREATMENT OF EMERGENCIES

As has previously been mentioned, annually in the UK, 14 500–18 000 deaths occur as a result of trauma (Driscoll et al 1993). A report by the Royal College of Surgeons of England (1988) identified that approximately one-third of these deaths were preventable and were often due to hypoxia, continuing haemorrhage and missed diagnosis. Driscoll et al (1993) describe a 'trimodal distribution' of death which identifies three peaks following trauma when casualties die as a result either of their injuries or of subsequent events (see Box 27.2). For these reasons it is important that any A&E department is fully prepared to receive any patient, no matter how severely injured, at any time of the day or night.

It is also vital that there is a predetermined system, such as the advanced trauma life support (ATLS) protocols (American College of Surgeons 1997), to guide personnel through the initial assessment of the patient, enabling them to identify any life-threatening conditions quickly and to treat them appropriately. Patients who are admitted with such injuries will be cared for in a resuscitation area which is designed to have the necessary equipment readily available and the space to enable a trauma team consisting of nurses, doctors and radiographers to care for the patient efficiently and effectively (see Fig. 27.1).

The resuscitation team

Effective staffing is as important as the organisation of equipment. Having too many people in the resuscitation room may be as dangerous as having too few, as overcrowding can lead to confusion and delays. A resuscitation team consists of an integrated group of nurses and doctors who are needed to ensure that there is an efficient and organised resuscitation approach. There should be a system of identifying, from the total nursing staff in the department,

Table 27.1 Priority rating guide in relation to ankle injuries. (Adapted from priority ratings used in the A&E department, Oxford Radcliffe NHS Trust, Oxford, UK)

Colour/number	*Priority*	*Nursing action*	*Signs and symptoms*
Red (1)	Immediate	Requires resuscitation by a trauma team	Patient has sustained multiple injuries including an ankle injury
Yellow (2)	Urgent	Immediate need for care. Nurse will have to assist with reduction of the fracture to prevent further damage to the limb	Circulation is impaired, the limb has no pulse Gross deformity of the ankle Obvious compound fracture
Green (3)	Semi-urgent	This injury needs treatment as soon as possible but a delay is permissible so long as the patient remains under close nursing supervision and continued assessment	Severe swelling of the ankle Some deformity Pain rated high using an assessment tool Patient is unable to take any weight on this foot
Blue (4)	Non-urgent	Patient is safe to wait for treatment and this will not be detrimental to his condition	Some swelling of the limb No deformity Some pain Able to take weight on the foot
Black (5)	Delay acceptable	Requires no intervention	Minimal swelling No deformity Vague pain Able to take weight on limb (Possibly an old injury)

Box 27.2 Trimodal distribution of death following trauma

First peak
Mortality during this peak occurs very shortly after the time of injury and usually at the scene of the incident. The person's injuries are so grave that no present-day technology would be able to resuscitate them. The primary way of preventing such deaths is through accident prevention programmes such as drink driving campaigns and seat belt legislation.

Second peak
Mortality occurs hours after the incidence of trauma and patients may die from airway, breathing and circulatory problems. Many of these deaths are preventable during this period, which is commonly known as the 'golden hour' and is the period during which the patient is in the resuscitation room of an A&E department.

Third peak
Mortality occurs days or weeks following the initial incident and patients may die from multi-organ failure, acute respiratory disease syndrome (ARDS) or sepsis.

a group of at least three nurses who will contribute to the team in the resuscitation room. Both a nurse and medical team leader lead the team. The aim of the resuscitation is to stabilise the patient, identify his injuries and initiate a definitive management plan. It has been shown that the most efficient resuscitation will occur if a 'horizontal organisation' approach is adopted (Driscoll et al 1993). This is when each member of the team carries out individual tasks simultaneously rather than sequentially. This reduces the time taken to resuscitate a patient and initiate life-saving procedures, which will improve the patient's chances of survival. For this to be successful, each member of the team must be aware of his or her precise role, which will have been designated by the team leader. The size of the team will depend on the size of the individual department. As well as the designated nurses, there will be either an A&E consultant or a senior doctor from A&E and an anaesthetist and surgeon on call. An example of the responsibilities of each nursing team member can be seen in Box 27.3. In order to give everyone this experience, the team can be changed on a daily, or shift, basis. On the patient's arrival an initial history will have been received from the ambulance crew, but further information may become available with the arrival of relatives or friends. Collecting this information should, where possible, be the responsibility of a fourth nurse who can act as liaison between the resuscitation team and the patient's family or friends. The paramedics routinely leave a copy of their clinical documentation for the patient with the A&E department.

The ATLS system

To care effectively for a seriously injured patient, he must be rapidly assessed, his injuries identified and any life-threatening conditions immediately treated. Within the A&E environment, this includes completing a primary and, where possible, a secondary survey to ensure a full assessment is made. Within the primary survey, an ABCDE process is followed to ensure that logical and sequential treatment priorities are identified:

A — Airway maintenance with protection of the cervical spine
B — Breathing and ventilation
C — Circulation with haemorrhage control
D — Disability, which involves a neurological assessment
E — Exposure of the patient ensuring that the environment is optimal to prevent further hypothermia.

If any life-threatening condition is identified during the process, it is treated before moving on to the next stage, e.g. if the patient is found to have a compromised airway, this is stabilised before the patient's breathing and ventilation are assessed.

The secondary survey is only started when the primary survey is completed and the patient's condition is stabilised. If the patient

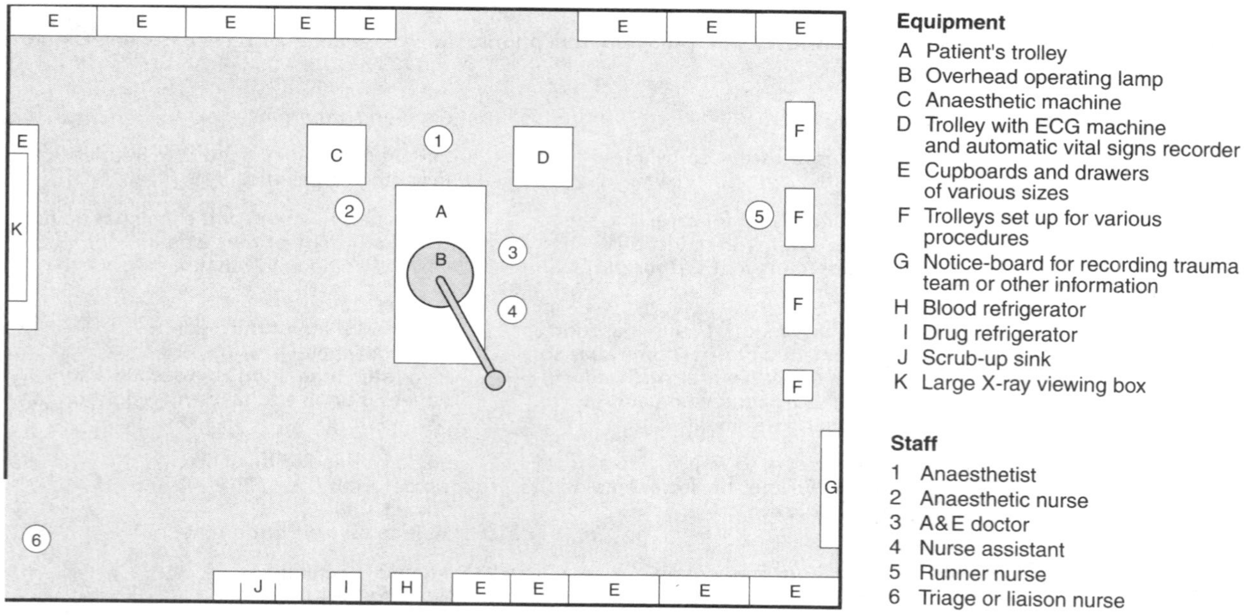

Fig. 27.1 Organisation of the resuscitation room.

Box 27.3 Responsibilities of nursing members of a trauma team

Nurse one
This nurse will coordinate the team. She will also assist the other nurses by preparing appropriate equipment as necessary for procedures, etc., and recording any clinical observations and laboratory findings.

Nurse two
This nurse is often referred to as the airway nurse and has two key responsibilities: firstly, to assist the anaesthetist in securing and maintaining the patient's airway whilst protecting the patient's cervical spine; and secondly, to establish a rapport with the patient, giving psychological support whilst in the resuscitation room. Ideally, all information should be relayed through this nurse.

Nurse three
This nurse may be referred to as the circulation nurse. Her responsibilities include removing the patient's clothes, attaching the patient to monitors and measuring the patient's clinical vital signs. Following this, she will ensure that i.v. access has been established and will be responsible for the patient's fluid requirements. Furthermore, she will assist with any procedures, e.g. catheterisation, insertion of a chest drain, etc.

is critically injured then this may not take place in A&E as the patient is likely to require surgical intervention to stabilise his condition. However, if the patient's condition does permit, then the secondary survey involves a full head-to-toe examination and gives the nurse the opportunity to complete a thorough set of clinical observations, including neurological observations.

The resuscitation room

It is important that the resuscitation area is designed to complement both the assessment principles (e.g. the ATLS protocols) that are going to be applied when examining the patient and the team who have to work within its environment. Usually staff are given some warning via their local ambulance service that a patient with severe or life-threatening injuries will be admitted shortly. This may mean that there is little time for preparation before the patient is rushed into the department. It is vital that the resuscitation area is always prepared for such emergencies and it is the nurses' responsibility at the beginning of each shift to ensure that all areas are fully stocked and the equipment is in working order. It is also vital that health and safety issues are considered to prevent staff becoming inadvertently injured during the haste of a resuscitation and to prevent any further harm occurring to the patient. This includes the availability of large plastic aprons, disposable gloves and protective goggles for all staff. Most resuscitation rooms have large trolley areas, allowing a greater space for the team to work in. A policy of keeping 'a place for everything and everything in its place' should be followed, so that staff can learn the location of every item and find anything that is needed immediately. Certain items may be prepared in advance. For example, the ECG monitor may have its chest electrodes attached, and receivers with the most commonly used blood sample bottles, corresponding forms and large syringes may be kept ready. Clipboards with the usual documentation may also be prepared in advance. As well as the technical life-saving equipment, it is important to ensure that sharps boxes and clinical waste bins are strategically placed so that nurses or doctors do not have to wander far to dispose of their needles etc. Furthermore, patients vary in size and weight. It is therefore important that ranges of appropriate sizes of all equipment are stored within the resuscitation area. The arrangement of the resuscitation room and its cupboards should not be changed unless all staff are informed. Moreover, staff must continually update their knowledge of the procedures that may be performed. It is easy to forget skills that are used infrequently, but patients' lives may depend on the rapidity with which certain measures are undertaken. When equipping the resuscitation area it is useful to consider the above assessment process.

Airway maintenance with protection of cervical spine

Equipment that will help to clear and maintain a patient's airway should be readily available at the head end of the patient trolley. On arrival, the patient's airway should be examined for any type of obstruction and appropriate steps taken to clear it if necessary. Piped suction with a rigid catheter attached will facilitate this process. If the patient is unable to fully maintain his own airway, the airway nurse can try several manoeuvres. Manual procedures such as a jaw thrust or chin lift can be done in the immediate instance but will mean that the nurse is unable to assist the rest of the team. Using adjuncts such as oropharyngeal or nasopharyngeal airways will free the nurse and may be all that is required in the patient who has an altered level of consciousness. A useful place to store this equipment is attached to the wall at the head of the patient. For patients who have more serious injuries, it may be necessary to definitively protect their airway. This is done by an anaesthetist who will intubate the patient using a laryngoscope and endotracheal (ET) tube. Again if this has to be done as a life-saving measure, the equipment has to be to hand. Occasionally it will be necessary to sedate and paralyse the patient to facilitate this process. The anaesthetist will require a range of drugs and the airway nurse should ensure that she is familiar with the current drugs used and have them ready for immediate use. Once the ET tube is in place, a mechanism for ventilation will be required which must be attached to a high percentage of oxygen via a piped oxygen supply. Ideally all this equipment should be pre-prepared for rapid use. In cases where the patient has sustained massive facial injuries, a surgical airway may be the only way of adequately oxygenating him. This requires specialist equipment which, again, should be pre-prepared and ready for immediate use.

Patients who present with multiple injuries have often been involved in high-velocity accidents, e.g. RTAs or falls from a height. It is vital that the patient's cervical spine is protected in in-line immobilisation until the resuscitation team is sure that the neck is uninjured. This requires the nurse either to support the patient's neck manually or to place a semi-rigid collar around it. Further support is then achieved by placing a sandbag by each of the patient's ears and applying tape across his forehead to the sides of the trolley. The airway nurse must be vigilant in observing the patient for any signs of nausea or vomiting. With the spine immobilised, the patient is unable to move. If he is likely to vomit then the team would have to log roll him (see p. 839) to protect his spine and assist him with suction apparatus.

Breathing and ventilation

The patient's respiration rate must be measured and recorded and this should include the rate, depth and use of any ancillary muscles. However, it is also important to note how effectively the patient is ventilating, i.e. that there is effective gas exchange taking place at the alveolar capillary membrane. All patients who have sustained significant injuries should receive a high flow of oxygen. This can be delivered via a mask with a reservoir bag with a flow rate of 12–15 L/min (American College of Surgeons 1997). Using pulse oximetry enables the nurse to continually monitor the patient's oxygenation saturation of arterial blood so a pulse oximeter should be situated by the trolley side. Usually this is part of an extensive monitoring system that is able to monitor the patient's heart rate, blood pressure, respiration rate and oxygen saturation continuously and simultaneously.

There are six immediately life-threatening chest conditions — airway obstruction, cardiac tamponade, tension pneumothorax, massive haemothorax, open chest wound and flail chest (Driscoll et al 1993). If the patient has sustained any of these injuries, he will require immediate treatment. It is vital therefore that the necessary equipment for chest drain insertion (see Ch. 3, p. 80) or pericardiocentesis (aspiration of fluid from the pericardial sac) is easily accessible. This type of equipment is usually pre-packed in sterile trays ready for use at a moment's notice. It is the nurse's responsibility to familiarise herself with the contents of these trays so that she is able to assist the medical staff with any necessary procedures.

Circulation with haemorrhage control

In severely traumatised patients, the most common circulatory problem is hypovolaemia (see Ch. 18, p. 638). Any overt bleeding should be controlled by direct pressure using absorbent dressings and bandages. Emergency treatment consists of restoring the circulatory volume as rapidly as possible by the infusion of intravenous (i.v.) fluids. One of the methods of estimating the amount of fluid a patient has lost, or is continuing to lose, is to monitor his clinical vital signs. This includes regular measurement and recording of the patient's heart rate, blood pressure and respiration rate, which can be done using the technical equipment described above. Simply observing the patient's skin colour can provide some indication of how shocked he is, whilst talking to him will indicate his current mental status. The greater the blood loss, the paler the patient will look, and as oxygen availability decreases in the blood supply, he will become increasingly confused and perhaps agitated (Driscoll et al 1993). Once 50% of his total blood volume is lost then the patient will become unconscious. A further guide is the patient's urine output. A catheterisation tray should be readily available and, if the patient has been catheterised, the urine output should be measured at regular intervals using a urometer. The normal urine output for an adult is 30–50 mL/h.

To prevent any deterioration as a result of hypovolaemia, the circulation nurse should ensure that two wide-bore peripheral cannulae are inserted simultaneously into large veins such as the antecubital fossa found over the elbow joint. In some A&E units, it is the nurse who has developed the clinical skills to carry out this procedure, ensuring that she withdraws enough blood for the necessary laboratory investigations to assess the patient's condition. To facilitate this process, sample bottles, forms and large syringes should be prepared and a policy should be in place for the quick transport of samples to the laboratory. Once the peripheral lines have been established, replacement fluids, either crystalloids or colloids warmed to approximately 39°C (American College of Surgeons 1997), must be administered. If the patient appears severely compromised, it may be necessary to use a mechanical pump, e.g. the Level One Blood Warmer, to infuse the fluid more quickly. However, by the time the patient reaches hospital, his peripheral circulation may be 'shut down' (see Ch. 18). This occurs in hypovolaemia as a result of the body's attempt to preserve the vital organs by constricting the peripheral blood vessels and redirecting the available blood to the major organs. Therefore it may be impossible to insert an i.v. cannula in a surface vessel and it may be necessary to perform an i.v. cutdown procedure. This involves making an incision in the skin and subcutaneous tissues and locating a deeper vein in which to insert a cannula. Again, the necessary equipment should be ready.

In order to monitor the patient's progress, it is important that all findings are recorded at regular intervals. In the initial stages of the resuscitation this may be as frequently as every 5 min. The appropriate charts should be available for the recording of vital signs and fluid balance.

Disability: neurological assessment

It is important that a rapid assessment is made of the patient's neurological status. On arrival it is easy for the airway nurse to determine if the patient is alert, i.e. eyes open and responding, or if he responds only to voice. If the patient does neither of these then the nurse needs to assess if the patient responds to painful stimuli. If not, the patient is considered to be unconscious. Concurrently, the nurse should use a torch to assess the patient's pupils to see if they are equal in size and react to light. Again this should be documented as a baseline for future comparison. For a more in-depth neurological assessment, the Glasgow Coma Scale will be used (see Ch. 28, p. 857).

Exposure ensuring environmental control

Whilst the patient's dignity should, of course, be preserved as much as is possible, it is essential that all clothing is removed so that the entire body can be examined from head to toe, front and back, to ensure that no injuries are missed. It is important to remember that exposed trauma patients can lose body heat rapidly, so it is vital that the resuscitation room temperature is warm enough to preserve the patient's body temperature. The use of warmed blankets, which must be replaced between any procedure or examination, will also prevent further temperature drop. The log roll technique (see Fig. 27.2) should be used to enable full examination of the patient's spine. To ensure total spinal immobilisation, a coordinated approach using a team of at least four people is required. The leader of the team will manually immobilise the patient's cervical spine, whilst the three assistants will control the patient's thorax, pelvis and legs.

Q **27.1** Find out from your teacher how to carry out a log roll safely and effectively. Practise this with your fellow students in your clinical laboratory.

A PATIENT WITH MULTIPLE TRAUMA

Assessment and immediate treatment

In Case History 27.1, the ambulance team have informed the A&E department by radio patch of J's condition and given an estimated time of arrival of 10 min. The resuscitation team and radiographer have been summoned and the resuscitation room prepared. Due to the nature of the accident the paramedics have immobilised J on a spinal board with full cervical spine immobilisation after safely removing his helmet.

On arrival, J is transferred onto a trolley which allows X-rays to be taken without moving him. At the same time the paramedics provide a verbal handover outlining the mechanism of the accident, i.e. speed, involvement of any other vehicles or any other injured patients, and an overview of J's clinical condition during his transportation to hospital.

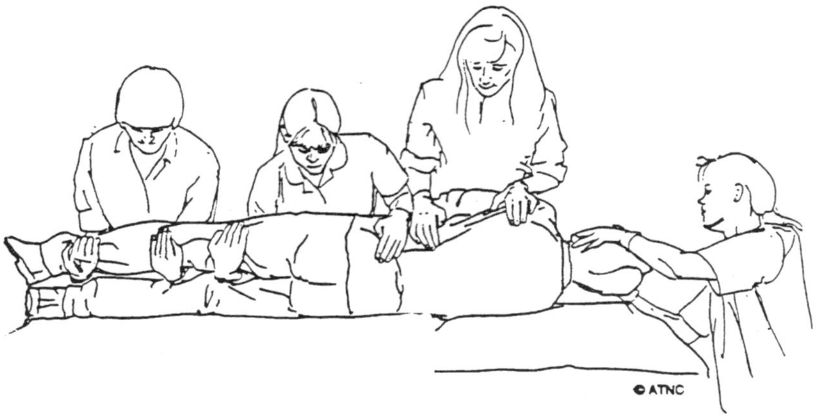

Fig. 27.2 The log roll technique (Reproduced with kind permission from ATNC.)

Case History 27.1 J

J is an 18-year-old man who has been knocked off his motorcycle while travelling at high speed. He was wearing a crash helmet but is brought into the department unconscious by ambulance. He has an oropharyngeal airway in situ and has been given oxygen by the paramedics. His left leg is splinted from the groin to the toes and a closed fracture of the femur is suspected. The police who were called to the scene of the accident have succeeded in finding identification and are now trying to contact J's family.

Once transferred, the airway nurse assesses J's airway. She notes that J is more alert and trying to remove the oropharyngeal airway which is causing him to gag. His airway is clear and there is no overt evidence of facial injuries. J is responding to her voice. Whilst reassuring him, she applies an oxygen mask with reservoir bag attached to 15 L/min of oxygen. She continues to explain to J what is happening to him. Meanwhile the circulating nurse removes J's clothes by carefully cutting them. This allows her to attach the monitor which will record J's pulse, blood pressure and oxygen saturation, whilst one of the doctors looks, listens to and feels J's chest. The nurse counts J's respiration rate, noting the depth of each breath. All clinical observations are passed to the team leader who records them on a trauma chart. J's breathing appears rapid (24 breaths/min) and laboured and, on inspection, it is found that the left side of his chest is not inflating. His oxygen saturation is 91% despite the high-flow oxygen administration. Palpation of the chest wall reveals swelling and crepitus on the left side, indicating possible fractured ribs and a possible pneumo/haemothorax. To ensure adequate gaseous exchange and tissue perfusion, a chest drain must be inserted (see Ch. 3, p. 80). This will also prevent mediastinal shift. Whilst the equipment is being prepared by the team leader and the radiographer is taking chest X-rays, the circulating nurse ensures that two wide-bore cannulae are inserted in J's arms and 2 L of Hartmann's solution warmed to 39°C are administered rapidly. The blood taken from one of these lines is sent directly to the laboratories for a full blood count, urea and electrolytes, and group and cross-match for at least 6 units of blood. The equipment is prepared and the chest X-ray confirms a haemothorax and three fractures of the lower ribs on the left side. The chest drain is inserted using local anaesthetic and strict asepsis. Its placement is confirmed by X-ray and by visible oscillations in the drainage tube. The amount of blood drained from the chest is carefully measured and recorded. Continued observation of respiratory rate, rhythm and depth reveals that J's respiration rate has improved (18 breaths/min), with fairly good expansion on both sides. His oxygen saturation is increasing (now measuring 95%). His colour is pale but not cyanosed.

(Note — motorcyclists often wear expensive leather protective clothing. Conscious patients will frequently forbid this clothing to be cut, preferring to suffer pain rather than have their leathers damaged. In a situation such as the one described here, the clothing must be cut to prevent further injury. Care should be taken, however, to cut clothing along the seams if at all possible, so that it can be repaired later. However, the patient's condition will dictate the urgency with which clothing should be removed.)

As J's breathing has stabilised, the circulating nurse is able to palpate J's radial pulse. She notes its rate, which is rapid (120 beats/min); rhythm, which is regular; and strength, which is thready. At the same time she notes that J's skin is cool, clammy and pale. The monitor displays that J is also hypotensive, with a blood pressure of 70/30 mmHg. These recordings show evidence of hypovolaemia (see Ch. 18, p. 638). There is no overt sign of haemorrhage, although there appears to be an obvious closed fracture to J's left femur and right wrist. J's clinical findings indicate that he may be bleeding internally. Simultaneously, the radiographer has completed pelvic X-rays, and these show no fracture. However, there is bruising over the left upper quadrant of J's abdomen and he is tender on palpation. A ruptured spleen is suspected, as this is often associated with left lower rib fractures. As the spleen is a highly vascular organ, the likelihood is that J has lost a considerable amount of blood into the abdominal cavity. A nurse contacts the general surgeon on call. Further assessment is carried out while the team waits for the surgeon.

Whilst the circulation nurse has been attending to J's circulatory status, the airway nurse has determined that J responds to her voice. He knows who he is, where he is and what month it is. He is complaining of severe pain in his left leg and right wrist. His pupils are checked and found to be equal, within normal limits (2–5 mm) and both react to light. The nurse informs the medical team leader of J's distress, who then decides to apply a Thomas splint to J's left leg and prescribe i.v. morphine to relieve J's pain, plus an antiemetic to prevent any nausea or vomiting. The splint will provide some pain relief as it realigns the fractured bone. Pre- and post-application of the splint, J's dorsalis pedis pulse is checked and is easily palpable.

Using both members of the medical and nursing team, J is now 'log rolled' so that his back and spinal column can be examined. Since his known major injuries are on the left side, he is rolled to the right. Spinal injury has not yet been ruled out, so great care is taken to keep his spine in anatomical alignment. The spinal column is palpated for loss of normal continuity and abnormal curves or 'dips'. J is asked to indicate any areas of pain. No abnormality is detected and J reports no back pain. After preparing J, a rectal examination is performed to check for a high riding or absent prostate gland, which may indicate urethral damage, prior to passing a urinary catheter (American College of Surgeons 1997). Other signs of urethral damage include blood around the external urinary meatus and scrotal haematoma in the male patient.

The blood has now arrived and the rapid infusion of two units is commenced. The appropriate care and observations for a blood transfusion are maintained (see Ch. 11, p. 441). The urinary catheterisation set is ready, and after explaining why it is important to monitor J's urine output the catheter is inserted and a urometer attached. A plaster of Paris backslab is applied to support J's wrist. The surgeon arrives and agrees that J needs immediate transfer to theatre for a laparotomy. Once this has been done and J's condition has further stabilised, the orthopaedic surgeon will reduce and immobilise the fractures more definitively while J is still anaesthetised. The operating staff are informed and a theatre will be prepared. A ward is identified for J's subsequent admission, but in the meantime J's clinical condition continues to be monitored at 15-min intervals.

Care of relatives

J's mother, Mrs S, has now arrived in the department. She has been met by the triage nurse and brought to the relatives' room. Ideally, each department should have a quiet room where the family and friends of seriously ill or injured patients may wait. This room should have comfortable chairs (waiting may often be long), facilities for making tea or coffee, and a telephone, so that other family members or friends can be contacted (British Association for A&E Medicine & RCN 1994). A nurse should, if at all possible, stay with the relatives. People who are in a strange and, in this case, threatening environment are often unsure of how to behave and what is expected of them. They may have questions to ask, such as where the toilets are located, but may be reluctant to leave the room they have been shown into in case they miss some vital information about their loved one. They may also feel that if they come out and ask questions they are depriving their relative of a key member of staff who is essential to the team. Clearly, much anxiety and distress can be avoided if a member of staff remains with the family. Where pressures of work or staff shortages make this impossible, the family should be reassured that their relative is being constantly monitored and is never left alone. They should also be introduced to a nurse who will act as their contact, told where she can be found, and encouraged to approach her with any queries or problems. This nurse should be responsible for seeing the relatives every 15 min or so in order to bring them up to date with developments.

Mrs S has not had the opportunity to contact her husband, as she has come straight to the hospital with the police. She is offered the use of a telephone to get in touch with him but requests that a member of staff does this for her instead. She is given details about her son's condition. These details are truthful, conveying the seriousness of J's condition. It is neither helpful nor compassionate to reassure people falsely in such circumstances. They need time to adjust their feelings in order to cope with what may be very bad news. If relatives are falsely reassured that everything will be all right, they will understandably feel cheated, and trust will be lost, if the outcome is not a happy one. At the same time, all hope should not be destroyed. In encounters such as this, it is essential that the nurse is an experienced communicator, since there is a fine line to be drawn between giving false hope and causing unnecessary anguish. Relatives also have needs at such a stressful time, which the nurse must assess before embarking on lengthy explanations. Mrs S, for example, may have preferred to wait until her husband arrived before being given any information. Breaking bad news thus requires distinct skills, which nurses must learn and practise.

The police have already told J's mother of the circumstances of the accident. She wishes to 'know the worst' about his condition and is now informed of his injuries and the treatment he has received so far. The fact that he has a chest drain and is receiving i.v. fluid is explained, so that she is not alarmed by the presence of this equipment. Mrs S is told that a surgeon has been called and that J is at present being prepared for theatre, but that she may see him if she wishes. The resuscitation team need not interrupt their treatment of J to allow his mother to see him. The team's first priority is, obviously, the patient's physical condition, and they may become so caught up in this that other considerations are forgotten. Often, all that is necessary to reassure relatives and patients is that they can see each other briefly. Family members will be more content if they can see that the patient is actually alive, and it will comfort the patient to know that his family is present. As Mrs S is keen to see her son, she is taken to the resuscitation room accompanied by the same nurse. She is encouraged to stand by the airway nurse and speak to her son. Everything that is happening is explained to both J and Mrs S. The surgeon has now arrived and J's mother returns to the relatives' room with the nurse to wait for her husband. She asks if J's brother, sister and girlfriend should be contacted, and is told that it may, in fact, do everyone good if they are all together at this time of family crisis.

J's vital signs continue to be recorded at regular intervals. It is found that his pulse and blood pressure have stabilised, remaining at 100 beats/min and 90/50 mmHg, respectively. The doctor now has time to spend with J's family, who have now arrived, and explain in more detail the implications of J's injuries. Meanwhile, in the resuscitation room all documentation is assembled. J's clothing and valuables have already been placed in property bags and are now given to his mother. Departments differ as to policy for dealing with property; some record details in a property book, while others leave this task to the admitting ward.

(Note — in certain circumstances, notably in cases of violent assault such as shootings, stabbings or rape, the victim's clothes should be carefully bagged, recorded and given to the police for forensic examination. This may also apply in the case of hit-and-run accidents. It is preferred that items are bagged separately, so that one item does not contaminate another. If property is given to the police, it is important that a police officer signs the property book as receiver of the property and that the nurse who hands it over also signs so that future queries from any source can be readily answered.)

J is now ready to be taken to theatre (see Ch. 26). His family and girlfriend are called to accompany him. They will be able to talk to him along the way and to say their goodbyes when he reaches theatre. The theatre staff are informed that J's family are going to wait, so that they can be kept informed of his progress and be notified when he is returned to the recovery ward. The family is taken to a relatives' room beside the wards, and theatre staff are told where they can be contacted.

It is likely that J will make a full recovery; however, what would have happened if he had died in the A&E department? The following section deals with the nurse's role in supporting relatives who are bereaved by the sudden death of a loved one.

DEATH IN A&E

A very difficult dilemma for A&E staff may arise when they begin to realise that resuscitative measures are not going to succeed. If staff know that the resuscitation attempts are likely to be futile and the family has arrived, it is important that the relatives are gently made aware of the situation by the nurse caring for them, who can outline the gravity of the situation. This provides the family with time, even just a few minutes to internalise the seriousness of the situation. The decision to stop resuscitation efforts is a difficult one, and one that should be made after considering individual team members' views. If the relatives have arrived in A&E, it may be possible to offer them the option of seeing their loved one to say goodbye before the resuscitation efforts are stopped.

All bereavement is traumatic, but sudden death is recognised as one of the most traumatic of experiences (Wright 1996). The deceased was usually last seen alive and well and the fact that he is now dead is very difficult for loved ones to comprehend, as they have had no opportunity to prepare for grief. Feelings of guilt may also prevail if the bereaved person begins to reflect upon things he or she failed to say or do when the loved one was still alive. Caring for distressed relatives in these sorts of circumstances is one of the most draining of nursing interactions (Scott 1995) and it is important that the nurse is prepared for a wide range of emotional reactions. It is also important that the nurse is aware of the individual's religious and cultural beliefs, particularly concerning the disposal of the body following a sudden death. Each A&E department should have direct access to religious ministers from different faiths who can either offer advice or, if the family members request it, be present to support them during this difficult period.

If relatives wish to see their loved one, nurses can do much to help. If possible, those parts of the body that are exposed should be washed. One or (if possible) both of the deceased's hands should be left outside the sheets. The head of the trolley should be slightly raised, otherwise the face may seem distorted when the family first sees the body. False teeth should be replaced for the same reason and the hair combed or smoothed. Where there are severe head injuries, bandages should be left in place and perhaps covered with a clean outer layer. A nurse should initially accompany the relatives, and if they seem hesitant she may indicate that it is all right for them to touch the body, perhaps by doing so herself or by asking the family members if they wish to hold the loved one's hand. The nurse should then offer to withdraw. Not everyone will want to be left alone, but some may have private words of parting to say and should be given the opportunity to do so. Where a whole family is present, this chance should be given to each person individually. One family member may not feel able to ask for this for himself, but when it is suggested by the nurse, he may gratefully accept. Relatives should also feel free to hug or kiss the body; in the case of a dead child, the parents should be able to take the child in their arms. This seems to help people to cope with the denial stage of grieving, especially in cases of sudden death (Kubler-Ross 1984).

Following this period, some relatives may find it difficult to leave the department and may need some assistance. Part of the concluding process may be to give the relatives information relating to the immediate future. Relatives should be made aware that where death has occurred as the result of trauma, a postmortem is always required and that there will probably be an inquest at a later date (HMSO 1993). Providing a card with the departmental phone number allows the relatives to ask any further questions. It is particularly helpful to provide the name of the liaison nurse who cared for them as this provides some continuity. At the same time, it is important to determine how the relatives are going to get home and arrange transport if necessary. On their departure it is wise to inform the family GP, so that she can offer any assistance. Families may also be directed to a variety of support groups such as CRUSE or Compassionate Friends (see 'Useful addresses', p. 849). Most groups have local branches and it is helpful if the department can supply their addresses and telephone numbers. Many organisations produce leaflets or other information that may be beneficial to the bereaved.

Organ donation

If it has become clear that resuscitation will not be successful, it may be possible to approach the family regarding the question of organ donation. Organs and tissues which may be used for transplantation may come either from the 'beating heart' donor — when the patient will usually be admitted to an intensive care unit until brain stem death tests (see Ch. 28, p. 868) are completed — or from patients who have died, i.e. when cessation of circulatory and respiratory function has occurred within A&E. In both instances, the subject may be broached in A&E, so that the family have time to consider their decision. However, it is important that nurses have a sound knowledge base about the different aspects of donation and transplantation, together with their own fears surrounding death, to give them greater confidence in communicating with potential donors. This may seem a cruel intrusion at a time of great grief, but in the long term the donation of the organs of the deceased may help the family to come to terms with their tragedy. By helping someone else to live, their loved one's death may come to seem less futile (Solursh 1990).

Sudden infant death syndrome

The parents of babies who have died from sudden infant death syndrome (SIDS) are particularly vulnerable. This is when an apparently healthy baby has died unexpectedly for no apparent reason (Foundation for the Study of Infant Death 1995). The parents will be asked to identify their baby in the presence of a police officer, before the postmortem examination. This may produce great anxiety and distress, as the parents may feel that they are being accused of causing their child's death. The police are very sensitive to this situation and extremely supportive of parents, but if staff forewarn the parents of this formality they can be saved much anguish. A further supportive measure that may be offered to these parents is to take a photograph of their baby and/or a lock of the baby's hair or a hand/footprint. Sometimes this is not wanted at the time, but the parents should be reassured that they can collect it at any time in the future. Most importantly, parents need time with their baby and they should be encouraged to hold him. Parents are going to need help and support at this difficult time and they should be given information such as the address of the Foundation for the Study of Infant Death (see 'Useful addresses', p. 849).

Staff grief

It is very difficult for staff to have worked hard to save a life without success. Feelings of inadequacy and failure may arise, especially when the patient is young or when the circumstances of the accident seem senseless. Caring for patients and relatives in these circumstances repeatedly may take its toll both emotionally and physically, which means that the care-givers themselves may become casualties. It is important, therefore, to consider the grief that will be felt by staff who have been involved with the patient or his relatives. There should be a forum for expressing feelings and anxieties within the department. One method is a 'defusing' session which can be described as a short type of crisis intervention for staff involved in such an incident (Wright 1996). It allows staff to talk with one another about the experience in a relaxed atmosphere and provides an opportunity to give all staff the key information relating to the whole episode of the incident. This ventilation of feelings and re-run of events can be of benefit in two ways: it can allow staff to express their emotions, and it can highlight defects in the system or ways of improving practice in the future. For particularly distressing incidents, a more formal type of debriefing may be required. Critical incident stress debriefing (CISD, Mitchell 1988) is a session which may be facilitated by someone who has knowledge of counselling skills. It usually takes place 24–48 h after the event and follows a structured format that focuses on the emotional consequences for staff involved in these types of resuscitation. Most importantly, staff should be prepared to help them cope with these types of stresses. Knowledge about stress and coping mechanisms will help staff to recognise their own limitations and to know when they themselves need help (see Ch. 17).

A PATIENT WITH MINOR TRAUMA

Development of the emergency nurse practitioner role

A&E departments and minor injury units (MIUs) have seen the development of an enhanced nursing role. Within the A&E environment these nurses are often referred to as emergency nurse practitioners (ENPs). To date, over 60% of A&E departments offer a service which includes the role of an ENP (Tye et al 1998). One of the fundamental rationales for these rapid developments is the need to reduce waiting times for patients who have suffered minor trauma (Hunt & Wainwright 1994, Crinson 1995). Nurses who practise in this role will have received some formal post-basic education in:

- holistic assessment
- physical diagnosis
- prescription of treatment
- promotion of health.

They will also be working within pre-arranged guidelines as recommended by the RCN (1992). A generally accepted definition of a nurse working within this role describes the practitioner who is able, without any reference to a doctor, to see a patient and elicit data which enable her to reach a diagnostic conclusion and make decisions about the patient's treatment (Hunt & Wainwright 1994, Walsh & Ford 1994, Cable 1995). Despite this definition, there are no nationally accepted boundaries of practice for ENPs to work within. The UKCC's *Scope of Professional Practice* (1992a), which provides guidelines for any nursing role expansion, requires that the nurse accept full responsibility and accountability for her actions. It further requires that any developments within nursing practice must maintain the continuity of patient care whilst meeting the needs and serving the interests of the patient. These guidelines are broad and unspecific, but have enabled A&E departments and MIUs to develop the ENP role to meet the needs of patients presenting with minor injuries. Generally ENPs are able to see, assess, diagnose and treat or refer patients who present with injuries that are considered to fall under the umbrella title of minor trauma. This ensures that the ENP is working within the *Scope of Professional Practice* in that she uses her expanded skills to ensure the continuity of care and, in many cases, to treat the patient's entire injury episode (UKCC 1992a). Examples of some common areas of practice can be seen in Box 27.4.

Box 27.4 Common areas of practice within the emergency nurse practitioner role. (Adapted from Oxford Radcliffe NHS Trust 1995)

- Assessment, examination and treatment of uncomplicated:
  —laceration and wounds
  —hand/wrist/arm/shoulder injuries
  —lower limb injuries
  —minor scalds and burns
  —specified dental, ophthalmic and ENT problems
- Assessment, examination and referral of the above, if there is evidence of any neurovascular or tendon injury or other complications that require specialist intervention
- The requesting of X-rays
- The removal of foreign bodies
- The issue of specified drugs, e.g. tetanus, antibiotics, analgesics, within identified protocols

Assessment and treatment

In Case History 27.2, Mrs N is seen by the triage nurse who assesses her injury using the SOAP model of assessment shown in Box 27.1. Mrs N is able to provide the subjective information and describes how her finger was cut whilst she was washing up some dishes. The water was fairly clean, as she had just put some glasses in to soak. She felt the wound had bled a fair amount since the accident happened approximately 30 min ago and became concerned because the wound looked deep and began to bleed again every time she bent her finger. On examining the wound, the nurse obtains objective information, i.e. there appears to be no evidence of neurovascular compromise as Mrs N's finger is pink and warm to touch and she can feel light touch at the end of her finger. The bleeding can now be described as a controllable minor haemorrhage. Mrs N states that she is usually fit and well and has no other illness or conditions that may complicate this injury. Using this information, the nurse considers the severity of her condition and decides that with the appropriate first aid she can safely wait for a short period for her treatment. As such, she is rated as a non-urgent priority category and the triage nurse documents her assessment on the triage form (see Fig. 27.3). In the interim period it is important

Case History 27.2 Mrs N

Mrs N is a 44-year-old mother of four. She lives with her family and her husband has brought her to the A&E department. Whilst washing up, she 'cut' her left ring finger on a broken glass. This has produced a wound that is still bleeding.

NAME	Mrs N	DATE		CUBICLE Minor 2 MIN/MAJ	PRIORITY LEVEL Non urgent
		ARRIVED	HRS		
AGE	44	ASSESSED	HRS		

NAMED NURSE: ENP

NISCM	A&E	MEDICAL	TRAUMA	SURGICAL	PAEDS	OTHER

PATIENT DEMAND			
Time	Cat		
0800		SUBJECTIVE	ATT STATUS 3 years ago
0900		washing up in clean water, cut (L) ring	OBSERVATIONS
1000		finger on glass - wound continues to bleed	TEMP
1100		OBJECTIVE	
1200			PULSE
1300		O/E Laceration over joint of finger–	
1400		circulation & sensation intact - not	BP
1500		actively bleeding	
1600			RESPS
1700			
1800		TREATMENTS	O_2 SATS
1900			
2000		FIRST AID - Dry dressing, high arm sling	PUPILS
2100		NB wedding ring removed and returned to Mrs N	
2200			G.C.S.
2300			
2400			BM STIX
0100			
0200			ECG
0300			
0400			URINALYSIS
0500			
0600			WATERLOW SCORE
0700			

RELATIVES	Accompanied by husband	PHONE NUMBER	
TIME BED REQUESTED		INITIAL NURSING ASSESSMENT	LACERATION LEFT RING FINGER
TIME Pt READY FOR TRANSFER		EXPECTED WAITING TIME 1 hour	SIGNATURE J Smith
TIME BED IDENTIFIED			

TIME DISCHARGED/ ADMITTED	DESTINATION	SIGNATURE

Fig. 27.3 Completed triage sheet (Mrs N).

Box 27.5 Key factors to consider in the assessment of wounds

History
- How did the injury occur?
- When did the injury occur?
- What environment did it occur in?

Examination
- What size is the wound?
- What type of wound is it?
- How deep is the wound?
- What is the associated neurovascular status?

Investigations
- X-ray for any foreign bodies
- Consider the possibility of infection — bacteriology

that the nurse ensures that no further harm is caused, and she therefore removes Mrs N's wedding ring because of the possibility of swelling and the potential of impairing the circulation to her finger. A pressure dressing is applied to the finger and Mrs N's arm is placed in a high arm sling to stop the bleeding and prevent any further swelling. Mrs N is then informed of the likely waiting time and asked to sit in the waiting area where the triage nurse can observe her. Her husband decides to return home to care for the children.

Mrs N is called through to the treatment area by the ENP, who begins to gather a thorough history and complete an extensive assessment of the injury, an outline of which can be seen in Box 27.5. Using a more in-depth examination technique, the ENP confirms that there is no neurovascular damage and that the finger can be moved within its full range of movement which indicates that there is no injury to the underlying tendons.

If there was evidence of damage to the vessels, nerves or tendons, the ENP would refer Mrs N to the relevant medical specialist team, e.g. the plastic surgery team or orthopaedic team who specialise in hand injuries. The ENP requests an X-ray to identify if there is any glass present in the wound. The result of this is that there is no glass visible. Despite this it is still important that the wound is explored thoroughly under local anaesthetic. Mrs N is transferred to the minor theatre where she is asked to lie on a trolley. The wound that she has sustained can be described as a laceration. The edges are jagged and the wound crosses over a joint, and so it gapes open every time Mrs N bends her finger. Because of this Mrs N requires some sort of primary wound closure. The purpose of this is to approximate the wound edges accurately, thus creating the right conditions to enable an epithelial covering to form over the defect and result in a thinner scar line (Wardrope & Smith 1996). The most common methods of wound closure used within A&E departments are plastic adhesive strips (Steri-Strips), staples, tissue glue and sutures. Whilst the first three of these methods are less invasive for Mrs N, they are usually used for wounds where the edges come together easily and preferably not over a joint. In Mrs N's case the wound edges are jagged and do not oppose easily, and therefore the most appropriate method to ensure adequate wound closure is to insert sutures which will keep the edges firmly opposed during the healing process. The ENP firstly infiltrates the wound with lignocaine using a needle and syringe; this is the most common local anaesthetic used in A&E (Wardrope & Smith 1996). It is important that approximately 5 min is allowed to ensure full effect, so the ENP prepares the equipment that is needed to insert some sutures into the wound whilst the local anaesthetic is being absorbed by the surrounding tissues. Following aseptic procedures throughout, the wound is cleaned using a sodium chloride solution and the ENP explores the wound carefully. Not only is it necessary to explore the wound for any contamination or foreign bodies, but it is also important to examine the underlying structures to ensure that they are fully intact. There is no evidence of any foreign bodies and the wound is not contaminated. The ENP then inserts four interrupted sutures using an aseptic technique and explaining all her actions to Mrs N. Once this is finished and the ENP is sure that there is no further bleeding, a dry but non-adhesive dressing is applied over this to ensure that the wound is kept clean and dry. Again a high-arm sling is placed on Mrs N's arm to minimise any swelling and prevent any further bleeding. The ENP has ascertained that Mrs N has recently had a tetanus vaccination and so does not require further cover.

Health education and discharge advice

For A&E staff, the main involvement in health education activity is in primary health education concerning accident prevention and secondary health education involving first aid and discharge advice (McConnell 1997). The aim of health education in A&E is to empower patients to take responsibility for their recovery and future health status. Patients require practical, achievable solutions to help them cope with their injury. Discharge advice can, if understood and followed, hasten the patient's recovery and prevent complications, but they may require the patient to change some aspects of his usual daily activities. As well as completing a full physical assessment, it is important that the ENP complete a psychosocial assessment. In the case of Mrs N, she has good family support and her children are old enough to contribute to the running of the family home. It is important that Mrs N keeps this finger clean and dry for at least 48 h after primary suture to allow epithelial cover over the wound (Wardrope & Smith 1996). She will need to keep the sling on for approximately 24 h. This may have been difficult if she had had young children to care for, with no one to help her with, for example, the cooking and washing up. Mrs N should also be warned against driving until her injured finger is completely healed. Were she to do so, she might not have complete control of the steering wheel. In addition, if she were to be involved in an accident through no fault of her own, normal car insurance would be unlikely to provide cover for her if it became known that she had an injured finger. It is important that she can get transport home. If necessary, she should be given the opportunity to phone her husband to ask him to collect her. Mrs N should be told that if, during the healing period, the wound becomes increasingly painful, or red and inflamed, she should seek further medical help as she may be developing an infection. A relatively recent innovation is the use of computerised discharge plans for A&E patients; these, whilst being quick and easy to use, allow patients to be given printed, individualised instructions (McKenna 1994). Mrs N is given instructions that remind her to have the sutures removed in 10 days' time (Wardrope & Smith 1996) and reiterate the signs and symptoms of potential infection. Mrs N is advised to have the sutures removed by the practice nurse at her GP's surgery and either to visit the surgery or return to the A&E department if she has any problems. The ENP completes the relevant documentation (see Fig. 27.4) which includes a discharge letter to Mrs N's GP so that there is a complete record of Mrs N's medical history.

PC Laceration to left finger
HPC washing up in clean water (approx 30 mins ago) - cut left finger on broken glass. Since then difficult to stop bleeding, especially when bending finger (NB right handed)
O/E 1.5 cm long laceration, approx 0.25cm deep over DIPJ palmar aspect of left ring finger, Edges of wound jagged and not easily opposed
F.R.O.M.- against resistance - FDP FDS intact
Circulation intact - finger warm and pink
Sensation - 2 point discrimination 4 mm
Not actively bleeding
PMH - fit & well – no illnesses
DH - nil - last tetanus 3 years ago
Allergies - nil
SH - mother of 4 children - youngest 14 years and independent - no particular hobbies
PLAN 1) x-ray (L) ring finger to exclude FB
2) No FB seen Clean, explore and suture wound

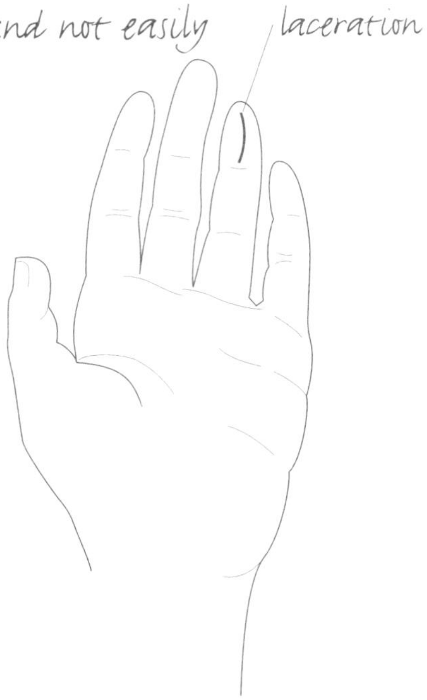

TREATMENT
Lignocaine 1% - 2.5 mls infiltration
Wound explored - no FB, tendons intact
Wound cleaned with n/saline
Wound closed - 3 x 4/0 ethilon(TM) sutures
Dry dressing + high arm sling applied
Advice given Re: removal of sutures in 10 days / with GP
signs of infection

Husband contacted
GP letter sent

J Smith

Emergency Nurse Practitioner

DRUGS /TREATMENT

DATE	DRUGS /TREATMENT	DR's INITS	NURSE	TIME

Fig. 27.4 Completed documentation by ENP (for Mrs N).
DH, Drug history; DIDJ, Distal inter-phalangeal joint; FB, Foreign body; FDP Flexor digitorum profundus; FDS Flexor digitorum superficialis; FROM, Full range of movement; HPC, History of presenting complaint; PC, Presenting complaint; PMH, Past medical history; SH, Social history

AGGRESSION AND VIOLENCE IN A&E

Our changing society

A&E is a challenging and rewarding area in which to work. The dynamic nature of the job means that one never knows what will happen next. One minute the nurse may be required to comfort an elderly gentleman who has unexpectedly lost his partner of 50 years, and the next to support a mother who has unexpectedly gone into labour and is about to deliver her baby. Likewise, caring for patients with minor injuries ranges from caring for a child who has fallen off his bike, to irrigating a patient's eyes as a result of a chemical splash incident whilst at work. As a result, nurses are able to practise a wider range of skills than are perhaps used in other clinical settings. However, there are drawbacks to operating an 'open door' policy. It means that nurses will be required to care for patients with a range of conditions and problems. The nature of these events may put the individual concerned into a sudden state of crisis that may produce various types of stress reaction. These include the intense emotions, e.g. fear, anxiety, confusion and loss of control, all experienced as a result of the uncertainty of the situation. On occasion this may display itself in the form of aggression and, in extreme cases, physical violence. The Health & Safety Commission (1997) defines violence against staff as 'any incident in which a person working in the healthcare sector is verbally abused, threatened or assaulted by a member of the public in circumstances relating to his or her employment'. It should be noted, though, that verbal abuse and threats are the most common types of aggression. A&E nurses face perhaps more verbal and physical abuse than any other nursing group (Health and Safety Commission 1997). A recent study (see Research Abstract 27.1) identified two frequently influential factors with regard to the occurrence of violence: the presence of alcohol or other drugs, and levels of perceived frustration of the aggressor (Harkness 1997). Within the A&E environment, patients are often treated for injuries that are alcohol-related or that have been self-inflicted, e.g. drug overdoses. Added to this is the frustration experienced by many patients over long waiting times. As a result of government initiatives such as the *Patient's Charter* (DoH 1991), patients are more aware of their rights, and sometimes their expectations to be seen and treated quickly exceed what the A&E department can provide. Whatever the predisposing factor, it is important that nurses working in this environment are able to anticipate possible situations and prevent them from escalating to a point where potential harm may be caused.

Research Abstract 27.1
A study of violence at work

Violence in the workplace is a growing concern for both employers and employees. A study which considered two service sector groups, including hospital staff, investigated the incidence of violence, observed the nature of violent incidents and observed the antecedents of any reported violent incidents, the actual behaviour and how the incident ended. Key findings identified that 24% of hospital staff had experienced aggressive physical contact and 69.8% had experienced verbal abuse in the preceding 12 months. Antecedents included patients questioning medical/nursing procedures, and individuals thought to be under the influence of alcohol. The most common methods of bringing an incident to a close included reassurance, discussion and walking away, although in 18% of cases hospital security was called and in 3% the police were called to intervene. The report concluded that training can help to equip an employee to be more competent in a range of situations.

Harkness L 1997 Part of the job? A study of violence at work. Occupational Health Review 65: 25–27.

Defusing a potentially aggressive situation

Nurses should remember that aggression is seldom directed towards them personally. It is important that they are able to recognise the factors that influence aggression in an A&E situation. These include a lack of information either about the condition of a relative or about the excessive waiting times. Waiting rooms that have poor facilities can contribute to an individual's level of frustration, e.g. a phone box that does not work, uncomfortable seating and an unwelcoming decor. The attitude of staff to patients, particularly if it appears judgemental and unsympathetic, may contribute to the development of a confrontation between patient or relative and nurse. However, it must be acknowledged that not all aspects of aggression are avoidable within the A&E environment. Sometimes the aggression is a result of metabolic disorders which cause acute confusional states, e.g. hypoxia or diabetes, or a result of head injury. In these situations the patient has no control over his actions. However, there are usually warning signs, such as those given in Box 27.6, and it is essential that nurses are able to recognise these if they are to prevent the situation escalating. Other strategies that help to defuse difficult situations include the use of good verbal and non-verbal communication and the adoption of a calm non-threatening approach.

Body posture

Trying to resolve situations within large groups often increases the aggression so it is preferable to invite the aggressive individual to a separate area. Ideally this should be in a private place, but this should not compromise the safety of the member of staff. Adopting an oblique posture is less confrontational and, if standing, the nurse should position her feet slightly apart with her body weight on the slightly flexed back leg. The nurse should be aware of the individual's personal space and it is recommended that she remain at least an arm's length away. These actions serve two

Box 27.6 Warning signs of aggression

Emotional
- Individual appears agitated and tense
- Individual's voice increases in volume and pitch, which is apparent in the way he abruptly responds to questions
- Individual may use sarcasm and obscenities when talking to staff

Behavioural
- Body posture may reveal muscular tension in face and limbs
- Individual may be making fists with hands, banging fists or hitting out at objects

Physiological
- Pupils may be dilated, although this may be difficult to observe

purposes: they are less threatening and allow a quick escape should the need arise (Neades 1994). The nurse must demonstrate that she is genuinely interested in what the individual has to say. Direct eye contact may be interpreted as being provocative, but completely avoiding eye contact may be perceived as dismissive and suggestive of disinterest, so it is better to focus away from the face, just below the larynx area.

Listening to aggressive patients

The nurse should listen carefully to the complaint and offer an explanation. It is difficult not to shout back when being shouted at, but it is more effective if the pitch, tone and volume of the nurse's voice remain within a normal conversational range (Neades 1994). The nurse should be sensitive to the individual's circumstances and a sympathetic approach may avoid the escalation of the aggressive confrontation. If the individual is confused for any reason, the nurse may have to repeat what is being said several times before being understood. If possible, she should agree a plan of action with the individual to resolve the situation. It is unwise to give false information or agree on solutions that are unachievable as this will result in trust being lost and may cause further aggression at a later stage.

Avoiding physical danger and attack

Unfortunately there are times when, despite all the strategies, violence does occur and it is vital that the nurse considers this possibility in all encounters with abusive patients. For this reason, nurses should never place themselves in a situation where they are trapped in an enclosed area. If interviewing an aggressive individual alone in a private room, the nurse should ensure that the area is free of objects that may be used as weapons and that the door is not lockable. Potential weapons include equipment such as scissors and stethoscopes carried by the nurse which, if grabbed, could be used to threaten her. The safety of the staff and the other patients is of paramount importance. If it appears that violence is going to erupt, the nurse should slowly back away from the situation and not attempt to restrain the individual. Help should be summoned using agreed departmental procedures. Most A&E units have panic buttons that either summon help from other A&E staff or security officers, or are connected direct to the local police station. Until help is available, the nurse should make every attempt to avoid physical contact. This may involve the use of hospital equipment to create space between herself and the aggressive individual. It is preferable that hospital equipment is damaged rather than people hurt.

It is important that, following any incident of aggression or violence, whether verbal or physical, an incident form is completed and that this is reviewed by the hospital's health and safety officer or risk management team. This monitors the escalating problem and may reveal patterns of aggression in the workplace, thereby allowing preventive strategies to be formulated. These may include extra training opportunities for the staff or an increase in staffing levels. If it is apparent that there is an increase in violent and aggressive situations, statistical evidence is useful when making a bid to management for more security staff or better protection.

Q

27.2 Find out about the procedure to follow in your hospital/health centre should a member of staff be injured. What documentation is required? Who should complete it and where should any forms be sent?

A&E and the law

Due to the nature of A&E work, nurses are, on occasion, required to work in close collaboration with the local police force. Sadly, victims of crime and those who have committed an offence may require hospital treatment and the medical findings are used as evidence in a court of law. If a death has occurred under suspicious circumstances, the police may require that forensic evidence be collected to assist them with their enquiries. This sometimes creates a conflict in the nurse's professional practice. All patients are entitled to confidentiality in respect of information about them and it is the nurse's responsibility to ensure that this right is respected (UKCC 1992b). However, there are exceptions to this which particularly arise within the A&E environment — e.g. if a person has been involved in an RTA then the law requires that any relevant information should be given to the police. Other examples are outlined in Box 27.7. As part of this process, the nurse may be required to make a statement which will form part of the police investigation, especially if she was a witness to an event such as a violent incident within the department. It should be noted, though, that it may be several years before a case, whether criminal or civil, comes before the courts and the nurse is asked to write the statement. For this reason it is important that careful attention is paid to accurate documentation within the patient's nursing and medical records.

MAJOR INCIDENTS

There is no one standard definition of a major incident. For the purpose of guidance, the NHS Management Executive (1990) states that a major incident arises when any occurrence presents a serious threat to the health of the community, disruption to a service, or causes or is likely to cause such numbers of casualties as to require special arrangements by the health service. This definition is deliberately unspecific, because what constitutes a major incident for a small rural hospital may have minimal impact in a large inner city general hospital. Similarly a large-scale disaster may affect only one hospital or may require the services of several hospitals within a region. The purpose of emergency planning for such situations within the NHS is to ensure that all the emergency services are able to work collaboratively and provide an effective response to any type of incident.

Major incident planning

It is essential that every hospital has a major incident plan. The A&E department plays a major role in this, as it is required to provide the initial response, often within a short period of time.

Box 27.7 Exceptions to the duty of confidentiality

- Consent of a patient
- Best interests of the patient
- Court orders
  —subpoena
  —Supreme Court Act (1981)
- Statutory duty to disclose
  —Road Traffic Act (1982)
  —Prevention of Terrorism Act (1984)
  —Public Health Act (1984)
  —Misuse of Drugs Act (1971)
- Public interest

To enable the A&E department to manage effectively in such a situation, it is vital that the department has the support of all other services within the hospital. Extra equipment will be needed, patients will have to be moved quickly and it should be anticipated that more staff will be needed than usually work on a shift. For this reason it is important that all hospital departments, including portering, catering staff, cleaning staff, as well as other clinical support areas, are involved in the development of the major incident policy. The essence of any plan is that it is flexible enough to cater for any situation, which may include chemical contamination incidents, a large number of patients with multiple injuries or thermal injuries.

In the event of an incident, the A&E department will be notified by the local ambulance service. It will have to prepare quickly to receive the predicted number of patients. This is achieved by clearing the department as quickly as possible and restocking principal areas with extra equipment whilst calling in extra staff. The A&E department may be asked to provide an on-site mobile medical team, which should consist of nurses and doctors, to assist the ambulance service with patients who are trapped in wreckage for long periods. It is vital that these staff are adequately equipped with warm and protective clothing, as they will be required to support the ambulance service in difficult and potentially dangerous environments. Casualties are predominantly brought into the department by ambulance, although 'walking wounded' patients will often be ferried in by local people not involved in the incident.

Due to the volume of patients, it is important that careful attention is paid to adequate identification of all individuals. The police will operate a casualty bureau to keep the general public informed. The A&E staff will have to keep this unit updated with details of patients, and this is done via a police documentation team, which will be based in the hospital. Many relatives will arrive at the hospital demanding information and, as in all public interest events, the media will require regular press statements. It is important that this does not interrupt the staff's care of the patients. The hospital will need to ensure adequate facilities and support staff to care for the friends and relatives waiting to see the injured, whilst establishing separate communication networks for the media. Once all the casualties have been cared for and transferred to other areas for their definitive care, the A&E department must resume its customary work as soon as possible.

Because of the relative infrequency of major incidents and the pattern of staff changes, it is recommended that hospitals exercise jointly with the ambulance and other emergency services at regular intervals to ensure a rapid and effective response (NHS Management Executive 1990).

Q **27.3** Where is the major incident plan held in your hospital? Ask your tutor or mentor if you may see it and discuss it during a seminar.

Post-traumatic stress disorder

It has become apparent in recent years that the survivors of major incidents may suffer from a range of long-term psychological and physical symptoms unrelated to injuries sustained at the time. These may include feelings of desperation, helplessness, guilt at having survived where others have died, and shame at the loss of control. The survivors may also experience anger, feelings of loss and profound sadness, and may be unable to put the incident out of their minds. Physical symptoms may include insomnia, nausea, diarrhoea, dizziness and palpitations, to name only a few (Sowney 1996; see also Ch. 17). It is important for survivors to realise that these manifestations are normal reactions to a terrible tragedy and that they are not 'losing their minds'. However, if these symptoms persist and start interfering with the individual's normal daily living then it may be that they are suffering from what has been described as 'post-traumatic stress disorder'. In these instances, some of the victims will require prolonged counselling in order to come to terms with their feelings and anxieties, and members of their families may also need to be included in counselling sessions. Witnesses of disasters may also be deeply affected. Following the Lockerbie air disaster in 1988, when as a result of a terrorist bomb, a Pan American aircraft disintegrated over a small town in Scotland, killing 259 passengers and 11 town residents, more than 100 residents were referred to community psychiatric nurses. O'Byrne (1989) reported: 'The brush with death had forced many of the town's inhabitants to re-evaluate what they were doing with their lives'. Close media coverage of such events may give those who were not involved, but who were bereaved as a result of the incident, the feeling that they were present when it happened. These people may also experience the feelings of guilt suffered by the actual survivors. This will naturally involve the families of the victims but may also include a much wider range of people. One example of this was when more than 200 people drowned in the Zeebrugge car ferry disaster in 1987 — 160 off-duty crew members of the *Herald of Free Enterprise*, some of whom had swapped duties with their shipmates, were among the circle of people requiring counselling and support (Johnston 1989).

Rescue workers, A&E staff and other personnel involved in the event are also vulnerable to serious emotional disturbances following such incidents (Scott & Stradling 1994). Even with good deployment of staff, disasters provoke an 'all hands on deck' situation. Staff may need to be called in from off duty, and others will volunteer after hearing about the incident on the news. Staff will be required to work long hours under difficult conditions, especially if they are part of an on-site team. Some victims will not be saved and this may produce feelings of inadequacy or guilt. Because of the need for the department to return to normality as soon as possible so that it can deal with other patients, there may be insufficient time for staff to rest before returning to more routine jobs. A rush of adrenaline will keep everyone going at the time, but afterwards they may display emotions ranging from anger to guilt or deep sorrow.

It is apparent that following major incidents a range of facilities must be made available to staff (Scott & Stradling 1994, Robson et al 1995). The nature of these facilities may differ from place to place, but they should include educational programmes and a support network for all staff, and should ideally be in place before any such incidents occur. Where these networks are available and accepted, staff may be less inclined to feel stigmatised if they make use of them when the occasion arises. Now that it is recognised that staff of all disciplines who are involved in disaster situations may suffer from post-traumatic stress disorder, it is essential that provision should be made in disaster planning for the support of these carers following a traumatic event.

REFERENCES

American College of Surgeons 1997 Advanced trauma life support program for physicians. American College of Surgeons, Chicago
Audit Commission 1996 By accident or design: improving A&E services in England and Wales. HMSO, London
Blythin P 1988 Triage in the UK. Nursing 3(31): 16–20
British Association for Accident & Emergency Medicine (BAAEM) and Royal College of Nursing (RCN) 1994 Bereavement care in A&E departments: report of the working group. RCN, London
Cable S 1995 Minor injuries clinics: dealing with trauma. British Journal of Nursing 4(20): 1177–1182
Central Statistics Office 1994 Social trends 24. HMSO, London
Chandler E 1993 Can post-traumatic stress disorder be prevented? Accident & Emergency Nursing 1(2): 87–91
Crinson I 1995 Impact of the patients' charter on A&E departments 2: the emergency nurse practitioner. British Journal of Nursing 4(22): 1321–1325
Department of Health 1991 The patient's charter: a summary. HMSO, London
Department of Health 1994 Hospital episode statistics, vol 2, England: financial year 1990–1991. HMSO, London
Driscoll P, Gwinnutt C, LeDuc Jimmerson C, Godall O 1993 Trauma resuscitation: the team approach. Macmillan, London
Fiest J, Brannon L 1988 Health psychology: an introduction to behaviour and health. Waddesworth, Belmont
Foundation for the Study of Infant Death (FSID) 1995 Sudden infant death: a workbook for professionals. FSID, London
Harkness L 1997 Part of the job? A study of violence at work. Occupational Health Review 65: 25–27
Health and Safety Commission 1974 Health and Safety at Work Act 1974. HMSO, London
Health and Safety Commission 1997 Violence and aggression to staff in health services. HSE Books, Suffolk
Hill M 1990 Trauma prevention: puzzlement or possibility? AAOHN Journal 38(10): 465
HMSO 1993 What to do after a death. HMSO, London
Hnott E, Davis D 1984 Triage problem orientated documentation reflects quality of care. Points of View Ethicon 21(2)
Hunt G, Wainwright P 1994 Expanding the role of the nurse: the scope of professional practice. Blackwell Science, Oxford
Johnston J 1989 Haunted by memories. Nursing Times 85(11): 56–58
Kubler-Ross E 1984 On death and dying. Tavistock, London
McConnell D 1997 Health promotion for A&E practice. Emergency Nurse 5(7): 19–22
McKenna G 1994 The scope for health education in the accident & emergency department. Accident & Emergency Nursing 2(2): 94–99
Manchester Traige Group 1997 Emergency triage. BMJ, London
Mitchell J 1988 Developments and functions of a critical incident stress debriefing team. Journal of Emergency Medical Services 13(12): 42–46
Neades B 1994 How to handle aggression. Emergency Nurse 2(2): 23–24
NHS Management Executive 1990 Emergency planning in the NHS: health services arrangements for dealing with major incidents. NHS Management Executive, London
O'Byrne J 1989 Talking through the pain. Nursing Standard 3(25): 12
Oxford Radcliffe NHS Trust 1995 Specialist skills practitioner (SSP) protocols (unpublished). Oxford Radcliffe NHS Trust, Oxford
Robson R, Mitchell J, Murdoch P 1995 The debate on psychological debriefings. Australian Journal of Emergency Care 2(4): 6–7
Royal College of Nursing Emergency Nurse Practitioners' Group 1992 Guidance notes. RCN, London
Royal College of Nursing 1994 The care of sick children: a review of the guidelines in the wake of the Beverly Allitt inquiry. RCN, London
Royal College of Surgeons of England 1988 The management of patients with major injuries: report of a working party. Royal College of Surgeons of England, London
Sbaih L 1992 Accident & emergency nursing: a nursing model. Chapman and Hall, London
Scott T 1995 Sudden death in A&E. Emergency Nurse 2(4): 10–13
Scott M, Stradling S 1994 Counselling for post traumatic stress disorder. Sage, London
Solursh D S 1990 The family of the trauma victim. Nursing Clinics of North America 25(1): 155–162
Sowney R 1996 Stress debriefing: reality or myth? Accident & Emergency Nursing 4: 38–39
Tye C, Ross F, Kerry S 1998 Emergency nurse practitioner services in major A&E departments. Journal of Accident & Emergency Medicine 15: 31–34
United Kingdom Central Council for Nursing, Midwifery and Health Visiting 1992a The scope of professional practice. UKCC, London
United Kingdom Central Council for Nursing, Midwifery and Health Visiting 1992b The code of professional practice. UKCC, London
Walsh M, Ford P 1994 New rituals for old: nursing through the looking glass. Butterman & Heinemann, Oxford
Wardrope J, Smith J 1996 The management of wounds and burns. Oxford University Press, Oxford
Wright B 1996 Sudden death: a research base for practice. Churchill Livingstone, Edinburgh

USEFUL ADDRESSES

CRUSE
Bereavement Care
126 Sheen Rd
Richmond
Surrey TW9 1UK

CRITEC
Crisis Counselling, Training, Education, Support

CRITEC Office
Leeds General Infirmary
Great George St
Leeds LS1 3EX

Foundation for Study of Infant Deaths
35 Belgrave Square
London SW1X 8QB

THE UNCONSCIOUS PATIENT

28

Lesley Pemberton

INTRODUCTION

The unconscious patient presents a special challenge to the nurse. Her medical management will vary according to the original cause of her condition, but her nursing care will be constant. The unconscious patient has no control over herself or her environment. She is therefore dependent upon the nurse to accept responsibility for the management of her activities of living and for monitoring her vital functions.

The quality of nursing care is of crucial importance if the patient is to relearn to perceive herself and others, to communicate, to control her body and her environment and to care for herself.

The responsibility placed on the nurse is considerable and can be a source of anxiety, even for experienced nurses (see Ch. 17). It is therefore essential that the nurse has a firm understanding of the mechanisms causing altered states of consciousness as well as a sound knowledge of the potential and actual physiological, psychological and social problems that these patients face. Skills training, exploring attitudes and using support systems can all help the nurse to overcome his anxiety and take up the challenge.

To nurse an unconscious patient back to recovery must be one of the most rewarding aspects of nursing; however, even with all the medical advances made recently, not all patients can hope for complete recovery. Some may not survive and others may be left with a residual mental and/or physical handicap. These patients and their families will need strong emotional support and reassurance. The nurse, who is with the patient more than other members of the multidisciplinary team, is often in the best position to give this support.

Defining consciousness

Normal conscious behaviour is dependent on an intact brain function. Impaired, reduced or absent consciousness implies the presence of brain dysfunction and demands urgent medical attention if potential recovery is to be expected. In order to appreciate the importance of altered states of consciousness an understanding of consciousness itself is required.

Hickey (1997, p. 134) defines consciousness simply as ‘a state of general awareness of oneself and the environment’ and includes the ability to orient toward new stimuli. The individual is wakeful, alert and aware of her personal identity and of the events occurring in her surroundings. Deep coma can be defined as the opposite — unrousable and unresponsive to external stimuli — and there may be varied states of altered consciousness in between the two extremes. The difference between sleep and coma is that, in sleep, the individual can be aroused by external stimuli, whereas in a coma this cannot be done. Consciousness therefore depends on whether the person can be aroused to wakefulness. Different stages of consciousness will be discussed later in this chapter.

ANATOMICAL AND PHYSIOLOGICAL BASIS FOR CONSCIOUSNESS

The reticular formation (RF) and the reticular activating system (RAS) are responsible for collating and transmitting motor and sensory activities and controlling sleep/waking cycles and consciousness (see Fig. 28.1 and Ch. 25).

The reticular formation

The RF is a network of neurones in the central core of the brain stem (Wilson & Waugh 1996). These neurones connect with the spinal cord, cerebellum, thalamus and hypothalamus. The RF is involved in the coordination of skeletal muscle activity, including voluntary movement, posture and the maintenance of balance. It is also concerned with automatic and reflex activities and it has links with the limbic system. All sensory pathways, including those of the special senses, link into the RF (Fitzgerald 1996). Neurones which produce aminergic neurotransmitters are embedded within the RF. Some of these have a stimulating effect and some an inhibitory effect on other neurones, although their exact functions are not fully understood at present.

The reticular activating system

The RAS is a physiological concept of the RF and the neurones which project (or radiate) to ocular motor nuclei and to the cerebral cortex via the thalamus and hypothalamus. It is concerned with the arousal of the brain in sleep and wakefulness (Fitzgerald 1996).

Two main parts of the RAS have been identified (Guyton 1991):

- the mesencephalon
- the thalamus.

The mesencephalic area is composed of grey matter in the upper pons and midbrain of the brain stem. Stimulation of this area causes a very diffuse flow of nerve impulses which pass upwards through the thalamus and hypothalamus. The impulses then radiate out to wide regions of the cerebral cortex (see Fig. 28.1). This causes a generalised increase in cerebral activity and general wakefulness.

The thalamic area is composed of grey matter within the thalamus (see Fig. 28.1). It differs from the mesencephalic part in that stimulation of this area activates localised areas of the cerebral cortex. Signals from specific parts of the thalamus initiate activity in specific parts of the cortex, rather than activating the whole cortex. This selective stimulation prevents the cortex from receiving too much information at once and may play a part in directing one's attention to specific mental activities.

The reticular nucleus, which receives impulses from the RF, surrounds the front and sides of the thalamus. It is this nucleus that sends inhibiting messages back to thalamic nuclei via a neurotransmitter called gamma-aminobutyric acid (GABA). In animal experiments it has been demonstrated that thalamocortical neurones are inhibited by the reticular nucleus during sleep (Fitzgerald 1996).

The arousal reaction

In order to function, the RAS must be stimulated by input signals from a wide range of sources via the spinal reticular tracts and various collateral tracts, such as the specialised auditory and visual tracts and therefore all the modalities of sensation (see Ch. 9). The RAS is also stimulated by signals from the cerebral cortex, i.e. the

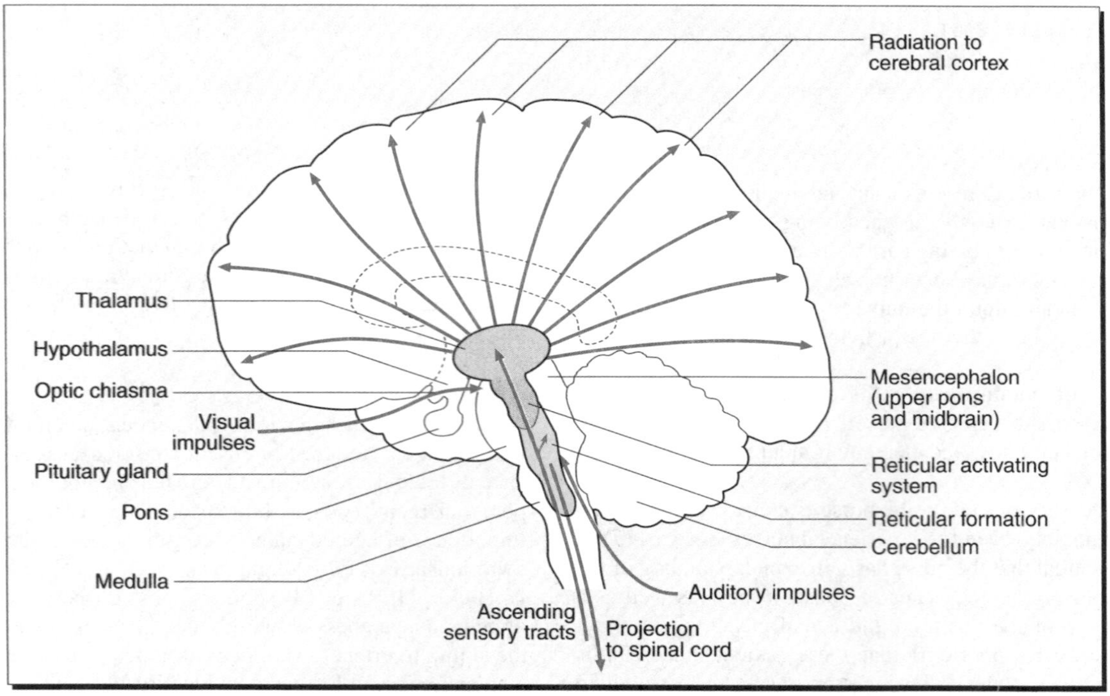

Fig. 28.1 The mid-sagittal section of the brain, showing the reticular activating system and related structures.

RAS may first stimulate the cerebral cortex and the cortical areas responding to reason and emotion may 'modify' the RAS either positively or negatively according to the 'decision' of the cerebral cortex. The RAS transmits and filters information (habituation).

For instance, when an individual is in a deep sleep, the RAS is in a dormant state. Almost any type of sensory signal, however, can immediately activate the RAS and waken her, e.g. pain stimuli or unaccustomed noise. This is called the 'arousal reaction' and is the mechanism by which sensory stimuli wake us from deep sleep (Guyton 1991) (see Ch. 25).

Sleep is induced by a substance called melatonin. This is synthesised from serotonin in the pineal gland. The normal arousal from sleep occurs as it gets light. Daylight is detected by the retina of the eye which sends impulses to the suprachiasmatic nucleus of the hypothalamus. This activates sympathetic nerve fibres which inhibit the secretion of melatonin in the pineal gland. There is also evidence from animal experiments that histamine, produced in the posterior hypothalamic area, activates the cerebral cortex. Lesions in this area can cause excessive sleepiness or even coma (Fitzgerald 1996).

There are numerous pathways to both mesencephalic and thalamic portions from the sensory and motor cortex and from cortical areas that deal with the emotions. Whenever any of these areas becomes excited, impulses are transmitted into the RAS, thus increasing the activity. This is termed a 'positive feedback response' (Spence & Mason 1987).

The feedback theory

Magoun (1963) claimed that the cerebrum regulates incoming information by a positive feedback mechanism (Fig. 28.2). A second feedback cycle that stimulates proprioceptors is also shown in Figure 28.2.

After a prolonged period of wakefulness, the synapses in the feedback loops become fatigued, the RAS becomes dormant and sleep is induced (Spence & Mason 1987). The degree of wakefulness and consciousness is normally dependent on the number of feedback loops activated (Guyton 1991). Figure 28.2 illustrates a number of activating pathways passing from the mesencephalon upward through the thalamus to the cortex. If only one of these becomes activated, the degree or level of consciousness is minimal. Conversely, if all pathways are activated simultaneously, a high level of consciousness ensues.

The return to consciousness demonstrates that the RAS is still functioning and capable of screening and discrimination.

The content of consciousness

The content of consciousness refers to the sum of cognitive and affective mental functions. It is dependent upon relatively intact functional areas within the cerebral hemispheres that interact with each other as well as with the RAS.

Injury to, or disease of, the cerebral hemispheres, resulting in diffuse damage, can inhibit or block the signals from the RAS and consciousness cannot be completely maintained. The damaged cortex is unable to interpret the incoming sensory impulses and therefore cannot transmit them to other areas for action.

Localised damage to the cerebral hemispheres can also diminish the content of consciousness to a lesser degree (Plum & Posner 1980). For example, a patient who has suffered a stroke causing aphasia may appear awake and alert. Her inability to understand or to use language, however, decreases her full awareness of herself and her environment. Such localised defects are not generally regarded as a true altered state of consciousness, but this example highlights the difficulties in defining true conscious behaviour.

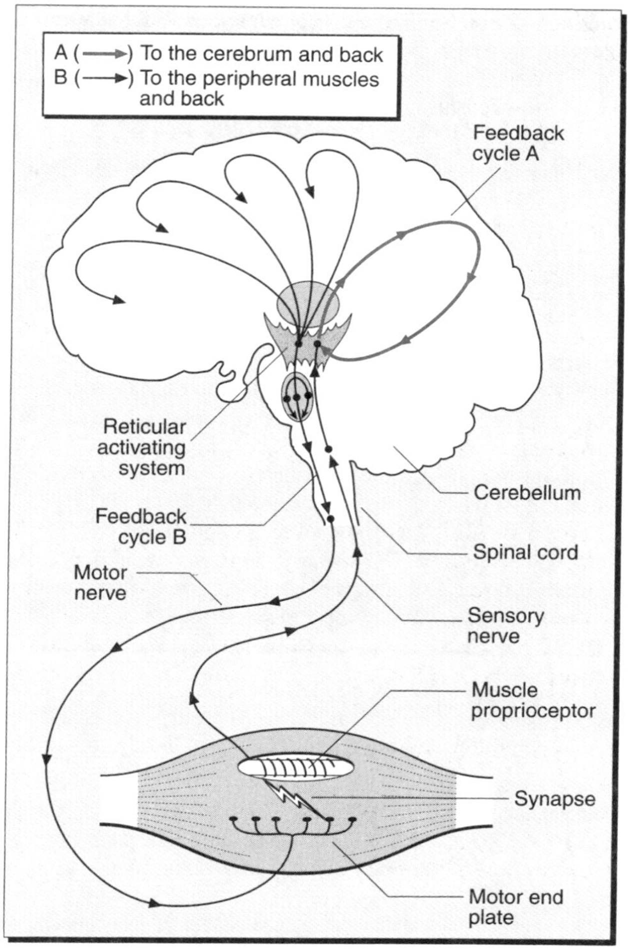

Fig. 28.2 The feedback mechanism, showing two feedback cycles passing through the RAS. In cycle A, the RAS excites the cerebral cortex and the cortex in turn re-excites the RAS. This initiates a cycle that causes continued intense excitation of both regions. In cycle B, impulses are sent down the spinal cord to activate skeletal muscles. Activation of the muscle stimulates proprioceptors to transmit sensory impulses upward to re-excite the RAS. Consciousness results when the RAS, in turn, stimulates the cerebral cortex.

STATES OF IMPAIRED CONSCIOUSNESS

There is no international definition of levels of consciousness but, for assessment purposes, differing states of consciousness can be considered on a continuum between full consciousness and deep coma (Hickey 1997 pp. 137–138). Consciousness cannot be measured directly but can be estimated by observing behaviour in response to stimuli. The Glasgow Coma Scale (GCS) is widely used as an assessment tool and helps to reduce subjectivity during assessment. The GCS is explained on pages 856–859.

Signs of deterioration in a patient's level of consciousness are usually the first indications of further impending brain damage. The nurse must be able to accurately assess and observe the patient so that appropriate intervention can be instituted if the level of consciousness changes. (Sleep is considered a normal phenomenon and is discussed in Ch. 25.)

Impaired states of consciousness can be categorized as acute or chronic. Acute states are potentially reversible, whereas chronic states tend to be irreversible as they are caused by destructive

Box 28.1 Continuum of levels of consciousness. (Adapted from Hickey 1997)

- *Full consciousness* — awake, alert, oriented, cognitive (mental) functioning intact
- *Confusion* — disoriented to time/place/person, short attention span, memory problems, may be agitated/restless/irritable
- *Lethargy* — oriented, slow speech, slow mental processes, slow motor activities
- *Obtundation* — rousable with stimulation, responds verbally with one or two words, follows simple commands, very drowsy
- *Stupor* — quiet, minimal movement, generally unresponsive except to vigorous stimuli, responds in normal way to painful stimuli
- *Coma* — unrousable, no verbal sounds, inappropriate or no response to stimuli

It is difficult to classify levels of consciousness exactly, but this is a useful guide to help to describe various levels.

brain lesions. The following definitions of impaired states of consciousness can be used as broad guidelines to describe the patient's condition. Individual patients are unlikely to exhibit all the stages noted on the continuum (see Box 28.1), even if they pass from full consciousness to coma or vice versa. Deterioration or improvement will depend on a number of factors such as type, extent and site of injury, age, previous state of health, length of coma and whether or not the altered level of consciousness is a result of acute or chronic insult.

Acute states of impaired consciousness

The acute states are caused by intracranial diseases and metabolic upsets, such as hypoglycaemic coma or drug overdose, which alter brain function. The acute states are:

- clouding of consciousness
- delirium
- illusions
- hallucinations
- delusions
- stupor
- coma.

Clouding of consciousness

Clouding of consciousness refers to changes of conscious activity where the patient's awareness is reduced. It reflects generalised brain dysfunction, as seen in systemic and metabolic disorders (see Fig. 28.3). These disorders have interfered with the integrity of the RAS, thus affecting the arousal response.

In its early stages, clouding may include hyperexcitability and irritability, alternating with drowsiness (Plum & Posner 1980).

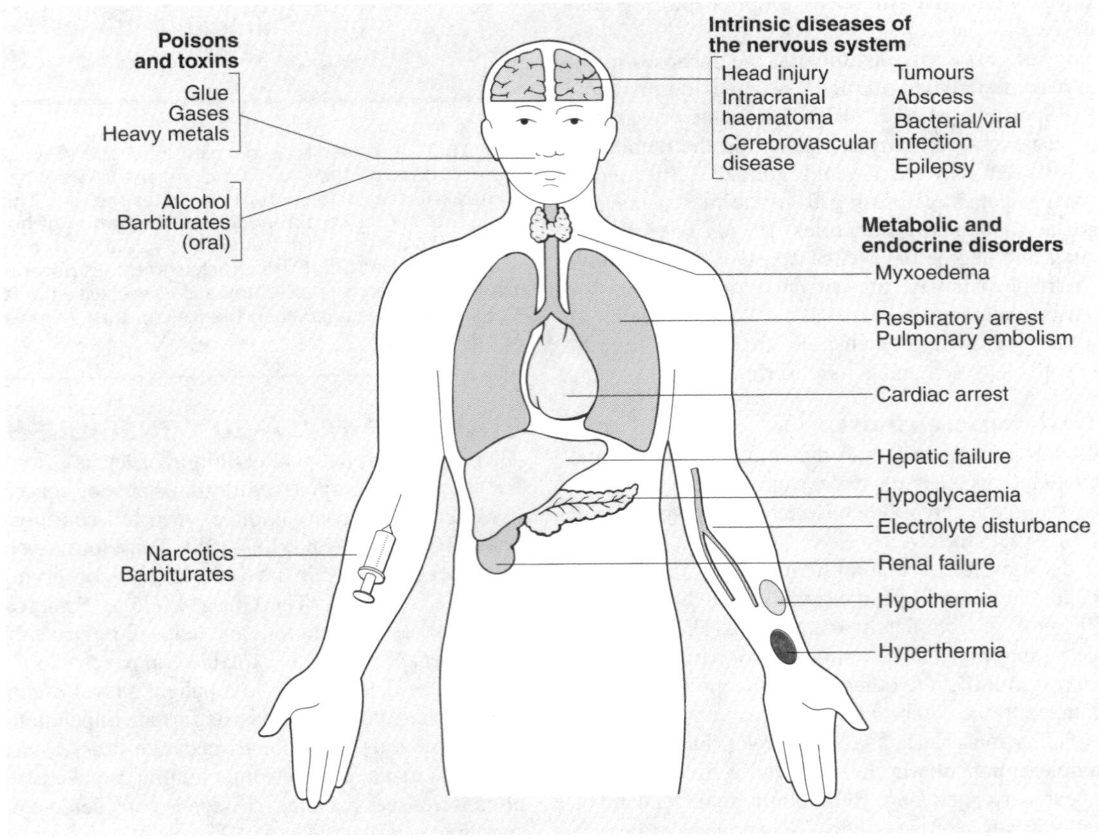

Fig. 28.3 Common causes of unconsciousness.

More advanced clouding produces a confused state in which stimuli are more consistently misinterpreted. The patient is bewildered and often has difficulty in following commands.

Signs of clouding may be reflected in subtle changes in the patient's behaviour. Minor disturbance of consciousness can easily go undetected if attention is not paid to what the patient says and does. If a normally placid and cooperative patient becomes irritable and aggressive, this should denote a behaviour change that requires further investigation. Similarly, comments from a relative such as 'she does not seem to recognise me today' should alert the nurse to the fact that something is not quite right with the patient. Martin (1994) suggests that nurses who are expert in the care of head-injured individuals can identify cues to indicate behavioural, cognitive, motor and sensory changes even in mild head injury.

Any change in the patient's behaviour must be reported to the appropriate nursing or medical staff, particularly if she has not previously exhibited any of these signs. The patient's nursing care plan will also need to be evaluated and a new goal for care set.

Cognitive disabilities, e.g. poor concentration and memory changes, may only become apparent when a patient returns home. These can cause emotional distress for both the patient and her family if they go unheeded and help is not provided. Hemingway & McAndrew (1998) suggest that the community mental health nurse could have a role in supporting people with acquired brain injury, and their families, in the early stages following injury and through to long-term community care.

Delirium

Delirium is often described as a form of clouding. It refers to a fluctuating noticeable mental state characterised by confusion, disorientation, fear and irritability. The patient is usually loud, talkative, offensive, suspicious and agitated (Plum & Posner 1980). This behaviour reflects generalised brain dysfunction due to interference with the RAS, affecting arousal. The causes and manifestations of delirium are listed in Box 28.2.

Illusions are defined as misinterpretations of sensory material in the patient's environment. A shadow on the wall is seen as an animal or a person, for example, or noises are misinterpreted as voices of strangers who have come to do harm.

Hallucinations are normally defined as seeing or hearing something in the absence of any sensory stimuli; for example, the patient will hear voices when no-one is present or see objects that do not exist in her environment (Trimble 1979). Other senses, such as touch, taste or smell, can be affected, but with acute disorders of the brain, hallucinations are usually visual (Plum & Posner 1980).

Delusions are defined as persistent misperceptions that are firmly held by a person, even though they are illogical or contrary to reality.

Illusions and hallucinatory experiences are common in temporal lobe epilepsy (see Ch. 9). Perceptual disturbances and delusions can also occur in patients exposed to sensory deprivation or overload, e.g. in intensive care units or in sleep deprivation (Phipps et al 1999). Therefore, when undertaking an assessment, it is important to consider the environment as well as the patient's physiological state.

Box 28.2 Causes and manifestations of delirium

- Toxic disorders of the nervous system, e.g. acute poisoning by:
  - —metals
  - —gases
  - —drugs
  - —alcohol
- Metabolic disorders, e.g.:
  - —renal failure
  - —hepatic failure
  - —encephalitis
- Severe head injury
- Psychological manifestations
  - —illusions
  - —hallucinations
  - —delusions

Stupor

The term stupor describes a state whereby the patient is quiet and tends not to move except in response to vigorous and repeated noxious stimuli (Hickey 1997).

Coma

Coma is an impaired state where the patient is totally unaware of herself and her environment. It may vary in degree, and in its deepest stages no reaction of any kind is obtainable. Some authors refer to differing grades of coma in relation to motor responses to painful stimuli.

For further reading, see Hickey (1997), Chapter 8.

Chronic states of impaired consciousness

The chronic states of impaired consciousness are:

- dementia
- vegetative
- locked-in syndrome.

Dementia

This condition is caused by a generalised and progressive loss of cortical tissue from the brain. Mental functions decline progressively. There is global deterioration of memory, thinking, motor performance, emotional responsiveness and social behaviour, but arousal remains intact.

As the condition develops, speech may become hesitant with eventual aphasia. Behaviour becomes increasingly unreasonable and often disruptive, until control of basic and vital processes is disorganised. There are numerous causes of progressive dementia. The most prevalent type is Alzheimer's disease.

Dementia is usually an irreversible condition. However, there are some occasions when the decline in cognitive functions can be halted and even partially reversed, e.g. in normal pressure hydrocephalus which can be treated by insertion of a ventricular shunt (Hickey 1997).

Vegetative

Vegetative state is a term used to describe a condition that can occur following severe brain injury. It is often referred to as persistent vegetative state (PVS) and is sometimes described as a coma vigil or irreversible coma.

The patient has sleep/waking cycles and will open her eyes when awake. However, there is no awareness of self or the environment and no cognitive function. Physiologically, the brain stem is functioning but the cerebral cortex is not. Patients can survive for many years in this condition and require full-time care.

Recently, there has been a considerable amount of debate, both in the UK and in other countries, about the moral, ethical and legal issues surrounding the care and treatment of these individuals (e.g. British Medical Association 1993, Multi-society Task Force Report on PVS 1994, Day et al 1995, Grubb et al 1996, Royal College of Physicians 1996, Smith 1997). Cases such as Bland (1993) in England and Cruzan (1990) in the USA brought the dilemma of 'the right to die' to media, and thus public, attention. Research into the views of doctors and nurses in Europe on PVS has been conducted by a project committee headed by Professor Andrew Grubb, Centre of Medical Law and Ethics, King's College, London (Grubb et al 1996).

Locked-in syndrome

This condition results in paralysis of voluntary muscles without interfering with consciousness and cognitive functions. The patient is unable to speak and is sometimes unable to breathe spontaneously. She is able to control vertical eye movements and blinking and may be able to use these movements to develop a simple communication system.

The pathological basis for this condition is damage to the pons in the brain stem, which may result from cerebral vascular disease or trauma.

It is important to remember that the patient is aware of her surroundings even though she appears to be mentally and physically inert.

Unfortunately, limited space prevents more detailed discussion of these issues within this chapter. The nurse should be aware of current debate and future developments regarding PVS and locked-in syndrome.

For further reading, see Royal College of Physicians (1996), Randall (1997), and Smith (1997).

28.1 What implications may there be for the patient and family if PVS is misdiagnosed?

ASSESSMENT OF THE NERVOUS SYSTEM

Nurses must be competent to monitor the conscious level for signs of deterioration, improvement or stability and they must understand what the observations mean. The need to assess conscious level may arise in any ward in any hospital. Ambiguities and misunderstandings can result when passing on information about the patient's state to other staff (Teasdale 1975). There is clearly a need for a standardised system of assessing the conscious level, so that different nurses and doctors will make similar observations on the patient at any one time. The system must encompass enough detail to determine changing status so that appropriate action can be taken.

The Glasgow Coma Scale (GCS) (Teasdale & Jennett 1974) is commonly used as an assessment tool (see Fig. 28.4).

The Neurological Observation Chart

The Glasgow Coma Scale

The Glasgow Coma Scale was designed by nursing and medical staff at the Institute of Neurological Sciences of the Southern General Hospital in Glasgow (Teasdale & Jennett 1974). It is widely used throughout the UK and in many other countries around the world. Its application is as follows.

In monitoring the patient's conscious level, the functional state of her brain is assessed as a whole. The nurse observes and describes three aspects of the patient's behaviour:

- eye opening
- verbal response
- motor response.

Each of these is independently assessed and recorded on a chart (Fig. 28.4). Each aspect shows a variety of responses. The patient's response is recorded by placing a dot in the appropriate square. The dots are joined to form a graph, making the chart easier to read. The decision about the time intervals between recording the assessments will be based on the patient's condition. The best response for each of these three aspects is recorded as a numerical score. In the case of eye opening, the best response scores 4, and the best verbal and motor responses each score 5. The lowest response for all three parameters is a score of 1.

The scores can be added together to give a total which could range from 3 to 14. The higher the score, the better the patient's condition; a score of 7 or less is generally considered to indicate that the patient is in a coma. However, it is important to consider each of the three aspects (eye opening, verbal response and motor response) separately as well as together. A patient may be blind, deaf, mute or have paralysis unrelated to her current condition and these would affect the scoring. In some wards/hospitals, the numerical scores are not recorded. It is also worth noting that, although the GCS is widely used, there may be some slight variations in the assessment chart in different hospitals.

The Neuroscience Nurses' Benchmarking Group (NNBG) recommends that the technique for assessment and recording should be in accordance with Frawley (1990) (see 'Note and useful address', p. 871).

Eye opening. The degree of stimulation required to make the patient open her eyes is observed and recorded using the following categories.

Spontaneously. The patient opens her eyes when she is first approached, which implies that the arousal response is active. This response is given a score of 4. Allowance must be made if the patient is in a natural sleep.

To speech. The patient's eyes are not open when she is first approached. The nurse should speak to her by calling her name and then ask her to open her eyes. It may be necessary to shout or shake the patient gently. A successful response scores 3.

To pain. A painful stimulus is applied if the patient fails to open her eyes spontaneously or to speech. Pressure is applied to the proximal side of the patient's fingernail using a pen or pencil (Fig. 28.5). This response scores 2 on the coma scale. Care must be taken not to exert pressure on the patient's cuticle as this will damage the nail bed.

None. If the painful stimulus does not cause the patient to open even one eye, then she is recorded as having no eye-opening response. This indicates a deep depression of the arousal system and is scored as 1 on the scale.

Possible assessment problems. The patient who is in a deep coma with flaccid eye muscles will show no response to stimulation. If the eyelids are drawn back, however, her eyes may remain open. This is very different from spontaneous eye opening and should be recorded as 'none'.

The nurse needs to be aware if the patient has any hearing deficits as, if her eyes are closed, this could affect her initial response. Congenital deficits of the eye or previous removal of the eye should also be taken into account.

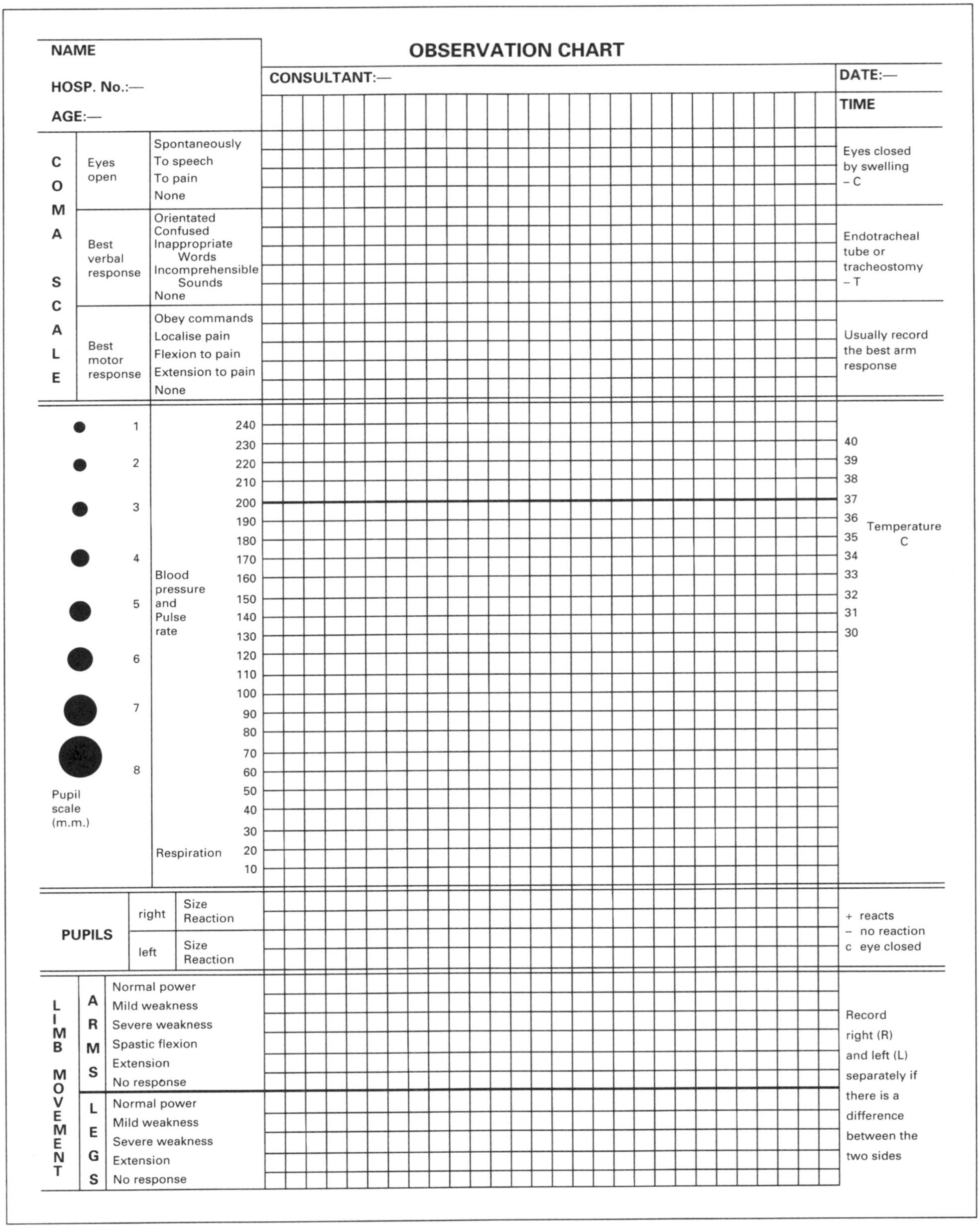

NAME

HOSP. No.:—

AGE:—

OBSERVATION CHART

CONSULTANT:—

DATE:—

TIME

COMA SCALE			
Eyes open	Spontaneously To speech To pain None		Eyes closed by swelling – C
Best verbal response	Orientated Confused Inappropriate Words Incomprehensible Sounds None		Endotracheal tube or tracheostomy – T
Best motor response	Obey commands Localise pain Flexion to pain Extension to pain None		Usually record the best arm response

Pupil scale (m.m.): 1, 2, 3, 4, 5, 6, 7, 8

Blood pressure and Pulse rate: 240, 230, 220, 210, 200, 190, 180, 170, 160, 150, 140, 130, 120, 110, 100, 90, 80, 70, 60, 50, 40

Respiration: 30, 20, 10

Temperature C: 40, 39, 38, 37, 36, 35, 34, 33, 32, 31, 30

PUPILS			
right	Size Reaction		+ reacts – no reaction c eye closed
left	Size Reaction		

LIMB MOVEMENT			
ARMS	Normal power Mild weakness Severe weakness Spastic flexion Extension No response		Record right (R) and left (L) separately if there is a difference between the two sides
LEGS	Normal power Mild weakness Severe weakness Extension No response		

Fig. 28.4 The Neurological Observation Chart, including the Glasgow Coma Scale. (Reproduced with kind permission from *Nursing Times* where this figure first appeared on 19 June 1975.)

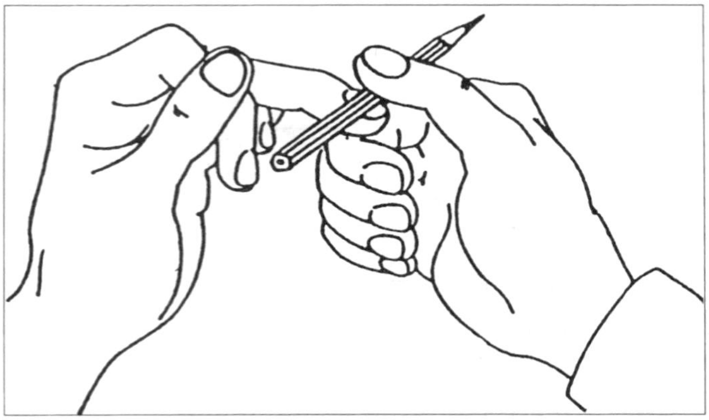

Fig. 28.5 Applying a painful stimulus: fingertip stimulation. (From Teasdale 1975. Reproduced with kind permission from *Nursing Times* where this figure first appeared on 12 June 1975.)

After trauma or surgery, eyelid swelling occasionally prevents eye opening, as does tarsorrhaphy where upper and lower eyelids are sutured together. A condition such as ptosis (nerve palsy) will also have this effect, although this seldom results in complete closure of both eyes. Enforced closure of the eyelid(s) should be recorded as 'C' on the chart.

Opening of the eyes implies arousal but it must be remembered that this does not necessarily mean that the patient is aware of her surroundings. This can be misleading and be a source of false optimism in relatives.

Verbal response. The patient's best achievement in respect of verbal response is observed and recorded using the following categories.

Oriented. The patient is recorded as oriented if she can state her name, where she is and what the year and month are. This is orientation in person, place and time, respectively, and is given a score of 5. Questions can be varied but they must be kept simple; for example, the date and even the day are not easily remembered, especially after a period in hospital.

Confused. If the patient is capable of producing phrases or sentences but the conversation is rambling and inappropriate to the questions about orientation, it is a confused verbal response and scores 4.

Inappropriate words. The patient will only speak one or two words, usually in response to physical stimulation. The words and phrases make little or no sense and may be obscenities. On occasions, the patient will shout out obscenities or call a person's name for no apparent reason. These all indicate a lower level of responsiveness and score 3.

Incomprehensible sounds. The patient will moan or grunt in response to physical stimulation. The verbal response may contain indistinct mumbling but no intelligible words. The response scores 2.

None. The patient will not produce any verbal response even when prolonged and repeated stimulation is given. This scores 1.

Possible assessment problems. The patient may be unable to understand the nurse's commands because she does not understand the language or has a hearing defect. The patient's verbal response may be impaired as a result of a speech defect such as dysphasia. If appropriate, written instructions and replies can be used to assess the patient's language ability. As well as noting the level of the response, the chart should be marked 'D' where the impairment is thought to be due to dysphasia.

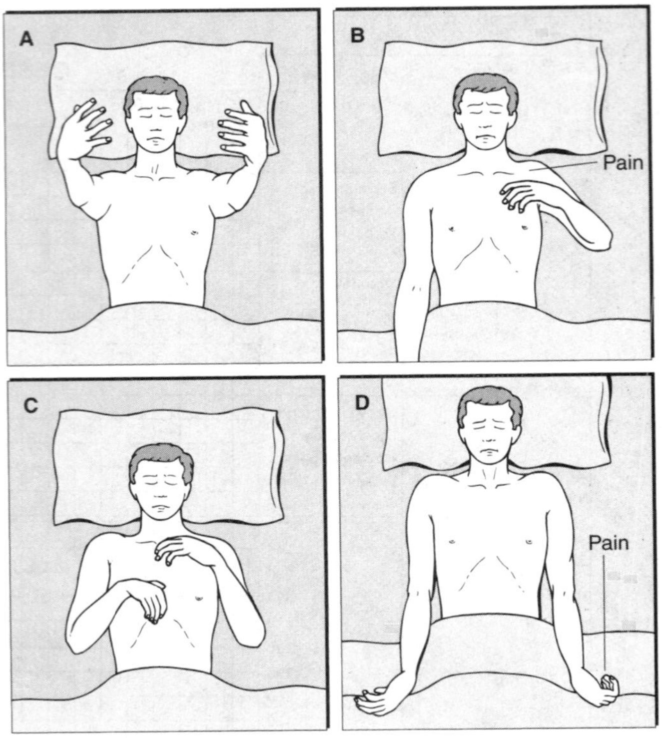

Fig. 28.6 Motor responses. A: Obeys commands ('lift up your arms'). B: Localising to pain. C: Flexing to pain. D: Extending to pain.

The verbal response may also be compromised by the presence of an endotracheal or tracheostomy tube. This is indicated on the patient's chart as 'E' or 'T'.

Motor response. The patient's best motor response is observed (see Fig. 28.6). Only upper-limb responses are recorded, as leg responses to pain are less consistent and inappropriate spinal withdrawal reflexes occur more readily in many patients who would otherwise show a total absence of brain function.

Obeys commands. The patient has the ability to appreciate instructions (Fig. 28.6A). These are usually given by verbal commands such as, 'Put out your tongue, please' or 'Lift up your arms, please'. If the patient obeys these instructions, she is given a score of 5.

Localises to pain. If the patient does not obey commands, a pain stimulus is applied. Using the trapezium pinch is the safest method. The patient's shoulder is partially exposed and the trapezius muscle is grossly pinched (Frawley 1990). The patient is recorded as 'localising to pain' when she moves her arm to locate the pain, in an attempt to remove the source of it (Fig. 28.6B). This response scores 4.

During the course of the day, the patient may display a localising response to other sources of irritation, e.g. attempts to remove her oxygen mask, nasogastric tube or urinary catheter.

Flexion to pain. After painful stimulation of the proximal side of the patient's fingernail, the patient responds by bending her elbow and withdrawing her hand, but no attempt to localise is made. The response may include a spastic flexion of the wrist and finger joints across an adducted thumb (Fig. 28.6C). This is 'flexion to pain' and scores 3.

Extension to pain. After painful stimulation, the patient responds by straightening her elbows. The response usually includes spastic hand and wrist movements, with an inward rotation of the shoulders and forearms (Fig. 28.6D). The legs are generally straight, with the feet pointing outwards. This response scores 2.

None. This response is recorded when repeated and varied stimulation provokes no detectable movement of, or change of tone in, the limbs. It scores 1.

Decortication and decerebration. Painful stimuli can initiate abnormal postures if motor nerves are interrupted at specific cerebral levels. A patient with severe brain damage may exhibit one or a combination of these postures without any stimulation (see the Glossary, p. 1057, for definitions of these terms).

Possible assessment problems. Variations in the motor response may occur during the assessment. Therefore, it is the best response that should be scored; for example, if the patient localises to pain on her left side but flexes to pain on her right, the localising response is recorded. Asymmetrical responses are significant, indicating that a focal neurological deficit is present, but overall brain function is more accurately reflected by the level of best response on the better side (see 'Limb movement' below).

When applying a painful stimulus, it is important to explain to relatives what you are about to do and why you are doing it, otherwise they may feel that unnecessary trauma is being inflicted on their loved one.

Recording other measurements

The Neurological Observation Chart is used to record additional measurements (see Fig. 28.4) as follows:

- vital signs
  - —blood pressure
  - —heart rate (pulse)
  - —respirations
  - —temperature
- pupil size and reaction
- limb movements.

Vital signs

Blood pressure and pulse. The famous neurosurgeon Harvey Williams Cushing (1869–1939) noted that a rise in intracranial pressure (ICP) led to a rise in blood pressure (elevated systolic pressure and widening pulse pressure) and a slowing pulse (see Ch. 9). 'Cushing's response' does not occur until the later stages of raised ICP, however, and the Glasgow Coma Scale will show evidence of deterioration much earlier.

Changes in the blood pressure and pulse can indicate injury or disease elsewhere in the body; for example, falling blood pressure and a rapid and weak pulse are indicative of haemorrhage and shock (see Ch. 18).

Respiration. Conditions that impair consciousness may also cause respiratory changes. The pattern and rate of respiration may be directly affected by brain damage. The rate of respiration is recorded on the chart, but it is also important for the nurse to observe the depth, rhythm and characteristics of respiration. Deep lesions in the cerebrum tend to produce a periodic pattern such as Cheyne–Stokes respiration. Lesions affecting the pons and medulla cause more irregular patterns. If the patient is being artificially ventilated, abnormal respiratory patterns will not be evident.

Temperature. Impaired brain function seldom causes significant changes in body temperature unless there has been direct damage to the temperature-regulating centre in the hypothalamus (see Ch. 22) when temperature can rise rapidly. A gradual elevation is likely to be an early sign of infection in the lungs or urinary tract, or in a wound. Each rise in degree of temperature increases the brain's metabolic rate, and therefore hyperthermia must be treated to prevent further neurological deterioration.

Pupil size and reaction

The size of both pupils is measured by comparing them with a series of circular millimetre measures on the chart (Fig. 28.3) or by descriptive terms (Hickey 1997). Reaction to light is scored by a plus (+), and no reaction is recorded by a minus (–). Pupil reactions should be assessed in dim surroundings, using a small bright flashlight. To elicit the direct-light reflex, the nurse holds each of the patient's eyelids open in turn, brings the light from the outer side of the eye and shines it directly into the eye. This should cause a brisk constriction of the pupil, and withdrawal of the light should produce brisk dilatation of the pupil. The size and reaction are observed and recorded on the chart. The shape of the pupils should also be assessed.

Abnormal pupillary size and reaction can indicate brain dysfunction and/or raised ICP. It is important to note any changes, particularly if they occur in conjunction with other changes in the neurological observations.

For further information on the assessment of pupillary signs and other neurological observations, see Hickey (1997), Ch. 8.

Limb movement

Disturbances of limb movement indicate localised or focal brain damage and vary according to the site and extent of the damage; for example, the right arm and leg will be affected by a lesion in the left cerebral hemisphere. More diffuse brain damage will result in a greater disturbance of movement.

When no localised brain damage is suspected, such as in metabolic or drug coma, the best motor response on the coma scale is usually sufficient for monitoring responses. When localised brain damage is suspected, an additional detailed assessment of each limb is necessary (see Fig. 28.4).

The nurse examines the arms and legs for movement and strength, and compares the right and left sides. When the two sides are the same, recordings are made in the standard manner (see p. 858). When differences exist, right and left are recorded independently, using 'R' for right and 'L' for left. Responses can be elicited by verbal commands, such as asking the patient to grip the nurse's hand as tightly as possible, to lift up her arms or to bend her knees. To test strength, the nurse may need to provide some form of resistance, such as pressing down on the patient's knee when the patient is trying to bend it.

Painful stimuli may be applied to the appropriate limb if verbal comments fail to elicit a response.

CAUSES OF UNCONSCIOUSNESS

The major causes of unconsciousness are shown in Figure 28.3.

Unconsciousness occurs when the RAS is damaged or its function is depressed so that there is an interruption of the normal arousal mechanisms. This may be caused by a primary or secondary insult to the nervous system. Primary insults are commonly caused by intrinsic diseases of the brain. Secondary involvement is most often caused by metabolic, endocrine or toxic conditions, where the critical insult is manifested elsewhere in the body.

Information on some of the conditions which can result in loss of consciousness can be found in Chapters 5 and 9.

EMERGENCY CARE OF THE UNCONSCIOUS PATIENT

Whatever the cause of unconsciousness and wherever the event occurs, the patient's life depends on the knowledge and skills of those who find her. The first aid and care that she receives until she regains consciousness (if this is achievable) will help to determine the outcome for the patient (see Box 28.3).

A hospital emergency

In a hospital ward or department, an individual can be rendered unconscious by any of the causes shown in Figure 28.3. The victim does not necessarily need to be a patient; visitors and members of staff are also at risk from events such as cardiac arrest, cerebrovascular accident or falls resulting in head injury. The measures a nurse should take if he finds someone collapsed are as follows:

Box 28.3 First aid for an unconscious patient

N.B. If alone, the first action normally is to seek help.

1. Check the victim's breathing and pulse. If she is not breathing and a pulse is not felt in the carotid artery, turn her onto her back and initiate cardiopulmonary resuscitation (see Ch. 2). If possible, get help to do this.
2. Clear the victim's airway with your finger. Remove dentures or dental plates, if possible, and keep them in a safe place.
3. Send someone to telephone for an ambulance. Make sure that the person knows the location and has some details of the victim. Ask the person to return to confirm that the telephone call has been made.
4. If the victim is breathing and has a pulse, loosen her clothing at the neck, chest and waist. Keep bystanders away from the victim. If necessary, and if possible, move her to a safer place.
5. Check for any other injuries or bruises and stem any bleeding.
6. Place the victim in the semi-prone or recovery position, as follows:
   (a) Kneel beside her and place her arms alongside her body.
   (b) Cross the ankle furthest away from you over the one nearest to you.
   (c) Cushion her head with your hand.
   (d) Place your other hand on the hip furthest from you and roll her gently towards you.
   (e) Maintain a clear airway by grasping under her jaw and moving her chin upwards and backwards. This extends the neck and prevents the victim's tongue from blocking her throat.
   (f) Pull up the arm nearest to you so that the point of the elbow is in line with the victim's shoulder.

   This position prevents the victim's tongue from falling into the back of her throat and blocking the airway. It also allows fluid, such as blood or vomit, to drain from her mouth.

   Note: The position is contraindicated in victims with suspected spinal injury, when movement risks further damage to the spinal cord (see Chapters 10 and 27).
7. Stay with the victim until the ambulance arrives. Give a detailed account of events to the ambulance attendants. This should include how the victim was found and what resuscitative measures were taken.

1. Shout for assistance and press the nurse call button.
2. Move the person into a wider space if this is possible.
3. Initiate CPR if the individual is not breathing and the carotid pulse is absent. The cardiac arrest team should be called at this point.
4. If the person is breathing and a pulse is present, place her in a semi-prone (recovery) position. Do not move the person or place her in the semi-prone position without keeping the head, neck and spine in alignment if spinal injury is suspected. In the hospital setting it may be possible to quickly obtain a cervical collar or spinal board if necessary. Stay with her until assistance arrives and she can be moved to an appropriate place for further treatment and investigation.

Planned admission

When an unconscious patient is to be admitted to a ward or department, the following measures must be taken:

- Remove the top bedclothes and the head of the bed to facilitate easy access to the patient.
- Check that the oxygen supply and suction apparatus are functioning and that there is an adequate supply of relevant equipment.
- The necessary equipment should be available for immediate use:
  (a) a resuscitation trolley containing the following:
    —Guedel airways (usually size 3 or 4 for an adult)
    —Ambu resuscitator (commonly called an 'ambu bag') with universal catheter mount
    —laryngoscope and selection of endotracheal tubes
    —lubricating jelly; strapping or tape; 5 mL syringe to inflate the endotracheal tube cuff
    —emergency drug box or pack
    —a mechanical ventilator, if possible. (Not all wards will have this facility. If the patient is unable to breathe on her own, she is ventilated manually via an endotracheal tube, using an Ambu resuscitator until she can be transferred to an intensive care unit.)
  (b) an intravenous infusion stand
  (c) equipment for the passage of a nasogastric tube to aspirate the stomach contents
  (d) a neurological examination tray
  (e) the appropriate charts and admission forms.

Priorities of nurse management

The following checklist itemises the priorities of nurse management in an emergency situation, in order to sustain the patient's vital functions:

1. Maintenance of a clear airway
   (a) the patient's position
   (b) artificial airways
   (c) suction
   (d) oxygen
   (e) nasogastric tube.
2. Assessment of the central nervous system
   (a) Glasgow Coma Scale
   (b) vital signs
   (c) pupillary reactions
   (d) limb movements.
3. Maintenance of fluid balance
   (a) intravenous infusion
   (b) catheterisation of the urinary bladder, if necessary.
4. Care of relatives.

Measures to sustain the vital functions of the patient must take priority over anything else. Anyone accompanying the patient, e.g. relatives, must also be considered. A nurse who is not involved in the immediate care of the patient should be allocated to take care of them. The nurse should provide them with written information regarding hospital procedures and explain the investigations related to the patient's condition. At the same time the nurse will be able to gather the patient's biographical data and other information to help in planning the patient's nursing care.

Medical management

An unconscious patient is a medical emergency, unless the unconscious state represents the terminal state of a progressive and not specifically treatable disease. The cause of the unconscious state must be determined before the appropriate treatment can be given, although life support measures have priority over anything else. These measures include establishment of an adequate airway, control of haemorrhage, and fluid or blood replacement. Gastric lavage may be indicated when the victim has ingested an overdose of drugs, although this is controversial (Bates et al 1997). An unconscious patient must be intubated before gastric lavage is carried out because of the risk of aspiration of fluid into the lungs.

For further reading on the management of acute poisoning, see Bates et al (1997).

28.2 What are the guidelines and protocols in the A&E department of your hospital for management of unconscious patients suspected of ingesting drugs or toxic substances?

The medical history

A doctor or an experienced nurse will need to find out information about the patient. It is important, if an appropriate person has accompanied the patient to hospital, that this person does not leave until the doctor or nurse has had an opportunity to question him or her about the medical history and the circumstances preceding and surrounding the onset of the unconscious state.

The physical examination

The general physical examination of the unconscious patient will include special attention to the patient's:

- vital signs
- pattern of respiration
- signs of trauma
- skin colour and texture
- breath odour.

The signs and symptoms listed in Table 28.1 can provide clues to the cause of the unconscious state.

Table 28.1 Clues to the cause of unconsciousness on general physical examination

Sign or symptom	*Possible cause*
Elevated temperature	Infection Heat stroke
Subnormal temperature	Dehydration Excessive intake of alcohol Barbiturate intoxication Myxoedema Exposure to the cold
Bleeding from the mouth	Epileptic seizure Trauma
Pulse irregularities	Hypoxia from inadequate cardiac output
Slow, regular respirations	Myxoedema Morphine or barbiturate intoxication
Cheyne–Stokes respiration	Bilateral cerebral dysfunction Late stages of increased intracranial pressure Severe cardiopulmonary disease
Ataxic, irregular (cluster) respirations	Lesions of the brain stem — signifies impending apnoea
Breath odour	Excessive intake of alcohol Hepatic dysfunction Renal dysfunction Ingested poisons Diabetes mellitus
Skin	
Jaundice	Hepatic dysfunction
Cyanosis	Cardiopulmonary problems
Rash	Infection; reaction to medication
Needle puncture marks	Drug abuse
Hypertension	Raised intracranial pressure Intracranial haemorrhage
Hypotension	Blood loss Septicaemia Myocardial infarction Pulmonary embolism

The doctor will also carry out a neurological examination of the patient. This will include assessment of the cranial nerves, motor and sensory function, and the patient's reflexes. A nurse should be present at the initial neurological assessment so that any future changes in the patient's condition can be monitored in relation to her initial state.

Laboratory tests

Laboratory tests in unconscious patients usually include a complete blood count, blood glucose levels and blood urea, and electrolyte estimation. Blood gas analysis is obtained when the patient's respiratory and/or cardiovascular state are compromised. Screening tests of blood and urine are carried out if drug intoxication or ingestion of poison or alcohol are suspected. The patient's urine may be checked for glucose, acetone, blood and infection.

Radiological studies and imaging

Radiological tests are carried out once the patient has been resuscitated and her condition stabilised. Skull and cervical spine X-rays are obtained when head trauma is obvious or is suggested from neurological signs (possible injury to the cervical spine should always be suspected in cases of head trauma).

If other injuries are apparent or suspected, X-rays will be taken as appropriate. Angiography, computed tomography (CT) or magnetic resonance imaging (MRI) scans may be undertaken if further investigation is considered to be necessary.

Further investigation

Further investigations may be undertaken to aid diagnosis, e.g.:

- electroencephalogram (EEG)
- lumbar puncture (LP)
- electrocardiogram (ECG)
- Doppler (ultrasonic) studies.

NURSING MANAGEMENT OF THE UNCONSCIOUS PATIENT

The activities of living model described by Roper et al (1996) is used to illustrate the nursing management of the unconscious patient. This model is based on 12 activities of living. The author has expanded this to include a 13th activity, spiritual care, which is taken from the work of Virginia Henderson (1960).

Breathing

Oxygen is essential for the survival of all body cells. Irreversible damage to the brain cells will occur if they are deprived of oxygen, even for a few minutes. Consequently, all activities of living and life itself are entirely dependent on breathing, and the establishment and maintenance of a patent airway are essential for the unconscious patient.

Any obvious obstructions such as dentures or dental plates should be removed. The nurse also needs to be aware of the presence of loose teeth, caps or crowns, as these could become detached and obstruct the airway. Bleeding into the oropharynx from head or facial injuries may also cause obstruction. Vomiting presents another hazard. The insertion of a nasogastric tube in the initial stages of coma will facilitate the emptying of the stomach, thus helping to avoid the potential aspiration of gastric contents into the respiratory tract.

Position of the patient

The patient should be nursed in a semi-prone or lateral recumbent position with the head of the bed tilted slightly upwards (10–30°). This prevents the tongue from obstructing the airway, encourages the drainage of respiratory secretions and saliva and therefore reduces the danger of aspiration into the lungs. Pillows positioned at the patient's back and between her knees help to maintain the position. At no time should an unconscious patient be flat on her back, except to facilitate procedures such as intubation or radiological studies, or if she is ventilated.

Artificial airways

The unconscious patient's cough reflex is depressed or absent, so she is unable to cough and clear her own airway. The use of artificial airways and suctioning may be required.

Oropharyngeal airway. The Guedel airway is the oropharyngeal airway most commonly used in UK hospitals. These have the advantage of relatively easy insertion and are available in varying sizes to facilitate the needs of individual patients. The airway is designed to lie over the tongue and permit the passage of air into the pharynx (Fig. 28.7). It keeps the patient's tongue from obstructing her throat and it has a passage that allows the patient to breathe through the device. It also allows easier access to facilitate suction of the oropharynx and trachea.

Endotracheal tube. An endotracheal tube is indicated if the Guedel airway proves inadequate. The tube is usually made of plastic and has an inflatable cuff (Fig. 28.8). The tube is inserted through the mouth or, occasionally, through the nose of the patient by a doctor or a nurse who is competent to carry out the procedure. It is then passed into the trachea to a point above the bifurcation which is proximal to the bronchi. This permits deep suctioning. Breath sounds are determined immediately after insertion to make certain that the tube is properly positioned and is not obstructing one of the primary bronchi. The cuff of the tube is then inflated with air. The inflated cuff provides an airtight seal, particularly when mechanical ventilation is required. It also prevents the aspiration of material from the digestive tract. The tube is secured in position externally using hypoallergenic tape or tied with ribbon gauze. It is the nurse's responsibility to check the patency and position of the tube at regular intervals.

In some hospitals, the practice of deflating the cuff for a few minutes each hour is employed in order to minimise the occurrence of erosion of the tracheal wall. The nurse must adhere to local policy on this practice.

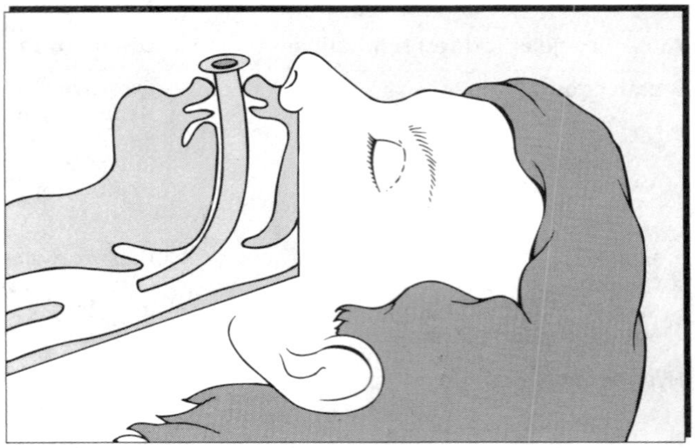

Fig. 28.7 A Guedel airway in situ.

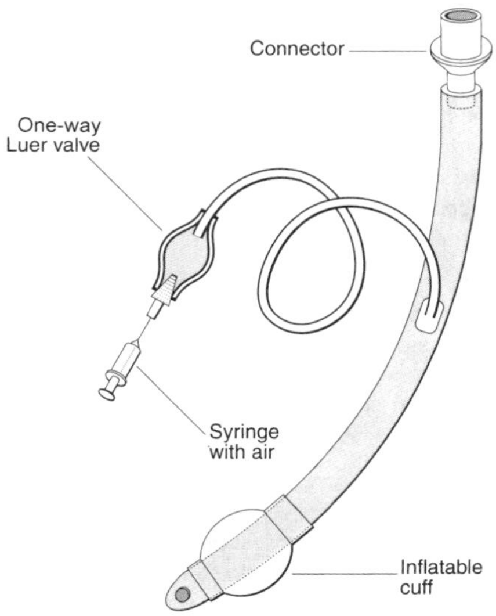

Fig. 28.8 Endotracheal tube.

Tracheostomy tube. The tracheostomy bypasses any obstruction in the upper airway and facilitates suctioning of bronchial secretions (see Ch. 14). Tracheostomy is usually indicated if endotracheal intubation is to be prolonged. An endotracheal tube is not usually left in place for more than 3–4 days.

An incision is made into the trachea through the second and third, or third and fourth, tracheal rings. The tube is inserted and secured externally with tape. The tubes are made of silver, plastic or nylon and may be cuffed or uncuffed.

Most tubes consist of three parts: an obturator in place when inserting the tube, an outer cannula and an inner cannula. The advantage of a tube with an inner cannula is that this can be removed every 2–4 h for cleaning, and then replaced. This prevents the potential danger of obstruction with secretions. The procedure can also be carried out without disturbing the outer tube. This reduces the frequency of outer tube changes, thus minimising the risk of trauma to the stoma and trachea.

Infection is a potential problem and the tracheal stoma should always be treated as an open wound. The incidence and severity of infection may be minimised by keeping the wound area free of secretions that collect around the tube. The nurse cleans the stoma using an aseptic technique, and a sterile absorbent, non-adherent dressing may be applied.

The NNBG (see 'Note and useful address', p. 871) recommends the following for best nursing practice:

- use of proprietary stoma dressings which should be changed at least once a day
- tracheostomy tubes should be changed in line with manufacturer's guidelines.

Harkin (1998) suggests that the cuff should be inflated slowly until no air flow around the cuff is detected in the upper airway.

Suctioning

The nurse carries out suctioning to remove potentially dangerous secretions from the oropharynx, trachea and bronchi. The nurse's assessment of the patient's colour, her respiratory rate and pattern will indicate how often this is required. Specific indicators include one or more of the following:

- signs of cyanosis
- increased and irregular respirations
- noisy, gurgling respirations.

The following equipment is required:

- a piped source of vacuum pressure, indicating calibrated pressures, or a portable suction device
- a collection jar and disposable connecting tubing
- disposable plastic sterile suction catheters of the correct size for the patient (usually 12–14 French gauge for an adult); the catheter should be no more than one-half the diameter of the tracheostomy/ET tube
- disposable plastic gloves
- bowl of sterile normal saline
- masks (optional).

The NNBG recommends the use of a closed suction catheter system and disposable suction equipment if possible.

Procedure. Each ward will have its own policy regarding suctioning but the procedure described by Allan (1988a), as follows, provides a general example. The NNBG based some aspects of what it considered to be best nursing practice on Clarke's (1995) discussion of tracheostomy care.

1. Explain the procedure to the patient.
2. Assemble the equipment needed (masks are advocated in some units for the nurse's protection). Turn on the suction device to 80–120 mmHg.
3. Wash hands and pour the saline into a sterile bowl.
4. Administer oxygen to the patient, if necessary.
5. Open the packet containing the sterile catheter and put the glove on the dominant hand.
6. Attach the catheter to the connecting tube, taking care not to contaminate the catheter.
7. Insert the catheter into the airway without applying suction.
8. Advance the catheter as far as it will easily pass, until resistance is met.
9. Withdraw the catheter 1 cm. Suction is applied intermittently as the catheter is slowly withdrawn, using a rotating action.
10. As many secretions are removed as possible within a time limit of 10 s.
11. The catheter is removed and discarded and the tubing is rinsed through with saline. The patient is given at least 60 s to recover before suctioning again. Oxygen is given again, if required.
12. If all the secretions have not been removed, the procedure is repeated using a new sterile catheter.
13. Using a separate catheter, the patient's mouth and nose are suctioned at the end of the procedure if necessary. Nasal suction is contraindicated if the patient has sustained a frontal skull fracture or has nasal leakage of cerebrospinal fluid (CSF rhinorrhoea). The passage of a suction catheter through the nose could lead to damage to brain tissue and infection.
14. If a disposable system is not available, collection jars should be emptied and disinfected at least once every 24 h during regular use; cleaning should be according to local policy.

Immediately before suctioning, some units advocate the instillation of 5–10 mL of sterile normal saline into the airway in order to loosen the secretions; however, the value of this technique is questioned (Ackerman 1996). Ackerman argues that this practice can irritate the mucosa and has little or no value in thinning, mobilising or removing dried secretions. The use of a saline nebuliser is a preferred option.

Humidification

Normally the air drawn into the lungs is warmed, moistened and filtered through the nose and upper respiratory tract. If the patient has an endotracheal or tracheostomy tube, the air is dry and so a humidifier must be used, otherwise irritated mucous membranes and dried tenacious secretions soon result.

Oxygen

The amount of oxygen prescribed depends on the respiratory status of the patient and the laboratory evaluation of her arterial blood gases. A specimen of arterial blood is taken to ascertain the pH and partial pressures of oxygen (P_aO_2) and carbon dioxide (P_aCO_2). Deviations from normal may be corrected by an increase or decrease in the amount of oxygen delivered. Mechanical ventilation may be indicated to ensure adequate oxygenation.

There are various methods of administering oxygen and the doctor's prescription will include instructions about the rate of flow, duration of therapy and type of equipment to be used. The nurse must monitor the administration of oxygen and observe the patient for complications. The reader is referred to Chapter 3 for a more detailed account of the administration of oxygen and mechanical ventilation. The ventilated patient is usually cared for in an intensive therapy unit or a high-dependency unit.

Nursing and physiotherapy

The prevention of respiratory complications is a priority in the nursing management of the unconscious patient, but infection may occur despite every precaution being taken. Antibiotics can be effective against organisms but the patient could drown in her own purulent secretions unless these are removed. Effective respiratory management is dependent on the skill and cooperation of the nurse and physiotherapist.

Communicating

The patient

There is much anecdotal evidence of patients recalling, with startling accuracy, conversations they have overheard whilst unconscious. It is only in more recent years that research has been undertaken, albeit with small numbers of people, into experiences and recollections of impaired consciousness (see Research Abstract 28.1). Conversations not intended for the patient should not be held in her presence, as unguarded or misinterpreted expressions can cause distress.

It is imperative that the nurse explains clearly and simply to the patient every aspect of her care, whether it is related to the associated equipment or to the patient's progress. The explanations and reassurances need to be repeated whenever a procedure is carried out. With the advent of ICP monitoring, several studies have been undertaken to determine the effects of verbal and physical interactions on ICP (e.g. Treloar et al 1991, Chudley 1994). Some situations cause a rise in ICP, some a decrease and some no change. However, authors of such studies have advocated a need for further research.

For further reading, see Treloar et al (1991) and Chudley (1994).

Patients may be helped to recover with sensory stimulation, e.g. with common smells, distinctive flavours, soft or harsh fabrics, visual stimuli such as light from a torch, and certain types of sound, such as favourite music.

Research Abstract 28.1
The unconscious experience

A small pilot study was carried out in the USA (Podurgiel 1990) involving patients who had been unconscious and returned to consciousness and nurses who had talked to such patients. The study describes how people consistently reported on four particular states:

- near-death — at peace, leaving the body, seeing a light, returning to life
- unconsciousness — no perception of external environment
- semi-consciousness — aware of external and own internal environment but unable to communicate
- dreams and nightmares.

There appeared to be movement back and forth between these states, rather than progressive stages, and patients were able to respond emotionally to what was happening to them. Warm, caring, personal contacts were noted as positive. Some procedures and negative statements the patients overheard had a more detrimental effect.

Podurgiel M 1990 The unconscious experience: a pilot study. Journal of Neuroscience Nursing 22(1): 52–53.

The family

Relatives and other visitors will be bewildered when they see the unconscious patient with her associated equipment, particularly for the first time. Time should be spent with them before they see the patient in order to explain what is happening and what the patient looks like. A brief explanation of the immediate environment and the function of any equipment is provided and relatives should be encouraged to speak with and touch the patient. The family should be given an opportunity to ask any questions and should be able to speak with the doctor and nurse in charge about the patient's progress. Many misconceptions about coma have developed, particularly through the media. The nurse should gently explore the relatives' or significant others' understanding of the patient's condition and correct any misconceptions.

Q **28.3** Can you think of any of these misconceptions? How might you correct them?

For further reading, see Johnson & Roberts (1996) and Hemingway & McAndrew (1998).

Rest and sleep

Providing adequate rest for a patient is one of the most difficult problems confronting the nurse and it is doubtful whether it is ever achieved with the associated hospital background noise. More information on sleep can be found in Chapter 25.

It must be borne in mind that the unconscious patient has a dysfunctional RAS — the system that is normally responsible for the sleep/waking cycle. Therefore it could be assumed that a normal sleep/waking pattern is not possible in the unconscious patient. However, patients whose level of consciousness fluctuates may experience periods of sleep and periods of wakefulness even though they may not be responsive to external stimuli. Podurgiel (1990) reported that some patients recalled dreams and nightmares (see Research Abstract 28.1). It has also been noted earlier in this chapter that patients in vegetative states exhibit sleep/waking cycles.

Treloar et al (1991) and Chudley (1994) mention the need to provide rest periods for patients between nursing and other activities. However, there does not appear to be any conclusive evidence in the current literature about the need for sleep and rest in the patient with an altered level of consciousness. Nurses should consider this potential need when planning care. It could be detrimental to patients to be stimulated constantly by nurses undertaking frequent observations and procedures, along with other members of staff attending to the patient.

Eating and drinking

The unconscious patient will be unable to eat or drink in the normal way and will need to receive nourishment and fluids by an alternative method. An adequate fluid intake also helps to prevent dehydration, which can cause drying and thickening of secretions, making suctioning difficult and creating a breeding ground for bacteria.

In any very stressful situation, whether physical or emotional, calorie intake should be increased to meet an increased metabolic rate. For example, a severely head-injured patient may require 4000–5000 calories/day in the acute stages (Hickey 1997).

Fluids

The most common method of administering fluids to an unconscious patient is intravenously, either peripherally or via a central line, usually placed in the subclavian vein. Intravenous (i.v.) fluids are also given to:

- administer medications, such as antibiotics
- administer additional electrolytes, such as potassium, to correct imbalances.

Intravenous fluids are normally prescribed by medical staff, following estimation of the patient's serum electrolyte levels which are measured on a daily basis. Fluids are usually prescribed for the following 24 h, although in seriously ill patients, prescriptions may be adjusted more frequently. It is essential that the correct fluids are administered at the prescribed rate to maintain fluid balance and metabolic needs. Fluids may be restricted if cerebral oedema is suspected (see Ch. 9).

Multiple lines and ports can be labelled with different colours to distinguish them. The patient may also have an arterial line, which looks very similar to an i.v. cannula and could easily be mistaken for one. An arterial line must therefore be clearly identified.

An infusion pump will be used to ensure accurate flow rates in the seriously ill patient (see Chs 20 and 21 for more information).

Nutrition

Provision of adequate nutrition is important in the unconscious patient. Malnourishment will result in weakening of the body's immune system and loss of muscle mass and energy, both of which are essential for recovery.

Intragastric tube. The easiest and most economical way to provide an alternative means of feeding is via an intragastric tube, passed either nasally or orally. Intragastric tube feeding is the most frequently used method in the unconscious patient and, provided the patient's alimentary tract is functional, is the preferred method to provide total nutritional support. The patient's nutritional requirements should be assessed and the appropriate dietary solutions prescribed with the help and advice of the dietician. The patient's nutritional status must be reappraised at regular intervals.

Daily nutritional requirements are usually calculated on the basis of body weight, gender, height and age. However, it may not be possible to weigh the unconscious patient unless a bed with a weighing scale incorporated into it is available.

Care must be taken when inserting an intragastric tube via the nose or mouth of an unconscious patient as it may not be possible to elevate the patient's head. Insertion is more difficult if the patient is not able to sit up. There is also a higher risk of aspiration of stomach contents into the trachea and lungs if the patient is in the lateral recumbent position. The patient must be observed carefully for any sign of aspiration which will compromise respiration. Suction equipment must be at hand and ready for use at all times.

Parenteral feeding is delivered through a central venous line. It should be used only in areas where staff are familiar with the technique as it can be problematic and hazardous (see Ch. 21). Unconscious patients who may benefit from parenteral nutrition include:

- multiple trauma patients, particularly if there are gastrointestinal and/or facial injuries
- malnourished patients
- patients with sepsis
- patients in prolonged coma who are unable to tolerate intragastric feeding.

Whenever possible, it is preferable to deliver food directly into the gut to prevent the risk of infection.

Long-term feeding may be better achieved by using a percutaneous endoscopic gastrostomy (PEG) tube. This is easier to manage and relatives/carers can be taught how to administer feeds through the tube. PEG tubes are particularly useful if the patient is later cared for at home.

When the patient recovers consciousness, it is essential to ensure that gag, coughing and swallowing reflexes are present before giving oral fluids or food. The speech and language therapist may assist in assessing individual patients for any swallowing difficulties. (For further information on enteral feeding and parenteral nutrition, see Ch. 21.)

Elimination

The normal means of elimination of urine and faeces are altered by confinement to bed and the ability of the patient to urinate or defaecate is impaired by her altered level of consciousness.

The unconscious patient will not be able to indicate when she requires to pass urine or defaecate, although she may become restless. Despite the acknowledged dangers of urinary tract infection and calculi, if the patient is unconscious for more than 24–36 h, catheterisation should be considered. This helps to retain the patient's dignity, avoid the embarrassment of incontinence and prevent skin breakdown. An accurate measurement of urinary output may also be required. A closed urine collection system helps to reduce the risk of infection. Local protocols should be followed with regard to catheter care (see Ch. 8).

Not all unconscious patients need to be catheterised. Many male patients can be managed with external penile collection devices such as uri-sheaths. This is useful once the initial acute period is over and the patient is stabilising.

There is no ready solution for the management of defaecation. The patient's bowel movements should be monitored, particularly if she is receiving tube feeding. Hospital protocols should be followed for the prevention and management of constipation and diarrhoea. If necessary, prophylactic stool softeners may be needed in order to produce a stool every other day. It is important for the patient to avoid straining to pass a stool as this will raise intracranial pressure.

Personal cleansing and dressing

The unconscious patient is dependent upon the nurse to attend to all aspects of personal cleansing and dressing, but still has the right to have these procedures performed in privacy. This is especially important when performing intimate procedures such as the provision of personal hygiene in the menstruating female or in giving urinary catheter care.

Bathing in bed is necessary for any totally dependent patient, but when turning the unconscious patient there is a danger that the airway may become compromised and the patient's chest movement may be impeded. To avoid this, turning should be planned and requires a minimum of two nurses to execute it safely. If an Arjo bath is available, the patient can be bathed using this. Bathing, hair and nail care should all be performed as often as necessary. Hair washing can be difficult and, if the use of wet shampoos is impossible, a dry shampoo may be used. Nails should be kept short and clean. Male patients may require a daily facial shave and an electric razor is recommended. If the patient has a moustache/beard, this should be trimmed as necessary.

Eye care is carried out on a regular basis to prevent damage to the cornea. In some unconscious patients the eyelids may remain open. Unconscious patients do not blink periodically, and therefore the corneas become dry.

The eye and the immediate surrounding area are cleaned with sterile normal saline, followed by the instillation of artificial tear drops. If the patient's eyelids do not close naturally, tape may need to be applied. If tape is used, the delicate skin of the eyelid will need to be closely observed for excoriation. This can be minimised by using hypoallergenic tape and regularly altering the position of the tape. Alternatively, the eyes could be protected by gauze pads, eye shields or eye patches. If the area around the eyes is swollen or bruised, ice packs or cold and warm compresses may be used. Local protocol should be followed.

Oral hygiene should be maintained following initial and ongoing assessment of the individual patient (Turner 1996). A number of authors note that mouth care tends to be based on traditional and ritualistic practices rather than being scientifically or research-based (e.g. Moore 1995, Holmes 1996, Pearson 1996). These authors and others note that evidence suggests that a toothbrush is the most effective tool, whereas foam sticks tend to be popular amongst nurses for cleaning a patient's mouth (Buglass 1995).

The unconscious patient may present with particular problems such as a dry mouth and difficult access to the oral cavity if an artificial airway or ET tube is in place.

The NNBG recommends using a small, soft toothbrush to clean the teeth, tongue and gums (with care) with a small amount of fluoride toothpaste or plain water. Many oral care products are available — for example, hydrogen peroxide or sodium bicarbonate can help to remove debris and tenacious mucus, and chlorhexidine mouthwash helps to reduce plaque and has an antimicrobial effect (Buglass 1995). If solutions such as these are used, the nurse must be aware of correct dilution for effective use. Vaseline is widely used to prevent dry lips, although there appears to be no research evidence as to its effectiveness (Holmes 1996, Turner 1996). Dentures can be stored dry, after being cleaned, and should be cleaned again (rinsed in cold water) before insertion. Some nurses may prefer to store a patient's dentures in water or a proprietary denture solution, particularly if relatives request this. Local protocols should be followed.

It is obvious from the research into and studies of oral hygiene that this is an area of practice that nurses should re-examine and change if necessary (see Ch. 15).

Maintaining a safe environment

The unconscious patient is vulnerable to many threats and nursing staff must always be alert to the need to maintain a safe environment.

Prevention of pressure sores

The prevention of pressure sores is important for the comfort of the patient and is good practice. Regular alteration of the patient's position is the main factor, particularly in the unconscious patient, who may be immobile (see Ch. 23).

Q **28.4** Apart from direct pressure on the skin, what other factors can contribute to the development of pressure sores? Can you think of any additional hazards that may cause tissue damage in the unconscious patient?

Infection

The unconscious patient is particularly at risk of infection occurring in the chest and bladder. Wounds and drains, e.g. external ventricular drains, are also potential sites for infection. The most commonly acquired infection associated with respiratory therapy is Gram-negative bacillary pneumonia (Mims et al 1993), the causative organism of which is constantly present in the environment. Most people are resistant to it, but certain factors contribute to the breaking down of physiological and immunological defences and the unconscious patient is exposed to many of these, including endotracheal intubation and the presence of invasive lines such as i.v. cannulae and urinary catheters. Antibiotic-resistant infections have become a problem in some hospitals. For example, methicillin-resistant *Staphylococcus aureus* (MRSA) is potentially a life-threatening organism, particularly in vulnerable patients. In areas where patients are at high risk of acquiring MRSA, staff should be screened to determine if they are carrying the organism (Mackenzie 1997).

The mechanism of infection. Infection will occur if a sufficient number of microbes reaches the lower respiratory tract or urinary bladder. The likelihood of infection occurring depends on the virulence of the organism and the susceptibility of the patient. Ironically, the original source of the Gram-negative bacilli is often the patient herself. Infection can spread from the digestive tract, its usual home, into the lungs or bladder. Endotracheal or tracheostomy tubes, which bypass the normal protective mechanism of the nose, encourage the spread of infection, and a depressed cough reflex encourages pooling of secretions within the lungs, resulting in stasis. Urinary bladder catheterisation provides a ready entry route to the bladder. Preventive measures, in which the nurse plays a major role, include:

- unit design, e.g. facilities for handwashing, facilities for cleaning and disposal of equipment, provision of single/isolation rooms
- a control-of-infection policy
- aseptic techniques.

The nurse needs to be aware of and conscientious about implementing universal precautions and local policies with regard to prevention and treatment of infection (see Ch. 16).

Medication

The hazards of administering medication to patients are well documented, but the risks are increased in the unconscious patient for two reasons.

- The routes that are used carry a greater risk for the patient. The simpler and safer oral route is contraindicated. Other methods of administration have to be utilised, including intramuscular injections, i.v. infusions, via an intragastric tube, and per rectum.
- The patient cannot confirm her identity, so the nurse must be vigilant in ensuring that the medication is being given to the correct patient via the correct route.

The types of medication most commonly used in the unconscious patient include analgesics, anticonvulsants, antibiotics and laxatives, depending upon her condition and individual requirements.

Motor and sensory loss or impairment

The motor and sensory loss experienced by unconscious patients may be drug-induced or part of the underlying disease process. Whatever the cause, the nursing intervention remains the same.

Motor loss. See 'Mobilisation' below.

Sensory loss. The sensory system is part of the body's defence system and the unconscious patient is unable to process sensory information. It is imperative that the patient is not exposed to extremes of temperature, particularly in a localised area of the skin, e.g. if heating or cooling devices are used.

Care must be taken when moving and positioning the patient as she will not be aware of friction or pressure.

Seizure

The role of the nurse (or onlooker) when a patient has a seizure is to ensure that the patient does not harm herself (see Box 28.4). As much information as possible should be noted by the nurse (see Ch. 9 p. 378).

Box 28.4 Dealing with a seizure (from Lindsay 1988)

What to do when someone has a seizure

- Stay calm. Do not try to restrain or revive the person.
- Help the person into the recovery position on the floor (or in bed) and put something soft under her head.
- Remove glasses and loosen any tight clothing. Remove hazards, such as hard objects that could cause injury if the person falls or knocks against them.
- If respiration continues to be laboured after the movements have stopped, gently check that saliva, vomit or dentures are not blocking the airway.
- There will be no memory of the seizure and the person should not be left alone until fully alert. Some people are quite able to resume their normal routines after a period of sleep or quiet rest. Calm reassurance is needed as the person may feel embarrassed or disoriented after an attack.

What not to do

- Do not try to revive the person. A seizure cannot be stopped once it has begun.
- Never attempt to force anything between the teeth. It is impossible to 'swallow the tongue', and cut tissue on the lips and tongue heals, but broken teeth are a social embarrassment.
- There is no need to call a doctor or ambulance if the seizure ends in under 15 min, if consciousness returns without further incident and if there are no signs of injury, physical distress or pregnancy.
- Do not give the person anything to drink until she is fully awake.

Mobilisation

The nursing management of mobilisation and activity remains the same whatever the cause of the unconsciousness. Lack of attention to mobilisation could lead to the development of:

- contractures
- muscle atrophy
- pressure sores
- postural hypotension
- deep vein thrombosis
- hypostatic pneumonia.

Any one of these hazards will delay the patient's rehabilitation and result in additional pain.

Range-of-movement (ROM) exercises

Whilst the patient remains dependent, the nurse is responsible, along with the physiotherapist, for ensuring that the patient's limbs are put through a range-of-movement (ROM) exercise programme, which exercises each joint through its full movement range.

Stages of ROM exercise. There are three levels:

- passive
- active–assistive
- active.

Passive. Initially the nurse makes all the effort during ROM exercises, i.e. without the cooperation of the patient.

Active–assistive. As the patient improves, she may be able to cooperate. The exercises then become 'active–assistive', i.e. the movement is initiated by the patient but with the assistance of another person.

Active. The final stage is 'active', with the patient making all the effort. Patients with an altered level of consciousness will not be able to undertake active exercise.

Procedure. ROM exercises should be performed at 4-hourly intervals, over a 24-h period. They are not just performed by the physiotherapist; a schedule should be agreed for each individual patient and implemented by all concerned with the patient's care. The exercises should not be performed if the affected limb is injured or if contraindicated by medical treatment.

To perform ROM exercises, one hand is placed above the joint to provide support against gravity and prevent any unwanted movement. The joint is then exercised by smooth, slow, rhythmical movement through its range. The movement should stop at its normal extreme but sooner if the patient expresses pain or the nurse feels resistance. To carry out the procedure proficiently, the nurse should adopt a good upright stance to maintain his own posture. The usual pattern of exercises consists of five repetitions of movement for each limb, gradually increasing to a maximum of 10 as the patient's toleration increases. Relatives can be taught to carry out these exercises for the patient as a way of becoming involved in her care.

Correct positioning of the patient is also important and the following should be considered:

- body alignment, especially if spinal injury is suspected
- use of aids such as pillows, foam pads or splints, if required, to help to support the patient
- avoidance of pressure, e.g. an arm trapped under the body, the pinna of the ear bent forward, bedclothes too tight
- avoidance of friction when moving the patient
- changing the patient's position; this should be done frequently — at least every 2 h is recommended
- careful handling of joints and paralysed or weak limbs
- safety — e.g. if the patient is restless, padded cot sides may be required.

Recovery from coma

Patients who have been nursed in bed for just a few days often experience dizziness and light-headedness due to postural hypotension when they sit up for the first time. The patient recovering from coma, who may also have some motor weakness, is no exception. It is advisable to nurse the patient in a sitting position in bed for a day or two, before progressing to sitting in a chair. This will help the patient to get used to the position and will give her a psychological boost.

On first raising the patient to a sitting position, the nurse should check the patient's vital signs and colour, and ask whether she is experiencing any untoward symptoms. If she is, the mobilisation programme should be implemented at a slower rate.

Q **28.5** What are the causes of postural (orthostatic) hypotension?

The patient will be very unsure and frightened of altering her position, so repeated explanations of what is expected of her will provide the necessary reassurance.

If the patient has not suffered any ill effects, she can progress to sitting on the edge of the bed. This will require the patient's full cooperation and the assistance of two, preferably three, nurses. On the first occasion, the patient should sit for no more than 10 min. The patient's colour and vital signs should be observed, as outlined earlier. If the patient's respiratory status is not compromised, the length of time and frequency of sitting can be gradually increased.

The patient can then progress to sitting in a chair. The procedure is as already outlined, ensuring that the patient does not suffer any ill effects. The patient with motor loss or impairment can sit up if given a high-backed chair, provided that adequate support is provided. Once in the chair, any equipment which the patient is able to use, such as a call bell, drinks, radio or newspapers, should be readily available to her. The amount of time that the patient is up in the chair should be noted; it is more beneficial for the patient to sit up for several short intervals in one day rather than for one long period (see Ch. 34).

An individualised mobility rehabilitation programme should be devised in conjunction with the physiotherapist.

Controlling body temperature

Body temperature must be maintained within a relatively constant range to sustain life, i.e. 36–37.5°C. It is controlled by the heat-regulating centre in the hypothalamus, which acts like a thermostat (see Ch. 22). Pyrexia, an abnormally high temperature, is more commonly seen in the unconscious patient than is hypothermia, an abnormally low temperature (although hypothermia may be the primary cause of unconsciousness) (see Ch. 22).

Pyrexia may be due to damage to the heat-regulating centre in the hypothalamus or to an infective process or metabolic disorder. The danger is that for each degree of temperature over the normal range, a proportionately greater amount of oxygen is utilised from the patient's often diminishing reserves, which may have serious implications for recovery.

The nursing interventions remain similar irrespective of the cause of pyrexia.

Measurement of temperature (see also Ch. 22)

Important considerations when assessing the temperature of an unconscious patient are as follows:

- The nurse must stay with the patient whilst the thermometer is in place.
- If using a glass mercurial thermometer, temperature should be taken in the axilla or groin, never in the mouth.
- Alternatively, a rectal thermometer may be used.
- Other types of thermometers, if available, may be safer and more accurate, e.g. electronic, infrared (tympanic) and liquid crystal thermometers.

Dying

Skilled care of the unconscious patient often saves life, but some patients will die despite all measures taken. Active treatment may have been continued right up until the last moment or it may have been decided that no further active intervention would benefit the patient. The emphasis would then move from curative to terminal care. A third possibility is that the patient fulfils the criteria for brain stem death.

Brain stem death

Some patients in apnoeic coma can suffer severe and irreversible brain damage but continue to have their blood pressure, heartbeat and respirations artificially maintained for a period of time by ventilation, drug therapy and other life support interventions. However, some of these patients will never recover and the brain stem death criteria have been developed to identify those patients, in order that therapy can cease.

Brain stem death may be clinically diagnosed by following a set of guidelines issued by the Working Group of the Conference of Medical Royal Colleges and their Faculties (1976, with revisions in 1979) and according to the concept of death endorsed by this Working Group in 1995. These consist of a number of tests that can only be applied after a series of preconditions have been fulfilled (see Fig. 28.9).

Preconditions. These include positively diagnosed structural brain damage that is irremediable and that the patient is unresponsive and on a ventilator. The examiner must satisfy himself that any reversible causes of coma have been eliminated, including:

- drug intoxication, e.g. as the result of an overdose or the administration of a neuromuscular blocking agent such as Pavulon to facilitate passage of an endotracheal tube
- primary hypothermia
- metabolic or endocrine imbalances such as uncontrolled diabetes.

Testing brain stem function. Once satisfied that the preconditions have been fulfilled, the testing of brain stem function can be performed. Two doctors should carry out the tests. Usually one is the consultant responsible for the patient and the other is of at least senior registrar status. If organ donation from the patient is being considered, neither doctor must be a member of the transplant team. The doctors may carry out the tests separately or together.

Diagnosis to be made by two doctors, one a Consultant and the other a Consultant or Senior Registrar.

Diagnosis should not be considered until at least 6 hours after the onset of Coma; 12-24 hours will be more usual.

NAME: .... UNIT NO. ....

PRE-CONDITIONS

Time of event leading to coma

Nature of irremediable brain damage

Dr A ....

Dr B ....

Do you consider that Apnoeic Coma is due to:

	Dr A	Dr B
Depressant Drugs		
Neuromuscular Blocking (relaxant) drugs		
Hypothermia		
Metabolic or Endocrine Disturbances		

TESTS FOR ABSENCE OF BRAIN STEM FUNCTION

Is there evidence of:

	Dr A	Dr B
Pupil reaction to light		
Corneal reflex		
Eye Movements with Cold Caloric Test		
Cranial Nerve Motor Responses		
Gag reflex		
Respiratory movements on disconnection from Ventilator to allow adequate rise in $PaCo_2$		

Date and time of First Testing ....

Date and time of Second Testing ....

	Dr A	Dr B
Signature	....	....
Status	....	....

Fig. 28.9 Criteria for the diagnosis of brain stem death (Allan 1987). (Reproduced with kind permission from *Professional Nurse*, where this figure first appeared in 1987.)

There are six parts to the test:

1. The pupillary response to light is tested, using a bright torch. Absence of response indicates loss of function, although the examiner should be satisfied that a non-responsive pupil is not due to the instillation of paralytic eye drops or damage to the third cranial nerve.
2. The integrity of the corneal reflex is tested by drawing a wisp of cotton wool across the exposed cornea. Absence of a blink response indicates loss of function, although the examiner should be satisfied that the presence of corneal oedema is not preventing the normal blink response.
3. Cranial nerve motor responses are tested at several sites, including the head and face, in case the patient has a cervical cord injury. Again, no response indicates loss of function, although spinal reflexes can remain intact even in a brain-dead patient (Mandefield 1993).
4. The cough and gag reflexes are tested by moving the endotracheal tube back and forth or by applying suction and observing the patient's throat muscles for movement. No response would indicate loss of the pharyngeal and laryngeal reflexes.
5. Absence of the oculovestibular reflex rules out the existence of normally functioning anatomical pathways within the brain stem and is a very sensitive test of brain stem function. It is tested by syringing 20 mL of ice-cold water into each of the patient's ears in turn and noting any eye movement in response. This is called 'cold caloric testing'. Before testing, the examiner should use an auriscope to look directly at the tympanic membrane to ensure that it is intact and that there is no obstruction preventing the water from making contact with the membrane.

6. The final test is that for apnoea. Arterial blood gases are checked and P_aCO_2 should be 5.33–6.00 kPa (40–45 mmHg). The patient is disconnected from the ventilator after providing a continuous flow of 100% intratracheal oxygen for 10 min. The patient's chest wall is observed closely for any respiratory movement and the P_aCO_2 is allowed to rise above threshold level to stimulate breathing, usually to at least 6.65 kPa (50 mmHg). The time taken to achieve this will vary, but is no more than 10 min for most patients (Mandefield 1993).

The entire process is repeated after a minimum of 30 min (in practice, usually longer) before the patient is declared brain dead. Although the second set of tests is not required by law, for medicolegal purposes the completion of the second testing determines the time of death and the patient is normally disconnected from the ventilator by medical staff. It may previously have been indicated that this patient wished to donate organs and/or tissues for transplantation, and if so, following the usual preliminary procedures, the patient would remain ventilated until the organs were removed.

Although not a legal requirement, it is usual protocol for the doctor or transplant coordinator to obtain permission from the patient's next of kin before taking organs and tissues. The transplant coordinator will offer counselling to the patient's relatives or those who have a significant relationship with the patient.

For further reading on brain stem death, see Pallis & Harley (1996).

Physical and psychological care

The patient. The principles of care for the dying unconscious patient are the same as those for the terminally ill patient (see Ch. 33).

The family. Psychologically, this is a traumatic and emotionally distressing period for the patient's family, friends and/or those who have a significant relationship with the patient. They have perhaps spent the last few days (and in some cases, much longer than that) watching the patient in the technical surroundings often used to support the unconscious patient and may be relieved that some sort of ending has been achieved. Often the patient's appearance has changed so much that the relatives do not recognise her any more.

The support of a religious adviser may be appreciated. The nurse should ascertain if this is desired and arrange it if the relatives request her to do so.

A coherent strategy for caring for the relatives is needed. The nurse should know what information has been given to the relatives by other members of staff, including doctors. This will enable the nurse to reinforce what has been said and avoid confusing them at a time when their ability to process information is drastically reduced. Allan (1988b) emphasises the need for the relatives to see the patient — unconscious and unresponsive as she is — being treated as a person through a humane, caring attitude on the part of the nurse.

Some relatives may be helped by being encouraged to perform simple acts of care for the patient such as bathing her or, providing her head is not shaved or bandaged, combing her hair. This reduces their feelings of passivity and helplessness in the strange, alien world of the hospital and in a situation in which they are unlikely to be able to draw on previous experience.

Inevitably, this chapter has focused on the care of unconscious people in hospital because, at the present time, only a very small minority are cared for at home. This may change in the future, at least to some extent, as new technology is developed. Where the outcome is death, some families may cope more easily with the stress and sadness in the familiar surroundings of the home. Wherever the location of care, it is important for nurses to be sensitive to the fundamental changes the unconscious patient has wrought in the lives of those who know her as a responsive being. Not only is the patient totally reliant upon the nurse, but the family and/or carers also require a great deal of support.

As noted at the outset of this chapter, caring for the unconscious person is a major challenge for nurses. Whatever the outcome, be it death, permanent disability or complete recovery, meticulous attention to nursing observations and careful nursing care are vital.

REFERENCES

Ackerman M H 1996 A review of normal saline installation: implications for practice. Dimensions of Critical Care Nursing 15(1): 31–38

Allan D 1987 Criteria for brain stem death. Professional Nurse 2(11): 357–359

Allan D 1988a Making sense of suctioning. Nursing Times 84(10): 46–47

Allan D 1988b Nursing and the neurosciences. Churchill Livingstone, Edinburgh

Bates N, Dines A, Volans G 1997 Acute poisoning: initial management and sources of information. Emergency Nurse 5(3): 20–24

Bland 1993 Airedale NHS Trust v. Bland E. AC 789. House of Lords

British Medical Association 1993 Guidelines on the treatment of patients in a persistent vegetative state. BMA

Buglass A 1995 Oral hygiene. British Journal of Nursing 4(9): 516–519

Chudley S 1994 The effect of nursing activities on intracranial pressure. British Journal of Nursing 3(9): 454–458

Clarke L 1995 A critical event in tracheostomy care. British Journal of Nursing 4(12): 676–681

Cruzan 1990 Cruzan v. Director, Missouri Dept of Health. 110 S Ct 2841. US Supreme Court

Day L, Drought T, Davis A J 1995 Principle-based ethics and nurses' attitudes towards artificial feeding. Journal of Advanced Nursing 21: 295–298

Fitzgerald M J T 1996 Neuroanatomy – basic and clinical, 3rd edn. WB Saunders, London

Frawley P 1990 Neurological observations. Nursing Times 86(35): 29–34

Grubb A, Walsh P, Lambe N, Murrells T, Robinson S 1996 Survey of British clinicians' views on management of patients in persistent vegetative state. Lancet 348: 35–40

Guyton A C 1991 Physiology of the human body, 5th edn. WB Saunders, Philadelphia

Harkin H 1998 Tracheostomy management. Nursing Times 94(21): 56–58

Hemingway S, McAndrew S 1998 Acquired brain injury: identifying emotional and cognitive needs. RCN Continuing Education Article 923. Emergency Nurse 5(10): 29–38

Henderson V 1960 Basic principles of nursing care. International Council of Nurses, Geneva

Hickey J V 1997 The clinical practice of neurological and neurosurgical nursing, 4th edn. J B Lippincott, New York

Holmes S 1996 Nursing management of oral care in older patients. Nursing Times 92(9): 37–39

Lindsay M D 1988 Care of the patient with epilepsy. In: Allan D (ed) 1988 Nursing and the neurosciences. Churchill Livingstone, Edinburgh, ch 16

Mackenzie D 1997 MRSA: the psychological effects. Nursing Standard 12(11): 49–53
Magoun H W 1963 The waking brain. Thomas, Springfield, IL
Mandefield H 1993 Making sense of brainstem death. Nursing Times 89(35): 32–34
Martin K M 1994 When the nurse says 'He's just not right': patient cues used by expert nurses to identify mild head injury. Journal of Neuroscience Nursing 26(4): 210–218
Mims C A, Playfair J H L, Roitt I M, Wakelin D, Williams R 1993 Medical microbiology. Mosby, London
Moore J 1995 Assessment of nurse-administered oral hygiene. Nursing Times 91(9): 40–41
Multi-society Task Force Report on PVS 1994 Medical aspects of the persistent vegetative state. New England Journal of Medicine 330: 1499–1508, 1572–1579
Pearson L S 1996 A comparison of the ability of foam swabs and toothbrushes to remove dental plaque: implications for nursing practice. Journal of Advanced Nursing 23: 62–69
Phipps W J, Sand J K, Marek J F (eds) 1999 Medical-surgical nursing: concepts and clinical practice, 6th edn. Mosby, St Louis
Plum F, Posner J B 1980 The diagnosis of stupor and coma, 3rd edn. E A Davies, Philadelphia
Podurgiel M 1990 The unconscious experience: a pilot study. Journal of Neuroscience Nursing 22(1): 52–53
Roper N, Logan W, Tierney A 1996 The elements of nursing, 4th edn. Churchill Livingstone, Edinburgh
Royal College of Physicians 1996 The permanent vegetative state. Journal of the Royal College of Physicians 30: 119–121
Smith S 1997 The outer edge of consciousness. Nursing Times 93(39): 28–32
Spence A P, Mason E B 1987 Human anatomy and physiology, 3rd edn. Cummings, Menlo Park
Teasdale G 1975 Acute impairment of brain function: assessing conscious level. Nursing Times 71(24): 914–917
Teasdale G, Jennett B 1974 Assessment of coma and impaired consciousness. Lancet 2: 81
Treloar D M, Nalli B J, Guin P, Gary R 1991 The effect of familiar and unfamiliar voice treatments on intracranial pressure in head-injured patients. Journal of Neuroscience Nursing 23(5): 295–299
Trimble M 1979 Altered consciousness. Nursing, 1st Series (8): 344–348
Turner G 1996 Oral care. RCN Continuing Education Article 330. Nursing Standard 10(28): 51–54
Wilson K J W, Waugh A 1996 Ross & Wilson anatomy and physiology in health and illness, 8th edn. Churchill Livingstone, Edinburgh
Working Group of the Conference of Medical Royal Colleges and their Faculties in the UK 1976 Diagnosis of death. British Medical Journal ii: 1187–1188
Working Group of the Conference of Medical Royal Colleges and their Faculties in the UK 1979 Diagnosis of death. British Medical Journal i: 3320
Working Group of the Conference of Medical Royal Colleges and their Faculties in the UK 1995 The criteria for the diagnosis of brainstem death. Journal of the Royal College of Physicians (London) 29: 1985–1990

FURTHER READING

Bates N, Dines A, Volans G 1997 Acute poisoning: initial management and sources of information. Emergency Nurse 5(3): 20–24
Chudley S 1994 The effect of nursing activities on intracranial pressure. British Journal of Nursing 3(9): 454–458
Hemingway S, McAndrew S 1998 Acquired brain injury: identifying emotional and cognitive needs. RCN Continuing Education Article. Emergency Nurse 5(10): 29–38
Hickey J V 1997 The clinical practice of neurological and neurosurgical nursing, 4th edn. J B Lippincott, New York
Johnson L H, Roberts S L 1996 Hope facilitating strategies for the family of the head injury patient. Journal of Neuroscience Nursing 28(4): 259–266
Pallis C, Harley D H 1996 ABC of brain stem death, 2nd edn. BMJ Publishing Group, London
Randall P 1997 A stranger in the family. Nursing Times 93(39): 32–33
Royal College of Physicians 1996 The permanent vegetative state. Journal of the Royal College of Physicians of London 30(2): 119–121
Smith S 1997 The outer edge of consciousness. Nursing Times 93(39): 28–32
Treloar D M, Nalli B J, Guin P, Gary R 1991 The effect of familiar and unfamiliar voice treatments on intracranial pressure in head-injured patients. Journal of Neuroscience Nursing 23(5): 295–299

NOTE AND USEFUL ADDRESS

The Neuroscience Nurses' Benchmarking Group (NNBG)

The NNBG was established in 1995. It consists of nurses from a number of neuroscience units in the UK and Eire, and membership is open to any neuroscience nurse who is interested. The group meets every few months to share ideas and information. A benchmarking system is used 'to identify and achieve continual improvement in best nursing practice'. Literature reviews, research and evidence-based practice are discussed to reach a consensus between the members on best practice relating to a specific aspect of nursing. The specific nursing activity is then 'tested' against the benchmark in the nurses' own areas of practice and comparisons made at the next meeting. The benchmarks are not static and are reviewed in the light of changing practice and updated as necessary.

Contact:
Mr John Pauls
Project Nurse
Worthington House
Hope Hospital
Salford
Manchester M6 8WH

THE CRITICALLY ILL PATIENT

Catriona E. Fulton

29

INTRODUCTION

The term 'critically ill' is used to describe people who have acute life-threatening conditions but who might recover if they are given prompt, appropriate, effective and often highly technical nursing and medical care. Critically ill patients, the conditions from which they suffer and the care and treatment they need are so varied that elements from every chapter in this book are relevant to their care.

Patients who present in a critically ill state can be considered in three main categories:

- those who have never before had a significant illness and who have suffered a sudden, acute life-threatening event, e.g. extensive trauma, severe burns, near drowning, major childbirth complications or deliberate self-harm
- those who suffer from chronic illness, perhaps involving frequent previous hospital admissions, e.g. chronic obstructive airways disease (COAD) or chronic pancreatitis, and who present as critically ill as a combination of their chronic illness with a life-threatening event
- those who have become critically ill as a result of surgery — in some cases, the life-threatening situation is not expected, while in others, postoperative intensive care is a recognised necessity.

Increasingly nowadays, the major health issues and inequalities in our society will be underlying factors with varying degrees of significance in the presentation of the critically ill patient, e.g. drug, alcohol and other substance abuse or dependence, smoking, poor dietary habits, lack of exercise and mental health concerns.

Because most of these patients will be nursed in specialised units, such as an intensive care unit (ICU), their treatment and nursing care will be viewed primarily within that context. Criteria for admission to an ICU vary from hospital to hospital, but in most general ICU settings, the main admission criteria are the patient's respiratory status and its maintenance. Intensive care has been defined as 'a service for patients with potentially recoverable diseases who can benefit from more detailed observation and treatment than is generally available in the standard wards' (Spiby 1989). Duration of stay in an ICU will vary greatly, from the overnight ventilation support that may be required postoperatively to months of intensive therapy required by multiple trauma victims. In recent years there has been considerable progress in the management of many acute life-threatening conditions and consequently there has been a substantial growth in both the number and size of such units.

The nursing care of the critically ill patient is an extensive area and one that will not be covered fully in this chapter. It is therefore expected that those interested in this field will refer both to relevant chapters within this textbook and to more specialised texts and journals.

For further reading, see Hinds & Watson (1996) and Oh (1997).

The Mead model for nursing

The primary responsibility of the nurse in the ICU setting is to provide care to patients with life-threatening illnesses requiring continuous monitoring and life support, embracing a holistic approach. Any model used to guide intensive care nursing must therefore be flexible and allow for creativity. This chapter introduces the Mead model for nursing (McClure & Franklin 1987) developed by staff at St Thomas' Hospital, London (Mead ward), specifically to guide the nursing care of critically ill patients. It is seen in practice in an increasing number of ICUs. Adapted from Roper et al's (1996) activities of living model (AL), the Mead model places the patient at the centre of all activities. Those factors which influence the ALs are given a higher profile and are used as a framework for care. Unlike Roper et al's model, the Mead model places explicit emphasis on the physical aspects of critical care nursing, such as the status of the respiratory, cardiovascular, neurological and other body systems. Generally, it is these physical needs that take priority, often reflecting the patient's reason for admission. However, the Mead model also addresses the important contextual factors that can affect the patient, his care and the eventual outcome of that care (see Nursing Care Plan 29.1). The aim of using this care plan format is to provide a structural framework for application of the nursing process (assessment, planning, intervention and evaluation) and to document this in such a way as to help others to find out about a patient's individual care easily, without working through irrelevant information, much of which is documented elsewhere (e.g. 24-h chart, drug prescription chart). The development of the Mead model for nursing demonstrates that the nurse should be free to select from a model those elements that are appropriate to that situation.

For further reading on nursing models in ICUs, see Robb (1997).

MEETING THE PHYSICAL NEEDS OF THE CRITICALLY ILL PATIENT

RESPIRATORY NEEDS AND CARE

Intensive care units became established when life could be supported and maintained by means of artificial ventilation (Hinds 1992). While many disease processes may lead to the need for mechanical ventilation (Box 29.1), it is most clearly indicated in the treatment of patients with severe respiratory failure who do not respond to conventional forms of medical treatment. Mechanical ventilation is the artificial support of or assistance with breathing when adequate gaseous exchange and tissue perfusion can no longer be maintained (see Ch. 3). Modern ventilation enables therapy to be specifically directed at a wide range of respiratory disorders and can do far more than just maintain vital functions.

Nursing priorities and management:

Goal: to ensure optimal gaseous exchange and tissue perfusion.

Plan:

- monitor and maintain safe ventilatory support
- assist with physiotherapy and the removal of tracheal secretions
- wean from ventilatory support when appropriate.

Monitoring respiratory function and maintaining safe ventilation

It is the nurse's responsibility to understand both normal and abnormal respiratory function, therapeutic modes of ventilation, how to maintain safe ventilatory support and how to respond appropriately to any problems that might occur. Ashworth (1990) suggests that advanced technology is only ever as good as those who use it.

29.1 Describe the general principles of respiratory physiology.

Ventilators

Consideration of the patient's specific needs and diagnosis will determine the most appropriate mode of ventilation for the patient. Positive pressure ventilators are those most commonly used, and the positive pressure, volume-cycled ventilator is that most widely seen in general ICUs. This type of ventilator exerts positive pressure on the airway, delivering a predetermined volume of gas and allowing limits to be set for pressure and time. Specific considerations in the choice of ventilator for those requiring respiratory support include:

- the delivery of accurate predetermined oxygen concentrations of 21–100%
- a wide range of modes (see Table 29.1)
- the delivery of preset volumes, despite lung characteristic changes
- the facility to monitor respiratory variables
- the appropriate alarm limits with electrical and gas safety features and a back-up system
- minimal circuit resistance allowing effective spontaneous breathing modes
- cost and user-friendliness
- reliable sterilisation and maintenance of the ventilator parts (Oh 1997)
- the use of heated bacterial filters
- the effective and safe provision of humidification and nebulised drugs.

Nursing Care Plan 29.1 The Mead model

Name: Iver HART **DOB:** 10/12/20 **Date:** 24/05/98

DIAGNOSIS: Repair of abdominal aortic aneurysm (AAA), ischaemic heart disease, peripheral vascular disease, respiratory failure, acute renal impairment

24 HOUR SUMMARY
Second day postop following AAA repair: respiratory function improving, continues on dopamine for renal impairment

Assessment ***Day/night***	***Goals and planned care***
RESPIRATORY	
SIMV: 10 × 700, ASB: 20, PEEP: 5, $F_{i}o_{2}$: 0.6 $S_{a}o_{2}$: 95–97%, RR: 15–20 Air entry R = L, quiet at bases minimal up on tracheal suction ABGs: Po_2 9.6, Pco_2 6.2	*Goal*: To optimise gaseous exchange and tissue perfusion *Plan*: Continue with ventilatory support; assist with physiotherapy and the clearance of secretions; position for optimal lung expansion; repeat ABGs
CARDIOVASCULAR	
HR: 95–110, irregular with ventricular ectopics BP: 180/95–210/100 Temperature: 37.5–38°C K^+: 4.3, Hb: 8.9 Peripherally cool, feet mottled with pedal pulses present	*Goal*: To promote and maintain cardiovascular stability *Plan*: Monitor vital signs hourly, reporting any abnormalities; control hypertension with GTN infusion; transfuse with 2 units of RCC; continue with antibiotic therapy; monitor K^+, 12-lead ECG
RENAL	
Hourly urine output: 25–55 mL/h CVP: +12–14 cm Maintenance fluid running at 30 mL/h + previous hour's urine output, slight peripheral oedema Urea: 12.5, Creatinine: 210 Dopamine infusion: 4 mg/mL, at 3 mL/h	*Goal*: To optimise renal function and maintain adequate hydration *Plan*: Record hourly urine output; continue with dopamine infusion at 3 mL/h; monitor urea and electrolytes; involve renal physicians if necessary; continue with maintenance fluids as is
NEUROLOGICAL	
GCS: 9, PEARL, size 3 Sedated on midazolam 2 mL/h (1 mg/mL) Morphine at 3 mL/h (1 mg/mL) Pain score: 0–1 Sedation score: 3	*Goal*: To maintain neurological integrity and maintain pain-free *Plan*: Assess neurological status at regular intervals; monitor sedation and pain scores hourly; continue with sedation and analgesia as is
NUTRITION/GI	
4-hourly NG aspirates minimal, on free drainage 50–85 mL/h bile-coloured fluid, no bowel sounds present, blood sugars: 6–12 mmol/L, i.v. antacid prescribed BD, no bowel movements	*Goal*: To optimise nutritional support and maintain GI integrity *Plan*: Aspirate NG tube 4-hourly; discuss on ward round about commencing enteral feeding as per protocol; monitor blood sugars 4–6 hourly, assessing the need for insulin therapy
HYGIENE/MOBILITY/WOUND CARE	
Pressure areas intact, feet mottled, especially left big toe, mouth dry due to open mouth breathing, eyes slightly sticky, tolerates side lying, abdominal wound left intact, minimal leakage	*Goal*: To promote and maintain personal hygiene and maintain skin integrity *Plan*: Give all care as required; assess pressure area score daily; assess wound and re-dress as per wound care protocol
PSYCHOSOCIAL	
Mr Hart appears to be a very anxious man. His wife and their two sons and their families keep in close touch and visit on a regular basis	*Goal*: To minimise the stress/anxiety of the ICU environment *Plan*: Offer adequate reassurance and encouragement and explain all procedures prior to them being carried out; keep Mr Hart's family well informed as to his condition

ABG, Arterial blood gases; CVP, Central venous pressure; ECG, Electrocardiograph; GCS, Glasgow Coma Scale; GTN, Glyceryl trinitrate; HR, Heart rate; K^+, Potassium; NG, Nasogastric; PEARL, Pupils equal and reacting to light; RCC, Red cell concentrate; SIMV, Synchronised intermittent mandatory ventilation

(cont'd)

Nursing Care Plan 29.1 *(contd)*

PROGRESS/EVALUATION REPORT

Day: Tuesday **Time**: 19.30	**Night**	**Time**
Ventilatory settings unchanged; gaseous exchange slightly improved, maintaining S_aO_2 95–97%; spontaneous respiratory effort minimal 2–5 breaths; tracheal secretions now mucopurulent; specimen sent to bacteriology. Tolerated manual hyperinflation with physiotherapy		
HR remains irregular, rate 100–135; BP about 180/90; continues on a GTN infusion; remains pyrexial; antibiotics discontinued; WBC up to 12.6 Transfused 2 units of RCC; 12-lead ECG shows AF started on i.v. digoxin; K^+ checked at 16.00: 3.9 Peripheral circulation remains the same; seen by the surgeons who seem content with his progress		
Urine output: 65–100 mL/h, on dopamine 3 mL/h CVP: + 10 to + 14 cm; remains slightly oedematous peripherally; maintenance fluids as before; urea and creatinine remain elevated; renal physicians to be consulted		
GCS 9, PEARL size 3; morphine at 3 mL/h and midazolam at 2 mL/h; responds to speech, and will obey commands		
NG aspirates nil; commenced on enteral feed at 25 mL/h, to continue as per enteral feeding protocol; blood sugars stable; i.v. antacid discontinued; no bowel movements		
All care given as required; pressure areas intact; abdominal wound left exposed, as no leakage		
Mr Hart requires a lot of reassurance. Mr Hart's wife and sons visited this afternoon for a short while; they seemed pleased with his progress		

Modes of ventilation are as follows (Table 29.1):

- intermittent positive pressure ventilation (IPPV)
- synchronised intermittent mandatory ventilation (SIMV)
- assisted spontaneous breathing/pressure support (ASB/PS)
- positive end-expiratory pressure (PEEP) — used as an adjunct to IPPV, SIMV and ASB/PS
- continuous positive airway pressure (CPAP).

Weaning modes (in order of decreasing ventilatory support) are:

- SIMV/ASB
- ASB
- CPAP.

During the weaning phase, patients may alternate between these three modes until they are able to cope continually on a reduced mode.

Assessment of respiratory function

The assessment of respiratory function will focus heavily on physical examination (such as chest auscultations, breathing rate and pattern), pulse oximetry and diagnostic findings from chest X-ray and arterial blood gas analysis. This, together with the patient's underlying medical condition, age and weight, will contribute to the doctor's chosen mode of ventilation. Monitoring and maintaining safe ventilation is the nurse's responsibility and, once the patient is intubated (see Ch. 28) and receiving ventilation support,

Box 29.1 Causes of respiratory failure. (Adapted from Weilitz 1993)

Acute respiratory failure without respiratory distress
- Central airway obstruction
- Decreased level of consciousness
  —head injury
  —sepsis
  —drug overdose
- Neuromuscular pathway
  —Guillain–Barré syndrome
  —myasthenia gravis
  —postoperative diaphragmatic paralysis
  —trauma
- Cardiovascular
  —acute myocardial infarction
  —cardiogenic shock

Lung parenchymal disease
- Asthma
- Pneumonia
- Adult respiratory distress syndrome (ARDS)

Acute or chronic respiratory failure
- Exacerbation of chronic obstructive airways disease (COAD)
- Chronic neuromuscular disease

Table 29.1 Modes of mechanical ventilation: IPPV, intermittent positive pressure ventilation; SIMV, synchronised intermittent mandatory ventilation; ASB/PS, assisted spontaneous breathing/pressure support; PEEP, positive end-expiratory pressure; CPAP, continuous positive airway pressure

Mode	*Advantages*	*Disadvantages*	*Uses*
IPPV — also referred to as volume control, it delivers a preset volume of air at a certain rate regardless of the patient's own attempts to breathe (Oh 1997)	Complete control over ventilation; improves CO_2 elimination and improves oxygenation	Provides only full ventilation; sedation and/or paralysing agents required for the patient to tolerate it; barotrauma; decreases cardiac output; water retention; atelectasis; reduced lung compliance	Failure of ventilation (e.g. neuromuscular disease) To facilitate CO_2 excretion To reduce cerebral blood flow in patients with cerebral oedema secondary to head injury To reduce the work of breathing in patients with cardiorespiratory failure (Hillman & Bishop 1996)
SIMV — the patient's positive pressure breaths are synchronised with the inspiratory effort. If no inspiration time is sensed, a mandatory breath is delivered at a predetermined interval (Hinds 1992)	Provides both partial and full ventilation support; minimises mean airway pressure; allows spontaneous unassisted breathing; synchronises positive pressure breaths with the patient's effort (Hillman & Bishop 1996)	General hazards of artificial ventilation	As above SIMV provides the most therapeutic mode of ventilation
ASB/PS — not found on older models of ventilators, this mode senses each breath and assists breathing with a preset amount of positive pressure (Rainbow 1989)	Aids the transition from ventilation support to spontaneous breathing; can be used on its own as a mode or in conjunction with ventilator breaths (SIMV mode)	Does not control ventilation	Facilitates weaning Used to encourage spontaneous breathing
PEEP occurs when, instead of allowing airway pressures to reach atmospheric pressure between breaths, an end-expiratory pressure is applied, enabling diffusion of more O_2 from the alveoli into the pulmonary capillaries and thus optimising gaseous exchange. Not used on its own (Hillman & Bishop 1996)	Improves oxygenation; recruits alveoli for ventilation	Decreases venous return; decreases cardiac output; can cause pulmonary barotrauma; decreases extrathoracic organ blood; increases the work of breathing; pulmonary overdistension	Patients with ARDS, LVF, pulmonary oedema, atelectasis or profound hypoxaemia may benefit greatly from the addition of some PEEP (MacKenzie 1992)
CPAP is an option which delivers gas to the airways at a constant pressure, allowing for inspiratory pressure as well as providing PEEP. Can be used on its own	Recruits alveoli; low intrathoracic pressures compared with full ventilation; improves oxygenation; increases lung compliance; decreases the work of breathing; decreases cardiac preload and can be delivered via the ventilator or through a plastic face mask, avoiding the need for intubation	Potentially has the same disadvantages as PEEP and artificial ventilation; however, pressures are lower and so, therefore, are the risks	Used to support spontaneous breathing

Box 29.2 Potential complications of mechanical ventilation

- Damage to the airways/lung parenchyma
- Barotrauma, tension pneumothorax, disconnection/occlusion of the ET tube
- Mechanical failure
- Subcutaneous emphysema
- Hypo/hyperventilation
- Pulmonary oedema/pleural effusions
- Nosocomial infection, consolidation
- Low cardiac output
- Cardiovascular depression
- Arrhythmias
- Water retention
- GI haemorrhage, aspiration of stomach contents, paralytic ileus
- Impairment of CNS, kidneys and liver function
- O_2 toxicity
- Altered body image
- Sleep deprivation
- Tracheal injury

constant and thorough observations are required as there are many associated complications (see Box 29.2) (Rippe et al 1995, Hillman & Bishop 1996).

Nursing priorities for maintaining safe ventilation

Chest auscultation. This should be performed at the start of a shift, as a baseline, and thereafter at the discretion of the nurse. It can offer a wealth of information about your patient's air entry — from an expiratory wheeze requiring treatment with a bronchodilator, to areas of reduced air entry due to secretion retention, consolidation or pulmonary oedema. Using a systematic approach, this can spotlight trouble early and assure appropriate intervention (Stiesmeyer 1993).

Maintaining a patent airway. This involves endotracheal suctioning at intervals of no more than 2–3 h. While it is essential to keep the airway clear of secretions, it is also just as important not to oversuction and thereby cause unnecessary trauma, irritation and hypoxia (Chang 1995).

Humidification. The oxygen used to ventilate the patient must be warmed, humidified and filtered artificially as the endotracheal tube bypasses these natural processes inherent to the nasal passages (Jackson 1996). Exposing the lungs and airways to cold gas has a number of potentially harmful effects: it can increase mucus viscosity, depress ciliary activity and obstruct the airways due to the build-up of the tenacious secretions. Temperature-controlled water humidifiers are used while disposable filters are changed daily.

Ventilator and endotracheal (ET) tubes. The ventilator tubes must not be allowed to become kinked in any way that would reduce the desired respiratory effect. Patient comfort must be balanced with the safe and secure position of the ET tube in the patient's mouth. This is achieved by tying crepe bandage or non-allergic adhesive tape (to decrease the risk of raised intracranial pressure in the case of a patient with a head injury) around the patient's mouth, in order to prevent movement of the ET tube. Care should be given to the prevention of mouth sores and the position of the ET tube can be changed daily to facilitate this. Ventilator tubes must not be allowed to drag, pulling on the ET tube and thereby applying pressure to the lips. Ventilators usually have an 'arm' which will support the weight of the tubes. It is important that the tubes slope downward from the patient towards water traps so preventing water from condensation entering the ET tube and the lungs. Care should always be taken to ensure that ET and ventilator tubes are guarded and supported when turning the patient.

Endotracheal cuff pressures. These need to be checked regularly using an endotracheal cuff manometer. While cuff pressures of 30 mmHg are recommended, pressures of 17–23 mmHg have been shown to be adequate. Complications arising from prolonged excessive ET cuff pressures include tracheal oedema, loss of mucosal cilia, ulceration, ruptured tracheo-oesophageal fistula, stenosis, necrosis, sore throat and hoarseness (Rippe et al 1995). Prevention of these complications is part of the rationale behind re-siting the airway and the fashioning a tracheostomy after 12–14 days of oral intubation.

Level of sedation. If patients are too alert when the mode of ventilation used prevents/reduces their opportunity to trigger a break, e.g. IPPV, they may fight against the work of the ventilator, so preventing the desired therapeutic treatment being carried out; in these cases, sedation becomes necessary. Other patients may clamp down on the tube, preventing ventilation and clearance of secretions. It is also not uncommon for patients to bite through the ET tube completely. On the other hand, oversedation will inhibit patient progress if weaning from the ventilator and spontaneous breathing are the goals. Maintaining the appropriate level of sedation is important.

Ventilator observations. Continual observations should include the patient's colour (to see if he is well perfused or cyanosed), oxygen saturations ($Sa\text{O}_2$), the patient's level of consciousness (if on sedation, is he drowsy due to CO_2 retention?) and chest movements (are both lungs being ventilated?). It is essential that the fraction of inspired oxygen ($Fi\text{O}_2$), the prescribed ventilatory setting, the expired minute volume, the patient's airway pressures and respirations (spontaneous and ventilator breaths) and the temperature of the humidification chamber are all recorded hourly, allowing for continual respiratory assessment and the early detection and treatment of any problems (Robb 1993).

Vital signs. Changes in a patient's vital signs can immediately indicate problems with ventilation. Blood pressure, heart rate and rhythm, temperature, and respiratory rate and pattern should all be closely monitored.

Arterial blood gases (ABGs). Regular analysis of ABGs (see Ch. 3) will most accurately reveal a patient's respiratory progress or deterioration and the adequacy of ventilation support.

Assisting with physiotherapy and the removal of tracheal secretions

Physiotherapists are invaluable members of the multidisciplinary team. Their main role in relation to the respiratory needs of the critically ill patient is to aid the clearance of tracheal secretions, preventing collapse, atelectasis or consolidation of the lungs and generally optimising ventilatory efficiency through good positioning, manual hyperinflation and ET suctioning. Modern physiotherapy methods are both prophylactic and therapeutic (Pearson & Parr 1993).

Positioning

Depending on where the pulmonary abnormality is, the patient should be positioned to maximise the matching of ventilation and perfusion. If a patient has a left lower lobe collapse, it may be helpful to nurse him on his right side, thereby optimising the treatment to the affected area. Regularly turning patients will not only assist in the prevention of pressure sores but also facilitate pulmonary postural drainage. When a patient's oxygenation remains extremely poor despite high oxygen delivery and high PEEP levels, it may be decided to turn him to the prone position. Studies have shown that significant and dramatic improvements in arterial blood oxygenation can be achieved through the use of the prone position (Canter 1987), especially in the treatment of patients with adult respiratory distress syndrome (ARDS). In ARDS patients, fluid tends to fill the alveoli predominantly in the posterior lung bases due to the effects of gravity and the usual supine positioning. These patients exhibit improved oxygenation when positioned prone because this position allows increased perfusion of the better ventilated antero-apical regions. Physiotherapy will be severely limited in this situation.

Once positioned and ready for physiotherapy with the most affected lung uppermost, manual hyperinflation (hand ventilation) is likely to be the method adopted, unless the patient's condition proves too unstable to tolerate it.

For further reading on the care of ARDS patients, see Kollef (1997) and Mulnier & Evans (1995).

Hand ventilation (manual hyperinflation)

This is a manual form of positive pressure ventilation which is not without severe adverse effects (see Box 29.3). It is used primarily to stimulate a cough in patients with either a poor or absent cough reflex, or when there is atelectasis or excessive bronchial secretions. It may also be necessary when there is a ventilator fault, or more obviously during cardiopulmonary resuscitation, or as part of the treatment of those with raised intracranial pressure. It may also be the method used during short transfers from theatre to ICU.

Endotracheal suction

Together with hand ventilation, ET suctioning is a procedure used to facilitate the clearance of secretions when a patient's normal cough mechanism is either inadequate or disrupted, e.g. where there is underlying respiratory or neurological disease or when the cough reflex is suppressed by sedation, muscle relaxants or anaesthetic agents during IPPV. Its purpose is the removal of pulmonary secretions, thereby avoiding any of the problems associated with their retention (Ashurt 1992), such as increased airway pressures, pneumothorax, cardiovascular instability, lobar consolidation, ventilation–perfusion mismatch, pneumonia, hypoxaemia and atelectasis. However, suctioning is not a benign procedure (Riegel & Forshee 1985) — it carries with it hidden risks (see Box 29.4). In order to minimise these risks, certain principles should be adhered to; these are discussed in Chapter 28.

Box 29.3 Some adverse effects of hand ventilation

Respiratory effects
- Pneumothorax
- Loss of the effect of PEEP
- Bronchospasm
- Decreased respiratory drive
- Rebreathing CO_2

Cardiovascular effects
- Decreased blood pressure due to decreased venous return caused by the IPPV of hand ventilation
- Increased blood pressure due to inadequate sedation or inadequate hand ventilation
- Vagal stimulation (causing bradycardias)

Weaning from ventilatory support

Weaning is the term employed for the gradual transition from mechanical to spontaneous ventilation (self-ventilation). It should be individually tailored and begun as soon as it is established that the patient is physically capable of maintaining respiration. Weaning is most successful when the underlying clinical condition predisposing the patient to require ventilation support has first been corrected. Such factors as a disturbed acid–base balance, electrolyte abnormalities, arrhythmias or altered state of consciousness may severely hinder the chances of successful weaning.

Before attempts are made to wean a patient, certain criteria must be met (Geisman 1989):

- stable physiological status
- stable psychological status
- adequate nutritional status.

The nurse must be able to recognise these signs and to monitor and offer support to the patient throughout the weaning process (Henneman 1991). The main underlying principle in weaning is that of 'minimising the work of breathing' (Weilitz 1993). Box 29.5 sets out how this may be done.

Box 29.4 Potential hazards of endotracheal suctioning

- Tracheal mucosal damage
- Hypoxaemia
- Atelectasis
- Arrhythmias
- Infections
- Excessive coughing
- Stress response
- Pain
- Aspiration of stomach contents

Box 29.5 Minimising the work of breathing in relation to weaning from ventilatory support

The nursing aims should be to:
- Prepare the patient psychologically
- Treat the underlying disease
- Reduce airway secretions
- Position for optimal lung expansion
- Reverse bronchospasm
- Maintain haemoglobin levels within normal limits
- Maintain cardiovascular stability
- Correct fluid and electrolyte imbalances
- Limit CO_2 production
- Maintain arterial blood gases within normal limits (all other aspects considered)
- Ensure optimal nutritional support
- Facilitate sleep
- Ensure neurological integrity
- Optimise pain control

Box 29.6 Indicators of poor tolerance to weaning

- Respiratory rate increases, exceeding 45/min, or 10 above the baseline, climbing over three consecutive half-hours
- Heart rate increases, exceeding 130 beats/min
- Hypoxia develops
- Hypercarbia develops
- Conscious level deteriorates
- Systolic blood pressure increases or decreases 20 mmHg
- Diastolic blood pressure increases or decreases 10 mmHg
- Poor tidal volumes (250–300 mL)
- Significant arrhythmias
- Significant changes to arterial blood gas analysis
- Shallow breathing/use of accessory muscles
- Desaturates (S_aO_2 decreases to an unacceptable level):
  —100–95%: acceptable
  —95–90%: acceptable*
  —90–80%: requires to be treated*
  —75%: life-threatening
- Cyanosis
- Profuse sweating
- Altered breath sounds

*Depending on past medical history, i.e. COAD.

Close monitoring is essential during the weaning process. Should signs of poor tolerance to weaning be evident (see Box 29.6), ventilation support may need to be resumed (Weilitz 1993).

Q **29.2** Discuss the measures used to wean a patient from ventilatory support.

Extubation

When spontaneous respiration is successfully maintained, the next step is the removal of the ET tube, a procedure known as extubation (Box 29.7). Prior to this procedure, ABGs, oxygen saturations, tidal volumes, respiratory rate and pattern, vital signs, any evidence of tiring, and the presence of a gag reflex together with a strong cough reflex must all be reviewed. Extubation should not be considered unless the patient can cough, swallow and protect his own airway, and is sufficiently alert to be cooperative. If possible, a planned extubation early in the day is ideal, with plenty of staff around. Emergency equipment should be available in case rapid reintubation is necessary.

Box 29.7 Extubation procedure (Hinds 1992, Rippe et al 1995)

1. Position the patient well, preferably as upright as possible, for optimal lung expansion.
2. Explain the procedure to the patient, as this will minimise anxiety and maximise cooperation.
3. Any sedation in use should be discontinued prior to extubation as it may hinder successful unassisted spontaneous breathing.
4. Clear the airway, both oral and tracheal, via endotracheal (ET) suction.
5. Deflate the cuff on the ET tube, cut the tape securing the ET tube, repeat ET suction and removal of the suction catheter, and then remove the ET tube.
6. Immediately replace ET tube with an appropriate percentage of O_2 via a face mask.
7. Be aware of the patient's vital signs.
8. Record oxygen saturations with the face mask in situ.
9. Clear any oral secretions.
10. Ask the patient to cough and encourage regular deep breathing post-extubation.
11. Listen to air entry.
12. Pain control may need to be reassessed following extubation, especially in the case of postoperative patients.

CARDIOVASCULAR NEEDS AND CARE

The cardiovascular system is a closed system with haemodynamic pressures existing within the heart and arterial system. Pressure changes occur because of altered circulating volume, vessel radius or blood viscosity and because of changes in the efficiency of the cardiac pump. In intensive care settings, monitoring systems are essential in order to evaluate any potentially fatal physiological derangements and to allow timely treatment to correct any abnormalities. The cardiovascular system can be monitored by the measurement of volume, flow, pressure and resistance in different areas. Chapter 18 covers haemodynamic monitoring and should be referred to in relation to this section.

Nursing priorities and management:

Goal: to maintain haemodynamic stability and optimal perfusion.

Plan:

- monitor heart rate and rhythm
- monitor arterial blood pressure
- monitor central venous pressure
- monitor pulmonary artery pressure
- monitor temperature control.

Monitoring heart rate and rhythm

The amount of information which can be gleaned from a three-lead ECG must never be underestimated and a sound understanding of the heart's electrical activity facilitates this. Cardiac arrhythmias are commonplace in the ICU. In general, hypoxia, shock, electrolyte abnormalities, sepsis, vagal stimulation from ET suctioning, irritation from central venous or pulmonary artery catheters, and medication are responsible for the majority of cardiac arrhythmias; however, some will be the result of myocardial ischaemia in patients with underlying heart disease. Accordingly, where possible, the nurse needs to be aware of any cardiac impairment the patient may have. Monitoring should be continuous, to enable early detection and prompt treatment of underlying problems (Hillman & Bishop 1996). For details on the conduction pathways of the heart, arrhythmias and their management, see Chapter 2.

Monitoring arterial blood pressure

Patients admitted to the ICU will routinely have an arterial line inserted for the accurate measurement of arterial blood pressure and easy access to arterial blood for blood gas analysis. Common sites for the insertion of arterial lines are (in order of preference):

- radial artery
- brachial artery
- femoral artery
- dorsalis pedis artery.

Being an invasive monitoring device, it is inserted aseptically and should be sutured in place and the site covered with a transparent dressing. The arterial line catheter is then attached to a flush system (see Ch. 18), keeping the line patent with 3 mL/h of 0.9% sodium chloride and thus preventing clotting of the cannula.

Box 29.8 Complications associated with arterial lines

- Infection/potential sepsis
- Haemorrhage due to disconnection of the line
- Air embolism
- Vascular occlusion/thrombosis (distal circulation should be assessed regularly)
- Ischaemia
- Poor reading
- Spasm of the artery

Arterial blood pressure monitoring is necessary in those patients who are haemodynamically unstable, requiring inotropic support, those who have cardiopulmonary failure or when a non-invasive blood pressure is unobtainable. When recording the arterial blood pressure, the mean arterial pressure (MAP) is also noted. The MAP is the measurement of perfusion pressure over the majority of the cardiac cycle. A MAP below 50 mmHg is not desirable as it is inadequate to perfuse vital organs and tissues; 65–85 mmHg is generally the acceptable range. Complications can and do arise associated with arterial lines (see Box 29.8).

Monitoring central venous pressure (CVP)

In the ICU setting, central venous access is often preferred over peripheral access, with the obvious benefit of being able to assess the patient's circulating blood volume as well as allowing the administration of those intravenous drugs that can only be infused centrally (i.e. all inotropes, specific antibiotics/antifungals and certain electrolyte supplements). Monitoring the CVP also allows for the assessment of the tone of the vascular system and the ability of the right side of the heart to accept and expel blood, which is itself influenced by left ventricle function. As with all invasive procedures, the insertion sites are at risk of infection. Air embolus is another complication associated with central lines. During insertion of this line, there is a risk of causing a pneumothorax or misplacing the catheter in the right ventricle. In the ICU the distal lumen of the central line is always reserved for the monitoring of CVP and a flush system is used to maintain patency; a transducer provides a continuous waveform and reading of the CVP. Readings are taken when the transducer has been levelled with the sternal angle (or the mid-axillary line). The trend in these readings along with other clinical information is more important than any one reading on its own.

Monitoring pulmonary artery pressure

A pulmonary artery catheter is an important tool in the care of the critically ill patient, enabling the rapid treatment of potentially life-threatening cardiac dysfunctions. It assesses the functioning of the left ventricle and very often becomes part of the monitoring profile in situations causing either circulatory failure or acute respiratory failure. Its use is considered when information is required about fluid status, cardiovascular function or oxygen delivery (Hagland & Wilkinson 1993). It provides information which guides the therapy of those patients on mechanical ventilation, circulatory assist devices or inotropic drug therapy (see below).

Insertion of a pulmonary artery catheter into the subclavian, external jugular or antecubital vein is not without its complications and patients may be susceptible to arrhythmias during the procedure; therefore access to continuous ECG monitoring is essential (see Ch. 18 for more detail on working with pulmonary artery catheters).

Box 29.9 Haemodynamic cardiac profile — normal readings (Coombs 1993)

- Pulmonary artery pressure (PAP)
  —systolic: 15–25 mmHg
  —diastolic: 8–15 mmHg
- Pulmonary artery wedge pressure (PAWP): 6–12 mmHg
- Cardiac output (CO): 4–8 L/min
- Cardiac index (CI): 2.5–4.2 L/min per m^2
- Systemic vascular resistance (SVR): 900–1600 dyn/s per cm^5 (this measurement relates to the resistance to flow in the whole systemic circulation)
- Mixed venous oxygen saturations (S_vO_2): 65–75%

The pulmonary artery wedge pressure (PAWP) or 'wedge' gives a more accurate indication of the fluid status of the patient. Elevated PAWPs may arise as a result of volume overload, left ventricular failure (LVF), mitral stenosis or regurgitation and cardiac tamponade, whereas abnormally low readings may relate to hypovolaemia.

The frequency of haemodynamic measurements depends on the patient's condition and, as with all invasive monitoring, actions should be supported by clinical findings (see Box 29.9).

29. 3 How could an atypical pneumonia cause multisystem failure in a 65-year-old woman admitted to ICU following a respiratory arrest in a medical high-dependency unit? Discuss her nursing care and what haemodynamic monitoring may be necessary.

Inotropic drugs

A pulmonary artery catheter is often inserted in order to guide inotropic therapy, as it clarifies whether there is a pressure problem (i.e. reduced blood pressure), a problem with the flow (i.e. decreased cardiac output) or a problem with oxygen delivery and consumption. Cardiac contractility can become impaired either as a direct result of cardiogenic shock or secondary to hypovolaemic and septic shock. In such cases, inotropic drugs such as adrenaline, dopamine and dobutamine, which improve cardiac contractility, are frequently used to support the patient until such time as definitive treatment is administered or the patient recovers (Hillman & Bishop 1996). Administration is always through a central vein and the effects of inotropic therapy are always monitored closely. Different combinations of inotropic drugs may be advocated in order to arrive at the desired effect. It is common practice to titrate inotropic therapy against MAP, generally aiming for a MAP of between 65 and 85 mmHg; inotropic drugs are always titrated down 1 mL at a time before discontinuation.

For further reading on the inotropes dopamine and dobutamine, see Gibson (1998).

Monitoring temperature control

Despite a wide variety of heat-producing metabolic processes and the range of ambient temperatures to which the human body may be exposed, core body temperature is maintained with remarkable stability. However, critical illness can disturb temperature control, producing temperatures at either end of the spectrum, i.e. hypothermia (>35°C) or hyperthermia/hyperpyrexia (<38.5°C). Chapter 22 explores temperature maintenance in depth.

RENAL/FLUID BALANCE NEEDS AND CARE

The kidneys are very sensitive organs and it is not uncommon for an abrupt decline in renal function to occur in the presence of other systemic illnesses. This is particularly so if the cardiovascular or respiratory systems become compromised. Renal function is especially susceptible to the effects of underperfusion and hypoxaemia, mainly because of the large renal blood supply and metabolic activity. The kidneys process about 180 L of blood chemical fluid daily and use 20–25% of all the oxygen used by the body at rest (Manes 1995). In the critically ill patient, acute renal failure (ARF) is a relatively common complication resulting from an isolated incident of severe hypotension or drug toxicity, or more frequently as a consequence of overwhelming sepsis and multisystem organ failure (MSOF). However, it is usually multifactorial — 'ARF can be defined as a sudden (and usually reversible) failure of the kidneys to excrete the waste products of metabolism and may be broadly categorised as prerenal, renal or postrenal' (Hinds 1992). The treatment of ARF is predominantly one of support until recovery occurs.

Nursing priorities and management:

Goal: to maintain indices of renal function within the patient's own normal limits.

Plan:

- monitor and maintain optimal fluid and electrolyte balance
- provide appropriate renal replacement therapy.

Monitoring and maintaining optimal fluid and electrolyte balance

In the susceptible patient, the primary goal must always be the prevention of renal impairment. This involves knowledge of the causes of ARF, meticulous monitoring and clinical assessment of the patient. The causes of ARF fall into three categories: prerenal, renal and postrenal (see Ch. 8, p. 343); the first two are largely responsible for the development of ARF, but elements of all three may coexist in the critically ill patient. ARF can be divided into phases, or stages (see Ch. 8, p. 343), as follows:

- the onset phase — the time between the precipitating episode and oliguria or anuria developing
- the oliguric phase (diminished urine output) — can last from 7 to 21 days
- the diuretic phase — characterised by an increase of urine output over several days
- the recovery phase — follows the gradual improvement of kidney function and usually occurs over 3–12 months.

A whole host of systemic manifestations may accompany the development of renal insufficiency, as outlined in Box 29.10 (Vander 1991).

Box 29.10 Systemic manifestations of acute renal failure

Respiratory
- Pulmonary oedema
- Suppressed cough reflex
- Kussmaul respiration

Cardiac
- Congestive cardiac failure/overload
- Arrhythmias
- Uraemic pericarditis

Vascular
- Hypertension
- Fluid overload, increased CVP, decreased urine output
- Electrolyte imbalance
- Metabolic acidosis

Haematopoietic
- Anaemia (as a result of reduced erythropoietin production)
- Coagulopathy (platelets have a reduced life span due to the uraemic toxins)
- More prone to infections (as a result of uraemic toxins)

Neuromuscular
- Electrolyte imbalance
- Uraemic encephalopathy

Gastrointestinal
- GI bleeding
- Nausea
- Uraemic halitosis
- Bowel changes

Skin integrity
- Purpura rash (due to coagulopathy)
- Yellowness (uraemia)
- Dry skin (due to decreased sweat production as a result of uraemic toxins)

Q **29.4** Discuss the key regulatory functions of the renal system.

Nursing priorities in monitoring and maintaining optimal fluid and electrolyte balance

Urine output. In addition to the monitoring of all fluid intake, hourly urine output volumes must be recorded, together with an accurate 24-h fluid balance, of all fluid gains and losses. While a urine output of 400 mL or less (oliguria), over a 24-h period is indicative of ensuing renal failure, it is also acknowledged that ARF can occur in the absence of oliguria (non-oliguric ARF).

Urea and electrolytes. Daily assays of urea and electrolytes will indicate the degree of renal insufficiency present. Urea, creatinine and some electrolyte levels rise with developing ARF, leading to varying degrees of metabolic acidosis. It should be noted, however, that elevated urea on its own may indicate merely that the patient is dehydrated.

The nurse must know the normal plasma values for urea, creatinine and the more common electrolytes and the significance of any deviations, as some electrolyte abnormalities can produce life-threatening arrhythmias (Huddleston & Ferguson 1990).

Fluid therapy. Intravenous fluid therapy should be considered carefully in the management of the critically ill patient. This is particularly so in conditions of sepsis, ARDS or systemic inflammatory response syndrome (SIRS). In such situations, the permeability of capillary endothelial cells increases and the vessels become 'leaky', allowing large protein particles to pass into the interstitial space and thus reducing the capillary osmotic pressure. This then facilitates the movement of water together with further protein molecules into the interstitial space, depleting intravascular volume and impairing gaseous exchange. This will result in peripheral oedema and, within the lungs, pulmonary oedema, causing hypoxaemia and consequently diminished oxygen delivery and consumption by peripheral tissues. The vascular volume must be restored. The three main groups of volume-expanding fluids are crystalloids, colloids and blood. Crystalloids are made up of non-ionic solutes such as sodium chloride added to water; they do not contain oncotic particles and will therefore move out of the vascular component (see Ch. 20). These fluids, unlike colloids, are cheap to produce and are not associated with immunologically mediated reactions. Conversely, colloids which contain oncotic particles, thus generating oncotic pressure, are mainly confined to the intravascular space, at least when they are first administered. Blood and blood products also exert an oncotic pressure due to the large protein particles they contain and so are less likely to contribute to interstitial oedema.

Clinical assessment. A careful clinical assessment is necessary, observing for signs of worsening pitting oedema, notably at the ankles and sacrum. Chest auscultation may reveal widespread coarse crackles and suggest fluid overloading and pulmonary oedema.

Cardiovascular status. The cardiovascular status directly affects renal perfusion. It is recommended that the MAP be above 60 mmHg for renal perfusion to take place (Beale & Bihari 1992). Regular monitoring of the CVP, cardiac output and PAWP will together indicate whether fluid input or inotropic support is required. Increasingly, peaked T waves are suggestive of a rising plasma potassium level.

Nephrotoxic drugs. The use of nephrotoxic drugs should be avoided in those with impending renal failure or in those whose renal function is precarious (Hillman & Bishop 1996).

Immediate management of diminishing renal function

- Optimise fluid balance either by giving a fluid challenge if vital signs indicate hypovolaemia or by using diuretic therapy if clinically there are signs of fluid overload. Frusemide is the diuretic of choice, but mannitol therapy may also be employed (Hinds 1992).
- Administer low-dose dopamine. Dopamine, depending on the dose, may be vasodilatory or vasoconstrictive. In low-dose use, its renal effect is vasodilatory. While its use in patients with diminishing renal function may suggest benefit by inducing, via improved perfusion, diuresis and sodium excretion, its use in those with well established renal failure is not thought to have any therapeutic value (Corwin & Bonventre 1988).
- Correct electrolyte imbalances as necessary.
- Maintain haemoglobin within the normal range.
- Assess nutritional input, with particular attention to a low-protein, high-carbohydrate content. Generally nutritional support is provided via the enteral route unless otherwise contraindicated. The dietician will make an important contribution to the team approach to care.
- Remove any known causative factors, e.g. nephrotoxic drugs
- Exclude obstruction, i.e. make sure that the urinary catheter has not become blocked with sediment.

If this is not enough to resolve renal impairment then continuous renal replacement therapy (CRRT) will be required.

Renal replacement therapy

In unresolving ARF, the management focuses on supportive renal replacement therapy and the control of metabolic derangements arising from renal failure. Rapid commencement of CRRT is essential in situations where the patient is severely hyperkalaemic, grossly overloaded or suffering from uraemic complications or pericarditis, or where ARF has been drug-induced. Forni & Hilton (1997) believe CRRT to be an effective and efficient way of controlling the problems caused by ARF and, while it will not provide a 'cure', it enables the critically ill patient to be supported until he recovers from the underlying disease process or injury.

Caring for patients with CRRT is deemed part of the professional practice of experienced nurses working in the ICU (UKCC 1992). They must therefore have a thorough knowledge of the reasons for its use, the equipment involved, the problems that can arise and how to respond to them.

Haemofiltration

Traditionally, the recognised form of treatment for critically ill patients with ARF was peritoneal dialysis or haemodialysis. However, dialysis has not always produced a beneficial outcome, haemodialysis often inducing severe hypotension and peritoneal dialysis impairing ventilation. For some decades now, there has been an increasing use of a less aggressive form of renal replacement therapy, haemofiltration. This is a relatively straightforward form of CRRT by which excess fluid and solutes are removed by passing the patient's blood through a haemofilter. By creating a positive pressure gradient within this haemofilter, fluid removal from the blood by ultrafiltration is facilitated. For the clearance of solutes, a large amount of fluid must be filtered. To prevent dehydration, replacement fluids must be carefully monitored (Hagland 1993).

Continuous venovenous haemofiltration (CVVH). This is generally the mode of choice in haemofiltration, as it allows the slow steady removal of fluid volume. It also gives the venous system time to compensate for fluid lost from the interstitial spaces. Most importantly, it avoids the rapid shift of solutes and electrolytes, thereby preventing the risk of cardiovascular instability. It is the only safe line of treatment in the management of ARF in those with haemodynamic instability and/or MSOF, where the removal of fluid and waste products is vital. A further advantage of CVVH is that it does not require arterial access. Access for CVVH is via a double-lumen catheter, often referred to as a Quinton line. This line is inserted into a main vein — the femoral, subclavian or internal jugular. When not in use, the lumens of this line are injected with heparin, a process known as 'hep-locking', which prevents clot formation and the release of emboli.

Nursing responsibilities in haemofiltration

Fluid balance. Accurate measurement of input and output of fluid is essential, and renal replacement therapy should be reviewed daily by the renal physicians. The nurse responsible for the patient should adjust filtration rates in accordance with the medical prescription.

Vital signs. The recording of vital signs is imperative. At the start of CVVH, the patient's blood pressure may fall, as approximately 200 mL of blood is removed from the circulating volume. However, this can be pre-empted and is easily corrected by giving volume expanders. The patient's temperature is also altered. It is generally believed that body temperature drops by 1°C with CVVH in process. It is therefore not uncommon for a patient to become slightly hypothermic. To prevent this, replacement fluid is passed through a blood warmer. It should be noted that CVVH may mask developing sepsis, as a recorded temperature of 37°C may equate to a patient temperature of nearer 38°C.

Urea, electrolytes and ABGs. Regular assessment of urea, electrolytes and ABGs is necessary in order to assess acid–base balance. Electrolyte supplements are often required and potassium is usually added to the replacement fluid being administered via the filter. It is common to see 9–18 mmol of potassium chloride added to each 4.5 L bag of haemofiltrasol depending on the patient's serum potassium level. Initially, no potassium may be required as hyperkalaemia may be the very reason for commencing haemofiltration. Other electrolyte supplements such as calcium and phosphate can be administered intravenously or nasogastrically.

Monitoring the activated clotting time (ACT). The ACT is the time it takes for 2 mL of blood to clot and is generally maintained between 120 and 140 s. It is of particular importance if the patient is receiving heparin as anticoagulation therapy while on the haemofilter. Heparin, the anticoagulant of choice, is administered to prevent clotting of the extracorporeal circuit. Patient coagulation (and therefore the demand for heparin) will vary greatly depending on the underlying disease process. However, a concentration of 250 IU/mL at a rate of 1–6 mL/h is normally administered. Some patients will not be able to tolerate the effects of heparin, as it is known to disrupt the intrinsic coagulation cascade and promote platelet aggregation. This is seen particularly in liver failure. In such cases, prostacyclin can be used as it preserves platelet function and number. It does, however, have strong side-effects, noticeably vasodilatation, causing facial flushing and significant hypotension. ACT is not required with prostacyclin as the normal clotting process is not so severely altered.

Preventing infection. Preventing infection and maintaining an aseptic technique are vital. Patients on haemofiltration are often immunocompromised and therefore are more susceptible to infection. Residual catheterisation is performed every 2–3 days, preventing stasis of urine in the bladder, a potential source for infection. If urine volume is ≥250 mL, the catheter is normally left in situ, as this can be indicative of the return of renal function.

Patient safety. Maintenance of patient safety is the nurse's responsibility. If access is via the femoral vein, the limb should be carefully observed for signs of poor perfusion (Woodrow 1993). Furthermore, the prevention of air emboli, infection or haemorrhage as a consequence of heparin use should all be borne in mind. Generally haemofilters remain functional for 72 h, but clotting problems will markedly reduce the life span. A pump speed of 150–200 mmHg and a venous pressure of 100–120 mmHg are recommended to ensure adequate and effective removal of filtrate. CVVH normally operates in cycles of 1 L in and 1 L out, but may be adjusted depending on the status of the patient (e.g. if a patient is overloaded it may be decided that 950 mL be infused in with 1 L removed, thus correcting the problem of fluid overload).

Psychological care. Providing psychological support and reassurance to the patient receiving CVVH is all-important, as is true for any procedure carried out on the critically ill patient. Extended body image is an issue not widely written about, but some (e.g. Smith 1989) have studied its implications in relation to the critically ill patient with particular reference to the ventilation tubing and dialysis lines. The nurse responsible for the patient undergoing CVVH must be aware and sensitive to this issue.

High-volume haemofiltration (HVHF) and haemodialysis

When a patient stabilises, HVHF or haemodialysis may then become an option. It facilitates the rapid clearance of waste products over a period of 3–4 h. Daily or alternate-day treatment may be necessary until the kidneys recover completely. Full renal recovery is entirely possible in patients with no prior history of renal impairment.

NEUROLOGICAL NEEDS AND CARE

A number of conditions predispose critically ill patients to altered states of consciousness. These include (Goldhill & Withington 1997):

- Intracranial pathology, such as intracranial haemorrhage, cerebral hypoxia, tumours and abscesses
- Systemic disease affecting the cerebral blood supply or oxygenation, such as sepsis, metabolic encephalopathy, hypoglycaemia, hepatic failure (hepatic encephalopathy), renal failure, pancreatitis, respiratory failure or hypo/hyperthermia
- Exogenous agents, such as drugs and toxins, and drug withdrawal.

Neurological functioning is an important part of the overall clinical assessment and continuous care of those being nursed in the ICU. The use of a standardised neurological assessment tool such as the Glasgow Coma Scale (GCS) is essential, enabling early detection of any deterioration and facilitating prompt treatment. In addition, invasive neurological monitoring of intracranial pressure (ICP), which facilitates the monitoring of the cerebral perfusion pressure (CPP), is often indicated in patients who demonstrate a GCS of 8 or less, and/or a grade 3 or 4 encephalopathy (see Box 29.11). As with the majority of clinical observations, it is the trend that is of greatest significance when monitoring ICP and CPP.

Nursing priorities and management:
Goal: to maintain neurological status.
Plan: monitor neurological function.

Monitoring neurological function

The Glasgow Coma Scale. The GCS is the standard tool used in assessing neurological function. It is an objective way of measuring levels of consciousness (LOCs) and is set out in detail in Chapters 9 and 28.

Cerebral function analyser monitor (CFAM). This comprises a visual display unit and printer which allows the continual monitoring and display of cerebral activity. This activity is picked up by five electrodes: two are situated over each hemisphere and one ground electrode allows both hemispheres to be compared. This system is better than the conventional EEG. It is used continuously by the bedside to assess whether the patient is appropriately sedated or fitting. It is commonly used with patients receiving paralysing agents in order to detect whether or not they are having seizures.

Computed tomography (CT) scan. In relation to neurological functioning, CT scanning is usually performed in order to detect cerebral haematomas, oedema, infarctions, atrophy, hydrocephalus and tumours.

ICP monitoring. Intracranial pressure is the pressure exerted by the intracranial contents against the skull. Normally, brain tissue constitutes 80%, cerebrospinal fluid (CSF) 10% and blood volume 10% of the intracranial contents. It becomes necessary to monitor the ICP in the critically ill when a patient displays signs of raised ICP manifested as severe encephalopathy (see Box 29.11). For

Box 29.11 Grades of encephalopathy

1. Mild confusion, poor concentration, but fully coherent when awake
2. Increasingly confused, disoriented, yet remains rousable
3. Very drowsy, may be agitated or aggressive when roused to command
4. Responsive to painful stimuli, not rousable to command. May display signs of pupil and limb changes, abnormal breathing and extensor plantars

patients who do not progress any further than a grade 1 or 2 encephalopathy, the prognosis is good. Severe head injuries remain the most common cause of raised ICP, but it may also occur in patients presenting with problems such as hepatic encephalitis due to fulminant hepatic failure (Hawker 1996).

For a case study of paracetamol poisoning, see Leighton (1995).

ICP monitoring can be used to help minimise neurological damage in those patients predisposed to neurological problems, as such monitoring will demonstrate neurological changes before they present clinically and thus greatly assist clinical observation. For further discussion of raised ICP, see Chapter 9 (p. 361).

Cerebral perfusion pressure (CPP). The value of monitoring the ICP is that it allows the CPP to be calculated. This is done by subtracting the ICP measurement from the mean pressure of circulating blood within the cranial cavity (i.e. CPP = MAP – ICP). Generally the aim is to maintain CPP above 70 mmHg, thus preventing underperfusion of the cerebral tissue.

Jugular bulb oximetry (S_jO_2). This is not a very common invasive monitoring system, but may be used to provide information about global cerebral oxygen consumption (Oh 1997).

The immediate management of elevated ICP

It is usually decided at what level of raised ICP a treatment regimen will be necessary. This level depends on the patient's condition, but it is often set at around >15 mmHg. Drugs of choice include mannitol 20% initially and then subsequent administration of frusemide, which both enhances its effect and produces a faster diuresis (it is important to be aware of the patient's renal status prior to administration of these drugs, i.e. is there a significant degree of renal impairment?). In order to counteract any sudden electrolyte changes due to induced diuresis, plasma protein solution (PPS) is also part of the treatment protocol. This line of treatment can be considered at 4- to 6-hourly intervals; if ineffective, barbiturate therapy may be necessary. Barbiturates exert their effect on ICP by reducing cerebral oxygen consumption and thereby producing vasoconstriction and reduction in ICP. Another useful agent is thiopentone which lowers ICP by reducing metabolism to a minimum as well as lowering blood pressure by reducing venous and arterial tone, thus reducing cerebral perfusion.

Nursing activities and ICP

- Perform ET suction only as required (i.e. in response to secretions). Retention of secretions will increase ICP, just as frequent suctioning can be detrimental. The maintenance of adequate ventilatory support is essential as hypercapnia and hypoxia will increase cerebral vasodilatation, causing raised ICP. It may be necessary to continually monitor the end-tidal CO_2.
- Secure the ET tube with adhesive tape, thus not restricting cerebral drainage.
- Ensure good head alignment, elevating the head of the bed to promote cerebral drainage.
- Keep all nursing procedures to a minimum.
- Check pupils hourly and following all nursing and medical procedures.
- Maintain an accurate fluid balance chart. Monitor and be aware of electrolyte levels (e.g. both hypo- and hypernatraemia can contribute to raised ICP).
- Prevent cerebral ischaemia and maintain CPP above 60 mmHg.
- Provide adequate nutritional support. Patients with ICP problems are often in a hypercatabolic state.
- Assess the need and extent to which pressure area care is appropriate (Chudley 1994).

29.5 Describe the nursing care of a patient following an overdose of tricyclic antidepressants.

SEDATION AND PAIN CONTROL

Nursing priorities and management:

Goal: to maintain the optimal level of sedation and pain control.
Plan: assess the need for sedation and analgesia.

Assessing the need for sedation and analgesia

Pain has been identified as a major problem for patients in the ICU. Pain is a subjective experience and the control of pain will require regular assessment and clear documentation. The challenge is always to provide the most appropriate form of pain relief. Pain control is covered extensively in Chapter 19 and therefore this section will focus primarily on the assessment of sedation required.

Most patients admitted to the ICU will, at some point during their stay, require sedation and/or analgesics. Views and practice have changed considerably over the years from the belief that patients should be heavily sedated and unaware of their surroundings to the now preferred state of lighter sedation while maintaining an optimal state of comfort (Shelley 1992). Patient comfort may be achieved by creating a supportive environment, through constant reassurance and explanation prior to all procedures together with the maintenance of some sort of diurnal rhythm. However, drug therapy may be required to produce the respiratory depression necessary to facilitate adequate ventilation, to aid tolerance of the presence of the ET tube or to decrease anxiety in general. Shelley (1992) suggests that patient comfort is a better term than sedation, as sedation is only one of the desired effects.

Sedation and analgesics can be administered continually or as a bolus, the prescribed regimen being tailored to the needs of each patient. The nurse must constantly assess the sedation level (a number of sedation scaling systems exist — see Box 29.12) and therefore should display a sound knowledge of the issues surrounding sedation in the ICU, i.e. sensory overload, sensory deprivation, ICU psychosis and psychological support. Carroll & Magruder (1993) suggest that the goal of sedation is to decrease anxiety, fear and restlessness and to increase cooperation and compliance. Optimal sedation should enable the patient to be rousable on stimulation but able to sleep/rest when undisturbed — 'Keeping the patient comfortable is a balance between undersedation and oversedation' (Shelley 1992).

Box 29.12 Sedation scale (Cohen & Kelly 1987)

0 Asleep, no response to tracheal suction
1 Rousable, coughs with tracheal suction
2 Awake, spontaneously coughs or triggers the ventilator
3 Actively breathes against the ventilator
4 Unmanageable

Patient comfort

Four main groups of drugs can be enlisted to enhance patient comfort:

Sedatives. Benzodiazepines are probably the most commonly used drugs in ICUs, with midazolam used widely. Its properties include sedative, anxiolytic and amnesic effects.

Propofol administered either as a bolus or continuous infusion has anaesthetic properties and is commonly used to sedate patients requiring short periods of mechanical ventilation. It is widely used, as it provides a controllable level of sedation which is easily maintained and recovery is rapid, allowing weaning from the ventilator to progress.

Analgesics. Morphine provides safe analgesic but should be used with caution in those with liver and renal impairment. Non-steroidal anti-inflammatory drugs (NSAIDs) and local analgesics in the form of nerve blocks may also be considered.

Alfentanil is a valuable analgesia used in the ICU especially when short-term analgesic supplementation is required. It is short-acting with a short half-life.

Neuromuscular blocking agents. The use of these agents has been reduced, partly as a result of the more effective use of sedatives, but also because of improved ventilator design. A muscle relaxant will be administered initially to most patients admitted to ICU, in order to facilitate intubation and line insertion e.g. suxamethonium has a rapid onset and offset action, but is not suitable for prolonged administration (Goldhill & Withington 1997). Longer administration may be required to aid ventilation control, reduce O_2 consumption in patients who have developed ARDS, and lower ICP in head injury — in such cases, a neuromuscular blocking agent such as atracurium is often used.

Antidepressants (e.g. amitriptyline). Antidepressants are often prescribed in those showing depressive behaviour (often patients who have been critically ill for weeks, where weaning from the ventilator is slow, or those with previous depressive illness) and, as well as improving mood, can help to normalise the sleep pattern.

NUTRITIONAL/GASTROINTESTINAL NEEDS AND CARE

The nutritional status of patients in hospitals has been the topic of much research over the years. It is well documented that malnutrition contributes to immunosuppression, increased postoperative complications, delayed wound healing and consequently longer stays in hospital (Deitch et al 1992). Chapter 21 covers nutritional support thoroughly and should be studied in relation to nutrition and the critically ill. Patients in hypercatabolic states are particularly susceptible to malnutrition, which can adversely affect their outcome. It is now believed that the gut has an extremely important and active role to play in the treatment of the critically ill patient (Singer & Carr 1996). Well recognised for its role in absorbing and digesting nutrients, the gut also has a vital function to play as a barrier to microorganisms and endotoxins. This defence mechanism is preserved by the normal epithelial cells and is supported by a series of immunological mechanisms. In the critically ill, this barrier is often severely compromised and as a result the bowel, which acts as a reservoir for organisms, facilitates the process of gut translocation of bacteria. This practice allows the transfer of endotoxins and pathogens into the portal and systemic circulation and may add to the risk of sepsis (Horwood 1992). Consequently, it is imperative that, where possible, optimal GI function should be maintained. In the past, nutritional support was often not considered an immediate priority in the management of critically ill patients, but it is now widely acknowledged that early assessment and optimal nutritional support are vital components in the overall treatment of such patients (Raper & Maynard 1992).

Q **29.6** Identify physiological changes caused by inadequate nutritional support.

Nursing priorities and management:

Goal: to minimise weight loss and maintain normal gastrointestinal (GI) function.

Plan:

- establish nutritional support
- maintain GI integrity.

Establishing nutritional support

Nurses are responsible for assessing nutritional needs, administering nutritional therapy, monitoring its effects and complications, and evaluating its effectiveness. There are basically two clinical routes for maintaining nutritional support: parenteral and enteral (see Ch. 21).

Parenteral nutrition

Until recently, parenteral nutrition (PN) was the accepted form of nutritional support for the critically ill. However, evidence now suggests that using the parenteral route may not only increase the risk of sepsis from complications associated with its administration (see Ch. 21), but also (because gut function is not maintained) result in mucosal atrophy and the facilitation of bacterial translocation (Raper & Maynard 1992). Microorganisms and endotoxins cross into the blood, sepsis/SIRS results and can lead to multisystem organ failure, as illustrated in Figure 29.1., PN, which requires administration via a large central vein, is an unnatural method of feeding that is, however, justified in certain situations where the use of the gut is either impossible or inadequate. Because of the well recognised complications arising from PN administration (as well as its cost), enteral feeding is preferred in the treatment and support of the critically ill patient.

Serum electrolytes. Monitoring electrolyte levels to prevent imbalances is essential. This in fact pertains to both routes of nutritional support, but is especially the case in PN. It is necessary to check regularly the patient's blood glucose level, monitoring for hypo/hyperglycaemia and consequently assessing the need for insulin therapy. Patients requiring inotropic therapy in the form of adrenaline also need their blood sugar levels monitored closely, as adrenaline, especially at higher doses, affects the utilisation of glucose from the cells.

Enteral nutrition

Besides being relatively inexpensive and safe to use (Perry 1993, see also Ch. 21), enteral feeding offers a protective effect on the GI tract, reducing bacterial translocation and maintaining mucosal integrity. It is also believed to maintain the autoregulation of blood flow to the gut. Most patients in the ICU can be fed enterally, the only absolute contraindication being true gut failure. Relative contraindications include bowel anastomosis distal to the feeding tube, pancreatitis or small bowel disease. Gut function may be decreased and an ileus develop as a result of IPPV or the use of opiates; however, the small bowel retains motility and absorptive functions in most critically ill patients. Feeding is usually via the nasogastric or nasoenteral route — nasoduodenum or nasojejunum — however a jejunostomy tube may be fashioned.

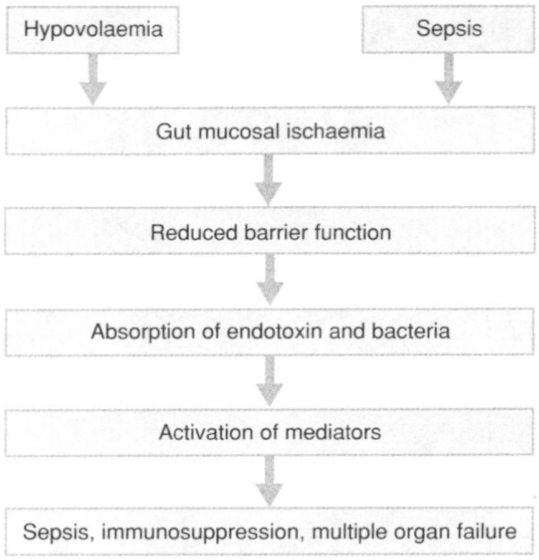

Fig. 29.1 The role of the gut in multiple organ failure. (Adapted from Raper & Maynard 1992.)

Feeding via the enteral route. On introducing enteral feeding, a protocol should be followed (Fig. 29.2) and this, together with competent nursing practice and perseverance, will enable most critically ill patients to be fed by this method. Lack of bowel sounds is not a contraindication to enteral feeding. Patients who are ventilated often swallow less air than normal, therefore reducing their main source of gas, and hence bowel sounds do not always correlate with gastric absorption. The feed should be administered preferably using an infusion pump at a constant rate, helping to reduce the incidence of diarrhoea. As well as aspirating the nasogastric tube every 4 h, as per protocol, it is recommended that a resting time of 4 h be allowed in a 24 h period (Raper & Maynard 1992).

A number of standard formula feeds exist and, while a polymeric feed is usually satisfactory for most patients, special feeds may be required to meet the excessive metabolic demands of the critically ill. Some examples of special properties are:

- high-protein, low-osmolarity feeds, e.g. Osmolite — commonly used in ICUs
- fibre/bulking agents
- low-carbohydrate, high-fat content — for those producing too much CO_2, inhibiting weaning from the ventilator
- low-protein, high-calorie content with reduced potassium — for those with renal or liver impairment
- constituents targeted specifically at critically ill patients (multiple trauma, sepsis, general states of catabolic stress), e.g. omega-3 fatty acids, glutamine — glutamine, in particular, is thought to increase the gut's ability to accept food during critical illness (Verity 1996), enhancing gut mucosal integrity and enabling proliferation of both lymphocytes and macrophages, correlating with a boost in the immune system.

For further reading on the benefits of glutamine, see van der Hulst et al (1993).

Maintaining GI integrity

As well as providing nutritional support, the assessment and alleviation of GI problems must be given due consideration. These can range from delayed gastric emptying, abdominal distension, diarrhoea or constipation to the presence of stress ulcers (see Ch. 4, p. 97).

Delayed gastric emptying

This may be alleviated through the use of a wide variety of pharmacological stimulants or direct irritants, e.g. cisapride, a drug whose action is known to enhance gastroduodenal motility (Spaden et al 1995). Similarly, metoclopramide stimulates gastric emptying, while Weber et al (1993) demonstrated that erythromycin, a motilin agonist, increases gastric motility. In extreme cases, when pharmacological stimulants/irritants are not enough, feeding via a distal tube, e.g. a jejunum tube, may be considered. In this way gastric emptying is bypassed.

Abdominal distension

This is associated with malabsorption of enteral feed and, in this case, feeding should be reduced or stopped for a few hours and the enteral feeding regimen reviewed.

Diarrhoea or constipation

This is not uncommon in the critically ill patient. However, it cannot be assumed automatically to be the result of enteral feed intolerance. Many factors can induce diarrhoea, not least antibiotic therapy or infection (*Clostridium difficile* being a common causative agent).

Rarely is feeding stopped because of feed-induced diarrhoea. On occasions, contamination of the feed may be the root cause, highlighting the need for an aseptic technique during the handling of feeding equipment (Weenk et al 1993). At the other end of the spectrum, it is also necessary to review the need for aperients.

Stress ulceration

This may develop due to damage to the mucosal layer, often during a period of ischaemia as a result of an episode of shock. In addition, impaired production of gastric mucus, reduced epithelial renewal, disturbed acid–base balance, reflux of bile acids and the presence of uraemia all predispose the patient to gastric ulceration.

Enteral feeding acts as prophylaxis; however, in patients being supported by PN, prophylactic medication should be prescribed. Antacids, H_2-receptor blockades or an aluminium hydroxide salt (e.g. sucralfate) are all thought to be equally effective as prophylactic agents for stress ulcers.

HYGIENE AND MOBILITY NEEDS AND WOUND CARE

Caring for the critically ill patient requiring mechanical ventilation is both a medical and nursing challenge. Many patients in the ICU setting are fully dependent on the provision of all care. Meticulous nursing care is required in order to maintain optimal body tissue integrity and organ function. Individualised care tailored to the needs of the patient is a prerequisite with regular assessment and evaluation of the effectiveness of care chosen.

Nursing priorities and management:

Goal: to provide optimal personal hygiene and to maintain skin integrity.

Plan:

- maintain personal hygiene, preventing infection
- maintain skin integrity and promote wound healing
- promote and maintain normal tone, power and movement of the musculoskeletal system.

Maintaining personal hygiene and preventing infection

Personal hygiene

Assisting with the maintenance of personal hygiene not only promotes comfort and dignity but also represents an opportunity for thorough assessment of the patient, including skin integrity, any

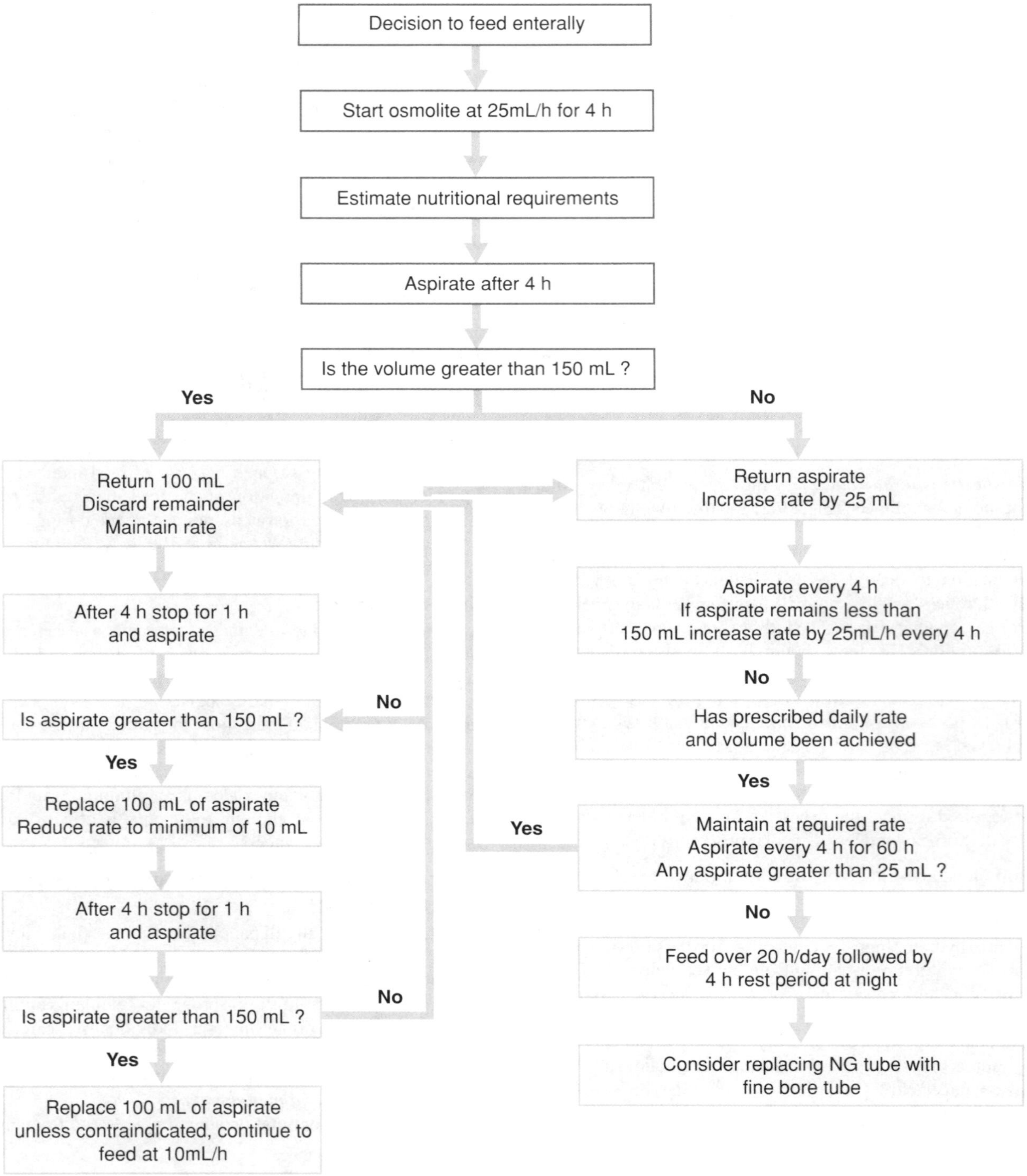

Fig. 29.2 Enteral feeding protocol. (Adapted from Raper & Maynard 1992.)

potential sites of infection (e.g. red or inflamed cannula insertion sites) and the peripheral circulation. The critically ill patient will be dependent on the nurse at all times to maintain his dignity.

Oral hygiene

Most seriously ill patients will encounter mouth problems, some specific to the disease and others associated with the medication. There is, for example, an increased risk of mouth ulcers, dry, cracked oral mucosa or yeast growth in those with diabetes mellitus, acute or chronic breathing difficulties and thyroid dysfunction.

Furthermore, with the use of certain antibiotics, diuretics or morphine and procedures such as intermittent suction, the potential for oral hygiene problems is heightened. Knowledge of the factors which contribute to poor oral health is important in order to maintain hygiene (Thurgood 1994) (see Ch. 15 for further detail on oral hygiene).

Eye care

Eye care is a very necessary procedure for those patients who are unconscious/paralysed or sedated, who lack a blink reflex, who have an inability to close their eyes or who experience dry eyes. It facilitates (Lloyd 1990) maintenance of healthy eyes, comfort and the prevention of infection.

Effective eye care is vital to prevent ocular complications; the main ones to consider in the care of the critically ill patient are:

- exposure keratopathy — incomplete closure of the eyelid
- dry eyes
- infection, e.g. conjunctival
- 'ventilator eye' (oedematous eyes)
- corneal ulcerations.

(Ch. 13 discusses the disorders of the eye in depth.)

The critically ill patient is more susceptible than most patients to developing eye problems, for the following reasons:

- Mechanical ventilation leads to the retention of body fluid, which in turn leads to increased venous pressure, producing oedematous eyes often referred to as 'ventilator eye' (Lloyd 1990).
- Drugs used during intubation can lead to intraocular pressure, predisposing the patient to ocular damage.
- Paralysing and sedation agents prevent patients from carrying out important physiological eye protection mechanisms. The blink mechanism becomes diminished with the consequence that tears are not effectively dispersed over the eye, if indeed they are produced at all. Tear production and dispersion are important in the prevention of infection and the maintenance of the structural integrity of the eye. In addition, those patients being ventilated artificially are at risk of eye infections arising from poor ET suctioning procedures (i.e. cross-contamination from droplets sprayed out of the ET tube during suction).
- The side-effects of some drug therapies are known to contribute to dry eyes, including atropine, some antihistamines and tricyclic antidepressants.
- The patient who is critically ill will often be immunocompromised and thus more susceptible to infection. As with all procedures pertaining to patient care, strict and thorough handwashing must be adhered to.

For further reading on preventing infection in the ICU, see Sproat & Inglis (1992).

Maintaining skin integrity and promoting wound healing

A sound knowledge of the factors involved in successful wound healing and those that adversely affect its progress is necessary (see Ch. 23). The main types of wound encountered in the ICU are surgical wounds (see Chs 23 and 26), traumatic wounds and pressure sores (Chs 23 and 30).

Pressure sores

Prevention is always better than cure and this is certainly the case when it comes to pressure sores. However, with the critically ill patient, the main priority is ultimately to maintain haemodynamic stability and optimise ventilation, and in some cases this may be jeopardised by turning or rolling the patient. Therapeutic beds are regularly requested for the maintenance of skin integrity. The past 5–10 years have witnessed many developments in the design of specialised beds, from temperature regulatory devices to beds specifically for cardiac or respiratory patients providing rotation and percussion, as well as devices to assist with the movement of patients and the nursing of patients in the prone position.

There is also a risk of tissue damage due to pressure from equipment, such as an ET tube pressing on the lip, a tightly taped three-way tap or tube pressing on the skin, or even an overinflated tube cuff, which has been shown to cause necrosis through the tracheal wall into the oesophagus (Rippe et al 1995).

Pressure sores may delay recovery, pose increased infection risks and entail much discomfort for the patient. Assessment of the patient's risk of developing a pressure sore should be undertaken daily using a standardised tool such as the Waterlow pressure sore prevention/treatment policy (see p. 754).

Promoting and maintaining normal tone, power and movement of the musculoskeletal system

As well as regularly positioning the patient to optimise air entry, ventilation and maintain skin integrity, passive and active exercises should be carried out. In patients who have limited movement or who are unable to move at all, a regimen of passive movements can be implemented which will progress to active/assisted movements as the patient's condition improves. This can counteract some of the effects of bed rest, namely deep venous thrombosis (DVT), contractures and foot drop.

MEETING THE PSYCHOSOCIAL, CULTURAL AND SPIRITUAL NEEDS OF THE CRITICALLY ILL PATIENT

PSYCHOSOCIAL NEEDS

Everyone who becomes critically ill is first and foremost a person. 'Patient' is only one of their current subsidiary roles in life. It is sometimes difficult to remember this when immersed in life-saving procedures on the body of someone unknown.

Critical illness may be caused by trauma, infection or other pathophysiological state, possibly complicated (at least initially) by major surgery, and may affect any or all of the body systems and vital organs. Malfunction of one organ or system is likely to affect others and progress to multiple organ failure. Patients may be fully conscious and able to talk and move, or totally unconscious or paralysed. Each person has a unique combination of age, sex, personality, ethnic origin, social and cultural background, general health and other experiences, which may result in different physical and psychological responses (Clark 1987).

Nursing priorities and management:

Goal: to support the patient psychologically, interacting in order to minimise the stress of the ICU environment.

Plan:

- provide adequate information, reassurance and encouragement
- prevent sensory overload or sensory deprivation
- maintain natural biorhythms/sleep patterns.

Providing adequate information, reassurance and encouragement

Nichols (1993) has identified informational care, emotional care and counselling as the essential components of good psychological care in illness. All are dependent on communication. Similarly, 'reassurance' and 'encouragement' are often identified as important to nursing, particularly in intensive care, but they are often not defined in practical terms. The difficulties of communicating with intubated patients and the theoretical reasons why communication is essential have long been known (Ashworth 1980). Good communication may enable patients to see monitoring equipment as helpful rather than frightening, even if they do not always remember being told about it. Support for each patient is most likely to be optimised when nurses, visitors and the patient collaborate to achieve effective and sensitive communication.

Preventing sensory overload/sensory deprivation

The sensory environment of an ICU is abnormal, compared with the environment in which people usually live, and can be disturbing even to those who are healthy. Sounds of ventilators, tracheal aspiration, equipment warning signals, the movement of trolleys and the like all combine to provide an auditory environment which may both bewilder and provoke anxiety. Patients may also experience other unusual stimuli, such as bright lights and strange equipment, and sensations of heat or cold, of being handled by other people, and of being attached to tubes and wires. There may also be a fear of falling out of bed during a change of position while paralysed, discomfort from wet tapes holding the ET tube in situ, and pain. Sometimes there is a lack of body privacy and a sense of humiliation (Ruiz 1993). Boredom, powerlessness and fear that essential machinery might fail are commonly reported (Uprichard et al 1987).

Critically ill patients may suffer sensory overload or sensory deprivation, or a combination of these. Many years ago, Goldberger (1966) identified five areas of investigation related to sensory alteration:

- reduction of stimulus input variables — an absolute reduction in the variety and intensity of stimuli
- reduction of stimulus variability — the quantity of stimuli is the same but there is reduced patterning, imposed structuring and homogeneous stimulation. When light is diffuse, sound is muffled and body sensations are non-distinct and difficult to interpret, this is referred to as perceptual deprivation
- social deprivation — isolation from people and familiar environment
- confinement — immobilisation or restriction of movement
- increased sensory input — input via a number of senses at greater intensity than normal.

All of these can be found in individual or collected accounts of the experience of critically ill patients, as can accounts of nightmare auditory and visual hallucinations, delusions and paranoid feelings about staff and the environment (Heath 1989).

Patients may also experience depersonalisation, disturbed body image and extension of body boundaries, so that they regard machinery such as the ventilator as part of themselves (Smith 1989). One factor which is important in determining a patient's responses to a critical care environment is the nature of the human environment. Psychological as well as physical stimuli can be stressful and cause physiological reactions that may be harmful to critically ill patients. Such stimuli may result from deficiencies in the human environment. Nurses are an important part of the sensory and human environment of patients, and vice versa. Nurses affect the internal environment and responses of patients, and are in turn affected by them (Ashworth 1980). Many ex-patients say that a caring staff member (usually a nurse) who they trusted was essential to their confidence and sense of security (Douglas 1982).

Psychological and behavioural problems

Mental health problems in the ICU can be divided into three categories:

- organic brain disorder, e.g. dementia, delirium
- psychological reaction to illness, i.e. depressive illness
- previous mental illness.

Delirium is common among critically ill patients within the general ICU setting; post-anaesthetic states, hypoxia, systemic infections, drug intoxication, alcohol withdrawal and metabolic derangement also contribute to states of delirium. Symptoms vary considerably and, prior to medical intervention, the patient should be assessed clinically, establishing haemodynamic stability and, where possible, the probable cause of delirium.

Haloperidol is usually the drug therapy of choice but should not be given before first assessing the patient's vital signs, clinical condition and the underlying cause of his behaviour.

Maintaining natural biorhythms/sleep

Human beings have biological or circadian rhythms that are normally related to the sleep/wake cycle, including fluctuations in body temperature, blood pressure, heart rate and plasma levels of various hormones (see Ch. 25).

In critical care units, there is always a danger that activity and lighting may be more or less constant, because of the need for constant observation and frequent treatment, leading to lack of sleep and disturbance of the biological rhythms and contributing to the sensory–perceptual alterations and delirium known to affect a considerable proportion of critically ill people. Diminishing light, noise and disturbance as far as possible at night can help to minimise such potential problems. It is clear that nursing requires the application of sound knowledge, judgement and skill.

Practice must be sensitive, relevant and responsive to the needs of the individual and nowhere more so than when preventing sleep deprivation.

For further reading on 'ITU syndrome', see Dyer (1995, 1996).

CULTURAL NEEDS AND SPIRITUAL CARE

Nursing priorities and management:

Goal: to meet the spiritual and cultural needs of the patient and his family.

Plan: ensure that the spiritual beliefs of the patient and his family are upheld.

Spiritual health relates to having a sense of meaning, hope and purpose in life, not simply to having a religious faith. Cultural and personal values are very relevant to purpose in life and should be considered in assessment and care (Lanara 1988, Parfitt 1988).

Some critically ill patients lose hope and 'give up', ceasing to fight for life, particularly when ill for days or weeks, and this can contribute not only to their current physical and emotional experience but also to the outcome of the illness. Many nurses feel helpless, unable to do anything to relieve the patient's suffering (Engberg 1991). Anything a nurse can do, either directly or with the help of the patient's family or friends, to help the patient draw on his usual resources and sources of support must be helpful. Simsen (1986) found that many patients needed to learn the skills of 'knowing', 'hoping' and 'trusting' in order to make sense of the experience of illness and in order to 'get through it'. Helping people to continue the practices important to them in life can enable them to do so, and there are a variety of ways of doing this. Many former patients have indicated that faith can be an important part of a person's life and a comfort in a crisis (Ashworth 1987).

The role of family and friends

Family and friends play an important role in relieving social isolation, depersonalisation and disorientation for patients. Indeed, this is often emphasised by former patients (Clark 1985, Heath 1989, Chen 1990). Yet family and friends are unable to be of maximum help to patients unless they themselves receive help from the nurses in the form of access, information and emotional support. Nurses have a great influence on the extent to which family and friends can support the sick person during intensive care, after transfer to a ward and then home. Family and friends can only provide optimum support if their own needs are met and nurses have an important role to play here. Some of the major expressed needs that have been identified from a number of studies are the need to reduce anxiety, the need for information, the need to be near the patient and the need to be helpful.

For further reading on the needs of family members of ICU patients, see Wilkinson (1995).

SUMMARY

Care of the critically ill patient is a diverse and ever-expanding field, as medicine and technology collaborate to support patients through increasingly acute life-threatening situations. It is often viewed only as a highly technical arena. However, the same general principles of care apply, be it in an ICU, a general hospital ward or the community setting. To be effective, nurses must have a sound knowledge and understanding of physiology and other sciences, of how the body works in health as well as in illness; of technical equipment and its functions and of how people behave in and respond to health and illness. The expertise, however, is to be able to use this knowledge to generate competent skills and the judgement necessary to achieve the best possible outcomes for patients and their families.

This chapter has only touched upon some of the fundamental concerns surrounding the nursing care of the critically ill patient. It has to be said that, as medicine strides forwards to maintain life in increasingly fragile states, it does indeed create its own ethical dilemmas, and while it is not possible to cover these issues in this chapter, it is important to consider the ethical implications that critical care nursing may encounter.

For further reading on ethical matters in intensive care, see Jones (1995), Pace & McLean (1996) and Morgan (1998).

REFERENCES

Ashurt S 1992 Suction therapy in the critically ill patient. British Journal of Nursing 1(10): 485–489

Ashworth P 1990 High technology and humanity in intensive care. Intensive Care Nursing 6(3): 150–160

Ashworth P 1980 Care to communicate. Scutari, Harrow

Ashworth P 1987 The needs of the critically ill patient. Intensive Care Nursing 3(4): 182–190

Beale R, Bihari D 1992 The management of acute renal failure in the intensive care unit. Current Anaesthesia and Critical Care 3: 146–149

Canter C 1987 Nursing mechanically ventilated patients in the prone position. Care of the Critically Ill 3(3): 70–71

Carroll K C, Magruder C C 1993 The role of analgesics and sedatives in the management of pain and agitation during weaning from mechanical ventilation. Critical Care Nurse Quarterly 15(4): 68–77

Chen Y C 1990 Psychological and social support systems in intensive and critical care. Intensive Care Nursing 6(2): 59–66

Chudley S 1994 The effect of nursing activities on intracranial pressure. British Journal of Nursing 3(9): 454–459

Clark K J 1985 Coping with Guillain–Barré syndrome (a personal experience). Intensive Care Nursing 1(1): 13–18

Clark S 1987 Nursing diagnosis: ineffective coping, I. A theoretical framework: II. Planning care. Heart and Lung 16(6): 670–685

Cohen A, Kelly D R 1987 Assessment of alfentanil by intravenous infusion as long-term sedation in intensive care. Anaesthesia 42: 545–548

Coombs M 1993 Haemodynamic profiles and the critical care nurse. Intensive and Critical Care Nursing 9: 11–16

Deitch E A, Dazhong X, Specian R D, Berg R 1992 Protein malnutrition alone and in combination with endotoxin impairs systemic and gut-associated immunity. Journal of Parenteral and Enteral Nutrition 16: 25–31

Douglas A M 1982 Where am I? In: Noble M A (ed) The ICU environment: directions for nursing. Reston Publishing, Reston, ch 10

Engberg I B 1991 Giving up and withdrawal by ventilator-treated patients: nurses' experience. Intensive Care Nursing 7(4): 200–205

Forni L G, Hilton M D 1997 Continuous hemofiltration in the treatment of acute renal failure. New England Journal of Medicine 336(18): 1303–1309

Geisman L K 1989 Advances in the weaning from mechanical ventilation. Critical Care Nursing Clinics of North America 1: 697–705

Goldberger L 1966 Experimental isolation: an overview. American Journal of Psychiatry 122: 774–782

Goldhill D R, Withington P S 1997 Textbook of intensive care. Chapman and Hall, London

Hagland M 1993 The management of acute renal failure in the intensive therapy unit. Intensive and Critical Care Nursing 9: 237–241

Hagland M, Wilkinson B 1993 Making sense of Swan–Ganz monitoring. Nursing Times 89(40): 26–28

Hawker F H 1996 Intensive care management of fulminant hepatic failure. In: Dellinger R P, Burchardi H, Dobbs G J, Bion J (eds) Current topics in intensive care, No. 3. WB Saunders, London, ch 9

Heath J V 1989 What the patients say. Intensive Care Nursing 5(3): 101–108

Henneman E A 1991 The art and science of weaning from mechanical ventilation. Focus on Critical Care 18(6): 490–501

Hillman K, Bishop G 1996 Clinical intensive care. Cambridge University Press, Melbourne

Hinds C J 1992 Intensive care: a concise textbook. Baillière Tindall, London

Horwood A 1992 A literature review of recent advances in enteral feeding and the increased understanding of the gut. Intensive and Critical Care Nursing 8: 185–188

Huddleston S S, Ferguson S G 1990 Critical care and emergency nursing. Springhouse, Pennsylvania

Lanara V 1988 Cultural value – influnce on the delivery of care. Intensive Care Nursing 4(1): 3–8

Lloyd F 1990 Eye care for ventilated or unconscious patients. Nursing Times 86: 36–37

MacKenzie S J 1992 Clinical use of PEEP. Indications, effects and practicalities. British Journal of Intensive Care, October: 335–340

McClure B, Franklin K 1987 The Mead model for nursing – adapted from the Roper/Logan/Tierney model for nursing. Intensive Care Nursing 3: 97–105

Manes E N 1995 Human anatomy and physiology, 3rd edn. Benjanmin/Cummings, California

Nichols K 1993 Psychological care in the physical illness, 2nd edn. Chapman and Hall, London

Oh T E 1997 Intensive care manual, 4th edn. Butterworth-Heinemann, Oxford

Parfitt B A 1988 Cultural assessment in the intensive care unit. Intensive Care Nursing 4(3): 124–127

Pearson S, Parr S 1993 Physiotherapy in the critically ill patient. Care of the Critically Ill 9(3): 128–131
Perry L 1993 Gut feelings about feeding: enteral feeding for ventilated patients in a district general hospital. Intensive and Critical Care Nursing 9: 171–176
Rainbow C 1989 Monitoring the critically ill patient, patient problems and nursing care. Butterworth-Heinemann, Oxford
Raper S, Maynard N 1992 Feeding the critically ill patient. British Journal of Nursing 1(60): 273–280
Riegel B, Forshee T 1985 A review and critique of the literature on preoxygenation for endotracheal suctioning. Heart and Lung 14(5): 507–512
Rippe J M, Irwin R S, Fink M P, Cerra F B, Curley F J, Heard S O (eds) 1995 Procedures and techniques in intensive care medicine. Little Brown, New York
Robb J A 1993 An overview of ventilator observations. Intensive and Critical Care Nursing 9: 201–207
Roper N, Logan W, Tierney A J 1996 The elements of nursing: a model of nursing, based on a model of living, 4th edn. Churchill Livingstone, Edinburgh
Ruiz P A 1993 The needs of the patient in severe status asthmaticus: experiences of a nurse–patient in an intensive care unit. Intensive and Critical Care Nursing 9(1): 28–39
Shelley M P, Sneyd R 1992 Sedation in intensive care. British Journal of Intensive Care 2: 323–332
Simsen B 1986 Nursing the spirit. Nursing Times 84(37): 31–33
Singer M, Carr C 1996 Early enteral feeding: benefits and mechanisms. In: Dellinger R P, Burchardi H, Dobb G D, Bion J (eds) Current topics in intensive Care, No. 3. WB Saunders, London, ch 6
Smith S 1989 Extended body image in the ventilated patient. Intensive Care Nursing 5(1): 31–38
Spaden H D, Duinslaeger L, Diltoer M et al 1995 Gastric emptying in critically ill patients is accelerated by adding cisapride to a standard enteral feeding protocol: results of a prospective study. Journal of Parenteral and Enteral Nutrition 16: 59–63
Spiby J 1989 Intensive care in the UK: report from the King's Fund panel. Anaesthesia 44: 428–431
Stiesmeyer J K 1993 A four-step approach to pulmonary assessment. American Journal of Nursing 93(8): 22–28
Thurgood G 1994 Nurse maintenance of oral hygiene. British Journal of Nursing 3(7): 332–353
UKCC 1992 The scope of professional practice. UKCC, London
Uprichard E, Martin A, Evans S 1987 Guillain–Barré syndrome: patients' and nurses' perspectives. Intensive Care Nursing 2(3): 123–134
Vander A 1991 Renal physiology. McGraw-Hill, Singapore
Verity S 1996 Nutrition and its importance to intensive care patients. Intensive and Critical Care Nursing 12(2): 71–78
Weber F H Jr, Richards R D, McCallum R W 1993 Erythromycin: a motilin agonist and gastrointestinal prokinetic agent. Am J Gastroenterol 88: 485–490
Weenk G H, Kemen M, Werner H P 1993 Risks of microbiological contamination of enteral feeds during the set up of enteral feeding systems. Journal of Human Nutrition and Dietetics 6: 307–316
Weilitz P B 1993 Weaning a patient from mechanical ventilation. Critical Care Nurse 13(4): 33–40
Woodrow P 1993 Resource package: haemofiltration. Intensive and Critical Care Nursing 9: 95–107

FURTHER READING

Bartlett E M 1996 Temperature measurement: why and how in intensive care. Intensive and Critical Care Nursing 12: 50–54
Buckley P M, Mac Fie J 1997 Enteral nutrition in critically ill patients – a review. Care of the Critically Ill 13(1): 7–10
Dyer I 1995 Preventing the ITU syndrome or how not to torture your patient. Part 1. Intensive and Critcal Care Nursing 11(3): 130–139
Dyer I 1996 Preventing ITU syndrome or how not to torture your patient. Part 2. Intensive and Critical Care Nursing 11(4); 223–232
Hinds C J, Watson D 1996 Intensive care: a concise handbook, 2nd edn. WB Saunders, London
Jones J 1995 Ethical dilemmas in intensive care: a case history. Intensive and Critical Care Nursing 11(1): 32–35
Kollef M H 1997 Inhaled nitric oxide for severe acute respiratory distress syndrome: a blessing or a curse? Heart and Lung 26(5): 358–362
Leighton H 1995 Paracetamol poisoning: a case study. Intensive and Critical Care Nursing 11(6): 280–282
McMahon-Parkes F, Cornock M 1997 Guillain–Barré syndrome: biological basis, treatment and care. Critical Care Nursing 13(1): 42–48
McMahon K 1995 Multiple organ failure: the final complication of critical illness. Critical Care Nursing 15(6): 20–28
Manji M, Bion J 1997 Transporting the critically ill patient. In: Goldhill D R, Withington P S (eds) Textbook of intensive care. Chapman and Hall Medical, London, ch 6
Mulnier C, Evans T 1995 Acute respiratory distress in adults (ARDS). Care of the Critically Ill 11(5)
Oh T E 1997 Intensive care manual, 4th edn. Butterworth-Heinemann, Oxford
Pace N, McLean S A 1996 Ethics and the law in intensive care. Oxford University Press, Oxford
Plowright C 1995 Auditing quality of nursing care. Intensive and Critical Care Nursing 11: 354–359
Robb Y A 1997 Have nursing models a place in intensive care units? Intensive and Critical Care Nursing 13: 93–98
Sproat L J, Inglis T J J 1992 Preventing infection in the intensive care unit. British Journal of Intensive Care, September
Sutcliffe L 1994 Philosophy and models in critical care nursing. Intensive and Critical Care Nursing 10: 212–221
van der Hulst R R W J,van der Kreel B K, von Meyenfeldt M F et al 1993 Glutamine and the preservation of gut integrity. Lancet 341: 1363–1365
Waterlow J A 1995 Pressure sores and their management. Care of the Critically Ill 11(3): 121–125
Wilkinson P 1995 A qualitative study to establish the self perceived needs of the family members of patients in a general intensive care unit. Intensive and Critical Care Nursing 11(1): 77– 86

THE PATIENT WITH BURNS

30

Frances M. Davidson

INTRODUCTION

Imagine for a moment having lost everything: your loved ones; your home and possessions, including mementoes from the past; your health and ability to function normally; your appearance — in other words, yourself. This not infrequently occurs when people are victims of a house fire.

Most people are burned more than once in their lifetime but few have any conception of the horror associated with severe burns injury. Extensive burns injury is catastrophic, both physically and psychologically, for the patient and her family. It is also one of the most challenging and arduous types of injury to treat. In order to help the patient and her family to achieve optimum function, the responsibility of care must be distributed throughout the multidisciplinary team. However, the nurse, being the only professional in 24-h attendance, will play an especially important role. Nurses also attend to many patients whose burns are not extensive, providing care in the community, in accident and emergency (A&E) departments and in general surgical wards. This chapter aims to provide information which will help the nurse care for patients with burn injuries in any of these settings.

PREVENTION OF BURN INJURIES

Burns are frequently described in the literature as being among the most serious of injuries because of the long-term physical and psychological problems which are often associated with them. Advances in treatment and improved facilities have led to a reduction in mortality rates, but the morbidity resulting from burns is such that prevention must be viewed as the responsibility of all health care personnel.

The first of the five aims stated in the constitution of the International Society for Burn Injuries (ISBI), formed in 1965, is 'to disseminate knowledge and to stimulate prevention in the field of burns' (ISBI 1979). Bouter et al (1990) emphasise that, in order to be effective, a burn prevention programme must involve assessment of the incidence of burn injuries followed by the planning, implementation and evaluation of appropriate interventions.

Assessment

This includes identifying the extent of the problem, its causative agents and any predisposing factors.

The extent of the problem

As yet, there are no national data on the incidence of burns. The Australia & New Zealand Burn Association (UK) (1996) estimates that, in the UK, 100 000 people are burned each year, that 50 000 will suffer some daily living restriction, 10 000 will be hospitalised, and 1000 will have life-threatening injuries. Due to advances in treatment, burn mortality rates have fallen over the last two decades (Rose & Herndon 1997). Linares & Linares (1990) make the point that although statistical data on burn mortality are generally available, the incidence of burn morbidity is difficult to estimate. Bouter et al (1990) identify the problem as being substantial in terms of morbidity, medical consumption and absence from work.

Causative agents

A more or less equal number of studies report that either scalds or flame burns are the most common type of burn injury. Contact burns (from touching hot objects) also have a high incidence. Chemical and electrical burns occur less frequently.

The Central Statistical Office (1991) identifies the most common cause of death in domestic fires as careless handling of fire and hot substances, mainly smokers' materials. Non-fatal burn casualties result from the misuse of equipment or appliances, most commonly cooking appliances (see Case History 30.1). In the case of scalds, the electric kettle is recognised as a major cause of injury, usually in children of pre-school age (Lawrence & Cason 1994). Hot water in plumbing systems is also a considerable cause for concern in countries where there is no legislation governing the upper limit of plumbed water temperature. Although many authorities advocate a temperature of 50ºC (which would take 2–3 min to cause a burn), because of altered sensation and reduced mobility in older people this figure has been reduced to 43ºC in residential accommodation for the elderly (Harper & Dickson 1995) (see Box 30.1 for advice on reducing the risk of scalds).

Predisposing factors

All epidemiological studies identify toddlers as being at greatest risk of burn injuries, with scalds accounting for most of these.

Case History 30.1 Ms C

Ms C (aged 24) returned home after a night out with her friends and, feeling hungry, decided to have some chips. She put the chip pan on the stove, leaving the fat to heat whilst she got ready for bed. Smelling smoke, she rushed back to the kitchen to find the saucepan in flames. In her panic she tried to douse the flames by smothering them with a dry towel, which promptly caught fire. She then remembered to put the lid on and turn off the stove. Her screams alerted the neighbours, who phoned for an ambulance. Ms C was rushed to the nearest casualty department, where, on examination, she was found to have a total of 8%, mainly superficial, burns to her hands, forearms, chest and face.

Box 30.1 Reducing the risk of scalds

- Water does not have to be close to boiling point to cause severe injury.
- A cup of freshly made tea or instant coffee takes 20 min to reach a temperature which will not damage the skin and 15 min if milk is added (Mercer 1988). The same study found that the contents of a newly boiled kettle containing 1.5 L of water will take 1 h to reach a safe temperature.
- Water at a temperature of 66°C will cause a full-thickness scald after 2 s contact and, at 60°C, after 6 s (Moritz & Henriques 1947). Many authors advocate the reduction of plumbed hot water temperatures to 50–55°C (Walker 1990, Adams et al 1991).
- Setting the hot water thermostat to a lower temperature will help to reduce fuel bills.

Adult high-risk groups include those with epilepsy (Spitz et al 1994) and those who smoke tobacco, drink alcohol to hazardous levels and take prescribed psychotropic medications (Duggan & Quine 1995) (see Case History 30.2). Haum et al (1995) found that patients with positive blood alcohol levels had a significantly higher fatality rate than those with negative blood alcohol levels. Elderly people have also been identified as being more susceptible to burn injury and as having a higher mortality rate following injury (Sarhadi et al 1995). Studies agree that males of all ages are at higher risk than females.

The main common denominator of predisposition to burn injury, therefore, appears to be a combination of reduced awareness of danger and decreased mobility.

Planning and implementation

Planning for a burns prevention programme must be realistic. While Van Rijn et al (1989) accept that it is impossible to manipulate some of the risk factors, e.g. sex and age, they argue that having identified the groups most at risk, it should be possible to alter some of the related predisposing factors.

In the past, most burn prevention programmes were based on education of the public, but recent studies indicate that, on its own, this is not an effective method.

Q **30.1** What is your personal attitude to health education?

McLoughlin (1995) advises the use of the 'Public Health Model' which considers three factors: the host or person at risk, the agent, and the environment. With regard to the host, Adams et al (1991) found that recognition of potential danger did not alter the behaviour of adult high-risk groups. There are already numerous health education campaigns aimed at persuading the public not to smoke and to drink alcohol only in moderation. It seems unlikely that those who do not comply would be influenced by the knowledge that smoking and drinking increase their risk of burn injuries. Tones et al (1990) point out that, unlike the promotion of commercial products, which is based on enhancing pleasure and promises immediate gratification, health promotion usually urges people to stop doing something which they find pleasurable in the hope of long-term gratification. They also state that the public have a right not to be 'unreasonably frightened'. Blatant shock tactics are therefore unacceptable and are only likely to make people 'switch

Case History 30.2 Mr M

Mr Robert M (aged 47) regularly abused alcohol and was a heavy smoker. One evening he fell into an alcoholic stupor, dropping his cigarette onto the horsehair sofa on which he was resting. The material smouldered, but did not burst into flames or produce toxic fumes. Robert was lying on his left side with his right hand resting on the sofa. He was eventually found by his brother, who dragged him off the sofa, extinguished the flames and called for an ambulance. On admission to the burns unit, Robert was found to have sustained full-thickness burns to the left side of the face and chest. There was no circulation through his left hand and arm (which required above-elbow amputation) and the fingers of his right hand were burned down to the bone. The total body surface involved was estimated at 20%.

off'. More subtle messages may be conveyed, e.g. by incidental reference in popular television series.

Identification of the agent or energy source results from epidemiology studies. It may be a result of poor design of equipment such as the hot water jug which has a higher centre of gravity than a kettle, or a stove or radiator which produces a high surface temperature. Once the problem has been recognised, modification of design may be sufficient to eradicate the danger.

Product modification may be carried out voluntarily by manufacturers; however, legislation is often required. Since 1990, it has been against the law to sell new or re-upholstered soft furnishings which are padded with foam that is not combustion-modified or which are covered with fabric that does not resist ignition tests for both smouldering cigarettes and match-like flames. Currently, cigarettes contain an additive which allows them to smoulder for 28 minutes, and in many developed countries there is interest in introducing a regulation to reduce the ignition propensity of cigarettes (Harper & Dickson 1995, McLoughlin 1995).

Previous legislation and regulations include the prohibition of the sale of highly flammable children's nightwear and the requirement that all new gas or electric fires and radiant oil-burning stoves are fitted with a fire guard which passes British Standards specifications.

With regard to the environment, probably the greatest single factor in reducing death and injury by fires in the home has been the introduction of smoke detectors/alarms. In North America, their installation into both new and established domestic properties is legally required in many states. In the UK, legislation is less arbitrary and installation into established properties is voluntary. Because of their sensitivity, smoke detector alarms may be set off by cooking fumes (e.g. burning toast) and there have been numerous reports of people consequently removing the batteries from smoke detectors in council-owned properties where they have been installed. Some detectors have a temporary 'silence' button which may solve the problem of false alarms; however, as the ceiling is the recommended site for mounting, the detector may be out of easy reach.

It must be accepted that the groups at highest risk of injury from burns, i.e. the elderly or disabled, will be less able than others to purchase the new, safer soft furnishings and heating appliances. Smoke detectors may be bought for as little as £5, but their fitting, although simple for the able-bodied, may be impossible for elderly or disabled individuals.

Health care workers therefore not only have a responsibility to disseminate information on the prevention of burn injuries but must also work closely with other interested groups such as the fire brigades, The Royal Society for the Prevention of Accidents and both local and national government offices in order to lobby for more effective legislation and regulations. Nurses working in the community have special opportunities to observe the environment and to give specific advice relating to burns prevention.

FIRST AID TREATMENT OF BURNS

Burn injuries result from the transfer of energy from a source of heat to vulnerable tissues. The higher the temperature of the heat source and the longer it is in contact with the tissues, the greater will be the destruction.

The first priority of first aid treatment is to remove the individual from the source of heat. If the causative agent is electricity, it is important to switch off the supply, if possible, or to use non-conducting material, such as a sling made out of dry clothing, to rescue the person.

Frequently there is a continuing source of heat in the form of the individual's clothing, which may be on fire or saturated by a hot liquid. The most effective way to remove this continuing heat source is to throw cool liquid (which is neither flammable nor corrosive) over the affected material, thus dousing the flames or reducing the temperature of the scalding liquid. If no such cool liquid is immediately to hand, rapid removal of hot saturated clothing will arrest the heat transfer. Where clothing is on fire, it is important to stop the person running around as this will fan the flames. The person assisting should lie the victim on the ground and use heavy material such as a coat or blanket to smother the flames. If chemicals are the causative agent, prompt sluicing with copious amounts of water will dilute the strength of the agent and limit the penetration of the chemical into the skin, where it will continue to cause damage for many hours. Herbert & Lawrence (1989) emphasise the advantage of taking this universal first aid measure rather than taking time searching for specific neutralising agents. (In the clinical situation a useful means of identifying whether a chemical is acid or alkaline is to apply a Multistix, normally used for urine testing, as this will give a pH reading.)

Having taken steps to remove the heat source from the skin, the next measure is to cool the superheated tissues. The easiest means of doing this is to place the affected part (obviously not the face, to which cold soaks should be applied) in cold water. Lawrence & Wilkins (1986) demonstrated that when cold water was applied 5 s after experimental burning (by the application of a metal block at 100ºC for 10 s), the subdermal temperature returned to normal in approximately 25 s, whereas untreated tissue took approximately 4 min. This experiment was carried out on laboratory animals and it is accepted that the length of time that the cold tap water treatment should be continued in humans is up to 10 min (Lawrence 1996a). The application of ice or chilled water below 5ºC is contraindicated, as Sawada et al (1997) found this was associated with increased likelihood of tissue damage, possibly due to vasoconstriction. There is no doubt that continuing application helps to reduce pain from the burn wound, but if a large area of the body surface is involved there is a risk of hypothermia.

Ellis & Rylah (1990) advise against using cold soaks or ice packs during the transfer of patients to hospital, especially if the journey will take some time. In a recent case, a 10-year-old girl sustained 12% burns on her back when her shirt-tail came into contact with a gas flame. Her brother, with whom she was playing, threw the contents of a jug of lemonade over the flames; then she was placed in a bath by her mother, who repeatedly scooped cold water over the burned area. She then wrapped her daughter in a clean sheet and took her to the local hospital. From there, the child was transferred to a specialist unit, a journey of more than 1 h. During the period of transfer she was lying prone on a stretcher lined with incontinence pads, absorbent surface up; the escorting nurse carried out her instructions, which were to continually irrigate the saline soaks which had been placed on the girl's back with cold saline from a cool-pack. When the patient arrived at the specialist unit, rectal temperature was recorded at 34.8ºC. Steinmann et al (1990) have noted the high mortality related to trauma patients who have core temperatures of less than 35ºC at the time of their admission to hospital. Fortunately, in the case described, the child survived. (NB — patients with extensive burns clearly have problems in retaining body heat. The use of space blankets or other heat-retaining coverings is advised during the period of transfer.)

Many burns units in the UK are now advising that the temporary wound dressing of choice is polyvinyl chloride film, e.g. clingfilm (Lawrence 1996a). The reasons for this are as follows:

Case History 30.3 Miss K

Miss K (aged 53) suffers from diabetes and lives alone. One morning she awoke to find that she had blistering on her left lower leg. She assumed this had been caused by contact with her hot water bottle. As there was no pain, she did not contact her doctor but dressed the burn herself, using an antiseptic cream and a bandage. A week later she attended the local health centre as the wound was now very inflamed and producing pus.

- the film is sterile on the inner rolled surface
- it does not adhere to the wound surface and cause pain on removal
- it conforms closely to the body contours and excludes air, thus reducing pain
- a succession of personnel can view the wound without removal of the transparent film.

This kind of material is often available in the home but, if not, a clean cloth should be used as temporary cover. The use of ointments, lotions and powders should be avoided as they may change the appearance of the wound and thus cause difficulty in the assessment of wound depth.

Practice and treatment room nurses often see people with severe sunburn that has been unsuccessfully self-managed and has become infected. This can also happen with other types of burns, as in Case History 30.3.

To summarise, first aid treatment of burn injuries consists of:

- Separating the individual from the source of injury
- Immersion of the affected part in cold water for 10 min (cold soaks to face)
- Application of polyvinyl chloride (cling) film or a clean cloth to the wound (cold soaks may be used for wounds which are not extensive).

ASSESSING THE SEVERITY OF BURN INJURIES

The majority of patients with burn injuries do not require hospital in-patient care. Gowar & Lawrence (1995) identify the categories of patients for whom admission or referral to a regional burns unit is advisable:

- those whose burns exceed 5% of the body surface area
- those with burns on functionally important areas such as face, hands, feet, perineum, joints or flexor surfaces
- those with infected wounds or evidence of infection
- those with small, full-thickness burns which would benefit from early excision and grafting
- those whose injury limits their capacity to care for themselves at home
- those with associated injuries, e.g. smoke inhalation or electric shock
- those with other medical conditions, e.g. epilepsy
- where there is doubt, either suspected non-accidental injury or uncertainty about the depth of the burn.

For patients who do not fall into any of these categories, relief of pain and local treatment of the burn wound are generally all that is required. Both interventions will be described later in the chapter (see p. 903).

Assessment of the severity of the burn injury involves estimation of:

- the extent of body surface area involved
- the depth of tissue damage
- the probability of associated respiratory tract injury.

Knowledge of the circumstances of the accident (e.g. whether electricity was involved) and information about the individual's general health and domestic situation will help in deciding whether the patient may or may not be managed by the primary health care team.

Extent of burn

Whenever body tissues are traumatised, the inflammatory response is stimulated, resulting in increased circulation to the area (hyperaemia) and increased movement of fluids from intravascular to interstitial compartments. If this occurs in a small area, i.e. over less than 5% of the body surface, the effects are localised. However, when a larger percentage of the body surface is injured, there is a massive shift of fluids into the tissues with a corresponding reduction in circulating volume. It is generally accepted that children with burns greater than 10% and adults with burns greater than 15% of body surface area will suffer from hypovolaemic shock unless there is prompt intravenous replacement of fluid (see Ch. 18).

In order to estimate the percentage of body surface affected, the simplest and most easily remembered method is the 'rule of nines' introduced by Wallace (1951) (see Fig. 30.1). In this method, the head and each upper limb equals 9%, while the anterior trunk, the posterior trunk and the lower limbs each equal 18%. The remaining 1% is usually applied to the perineum. Another rapid approximation of percentage can be made by using the palmar aspect of the patient's hand (with fingers together) as 1.5% of the body surface area.

The rule of nines should never be used for estimating burn percentage in young children as it does not allow for the different proportions of head and lower limbs in infants and toddlers. Under

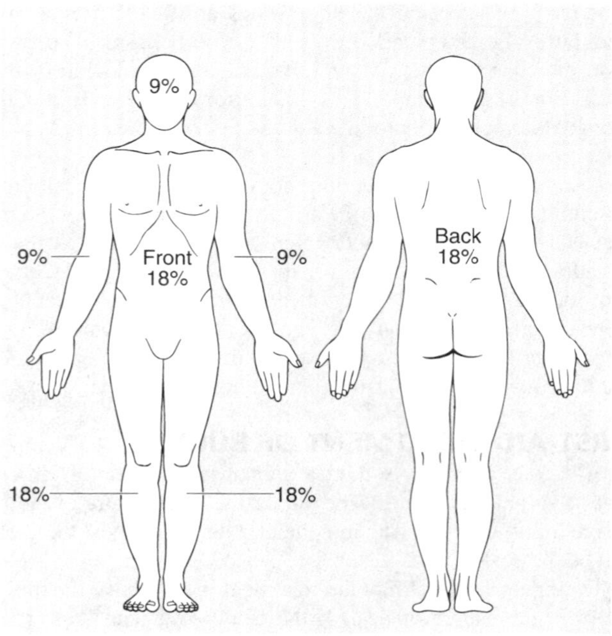

Fig. 30.1 Wallace's rule of nines.

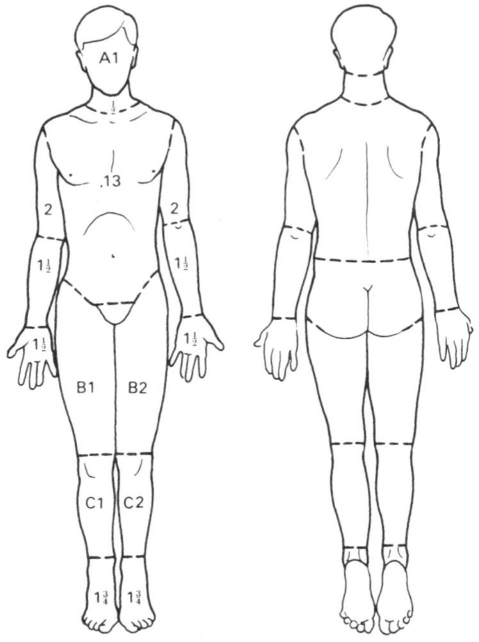

Percentage of body surface at various ages

Percent of areas affected by growth

	0	1	5	10	15	Adult age
A = ½ head	9½	8½	6½	5½	4½	3½
B = ½ one thigh	2¾	3¼	4	4¼	4½	4¾
C = ½ one leg	2½	2½	2¾	3	3¼	3½

To estimate the total of the body surface area burned, the percentages assigned to the burned sections are added. The total is then an estimate of the burn size.

Fig. 30.2 The Lund & Browder burn chart.

the age of 1 year the child's head equals 19% of the body surface area and the lower limbs are correspondingly smaller. A more accurate chart which allows for the changing proportions of different age groups and which shows percentages applicable to smaller, more specific areas of the body surface is the Lund & Browder (1944) burn chart (see Fig. 30.2). This is generally in use in specialist units and is available in A&E departments throughout the country.

Burn depth

The depth of a burn influences the rate at which the wound will heal spontaneously. The longer the wound takes to heal, the greater the probability of infection and the worse the scarring and loss of function (see Ch. 23). There are a number of methods of classifying burn depth. In the UK, the most popular is to differentiate between partial-thickness and full-thickness skin destruction. Partial-thickness burns involve the epidermis and part of the dermis. Full-thickness burns destroy the epidermis and all of the dermis. Full-thickness burns may also involve deeper structures such as fat, muscle and bone. Partial-thickness burns are classified as 'superficial' or 'deep', depending on the amount of dermis involved. As a general rule, deep partial-thickness and full-thickness burns require surgical enhancement of healing in the form of skin grafting.

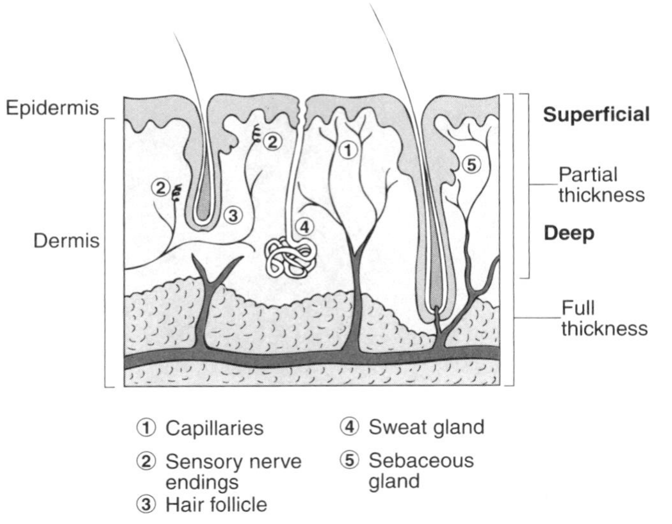

Fig. 30.3 Classification of burn depth.

As may be seen from Figure 30.3, the more superficial the injury, the greater the number of surviving epithelial sources from which cells will undergo mitosis and migrate across the wound surface; thus a more superficial burn heals more rapidly and causes less wound contraction. The effects of superficial partial-thickness burns and full-thickness burns are described below and in Table 30.1.

Superficial partial-thickness burns

These burns are very painful as the sensory nerve endings are stimulated by the injury or exposed to air. They are characterised by oedema, blister formation and serous exudate where the blisters burst. The blistering results from the increased permeability of the capillary walls, with fluid leaking into the interstitial spaces and from the wound surface (this fluid collects into blisters beneath the non-germinating layers of the epidermis). Heat radiates from the wound surface due to arteriolar dilatation and increased blood flow and as part of the inflammatory response. This also causes the typical bright pink appearance of the wound, which will blanch on pressure. On removal of the pressure the hyperaemia is restored.

Full-thickness burns

These burns are painless, as the sensory nerve endings have been destroyed. There is no blister formation and the wound surface is dry. There is no overt oedema, the wound surface is cool to the touch and the colour may be white, brown or bright red (with no blanching on pressure). These characteristics are all due to the fact that there is no surviving circulation within the dermis. The brown or red colour is due to the release of haem pigments from destroyed red blood cells. The area may appear translucent with thrombosed vessels being apparent. It is important to recognise that there is an inflammatory response in the deeper tissues affected, but this is masked by overlying necrotic tissue. High temperatures (greater than 60°C) cause coagulation of the tissue proteins and water is lost from the cells, interstitial spaces and blood vessels, resulting in a degree of contraction of the affected tissues. Destruction of the dermis renders the skin inelastic and the texture becomes firm and leathery. This destroyed tissue is known as eschar (see Box 30.2).

Table 30.1 Indications of burn depth

Depth	*Signs and symptoms*	*Related anatomy/physiology*
Superficial partial-thickness burns	Very painful	Sensory nerve endings in the dermis are stimulated by the injury and/or exposed to air
	Oedema, blister formation, serous exudate where blisters have burst	As a result of the inflammatory response, the capillary walls are more permeable and fluid leaks into the interstitial spaces of the dermis, collecting below the non-germinating layers of the epidermis or exuding from the wound surface
	Wound surface warmer than unburned skin	Also due to the inflammatory response; arteriolar dilatation causes increased blood flow
	Wound appears bright pink and blanches with pressure	Due to increased blood flow. Pressure greater than capillary blood pressure occludes the flow of blood
Full-thickness burns	Painless, no sensation	Sensory nerve endings in the dermis are destroyed
	Wound surface dry. No blistering	Cessation of blood flow through dermal capillaries
	No overt oedema	Necrosis of dermis renders it inelastic
	Wound surface cooler than unburned skin	Cessation of blood flow through dermal capillaries
	Wound colour may be white, brown, translucent showing thrombosed vessels, or bright red (does not blanch on pressure)	Cessation of blood flow through dermal capillaries. Brown or red appearance is caused by release of haem pigments from destroyed red blood cells

Box 30.2 Escharotomy

Where full-thickness burn injury occurs circumferentially around a limb, the combination of a firm inelastic eschar and the covert inflammatory response in the subcutaneous tissues will cause compression of the deeper structures, especially the blood vessels. Incisions through the eschar to allow decompression are carried out by the surgeon and are termed escharotomy.

Escharotomy may also be carried out when full-thickness burn injury of the chest and upper part of the abdomen inhibits rib or diaphragmatic movement, causing respiratory difficulty.

Nursing note. Monitoring of circulation to distal parts of limbs involved or of respiratory ease is required when full-thickness burns are suspected in either site.

Deep partial-thickness burns

As the depth of destruction in this type of burn is between those of superficial partial-thickness and full-thickness burns, the presenting signs and symptoms indicate moderation of the extremes in sensation, blistering, temperature and colour.

Problems in assessment

The assessment of burn depth is not an exact science, although much work has been carried out to make it more so in recent years. The use of a hypodermic needle to test for pinprick sensation was first described by Bull & Lennard-Jones (1949), and Settle (1996) admits that, although not an absolute test for viability, it is still useful. Wyllie & Sutherland (1991) found that temperature sensors, which are available in most anaesthetic departments, may be used successfully with minor adaptation in aiding diagnosis of burn depth in some areas of the body. Frequently, assessment of burn depth is dependent on the characteristics of the wound, the information given regarding the circumstances of the accident, the agent involved and the first aid measures carried out.

Burn-associated respiratory tract injury

Inhibition of respiratory function may result from thermal injury to the skin of the trunk and neck. Covert oedema formation below the leathery, inelastic eschar of circumferential full-thickness burns causes pressure on the deeper structures. In deep burns of the neck, this may cause compression of the trachea and, if there is involvement of the chest and upper abdomen, will inhibit expansion of the thoracic cavity. Decompression by escharotomy will be required (see Box 30.2).

Inhalation of smoke and hot toxic gases is frequently associated with burn trauma. The potent synergistic effects of burns and smoke inhalation are noted by Beeley & Clark (1996), who state that for victims of smoke inhalation who are unburned and alive on arrival at hospital the mortality rate is low, whereas for those who are also burned the mortality rate associated with the extent of burn is substantially increased.

The main causes of inhalation injury are:

- intoxication and hypoxaemia
- thermal damage to the airways
- respiratory tract injury due to irritants.

Intoxication and hypoxaemia

Intoxication and hypoxaemia most commonly result from inhalation of carbon monoxide and/or hydrogen cyanide produced by burning plastics.

Carbon monoxide (CO), produced by the combustion of carbon and organic materials in a limited oxygen supply, has an affinity for haemoglobin many times that of oxygen. Therefore, following inhalation of CO there is displacement of oxygen on the haemoglobin molecules and the production of carboxyhaemoglobin (COHb) with resulting generalised hypoxia. The symptoms of CO poisoning are related to the concentration of the inspired gas and to COHb levels and are recognised as mild headache, dizziness, confusion, irritability, nausea, vomiting and fainting. At higher levels there will be convulsion, coma, respiratory failure and death. Diagnosis is suggested by the typical cherry pink appearance of the patient and confirmed by checking COHb levels. The formation of carboxyhaemoglobin can be reversed by the administration of high concentrations of oxygen.

Cyanide is rapidly absorbed through the lungs and binds readily to the cytochrome system, inhibiting cell function and resulting in metabolic acidosis. It causes loss of consciousness, neurotoxicity and convulsions. However, over a period of time it is gradually metabolised by the liver enzyme rhodenase (Australia & New Zealand Burn Association Ltd (UK) 1996).

Thermal damage

The upper airway may be damaged by the inhalation of hot gases, hot vapours or combustible gas mixtures. Mucosal oedema will narrow the lumen of the airway. The diagnosis is suspected where there is a history of explosion, burns of the face, singed nasal hairs, erythema and ulceration of the oropharynx. Hoarseness and inspiratory stridor may present later. As signs of upper airway obstruction may take several hours to become apparent, constant supervision is advised.

Hot, dry air seldom causes burns of the airway below the level of the epiglottis as the respiratory tract has an excellent heat exchange capability. Injury to the lower airway is most commonly caused by inhalation of toxic chemicals.

Inhalation of irritant chemicals

The combustion of various materials produces a wide spectrum of irritant chemicals, including chlorine, ammonia, formaldehyde and phosgene. The extent of the resultant damage to the respiratory system will be determined by the density of the smoke and the duration of exposure. Patients who are asleep or under the influence of drugs or alcohol at the time of the fire will tend to have a longer exposure time, as will those who have restricted mobility, e.g. the elderly or disabled.

When irritant chemicals bound to carbon particles settle on the respiratory endothelium, the following reactions occur:

- the inflammatory response — this causes increased secretions and narrowing of the lumen of the trachea, bronchi and bronchioles
- inflammation of the alveolar capillary membrane — this interferes with gaseous exchange, and capillary exudate will leak into the alveoli
- bronchospasm — this causes further narrowing of the lumen of the airway
- chemical denaturation of all protein, which leads to:
  - —necrosis and ulceration of the epithelial tissue, with an increase in cellular debris
  - —cessation of ciliary activity, inhibiting removal of secretions and cellular debris
- loss of surfactant production by type II alveolar cells.

Surfactant normally lowers the surface tension of the walls of the alveoli, thus preventing collapse, and also prevents the transudation of fluid from capillaries into the alveoli. Loss of surfactant production will therefore lead to atelectasis (see Ch. 3).

In summary, the pathophysiological results of inhalation of irritant chemicals may include tracheobronchitis, pulmonary oedema, atelectasis and airway obstruction. These are frequently compounded by infection.

In cases where the patient survives long enough for admission to hospital, the respiratory damage related to inhalation of smoke may take several hours or even days to become manifest. Suspicion should be aroused where:

- the fire occurred within an enclosed space, especially at night
- there is a history of exposure to smoke, especially if the patient required bodily rescue
- the patient's breath and clothing smell of smoke
- there is inflammation of the conjunctivae
- carbon particles are present in clothing, wounds, nose, mouth and sputum.

Other injuries

The appearance of a patient with extensive burns may be so visually dramatic as to distract the assessor from checking for other, less obvious, injuries. Fractures, internal injuries and spinal cord damage may have been sustained, especially if the burn was a result of a road traffic accident, an explosion or high tension electricity, or if the patient jumped from a burning building.

THE PATIENT WITH EXTENSIVE BURNS

Early problems and nursing care

The patient with extensive burns has multiple problems, the relative urgency of which will vary during the perhaps very prolonged period following injury. In recent years there has been an increasing awareness that extensive burn injury causes a systemic inflammatory response in which there is widespread disorganisation of the immune system, eventually resulting in multiple organ dysfunction syndrome (Sparkes 1997). Sparkes attributes this to a lipid protein complex associated with burned skin.

During the first 36–48 h, however, the most life-threatening problem (except where inhalation injury is present) will be burns shock. The subject of shock is covered in Chapter 18, but a summary of events which have particular relevance to burns injury is given here (see Table 30.2).

The initial physiological response to a burn injury results in plasma loss from the circulation (see p. 896). This in turn is accompanied by:

- *Gross oedema* of the affected tissues.
- *Hypovolaemia.* As in all types of shock, this results in decreased circulation of the skin, muscle and internal organs. Cerebral and coronary perfusion, being of greatest priority, are temporarily maintained.
- *Haemoconcentration.* Unlike the hypovolaemia which results from haemorrhage, the loss of plasma alone from the intravascular compartment causes an increase in the ratio of blood cells to plasma in the circulation (raised haematocrit). This increases the viscosity of the blood, further reducing the flow through the capillaries.

In addition to suffering from burn shock, the patient may be emotionally shocked, in great pain and have extensive destruction of the skin and, possibly, deeper structures. There may be associated injuries, especially inhalation of smoke, and a pre-burn illness may be present.

Table 30.2 Pathology and related clinical features of burn shock

Pathological condition	*Clinical signs and symptoms*
Hypovolaemia	Thirst Rapid, weak pulse Hypotension Peripheral and splanchnic vasoconstriction
Peripheral vasoconstriction	Pale skin and mucosa Extremities feel cold Patient complains of feeling cold
Reduced perfusion of kidneys	Oliguria, anuria Impairment of renal function Metabolic acidosis Renal failure may occur
Red cell haemolysis	Haemoglobinuria Renal failure may occur
Reduced perfusion of lungs	Rapid, shallow breathing Air hunger — gasping
Reduced perfusion of gastrointestinal tract	Reduced absorption and intestinal stasis Vomiting, loss of electrolytes Paralytic ileus, lack of bowel sounds Bacterial translocation through mucosa
Hypoxaemia/electrolyte imbalance	Restlessness, disorientation, confusion May lead to coma and death

Box 30.3 Haemoglobinuria

This is a potential complication of extensive burn injury which may result in acute renal failure.

As haemoglobin has the molecular weight of 68 000 mol, it may be filtered through the glomerulus and pass into the renal tubules. Under normal circumstances, haemoglobin is not free in plasma, because when erythrocytes degenerate they are processed by the mononuclear phagocytic system. If pathogenic haemolysis does occur intravascularly, the haemoglobin is usually combined with the plasma protein haptoglobin, a mechanism for iron conservation, which forms a molecular complex too large to pass through the glomerulus.

However, if intravascular haemolysis is extensive there will be exhaustion of the haptoglobin and therefore free haemoglobin will be present in plasma. The reason why haemolysis occurs in extensive thermal injury appears to be more complicated than the direct effect of heat on the erythrocytes (Yuan et al 1988). Animal studies indicate that one of the mechanisms involved is the release of toxic oxygen metabolites, e.g. superoxide and hydrogen peroxide from activated neutrophils (Hatherill et al1986). The red blood cell changes include increased osmotic fragility and decreased membrane deformability (Endoh et al 1992). Brady et al (1996) note that there is uncertainty as to the means by which free haemoglobin (and myoglobin from damaged muscle) causes damage to the renal tubules and suggest that it may be due to metabolites of the compounds, other toxins from red blood cells/muscle or the coexistence of other renal insults such as hypovolaemia.

Haemoglobinuria may develop in patients who have been badly burned. This is described in Box 30.3.

The accident and emergency department

Ellis & Rylah (1990) highlight the fact that, to those who are unfamiliar with burns, the patient with extensive burns may not appear to be critically ill. The loss of plasma from the circulation is less rapid than haemorrhage from ruptured vessels and the patient may appear quite well. Inexperienced staff should consult with the regional burns unit to ensure that treatment is appropriate to the severity of the injury.

The Australia & New Zealand Burn Association Ltd (UK) (1996) identifies the following principles of primary assessment and management by medical personnel:

A Airway maintenance and cervical spine control
B Breathing and ventilation
C Circulation; cardiac status, with control of haemorrhage if present
D Disability, neurological status
E Exposure with environmental control; evaluation of extent and depth of injury, including removal of jewellery and keeping the patient warm
F Fluid resuscitation; i.v. fluid replacement, including introduction of urinary catheter for monitoring output, and insertion of nasogastric tube.

These are followed by X-ray of the cervical spine, chest and pelvis to exclude associated injury.

After life-threatening conditions have been excluded or treated, the secondary survey should be commenced. This includes a patient history, description of incident and complete examination.

Except in instances where nurses are specially trained, the role of nursing staff is to assist with the above procedures, to support the patient and her relatives and to keep meticulous records of fluid balance and of drugs given.

Transfer of the patient with extensive burns

The patient should be prepared for transfer with the application of a temporary wound dressing, preferably clingfilm, and covered with a space blanket or layers of ordinary blankets. As described earlier, there is a high risk of hypothermia, especially during transfer, and wet dressings should not be used. The patient will need to be accompanied by an experienced nurse, as well as by a member of the medical staff if there are airway problems. Monitoring of vital signs and maintenance of the intravenous fluids is usually carried out by the nurse. The speed of travel is frequently rapid, which will make the task of monitoring and recording fluid balance and vital signs very difficult; nonetheless these records are important and should be given, along with the A&E file, to the staff of the burns unit on arrival.

Admission to a regional burns unit

The burns unit staff are usually informed in advance of the imminent admission of a patient with extensive burns. The time between their notification and the actual arrival of the patient, depending on the distance from the referral centre, is used to prepare the environment and to get the necessary equipment ready.

Reception of the patient

When the patient arrives at the unit, she should be greeted and orientated as to place, as many regional burns units receive patients from a wide catchment area. One nurse should be designated to receive the patient from the escorting nurse. Where possible, the patient should be reassured and given a simple explanation of what is being done at every stage of the admission procedure — and thereafter, throughout her stay in the unit. The appearance and smell of the burn wounds may be very upsetting for inexperienced staff, but it is important to appear calm and confident.

The receiving staff must wear protective clothing, e.g. waterproof gowns, plastic aprons or tabards and gloves. This is to protect staff against contact with wound exudate and blood (Locke 1993) and the patient against wound contamination.

The patient should be received into a single room warmed to a temperature of 28°C, as heat loss from the inflamed wounds in addition to evaporative heat loss from the wound exudate can be extensive.

Maintaining the airway

If the patient has inhalation injury, endotracheal intubation and assisted ventilation may have been instituted in the A&E department or may be required at the time of admission to the unit. In any case, all nursing care and observations relative to this treatment must be carried out (see Ch. 3).

Constant observation of respiratory rate and ease, and of the colour of unburned skin and mucosa, must be carried out and recorded. Humidified air or oxygen administered by face mask or nasal catheter may be required.

Weighing the patient

If possible, an accurate body weight in kilograms should be obtained as this is one of the baseline measurements on which the volume of fluid replacement is calculated. Estimation of weight is sometimes carried out but, unless the person doing so is experienced in this, gross over- or undertransfusion may result. In many units the patient is weighed, on a special bed or sling, still covered in the blankets and temporary dressings used for the transfer; these are then gently removed and the patient laid on and covered with sterile sheeting (linen, foam or clingfilm). The original coverings are then weighed and their weight subtracted from the total in order to get a naked weight. It is important to record the weight immediately as the exact figure may easily be forgotten if there is a great deal of activity in the room.

Wound assessment

The medical staff will estimate the depth of the burn wounds and chart their position and extent. Colour photographs may also be taken for recording purposes. In addition to being useful baseline records of wound appearance and distribution, the photographs may, with the patient's permission, be used in evidence in criminal or civil proceedings. Whilst the wounds are exposed, the nurse can take swabs for bacteriological examination from each wound site, e.g. right hand, left hand, chest, neck. This reduces the possibility of wound contamination and the discomfort and possible loss of dignity suffered by the patient during repeated removal of the coverings. The initial wound swabs usually show no bacteriological contamination but provide a useful baseline for further monitoring. The wounds are then covered with a temporary dressing. Specific care will be carried out once the patient's condition has been stabilised.

Bacteriology swabs from nose and throat are also obtained in order to identify commensals which may act as wound pathogens.

Analgesics

It is unusual for patients to complain of pain at this stage, even if their wounds are of partial thickness. If pain is felt, however, intravenous analgesics, usually in the form of morphine, are administered by infusion pump (after the loading dose) at an hourly rate of 20–30 μg/kg. The intramuscular route should never be used if the patient is shocked, as the drug will not be absorbed owing to the peripheral vasoconstriction.

Intravenous fluid replacement

Once an accurate body weight has been obtained and the percentage area of the burn estimated, the medical staff will calculate the volume of intravenous therapy required. There are a number of different formulae in current use but most depend on these two parameters for calculation of the volume to be infused. Regulation of the rate of flow and recording of the volume transfused as well as care of the intravenous site is the responsibility of the nurse. It is usual to use a volumetric intravenous pump to aid accuracy in intravenous infusion as the volumes required in each period may be very large.

Monitoring urine

If this has not been carried out in the A&E department, an indwelling urinary catheter is passed, the bladder emptied and the urine volume measured. A specimen is tested for specific gravity and analysed using a Multistix. The appearance is noted. A urimeter which allows hourly measuring and sampling whilst maintaining a closed system is attached to the catheter. Settle (1996) emphasises the importance of monitoring renal function through regular, frequent measurement of volume and composition of the urine. A volume of 0.5–1.0 ml/kg body weight is generally accepted as indicating that intravenous fluid replacement is satisfactory, although urine concentration (measured by specific gravity or osmolality) must also be estimated in order to assess renal function.

The appearance of the urine is monitored for indications of haemoglobinuria (see Box 30.3) and, if this is present, for indications that it is diminishing. It is important that the nurse inform the medical staff at the first indication of haemoglobinuria, as it is usual for a solution of sodium bicarbonate and an osmotic diuretic (e.g. mannitol) to be prescribed in order to clear the pigments.

Monitoring vital signs

Pulse. If the patient is shocked, the pulse will be rapid and weak; this, combined with generalised oedema, can make manual counting very difficult and mechanical aids such as the pulse oximeter are normally used.

Blood pressure. Where all four limbs have been burned, it has not always been usual practice to record blood pressure. Indeed, even if one limb is unaffected it has been considered more important to ensure effective intravenous replacement than to repeatedly constrict the vessels with a blood pressure cuff. Bainbridge et al (1990), however, found that it is possible to monitor mean arterial pressure by using oscillometric automatic blood pressure monitors with the cuff applied over bulky dressings and this method is useful for monitoring blood pressure in limbs with burns.

The routine measurement of central venous pressure or of arterial pressure is not recommended in most British burns units because of the risk of systemic infection associated with such techniques, especially if the site of entry of the catheter is close to the burn wound. Settle (1996) advises that invasive monitoring should be employed if there has been a delay in starting fluid replacement or if severe respiratory, renal or cardiac impairment exists. However, Schiller & Bray (1996) found that the routine use of the pulmonary artery catheter in patients with extensive burns facilitated optimum levels of fluid replacement and was associated with a significant decrease in overall mortality

Temperature. A good indicator of the state of peripheral perfusion is the difference between core and shell temperatures (see p. 720). In the normal person, under warm conditions, the temperature of a toe is 1–4°C lower than rectal temperature, but in the patient suffering hypovolaemic shock the vasoconstriction is such that the difference may be as much as 15°C. Temperature monitoring is usually facilitated by the use of thermistor probes in preference to the repeated insertion of a rectal thermometer. In some units, a specially designed probe is inserted into the external auditory meatus in preference to using the rectum (see Ch. 22, p. 721). If thermistor probes are not available, it is possible to gauge the shell temperature by feeling the temperature of the peripheries, especially the toes or the tip of the nose.

In addition to monitoring the difference between a normal core temperature and changes in the shell temperature, measuring the core temperature will, of course, also indicate a trend towards hyperpyrexia or hypothermia (see Ch. 22).

Oral intake

Because of the reduction in gastrointestinal tract perfusion which results from hypovolaemia, it is necessary to restrict the volume of oral fluids initially, even if the patient is very thirsty, until it has been established that there is no nausea or vomiting. If there is persistent vomiting, a nasogastric tube is passed and is either allowed to drain freely or aspirated hourly before small amounts of water are given. In some units, a tube is passed routinely in all patients with burns greater than 35% of the body surface. However, studies have shown that early (within 6 h) introduction of intragastric feeding is beneficial in reducing both mortality (Raff et al 1997b) and gastrointestinal ulceration (Raff et al 1997a).

Patient behaviour

In addition to recording clinical measurements as described above, it is useful for the nurse to keep a record of the patient's behaviour, noting restlessness, confusion, distress, apathy, etc., as these along with the measured recordings will give a more complete picture of the patient's condition. If there is cause for concern, monitoring of neurological status is facilitated by use of the Glasgow Coma Scale (see Ch. 28).

The post-shock phase

After the first 36–48 h following injury, the fluid in the interstitial spaces is reabsorbed into the circulation and, although there is continuous fluid loss through exudate and evaporation from the wound surface, there is normally no longer a need for intravenous replacement of fluids. Unless complications arise (see Box 30.4), the intermediate stage of management will have been reached.

Nursing management during the intermediate stage of burn injury recovery follows the basic principles of burn care whatever the extent of body surface involved. Thus nursing priorities include:

- hydration and nutrition
- prevention of infection and local wound care
- pain relief
- psychosocial support for patients and relatives.

Box 30.4 Complications of burn injuries

In some patients with extensive burns, recovery from the initial injury may be complicated by episodes of severe illness such as septicaemia, adult respiratory distress syndrome (ARDS) and/or disseminated intravascular coagulation (DIC), causing them to fluctuate between a satisfactory and a critical condition, perhaps for many weeks. This is especially distressing for the relatives who are trying to cope with the altered appearance of their loved one and who can be given no assurance of eventual recovery; their hopes are raised and dashed repeatedly by their own observations of the patient's condition. Less life-threatening complications include gastrointestinal ulceration and haemorrhage; systemic infection of the respiratory system or urinary tract; wound infection; and wound contraction and scar formation.

Hydration and nutrition

Until wound closure is complete, there will be continuous loss of the water, protein and electrolytes which comprise the wound exudate. In addition, nutritional requirements will be increased because of the elevation in the metabolic rate resulting from trauma, as well as the cellular requirements of wound healing. In patients whose burn area is less than 20% of the body surface, oral intake of a normal diet, perhaps supplemented with high-protein, high-calorie drinks, should be all that is required. Dietary intake should be monitored to allow assessment by the dietician and the patient should be weighed weekly. The patient should be encouraged to take fluids when she is awake and fluid balance should be charted.

In more extensive burns, metabolic requirements will be hugely increased, making enteral nutrition via a nasogastric tube necessary. As a fine-bore tube is used to facilitate patient comfort and reduce trauma, there may be difficulty aspirating gastric contents to ensure correct placement; X-ray confirmation of the position of the tube will therefore be required. There are a number of proprietary preparations of enteral feeds available and the dietician will prescribe the type, volume and rate of administration for each individual. Many manufacturers of enteral feeds produce their own giving sets and volumetric pumps; their instructions should be followed in the use of this equipment. Diarrhoea, nausea and vomiting may complicate enteral feeding. Raff et al (1997a) advise that, rather than commencing with diluted feeds, patient tolerance is best developed by introducing the feed at a slow drip rate and gradually increasing until the required rate is reached. If there is a problem with using the nasogastric route, percutaneous endoscopic gastrostomy (PEG) may be performed; Patton et al (1994) found that the placement of PEG tubes through wound areas did not result in wound complications. Parenteral nutrition is reserved for patients who are unable to achieve adequate nutrition by the enteral route because of the danger of infection associated with the introduction of central lines; peripheral lines are usually impractical because of the limited availability of peripheral veins.

Prevention of infection

Both non-specific and specific mechanisms of the immune system are impaired in patients with extensive burns.

Because of the large areas of skin destruction and the presence of exudate and necrotic tissue, burn wounds rapidly become colonised with bacteria. It has been found that most of the bacteria are acquired from other patients in the ward or unit (Lee et al 1990) and that meticulous attention must be paid to the prevention of cross-infection (see Ch. 16). When possible, the patient should be nursed in a single room and isolation techniques implemented. Muir et al (1987) emphasise that once the patient's wound becomes colonised with an organism, it will soon be found on her bedclothes, personal clothing and on the surface of dressings. Protective clothing must be worn whenever the patient is attended to; this normally consists of plastic tabards or water-resistant gowns. Disposable water-resistant gowns are expensive but are necessary in the care of patients with major burns, as bodily contact between nurse and patient extends well beyond the confines of an apron when handling and moving procedures are carried out or when dressings are being changed. The wearing of masks and caps is usually not necessary except when the wound is exposed. Gloves should be worn during any direct contact with the patient and her immediate surroundings; clean (rather than sterile) gloves may be used for most procedures, apart from those requiring an aseptic technique. Adherence to good handwashing practice requires frequent emphasis, as Lee et al (1990) found that compliance with the correct procedure declines over a period of time following education.

The bacteriological status of the wounds should be monitored regularly by obtaining wound swabs during dressing changes.

THE BURN WOUND

As for any wound, the aim of management is to provide the optimum environment for the natural healing processes to take place (see Ch. 23). However, most burn wounds involve larger areas of the body surface than is common in other types of wound; this in itself presents many problems in wound management.

Most burn wounds exude copious amounts of fluid. This is evident in superficial partial-thickness wounds right from the start, but in deeper wounds the surface is initially dry and, depending on the depth of tissue destruction, it may take days before the eschar becomes saturated with fluid leaking from the damaged capillaries in the deeper tissues. The volume of exudate has been calculated to be as much as 5200 g/m^2 per day in some burn wounds (Lamke et al 1977) and the evaporative water loss may be as much as 20 times the rate of that from normal skin (Quinn et al 1985).

Unless the superficial partial-thickness burn wound becomes infected or is subjected to further trauma, it should re-epithelialise in 7–10 days. As migration of the epithelial cells occurs, the exudate will gradually diminish. Bayley (1990) describes the major aim in burn wound care as obtaining wound closure as soon as possible. In order to meet this goal, management must entail:

- meticulous cleansing and debridement of devitalised tissue in order to prevent infection
- facilitating re-epithelialisation or granulation in preparation for wound grafting
- reducing contractures and scarring
- promoting patient comfort.

Pain control

It is generally agreed that patients with burns experience the greatest pain during therapeutic procedures (Kinsella & Booth 1991). Pain-relieving strategies used in wound care include:

- the administration of morphine and other similar opioids timed to ensure optimum cover during the procedure
- patient-controlled analgesia by intravenous or inhalation methods, e.g. Entonox
- relief of anxiety through explanation, hypnosis and other psychological coping strategies.

The degree of discomfort the patient experiences will be strongly related to the skill of the dresser and to his/her ability to recognise and appreciate the individual's pain tolerance level. Examples of useful pain assessment tools are given in Chapter 19.

Wound cleansing and debridement

The following procedures must be carried out using strict aseptic technique. If done correctly, they may be very time-consuming and, where wounds are extensive, will require a number of staff. In some units, patients with extensive burns will have dressings changed under general anaesthesia with the involvement of a full surgical team.

A number of different methods are currently in use for burn wound cleansing. As long as the wound surface comprises non-viable tissue, the method of choice may be to use saturated gauze or foam pads, although physical cleansing is contraindicated in wounds which are granulating or epithelialising. Depending on the size and site of the wound, less traumatic methods include irrigation via a syringe, showering or immersion in a special tub. There is still debate over the type of solution to be used. The use of sterile normal saline is generally advocated for wound cleansing, but many authors advise the use of antiseptics such as povidone-iodine (Fowler 1994a), Savlon (Settle 1996) or aqueous chlorhexidine 0.1–0.2% (Australia & New Zealand Burn Association (UK) 1996) for the initial cleansing of burns; however, as no rationale is given for the use of the antiseptics, local policy is best adhered to. What is important for both patient comfort and to limit heat loss, especially when the wounds are extensive or on the trunk, is to ensure that the solution used is warmed to body temperature.

Following cleansing, loose devitalised tissue is trimmed using sharp scissors. Specialists vary in their approach to the management of blisters: Bayley (1990) advises that they be left intact unless they appear contaminated or restrict joint movement, while Fowler (1994a) advocates that blisters be punctured. A postal survey (F M Davidson, unpublished work, 1993) found that, out of 32 burns units in the UK, the former method was usual practice in three units, the latter in seven, and that in the large majority (22) it was usual practice to totally debride loose epithelium, including removal of the overlying skin from blisters in order to prevent wound infection. This method is not supported by research and significant pain is experienced when the debrided wound surface is exposed to air. On the other hand, components of blister fluid have been found to inhibit the healing process (Rockwell & Erlich 1990) and to promote wound contraction (Wilson et al 1997). It would therefore appear that evacuating the fluid from intact blisters, allowing the 'roof' of the blister to come into contact with the wound surface and act as a biological dressing, is the most logical approach.

As hair harbours bacteria, it should be clipped short in the area of the wound and a surrounding margin of about 5 cm. Shaving is not advised as it can be painful and cause further wound trauma. Long hair which may encroach on the wound should be restrained with elastic bands or adhesive tape.

Promotion of re-epithelialisation or granulation and the prevention of wound contamination may be facilitated either by exposing the wound or by applying dressings.

Exposing the burn wound

This method is currently most commonly used for burns of the face and occasionally for burns of the perineum. The aim of the exposure method is to provide a dry, intact scab under which re-epithelialisation will take place. Relevant nursing management is described in the section dealing with burns of the face (see p. 904).

Dressing the burn wound

One of the main problems presented by the burn wound is the copious amount of exudate it produces. This strongly influences the choice of dressing material used. Many modern materials are designed to create the optimum environment for healing, i.e. warmth and moisture, but to remove excess exudate. This may be accomplished by highly absorbent materials, such as alginates, hydrocolloids or hydrophilic foams, or by materials which allow rapid transmission of water vapour (e.g. Lyofoam). These types of dressing can be used successfully in burns which are of a relatively small area, but they require a substantial margin to be in contact with unburned skin to prevent leakage of exudate. Thus their use is often not feasible for large wounds.

For extensive burns, no materials have yet been found to exceed the benefits of conventional dressings (Lawrence 1996b). These comprise an inner layer of mesh, usually impregnated with paraffin or water-miscible cream, which may or may not provide a base for antibacterial agents; layers of cotton gauze or sterile J cloths (Fowler 1994b); cotton wool or Gamgee. The materials may be retained with cotton conforming bandages, or on the trunk by stitching or stapling. The aim of conventional dressings is to allow exudate to filter through the layers and for water to evaporate from the surface of the dressing, thus preventing maceration of the wound. It is important, therefore, that the surface of the dressing is not occluded with a non-porous material such as many of the adhesive tapes used to retain bandages. Other non-porous materials which may come into contact with the surface of the dressing include plastic mattress and pillow covers; such contact should be avoided by the use of foam wedges, slings and special mattresses or beds. If the outer surface of the dressing does become moist, the outer layers only are changed under aseptic conditions. To change the whole dressing unnecessarily exposes the burn to contamination from the atmosphere and may disrupt healing if the innermost layer has become adherent.

The frequency of scheduled dressing changes depends on the depth and state of the wound and on the properties of any medication incorporated in the innermost layer. Superficial partial-thickness burns may have their dressings left undisturbed for 7–10 days (estimated time of healing) unless there are indications for investigating the wound, such as signs of infection. More frequent changes (daily, every second day or twice weekly) are required in deeper burns as the presence of necrotic tissue increases the likelihood of bacterial growth. In such cases, antibacterial agents are normally used. For many years, silver sulphadiazine cream (in the UK, Flamazine) has been a popular antibacterial application for burn wounds throughout the developed world. However, because of its tendency to change the appearance of the wound and to macerate non-viable tissue (making surgical excision difficult), current interest is being expressed in silver sulphadiazine with cerium nitrate (Flammacerium). In addition to its antibacterial effects, Sparkes (1997) found that cerium nitrate inhibits the release of toxins from the burn eschar.

The ideal wound cover is the patient's own skin in the form of a graft (autograft) which 'takes' to provide wound closure. Other types of skin graft, i.e. from other humans (allograft) or from animals (xenograft), provide only temporary cover except in the case of identical twins. Sheets of epidermal cells (keratinocytes) may be cultured from the patient's own skin but it may take some weeks before sufficient material is available and current research indicates that, for optimum survival and growth when applied to the wound, they require a collagen-based carrier (Shakespeare 1993). Clinical trials of a number of types of collagen-based sheets, e.g. Dermagraft (Morgan 1997) and Integra (Cameron 1997), are currently in progress.

Care of burn wounds prior to skin grafting

The necrotic tissue has to separate from the wound bed before granulation tissue, suitable for skin grafting, is produced. This process of separation may take many weeks and is aided by judicial trimming of loose slough at each dressing change. In relatively small wounds, the process may be accelerated through the use of hydrogels or hydrocolloids.

Surgical removal of necrotic tissue may be carried out, usually within the first 4 days following injury. The tissue is either excised with a scalpel or shaved down to a viable (bleeding) surface with a skin grafting knife. This procedure can result in extensive blood loss, and multiple transfusion may be required. The freshly prepared bed is usually skin grafted immediately, but if the bleeding is difficult to control, the skin grafts will be harvested and stored in order that they can be applied without a second operation, usually within the following 48 h.

A skin graft 'takes' by the ingrowth of capillaries from the wound into the graft, a process which takes only a few days. This will be disrupted if there is any blood, serum or pus preventing contact between graft and wound. Other factors which can cause disruption of the graft include any shearing of the graft/wound interface and the presence of β-haemolytic *Streptococcus*, group A (*Strep. pyogenes*) which produces streptokinase, an activator of plasmin which is fibrinolytic. Sometimes the surgeon will choose not to apply a dressing to a newly grafted area. Nursing staff will be responsible for ensuring that there is no collection of fluid under the graft. This is done by gently rolling a rolled-up swab from the centre to the margins of the graft, thus expressing any blood or serum. An aseptic technique is employed and great care is required to prevent the graft shearing on its bed.

The skin graft donor area is a very superficial wound and as a result can be very painful. For the first 48 h or so it produces large amounts of bloodstained exudate and is usually dressed with calcium alginate followed by a conventional dressing which is managed in the same way as that covering a superficial burn. The speed of re-epithelialisation depends on the depth of dermis removed along with the epidermis but is normally between 10 days and 2 weeks.

Ideally, the dressing is left intact until it falls off. Injudicious early investigation will cause further trauma and delay healing. The alginate dressing dries out as epithelialisation occurs but readily regains its gel consistency when soaked with normal saline.

Care of special areas

The face. The most common method of managing facial burns is that of exposure. Bulky absorptive dressings which extend well beyond the wound margin are liable to encroach on the facial features, which should not be covered.

The face becomes very oedematous and the head should be elevated as soon as the patient's condition allows. Drying out of the exudate is encouraged in order to produce a thin scab. The longer the wound exudes, the greater is the build-up of serum; this will produce a thick crust which may never completely dry out and is more likely to crack. Rapid drying may be facilitated by regular aseptic application of well wrung-out saline swabs which quickly absorb the exudate and are then removed (barely damp material absorbs liquid more effectively than dry material). Careful use of a hair dryer on a cool setting will also speed the drying process but care should be taken that the patient is able to achieve complete closure of the eyelids before such air flow is directed at the face.

Once the scab has formed, it will be similar to a cosmetic face mask and greatly restrict facial movement. Because of this it is usual practice in some units to apply a thin layer of liquid paraffin to the areas around the eyes and mouth, as mobility of these areas is most important (Wilding 1990). The resultant stickiness may allow adherence of debris and it is important to cleanse these areas gently with saline on a regular basis.

Oedema of the periorbital region can cause closure of the eyelids. This is very frightening for the patient, who may think the blindness is permanent. The nurse should warn the patient that eyelid closure may occur and assure her that the swelling will lessen in a few days. Eye drops or ointment will be prescribed in order to reduce the possibility of conjunctivitis. The use of artificial tears will make the patient more comfortable.

Oedema of the lips may cause eversion of the oral mucosa, which should not be allowed to dry out. The skin of the lips should be kept lubricated with yellow soft paraffin and care must be taken when oral hygiene is being performed. The use of a small child's toothbrush, by patient or nurse, will help to maintain normal mouth care and, if the patient is unable to eat, regular mouthwashes should be given. If oral intake is allowed the patient may experience difficulty in drinking from a normal cup; a feeding cup with a spout is preferable to using a straw as the patient may find it difficult to exert just the right pressure to allow suction without collapsing the straw.

Oedema of the ears may cause them to jut out at right angles to the head, making them more susceptible to further trauma. If the pinna produces exudate, this is liable to trickle into the external auditory meatus, where it will collect and dry out at the level of the ear drum, reducing the patient's ability to hear. This may not be detected until some time later in which case it may prove very difficult to evacuate the plug. It is easy to avert this problem by inserting a small piece of gauze just at the opening of the meatus to absorb the exudate, changing it as necessary. The ears may be dressed lightly with a conventional dressing or have gauze spread with an antibacterial ointment (e.g. Flamazine) gently applied. The ears will be very painful when touched and it is useful to elevate the head slightly off the pillow, using either a well-padded foam ring or a foam wedge, as this will reduce the possibility of the ears coming in contact with the pillow.

The lower nostrils should be kept free of exudate build-up by regular cleansing with a dampened cotton bud. If exudate dries on the nasal hairs, the crust will occlude the nostrils and its removal will be very painful indeed. This problem may be prevented by the application of a light smear of soft yellow paraffin just inside the nostrils.

The beard in male patients also becomes incorporated in the crust as it grows. This does not usually present problems until the scab is separating from the newly epithelialised facial skin (in the case of deep burns, the hair follicles will be destroyed and no hair growth will occur). Once the scab starts to lift it may be rehydrated using a moisturising lotion or hydrogel; this causes swelling of the scab, which will then no longer fit the contours of the face, and softens it to allow painless removal. Many men prefer to keep their beard for a time, but if they wish to be clean-shaven, the use of an electric razor is preferable as it causes less trauma to the skin.

Scab removal. As the scab lifts on the rest of the face, loose areas should be trimmed with care. There may be a strong temptation on the part of both nurse and patient to remove as much as possible, as the satisfaction of revealing nice pink skin can prove irresistible. However, it must be borne firmly in mind that removing adherent crust causes trauma and may increase the possibility of scar formation. Newly epithelialised skin needs to be moisturised regularly with a bland cream to keep it from drying out (see Box 30.5).

Box 30.5 Care of newly healed skin

Care of newly healed skin consists of washing with mild soap, rinsing well, patting dry and applying a moisturising cream. Newly healed skin does not produce sufficient sebum to prevent it from drying out or cracking on the surface; neither does it produce enough melanin to prevent burning if exposed to sunlight. It must therefore be protected by covering with clothing or by high protection factor sun creams for at least a year.

The hands. Burns of the hands are most commonly treated by the application of polythene bags or gloves (with or without the addition of an antibacterial cream) in order to facilitate movement and thus prevent joint stiffness and allow the patient a degree of independence. Because the polythene does not allow evaporation of water, the wound environment is very moist and the non-burned skin will become macerated. As large volumes of exudate will collect, it is usual to apply several layers of gauze around the wrist before applying the bag to absorb some of the exudate. The bags should be changed on a daily or more frequent basis, and the hand gently cleansed at each change.

In recent years there has been increased interest in the use of vapour-permeable gloves or bags. Gore-tex material made into draw-string bags has been found to produce less maceration, less weight from the accumulated exudate to restrict mobility, and to have fewer problems associated with leakage of exudate. The material is much stronger than polythene and can be washed and autoclaved (Muddiman 1989). Terril et al (1991) found that the opacity of the material was preferred by patients and their visitors and that the material allowed a more secure grip. However, the Gore-bag is no longer manufactured and the alternative, disposable expanded polytetrafluoroethylene (PTFE) membrane gloves have been found to be less cost-effective (Hall 1997).

Limbs. In order to reduce oedema formation, burned limbs are elevated and exercised on a regular basis, unless freshly laid skin grafts preclude movement.

Joints. Wound contraction is an integral part of the healing process, but excessive contraction leads to dysfunction and deformity. As flexor surfaces are more liable to contract, joints must be correctly positioned, with compensatory hyperextension especially of the wrists and neck. Physiotherapy should be carried out regularly, with adequate analgesic cover, to maintain a full range of movements of all joints. However, splinting may be necessary to arrest or correct contracture formation.

Scar formation

Scar formation is part of the maturation phase of the healing process. In wounds healing by secondary intention, the scar often appears red and is raised above the level of the surrounding skin (hypertrophic). Hypertrophic scarring is a well known complication following burn injury and the resulting disfigurement causes great distress. The most common means of prevention is the application of external pressure, usually effected by the use of specially designed elasticated garments which can be made to fit any anatomical part. The garments should be worn, apart from bathing and skin care, for 24 h/day; treatment should continue for at least 9 months and a pressure of at least 24 mmHg is necessary for the treatment to be effective. Patients are provided with at least two sets of garments, which are alternately washed and worn.

Elastic garments are not very effective for applying pressure to concavities on the body surface, especially on the face around the nose and mouth. For treatment of these areas, a rigid, or semi-rigid, transparent face mask can be made. One technique which does not rely on pressure to reduce the hypertrophy and redness of scars is the use of silicone gel sheets (Hurren 1995). These need to be retained in place with light bandages or adhesive tape and must be removed regularly for washing as they are reusable for a few applications. The sheets are relatively expensive and tend to be used only when problems arise in pressure therapy. A cheaper and more practical method described by Davey (1997) is the use of adhesive tapes such as Hypafix and Mefix applied directly onto florid scars, with the application of Silastic elastomer on areas when early thickening is detected.

PSYCHOLOGICAL EFFECTS OF BURN INJURIES

The disfigurement and impaired function which result from wound contracture and scar formation are generally accepted as the major sequelae of burn injuries, causing great distress and psychological problems for the patient and her loved ones. This, however, describes the long-term view and does not consider that for the patient and her family the psychological effects start at the time of injury.

Partridge (1990) gives a graphic account of his experiences when he sustained burns in a road traffic accident and notes that 'being on fire is unforgettable, you will recall those seconds with crystal clarity for the rest of your life'. Many patients voice their relief at being alive in the immediate period following the accident, but as the implications of their injury sink in, their emotions and behaviour may begin to go through a series of changes.

Bereni-Marzouk et al (1981) describe four psychological phases experienced by patients hospitalised following burn injuries:

- critical
- stabilisation
- recovery
- pre-discharge.

This categorisation will be adopted in the following discussion of the problems commonly encountered by individuals with burn injuries.

The critical phase

During the early stages of treatment, the patient will be preoccupied by bodily feelings and by the care provided by nursing and medical staff. If her wounds are extensive and complications arise she will require constant attendance, perhaps for lengthy periods of time, which may result in intensive care psychosis (see Ch. 29, p. 890). Briggs (1991) emphasises the need for nursing staff to be aware of the harmful effects of intensive care, providing communication and controlling environmental factors in order to promote sleep and sensory balance. Nightmares associated with the accident are common at this stage, as are fears of dying. Constant reassurance and reorientation will be necessary.

Stabilisation

When the patient reaches this stage, anxiety related to survival is replaced with fears for the future, both short and long term. In the short term, stress is related to anticipation of pain and many patients become depressed or are hostile towards the nursing staff. They may regress in their ability to cope with activities of living and demand care and attention. This is perhaps the most difficult phase for the unit staff to cope with. Pain control helps to reduce patient anxiety related to wound care, and physiotherapy and monitoring of pain should continue throughout the period of hospitalisation.

Although there is a tendency to expect that there will be more pain the greater the injury and that pain will reduce in time, in their study Choiniere et al (1989) found no correlation between pain scores and the time elapsed following injury, or between pain scores and size of burn.

Longer-term anxieties include the fear of disfigurement and of losing function and former roles. Nursing staff can help the patient come to terms with her changed situation by being honest and supportive and allowing her to grieve. The first look in the mirror should not be accidental but a planned occasion with the patient making the choice whether to be alone or to be accompanied by nursing staff or loved ones. Although she may have some idea of her changed appearance from watching the reactions of her visitors, she will see the true extent of her disfigurement only when she first looks in a mirror. Some patients have glimpsed their reflection in the spectacles of attendant personnel, in darkened windows or in plate glass doors and later reported that they were able to deny their appearance, attributing it to a flaw in the glass. If the hands are not injured, the patient may gauge contour and textural changes through touch, but the reality of her changed appearance will still be a great shock.

Manifestations of hostility may range from refusal to cooperate with treatment, through cursing and swearing, to actual bodily assault. Sometimes the hostility is directed only towards certain nurses and the patient may manipulate the situation to create discord among the staff. Care should be planned to ensure a consistent approach by all staff but, especially if primary nursing is practised, it may be necessary to reallocate staff. If the patient's behaviour is uncooperative to the extent that it will interfere with her recovery, behaviour modification techniques may be in order. A contract may be drawn up specifying the type of behaviour expected of the patient and describing the rewards which will be given or withheld accordingly. Many such contracts exist informally, e.g. the patient may be allowed a small aperitif if she eats all her supper, but Wallace (1987) advocates a more formal agreement.

Q **30.2** To what extent do we modify the behaviour of others in our daily lives?

Regression in physical ability may also be managed by behavioural modification, with the patient being set easily achievable tasks such as pouring a drink from her own water jug and being encouraged to feel a sense of achievement when she does so. Many patients regress when there is a sudden, unexplained reduction in the amount of nursing care they receive. Explanation about their improving condition, and patient involvement in identifying needs and planning the reduction of care can help to alleviate this problem.

Recovery

This phase is marked by the patient beginning to rediscover former interests and pleasures. She may, for example, take more notice of the goings-on in the unit and of the other patients. When possible, mixing with the other patients should be encouraged; the patient's involvement in small tasks such as distributing newspapers will also aid independence and self-esteem. When disfigurement is highly visible, such as on the face and hands, the patient may not wish to mix with others and will require a great deal of support from staff as well as from visiting family and friends. Griffiths (1989) offers the following list of coping strategies which the nursing staff can explore with the patient:

- Do not give in to fear.
- Learn to control fear and anxiety.
- Practise positive self-talk.
- Concentrate on relevant pieces of information.
- Do not interpret discomfort as rejection.
- Find your own way of acknowledging the disfigurement.
- Congratulate success.

The pre-discharge phase

Patients frequently experience ambivalence about leaving the safe confines of the unit where they are known and accepted. The actual discharge may be graduated by the introduction of progressively longer visits home and by giving the patient the opportunity to discuss the pleasures and problems she encountered. Williams & Griffiths (1991) emphasise the patient's need for practical advice in the form of staff-led discussions during the period prior to or immediately following discharge from hospital in order to reduce the psychological sequelae of burn injuries. Liaison with the primary health care team will ensure continuity of care, and involvement of the social work department and occupational therapists in the community will provide financial and practical help in the resumption of home life.

After discharge

It is possible that the patient will need to return to hospital for clinic appointments and, later on, for plastic surgery to improve appearance and function — a process which may involve many operations over a number of years. Many patients suffer long-term psychological problems including depression, anxiety and other post-traumatic stress symptoms. In 1988, Wallace found that the provision of continuing support was inadequate and there is no evidence that this has improved with regard to the NHS; it would therefore appear that there is a growing need for voluntary groups such as Changing Faces.

No matter how high the standard of care provided, the patient who suffers extensive burns may never return fully to her former physical or emotional functioning — a fact which can only serve to emphasise the need for greater effort in the field of burn prevention.

REFERENCES

Adams L E, Purdue G F, Hunt J L 1991 Tap-water scald burns: awareness is not the problem. Journal of Burn Care and Rehabilitation 12(1): 91–95

Australia and New Zealand Burn Association Ltd (UK) 1996 Emergency management of severe burns course manual. UK version for The British Burn Association

Bainbridge L C, Simmons H M, Elliot D 1990 The use of automatic blood pressure monitors in the burned patient. British Journal of Plastic Surgery 43: 322–324

Bayley E W 1990 Wound healing in the patient with burns. Nursing Clinics of North America 25(1): 205–221

Beeley J M, Clark R J 1996 Respiratory problems in fire victims. In: Settle J A D (ed) Principles and practice of burns management. Churchill Livingstone, Edinburgh

Bereni-Marzouk T, Giacalone L, Thieulard L et al 1981 Behavioural changes in burned adult patients during their stay in hospital. Burns 8(5): 365–368

Bouter L M, van Rijn O J L, Kok G 1990 Importance of planned health education for burn injury prevention. Burns 16(3): 198–202

Brady H R, Brenner B M, Lieberthal W 1996 Acute renal failure. In: Brenner B M (ed) The kidney, vol II, 5th edn. WB Saunders, Philadelphia

Briggs D 1991 Preventing ICU psychosis. Nursing Times 87(19): 30–31

Bull J P, Lennard-Jones J E 1949 The impairment of sensation in burns and its clinical application as a test of the depth of loss. Clinical Science 8: 155

Cameron S 1997 Changes in burn patient care. British Journal of Theatre Nursing 7(5): 5–7

Central Statistical Office (CSO) 1991 Social trends 21. HMSO, London

Choiniere M, Melzack R, Rondeau J et al 1989 The pain of burns: characteristics and correlates. Journal of Trauma 29(11): 1531–1539

Davey R B 1997 The use of contact media for burn scar hypertrophy. Journal of Wound Care 6(2): 80–82

Duggan D, Quine S 1995 Burn injuries and characteristics of burn patients in New South Wales, Australia. Burns 21(2): 83–89

Ellis A, Rylah L T A 1990 Transfer of the thermally injured patient. British Journal of Hospital Medicine 44: 206–208

Endoh Y, Kawakami M, Orringer E P, Peterson H D, Meyer A A 1992 Causes and time course of acute haemolysis after burn injury in the rat. Journal of Burn Care and Rehabilitation 13: 203–209

Fowler A 1994a Nursing management of a patient with burns. British Journal of Nursing 3(21): 1105–1112

Fowler A 1994b Burns care and management. Journal of Tissue Viability 4(1): 3–9

Gowar J P, Lawrence J C 1995 The incidence, causes and treatment of minor burns. Journal of Wound Care 4(2): 71–74

Griffiths E 1989 More than skin deep. Nursing Times 85(40): 34–36

Hall M 1997 Minor burns and hand burns: comparing treatment methods. Professional Nurse 12(7): 489–491

Harper R D, Dickson W A 1995 Reducing the burn risk to elderly persons living in residential care. Burns 21(3): 205–208

Hatherill J R, Till G O, Bruner L H, Ward P A 1986 Thermal injury, intravascular haemolysis, and toxic oxygen products. Journal of Clinical Investigation 78(3): 629–636

Haum A, Perbix W, Hack H J, Stark G B, Spilker G, Doehn M 1995 Alcohol and drug abuse in burn injuries. Burns 21(3): 194–199

Herbert K, Lawrence J C 1989 Chemical burns. Burns 15(6): 381–384

Hurren J S 1995 Rehabilitation of the burned patient. Burns 21(2): 116–126

International Society for Burn Injuries (ISBI) 1979 Constitution.

Kinsella J, Booth M G 1991 Pain relief in burns. Burns 17(5): 391–395

Lamke L O, Nilsson G E, Reithner H L 1977 The evaporative water loss from burns and the water vapour permeability of grafts and artificial membranes used in the treatment of burns. Burns 3: 159–165

Lawrence J C, Cason C 1994 Kettle scalds. Journal of Wound Care 3(6): 289–292

Lawrence J C, Wilkins M D 1986 The epidemiology of burns. In: Lawrence J C (ed) Burncare, a teaching symposium arranged by the British Burn Association. Smith & Nephew, Hull

Lawrence J C 1996a First aid measures for the treatment of burns and scalds. Journal of Wound Care 5(7): 319–322

Lawrence J C 1996b Dressings for burns. In: Settle J A D (ed) Principles and practice of burns management. Churchill Livingstone, Edinburgh

Lee J J, Marvin J A, Heimbach D M et al 1990 Infection control in a burn centre. Journal of Burn Care and Rehabilitation 11(6): 575–580

Linares A Z, Linares H A 1990 Burn prevention: the need for a comprehensive approach. Burns 16(4): 281–285

Locke G 1993 Infection precautions in a burns unit. Nursing Standard 7(48): 25–29

Lund C C, Browder N C 1944 The estimation of areas of burns. Surgery, Gynaecology and Obstetrics 79: 352–354

McLoughlin E 1995 A simple guide to burn prevention. Burns 21(3): 226–229

Mercer N S G 1988 With or without? A cooling study. Burns 14(5): 397–398

Morgan D A 1997 Formulary of wound management products, 7th edn. Euromed Communications, Surrey

Moritz A R, Henriques F C 1947 Studies of thermal injury: the relative importance of time and surface temperature in the causation of cutaneous burns. American Journal of Pathology 23: 695–699

Muddiman R 1989 A new concept in hand burn dressing. Nursing Standard 52(3): 1–3
Muir I F K, Barclay T L, Settle J A D 1987 Burns and their treatment, 3rd edn. Butterworths, London
Partridge J 1990 Changing faces: the challenge of facial disfigurement. Penguin, London
Patton M L, Haith L R, Germain T J, Goldman W T, Raymond J T 1994 The use of percutaneous endoscopic gastrostomy tubes in burn patients. Surgical Endoscopy 8(9): 1067–1071
Quinn K J, Courtney J M, Evans J H et al 1985 Principles of burn dressings. Biomaterials 6(6): 369–377
Raff T, Germann G, Hartmann B 1997a The value of early enteral nutrition in the prophylaxis of stress ulceration in the severely burned patient. Burns 23(4): 313–318
Raff T, Hartmann B, Germann G 1997b Early intragastric feeding of seriously burned and long-term ventilated patients; a review of 55 patients. Burns 23(1): 19–25
Rockwell W B, Ehrlich H P 1990 Should burn blister fluid be evacuated? Journal of Burn Care and Rehabilitation 11(1): 93–95
Rose J K, Herndon D N 1997 Advances in the treatment of burn patients. Burns 23(suppl 1): S19–26
Sarhadi N S, Kincaid R, McGregor J C, Watson J D 1995 Burns in the elderly in the South East of Scotland: review of 176 patients treated in the Bangour burns unit (1982–91) and burns inpatients in the region (1975–91). Burns 21(2): 91–95
Sawada Y, Urushidate S, Yotsuyanagi T, Ishita K 1997 Is prolonged and excessive cooling of a scalded wound effectve? Burns 23(1): 55–58
Schiller W R, Bray R C 1996 Haemodynamic and oxygen transport monitoring in management of burns. New Horizons 4(4): 475–482
Settle J A D 1996 General management. In: Settle J A D (ed) Principles and practice of burns management. Churchill Livingstone, Edinburgh
Shakespeare P 1993 Burn wound healing. Journal of Tissue Viability 3(1): 16–21
Sparkes B G 1997 Immunological responses to thermal injury. Burns 23(2): 106–113
Spitz M C, Towbin J A, Shantz D, Adler L E 1994 Risk factors for burns as a consequence of seizures in persons with epilepsy. Epilepsia 35(4): 764–767
Steinmann S, Shackford S R, Davis J W 1990 Implications of admission hypothermia in trauma patients. Journal of Trauma 30(2): 200–202
Terril P J, Kedwards S M, Lawrence J C 1991 The use of Gore-tex bags for hands. Burns 17(2): 161–165
Tones K, Tilford S, Robinson Y K 1990 Health education. Chapman and Hall, London
Van Rijn O J L, Bouter L M, Meertens R M 1989 The aetiology of burns in developed countries: review of the literature. Burns 15(4): 217–221
Walker A R 1990 Fatal tapwater scald burns in the USA, 1979–86. Burns 16(1): 49–52
Wallace A B 1951 The exposure treatment of burns. Lancet i: 501–504
Wallace L 1987 Behavioural contracts. Nursing Times 83(47): 33–34
Wallace L 1988 Abandoned to a social death. Nursing Times 84(10): 34–37
Wilding P A 1990 Care of respiratory burns: hard work can bring spectacular results. Professional Nurse 5(8): 412–419
Williams E E, Griffiths T A 1991 Psychological consequences of burn injury. Burns 17(6): 478–480
Wilson A M, McGrouther D A, Eastwood M, Brown R A 1997 The effect of burn blister fluid on fibroblast contraction. Burns 23(4): 306–312
Wyllie F J, Sutherland 1991 Measurement of surface temperature as an aid to the diagnosis of burn depth. Burns 17(2): 123–128
Yuan Y, Fang Z Y, Zhang Z H 1988 Changes in the rate of haemolysis during the early stage after burns in the rabbit. Burns 14(5): 365–368

USEFUL ADDRESS

Changing Faces
1 & 2 Junction Mews
Paddington
London W2 1PN

THE PATIENT WITH CANCER

Bernadette M. Byrne

31

INTRODUCTION

Cancer is a disease with a profound effect on every aspect of life, whether physical, psychological, social or spiritual. There are two principal reasons for this. First, cancer is often associated with suffering and death. Secondly, despite improvements in cure rates, many uncertainties persist concerning the nature and causes of cancer and the methods of prevention and cure. This uncertainty serves to perpetuate various myths and fears surrounding the disease, some of which are described in Box 31.1.

Q **31.1** (a) What words come to mind when you think of the word 'cancer'?
(b) Ask the same question of a few friends, or a member of your family.
(c) How do their responses compare with yours?
(d) Is their overall attitude one of optimism or of pessimism?

Indeed, cancer is a serious social problem, costing much in human and financial terms. One in 3 people in the UK will develop cancer in their lifetime, and 1 in 4 deaths are caused by cancer (Cancer Research Campaign 1999a). Incidence also appears to be rising, and cancer has now overtaken heart disease as Scotland's number one killer (Cancer Research Campaign 1998). Globally, by 2020, there are likely to be 20 million new cancer patients each year, double the present number (Oliver 1999). While statistics present a bleak picture, nurses and other health professionals should be aware that there are reasonable grounds for a positive approach that will foster realistic hope in their patients. Sikora (1999), as chief of the WHO cancer programme, believes that 25% of cancers could be prevented using existing knowledge, and 33% cured with today's technology, rising to 50% in the next 25 years (Sikora 1999).

Before reading further, consider your own knowledge and attitudes towards cancer by carrying out the following exercise.

Box 31.1 Sociohistorical perspectives

In medieval times, cancer was believed to be contagious, caused by lack of cleanliness and even by a form of demon possession (Nery 1986).

Society

The cultural legacy of historical beliefs is the aura of fear and shame that surrounds the disease even today. Benner & Wrubel (1989) examine the phenomenon of cancer from a sociocultural rather than a medical perspective and examine the highly metaphorical language in which the disease process is described — for example, in terms of 'decay' and 'disintegration' or of an 'invasion' by an 'alien army' of 'colonising' cells.

This tendency to view cancer symbolically is also evident in the causes to which many patients attribute their disease, ranging from divine retribution to a stressful life event, a fall or physical blow, dirt or, very commonly, personal failing (Walker 1990).

Cancer stigma

Fitzpatrick et al (1984) define 'stigma' as the disgrace associated with some condition or behaviour which 'breaks the rules' of society, even if unintentionally. A study by Mathieson & Stam (1995) reported that all but two persons they interviewed spontaneously mentioned stigma-related issues, despite the fact that a question about stigma was never asked. One patient commented that she felt as if she had 'leprosy' and was no longer 'part of the human race'.

For individuals with cancer, insurance cancellations or refusal, job discrimination and problems with reintegration into school or the workplace are manifestations of the persistent social stigma of cancer.

In favourable circumstances, most people are not conscious of these underlying social attitudes. However, a person with cancer may soon become painfully aware of the degradation and isolation which accompanies his disease. Family and friends may struggle to maintain a relationship with the person at the same time as they avoid confronting the crises precipitated by his illness.

Media coverage and the widespread availability of accurate information about cancer may be slowly replacing such negative attitudes with a more realistic and helpful public awareness. However, cancer remains a taboo subject, as anyone who tries to discuss it in social gatherings will discover.

Patients and their families bring these attitudes and beliefs into their cancer experience. Assessment of their perception of the situation is an essential first step in the provision of supportive care.

31.2 Consider the following statements. Decide whether they are true, partly true, or false:

(a) Everyone with cancer dies from the disease.
(b) Cancer is the cause of the highest number of deaths per year in the UK.
(c) Cancer is the result of a person's lifestyle.
(d) Cancer is hereditary.
(e) Certain personality types are more prone to cancer than others.
(f) Some forms of cancer are contagious.
(g) Most persons with cancer are disfigured in some way by the disease.
(h) Cancer patients can enjoy many years of normal, productive life.

31.2 *(cont'd)*

(i) A cancerous growth is a collection of cells that are foreign to the body.
(j) The side-effects of all cancer treatments are particularly severe.
(k) Everyone with cancer suffers pain at some point during the disease.

Oncology as a speciality

The publication of the Calman-Hine/Calman report has provided a policy framework for the commissioning of cancer services across the UK, heralding fundamental changes in the organisation and provision of cancer care (Department of Health 1995, Morris et al 1998). This restructuring has been in response to concerns regarding variable patterns of care and disappointing death rates — noticeably in breast cancer — in comparison with other countries. In some parts of the UK, patients with cancer remain predominantly cared for by general clinicians in general wards.

The principles upon which this framework is based include:

- the need for an integrated service encompassing primary care, designated cancer units and centres
- the delivery of a uniformly high level of cancer care based on a collaborative network of expertise comprising primary, secondary and tertiary care
- the provision of care as close to the patient's home as possible
- a commitment to patient-centred care with a clear statement that services should address psychosocial as well as medical needs.

The vision of the Calman report is that care is focused around the patient and his family, care being delivered by coordinated services in genuine partnership with each other. For this vision to become a reality, effective communication is the key, with smooth systems for patient referral to the hospital, community and voluntary sectors. Patients should have access to all available services, fulfilling their needs and supporting them through their cancer experience.

Acknowledgement is also given to the need for investment in education, research and professional development of all health professionals. Core skills in communication, teamwork and palliative care are advocated. Students and newly qualified health professionals need to understand the multidisciplinary nature of cancer management within and outside the hospital, appreciating the roles of all persons providing patient care (Department of Health 1995, RCN 1996a,b).

The cancer process

The process of cancer or carcinogenesis has many stages and occurs over time. Cancer develops when cells grow and divide uncontrollably outside the normal cell regulatory mechanisms. These cells have no specific tissue function, but are able to spread from the site of origin to distant tissues. The last two decades have seen the field of molecular biology making great progress in unravelling the steps involved in this process. However, there still remain many unanswered questions.

A critical component in understanding the cancer process and rationale for treatment is a knowledge of the structure and function of cells, the role of DNA and the reproductive cell cycle — see Russell (1994) Tortora & Grabowski and (1996) for further reading.

When a cell divides, a chain of chemical signals controls the process. The links are proteins such as growth factors, receptors, cytoplasmic message-carrying proteins and cell nucleus regulatory proteins. Specific genes in the cell DNA express these proteins during protein synthesis. The basic cause of cancer is damage to one or more of these genes. Such damage may occur from either errors in DNA replication during mitosis or exposure to environmental agents. In the transformation to a cancerous growth, there is a progressive series of mutations of genes regulating cell division and differentiation.

Exciting research into these cell regulatory genes over the past two decades has discovered that 'proto-oncogenes' promote cell division ('on switch') and 'tumour suppressor genes' inhibit cell division ('off switch'). The p53 tumour suppressor gene is mutated in at least 50% of human cancers (Carson & Lois 1995). The protein from a normal p53 gene halts the cell cycle in the G1 phase at a control checkpoint before DNA replication occurs. This allows the cell to repair any DNA damage identified. If, however, genomic damage is excessive, the cell undergoes a programmed cell death (apoptosis). For this reason, p53 is often referred to as the 'guardian of the genome'. When p53 is mutated, cells do not repair defective DNA and continue to replicate. Changes in p53 are not a direct cause of cancer, but cells lacking in p53 are at high risk of malignant transformation (Sikora 1994).

Cancer cells therefore grow in an erratic and uncoordinated way because of an alteration in cell regulatory mechanisms. As tumours grow by repeated cell divisions, their rate of growth is often defined in terms of 'doubling time'. Tumours vary greatly in their doubling time but, contrary to popular belief, their growth is not as rapid as that of certain normal tissues. For a tumour growth to exceed 1 or 2 mm, it requires a blood supply for survival; therefore a capillary network from the surrounding host tissue is initiated by proteins or angiogenic factors, e.g. fibroblast growth factor (FGF) and tumour necrosing factor (TNF) (Fidler 1997, Franks & Teich 1997).

At any one time, a tumour consists of a mixture of cells, some dividing or growing, some dying or dead. Tumour cells appear to have the capacity to develop various strains within one tumour, each with different properties and, unfortunately, different levels of resistance to anticancer treatments.

Tumour histology

Histology is the study of types of tissue, both normal and diseased. A definitive cancer diagnosis is usually made by histological examination of tumour cells under a microscope.

Histology reports often refer to the degree of differentiation of tumour cells. Well-differentiated tumour cells bear considerable resemblance to the host tissue in structure and function. These tumours are usually slower-growing and are less likely to metastasise (spread); they often respond well to treatment. Undifferentiated, or anaplastic, tumour tissue has lost all resemblance to the corresponding normal tissue. It grows and disseminates (spreads) more rapidly than differentiated tissue and usually responds poorly to treatment.

Malignant and benign tumours. The word 'cancer' is a general term used to describe all malignant neoplasms (i.e. a new growth of tissue, or tumour). A tumour may be benign or malignant, although this distinction is not always clear. Brain tumours, for example, may be benign in nature (e.g. meningioma) but because of their location within a limited space may prove to be fatal.

In general, benign tumour cells are well differentiated and slow-growing and do not invade surrounding tissue or form metastases in distant tissue. Once removed, they rarely recur. Malignant tumours have the opposite properties, albeit to varying degrees. A malignant tumour poses a threat to life mainly because of its ability to proliferate destructively into surrounding tissue and to metastasise to other parts of the body.

Tumours are named according to their tissue of origin (see Table 31.1). Tumours of one organ may be of various tissue types with varying behaviours and prognoses. For example, adenocarcinoma of the lung behaves in a much less malignant way than small cell carcinoma of the lung, which carries a very poor prognosis.

Cancer is therefore not one disease but many, each type behaving in a very different way from the others. This must be taken into account in all discussions about cancer and in all relationships with cancer patients.

The spread of cancer (see Fig. 31.1)

The term 'carcinoma in situ' refers to cancer before it has become invasive. The exact manner in which invasion occurs is unknown but is thought to be partly due to physiological changes occurring in tumour cell membranes which reduce their adhesion to other cells. Tumours also produce proteolytic enzymes (protein-dissolving) which may assist the invasion of normal tissue. Malignant cells also seem to lose 'contact inhibition', failing to recognise their boundaries and cease growth on meeting a different tissue type. For example, tumours of glandular lung tissue may continue invasion through the pleura to the chest wall. Once local invasion has occurred to any degree, metastases may develop in distant tissue. Metastatic spread (dissemination) may occur in one of four ways:

- via the lymphatic system
- via the bloodstream
- via serous cavities
- via the cerebrospinal fluid (CSF).

Lymphatic spread. Tumour cells may invade the lymphatic vessels and grow in clumps and cords, establishing themselves en route in local lymph nodes. This is termed 'regional spread'. It causes lymph node swelling, which may be painful, and may prevent local tissue fluid drainage, causing lymphoedema. This is common in the arms of patients with breast cancer. Eventually, distant lymph nodes are also involved.

Arteriovenous spread. Tumour cells enter blood vessels near the primary tumour or are shed into the blood via the thoracic lymph duct. They then become enmeshed in the next capillary network they encounter. Hence cancer of certain organs has a certain pattern of spread; gastrointestinal tumours, for example, typically spread via the portal venous system, initially to the liver.

Serous cavity spread. Serous membranes (e.g. the pleura or peritoneum) may be invaded by tumours, either locally from the primary tumour or from nearby metastases. Resulting irritation causes excess serous fluid to be produced which can distribute cancer cells widely in the serous cavity. This process is called 'seeding'. The excess fluid forms malignant pleural effusions or ascites.

CSF spread. Similarly, tumour cells may spread directly in the CSF. Some brain tumours metastasise along the spinal cord in this way.

The most common sites of metastatic deposit are the lungs, bones, brain and liver. Two-thirds of patients develop metastases; in half of these, dissemination occurs before diagnosis, and often before symptoms arise.

Table 31.1 Classification of malignant tumours

Tissue of origin	*Malignant tumour*
Epithelium	Carcinoma
Surface epithelium, e.g. skin, cell lining and covering, body cavities, organs and tracts	Squamous cell carcinoma, e.g. of the skin, lung, stomach
Glandular epithelium, i.e. glands or ducts in the epithelium	Adenocarcinoma, e.g. of the breast, lung
Basal cell layer of the skin	Basal cell carcinoma, often termed 'rodent ulcer'
Transitional cells, e.g. of the bladder lining	Transitional cell carcinoma, e.g. of the bladder
Connective tissue	Sarcoma
Bone	Osteosarcoma
Cartilage	Chondrosarcoma
Fatty tissue	Liposarcoma
Fibrous tissue	Fibrosarcoma
Muscle	Myosarcoma
Smooth muscle	Leiomyosarcoma
Striated muscle	Rhabdomyosarcoma
Endothelium	
Blood vessels	Angiosarcoma
Meninges	Meningioma
Mesothelium: cells covering the surface of serous membranes, e.g. of the pleura, peritoneum	Mesothelioma
Haemopoietic and lymphoid tissue	
Bone marrow	Myeloid leukaemias
	Multiple myeloma
Lymphoid tissue	Lymphocytic leukaemias
	Lymphoma
Nervous tissue	
Nerves	Neuroblastoma
CNS supporting tissue	Glioma, e.g. astrocytoma, oligodendroglioma
Germ cells	
Testes or ovary	Seminoma, teratoma

The effects of cancer

The manifestations of cancer depend directly or indirectly on the location, size and type of tumour involved and on the extent of any metastases. The medical and nursing problems associated with cancers of particular body systems are covered in preceding chapters. Revise your knowledge of two cancer types before reading further.

Direct tumour effects. Symptoms may be due to the following direct tumour or metastatic effects.

Occupation of limited space. Because it takes up space within the body, the tumour can cause the following effects:

- obstruction of passageways, e.g. the oesophagus, causing dysphagia
- compression of major blood vessels — e.g. tumours at the apex of the lung or metastatic mediastinal lymph nodes may compress the superior vena cava, causing ischaemia, oedema of the head, neck and right arm, and dyspnoea
- compression of neighbouring tissues and organs — e.g. brain metastases may cause pressure and local oedema, which can compromise brain function and consciousness, depending on the area of brain tissue involved
- pressure on regional nerves, causing pain and/or paralysis — e.g. metastases in the spinal vertebrae may compress the spinal cord and result in pain or loss of sensation and paralysis from the level of the lesion downward
- invasion and replacement of normal tissue — e.g. gastric tumours often spread diffusely across the gastric mucosa, compromising its digestive function.

Haemorrhage. Tumours may invade small local blood vessels, causing chronic haemorrhage and anaemia. Occasionally haemorrhage may be sudden and fatal, as when a major blood vessel such as the carotid artery is eroded.

Ulceration. Tumour tissue growth may outstrip local blood supply, causing necrosis, or ulceration, of part of the tumour and adjacent normal tissue. This ulceration may be internal or external. Advanced breast tumours may cause surface ulceration. Due to their appearance, these lesions are often termed 'fungating'.

Infection. This is very common, being attributed as a cause of death in 50% of patients with metastatic cancer. Increased susceptibility to infection is caused by malnutrition, cancer treatments and, sometimes, by metastatic invasion of the bone marrow, compromising haemopoiesis. Eroded or ulcerating tumours are prone to local infection, which may become systemic.

Metabolic imbalances. These are numerous and tumour-specific and may become widespread with advancing disease. Tumours of the pancreas may cause disturbance in glucose metabolism. Liver metastases may alter ability to metabolise essential drugs. Renal tumours cause progressive renal failure, leading to fluid and electrolyte imbalance.

Hypercalcaemia is a common and serious manifestation of advanced cancer of the breast, bone, lung and kidney and is caused by bone destruction due to metastases or by the tumour's production of substances causing bone dissolution.

Indirect tumour effects. These are sometimes termed 'paraneoplastic' effects (or syndrome) and may be the presenting features before diagnosis. They may include skin changes, peripheral neuropathy, myopathy, cerebral degeneration, anaemia, white blood

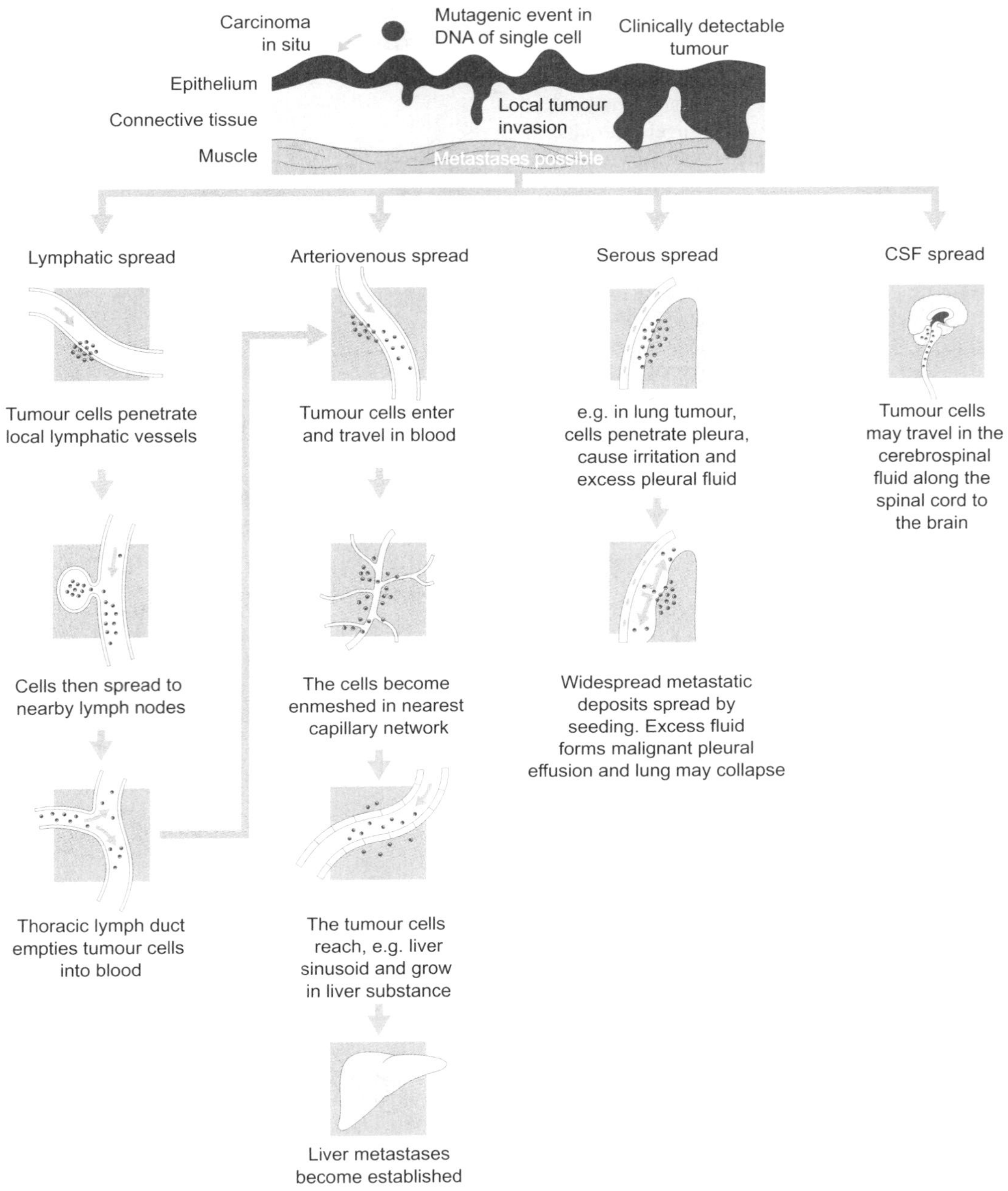
Carcinoma
in situ
Mutagenic event in
DNA of single cell
Clinically detectable
tumour
Epithelium
Connective tissue
Muscle
Local tumour
invasion
Metastases possible
Lymphatic spread
Arteriovenous spread
Serous spread
CSF spread
Tumour cells penetrate
local lymphatic vessels
Tumour cells enter
and travel in blood
e.g. in lung tumour,
cells penetrate pleura,
cause irritation and
excess pleural fluid
Tumour cells
may travel in the
cerebrospinal
fluid along the
spinal cord to
the brain
Cells then spread to
nearby lymph nodes
The cells become
enmeshed in nearest
capillary network
Widespread metastatic
deposits spread by
seeding. Excess fluid
forms malignant pleural
effusion and lung may collapse
Thoracic lymph duct
empties tumour cells
into blood
The tumour cells
reach, e.g. liver
sinusoid and grow
in liver substance
Liver metastases
become established

Fig. 31.1 The cancer process.

cell abnormalities, fever, and generalised endocrine and metabolic disturbances. These effects are relatively common but vary with tumour type and are usually more marked with advanced cancer. In recent years, much insight has been gained into the causes of these syndromes (Souhami & Tobias 1998). Early detection is important as these symptoms can often be alleviated even when the primary tumour cannot be controlled.

Cancer cachexia. Approximately two-thirds of cancer patients suffer some degree of cancer cachexia. This syndrome has been termed 'a physical fading of wholeness' (Costa 1977). It involves progressive and extreme weight loss and muscle wasting. The resulting weakness can be very severe and death may eventually ensue due to exhaustion of the respiratory muscles. This is most common in patients with gastrointestinal and lung tumours. The causes are many, some directly related to the tumour and some not. Research has demonstrated increased basal metabolic rate and disturbed fat, protein and carbohydrate metabolism, with accompanying anorexia and altered digestion and absorption of nutrients (Skipper et al 1993). Many of these effects are thought to be caused by a substance called cachectin produced by the tumour.

Prognosis and the cause of death. Overall, there has been little change in 5-year disease-free survival rates for most common cancers (Souhami & Tobias 1998). The calculation of these rates is used to estimate possible cures, since for many tumours, recurrence is less likely should the patient survive for 5 years following treatment. Nevertheless, the term 'cure' must be used cautiously; indeed, some health care professionals prefer the phrase 'complete remission'.

This bleak outlook can probably be explained by the fact that malignant cells, which are often undetectable by current diagnostic techniques, frequently persist despite treatment and in time cause local recurrence of the tumour and/or metastases. Many factors intervene, however, such that no patient's prognosis can be calculated with certainty. In general, younger patients in good health and with a positive outlook have better survival rates, whatever the tumour site.

It may seem obvious that any of the effects of cancer (described on p. 912) may result in or contribute to death. While this is the case, the immediate cause of death is often uncertain, in which case it is generally presumed to be the subtle interplay of the failure of different body systems. The significance of psychological and social factors in determining prognosis cannot be underestimated. Depression and loss of hope may result in loss of the will to live (Stoll 1979).

It is now widely accepted that quality of life in cancer patients may be improved by psychological interventions (Devine & Westlake 1995, Meyer & Mark 1995). Prolongation of life, however, is more controversial, but this has opened up a new area known as immunopsychology. The last decade has seen increasing speculation in the psychosocial literature on whether intervention groups can lead not only to good outcomes with respect to mood but also to improved chances of survival (Fox 1995, Greer 1995). Preliminary evidence from research by Spiegel et al (1989) indicates that cancer support groups may foster positive changes in immune function, which may influence tumour growth rate, thus promoting survival (Fawzy et al 1993). Caution is advocated, however, as it is difficult to prove this type of relationship, and attributing physical deterioration to the patient's emotional state is not justified (Bottomley 1998). Research has also indicated that social deprivation and life crises may have a negative impact on prognosis (Barraclough 1994). A good social support system and elements of spirituality and religious belief appear to be consistent predictors of quality of life (Creagan 1997). It is therefore clear that the expected time of death is often uncertain; a specific prediction of prognosis is therefore unwise and may even lead to loss of hope.

Q

31.3 Consider patients you have cared for who have died with cancer. Do you know what was the immediate cause of death? Ask a doctor involved if you are unsure. Is he or she certain of this cause? Were psychological and social factors important?

31.4 It is common for relatives to want to know the details and exact cause of death of the patient. Discuss with other students why you think this need is so common. Relate any experiences of being with the recently bereaved. What do you think is the nurse's role in the face of this uncertainty? What are the ethical issues involved?

Epidemiology of cancer

Epidemiological studies have given rise to theories about the possible causes of different forms of cancer and hence to strategies for cancer prevention and for the screening of high-risk population groups for early-stage, treatable disease. Figure 31.2 shows the incidence of the 10 most common causes of cancer mortality in the UK.

Across the world, populations are ageing and age is one of the major risk factors for developing cancer. More than 50% of all cancer cases diagnosed are over 65 years old (Redmond & Aapro 1997). Although cancer is very rare in children, it is the third most common cause of childhood death, despite the fact that childhood tumours respond to treatment far more readily than those in adults.

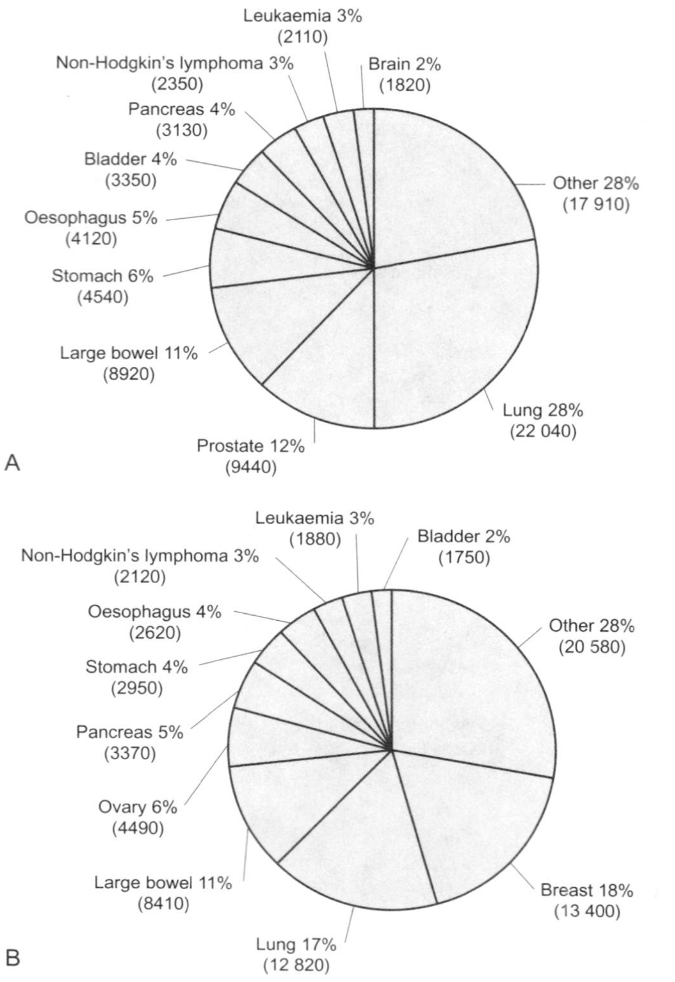

Fig. 31.2 Incidence of the 10 most common causes of cancer deaths in the UK in 1997 (Cancer Research Campaign 1999b). A: Men; total number of cancers = 79 730. B: Women; total number of cancers = 74 390. *, Non-Hodgkin's lymphoma. Variations in the cancer mortality between the sexes reflect, as well as anatomical differences, different behavioural and environmental factors. For example, the prevalence of lung cancer in men reflects the fact that many men began to smoke during World War I; the result was a rapid increase in lung cancer in these men, who are now elderly. Women began to smoke in large numbers during World War II; hence, lung cancer in women has begun to overtake breast cancer in incidence. In Scotland this has already occurred.

See Foley et al (1993) for a discussion of the specialist treatment of paediatric cancer care.

The incidence of cancer in the UK is one of the highest in the Western world. Predominantly, cancer is a disease of the rich, although the pattern is shifting and many developing countries will triple their cancer incidence over the next two decades (Parkin et al 1997, IARC/WHO 1998). The greater incidence in Western society may be partly attributed to the more sophisticated screening, diagnostic and reporting procedures. Also with the eradication of smallpox, polio and other diseases, life expectancy is greater. Western diet, industrial pollution and behaviours such as smoking and excessive alcohol consumption are chief environmental causes of cancer.

Geographical variations in the incidence of cancer provide fascinating clues to the causes of the disease. In Mozambique a high incidence of liver cancer is thought to be associated with aflatoxin from mould found on stored peanuts. Since the introduction of more appropriate storage practices, the incidence of liver cancer has been falling (Souhami & Tobias 1998). The Japanese have a low incidence of breast cancer but a high incidence of stomach cancer, which is thought to be partly related to the consumption of large quantities of salted food. However, within one or two generations, Japanese immigrants to Hawaii showed the American pattern of a high incidence of breast cancer and a moderate incidence of stomach cancer (Haenszel & Kurihera 1968). This is thought to be due to the adoption of an American diet that is high in fat and protein. These and other similar studies indicate that geographical variations in cancer incidence are attributable to environmental rather than genetic factors; however, there may be an interaction with genetic disposition.

Epidemiological investigation of genetic predisposition to cancer is fast growing as developments in molecular biology make it possible to study genetic markers in large populations. The ongoing Human Genome Project (see Box 31.2) is almost certain to accelerate this work with the discovery of such markers (Williams 1997).

The causes of cancer

Many questions remain to be answered regarding the mechanisms involved in the cellular mutations that lead to cancer. However, epidemiological studies have identified certain causative factors, termed 'carcinogens'. Knowledge of identified carcinogens is essential for:

- the development of prevention and screening strategies
- the provision of accurate information for patients, allaying the myths surrounding cancer causation.

Carcinogenesis involves a sequence of specific genetic events, the order of which may vary. Causation is multifactorial and factors may enhance or inhibit the process. Stages include:

- *initiation* — a mutagenic event occurs in the DNA of a single cell; this may, for example, be radiation-induced
- *promotion* — repeated exposure to carcinogenic agents may or may not cause this initiated cell to proliferate to form a tumour.

Box 31.2 Human Genome Project

In the mid-1980s, it was first suggested that the fundamental problem of cancer could be addressed by studying the sequence of the entire human genome (Dubecco 1986). Initiated in 1988, the specific aim of the International Human Genome Project (HGP) is to map the estimated 50 000–1 000 000 genes and determine the sequence of nucleotides that make up the human genome. It is predicted that the mapping and sequencing of components will be completed by 2005 (Williams 1997).

The HGP will also consider the ethical, legal and social implications of new genetic knowledge to maximise potential benefit and minimise potential harm.

A long latency period may exist between carcinogen exposure and cancer development. Carcinogenic factors and substances can be divided into those that are intrinsic and those that are extrinsic to the individual.

Intrinsic factors

Heredity. Some genetic disorders predispose the individual to cancer. There is, for example, a high incidence of acute leukaemia in individuals with Down's syndrome, and childhood tumours such as retinoblastoma are due to inherited chromosomal abnormalities.

Inherited susceptibility to adult cancers is a promising area of research, with the identification and cloning of certain genes which predispose to cancer. Cancer susceptibility genes are implicated in about 5–10% of all breast and ovarian cancers. Two genes, BRCA1 and BRCA2, have been identified in breast cancer. Approximately 85% of women who carry the BRCA1 mutations develop breast cancer by the age of 80 (Futreal et al 1994, Calzone 1997) (see Ch. 6 for more details regarding genetics and the implications for individuals with cancer).

Hormones. Excessive amounts of certain hormones are thought to promote some tumours. Early menarche, late menopause and nulliparity are all associated with a high incidence of breast cancer, implying that prolonged exposure to oestrogen is a causative factor (Toniolo et al 1995). Endometrial cancer risk increases with exposure to 'unopposed' oestrogen, i.e. HRT, obesity, the sequential use of oral contraceptives and a late menopause. High levels of gonadotrophins are associated with an increased risk of ovarian cancer and it is a possibility that high testosterone levels are related to prostate cancer, although further research is required in this area (Henderson et al 1997).

Immunity. Individuals with impaired immunity are more prone to cancer than others; for example, people with AIDS have a high incidence of Kaposi's sarcoma. This does not mean that cancer is an infectious disease. Immunosuppression may predispose to certain infections, which may then contribute to the cancer process.

Pre-existing disease. Any tissue subjected to constant irritation or to some disease process has an increased susceptibility to malignant change. Hence, ulcerative colitis may precede colonic carcinoma.

Age. The rising incidence of cancer with age is thought to be attributable to:

- prolonged exposure to carcinogens
- decreased resistance to carcinogens
- hormonal changes that occur with age.

Stress. Increasing interest has been shown in the role of life stress in cancer causation; for example, the number of deaths due to cancer has been shown to be increased in recently bereaved men (Parkes et al 1969). In general, however, evidence is limited, although there is some reason to believe that stress may alter the growth rate of a tumour (Barraclough 1994, Creagan 1997). The role of psychological factors in cancer growth remains unclear.

Extrinsic factors

The fact that 70% of cancers occur in epithelial cells that are constantly exposed to external, ingested or inhaled substances implies that extrinsic factors related to lifestyle and the environment are by far the most important in carcinogenesis. These factors may be considered under the following headings:

- physical agents
- chemical agents
- viruses
- diet.

Physical agents

Radiation is known to cause cellular mutations and cancer. Survivors of the atomic bomb explosions in Hiroshima and Nagasaki experienced a high incidence of leukaemia and skin cancer. Recent research has shown an apparent increase in the incidence of leukaemia among the children of fathers working in the nuclear industry, possibly due to germ cell mutations (Gardner et al 1990). Repeated exposure to therapeutic doses of radiation is not thought to be harmful, although stringent precautionary regulations should be followed for the protection of all exposed workers. Therefore, it is not routine discharge of radioactivity by the nuclear industry that should be feared, but rather the catastrophic event, such as occurred at Three Mile Island and Chernobyl. In the former accident, radioactive noble gases were released into the atmosphere. By the worst estimate, there will be one radiation-induced cancer death in the 2 million people living around the reactor. Chernobyl, however, released much of its radioactive core into the atmosphere and will account for an increase of 2–3% in related cancer deaths (Hall 1997).

UV light. There is overwhelming evidence that chronic repeated exposure to solar UV light is the primary cause of basal and squamous cell carcinoma. Data establishing a direct causal relationship with sunlight are more complex, but suggest a promotional role of sunlight in the cause of melanoma. Fair-skinned or freckled individuals who are unable to manufacture sufficient protective melanin are particularly at risk (see Ch. 12).

Electromagnetic fields have recently been added to the list of environmental agents. Low-frequency electric and magnetic fields around electric power transmission lines and magnetic resonance have been implicated in the causation of brain tumours, but studies have proved inconclusive due to confounding variables (Kheifets et al 1995).

Chemical agents. Ninety per cent of all lung cancer cases can be attributed to tobacco smoking. The temporal relationship between smoking and lung cancer was defined in the 1950s by studies undertaken by Doll & Hill (1954). It has been estimated that smoking is responsible for 35% of all cancer deaths, as it is also a contributing factor in cancers of the mouth, pharynx, larynx, oesophagus, bladder and cervix. High-tar cigarettes carry the highest risk, although risk is more dependent on duration of smoking than on consumption. Smoking 20 cigarettes a day for 40 years is eight times more hazardous than smoking 40 cigarettes a day for 20 years. Risk is reduced by ceasing to smoke; within 10 years, an ex-smoker's risk of cancer returns to almost that of a non-smoker (Shopland 1995). Recent research showed that non-smokers are at risk by exposure to other people's smoke: one-quarter of lung cancer cases in non-smokers are estimated to be due to passive smoking (Trichopoulos et al 1981, Valanis 1996).

Excessive alcohol, ingested over long periods of time, contributes to cancers of the mouth, pharynx, oesophagus and liver. Those who drink spirits as opposed to wine and beer and those who smoke as well as drink are particularly at risk.

Many other chemicals, whether inhaled, ingested or absorbed through the skin, have been shown to cause cancer. Lung cancer in non-smokers is most prevalent in large cities where traffic fumes and chimney smoke raise atmospheric levels of polycyclic hydrocarbons, the same chemicals present in cigarette smoke.

Other carcinogenic chemicals present occupational hazards. Some of these, but by no means all, are now subject to government control or ban. These controlled substances (and associated cancer sites) include:

- asbestos (lung)
- vinyl chloride (liver)
- certain chemical dyes (bladder)
- arsenic (lung and skin)
- some hardwood dusts (nasopharynx).

Viruses. Although cancer is not contagious, viral infections account for 1 in 7 human cancers worldwide (Poeschla & Wong-Staal 1997). The Epstein–Barr virus causes a systemic infection that may precede Burkitt's lymphoma, a malignant disease common in parts of Africa. Patients with chronic hepatitis B are more susceptible than others to liver cancer. The human papilloma virus, which may be sexually transmitted, is associated with cervical cancer.

Diet. Epidemiological studies that isolate diet as a causal factor in the development of cancer are extremely problematic to undertake. Nevertheless, dietary factors have been implicated as a major cause of the high incidence of cancer in the West. Countries where the average diet is high in fat and protein appear to have a high incidence of breast cancer, and low-fibre diets are thought to contribute to bowel cancer. Some food additives have been found to be carcinogenic and have been removed from the market, although many others have not yet been fully investigated.

Cancer prevention and screening

Prevention of human cancers is a major focus of research and education. The principal hope of achieving desired outcomes lies in the rigorous application of prevention and screening programmes. The goal of primary prevention is to reduce the risk of the healthy population developing cancer. Secondary prevention aims to detect early-stage, curable, cancer. Primary prevention is therefore the most effective and economic method of controlling cancer.

Nurses now have a much wider role, incorporating health promotion, health education and disease prevention as well as the care of those who are ill. This wider role is reflected in their initial education and in post-basic education. Many health visitors, district nurses and practice nurses working in community health centres offer innovative health promotion programmes as well as screening for ill health. Antenatal care, well-woman or well-man clinics, family planning centres and other health screening clinics all provide opportunities for the promotion of cancer prevention.

Primary prevention

Primary cancer prevention is true health promotion and includes such activities as:

- identifying risk factors in individuals or groups
- counselling high-risk persons to promote behaviour modification
- genetic screening
- implementation of new cancer prevention programmes, e.g. smoking cessation, healthy eating.

Cancer prevention programmes that use fear of the disease to motivate compliance are counterproductive (Walker 1990). Media reporting of cancer risk development requires cautious interpretation and should be put into perspective by reference to the original studies on which they are based. It is important to remember, for example, that substances that are carcinogenic in animals are by no means always so in humans. Moreover, everyday exposure to some of the substances implicated is so minimal as to make risk insignificant. Some of these media scares do little to promote health; fear of cancer, after all, is one of the most common reasons why people avoid screening or fail to present with symptoms.

Box 31.3 Europe's 10-point code against cancer for a healthy life (Cancer Research Campaign 1997)

1. **Breathe clean air.** Don't smoke.
2. **Drink sensibly.** Don't drink too much alcohol.
3. **Eat plenty of fruit and vegetables** and high-fibre foods.
4. **Be active.** Avoid getting overweight.
5. **Protect yourself in the sun.** Don't burn.
6. **Take care with chemicals.** Follow health and safety instructions.
7. **See your doctor** about unusual lumps, moles, sores or bleeding.
8. **See your doctor** about persistent constipation or diarrhoea, hoarseness, unexplained weight loss, coughs, indigestion or loss of appetite.
9. **Check yourself out.** Be aware of changes in your breasts or your testicles.
10. **Get checked regularly:** breast clinic, health centre, surgery, invitation to have your cervical smear test, local screening services.

Health promotion programmes. Box 31.3 lists 10 actions that people can take to reduce their risk of cancer. Obviously, observing this code will result in a healthy lifestyle with a low risk of many health problems including cancer. Health promotion programmes should explore practical and realistic ways of assisting people to integrate such generally healthy behaviours into their daily lives.

Health education programmes have been shown to have some measure of success (Ewles & Simnett 1999). The Community Intervention Trial for Smoking Cessation (COMMIT) funded by the National Cancer Institute (NCI) was designed to test the effectiveness of a multifaceted, 4-year community-based intervention programme to help smokers achieve and maintain cessation. Twenty-two matched communities (20 in the USA, two in Canada) were randomly assigned to either intervention or control. The results showed the intervention programme to have a positive effect on light to moderate smokers; however, there was no significant impact on the 'heavy smokers' group beyond any favourable transient trends (The COMMIT Research Group 1995). These results are both positive and disappointing. This large study, however, has provided important information regarding future cessation programmes. Dissemination of knowledge, it appears, is not in itself sufficient to motivate changes in behaviour.

The White Paper *Towards a Healthier Scotland* (Scottish Office Department of Health 1999) promotes 'The Cancer Challenge', which includes new measures to combat the cancerous effects of smoking. The Scottish Office and Health Education Board for Scotland (HEBS) are working in partnership with health boards, local councils, the voluntary sector and the mass media to stimulate a 'pro-health' culture.

Attitudes. Many factors other than knowledge deficit are known to affect a person's health attitudes. Psychologists have developed a Health Belief Model (as summarised by Niven 1994) to predict an individual's preventive health behaviour and account for some of the factors which determine attitude.

The Health Belief Model states that an individual feels vulnerable to a disease if he believes himself susceptible to developing it and believes the disease to be serious. Furthermore, preventive action will be taken only after the individual has balanced the benefits of that action against its physical, psychological and financial costs (Frank-Stromborg & Cohen 1993).

Despite being taught about the risks of smoking, a teenage smoker may consider himself to be young and healthy and therefore not 'at risk'. Young people in general are motivated by short-term rather than long-term rewards. Smoking in some subcultures and families is associated with attributes such as maturity or rebelliousness, which the young person and his peer group may value. Later, the physical addiction to nicotine becomes a coping mechanism for life's stresses and social deprivation. For such people, possible avoidance of lung cancer is not worth the cost of surrendering the immediate gratification and social status offered by smoking.

Clearly, consideration of the wider causes of individual behaviour would lead those involved in health promotion to an awareness of the social and political action necessary. Most cancers are more common in lower socioeconomic groups than in more affluent groups, yet uptake of preventive and screening services is lower in the former. The causes of social deprivation need to be considered alongside individual behaviour. Preventive services must be readily accessible and based on the expressed needs of the community, e.g. on the principle of client-centred care (Department of Health 1998a). Political action as outlined in the White Paper *Smoking Kills* (Department of Health 1998b) aims over 3 years to assist existing smokers to quit and prevent youngsters from starting to smoke. Proposals include further restrictions on tobacco advertising, the setting up of new 'stop smoking clinics' and free nicotine patches for the impoverished. More legislation is required, however, regarding the control of tobacco sales, occupational exposure to carcinogens and regulation of food additives.

The concepts of health and ill health are open to wide interpretation. An essential aspect of communication is that everyone understands and attaches the same meaning to language used. Nurses need to understand an individual's personal health beliefs and how information is interpreted (Wilkinson 1999) if compliance with health care programmes is to be achieved.

Q

31.5 Using the Health Belief Model, consider the factors that would be taken into account by a practice-based health visitor working in liaison with an area health promotion officer in devising a cancer prevention programme in the following community health centres:

(a) An inner city practice in which 50% of the population are first- and second-generation immigrants from the Indian subcontinent. The remaining 50% consist of students in rented housing, young professional people in their first jobs and homes, and workers in a local petrochemical industry.

(b) A new town practice covering a large area of farmland. The new town housing estates accommodate a large percentage of single, unemployed parents. The nearest large hospital is 20 miles away.

Discuss this question as a group. Also consider how community nurses in each centre might incorporate cancer prevention into their practice.

Secondary prevention: screening

The prognosis of patients with most types of cancer is very much improved if the tumour is detected at an early stage. Often, complete cure can be assured if pre-cancerous tissue can be identified and treated, as in the case of cervical intraepithelial neoplasia (CIN).

Problems in cancer screening. The development of accurate and cost-effective methods of screening at-risk sections of the population is problematic for several reasons (Skrabanek 1990a). The test must have a high degree of sensitivity (reducing the risk of false-negative results) and specificity (reducing the psychological trauma and expense of treating false-positive results). It must be possible to identify an at-risk group; otherwise, the cost of screening becomes prohibitive. Finally, and most problematically, it must be determined whether detecting the cancer type at an early stage will actually prolong life. In the case of small cell lung cancer, for example, early detection with existing tests would simply mean that patients would have an earlier knowledge of their diagnosis, but still live for the same number of years (see Ch. 3).

Two standard screening methods concern cancers affecting women:

- breast cancer screening
- cervical screening.

Breast cancer screening. Widely accepted techniques include mammography, clinical breast examination and breast self-examination. Despite over 30 years of trials, questions remain unanswered regarding the age and appropriate interval at which women should be screened. Eight randomised international trials conducted in New York, Sweden, Edinburgh and Canada vary greatly in their results (Tabar et al 1992, Fletcher et al 1993, Alexander et al 1994). However, it is generally agreed that there is clear benefit in screening women over the age of 50 years, with a consequent reduction in mortality. As controversy surrounds the value of screening women of 40 years or younger, professional clinical judgement and a woman's choice should guide decision-making. The denser breast tissue of premenopausal women makes mammograms difficult to interpret in this age group. Genetic screening may be of great benefit in this situation.

Cervical screening by the Pap (Papanicolaou) smear test has been available for over 20 years. It has been estimated that screening would reduce mortality by 90% (Hakami 1993). However, reduction in mortality in the UK has not been achieved. This is due mainly to the following:

- Progression of cervical cancer is still not understood, and hence the value of cervical screening is uncertain and, indeed, disputed by some (Skrabanek 1990b). It is ethically important that women are informed about this uncertainty and of the possibility of a false-negative or false-positive result.
- Uptake of the service by the group at highest risk, i.e. women over the age of 40 and of lower socioeconomic status, has been poor. Research shows that two-thirds of patients with cervical cancer have never been screened (Walker 1990). A South Tees-based study showed that many women and their partners hold negative attitudes towards cervical screening, based in part on the possible link between cervical cancer and multiple sexual partners (McKie & Gregory 1989).

A similar early study showed that judgemental attitudes of health professionals and a lack of privacy and supportive care in clinics might exaggerate resulting feelings of guilt and embarrassment. Staff working in screening services need training in communication skills, and clinic schedules should allow time for necessary counselling (Quilliam 1989).

Intervention strategies based on individual respect, health care provider relationships and inclusion of significant others may increase adherence to cancer screening guidelines (Burnett et al 1995).

In recent years, there has been much controversy regarding the reliability and accurate detection of abnormal smears. This has led to a review of practices and the need for quality assurance (Beecham 1998). Unfortunately, media reports of deaths following initial false reporting of abnormal smears has undermined public confidence and increased the need for appropriate support from health professionals to encourage women to comply with screening (Oliver 1997) (see Ch. 7).

Screening for other cancers. Screening programmes for other cancers are now under scrutiny, including:

- prostate cancer
- colon cancer.

Prostate cancer. There is at present no consensus regarding the most appropriate screening method. There are three main screening modalities; digital rectal examination (DRE), serum prostate-specific antigen (PSA) and transrectal ultrasonography (TRUS). There are wide ranges in the estimates of sensitivity and specificity. Interest in PSA (a blood test) came about in the late 1980s when it was shown that, post-prostatectomy, previously abnormal PSA levels reduced by half (Catalona et al 1991). However, PSA is often elevated in men with non-cancerous conditions. There is no evidence that prostatic screening improves clinical outcomes; in fact, there are issues of uncertainty surrounding the appropriateness and type of treatment for men with early-stage prostatic cancer, since it has a long asymptomatic latency period. It is therefore important to consider that there might be an adverse psychological impact as a result of prostate screening.

Colon cancer. The natural history of colon cancer with the relatively long time from biological onset to the development of cancer makes it a good candidate for screening. Sigmoidoscopy and faecal occult blood (FOB) are the two methods used. Campaigns promoting greater awareness of the early warning signs of colon cancer are underway. A demonstration screening project as part of 'The Cancer Challenge' is to be established in Scotland to test the feasibility of a national programme to detect colorectal cancer. The value and sensitivity of FOB testing as a screening measure are to be examined (Scottish Office Department of Health 1999). Once again, questions need to be answered regarding the population to be targeted and appropriate intervals for screening.

Screening in the future. Many new challenges for health professionals lie ahead in the area of screening. With the discovery of susceptibility genes, cancer prevention will become a more prominent area of cancer care. The provision of psychological support for compliance and for decision-making regarding treatment in cases with a positive diagnosis requires considerable knowledge, skill and sensitivity on the part of nurses and team colleagues.

Q **31.6** Consider the role of (a) school nurses and (b) occupational health nurses in the primary and secondary prevention of cancer. Try to arrange to spend a day with one of these practitioners, and identify the elements of her role which could be further expanded to fulfil this function.

MEDICAL INTERVENTION AND THE NURSE'S ROLE

Diagnosis and staging

Patients present with cancer in a wide variety of ways. Consider the different physical and psychosocial care needs of the three patients in Case Histories 31.1–31.3.

Patients may present at any point in the disease process, ranging from the premalignant to the metastatic phase. Staging is the process whereby the extent of the disease is established; this involves a varied number of tests for each patient (see the appropriate chapter for a given tumour site). Diagnosis and staging are carried out in a variety of settings, depending on the patient's presenting signs and symptoms. This process can be long, complex and tedious for the patient, raising many issues of uncertainty. However, accurate staging of the extent of the disease is vital for the following reasons:

- Certain modes of treatment are known to be effective at specific disease stages. For example, thoracic surgery for Mr H (see Case History 31.3) would be inappropriate given the dissemination of his disease. Staging spares the human and financial cost of inappropriate treatment.
- The prognosis can be estimated according to the disease stage.
- Staging information is valuable for cancer research, for statistical analysis and in considerations of the patient's eligibility to enter a trial of a new treatment.

The TNM system

The most common internationally used method of defining disease stages is the TNM system, in which:

- T denotes the size or extent of local invasion of the primary tumour
- N refers to the spread to local lymph nodes
- M refers to the presence of metastases.

Case History 31.1(A) D

D, a 22-year-old student, discovered a testicular swelling but chose to ignore it, initially because he misinterpreted it as a sports injury, and later because he felt embarrassed. Nine months later he presented to the student health centre because he was becoming breathless far more readily than usual and suffered a constant backache. These symptoms were due to lung metastases and referred pain caused by metastases in the para-aortic lymph nodes.

Case History 31.2 Mrs F

Mrs F is 54, married and has three grown-up children. She is very health conscious and presents herself every 2 years for a cervical smear at the occupational health centre of her workplace. On this occasion, she is informed that her smear is positive. Subsequent colposcopy reveals carcinoma in situ, i.e. a pre-invasive cancer of the cervical cells that is curable by cone biopsy or laser therapy.

Case History 31.3 Mr H

Mr H is a 76-year-old widower. A heavy smoker, he has suffered from chronic bronchitis for 30 years. His respiratory symptoms have seemed more troublesome lately, but it is pain in the ribs and back (due to bone metastases) which finally cause him to consult his GP. These pains are initially considered to be arthritic in nature, causing further delay in the eventual diagnosis of disseminated small cell bronchogenic carcinoma.

Box 31.4 illustrates the use of the TNM system in non-small cell carcinoma of the lung. Some types of cancer — usually those that are disseminated at presentation — cannot be effectively staged with the TNM system and have necessitated the development of other systems. Box 31.5 shows the staging system generally used in the UK for testicular tumours. During the course of their illness, patients may be restaged in order for their response to treatment, or the extent of disease recurrence, to be assessed. Case History 31.1(B) illustrates the experience of staging for a patient with testicular cancer.

Psychological impact of diagnosis and staging

Confirmation of diagnosis. It is very common for patients to be aware that they have cancer before they are told formally of their diagnosis. This awareness derives from their experience of symptoms, tests and, in some cases, surgery and from the non-verbal communication of staff or relatives. Whether to inform patients in full of their diagnosis, and when and how this should be done are issues of ethical debate (see Box 31.6).

Even if they suspect their diagnosis, patients often cling to hope or use denial as a coping mechanism. These are the early emotional reactions experienced by people facing any actual or potential life crisis or loss, as described by Kübler-Ross (1973).

For further reading, see Niven (1994), Chapter 5.

For most patients, confirmation of their fears comes as a devastating shock; this is often followed for varying periods by a normal stress reaction, which may include anxiety, depression, insomnia and poor concentration. This stressful time is one of great emotional confusion, during which the patient attempts to adjust to a shattered

Case History 31.1(B) D (cont'd from Case History 31.1(A)

D was admitted to a surgical ward, where a biopsy under general anaesthesia was performed. A frozen section taken for histology showed a testicular teratoma. A left orchidectomy was then performed.

Following postoperative recovery, D was taken to an oncology ward for staging. D lived too far away to travel to the department each day; otherwise, the necessary tests could have been performed while he was an outpatient. The tests were carried out and their results were as follows:

- chest X-ray: showed multiple lung metastases
- thoracic CT scan: confirmed lung metastases
- abdominal CT scan: showed a large para-aortic lymph node and no liver metastases
- blood samples for full blood count, urea, creatinine and electrolytes, liver function and tumour markers (AFP and HCG).

These tests showed that D had stage IV testicular teratoma. But even in such extensive disease, the cure rate with cisplatin-based chemotherapy is approximately 70% (Souhami & Tobias 1998). Accordingly, this was the treatment course chosen.

Creatinine clearance is calculated from the serum creatinine to establish baseline measurements for subsequent assessment of any nephrotoxicity induced by platinum compounds.

Box 31.4 TNM staging system for non-small cell lung cancer. (Adapted from UICC 1987)

T (primary tumour)
T1 Tumour ≤3 cm in diameter. No local invasion
T2 Tumour >3 cm in diameter, or invading pleura
T3 Tumour of any size with chest wall invasion, or tumour causing lung collapse or pleural effusion

N (lymph nodes)
N0 Nodes negative
N1 Positive nodes in hilum of affected lung
N2 Positive mediastinal nodes

M (distant metastases)
M0 No metastases
M1 Metastases present

The disease is then staged using the above information, as follows:

Stage I	T1	N0	M0
	T2	N0	M0
Stage II	T1	N1	M0
	T2	N1	M0
Stage III	Any	T3	M0
	Any	N2	M0
Stage IV	Any	M1	

Box 31.5 UK staging system of testicular tumours

Stage I	Tumour confined to testes
Stage II	Pelvic and abdominal lymph node involvement
Stage III	Mediastinal and/or supraclavicular lymph node involvement
Stage IV	Distant metastases, e.g. lung

world. Relatives and friends also experience a conflict between their desire to be supportive and their fear of impending change and loss. The following words summarise the feelings of one patient immediately after she was told of her diagnosis (Evans 1989):

> *Then he mentioned cancer. I suddenly went numb, rooted to the spot. The only thing that I could think of was that I was going to die. With that one word he had shattered my well ordered world. I felt my life was closing in on me. I wanted to cry but the tears would not come. I wanted to laugh but it was not funny. Shock and fear invaded my mind. Did I really hear correctly what he had said? I wondered what on earth I was going to do. I turned to my husband and looked into his eyes, hoping to find the much needed help and support. All I could see was my own disbelief, horror, and fear mirrored back at me. I knew I was on my own.*

At the same time, this patient expressed relief at having a label for her symptoms and knowing that treatment could now proceed.

The discovery that the disease has recurred after a symptom-free period has been shown to provoke even greater psychological disturbance, for the patient's hopes of cure have been disappointed (Moorey 1988). In any event, most newly diagnosed or re-diagnosed patients will be anxious to proceed with treatment as soon as possible, and many will become frustrated with the staging process. The period of waiting for test results is one of great anxiety; the patient is often afraid of the verdict but nonetheless desperate to know it.

Box 31.6 Informing patients of their diagnosis: ethical considerations

Two ethical principles are central to the discussion of whether it is always right to tell a patient the whole truth about his diagnosis: these are the principles of autonomy and of beneficence (for a fuller discussion see Thompson et al 1994).

Autonomy
Patients have a right to autonomy, or self-determination. They cannot make decisions about their treatment or the future if they are not fully aware of their diagnosis. Nevertheless, research implies that some patients adapt better if they can deny certain information about the seriousness of their disease (Haes 1989). Although there is some consensus that patients should be told their diagnosis, discussion of prognosis, which is very often a medical uncertainty, should be considered individually. Stoll (1979) claims that prognostication may deprive patients of hope, and even give rise to self-fulfilling prophecies of death. Some patients demand to know their prognosis so that they can order their lives and affairs accordingly. Others make it clear that they do not want to know. Still others do not need to be told.

Beneficence
The principle of beneficence obligates health care professionals to prevent harm and 'do good' for their patients. It may seem obvious that to tell lies or withhold the truth is wrong. The patient may suffer severe psychological problems if he continues to feel unwell despite the optimistic messages he receives from others, and may even blame himself for his symptoms. He may also lose trust if and when he discovers the 'conspiracy'.

Discussion
The matter is seldom as simple as the choice between lying and truth-telling, and each case must be considered individually. Relatives may ask that their family member be protected from the whole truth. In most instances, respect for the patient's autonomy should override such a request, especially if the patient is able to ask direct questions of staff.

Tension can arise within the health care team when medical staff fail in their responsibility to disclose diagnosis and prognosis to those patients who clearly wish to know them. Other staff — nurses in particular — who spend more time with patients become frustrated in their attempts to meet the psychological needs of individuals who lack awareness of the reality of their situation. There must be an open staff forum for the discussion of such problems.

In most cancer centres, the issue is not whether, but how and when, to inform patients of diagnosis and prognosis. A study by Walker (1990) showed that patients feel they need time to take in the full implications of what they are told, and then to be given a 'second chance' to ask questions of the doctor when they are less 'shell-shocked'. It would seem appropriate that a nurse is present at such discussions because she can follow up the conversation and help the patient to strike a balance between realistic hope and the acceptance of reality.

Psychological support. Aside from providing the necessary nursing care prior to and following each test, the nurse must act as communicator. It is important for her to know why each test is being performed and what it will entail for the patient so that she can provide explanations and reassurance. The nurse should also act as facilitator, ensuring that the doctor explains test results and their significance to the patient as soon as possible, preferably with a nurse present (see Box 31.6). Many fears for the future, both rational and irrational, arise at this time. These need to be discussed openly, and it is the nurse who is most suitably placed to do this.

Q **31.7** (a) Consider D's needs for information and emotional support during the staging process (see Case History 31.(1B)). Devise a care plan showing how you would meet these needs.
(b) Mr H (see Case History 31.3) has been discharged home following palliative radiotherapy to his ribs and spine. One day he asks his district nurse how long it will be before his strength returns. Consider the other questions he may be implying by asking this. What information would the nurse need and how might she reply?

Aims of treatment

Cancer treatments can be described in terms of the following categories:

- curative — often termed 'radical' treatment
- palliative — given with the intention of controlling the disease and distressing symptoms

The transition from radical to palliative therapy need not be presented to the patient as a major or sudden change of direction, as this may lead to feelings of abandonment and hopelessness. Often, several forms of treatment are given in combination; this is termed 'multimodal therapy'. Usually one therapy is the primary therapy while the others are termed 'adjuvant' therapies, as in the case of adjuvant radiotherapy following breast surgery.

Response to treatment

Changes in the size of a tumour following treatment are termed 'response rates'. These may be complete, partial (≥50%), minor or absent (in which case the disease is termed 'progressive').

A good tumour response does not necessarily prolong the patient's survival, but it may, in any event, significantly improve quality of life. Unfortunately, cancer treatments can have considerable side-effects, which may seriously reduce quality of life. Thus, the decision to treat a patient must be based upon a careful balancing of the costs and benefits of treatment and should, ideally, be taken jointly by the health care team and the patient.

Treatment modalities

The principal forms of cancer treatment are:

- surgery
- radiotherapy
- chemotherapy.

Surgery

Surgery is the oldest form of treatment for cancer and remains the most successful method of achieving long-term survival for patients with various types of localised tumour. Surgical removal of tumours of the skin (non-melanoma), thyroid gland, uterus, colon and rectum (early stage) are associated with an excellent chance of cure. Certain other tumours, particularly those disseminated at presentation such as small cell carcinoma of the lung, are inoperable.

Surgical procedures are not always performed with curative intent. Surgery may be used adjuvantly with other treatments, e.g. in the resection of diseased bone after radical chemotherapy for osteosarcoma. Palliative surgery can improve the quality of the patient's remaining life; for example, a bypass of the common bile duct can be performed to relieve jaundice in cancer of the head of the pancreas.

In the case of some cancers, diagnostic methods are not accurate enough for thorough staging; hence, 'second look' laparotomies may be necessary to assess response following chemotherapy in, for example, ovarian cancer.

Psychological support. Surgical techniques, pre- and postoperative nursing care, and the psychological problems associated with undergoing surgery are discussed in Chapter 26. The patient with cancer has all of the usual problems of the surgical patient to contend with, together with the stigma of cancer and the fear and uncertainty of an unknown outcome. Frequently, it is during the perioperative period on a general surgical ward that the patient is told of his diagnosis. There is a need for the nurses on these wards to be aware of the particular problems and needs of the cancer patient.

Radiotherapy

Radiotherapy is the use of ionising radiation to destroy cancer cell populations. Approximately half of all patients with cancer receive radiotherapy during the management of their disease.

Radiation physics and biology are complex topics which are subject to intense research and development. More comprehensive accounts can be found in Groenwald et al (1997), Holmes (1996) and Dow et al (1997).

There are two kinds of radiation:

- *particle radiation*, e.g. alpha particles and beta particles; beta particles are electrons
- *electromagnetic radiation*, i.e. gamma (γ) rays and X-rays — these are similar to light or radioactive rays, but have a very much higher energy level.

Alpha particles are of low energy; they can be absorbed by a sheet of paper and are too weak to kill cancer cells. Electrons are of higher energy and can penetrate anything up to the density of wood. They are occasionally used in radiotherapy, e.g. in the form of radioactive phosphorous. Gamma rays are short, very powerful waves that require lead or concrete to absorb them. They are widely used in radiotherapy due to their ability to penetrate deeply into the body tissues.

The most common form of radiotherapy is now the X-ray. These rays are artificially manufactured in an X-ray tube in which electrons are transmitted using a high-voltage current. These electrons, on colliding with a tungsten target, emit energy in the form of electromagnetic rays. These rays are termed X-rays and behave in exactly the same way as gamma rays.

Radioactivity. Understanding ionising radiation requires a basic understanding of atomic and molecular structure. All matter is made up of atoms, which consist of a central nucleus composed of positively charged protons and uncharged neutrons, orbited by negatively charged electrons (see Fig. 31.3). The atom maintains a stable state through the balance between the number of protons (+) and electrons (–). Strong nuclear forces, provided in part by the neutrons, are required to overcome the electrostatic forces, which push the charged protons apart.

The atom in Figure 31.3 is stable. However, as the number of protons increases, an excess number of neutrons is required in order to hold the nucleus together. This imbalance of neutrons and protons causes the nucleus to become unstable and liable to emit gamma rays and particulate radiation.

Some elements exist in a variety of states, depending on the number of neutrons in the nucleus. These are termed the isotopes of an element. Two isotopes of iodine, for example, are ^{127}I and ^{131}I. The latter is a radioisotope, i.e. it is unstable, because the nuclei of its atoms have a disproportionate number of neutrons. Radioisotopes may be naturally occurring, such as radium-226 (^{226}R), which is now seldom used in radiotherapy, or artificially manufactured by bombarding elements with neutrons in a nuclear reactor, e.g. cobalt-60 (^{60}Co).

The effects of radiation. Cellular response to radiation is not yet fully understood. Radiation causes ionisation of atoms and molecules in living cells. During ionisation, electrons are 'knocked off' one atom and may be taken up by another, creating one positively and one negatively charged atom, both of which will be unstable. The main target of radiation is DNA, which is altered either directly by ionisation of its own molecules or indirectly by changes in the chemical environment of the cell, caused by ionisation of other molecules, particularly water. Although the exact mechanism is not fully understood, oxygen increases the number of free radicals (a very reactive atom with an unpaired electron) in the cell, which triggers chemical changes. This ultimately stimulates a chain of events that leads to biological damage, irreparably damaging DNA, which retards cell metabolism and causes cell death. Cells are therefore most sensitive to radiation-induced damage towards the end of the G1 phase, in the G2 phase and in the M phase of the cell cycle.

To revise your knowledge of the cell cycle, see Tortora & Grabowski (1996).

Radiosensitivity of a given tumour is closely related to cell proliferation activity; however, this does not necessarily correlate with radioavailability. As malignant cells are constantly dividing, they are all radiosensitive, although to varying degrees. Unfortunately, rapidly dividing healthy cells, such as those of the skin, the epithelium of the gastrointestinal and urinary tracts, the gonads and the bone marrow, are also vulnerable to radiation damage; this accounts for the unwanted side-effects of radiotherapy. Figure 31.4 explains the difference between the radiation responses of tumour cells and normal cells. In theory, all tumour cells could be eradicated by radiotherapy, but some would require such high doses that normal cell damage would be irreversible; such tumours, e.g. malignant melanoma, are termed 'radioresistant'.

Radiotherapy is prescribed as an 'absorbed dose'. The unit used is the gray (Gy), where 1 Gy = 1 joule as absorbed by 1 kg of body tissue. The dose will vary for each patient, depending on whether he is receiving radical or palliative treatment and on the radioresponsiveness of the particular tumour.

Sources of radiation. Radiotherapy is given in a variety of ways, according to tumour type and stage and, occasionally, the patient's condition. Teletherapy (from the Greek *téle* — 'far'), sometimes called 'external beam therapy', is the most common method of treatment. Brachytherapy (from the Greek *brachys* — 'short') is administered via radioactive sources placed within, or on the surface of, the body.

Teletherapy. External beam radiotherapy is administered by X-ray machines which are categorised according to the amount of energy produced and depth of penetration to the target area (kilovoltage, orthovoltage, megavoltage, cobalt machine). The 'linear accelerator' or 'linac' is the predominant teletherapy equipment in use throughout the world. Machines delivering lower voltages are still used to treat superficial lesions, such as skin carcinomas. The total prescribed radiation dose, if administered in one session, would be far too toxic to normal tissue and possibly

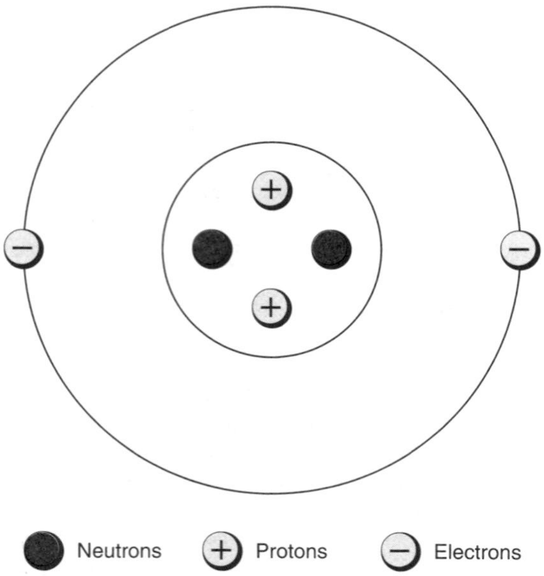

Fig. 31.3 The stable atom. The nucleus of this atom is stable because the number of neutrons and protons are in balance. The neutrons counteract the electrostatic forces pushing the protons apart.

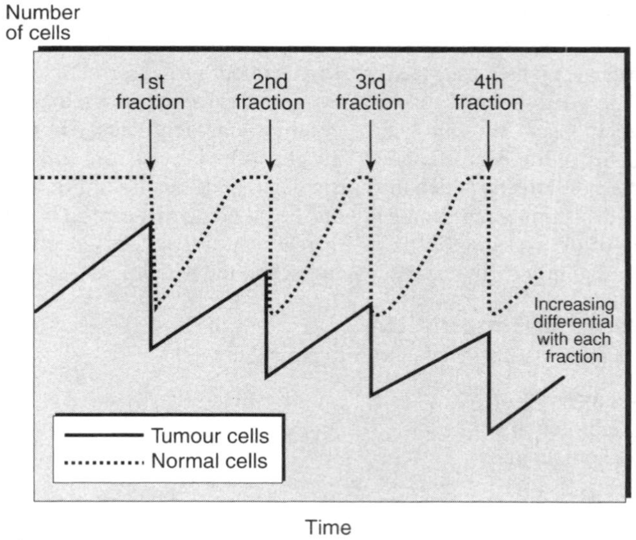

Fig. 31.4 The difference between normal and tumour cell kill and recovery in radiotherapy. Normal cells have the capacity to recover to their previous population level more rapidly than malignant cells. Therefore, successive treatments given after normal cell population recovery but before malignant cell population recovery will result in minimal damage to normal tissue but successive reductions in tumour size.

even fatal to the patient. Hence treatment is administered in daily 'fractions' of the total dose, so as to take advantage of the four Rs of radiobiology — repair, reproduction, redistribution and reoxygenation. Repair of sublethal cell injury generally occurs within 24 h, but possibly in as little as 4 h. Normal cells can therefore repair between daily doses of radiation. Tumour cells may do so initially but become less capable as treatment is protracted. The single most important advantage of fractionation is the opportunity it provides for reoxygenation of the tumour cells.

The patient's initial visit to the department involves a planning session (simulation) which may take several hours.

Extreme accuracy in devising a unique individualised plan for each patient is vital, the aim being adequate dosage to the tumour and minimum exposure of healthy tissues and organs. A machine called a 'simulator' is used in planning. This mimics the treatment machine and is equipped with tumour visualisation facilities. The treatment field is marked out on the patient's skin using ink, which must not be washed off, or very small tattoos, which are permanent.

Radiation to the head or neck involves the manufacture of a Perspex shell, which can be fixed to the treatment table in order to ensure the accuracy necessary and to avoid marking the skin on the patient's face. This may be a little claustrophobic for the patient.

Brachytherapy. This form of treatment is less common than teletherapy. It is the temporary or permanent placement of a radioactive source either on or within a tumour. It offers the advantage of delivering a high dose of radiation to a specific tumour volume. The most common methods used include interstitial implants, intracavitary treatment and systemic therapy. In an interstitial implant, the radioactive source is contained in the form of a needle, seed, wire or catheter that is implanted directly into the tumour (e.g. iridium — breast, prostate, head and neck cancer). In an intracavitary treatment, the radioactive source is placed directly into the body cavity and held in place by an applicator (e.g. caesium — cervical, endometrial, vaginal and lung cancer). In systemic therapy an unsealed radioactive source is given orally or intravenously (e.g. iodine — hyperthyroidism). Nurses caring for patients receiving brachytherapy are advised to use a specialist text (e.g. Holmes 1996, Dow et al 1997).

Types of radiotherapy treatment. Radiotherapy may be:

- radical
- adjuvant
- palliative.

Radical radiotherapy is used as a local treatment modality and is often the treatment of choice for early-stage, localised malignant disease, such as tumours of the head and neck, early-stage carcinoma of the breast and cervix, and stage I and II Hodgkin's disease. Tumours vary in their radioresponsiveness and, therefore, their curability. Approximately 80–90% of stage I and II Hodgkin's disease patients are cured by radiotherapy. The curability of early-stage seminoma (a germ cell tumour, usually testicular in origin), skin cancer and breast cancer (postoperatively) is also high. Later-stage breast cancer, small cell lung cancer and thyroid cancer have poor response rates.

Adjuvant radiotherapy. Radiotherapy is commonly used as adjuvant treatment to ensure local control, usually either pre- or postoperatively, or, increasingly, with chemotherapy. Early-stage carcinoma of the larynx, for example, is treated by radiotherapy alone, with a cure rate of 95%. Later-stage disease is treated by a combination of surgery and radiotherapy, i.e. either with emergency surgery followed by postoperative radiotherapy to ensure control of local lymph nodes, or with 4 weeks of planned radiotherapy followed by surgery.

Palliative radiotherapy constitutes 50% of all radiotherapy treatments given (Dow et al 1997) and involves much lower doses than either radical or adjuvant therapy. Its aim is to achieve symptom relief with minimum side-effects. Again, radiotherapy is effective primarily in the control of local problems, such as local recurrence of breast cancer, pain, compression of adjacent structures by metastases and bleeding (e.g. haemoptysis in carcinoma of the lung or rectal bleeding in carcinoma of the rectum). Spinal cord compression and superior vena cava obstruction, for example, often present as emergencies, and the treatment is usually immediate radiotherapy.

When the intent is palliation, generally a shorter course of radiotherapy is enough to accomplish symptom control without undue side-effects. It is important that quality of life is maximised for a shorter life expectancy.

Large field radiotherapy. Occasionally, radiotherapy is given to much larger areas of the body. Total body irradiation is used for some patients with leukaemia to eradicate all tumour cells from chemotherapy-resistant tissues. This treatment must be followed by bone marrow transplant to restore bone marrow function (see Ch. 11).

Hemi-body (half body) radiation provides effective palliation for patients with extensive bone metastases, as are common, for example, in prostatic cancer.

The decision-making and planning surrounding any course of radiotherapy involve a team approach. Informed consent is essential as is patient and carer education. Incorporation of the principles of physics, radiobiology, dosimetry, treatment technique, anatomy, physiology, psychosocial and patient/family care requires a multidisciplinary approach.

Radiation protection. There is much fear and misconception amongst both professionals and lay people about the dangers of radiation exposure. Indeed, radiation is potentially extremely hazardous, and exposure to high doses can cause all of the side-effects itemised in Table 31.2 together with cell mutations that may lead to carcinogenesis, or to congenital abnormalities if pregnant women are exposed.

Every institution dealing with radiation is legally obliged to appoint a radiation protection officer and to follow stringent guidelines for radiation monitoring and protection. If these are adhered to, radiation damage risk is minimal. Staff most at risk are those working constantly in the radiotherapy or X-ray department and nurses caring for patients receiving brachytherapy, particularly from unsealed sources. These staff should wear badges in which radiographic film records the cumulative amount of radiation exposure per month.

Q

31.8 Arrange to visit a radiotherapy department. Where is it located in the hospital, how is it designed, and why? Ask what kinds of machines are in use and what kind of treatment each is used for. Ask who the radiation protection officer is, and ask to see a copy of the local policy. Try to imagine how a patient might feel arriving at the department for his first treatment. Compare your impressions with that of another student.

Side-effects of radiotherapy. Side-effects occur when normal tissue is irradiated and subsequently destroyed. The management of side-effects forms a major part of the nursing role in the radiotherapy department (see Table 31.2). Manifestation of side-effects varies greatly from patient to patient, depending on the location and amount of tissue being irradiated, the dose and its fractionation,

Table 31.2 Nursing management of the side-effects of radiotherapy

Irradiated body part/organ	*Radiation effect*	*Nurse intervention*	*Rationale*
General	Fatigue	Reassure the patient that this is normal Encourage extra rest but also maintenance of as normal a life as possible	Patient may otherwise fear disease progression To prevent feelings of social isolation and depression
Skin, particularly thinner skin and/ or moist areas, e.g. skin folds, axilla, groin. Fair skin is especially radiosensitive	Three-stage reaction: 1. Erythema: redness, heat, itchiness	No metal-containing skin preparations Washing if permitted, must be with tepid water and gentle patting, not rubbing If itchy, apply 1% hydrocortisone cream as prescribed Avoid exposure to the sun and extremes of heat and cold Encourage non-constrictive clothing in light, natural fabrics; no tight bras or elastic	Metal intensifies radiation reactions Friction causes irritation Ink marks must not be washed off, but there is evidence that washing causes damage Cream is soothing and reduces friction Ultraviolet light may intensify any reaction Reduces sweating and friction
2. Dry desquamation;	1% hydrocortisone or lanolin dryness, scaliness, tight feeling, pain on movement	Soothing, emollient and/or cream (centres vary in their recommendations) Expose skin to fresh air or cool fan For moderate–severe reaction, or if skin folds involved, consider application of Hyperfix dresssing	anti-inflammatory Cooling, with an analgesic effect Thin aerated self-adhesive dressing which may be left in situ until the end of treatment — prevents friction and promotes wound healing
	3. Moist desquamation: blisters, loss of surface epithelium, pain, susceptibility to infection. Occasionally progresses to necrosis	A break in treatment may be necessary Analgesia Observation for signs of infection; topical antibiotics as prescribed Hydrogel dressing Absorbant, non-adherent dressing if area cannot be exposed	Infection exacerbates skin damage and may become systemic To promote wound healing To prevent exudate adhering to clothing and reduce friction to skin surfaces
Scalp	Alopecia (in treatment field only). Loss of any body hair occurs from weeks 2–3	Reassure the patient that hair will usually grow back in 2–3 months, although it may be of a different texture and colour Organise provision of a wig Assist patient to arrange remaining hair to cover bald patches Wearing of scarf/turban at night	Hair loss poses a very stressful threat to body image, especially for women Prevents distress of hair on pillow
Brain	Cerebral oedema (within week 1 of treatment): altered mental state, restlessness, irritability, headaches, nausea, ↑ BP, ↓ P, ↓ respirations	Administer prescribed steroids Observe and report alterations in mental status Ensure patient safety	Anti-inflammatory Enables prompt medical intervention
Mouth	1. Mucositis due to damaged, sloughed oral mucosa Opportunistic infection may ensue, e.g. *Candida albicans*	Regular oral assessment Teach and assist with frequent, gentle oral hygiene using a soft toothbrush Use antibacterial/antifungal preparations prophylactically, e.g. chlorhexidine, nystatin Analgesia: topical, e.g. benzydamine, and systemic; occasionally opiates are necessary Observe for signs of dehydration and inadequate nutrition	To prevent further damage and infection which may become systemic Oral pain is excruciating and always to the forefront of consciousness Prompt parenteral hydration and dietary supplements or enteral feeding may be commenced
	2. Xerostomia (dry mouth) due to altered salivary gland function. May be permanent. Causes difficulty in chewing, swallowing and talking	Frequent mouth rinses with water Artificial saliva Avoid spices, alcohol, smoking, extremes of temperature	Comforting, aids swallowing These are mucosal irritants

Table 31.2 (*cont'd*)

Irradiated body part/organ	*Radiation effect*	*Nurse intervention*	*Rationale*
Mouth (*cont'd*)	3. Taste changes due to xerostomia and damaged taste buds	Assist patients to experiment with other foods	Only certain tastes are altered (see Holmes 1996, p. 91)
	4. Dental decay/due to xerostomia and radiation gingivitis	Pre-treatment dental referral	Any caries will be exacerbated by radiation and form foci for infection
Neck area	1. Pharyngitis, laryngitis, causing pain, hoarseness, loss of voice, dry cough and occasionally respiratory stridor	Discourage smoking Encourage patient to rest voice Observe respiratory status and colour	Mucosal irritant Medical intervention in the form of steroids or even a tracheostomy may be necessary
		Linctus as a cough suppressant	Prevents mucosal irritation caused by coughing
		Topical analgesia prior to food, e.g. aspirin gargles, anaesthetic throat spray; systemic analgesia	Promotes comfort and aids swallowing
	2. Oesophagitis (upper one-third) causing dysphagia	Maintain nutrition. Soft diet and dietary supplements. Avoid irritant foods, strong alcohol and smoking	These patients are often already malnourished
Thorax	1. Oesophagitis (lower two-thirds) causing 'heartburn'-type pain	As above; also administer antacids prior to food (some antacids contain topical anaesthetics)	Lines oesophagus and prevents pain and trauma of swallowing and from gastric acid reflux
	2. Pneumonitis due to inflammation of bronchioles and alveolar lining. May cause dsypnoea, productive cough and haemoptysis	Discourage smoking Observe for signs of infection: pyrexia, purulent sputum Oxygen as prescribed (see Ch. 3)	Enables prompt commencement of antibiotics
	3. Dyspepsia, nausea and vomiting (less severe than with abdominal radiation)	(See below)	
Abdomen and pelvis	1. Nausea and vomiting. Due to inflammation of gastrointestinal epithelium; also a generalised radiation reaction	Encourage a small meal 3 h before treatment and light snacks after Regular antiemetics: systematically try various kinds and routes	Some patients are unable to eat after treatment due to nausea Regular administration required to prevent and relieve nausea
		Distraction/ relaxation techniques	There may be a contributing psychological factor in nausea (Holmes 1996)
		Monitor fluid and food intake	To avoid dehydration
	2. Diarrhoea, possibly accompanied by rectal bleeding	Maximise privacy Administer antidiarrhoeals as prescribed Low-residue, bland diet Observe for dehydration Maintain high fluid intake	
		Observe perianal skin: gently apply barrier cream after washing if necessary	To prevent skin excoriation
	3. Cystitis due to inflammation of urinary tract. Predisposition to urinary tract infection	Encourage high fluid intake (3 L daily)	Prevents stasis of urine and sloughed epithelium
		Encourage and/or assist with personal hygiene	Helps prevent ascending urinary tract infection
		Regular collection of urine specimens for microbiology	Enables prompt antibiotic treatment of urinary tract infection
	4. Altered sexual function (degree depends on exact treatment site and dosage)	Psychological support and counselling (see Holmes 1996)	Loss of any degree of sexual function is very threatening to most people's self-image; opportunity to talk this through is vital
		Include partner in discussion if patient wishes	To gain understanding and support and minimise body image problems

(cont'd)

Table 31.2 ***(cont'd)***

Irradiated body part/organ	*Radiation effect*	*Nurse intervention*	*Rationale*
Abdomen and pelvis (*cont'd*)	*Men*: Impotence (usually temporary) Sterility (usually permanent)	Offer pre-treatment sperm banking if appropriate	To enable sperm to be used for artificial insemination
	Women: Sterility (if ovaries are irradiated). May be temporary or permanent	Advise continued contraception during and for several months after treatment	Fertility is not always immediately affected and any pregnancy may not be viable
	Dyspareunia due to vaginal fibrosis and dryness	Advise use of vaginal lubricant Discourage intercourse during treatment and for 2–4 weeks afterwards Provide vaginal dilator after treatment, especially brachytherapy	 Intercourse would exacerbate vaginal inflammation Prevention of vaginal fibrosis, eases future intercourse and internal examination
	Loss of libido	Sensitively explain that this is not uncommon and is usually temporary	
	Premature menopause (if ovaries irradiated)	Inform of possibility Administer hormone supplements if prescribed	To prevent menopausal symptoms

and the patient's physical and psychological state. Treatment techniques are constantly being developed to improve accuracy of delivery and to reduce side-effects, particularly to the skin. Alternative fractionation schemes continue to receive attention as the search continues to achieve greater cell kill and tumour control. Two strategies have been developed involving multiple fractions per day: hyperfractionation and accelerated hyperfractionation (CHART). In both approaches, 4–6 h between doses must be allowed for repair of sublethal damage from the first dose before the second is given (Hall & Cox 1994). Hyperfractionation is the use of several smaller than standard doses given two to three times daily. The accumulative daily and total doses are usually greater than for conventional treatment. Accelerated hyperfractionation refers to an overall shortened treatment time, achieved by increasing the number of fractions per day.

With the advancement of computer technology, conformal radiotherapy has been further developed. Conformal therapy is defined as the integration of computed tomography (CT) with the planning computer to determine a beam configuration that conforms precisely to the target organ or site. The ability to be more precise restricts doses to surrounding tissues.

In the field of brachytherapy, stereotactic radiotherapy has been developed to implant radioactive sources into brain tissue (see Kreth et al 1995 for more details).

Patients may suffer from systemic side-effects such as fatigue, lethargy, nausea, anorexia and headaches. This syndrome, termed 'radiation sickness', may be due to the circulation of tumour breakdown products. In general, however, radiotherapy affects only those tissues in the area being irradiated. For example, a patient receiving treatment for bladder carcinoma will not lose the hair on his head.

Side-effects may be 'early', occurring 10–14 days after commencement of treatment, or 'late', usually presenting 18 months to 2 years after treatment. Acute problems manifest in areas of rapid cell growth and division and are usually reversible. The nursing management of the most common of these is discussed in Table 31.2. The effects of radiation on the bone marrow have not been included as it is rare for bone marrow to be irradiated to the extent of serious compromise of haemopoiesis, except in the case of total body irradiation.

Late side-effects occur as (due to DNA damage) slowly dividing cells fail to replicate. Problems are most often a consequence of damaged vasculature and are usually permanent. Examples include fibrosis of the lung, chronic bowel inflammation, and lymphoedema resulting from lymph node damage.

Psychological support. Radiotherapy patients are often perceived as the self-caring 'walking wounded'. Their needs are often less obvious and treatment is mostly on an outpatient basis (Wells 1998a). It is important to remember that radiotherapy treatment is not always an isolated event but usually precedes or follows other forms of cancer treatments. Although it brings its own problems and side-effects, its impact needs to be considered in the context of the patient's overall experience. That experience may also be coloured by existing psychosocial, physical and functional needs related to other existing disease or to financial or social disadvantage. Several studies have shown that patients have many fears, misconceptions and high levels of psychological distress, and more often than not are given insufficient information pre- and post-treatment (Peck & Boland 1977, Eardley 1985, Wells 1998b) (see Research Abstract 31.1).

A particularly vulnerable time for a patient is at the end of treatment, when side-effects are often at their peak and professional support is not always accessible. Patients may experience considerable uncertainty and vulnerability.

Myths and fears. Few therapeutic modalities in medicine induce more misunderstanding, confusion and misapprehension than radiotherapy (Rotman et al 1977). For many patients, the news that they are to receive radiotherapy comes soon after knowledge of their diagnosis and hence when they are already coping with multiple stresses and feelings of loss. Compounding these stresses are the many myths and fears that surround radiotherapy. Hammick et al (1998) looked at the patient's knowledge and perceptions of radiotherapy and radiation. Outside of medical usage, radiation was commonly perceived in terms of the atom bomb. Media coverage was also perceived to be negative, often highlighting problems in terms of overdosages, burns and permanent damage. From observations in clinical practice it is apparent that media reports do influence patients' anxiety levels regarding treatment. This became evident at the time of publicity surrounding patients belonging to RAGE (Radiation Action Group Exposure), where

Research Abstract 31.1

This descriptive American research, carried out by psychologists, was the first study to examine the information that is given to radiotherapy patients, and how that information influences emotional response. Fifty patients, most of whom were receiving radical radiotherapy, were interviewed before and during radiotherapy. The majority had many unanswered questions about their disease and about radiotherapy and its side-effects. They also regarded the prescription of radiotherapy as bad news, rather than as a postoperative attempt at cure. The fear of losing the doctor's goodwill by asking questions was described by several respondents, and these particular patients reported a high level of anxiety and depression.

The anxiety level was found to be 60% before and 80% during treatment. Depression levels were similar. This is an American study, however, and the diagnostic definitions of 'anxiety' and 'depression' used in this research vary considerably from the application of those terms in the UK. Criticisms of the study include the fact that 74% of the sample were women, and 22% had a pre-existing psychiatric disorder, leading to some difficulty in making generalisations from these results.

It is possible that, with increasing awareness of patients' needs, the picture has changed since 1977, although a later UK study indicated that provision of information and support for radiotherapy patients was still inadequate (Eardley 1986). While Peck & Boland (1977) imply that the problem lies with the doctor's lack of time, Eardley argues that information in written form is needed as soon as a patient discovers that he needs radiotherapy, rather than when he arrives, in an extremely anxious state, for treatment. Neither study considers the role of nurses, who, according to Strohl (1988), are ideally placed and skilled to provide the kind of support that radiotherapy patients need.

Peck A, Boland J 1977 Emotional reactions to radiation treatment. Cancer 40: 180–184.

women had developed long-term toxicity as a result of radiotherapy to the brachial plexus following treatment for breast cancer. Health care professionals need to be aware that patients may have many anxieties following public information releases and that it is important to place these reports into perspective.

As Mackenzie (1996) points out, it is not surprising that patients find it confusing that radiation, which causes cancer (e.g. following Chernobyl), can be both curative and survivable.

The nurse's role. Nurses can do much to alleviate the patient's fears and make the experience of radiotherapy tolerable. In a study by Johnson et al (1989), 42 patients with prostatic carcinoma who were given systematic, descriptive explanations of all stages of their radiotherapy showed a significantly improved quality of life compared with a control group who did not receive such information.

The patient's greatest need is for information. Nurses are responsible, therefore, for becoming accurately informed themselves — about radiotherapy in general, and about each patient's individual treatment plan and likely side-effects in particular. A study by Slevin et al (1996) indicated that written material about cancer and its treatment was considered to be more satisfactory and popular than information from the media. Verbal information, however, was viewed to be of greater importance. The last few years have seen the development of a comprehensive patient information strategy, with all members of the multidisciplinary team producing balanced and holistic material. A patient survey (Lauer et al 1982) found that the information most desired, in rank order, concerned:

- the purpose of the treatment
- the action of radiotherapy
- the treatment schedule
- likely side-effects
- a description of the experience of treatment planning and administration.

The majority of patients receive radiotherapy as outpatients and thus must cope with the added stress of daily travel to and from the department. Their needs for information and counselling are often greater than those of in-patients because they and their carers must cope with side-effects and anxieties at home.

Nurses in Europe, in comparison with their American colleagues, have been slower to realise their contribution to radiotherapy care. However, this is changing, with nurses being given designated roles within radiotherapy departments. The central components of this role include assessment, education, knowledge and prevention of side-effects, psychosocial support, liaison with other health care professionals and rehabilitation. Some centres are now employing nurse specialists who provide information and counselling services, nurse-led review and follow-up clinics, telephone follow-up and nursing interventions for side-effects (James et al 1994, Dodwell et al 1997, Faithful 1997). The future holds many challenges for nurses working in this field to improve quality of care for patients undergoing radiotherapy treatment.

Q

32.9 Use the above information together with supplemental reading to devise an explanation of external beam radiotherapy and its effects that would be suitable to give to a patient prior to treatment. Draw upon available patient literature, such as that published by BACUP (British Association of Cancer United Patients), and your own impressions during your visit to the radiotherapy department. Avoid technical terms and emotive words such as 'burn' or 'blast', and bear in mind that patients need to know what they will actually experience.

Chemotherapy

The word 'chemotherapy' literally means 'treatment with chemicals' and therefore can refer to any form of drug therapy. Cytotoxic (literally 'poisonous to cells') chemotherapy involves the use of drugs to disrupt the cell cycle and thus ultimately kill malignant cells. Other drugs, which are not necessarily cytotoxic, are also used in cancer management and will be discussed briefly on page 932.

How cytotoxic chemotherapy works. Cytotoxins are termed 'antiproliferative'; like radiation, they are toxic to dividing cells, both healthy and malignant. There are many different types of cytotoxic agent, which have various modes of action and therefore work at different phases in the cell cycle (see Tortora & Grabowski 1996 for a description of the cell cycle.) Cytotoxic drugs are usually classified according to their chemical structure, cell cycle activity and primary mode of action. The classic categories include:

- alkylating agents
- antimetabolites
- antitumour antibiotics
- plant alkaloids.

The action of each of these is described in Box 31.7.

Modes of cytotoxic chemotherapy treatment. Cytotoxic chemotherapy differs from radiotherapy in that it is a systemic rather than a localised treatment modality. It is therefore particularly useful for the treatment of haematological malignancies, which are by their very nature usually disseminated or metastatic in nature. These drugs are a relatively recent development, the first being discovered in the 1940s, and their use has become widespread only in the last 40 years. Despite their great potential, results have been disappointing to date because it has been mainly the rarer tumours that have responded well. Childhood leukaemia is particularly responsive, with approximately 70% of children being cured. Complete responses are also being achieved in adults with Hodgkin's disease. Very few solid tumours are as responsive, the exception being some childhood tumours and testicular teratoma, in which cure rates of 80–90% have been achieved. Sadly, these potentially curable malignancies represent approximately 5% of patients with cancer.

Adjuvant and palliative chemotherapy. For the most part, chemotherapy is used:

- as the sole (or most important) treatment
- as a means of reducing the size of the tumour to aid the success of subsequent surgery or radiotherapy, i.e. 'debulking' of tumours, such as those of the head, neck and bladder
- following radiotherapy or surgery to eliminate remaining tumour cells or micrometastases; adjuvant postoperative chemotherapy is commonly used after surgery for cancer of the breast or ovary to improve disease-free survival
- to treat a relapse after initial treatment
- for palliation of symptoms — some tumours are partially chemoresponsive, so that treatment may relieve symptoms and improve the quality of, and possibly lengthen, life
- for investigation of the usefulness of a new drug.

Combination chemotherapy, which uses a variety of agents, has been found to be far more effective than single-agent chemotherapy. At any given time, the cells of one tumour will be at different phases of the cell cycle: a combination of agents acting on those various phases will therefore kill more cells than a single agent. A lower dose of each agent is given, thus reducing the side-effects of each. Tumour cells unfortunately have the capacity to acquire resistance to single agents, and therefore giving intermittent high doses of drugs, alternating drugs and minimising the intervals between treatments are the major factors used to prevent acquired drug resistance.

Administration of chemotherapy. Chemotherapy is usually given in 'intermittent' doses, sometimes called 'pulses' or 'cycles', the principle being similar to that of fractionation in radiotherapy. Chemotherapy is toxic to rapidly dividing healthy cells, although these have the capacity to recover more quickly than tumour cells. A graph similar to Figure 31.4 could be drawn to illustrate this principle. Hence, most chemotherapy is organised into 'regimens', which are sometimes called 'protocols' if the treatment is part of a research trial.

Chemotherapy may be administered systemically or regionally and by several routes.

Systemic chemotherapy. The goal is to provide a concentration of the drugs that is sufficient to achieve a therapeutic cytotoxic effect without causing too much toxicity to normal cells. Routes of administration include oral, subcutaneous, intramuscular and intravenous. Intravenous administration may be delivered either as a 'bolus' or infusion. Continuous infusions may be delivered using a computerised drug delivery pump via a vascular access device (VAD) such as a skin-tunnelled catheter (STC), a totally implanted port (TIP) or a peripherally inserted central catheter (PICC).

These devices have permitted safe and reliable access to the venous system and patients are now able to spend longer periods at home while receiving continuous infusions of chemotherapy. The development of such devices has enhanced the lives of cancer patients but their use poses challenges for patients and health care professionals. Concerns include psychosocial issues, care of the device to prevent potential complications, and management of any complications which may occur. Some of these complications may be life-threatening and require immediate and effective intervention.

Box 31.7 Classification of cytotoxic drugs

Alkylating agents

Alkylating agents are highly reactive and are cell cycle non-specific. Their primary mode of action is to join together or cross-link the two strands of DNA, preventing them from separating and therefore replicating. Cyclophosphamide is an example of a cytotoxic which acts in this way. Another group of alkylating agents are platinum-based compounds, e.g. cisplatinum and carboplatin, which cause interstrand and intrastrand linkages.

Antimetabolites

These drugs are cell cycle specific, exerting their effect in the S phase. These drugs are structural analogues of normal intracellular metabolites essential for cell function and replication and so are used to disrupt cellular metabolism. Methotrexate, for example, inhibits the enzyme necessary for the conversion of folic acid to folinic acid. Folinic acid is necessary for the formation of purines and pyrimadines, which are components of DNA. Folinic acid rescue (in the form of folinic acid replacement) is necessary 12–24 h after the administration of methotrexate to prevent the death of too many healthy cells. Other antimetabolite drugs include 5-fluorouracil (5-FU) and cytosine arabinoside.

Plant alkaloids

Many plants and plant extracts continue to be screened to identify new cytotoxic drugs. Drugs to date include the vinca alkaloids, taxanes and topoisomerase inhibitors.

Topoisomerase inhibitors (etoposide, tenoposide, irinotecan and topotecan) interfere with DNA replication by binding to DNA and the topoisomerase enzymes. Mitotic inhibitors include vincristine, vindescine and vinblastine, which are cell cycle specific acting in the mitosis phase. They bind to microtubule proteins, blocking spindle formation and preventing cell separation. The taxanes, taxol and taxotere, on the other hand, promote assembly of the microtubule which results in a very stable microtubule that is non-functional.

Antitumour antibiotics

Some classes of antibiotic have been found to be cytotoxic. In general, they are cell cycle non-specific and interfere with DNA function, although several other mechanisms of action may occur, such as alteration of the cell membrane or inhibition of certain enzymes. The most widely used is doxorubicin because it has a broad spectrum of activity; others include mitoxantrone and bleomycin.

Cytotoxic drugs are constantly being researched and developed. There are several which do not fit into the above categories and whose action may not be fully understood.

See *Seminars in Oncology Nursing* (1995), vol. 11, no. 3, for more information about VADs. This issue covers appropriate usage, insertion techniques and the management of associated complications, both common and rare.

Regional chemotherapy. The goal of regional chemotherapy is localisation of effects by delivering chemotherapy drugs directly into blood vessels supplying the cavity containing the tumour or into the tumour itself. Such routes include intrahepatic, intra-arterial, intrapleural, intraperitoneal and intrathecal.

Many patients receive chemotherapy as outpatients, on a day unit, and so need a considerable amount of support and teaching in order to be able to cope with the side-effects they experience at home. There is agreement that although this represents role extension, trained nurse specialists are the best people to fulfil this role and to give chemotherapy (Souhami & Tobias 1998) (see Box 31.8).

Side-effects of chemotherapy. As seen with the examples given in Table 31.3, each cytotoxic agent causes different side-effects, varying in intensity with dosage and method of administration. Nursing management of the potential side-effects requires an in-depth knowledge of the common and uncommon toxicity profiles of each drug given in the regimen (see Fischer et al 1997).

Physical and emotional responses to chemotherapy vary greatly between patients. Studies by Sitzia & Wood (1998) and Tanghe et al (1998) have shown that the nurse's interpersonal skills and manner influence patients' coping mechanisms. In both studies, nurses underestimated the distress caused by chemotherapy and overestimated the patients' ability to cope. Nurses reported common side-effects, such as alopecia and nausea and vomiting, as being the most distressing toxicities for patients. However, interestingly, a large number of patients reported fatigue, mood disturbances, altered appetite, restlessness, mouth problems, bowel elimination and temperature changes as causing the most distress. These findings have implications for nurses assessing patient side-effects and delivering appropriate therapeutic interventions. The following is a very brief summary of some of the potential physical side-effects of chemotherapy.

Sexual dysfunction may occur due to vascular changes and hormonal imbalance. Amenorrhoea and menopausal symptoms may be induced due to ovarian failure and follicle destruction. Women under 40 years have a greater chance of resumption of the menses on completion of treatment; however, this may not occur for 6–12 months.

Infertility may occur, depending on the drug, its dosage, the patient's age and sex, and other unknown factors. Infertility may be temporary or permanent. Alkylating agents such as cyclophosphamide, chlorambucil and the nitrosurea compounds are certain to induce infertility (McInnes & Schilsky 1996). This variability must be stressed when patients are informed about potential side-effects. Barrier methods of contraception are encouraged, as the exposure of an unborn fetus to cytotoxic drugs may result in deformities or an unviable fetus.

In certain circumstances, some patients may receive counselling for sperm banking or oocyte harvesting. These options raise emotional and ethical dilemmas which may compound patients' existing stress concerning their diagnosis and treatment. This is an area of nursing that provides new challenges in terms of psychological support for patients and their partners.

Myelosuppression is not only the most common dose-limiting toxicity of chemotherapy but also potentially the most lethal. To understand the potential damage that chemotherapy may cause to the bone marrow, it is helpful to review normal blood cell development (see Ch. 11). The suppression of the production of blood constituents by the bone marrow occurs to varying degrees after almost all types of cytotoxic chemotherapy. Cell cycle specific agents (e.g. antimetabolites, natural products) tend to cause a rapid decline to a low point (nadir) in the marrow cells usually 7–10 days after drug administration, although with some drugs the nadir may be reached earlier. Cell cycle non-specific drugs (doxorubicin, cisplatin) have nadirs around 10–14 days, while the nitrosureas' nadir is 26–30+ days. Such factors need to be considered in the planning of treatment regimens. The resultant three problems of leucopenia/neutropenia, anaemia, and thrombocytopenia are far more severe in the case of chemotherapy for haematological malignancies (see Ch. 11). Since the prime function of neutrophils is phagocytosis,

Box 31.8 Safe administration of chemotherapy

Cytotoxic agents can be dangerous if they are not handled appropriately. A joint proposal to develop national guidelines for the administration of chemotherapy has been funded by the NHS Executive (1995) and the final document is awaited (Goodman 1998). These guidelines are to assist practitioners in defining and demonstrating high standards of practice, reducing unacceptable variations.

Extravasation

Some cytotoxic agents, e.g. doxorubicin and vincristine, are termed 'vesicants' and can cause severe burns and tissue damage if they leak from the vein into the subcutaneous tissue. Figure 31.5 shows the possible result of extravasation. If extravasation is suspected, the infusion should be stopped and an experienced clinician informed immediately. There are various antidotes available, but more scientific research is required (see How & Brown 1998 for more details).

Staff protection

Exposure to cytotoxic agents remains controversial. Sufficient scientific evidence exists, however, to support the need for staff handling these drugs to do so with extreme caution. It is known that at therapeutic doses these substances can cause carcinogenesis, cell mutations and fetal damage. Staff handling cytotoxic drugs should be educated about exposure risks, safe handling procedures and appropriate clothing, i.e. aprons and latex gloves. More research is required to evaluate occupational surveillance. A register for those at risk should be kept and safe practice needs to be regularly audited. Chemotherapeutic agents should be prepared in a specially designed pharmacy unit (laminar air flow/isolator). Staff should always wear gloves when handling oral preparations and should mop up spillages immediately, using large amounts of water and wearing protective clothing. Spillage kits should be available in all the areas where chemotherapy is administered. On seeing the precautions necessary, patients may be alarmed that such dangerous substances are required to control their disease. They should be reassured that these measures are necessary to protect those who are constantly dealing with cytotoxic agents.

Handling body fluids

Many cytotoxic agents are excreted unchanged in urine and faeces and both should be treated as hazardous for at least 48 h. However, Cass & Musgrove (1992) highlight that some excreta may be contaminated for as long as 7 days. It is therefore important to wear gloves when handling the body fluids of patients receiving chemotherapy, and also to teach patients and their families to take precautions.

Table 31.3 Cytotoxic agents and common side-effects

Cytotoxic	*Action*	*Common use*	*Side-effects*
Methotrexate	Antimetabolite (folic acid antagonist)	Wide spectrum Acute lymphocytic leukaemia Non-Hodgkin's lymphoma Breast cancer Osteosarcoma	Myelosuppression Stomatitis Diarrhoea Renal failure (HD) Occasional nausea
5-Fluorouracil	Antimetabolite	Breast cancer Colonic cancer	Myelosuppression Diarrhoea (HD) Stomatitis Vein discoloration Occasional nausea
Cytosine arabinoside (Ara C)	Antimetabolite	Acute myeloid leukaemia Acute lymphoblastic leukaemia (low dose often given subcutaneously)	Severe nausea and vomiting (HD) Myelosuppression Flu-like symptoms Stomatitis Corneal ulceration
Cyclophosphamide	Alkylating agent	Wide spectrum Small cell carcinoma of the lung Cancer of the breast, ovary and bladder Acute leukaemias	Nausea and vomiting (HD) Myelosuppression Haemorrhagic cystitis Alopecia (HD) Infertility (especially in men)
Melphalan	Alkylating agent	Myeloma Cancer of the breast, ovary	Nausea and vomiting (HD) Alopecia (HD) Myelosuppression
Doxorubicin	Antitumour antibiotic	Wide spectrum Lymphomas Small cell carcinoma of the lung Cancer of the ovary, breast, stomach, bladder	Severe stomatitis Severe nausea and vomiting Cardiotoxicity Myelosuppression Alopecia Vesicant if extravasated
Mitoxantrone	Antitumour antibiotic	Similar to doxorubicin Metastatic breast cancer Leukaemias Lymphomas	Cardiotoxicity Mild nausea and vomiting Myelosuppression Minimal alopecia Green discoloration of urine (persists ~24 h)
Vincristine (Oncovin)	Vinca alkaloid Spindle poison	Acute lymphocytic leukaemia Lymphomas Small cell carcinoma of the lung Breast cancer	Peripheral neuropathy: numbness, tingling and loss of function Constipation due to neurotoxicity Alopecia (HD) Vesicant if extravasated
Etoposide (VD 16)	Action uncertain Similar to spindle poison	Testicular cancer Small cell carcinoma of the lung Lymphomas Acute lymphocytic leukaemia	Myelosuppression Stomatitis (HD) Alopecia Hypotension if infused rapidly
Cisplatin	Action uncertain Similar to alkylating agent	Small cell carcinoma of the lung Cancer of the testes, ovary, bladder Tumours of the head and neck Lymphomas	Severe nausea and vomiting Metallic taste during infusion Diarrhoea (HD) Myelosuppression Hearing changes and loss (due to damage to eighth cranial nerve) Peripheral neuropathy
Irinotecan (CPT11)	Topoisomerase I inhibitor Spindle poison	Colorectal cancer	Myelosuppression Acute cholinergic syndrome Delayed diarrhoea Nausea and vomiting Alopecia
Paclitaxel (Taxol)	Plant alkaloid Spindle poison	Ovarian cancer Breast cancer	Myelosuppression Hypersensitivity — urticaria, abdominal cramping, anaphylaxis Alopecia Peripheral neuropathy Myalgia/arthralgia — joint and muscle pains
Fludarabine	Purine antimetabolite	Chronic lymphocytic leukaemia Low-grade non-Hodgkin's lymphoma	Myelosuppression Nausea and vomiting Flu-like symptoms Central nervous system toxicities (HD)

HD, high dose.

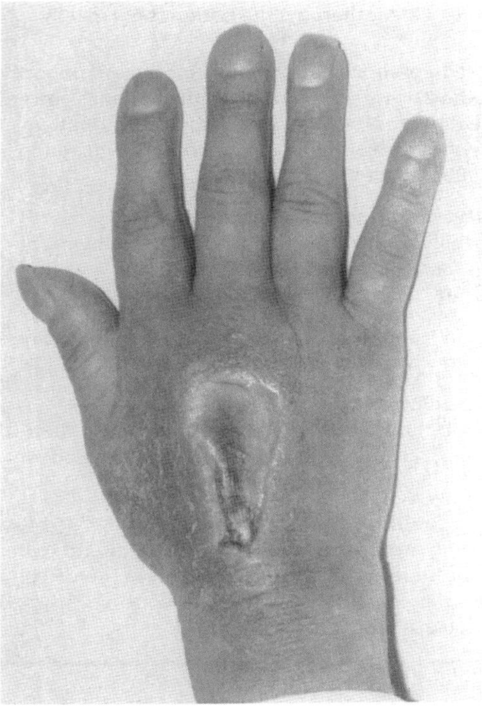

Fig. 31.5 Skin damage caused by extravasation of vesicant cytotoxins. This photograph shows a moderate degree of damage; in some cases there may be nerve and blood vessel damage, progressing to necrosis and requiring skin grafting or even amputation. The key factor in avoiding this situation is vigilant, regular observation of cannulation sites during injection or infusion. The patient should also be asked to report any altered sensation in the area, e.g. wetness, coldness, heat, tingling, numbness or swelling. Should extravasation occur, the infusion should be stopped immediately, the cannula removed, a doctor informed and a pharmacist consulted for advice. There is a lack of research to guide treatment for extravasation; however, pharmacy departments usually issue local guidelines. It is most important to avoid concentrating only on the affected limb whilst ignoring the stress generated for the patient in this situation.

neutropenia eliminates one of the body's prime defences against bacterial infection. The longer the nadir period, the greater the frequency and severity of infections which are invasive or due to overgrowth of pathogenic microbes. Thrombocytopenia is usually delayed and, if active bleeding occurs, transfusions of platelets may be given. For all patients, myelosuppression may compound other side-effects such as stomatitis.

In view of the significant problems associated with bone marrow suppression, much attention has been focused on the therapeutic use of haemopoietic growth factors such as granulocytic colony-stimulating factor (GCSF) and granulocytic macrophage colony-stimulating factor (GM-CSF). Studies have shown that these factors can significantly reduce or prevent myelosuppression induced by chemotherapy (Trillet-Lenoir et al 1993). It is hoped that with the support of GCSF/GM-CSF, higher doses of chemotherapy will be able to be given, whilst minimising the effects on the bone marrow.

Therapeutic interventions for myelosuppression are aimed at the prevention and active treatment of infection and bleeding.

Stomatitis/mucositis induced by chemotherapy is the result of a two-stage process. First, some cytotoxic agents have a direct effect on the oral mucosa, causing thinning and ulceration within 4–7 days of administration. Patients may experience mild erythema and oedema along the mucocutaneous junction of the lip, mouth dryness and a burning sensation in the lips (Dose 1995). Nausea, vomiting and a reduced food and fluid intake compound this effect, making the mucosa an ineffective barrier to opportunistic infection. Within 10–16 days, myelosuppression causes the already compromised mucosa to be even more susceptible to infection and haemorrhage. Nursing care is similar to that for the patient with radiation stomatitis, described in Table 31.2, see p. 924. Chlorhexidine mouthwash has been shown to be useful in the immunocompromised patient, particularly in inhibiting bacterial and fungal infections. With prolonged usage, however, it can cause brown discoloration of the teeth and altered taste (Rutkauskas 1993). Patients receiving chemotherapy require very thorough prophylactic oral assessment and care (see Dose 1995).

5-Fluorouracil (5-FU) commonly causes mucositis. Oral cryotherapy or sucking on crushed ice during the administration of 5-FU has been shown to reduce the frequency and severity of resulting mucositis. However, further clinical evaluation of this approach is needed (Casanu et al 1994).

Nausea and vomiting induced by chemotherapy can be particularly troublesome, especially with agents such as adriamycin and cisplatin. These drugs activate the chemoreceptor trigger zone in the brain, which in turn stimulates the centre in the brain stem that controls nausea and vomiting. It is important to remember that persistent nausea is often more unbearable than vomiting, which may relieve nausea. The problem may be severe enough to trigger 'anticipatory vomiting' at the sight of the hospital or any stimulus related to chemotherapy. During the past decade, with the advent of new antiemetics, the management of chemotherapy-related nausea and vomiting has vastly improved. This includes the effective use of 5-HT3 antagonists such as ondansetron, tropisetron and granisetron. These drugs have their own side-effect profile, which includes constipation and headaches. Steroids such as dexamethasone potentiate the effect of these antiemetics and are most effective in delayed emesis. Again they have their own toxicity profile, such as indigestion, hyperactivity and mood disturbance, and may mask signs of infection in myelosuppressed patients. Relaxation, meditation and sedatives such as lorazepam have also been found to be helpful for some patients.

Alopecia is caused by some agents (e.g. adriamycin, taxanes, topoisomerase inhibitors) and may range from slight thinning to total loss of hair. The degree and duration of alopecia are dependent on the drug, or combination of drugs, dosage and route of administration. It usually occurs approximately 2 weeks after therapy has started and is temporary, with hair regrowth occurring about 6 weeks after the completion of treatment. Hair may grow back a different texture and colour, something patients need to be warned about. Patients should be offered the choice of a wig before they experience hair loss in order to enable close matching to their own hair. Advice on minimising or delaying hair loss and the use of fashion accessories should be given.

Scalp cooling techniques have been developed with varying degrees of success (Tierney 1987). Earlier scalp cooling techniques involved wetting the scalp and applying ice packs, but more sophisticated refrigeration systems are now available which offer a more uniform cooling at a constant rate (Adams et al 1992). Observations from clinical practice suggest that scalp cooling can slow down the rate of hair loss when used with single-agent drugs with a short half-life at low dosages, e.g. adriamycin, cyclophosphamide, taxotere. It may also be effective with such regimens as FAM (5-fluorouracil, adriamycin, mitomycin C) and CMF (cyclophosphamide, methotrexate, 5-fluorouracil).

Other side-effects. It is not possible to address all the potential side-effects of chemotherapy in this chapter. However, apart from the more common ones mentioned above and those in Table 31.3, it is important to remember the more generalised effects, e.g. fatigue, anorexia, general malaise, mood disturbances and lack of concentration. Recently, nursing research has focused on fatigue and the need to develop positive interventions such as energy conservation (Richardson 1995).

Q **31.10** Choose a patient who is about to receive combination chemotherapy. Find out whether the doses or drugs in the regimen are low or high. List the side-effects you may expect to see and those that actually occur. For information, consult the manufacturers' instructions, your hospital pharmacy cytotoxic manual and texts on chemotherapy, e.g. Holmes (1997), Fischer et al (1997).

Psychological support during chemotherapy (see Box 31.9). There is increasing recognition, supported by research, that chemotherapy, particularly the highly toxic regimens, can cause severe psychological distress (Barraclough 1994). Postoperative adjuvant chemotherapy for breast cancer is associated with an increase in depression, anxiety and sexual problems, possibly because patients see no tangible improvement in their condition to outweigh the distress of the side-effects (Maguire et al 1980).

As with radiotherapy, the key to effective support for these patients is to provide written and verbal information in a suitable, individualised form. Nurses in most oncology centres and some cancer units have their own patient caseload. Treatment management includes cannulation and administration of bolus and i.v. chemotherapy, coordinating the chemotherapy regimens in collaboration with the clinician. The continuity of care engendered by this approach allows a trusting supportive relationship to be built between nurse and patient.

A more recent development in the UK is home chemotherapy. Specialised nurses, who may be hospital- or community-based, deliver chemotherapy to patients in the comfort of their own homes. Many of these projects are being set up and cost–benefit evaluation is awaited (Watters 1997).

Q **32.11** The patient receiving palliative chemotherapy may find travelling exhausting and feel that staying at home is far preferable to spending precious time in hospital. Richardson (1989) describes a scheme in which Macmillan nurses give single-agent palliative chemotherapy in the patient's home. What problems can you foresee for the patient, the family and the nurse? On balance, do you think this is a worthwhile scheme?

Non-cytotoxic chemotherapy

Agents other than cytotoxic drugs are used to control, but as yet not to cure, cancer. Tumours that arise in tissues under the control of hormones have been found to respond to hormone manipulation. This may mean surgical removal of the ovaries (oophorectomy) or testes (orchidectomy) to reduce the growth stimulus to tumours of the breast and prostate provided by oestrogen and testosterone, respectively. Recently, however, similar control has been achieved using drugs. Tamoxifen blocks the effect of oestrogen by binding to oestrogen receptor sites on tumour cells. Various forms of oestrogen can inhibit the production of testosterone by the testes.

Box 31.9 Chemotherapy: the patient's perspective

The need for information and emotional support during chemotherapy varies according to the patient's perception of the treatment. The following responses by patients to the discovery that they required chemotherapy (cited in Tierney et al 1989) reflect this variability.

Negative feelings

I can't tell you how terrified I am...it's like being put into a dark room...you've no idea what to expect and you're really frightened.

The word 'chemotherapy' sends shivers up my spine — you hear so much about how awful it is.

Mixed feelings

I do want it, but I don't. I feel really nervous....Butterflies in my tummy all the time...and then I tell myself not to be silly....You'll manage, I say.

Positive feelings

I'm making myself feel positive because I intend to do everything possible to survive. That never occurred to me before...the idea of survival...but your priorities change when you are faced with a disease like this.

Steroid hormones, such as prednisolone and dexamethasone, are also widely used, the former in conjunction with cytotoxic drugs as primary treatment (usually for lymphomas) and the latter for its anti-inflammatory action in symptom control and the control of emesis.

Symptom control forms a major part of both the nursing and medical roles in oncology (see Ch. 33).

New developments in cancer treatment

Despite an enormous amount of worldwide investment in research, cancer remains on the whole an incurable disease. Most cancer centres are involved in multiple research trials, and nurses should be familiar with the format of these trials in order to understand the implications for patients and for their nursing care and to consider the ethical dilemmas which arise around all experimental therapy.

Following laboratory testing, new treatment methods are tested on consenting patients by means of a series of trials termed phase 1, 2 and 3 trials. During phase 1, the maximum tolerable dose is established and information is obtained about the drug's toxicity profile; phase 2 trials discover which type of cancer is most responsive; and finally, phase 3 trials discover the extent to which the treatment improves survival. In phase 3 trials, patients from the target group are randomly selected to receive either the new treatment or the best established one. Survival rates are then compared.

New approaches to established radiotherapy and chemotherapy treatments are constantly being tested in this way. In addition, some centres are involved in trials of totally new modes of treatment.

Biological therapy, often referred to as the fourth treatment modality, involves the therapeutic use of substances known to occur naturally in the body. Most of these are involved in some way in the immune response, controlling cell-mediated and humoral responses; hence some of these new developments are termed 'immunotherapies'. The theory behind these new treatments is that it may be possible to manipulate the immune system such that it recognises tumour cells as antigens and causes the body to reject them. Indeed, genetically identical laboratory mice with transplanted tumours have been found to develop resistance to further tumour transplants.

Biological therapies were prematurely hailed as 'miracle cures' for all cancer types. In fact, the response of the immune system to tumours has been found to be far more subtle and complex than the response to microbes, and results have been far from dramatic. Nevertheless, several substances, mostly created by recombinant DNA technology, have been developed. Although research is still at a very early stage, tumour response, however transient, has been achieved for some cancer types.

Cytokines are substances released from an activated immune system. Interferon, for example, is a cytokine that protects host cells against viruses. It has been found to maintain remission in hairy cell leukaemia and is being used with some success in certain patients with renal cell carcinoma and melanoma. Side-effects include flu-like symptoms and mood disturbances, which may be very unpleasant. Other similar substances include tumour necrosis factor (TNF) and interleukin 2.

Haemopoietic growth factors include GCSF and GM-CSF, which stimulate the proliferation of leucocytes. Used appropriately, these factors may reduce the number or degree of myelosuppressive episodes, prevent treatment delays and allow high doses of treatment to be given. Erythropoietin is another stimulating factor used in the treatment of anaemia, e.g. in end-stage renal disease. The number of blood transfusions may be reduced and symptoms of fatigue minimised, thus enhancing quality of life.

A limiting factor in effective cancer therapy is its current lack of specificity. During the 1980s, significant strides were made in the field of antibody therapy, which promotes specific targeting of cells through an antigen–antibody response. Tumours have been found to possess antigens on their surface, and monoclonal antibodies to these antigens can now be manufactured in laboratories. However, monoclonal antibodies have yet to live up to their expected potential.

Understanding the molecular biology of cancer has led to some optimism about incorporating this knowledge into cancer screening, diagnosis, prognosis, relapse monitoring, treatment and genetic susceptibility testing. Gene therapy is a treatment in its infancy, the principle being to correct the gene alteration in affected cells in order to achieve a permanent correction of the mutated gene. Preliminary trials are taking place using viral vectors to transfer the gene. Non-viral methods of transfer rely on chemical methods, e.g. liposomes (Peters 1997, Bradley 1999).

Another method of gene therapy currently under investigation in phase 2 trials involves patients being exposed to specific segments of DNA, or 'antisense' molecules, which block the oncogenes ('on' switch) thereby suppressing the growth of tumour cells.

It is hoped that future use of these approaches in conjunction with cytotoxic chemotherapy will have an impact on the treatment of cancer. These therapies have quite different toxicity spectra from that of chemotherapy and nurses need to be aware of these in order to support their patients.

Laser beam therapy. A laser beam is an intensified form of light that can be focused on a spot the size of a pinprick and which is capable of vaporising tumour tissue. Apart from its use in removing premalignant or neoplastic cells from the cervix, to date this treatment has mainly been used as a palliative measure, as tumour tissue tends to regenerate. Intraluminal tumours of the oesophagus, for example, can be reduced in size to relieve dysphagia and malnutrition.

Complementary therapy. The outcome of conventional medical cancer treatments is a matter of great uncertainty for patients. For many, cancer will become a chronic illness that affects every area of their lives. For these reasons, there is increasing interest in complementary therapies, such as therapeutic touch, aromatherapy, relaxation techniques, yoga, hypnotherapy and special diets.

Little research exists to justify the use of any of these therapies as alternatives to orthodox treatments (Fitch et al 1999). Evidence for the value of complementary therapy is conflicting. Bagenal et al (1990) found that certain therapies, particularly extreme dietary control, may be detrimental to survival. However, a study of 86 patients with metastatic breast carcinoma showed that those who were taught self-hypnosis for pain control and were involved in supportive group therapy lived an average of almost 18 months longer than the control group, even though they received the same orthodox treatment (Spiegel et al 1989).

Recent discoveries of neurotransmitters connecting the brain, body and immune system suggest a physiological basis for this finding. It is also possible, however, that the extra time, attention and caring mediated by therapists in the course of complementary treatments are factors in the client's feeling of well-being. Many of these therapies also focus on the 'holistic' approach to health, in which the individual is encouraged to take control of his own life, both mentally and physically. It is well established that, when patients feel in control, they have a positive attitude, comply more willingly with medical treatment and, most importantly, experience subjectively a better quality of life.

Problems in complementary therapy. Problems associated with some complementary therapies include the fact that an overemphasis on 'taking control' may lead to feelings of guilt and failure when disease problems recur. Some therapies, such as hypnosis, must only be practised by experts. More basic techniques such as aromatherapy and massage may be incorporated into the nursing care plan, but nurses practising these must be taught to do so by experts. Caution is also required when using natural oils as there is insufficient research-based evidence regarding their safety. There is a risk that they may interact with conventional treatments. Certain complementary therapies are contraindicated for some patients: for example, all but the gentlest massage may be detrimental for those with bone metastases, where fractures occur easily. It is a good idea to discuss any planned complementary therapy with the whole health care team as well as with the patient.

NURSING PRACTICE IN CANCER CARE

The cancer nurse

Cancer and its treatment have a unique impact on an individual's life. Although the physical problems experienced by cancer patients may be similar to those of patients with many non-malignant conditions, the combination of these problems with the chronic nature of cancer, the highly toxic effects of treatment and the profound psychological impact of the disease means that cancer nurses require specialised knowledge and skills. The key skills in cancer nursing are those that help the cancer patient and his carers to adapt to the reality of living with cancer while maximising quality of life.

Hospital–community liaison

Cancer is a chronic illness characterised by remissions, exacerbations and slowly progressive physical changes. More patients with cancer are living longer. Health professionals caring for cancer patients should view care as a continuous process whether it takes place in the hospital or in the community setting. Supporting the patient through the cancer journey requires the skills of all members of the multiprofessional team in conjunction with the patient and family. If care is to be a truly continuous process then the importance of sharing the care between hospital and community needs to be acknowledged (Owen & Black 1996). Shared care protocols are a relatively new concept in cancer care which have come about in response to the recognition of unfulfilled needs of patients receiving active treatments at home, e.g. immunotherapy or continuous chemotherapy infusions. Treatment is initiated in hospital and continued in the community. Shared care protocols will develop and enhance patient care whilst promoting the philosophy of continuity of care between hospital and community. Effective communication and discharge planning are essential to optimal care. Without proper coordination and integration of services, the cancer patient's 'journey' through the health care system can be a bewildering and demoralising experience. The example of Mr A in Case History 31.4 illustrates the need for good discharge planning and liaison between hospital and community nurses.

Cancer patients spend most of their lives at home, interrupted by short hospital admissions. As a result, the psychological and physical adjustment to cancer takes place at home. Community initiatives and services are set up to support patients, their families and other carers from diagnosis to terminal illness, helping patients in decision-making and achieving optimal independence and quality of life.

Cancer care in any setting can be very satisfying; it can also be stressful and nurses working in this speciality will need to develop healthy and effective coping strategies (see Box 31.10).

Cancer care in the community

Community nursing staff are involved in cancer care during four phases:

- prevention programmes
- treatment-related support
- rehabilitation following initial cancer treatment
- palliative care.

It is mainly practice nurses and health visitors who are involved in prevention schemes. Some health visitors may visit patients recently discharged from hospital in order to assess how they and their families are coping and their needs for care and emotional support. District nurses coordinate and carry out nursing care for patients throughout their time in the community. In some areas, new initiatives are being developed to support patients in the community at diagnosis and during treatment with the introduction of community cancer care nurses with specialist oncology knowledge and skills. Towards the later stages of the disease, symptoms may become more problematic and place more strain on carers; at this stage, Macmillan or home care nurses may become involved. These nurses have in-depth knowledge of symptom control, additional training in counselling skills, and time to assess each patient and to plan care in conjunction with the district nurse. They also have close links with hospice and hospital palliative care teams. The fostering of links with the Macmillan service as early as possible, when a patient is still able to discuss his hopes, fears and goals, assists in the establishment of a supportive relationship. The role of Macmillan nurses is further discussed in Chapter 33.

The role of the district nurse. The role of community staff is one of partnership with the patient and his family, who constitute the main 'unit of care'. Providing information, support and advice is often as important as assistance with physical care.

Case History 31.4 Mr A

Mr A, a 58-year-old head teacher, was married with two children: a daughter in Australia and a married son with two small children who lived nearby.

He presented to his GP with urinary hesitancy and frequency. Examination and subsequent referral to a urologist revealed a T3 adenocarcinoma of the prostate (a locally invasive tumour with no metastases). A biopsy of the tumour and a bone scan were performed with Mr A as an outpatient. Mr A opted for 4 weeks of radical radiotherapy rather than a prostatectomy. Because he lived in a small town 50 miles away from the nearest radiotherapy department, he became an in-patient, going home at weekends. During his recovery at home, a health visitor visited twice.

Two years later, 1 week after his retirement, rib pain necessitated a further bone scan. This showed metastatic deposits in the ribs and spine. At Mr A's local hospital, a bilateral orchidectomy was performed to reduce hormonal stimulation of tumour growth. Mr A was then readmitted to the radiotherapy department. One week of palliative radiotherapy and the commencement of opiate analgesics enabled discharge and 6 months of reasonably independent life.

However, a fall whilst Mr A was gardening resulted in the collapse of the third thoracic vertebrae, with resultant severe pain and paraplegia due to spinal cord compression. Emergency radiotherapy and intensive physiotherapy restored some function, but Mr A was now confined to a wheelchair and had no bladder or bowel control.

Mrs A was fit and was very determined to cope at home with the help of her son and his wife. Prior to Mr A's discharge, the community occupational therapy department oversaw the installation of a wheelchair ramp, bath aids and a hoist in the A's bungalow. District nurses visited daily, and the Macmillan nurse weekly.

Within 6 weeks a further admission, this time to the local hospital, was necessary due to hypercalcaemia. Following this, Mr A was generally too weak to get out of bed. District nurses now visited him twice a day, and the Macmillan nurse every second day as the control of pain and nausea became a problem. It was arranged for Marie Curie nurses to care for Mr A at night, in order to give the family a rest. Mr A died peacefully at home with his family, 10 days after discharge.

Another major role of the district nurse involves coordination of the primary care team and integration of statutory and non-statutory services. Because of the nature of cancer, the need for these services is considerable. The statutory services available include all of those necessary for the care of the chronically ill in the community (see Ch. 32).

Non-statutory services in the community. Non-statutory services for cancer patients are particularly comprehensive in their provision and include the following.

Support and self-help groups. Such groups can reduce the isolation of the cancer experience. The sharing of feelings and experiences provides emotional support, fosters hope and encourages a sense of self-worth and purpose. Many local groups exist for patients and/or their carers; a directory is published by Cancerlink (see 'Useful addresses', p. 943).

Support centres are now being developed which are resources for information to enable decision-making. They often provide

Box 31.10 Stress in cancer nursing

Speck (1988) states that the most important ethical choice made by cancer nurses is whether or not to engage in 'an intense, personalised involvement' with their patients in response to human need. A degree of emotional involvement is inevitable, and even necessary, to achieve excellence in cancer care. But such involvement, particularly as it may be terminated by the patient's death, results in considerable occupational stress. Community staff are particularly vulnerable because they often work in isolation and build up relationships with cancer patients over longer periods of time than do hospital nurses.

Bailey & Clarke (1989) describe 'indirect' coping methods as more constructive ways of dealing with this inevitable stress than 'palliative' methods (e.g. smoking, excess alcohol consumption, work absenteeism). Indirect coping involves achieving personal awareness and control under stress. Bailey & Clarke give practical guidelines to such methods, which include relaxation, desensitisation and assertiveness training.

The constructive expression of emotions is as important as stress control. A work atmosphere in which it is safe to admit to colleagues feelings of inadequacy, grief and guilt, and even personal fears about cancer and death, is beneficial in relieving stress. Such support should also be provided on an organised basis in the form of support groups and counselling services (Tschudin 1996). An active life and supportive relationships outside of work are also vital in maintaining a realistic perspective on life. Without external interests, it may be easy for the nurse to imagine that cancer is far more prevalent than it is.

A study of cancer nurses by Wilkinson (1990) showed that feelings of inadequacy and lack of knowledge and skill, particularly in communication, were major stressors. A commitment to continuing education by nursing management is therefore essential in stress control. However, as Tschudin (1996) concludes: 'nurses themselves need to take on more direct responsibility for their own psychological care', and in campaigning for support and education.

Areas of high stress in nursing often correlate with high job satisfaction (Bailey & Clarke 1989). Wilkinson's (1990) study confirms this: 96% of the sample claimed that they would choose cancer nursing as a career again.

complementary therapies and sometimes formal/informal psychological support. Their philosophy is based on the fostering of positive coping mechanisms and self-help and is grounded in research by psychologists who have shown that positive adaptation to the cancer situation may improve survival.

Counselling services. Counselling may be necessary to assist the patient and his family to adapt emotionally to cancer and can help to relieve anxiety and depression. BACUP is one example of an organisation which provides this service by telephone and in person and advises about other local counselling services.

Information services. Information fosters independence in decision-making and can be supportive in itself. Examples of organisations for particular groups of cancer patients include Breast Cancer Care, The British Colostomy Association and the Leukaemia Care Society.

Financial aid. The Cancer Relief Macmillan Fund (CRMF) can provide financial aid to meet the cost of aids, appliances, heating, bedding, holidays and other special needs.

Nursing services. Macmillan or home care nursing services are discussed above. The Marie Curie organisation provides nursing staff, including a night nursing service, to allow carers some respite or sleep.

Choosing a nursing model for cancer care

No one model of nursing can be suitable for every cancer patient or care setting. It is important to adapt and combine models and approaches to provide a workable framework of care for each patient.

Activities of living model

Cancer may affect every activity of living. Because cure is often not possible, the emphasis in care is on maximising quality of life. This includes promoting as much independence as possible. The basic framework of the Roper et al (1996) activities of living model can be used here. This model focuses on three components of nursing activity — preventing, comforting and assisting — in relation to each of 12 activities of living (ALs). Any one of these components may become particularly relevant at different stages in the cancer process.

As with any nursing model, the AL model is not applicable to cancer care in every respect. Most people with cancer live with the disease as a chronic illness and many will find it impossible to regain or maintain independence in every AL; yet some of these individuals may be described at a given point as healthy because they have learned to cope with their limitations. Another shortcoming of the model is that 'communication', one of the ALs, is not a sufficiently comprehensive category to encompass the whole range of psychological and emotional needs and responses that the cancer patient will experience.

Roy adaptation model

Some aspects of the Roy adaption model (Roy 1989) may be more applicable to the nursing care of cancer patients, particularly in a community or rehabilitative setting. Roy sees the cancer as a stimulus to which the patient and his family must be assisted to adapt. The nurse either manipulates the stimulus and its symptoms, or promotes the coping abilities of the patient and his family. This inclusion of the family is especially important in any chronic disease.

A combined model

A suitable nursing approach for many cancer care settings would be to combine those aspects of both the AL and Roy models that are especially relevant, giving particular emphasis to the communication needs of the patient, as these would now be defined more broadly. Whatever model is selected or devised will attempt to outline the nurse's unique contribution to care. It should be stressed, however, that in many situations, particularly those where cure is not possible, it would be artificial to think in terms of separate approaches by nursing and medical staff. Here, a teamwork model is required which will allow the nurse's role to overlap greatly with that of other team members, but which acknowledges and makes provision for the special contributions of the nurse, such as her role in ensuring continuity, consistency and coordination of care.

Cancer patients may have multiple problems that require nursing intervention. Four such areas of potential difficulty have been selected for discussion in the following sections. The first, family coping, is a problem of adaptation. The others — eating and drinking, expressing sexuality, and communication — are three of the ALs. For each, various considerations relevant to assessment are listed, followed by a set of possible nursing interventions to aid the patient in adapting to his situation.

Family coping

A cancer diagnosis can have a drastic effect on the patient's family and loved ones in the following ways:

- Cancer can disrupt patterns of familial and other interpersonal interaction. Those who are close to the patient are usually perplexed as to how to relate to him in the most helpful way. Reactions vary from overprotection and excessive vigilance to distancing behaviour and even the complete breakdown of relationships. Many patients, especially in the early stages of the disease, find they have to be the strong one emotionally, supporting and holding the family together (Evans 1989). Under such strain it is no wonder that cancer can (and does) precipitate partnership and marital breakdown. Most at risk are those whose relationship is already unstable. In a study by Barraclough (1994), however, a majority of married people stated that they actually felt closer to their partners in the few months following a cancer diagnosis.
- Cancer disrupts planning for the future. An experience with cancer may last for many years. The uncertainty involved disrupts family plans and dreams — for holidays, retirement, parenthood and so forth. Roles within the family change, particularly if the patient is a breadwinner or parent. Such change is stressful and can undermine the patient's sense of self-worth and purpose. Loss of income and increased expenditure due to the illness can create financial strain.
- Cancer alters the interaction of the family with external groups. Patients and their families may become isolated as a result of the social stigma of cancer, financial hardship and any residual disability. For some, however, involvement in self-help groups and cancer charities expands social interaction.

Nursing interventions. After assessment of family dynamics and needs, the following nursing interventions may help to alleviate some of the above problems:

- Providing regular information about the patient's status and plans for care, preferably with the patient and his family together to facilitate open communication. Studies show that relatives may feel they are not entitled to information, yet nurses usually leave it to them to take the initiative in asking for it (Bond 1982).
- Encouraging relatives to express their feelings of fear, loss, guilt and exhaustion.
- Encouraging realistic, mutual goal-setting, e.g. the timing and planning of holidays.
- Encouraging family members to adapt the patient's role within the family to maintain his sense of belonging and of worth, e.g. by exchanging physical tasks for clerical ones.
- Referring families promptly to the social work department for financial assistance and, if necessary, rehousing.
- Recognising signs of exhaustion in carers, giving them 'permission' to take time off and arranging respite care or hospital/hospice admission for the patient if necessary.
- Encouraging continued social involvement, suggesting appropriate activities if necessary.
- Suggesting referral to a psychologist or marriage guidance counsellor if family relationships appear to be breaking down.

Eating and drinking

Malnutrition accompanied by varying degrees of weight loss affects up to two-thirds of cancer patients at some stage in their disease, many cancer patients having a deficient intake of protein and calories (Kern & Norton 1988).

Cancer cachexia is described by Foltz (1997). Although not all patients suffer from this in the extreme, the associated weight loss can have a very negative effect on a patient's body image and sexuality, and serves as a constant reminder of the disease.

Malnutrition in cancer patients is associated with a poor prognosis, reduced response to anticancer treatments and prolongation of treatment side-effects (Holmes 1996). Causes of malnutrition and weight loss in cancer patients are numerous and interrelated. They include:

- Reduced food intake due to:
  —anorexia: multiple causes, but may be partly due to cachectin, a substance produced by some tumours
  —taste changes: may occur in any cancer patient (Stubbs 1989); they are commonest following radiotherapy to the head or neck due to destruction of salivary tissue. Usually involve lowered threshold for bitter tastes, and therefore aversion to meat; raised threshold for sweet tastes, and hence many foods taste bland and 'cardboard-like'; alteration of the taste of tea and coffee
  —early satiety: a premature feeling of fullness, usually progressing over the day
  —other symptoms, such as pain, nausea, vomiting and drowsiness
  —physical difficulties due to the tumour or its treatment, e.g. stomatitis, or dysphagia due to oesophageal obstruction
  —anxiety and depression.
- Malabsorption due to:
  —tumours of the GI tract
  —impairment of nutrient absorption resulting from chemotherapy and abdominal radiotherapy.
- Excess expenditure of nutrients, due to:
  —(in many patients) raised basal metabolic rate, partly due to the demands of the tumour
  —excessive loss of body protein due to vomiting, diarrhoea, haemorrhage, oedema, and exudates from stomas, fistulae and ulcerations.

Nursing interventions. Actions that the nurse can take to help the patient overcome or manage difficulties with eating and drinking include the following:

- Carrying out an initial assessment of the patient. This should include a thorough nutritional assessment which is repeated at regular intervals. Weekly weighing is adequate; more frequent weighing may cause the patient to become anxious about and demoralised by continued weight loss.
- Identifying the major factors from the list above that contribute to the nutritional deficit.
- Referring all at-risk patients to a dietician.
- Enlisting the help of relatives and friends in providing encouragement and supplying the patient's favourite foods. The nurse should explain, however, that there are very real reasons for the patient's reluctance to eat.
- Encouraging the patient to eat, whilst respecting his autonomy. It may be necessary to encourage the patient temporarily to regard food as a necessary medicine.
- Offering frequent, small, attractive meals; negotiating with the catering department for flexibility in portion size and for a supply of nutrient-rich foods to be kept at ward level.
- Encouraging patients to take fluids in the form of high-energy drinks; discouraging drinking at mealtimes, to avoid early satiety.
- Reassuring the patient that taste changes are normal and may disappear in time; offering taste-enhancing herbs and spices and alternatives to tea and coffee.

- Encouraging, if appropriate, consumption of a small amount of alcohol with meals as an appetite stimulant.
- Controlling other symptoms. Antiemetics should be administered 30 min before meals. Patients with a painful mouth or throat may be given topical anaesthetic mouthwashes immediately before eating.
- Providing dietary supplements in liquid form between meals and as powdered additives with meals. A study by Parkinson et al (1987) showed that Polycal and Protifar were the most palatable additives for a group of cancer patients. Their use achieved a significant increase in calorie and protein intake in 30 patients. Other dietary supplements available include Maxijule, Maxipro, Calsip, Ensure and Build up.
- Eliminating nauseating environmental stimuli at mealtimes, such as bedpans, odours and disturbing procedures.
- If intake is consistently inadequate and/or weight loss continues, commencing other forms of feeding: nasogastric if absorption is adequate; parenteral if not.
- Once the patient is well, encouraging a healthy, well-balanced diet, similar to that recommended for preventing cancer (see Box 31.3); discouraging faddish or drastic diets, particularly those involving prolonged fasting.

Expressing sexuality

Following treatment for cancer, up to 50% of patients who were sexually active before the illness report some reduction in sexual interest or activity (Barraclough 1994). Health care professionals in general fail to take the initiative in discussing their patients' sexual problems. Wilson & Williams (1988) demonstrated a discrepancy between nurses' attitudes towards the need for assessment of sexual problems and their actual behaviour. The reticence of some nurses may be due to embarrassment, but a lack of relevant knowledge and counselling skills has also been reported.

Sexuality involves more than sexual intercourse. It includes self-image in relation to gender, role behaviour within a partnership, and many forms of love and affection between partners. A cancer patient's sexuality may be altered for many reasons, including:

- The physical effects of the tumour — e.g. lesions of the spinal cord may interfere with the nerve pathways necessary for sexual sensation or motor function
- Symptoms caused by the tumour — e.g. pain, immobility and fatigue all decrease libido and performance
- The physical effects of treatment — hormone manipulation may alter sexual function; surgery may alter the anatomy (e.g. a prostatectomy may cause pelvic nerve damage resulting in impotence); pelvic irradiation may reduce vaginal lubrication causing dyspareunia (painful intercourse)
- Body image problems, e.g. post-mastectomy or following stoma formation. Less obvious changes may also contribute, e.g. varying degrees of weight loss or hair loss
- Anxiety and depression related to the cancer diagnosis resulting in low self-esteem.

Nursing interventions. The nurse can provide support for the cancer patient experiencing problems with the expression of sexuality in the following ways:

- Initiating discussion in order to give the patient 'permission' to voice his concerns. Once the discussion is initiated, the patient will indicate whether or not he wishes to pursue the topic.
- Anticipating problems before treatment: explaining how long they will last and that they are to be expected; describing measures that can be used to relieve them. See Table 31.2 for examples of interventions for radiotherapy patients.
- Opening discussion with non-threatening subjects such as contraceptive advice or the alterations in partnership roles due to illness. This will aid progression to potentially more embarrassing issues.
- Discovering and using the patient's own language in relation to his sexuality.
- Ensuring that anxiety and depression are treated and body-image problems addressed. Severe body-image problems may require desensitisation therapy by a psychologist.
- Involving partners in discussion and physical care as appropriate.
- Facilitating the privacy of couples in hospitals.
- When appropriate, discussing ways in which a couple may share sexual pleasure that does not involve intercourse. Cancerlink and BACUP provide information that describes such methods.
- Referring patients and partners with severe problems to a psychologist or sexual counsellor as appropriate.

Communicating

From the cancer patient's perspective, communication can be the most important aspect of treatment, in part because of its capacity to exacerbate or allay the fear that often accompanies cancer (Thorne 1988). Communication can be divided into three areas of activity, which may be described as:

- cognitive — the giving and receiving of information
- emotional — the feeling and expression of psychological responses
- spiritual — the expression and feeling of thoughts relating to existential issues beyond the self.

Although this division can help us to identify specific nursing activities, the three areas are very much interrelated. Providing information in a sensitive, caring manner affords emotional support, and many people do not consciously make the distinction between the emotional and spiritual dimensions.

Cognitive activity. The patient's need for information in relation to diagnosis and treatment has been examined in earlier sections of this chapter. To this discussion the following observations may be added:

- Information is power: power to enable independence, autonomous decision-making and realistic goal-setting for patients and their families. Information promotes the patient's sense of control over his life.
- Studies of patients' perceived needs rank information as the highest need (Peck & Boland 1977, Eardley 1986).
- Lack of information can deepen a depressive reaction to a cancer diagnosis.
- Cassileth et al (1980) showed that specific information about diagnosis and prognosis can encourage active participation by patients in their own care, and in fact generates rather than negates hope.
- Patients have traditionally expected their needs for information to be met by doctors, and their needs for support to be met by nurses (Thorne 1988). However, in practice, particularly with the evolution of specialist nurses, this is changing. Patients will choose the person they wish to obtain information from depending on their needs. Doctors are recognising the need to develop appropriate communication skills in order to support their patients when information is given. Communication courses are

now available for all levels of clinicians and communication is now an integral part of the medical undergraduate course.

- Studies show that patients seldom take the initiative in seeking information, mainly because staff appear busy and unavailable (Bond 1982, Wells 1998b).
- A nurse who is behaving in an unavailable manner may be too busy to answer questions at that particular time. She may also lack the information the patient is seeking, or fear that information-giving may lead to an emotional unburdening by the patient, for which she may lack the personal resources necessary to cope.
- Patients and their families need information on the cause of their cancer, the possible course of their disease, treatment options, the role of the health care team, available services, and sources of further information.
- Patients vary greatly in their desire for, and receptivity to, information. For example, patients who actively deny their cancer are unlikely to listen to information about community nursing support on discharge, and patients with a fatalistic attitude may not be interested in information about self-help groups or complementary therapy.

Nursing interventions. The following advice may assist the nurse as she strives to meet the patient's communication needs:

- Be equipped with the information that the patient needs. Be assertive in obtaining this information from other members of the health care team so that a consistent 'story' is given to the patient.
- Be present at as many interactions between the patient and the doctor as possible. Afterwards reinforce messages and ensure that the patient has understood.
- Find out what the patient already knows and has been told, and what he wants to know. In general, follow the patient's agenda.
- Discover the patient's principal fears and give information to correct any misconceptions.
- Bear in mind that when receiving information most people remember only three specific points; the first three points made are those most likely to be remembered.
- Avoid jargon: 'your white cell count will fall', for example, will mean nothing to most patients. Information about how they will feel and what they will experience is most important to patients.
- Document information given, together with an estimation of the patient's retention and reaction.
- Be prepared for the patient to forget or deny the information given.
- Reinforce verbal information with written information. BACUP and many oncology centres, e.g. the Royal Marsden, produce patient literature on a wide range of subjects.
- Be prepared for information-giving to lead to emotional issues. Allow time for this or promise to return at an arranged time.
- Give the patient and his relatives the same information. Give each the opportunity to receive this information both together and separately, so that personal anxieties can be expressed privately and within the family group.

Emotional activity. Enabling patients and their families to cope with the emotional impact of cancer demands effective listening skills and is an essential component of counselling (see Box 31.11). The following considerations should be borne in mind by the nurse as she addresses the cancer patient's emotional needs:

- During any stage of the disease, the cancer patient is suffering the effects of various actual or potential losses. These may include loss of a body part or function, loss of self-image, loss of work or leisure activities, loss of family or social role, loss of control over his life, loss of goals and dreams for the future, and, ultimately, loss of life itself. Loss is the predominant factor in all sadness and depression.
- There are many uncertainties involved in cancer; uncertainty leads to anxiety.
- While the majority of cancer patients adjust emotionally and cope reasonably well with loss and uncertainty, several studies document the prevalence of psychological distress and even psychiatric illness among this client group. For example, within the first 12–18 months of mastectomy, at least 1 in 5 patients develops an anxiety state or depressive illness. Even in the case of Hodgkin's disease, which has a good prognosis, up to one-third of patients develop psychiatric morbidity, particularly if chemotherapy and/or radiotherapy are used (Maguire 1985).
- A great deal of this emotional turmoil, anxiety and depression passes undetected and unrelieved. Rates of depression have been reported to have been as high as 75% in several psychiatric studies (Mathieson & Stam 1995). Maguire (1985) calculates that only one-fifth of patients with severe emotional problems are helped effectively.
- Some studies show that this lack of emotional support is not related to inappropriate communication by nurses, i.e. to the saying of unhelpful things, but rather to their lack of availability or willingness to communicate at all (Bond 1982, Wells 1998b).
- Emotional support is not a luxury in nursing care. Emotional distress may result in somatic symptoms such as confusion, immobility, insomnia and pain. Some research suggests that the patient's emotional coping ability and level of hope may even prolong life: patients who express their feelings of anxiety and anger, and who adopt a 'fighting spirit' with a degree of positive denial, have a better prognosis (Greer et al 1979).
- The growth of complementary therapies in cancer care represents a recognition that healing is a much wider concept than that of cure; indeed, healing can take place even in the absence of a medical cure. Healing involves psychological adaptation to living with cancer, a process of coming to terms with one's situation.
- Patients' reactions to cancer vary greatly, depending on personality, past experience and learned coping strategies.

Nursing interventions. The following strategies can be employed to give the patient support as he adjusts emotionally to his illness and treatment:

- Many patients cover up a great deal of their distress and assume that nurses do not have time to listen to them. Be alert to clues to this distress, such as constant information-seeking, manipulative behaviour and unrealistic goal-setting.
- Give the patient 'openings' to state what is on his mind, e.g. by concluding an information-giving session by asking him how he feels about the information, or by remarking upon a worried or sad expression.
- Do not be afraid of saying the wrong thing. A study by Thorne (1988) showed a strong association between 'perceived concern' and interpretation of a communication as helpful by patients. A desire to understand and an attitude of concern are the important factors.
- Learn and apply interviewing techniques used in counselling, e.g. reflecting a patient's question or statement back to him. This gives the patient the chance to realise what he has said and

Box 31.11 Communication skills: an example

This is an example of how one nurse offered her support to a young woman with acute leukaemia and her family. Notice the importance of following the patient's agenda and responding to the situation as it developed rather than imposing a preconceived structure for communication (cited by Benner & Wrubel 1989, pp. 298–308):

While waiting for confirmation of the diagnosis, I did a lot of listening. I listened to the expression of shock, fear and guilt. I did not negate their concerns or try to offer false assurances.

It was clear that one of the most useful things I could do for this distraught family, who were in a strange and overwhelming place, was to assist them, little by little, in gaining control over their experiences. This involved helping them to anticipate and be prepared for what was to come, for how it might feel or look physically or emotionally. It also involved helping them to continue in their usual roles as much as possible, and engaging them in the decisions affecting Lara's care.

Although she knew that she had less than a 50% chance of survival, she concentrated on the here and now; the pain associated with frequent i.v.s, bone marrows and lumbar punctures; the embarrassment of hair loss, the isolation from her friends, and the nausea and vomiting associated with her chemotherapy. I followed her lead by responding to her immediate concerns.

I used a variety of approaches in working with her, depending on what kind of day she was having. Sometimes we would just joke around; other times we would talk about more serious issues — not just her illness but her personal life, as well as my own.

I was always open with her, accepted her feelings, and never made light of them. I did not assure her that 'it would get better soon' or that 'I knew how she must be feeling' because I truly did not know whether she would get better or how she actually felt.

Lara was just plain miserable. All I could do with her was listen, acknowledge how awful it must be, and honestly say that she must feel like crying. Permission to cry was all she needed to let the tears flow. One day, she looked me directly in the eyes and said 'I'm so sick, am I going to die?'. Although it was a matter of seconds before I answered, it seemed like hours as my mind groped for the right words. I did not avert my gaze and answered from my heart 'I'm afraid Lara, that you are so sick that you could die'.

to expand on it, and the nurse time to reflect on what is meant. Remember, however, that constant reflection of questions will irritate patients. Once the patient's main concerns have been established, it may be time to give direct answers.

- Resist giving pat answers and false reassurances. Many of the dilemmas faced by cancer patients have no ready solution. Do not be afraid to admit that you cannot give answers to all the patient's questions about the future. Try, however, to leave the patient with some hope: help him to identify something positive in his situation on which to focus.
- Assist the patient in identifying realistic goals in order to foster hope. These goals should originate from the patient but often need an objective person to identify them. Examples may be the goal of fighting the disease, of living until a daughter's wedding, of returning to work part-time, and so on.
- A certain degree of worry and sadness is to be expected. Be alert to signs of disabling anxiety (somatic stress symptoms, lack of concentration, feelings of panic) or depression (a 'flat' mood, an exaggerated feeling of guilt and self-blame, suicidal ideation). If these are noted, refer the patient to a psychologist or psychiatrist. Anxiolytic and antidepressant drugs and various forms of psychological therapy may be required before other forms of counselling therapy can be effective (Moorey 1988).
- Patients may react to their disease with denial, anger, bargaining, depression and acceptance (Kübler-Ross 1973). Counselling cannot force the patient to move from one stage to another, but it does allow him to express feelings and perhaps make progress. The nurse should give the patient permission to express his feelings in any safe way he chooses and should not feel that she has failed when a patient becomes emotionally distraught. The expression of emotions is therapeutic and is an important part of psychological adaptation.
- Supporting patients and their families through the cancer experience is very demanding emotionally. It is important for nurses to recognise the resultant stress in themselves and their colleagues and to seek and offer active support (see Box 31.10).

Spiritual activity. A full consideration of the cancer patient's quality of life must recognise the spiritual dimension of his experience, which we might describe, in the most basic terms, as his search for meaning and purpose. Cancer has been described as 'a modern metaphor for human confrontation with existential uncertainty' (Goldberg & Tull 1983). Because spirituality involves the contemplation of things that affect us but lie beyond our control, cancer has the capacity to precipitate a spiritual crisis.

For many in modern society, the spiritual needs for love, hope, creativity and purpose are met in relationships with others and in their engagement with the material world. The person faced with a cancer diagnosis may feel such needs with particular acuteness and may be assisted by interventions similar to those described in the section on emotional activity (p. 938).

For some, whether or not death is likely, a cancer diagnosis creates a greater urgency to come to terms with concepts of God, the meaning of life, the problem of human suffering and the possibility of an afterlife. For others, religious conviction will provide a framework for such questioning and a vehicle for spiritual expression.

Nursing interventions. In acknowledging and addressing the cancer patient's spiritual needs, the nurse should bear in mind the following considerations:

- Spiritual issues are often not expressed as such by the patient. They may be expressed as anger and disbelief, doubts about self-worth, feelings of guilt and a fear of death. These feelings should be recognised as possibly stemming from spiritual questioning. The nurse should listen non-judgementally to the patient's views and acknowledge that some questions can never be answered.
- Patients of all faiths should be assisted to worship according to their custom. Nurses who share the patient's faith may find that a few minutes of prayer with him may be of more benefit than an hour of counselling.
- Even the most religious patients may express feelings of doubt, despair and anger against their God. This does not necessarily mean that they are losing their faith, but could indicate that they

are grappling with it. The nurse should acknowledge the patient's distress and, if the patient wishes, enlist the help of a spiritual counsellor or minister.

- Not everyone with cancer is dying. However, almost all cancer patients consider the possibility of death at some point. If the patient verbalises this possibility, and the timing is appropriate, he should not be denied the chance to begin the very necessary process of anticipatory grief. At the same time, all reasonable hope for the short-term future should be fostered and the patient's quality of life in the present should be enhanced by all means possible.

New directions for cancer care

Slevin et al (1990) point out that those who do not have cancer, whether they are lay people or professionals, have very little concept of the experience of cancer or of how the cancer patient perceives his quality of life, his future and the decisions that must be made. Cancer is a chronic illness and more patients are living with their disease than previously. These patients, as survivors, have needs and expectations — physical, psychosocial and spiritual. Cancer patients may survive but they may not necessarily thrive. In this situation, cancer rehabilitation is paramount to support patients in effectively managing their illness on a day-to-day basis. This new millenium will see an increase in self-care, with individuals, families and communities playing a larger role in determining and meeting their own health needs. The internet has empowered patients by providing access to information about their disease and treatment, and opening up communication links with fellow patients. Advances in molecular biology may lead to the identification of high-risk groups and better targeted prevention as well as treatment. New challenges lie ahead for nurses in all fields for role development, research and education to support patients and their families through the cancer experience.

REFERENCES

Adams L, Lawson N, Maxted K J, Symonds R P 1992 The prevention of hair loss from chemotherapy by the use of cold air scalp cooling. European Journal of Cancer Care 1(5): 16–18

Alexander F E, Anderson T J, Brown H K et al 1994 The Edinburgh randomised trial of breast cancer screening: results after 10 years follow up. British Journal of Cancer 70(2): 542

Bagenal F S, Easton D F, Harris E et al 1990 Survival of patients with breast cancer attending the Bristol Cancer Help Centre. Lancet 336: 606–610

Bailey R, Clarke M 1989 Stress and coping in nursing. Chapman and Hall, London

Barraclough J 1994 Cancer and emotion. A practical guide to psycho-oncology. Wiley, Chichester

Beecham L 1998 Cervical screening labs should be accredited (news). British Medical Journal 316(7131): 572

Benner P, Wrubel J 1989 The primacy of caring: stress and coping in health and illness. Addison-Wesley, Menlo Park, CA

Bond S 1982 Communication in cancer nursing. In: Colhoon M C (ed) Cancer nursing. Churchill Livingstone, Edinburgh, ch 1

Bottomley A 1998 Psychotherapy groups and cancer patient survival: choosing fool's gold? European Journal of Cancer Care 7(3): 192–196

Bradley A N M 1999 The contribution of molecular genetics to the understanding and management of cancer: potential future applications and implications for nurses. European Journal of Cancer Care 8(2): 97–103

Burnett C B, Steakley C S, Tefft M C 1995 Barriers to breast and cervical cancer screening in underserved women of the District of Columbia. Oncology Nursing Forum 22(10): 1551–1557

Calzone K A 1997 Predisposition testing for breast and ovarian cancer susceptibility. Seminars in Oncology 13(2): 82–90

Cancer Research Campaign 1997 Ten out of Ten: against cancer - for life. Europe's 10-point code against cancer. Comic Co, London

Cancer Research Campaign 1998 Factsheets 1.1–1.4. CRC, London

Cancer Research Campaign 1999a About cancer: the facts. Cancer Research Campaign pp. 1–3 http://www.crc.org.uk/cancer/Aboutcan_stats

Cancer Research Campaign 1999b Cancer stats: mortality–UK. CRC, London

Carson D A, Lois A 1995 Cancer progression and p53. The Lancet 346: 1009–1011

Casanu S, Fedeli S L, Catalano G 1994 Oral cooling (cryotherapy): an effective treatment for the prevention of 5 fluorouracil induced stomatitis. Oral oncology. European Journal of Cancer 30B(4): 234–236

Cass Y, Musgrove C F 1992 Guidelines for safe handling of excreta contaminated by cytotoxic agents. American Journal of Hospital Pharmacy 49: 1957–1958

Cassileth B R, Zupkis R V, Sutton-Smith K et al 1980 Information and participation preferences among cancer patients. Annals of Internal Medicine 92(6): 832–836

Catalona W J, Smith D S, Ratliff T L et al 1991 Measurement of prostate-specific antigen in serum as a screening test for prostate cancer. New England Journal of Medicine 324: 1156

Costa G 1977 Cachexia: the metabolic component of neoplastic disease. Cancer Research 37: 2327–2335

Creagan E T 1997 Attitude and disposition: do they make a difference in cancer survival? Mayo Clinic Proceedings 72(2): 160–164

Department of Health 1995 A policy framework for commissioning cancer services: a report by the Expert Advisory Group on Cancer to the Chief Medical Officers of England and Wales. HMSO, London

Department of Health 1998a A first class service: quality in the new NHS. HMSO, London

Department of Health 1998b Smoking kills. Stationery office. HMSO, London

Devine E C, Westlake S K 1995 The effects of psycho-educational care provided to adults with cancer: a meta-analysis of 116 studies. Oncology Nursing Forum 22(9): 1369–1381

Dodwell D, Cambell J, German L, Coyle C, Lane C 1997 Developing a model for nurse led clinics within a radiotherapy out-patient department. British Journal of Cancer 76(34)

Doll R, Hill A B 1954 The mortality of doctors in relation to their smoking habits. A preliminary report. British Medical Journal 1: 1451–1455

Dose A M 1995 The symptom experience of mucositis, stomatitis and xerostomia. Seminars in Oncology Nursing 11(4): 248–255

Dow K H, Bucholtz J D, Iwamoto R R, Fiefer V K, Hilderley L J 1997 Nursing care in radiation oncology. WB Saunders, Philadelphia

Dubecco R 1986 A turning point in cancer research: sequencing the human genome. Science 231: 1055–1056

Eardley A 1985 Patients and radiotherapy. 1. Expectations of treatment. 2. Patients' experience of treatment. Radiography 51: 324–326

Eardley A 1986 What do patients need to know? Nursing Times 82(16): 24–26

Evans J 1989 The cancer experience: a patient's view. In: Phylip Pritchard A (ed) Cancer nursing: a revolution in care. Macmillan, London

Ewles L, Simnett I 1999 Promoting health: a practical guide. 4th edn. Harcourt Brace, Edinburgh

Faithful S 1997 The management of radiation morbidity: can nursing make a difference? European Journal of Cancer 33(suppl 8): 1344

Fawzy F, Fawzy N, Hyun C, Elasheff R, Guthrie D, Fahey J, Morton D 1993 Malignant melanoma: effects of an early structured psychiatric intervention, coping, and affective states on recurrence and survival six years later. Archives of General Psychiatry 50: 681–689

Fidler I J 1997 Molecular biology of cancer: invasion and metastases. In: DeVita V T et al (eds) Cancer: principles and practice of oncology. Lippincott-Raven, Philadelphia, ch 7

Fischer D S, Knobf M T, Durivage H J 1997 The cancer chemotherapy handbook, 5th edn. Mosby Yearbook, St Louis

Fitch M I, Gray R E, Greenberg M, Labrecque M, Douglas M S 1999 Nurses' perspectives on unconventional therapies. Cancer Nursing 22(3): 238–245
Fitzpatrick R, Hinton J, Newman S et al 1984 The experience of illness. Tavistock, London
Fletcher S, Black W, Harris R, Rimer B, Shapiro S 1993 Special article: report of the international workshop on screening for breast cancer. Journal of the National Cancer Institute 85: 1644
Foltz A T 1997 Nutritional disturbances. In: Groenwald S L, Frogge M H, Goodman M, Yarbro C H (eds) Cancer Nursing: principles and practice. Jones & Bartlett, Massachusetts, ch 24
Fox B H 1995 Some problems and some solutions in research on psychotherapeutic interventions with cancer patients. Supportive Cancer Care 3: 257–263
Frank-Stromberg M, Cohen R F 1993 Assessment and interventions for cancer prevention and detection. In: Groenwald S L, Frogge M H, Goodman M, Yarbro C H (eds) Cancer nursing: principles and practice. Jones and Bartlett, Massachusetts, ch 8
Franks L M, Teich N M (eds) 1997 Introduction to the cellular and molecular biology of cancer. Oxford University Press, Oxford
Futreal P A, Liu Q 1994 BRCA1 mutations in breast cancer and ovarian cancer. Science 266(5182): 120–122
Gardner M J, Snee M P, Hall A J et al 1990 Results of case control study of leukaemia and lymphoma in young people near Sellafield nuclear plant in West Cumbria. British Medical Journal 300: 423–429
Goldberg R J, Tull R M 1983 The psychosocial dimensions of cancer: a practical guide for health care providers. Free Press, New York
Goodman I 1998 Development of national evidence based clinical guidelines for administration of cytotoxic chemotherapy. European Journal of Clinical Oncology 2(1): 43–50
Greer, S 1995 Improving quality of life: adjuvant psychological therapy for patients with cancer. Supportive Cancer Care 3: 248–251
Greer S, Morris T, Pettingale K W 1979 Psychological response to breast cancer: effect on outcome. Lancet 2: 785–787
Haenszel W, Kurihera M 1968 Studies of Japanese migrants: 1. Mortality from cancer and other diseases among Japanese in the United States. Journal of the National Cancer Institute 60: 545–571
Haes H 1989 Decision making in oncology: the role of patients and nurses. In: Phylip Pritchard A (ed) Cancer nursing: a revolution in care. Macmillan, London, pp 65–68
Hakami M 1993 Potential contribution of screening to cancer mortality reduction. Cancer Prevention and Detection 17: 513
Hall E J 1997 Etiology of cancer: physical factors. In: DeVita V T et al (eds) Cancer: principles and practice of oncology. Lippincott-Raven, Philadelphia, ch 10
Hall E J, Cox J D 1994 Physical and biologic basis of radiation therapy. In: Cox J D (ed) Moss' radiation oncology: rationale, technique, results, 7th edn. Mosby Yearbook, St Louis
Hammick M, Tutt A, Tait D M 1998 Knowledge and perception regarding radiation in patients receiving radiotherapy: a qualitative study. European Journal of Cancer Care 7: 103–112
Henderson B E, Bernstein L 1997 Etiology of cancer: hormonal factors. In: DeVita V T et al (eds) Cancer: principles and practice of oncology. Lippincott-Raven, Philadelphia, ch 11
Holmes S 1996 Radiotherapy: a guide for practice. Asset Books, Surrey
Holmes S 1997 Cancer chemotherapy: a guide for practice. Asset Books, Surrey
How C, Brown J 1998 Extravasation of cytotoxic chemotherapy from peripheral veins. European Journal Oncology Nursing 2(1): 51–58
IARC/WHO 1998 Cancer in five continents. Electronic database for cancer. International Agency for Research on Cancer, Lyon
James N, Guerrero D, Brada M 1994 Who should follow up cancer patients? Nurse specialist based out-patient care and the introduction of a phone clinic system. Clinical Oncology 6: 283–287
Johnson J E, Lauver D R, Nail L M 1989 Process of coping with radiation therapy. Journal of Consulting and Clinical Psychology 57(3): 358–364
Kern K A, Norton J A 1988 Cancer cachexia. Journal of Parenteral Nutrition 12: 286–298
Kreth F, Faist M, Wernke P C, Rossner R, Volk B, Ostertag C B 1995 Interstitial radiosurgery of low grade gliomas. Journal of Neurosurgery 82(2): 418–429
Kheifets L I, Afifi A A, Buffer P A, Zhang Z W 1995 Occupational electric and magnetic field exposure and brain cancer: a meta-analysis. Journal of Occupational and Environmental Medicine 37(12): 1327–1341
Kübler-Ross E 1973 Death, the final stage of growth. Prentice-Hall, New York
Lauer P, Murphy S, Pavers M 1982 Learning needs of cancer patients: a comparison of nurse and patient perceptions. Nursing Reseach 31(1): 11–16
Mackenzie C 1996 Patients' perceptions of radiotherapy treatment. In: Patterson A, Price R (eds) Current topics in radiography. WB Saunders, London.
McInnes S, Schilsky R L 1996 Infertility following cancer chemotherapy. In: Chabner B A, Lango D L (eds) Cancer chemotherapy and biotherapy: principles and practice. Lippincott-Raven, Philadelphia
McKie L, Gregory S 1989 Wasted lives. Nursing Times 85(18): 22–23
Maguire P 1985 The psychological impact of cancer. British Journal of Hospital Medicine 34(2): 100–103
Maguire P, Tait A, Brooke M et al 1980 Psychological morbidity and physical toxicity associated with adjuvant chemotherapy after mastectomy. British Medical Journal 281: 1179–1180
Mathieson C M, Stam H J 1995 Renegotiating identity: cancer narratives. Sociology of Health and Illness 17(3): 283–306
Meyer T J, Mark M M 1995 Effects of social intervention with adult cancer patients: a meta-analysis of randomised experiments. Health Psychology 14: 101–108
Moorey S 1988 The psychological impact of cancer. In: Webb P (ed) Oncology for nurses and health care professionals. Harper & Row, London, ch 2
Morris S, McIllmurray M B, Soothill K, Leadwith F, Thomas C 1998 All change: cancer services in transition. European Journal of Cancer Care 7(3): 168–173
Nery R 1986 Cancer: an enigma in biology and society. Croom Helm, London
NHS Executive 1995 A policy of framework for commissioning cancer services. Department of Health, London
Niven N 1994 Health psychology: an introduction for nurses and other health care professionals. Churchill Livingstone, Edinburgh
Oliver G 1997 Restoring confidence. Nursing Standard 12(6): 16
Oliver G 1999 WHO programme on cancer control: developing a global strategy for cancer, a review. European Journal of Cancer Care 8: 10–11
Owen J, Black C 1996 Supportive and shared care. In Hancock B (ed) Cancer care in the community. Radcliffe Medical Press, Oxford, ch 8
Parkes C M, Benjamin B, Fitzgerald R G 1969 Broken heart: a statistical survey of increased mortality among widowers. British Medical Journal 1: 740–743
Parkin D et al 1997 Cancer in five continents. VII. International Agency for Research on Cancer, Lyon
Parkinson S A, Lewis J, Morris R et al 1987 Oral protein and energy supplements in cancer patients. Human Nutrition: Applied Nutrition 41A: 233–243
Peck A, Boland J 1977 Emotional reactions to radiation treatment. Cancer 40: 180–184
Peters J A 1997 Applications of genetic technologies to cancer screening, prevention, diagnosis, prognosis and treatment. Seminars in Oncology Nursing 13(2): 74–81
Poeschla E M, Wong-Staal F 1997 RNA viruses. In: DeVita V T et al (eds) Cancer: principles and practice of oncology. Lippincott-Raven, Philadelphia, ch 8
Quilliam S 1989 Positive smear. Penguin, Harmondsworth
Redmond K, Aapro M S 1997 Cancer in the elderly. A nursing and medical perspective. European School of Oncology, Scientific Updates 2. Elsevier Science, Amsterdam
Richardson J 1989 The administration of chemotherapy in the patient's home: a new perspective. In: Phylip Pritchard A (ed) Cancer nursing: a revolution in care. Macmillan, London
Richardson A 1995 Fatigue in cancer patients: a review of the literature. European Journal of Cancer Care 4: 20–32
Risser N L 1996 Prevention of lung cancer: the key is to stop smoking. Seminars in Oncology Nursing 12(4): 260–269
Roper N, Logan W, Tierney A (eds) 1996 The elements of nursing. A model for nursing based on a model of living, 4th edn. Churchill Livingstone, Edinburgh
Rotman M, Rogow L, Delean G, Heskel N 1977 Supportive therapy in radiation oncology. Cancer 39: 744–750
Roy C 1989 The Roy adaptation model. In: Reihl-Sisca J (ed) Conceptual models for nursing practice, 3rd edn. Appleton & Lange, East Norwalk
Royal College of Nursing 1996a A structure for cancer nursing services. RCN Cancer Nursing Society, London
Royal College of Nursing 1996b Guidelines for good practice in cancer nursing education. RCN Cancer Nursing Society, London

Rutkauskas J S, Davis J W 1993 Effects of chlorhexidine during immunosuppression chemotherapy. Oral Surgery Oral Medicine Oral Pathology 76: 441–448

Scottish Office Department of Health 1999 White paper – towards a healthier Scotland. Stationery Office, Edinburgh

Shopland D R 1995 Tobacco use and its contribution to early cancer mortality with a special emphasis on cigarette smoking. Environmental Health Perspectives 103(suppl 8): 131–141

Sikora K 1994 Genes, dreams and cancer. British Medical Journal 308: 1217–1221

Sikora K 1999 Cancer – a global problem. Cancer Topics 10(12): 17–19

Sitzia J, Wood N 1998 Study of patient satisfaction with chemotherapy nursing care. European Journal of Cancer Care 2(3): 142–153

Skipper A, Szeluga D J, Groenwald S L 1993 Nutritional disturbances. In: Groenwald S L, Frogge M H, Goodman M, Yarbro CH (eds) Cancer nursing: principles and practice. Jones and Bartlett, Massachusetts, ch 27

Skrabanek P 1990a Screening for cancer. Update 40(4): 384–387

Skrabanek P 1990b Cervical cancer screening. Update 40(8): 868–872

Slattery M I, Kerber R A 1993 A comprehensive evaluation of family history and breast cancer risk. Journal American Medical Association 270: 1563–1568

Slevin M L, Nichols S E, Downer S M et al 1996 Emotional support for cancer patients: what do patients really want? British Journal of Cancer 74: 1275–1279

Slevin M, Stubbs L, Plant H et al 1990 Choices in cancer treatment: comparing the views of patients with cancer with those of doctors, nurses and the general public. British Medical Journal 300: 1458–1460

Souhami R, Tobias J 1998 Cancer and its management, Blackwell Science, Oxford

Speck P W 1988 Ethical issues in cancer care. In: Webb P (ed) Oncology for nurses and health care professionals, 2nd edn. Harper & Row, London, ch 3

Spiegel D, Kraemer H C, Bloom J R et al 1989 Effect of psychosocial treatment on survival of patients with metastatic breast cancer. Lancet 2(8668): 888–891

Stoll B (ed) 1979 Mind and cancer prognosis. Wiley, Chichester

Strohl R A 1988 The nursing role in radiation oncology: symptom management of acute and chronic reactions. Oncology Nursing Forum 15(4): 429–434

Stubbs L 1989 Taste changes in cancer patients. Nursing Times 85(3): 49–50

Tabar L, Faberberg G, Duffy S et al 1992 Breast imaging: current status and future directions: update of the Swedish two County program of mammographic screening for breast cancer. Radiology Clinics of North America 30: 187

Tanghe A, Evers G, Pandoens K 1998 Nurses' assessments of symptom occurrence and symptom distress in chemotherapy patients. European Journal of Oncology Nursing 2(1): 14–26

The COMMIT Research Group 1995 Community Intervention Trial for Smoking Cessation (COMMIT) II : changes in adult cigarette smoking prevalence. American Journal of Public Health 85(2): 193–200

Thomson I E, Melia K M, Boyd K M 1994 Nursing ethics, 3rd edn. Churchill Livingstone, Edinburgh

Thorne S E 1988 Helpful and unhelpful communication in cancer care : the patient perspective. Oncology Nursing Forum 15(2): 1647–1672

Tierney A J 1987 Preventing chemotherapy induced alopecia in cancer patients: is scalp cooling worthwhile? Journal of Advanced Nursing 12: 303–310

Tierney A J, Taylor J, Closs S J 1989 A study to inform nursing support of patients coping with chemotherapy for breast cancer. Nursing Research Unit, University of Edinburgh, Edinburgh

Toniolo P G, Mortimer L et al 1995 A prospective study of endogenous oestrogens and breast cancer in postmenopausal women. Journal of the National Cancer Institute 87(3): 190–197

Trichopoulus D, Kalandidi A, Sparros L, Macmahon B 1981 Lung cancer and passive smoking. International Journal of Cancer 27(1): 1–4

Trillet-Lenoir V, Green J, Manegold C et al 1993 Recombinant granulocyte colony stimulating factor reduces the infectious complications of cytotoxic chemotherapy. European Journal of Cancer 29A: 319–324

Tschudin V (ed) 1996 Nursing the patient with cancer, 2nd edn. Prentice-Hall, Hemel Hempstead, Herts

UICC (International Union against Cancer) 1987 TNM classification of malignant tumours. Springer-Verlag, Berlin

Valanis B G 1996 Epidemiology of lung cancer: a worldwide epidemic. Seminars in Oncology Nursing 12(4): 251–259

Walker A 1990 The problems of patients with cervical cancer. In: Faulkner A (ed) Excellence in nursing: the research route: oncology. Scutari, London, ch 3

Watters C 1997 The benefits of providing chemotherapy at home. Professional Nurse 12(5): 19–21

Wells M 1998a What's so special about radiotherapy nursing? European Journal of Oncology Nursing 2(3): 162–168

Wells M 1998b The hidden experience of radiotherapy to the head and neck: a qualitative study of patients after completion of treatment. Journal of Advanced Nursing 28(4): 840–848

Wilkinson S 1990 Nursing the patient with cancer. In: Faulkner A (ed) Excellence in nursing: the research route: oncology. Scutari, London, ch 6

Wilkinson J A 1999 Understanding patient health beliefs. Professional Nurse 14(5): 320–322

Williams J K 1997 Principles of genetics and cancer. Seminars in Oncology 13(2): 68–73

Wilson M E, Williams H A 1988 Oncology nurses' attitudes and behaviours related to sexuality of patients with cancer. Oncology Nursing Forum 15(1): 49–53

Yarbro J W 1993 Milestones in our understanding of the causes of cancer. In: Groenwald S L, Frogge M H, Goodman M, Yarbro C H (eds) Cancer nursing: principles and practice. Jones and Bartlett, ch 1, pp 3–16

FURTHER READING

Boot-Vickers M, Eaton K 1999 Skin care for patients receiving radiotherapy. Professional Nurse 14(10): 706–708

Brown J K, Radke K J 1998 Nutritional assessment, intervention, and evaluation of weight loss in patients with non-small cell lung cancer. Oncology Nursing Forum 25(3): 547–553

Dow K H, Bucholtz J D, Iwamoto R R, Fieler V K, Hilderley L J 1997 Nursing care in radiation oncology. WB Saunders, Philadelphia

Foley G V, Fochtman D, Mooney K H 1993 Nursing care of the child with cancer. 2nd edn. Association of Paediatric Oncology Nurses, WB Saunders, Philadelphia

Groenwald S L, Frogge M H et al (eds) 1993 Cancer nursing principles and practice. Jones and Bartlett, Massachusetts

Holmes S 1996 Radiotherapy: a guide for practice. Asset Books, Surrey

Neal A J, Hoskin 1998 Clinical oncology: basic principles and practice. Arnold, London

Niven N 1994 Health psychology: an introduction for nurses and other health care professionals. Churchill Livingstone, Edinburgh

Otto S E (ed) 1994 Oncology nursing. Mosby, St Louis

Russell P J 1994 Fundamentals of genetics. Harper Collins, New York

Seminars in Oncology Nursing 1995 11(3)

Tannock I F, Hill R P (eds) 1992 The basic science of oncology. McGraw-Hill, Toronto

Tortora G J, Grabowski S R 1996 Principles of anatomy and physiology. Harper Collins, New York

Varmus H, Weinberg R A 1993 Genes and the biology of cancer. Scientific American Library, New York

Vooght S 1996 A study to explore the role of a community oncology nurse specialist. European Journal of Cancer Care 5(4): 217–224

USEFUL ADDRESSES

Cancerlink
17 Britannia Street
London WC1X 9JN

CancerBACUP (British Association of Cancer United Patients)
121–123 Charterhouse Street
London EC1M 6AA

CancerBACUP Scotland
Cancer Counselling Service
Glasgow

Breast Cancer Care
Kiln House
210 New Kings Road
London SW6 4NZ

Breast Cancer Care Scotland
46 Gordon Street
Glasgow G1 3PU

Leukaemia Care Society
14 Kingfisher
Veny Bridge
Exeter
Devon EX2 5DP

OVACOME
St Bartholomew's Hospital
West Smithfield
London EC1A 7BE

THE CHRONICALLY ILL PERSON

32

Erica S. Alabaster

INTRODUCTION

The care of people with chronic illness has long been of concern to nurses, presenting many challenges and opportunities and demanding the use of a broad range of skills. In seeking to articulate the concepts which underpin the process of care, nursing theorists now define health in terms of an integrated state of wellness within which the individual achieves optimal physical, social, psychological and spiritual balance. This holistic approach therefore regards ill-health as a state of disequilibrium. Further, it does not rely solely on the application of a medically determined diagnostic label to legitimise nursing involvement and to dictate the direction this takes.

Chronic illness has significant consequences for the individual's social and psychological well-being. The nurse's role in caring for people who are chronically ill must be formulated within a broad context, which includes the nature of chronic illness, its impact on individual experience and functioning, prevalence, and the relationship between patients, informal carers and health care agencies. Perhaps the best place to begin in considering this role is with a practical definition of chronic illness.

THE NATURE OF CHRONIC ILLNESS

Terminology

Dimond & Jones (1987) note that a number of terms have been employed to describe illness 'that is of long-term duration, is not curable, and/or has some residual features that impose limitations on an individual's functional capabilities'. An analysis of such terminology is an essential starting point for any discussion of chronic illness. The way in which key terms are applied may reveal the existence of certain assumptions about the causation and prognosis of chronic conditions and about the individuals who experience them. Along with many other North American authors they refer to the definition of chronic illness agreed by the Commission on Chronic Illness in 1954 (cited by Daly 1993):

> All impairments or deviations from normal which have one or more of the following characteristics: permanency, leave residual damage, are caused by non-reversible pathology, require specialised training of the patient for rehabilitation, and/or require a long period of supervision.

This statement is still considered to have currency despite its ambiguity and biological emphasis. How, for example, is a 'normal' state to be defined? What constitutes 'damage'?

'Illness' and 'disease'

It is important to note that the definition of chronic illness above is orientated towards disease rather than illness. A distinction is made between these two terms by some writers such that 'disease' is a medical conception of pathological abnormality as indicated by its presenting features, whereas 'illness' is the subjective response by the individual to feeling unwell (Scambler 1991a, Armstrong 1994). Greaves (1996) argues, however, that although it is possible to feel ill without having a disease, and vice versa, 'illness' and 'disease' do not constitute discrete phenomena but, rather, operate at different levels of human experience. Their relationship is dependent on the nature and severity of the disease process and on coexisting psychosocial variables. Chronic illness is generally associated with the presence of a protracted disease process which is not amenable to treatment, is responsible for impairment or disability and so has a sustained influence on the functioning and lifestyle of the individual. In this view, the relationship between disease and illness is characterised by its complexity.

'Impairment', 'disability' and 'handicap'

Anderson & Bury (1988) demonstrate that biomedical classifications of disease do not necessarily account for the psychological and social consequences which accompany the conditions identified. This can be supported with reference to a study conducted by Williams (1993) to investigate the problems experienced by people diagnosed as having chronic obstructive airways disease (COAD). He concluded that psychosocial disabilities which could result in a reduction in quality of life were not associated with the nature of the underlying disease.

The terms 'impairment', 'disability' and 'handicap' are commonly employed in the literature with reference to chronic illness and are applied in a variety of ways, whether their definitions are stated explicitly or merely implied. Field (1993a) comments that the term 'impairment' is generally used to describe any disturbance or interference with body structure and function caused by disease processes. Impairment may also be influenced by extrinsic factors such as the manner in which the presenting condition is managed. Pressure sores, constipation, urinary tract infections and other complications of restricted mobility are examples of these.

The word 'disability', on the other hand, can be used to identify any long-term or permanent incapacity which is due to disease, injury, innate defect or old age. This is related to functional limitation but may in addition be defined in terms of behaviour, such as that arising from the individual's inability to perform activities which are expected of her (Nettleton 1995). The level of disability experienced by an individual reflects the severity and duration of impairment, taking into account concurrent disease, illness and the effects of the ageing process.

Dimond & Jones (1987) argue that it is constructive for people interested in the study of chronic illness to consider the notion of disability since this presents an opportunity to discuss a range of behavioural responses without concentrating on the diseases concerned. They explain that the term 'handicap' may be applied when limitation of activity persists as a residual effect of impairment, even following rehabilitative efforts to restore function. Handicap is not, therefore, merely the presence of disability and impairment, but the social, economic and environmental consequences of these. The individual is considered to be disadvantaged in so far as she is unable to participate in socially prescribed roles and relationships. Further, Locker (1991) suggests that handicap can have different implications for individual experience depending on the way in which social, cultural and economic values are applied to restricted role behaviour. In this way, 'handicap' can be interpreted as both more and less than 'disability'.

Issues surrounding the concepts impairment, disability and handicap are also explored in Chapter 34.

SOCIETAL ATTITUDES TOWARDS ILLNESS AND DISABILITY

The literature suggests, however, that attention is still clearly directed towards drawing associations between aspects of lifestyle and some chronic illnesses; for example, smoking is linked with lung cancer and a high dietary intake of saturated fats with coronary heart disease. Nettleton (1995) contends that a general awareness of these relationships may result in the individual being judged to be the cause of her own disease and related suffering. There is also an implication that the individual has failed to respond to preventive health education campaigns. Attribution of personal blame is shown to have a strong moral influence where an association has been made between disease and sexual behaviour, such as that alleged between HIV/AIDS and promiscuity (Eisenberg 1990, Pitts 1996).

Current beliefs concerning the origin of chronic illness and disability appear, therefore, to reflect a combination of moral ideology and scientific principles.

Q **32.1** Given the association between cigarette advertising and tobacco consumption (Smee 1992, Charlton et al 1997) and that tobacco companies appear to be accepting the addictive nature of their products, can individuals be blamed for their behaviour? What are the other forces influencing personal health choices?

Disability and unemployment

The individual's economic survival in a pre-industrial society largely depends on her capacity to engage in physical labour. Those who are restricted by the effects of protracted illness or impairment will thus have a limited function within their social group. This, together with their likely dependency on others, can result in the perception that disabled people are of less value than their able-bodied counterparts.

In an industrialised society, however, technological developments and diversification of working practices should create opportunities for people with a wide range of disabilities to gain employment. Nonetheless, discrimination is encountered by disabled individuals seeking to enter the labour market (Oliver 1990). It can be argued that The Disability Discrimination Act (1995) has not addressed this because it defines disability using a medical rather than a social model (Reid 1997) and does not assure full civil rights (Mahony 1997).

Governmental response to poverty is influenced by the way in which poor people are viewed by other members of society. The assumption that those living with chronic illness experience economic difficulties because they are unable to obtain employment as a direct result of their incapacity is not held universally. Some may take the view instead that such individuals are malingerers who choose not to work (Scambler 1991b). When this interpretation predominates, programmes for the alleviation of poverty concentrate on motivating individuals by reforming attitudes and offering retraining programmes and may appear to be punitive rather than benevolent.

Stigma

As Goffman (1963) points out, the word 'stigma' was originally used with reference to visible signs inflicted with the intent of branding individuals (including slaves or criminals) unfit for participation in normal social interaction.

The stigma attached to a chronic illness depends on the part of the body affected, the degree to which effects of the condition are visible, application of a diagnostic label and the likelihood of cure. People with a chronic illness may be so affected by the embarrassment or discomfort which their disorder creates in others that their stigmatising condition assumes primacy as they establish their social identity and manage relationships with others. Case History 32.1 gives some insight into the stigmatisation that may be suffered by an individual with an obvious skin condition.

Q **32.2** Have you ever been aware of being embarrassed or uncomfortable when you were with someone with an obvious skin disorder? What were your reactions?

Public awareness campaigns

A variety of groups have been established to raise public awareness of problems encountered by individuals with long-term illness and disability. Dimond & Jones (1987) recall that, in the USA, veterans of the First World War were successful in exerting large-scale efforts to obtain privileges and opportunities for disabled servicemen returning to civilian life. The amount of popular support such programmes receive is dependent upon whether the situations to which they are related are viewed positively. This can be illustrated with reference to American veterans of the Vietnam War, who endured stigmatisation by association with a controversial and unpopular conflict.

Other groups act to draw attention to named conditions and their effects on individual experience. These organisations function as a resource for sufferers and their families, campaign for issues such as open access to public buildings, and raise funds for facilities and research. It may be suggested that some groups encourage little active participation by disabled people themselves, and that aid programmes are consequently planned in relation to assumed more than actual need. In addition, activists within campaigns such as the British Council for the Organisation of Disabled People assert that national fundraising events merely serve to reinforce the notion that an automatic relationship exists between disabled people and charity. Members of these groups believe that sick and disabled people should avoid passivity and the socialised dependency which results. Their practice of self-advocacy, use of direct action and insistence upon parity rather than charity contrasts sharply with the conventional image of disabled people as recipients of care.

THE PREVALENCE OF CHRONIC ILLNESS

The prevalence of chronic illness or disease is difficult to establish in view of the many definitions and interpretations of these conditions offered by various agencies. Some indication of their prevalence may, however, be derived from a review of studies which take into account such variables as demography and disability.

Case History 32.1 Mrs I

Mrs I is 44 years old and is employed as a part-time receptionist. She lives in a terraced house with her husband and their three teenage children. Mrs I has had psoriasis for some years, involving much of her body surface.

Although prescribed treatment has controlled features of the condition to some extent, Mrs I has periods of exacerbation. Reddened raised patches sometimes appear on her face, and her scalp is often affected. Medical opinion varies as to whether this is actually due to psoriasis or to seborrhoeic dermatitis. Mrs I feels this distinction to be largely academic because she believes that neither condition is curable and the outcome for her remains the same. At present her scalp is covered in a thick, hardened layer of scales. When these areas are detached, her scalp surface weeps and becomes painful. Scales are also deposited continually on her clothing and in her immediate vicinity.

Mrs I finds that living with a skin condition is made more difficult by the reaction of others. She is often conscious that people stare at her and that they look at her affected skin rather than making eye contact during conversations. Mrs I remembers that when her children were small, one of them tried to prevent her from attending a school play. After a long discussion he admitted that it was because he was embarrassed by her appearance. Mrs I thinks that some people regard her condition to be contagious or to be caused by poor personal hygiene. She considers that this explains why passengers on the bus she takes to and from work rarely occupy the space next to her until the vehicle becomes crowded. Such behaviour still makes her uncomfortable but she has learned to accept it as something she must live with.

Mrs I feels that she has developed effective methods of coping with the problems resulting from her disorder. Since her job involves meeting the public, she has learned to project an outgoing and friendly image which she feels is stronger than the visual impression which her condition creates. She avoids wearing dark clothes likely to make her fallen scales more obvious and purchases her clothing by mail order or from shops which do not have communal changing rooms. She has learned by trial and error which chemicals or cosmetics irritate her skin and excludes them from the household. She takes her own prescribed shampoo to the hairdressers and never uses biological washing powder. Her friends and relations are aware that only selected toiletries are welcome as birthday and Christmas presents. Mrs I has also adapted her treatment regimen to account for exacerbations of her condition. She applies some creams only when she feels that she needs to, rather than at prescribed intervals. As some preparations require careful application due to possible staining of clothes and localised burning (see Ch. 12), Mrs I tries to restrict their use to days when she is not rostered to work. To prevent unnecessary soiling, she reserves specific bed linen for occasions when she needs to leave scalp ointment on overnight.

Improvements in public health in the UK since the turn of the century have resulted in the near-eradication of some infectious diseases, whilst others have been largely controlled by vaccination programmes (Galbraith & McCormick 1997). In addition, once contracted, infectious diseases are generally amenable to treatment. Chronic rather than infectious disease therefore remains the major cause of premature death and disability.

As Radley (1994) points out, however, it must not be assumed that infection has been eliminated from Western societies, nor that chronic disease cannot be infectious. AIDS is the result of infectious disease, yet to contract it then means living with a chronic illness.

It should also be recognised that patterns of infection are subject to continual change worldwide. The speed at which this occurs reflects the acceleration of human social, technical, environmental and population change. This has resulted in the appearance of new diseases and the re-emergence of others. For example, notifications of tuberculosis have risen in the UK since 1987 with an increase in drug-resistant isolates. It is thought that this is in part due to improvements in the system of notification, but the increase of pulmonary tuberculosis was genuine and associated with socioeconomic deprivation. Almost half of overall notifications were from immigrant communities and were most prevalent among young South Asians (Galbraith & McCormick 1997). Observations such as this have led to members of marginal groups being viewed prejudicially because they are perceived to be the cause of disease and thus a threat to wider society (Pitts 1996). Further, as shown by Smaje (1995), this gives rise to 'port health' thinking, associated with unreasonable fears of infection from abroad and a restrictive view of minority ethnic health issues.

The continuing decline in mortality from infectious disease is reflected in an increased expectation of life for all age groups, a trend which is predicted to continue (Charlton 1997). This has implications for the number of people afflicted by chronic disorders. Tinker (1996) concludes that the proportion of the population considered to be handicapped or impaired rises with advancing age. Confirmation of this relationship can be found in a report published by the Office of Population Censuses and Surveys (OPCS 1995) — now part of the Office for National Statistics (ONS) — using data from the annual General Household Survey (GHS) provided in 1993 by a sample of 18 492 people aged 16 years and over. Respondents were asked whether they had any long-standing illness, disability or infirmity and to state whether it served to limit their activities in any way. A long-standing illness was reported by 34.2% of the respondents and a limiting long-standing illness by 20.4%. A comparative measure of acute illness was obtained by enquiring whether participants had limited their usual activities as a result of illness or injury within the 2-week period prior to the interview. Only 14% of the sample fell into this category. The report concludes that in the period 1972–1993, rates of long-standing illness have increased, whilst the incidence of acute illness remained virtually unchanged. Although the reporting of long-standing disorders rose from 26% of those aged 16–44 years to 67% of those aged 75 years or more, fewer elderly men were found in this category.

In 1988–1989 the GHS included specific questions regarding types of illness or disability, and respondents declaring long-standing illness were asked to identify its source (Department of Health 1990). Musculoskeletal, circulatory, respiratory and digestive disorders were most frequently reported. Among these disorders, musculoskeletal conditions were the most common. A similar finding was obtained in the ONS disability survey by Martin et al (1988). Circulatory problems were the second most common form of chronic illness identified in the DoH report; these were reported by 2% of adults aged 16–44 years and approximately 25% of those aged 65 years or older. A summary of selected causes of death for the years 1951 and 1988 provides evidence to suggest that the incidence of circulatory disease is rising. Deaths from such disorders, including myocardial infarction and cerebrovascular accident (CVA), accounted for around one-third of all deaths in 1951 and almost half of all deaths in 1988 (Central Statistical Office 1990).

The DoH report records a striking similarity between the proportions of men and women experiencing various forms of chronic illness, with the following two exceptions. Firstly, 22% of men aged 75 years and above stated that they had a long-standing musculoskeletal disorder, compared with 40% of their female counterparts. This is thought to be due in part to the higher proportion of very elderly women who fall into this age category. Secondly, 13% of elderly males considered themselves to be suffering from a respiratory disease, whereas only 8% of women in the same age group characterised themselves in the same way. Differences in lifetime smoking behaviour are felt to be reflected here, although occupational factors may also be significant (Dunnell 1997).

The number of conditions identified per person increased with advancing age, being 1.2 for those aged 16–44 years and 1.7 for those aged 75 years and above. In this regard little variation was found between males and females.

The findings of these surveys support the notion put forward by Anderson & Bury (1988) that whilst chronic illness is widespread and involves a variety of conditions, only a proportion of those affected are appreciably disabled. A survey carried out in 1995 on behalf of the Department of Health revealed that, amongst adults aged 16 years and over, serious disabilities were most likely to be caused by arthritis and rheumatism, diseases of the nervous system (particularly Parkinson's disease and multiple sclerosis) and circulatory disease/stroke.

Q **32.3** Given that chronic illness is so widespread, think again about the meaning of health for different people. Can people with chronic disease be 'healthy'?

Cancer was reported as the cause of their disability by 2% of respondents (DoH 1997). According to Swerdlow et al (1997), cancer mortality has fallen during the last 20 years in men under 70 years and women under 50 years of age as a consequence of improved treatment and reduced risk. Data from the 1988 and 1989 GHS and ONS longitudinal survey indicate that cancer is the cause of long-standing illness in 1% of adults.

Q **32.4** Read Case History 32.2 and also refer to Chapter 31. Do all cancers result in chronic illness?

FEATURES OF CHRONIC ILLNESS

Whilst an analysis of the prevalence of long-standing disease is useful in predicting the demand for support services, it may be argued that it is of limited value in gaining an appreciation of the impact of such conditions on the daily lives of individual sufferers. An overemphasis on diagnosis and disease entities is also felt by Strauss et al (1984) to conceal psychological and social problems shared by people who are chronically ill. In this seminal work, the

Case History 32.2 Mrs F

Mrs F is 64 years old. She has been widowed for 9 years and has lived with cancer for the last 8. Mrs F can recall clearly the moment when she feels her life changed. She had dropped her soap whilst taking a bath and, when bending to retrieve it, she noticed a lump in her left breast. For a time it seemed to her that the world stood still, her immediate fear being of the likely diagnosis. Mrs F knew what her course of action should be but she postponed visiting her GP for a week. She felt as though hearing someone else voice her suspicions would make things worse and that somehow the lump would be more real.

Within a short time, Mrs F underwent a series of investigations and a lumpectomy. It seemed that she was on a merry-go-round and could not get off. Each appointment with a hospital department led to another and she joked that her social diary had never been so full. Once surgery was over Mrs F was unsure of herself. Her life was under immediate threat. She did not know how she was supposed to feel or what was normal behaviour in this abnormal situation. The sense of threat lessened as the period between follow-up appointments increased. Despite the surgeon's optimism, Mrs F feared the disease returning. Her drug regimen acted as a constant reminder but as time passed she wondered if she dared to believe that she was safe. Feeling it important to do something to occupy her time, Mrs F enrolled in adult education classes and began work for a local children's charity.

Two years later, further surgery was advised to remove diseased axillary lymph nodes. A course of radiotherapy followed. Mrs F coped by fitting appointments around her charity work but found that her condition was less easy to ignore than before. She was tired, her skin was sore and she found it difficult to use her left arm. Again, the medical team appeared optimistic. Mrs F wondered if they were telling her the truth and found herself looking for clues in their words and mannerisms. She recognised that the disease now posed more problems than ever. Until now she had described herself as healthy.

Mrs F gained some reassurance as the time between follow-up appointments increased as before and scans did not reveal further metastatic spread. The doctors always seemed to define survival in terms of a 5-year period. This assumed great importance for Mrs F. She felt as though it represented an almost magical goal, beyond which her existence was assured. In the meantime she managed her drug regimen and the side-effects of additional treatment. Every previously innocent ache, pain or cough she experienced took on a new meaning. Was it her arthritis, a chest infection or had the disease spread?

Increasing back pain led to Mrs F relinquishing her charity work and to the recent diagnosis of bony metastasis. She was offered a place at a hospice day centre but refused. Mrs F felt that accepting it confirmed that the cancer was now bigger than she. She also did not relish making new acquaintances there and then wondering who would be missing when she next attended. Mrs F thought the outcome of her illness was certain but was still unsure of what would happen on the way.

authors therefore developed a framework to enable the experience of chronic illness to be understood more clearly and empathically. To provide a basis for this, the seven features of chronic illness outlined below were identified. Only when they are aware of these features can nurses begin to appreciate the profound effect of chronic illness on individuals, their families and health care personnel.

Chronic illnesses are long-term by nature

The timespan for the treatment of acute illness contrasts markedly with that of chronic disease. Once contact with medical services is initiated and treatment commenced, the resolution of acute illness is generally achieved within a short period of time. The protracted nature of chronic illness results in repeated interactions between individuals and health care services, perhaps over a period of months or years. This leads to patients gaining familiarity with the organisations providing support and the personnel with whom they come into contact, and has implications for the development of complex social relationships between patients and carers as the illness progresses.

Adulthood is a dynamic period usually associated with autonomy and control. It is a time of life in which the individual expects to nurture others, rather than to be nurtured. The need for protracted nursing care conflicts with these expectations and can be damaging to the individual's self-esteem. Once admitted to caring facilities, people with chronic illness may be encouraged to relinquish whatever control they still possess in favour of control by the staff (Daly 1993). Failure to accept this may be regarded as active opposition to adopting the role of patient and may lead to the individual acquiring a reputation for being 'difficult'. Long-term admission to hospital does not necessarily enhance relationships between patients and nursing staff, despite the opportunity it presents for interpersonal development in the course of continued interactions (Stockwell 1972).

Chronic illness is uncertain

Mishel (1993) believes that living with chronic illness means living with uncertainty. Obtaining a diagnosis may be a lengthy process due to the ambiguity of symptoms experienced. Difficulty in establishing a prognosis for chronic illness with any degree of certainty is also a source of stress for sufferers and their carers. Strauss et al (1984) note that only the progress of the disease itself gives sufficient information to suggest a likely timescale of events for a particular individual.

Adulthood is associated with the achievement of socially and culturally specified tasks such as leaving the parental home, finding a partner and rearing a family (Kimmel 1990). The restriction, discomfort and possible dependence accompanying chronic illness may force the individual to forgo these roles and adopt an alternative lifestyle. Fear of dependence, which in itself causes uncertainty, is identified by Pinder (1990) as a fundamental human concern 'in a culture which values self-reliance and economic and physical independence'. Her study demonstrates that following a diagnosis of Parkinson's disease, this problem is shared to an extent by medical staff who must decide how much information to give the patient regarding the likely course of the disorder and difficulties of treatment. Although it is seen as important to provide patients with sufficient data to enable them to exert maximum control over their new situation, doctors are shown to question their own professional commitment in situations where purely medical solutions have only a limited effect.

Uncertainty is also present because of the inherently episodic nature of many chronic illnesses, in which recurrent unpredictable crises occur followed by periods of remission or control. Since the onset and duration of these crises cannot be anticipated, patients and their carers must constantly be alert for indications of impending difficulty and must be ready to respond at any time. This results in the restriction and reorganisation of lifestyle in an attempt to accommodate the sudden changes in behaviour which may be imposed. Social uncertainty thus exists for people with chronic illness and their families, who find it difficult to plan their activities in either the long or short term and may be excluded from full participation in community life as a result (Strauss et al 1984). (The difficulty that individuals with a degenerative illness may have in visualising the future is illustrated in Case History 32.3.)

In his study of the social context of multiple sclerosis, Robinson (1988) provides evidence to show that the occurrence of crises in chronic illness influences the way in which sufferers are perceived by others. People with multiple sclerosis felt that the consequences of living with a protracted disorder were largely ignored by others, who believed them to be directly affected by the disease only when it became visible through the exacerbation of physical symptoms. Variation in their ability to perform daily activities in periods of crisis and remission were therefore poorly understood.

Paradoxically, Mishel (1993) observes that uncertainty can be a positive experience for people with chronic illness. In a study of people receiving renal dialysis, higher levels of uncertainty were correlated with compliance whilst lower levels were related to non-compliance.

Q **32.5** In Case History 32.3, S obviously believes that her life course is being undermined and she has many anxieties about her long-term goals. Anxiety is a distressing experience in itself, but could interfere with her ability to function. If you were caring for S, how would you help her to deal with her situation?

Chronic illnesses require proportionately greater efforts at palliation

In view of the remote prospect of effecting a cure in chronic illness, the control of elements which influence the individual's quality of life assumes primary importance. More emphasis is placed on palliative measures, i.e. alleviating pain and discomfort, providing symptomatic relief and addressing the problems created by the restriction of activity. Strauss et al (1984) contend that palliation is of greater significance here than in acute illness because people with long-term disease must learn to live with both the features of their condition and the side-effects of treatment. The cooperation of patients, their families and close associates is necessary in order to achieve this. Since symptoms such as constant pain and nausea can compromise the ability of individuals to engage in a variety of activities, their treatment is seen to be desirable even though it will have little effect upon the disease process.

Decisions as to which palliative measures are selected for individual treatment are influenced by availability, acceptance by the medical profession, their perceived benefit to the patient and financial constraints. Improvements in quality of life following palliation are difficult to measure objectively, and this has implications for the allocation of resources.

Case History 32.3 S J

S J is 28 years old and works as a cook in an independent school for girls. She has been in this employment since leaving college and lives on the premises. Her social life revolves largely around sporting activities, an interest shared with her boyfriend, A.

S was diagnosed as having multiple sclerosis (MS) 2 years ago when she was admitted to hospital following a fall whilst playing tennis. She had been experiencing difficulty in focusing her eyes for some time, but had thought that this was due to overwork. She had also begun to find it difficult to coordinate her movements and became known for dropping and spilling things. These events were explained when the diagnosis was made and S found it strange that she had lived with the condition for so long without realising that something was seriously wrong.

After the diagnosis was confirmed, S felt compelled to visit a library to find out more about the condition and what it would mean to her. She resolved that her approach would be to get on with living despite the disease. Within a short period, however, her balance deteriorated and walking became difficult. She also found that she tired easily. S responded by opting out of strenuous activities. Having valued her physical fitness, she began to experience frustration at her loss of ability and function. She felt as though her body had betrayed her and she did not like to be seen walking with a stick. When S developed frequency and urgency of micturition, she began to avoid visits to public places where toilets would be difficult to reach or where queues were likely.

In private, S found herself increasingly reduced to tears of frustration and despair, believing that no one else could understand her experience. She chose not to share these feelings. She had always been able to manage her life independently and wanted to appear to be continuing to do so. S's boyfriend, A, tried to support her as much as possible, but maintaining a positive stance at all times was hard. His friends advised him not to remain in the relationship purely because of his concern for S, and his feelings for her were sometimes confused. He wondered if her reluctance to visit public venues was actually her way of avoiding him because she wanted their relationship to end.

S was preoccupied by questions about her future. How long would she be able to continue in her present post? Would it be possible to seek alternative employment? Giving up her job would mean giving up her home. Her parents wanted her to live with them but S was anxious to retain her autonomy and knew that her mother would try to protect her too much. However, it was her future with A that was her greatest concern. S loved him and had hoped that their relationship would lead to marriage. She wanted children of her own and already felt that time was running out. S felt it impossible to confront A about such a commitment, fearing that he would perceive this as pressure to make an immediate decision and that as a result she may lose him altogether. Her sad conclusion was that with MS she could no longer be sure of anything.

Individuals have considerable resources of their own and may first try to solve their health problems themselves before seeking professional and statutory help. Should statutory health services be unable to provide palliation, or if their efforts prove to be unsuccessful, people with chronic illness may seek alternative methods to resolve their symptoms. Coping strategies can be learned through experience and by sharing ideas with others through membership of support groups (Field 1993b). The use of complementary therapies is increasingly common among people with intractable disease who feel that conventional medicine has no further treatment to offer them and is supported by writers such as Sharma (1992) and Watkins (1996). This not only represents the individual's assumption of responsibility for her own well-being in the face of perceived medical impotence, but also reflects a desire to achieve control over an unpredictable illness (Montbriand & Laing 1991).

Chronic diseases are multiple diseases

According to Strauss et al (1984), the systematic and degenerative effects of a number of chronic diseases are such that in time the failure of one organ or physiological system leads to the involvement of others. In addition, long-term disability related to an existing chronic condition is likely to generate further disease. This can be illustrated with reference to complications associated with diabetes mellitus. Stewart (1990) explains that these include vascular damage, which may result in renal and visual dysfunction and an increased risk of myocardial infarction. Impaired circulation to the lower limbs also predisposes to the development of gangrene, the onset of which is in turn influenced by degeneration of the nervous system and greater susceptibility to infection. Amputation of an affected limb results in further alteration of physical, psychological and social functioning. Clearly, the disabling effects of chronic conditions are not merely confined to features of the disease process, but are compounded by the consequences of treatment used.

Efforts to adjust to the reduction in activity imposed by chronic disease are complicated by the multiplication of symptoms and the increasing disability that results (Strauss et al 1984). To be confronted with the inevitability of her condition worsening is an important psychological challenge for the individual and her carers, acting as an additional source of stress. Individuals may fear the prospect of total disability and regard any development of their disease with anxiety and anger, directing these emotions towards close associates and health care personnel. Carers are faced with difficulties in dealing with this, together with increased demands placed on them to compensate for the individual's failing abilities. These may include the need to seek information about treatment and services, learn new skills and accommodate more physical activity in the management of care. Such demands have a considerable impact on carers because care-giving is carried out in the context of other competing demands, such as employment, marriage and child-rearing (Bull & Jervis 1997).

Nursing and other staff may be perceived by the individual as being incapable of resolving certain problems or, in the case of problems resulting from treatment, actually being responsible for them. This has obvious implications for the quality of nurse–patient relationships, which must be characterised by mutual trust and cooperation in order to be genuinely therapeutic.

Chronic diseases are disproportionately intrusive

People with chronic illness may direct much of their lives towards monitoring symptoms and adhering to treatment regimens (Nettleton 1995). Strauss et al (1984) comment that this prompts a fundamental reorganisation of lifestyle and of personal commitments. In episodes of acute illness it is both feasible and acceptable for individuals to gain temporary exemption from normal social obligations. This is not always possible, however, for those who are chronically sick and must structure daily life such that persistent features of their condition and periods of crisis can be accommodated. It may be difficult for these patients and their families to enjoy a sense of continuity in their lives, as their capacity to pursue various activities will vary unpredictably over time.

Dimond & Jones (1987) consider this idea as they question the application of the notion of the 'sick role' to long-term illness. They point out that the conceptualisation of the sick role by Parsons in 1951 forms the dominant framework within which health professionals work, even though it has limited applicability to the management of protracted illness. The expectation implied in the concept of the sick role that individuals should be obliged to get well is not appropriate in the face of irreversible pathology.

Strauss et al (1984) assert that chronic illness often results in the imposition of changes to normal domestic routines to allow for physical limitations and requirements of the treatment regimen. Structural alteration of accommodation may also be required; it may be necessary to install equipment and reassign room space to allow access to household facilities. These adaptations, together with alterations in appearance and behaviour associated with the long-term disease, will have an impact on other members of the household and their relationship with the sufferer.

Chronic illness will also have economic implications. Even if not totally disabled, the individual may be unable to continue employment because of the demands which her condition and its treatment make upon her time, strength and stamina. Difficulty in adhering to work schedules and periods of absence during more acute phases of the disease can give employers the impression that people with chronic illness are unreliable. Individuals may be assigned less demanding positions and not be promoted readily because they are perceived to have a poor prognosis and are thus not deserving of the investment of training for more advanced work (Taylor 1995). Gaining employment may be problematic in itself; the prospect of incapacity and variable function may be seen by the employer to represent hidden costs, including lost production and redeployment of other workers. In a study of the consequences of living with renal failure, Morgan (1988) reveals that people with kidney disease seeking new work were frequently unsuccessful in their applications. They alleged that prospective employers labelled them as 'kidney patients' and identified them as an employment risk.

Chronic illness may also affect the individual's ability to participate in a broad range of social activities. The degree to which these activities are impeded will depend to some extent on whether the individual has learned to deal with the features of the disease process. For example, Lambert & Lambert (1987) explain that fear of frequent episodes of loose stools and the presence of odour are major social concerns for people with ulcerative colitis. The management of these features is particularly difficult in settings where toilet facilities are not readily available. Individuals may respond either by withdrawing from interaction or by planning their outings carefully, using known routes and venues with accessible lavatories. The accidental emission of faecal odour or diarrhoea during sexual encounters is an additional source of anxiety, which can be met either by avoiding intimate relationships or by instituting coping strategies such as keeping an absorbent towel unobtrusively at the bedside. Spontaneous sexual engagements are felt to be preferable by some, as these provide little opportunity to become preoccupied with the manifestations of the disorder (Lambert & Lambert 1987).

The nature of chronic disease is such that it impinges on domestic, work-related and recreational activities, and is liable to result in social isolation. This is recognised widely as a consequence of long-term illness and disability which affects both sufferers and their close associates (Fitzpatrick 1990). People who are chronically sick require sustained support from those around them to manage their conditions and treatment regimens. The daily activities of their families must therefore be centred around meeting these needs, and it may no longer be possible for them to pursue interests which they once enjoyed together. Anderson (1988) discusses this with regard to the quality of life experienced by patients and their supporters after a CVA. Carers found the restrictions placed on their social lives and their use of free time to be distressing, and they deeply regretted not being able to go for walks or enjoy holidays with the affected person as they had done previously.

Chronic diseases require a wide variety of ancillary services

McClymont (1985) comments that there is an abundance of statutory and voluntary agencies in the UK concerned with the care and support of people with long-term illness. Statutory support is provided in the main by the National Health Service, the Department of Social Security, the Department of Employment and the local authority social services. The responses of these agencies are not always effective, however, due to differences in priorities and administrative practices. Care within institutional and domestic settings requires the close collaboration of a wide range of representatives of these services, such as nurses, therapists, doctors, social workers, civil service employees and home care workers. This can be difficult to achieve given the number and variety of staff necessary to meet an individual's needs, and problems are sometimes compounded by poor interservice coordination and frequent transfers between care settings (Howkins 1995).

Roberts (1985) states that the relationship between disabled people, their families and public services stems from the claim which any citizen may make for collectively funded care or support when independence is not possible. The legal, bureaucratic and medical definitions adopted routinely by formal agencies to categorise individuals and allocate resources are not generally compatible with the experience of people with long-term illness. For example, assessment to determine eligibility for benefits and support services may fail to acknowledge variation in function during episodes of crisis; if the assessment is performed during a period of relative wellness, the type and level of support required at other times may not be apparent to the assessor.

Roberts (1985) argues that some people either fail to obtain statutory support or decline the support to which they are entitled because they perceive the organisation of services to be complex or somewhat arbitrary. Ineffective communication can present an obstacle when individuals who are entitled to benefits lack information or have difficulty interpreting the information they are given. In addition, some families may be reluctant to seek or accept help from formal or informal agencies because to do so would be at variance with their cultural values regarding responsibility and self-sufficiency.

Roberts (1985) further asserts that provisions of the Chronically Sick and Disabled Persons Act (1970), intended to ensure support for disabled people living in their own homes, have not been realised because implementation by local authorities varies according to economic and political pressures. Variation can again be found in the criteria used to define need and eligibility. The literature indicates that the overall provision of statutory services is structured in terms of perceived need and that individuals are expected to fit into the network of support already available, although Vigars (1995) demonstrates that the rationale of the NHS and Community Care Act (DoH 1989) was that assessment should be needs- rather than service-led. Carers are entitled to ask for a separate assessment of their needs, with their ability to continue caring taken into account, but this may not occur as many partners and family members do not define themselves as carers and it is expected that they have assumed the role willingly (DoH 1997). People with long-term illness and their families may not, therefore, receive the kind of help which they believe would be of greatest benefit to them in maintaining their desired way of life (Pitkeathley 1991, Finkelstein & Stuart 1996).

Chronic disease is expensive

The direct and indirect costs of chronic illness are high (Strauss et al 1984). While expensive technological intervention is not always required, any support given will be continuous and increase in intensity as the illness progresses. The chronically ill individual will have to make repeated contact with health agencies to monitor the effectiveness of treatment and rehabilitation programmes. This may involve regular encounters with members of the primary health care team and frequent visits to hospital-based outpatient clinics. People with chronic illness are likely to experience multiple pathology as a result of systemic and degenerative disease; and since contemporary medical services are organised by area of specialisation, patients will frequently need to attend a variety of clinics. An individual with diabetes mellitus, for example, may require referral to a physician in renal medicine, an ophthalmologist and a vascular surgeon.

The long-term prescription of medication to control or palliate features of chronic conditions has significant financial and ethical implications. Rationing of health care has become more explicit in the face of growing demand and the increased availability of treatment options, coupled with pressure to reduce expenditure. As a result, prescription is not based solely on clinical need. Limited resources mean that decisions regarding treatment options are concerned with identifying the potential benefit to the individual and justifying whether such expenditure on a single patient is warranted. For example, lipid-lowering drugs used to reduce the risk of dying from coronary artery disease in men with hypercholesterolaemia cost £400 000 per life saved (Page et al 1997).

Treatment intended to inhibit the development of underlying disease but which does not necessarily cure or save lives can also be costly. Individuals with relapse-remitting multiple sclerosis (a pattern of disease characterised by at least two attacks of neurological dysfunction over the preceding 2-year period, followed by complete or incomplete recovery) and who are able to walk unaided can be prescribed interferon beta-1b, to be administered by self-injection every other day (Reynolds 1996, Bourdette 1997). This may decrease the frequency of relapses and prevent the accumulation of neurological damage, although there is limited evidence that it improves clinical disability (Wiener et al 1997). Efficacy of treatment for longer than 2 years has not been demonstrated conclusively (Walker 1998). At current costs, treatment for one patient for this period would be around £19 619 net for medication alone (Joint Formulary Committee 1999).

New drugs can be licensed for use when the evidence of benefit appears insubstantial. Dent & Hawke (1997) comment that the advice of local therapeutics committees to restrict the use of a particular drug until the results of research can be scrutinised may be offset by the effects of manufacturers' marketing strategies and the demands of patient groups lobbying for access to treatment.

Additional medications may need to be introduced to the regimen as illnesses evolve and to compensate for side-effects of treatment or drugs already prescribed. Changes in the treatment programme may be initiated by episodes of crisis. This, and the increased use of health and social services during such times, is a source of considerable expense.

Repeated periods of admission for acute hospital care may be necessary to achieve management of crises. Interdisciplinary involvement will be desirable in view of the effect that chronic illness has on all aspects of the individual's life. Cost containment in health care has led to a reduction in the length of stay in acute care hospitals; however, the presence of acute illness superimposed on a chronic condition inevitably results in a longer stay (Daly 1993).

The cost of chronic illness in comparison with that of acute illness is very high in respect of lost employment, reliance on state benefits and cessation of social activities. The onset of disability may also pose a threat to the stability of marital relationships (Taylor 1995).

32.6 Where resources are limited, it could be argued that efforts should be directed towards patients for whom improvement can be assured rather than those who are chronically ill. Why should patients with a chronic illness be given equal consideration?

For further exploration of related ethical issues, see Thompson et al (1994).

A FRAMEWORK FOR UNDERSTANDING THE EXPERIENCE OF CHRONIC ILLNESS

The features of chronic illness detailed above are reflected in the framework subsequently presented by Strauss et al (1984) for understanding the experience of ongoing ill-health. This framework is built around the five components outlined in the following.

Key problems

Any disease has the potential to create multiple problems for individual sufferers, and these are liable not only to disrupt routine activities but also to lead to social isolation and attendant psychological and familial difficulties. For example, people with multiple sclerosis and their associates may have difficulty adjusting to the effects of variation in ability and fatigue experienced during swings to and from 'good' and 'bad' days or weeks. It may be difficult for them to make firm arrangements to attend social gatherings, and friends may eventually hesitate to extend invitations when the affected individual withdraws repeatedly from events due to fatigue. Family members may begin to feel some resentment as outings and social activities are curtailed.

Basic strategies

Patients and their associates need to develop a repertoire of methods or techniques for overcoming key problems. For instance, an individual with diabetes can learn to adjust her behaviour and treatment regimen when attending social occasions where food and drink are offered. Her selection from a menu or buffet table may be guided by her treatment regimen, rather than purely by desire, in terms of the type and quantity of foods taken. If she does not wish to bring her condition to the attention of others at this time, she might avoid alcoholic drinks on the pretext of wanting to 'keep a clear head'; or she may choose to amend the timing and dosage of insulin injections to allow her to indulge in the food and drink which she actually prefers. Creative non-adherence (Taylor 1995) to treatment regimens or 'intelligent cheating' (Pressly 1995) is common in chronic illness and, although not necessarily problematic, can result in errors. It tends to be adopted by individuals who adapt, within reasonable limits, aspects of their treatment schedule to fit in with their current lifestyle.

Agents

Any basic strategies employed require the assistance of family members, friends, acquaintances or strangers. These 'agents' may function in a variety of ways, for example by assisting the individual to maintain a treatment regimen or protecting her from harmful effects of the disorder. A person who has epilepsy may need help from colleagues such that, should an unexpected seizure occur in the workplace, she is eased to the ground and away from dangerous machinery (see Ch. 9).

Organisational or family arrangements

The strategies adopted to address key problems require the coordinated effort of the individual and agents involved. The establishment and maintenance of arrangements rely on trust, skilled interaction, sufficient resources and realistic negotiation of the roles, responsibilities and expectations of all concerned. Someone who is housebound due to long-standing arthritis may be able to enlist family members and neighbours to do shopping, pick up drug prescriptions and collect benefit monies. The continued success of such arrangements will depend on each person involved having a clear appreciation of what the sufferer actually requires as well as an understanding of his or her own contribution to the well-being of the individual in the context of the help given by others.

Consequences

The strategies and arrangements adopted by people with chronic illness and their associates to manage key problems may be successful in resolving them but can have implications for the agents taking part, thus creating further problems. For example, the paced schedule of activities that enables individuals with COAD to accommodate oxygen deprivation and recovery times between tasks may present little opportunity for flexibility. Events such as a visit to the hairdresser's can disrupt well-established routines, with implications for both the sufferer and carer alike. Both parties are also faced with developing a lifestyle structured by demands of the presenting condition within which spontaneity has no place (see Research Abstract 32.1).

The elements in Research Abstract 32.1 provide a means to think about the experience of chronic illness from the perspective of the people concerned. It is only through this that the impact of the condition for each individual can be truly appreciated. Coping with chronic illness is influenced by a number of interacting psychosocial variables. Radley (1994) explains that central to these is an awareness of loss of aspects of self which were previously taken for granted. Chronic illness prompts the construction of a new life shaped by the course of the disease, within which the 'old self' is reconfigured. For many people, physical suffering is mediated by a sense of loss of self. Factors contributing to a loss of self include:

- living a restricted life — as a direct result of either impairment or treatment; this promotes a retreat into a world governed by illness

Research Abstract 32.1
Carers of the chronically ill

A survey conducted by the Carers National Association (CNA) (1992) to establish both perceptions and experiences of its members revealed the following (*n* = 2916):

- 72% are female and 66% are over 55 years old
- 38% have been caring for more than 10 years and 22% for more than 15 years
- 79% had no choice in taking on the caring role
- 39% did not talk to anyone about taking on the caring role
- 33% get no help or support at all with their caring responsibilities
- 20% have never had any break from their caring responsibilities
- 47% have experienced financial difficulties since becoming a carer
- 65% say their own health has suffered from their caring responsibilities
- people cease being carers mainly because those they care for die (61%)
- for only 1% had someone else taken over the caring responsibilities

- social isolation — resulting from the restriction above or the responses of others
- discrediting definitions of self and related negative self-sentiment — perhaps arising from the hostility shown by others (see 'Stigma', p. 947)
- becoming a burden — by being unable to fulfil obligations and feeling useless.

Living with a chronic illness therefore involves developing methods of coping with the perceived consequences of the disease and adjustment in managing social relationships.

For more information about the social psychology of chronic illness, see Radley (1994), Chapter 7.

32.7 'Chronic illness is a lonely experience. It makes for a sense of uniqueness that often leads to a feeling of separateness and alienation. It tends to foster a perception that you are in a world of your own and cannot join the ranks of mainstream culture' (Klein & Landau 1992). Refer to this, or any self-help guide written for people with a chronic illness. Has this helped you to understand the experience of living with a chronic condition? If so, in what way? Why is the use of self-help groups of particular value to people with chronic illness?

NURSING INTERVENTION

Developments in the location and organisation of care

Nurses will encounter adults with chronic illness in both community and institutional settings. These can include the person's own home, residential and nursing homes, or hospitals providing acute or continuing care. Acute hospital care occurs in relation to the establishment of diagnoses and periods of crisis during which features of the illness are exacerbated. Acute care is also necessary when the disease process necessitates revision of treatment regimens in order to achieve stabilisation or palliation. Such contact is therefore intermittent and recurrent. In addition, it should be recognised that hospitalisation could result from the development of an unrelated acute condition.

In general terms, admission to a long-term care facility has always been seen as the last resort for people with chronic illness.

It could be argued that the pattern of care in long-stay facilities developed in response to the interests of the staff rather than to meet the needs of individual patients. An important study by Baker (1978) revealed that the completion of physical tasks assumed priority in the provision of care for elderly people and that nurses expected their own worth to be judged purely in terms of the amount of energy expended whilst on duty. Echoing ideas first expressed by Coser (1963), Reed (1989) and Waters (1994) demonstrate that adherence to routinised methods of working is a strategy used by nurses employed within an environment which cannot provide job satisfaction through the achievement of cure. Here, effort is diverted to aspects of housekeeping by which success is made visible and measured. Routine practices, however, can result in patients being socialised into dependency and can undermine philosophies of care which place emphasis on promoting optimum independence.

People admitted for continuing care are deprived of their familiar social environment and accustomed lifestyle. The quality of their daily lives while in hospital will depend upon the extent to which nursing staff recognise their adult status, enable them to exercise choice in their activities, and help them to preserve links with the wider social world.

An increasing commitment to the concept of community care by NHS management has been evident in recent years (DoH 1989). This policy is demonstrated by Benjamin (1997) to be the response made by the health, social and voluntary services to meet rising demands and provide an individualised service, whilst taking into account the shortcomings of long-term institutionalisation. The shift towards community care has resulted in the closure of a number of long-stay facilities; as a result, it is now more likely that nurses will come into contact with people with chronic illnesses who are being cared for in their own homes.

The foundation for the nursing role

It is important to recognise that formal health care personnel are of relatively little importance in the overall management of long-term illness. Whilst their contribution to care is crucial during periods of crisis and in the establishment of treatment regimens, the sufferer and her associates hold primary responsibility for day-to-day management of the condition (Strauss et al 1984).

McClymont (1985) explains that although the majority of people with chronic illness are able to manage their conditions with minimal and intermittent assistance from medical or nursing staff, a significant proportion are not able to function independently and require support from others. Responsibility for this level of caring for adults with chronic illness thus frequently rests with family members. The nursing role in relation to adults with chronic illness is therefore far from restricted to the delivery of direct care. For example, in order to develop effective self- and lay-care practices it is essential to investigate the capacity of individuals and their carers to take on this responsibility. It is also vital to ensure that the information that patients and their carers need in order to implement care regimens at home has been successfully communicated (see Case History 32.4). In pursuing the goal of optimum patient autonomy, the nurse must also be prepared to adopt a flexible approach to care. During some phases of long-term illness it may be necessary to act for patients and carers, whilst on other occasions support will be focused on monitoring the performance of self-care activities, imparting knowledge or teaching practical skills to facilitate coping behaviour. This means that nurses need to be committed to the idea of forming and maintaining collaborative relationships with clients, empowering them as described by McWilliam et al (1997).

The notion of empowerment has particular value for people living with chronic illness because they hold responsibility for day-to-day management of their condition; yet they are likely to have lost power, control and confidence in their own abilities, through the psychological effects of the illness or institutionalisation. Empowerment is an enabling process that enhances personal control and facilitates the process of recreating self. This strategy will, however, present difficulties for a nurse who feels that sharing information and skill constitutes a threat to his control of the caring situation or somehow undermines his professional role.

Q

32.8 After reading Case History 32.4, how do you think communication could have been enhanced to prevent the problems which occurred when Mr P was learning about his diabetes? The community nurse recognised the need to respond to Mr P's difficulties with language by involving a link worker. A number of different people could have been asked to perform this role in the hospital setting:

(a) a young female family member
(b) any member of the local South Asian community
(c) a member of the hospital catering staff who speaks the same language as Mr P
(d) a community link worker employed for this purpose on a sessional basis.

Q

32.8 *(cont'd)*
What are the advantages and disadvantages of using each of the above as an interpreter? You may like to think about issues relating to culture, age, gender, varieties of Asian language, availability and confidentiality.

The complexity of long-term illness and its impact on individual lifestyle and functioning have already been emphasised. It is all too easy for nurses to make assumptions about the problems experienced by individuals in their care on the basis of medical diagnosis alone. There are additional implications arising from the patient's classification as 'chronically ill'. The overuse of this label can leave the impression that people with long-standing illness or disability are members of an homogeneous group for whom care can be planned unilaterally.

Using models to guide practice

The case has already been made that although a variety of characteristics are shared by adults with chronic illness, there is considerable diversity in the way in which individuals are affected by ongoing ill-health. It is therefore advantageous to adopt an approach to the delivery of nursing care which recognises explicitly the uniqueness of each individual and enables the totality of her situation to be understood. The use of a formalised framework to guide practice is also valuable in that it presents a systematic prescription for action and encompasses a sound theoretical base.

A variety of nursing models have been constructed which serve to articulate beliefs about the essential components of nursing practice and the concepts and theories underpinning them. These conceptual models are intended to provide a descriptive representation of the reality of practice. Consideration of the individuals

Case History 32.4 Mr P

Mr P is 62 years old and lives with his wife and their son V in a suburban area of a large city. The family own and manage a successful video rental business and are active within the local South Asian community.

Mr P usually enjoys good health but had been feeling unwell during recent months, experiencing frequency of micturition and an increased thirst. He was eventually persuaded to visit his general practitioner and was admitted to hospital on her advice. A diagnosis of diabetes mellitus was made and medical staff decided that control could be achieved through a combination of prescribed oral hypoglycaemic agents and a restricted diet (see Ch. 5). In the 10 days which followed, stabilisation of blood glucose levels was achieved. Nursing staff and the ward dietician spent time with Mr P explaining the nature of his condition and his future role in its management. He seemed to listen carefully to what was said but did not ask questions of the staff. It was believed that this was an expression of his quiet and reserved nature which had been in evidence since admission. The dietician was anxious to speak to Mrs P about her husband's dietary requirements, but the latter was not able to visit the hospital during office hours. Mr P said that he had discussed his condition with his wife and was confident that he would be able to cope after discharge. He was very much looking forward to returning home.

The responsibility for Mr P's nursing care was transferred to staff outside the hospital by way of the community liaison sister. When the community nurse, N, visited to assess the level of support which would be needed, she was greeted by V. He told her that both he and his mother were concerned about Mr P, who now appeared to be little better than he had been before admission to hospital. N checked Mr P's blood glucose level and found it to be higher than expected. In an attempt to discover the likely cause of this problem she asked Mr and Mrs P what they knew of the condition and to describe the treatment regimen.

It soon became clear that Mr P had not understood the information given to him in the hospital. He felt that the staff had been kind and concerned for his welfare, but he had observed them to be busy and did not wish to detain them unnecessarily by asking what he feared were trivial questions. He also confided that he was a little deaf and could not always hear what was said to him. The nurses had spoken quietly and quickly but Mr P had been too embarrassed to ask them to repeat all the information given. Although his working knowledge of English is good, Mr P uses this as his second language in daily life. Unfamiliar vocabulary presented during his admission had not enhanced communication with hospital staff. N discovered that Mr P believed he should reduce only the amount of sugar in his diet. Apart from this his food intake was unaltered, being predominantly based on rice and foods high in fat and refined carbohydrate. N recognised that the specific support she could give was limited and decided to offer the family contact with a community link worker.

receiving nursing care, the environment in which they are placed, the meaning of 'health' and the role of the nurse is therefore central to any model of nursing practice (Fawcett 1995). The selection of a particular model by a team of nurses largely depends on the extent to which it reflects their own personal values and what they perceive their goals of work to be. Fawcett notes that several possible advantages can be gained when a nursing team achieves agreement as to their model of choice; not least among these are consistency and continuity of nursing action.

Whilst there are a number of models which have relevance for nursing adults with chronic illness, the three models discussed in this chapter may be of particular value and interest to nurses entering this field of care.

Orem's self-care model

It is likely that the model put forward by Orem (1995) would be favoured by nurses who consider that its emphasis on client autonomy and motivation is consistent with the aim of helping individuals to accept responsibility for themselves. This may be seen as an appropriate choice in view of the limited role of formal health care personnel in the day-to-day management of long-standing disease. There may be a tendency, however, for nurses to select this model simply because they feel it to be synonymous with the concept of self-care (Cavanagh 1991). As a result, it is possible that some would fail to recognise fully that this concept forms only part of the model and that it must be seen in the context of the other components in order for the underlying theory to be understood.

According to Gast (1996), Orem believes that self-care is the contribution made by adults to their own continued existence and involves the practice of activities to maintain health and well-being. The nurse acts to assist patients and their associates to achieve self-care, taking ability and need into account. Patient care is organised in terms of one of three nursing systems following negotiation involving all parties concerned. Intervention can be wholly compensatory, partly compensatory or supportive-educative — i.e. the nurse may perform activities for the individual, assist the individual in carrying out shared activities, or help her to develop the ability to act on her own behalf. The decision to use a nursing system or a combination of systems is not static but changes in response to patient need over time.

Orem's model therefore presents some advantages for the care of people with chronic illness in both hospital and community settings. The importance of the role of the patient and her lay carers is acknowledged and their involvement in the planning of nursing interventions is considered essential. Attention is given to the notion that patients and their families are active in learning to live with the effects of the condition, and it is assumed that they are motivated to do so. The variation in nursing activity necessary to address the range of problems likely to be experienced during the course of long-term illness is also accounted for.

Roy's adaptation model

Another model which may be applied to the nursing care of chronically ill individuals is that devised by Roy (Andrews & Roy 1991). In Roy's view, the behaviour of individuals is influenced by an interrelated set of biological, psychological and social systems. Each of these systems is directed towards achieving a state of relative balance which will, as far as possible, promote the regularity of function and the ability of each person to adapt positively to environmental stimuli. Roy identifies three types of stimuli to which individuals are exposed: focal, contextual and residual. A focal stimulus is something which has an immediate effect on the person; a contextual stimulus is a contributory circumstance; and a residual stimulus arises from beliefs or attitudes relating to past experiences. Walsh (1991) comments that a focal stimulus should be present for each patient problem identified, but that contextual and residual stimuli are not necessarily present.

Where the effect of any stimulus exceeds the capacity of the individual to make a positive response, maladaption is said to occur. This results in a threat to continued health and well-being. Roy's model accepts that each individual possesses a unique capacity to deal with stimuli, such that people react differently when faced with the same events. The ability to adapt thus varies from person to person.

Nursing intervention is needed when an individual's usual methods of coping with stressors prove ineffective. The role of the nurse centres on promoting adaptation both in maintaining health and during periods of illness, and is concerned with the manipulation of stimuli so that the patient is able to respond in a positive way. Roy emphasises that patients have an active responsibility to participate in their own care (Fawcett 1995).

This model would be of value in the treatment of long-term illness in a variety of care settings. Its focus is congruent with the idea that it is desirable for people with chronic illness to develop the ability to live with the effects of their condition. Nurses are encouraged to consider factors which influence the individual's total situation, not merely the immediate problems confronting her. In this way it is possible for them to appreciate the effects of the disorder on the patient's personal functioning over time and how she feels about this. The model assists nurses in identifying successful coping mechanisms which have been used in the past and elements likely to impede future adaptation, so that intervention may be planned with realisable goals. Care can therefore be tailored in relation to individual resources.

The Roper–Logan–Tierney model

A more detailed examination will be made here of the model for nursing put forward by Roper et al (1996). This model has been widely adopted to guide nurse education and practice in the UK, and is thus one with which many nurses are familiar. In addition, as Newton (1991) points out, it is based on ideas drawn directly from practice and is articulated in terms which may be readily understood. The representation of the reality of practice presented in the model by Roper et al (1996) is such that it can be identified as being 'for real nurses, nursing real people' (Newton 1991). Examples of how this model may be applied have already been given in earlier chapters.

The authors based their model for nursing on a model for living. This demonstrates that health status and lifestyle are closely related. It is also intended that an awareness of this relationship should help nurses to perceive that their role is broadly concerned with health maintenance as well as being disease-orientated. Their portrayal of an uncomplicated view of nursing is a deliberate attempt to provide a flexible framework which can be applied in a variety of settings. The stated purpose of this model for nursing is to equip practitioners with a means to plan and deliver individualised care. This refers mainly to nurse-initiated activity, but acknowledges the contribution of other members of the health care team. Roper et al (1996) explain that the model also offers a method of thinking about the beliefs, aims and practice of nursing in general terms.

The Roper–Logan–Tierney model for nursing has the following five components:

- the activities of living (ALs)
- lifespan
- the dependence/independence continuum
- factors influencing the activities of living
- individualising nursing.

These will now be considered in turn with reference to the care of adults with chronic illness.

Activities of living. Roper et al (1996) identify 12 activities of living as follows:

- maintaining a safe environment
- communicating
- breathing
- eating and drinking
- eliminating
- personal cleansing and dressing
- controlling body temperature
- mobilising
- working and playing
- expressing sexuality
- sleeping
- dying.

The authors incorporated these activities into their model of living in order to provide a description of behaviours involved in the process of engaging in daily life. Although Roper et al (1996) advise that the activities of living should be used as a framework for assessment when the model is applied to practice, there is a danger that some nurses may employ this component of the model simply as a checklist to guide the organisation of care, and that its other dimensions may be overlooked as a result (Price 1991). This would both restrict the model's usefulness and yield a limited understanding of the needs of patients and their families.

The focus of nursing intervention in this model is on assisting patients in the prevention, resolution and management of problems identified in relation to the activities of living. Problems are defined as actual or potential, as the nurse is not only concerned with problems which actually exist, but also seeks to prevent the development of others.

The performance of any of the activities of living requires the coordination of a complex pattern of behaviour. The ability to communicate, for example, relies on a number of skills, including the reception and interpretation of information and the formulation and transmission of appropriate verbal and non-verbal responses. This is influenced by many variables, such as the efficiency of physiological and psychological functions. There is thus considerable scope for errors to occur, and it is likely that people with chronic illness will experience a wide range of associated problems. For example, some individuals may discover that they cannot understand or express ideas verbally following a CVA, whilst others find no difficulty in this area but are unable to articulate words clearly (see Ch. 9). In either case, sufferers will be limited in their ability to make their thoughts and feelings known, and this will cause frustration for all concerned.

Speech deterioration also takes place in Parkinson's disease (see Ch. 9). In this condition, communication may be further inhibited by memory impairment and loss of facial expression. The latter provides the listener with poor feedback and results in the absence of important non-verbal cues. Alteration in physical appearance can also present a barrier to communication. People may be embarrassed when they encounter disfigurement and avoid casual social contact with someone whose appearance disturbs them. In addition, they may make unfair assumptions about the individual's mental state. Wheelchair users often comment that people tend to speak over their heads to anyone who happens to be accompanying them, even when it would be more appropriate for them to be addressed directly.

It is common for people with long-term illness to find that disruption in the performance of one activity of living leads to difficulty in the performance of others. For instance, someone who has COAD and experiences shortness of breath may discover that her capacity to walk, eat and drink, communicate and attend to personal hygiene is also compromised. The restriction in mobility associated with arthritis can also interfere with the performance of workplace, domestic and recreational activities. For example, the purchase of food may prove problematic due to an inability to carry shopping, and the preparation of meals may be made difficult by reduced physical dexterity.

Lifespan. This component of the model represents the passage of each person through life from conception to death. The progression along the lifespan is marked by continual change as the individual moves through a series of developmental stages, each of which is associated with the expression of different levels of physical, cognitive and social function. Roper et al (1996) acknowledge that adulthood is sometimes described in terms of three stages, i.e. young adulthood, the middle years and late adulthood.

As mentioned previously, adulthood is a period generally characterised by self-reliance which centres around occupational and family interests. There is, of course, great diversity in the lifestyle and behaviour exhibited by individuals in this stage of life. Awareness of an individual's chronological age does not give the nurse sufficient information to appreciate the likely impact of chronic illness. Rather, the nurse will need to gain an understanding of the developmental tasks which the individual has already achieved, those she aspires to and the value placed on them by the individual herself and by those who are close to her.

This kind of information, obtained during assessment, would reveal the existence of actual or potential problems requiring nursing intervention. For example, a woman who has multiple sclerosis may have to come to terms with the fact that becoming pregnant would threaten her own health and that her functional impairment would present difficulties in meeting the needs of an infant. If, despite her desire to become a mother, she decides not to have children, she may experience profound regret. Once the nurse identifies this as a source of emotional distress it can be accounted for in the subsequent planning and implementation of care.

The dependence/independence continuum. By including this element in their model Roper et al (1996) acknowledge that individuals are not always able to perform each of the activities of living independently. Some people have yet to acquire the necessary skills or do not have the means to develop them, whilst others lose abilities which they once had, possibly as a result of illness or trauma.

According to Roper et al (1996), there can be no single measure which reflects the capacity for independent function in all activities of living, since it can be argued that few, if any, people are truly self-sufficient. In addition, they concede that the concepts of dependence and independence have meaning only when considered in relation to each other. For these reasons, any form of assessment will have a subjective bias which is determined by the nurse's interpretation of the abilities of each individual in comparison with clinical, developmental and social norms (Newton 1991). Assumptions about the inevitability of global deterioration with age and chronic illness need to be questioned, for example.

Health professionals must not fall into the trap of labelling or stereotyping the older person. Take, for example, the case of a community nurse who was asked to perform a home-based 'over 75 years' assessment of a frail woman who had chronic arthritis. The nurse assumed her client would require support and services for health needs. To her astonishment she found herself being asked to find out about entrance requirements for the Open University — her client was planning to gain a degree!

The interactive nature of the activities of living has been mentioned earlier with reference to the way in which difficulty in carrying out one activity can affect adversely the performance of others. This notion also has implications for the maintenance of independent action in chronic illness. In recognition of this, it is essential that attention is paid to each of the activities of living when assessment of a patient's dependence/independence status is made.

Factors influencing the activities of living. Individual differences can be identified in the way in which the activities of living are performed, regardless of the point reached in the lifespan or the level of dependence held. As an aid to describing these differences, Roper et al (1996) include five groups of factors in this component of their model:

- biological
- psychological — incorporating intellectual and emotional factors
- sociocultural — incorporating spiritual, religious and ethical factors
- environmental
- politico-economic — incorporating legal factors.

These factors, acting singly or in combination, influence each of the activities of living to some degree. It is not always easy to distinguish the influence of one group of factors from that of another since they are interrelated and share several areas of concern.

Consideration of this range of factors during assessment provides the basis for a deeper understanding of the cause of difficulties experienced by individuals as well as indicating likely outcomes. This has particular relevance for chronic illnesses in view of the timescales involved, the multiple effects of these disorders and the cycle of deterioration that may be associated with them. For example, knowledge of normal anatomical structure and physiological function enables the nurse to appreciate the effects of disease processes. This is useful both in guiding immediate action to alleviate existing problems and in devising patterns of care to prevent the onset of anticipated complications. An exploration of psychological status will reveal what the individual comprehends about her condition. Her capacity and motivation to acquire further information and develop the skills necessary for self-management can also be identified.

The behaviour an individual exhibits in everyday life in relation to the promotion of health and the management of chronic illness has strong social and cultural determinants. The nurse should attempt to understand how the condition has affected the individual's accustomed roles and in what respect this has influenced that person's relationships with others. A male manual worker who has multiple sclerosis, for instance, may perceive that his role as head of the family group is threatened when he is no longer able to continue employment and requires help from his partner to perform basic living activities.

Environmental factors such as noise, climate and atmospheric pollution can affect the performance of each of the activities of living in protracted illness. People with COAD experience worsening of their symptoms during periods of poor air quality. They may also find it difficult to obtain adequate rest and sleep if their home is located in a noisy neighbourhood or following admission to a busy hospital ward.

The structure and layout of buildings in which activities are performed are also of interest here. Someone who suffers from arthritis and lives in a top-floor flat without a lift may not be able to negotiate the stairs easily in order to leave the building. These circumstances would serve to further reduce her mobility, limiting opportunities for social interaction and activities such as shopping for clothes and food. Access to health centres can be made difficult if they are sited at some distance from available public transport or situated on a steep incline. This may deter individuals from attending appointments with members of the primary health care team and result in inadequate monitoring of treatment regimens and a lack of attention to some features of the disease. Lastly, admission to hospital is a source of anxiety to people for whom the environment is unfamiliar. The distance between facilities and the need to share bathing and sleeping accommodation may interfere with the individual's routine performance of a number of activities of living.

The organisation of all public services such as education, housing and social welfare is subject to political and economic influences, and these factors therefore have a significant effect on the manner in which people conduct their daily lives. Despite the high cost of chronic illness in both direct and indirect terms (see p. 952), long-term illness is not always given high priority in the allocation of health care funding. This has implications for staffing levels and the provision of equipment and hence for the quality of nursing support that can be offered to patients as they strive to attain optimum functioning and independence in the activities of living. Poor resourcing has additional implications for individual lifestyles. If a chair of a suitable height cannot be obtained for someone who has arthritis and she is unable to rise to a standing position as a result, it will not be possible for her to obtain exercise or get to the toilet independently.

Individualising nursing. This component of the model reflects the fact that the way in which each individual carries out the activities of living is unique. This individuality arises from the complex interaction between the components described above and is apparent in the frequency, location and timing of activities, rationale for the use of particular practices, and the knowledge, beliefs and attitudes of the person concerned. An appreciation of such variables provides the foundation for individualised nursing. Roper et al (1996) employ the process of nursing as a vehicle to translate theory into practice and as a means of achieving the individualisation of care.

APPLYING THE ROPER–LOGAN–TIERNEY MODEL USING THE NURSING PROCESS

Assessment

This stage of the nursing process should be recognised as a dynamic and ongoing activity, rather than as a single event associated with the first encounter between nurse and patient. In protracted illness, an initial assessment is important because it presents the nurse with a structured method of data collection which will create a total picture of the individual and thus provide a baseline against which change can be measured (see Case History 32.5). It must be acknowledged, however, that in ongoing illness circumstances are seldom static and therefore continued assessment will be essential.

Roper et al (1996) advise that two forms of information should be gathered, i.e. that relating to biography and health and that concerning the activities of living. It is likely that these elements will

Case History 32.5 H

H is a 19-year-old nursing student who was diagnosed in early adolescence as having epilepsy. Since leaving home to take up his studies, H has become more acutely aware that he is in some way 'different' from other people. Although realising the importance of informing teaching and ward staff of his condition, should any seizures occur whilst he is working with equipment or patients, H feels as if he is introducing himself as an epileptic first and an individual second. He believes that people are more likely to remember him by his diagnosis rather than his personal qualities.

H's epilepsy had been generally well controlled by prescribed medication but recently he has become tired, vague and forgetful. He has experienced seizures in the student residences and in the hospital canteen and feels angry that he seems to be losing control of himself.

Although H's medication was changed following a visit to the outpatient department, the seizures have continued. Their onset is unpredictable and H finds that he is increasingly anxious about the uncertainty of his situation. He spends much of his time wondering when the next seizure will occur. He has not taken sick leave because he fears that this would detract from his image, which he considers to be already tarnished by his condition.

H has stopped riding his bicycle and limits his excursions to journeys within a small radius of the hospital campus. His friends do not seem to understand this change in behaviour. H had always been the first to suggest visits to the pubs and clubs in the city centre. They respond by going out without him and suggest that he is taking himself too seriously. H feels isolated and is annoyed by having to think before doing anything.

When he next visits the outpatient department H's unstable condition results in admission to hospital for monitoring of his seizures. U, H's allocated nurse, finds him to be aggressive during her initial assessment. As they talk, H tells her that he has always made every effort to take his medication at prescribed intervals and yet his difficulties persist. He thought that he had recognised the problems his current situation presents for his safety and had adjusted his activities accordingly. He now feels as though he were somehow being punished for this. H considers that he has done everything in his power to help himself and he expresses resentment towards hospital staff because he believes that they have failed him. H is also concerned that he will not be able to continue to cope with the demands of his studies. His sole ambition is to become a nurse. From what he says, U becomes aware that H has lost confidence and lacks self-esteem. Her assessment reveals that H's condition has more implications for his care than had at first been obvious.

be closely related in people who are chronically ill; for example, the perception which the individual and her lay carers have of her health status can shape the performance of some life activities. Efforts should therefore be directed towards obtaining a comprehensive assessment at any stage of the nurse–patient relationship.

A number of variables will warrant attention during the assessment of an adult with chronic illness, whether nursing care is to be delivered in an institutional or a domestic setting. Some are related directly to the disease process and include the type and duration of the presenting condition, methods already used for managing symptoms and the extent to which strategies have been developed to cope with the uncertainty generated. Details of the treatment regimen should also be collected to help the nurse ascertain how the individual deals with incorporating this into daily life.

In encouraging the review of biographical data, Roper et al (1996) provide an opportunity for nurses to explore the individual's previous lifestyle and to appreciate the changes imposed by long-term illness in this context. The impact of these changes should be reviewed with reference to the activities of living while the other components of the model are borne in mind. It is suggested that all the activities should be considered so that for each individual their specific relevance can be established and relationships between them identified. For instance, some people may be concerned that their disease presents them with the prospect of dying, while others may instead express profound grief at the loss of social function which has resulted from the gradual loss of personal and occupational roles.

The Roper–Logan–Tierney model (1996) prompts nurses to pay attention to the individual's abilities as well as disabilities in carrying out the activities of living through reference to the dependence/independence continuum. Any equipment used to assist independence in daily routines can be identified, and the involvement of statutory support services and of lay carers can be examined. This part of the assessment may well help to determine whether the individual has a realistic idea of her own abilities.

Although much of the data required for assessment may be obtained from the patient, other sources of information must not be ignored. The views of both formal and informal carers should be solicited in order to build up a more detailed impression of behaviour and events. For example, when a patient with motor neurone disease (MND) is admitted to hospital for respite care, a community nurse might communicate the observation to the caring team that during recent months there has been a marked deterioration in the relationship between the patient and her spouse, although the couple may strenuously deny that this has taken place. This could then be interpreted with reference to the features of MND and the key problems associated with this (see p. 1001), and borne in mind as a plan for care is drawn up.

Planning

A plan for care is formulated to address the actual and potential problems identified in the course of assessment. The priority accorded to each problem depends upon the situation in which the individual is placed. Roper et al (1996) accept that life-threatening problems must assume precedence over those with a less immediate impact. Aside from this, priority-setting in chronic illness should always be negotiated by the nurse, patient and main lay carer. An open discussion is useful in clarifying the meaning of each problem to the individual, determining how problems are related to each other and creating a shared awareness that certain difficulties exist. This helps to foster a collaborative relationship and enhances the motivation of all concerned.

The aim of the care plan is to assist the patient in preventing, solving, alleviating or managing problems as far as is possible. Goals are set for each actual and potential problem and appropriate activities devised to attain them. In chronic illness it is particularly important that the goals selected are realistic in terms of the capacity of the individual to achieve them and are consistent with her own values and priorities. The patient and relevant lay carers should therefore be involved in this process.

> **32.8** Sometimes a care plan has been well established prior to any nursing involvement at home or in hospital. In Case History 32.5, H had established his, with the previous help of his family. What might the implications of this be for H and his carers when the nurse as a professional carer becomes involved?

Both short- and long-term goals can be specified. However, given the instability of chronic illness, the selection of broad objectives for future achievement, such as adaptation to the features of the condition and total self-management, may not be appropriate. It is preferable to simplify these by dividing them into a series of short-term goals related to the performance of relevant activities of living so that some progress can be achieved. Goals must also be expressed in measurable terms so that their attainment can be seen.

This information should be articulated in the form of a care plan with prescribed nursing interventions described in detail. This provides a means of ensuring continuity of care and is of particular value in long-term illness; for example, it can help to prevent confusion when a patient is learning to develop a routine for renal dialysis in a domestic setting. Activities initiated by other members of the interdisciplinary team can also be integrated into the care plan. Developments in collaborative care planning, which formalise such integration, are therefore particularly appropriate for use with this client group.

Implementation

The actions proposed in the care plan are realised in this phase of the nursing process. It is tempting to believe, as Roper et al (1996) point out, that because the majority of nurses are familiar with the idea of carrying out practical activities they will experience little difficulty in this area. Whilst there may be some truth in this assumption, there is a tendency for ease of performance to conceal the depth of knowledge and the complex array of skills necessary to allow the nurse to meet the needs of an adult with chronic illness effectively.

The delivery of care in relation to the activities of living should be consistent with the way in which individuals usually behave, whether or not they normally require assistance. As in Orem's (1995) model, this may require the nurse to act for the patient, to supplement and develop her self-care capability or to help her develop an understanding of the promotion of health. In order to determine the emphasis to be placed on each of these activities in a given situation, nurses must be sensitive to the individual's experience of chronic illness in the light of the factors considered in the first part of this chapter, whilst being aware of the possibilities of their nursing role.

The development of a therapeutic relationship with patients and lay carers is a sound basis from which to work. It is important for nurses to gain their patients' trust and to recognise that under normal circumstances they have the responsibility for the management of their daily lives and features of the disease process. In both hospital and domestic settings, nurses must be mindful of their role in enabling these individuals to retain control of their situation rather than expecting them to conform to alien norms and expectations.

In chronic illness, nursing intervention is far from restricted to the delivery of physical care, although the value of this should not be underestimated. Assisting another person in carrying out any activity, such as washing and dressing, requires more than the ability to reproduce simple physical actions. Nurses working with people who are chronically ill need to be prepared to help patients to express their needs and, if necessary, to adopt the role of advocate in liaising with statutory and lay carers. The promotion of health and self-care capability requires an understanding of an individual's developmental level as well as effective teaching techniques. This involves the use of refined communication skills, as does the role of counsellor and supporter to both the patient and her family.

When helping an individual to adapt to the presence of a protracted degenerative disease, and the difficulties which this can cause, the nurse should present explanations honestly yet positively to foster realistic hope for the future. It is worth remembering that non-verbal communication, principally that of touch, can be a useful tool to strengthen a caring relationship (Tutton 1991). Some nurses consider it appropriate to extend their traditional skills in this direction. The provision of massage, for example, can be of value in assisting the individual to deal with stress, creating a sense of self-worth and achieving a palliative effect (Vickers 1996).

Evaluation

The effectiveness of nursing interventions can be judged by evaluating whether or not goals have been achieved. This phase of the nursing process thus lends meaning to the phases which precede it. The extent to which goals have been achieved should be measured objectively where possible. For example, successful self-management of insulin-dependent diabetes can be demonstrated by a pattern of stability in blood glucose readings (Coates & Boore 1995). It is also possible to identify movement on the dependence/independence continuum in response to teaching programmes or the handling of symptoms.

The evaluation of some aspects of care is, however, largely dependent upon subjective data. For instance, it is difficult to measure to what extent a patient has adapted to the idea of having a chronic disease. Evaluation in this area could be guided instead by questioning the individual and interpreting her responses in terms of known variables, such as evident interest in the management of the condition or avoidance of discussion of the illness and its related problems.

The achievement of any goal for care relies on a variety of situational variables. It is therefore sometimes difficult to identify whether nursing strategies have been successful or not. The contribution of staff and material resources, efforts made by lay carers and the emotional status of the patient can all influence outcome. Nurses should be prepared to recognise that not all interventions which they initiate will be effective for each individual, even if they have been used with success on previous occasions. This serves as a stimulus for reassessment, from which revised problem statements and new goals for care can be generated (Newton 1991).

The importance of the nurse's own self-evaluation must not be forgotten here. Caring for adults with chronic illness exerts considerable physical and emotional pressures on nursing staff as well as on principal lay carers. There are a number of reasons for this. Nurses sometimes find it difficult to work within the boundaries of their occupational role as their relationships develop with individuals and their families over time. They may find it difficult to accept the inevitability of the patient's decline in health and independence. It is also likely that they will identify with the experience of a patient, particularly if they occupy the same stage of the lifespan. Some nurses will be unable to form close protracted relationships with particular patients due to differences in personality, culture and attitude. Individual nurses must recognise that they cannot be all things to all people. They should develop their own strategies for coping with the stress of caring and be prepared to share this burden with other members of the nursing team (Burnard 1991).

CONCLUSION

Nurses encounter people who are chronically sick in a variety of settings. Effective care requires not only a full understanding of the patient's particular illness, but also a grounding in social and physical sciences so that the experiences of the individual and her family can be interpreted accurately. The nursing role is collaborative in nature and involves the expression of technological, clinical and interpersonal skills. In the long term, emphasis is placed on caring, a concept fundamental to the practice of nursing which has often been overshadowed by other considerations. Working with individuals with chronic illnesses presents nurses with the opportunity to reaffirm their unique contribution to health care.

Finally, it is suggested that a good foundation for the development of an effective nursing role is for the nurse, and indeed the interdisciplinary health care team, to avoid thinking about the individual in need of intervention as a chronically ill person, but rather as a person with a chronic illness.

REFERENCES

Anderson M P 1988 Stress management for chronic disease: an overview. In: Russell M L (ed) Stress management for chronic disease. Pergamon, New York, ch 1

Anderson R, Bury M (eds) 1988 Living with chronic illness: the experience of patients and their families. Unwin Hyman, London

Andrews H A, Roy C 1991 Essentials of the Roy adaptation model. In: Andrews H A, Roy C (eds) The Roy adaptation model: the definitive statement. Appleton & Lange, Norwalk, CT, ch 1

Armstrong D 1994 Outline of sociology as applied to medicine, 4th edn. Butterworth-Heinemann, Oxford

Baker D E 1978 Attitudes of nurses to the care of the elderly. PhD thesis, University of Manchester (unpublished)

Benjamin A E 1997 Home-care politics in the 1990s. In: Fox D M, Raphael C (eds) Home-based care for a new century. Blackwell/Milbank Memorial Fund, Malden, ch 3

Bourdette D 1997 Multiple sclerosis. In: Rakel R E (ed) Conn's current therapy. Saunders, Philadelphia, PA

Bull M J, Jervis L L 1997 Strategies used by chronically ill older women and their caregiving daughters in managing posthospital care. Journal of Advanced Nursing 25(3): 541–547

Burnard P 1991 Coping with stress in the health professions – a practical guide. Chapman and Hall, London

Carers National Association 1992 Speak up, speak out: a survey of carers. CNA Publications, London

Cavanagh S J 1991 Orem's model in action. Macmillan, Basingstoke

Central Statistical Office 1990 Social trends 20. HMSO, London

Charlton A, While D, Kelly S 1997 Boys' smoking and cigarette-brand-sponsored motor racing. Lancet 350(9089): 1474

Charlton J 1997 Trends in all-cause mortality: 1841–1994. In: Charlton J, Murphy M (eds) The health of adult Britain 1841–1994 (1). Office for National Statistics, Stationery Office, London, ch 3

Coates V E, Boore J R P 1995 Self-management of chronic illness: implications for nursing. International Journal of Nursing Studies 32(6): 628–640

Coser R L 1963 Alienation and social structure. In: Freidson E (ed) The hospital in modern society. The Free Press, New York

Daly B J 1993 Managing the hospitalized chronically ill. In: Funk S G, Tornquist E M, Champagne M T, Wiese R A (eds) Key aspects of caring for the chronically ill: hospital and home. Springer, New York, NY, ch 3

Dent T H S, Hawke S 1997 Too soon to market. British Medical Journal 315(7118): 1248–1249

Department of Health 1989 Caring for people: community care in the next decade and beyond. HMSO, London

Department of Health 1990 On the state of the public health 1989. HMSO, London

Department of Health 1997 On the state of the public health 1996. Stationery Office, London

Dimond M, Jones S L 1987 Chronic illness across the lifespan. Appleton-Century-Crofts, Norwalk, CT

Disability Discrimination Act 1995. HMSO, London

Dunnell K 1997 Are we healthier? In: Charlton J, Murphy M (eds) The health of adult Britain 1841–1994 (2). Office for National Statistics, Stationery Office, London, ch 25

Eisenberg L 1990 Health education and the AIDS epidemic. In: Doxiadis S (ed) Ethics in health education. Wiley, Chichester, ch 11

Fawcett J 1995 Analysis and evaluation of conceptual models of nursing, 3rd edn. Davis, Philadelphia, PA

Field D 1993a Social definitions of health and illness. In: Taylor S, Field D (eds) Sociology of health and health care. Blackwell Scientific, Oxford, ch 6

Field D 1993b Chronic illness and physical disability. In: Taylor S, Field D (eds) Sociology of health and health care. Blackwell Scientific, Oxford, ch 7

Finkelstein V, Stuart O 1996 Developing new services. In: Hales G (ed) Beyond disability: towards an enabling society. Open University/Sage, London, ch 17

Fitzpatrick R 1990 Social aspects of chronic illness. In: Hasler J, Schofield T (eds) Continuing care: the management of chronic disease, 2nd edn. University Press, Oxford, ch 3

Galbraith S, McCormick A 1997 Infection in England and Wales 1838–1993. In: Charlton J, Murphy M (eds) The health of adult Britain 1841–1994 (2). Office for National Statistics, Stationery Office, London, ch 15

Gast H L 1996 Orem's self-care model. In: Fitzpatrick J J, Whall A L (eds) Conceptual models of nursing: analysis and application, 3rd edn. Appleton & Lange, Stamford, CT, ch 7

Goffman E 1963 Stigma. Penguin, Harmondsworth

Greaves D 1996 Concepts of health and disease. In: Greaves D, Upton H (eds) Philosophical problems in health care. Avebury, Aldershot, ch 5

Howkins E 1995 Collaborative care: an agreed goal, but a difficult journey. In: Cain P, Hyde V, Howkins E (eds) Community nursing – dimensions and dilemmas. Arnold, London, ch 4

Joint Formulary Committee 1999 British national formulary (37). British Medical Association/Royal Pharmaceutical Society of Great Britain, London

Kimmel D C 1990 Adulthood and aging: an interdisciplinary, developmental view, 3rd edn. Wiley, New York, NY

Klein R A, Landau M G 1992 Healing the body betrayed: a self-paced, self-help guide to regaining psychological control of your illness. Chronimed, Minneapolis

Lambert C E, Lambert V A 1987 Psychosocial impacts created by chronic illness. Nursing Clinics of North America 22(3): 527–533

Locker D 1991 Living with chronic illness. In: Scambler G (ed) Sociology as applied to medicine, 3rd edn. Baillière Tindall, London, ch 6

McClymont M E 1985 Intervention and care. In: King K (ed) Long term care. Churchill Livingstone, Edinburgh, ch 4

McWilliam C L, Stewart M, Brown J B et al 1997 Creating empowering meaning: an interactive process of promoting health with chronically ill older Canadians. Health Promotion International 12(2): 111–123

Mahony C 1997 An act of contrition. Nursing Times 93(30): 18

Martin J, Meltzer H, Elliot D 1988 The prevalence of disability among adults (OPCS surveys of disability in Great Britain: report 1). HMSO, London
Mishel M H 1993 Living with chronic illness. In: Funk S G, Tornquist E M, Champagne M T, Wiese R A (eds) Key aspects of caring for the chronically ill: hospital and home. Springer, New York, NY, ch 6
Montbriand M J, Laing G P 1991 Alternative health care as a control strategy. Journal of Advanced Nursing 16(3): 325–332
Morgan J 1988 Living with renal failure on home dialysis. In: Anderson R, Bury M (eds) Living with chronic illness: the experience of patients and their families. Unwin Hyman, London, ch 9
Nettleton S 1995 The sociology of health and illness. Polity Press, Cambridge
Newton C 1991 The Roper-Logan-Tierney model in action. Macmillan, Basingstoke
Oliver M 1990 The politics of disablement. Macmillan, Basingstoke
OPCS 1995 General household survey. HMSO, London
Orem D E 1995 Nursing: concepts of practice, 5th edn. McGraw-Hill, New York, NY
Page C L, Curtis M J, Sutter M C, Walker M J A, Hoffman B 1997 Integrated pharmacology. Mosby, London
Parsons T 1951 The social system. Routledge & Kegan Paul, London
Pinder R 1990 The management of chronic illness: patient and doctor perspectives on Parkinson's disease. Macmillan, Basingstoke
Pitkeathley J 1991 Seen but not heard? Nursing Times 87(42): 22
Pitts M 1996 The psychology of preventive health. Routledge, London
Pressly K B 1995 Psychosocial characteristics of CAPD patients and the occurrence of infectious complications. ANNA Journal 22(6): 563–572
Price B 1991 Preface. In: Newton C (ed) The Roper-Logan-Tierney model in action. Macmillan, Basingstoke
Radley A 1994 Making sense of illness: the social psychology of health and disease. Sage, London
Reed J 1989 All dressed up and nowhere to go: nursing assessment in geriatric care. PhD thesis, Newcastle Polytechnic (unpublished)
Reid T 1997 Caught in the act. Nursing Times 93(28): 12–13
Reynolds J E F (ed) 1996 Martindale – the extra pharmacopoeia, 31st edn. Royal Pharmaceutical Society of Great Britain, London
Roberts I 1985 Social and economic implications of chronic illness: a British perspective. In: King K (ed) Long term care. Churchill Livingstone, Edinburgh, ch 5
Robinson I 1988 Reconstructing lives: negotiating the meaning of multiple sclerosis. In: Anderson R, Bury M (eds) Living with chronic illness: the experience of patients and their families. Unwin Hyman, London, ch 2
Roper N, Logan W, Tierney A J 1996 The elements of nursing, 4th edn. Churchill Livingstone, Edinburgh
Scambler G 1991a Health and illness behaviour. In: Scambler G (ed) Sociology as applied to medicine, 3rd edn. Baillière Tindall, London, ch 3
Scambler G 1991b Deviance, sick role and stigma. In: Scambler G (ed) Sociology as applied to medicine, 3rd edn. Baillière Tindall, London, ch 13
Sharma U M 1992 Complementary medicine today: practitioners and patients. Tavistock/Routledge, London
Smaje C 1995 Health, 'race' and ethnicity: making sense of the evidence. King's Fund Institute, London
Smee C 1992 Effects of tobacco advertising on tobacco consumption: a discussion document reviewing evidence. Department of Health, London.
Stewart T I 1990 Diabetes mellitus. In: Hasler J, Schofield T (eds) Continuing care: the management of chronic disease, 2nd edn. University Press, Oxford, ch 7
Stockwell F 1972 The unpopular patient. Royal College of Nursing, London
Strauss A L, Corbin J, Fagerhaugh S, Glaser B G, Maines D, Suczek B, Weiner C L 1984 Chronic illness and the quality of life. Mosby, St Louis, MO
Swerdlow A, Doll R, dos Santos Silva I 1997 Time trends in cancer incidence and mortality in England and Wales. In: Charlton J, Murphy M (eds) The health of adult Britain 1841–1994 (2). Office for National Statistics, Stationery Office, London, ch 7
Taylor S E 1995 Health psychology, 3rd edn. McGraw-Hill, New York
Tinker A 1996 Older people in modern society, 4th edn. Longman, New York, NY
Tutton E 1991 An exploration of touch and its use in nursing. In: McMahon R, Pearson A (eds) Nursing as therapy. Chapman and Hall, London, ch 7
Vickers A 1996 Massage and aromatherapy: a guide for health professionals. Chapman and Hall, London
Vigars C 1995 The boundaries between social work and community nursing. In: Littlewood J (ed) Current issues in community nursing: primary health care in practice. Churchill Livingstone, Edinburgh, ch 11
Walker G 1998 ABI compendium of data sheets and summaries of product characteristics 1998–99. Datapharm, London
Walsh M 1991 Models in clinical nursing: the way forward. Baillière Tindall, London
Waters K R 1994 Getting dressed in the morning: styles of staff/patient interaction on rehabilitation hospital wards for elderly people. Journal of Advanced Nursing 19(2): 239–248
Watkins A D 1996 Contemporary context of complementary and alternative medicine: integrated mind-body medicine. In: Micozzi M S (ed) Fundamentals of complementary and alternative medicine. Churchill Livingstone, Edinburgh, ch 4
Weiner H L, Olek M J, Hohol M J, Khoury S J, Dawson D M, Hafler D A 1997 Rational therapy in multiple sclerosis. In: Russell W C (ed) Molecular biology of multiple sclerosis. Wiley, Chichester, ch 17
Williams S J 1993 Chronic respiratory illness. Routledge, London

FURTHER READING

Brykczynska G (ed) 1997 Caring: the compassion and wisdom of nursing. Arnold, London
Ewles L, Simnett I 1995 Promoting health, 3rd edn. Wiley, Chichester, chs 1, 4
Hyde A 1990 What is health? Health studies in nurse education. Discussion paper 2. Health Education Board for Scotland, Edinburgh
Kaplun A (ed) 1992 Health promotion and chronic illness: discovering a new quality of health. WHO European Series No 44. WHO Regional Publications, Copenhagen
Miller J F 1992 Coping with chronic illness: overcoming powerlessness, 2nd edn. Davis, Philadelphia, PA
Radley A 1994 Chronic illness. In: Radley A (ed) Making sense of illness: the social psychology of health and disease. Sage, London, ch 7
Rankin-Box D F 1995 The nurses' handbook of complementary therapies. Churchill Livingstone, Edinburgh
Shanley E 1992 Health and chronic conditions. Health studies in nurse education. Discussion paper 6. Health Education Board for Scotland, Edinburgh
Thompson I E, Melia K M, Boyd K M 1994 Nursing ethics, 3rd edn. Churchill Livingstone, Edinburgh

33 THE PATIENT RECEIVING PALLIATIVE CARE

Helen A. S. Dougan
Margaret M. Colquhoun

INTRODUCTION

Palliative care is the term given to the approach adopted when cure is unlikely and it is expected that the patient will die in the foreseeable future. People of all ages die, in a range of settings — at home, in hospitals, in nursing homes and in hospices. They die of many different diseases. Some die suddenly and some die slowly. Palliative care has been developed to help those who are dying slowly or, as is often said, living with dying. Led by the hospice pioneers, this approach to care has a recent and inspiring history (Doyle et al 1998, Faull 1998, Clark & Seymour 1999).

Many reasons have been given as to why this speciality has developed quickly and comprehensively in the UK in the late 20th century. Among the most notable are:

- the improvements in medical care, which have lengthened the time from diagnosis to death
- the promotion of honesty and openness between doctor, patient and family regarding a life-threatening diagnosis and prognosis
- the intolerance of the physical and mental suffering witnessed by those caring for patients with cancer.

A useful definition of palliative care is (World Health Organization 1990):

> *The active total care of patients whose disease is not responsive to curative treatment. Control of pain, of other symptoms, and of psychological, social and spiritual problems is paramount. The goal of palliative care is achievement of the best quality of life for patients and their families.*

The need to apply the new, evidence-based knowledge to the care of people dying from diseases other than cancer has long been recognised, and since the Barcelona Declaration (1996), there has been a determined effort to do this.

At its best, palliative care is teamwork where the patient and family are part of the interdisciplinary team. The care is individual, sensitive, non-judgemental, detailed and time-consuming. Patients and their families are met where they are (i.e. the health professional should have no preconceived ideas about them); there is no such being as a typical dying patient. It is a style of care in which the successful outcome has been redefined to mean a good death — a death that meets the expectations of the patient first and foremost, but also those of the family and the health professionals.

Delivering good palliative nursing care requires knowledge and a wide range of skills and it draws on life experience, self-awareness and motivation. It requires the nurse to understand and respect the roles of all the interdisciplinary team members and to work together with them to achieve a comprehensive and consistent approach to care. It is a daily challenge, which can be harrowing and stressful; however, the ultimate reward of facilitating a good death is very satisfying and worth striving for.

In the UK and many other countries, specialist palliative care nurses (sometimes known as Macmillan nurses) and specialist palliative care teams are well established in the community, in some hospitals and in the hospices. These specialists provide expertise for patients and families with problems that are difficult to manage. They frequently advise health professionals from other areas of health care. The palliative approach to care, however, is the right of all patients, no matter what their diagnosis, lifestyle or age. It is essential, therefore, that all nurses develop the knowledge and skills to offer this style of care.

In this chapter, a model for palliative care is presented. The model is flexible in that it can be adapted to suit each individual and his circumstances, and therefore can guide the nurse to provide person-centred and family-centred care. The style of record-keeping used within a health care setting is often very personal to the interdisciplinary team; it may have been designed or adapted to their satisfaction. Therefore, the suggested model does not have a set written format; it may be used along with the established documentation.

The text has been structured by applying the model to the case studies of three patients. The first patient's care is used to outline the application of the model without exploring the necessary detailed knowledge required to implement the care. In contrast, the care of the second and third patients is given in more detail. Issues of communication, psychological theory, pathophysiology and symptom control are discussed, illustrating the application of theory to practice. A nurse's formal reflection, using the reflective cycle described by Gibbs (1988), is presented in relation to Case Study 2 (Box 33.3, p. 976).

A MODEL FOR PALLIATIVE CARE

In the busy world of health care, the sheer volume of information available to the nurse in relation to palliative care could be overwhelming. This is not a narrow speciality where the range of in-depth knowledge and specific skills is limited to a particular organ and its pathology. The knowledge base for palliative nursing care is necessarily broad and derived from many disciplines. The very diversity of the population who may benefit from palliative care demands a structured model which, although fixed in its parts, is totally flexible in its content.

The model in Figure 33.1 is presented as a guide for the clinical nurse at the beginning of the 21st century. This nurse, in the climate of continuous lifelong learning, is envisaged as a critical thinker, i.e. one who challenges assumptions and looks for creative and workable solutions to problems, who critically reads literature and appraises research, and in partnership with the interdisciplinary team implements reflective, evidence-based practice.

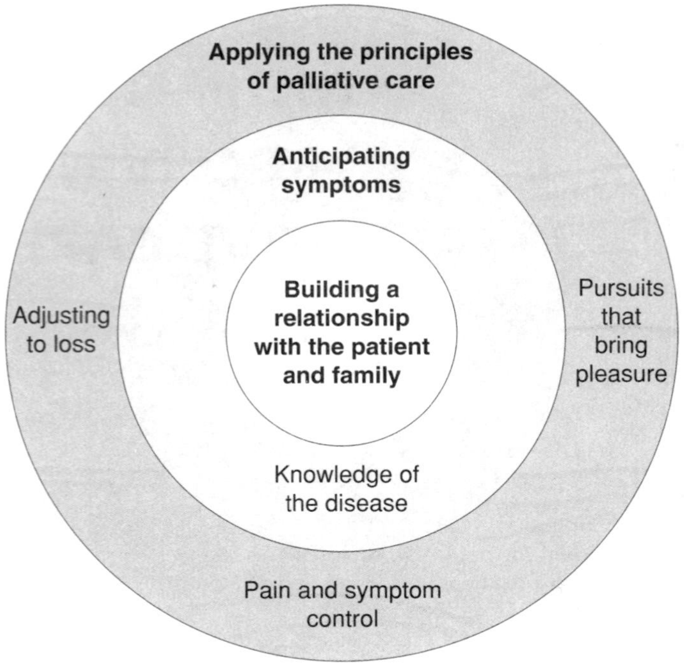

Fig. 33.1 A model for palliative care.

The three salient features of the model are presented. The order of their application should be interchangeable depending on individual circumstances. They are:

- *Building a relationship* with the patient and his family to explore their experience with the life-threatening illness and to become informed as to their functioning (i.e. their roles, bonds and coping strategies), as well as to ascertain their needs, priorities and wishes
- *Anticipating the symptoms* that may occur by using knowledge of pathophysiology and disease management
- *Applying the principles* of palliative care:
  —employing good control of symptoms
  —facilitating adjustment to losses and changes in lifestyle, of both the patient and his family
  —providing support to carry out pursuits that give pleasure for as long as possible.

Central to the model is the quality of life of the patient and his family. When a patient requires palliative care, his immediate problems are often overwhelming physical suffering, such as pain or nausea and vomiting. It is essential that these problems are tackled and the symptoms reduced before exploring the patient's psychosocial concerns.

Before embarking on the case studies, each aspect of the model will be considered in more detail.

Building a relationship and developing a profile

Communication is an essential feature of palliative care. This includes verbal, non-verbal and written communication with the patient and his family and within the interdisciplinary team. Particular emphasis is therefore placed on this aspect of the model at the outset.

When it is recognised that the intention of a patient's care has become palliative, this often means subjecting him to information-seeking interviews. However, one of the most commonly reported problems in the last few months of life is fatigue (Neuenschwander & Bruera 1998), and patients often complain that too many people ask them the same questions (Faulkner 1998). Therefore, effective communication within the team must be developed to protect these tired frail patients, without compromising opportunities for them to share their fears, problems and concerns.

Combined medical, nursing and paramedical written documentation in the form of patients' notes is being adopted by many teams. In addition, interdisciplinary team meetings are being held regularly at which the many different facets of patient and family problems may be discussed and shared goals set.

Patients and families need to feel secure that confidentiality will be maintained concerning matters revealed to the health care team. It is often believed that patients realise that they are being cared for by a team of staff and that they therefore implicitly agree that information given to one may be shared within the team. This should not be assumed. It is useful at times to remind patients and families that information is shared within the team and to emphasise that they do not have to talk about areas they prefer to keep private.

The ethics of confidentiality are beyond the scope of this text; readers wishing to explore this important area in more detail may refer to Randall & Downie (1996).

To implement the model, a great deal of information needs to be gathered in relation to the patient and his family. This section gives an example of a named nurse building a relationship and developing a profile.

Before embarking on an interview with the patient, the named nurse should ascertain what information is required, recognising that the patient profile will very likely be added to throughout the illness. The patient's notes should be read, as they may contain a great deal of the required information regarding diagnosis, treatment and other problems. However, it is wise to remember that the problems as perceived by the referring doctor or nurse, or the team currently caring for the patient, may be different from those causing the greatest concern to the patient (Heaven 1995). Communication with other members of the team may reveal that another interview is planned on the same day, and the team members may agree to sit down with the patient together. If not, one of the interviews should be postponed until the following day to prevent overtiring the patient.

An ideal situation for an assessment interview will be one in which privacy is provided without interruption. The nurse will give good eye contact, display warmth and respect, and the patient's physical comfort will be attended to. Skilful questioning will be utilised and blocking behaviour curbed. Many authors discuss sound communication and counselling skills (Faulkner & Maguire 1994, Kagan & Evans 1995, Faulkner 1998).

The patient should be engaged in a conversational interview (Brown 1995) by being encouraged to talk about his main current problems. It is then useful to enquire how each problem affects the patient's life and what expectations he has of getting help with these problems, i.e. what are his goals. Should the patient concentrate on physical concerns, it is useful to indicate that how he is feeling is also important. From this conversation, the named nurse should be able to appraise the patient's understanding of his illness (Heaven 1995, Silverman et al 1998). The patient may become tired or distressed during the interview, in which case the nurse must enquire if he wishes to stop. The distressed patient should not be abandoned. A cup of tea might be appreciated and the mood lightened by moving the conversation away from the difficult topic.

Box 33.1 Assessing a specific problem. (Adapted from Heaven 1995)

To assess a problem fully, be it physical or emotional, it is useful to structure your questions using the following framework:

- Nature — what is it like?
- Location (for a physical problem) — show me where you get it
- Severity — what is it like at its worst?
- Frequency — how often do you get this?
- Duration — how long does it last?
- Triggers — what starts it up or makes it worse?
- Alleviating factors — what helps?
- Impact on life — how does this affect your day-to-day life?
- Impact on patient — how does this affect how you are feeling in yourself?

The framework in Box 33.1 is suggested as a means of helping the patient to communicate fully about specific physical or emotional problems (Heaven 1995).

Having given the patient the opportunity to discuss his concerns, it is useful to move on to include the family. A family tree or genogram is a good method for gathering information in a form that is easily shared within the team (Fig. 33.2). Compiling the genogram may encourage the patient to talk about roles, relationships and personalities and to identify issues of concern. In addition, it demonstrates an interest in the patient's family, thus reinforcing the principle that family support is an integral part of palliative care (Murray Parkes et al 1996).

Following the interview, the named nurse will clearly and succinctly document the information and communicate any immediate issues to the appropriate team member.

Anticipating symptoms

Consideration now needs to be given to the nature of the life-threatening illness and any other existing medical problems from which the patient may suffer. For example, if caring for a person with cancer, the named nurse needs to know how that disease may spread. If the person has AIDS, it will be important to have an understanding of opportunistic infections or HIV-related malignancies that may occur. Complications of advanced disease can often be anticipated and, in some cases, effective management instigated. This can result in an improved quality of life for the patient and is therefore an important aspect of good palliative care. The named nurse may wish to update her knowledge of the specific disease process; the chapters in the first section of this book are a rich source of relevant information.

The named nurse is now in a position to prepare a summary of the patient's main problems, expectations and priorities and of his understanding of the illness and the problems that may occur.

Applying the principles of palliative care

Once the named nurse has developed a profile and identified the actual and potential problems that the patient may have, she is

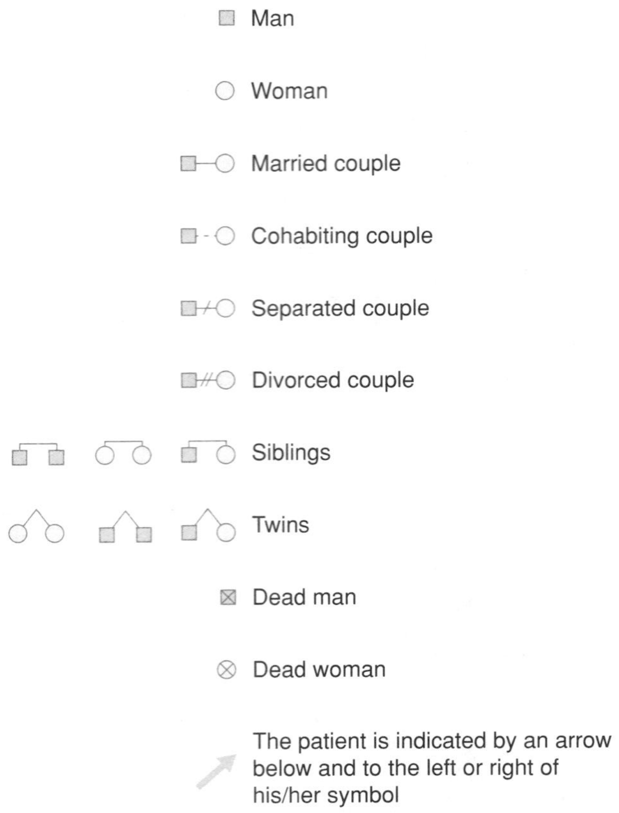

Fig. 33.2 A genogram is a code for recording a family, using the symbols shown (McGoldrick & Gerson 1985).

ready to devise a plan of care. This will be done with the patient, his family and the interdisciplinary team. In the plan, the principles of palliative care will be applied.

Pain and symptom control

The key components of good symptom control in palliative care are well described in Sims & Moss (1995) and Twycross (1997). In summary, the interdisciplinary team must work with the patient to:

- make a thorough assessment of each symptom
- discuss causes and treatment options
- plan symptom management in the light of the patient's expectations and priorities.

Attention to detail is also important, as is continuous review of the situation, because of the progressive nature of disease.

All of this must be underpinned by an understanding of the pathophysiology of the symptom.

Facilitating adjustment

Making the adjustment from thinking of oneself as a relatively healthy person who will die someday in the future to thinking of oneself as an ill person who is dying right now is a very big step. Many theorists have described the potential emotions and behaviours of people in this situation (Buckman 1992, Barraclough 1999). Many variables influence the responses of the dying patient and his family, the most notable being personal characteristics, level of social support, past experience of illness and death, age, culture, religious belief and the characteristics specific to the illness.

Loss is an abiding feature in the life of a person who is dying — loss of future, loss of role, loss of independence. This period in the palliative care patient's life has been compared to bereavement. Many of these patients perceive that the dying are shunned by health professionals because they cannot be cured. The nurse caring for the dying person needs to be acutely aware of this and must demonstrate the importance of the individual by displaying interest and respect, e.g. by consulting the patient about his needs, wants and priorities and thereby helping him to maintain his self-esteem.

It has been suggested that a useful starting point for understanding an individual's response to a life-threatening illness is to consider the question: 'What does this illness mean to this person?' (Barraclough 1999).

Supporting pursuits that give pleasure

Supporting the patient in carrying out pursuits that bring pleasure plays a vital part in maintaining hope and improving quality of life. One nurse in a research study (Degner et al 1991) describes this: 'It's helping [the patients] do things that are important to them, things that aren't really connected to their dying'.

This might be anything, from moving a patient's bed out into the hospice garden to enjoy the summer sunshine, to enabling a very frail patient to attend the performance of a play he particularly loves. The named nurse in palliative care needs to actively seek these opportunities.

Case Study 1 will briefly illustrate the model.

CASE STUDY 1 — MRS A

Building a relationship, developing a profile and anticipating symptoms

Mrs A was admitted to the community hospital yesterday. She was admitted by her general practitioner (GP) because of pain and rectal bleeding. The named nurse spends time building a relationship and developing a profile of the patient and her family:

- *Main problems.* The patient identifies these as a foul rectal discharge with some bleeding, pain at times in her bottom and a sensation of wanting to empty her bowels continuously. In addition, her husband, who has suffered a stroke, is already in the same hospital.
- *Expectations.* Mrs A is pleased to be in the hospital — 'my husband is so well looked after, and I am so tired and weary'. She does not expect that the smell will go away but she is sure the staff will not let her suffer.
- *Priorities.* The things that are most important to her are seeing her family, her faith, playing the piano, and having her clothes on during the day.
- *Understanding of illness.* Mrs A speaks openly about her cancer. She admits that she put off going to the doctor because of caring for her husband. When she was told her diagnosis, it was a relief to have it out in the open. It was a shock for the family. She is still trying to help them to come to terms with it, especially her eldest daughter.
- *Anticipated symptoms.* Because of her diagnosis of advanced rectal cancer, her main anticipated problems are pain, difficulty with defaecation, possible development of fistulae between the bowel, bladder and the vagina and a very small risk of catastrophic rectal haemorrhage.

Having obtained this information, the named nurse will liaise with the other members of the interdisciplinary team, in particular the family doctor, who will have completed a medical examination. A care plan will then be written. Towards the end of life, a patient's condition may change rapidly, and therefore the care plan should be reviewed daily and updated promptly.

Applying the principles of palliative care

The care plan for Mrs A, structured by the three principles of palliative care, will include the following.

Pain and symptom management

- Stop co-proxamol and commence 4-hourly oral morphine, to enable titration of the optimum daily dose of morphine required to control perineal pain. Also, begin on amitriptyline as adjuvant analgesia for the tenesmus.
- Continue the combined softening and stimulant oral laxative, co-danthramer.
- Emergency drugs have been prescribed, to be given in case of a catastrophic haemorrhage.
- Allow daily bath to soothe perineal area and dressing change as required.
- Install air freshening unit in room.

Adjustment to loss and change

- The named nurse will ensure that openings are given to Mrs A to talk about her feelings should she wish to. The patient has requested some time with her priest. This has been organised for today. A family meeting has been arranged for Friday at 15.00 h.
- Make it possible for the family to spend time together privately.

Pursuits that give pleasure

- Arrangements have been made for the patient to play the piano in the sitting room in the late afternoon; she may wish her visitors to accompany her.
- Ensure that the timing of help with personal hygiene does not prevent Mrs A going to the Sunday service in the chapel.

To demonstrate its flexibility, the model will now be applied more fully to two further case studies. The detailed content will include evidence-based theory and practice, providing a transferable body of knowledge as a basis for palliative nursing care practice in hospital, hospice, home or nursing home.

CASE STUDY 2 — MS M

Day 1. Ms M is a 39-year-old mother and company director who is separated from her husband. She has advanced breast cancer with metastases to bone, liver and brain. Ms M has been admitted to the hospice at her own request, having had a short admission 6 months previously for pain management. The referral from the GP requested admission for escalating pain, nausea and vomiting, and general deterioration.

On admission, Ms M is very pale and quiet. She is accompanied by her mother who looks distressed. Neither of them appears to recognise Sarah, the named nurse who cared for them on the previous admission. Quietly and without speaking much, Sarah (displaying warmth and concern in her non-verbal communication) settles the new patient into her bright comfortable single room. Together, she and one of the medical staff talk with Ms M about her immediate physical problems. The doctor carries out a brief examination. Having administered a subcutaneous (s.c.) injection of the analgesic diamorphine and an intramuscular (i.m.) injection of the antiemetic cyclizine, Sarah leaves her to rest. The doctor will return later to take a medical history and carry out a full physical examination. Some time is spent with the patient's mother listening to her concerns and reassuring her before arranging for a friend to take her home.

Using the model, Sarah has started to build a relationship with the patient and her family. It is not appropriate at this stage to tire the patient with a psychosocial interview. Pain and symptom control must take priority. Knowledge of the patient's disease, including the anticipated problems, is necessary, as well as knowledge of pain management to provide good palliative nursing care.

The anticipated symptoms of advanced breast cancer

In common with many patients suffering from advanced disease, patients with breast cancer may complain of insomnia, fatigue, anorexia, constipation or sore mouth. They may be at risk from pressure sores and infections. The causes of these problems are many and varied; observant and vigilant nursing care may alleviate or prevent these conditions. There are, however, symptoms associated specifically with advanced breast cancer and its spread. Fortunately, many of these can be anticipated and some can be managed to prevent unnecessary suffering.

Bone is generally considered the most common site for disseminated breast disease (Dixon & Sainsbury 1993, Hoskin & Makin 1998), followed by metastases to lung, liver and brain. It is important to remember that this is spread of the original disease. For example, when a patient with adenocarcinoma of the breast is diagnosed as having metastases in the femur, she has breast cancer in the bone not osteosarcoma.

Bone metastases

The bones most commonly affected by metastases are the ribs, vertebrae and pelvis, followed by the long bones, in particular the humerus and the femur. Patients often have metastases in more than one site.

The problems that may arise as a result are localised or neuropathic pain, pathological fracture and spinal cord or nerve root compression. In the past, hypercalcaemia would have been included in this list. Although this serious paraneoplastic disorder is associated with bone metastases, it is not now thought to be due directly to bone destruction. It will therefore be discussed separately.

The clinical diagnosis of bone metastases may be confirmed by X-ray. It is not unknown, however, for the X-ray to appear relatively normal, contradicting the clinical examination, and therefore a bone scan may be required to confirm the diagnosis. Radiotherapy, orthopaedic surgery, chemotherapy and hormone therapy are all used to manage this complication of cancer. Until these therapies can be organised, analgesia may give some relief.

A single dose of radiation is usually effective in relieving localised bone pain. Around 15–20% of patients will fail to respond to radiotherapy (Hoskin & Makin 1998). Patients should be warned that it can take 2–4 weeks for a response to be noticed. Side-effects from the treatment are usually minor. Hemibody radiotherapy is a useful treatment for scattered bone pain, but because of the associated potential toxicity, it has to be considered on a holistic basis for a patient with far-advanced disease.

Radiotherapy is an effective method of relieving bone pain and facilitating healing of a pathological fracture. It may be used as the sole treatment or in conjunction with surgery. Orthopaedic surgery in the form of surgical internal fixation of a long bone is an effective method of either preventing a pathological fracture or quickly relieving the severe pain when the fracture has occurred.

Chemotherapy may be a useful treatment for bone metastases, when the primary tumour is chemosensitive, and may be given in conjunction with local radiotherapy. Hormone therapy is often beneficial to relieve the pain of bone metastases in patients with hormone-sensitive cancer of the breast.

Spinal cord compression is a very serious complication of bone metastases in the vertebrae. Bone metastases will be the cause in approximately 85% of patients with this condition (Twycross 1997). The tumour may encroach on the spinal cord causing paralysis. This serious condition most commonly affects the thoracic vertebrae. However, for a significant minority, the site will be the lumbar region, and a smaller group will be at risk from quadriplegia because of tumour in the cervical vertebrae. Disease in more than one site is common. Spinal cord compression can be prevented, and therefore anticipation of this condition is of major importance.

Patients who are at risk of this complication, including patients with a diagnosis of breast cancer, must be warned to seek help immediately if they become aware of any of the following symptoms:

- a history of increasing back pain, which may radiate and be worse on movement and lying down
- sciatic-type pain in the lower back
- muscle weakness, which may make climbing stairs difficult and tripping-up common
- the sensation of weakness or a loss of feeling in the lower limbs or buttocks
- urinary hesitancy or retention, sphincter disturbance with incontinence of urine or faeces, or constipation.

In addition, neck pain, pain radiating to the shoulders and arms, or general weakness in the upper body should not be overlooked as this may be indicative of a cervical cord lesion.

Diagnosis is made on clinical examination and confirmed by an urgent magnetic resonance imaging (MRI) scan. Management must be considered immediately, as the progression to paralysis can be very rapid with significant implications for deterioration in the quality of life. Oral or intravenous (i.v.) steroids would be commenced. Analgesia such as oral morphine may also be required to provide some comfort for the patient.

Local radiotherapy is very effective and is usually the treatment of choice. However, some patients may benefit from surgery to stabilise the spine.

Lung metastases

The most common radiological abnormalities of lung metastases are multiple opacities in the lower lobes of the lungs. Lymphangitis carcinomatosis, the infiltration of the pulmonary lymphatics by tumour, may also be a problem. The severity of symptoms will depend on the number, site and size of the metastases. Dyspnoea may be caused by invasion of lung tissue, lymphangitis, pleural effusion or infection. Pain may also be caused by the pleural involvement. Haemoptysis and cough may be due to lobular collapse (Hoskin & Makin 1998).

Patients with breast cancer who have dyspnoea due to bronchial obstruction may respond to chemotherapy, radiotherapy or hormone therapy if these treatment options have not already been exhausted.

Respiratory symptoms are common in patients with advanced illness, with and without cancer (see Ch. 3). The management of acute breathlessness in chronic obstructive pulmonary disease is discussed in Case Sudy 3.

Liver metastases

Liver metastases indicate widespread dissemination of the disease and are therefore a poor prognostic sign. They may present as stretched capsule pain due to liver enlargement or be noticed on clinical examination of the abdomen. The diagnosis can be confirmed by ultrasound examination. Like the previous sites of secondary tumour discussed above, chemotherapy may be an option for the patient with breast cancer.

The enlarged liver may be the cause of a 'squashed stomach syndrome' with resultant nausea, vomiting, reduced gastric emptying and oesophageal reflux. The patient might also complain of dyspnoea, peripheral oedema and ascites. Liver function may be adequate until far on in the illness when liver failure may produce jaundice, pruritus, disturbances of homeostasis and eventually hepatic encephalopathy.

Corticosteroids are very useful in relieving the pain of a liver enlarged with advanced cancer. Cancerous cells are frequently surrounded by inflamed oedematous tissue; a steroid such as dexamethasone will reduce this swelling and therefore the overall dimensions of the tumour. The result is some relief of the pain (Penson & Fisher 1995).

Brain metastases

On occasion, secondary cancer in the brain is the presenting sign of a patient's cancer. It is, however, more commonly a sign of widespread disseminated disease with a poor prognosis. The main symptom of a severe headache is the result of local pressure produced by the tumour, associated haemorrhage or oedema of the surrounding brain tissues. The headache is often described as being like a tight band around the head, which is sometimes worse in the morning. It may be associated with visual disturbances, nausea and vomiting, confusion and altered consciousness.

Other signs and symptoms will depend on which area of the brain is affected, with many patients having tumours in multiple sites. Suspicion should be raised when the patient appears to have cognitive impairment, i.e. confusion, memory loss or personality change, or if he suffers from seizures, motor or sensory loss, or difficulty with balance.

The diagnosis may be confirmed by a brain scan. However, if the patient is very frail, a corticosteroid such as dexamethasone for a few days should confirm the diagnosis by relieving the symptoms. Radiotherapy to the whole brain is the usual method of treating cerebral metastases for patients who are strong enough and have a prognosis of longer than a few weeks. Steroids will be given to the patient to relieve the symptoms until the radiotherapy has an effect and to treat the potential increase in cerebral oedema, which may be a temporary result of the therapy. The patient must be warned of the likely hair loss.

Paraneoplastic disorders

These are generally thought to be due to substances produced by the tumour or by other cells in the body in response to the tumour. Some paraneoplastic disorders are life-threatening and many have a detrimental effect on the patient's quality of life. Therefore, when implementing this model of palliative care for a patient with a specific cancer, reference must be made to an oncology text. The paraneoplastic disorder most commonly associated with breast cancer is the metabolic disorder of hypercalcaemia.

Hypercalcaemia. Hypercalcaemia is an easily managed disorder and therefore knowledge of its symptoms is important in anticipating this life-threatening condition. Untreated hypercalcaemia can have a miserable effect on the patient's quality of life.

There was a time when it was believed that the high calcium in the blood was due to the mere presence of bone metastases. This theory has been superseded; it is now recognised that many patients with bone metastases do not develop hypercalcaemia and that some patients without bone metastases do. A simple outline of the present understanding will be given, as will the symptoms and management of the condition.

It would seem that various substances released from tumour cells cause tumour-induced hypercalcaemia. The most common of these is the parathyroid-related protein (PTHrP — not to be confused with the parathyroid hormone). PTHrP causes the reabsorption of calcium from bone and renal tubular reabsorption of calcium. Therefore, the presence of bone metastasis in a patient with breast cancer does not mean that hypercalcaemia is inevitable, unless the tumour is also producing PTHrP (Twycross 1997, Faulk & Fallon 1998, Faull & Barton 1998).

A high serum calcium will cause an osmotic diuresis, leading to polyuria, dehydration and thirst. The action on smooth muscle and the central nervous system may cause constipation, confusion and nausea. As this is a biochemical imbalance, it can stimulate the chemoreceptor trigger zone (CTZ) in the brain to cause vomiting.

The symptoms associated with rising calcium levels may therefore include the following: fatigue, lethargy, weakness, anorexia, thirst, constipation, polyuria, nausea, vomiting, delirium, drowsiness or coma. Death may be preceded by renal failure and/or cardiac arrhythmia in severe untreated hypercalcaemia.

Immediately a clinical diagnosis is made, treatment will begin by rehydration with i.v. normal saline. The drug treatment of choice is a biphosphonate such as i.v. pamidronate, which should normalise the serum calcium concentration within a week. This drug inhibits osteoblast activity and therefore inhibits bone absorption. It does not block PTHrP-mediated renal tubular reabsorption of calcium (Twycross 1997).

The effect on the patient is often dramatic. However, the condition will recur and the treatment will need to be repeated regularly for the remainder of the patient's life. This management alone may relieve the many symptoms associated with the condition, but until this reversal comes about, vigorous pain and symptom management will be necessary.

Building a relationship and developing a profile

Day 2. Ms M has had a settled night requiring further s.c. diamorphine at 04.00 h with good effect. Today her pains will be assessed and titration of the analgesics will be commenced. Simultaneously, other physical problems will be addressed, but first attention is given to total pain and suffering (see p. 970). It is known that pain and other symptoms are often difficult to manage because of psychological and emotional concerns. Therefore Sarah, the named nurse, has determined to carry out an initial interview with Ms M today, and later she will arrange to spend time with the patient's mother.

Sarah refreshes her memory by reading the patient's notes. Ms M's genogram constructed on the previous admission is useful (Fig. 33.3). She is also aware of the detailed clinical examination carried out by the consultant physician earlier this morning. To enable her to implement the model, Sarah will require to collect information from the patient, so that an-up-to-the-minute patient-centred care plan can be written. Ensuring the patient's comfort and that they will not be interrupted, Sarah gently encourages Ms M to talk about her situation and her feelings.

Gradually responding to Sarah's warm approach, Ms M confides that she has underestimated the emotional pain of leaving her children and that she is very worried about her mother. Ms M goes on to explain that her daughters Fiona, aged 9, and Katy, aged 5, have moved in on a permanent basis with their father, his new partner and their 2-year-old son. This seemed to be the most practical solution as he is a good dad and really loves them. It was, however, a terrible wrench: 'I cried and cried and really upset Mum. My mother is used to me being strong, all this is difficult for her.'

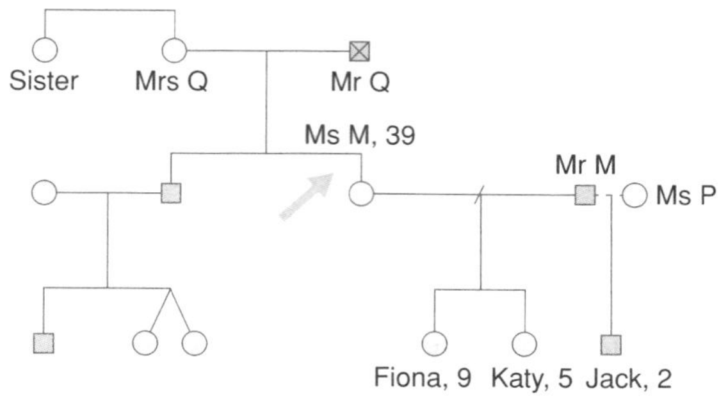

Fig. 33.3 Genogram for Ms M.

Ms M continues by repeating that she knew that this was the best for her children, and that their father's new partner is a real 'earth mother' type. She jokes about this having its good and bad points; that she as a career woman would have brought them up to be strong, independent women like herself. 'However, they know I am dying, we have talked and cried about it and read the right books. I have tried my best to prepare them.'

Note that Sarah asks Ms M what her main problems, expectations and priorities are. She does not ask her directly about her understanding of the disease or the anticipated problems, as that would have been insensitive. Sarah is able to document the information from the conversation; other members of the team will be consulted to add to this section of the assessment:

- *Main problems.* Initially, the patient identifies these as uncontrolled pain, nausea and vomiting, and sheer exhaustion. Following the above conversation, she admits to emotional pain, but wishes it to be recorded that she would only talk to Sarah about it.
- *Expectations.* Having had her pain brought under control on a previous admission, she hopes that the doctor will be able to help her again. She trusts him and is comforted by his determination; she knows he will not give up on her. She also expects to go home again.
- *Priorities.* Ms M identifies that she needs to rest. She requests not to be disturbed in the mornings until at least 10 o'clock. Getting her assets put in trust for her daughters has been a lengthy procedure. Fortunately, her lawyer and business partner will come to the hospice for final signatures sometime this week, and then she will be able to relax. It is very important for Ms M to see her daughters; she has, however, instructed her husband that the girls are only to visit at the weekend, as she does not want to prejudice their schooling. Her mother and her aunt will be in every day. They are her main carers and have a need to visit. Other people have been instructed not to come.
- *Understanding of illness.* Having read widely in relation to her disease, including searching the internet, Ms M has been involved in the decisions at every stage of her illness. She assures Sarah that it has been a conscious decision to come to

the hospice, as she liked what she had read about palliative care units. She is also aware of the complications that might come about because of her disease.

- *Anticipated symptoms.* Because of her diagnosis of advanced metastatic breast cancer, Ms M's main anticipated problems are pain at multiple sites, hypercalcaemia and spinal cord compression. Because she is on morphine, constipation must be prevented.

Having obtained this information, Sarah ensures that Ms M is not upset and is comfortable before writing up the assessment and the care plan. Ms M thanks Sarah for listening to her, saying with a wry smile: 'It has helped to talk, but I will not be making a habit of it.'

Later in the day, Sarah spends some time talking with Mrs Q, the patient's mother. From this conversation, she is made aware that the patient and her mother had a strained relationship before the daughter's illness. Mrs Q had at times found her daughter's forceful personality difficult, although she is very proud of her. She was very upset when the marriage broke down and continues to admire her son-in-law for his gentle, loving nature and his good parenting skills.

She cries when she tells Sarah of how the last few weeks have been so much better. It has been like 'having her little girl again', as she has helped her to shower and dress, and she talked about the past. Now she feels so useless and is dreading the next few weeks.

Sarah gently asks whom Mrs Q has to talk to, having noticed on the genogram that she has a sister. She is very relieved when Mrs Q speaks warmly of the support her sister is providing and the importance of her friends in the church.

Sarah reminds Mrs Q that the hospice staff are available to help families as well as patients. She also decides to ask the patient how she would feel about her mother coming in some days to help with her physical care.

Before moving on to care planning, the reader will realise that knowledge of suffering, pain assessment and management as well as nausea and vomiting are necessary to implement this patient's care.

Suffering

Pain and suffering are terms that are sometimes used as if they had the same meaning; this demonstrates a deep misunderstanding of human suffering. Physical pain can usually be controlled or reduced, whereas suffering is a much more complex phenomenon, which encompasses emotions and psychosocial concerns that may elude control (Chapman & Gavrin 1993, Gregory & English 1994, Roy 1998).

Patients and families may suffer because of unresolved issues from the past. There may be guilt, remorse, loss of hope and fear of the future. People who are dying have lost control over their future, have suffered multiple losses in relation to their previous lifestyle and are often witnessing their decline into total dependence on others. In addition, they may be suffering through observing the effect their imminent demise is having on their family, and may be worried about how their survivors will cope. The family members are suffering by watching their loved one's decline, feeling useless and unable to help. Previous bad experiences of poor symptom control in the dying may be the cause of considerable anxiety.

Coping styles have attracted much interest in the literature. There is no doubt that some people cope much better than others in stressful situations. Some individuals are flexible in being able to change their lifestyle to their new circumstances, to seek information, to be involved in the decision-making, to maintain hope and to preserve their self-worth. Others become helpless and hopeless and go into a steep decline (Murray Parkes et al 1996, Barraclough 1999).

Many factors are involved. These are as diverse as personality, the manner in which the bad news was broken, and the social support available. A previous coping style is not always useful in relation to facing a life-threatening illness. This can be very distressing for patients and families as they struggle to cope with the fearful situation. Changing coping styles is not generally an option. What is recommended is to provide extra coping strategies, to enable the individuals some relief from the suffering (Rowland 1990).

Realising the enormity of suffering, by both patient and family, can be daunting in palliative care. However, some help can be offered. By building up a relationship with the patient and the family, the nurse may gain some insight into what would be useful.

Daily communication with the family is a good method of giving support. The family members should never feel they have to search for someone to talk to, or that the nurse or doctor is too busy. A conscious effort must be made to give the family members respect by memorising their names and displaying warm body language towards them. Listening to their concerns is often useful, as is exploring who they have outwith the family to give support. Practical solutions may help, such as providing privacy for the patient and family to talk and for Ms M's mother to be involved in her daughter's physical care.

Mind and body are inextricably linked. The stresses caused by suffering may evoke physiological effects on the body. Therefore the individual may have an increased heart rate, blood pressure and muscle tension (Lang & Patt 1994). Complementary therapies may therefore be of great benefit to patients. Relaxation, massage, music therapy and other distracters may help to relieve the stresses of dying and should be available alongside mainstream medicine.

Whenever the patient seems to be very anxious or down, or when the usual pain management does not appear to be having the desired effect, the nurse caring for the dying must consider whether all avenues have been explored to assist the patient with the suffering. This may mean referring the patient to a social worker, counsellor, chaplain or a clinical psychologist.

The health care team may also suffer. Realising that clinical skills and knowledge are insufficient to relieve the patient's suffering may cause considerable distress (Cherny et al 1994). A culture of support must be developed by those caring for the dying, to enable them to realise, through maturity and experience, that there are limits to what can be achieved in relieving the suffering of some individuals.

Roy (1998) supports this, urging the health care team to 'realise your limits, there are some kinds of suffering that are so bound up in another person's uniqueness that they cannot be spoken away by other human beings, no matter how compassionate their words might be'.

Anxiolytic drugs such as the benzodiazepines, i.e. diazepam and midazolam, are frequently prescribed in palliative care. They can help the patient sleep at night and get some relief from inner torment (Twycross 1997).

In getting to know Ms M, Sarah recognises that the patient has trust in her hospice doctor because of her previous good experience of being helped with her pain. She also recognises that this is a lady who has what the psychologists call a 'high internal locus of control' (Murray Parkes et al 1996), i.e. she has a need to continue to have some control over her circumstances. Sarah will therefore ensure that the patient is consulted and informed as to any decisions being made about her care. Sarah is also realistic in knowing that she cannot take away the profound sadness that her patient feels at the loss of her future as a mother. She can empathise with her and provide her with openings to talk about it and pleasurable distractions, but she cannot remove that suffering.

One area of suffering that can generally be helped is the management of physical pain. When physical pain is relieved or reduced to a level acceptable to the patient, other areas of suffering can be explored. Before moving on to this section of the chapter, the reader is advised to read Chapter 19.

Pain assessment

Despite the complexity of pain, a vast amount of knowledge is available to manage pain effectively. However, pain that is not identified will not be treated, and pain will not be treated vigorously enough if its severity is underestimated (Vallerand 1997).

It has now been well accepted that the patient's self-report is the most reliable indicator of pain (McCaffery & Beebe 1994). Self-report of pain, however, is rarely an option in the confused or non-verbal elderly patient. Behaviour becomes the main method of assessing pain in these individuals. In addition, of course, there are many personality, attitudinal and cultural reasons why people do not reveal their pains. These range from being loath to admit to an increase in pain, as this may signify progression of their disease, to being unwilling to admit that the doctor's best efforts have been to no avail.

Patients who are dying have more than one pain, and therefore the nurse committed to helping her patient must systematically and regularly assess and document information about these pains.

The following information should be documented in relation to each pain:

- location
- severity
- radiation
- type (dull/acute)
- when started
- aggravating factors
- alleviating factors.

The nurse, having assessed the patient's pain, should then discuss this with the medical staff. It is essential this be done in an informed manner by giving a detailed description of the pain as outlined above. It is poor practice when requesting medical attendance to give the blank statement that the patient is in pain.

Pain management

An accurate diagnosis of new pains derived from observation, discussion and physical examination must be undertaken by a physician. This is essential, as the new pains may require laboratory or radiological investigations and other treatments as well as analgesia.

Analgesic drugs given regularly to prevent the recurrence of pain are central to effective pain management. It is essential that an adequate, regular dose is calculated and administered, enabling the patient to be as comfortable as possible without being drowsy. A list of analgesic drugs commonly used for cancer pain is given in Box 33.2.

Adjuvant drugs are frequently given along with analgesics in the effective management of pain. Some pains do not respond well to the analgesics codeine, morphine and the other drugs that are known collectively as opioids. Bone pain and neuropathic pain commonly require adjuvant therapy. A list of adjuvant analgesic drugs is in Table 33.1.

Principles have been established by the World Health Organization (WHO 1986) to guide medical staff in the management of chronic pain. Registered nurses must have a sound knowledge of these principles to promote good interdisciplinary understanding and patient confidence.

The WHO analgesic ladder

The key principles of the WHO approach are that analgesics be given by the mouth, by the clock and by the ladder.

By the mouth. This convenient and easy route of administration should be the route of choice for as long as possible. When the patient can no longer tolerate oral medicines, the s.c. route is frequently used by setting up a syringe driver.

Box 33.2 Analgesic drugs commonly used for cancer pain

Step 1 — non-opioids
Paracetamol or non-steroidal anti-inflammatories (NSAIDs)

Step 2 — mild opioids
Codeine or dextropropoxyphene, often combined with paracetamol, e.g. co-proxamol

Step 3 — strong opioids
Immediate release — Oramorph or Sevredol
Sustained release — MST Continus or MXL
Diamorphine by subcutaneous injection

Table 33.1 Adjuvant analgesics commonly used for cancer pain

Drug	*Example*	*Indications*
Non-steroidal anti-inflammatory (NSAID)	Diclofenac	Bone pain, soft tissue infiltration
Corticosteroids	Dexamethasone	Raised intracranial pressure Nerve compression Soft tissue infiltration Hepatomegaly
Tricyclic antidepressants Anticonvulsants	Amitriptyline Sodium valproate	Nerve compression or infiltration, paraneoplastic neuropathies
Bisphosphonates	Pamidronate	Bone pain

By the clock. Morphine solution is effective for 4 hours. Therefore, the drug *must* be administered regularly every 4 hours. The exceptions to this are the sustained-release preparations, such as MST Continus.

Persistent pain must be prevented; it is inhumane to allow pain to return before administering the next dose. In an in-patient setting, care must be taken, therefore, that the patient does not have to wait on a routine drug round for this analgesic. A more accurate timing of the drug administration may be achieved if it is given directly by the patient's named nurse or deputy, or by self-medication.

By the ladder. Having taken a careful history and carried out a physical examination, the doctor will now be in a position to prescribe medication for the patient's pains. This may be a combination of analgesics and adjuvant therapies.

If the patient's management starts on step one of the ladder, paracetamol will be given until the ceiling of 4 g in 24 h has been reached. That is the upper dose limit of this drug. If it does not control the pain then a drug on step two will be prescribed. Co-proxamol, a combination of the mild opioid dextropropoxyphene and paracetamol, is commonly used. It will be given up to the ceiling of two tablets 4-hourly, and when that ceases to control the patient's pain, a drug on step three will be prescribed.

The decision to use a strong opioid should be based on patient need, not the prognosis. The outdated practice of saving morphine for the last few weeks of life is misinformed.

An immediate-release oral preparation of morphine, such as Oramorph, Sevredol solution or Sevredol tablets, will be prescribed, with the intention of establishing a regimen that will relieve the pain without causing oversedation. This is known as titration. A common starting dose of immediate-release morphine is 5–10 mg, except in the elderly or the cachectic patient when 2.5 mg might be the starting dose. The drug will be prescribed to be taken 4-hourly round the clock, i.e. at 06.00, 10.00, 14.00, 18.00, 22.00 and 02.00 h. If sleeping, the patient should be wakened at 02.00 h, at least for the first few nights. Thereafter the doctor will probably prescribe a double dose at 22.00 h and the 02.00 h dose will then be omitted.

Should the patient be in pain between doses, a breakthrough dose equivalent to the standard 4-hourly dose will be given. If a breakthrough dose is given, the timing of the next regular dose must not be altered. For example, if a patient has Oramorph at 06.00 h and requires a breakthrough dose at 09.00 h, the dose due at 10.00 h will still be given on time.

Some common side-effects might be expected when a patient commences on strong opioids. Transitory effects may be sleepiness and nausea; these usually pass in a few days. More troublesome are constipation and a dry mouth. Constipation must be treated prophylactically; a laxative such as co-danthramer *must* be prescribed at the same time as the opioid.

When the dose of morphine has been stable for 24–48 h, the patient may be prescribed the daily dose of morphine in a slow-release preparation. For example, on her first admission, Ms M was stabilised on 10 mg of morphine 4-hourly, i.e. 60 mg daily. She was therefore discharged home on 30 mg of MST Continus twice daily (b.d.). She was also instructed to take a sixth of her daily dose, i.e. 10 mg, of quick-release morphine mixture for breakthrough pain if required.

Around 80–90% of pain due to cancer can be relieved with oral analgesics and adjuvant drugs following the WHO guidelines. The remaining percentage of pain can be difficult to manage (Sykes et al 1998).

For detailed information on difficult pain problems, refer to Twycross (1997), Fallon & O'Neill (1998) and Dymock & McConnachie (1999).

Fear of addiction

One barrier to effective pain control in palliative care is the fear that patients, families and some health care professionals have of addiction to opioids. This fear is unfounded when the patient has physical pain. The confusion frequently arises when the patient on opioids requires increasing doses to relieve the physical pain.

An understanding of the terms 'addiction', 'tolerance' and 'dependence' is useful to reassure the patient and family. Addiction, i.e. psychological dependence, is usually seen in individuals who are taking morphine in the absence of physical pain. In contrast, tolerance is an involuntary physiological response to opioids when, having taken the opioids for some time, the patient requires larger doses to benefit from the same analgesic effect. Physical dependence is another physiological response, which these patients may show when an opioid is suddenly stopped (Watt-Watson & Donovan 1992).

Tolerance and physical dependence are not the same as addiction. Less than 1% of patients receiving opioids for physical pain over many months will develop addiction. However, 75–100% of patients receiving opioids for some months will develop tolerance and physical dependence (American Pain Society 1992). Other authors consider that the requirement for increasing doses is due to disease progression and not pharmacological tolerance (O'Neill & Fallon 1998).

Assessing and managing Ms M's pain

Until recently, Ms M completed a pain diary on a daily basis. She found it a useful method of monitoring her pain management and of communicating with her doctors. In the last week, however, she has been too exhausted to continue this activity. She is therefore pleased that both the hospice physician and Sarah are systematically assessing her pains.

The doctor, using a body chart and writing directly into the patient's notes, has thoroughly documented the patient's description of her pains along with the findings of the physical examination.

Sarah has learned from past experience that very ill patients sometimes overlook communicating a feature of their pain when faced with a formal enquiry. She has therefore decided to carry out a pain assessment while bedbathing Ms M. Carefully observing the patient's non-verbal communication, Sarah asks Ms M to talk about her pains as she helps her to wash. She also encourages Ms M to use her hands to identify where she is sore.

Ms M identifies three pains. Firstly, she rubs the upper quadrant of her abdomen and states that a feeling of extreme pressure builds up from deep inside her body. It has been getting steadily worse over the last few weeks, especially if she tries to lie on her right side. Sarah recognises this as visceral pain because of a liver enlarged with metastases and a stretched liver capsule. Ms M has been prescribed the opioid analgesic diamorphine by s.c. injection and the adjuvant drug dexamethasone (a steroid) for this pain. Before admission, Ms M was trying to take MST Continus 60 mg b.d. for this pain, however nausea and vomiting affected compliance.

The reader may be interested to read the guidance for medical staff transferring patients from oral morphine to diamorphine in Dymock & MacConnachie (1999).

Secondly, Ms M places her hands around her head and describes the tight band of headache that is frequently worse on waking in the morning. The dose of dexamethasone already prescribed for her liver pain has been increased to reduce the cerebral oedema caused by cerebral metastases and to relieve this headache. The doctor has discussed with Ms M the role of palliative radiotherapy in treating this problem, if she can bear losing her hair again.

Lastly, Ms M grimaces as the skin over her right femur is washed. When encouraged, she points with her finger to a specific area of pain in the bone that is causing discomfort. (Extensive bone metastases were a considerable problem almost 1 year previously when they were successfully managed with hemibody radiotherapy.) Ms M is upset as she recognises that this may be a recurrence of bone pain. Sarah listens to her and then gently suggests that the doctor will want to know, as there is a group of drugs known as non-steroidal anti-inflammatory drugs (NSAIDs) which can bring considerable relief.

Having left her patient refreshed and comfortable, Sarah carefully documents a detailed pain assessment in the patient's notes. She then seeks out the doctor to discuss the pain in Ms M's right femur.

Managing nausea and vomiting

Nausea and vomiting are common symptoms in palliative care and are considered by some patients to be more distressing than pain. The pathophysiology of nausea and vomiting is complex and incompletely understood. There is no WHO antiemetic ladder to guide the interdisciplinary team, but efforts are being made to identify a logical approach to these symptoms (Twycross & Back 1998). This involves:

- understanding the pathophysiology
- assessment
- explanation
- individualising the plan of care
- attention to detail.

An understanding of the pathophysiology of nausea and vomiting (well described by Hawthorn 1995) is important for the named nurse, so that she can actively participate in planning care and explaining care to patients and their families.

In order for vomiting to occur, the body needs to have detectors (to identify the need to vomit), a coordinating centre and effectors (which make the vomiting take place). The main detectors of the need to vomit are in the gastrointestinal tract; in the chemoreceptor trigger zone (CTZ), a specialised area of the brain on the floor of the fourth ventricle; in the inner/middle ear; and in the higher brain centres.

Messages from each of these detectors are transmitted to the vomiting centre in the medulla, which coordinates vomiting. Transmission from the gastrointestinal tract to the vomiting centre is via the vagus nerve. As this nerve innervates other tissues, vomiting may be stimulated by disease or trauma to other organs, e.g. the pharynx, liver or bladder. Direct stimulation of the vomiting centre by pressure, trauma or disease may also cause vomiting.

In advanced cancer, therefore, the vomiting centre can be activated in a number of ways:

- Vagal stimulation caused, for example, by gastric or bowel distension, liver capsule stretch, mediastinal disease or genitourinary problems
- Stimulation from the CTZ caused by chemical abnormalities in the blood, e.g. uraemia, hypercalcaemia, drugs or bacterial toxins
- Stimulation from the inner/middle ear due to infection, movement, ototoxic drugs or local tumour
- Stimulation from higher central nervous system centres by anxiety, fear or revulsion
- Direct stimulation from raised intracranial pressure (Regnard & Comiskey 1995).

Many neurotransmitter receptors have been identified as playing a part in these vomiting pathways (Mannix 1998) and understanding of this is constantly changing. What is important in terms of patient care is to appreciate that particular antiemetics are thought to block messages about the need to vomit at specific points along the vomiting pathways. It is this action which produces improvement or control of nausea and vomiting. Some of the commonly used antiemetics in palliative care act centrally at the vomiting centre, vestibular centre and/or the CTZ. Some act peripherally in the gastrointestinal tract and some act at both levels (Twycross 1999). Specific antiemetics may therefore be selected for specific causes of nausea and vomiting.

Cyclizine, for example, acts centrally at the vomiting centre and in the inner or middle ear. It is, therefore, useful in managing the vomiting associated with raised intracranial pressure or motion. Haloperidol acts centrally at the CTZ and is an effective antiemetic for chemical causes of nausea and vomiting, such as hypercalcaemia or drug-induced vomiting. In contrast, metoclopramide has its principal site of action peripherally in the gastrointestinal tract, where it acts by improving gastrointestinal motility. It may therefore be used to treat motility problems such as gastric stasis or 'squashed stomach syndrome'. Levomepromazine (methotrimeprazine) is a broad-spectrum antiemetic that has activity at the vomiting centre, vestibular centre and CTZ. It is useful in vomiting of uncertain or mixed origin and when other antiemetics have failed. In situations where an antiemetic is required and a degree of sedation is appropriate, levomepromazine may be prescribed. Ondansetron and granisetron, although very effective in the vomiting associated with cancer chemotherapy, have yet to find a place in the management of nausea and vomiting in palliative care (Mannix 1998).

Careful assessment of nausea and vomiting is crucial. Working with the patient, the team puts together a detailed picture of nausea and vomiting. Information about the onset, nature, pattern and severity of the nausea and vomiting is required. The doctor's comprehensive physical examination of the patient is another important source of information. Blood tests may be organised to check serum urea, calcium and electrolyte levels. In the process of care, the named nurse may acquire an understanding of the meaning of this symptom to the patient.

Management of nausea and vomiting involves identifying the cause or causes of the symptoms and discussion with the patient. Only in this way can care be truly individualised. The named nurse is central to this process. Reversible causes, such as pain, oral infection or raised intracranial pressure, should be treated. The interdisciplinary team may consider non-drug measures as part of the plan. The potential benefits of non-pharmacological approaches such as transcutaneous electrical nerve stimulation (TENS), acupuncture and guided mental imagery are acknowledged in the literature (Mannix 1998), but more research is required. An appropriate antiemetic should be selected, either while reversible causes are treated or in the longer term. Because of the progressive nature of advanced disease, regular review of symptom control must be planned.

The challenge for the interdisciplinary team in caring for Ms M is to use these principles to tailor symptom management to Ms M's problems, expectations, priorities and wishes. A detailed history and physical examination are undertaken by the palliative care consultant. Blood tests are organised to measure urea, electrolytes and serum calcium levels. Sarah, the named nurse, learns from Ms M that during the week prior to admission, Ms M felt pressured by her mother to eat at mealtimes: 'It seemed so important to her that I should eat. Like a mother coaxing a child to clear her plate. She means it for the best….'

Identifying the cause or causes is vital to managing nausea and vomiting. In advanced disease, there may be more than one cause. For Ms M some likely causes might be:

- raised intracranial pressure due to cerebral metastases
- 'squashed stomach syndrome' because of an enlarged liver
- hypercalcaemia
- anxiety about pleasing her mother by eating at mealtimes.

The blood tests are satisfactory and the serum calcium is normal. The interdisciplinary team decide that Ms M's vomiting is most likely to be associated with her cerebral metastases. Cyclizine, an antiemetic directed principally at the vomiting centre, is selected. Cyclizine 50 mg i.m. is given to Ms M shortly after admission, as the oral route is best avoided until vomiting settles. The corticosteroid dexamethasone is increased to treat the raised intracranial pressure. It is acknowledged by Ms M and the team that not feeling pressured to eat may in itself improve the symptoms. The importance of Ms M deciding when she wants to eat and what she wants to eat is documented in the care plan.

On review next day, Ms M has not felt sick or been sick since admission. When this symptom is discussed with Ms M, she makes it clear to Sarah and the doctor that she does not want to start taking an antiemetic regularly if it is not required. It is agreed with Ms M that cyclizine be prescribed on an as-required basis in the meantime. Sarah or her deputy is to discuss this with Ms M on each shift and it is to be reviewed with the doctor each day.

Attention to detail is the key in assessing Ms M's nausea and vomiting, in planning its management with her and in reviewing its effectiveness.

The assessment and management of nausea and vomiting in palliative care are addressed in much more detail in Mannix (1998) and Twycross & Back (1998). In particular, discussion of the complex issues of managing nausea and vomiting in intestinal obstruction, not addressed here, can be found in Baines (1998) and Twycross (1997).

Applying the principles of palliative care (a care plan for Ms M)

It is useful to be aware that every day in this hospice ward, the named nurse or her deputy ensures that the patient's activities of living are met and reviewed and that care is tailored to the individual patient's capability on that day. A pressure area assessment, mouth assessment, manual handling assessment and a record of the care given are documented daily for the purposes of good team communication and to facilitate audit. In addition, however, the care plan for Ms M is structured by the three principles of palliative care. This part of her care plan, for the third day of her present admission, is given below.

Pain and symptom management

- Syringe driver to be set up at 11.00 h loaded with diamorphine 40 mg and dexamethasone 8 mg, scheduled to be delivered in 24 h; see prescription sheet. Accuracy of delivery should be checked every 6 h by measuring the length of the solution remaining and checking that the indicator light is flashing. A 6-hourly check should also be carried out at the site of the 22-gauge 'butterfly' cannula inserted subcutaneously in the left upper arm.
- These drugs are being given to relieve deep pain in the right upper quadrant of the abdomen (from the liver) and a tight band of headache. Constant attention should therefore be given to assessing these pains to ensure drug efficacy.
- When able to tolerate oral drugs, the NSAID Arthrotec (diclofenac misoprostol) will be prescribed for bone pain.
- As she is unable to tolerate co-danthramer at present and is complaining of rectal discomfort, one bisacodyl and one glycerine suppository should be given today.
- Do not disturb until 10.00 h, as she is very tired.
- Ms M should decide when to eat and what to eat. A supply of her favourite foods is kept in the patients' fridge in the kitchen. Topping up of this supply will be organised by Ms M.
- The antiemetic cyclizine 50 mg is prescribed, orally or i.m. on an as-required basis. This is to be reviewed each shift.
- The patient is performing her own mouth care with toothbrush and paste.

Adjustment to loss and change

- Ms M is a highly organised person who has coped with her illness and impending death in a practical fashion, by being informed and involved. She has made careful arrangements for those who will survive her. She is very private regarding her feelings. However, she has spoken to Sarah about her profound sadness. It is important to her that she is seen to be coping bravely. Sarah will provide her with opportunities to talk should she wish to. Ms M's estranged husband and her daughters are being helped by counselling arranged by their family doctor.
- Ms M is expecting her lawyer at 14.00 h today. This is an important meeting for which she requires to conserve energy. She would very much like to be helped to sit out in a chair and to be wearing a smart outfit.

Facilitating pursuits that give pleasure

- Ms M likes to have her radio tuned to *Classic FM* and does not watch television. She enjoys picking up and sending her own e-mail. She can do this in the day hospice if taken by wheelchair.
- It is very important for Ms M to get her *Financial Times* every day. As she is very tired, encourage one of the volunteers to ask her if she would like it read to her.
- Ms M's daughters, Fiona and Katy, are in a school concert this week. She is determined to go to the school and give the girls a surprise on Thursday afternoon. Having been seen at sports day last month in a wheelchair, she is sure she will not embarrass her daughters. Joan (a very capable nursing auxiliary) has agreed to go with Ms M. They will be taken in the hospice people carrier, which will wait for them, enabling them to return at any time.

This care plan is constantly being updated as the patient's circumstances change. Good written documentation is essential for good communication within the team and with the patient and family. It is an important element in high-quality care.

Sarah's reflection

Good staff support systems must be in place to enable nurses like Sarah to cope with caring for dying patients and their families. In the hospice ward in which she works there is a good culture of support. The senior staff make it explicit that they value their staff by involving them in important decisions, providing a pleasant working environment and granting generous study leave. The nurses and other members of the interdisciplinary team are quick to recognise when difficult situations are being encountered by their colleagues. They help each other by being flexible and by being available to listen to worrying concerns.

In addition to this, a system of formal clinical supervision is in place. Sarah uses a reflective diary to prepare herself for her monthly supervision. She also uses a formal model to help her learn from experience when an incident from work is very troubling. One such incident happened during this week in relation to caring for Ms M. Sarah broke down and cried when handing over to the patient's named nurse on night duty. Naturally, her colleague was very sympathetic; recognising that Sarah was very tired she listened to her and then encouraged her to get away home to her family.

Sarah was concerned at her behaviour and decided to try to make some sense of it by analysing the incident using Gibbs' (1988) reflective cycle (Fig. 33.4). This reflection (see Box 33.3) is written in the first person.

Sarah wrote this reflection on her day off. She found it a very cathartic experience. However, she felt relieved following the exercise and decided that she must care for herself more vigilantly. She therefore immediately arranged to go swimming and out for lunch with a friend.

Sarah will take this reflection to clinical supervision next week, as the wise counsel of the very experienced home care sister who is her supervisor is a major part of her professional support system.

CASE STUDY 3 — MR Z

Mr Z is being cared for at home by his wife, daughter-in-law and the primary care team. At the age of 75, this retired gardener wants to die in his own home surrounded by his family. He is very fortunate that his GP and the district nurses in the practice have extensive experience in palliative care. They occasionally seek help from the local hospice but that has been less necessary in recent years.

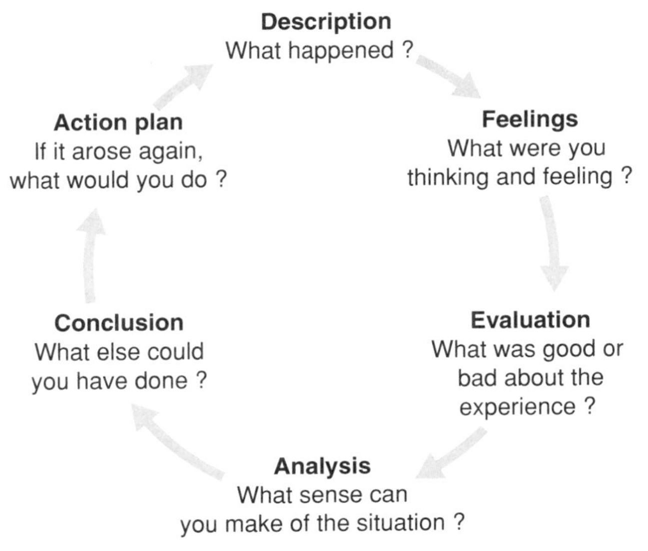

Fig. 33.4 The reflective cycle (Gibbs 1988).

Mr Z knows and is known to his doctor well, as his chronic obstructive pulmonary disease (COPD) has caused a gradual deterioration in his health for 6 years. Recently, Mary or Carol, the district nurses, have been visiting the house regularly to dress Mrs Z's varicose ulcer. They have discussed Mr Z's steady deterioration with Dr J and, along with the patient and family, have made plans for the patient's end-of-life care at home. Mary is concerned, however, that this will not be possible as Mrs Z, who is a few years older than her husband, is also in poor health.

Working closely with the social services, equipment has been installed to ensure patient comfort and carer safety. This comprises an adjustable-height bed, a hoist, a wheelchair and sliding sheets. Oxygen equipment, including a regular supply of cylinders, has been in place for a year. Fortunately, the house is all on the ground level, a walk-in shower was installed to replace the bath some years ago, and Mr Z has an upright adjustable armchair.

Although Mary knows this patient and family well, she recognises the importance of going back to the model of palliative care (Fig. 33.1) to ascertain that all aspects of care are being addressed.

Building a relationship and developing a profile

In reconsidering the relationship the primary care team have built up with the family, Mary studies the genogram that Dr J has drawn of Mr Z in the patient's notes (Fig. 33.5).

Mr and Mrs Z have two surviving sons and a daughter, having lost a third son in childhood. Their sons are both happily married and their daughter is divorced. All three have had two children of their own, so the Zs have six grandchildren. The oldest grandchild, Emma, whose wedding 3 years ago was the last social event Mr Z enjoyed, has recently had her first child Zoë.

The sons Jim and Paul and their respective wives Ann and Jenny all live in the same neighbourhood as Mr and Mrs Z. They are all patients of the same health centre and are regarded as a very close supportive family. Their sister lives in Minnesota; she has not been home since Emma's wedding.

This family is pulling together in stressful circumstances. They have open clear communication, flexible boundaries and roles, and yet they all have clearly designated responsibilities. Mr Z is always consulted on family matters. Although frail and the centre of care and attention, he is still the head of the family. Paul is beginning to take on his father's role, as he is looked on as the family representative when decisions have to be made. Jim, a quiet man, occupies himself by ensuring that heavy physical tasks are attended to. Ann is the listener and at times the peacemaker, and Jenny is the domestic wizard. Mrs Z is the coordinator and the communicator, although recently she has been very forgetful. The relationships within the family are warm and affectionate; they are tolerant of each other's idiosyncrasies.

Mary recognises these traits as being those of a well-functioning family (Bloch et al 1994, Davies et al 1994). She is aware, however, that the stress of nursing a dying relative at home has the potential to destabilise any family. Therefore, the primary care team must provide constant support, education and reassurance to enable this family to complete its task.

A district nurse is required to have a very wide knowledge base in many areas of health care. This depth of knowledge cannot always be easily remembered. Mary acknowledges this and has therefore developed her information-seeking skills, frequently using the local nursing library. In relation to this family, she recognises the need to revise her knowledge of the disease process of COPD, to enable her to anticipate the symptoms Mr Z may suffer from at the end of life.

Box 33.3 Sarah's reflective account

Description — what happened?
On Thursday evening, when handing over to the night staff, I managed to get to my last patient Ms M, when I could not continue as I started to cry. This had never happened before. I do occasionally cry at work, but it is normally done discreetly. It had been a very busy day, part of a difficult week. Two of my patients had died, one of whom I had known for many months. His family were extremely distressed at the end, especially his mother — after all he was only 35. I was glad I was on duty at the time as I had come to know them well.

After that family had gone home in the early afternoon, I had been auditing part of our admission standard. This involved accessing patients' notes from 6 months ago. The colleague who was supposed to help me with the audit was off sick. I went ahead without her because the secretary had looked out the notes, a considerable amount of work. Many of the patients whose notes had to be read have died since then; it was therefore a sad task.

Later in the evening one of my patients, Ms M, was talking about her daughters' excitement at performing in the school concert. It reminded me of when my daughters were young and I showed her a picture of my older daughter's graduation last month. Afterwards I wished I had not, as I saw the sadness come over her. I quickly changed the subject and some minutes later left the room.

I was tired when the night staff came on duty; however, that is a common experience. What was uncommon was for me to break down and cry.

Feelings — what were you thinking and feeling?
I was very embarrassed. My immediate thought was that my colleagues would think I was not coping. It was a distressing experience, especially as I cried all the way home and into the night. I felt better the next morning and was very grateful I was again on the late duty, as it gave me time to recover.

I know I am good at my job, and feel valued for my maturity and experience. I felt that I handled the young man's death well and really helped his family cope. Doing the audit was awful, I should have realised how it was affecting me and stopped. I have done a similar exercise before but always with a colleague.

I felt rotten at my lack of self-awareness in relation to Ms M. I know that her greatest source of emotional pain is in not being part of her daughters' future. Their graduation is potentially part of that. I like and admire Ms M and I do think she trusts me to do my best for her. I would be very upset to lose that trust. I also feel very guilty that I may have hurt her.

Evaluation — what was good and bad about the experience?
The good was that Mary, the night nurse I was handing over to, is a particularly valued colleague. She is wise and always helpful. On this occasion, she said, 'It is surprising we don't all break down more often, especially at the end of a harrowing day when we are exhausted like you are'. I felt supported and relieved to be going home.

The bad was my momentary lack of self-awareness, which meant that I might have reminded a patient of her emotional pain; also, that I left her room without giving her the opportunity to talk about it. Although in retrospect that was probably wise — because of my tiredness, talking at a deep emotional level with a patient would have been ill advised.

Analysis — what sense can you make of the situation?
That I have very high expectations of myself and therefore get very upset if I do not always get things right. That I need to continue to develop my self-awareness, particularly in recognising and taking appropriate action when I am stressed, such as in doing the audit unsupported. Also, that I need to be more vigilant with my communication, especially when tired.

That helping Ms M means a lot to me, I respect and admire her. I would be very upset if I lost her trust. I also feel I have a good understanding of her profound sadness, as I have had the joy of seeing my own two daughters into adulthood. Perhaps that was why I let her see the photograph.

Conclusion — what else could you have done?
I could have been open with Ms M and apologised for being insensitive. However, would that have benefited the patient or me? Ms M has acknowledged her emotional pain and indicated that she does not generally find it useful to talk about it. Perhaps I am being overly sensitive, as on the following day she asked me about my girls and asked me to bring in more pictures. She also indicated that she had asked her mother to bring in the photograph albums of her daughters so we could share them.

In relation to the audit, when I found it distressing I should have stopped and consulted the audit coordinator.

Action plan — if it arose again, what would you do?
I would indicate to the night staff that I had had a very emotional day and would be grateful if they would not be 'nice' to me as I might break down! I would give a brief report without any deep discussion and then I would go home. I would, of course, reassure them that a detailed report on each patient had been documented. In future, if an audit partner is off sick I will cancel the audit.

The anticipated symptoms of advanced COPD

Although there are many types of advanced pulmonary disease, of which Mr Z's diagnosis of COPD is one, the final problems are very similar. These are respiratory failure, cardiac failure and infection (Herbst 1996). COPD is a broad classification for a number of conditions in which there is a chronic obstruction to airflow entering and leaving the lungs. Usually these conditions are bronchitis, an excessive secretion of mucus within the airways, and emphysema, an increase in the size of the air sacs distal to the terminal bronchioles with a loss of alveolar walls and elastic recoil of the lungs.

Advanced COPD often progresses to produce hypertrophy and failure of the right ventricle (right-sided heart failure). This is the result of the lungs being deprived of oxygen, which causes hypoxaemia (decreased arterial saturation) and hypercapnia (increased carbon dioxide in the blood) resulting in ventilatory insufficiency. This in turn leads to increased resistance in the pulmonary circulation with subsequent pulmonary hypertension. It is the pulmonary hypertension that leads to the right-sided heart failure (Smeltzer & Bare 1996).

The anticipated symptoms of advanced COPD are extreme breathlessness and a productive cough. An increase in the decline of the patient's forced expiratory volume (FEV) has been shown to be a useful indicator of the terminal phase of the patient's illness (Burrows 1990). In addition, a drop in body weight due to increased metabolism from the effort of breathing and difficulty in

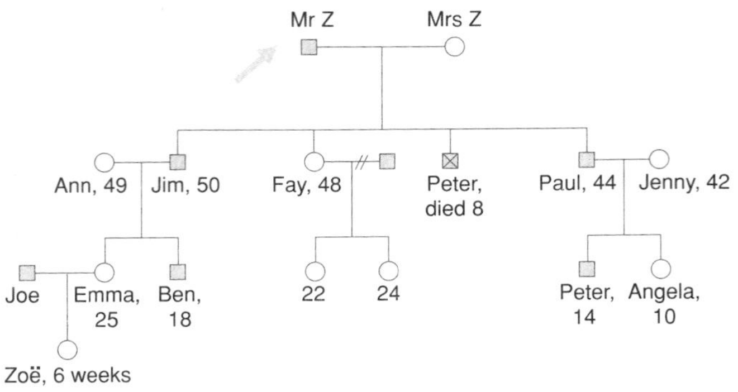

Fig. 33.5 Mr Z's genogram.

maintaining an adequate nutritional intake indicates a poor prognosis (Herbst 1996). Other symptoms that should be anticipated include generalised muscle weakness and osteoporosis due to prolonged steroid therapy, pain from the osteoporosis, and chest pain due to ischaemic heart disease. Pulmonary embolism is also a risk due to immobility.

As the right ventricle fails, it should be anticipated that venous congestion and impaired sodium excretion might cause oedema in the peripheral tissues. Venous congestion of the abdominal organs may cause anorexia and nausea, and hepatic congestion may cause abdominal pain from an enlarged liver. In addition, there may be distended neck veins, ascites or a pleural effusion. Headache, confusion and stupor may come about because of carbon dioxide retention.

The medical management of COPD includes the use of long-term oxygen. Studies done in the 1980s in both the UK and the USA (see Shee 1995) demonstrated that the use of long-term oxygen and cessation of smoking were the only actions that prolonged life in these chronically ill patients. Physiotherapy, including a gentle exercise programme and breathing exercises, is thought to improve the patient's quality of life.

Exacerbations of chest infections are usually treated with antibiotics. Inhaled drugs, such as the bronchodilators salbutamol and terbutaline, as well as the anticholinergic drugs ipratropium and oxitropium bromide, are useful in relieving breathlessness, if they are administered correctly. The nurse must educate the patient and family in how to do this; an explanation of this method of delivering drugs is given in Chapter 3.

Inhaled or oral corticosteroids may be prescribed for their anti-inflammatory effect. Oral corticosteroids may be prescribed to promote a feeling of well-being and increase the appetite (Shee 1995).

Severe breathlessness frequently responds to immediate-release oral morphine. It should be started at a low dose (O'Brien et al 1998). There is a slight risk that some patients may develop carbon dioxide retention (respiratory acidosis). Therefore, a patient with advanced COPD who is commenced on morphine should be observed for headache and disorientation. It is useful to remember that a laxative must be prescribed when opioids are commenced.

A low dose of an anxiolytic such as lorazepam may partially relieve breathlessness by helping the patient to relax. Diuretics and a reduction of oral fluids to 1500 mL a day can help to relieve oedema (O'Brien et al 1998).

Monday. In preparation for a team meeting on Tuesday at which the Z family will be discussed, Mary revised the pathophysiology of COPD in her local nursing library. She now feels prepared to seek information from Mr Z on which to plan care, i.e. based on his needs and priorities. She finds Mrs Z preoccupied making a fancy dress costume with her granddaughter, and takes the opportunity to speak to Mr Z on his own. Mary has structured her information-seeking guided by the headings suggested earlier in this chapter. In a short period, Mary skilfully gathers wide information to develop a profile and care plan. One potential problem she is aware of is constipation.

Constipation. Constipation is a very common problem for patients in the palliative phase of illness. It can cause abdominal discomfort, pain and embarrassment. It may lead on to other serious problems such as faecal impaction, overflow diarrhoea, urinary dysfunction, nausea, vomiting and even confusion (Fallon & O'Neill 1998). Careful assessment, management and documentation of this symptom may make the difference between the patient staying at home and hospital admission (Doyle 1994). The nurse's role in this is crucial.

In patients with advanced disease, many factors may work together to cause constipation. Sometimes constipation is disease-related. For example, in the patient with cancer, the site of the tumour or the presence of hypercalcaemia may be a cause. Eating very small helpings of food with little roughage, drinking considerably less than before and restricted mobility may all contribute to the development of constipation. When opioids are added to this scenario, constipation becomes a certainty. Opioids have a number of effects on the bowel. They reduce peristalsis, inhibit fluid secretion, increase sphincter tone and diminish sensitivity to rectal distension. In this way, the patient can quickly become constipated, struggling to expel small, dry, hard stools.

Anticipation and assessment of this symptom form the basis for effective management. In other words, the district nurse does not wait until the patient complains of constipation, but is constantly alert to this possibility, reviewing the situation at each visit. As part of holistic assessment of the patient, the nurse needs to take a careful and sensitive history. This will include enquiry about:

- past bowel habit
- the most recent stool (when it was passed; what it was like; any problems experienced)
- intake of diet and fluid
- compliance with laxative regimen
- other medications taken
- accessibility and acceptability of toilet arrangements.

Most important of all, the nurse needs to explore sensitively the patient's perception of the problem, i.e. his priorities and expectations. Where constipation is suspected, abdominal and digital rectal examinations are indicated. Depending on local policy, a nurse may perform a rectal digital examination if she fulfils the principles of the *Scope of Professional Practice* (UKCC 1992). A plain X-ray of the abdomen may be useful in assessing constipation.

The management of constipation is about more than prescribing and administering laxatives (Fallon & O'Neill 1998). It involves attention to the relief of pain and other symptoms, to fluid and diet and to adapting toilet facilities. Especially in the community, education of the patient and family may allow the patient to remain in control of this very personal and private aspect of his care. Most patients in palliative care will, however, require a laxative. An understanding of laxatives is vital, especially for the district nurse who may also be a nurse prescriber.

Oral and rectal laxatives may be classified as predominantly peristalsis-stimulating or stool-softening agents. Danthron and senna are predominantly stimulants. Examples of oral stool softeners are lactulose and docusate. Bulking agents are rarely used in palliative care because they are unpalatable, require to be taken with a large volume of fluid and may complete an incipient intestinal obstruction. There is evidence to suggest that the combination of a stimulant and stool softener (e.g. senna with lactulose, or co-danthrusate, or co-danthramer) gives the most favourable results, at an acceptable dose, with a minimum of unwanted side-effects (Sykes 1997). The dose should be titrated against patient response.

As the majority of patients prefer oral to rectal measures (Sykes 1997), the nurse should endeavour to keep the use of enemas and suppositories to a minimum. All rectal measures act, to a greater or lesser extent, by stimulating the anocolonic reflex. Enemas and suppositories, however, can also be classified as stimulants or softeners. For example, the stimulant bisacodyl suppository is useful for evacuating soft stool from the rectum. A microenema or phosphate enema may be effective in softening and evacuating more solid stool. Arachis oil enema or glycerine suppository may be used to soften hard stool, where this needs to occur before further treatment to evacuate the bowel will be possible. When rectal treatment is given, the doctor should review the oral laxative prescription and increase the dose if appropriate. Many teams will have devised a multidisciplinary protocol for the use of oral and rectal laxatives.

The management of constipation in palliative care patients is addressed in more detail in White (1995), Sykes (1997, 1998), Fallon & O'Neill (1998) and Maestri-Banks (1998).

Mr Z has never in his life had problems with constipation. When Dr J prescribed an opioid for Mr Z's increasing breathlessness, he simultaneously prescribed the laxative co-danthramer suspension 5 mL at night (a combined softener and stimulant). Mary emphasised to Mr Z and his wife the importance of taking this regularly (as prescribed), rather than waiting to see if constipation developed. Mr Z indicated that he could not bear the taste of the laxative, so Mary arranged for the doctor to change the prescription to co-danthramer one capsule at night. She also warned Mr Z that his urine may turn pink as result of taking co-danthramer, as this is a recognised side-effect of the laxative.

While gathering information for the profile, Mary asks Mr Z about his bowels. He says that although he has been taking the 'medicine', his bowels have not moved for 3 days. Until now, his bowels have moved daily. At first he was glad, because 'it's such an effort with this breathlessness' and he rationalised that as he was 'not really eating' it did not matter. However, people eating very little can still become constipated, because desquamation, gut secretions and bacteria mean that waste is still produced in the bowel (White 1995). Mary explains this to Mr Z. On further sensitive questioning, Mary learns that the last stool passed was small, as he 'hadn't the puff to push more out'. Mr Z is now beginning to experience rectal discomfort.

Together they discuss some options. Mary explains that a rectal examination would allow her to give appropriate treatment. Rectal examination is within the scope of Mary's professional practice and there is a local multidisciplinary protocol on the use of rectal laxatives in the community. As rectal examination is an invasive procedure, Mary carefully and thoughtfully discusses and negotiates the need for this with Mr Z. Because he is tired from his conversation with Mary, they agree that she will come and help with his care first thing tomorrow. If it is still required, she can treat his constipation then.

Tuesday morning. Before attending the multidisciplinary meeting, Mary goes to Mr Z's house. While assisting his daughter-in-law to wash Mr Z in bed, she notices that his abdomen is quite soft. There is no reason to suspect an intestinal obstruction (if there had been she would contact Dr J). Gentle rectal examination reveals that his rectum is loaded with fairly hard faeces. A microenema is given as indicated on the protocol. Mary documents this in his notes, and shortly afterwards she helps Mr Z to the toilet and his bowels move well. It is clearly an enormous effort for Mr Z to get to the toilet. He acknowledges that a commode may be useful, but 'not yet'. Mary decides to place an order for a commode to be ready if required. She also makes a note to discuss Mr Z's laxative prescription with Dr J at the meeting later. A small increase in oral laxative may be worth considering.

Before the extended multidisciplinary meeting, Mary writes the following summary into the patient's notes in preparation for updating the interdisciplinary care plan.

Main problems. Extreme breathlessness is Mr Z's main problem. It has been getting steadily worse for years. He now requires help with washing, dressing and going to the toilet. He uses continuous oxygen administered with nasal cannulae, which he describes as 'his lifeline'.

Eating is a problem, as he does not have the energy to lift the food to his mouth and his dentures are loose. He finds it embarrassing but his wife is now feeding him her good home-made soups and his favourite puddings. He is, however, still losing weight and that is upsetting as he already thinks he looks like 'a bag of bones'.

Breathlessness is also making it difficult to empty his bowels. It is very exhausting and therefore he has been pleased that recently bowel movements are infrequent. He has rationalised that this is because he is not eating. He has in fact become constipated and the reasons for this have been explained to him.

Expectations. Mr Z expects that soon he will not be able to get out of bed except when the nurses come and use the hoist. This is causing him some concern as the bedroom window looks out onto a brick wall whereas the sitting room has large windows onto the garden.

Doctor J has promised him he will die at home. That is all he is hoping for now. He is sure that everyone will rally round and he will try not to be too much bother to anyone: 'One day soon I will just stop breathing. I wouldn't say this to the family but it will be a relief, I am worn out with all of this being ill.'

Priorities. Mr Z has a beautiful garden, which he laid out over 30 years ago. It is maintained by his son Jim who lives with his wife and grown-up family in the next street. Mr Z tells Mary that watching the garden throughout the seasons is still his greatest pleasure. He impresses on her his need for the garden, although now he is just a spectator, not the worker he used to be. He jokes about how he used to rush back to it from the family holidays. Mr Z chuckles as he reminisces about this and then becomes serious again, anxious that Mary understands why he must die at home.

He insists that his only other pleasure is being with the family when they all gather round in the evening. This is why he wants to be able to continue to sit in his chair in his own sitting room.

Understanding of illness. Mr Z demonstrates a full understanding of his illness. He has shared with Mary how he expects to die. The actual process of dying does not appear to be worrying him; what he is concerned about is where the last days of his life will be spent.

Anticipated symptoms. Because of Mr Z's diagnosis of COPD and his long-term incapacity, he has many actual and potential problems. His skin is very friable due to long-term use of steroids, and recently he has lost 2 stone in weight. Nocturnal dyspnoea affects his sleep. His main anticipated physical symptoms are increasing oedema of the lower limbs, pressure sores, sore mouth, constipation, pain in the chest and/or the right upper quadrant of the abdomen, chest infection, pulmonary embolism and progressive respiratory and/or cardiac failure.

Mr Z may also become very anxious and frightened and may have a respiratory panic attack.

Applying the principles of palliative care

Pain and symptom management

- Mr Z has continuous oxygen by nasal cannulae at 2 L/min.
- He is helped by the family to take his medication regularly, continuing to take the bronchodilators salbutamol and ipratropium by nebuliser, oral prednisolone 10 mg daily and frusemide 80 mg daily for ankle oedema.
- The laxative co-danthramer suspension 5 mL has been changed to co-danthramer one capsule at night, as Mr Z hates the sickly taste. Rectal treatment (a microenema) was given today for constipation. The need to increase the oral laxative will be discussed with Dr J at the meeting. A commode has been ordered, so that it is ready when Mr Z wants it.
- For 2 weeks he has been taking oral morphine 5 mg 4-hourly to ease his severe breathlessness. This has been a useful addition to his pharmacological management, easing the dyspnoea especially at night.
- Mr Z insists that he has no pain, however he did admit that his chest felt more relaxed since commencing on the morphine and he is not breathing so rapidly.

Adjustment to loss and change

- Mr Z has suffered many losses throughout his long illness. He appears to have adjusted to his increasing incapacity in a positive fashion, although when he could no longer work in his garden he was angry with the doctors. He did not believe there was not a cure for his illness.
- Mr Z states that he is not a religious man but a man of the soil, observant of the life cycle as well as the seasons. He is sorry he will not see the snowdrops again but he recognises that his lifespan is ending. He has had a good life and has few regrets although he is worried about how his wife will cope with his death. She has suffered from depression regularly throughout her life and was in hospital on two occasions, once after they lost a son. The other occasion was when her elderly mother died.

Pursuits that give pleasure

- Mr Z has impressed on all of the health care team that being in his own home surrounded by his family looking out on his beautiful garden gives him the greatest pleasure. He cannot concentrate on television and is too weary to read.
- Obtaining a wheelchair 3 months ago from the social services has been a great success, as Mr Z can again be out in the garden, with the help of his family.

Tuesday (cont'd). Mr Z is the subject of a case conference at which the extended primary care team are present; Paul Z is also in attendance. Dr J leads the meeting, ensuring that all present have the opportunity to contribute. Two main issues arise which require discussion with the patient.

Mary tentatively raises the issue of moving Mr Z's adjustable-height bed from the master bedroom into the sitting room. This is accepted as sensible by Paul but he is not sure what his father's reaction will be to the suggestion. Mr Z has slept in the same room as his wife for over 50 years. Paul agrees to discuss the move with Mr Z.

Paul informs the team that his father has been incontinent of urine regularly in the mid-morning for a few weeks, but he will not tell the nurses. Dr J suggests that he would talk with Mr Z about this 'man to man' and suggest a urinary catheter.

Mary suggests that it is time for the care assistants Mabel and Kaye to assist the family with the patient's personal care on a daily basis.

Wednesday. Dr J visits Mr Z in the late morning, a time when patients' respiratory problems are often at their least troublesome. He finds Mr Z in his bed in the sitting room; the family made the move with their parents' consent on the Tuesday evening. After a short useful discussion, Mr Z thanks the doctor for his help and readily agrees to have a urinary catheter inserted. Dr J is very concerned that Mrs Z is looking very tired and frail. He records her blood pressure, which is slightly raised, and draws some blood for a full blood count.

Mary calls in the early evening on her way home to teach Jim and Paul catheter care, including emptying the closed system bag.

Friday. Jim Z pays an early morning call to his father, sharing a cup of tea before his mother rises. This is a routine for father and son especially in summer time. Before leaving to go to work, Jim becomes aware that his mother is not around, and on going to waken her he finds that she has died in the night. Shocked and unsure what to do, Jim is relieved when he sees Mary's car drawing up at the gate.

Mary immediately arranges for Dr J to come to the house. When he has certified Mrs Z as dead, the doctor, district nurse and Jim sit down together to make plans for sharing the bad news. Jim and Dr J will speak to the immediate family and call the undertaker. Mary will tell Mr Z.

Mary is very aware of the need for this communication to be sensitive and structures her approach following the framework advised by Buckman (1992). She starts by 'firing the warning shot': 'You know how your wife has been looking so tired and frail lately. Well, Dr J had noticed and did some tests on her. I am afraid I have a shock for you.' At this point Mary hesitates to ensure that Mr Z had heard and understood her communication. The patient nods his head. Mary continues, gently telling him in 'bite-sized pieces' what happened that morning. Mr Z reaches out towards her, holds her hands but says nothing. They sit for a few minutes. Mary then asks, 'What can I do for you?'. After a long silence, Mr Z says, 'It is for the best, she has gone before me'. After another long silence and a few tears, he asks to see Jim, and Mary leaves them together.

Monday, week 2. It has been a busy weekend for the Z family as they try to come to terms with Mrs Z's sudden death. There is a sense of unreality about what has happened as they arrange for the funeral, care for Mr Z and support each other. Many emotions and feelings are being experienced in this initial period of grief, as the impact of the event becomes a reality (Worden 1991, Murray Parkes et al 1996).

Wednesday week 2. Fay, the Z's daughter, arrived from the USA on Tuesday. She is causing some anxiety in the household, as she is very critical of her father's care, indicating that such an ill man should be in hospital. At Paul's request, Dr J and Mary have an appointment to see her in the health centre this morning. They will have to employ patience and understanding towards a family member who may be very insulting in her attitude about their care. This reaction has been described by Jenkins & Bruera (1998) as the 'daughter-from-California syndrome'. It refers to the reactions and behaviour of an absentee member of the family who returns during a serious illness.

Four characteristics are described:

- shock at the extent of the patient's deterioration
- unrealistic expectations regarding treatment options, because of lack of involvement in treatment decisions
- guilt about being absent at such an important time
- reassertion of role through conflict.

Friday, week 2. Mary has timed her visit to Mr Z to coincide with the time of his wife's funeral, knowing that it will be an emotional time, a time in which she can demonstrate her support by being there. Most of the family have gone to the crematorium. Mary enters by the garden, as she has many times before. Standing in the door, she witnesses an intimate family picture. Emma, the eldest granddaughter, is sitting by the bed breast feeding Zoë, and her husband Joe is at the other side of Mr Z's bed reading from the *Psalms*.

On approaching the bed, Mary realises that Mr Z is dying. His peripheral circulation is failing, he is covered in a drenching sweat, his skin feels cold and clammy and his extremities are blue. There is a Cheyne–Stokes pattern of breathing and he appears to be unconscious. Mary speaks to him but there is no response. She then concentrates on explaining to the young couple that their grandfather is dying. By the time the family return from the funeral, Mr Z has died — as he had wished, in his own home.

Wednesday, week 3. On the day following Mr Z's funeral, Mary and Dr J have arranged to meet the family to offer their condolences, answer any questions regarding their parents' deaths and offer bereavement support.

Bereavement. Talking with the health professionals who have become known and trusted by the family during the final illness may help the family in this early phase of grief to accept the reality of the loss. Discussing the death and answering questions can help to dispel anger and prevent needless guilt arising. It can give the family the opportunity to criticise the care provided. Relatives rarely feel able to do this when the patient is alive. It can also give the family the opportunity to thank the health professionals and therefore finish the experience of living with the terminal illness and move into the adjustment period of the bereavement (Murray Parkes et al 1996).

Case review

Part of the primary care team's support system is to hold a debriefing meeting following difficult situations. Mary and Dr J are pleased to hold such a meeting following the deaths of Mr and Mrs Z.

The interdisciplinary team members discuss the patients' illnesses and the care and management provided. The postmortem carried out on Mrs Z concluded that she had suffered a stroke. A lively discussion is held postulating the possible outcome had intervention been offered before the event. The successful conclusion to Mr Z's final illness allows the team to feel satisfied. Mary and Dr J are supported by their colleagues' praise for the organisation and hard work, which enabled Mr Z to die at home in very difficult circumstances.

Bereavement assessment is discussed. A leaflet containing information about the help available both in the health centre and from Cruse bereavement care has been left with the family. Mary is going on holiday for 2 weeks and has arranged to meet the family for a bereavement visit on her return.

CONCLUSION

Working in a hospice, one is often asked, 'What is so special about palliative care?'. This chapter has endeavoured to answer that question by demonstrating how this approach to care can be utilised in a hospital ward, in a hospice and in the home. It is never appropriate to say that 'there is nothing more that can be done'; what can be done is to implement a palliative care model, the focus being on the quality of life of the patient and his family in the time that they have left together.

ACKNOWLEDGEMENTS

The authors would like to thank Dr T. F. Benton, Medical Director, and Dorothy McArthur, Clinical Pharmacist, as well as many other members of staff at St Columba's Hospice Edinburgh.

REFERENCES

American Pain Society 1992 Principles of analgesic use in the treatment of acute pain and cancer pain, 3rd edn. American Pain Society, Skokie, IL

Barcelona Declaration on Palliative Care 1996 European Journal of Palliative Care 3(1): 15

Barraclough J 1999 Cancer and emotion. A practical guide to psychooncology, 3rd edn. Wiley, Chichester

Bloch S, Hafner J, Harari E, Szmukler G I 1994 The family in clinical psychiatry. Oxford University Press, Oxford

Brown S J 1995 An interviewing style for nursing assessment. Journal of Advanced Nursing 21: 340–343

Buckman R 1992 How to break bad news. Papermac, London

Burrows B 1990 Airways obstructive diseases: pathogenic mechanisms and natural histories of the disorders. Medical Clinics of North America 74(3): 547–559

Chapman C R, Gavrin J 1993 Suffering and its relationship to pain. Journal of Palliative Care 9(2): 5–13

Cherny R N, Coyle N, Foley K 1994 Suffering in the advanced cancer patient: a definition and taxonomy. Journal of Palliative Care 10(2): 657–670

Clark D, Seymour J 1999 Reflections on palliative care. Open University Press, Buckingham

Davies B, Reimer J C, Martens N 1994 Family functioning and its implications for palliative care. Journal of Palliative Care 10(1): 29–36

Degner L F, Gow C M, Thompson L A 1991 Critical nursing behaviours in care for the dying. Cancer Nursing 14(5): 246–253

Dixon J M, Sainsbury J R C 1993 Handbook of diseases of the breast. Churchill Livingstone, Edinburgh

Doyle D 1994 Caring for a dying relative – a guide for families. Oxford University Press, Oxford

Doyle D, Hanks G, MacDonald N (eds) 1998 Oxford textbook of palliative medicine, 2nd edn. Oxford University Press, Oxford
Fallon M, O'Neill B 1998 Constipation and diarrhoea. In: Fallon M, O'Neill B (eds) ABC of palliative care. BMJ Books, London
Faulk S, Fallon M 1998 Emergencies. In: Fallon M, O'Neill B (eds) ABC of palliative care. BMJ Books, London, ch 10
Faulkner A 1998 Effective interaction with patients, 2nd edn. Churchill Livingstone, Edinburgh
Faulkner A, Maguire P 1994 Talking to patients with cancer. Oxford Medical Publications, Oxford
Faull C 1998 The history and principles of palliative care In: Faull C, Carter Y, Woof R (eds) Handbook of palliative care. Blackwell Science, Oxford, ch 1
Faull C, Barton R 1998 Managing complications of cancer In: Faull C, Carter Y, Woof R (eds) Handbook of palliative care. Blackwell Science, Oxford, ch 12
Gibbs G 1988 Learning by doing: a guide to teaching and learning methods. Further Education Unit, Oxford
Gregory D, English J C B 1994 The myth of control: suffering in palliative care. Journal of Palliative Care 10(2): 18–22
Hawthorn J 1995 Understanding and management of nausea and vomiting. Blackwell Science, Oxford
Heaven C 1995 Communication skills in palliative care. The Cancer Research Campaign, Psychological Medicine Group, Christie Hospital, Manchester
Herbst L H 1996 Prognosis in advanced pulmonary disease. Journal of Palliative Care 12(2): 54–56
Hoskin P, Makin W 1998 Oncology for palliative medicine. Oxford Medical Publications, Oxford University Press, Oxford
Jenkins C, Bruera E 1998 Conflict between families and staff. In: Bruera E, Portenoy R K (eds) Topics in palliative care. Oxford University Press, New York, vol 2
Kagan C, Evans J 1995 Professional interpersonal skills for nurses. Chapman and Hall, London
Lang S S, Patt R B 1994 You don't have to suffer. Oxford University Press, New York
McCaffery M, Beebe A 1994 Assessment. In: Latham J (ed) Pain. Clinical manual for nursing practice. Mosby, London, ch 2
McGoldrick M, Gerson R 1985 Genograms in family assessment. W W Norton, New York
Mannix K A 1998 Gastrointestinal symptoms In: Doyle D, Hanks G W C, MacDonald N (eds) Oxford textbook of palliative medicine, 2nd edn. Oxford University Press, Oxford
Murray Parkes C, Relf M, Couldrick A 1996 Counselling in terminal care and bereavement. British Psychological Society, Leicester
Neuenschwander H, Bruera E 1998 Asthenia. In: Doyle D, Hanks G, MacDonald N (eds) Oxford textbook of palliative medicine. Oxford University Press, Oxford, ch 9.4
O'Brien T, Welsh J, Dunn F G 1998 Non-malignant conditions. In: Fallon M, O'Neill B (eds) ABC of palliative care. BMJ Books, London
O'Neill B, Fallon M 1998 Principles of palliative care pain control. In: Fallon M, O'Neill B (eds) ABC of palliative care. BMJ Books, London
Penson J, Fisher R 1995 Palliative care for people with cancer, 2nd edn. Edward Arnold, London
Regnard C, Comiskey M 1995 Nausea and vomiting. In: Regnard C, Hockley J (eds) Flow diagrams in advanced cancer and other diseases. Edward Arnold, London
Rowland J H 1990 Intrapersonal resources in coping. In: Holland J, Rowland J H (eds) Handbook of psychooncology. Oxford University Press, New York
Roy D 1998 Editorial. The relief of pain and suffering: ethical principles and imperatives. Journal of Palliative Care 14(2): 3–5
Shee C D 1995 Palliation in chronic respiratory disease. Palliative Medicine 9: 3–12
Silverman J, Kurtz S, Draper J 1998 Skills for communicating with patients. Ratcliffe Medical Press, Abingdon
Sims R, Moss V A 1995 Palliative care for people with AIDS, 2nd edn. Edward Arnold, London
Smeltzer S C, Bare B G 1996 Brunner and Suddarth's textbook of medical – surgical nursing, 9th edn. Lippincott, Philadelphia
Sykes N 1997 Constipation in palliative care. Palliative Care Today V(IV): 55–56
Sykes J, Johnson R, Hanks G W 1998 Difficult pain problems. In: Fallon M, O'Neill B (eds) ABC of palliative care. BMJ Books, London, ch 2
Twycross R 1997 Symptom management in advanced cancer, 2nd edn. Radcliffe Medical Press, Abingdon
Twycross R 1999 Guidelines for the management of nausea and vomiting. Palliative Care Today VII(IV): 32–34
Twycross R, Back I 1998 Nausea and vomiting in advanced cancer. European Journal of Palliative Care 5(2): 39–45
UKCC 1992 The scope of professional practice. UKCC, London
Vallerand A H 1997 Measurement issues in the comprehensive assessment of cancer pain. Seminars in Oncology Nursing 13(1): 16–24
Watt-Watson J H, Donovan M I 1992 Pain management – nursing perspective. Mosby Year Book, St Louis
White T 1995 Dealing with constipation. Nursing Times 91(14): 57–60
Worden J W 1991 Grief counselling and grief therapy, 2nd edn. Routledge, London
World Health Organization 1986 Cancer pain relief. WHO, Geneva
World Health Organization 1990 Cancer pain relief – palliative care. Technical Report Series 804. WHO, Geneva

FURTHER READING

Baines M J 1998 Nausea, vomiting and intestinal obstruction. In: Fallon M, O'Neill B (eds) ABC of palliative care. BMJ Books, London
Dymock B, MacConnachie A 1999 Relief of pain and related symptoms. The role of drug therapy. Scottish Partnership Agency for Palliative and Cancer Care, Edinburgh
Fallon M, O'Neill B (eds) 1998 ABC of palliative care. BMJ Books, London
Maestri-Banks A 1998 An overview of constipation: causes and treatments. International Journal of Palliative Nursing 4(6): 271–275
Mannix K A 1998 Gastrointestinal symptoms In: Doyle D, Hanks G W C, MacDonald N (eds) Oxford textbook of palliative medicine, 2nd edn. Oxford University Press, Oxford
Randall F, Downie R S 1996 Palliative care ethics, a good companion. Oxford Medical Publications, Oxford University Press, Oxford
Sykes N 1997 Constipation in palliative care. Palliative Care Today V(IV): 55–56
Sykes N P 1998 Constipation and diarrhoea. In: Doyle D, Hanks G W C, MacDonald N (eds) Oxford textbook of palliative medicine, 2nd edn. Oxford University Press, Oxford
Twycross R 1997 Symptom management in advanced cancer, 2nd edn. Radcliffe Medical Press, Abingdon
Twycross R, Back I 1998 Nausea and vomiting in advanced cancer. European Journal of Palliative Care 5(2): 39–45
White T 1995 Dealing with constipation. Nursing Times 91(14): 57–60
Working Party on Clinical Guidelines in Palliative Care 1997 Changing gear – guidelines for managing the last days of life in adults. The National Council for Hospice and Specialist Palliative Care, London

THE PATIENT IN NEED OF REHABILITATION

34

Margaret Harris

INTRODUCTION

Rehabilitation is an active process in which disabled people work together with professional staff, relatives, and members of the wider community to achieve their optimum physical psychological, social and vocational well-being (O'Kelly 1997).

This chapter devotes itself to a patient group for whom full recovery is not an option because, whether or not it has been possible to reverse the disease process, there are consequences which do not simply go away. For some, the development of these consequences is insidious; for many the onset will be sudden and traumatic; for all, there is a huge need for psychological adjustment.

As long ago as 1966, Henderson suggested a causal link between the assistance given by the nurse and the regaining of independence by the individual. The difference between 'I assist you because you cannot do it yourself' and 'I assist you in order that you may be able to do it yourself' lies in teaching and motivating in order to increase will and knowledge. These skills can be developed in rehabilitation nursing because time is not the enemy that it is in acute care. Often the value of nursing interventions cannot be evaluated because the period of patient–nurse contact is too brief. In rehabilitation nursing, there is an opportunity for the nurse to function in a different and rewarding way.

The standard ingredients of scientific nursing practice are still required (see 'Meeting self-care needs', p. 990), but distinctive priorities derive from the interdisciplinary approach to the tasks (see 'The process of rehabilitation', p. 986) and a different value system where wholeness as a human being involves looking forward to an adapted lifestyle rather than back to previous levels of health and achievement.

The nurse may require increased self-knowledge and perhaps personal growth before she can cope with disability. There may be a need for a different theoretical model within which to function. Certainly, the meaning of professionalism comes under scrutiny.

This chapter gives general, rather than prescriptive guidelines, so the final activities are important in guiding the students to apply the general principles to day-to-day practice.

What is rehabilitation?

Rehabilitation is about rebuilding lives: 'Acute care deals with a threat to life. Rehabilitation deals with a threat to living' (Pires 1989).

The notion that one should work to get better, rather than wait for recovery to occur, is quite modern. During the mid-20th century, rehabilitation became a speciality in its own right, concerning itself with problems that cross many diagnostic boundaries, continue after discharge and require teamwork to achieve success.

Rehabilitation takes place in three stages:

- preventing complications
- promoting independence
- maintaining independence.

Preventing complications. Earlier chapters have emphasised how nurses should intervene early in the disease or injury process to prevent avoidable complications. This is the first stage or principle of rehabilitation.

Promoting independence. The second stage is the active promotion and restoration of independence. It is a post-acute phase when patients need help to set personal goals and decide what should be done, by whom, where and at what pace. In this phase, patients regain control of their own lives and exchange their sick role for a health-seeking role.

In his seminal text, Parsons (1951) described the sick role as exempting the patient from:

- 'normal' social activities and responsibilities
- responsibility for her own condition.

The sick role is not compatible with rehabilitation, and the beginnings of successful rehabilitation occur when the sick role is abandoned in favour of self-determination. There is an unwritten contract between a professional who abandons paternalistic attitudes and a patient who abandons the sick role.

The focus of interest is no longer on disease but on an active person with health-seeking behaviour. According to the Helsingborg Declaration (WHO 1995), management of all aspects of disability should be planned in close collaboration with patients and their families and be sensitive to their needs.

Maintaining independence. Once an acceptable level of functioning has been established and social integration achieved, the third stage of rehabilitation is entered: management of problems that might cause the person to become dependent again.

Beyond this are the goals of rehabilitation as a social movement. It must include the education of all the professions involved in medical and supportive care in order to focus endeavours on human values rather than mere technical success.

According to Sim et al (1998), until the social model of disability is more widely accepted, disabled people will continue to find difficulty in gaining a successful response to needs which they have defined.

Who needs rehabilitation?

Rehabilitation skills are inherent in sound, scientific nursing practice and will have been described for specific conditions elsewhere in this book. The purpose of this chapter is to focus on the needs of a particular client group whose disease or disorder causes *continuing* functional disability, requiring professional involvement.

World Health Organization models and terminology

When the World Health Organization (1980) provided a medical model of illness-related phenomena, it was adequate for the many diseases that are self-limiting and amenable to prevention or cure. The model encompasses a search for cause, i.e. aetiology, the identification of pathology and the identification of signs and symptoms, i.e. manifestation. It then became obvious that in order to accommodate chronic, progressive or irreversible disorders, a different conceptual framework was required, and an international classification of impairments, disabilities and handicaps was added. Thus:

- impairment relates to deficiencies at the organic level
- disability relates to the functional consequences of organic impairment
- handicap relates to the social consequences of deficient ability.

Handicap is not inevitable and the state of being handicapped is relative to other people; for example, in 1997 a blind girl was enabled to take part in the Miss Italy beauty contest by her boyfriend, who directed her steps on stage through a radio transmitter hidden in her ear.

To summarise (Duckworth 1982):

- impairment — parts that do not work
- disability — activities that cannot be carried out
- handicap — roles that cannot be performed.

Whereas this classification remains a useful tool within the limitation of this chapter, it is acknowledged that it conserves notions of normality which are unacceptable to the British Council of Disabled People (Tyler 1992).

The main disorders resulting in a need for rehabilitation are listed in Box 34.1. This list is not exhaustive and is continually growing. Advances in medical technology not only prevent death but also provide new challenges regarding quality of life.

Research awareness

Research provides the foundation for good practice in any field, but the speed of change in rehabilitation poses a particular challenge. The obligation is not necessarily to do research but to be influenced by the relevant work of nurses, pharmacologists, psychologists, bioengineers and others. The current trend is towards

Box 34.1 Some examples of disorders causing functional disability

Neurological
- Paraplegia
- Tetraplegia
- Hemiplegia
- Head injury

Musculoskeletal
- Arthritis
- Osteoporosis

Cardiovascular
- Cerebrovascular accident (stroke)
- Intermittent claudication

Endocrine — metabolic
- Diabetes mellitus (complications of)

Sensory
- Visual impairment
- Deafness

Consequences of mutilating surgery
- Mastectomy
- Stoma
- Amputation

Consequences of progressive diseases (in remission)
- Multiple sclerosis
- Parkinson's disease
- Malignancy
- HIV/AIDS

high technology, which has improved quality of life with, for example, phrenic nerve pacers as aids to breathing and sacral stimulators as aids to continence. Other developments, such as electronically assisted walking, may raise false hopes and actually hinder realistic adaptation.

Research awareness should also provide knowledge of the extent of disablement problems. Chamberlain (1989) found that (statistics from OPCS 1988):

- some 6 million adults in the UK (1 in 7) have at least one disability
- current provision is documented as being chaotic, fragmented and piecemeal, with most disabled people receiving little practical help
- disabled adults with rheumatological diagnoses constitute the largest group with disabilities.

Finally, the role of the nurse in rehabilitation has come under close scrutiny in recent years and, particularly in specialist units, research is indicating that it has moved from the unglamorous 'Jack of all trades' image described by Booth & Waters (1995) to one which is innovative and rewarding (O'Connor 1996).

THE PSYCHOLOGY OF DISABILITY

Few would disagree with the statement that rehabilitation begins in the mind. Anything that assists in widening perceptions as to the enormous impact of emotional and psychological factors on the well-being of people with disabilities has to be welcomed.

It follows that an understanding of the psychology of disability provides the basis for the sustained therapeutic relationship which is crucial in the rehabilitation process. Understanding:

- promotes empathy
- predicts success
- analyses the effects on family members
- facilitates adjustment.

Stigma

In his review of research on handicap, Richardson (1976) remarked that physical disability is a 'powerful and pervasive' disadvantage in initial social encounters. Goffman (1968), in his seminal text, found that people view the person with a stigma as 'not quite human' and therefore accept treatment of the disabled that they would not tolerate for the able-bodied.

Hahn (1983) suggested that disabilities arouse anxiety by reminding people of departures from standards of beauty and perceived competence. It is assumed that beauty is accompanied by traits of sensitivity, kindness and amiability. The able-bodied may be embarrassed, made uncomfortable or even repulsed by the awkward or unusual. Rubin & Peplau (1975) point out that an encounter with a disabled person violates belief in a just world; for able-bodied people to maintain their belief in justice, people with disabilities are viewed as deserving the disability.

Aveyard (1997) asserted that, with very few exceptions, even the media stigmatise disabled people and, as a result, contribute to the discrimination of disabled people within society.

In a culture which prizes competence and autonomy, people with disabilities also evoke strong anxieties about loss, vulnerability and weakness. For most people, the sick role is a temporary experience of incompetence and dependency. It is too short for them to become familiar with the methods used by people with permanent disabilities to accomplish tasks of daily living and work. They may consequently treat disabled people as though they have no ordinary functions and no capacity for making decisions.

Nurses should be particularly sensitive to this when, for whatever reason, people with disabilities need to be cared for in an acute hospital setting. Biley (1994) found that nurses failed to value and utilise the patients' understanding of their own disability. This was described by Lonsdale (1990) as a typical trait of the arrogant professional in response to those who were simply expressing their own preferences about how their condition should be handled.

Grief

The impact of sudden disability is similar to that of bereavement. Kubler-Ross (1974) noted that, for some, facing death is easier than facing life with a serious disability. Grief is a normal reaction to the loss of abilities and should not be mistaken for a depressive episode. Symptoms of grief include:

- preoccupation with the lost object (a limb, a function, a status)
- somatic distress
- inappropriate behaviour
- hostility
- denial.

Ray & West (1987) describe five phases of coping behaviour:

- denial
- suppression
- resignation
- positive thinking
- independent assertiveness.

There are two dangers in describing these phases in order. First, it encourages the assumption that each will pass and give way to the next, leading to eventual acceptance. This is not always the case. Second, it may imply that each phase is discrete and, once passed, is over and done with. Again, this is not so. The phases are likely to interact in a dynamic and sometimes erratic flow.

Twelve years after her riding accident and leading a fully independent life, Spooner (1995) still doubts if psychological rehabilitation can ever be complete.

Stress

Engel (1964) identified three broad classes of psychologically stressful events:

- loss or threat of loss of psychic objects, people, possessions, ideals or anything that is of great importance for that individual
- real or threatened injury to the body
- frustration of drives.

On all three counts, the newly disabled are stressed (see Ch. 17).

Control

The concept of control, or perceived control, is particularly relevant to disability. Seligman (1975) described how feelings of helplessness produce depression, inertia and inability to learn. De Charms (1968) described people as 'originators' or 'pawns'. Those who consider themselves to be mere pawns in the hands of fate will see little point in making much effort, but those who feel they can control the outcome of what they initiate are more likely to succeed.

This is confirmed anecdotally by Jones (1997) who praises his mother for always letting him take control of his life — following his skiing accident, which resulted in tetraplegia, her prime aim was to empower him to take control again.

THE PROCESS OF REHABILITATION

Interdisciplinary teams

Rehabilitation is an interdisciplinary endeavour. The challenge to the organisation is to create a client-centred team structure which involves family and other carers, and concerns itself with quality of life. This is very different from each profession providing therapy, however skilled, in isolated units. The patient must be seen as the pivot or hub of the structure, while the nurse coordinates management of the patient's day. Teamwork is facilitated by interdisciplinary meetings during which rehabilitation goals are formulated and adapted. Team meetings are commonly chaired by the medical consultant, who also functions as team leader; however, it often happens that informal leadership occurs, and in a well-integrated team, leadership will be shared according to the task and the organic growth of relationships with and around the patient.

Some patients may find a multiplicity of therapists confusing, and require a stable relationship with one person who may be known as a coach, mentor or key worker. The person chosen will have leadership functions, but always as a contributor to the strategic plan.

Rehabilitation units

Rehabilitation units or hospitals tend to specialise in one type or group of impairments so that resources are concentrated, research is facilitated and professionals become very expert. 'Demonstration centres' and 'Professorial units' are centres of excellence from which all can benefit. Many take on a formal educational role, e.g. the Disabled Living Centre, Cardiff. All acknowledge that a key feature of the structure is adequate information resources. A great deal of help is available but people can only benefit if they know about it.

Statutory and voluntary bodies

For practically every form of disability, there is a statutory or voluntary body, e.g. the Partially Sighted Society, the Music Advisory Service, the Volunteer Stroke Scheme, the Disabled Drivers' Association, Different Strokes (for young stroke victims), The Horder Centre for Arthritics and The Winged Fellowship Trust. A full list is obtainable from the Disabled Living Centres Council (see 'Useful addresses', p. 998) and the Disability Rights Handbook (1997).

Many special training centres and colleges exist. Employment retraining centres provided one of the earliest forms of rehabilitation. There are now 'placement, assessment and counselling teams' (PACTs) and these have considerable powers to help people realise personal ambitions.

Sport and leisure

Practically everyone has heard of the Paralympics, but the British Sport Association for the Disabled tries to ensure that no-one is excluded from leisure pursuits due to disability. There is a charity called 'Holiday Care Service', and information is also provided by agencies such as Threshold Travel, The National Trust and British Airways (Care in the Air).

Q **34.1** Are the Paralympics a good or a bad idea? Debate this in your group.

Artificial aids

There are over 40 disablement services centres in the UK. Specialist nurses, with counselling skills, should ensure that aids are matched to needs. There are hundreds of items, from basic equipment in the kitchen to complex environmental control systems.

The manufacture of aids and appliances represents big business and mobility is a high priority. In the 1980s, invalid cars were phased out in favour of adaptations to conventional cars, and now manufacturers of 500 different cars are linked to the Motability scheme (see 'Useful addresses', p. 998).

Living accommodation

Living accommodation ranges from ordinary housing, through purpose-built individual properties, to residential hostels with full-time staff. Key features are described in Disabled Access to New Housing Regulations (HMSO 1995). During recent years, many political decisions have been based on the notion that all institutionalisation is bad and all rehabilitation to the community is good, yet many instances have been reported where a person's (admittedly impoverished) life in a hospital has been exchanged for greater loneliness and isolation at home. Good rehabilitation is only possible if society is willing to undertake its responsibilities, and if human, and therefore financial, resources are moved from acute medical care, with its emphasis on speedy cure, to services provided for those with lasting disability. Sim et al (1998) warn of the danger of people becoming institutionalised in their own homes if there is a lack of commitment to extend the definitions of need to the social environment.

Outcome of the rehabilitative process

The intended outcome is an optimal or an acceptable level of function. This will be highly individual but has been described by Kallio (1982) as one of the following:

- regaining premorbid function within the usual environment
- adapting function to enable the person to be effective in the usual environment
- modifying the environment to facilitate function, despite restricted abilities.

The aim is to reduce the negative impact on people's lives of physical, emotional and cognitive impairments (O'Kelly 1997).

Measurement of the success of the rehabilitation process is problematic. A crude, though useful, measure is lack of need for readmission to hospital (see Fig. 34.1).

Quality of life is not a luxury. The Black report (HMSO 1980) and other studies demonstrate that quality of life and health/illness status are linked. To strive to achieve the objective of improved quality of life can be justified not only on humanitarian grounds but also on economic grounds, as failure in this area will lead to medical complications, ill health and possibly readmission to hospital. This is not only disappointing, or even unacceptable, it is expensive.

ROLES

Patient–professional roles

The patient and significant others have been identified as being pivotal in the rehabilitation concept, but it must be acknowledged that the patient/professional interface is also of critical importance and quite complex.

The skills required by the patient will change and become redundant as the sick role is abandoned. The nurse, other professionals and the family must share the goals but tolerate movement of the goalposts. Professional input must be flexible, enabling change to occur.

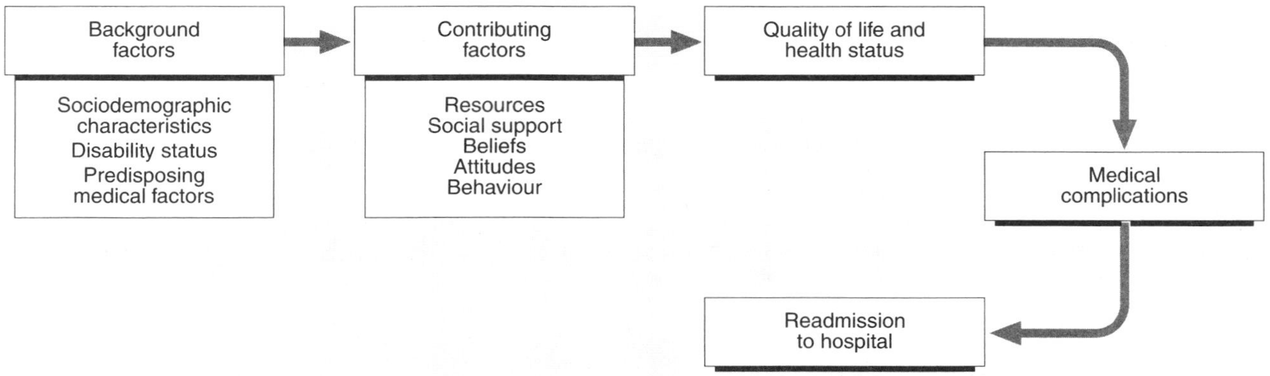

Fig. 34.1 A model of rehabilitation (adapted from Lawes 1984).

Major problems are as follows:

- the patient may have difficulty in setting goals and in coping with professionals who are reluctant, and indeed may refuse, to do this for her
- professionals may have difficulty in coping not only with an interdisciplinary team approach, but also with a situation where it is the patient's decision which is pivotal and not that of the professional.

The patient

Recently disabled people usually have little experience of disability, or of the options and opportunities available to them. Decision-making may be complicated by depression, hidden family dynamics and ambivalent feelings. Patients may try to avoid therapy sessions, for example, so staff may encourage, bargain with or even coerce patients into compliance. In the patient role, people are reassured and comforted by professional paternalism and professionals gain confidence from having their judgements respected.

The professional

In rehabilitation, professionals must learn to modify their judgements not only to take into account patients who may behave in an unpredictable manner at times, but in order to achieve a consensus with other team members. Just as the patients do, so the professionals bring their own values, moods and states of health to every situation. They must learn to separate their own needs from those of the patient and to respect the patient's wishes (Jennett 1987).

The role of the nurse (see Research Abstract 34.1)

Since its inception, nursing has relied on socio-scientific knowledge as an adjunct to practice, and for knowledge to be useful, it must be applied. Care should mean active therapeutic management, which requires:

- knowledge of the therapeutic use of self
- skill in ensuring that the patient's self-care needs are met
- attitudes that adapt and progress with the patient's increasing independence.

The Orem model

Orem (1995) described a self-care model of nursing that can be applied in rehabilitation. The beliefs on which this model is based are that:

- all individuals have self-care needs
- it is the right of individuals to meet these needs themselves, wherever and whenever possible
- self-care is given by oneself for oneself
- self-care is grounded in the belief that self-maintenance and self-regulation are valued as first-line strategies for effective human functioning in society (see Research Abstract 34.2).

It is not suggested that Orem (1995) provides the only model for rehabilitation nursing, but it does have the virtue of emphasising the need for progressive attitudes and behaviour on the part of nurses. Identifying the moment when facilitative intervention should give way to facilitative non-intervention is a high-level skill.

Research Abstract 34.1
Nurses' attitudes towards stroke patients in general medical wards

Gibbons' (1991) paper summarises a research study enquiring into the attitudes of qualified nursing staff and nursing auxiliaries towards stroke patients in general medical wards. The survey was undertaken on eight mixed-sex wards in a large teaching hospital. All wards were used for clinical nursing experience for nurses in training. Each of the wards, despite having a particular interest in one or more medical specialities, regularly admitted patients following stroke. All nurses were therefore familiar and in regular contact with this particular client group.

Results showed that nurses were largely ambivalent in their attitudes towards stroke rehabilitation. Nurses who had more positive attitudes about stroke patients considered that they had a role in stroke rehabilitation and valued the nursing contribution. Nurses with less positive attitudes saw stroke patients as uncooperative and demanding. All nurses and auxiliaries believed that the more they learnt about stroke rehabilitation, the more motivated they became to look after such patients.

The findings suggest the need for specific education regarding the role of the nurse as a rehabilitator and for further research to explore this role.

Gibbon B 1991 A reassessment of nurses' attitudes towards stroke patients in general medical wards. Journal of Advanced Nursing 16(11): 1336–1342.

Research Abstract 34.2

Patients who have had bowel surgery that results in the formation of a colostomy require to re-learn self-care skills in relation to elimination.

In this study, the nursing care provided for 12 such patients during changes of their colostomy appliance was observed and analysed within the framework of Orem's model of nursing. From the literature, nine elements of physical care which the patients had to accomplish in order to manage their appliance were identified: preparation of the equipment; preparation of the patient; removal of the old appliance; skin care; skin protection; selection of the new appliance; preparation of the new appliance; its application; and disposal of the old appliance.

The study, albeit on a small scale, demonstrated an uncoordinated approach to the process of preparing the patients for self-care and insufficient opportunities for these patients to practise all the steps in the physical management of their stoma. As a result, all were discharged without having demonstrated the necessary new self-care skills.

Given that containment rather than control of elimination is a key issue in the rehabilitation of such patients, the study concludes that, as the period of patients' postoperative hospitalisation becomes ever shorter, a planned approach to the development of self-care is required. Where continuation of self-care preparation is necessary after discharge, there should be an organised exchange of information between hospital and community staff.

Ewing G 1989 The nursing preparation of stoma patients for self-care. Journal of Advanced Nursing 14(5): 411–420.

ACTIVITIES FORMING THE NURSING ROLE

It is not intended in this chapter to describe in detail all the procedures appropriate to the physical needs of rehabilitation patients, because this would only repeat information that can be obtained more comprehensively from other chapters. The common need linking all these patients and their families is for personal growth, and what follows is an examination of eight activities which form part of the nursing role, given here in order to highlight nurses' potential to contribute to this process.

These activities are:

- control of the environment
- holistic assessment
- communication
- meeting self-care needs
- mobility
- social, emotional and economic self-sufficiency
- teaching
- preparing the patient for an unsympathetic environment.

Control of the environment

The nurse's role in the hospital setting is to care for 'whole' people over a 24-h period and to be responsible for the environment in which the activities of living take place. This is undoubtedly the most powerful tool he has at his disposal, because the psychological change and personal growth required to cope with disability will only occur in a proper therapeutic milieu. Florence Nightingale's supreme aim was to provide an environment in which the body could heal itself. She may not have been familiar with the term 'model of nursing', but it is possible to produce a simple diagram (Fig. 34.2) of the approach she took.

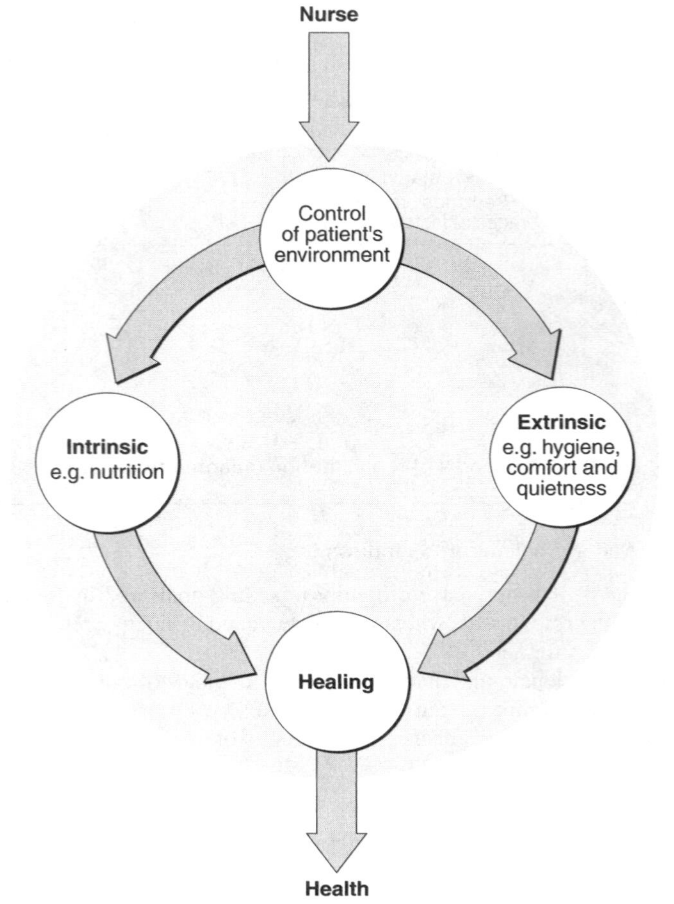

Fig. 34.2 A model of Florence Nightingale's approach to nursing (devised by Harris (1982)).

> **34.2** Identify ways in which the nurse could foster a therapeutic environment in the disabled person's home and community.

The nurse of the new millennium has many more tools at her disposal than did Florence Nightingale in the Victorian era, but in spite of that, the creation of an appropriate environment for the promotion of the rehabilitative process remains challenging. The distinctive atmosphere of a rehabilitation unit should be felt immediately on walking through the door. This will consist of:

- an ethos of warmth, acceptance, understanding, optimism, openness and cooperation
- posters, wallcharts, books and people, reinforcing the notion that information is not only available and free, but that it is worth having, because knowledge is power
- an open-door policy to family and friends of the patient
- involvement of community staff in establishing personal relationships and sharing expertise
- explanations of treatment and rationale so that learning opportunities are created out of practically every activity

- role modelling by those patients who are succeeding
- staff with a very flexible approach to role and status
- adaptations of physical layout with aids and appliances as appropriate.

Holistic assessment

Holistic assessment should consider the person in hospital, at home and in the work situation. Assessment must adopt a counselling approach in order to be person- and family-centred and individualised. Every nurse should attempt to be a good listener and to be sensitive to a patient's emotional state, but counselling is a high-level skill, the development of which requires intensive education and training. It should therefore be borne in mind that rehabilitation nursing will be practised at several different levels of skill by those who:

- are simply involved in such care
- have chosen to specialise in such care
- have become clinical nurse specialists appointed to senior posts comprising advanced-level practice in consultancy, liaison, innovation, research and education; these nurses are to be found in the increasing numbers of rehabilitation units, and are available to cascade their expertise (O'Connor 1996).

Nursing assessment, planning and intervention must be carried out in the light of the total rehabilitation assessment, however this is achieved.

The nursing plan

A plan that is coherent and integrated will only emerge from a functional profile of the patient to which the entire team, including the patient herself, have contributed. There are many frameworks for this, all basically similar, as all must take account of the common major life activities. Halstead & Grabois (1985) use the acronym 'PULSES' for this holistic assessment:

P Physical condition, including visceral, cardiovascular, gastrointestinal, genitourological, endocrinological and neurological disorders
U Upper-limb function upon which self-care activities depend, e.g. grooming, bathing, perineal care, drinking, feeding, dressing, applying braces and/or prostheses
L Lower-limb function upon which mobility depends, e.g. transferring, walking or negotiating stairs
S Sensory components relating to communication, i.e. speech, hearing and vision
E Elimination functions of the bladder and bowel
S Supportive components:
—intellectual ability
—emotional adaptability
—support from family
—financial capability.

In each of these areas, present abilities and limitations must be set against:

- previous level of functioning
- desired level of functioning
- predicted or realistic level of functioning.

Functional status and goals may be rated as:

1. dependent
2. requiring assistance
3. requiring supervision
4. independent.

Nurses are familiar with care planning that is compatible with the therapeutic plan described by the doctor. Planning to meet the goals of the total rehabilitation strategy is much more challenging. It may be necessary for the therapists to adapt their day so that nurse and patient can work with, for example, an occupational therapist for dressing, a physiotherapist for walking, and a speech therapist for feeding and communication.

Last, it must be stressed that the PULSES framework does not present functional abilities in order of importance. The supportive components are as vital as the physical ones, so emotional status, mood and motivation must be monitored and taken into account.

People must be allowed to grieve and should be given time and help to work through this process. Moments of optimism must be exploited. Motivation must be reinforced by positive feedback.

Communication

Brown (1954) wrote: 'They thought because I couldn't speak I had nothing to say.' No relationship, much less a therapeutic one, can commence without communication, yet health professionals do not have good reputations as communicators. In a study by Fallowfield et al (1998), it was found that bad communications were at the heart of the majority of complaints to the NHS ombudsman. A research grant was used to institute a training programme for nearly 200 specialists who admitted that experience and seniority had not improved their communication skills. Three months later, 95% demonstrated a positive shift in communication confidence.

Many nursing research studies, e.g. the seminal studies by Boore (1978) and Hayward (1975), have shown that patients want more information, that information is therapeutic in terms of reducing stress and pain, and that patients perceive themselves to have received less information than they have actually been given.

Patients also complain about information that is economical with the truth and gives false reassurance. Following a riding accident, Spooner (1995) was told she would regain 95% of her former ability. She assumed this would include walking. In fact, it did not. Also, when nerve root pain developed 3 weeks after the accident, she was told it was due to returning sensations. It was 2 years before someone admitted that this pain would be ongoing in nature, and explained that she would always need pain relief medication (see also Case History 34.1).

When speaking, writing instructions or interpreting those that already exist, it is important to recognise the patient's frame of reference. The nurse should restate, rephrase and reinforce information that needs clarification. Non-verbal communication is very powerful. Bad news cannot be merely accepted. It needs to be explored. The nurse should remember the evidence that coping behaviour begins with denial and suppression (Ray & West 1987).

It is an oversimplification to say that speech therapists simply help people regain the ability to talk. As nurses, and all involved,

Case History 34.1 Mr D

During his time in the ICU, unable to breathe unaided, bilaterally paralysed and unconscious most of the time, D was aware of someone patiently talking and explaining what was going on. The information included descriptions of the nature of a stroke and the efforts of the brain to make sense of its dilemma. He later discovered he had been listening to the voice of a night nurse, and, several years on, he is still grateful for that nurse's sensitive understanding of his need for lucid auditory input.

Research Abstract 34.3

Nieuwenhuis (1989) established group activities in a ward for long-stay patients with neurological deficits. She demonstrated that their communicative potential was greater than it had previously appeared and intragroup awareness was greatly raised, with people making an effort to compensate for each other's disabilities.

Nieuwenhuis R 1989 Breaking the speech barrier. Nursing Times. 85(15): 34–36

cooperate best with a patient's therapy if they are fully informed about what is taking place, multidisciplinary group activities in the ward should be organised so as to use time efficiently by allowing staff and patients to learn together. Such sessions can also help to build up confidence in social skills (see Research Abstract 34.3).

Patient choice

Good communication is also vital to patient choice and control and is essential to informed consent. A classic study by Maguire et al (1978) showed that up to one-third of women with breast cancer expressed dissatisfaction with the amount of information they received before surgery. Since that early work, Frank & Maguire (1988), in further research, have advocated frank and honest discussion of the treatment options, so that the trauma of mastectomy may be lessened. Not surprisingly, patient choice will also improve patient compliance with prescribed behaviours and use of aids and appliances. Ballard (1997) compared two alternating pressure mattresses (APMs) by taking patient comfort and quality of sleep into consideration. Whereas APMs have proved popular with medical staff in the prevention of pressure sores, anecdotal reports have described them as causing discomfort and nausea. The findings highlight the importance of taking patients' opinions into consideration when selecting pressure-relieving interventions, and can be applied to any other therapy which produces unpleasant side-effects.

Team liaison

Liaison work is sometimes delegated to the ward sister but may be the responsibility of specially appointed nurses whose task is to facilitate the transition from acute to rehabilitation units, then from hospital to community care. Early contact can be made with the community staff who will take over the post-discharge period (see Case History 34.2). They can be encouraged to come into the hospital, meet their patient, get to know the family and learn caring skills specific to the patient's needs. Patients who need long periods of rehabilitation may become institutionalised and anxious about discharge. Previous encounters with community staff will build up the patient's and the carer's confidence in them.

34.3 Review Case History 34.2 in the context of Orem's model for nursing and liaison between hospital and home. Try to do this with your classroom teacher and also with your mentor on community placement.

Access to information

Access to all types of information has been facilitated by the setting up of information services centres such as Dial UK, Derbyshire; Help for Health, Southampton; Action Aid, Newport; Health Search, Scotland; and all disabled living centres. A full list of these is given in the Disability Rights Handbook (1997). Nurses can make people aware of these resources and can also use them to raise their own levels of knowledge.

Case History 34.2 Mr A

A, an 18-year-old youth suffering from paraplegia, was totally unprepared emotionally for discharge when he was physically ready, but he was determined to go home.

He was given over to the care of a skilled, motherly community nurse, but he did not want mothering. It was only after he and his girlfriend had been unable to cope with his rehabilitation programme and he had nine pressure sores that he consented to receive care.

Case History 34.3 Mr C

C, a long-distance truck driver, fell asleep at the wheel of his cab and was involved in an accident, as a result of which he became tetraplegic and was unable to breathe independently. Despite very positive attitudes by community nurses, this prevented his discharge from hospital for over 12 months. His eventual return home was made possible because his loving wife learned new but essential skills in order to care for him. She undertook much of his care, including suction of his tracheostomy tube, during the 12 h of daytime support provided by the social services. A qualified night nurse covered the other 12 h. The present timetable gives her one afternoon off per week and 2 weeks' respite care every 6 months.

Meeting self-care needs

Breathing

Some patients who will be discharged home will require respiratory support for life. This is an area where allocation of resources and socioeconomic factors must be particularly carefully considered (see Case History 34.3).

For further information see Dettenmeier (1990).

Eating and drinking

Food may assume a greater-than-usual significance in the life of a disabled person, simply because other options are fewer. Maintaining nutritional status involves activities which may be impaired at any point in relation to the process of purchasing food, preparing meals, and eating and drinking:

- choosing food and drink
- responding to hunger
- balancing the diet
- gaining access to shops
- preparing food and drink
- conveying food and fluid into the mouth
- chewing and swallowing
- controlling weight.

Q **34.4** How many modifications would be needed to help a young tetraplegic man enjoy eating and drinking?

Pleasure and freedom in eating and drinking are areas of personal choice and control, but choice means having information, e.g. that alcohol consumption increases the risk of epileptic attacks. Physically disabled people who gain weight, especially those in wheelchairs, increase the load on their pressure areas and this may further reduce their mobility. Mutilating surgery, which can lead to comfort eating, may add obesity to an already unacceptable body image. Stroke victims who do not master their eating impairments may choose to become socially isolated or may experience rejection in social encounters.

For further information, see Gilbert (1986) and Bender & Brookes (1987).

Eliminating (see Case Histories 34.4 and 34.5)

Control of urinary and faecal elimination is not only a critical component of quality of life, but is often also vital to life itself. A regimen for the spinally injured, devised by Sir Ludwig Guttman in the 1940s, meant that 80% of such patients lived, whereas previously 80% had died within 2–3 years. The key differences in this regimen lay in the management of bladder, bowels and pressure areas in order to preserve the integrity of the renal tract, the gastrointestinal tract and the skin. Previously, a causal relationship had been demonstrated between urinary tract infections, renal failure and death. The nursing challenge was that if the urine could be kept sterile, life expectancy would be normal. This still holds good today (see Ch. 24).

Continence advisers refer to:

- education to maintain continence
- training to regain continence
- management to contain incontinence.

Case History 34.4 Mr P

P, a 19-year-old man with paraplegia, adapted to his wheelchair more successfully than to his leg bag, which he felt was the ultimate indignity. Learning self-catheterisation techniques made a vast difference to his self-image. Despite the discipline of 4-hourly catheterisation, he now feels 'free'. He attaches a leg bag only for long-distance travel or trips to the pub, where he drinks beer in pints rather than halves.

Case History 34.5 Mrs J

Mrs J, a 50-year-old woman, had suffered from diverticulosis for many years. Her social life was handicapped by dietary restrictions, pain and embarrassment. A sudden, life-threatening episode of peritonitis resulted in gut resection and the fashioning of a colostomy. Within a few months she had learned self-management and was particularly grateful for well-designed and individually prescribed stoma bags. She has no ambition to have the colostomy reversed.

The role of the hospital nurse in preparing the patient to live at home with a stoma is highlighted in Ewing (1989).

Q **34.5** Consider Case History 34.4. Does P fit neatly into any of the above categories? Does it surprise you that the leg bag was more of a problem than the wheelchair?

For further information, see Roe (1992).

Personal cleansing and dressing

Together with management of bladder and bowel, self-care in personal cleansing is the area where independence is likely to be most desired by the physically disabled (see Case History 34.6). For effective rehabilitation, the combined expertise of the nurse and the occupational therapist is often needed, e.g. in dressing techniques for stroke patients.

Hygiene and grooming are basic to self-respect and involve activities that are usually carried out in private. For those who cannot regain self-care abilities, a lack of attention to detail in areas formerly controlled by the patient greatly reduces self-esteem.

Q **34.6** Discuss the statement, 'There is no such thing as a menial task in nursing' (Castledine 1997).

Whereas intimate care-giving has probably always been the pivot of nursing activities, it is only since the publication of Henderson's (1966) seminal work that its value has been expressed in the literature. In 1963, Lydia Hall, Director of the Loeb Centre, New York, abandoned the notion of a hierarchy of procedures and instituted total patient care given by qualified nurses.

This philosophy has been adopted in the UK with varying degrees of commitment ever since, and became a crucial element in the *Patient's Charter* (Department of Health 1991) followed by the 'Named Nurse Initiative' (Hancock 1992). Whatever the perceived difficulties in terms of resources, it is particularly appropriate in rehabilitation nursing because it increases the potential for the nurse to create and sustain a therapeutic relationship (see Fig. 34.3).

Mobility (see also Ch. 35)

Mobility can be considered at two levels:

- any change of position that aids physiological function
- movement from one place to another, which is important for quality of life and also has benefits in terms of continence, shopping and travel.

Case History 34.6 Mrs B

Mrs B, a 53-year-old woman suffering from paraplegia, expressed a desire to be totally self-caring, i.e. free of the community nursing service. Despite having a husband and three supportive children, she was determined not to impose a physical burden on anyone.

Her two principal problems were incontinence due to urine bypassing her indwelling catheter and an inability to wash the lower half of her body. Although she appreciated the weekly bath given by community nurses, she wished to be able to shower herself. It required the efforts of the multidisciplinary team to provide the necessary aids and adaptations, but it was the nurse's initial help with catheter management and access to a shower that allowed Mrs B to meet her own goals for quality of life.

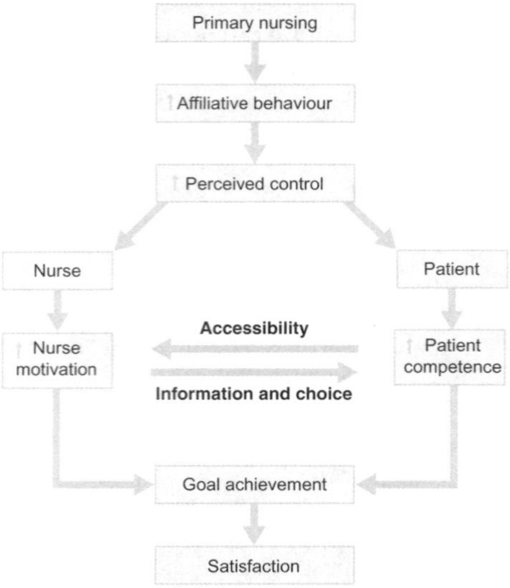

Fig. 34.3 A model of primary nursing (Harris 1982).

Changing position

Prolonged inactivity results in serious deterioration in functional capacities, known as 'immobilisation syndrome', in which practically all organs and systems of the body suffer the consequences of immobilisation. This can be avoided if early rehabilitation nursing provides:

- environmental stimuli
- regular passive movements of all limbs
- passive tilting
- regular turning and change of position
- breathing exercises
- adequate nutrition and hydration
- skin care.

Movement

It is important for nurses to learn from and cooperate with other professionals in the training of patients and carers, as, when there is little or no coherence between the aims and objectives set by various health care professionals, the negative effects on the patient are considerable. Furthermore, unsuitable transfers can cause actual pain and injury. All health care professionals must comply with the *Manual Handling Regulations* (HMSO 1993). Risk assessments are required and the use of lifting/handling aids is mandatory. These are intended to protect both patient and nurse, but the goals of maximum independence and prevention of complications remain paramount.

For further information, see Jamieson et al (1997).

Available techniques and aids include:

- lifting in a safe manner
- pivot transfers
- hoists, sliding and turning equipment
- walking with a stick
  —crutches
  —quadrupeds
  —frames
- getting about in a wheelchair
  —self-propelled
  —powered
- shopmobility schemes
- motability allowances
- adaptations that facilitate access and manoeuvre.

34.7 Assess the ease of access to public buildings in your community.

Social, emotional and economic self-sufficiency

The nurse has a role in the sharing of information obtained from formal assessments and in the ongoing monitoring of interpersonal relationships, emotional status and future plans.

Family relationships

The onset of a disability is not only a crisis for the individual — it is also likely to instigate a family crisis. It inevitably changes the nature of the marital relationship between partners. The spouse may feel the strain of assuming more family obligations. The range of sexual activities may be limited and fertility threatened (see Case History 34.7). There are a number of barriers that impede the delivery of effective sexual rehabilitation to disabled people. Two of the most common are negative attitudes about sexuality and lack of information about normal sexual function in the presence of a specific impairment. Nurses often find themselves in the role of sexual counsellor because of their intimate care-giving functions, although referral to a family therapist is ideal and doctors can advise on the functional limitations.

Misunderstanding by the patient and her family about the severity, prognosis and recovery process of the impairments can lead to high anxiety and impede progress. Consistency and openness in discussions foster realistic adjustment (see Case History 34.8).

Case History 34.7 — Mr and Mrs P

P and his wife were involved in a road traffic accident which resulted in a closed head injury for her, and tetraplegia for him. They had been hoping to start a family so, as soon as was feasible after his injury, P's healthy sperm were collected and frozen. When completely recovered, his wife submitted herself to fertility tests and was found to have low hormone levels. Two years after hormone therapy and several attempts at artificial insemination with her husband's sperm, she gave birth to a healthy baby girl.

Case History 34.8 — Mr M

M had always been the organiser in his marriage, not only planning budgets and holidays, but actually doing household repairs and car maintenance. Following a head injury, all that stopped. Neither he nor his wife talked about their feelings of insecurity and a lot of unresolved anger was waiting to become manifest in both partners. The crisis was absurd. A simple plumbing problem caused the wife to move out and return to her parents. Both eventually realised the need to adjust the balance in the relationship and, with patience and professional help, were eventually successful.

The stages of the family's emotional reaction to disability have been graphically described by one wife of a head-injured man (Powell 1994):

1. Shock, panic, denial — 'Please God, let him live'.
2. Relief, elation, denial — 'He's going to be fine'.
3. Hope — 'He's still making progress, but it's slow'.
4. Realisation — 'He's not going to get back to his old self'. (Anger, depression, mourning.)
5. Acceptance, recognition — 'Our lives are now very different'.

Employment

Economic self-sufficiency is usually dependent on employment, and many people obtain their self-image and primary sources of satisfaction from their work. The implications of disability for employment will depend on the previous employment and the types of impairment.

Social, emotional and economic self-sufficiency are fluctuating states that require empathy at all times; emotional support must be given as and when the need arises, rather than being parcelled out in hourly sessions. Not all units have psychologists or family therapists on site and visits by the placement, assessment and counselling team (PACT) will only be occasional. The nurse offers a more constant presence, enabling a therapeutic relationship to develop. Liaison with, and referral to, the appropriate experts can then occur as needed.

34.8 A young man of 17 and another man of 41 have both suffered traumatic amputations, the former as a result of foolhardy behaviour and the latter due to an industrial accident. The youth may not have achieved independence from his parents, trained for a job or completed self-development. His self-image and intended lifestyle may be shattered. The 41-year-old man may have a wife and family to support him, an offer of his job back or something lighter if preferred, and perhaps industrial compensation.

Consider whether one man's needs are greater than the other's. Is that too simplistic a viewpoint? Think about the differences in their rehabilitation needs.

Teaching

Teaching is ongoing and for all; professional knowledge must not be jealously guarded. Formal, informal, individual and group approaches can be used to educate the patient, family, friends and community carers. Preventable complications may be caused by episodes of depression, indiscretion or neglect but should not be allowed to occur because of ignorance.

Family

Whereas patient teaching will be viewed as a part of the rehabilitation process, the involvement of family and others must be timed and handled with sensitivity, since it represents an acknowledgement that the patient needs the help of others to manage or improve, and that the disability is not going to disappear overnight.

Planning a programme

The structure of educational programmes should be as carefully organised as any in a formal educational setting. Individual educational needs should be assessed (using a counselling approach). Plans should take account of available:

- time
- place
- resources.

Implementation methods should be varied to include:

- demonstrations
- videos
- discussions
- experiential roles.

Evaluation should require feedback which demonstrates:

- understanding
- acceptance
- competence.

All nurses should be involved in the health-promotion aspects of rehabilitation. A study by Rutherford (1990) demonstrates the benefit of exercise in preventing osteoporosis (see Ch. 7, p. 236). Pre-retirement courses commonly take on the concepts of 'fitness, fun and finance', all relevant to preventing disability in old age. Young (1994) found that community nurses can provide relevant and useful information on the prevention and management of leg ulcers in the home setting (see Ch. 23, p. 755).

For further information, see Pike & Forster (1995).

34.9 During your community placement, assess how many patients have leg ulcers. Select one of these patients, decide on a suitable model of nursing, and with the help of the district nurse and the patient plan a programme that includes short-term, intermediate and long-term goals.

Preparing the patient for an unsympathetic environment

The physical environment

Shearer (1981) says, 'What I feel the able-bodied person does not realise is the tremendous self discipline the disabled life entails… travel is limited, shopping difficult, entertainment has to be planned like a campaign. Just getting there in a wheelchair is a major hurdle'.

The social environment

When one reads disabled people's accounts, one quickly discovers that it is more often the attitudes of others, and the frustrations of discrimination, rather than the intrinsic effects of impairment, which produce trauma (Marks 1997) (see Box 34.2).

For the individual, discharge from hospital can be very threatening rather than being a joyous experience. Visits home, gradually increasing in length from a few hours to a few days, help to prepare the patient by building up confidence and highlighting any problems, although, where home adaptations are necessary, it is rare for these to be completed before the discharge date.

Given that the environment is often unsympathetic, or even hostile, it may be that more psychological training strategies should be built into rehabilitation programmes. These might include:

- assertiveness training
- relaxation techniques
- cognitive therapy
- coping skills.

Box 34.2 Friend or foe? (Reproduced with kind permission from New Internationalist (1992; 233: 14–15)

Ask exactly what you can do if you want to help a disabled person — and listen to the reply. We know our needs best. Never help us without asking first whether your help is wanted. And don't expect us to be eternally grateful to you for the help you do offer...

Acknowledge our differences. For many disabled people, our difference is an important part of our identity. Don't assume that our one wish in life is to be 'normal' or imagine that it is 'progressive' or 'liberal' to ignore our differences.

Respect our privacy and our need for independence. Don't assume that because we are disabled you can ask us more personal questions than you would a non-disabled person.

Think about the way society creates barriers for us. Take account of the social and economic context in which we experience our medical condition. But don't reduce us to our medical conditions. Why should it matter to you what our condition is called? Challenge patronising attitudes towards us. We want your empathy not your pity. Putting us on a pedestal or telling us how 'wonderful' and 'heroic' we are does not help. This attitude often conceals the judgement that having an impairment is tolerable — which is very undermining for us.

Recognise our existence. A gaze can express recognition and warmth. Talk to us directly. Neither stare at us — nor immediately look away either. And never talk about us as if we weren't there.

Realise that we are sexual beings, with the same wishes, needs and desire for fulfilling relationships as non-disabled people. Don't assume that we will never have children. And if a disabled person has a non-disabled lover, don't jump to the conclusion that the latter is either a saint or has an ulterior motive.

Appreciate the contribution that we make to society in the fields of work, politics and culture. We engage in these activities for the same reasons as you do — but we may have some different insights to offer. Don't assume that we are passive — or that our activities are a form of 'therapy' to take our mind off our disability. Most disabled people are financially hard up and so we may have a greater need to earn a living than you.

Fig. 34.4 Professions commonly involved in assessment of patients (adapted from Williams et al 1994).

34.10 Discuss with your fellow students the pivotal importance of the loving support of family and friends in the rehabilitation of a severely disabled patient.

QUALITY OF LIFE IN THE COMMUNITY

Comprehensive assessment of the patient in the home situation is an integral feature of discharge and community care (see Fig. 34.4). Specific goals must be identified and agreed by the professions involved so that collaborative care planning can ensue. Even so, this should only be regarded as an interim assessment. Rehabilitation is rarely completed in hospital and adjustment to disability may be a painful, prolonged and difficult process. The self-image of a mastectomy patient, the sex life of a crash victim and the employment status of a person following a stroke can only be monitored over a period of time.

For some patients, e.g. those with severe head injury or paraplegia (see Ch. 9), follow-up is particularly important as they can improve very slowly over a long period of time. They may 'plateau' for a period, but may then progress again later. The possibility of further improvement should never be forgotten.

Following discharge, disability may improve, deteriorate or fluctuate slightly. Mayon et al (1993) found that mood disorder and horrific intrusive memories, sometimes accompanied by phobic travel anxieties, were still affecting people 1 year after road traffic accidents. The goals of care are:

- to prevent deterioration
- further improvement of functional status
- possible discharge from professional care.

In a longitudinal study charting the social integration of 129 stroke survivors, Belanger et al (1988) found that, whereas 73% of patients were able to return home and over 60% were autonomous in self-care and mobility, many had deteriorated after 6 months. About 25% had problems with psychological well-being and complained that these had not been addressed during their rehabilitation programme. In contrast to this, even where functional abilities showed no improvement, social outcomes were demonstrably improved by the use of volunteer stroke schemes (Geddes & Chamberlain 1994).

The model of rehabilitation in Figure 34.1 (see p. 987) can be applied here.

The background factors are independent variables or facts of life that have to be accepted, e.g.:

- geographical location
- type of family and job
- previous personality
- marital status
- age
- sex
- nature and extent of the functional impairments.

The contributory factors are those which it should be possible to alter.

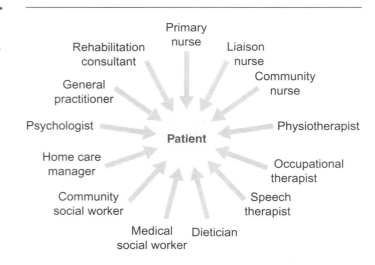

Resources include:
- professional and lay carers
- aids
- adaptations
- environmental design.

Social support:
- friends
- clubs
- mobility
- accessibility.

Beliefs, attitudes and behaviour are modified by:
- education
- training
- the mass media
- legislation
- cultural developments.

Professional and political implications arise here. Many of the problems relate to human relationships, economics and bureaucracy, areas over which people perceive themselves to have little control. Nurses have a significant role in promoting the autonomy of disabled people by increasing their understanding of their rights and helping them to self-advocate effectively.

A holistic nursing assessment might group these concerns into the following categories:

- personal care
- physical activity
- role fulfilment
- mental health status
- medical status
- economic productivity.

Personal care

The delivery of personal care may be in the hands of many, e.g. family, friends, volunteers, neighbours, other professionals and the patient herself, i.e. self-care. Standards must be maintained but needs will not be constant; for example, the normal care of pressure areas may be quite inadequate during a chest infection, and self-care in personal hygiene may be quite impossible outside the patient's specially adapted home. Respite care may make life at home, rather than in an institution, possible. The care-givers' needs should always be considered; care-givers, who are a prime resource, should be cherished (see Case History 34.3, p. 990)

Physical activity

Physical activity is made possible, to a varying extent, by a sympathetic environment. Home adaptations may not be completed before discharge and situations that are acceptable for a short period become major causes of emotional trauma if they continue for a long time. The local environment usually also presents some insurmountable barriers and it is not surprising that some people feel discriminated against. Some problems can be solved in personal ways, e.g. a local landlord may provide ramped access to his public house, but in general terms adaptations that promote the interest of some disabled people may handicap others. Curb cuts, for example, may help wheelchair users, but cause difficulties for blind people. Access to public buildings is a statutory right, but the ideal of a perfect environment is illusory (Marks 1997).

34.11 Analyse possible reasons for the delays mentioned above. How might the nurse adopt an advocacy role for the person?

Role fulfilment (see Fig. 34.5)

Role fulfilment depends on the breaking down of barriers between the able-bodied and the disabled; not just physical barriers but ignorance, prejudice and fear. People usually have many different roles, which enrich their lives. Being reduced to a single role and labelled 'disabled' diminishes the quality of life. Disability may mean that while some roles are actually lost, new ones can be gained. Beethoven is one example of this. His prestige as a solo pianist was at its zenith when he became deaf but he subsequently poured more energy into composing. People may hold exaggerated notions of the degree to which disability limits them. The newly disabled must also decide whether or not to identify with other disabled people; for example, those who go deaf as adults may choose to suffer extreme isolation and curtailment of their social lives rather than learn sign language. Ideally, people should benefit from mutual support groups while enjoying integrated activities in other ways.

Mental health status

All newly disabled people have to cope with stigma and find it is the task of the stigmatised to put others at their ease. Many need help in the early days if they are to be prevented from segregating themselves and becoming hermits. The truly fortunate receive sufficient empathic encouragement from their families, but the community nurse may be the only professional in a position to assess whether the disabled person needs extra help or even psychotherapy. Early detection of depression is very desirable since it can cause, and be intensified by, handicap in a way that is vicious and circular (Marks 1997).

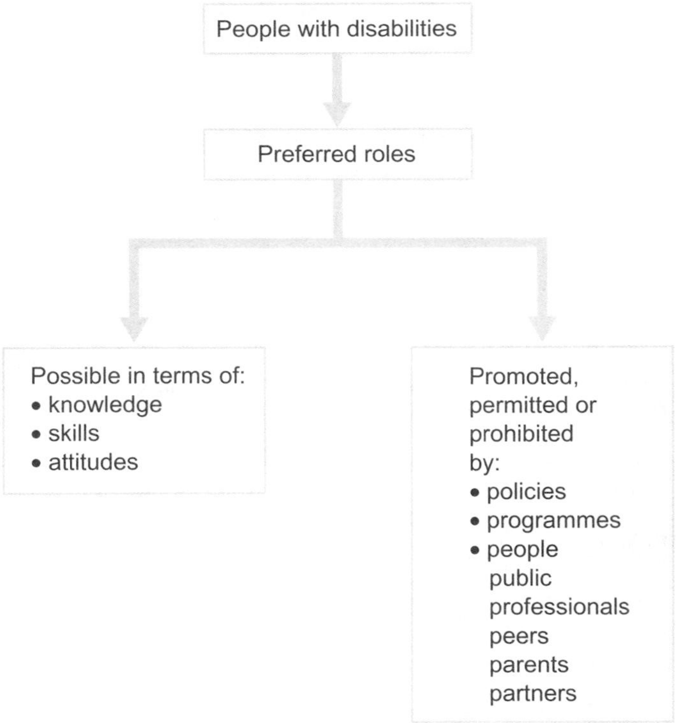

Fig. 34.5 Factors affecting role fulfilment.

As part of their educative role, nurses must involve themselves actively in attempting to change social attitudes. However, problems are highly individual and need to be handled as and when they occur.

34.12 Consider Case History 34.6. Discuss in your group whether Mrs B is exercising her rights of choice and personal control, or whether she is being grossly unfair to her caring husband and manifesting a negative mental health status that should be investigated and treated?

Medical status

Traditionally, the medical status of the disabled person, once discharged into the community, is assessed by self-referral to a general practitioner when a problem already exists or by checking into an outpatient department at intervals increasing in length and ranging from 3 months to 1 year. Neither system allows for the early detection of potential problems.

Departments of rehabilitation have been given the task of breaking down barriers between hospital and primary health care teams, so 'demonstration' centres have been created and resettlement or liaison nurses appointed. A demonstration centre should function not only as a centre of excellence in rehabilitation but also as a resource to the community, providing information, education, equipment and problem-solving of many kinds. Changes in the medical status of patients can be reported and discussed on a day-to-day basis and, ideally, prompt interventions may avoid the need for readmission to hospital.

Economic productivity

Occupational therapy units may prepare the disabled for community life by teaching driving, computer and other technical skills, but the post-discharge picture for many has been quite bleak.

It is hoped that the Disability Discrimination Act 1996 is now being applied with vigour and will improve this picture.

This Act requires employers to:

- operate anti-discriminatory measures in recruitment
- provide better conditions of employment for the disabled
- fund adaptations to the physical environment
- take all reasonable steps to maintain the employment of the newly disabled worker.

In 1981, the Independent Living Movement described the ability to live productively, not only in terms of gainful employment, but also in terms of other contributions made to community and family life. There are many examples of people quoted in this chapter who have done just that on an impressive scale.

CONCLUSION

This chapter has shown that success in rehabilitation depends on many factors: social, political, economic, environmental and personal. Attitudes are crucial. The able-bodied have been described as friends or foes, as allies of disabled people or as patronising oppressors. In their own words (see Box 34.2, p. 994), disabled people are presenting us, individually and collectively, with many challenges. Where do you stand: friend or foe?

34.13 (a) Investigate rehabilitation provision in your locality. Visit a disabled living centre or an employment retraining centre.
(b) Study the role of several specialist rehabilitation nurses, e.g.:
- mastectomy nurse
- stoma nurse
- spinal injury liaison nurse
- neurorehabilitation nurse.

(c) Study disability experientially, e.g.:
- wear special lenses that simulate a visual impairment
- go shopping in a wheelchair
- eat, using only one hand — your left, if you are right-handed; your right, if you are left-handed
- try washing and dressing using only one hand.

(d) Critically evaluate the patient-versus-client role.
(e) Work with other professionals in the multidisciplinary team.
(f) Attend a multidisciplinary team meeting.
(g) Attend a care conference.
(h) Secure a relationship with a family which contains a disabled member.
(i) Lobby your MP or councillor about any handicapping situations that become apparent.
(j) Read a biography of a severely disabled person, e.g.:
- Hurley G (1983) Lucky break? Milestone Publications, Horndean
- Hahn D (1984) The story of Margaret Price. Barker, London
- Chevigny H (1962) My eyes have a cold nose. Yale University Press, New Haven
- Jones T (1997) Walking on air. Heinemann.

REFERENCES

Aveyard B 1997 Stigma and the media. Assignment 3(2): 23–28
Ballard K 1997 Pressure-relief mattresses and patient comfort. Professional Nurse 13(1): 27–32
Belanger L, Boldue M, Noel M 1988 Relative importance of after-effects, environment and socio-economic factors on the social integration of stroke victims. International Journal of Rehabilitation Research II(3): 251–260
Biley A M 1994 A handicap of negative attitudes and lack of choice: caring for patients with disabilities. Professional Nurse 9(12): 786–787
Boore J R P 1978 Prescription for recovery. RCN, London
Booth J, Waters K R 1995 The multi-faceted role of the nurse in the day hospital. Journal of Advanced Nursing 22(4): 700–706
Brown C 1954 My left foot. The childhood story of Christy Brown. Pan, London
Castledine G 1997 Castledine column. British Journal of Nursing 6(7): 407
Chamberlain M A 1989 Editorial: what is rehabilitation? British Journal of Hospital Medicine 41(4): 311
De Charms R 1968 Personal causation. Academic Press, New York
Department of Health 1991 The patients' charter. HMSO, London

Disability Discrimination Act 1996 HMSO, London
Disability Rights Handbook 1997 Disability Rights Alliance, London
Duckworth D 1982 The classification and measurement of disablement. HMSO, London
Engel G 1964 Grief and grieving. In: Schwartz L, Schwartz S (eds) The psychodynamics of patient care. Prentice-Hall, New York
Ewing G 1989 The nursing preparation of stoma patients for self-care. Journal of Advanced Nursing 14(5): 411–420
Fallowfield L, Lipkin M, Hall A 1998 Teaching senior oncologists communication skills: results from phase I longitudinal programme in UK. Journal of Clinical Oncology 16(5): 1961–1968
Frank A O, Maguire G P 1988 Disabling diseases. Heinemann, Oxford
Geddes J M L, Chamberlain M A 1994 Improving social outcome after stroke: an evaluation of the volunteer stroke scheme. Clinical Rehabilitation 8: 116–126
Gibbon B 1991 A reassessment of nurses' attitudes towards stroke patients in general medical wards. Journal of Advanced Nursing 16(11): 1336–1342
Goffman E 1968 Stigma. Penguin, London
Hahn H 1983 Paternalism and public policy. Society (March–April): 36–46
Halstead L S, Grabois M (eds) 1985 Medical rehabilitation. Raven Press, New York
Hancock C 1992 Named nurse initiative. Nursing Standard 6(17): 16–18
Harris M 1982 Unpublished MSc thesis. University of Wales, Cardiff
Hayward J C 1975 Information: a prescription against pain. Royal College of Nursing, London
Henderson V 1966 Basic principles of nursing care. International Council of Nurses, Geneva
HMSO 1980 (Chairman: Black D) Inequalities in health. HMSO, London
HMSO 1993 Manual Handling Regulations. HMSO, London
HMSO 1995 Disabled Access to Housing Regulations. HMSO, London
Jennett B 1987 Decisions to limit treatment. Lancet 8562(2): 787–789
Jones T 1997 Walking on air. Heinemann, Oxford
Kallio V 1982 Medical and social problems of the disabled. Euro Reports, WHO, Copenhagen
Kubler-Ross E 1974 Questions and answers on death and dying. Macmillan, New York
Lawes C 1984 Pressure sore readmission for spinal injured people. Care 4(2): 4–8
Lonsdale S 1990 Women and disability. Macmillan, London
Maguire G P, Lee E G, Bevington D J, Küchemann C S, Crabtree R J, Cornell C E 1978 Psychiatric problems in the first year after mastectomy. British Medical Journal 1: 963–965
Marks D 1997 Models of disability. Disability and Rehabilitation 19(3): 85–91
Mayon R, Bryant B, Duthie R 1993 Psychological consequences of road traffic accidents. British Medical Journal 307(6905): 647
Nieuwenhuis R 1989 Breaking the speech barrier. Nursing Times 85(15): 34–36
O'Connor S 1996 Stroke units: centres of innovation. British Journal of Nursing 5(2): 105–109
Office of Population and Census Studies (OPCS) 1988 Survey of disability in Great Britain. HMSO, London
O'Kelly D 1997 Rehabilitation – the different strokes way. Different Strokes Annual Review, London
Orem D E 1995 Nursing: concepts of practice. McGraw-Hill, New York
Parsons T 1951 The social system. The Free Press, Glencoe, IL
Pires M 1989 Ethical perspective: a nursing reaction to 'Tom's story'. Rehabilitation Nursing 14(5): 255–256
Powell T 1994 Head injury. A practical guide. Headway and Winslow, UK
Ray C, West J 1987 Spinal cord injury. The nature of its implications and ways of coping. International Journal of Rehabilitation 6: 364–365
Richardson S A 1976 Attitudes and behaviour towards the physically handicapped. Birth Defects, Original Article Series 12: 15–34
Rubin Z, Peplau L 1975 Who believes in a just world? Journal of Social Issues 31: 65–89
Rutherford O M 1990 The role of exercise in prevention of osteoporosis. Physiotherapy 76(9): 522–526
Seligman M E P 1975 Helplessness. Freeman, San Francisco
Shearer A 1981 Disability: whose handicap? Blackwell, Oxford
Sim A J, Milner J, Love J, Lishman J 1998 Definitions of need: can disabled people and care professionals agree? Disability & Society 13(1): 53–74
Spooner A 1995 A personal perspective. The psychological needs of the spine injured patient. Professional Nursing 10(6): 359–366
Tyler A 1992 Political cripples. New Statesman and Society 5(206): 21–22
Williams C, George L, Lowry M 1994 A framework for patient assessment. Nursing Standard 8(38): 29–33
World Health Organization 1980 International classification of impairments, disabilities and handicaps. WHO, Geneva
World Health Organization 1995 Helsingborg Conference Pan European Consensus on Stroke Management. WHO, Sweden
Young T 1994 Treatment of mixed aetiology leg ulcers. British Journal of Nursing 3(12): 598–601

FURTHER READING

Bender A E, Brooks L J 1987 Body weight control. Churchill Livingstone, Edinburgh
Chevigny H 1962 My eyes have a cold nose. Yale University Press, New Haven
Department of Health 1996 Practical guide for disabled people (free). Department of Health, Ref. HB6, Wetherby
Dettenmeier P A 1990 Planning for successful home mechanical ventilation. Critical Care Nursing 1(2): 267–279
Gilbert S 1986 The psychology of eating: psychology and treatment. Routledge & Kegan Paul, London
Hahn D 1984 The story of Margaret Price. Barker, London
Hurley G 1983 Lucky break? Milestone Publications, Horndean
Jones T 1997 Walking on air. Heinemann, London
Heslop A P, Bagnall P 1988 A study to evaluate the intervention of a nurse visiting patients with disabling chest disease in the community. Journal of Advanced Nursing 13(1): 71–77
Jamieson E M, McCall J M, Blythe R, Whyte L A 1997 Guidelines for clinical nursing practices, 3rd edn. Churchill Livingstone, Edinburgh
Johnstone M 1987 Home care for the stroke patient. Churchill Livingstone, Edinburgh
Lake T, Acheson F 1988 Room to listen: a beginner's guide to analysis, therapy and counselling. Bedford Square Press, London
Newton T, Butler N M, Dawson J 1989 Engagement levels on a unit for people with a physical disability. Clinical Rehabilitation 3: 299–304
Oliver M 1988 Flexible services. Nursing Times 84(14): 25–29
Pentland B, Miller J D 1988 Head injury rehabilitation: 4 years' experience in Edinburgh. British Journal of Neurosurgery 2(1): 61–65
Pike S, Forster D 1995 Health promotion for all. Churchill Livingstone, Edinburgh
Roe B (Ed) 1992 Clinical nursing practice: the promotion and management of continence. Prentice-Hall, New York
Royal College of Nursing 1991 The role of the nurse in rehabilitation of elderly people. Scutari, London
Shearer A 1981 Disability: whose handicap? Blackwell, Oxford
Waters K 1987 The role of nursing in rehabilitation. Care Science and Practice 5(3): 17–21

USEFUL ADDRESSES

Disabled Living Centres Council
286 Camden Road
London N7 0BJ

Holiday Care Service
2 Old Bank Chambers
Station Road
Horley
Surrey RH6 6HW

RADAR (Royal Association for Disability and Rehabilitation)
12 City Forum
250 City Road
London EC1V 8AF

SPOD (Association to Promote the Sexual and Personal Relationships of People with Disabilities)
286 Camden Road
London N7 0BJ

MOTABILITY
Goodman House
Station Approach
Harlow
Essex CM20 2ET

THE OLDER PERSON

35

Elizabeth S. Farmer

INTRODUCTION

> For the complete life, the perfect pattern includes old age as well as youth and maturity. The beauty of the morning and the radiance of noon are good, but it would be a very silly person who drew the curtains and turned on the light in order to shut out the tranquillity of the evening. Old age has its pleasures, which, though different, are not less than the pleasures of youth (W. Somerset Maugham, *The Summing Up*).

This chapter is based on the view that learning in nursing is a journey which starts with personal experiences of life and is facilitated by human caring. Teachers therefore need to be problem-posers, consultants and nurturers of curiosity, inquiry, caring and interpretation (Bevis & Watson 1989, Higgins 1996, Dillon & Stines 1996). Students should not expect from this chapter a prescriptive account of how to nurse elderly people, for nursing care cannot be fully prescribed apart from the situation and the moment in which it is to be offered. It is, however, possible to identify likely patterns of caring and to describe these by means of narrative accounts of patients' experiences and of the nursing interventions taken in response to those experiences.

The first sections of the chapter set out the general principles of caring which inform holistic nursing practice. The second half of the chapter demonstrates through a series of case histories and accompanying commentaries how those principles might be applied. Throughout the chapter it is argued that the essential needs of elderly people are no different from those of any other group. But if the adoption of humanistic nursing practice seems a matter of particular urgency for elderly patients, perhaps it is because older people have typically been marginalised within a society that tends to view old age as an illness and to value cure above care.

CARING

Caring is the essence of holistic nursing practice. It implies relating to patients as complex persons with intrinsic worth, rather than as a collection of disorders and disabilities. The intention in this chapter is to focus on those aspects of nursing which have enormous healing power but which tend to be devalued in a society dominated by technology and economics. Love, hope, empathy, compassion, conscience and commitment are some of the elements of holistic nursing which this chapter will try to highlight through accounts of caring in action.

Watson (1988) defines caring as:

> the moral ideal of nursing whereby the end is protection, enhancement, and preservation of human dignity. Human caring involves values, a will, and a commitment to care, knowledge, caring actions, and consequences. All of human caring is related to intersubjective human response to health–illness; environmental–personal interaction; a knowledge of the nursing caring process, self knowledge, knowledge of one's power and transaction limitations.

According to Benner (1985), caring reflects interpersonal concern and liking so that the other person's plight and fate matters to the one who cares. Caring is possible only from a position of engagement, attachment and concern, which create the conditions for significant details to be noticed and appropriate help to be offered. Caring by its nature does not seek to control or master, but to facilitate understanding and uncover possibilities inherent in the situation. Caring is thus contextual and empowering (Minick 1995, Strickland 1996, Watson 1997).

The disciplines of natural science reduce life to separate variables and processes, any of which can be studied apart from the others. Humanistic science, on the other hand, views life as a composite of multiple, inseparable realities that are irreducible and can only be studied holistically (Kikuchi & Simmons 1993). Nursing practice synthesises natural and humanistic science in its response to human experiences. In her seminal work, Carper (1978) expresses this view through her argument that nurses need four types of knowledge, namely:

- scientific knowledge of human behaviour in health and illness
- the aesthetic perception of significant human experiences
- a personal understanding of the unique individuality of the self
- the capacity to make ethical choices within concrete situations involving particular moral judgements.

Nurses generally have no difficulty describing the biological components of their discipline, but often have trouble defining and describing the aesthetic, ethical and personal elements. Peplau (1988) has described the blending of these components of nursing in the following way:

> Art is always an expressive response, a statement of what the artist sees, said in the artist's way, with great pride in the necessary craftsmanship, and in the case of nursing, often for an audience of one. The unique blend of ideals, values, integrity, and commitment to the well-being of others, expressed in a nurse's self-presentation and responses to clients, makes each nurse a one-of-a-kind artist in nursing practice. Thus, the art of nursing is always pluralistic, characterized by great diversity and variety of nurse in action, and in this aspect is not replicable, from one situation to another, even by the same nurse.
>
> The art of nursing is highly personal, always imprecise, and nonscientific. Its language is behavior, ideally directed by the highest values of the human community, internally held by the nurse. Art is not bound by limits except for the nurse's conscience and the profession's ethics. A nomenclature to classify nursing's art is not possible. This aesthetic component is influenced by the style, taste, personality, and habits of both nurse and client and by the reactions of each to the expressions of the other.

Exploration of the art and science of nursing has continued relentlessly, with particular emphasis on the concept of caring (Omery et al 1994, McCance et al 1997, Crigger 1997, Davis 1997). Caring in nursing is concerned with relieving the vulnerability experienced by individuals as a consequence of illness, injury and disability (Gadow 1988, Leininger 1988, Chipman 1991, Fosbinder 1994, Pearson et al 1997, Sherwood 1997) as well as with promoting health. As Carper (1978) has suggested, the care which is provided should result from the sensitive blending of knowledge from both humanistic and natural science. Thus, optimism, compassion and empathy can be called upon to moderate actions that might otherwise be based solely on empirical data or motivated by ritual adherence to idealised norms. To develop the 'artistic' and 'ethical' components of nursing demands, of course, the engagement of the nurse's self as expressed through body movement, tone of voice, eye contact, facial expression and touch (Benner & Wrubel 1989, O'Berle & Davies 1992, Lovgren et al 1996).

Gaut (1991) argues that caring is a stance of respect for all living things that requires knowledge, trust, hope, honesty and courage:

> If you define yourself as a caring person, then your responsibility is to develop your capacity to experience the other person and be receptive to that person's needs. Caring is a natural way to relate to another human being, and in that relating, both persons become more human.

Storytelling

Somerset Maugham's perspective on old age, expressed in the introductory quotation, points to a conception of life as a continuous narrative in which the meanings we attach to our experiences are crucial to how we exist in the world and to the effectiveness of the relationships we have with significant persons in our lives. In this view, life experiences are intelligible only in terms of the personal biography of the individual. As this living narrative unfolds, past and present experiences illuminate one another and give new meaning to the whole; thus, there can be no separation of persons into parts or of lives into stages. When this view is applied to holistic nursing practice, prediction and explanation do not *precede* caring, but *evolve* from the sensitive practice of nursing.

Human virtues (such as courage, strength and honesty) underpin human activity, inquiry and practice. These virtues dispose us to act and feel in particular ways within a given context, i.e. within the flow of events — the enacted story — which constitutes every human life (Macintyre 1981). The virtues exhibited by an individual's character and actions constitute a complex moral unity which must be considered as a whole. They must also be considered within a wider sociocultural context: some qualities are prized more than others, depending upon culture and related social structures. Human behaviour cannot be characterised independently of the settings which make an individual's intentions intelligible both to himself and to others (Macintyre 1981, Kitwood 1997).

We make sense of human experience by framing events and experiences in terms of a history or narrative. Narrative accounts of events are the chief means of moral education (Macintyre 1981) and are of critical importance for the interpretation of human behaviour. The growing emphasis on storytelling and the use of metaphor in nursing marks a movement away from scientific reductionism, which views persons as no more than the sum of their parts, towards relativism and holism (Sandelowski 1991, Downie 1994, Ryan & McAllister 1996, Watson 1997). In the context of health care provision, this shift in perspective demands that the problems which patients encounter are no longer seen in the narrow terms of the biomedical model. From this shift also emerges an important distinction between 'disease' and 'illness'.

Disease refers to pathophysiological processes. Illness refers to the innately human experience of symptoms and suffering which are manifestations of disease. As Kleinman (1988) notes:

> When chest pain can be reduced to a treatable acute lobar pneumonia,...biological reductionism is an enormous success. When chest pain is reduced to chronic artery disease for which calcium blockers and nitroglycerine are prescribed, while the patient's fear, the family's frustration, the job conflict, the sexual impotence, and the financial crisis go undiagnosed and unaddressed, [the biomedical model] is a failure.

An individual's experience of illness will, in part, be determined by culture. Within his social environment, certain expectations will prevail as to how someone who is ill will or should behave. At the same time, the individual's responses will be shaped by his personal biography and by his unique character (Kleinman 1988).

Illness can be brief and minimally disruptive, or long-term and much more threatening. In either case, illness results in vulnerability and loss of control. Nursing is concerned with reducing the patient's vulnerability, primarily through understanding the significance that his illness has for him and reducing the frustrating consequences of disability. This can be achieved through strengthening contact with social support, rekindling hope and aspirations, and enhancing independence (Roach 1987, Gadow 1988, Kleinman 1988, Dancy & Wynn-Dancy 1995, Strickland 1996). This is particularly important in chronic illnesses, which offer little or no hope of cure and challenge the individual to find new and satisfying ways of being in the world.

Our personal life histories influence our perceptions of situations and give meaning and intelligibility to our experiences and our interactions with others. It is the nurse's task to be sensitive to the reality that has been created by each patient's personal biography, and to help him make sense of the experience of illness within his evolving view of the world.

Caring for older persons

An understanding of the lived experience of growing older is crucial to our ability to care for elderly patients. Lacking the direct experience of ageing herself, the student nurse may nonetheless gain invaluable insight by reading fictional accounts of old age. Wolf (1987) commends May Sarton's depiction of the experience of ageing in her novel *Kinds of Love*, which tells the story of a group of individuals facing the challenges of shared personal growth, creativity and mortality. One particularly sensitive passage describes a conversation between two elderly people, Christina and Eben. Eben declares that Christina 'grows more beautiful every day'; Christina, in response, says that she 'is getting to be a wrinkled old apple'. Christina's self-perception is not shared by Eben, who tells her: 'Don't look into mirrors, look into people's eyes....After a certain age mirrors lie...they give the bare facts all right, but they leave out the poetry.'

In caring for older people, the nurse must endeavour not to 'leave out the poetry'; she must always bear in mind that the frailty of the flesh is often at odds with the spirit within. As St Exupery's (1943) Little Prince learned: 'It is only with the heart that one sees rightly, what is essential is invisible to the eye'.

A social problem?

Census data show that there has been a gradual ageing of the UK population since the turn of the century. Decreased mortality and fertility rates are responsible for this change, which is in fact a feature of all Western societies. In the UK, 9% of the population falls within the age group 65–74 years and 7% are 75 years and over. This figure is set to rise over the next decade while the number of people in the wage earning groups will fall (CSO 1997).

In the face of this demographic shift, there has been an unfortunate tendency in Western society to view its elderly population as a social problem rather than as an asset. Largely for economic reasons, society has attached chronological markers to the process of ageing, with old age being that part of the life cycle which begins at the statutory age of retirement. Age has become an important criterion for establishing social status and, implicitly, rights and obligations. Social status is defined largely by wealth, power and prestige (Redfern 1997). It has been argued that the close association between wealth and power means that elderly people have little impact on social trends and limited ability to control their own destinies and lifestyles (Victor 1994). Because the ability to work and to generate wealth is a major determinant of prestige, enforced retirement consigns elderly people to a low position in the social pecking order (Victor 1994).

The majority of elderly people in the UK are on low incomes, and it is unfortunate that the greatest material poverty is associated with extreme old age, a period when, paradoxically, expenses tend to be greatest (Evers 1991). The prevailing image of the elderly person is of a dependent individual lacking social autonomy — a person who is powerless, unloved and neglected, and a burden on society because he consumes scarce resources but contributes nothing to the creation of wealth (Redfern 1997, Victor 1994). This view of old age as a period of stagnation and decline has been challenged by, among others, Altschul (1986), who decries the belief that elderly people are a burden on society. Rather, she argues, the current 'young elderly' provide a pool of unpaid carers for the oldest old, represent a large consumer group in commerce, travel and education, and are the mainstay of many voluntary organisations. What would happen, Altschul (1986) asks, if the young elderly unpaid carers withdrew their charitable services and invested their time and energy campaigning for more rights and better pensions? Who would fill the gaps created by the unpaid labour force? How would a switch from voluntary to paid care be financed? What effect would increased spending power of elderly people have on health, welfare and the economy? It is clear that prevailing notions of the 'dependent' status of the elderly population need to be re-examined.

The nurse should bear in mind that by stereotyping elderly people she will distort the professional–patient relationship and inhibit her ability to act therapeutically. She should also consider whether her attitudes towards elderly people reflect a personal fear of growing old. For many people, old age conjures up images of disease, disability, powerlessness, uselessness and death. Age need not, however, be a barrier to health and well-being. In spite of social and political discrimination, most elderly people live independent lives in the community.

Promoting health

In 1988, the World Health Organization (WHO) and the International Council of Nurses (ICN) produced a joint publication setting out programmes for nursing and health promotion for elderly people. In this document it was stressed that when the societies in which older people live have negative views about ageing and being old, the older people themselves are likely to have negative perceptions of themselves and their social roles. One of the main tasks of nursing is therefore to promote, primarily through caring, unconditional positive regard for elderly people.

The WHO/ICN (1988) report works from a definition of health as a state of complete physical, mental and social well-being rather than merely the absence of disease. It could be argued that if this definition were applied within the context of the biomedical model it would effectively mean that no-one is healthy. It is important to appreciate that health is a relative concept and, as such, has personal meanings. The WHO/ICN report also tends to define the needs of elderly persons with reference to what they cannot do rather than what they can do. There is a danger that this approach will reinforce negative attitudes towards elderly people and overlook the potential for personal growth in old age.

Caution should also be exerted in any attempt to define health needs in elderly persons in terms of functional capacity using scales which aim to identify and measure deficits in physical and mental ability and the relationship of these to social functioning.

In this approach, norms are established for activities such as eating, dressing, walking, standing and eliminating (Robinson et al 1986, Bucks et al 1996). Needs are assumed from the manifestation of certain behaviours relative to these norms. While this approach has some value in shifting the focus from disease to the impact of the disease on the person's lifestyle, it can have the effect of emphasising deficits rather than identifying possibilities for the enhancement of quality of life. Moreover, if an older person fails to perform at the expected level on a particular scale then he is described as disabled and is labelled accordingly. Diagnostic labels are often a means of identifying those individuals who are eligible for financial benefit. But labels can disempower individuals by implying that they occupy a marginal position within society and can therefore be given low priority in the provision of resources.

The requirements for well-being among older people are not necessarily different from those that apply to persons in other age groups. Family and community support, appropriate housing, adequate income, nutritious food in appropriate amounts, and screening and basic health services are identified in the joint WHO/ICN (1988) report as being of critical importance for health for everyone. The health of individuals within a society is, in large measure, determined by standards of, for example, nutrition, education, housing and income. There is a prevailing notion, nonetheless, that the individual, not society, is responsible for health, i.e. that illness is somehow a failure of the individual to stay well regardless of all the socioeconomic and environmental influences on his well-being (Gott & O'Brien 1990). Rather than regarding ill-health as a personal failure, however, it is more productive to assist individuals to attain or maintain good health through the provision of appropriate resources, including knowledge on how to achieve and maintain healthy lifestyles. Over the years, increasing emphasis has been placed on health promotion among older people through such means as individual counselling on diet and exercise, social clubs, keep-fit classes, art, dance and drama classes, and further education programmes.

Health is contextual; it cannot be viewed solely as an individual achievement. Changing unhealthy lifestyles requires an examination of existing concerns, habits and skills within a social context in order to understand the relevant issues and any existing barriers to change. Health promotion also involves an exploration of the potential strengths and possibilities offered by the person's perspective on his own situation (Dancy & Wynn-Dancy 1995).

Older people have essentially the same needs as others in society. Biological changes that occur with ageing may not of themselves be problematic; it may be only when disease is superimposed on such changes that vulnerability is experienced. Assessment of needs for nursing care should take account of these changes but they should be kept in their proper perspective — being old is neither a disease nor an illness.

For descriptions of the changes associated with ageing see Redfern (1997) and Carnevali (1993).

A caring community?

Community care is defined (Griffiths 1988) as providing the services and support which people who are affected by problems of ageing, mental illness, mental handicap or physical or sensory disability require to be able to live as independently as possible in their own homes or in home-like settings in the community. The NHS and Community Care Act (1990), which resulted from the Griffiths (1988) report, had six key objectives for service delivery:

- to promote the development of domiciliary day and respite services to enable people to live in their own homes wherever this is feasible and sensible
- to ensure that service providers make practical support for carers a high priority
- to make proper assessment of need and good case management the cornerstone of high quality care
- to promote the development of a flourishing independent sector alongside good quality public services
- to clarify the responsibilities of agencies and to make it easier to hold them to account for their performance
- to secure better value for taxpayers' money by introducing a new funding structure for social care.

While it would be difficult to argue against the principles implicit in the Griffiths (1988) report, many questions were posed about how its objectives could best be met. The most important of these was whether or not there would be sufficient funds to implement the proposals. How would needs be assessed and by whom? What role would charitable organisations and families be expected to play in meeting any financial deficits? How would care provision be monitored? Experience of implementing these proposals has heightened the anxieties underpinning these questions. For example, following a study to assess community care management in operation, Newham et al (1996) concluded that local authority funding falls significantly short of meeting the needs of dependent elderly people who require institutional care. Furthermore, nursing homes favour privately funded residents with low dependency levels, leaving those with greater dependency and in need of local authority funding occupying NHS acute service beds. The major deterrents to the effective implementation of the NHS and Community Care Act (1990) appear to be the lack of funds and major disagreements among professionals about what constitutes need and how needs can be assessed. Consequently, demand consistently outstrips the allocated resources, causing considerable stress among carers and those in need of care. For example, Thompson & Dobson (1995) highlighted the plight of five disabled elderly people who raised a court action against Gloucestershire County Council claiming that the council had indiscriminately cut its community care services. While the judge upheld the claim brought by the elderly people, he ruled that it was appropriate to take resources into account in the assessment of need. Griffiths (1988) argued that community care should be driven by need, not money. Thus, while the five elderly people had won a battle, the war was lost.

Rationing of care has become a major concern of professionals (Obeid & Ridout 1997) which is linked to issues of who should assess need and how this should be done. The need for multidisciplinary clinical assessment was highlighted by Sharma et al (1994) but this has apparently not happened. The assessment and allocation of community care resources are the responsibility of social workers who, when faced with inadequate budgets to meet the demand, are placed in an unenviable position of rationing care largely on monetary grounds (Dowson 1995, Herd & Stalker 1996).

While stressing the importance of families in providing care for dependent elderly people, the WHO/ICN (1988) report highlights the fact that in Western societies families are small and often scattered. This means that responsibility for care will necessarily extend beyond family affiliations. In any case, as Dalley (1996) has argued, the familial mode of care may be somewhat idealistic. Divorce, marriage and cohabitation have produced many complex relationships and living arrangements. Dalley argues that there is a need for a societal alternative to the family unit which could provide care without self-sacrifice and which would be flexible and responsive to individual needs. Dalley also argues that certain beliefs about the caring processes need to be re-examined in order to avoid major errors in policy and planning. In this connection, a distinction must be made between 'caring for' (tending another) and 'caring about' (having feelings for another). Dalley holds that these two processes are not necessarily equivalent or mutually exclusive. Caring about a dependent loved one does not necessarily imply a willingness to perform certain caring tasks for him. In support of this argument, Dalley refers to Ungerson's (1983) work which proposes that caring functions often require a transgressing of gender, age and sexual boundaries, creating tensions in relationships and disturbing the sensibilities of all involved.

According to Dalley (1996), the confusion between 'caring for' and 'caring about' may have devastating consequences. On the one hand, she argues, love often becomes fractured and distorted by feelings of obligation, burden and frustration, while on the other, the assumption that kinship is a precondition for caring implies that professional carers are unable to 'care about' as well as 'care for' dependent people.

Q **35.1** Would you agree that Dalley's (1996) view runs counter to the humanistic philosophy of caring, which stresses connectedness, not individuality, and our moral obligation to care for one another? Justify your answer.

CARING IN ACTION

The foregoing discussion provides a basis for analysis of the examples that follow, which describe the nursing care of elderly people. These case histories will illustrate the complexity of caring for older people who have been made vulnerable by chronic illness and highlight the need for the four types of knowledge described by Carper (1978; see p. 1000) and others. At the beginning of this chapter, students were urged to view their learning as a journey. What has been provided here is barely a route map. The exploration that is part of the journey of learning to care for elderly people demands that students read widely as well as developing the skills of 'presencing' (Osterman & Schwartz-Barcott 1996), i.e. sharing with elderly people their illness experience.

Case History 35.1 Miss W

Miss W is 76 years old and unmarried. She was admitted for respite care to a 30-bed ward in a continuing care unit for elderly people. Her admission had been arranged over the telephone by her general practitioner (GP) and the consultant physician in geriatric medicine. Miss W had lived for a year with her widowed sister, who was 80 years old and who had a married daughter living nearby and a son living some 400 miles away. Miss W had a history of hypertension which did not warrant medication and was prone to dizzy spells. She also suffered from osteoarthritis and walked with the aid of a stick. The arthritic pain was controlled through the administration of ibuprofen 400 mg three times daily.

Miss W had gone to live with her sister because she was having difficulty getting out of the house and generally coping with the day-to-day activities of living. Increasingly in the 6 months prior to admission she had become verbally abusive towards her sister, had wandered about the house incessantly, was neglectful of her personal care, and had developed nocturnal urinary incontinence (see Carnevali 1993 and Redfern 1997 for discussions of these problems). The GP prescribed night sedation, but this had little effect and appeared to increase the behavioural symptoms. Offers of community nursing services had been rejected.

Miss W was driven to hospital by her niece. On arrival in the ward, she was verbally abusive and lashed out at the nurses with her stick. It very quickly became clear that she had not been told she was going to hospital for respite care. She thought she was only going to the hairdresser. The medical staff were summoned to the ward and, during discussions, Miss W's niece made it clear that she would not take her aunt home because of the adverse effect her behaviour was having on her mother's health. Consequently, it was decided that Miss W should be persuaded to stay so that medical screening could be undertaken and so that her sister might have a much-needed rest.

For some hours after admission, Miss W walked up and down the ward looking for a way out and demanding that an ambulance take her home. The nurses gently steered her away from the doors, tried to engage her in conversation and offered refreshments to try to reduce her perception of threat. Some hours passed before Miss W was finally persuaded to have a little food and drink, by which time darkness had fallen and Miss W had agreed to stay overnight. She slept through the night, apparently exhausted by the day's experiences.

Miss W made it clear that she perceived her situation to be the consequence of a wicked deception. She believed she had been abandoned in what she referred to as the 'workhouse'. This perception was reinforced in her declaration that 'no matter what they [the nurses] do to me, I'll not do a hand's turn for them'. The nurses felt that the immediate need was to manage Miss W's aggression, primarily to reduce her energy demands. This was achieved by:

- staying calm
- respecting Miss W's personal space
- keeping a safe distance and allowing Miss W to remain in her position as long as her safety was not compromised
- encouraging Miss W to express feelings, perceptions and fears
- being flexible and accepting, not rigid or rejecting
- communicating to Miss W that staff members were accessible
- offering Miss W alternative coping strategies.

In the immediate post-admission period, staff reinforced the reasons for Miss W's admission to hospital and engineered social activities so that, although she did not initially participate, she was at least exposed to them. They did ensure that she had her hair done — that was, after all, why she left home that fateful day.

Case History 35.1 *(cont'd)* Miss W

Establishing trust

Three days passed before sufficient trust was established to enable Miss W's symptoms to be fully explored. There were two main aspects of nursing intervention: organisation of care through primary nursing, leading to acceptance of physical care through the expression of concern within the person-to-person relationship stressed in primary nursing (see Pearson 1988). Primary nursing gives to designated, experienced, first-level nurses total responsibility for the planning, delivery and evaluation of care for a specific number of patients for the duration of their stay. In view of the complexity of Miss W's situation, the ward sister took on the role of the primary nurse and selected associates from the nurses and nursing auxiliaries who would be continuously available for a few days following Miss W's admission. This meant that meaningful relationships could be established while the number of people involved in care, and hence the potential for confusion, was reduced.

By the end of the third day, Miss W was lucid and well orientated, experiencing only minor lapses of short-term memory. She ate and drank well, was attentive to other patients and staff and attended to her personal hygiene without prompting, needing help only to get in and out of the bath. During the 2-week respite period, a toileting programme was developed which restored continence. Such a regimen is described in Rooney (1987). This programme used the times of nocturnal wakefulness for bladder management, effectively turning a negative experience into a purposeful activity. A bond developed between Miss W and the ward sister, and in the course of many conversations it became clear that Miss W resented having to give up her home and her friends because of 'memory lapses'. She was aware that on occasion she forgot to turn off the gas appliances and that she was finding shopping and cooking difficult because of her poor memory and the distance she had to go to the shops, and agreed that she needed someone to be with her most of the time. She and her sister had always been on good terms and it had seemed like the ideal solution for them to live together. However, they had never had to live together as adults, and the strain was 'getting to both of them'. Miss W confessed to some jealousy over her sister's familial relationships and felt that she was looked upon as a visitor rather than as part of the family.

The challenge for the nursing team was to create a new perception of well-being for Miss W in the context of her changed situation. This involved the significant people in Miss W's life — most importantly, her sister. Soon after Miss W's admission, the ward sister contacted the health visitor, who began addressing the needs of the carers. Following discussions with Miss W's sister and niece, arrangements were made for respite care for 2 weeks every 3 months and for day hospital care 1 day each week while Miss W was at home. The offer of home-help services was rejected, as Miss W's sister could not reconcile herself to the idea of a 'stranger' in her home. The arrangement reached with Miss W's sister was communicated to the ward sister and through her to Miss W, who then had the opportunity to visit the day hospital while she was in respite care. These services were offered in the context of introducing new social contacts and creating new opportunities and new meanings in life for both Miss W and her family.

Until her death, some 5 years after the incident described, Miss W remained happily at home with her sister, enjoyed her outings to the day hospital and looked forward to her regular 'holidays' in the ward where she had 'many friends'. Her sister was also content, felt that she had been given adequate support and was free of the guilt which she said she would have experienced had her sister remained permanently in care.

CONFUSION AND VULNERABILITY

Commentary: Case History 35.1

Reducing vulnerability

From a strictly biomedical perspective, the immediate concerns relating to Miss W's condition were:

- confusion
- alteration in the pattern of micturition
- altered mobility
- altered sleep patterns.

These problems resulted in maladaptive coping and in impairment of self-care responses and home management.

Confusion is a term which is often applied in nursing to describe patients whose behaviour does not conform to social expectations. In applying this term, however, the nurse should remember that behaviour can only be understood in context. It has been argued that confusion is a term which should be limited to the description of conditions which are temporary, have an identifiable cause and are reversible (Open University 1988). The causes of confusion in older people are many and include brain injury, certain medications, sudden loss, environmental change and system disorders such as respiratory infection, cardiac failure and renal disease. The distinction between acute and chronic confusional states is usually made in terms of time of onset. Acute confusion has a relatively sudden onset (days or weeks), whereas chronic confusional states develop more slowly (over months or even years).

In Miss W's situation, the classification is difficult to apply, which once more highlights the danger of labelling patients (see p. 1001). The GP suspected dementia and responded with sedatives while awaiting expert advice. Dementia is a clinical syndrome in which there is acquired persistent intellectual impairment with compromise in at least three of the following spheres of activity (Cummings 1980):

- language
- memory
- visuospatial skills
- personality/affect
- cognition (abstraction, judgement, mathematics, etc.).

The emphasis on dementia as a clinical syndrome reinforces the idea that it is not a specific diagnosis but a constellation of signs of intellectual compromise that must be investigated to rule out irreversible as well as reversible causes (Shapira et al 1986). The two most common forms of dementia are Alzheimer-type (in which there is extensive brain cell loss, the causes of which are not yet known) and multi-infarct-type (which, as the name suggests, is caused by interruption of the blood supply resulting in multiple small infarcted areas of tissue throughout the cerebral cortex).

For a description of the care required by patients suffering from these disorders see Norman (1997) and Jacques (1992).

'Taking care of patients'

Since to give care to patients against their will is to commit the offence of battery, the time spent persuading Miss W to stay and steering her away from the door has to be examined carefully. In their guidelines, the Mental Health Act (1983) Commissioners have tried to steer a middle course between the principle of the inviolable nature of the human body and the protection of the incompetent patient's interests. This position, however, is not at all clear-cut. Each situation needs to be judged as it arises by the professionals involved.

Hirsch & Harris (1988) have argued that respect for persons, which underpins nursing practice, has two dimensions, namely concern for the individual's welfare and respect for his wishes. These two dimensions are usually complementary, but tension may arise between them, creating a dilemma. As Hirsch & Harris (1988) see it:

> The problem for all who care about others is how to reconcile respect for the free choices of others with real concern for their welfare when their choices appear to be self-destructive or self-harming.

This emphasis on autonomy would be interpreted by Benner & Wrubel (1989) as extreme individualism posing a threat to health. This alternative view is based in the belief that the ultimate goal in human development is to care and feel cared for and that this caring implies involvement and interdependence.

The law is faced with the challenge of reconciling these opposing concerns for the autonomy of individuals on the one hand and for their protection on the other. In law, 'the fundamental principle, plain and incontestable, is that every person's body is inviolate' (Sullivan 1988). The courts would disavow this principle only if they were satisfied that sufficient measures had been taken to protect the person's interests within the limits imposed by his incapability (Sullivan 1988). Common law is supplemented by statute law, which defines the circumstances under which consent for treatment, as defined in the Mental Health Act 1983, may be dispensed with. Murphy (1988) argues that the legalistic approach to the dilemmas of professional practice of caring for people judged to be incompetent gives no practical help in the day-to-day problems of treating incapable patients.

There are a number of important factors in Miss W's situation which influenced the giving of nursing care. In the first instance, fragmentation of services and poor communication among disciplines has left considerable gaps in knowledge of Miss W's life. The medical notes, containing only a brief introductory note from her GP, arrived in the ward only on the morning of admission. Only the briefest biographical history had been given to the ward sister by the niece, who made it clear that her mother was not fit to cope with her sister, Miss W, any longer and must have a rest. The niece's interpretation of Miss W's behaviour, and her subsequent actions, were based on the GP's provisional diagnosis of 'dementia'. Also, Miss W had been told that she was going to the hairdresser. It is hardly surprising that she reacted as she did on arrival in the ward. Miss W's experience of hospitals can be inferred from her comments about the 'workhouse'. She perceived the situation as a threatening one, and in that context her behaviour could be considered quite reasonable.

Respect for persons

'Taking care' of people does not necessarily amount to genuine caring. In providing only physical care it is possible to view the person as an object: 'the CVA', 'the coronary', 'the dementia'. Caring, on the other hand, involves 'presencing' as described by Marcel (cited in Reimen 1986):

> When someone is present to me, I am unable to treat him as if he were merely placed in front of me: between him and me there arises a relationship which surpasses my awareness of him; he is not only before me, he is also with me.
>
> The person who is at my disposal is the one who is capable of being with me with the whole of himself when I am in need; while the one who is not at my disposal seems merely to offer me a temporary loan raised on his resources. For the one I am a presence; for the other I am an object.

The account of Miss W's care in Case History 35.1 illustrates that the nursing staff had respect for her as a person. In biomedical terms, Miss W presented as 'confused', and if her behaviour had been separated from her life history she would have been 'taken care of' paternalistically by means of sedatives and permanent hospitalisation. This would have resulted in depersonalisation and learned helplessness. Paternalism claims a right to order the lives of others on the grounds that it is immoral to act against one's own general welfare (Hirsch & Harris 1988). In the first instance, a paternalistic approach was used by the ward sister, but only in order to ensure Miss W's safety and to buy time to get close enough to be 'present' for her. The ward sister knew from experience that she had to gain access to Miss W's world, to see things as she saw them. This is caring. Without shared meanings, the situation might have evolved into that which is sensitively described in the following poem by Fiona Sinclair (1991):

Confused

If my confusion
Is your confusion
Then how confused you must be
For my confusion
Confuses me
To the point where I can't see
And if your confusion
Confuses me
As mine confuses you
Then the two of us
Must be confused
As to who's confusing who!

When there is no shared understanding, the potential for cruelty, however unintentional, is enormous. The ward sister knew that Miss W was not pathologically confused: she simply had no markers to help her to interpret a new experience (this point is stressed by Kitwood 1997).

Knowledge of persons requires openness, participation and empathy. Holistic caring is not possible otherwise. Miss W's usual lifestyle was compromised by disease (arthritis) and by a phenomenon of ageing (short-term memory lapse). This combination of factors produced anxiety, which can result in a withdrawal from the outside world (Carnevali 1993). Thus, anxiety triggers a vicious circle of dulled memory and judgement, emotional lability and impaired social, psychological and physical reactions. Caring is not a fall-back position to be adopted when curing is not possible: caring is at all times primary. Through the caring relationship established between Miss W and the wardsister, it was possible to turn problems into possibilities and to establish new patterns. The use of nocturnal wakefulness to manage urinary incontinence is one example of this. Altered sleep patterns are not uncommon among older people but they can cause anxiety if it is not explained that they are a natural phenomenon. Imparting knowledge and offering explanations form part of health promotion. In Miss W's situation, the sleep disturbance which was originally perceived negatively became a new and purposeful pattern in her life — an opportunity to become continent was created. This is what Carper (1978) refers to as the artistic component of nursing.

Nursing care should be contextual, taking account of the person's environment and the way in which he perceives the situation which threatens his established patterns of living. Services should be well coordinated and supportive, and staffing levels must allow time and opportunity to implement and maintain the care plan negotiated with the person. Activities need to be purposeful and meaningful and to have some immediate goals. Thus, therapies should be built into activities of daily living. For example, stretching of limbs can be more easily encouraged by placing cutlery on a table at a slightly greater distance from the patient than would normally be expected, so encouraging him to reach out for it. The simplicity and regularity of such an exercise, the opportunity for increasing the degree of difficulty attached to the activity, and the immediacy and relevance of the goal combine to create a formula much more likely to maintain flexibility of limbs than irregular programmes of apparently purposeless exercises requiring a degree of motivation. This is particularly important where there is cognitive impairment: activities have to be centred on the living skills which are retained. Similar observations have been made by McMahon (1988) with regard to reality orientation programmes. The traditional brief therapy sessions have been shown to have little effect on patients, and McMahon has argued that a 24-h reality approach, in which orienting is part of every interaction, is more person-centred and respectful.

The nursing care provided for Miss W required a skilful blending of the four types of knowledge identified by Carper (1978): scientific, aesthetic, personal and ethical (see p. 1000). Through the understanding and dialogue implicit in caring, Miss W and the significant persons in her life were able to establish different and meaningful lifestyles.

THE RIGHT TO INDEPENDENCE

Commentary: Case History 35.2

The caring dilemma

The primary care team had agonised over the decision to try to support Mrs A in her home as she wished. The health visitor described the whole experience as 'walking on eggshells'. When pressed to explain this statement, she described the feeling of being torn between wanting to provide safe and continuous care and recognising that these goals had to be reconciled with the patient's values. Whether or not this was achieved in the end is a matter for debate.

The disease-oriented model of care is dominant in the description of the care provided for Mrs A. This model views situations in terms of problems or deficits and, for Mrs A, identified a set of problems which included non-compliance with a drug regimen, social withdrawal, impaired mobility worsened by excess weight, urinary incontinence, risk of injury, inability to attend to personal care independently, and impaired home management. This model assumes the dominance of the professionals concerned and confirms their problem-solving role. From the point of view of the patient, however, it can create increased dependence and reinforce a feeling of powerlessness.

Conversely, Kleinman (1988) and Dancy & Wynn-Dancy (1995) have argued that the role of health professionals is to empower the persons for whom they care by helping them to assert what is important to them in their lives and in their care. This view is supported by Watson (1979) who identified 10 aspects of caring in nursing:

- formation of a humanistic–altruistic system of values
- instilling of faith/hope
- cultivation of sensitivity to one's self and others
- development of a helping/trusting relationship
- promotion and acceptance of the expression of positive and negative feelings
- systematic use of the scientific problem-solving method for decision-making
- promotion of interpersonal teaching/learning
- provision of a supportive, protective or corrective mental, physical, sociocultural and spiritual environment
- assistance with the gratification of human needs
- efforts to understand persons in concrete lived situations and moments, and the responses to these.

There is nothing in the NHS and Community Care Act (1990) which in principle prohibits sensitive caring. The difficulties arise primarily from practical limitations, such as the setting of predetermined cash limits as an incentive to obtain value for money, disagreements on how best to assess needs, and fragmentation of services resulting in delays in intervention. One of the ways in which the government seeks to remove potential difficulties is through the case worker principle or brokerage (Moore 1992). As this advocacy role has, in the context of community care, been given to the social worker, it is clear that social security policies must be aligned with community care policies if choice and adequacy of care are to be a reality.

Harmonising curing and caring

What can be identified from the account of Mrs A's care in Case History 35.2 is the importance of the patient's biographical details. During her first period of hospitalisation, the focus of treatment was on correcting Mrs A's heart failure. Unfortunately, the therapeutic regimen implemented had an undesirable effect on Mrs A's mobility, continence, safety and general capacity for independent living. She was, not unnaturally, distressed and one wonders if the effects of the drug therapy had been explained to her in advance. Mrs A expected to get better, not worse; given the amount of persuasion needed for her to accept hospitalisation, it would have been perfectly understandable if the bond of trust between the health visitor and the patient had been irreparably damaged by the fact that the latter's expectations were not immediately met.

Knowledge of the pathological effects of excess weight resulted in dietary restrictions which were not acceptable to Mrs A and clearly were not adhered to on discharge. She was 83 years old and had an established dietary pattern. The medical aim was clearly to preserve life without regard for what would constitute an acceptable quality of life for Mrs A. Changes in the way in which a person leads his or her life can be made only if they are valued by that person.

Another contributing factor in Mrs A's distress in hospital was the fragmentation of care; she was not accustomed to this at home. It can be argued that there is a need for multicompetent practitioners to replace the host of specialists whose services have not been properly evaluated (Beachey 1988). If services are broken into a series of tasks, it is unlikely that they will amount to genuinely holistic care. That said, however, increasing flexibility within the professions, cross-training and the ability to perform

Case History 35.2 Mrs A

Mrs A was an 83-year-old widow who lived in a socially deprived urban area. She had no children and her nearest relatives lived on the other side of the city, visiting on average once a week. She lived in a one-bedroom flat in a four-storey building. Mrs A was described in her medical record as arthritic, obese and reluctant to venture out of doors. She had an obliging neighbour who paid all her bills, collected her pension from the post office and did all her shopping. Otherwise, Mrs A managed her housework and her personal care independently.

Mrs A's local practice team of GP, health visitor and district nurse had a well-developed screening and support programme for the elderly people registered with the practice (as described, for example, in Littlewood & Scott 1990). This programme was based on agreed criteria for identifying those at risk. The programme worked well, with admissions to hospital or other care facilities being fairly low compared with patients with similar characteristics in other practices within the area.

During a particularly severe winter, in which the threat of hypothermia intensified the visiting programme, Mrs A appeared content and was coping well with her preferred lifestyle. She liked to be visited by people she knew but was reluctant to go out, partly because she found the stairs too much, but mainly because she did not mix well with strangers. The health visitor offered to make arrangements for her to attend the local pensioners club but this was refused. Mrs A got through the winter with no major problems and 6 months later was still coping well.

A further 6 months on, the health visitor found a different situation. She noted that the house was unkempt and that Mrs A's personal appearance had deteriorated. After much persuasion, Mrs A agreed to have the district nurse visit weekly to give assistance with personal hygiene. Arrangements were also made for home-help services 3 days per week. The amount of persuasion needed to get Mrs A to agree to a home-help prompted the health visitor to liaise with the home-help organiser more closely than usual in the hope of finding 'just the right person'. (Very often, a concerned relationship will develop between a client and home-help which usually means that more of the 'self' will be given than would be expected within the carefully prescribed job description of the home-help.) The 'right person' was duly found, Mrs A's situation improved 'practically overnight', and this new level was maintained for about 6 months, until the doctor was called because of Mrs A's increased breathlessness. A diuretic was prescribed which, while it relieved her breathlessness (diagnosed as cardiac failure), created a problem with urinary incontinence. Also at this time, Mrs A's mobility deteriorated. Previously able to get about with a stick, she needed a Zimmer aid to get about her flat. Additionally, she had been found on the floor by her home-help on two occasions.

The GP, health visitor and Mrs A's relatives combined forces to persuade her that a period in hospital was necessary to sort out her problems. She was subsequently admitted to an assessment unit for elderly people. This period of hospitalisation was described by the health visitor as a 'disaster' for Mrs A, who became confused and had great difficulty adjusting to her new drug regimen of digoxin and long-acting, potassium-sparing diuretics (Royle & Walsh 1992). During the month in hospital, Mrs A was seen by a dietician and subsequently commenced on a 1000-calorie diet. She agreed to this only because she thought it was expected of her. Physiotherapy was also introduced to try to improve her mobility, with no great success. Mrs A was also seen by the occupational therapist, who assessed dressing and walking ability and the need for bathing aids and a commode for night use. Finally, the social worker was summoned to consider Mrs A's social circumstances to determine the capacity for independent living. Despite this well-intentioned care, the health visitor found Mrs A confused, generally feeling helpless and hopeless, and pleading to be allowed home.

Mrs A was, after much pleading, discharged home, whereupon she abandoned her diet and, it seems, her diuretics. Her home-help was recommenced and the district nurse called three times each week to attend to her personal hygiene. About 1 month after her discharge from the assessment unit, Mrs A again became unwell and her GP suspected a cerebrovascular accident (CVA) because of left-sided weakness. Mrs A refused to return to the assessment unit and after a great deal of persuasion was admitted to an acute medical ward where she stayed for 2 months. Compared with her previous time in hospital, this was a very positive experience. When asked what was different, Mrs A said the nurses had let her be herself and did not make her do things she did not want to do. In particular, she had the same food as all the other patients, albeit in smaller portions.

Mrs A made a full recovery from what appeared to have been a transient ischaemic attack. While in hospital it was put to her that she could no longer live safely at home and should consider a nursing home. With great reluctance, Mrs A agreed to a 3-month trial in a local nursing home. During her time there, the health visitor called to see how she was settling in. On both occasions, she was described as 'weeping and miserable' and expressing a wish to die. Following a meeting with the GP and the district nurse, it was agreed, to Mrs A's delight, that she should go back home.

At home, the previous services were restored and a 'tuck-in' service was introduced whereby a nursing auxiliary visited in the evening to help Mrs A get to bed safely. A commode was placed by her bed to avoid falls en route to the toilet and a supply of incontinence pads was provided to relieve the anxiety associated with possibly not making it to the toilet on time. In view of her previous reluctance to take her diuretics (deemed necessary to control her heart failure), the health visitor explored further the reasons for Mrs A's non-compliance with her drug regimen relative to the pattern of falls (occurring mainly at night) and the incontinence. The health visitor concluded that postural oedema developing during the day was being corrected through rest on retiring for the night, with a resulting improvement in diuresis. Consequently, the tuck-in service would not be as effective as it might be because Mrs A would still need to get out of bed to use the commode, thus increasing the risk of falls. The health visitor therefore suggested that the patient should lie on her bed between 17.00 and 19.00 h so that the improved diuresis would occur before the nursing auxiliary came to see her safely to bed at 20.30 h and she would be less likely to have to get up again to use the commode.

The strategy was very successful, and for about 3 months Mrs A was happily maintained at home. Sadly, one morning, the home-help arrived to find that Mrs A had died in bed sometime during the night.

duties in more than one discipline will not of themselves produce holistic care (Farmer 1994). What is needed is a shared view of the priorities of care for any given patient. Care plans need to be tailor-made in the light of the values, motivation and residual capacities of the patient. Thus, following Mrs A's second admission to hospital, the goal of medical and nursing interventions was to enable her to be all she could be and not to make her what the medical model would consider 'normal'.

The short time in the nursing home was equally disastrous and again demonstrates the consequences of the dominance of professional goals which are not shared by patients. A residential home might have been a more acceptable alternative. On a positive note, what is perhaps most striking about the account of Mrs A's care is the sensitivity of the health visitor and her expert and skilful blending of the artistic and scientific elements of caring.

THE CHALLENGE OF SEVERE DISABILITY

Commentary: Case History 35.3

The purpose of nursing is to reduce the vulnerability of persons who are facing particular challenges in their lives. If we are to help our patients to see new possibilities in otherwise hopeless situations, there needs to be commitment and involvement. The nursing team involved in Mrs R's care demonstrated this involvement by addressing her physical difficulties in a way that reflected an understanding of the implications of those problems for her social and emotional well-being. Good seating arrangements, for example, can enhance the individual's cognitive and communication skills and can influence for the better the attitudes and approaches of other people to the disabled person. The optimal sitting position for all persons is with the hips, knees and ankles flexed to 90°. Weight should be evenly distributed under the buttocks and thighs, with the feet firmly planted on the ground and forearms resting at elbow height on an armrest. In achieving proper positioning, attention should be directed first to the pelvis, followed in order by the buttocks and thighs, trunk and head (Fraser et al 1987).

Optimal positioning remains the goal for all persons with multiple handicaps, even though its achievement is rarely possible. To even approximate this goal, seating systems need to be adapted to provide comfort and security, maximise function, prevent, minimise or delay contractures, inhibit abnormal reflex activity and facilitate movement (e.g. from chair to bed). The careful use of positioning techniques in patients with athetoid movements may bring about some control in upper extremity movement and even provide a stable base for purposeful arm movements, however limited. When, as in the case of Mrs R, the problems of athetoid movements are compounded by tongue thrust, good positioning is absolutely essential if eating and drinking are to be assisted in a pleasurable, dignified manner. The critical factor is positioning of the head in flexion in a static midline position to give more control when assisting the patient to eat and drink (Fraser et al 1987).

In caring for people like Mrs R, nurses need to be sufficiently committed and involved to overcome enormous obstacles, not least of which is the cost of equipment. Additionally, in an era of cost containment and centralisation of services, central purchasing of equipment may militate against the provision of appropriate items for individual patients. Nurses must therefore insist on being involved in making choices to meet particular needs, especially when patients are themselves unable to communicate their preferences. To do this work effectively, nurses need to have some knowledge of ergonomics and anthropometrics, and often they will need to negotiate priorities with physiotherapists who may not perceive a patient's situation in quite the same way as they do.

Hobson & Molenbroek (1990) and Ward et al (1995) have highlighted the lack of anthropometric resource data appropriate for use in individuals with specific disabilities, and have identified important qualitative and quantitative factors influencing the design of seating and mobility devices for a specific segment of the population. The data generated by these authors is very different from that gathered from able-bodied subjects, which is generally employed in the design of seating and other equipment which may be used by disabled people. This work clearly indicates the need for a resources database specific to people with particular disabilities. Through observation and careful documentation of experiences, nurses could make a significant contribution to the development of databases for people with particular needs.

Caring should not focus on the pursuit of short- or long-term goals while disregarding the individual's state of mind in the present. To put this another way, interventions must support being as well as becoming. This may entail constructing imaginative and innovative ways of helping. Passant (1990), for example, has given a very sensitive account of her use of complementary therapies in the care of elderly people. Therapeutic touch, massage, aromatherapy and herbal remedies have brought great comfort and pleasure to many elderly people who were previously sad and unresponsive (Francis 1995).

Spiritual caring

Before her illness, Mrs R regularly attended church, yet no mention is made in Case History 35.3 of her spiritual needs. The spiritual dimension of caring has become increasingly prominent in the literature relative to advances in science and how these impact on our understanding of the world and our place within it. In general, nurses may feel ill-equipped to enhance the spiritual well-being of patients. However, this aspect of caring does not depend upon religious belief *per se*. It depends upon our understanding of what constitutes wholeness for individuals. Creating space and quiet and using poetry and music are ways of nourishing the soul and replenishing the spirit. As nurses, we are not asked to enter into theological debate with patients, but in caring we can demonstrate love in action and in so doing help to provide spiritual comfort and peace.

Q

35.2 The ward sister believed that Mrs R knew that she was loved, respected and wanted. Does this, however, constitute an acceptable quality of life? Contemporary medicine goes to great lengths to keep people alive, sometimes even against their will. The moral and economic implications of this have put the subject of euthanasia on the legislative agenda of the Western world (Billings 1996, Dunstan 1996). In the majority of cases, the motive for precipitating death is to end suffering and to preserve dignity. These motives must sit unhappily with the notion of caring as the essence of nursing. Discuss with your colleagues the following questions related to the debate on euthanasia:

- Can nurses reconcile mercy killing with their ethical codes (UKCC 1992), which are concerned with doing good and avoiding evil?
- How does the principle of the patient's autonomy operate in the context of withholding treatment?
- What happens to those who cannot communicate, or who are incapable of making decisions on their own?
- Is it likely that, in an era of increasing economic pressures, legalised euthanasia would be subject to grave abuse?

Case History 35.3 Mrs R

A student nurse came on duty in a continuing care unit for elderly people. She learned that a patient she had been caring for had died during the night. The permanent members of staff were clearly saddened by the loss and the student nurse could not understand why. The patient, Mrs R, was 72 years old and had been a patient in the hospital for 6 years because of a CVA resulting in athetosis (see Ch. 9) with an accompanying spasticity and loss of verbal communication skills. Prior to her transfer to long-term care, Mrs R had spent nearly 1 year in an acute care facility where she developed contractures of her hip and elbow joints. An additional complication was tongue thrust, a reflex pushing out of the tongue which makes eating and drinking difficult (for information on tongue thrust and its management, see Fraser et al 1987).

Mrs R had a devoted husband who visited every day. The couple had no children, and friends had ceased to visit, largely because of her inability to communicate verbally and their feelings of awkwardness in trying to express their care. Consequently, her only other visitor was the minister of the church where Mrs R had been an active member.

The ward in which Mrs R was cared for was of the Nightingale style and she was one of 30 patients with equally complex illnesses. Taking a problem-oriented view of Mrs R's situation, the challenges for nursing could be listed as follows:

- inability to communicate verbally
- impaired non-verbal communication
- disordered motor activity with potential for injury and total lack of purposeful movement
- eating disorder threatening her nutritional status
- inability to perform personal care
- uncontrolled voiding of urine and faeces
- imbalance between solitude and social interaction
- imbalance between activity and rest
- alteration in role
- potential alteration in perception and self-esteem
- possible pain of loss, loneliness, emptiness.

It was not possible, even after multidisciplinary assessment, to make a definitive statement about Mrs R's comprehension. She could make eye contact and turned toward sounds. Attempts to initiate eye signalling had all failed. Mrs R was, in effect, wholly dependent on others for all aspects of living and the student nurse could not understand why the staff should mourn the passing of someone she would describe as a 'vegetable'.

The humanistic perspective taken by the ward sister, however, drew attention away from the deficits listed above towards the need for Mrs R to find new meaning in life and to be empowered through the relationships and care offered by others. It is worth repeating that if a patient's situation is always viewed as a cluster of problems, opportunities for positive and healing interventions will be lost. The ward sister carefully explained to the student nurse the therapeutic use of self, by which she meant the ability to project oneself into a situation to achieve results no matter how small they may appear to be. In the first place, the sister argued, Mrs R did have some comprehension. In spite of her athetoid movements, Mrs R followed with her eyes the significant persons in her life. Also, she would turn her head away from or towards people in rejection or approval of some act or comment.

Sister argued that Mrs R knew she was cared for. Through the use of primary nursing, Mrs R had her own, clearly identifiable, supporters who were sufficiently committed to act on her behalf. To care for Mrs R, each of her carers had to have a great breadth and depth of knowledge and a willingness to use this to help Mrs R to find a way of being in the world. Sister gave the student the following examples of the challenges which the nurses had to meet in caring for Mrs R.

Mrs R had very little physical mobility. She could not make purposeful or coordinated movements, had limb spasticity and could not weight-bear or sit completely upright or unsupported. The challenge was to find a supported sitting position which would be comfortable and also fulfil certain other benefits such as facilitating cardiopulmonary and gastrointestinal function. Mrs R's care was complicated by limb contractures acquired in the acute care setting from which she was transferred. In addition to preventing pressure sores, the plan for Mrs R was to try to control disturbing movements for energy conservation, aesthetic purposes and, not least, for comfort. Good positioning was especially important at mealtimes. Mrs R's tongue thrust made it difficult for a spoon to be inserted into her mouth. This was accommodated by using slight downward pressure on the tongue with a spoon and the spout of a feeding cup to inhibit the tongue thrust and to encourage lip movement. Mrs R had no teeth and had not worn dentures since the time of her stroke. The tongue thrust made it impossible to consider a prosthetic device of any kind, primarily for reasons of safety. This presented an additional challenge in the selection of food. Nonetheless, the sloppy soft diet that tends to be standard provision for patients who require assisted feeding was not resorted to. With good tongue and lip movements, Mrs R was able to manage most foods. She was particularly fond of fish and chips; this was confirmed by her husband and evidenced by the fact that she always cleared her plate!

The process of eating took into account Mrs R's social environment. She ate in the same area as the other patients and her need for assisted feeding gave her the individual attention of a nurse for about 45 minutes three times each day, in addition to 15 minutes every 2 h for additional fluids.

Re-peopling Mrs R's world meant introducing her to all the other patients in the ward and sharing with her the general events affecting the lives of all the patients as well as the special things such as a new grandchild or a birthday. Much time was spent by the nurses with Mrs R's husband initially; they got to know his wife through him and subsequently involved him in the decisions affecting her life. In this way, clothing reflecting her personality and preferences could be selected. Consideration was also given to special needs such as slight oversizing of garments to accommodate contracted limbs, and selecting fibres that were warm, comfortable and helped to manage the excessive perspiration produced on occasion by the athetoid movements.

The hospital had large attractive grounds with patios and verandahs for those who were unable to make use of the gardens. These facilities were available to Mrs R, and the nurses believed she took pleasure from her time out of doors. Mrs R's husband became very much a part of the team and had daily opportunities to discuss his own feelings, hopes and desires. Thus, an extended caring role evolved.

CARING AND THE FAMILY

Commentary: Case History 35.4

Attitudes toward death

Some nurses may be uncomfortable with the idea of death, seeing it as a failure, or possibly as a relief when life is perceived as meaningless. The death wishes of patients are seldom explored, and valuable insight into individuals' perspectives and values is lost as a result. The charge nurse in Case History 35.4 did not, however, dismiss the issue of death but used the opportunity to help Mr F discover new strengths and possibilities.

Benner & Wrubel (1989) have argued that ours is a future-oriented, death-denying society which is preoccupied more with achieving than with being. These authors further argue that one of the ways in which we cope with death is to identify it as a process with progressive stages and then to turn the process into a developmental achievement. Kubler-Ross's (1970) work on death and dying identifies stages of denial, anger, rejection, bargaining and acceptance. This work has been cited by Benner & Wrubel (1989) as a prescription for a 'healthy way to die', and an example of society's obsession with goal orientation even in dying.

Family care-giving

Larson & Dodd (1991) have defined caring as the intentional actions and attitudes that convey physical care and emotional concern and promote a sense of safeness and security in another. Mr F's age and chronic illness combined to classify him as being in need of continuing care. Hospitalisation was seen as the only response to this and, in the absence of more suitable accommodation, Mr F found himself in a unit specialising in the care of elderly people. This is yet another example of the consequences of stereotyping. Mr F did not consider himself as elderly, and, indeed, in terms of chronological age he was not. Persons with chronic illnesses (see Ch. 32) and older people share an unenviably marginalised position in society.

The power of the professionals involved in Mr F's acute care to make decisions without consultation is evident in the description of the bewilderment of both Mr and Mrs F and their ensuing anger and sense of hopelessness. Community nursing services might have been a more acceptable way of providing care in the post-acute phase of the illness and would at least have taken account of established family patterns of caring. Larson & Dodd (1991) have noted that, although caring within a family may be inherently valuable, during a crisis appropriate care cannot always be given without support from outside the family. It appeared to Mr and Mrs F that the staff in the acute care setting did not care sufficiently to explore the possibility of alternative arrangements for caring. The emphasis of the professionals upon cure obscured the need for care.

By supporting the carers within a family, professionals can help to create a sense of togetherness, reciprocity and networking (Larson & Dodd 1991). Mr F's family had a well-established pattern of support and of physical caring which was disrupted and, in the acute area, apparently discounted. It would have been more helpful for the professionals concerned to investigate the established patterns by which Mr F's family functioned. The history of family relationships needs to be taken into account in helping patients and their families to establish new coping strategies when usual patterns are disrupted. Swimming against the tide of established caring practices is often counterproductive, if not futile. The artistry of the nurse is required in choosing interventions and approaches which are congruent with the family's perceived needs (Friedemann 1991).

The context of caring

Mr F had been moved from a high-technology area in a modern, purpose-built hospital to a Victorian building which, at first sight, added to his sense of hopelessness. However, Mr F soon discovered that buildings were not the best indicators of the care which could be expected within. The account of Mr F's care in Case History 35.4 illustrates the establishment and effective use of a healing relationship in the context of nursing. There is a clear indication of the use of dialogue and active listening to mobilise hope and to preserve personhood and dignity. Information was given to relieve anxiety, and family care-giving was enhanced through emotional support and the mobilisation of collective strength, drive and desire. This approach helped to relieve Mr F's sense of alienation from the treatment and recovery process which was unwittingly created in the acute care setting. By being encouraged to set realistic and achievable goals, the family members were helped to find a new but comfortable way of relating to one another in the context of caring.

CONCLUSION

In this chapter, an attempt has been made to illustrate that the four types of knowledge identified by Carper (1978) — scientific, aesthetic, personal and ethical — are necessary for the practice of nursing. Nursing practice synthesises subjective and objective data in the systematic study of human experiences of illness, injury or disease. Focusing on a disease-oriented model can result in interventions based on idealised clinical norms which often bear little relation to the needs of individual persons.

The case histories focus on aspects of caring in nursing. Developing competencies is of course an important aspect of nursing practice and references for further reading have been provided to enable students to learn about the signs, symptoms and treatments associated with specific diseases. While the importance of disease phenomena cannot be denied, the concern in this chapter has been to stress the person- and situation-specific nature of the challenges to well-being created by illness experiences.

Growing old is not a disease. Social constructs tend to set older people apart and cause policy-makers to look upon them as a homogeneous group — which clearly they are not. Like any other person, the older individual is distinguished by a personal biography and by the meanings which he attaches to particular circumstances in his life at particular times. The introduction of the arts and the humanities in nursing education will perhaps help to create a balance between art and science in nursing. Of equal importance is the need for nurses, and others who are privileged to be with individuals in times of joy and sadness, to care for each other. Cassidy (1988) writes:

> I have discovered that the world is not divided into the sick and those who care for them, but that we are all wounded and that we all contain within our hearts that love which is for the healing of the nations. What we lack is the courage to give it away.

It is hoped that this chapter will help to enrich the learning experiences of students and create opportunities for shared personal growth for them as nurses and, especially, for the older persons whose worlds they must enter in order to care.

Case History 35.4 Mr F

Mr F is a 62-year-old previously self-employed timber merchant who for 3 years had suffered from motor neurone disease — characterised by spasticity and weakness of the limbs, loss of fine movements and, as the disease progresses, impaired speech, swallowing and respiration (see Walsh 1997). During the course of his illness, Mr F had been cared for at home by his wife with support from his son and daughter, both of whom were married and jointly ran the family business. Mr F developed a severe respiratory illness and had to be admitted to an acute care unit in a modern district general hospital, where he stayed for 3 weeks prior to his transfer to a continuing care hospital for elderly people. The charge nurse had been notified of his admission.

Mr F arrived on the ward looking very apprehensive. He was accompanied by his wife, who explained that her husband had had a harrowing experience in hospital wherein he had gone from being a unique, dignified person to a dependent, dejected shell of his former self. Their well-established routines at home had been completely rejected and Mrs F's advice on ways of managing particular tasks was 'unwelcome'. The move to long-term care was seen as the last straw. The dilemma was that while it was felt that Mr F was not well enough to be managed at home, he had no desire to remain in the acute setting, nor did he want to be in a 'geriatric' ward. The beds in the acute care unit were needed, no option was given, and resentment and anger ensued.

The charge nurse welcomed Mr F onto the ward. At first sight, he was pale, anxious and breathless. He was settled in bed and the charge nurse sat down beside the couple and, over a cup of tea, described the care that could be expected in the unit. It was clear that the patient had not fully recovered from the respiratory illness and, from the medical notes and the information provided largely by Mrs F, the following problems emerged:

- activity intolerance
- inefficient respiratory function
- impaired communication
- disrupted family relationships
- feelings of hopelessness
- fluid volume deficit
- constipation
- change from chronic to acute illness
- insufficient intake of nutrients
- alteration in the usual pattern of personal care
- urinary retention with overflow incontinence
- threat to skin integrity at pressure points.

Problems or possibilities?

Insofar as it reflected a deficit model of care, the above list could have obscured the possibilities for positive intervention. In view of Mr F's negative experience in the previous situation, and the complexity of his problems, the charge nurse decided to take the role of primary nurse. This was explained to Mr F and his wife, who was encouraged to visit as and when she wished. It was also put to Mrs F that while her need to satisfy herself about the standards of care her husband would receive was understood, she should also try to rest and share the visiting with her family. An alternative offer of visitor's accommodation was made.

Mr and Mrs F were aware of the poor ultimate prognosis. They had a loving marital relationship and a fierce determination to protect and nurture one another. For Mrs F, the most upsetting part of the experience in the acute care unit had been her husband's expressed wish to die. Although they had from time to time spoken of separation, this had always been referred to as a distant event. These feelings were explored by the charge nurse, who discovered that the nature of the acute illness had not been fully explained to Mr F. Accordingly, arrangements were made for the couple to have an early meeting with the doctor. As a way of offering immediate support and comfort, the charge nurse explained that, with good care, there was every reason to believe that things would improve. He suggested that they start planning for discharge home and consider regular respite admissions to maintain optimum wellness. The idea that it was appropriate to make plans had a dramatic effect on the couple.

Mr F's value as a husband, father, grandfather and business advisor were explored in the context of his changed situation. In the process of the conversations, the charge nurse learned how the couple had coped with the illness thus far and used this information to structure the care plans so that no unnecessary disruption of routine occurred.

The charge nurse and Mr and Mrs F agreed to set out a plan that would celebrate life and to work at this by devising acceptable ways of dealing with the difficulties of the immediate situation. Within 3 weeks of admission, Mr F could transfer from bed to chair or chair to chair with the assistance of one person and could walk a few steps with the support of two people. His respiratory infection had resolved, his bowel function was restored to the previous pattern, he had gained weight, and fluid and electrolyte balance were maintained at appropriate levels. Mrs F had regained her strength and vitality and felt she was ready to take her husband home. As planned, discharge was arranged with district nurse support for bathing, maintenance of the urinary catheter, controlling urinary retention and general surveillance. It was arranged that respite care would be given for 2 weeks every 3 months.

REFERENCES

Altschul A T 1986 The elderly make the world go round. Geriatric Nursing 6(2): 26–27

Beachey W 1988 Multicompetent health professionals: needs, combinations, and curriculum development. Journal of Allied Health 17(4): 319–329

Benner 1985 Preserving caring in an era of cost-containment, marketing and high technology. Yale Nurse August: 12–20

Benner P, Wrubel J 1989 The primacy of caring. Addison-Wesley, Menlo Park

Bevis E O, Watson J 1989 Toward the caring curriculum: a new pedagogy for nursing. National League for Nursing, New York

Billings J 1996 A review of physician-assisted suicide: where do you stand? Journal of Holistic Nursing 14(3): 206–222

Bucks R S, Ashworth D L, Wilcock G K, Siegfried K (1996) Assessment of activities of daily living in dementia: development of the Bristol activities of daily living scale. Age and Ageing 25: 113–120

Carnevali D L 1993 Nursing management for the elderly, 2nd edn. Lippincott, Philadelphia

Carper B A 1978 Fundamental patterns of knowing in nursing. Advances in Nursing Science 1(1): 13–23

Cassidy S 1988 Sharing the darkness: the spirituality of caring. Darton, Longman & Todd, London
Central Statistical Office (CSO) 1997 Social trends, 1997 edn. HMSO, London
Chipman Y 1991 Caring: its meaning and place in the practice of nursing. Journal of Nursing Education 30(4): 171–175
Crigger N J 1997 The trouble with caring: a review of eight arguments against an ethic of caring. Journal of Professional Nursing 13(4): 217–221
Cummings J L 1980 Reversible dementia. Journal of the American Medical Association 243: 2434–2439
Dalley G 1996 Ideologies of caring, 2nd edn. Macmillan Education, Philadelphia
Dancy J Jr, Wynn-Dancy M L 1995 The nature of caring in volunteerism within geriatric settings. Activities, Adaptation & Aging 20(1): 5–12
Davis R 1997 Community caring: an ethnographic study within an organizational culture. Public Health Nursing 14(2): 92–100
Dillon R S, Stines P W 1996 A phenomenological study of faculty-student caring interactions. Journal of Nursing Education 35(3): 113–118
Downie R S (ed) 1994 The healing arts. Oxford University Press, Oxford
Dowson S 1995 Means to control. A review of the service brokerage model in community care. Values In Action, London
Dunstan E 1996 …And a time to die: the medicine of old age. British Medical Bulletin 52(2): 255–262
Evers H K 1991 Care of the elderly sick in the UK. In: Redfern S (ed) Nursing elderly people, 2nd edn. Churchill Livingstone, Edinburgh, pp 417–436
Farmer E S 1994 Multicompetence in professional caring. In: Harris J, Corbett J (eds) Training and professional development: an interdisciplinary perspective for those working with people who have severe learning disabilities. British Institute Of Learning Disabilities, Kidderminster
Fosbinder D 1994 Patient perceptions of nursing care: an emerging theory of interpersonal competence. Journal of Advanced Nursing 20: 1085–1093
Francis J 1995 Healthy alternatives. Community Care 1078: 20–26
Fraser B A, Hensinger R N, Phelps J A 1987 Physical management of multiple handicaps. Paul Brookes, Baltimore
Friedemann M-L 1991 Exploring culture and family caring patterns with the framework of systematic organization. In: Chinn P L (ed) Anthology on caring. National League for Nursing Press, New York
Gadow S 1988 Covenant without cure. In: Watson J, Ray M A (eds) The ethics of care and the ethics of cure. National League for Nursing Press, New York, pp 5–14
Gaut D A 1991 Caring and nursing: explorations in feminist perspectives. Introductory remarks. In: Neil R M, Watts R W (eds) Caring and nursing: explorations in feminist perspectives. National League for Nursing, New York
Gott M, O'Brien M 1990 The role of the nurse in health promotion (unpublished). RCN Research Society Conference, University of Surrey
Griffiths Sir Roy 1988 Community care: agenda for action. A report to the Secretary of State for Social Services. HMSO, London
Herd D, Stalker K 1996 Involving disabled people in services: a document describing good practice for planners, purchasers and providers. The Social Work Services Inspectorate, Edinburgh
Higgins B 1996 Educational innovations. Caring as therapeutic in nursing education. Journal of Nursing Education 35(3): 134–136
Hirsch S R, Harris J 1988 Consent and the incompetent patient: ethics, law and medicine. Gaskell, London
Hobson D A, Molenbroek J F M 1990 Anthropometry and design for the disabled: experiences with seating design for the cerebral palsy population. Applied Ergonomics 21(1): 43–54
Kikuchi J, Simmons H (eds) 1993 Developing a philosophy of nursing. Sage, London
Kitwood T 1997 Dementia reconsidered. The person comes first. Open University Press, Buckingham
Kleinman A 1988 The illness narratives: suffering, healing & the human condition. Basic Books, New York
Kubler-Ross E 1970 On death and dying. Tavistock, London
Larson P J, Dodd M J 1991 The cancer treatment experience: family patterns of caring. In: Gaut D A, Leininger M M (eds) Caring: the compassionate healer. National League for Nursing, New York, pp 61–78
Leininger M M (ed) 1988 Caring, the essence of nursing and health. Wayne State University Press, Detroit
Littlewood J, Scott R 1990 Screening the elderly. Health Visitor 63(8): 268–270
Lovgren G, Engstrom B, Norberg A 1996 Patients' narratives concerning good and bad caring. Scandinavian Journal of Caring Sciences 10(3): 151–156
Macintyre A C 1981 After virtue: a study of moral theory. Duckworth, London
McCance T V, McKenna H P, Boore J R 1997 Caring: dealing with a difficult concept. International Journal of Nursing Studies 34(4): 241–248
McMahon R 1988 The 24-hour reality orientation type approach to the confused elderly: a minimum standard for care. Journal of Advanced Nursing 13: 693–700
Maugham W S 1938 The summing up. Garden City, New York, p 290
Mental Health Act 1983 HMSO, London
Minick P 1995 The power of human caring: early recognition of patient problems. Scholarly Inquiry for Nursing Practice 9(4): 303–317
Moore S 1992 Case management and the integration of services: how service delivery systems shape case management. Social Work 37(5): 418–423
Murphy E 1988 Psychiatric implications. In: Hirsch S R, Harris J (eds) Consent and the incompetent patient: ethics, law, and medicine. Gaskell, London, pp 65–76
National Health Service and Community Care Act 1990 HMSO, London
Newham D M, Berrington A, Primrose W R, Seymour D G 1996 Self-funding and community care admissions to nursing homes in Aberdeen. Health Bulletin 54(4): 301–306
Obeid A, Ridout S 1997 Rationing elderly care. Journal of Community Nursing 11(1): 18–20
O'Berle K, Davies B 1992 Support and caring: exploring the concepts. Oncology Nursing Forum 19: 763–767
Omery A, Kasper C E, Page G G (eds) 1994 In search of nursing science. Sage, London
Open University 1988 Handbook of mental disorders in old age. The Open University Press, Milton Keynes
Osterman P, Schwartz-Barcott D 1996 Presence: four ways of being there. Nursing Forum 31(2): 23–30
Passant H 1990 A holistic approach in the ward. Nursing Times 86(4): 26–28
Pearson A (ed) 1988 Primary nursing: nursing in the Burford and Oxford nursing development units. Croom Helm, London
Pearson A, Borbasi S, Walsh K 1997 Practising nursing therapeutically through acting as a skilled companion on the illness journey. Advanced Practice Nursing Quarterly 3(1): 46–52
Peplau H E 1988 The art and science of nursing: similarities, differences, and relativities. Nursing Science Quarterly 1(1): 8–15
Redfern S J (ed) 1997 Nursing elderly people, 2nd edn. Churchill Livingstone, Edinburgh
Reimen D 1986 The essential structure of a caring interaction: doing phenomenology. In: Munhall P, Oiler-Boyd C (eds) Nursing research: a qualitative perspective. Appleton-Century-Crofts, Norwalk, pp 85–106
Roach S 1987 The human act of caring: a blueprint for the health professions. Canadian Hospital Association, Ottowa, Ontario
Robinson B, Lund C, Keller D, Cuervo C A 1986 Validation of a functional assessment inventory against a multidisciplinary home care team. Journal of the American Geriatric Society 34: 851–854
Rooney V M 1987 Toileting charts. Nursing 22: 827–830
Royle J A, Walsh M 1992 Watson's medical-surgical nursing and related physiology, 4th edn. Baillière Tindall, London
Ryan M, McAllister M 1996 The good samaritan: a revitalised narrative for nursing. Australian Journal of Holistic Nursing 3(1): 12–17
St Exupery A de 1943 The little prince. Harcourt, Brace & World, New York
Sandelowski M 1991 Telling stories: narrative approaches in qualitative research. Image: Journal of Nursing Scholarship 23(3): 161–166
Shapira J, Schlesinger R, Cummings J L 1986 Is it cortical or subcortical dementia? The answer makes a difference in nursing interventions. American Journal of Nursing 86(6): 699–702
Sharma S S, Aldous J, Robinson M 1994 Assessing applicants for Part III accommodation: is a formal clinical assessment worthwhile? Public Health 108(2): 91–97
Sherwood G D 1997 Meta-synthesis of qualitative analyses of caring: defining a therapeutic model of nursing. Advanced Practice Nursing Quarterly 3(1): 32–42
Sinclair F 1991 To touch your heart. Clay Pot, Edinburgh
Strickland D 1996 Applying Watson's theory for caring among elders. Journal of Gerontological Nursing 22(7): 6–11
Sullivan D 1988 The incapable patient and the law. In: Hirsch S R, Harris J (eds) Consent and the incompetent patient: ethics, law, and medicine. Gaskell, London, pp 1–8
Thompson A, Dobson R 1995 Death of an ideal. Community Care 1075: 20–21
UKCC 1992 Code of professional conduct for the nurse, midwife and health visitor, 3rd edn. UKCC, London

Ungerson C 1983 Women and caring: skills, tasks and taboos. In: Gamarnikov E et al (eds) The public and the private. Heinemann, London
Victor C R 1994 Old age in modern society: a textbook of social gerontology, 2nd edn. Chapman and Hall, London
Walsh M (ed) 1997 Watson's clinical nursing and related sciences, 5th edn. Baillière Tindall, London
Ward J, Rogers N, Brown R, Jeffries G, Wright D 1995 Techniques in anthropometry applied to disabled and elderly populations. Biomedical Sciences Instrumentation 31: 281–285
Watson J 1979 The philosophy and science of caring. Little Brown, Boston
Watson J 1988 Nursing: human science and human care: a theory of nursing. National League for Nursing, New York
Watson J 1997 The theory of human caring: retrospective and prospective. Nursing Science Quarterly 10(1): 49–52
WHO/ICN 1988 The age of aging: implications for nursing. World Health Organization, Copenhagen
Wolf M A 1987 Human development, gerontology and self-development through the writings of May Sarton. Educational Gerontology 13(4): 289–295

FURTHER READING

Benner P 1984 From novice to expert. Addison-Wesley, Menlo Park, CA
Carnevali D L 1993 Nursing management for the elderly, 2nd edn. Lippincott, Philadelphia
Chinn P L (ed) 1991 Anthology on caring. National League for Nursing Press, New York
Farmer E S (ed) 1996 Exploring the spiritual dimension of care. Quay Books, Salisbury
Ford P, Heath H 1996 Older people & nursing. Issues of living in a care home. Butterworth-Heinemann, Oxford
Jacques A 1992 Understanding dementia, 2nd edn. Churchill Livingstone, Edinburgh
Lawler J 1997 The body in nursing. Churchill Livingstone, Melbourne
Norman A 1991 Room for a view. Health Visitor 64(4): 103
Norman I F 1997 Mental health care for elderly people: assessment and planning. In: Redfern S (ed) Nursing elderly people, 2nd edn. Churchill Livingstone, Edinburgh
Redfern S J (ed) 1991 Nursing elderly people. Churchill Livingstone, Edinburgh
Stotter D 1995 Spiritual aspects of health care. Times Mirror International, London
Veatch R M, Fry S T 1987 Case studies in nursing ethics. Lippincott, Philadelphia

PEOPLE WHO USE AND ABUSE SUBSTANCES

David B. Cooper

36

INTRODUCTION

Q

36.1 In preparation for reading this chapter, carry out the following exercise:

(a) List as many legal and illegal substances you can think of. Beside each, briefly write your feelings, positive or negative, relating to these substances. For example, are they acceptable/attractive/frightening?
(b) Write a brief description of your feelings in relation to:
- illegal substance use and substance users
- alcohol use and problem drinkers
- tobacco use and smokers
- legal substances (e.g. prescribed medication, tea, coffee) and their users.

This chapter offers a basic introduction to substance use and substance use problems and outlines the important contribution that nurses can make to the care of people with such problems. The term 'substance' is used to refer both to legal substances (i.e. alcohol, tea, coffee, tobacco and prescribed medications) and to illegal substances such as cannabis, cocaine, opiates and opioids. Throughout the chapter it is emphasised that whatever the nature of substance use, it must be considered in the context of the individual's personal history and circumstances; stereotypes of the substance user must be abandoned in favour of a more individualised and holistic understanding of the person. As in all areas of nursing, interventions on behalf of patients with substance use problems must be based on thorough assessment and should involve the individual to the greatest degree possible, as a partner in care.

Because substance use will have physical, mental, emotional, social and economic implications for the individual, a multidisciplinary approach to treatment will help to ensure that all dimensions of the patient's situation are considered as she makes the difficult adjustments necessary to resolve a substance use problem (DoH 1995). Prochaska & Di Clemente's (1986) integrative model of change is outlined as one which will be especially relevant to nurses working in this area of care.

The importance of early detection cannot be overstressed. To assist nurses in all fields in recognising the signs and understanding the long-term effects of excessive or inappropriate substance use problems, the second half of the chapter outlines the physical and psychological effects of a range of legal and illegal substances. Alcohol use problems are discussed at some length in recognition of the high prevalence of alcohol-related illness in the UK. This is in keeping with Saunders & Marsh's (1999) suggestion that it is misleading to consider alcohol and drug misuse as separate entities given the many similarities between their social, psychological and medical implications.

In view of the wide range of psychoactive substances that can be obtained by legal or illegal means, and the wide range of therapies that are available to individuals who seek help, this chapter cannot hope to be comprehensive. Readers are urged to consult the 'Further reading' list when pursuing any topics of special relevance to their area of practice.

'Understanding drug use' is an interactive CD-ROM that provides an excellent overview of substance use problems and helps to put problematic substance use in perspective. Contact: The Drug and Alcohol Coordinator, Southern Public Health Unit, Bunbury, Western Australia (tel: +61 (08) 9792 2500; e-mail: raquel.willis@health.wa.gov.au).
Alcohol Use (Cooper 2000) offers an overview of alcohol use.

Definitions

Dependency and addiction

Drug dependency is described by the World Health Organization (WHO 1969, personal communication) as:

> …resulting from the interaction between a living organism and a drug, characterised by behavioural and other responses that always include compulsion to take the drug on a continuous or periodic basis in order to experience its psychic effects and sometimes avoid the discomfort of absence. Tolerance may or may not be present. A person may be dependent on more than one drug.

Dependency may be psychological or physical, or both:

- *Psychological dependency* is 'a condition in which a drug produces a feeling of satisfaction and a psychic drive that require periodic or continuous administration of the drug to produce pleasure or to avoid discomfort' (WHO 1974, personal communication).
- *Physical dependency* is 'an adaptive state that manifests itself by intense physical disturbances, i.e., the withdrawal or abstinence syndromes, which are made up of specific arrays of symptoms and signs of a psychic and physical nature that are characteristic for each drug type' (WHO 1974, personal communication).

Thus, dependency may develop when an individual becomes physically, socially or psychologically reliant on a substance such that life without it becomes intolerable. Dependency is not automatic. Any substance can be used without the user becoming dependent on it. At the same time, dependence on a substance does not necessarily lead to substance abuse (Saunders & Marsh 1999).

During the 1960s, many experts tried in vain to clarify the distinction between addiction and habituation. These two terms were subsequently abandoned in favour of dependence. It is therefore safe to assume that 'dependence' and 'addiction' refer to the same thing. However, an increasing number of professionals working within the substance use field believe that such labels as dependence and addiction are, at best, unhelpful in the treatment setting.

Other terms

Drug. The WHO Expert Committee on Drug Dependence describes the word 'drug' as 'a term of varied usage'. As a medicinal product, 'drug' can refer to 'any substance in a pharmaceutical product that is used to modify or explore physiological systems or pathological states for the benefit of the recipient' (WHO 1985). The term is also used to refer to substances of abuse, among which some people include alcohol, tobacco and caffeine.

Tolerance and cross-tolerance are generally understood in pharmacology as 'a decrease in response to a drug dose that occurs with continued use' and 'the development of tolerance to another substance, which the individual has not previously been exposed to, as a result of acute or chronic intake of a substance', respectively.

Drug abuse refers to the 'persistent or sporadic excessive use [of a drug] inconsistent with or unrelated to acceptable medical practice' (WHO 1969, personal communication).

Detoxication. This is a process of removing from the body the substance on which the individual is physiologically dependent. During this process, medication may be given and the patient is assisted in making adjustments to her lifestyle such that the substance is no longer needed. Detoxication is increasingly undertaken in the patient's home environment. Only severe cases in which complications have been identified require hospitalisation (Cooper 1994).

Withdrawal symptoms. These are best described as psychological and/or physiological reactions to the reduction or complete withdrawal of the substance of use. How long withdrawal lasts often depends on the previous use of the substance and on the nature and extent of both physiological and psychological dependence (Cooper 1994).

A MODEL FOR CHANGING ADDICTIVE BEHAVIOURS

As many as 250 different therapies are now available to individuals with substance use problems (Parloff 1980). In 1984, a conference held in Scotland aimed to 'develop a more comprehensive model of change for the treatment of addictive behaviours' (Prochaska & Di Clemente 1986). It was agreed that any model developed should be applicable to the many different ways in which people change, i.e. ranging from those requiring maximum intervention (in-patient care) to those needing minimal intervention, e.g. self-help manuals (Prochaska & Di Clemente 1986). This model also had to be applicable to the variety of dependency behaviours that individuals wish to change and, at the same time, to advance the understanding of how people change their behaviours, from the stage at which a problem is recognised to the point at which it is resolved.

Prochaska & Di Clemente (1986) proposed a model of change which is now widely accepted. This model provides a framework which can assist professionals in organising their knowledge and in making case management decisions. Prochaska & Di Clemente felt that this model should take account of the person who self-changes as well as the individual progressing through therapy and that it should be applicable to the wide range of dependency problems that exist. It should also help the therapist to synthesise the various treatment methods presently available.

The Prochaska & Di Clemente (1986) model is 'three-dimensional', integrating changes, processes and levels of change. The model comprises four stages — pre-contemplation, contemplation, action and maintenance — which may be conceived of as cyclical, thus allowing the individual to join or leave the process of change at any given stage (see Fig. 36.1). This model can be referred to as 'the integrative model of change' or 'the motivation to change model'. Its stages may be described as follows:

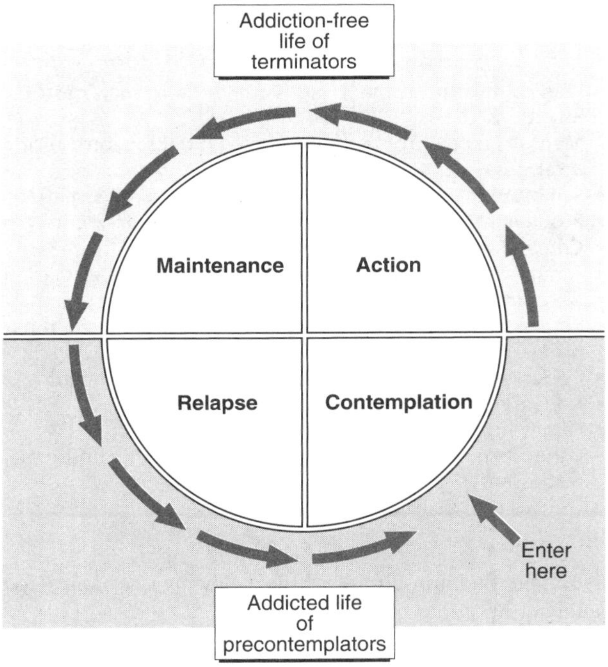

Fig. 36.1 The integrative model of change. (Reproduced with permission from Prochaska & Di Clemente 1986.)

- *Pre-contemplation stage.* At this stage the individual is not aware of her dependency. This could be because of ambivalence, denial or selective exposure to information. As the individual becomes aware of her problem, progression to the next phase is made possible.
- *Contemplation stage.* At this point the individual admits that something is wrong and begins to think seriously about changing her behaviour. This stage may last for a period ranging from a few weeks to many years, and some individuals never progress beyond this point.
- *Action stage.* Here, the individual makes a commitment to alter her problematic behaviour. This is a brief stage, as when the decision has been made the individual progresses to the next stage.
- *Maintenance stage.* At this point, new behaviour is strengthened and develops into self-efficacy; the individual's feeling of being in control is maximised. This stage affords the exit point to termination.

At the maintenance stage, the individual may temporarily lapse as a result of the extreme effort required to maintain the change in behaviour. Occasionally this extends to relapse, in which case the individual often goes back to the pre-contemplation stage before rejoining the cycle. Prochaska & Di Clemente (1986) suggest that 84% of 'relapsers' progress back into the contemplation stage. It would also appear that the typical self-changer makes three serious revolutions of the change cycle before exiting into a relatively dependency-free life (Schacter 1982, Prochaska & Di Clemente 1983). Some individuals do, however, become arrested at one particular stage.

It is essential that the individual and the professional are in agreement as to which stage of change is relevant at a given time. Any resistance to therapeutic interventions often comes as a direct result of the therapist and client working at different stages of the change process. Prochaska & Di Clemente (1986) explain the importance of this as follows:

> The more directive, action-orientated therapist would find a client who is at the contemplation stage to be highly resistive to therapy. From the client's perspective, however, the therapist may be seen as wanting to move too quickly....A therapist who specialises in contemplating and understanding the causes of problems will tend to see the client who is ready for action as resistive to the insight aspect of therapy. The client would be warned against acting impulsively. From the client's perspective...the therapist might be warned against moving too slowly.

In giving the Prochaska–Di Clemente integrative model of change practical application in their interventions with substance-using patients, nurses should never hesitate to seek help and advice from more experienced or knowledgeable practitioners. At the same time, nurses should strive to be well informed about all aspects of substance use. Nurses of all levels and specialities have contact with people with substance use problems and therefore need to be aware of the physical, social, psychological and legal consequences of dependency and the implications of these for the individual, her family and the nurse (English National Board (ENB) 1995, 1996a,b).

All nursing assessments should include investigations addressing substance use. While nurses become accustomed to asking about the most intimate details of bowel action or sexual function, many feel uncomfortable about broaching the subject of substance use. This may reflect a lack of basic knowledge, as well as a need to make such questioning routine. The following section is devoted to the question of how nurses can enhance their ability to recognise drug-related problems and initiate appropriate interventions.

THE ROLE OF THE NURSE

Even though our understanding of substance use problems has improved in recent years, there is still a tendency for nurses and other professionals to shy away from substance-using individuals as a client group. *Tackling Drugs Together* (DoH 1995) calls for all services to work together in an effort to supply effective interventions for those with substance use problems. A training needs analysis undertaken by the ENB (1995) identified a lack of pre- and post-basic nurse education and training, which resulted in the publication of the guidelines for curriculum development and education and training programmes currently being implemented in the UK (ENB 1996a,b).

Unfortunately, despite continued efforts by specialist workers, one still hears nurses make comments such as these:

- 'It's not right her being here; it's different when people have to come in through no fault of their own.'
- 'He's always coming in and out; never changes.'
- 'They're all psychopaths.'

Such statements are often offered as justification for inaction. The following exercise might help the nurse to imagine himself in the problem substance user's place.

Q **36.2** For 1 week, stop using your favourite substance, e.g. tea, coffee, alcohol, chocolate, tobacco. At the end of the week, make a few notes on the following:
(a) How easy did you find it to live without the substance?
(b) Was your mood affected? If so, in what way? Did you experience cravings?
(c) What strategies did you use to avoid temptation?

In his interactions with individuals with a substance use problem, it is important for the nurse to realise that the substance used forms only a small part of the problem. Each patient will present with a unique set of concerns, which may have caused, contributed to, or interacted with the development of the overall problem.

Those individuals experiencing substance use problems often change their behaviour as a direct result of a major life event, such as a change in an important relationship, an accident or illness, redundancy, a birth or a death. Such events can curtail, neutralise or enhance the nurse's endeavours with an individual (Davidson 1991) and must be taken into account in the formulation of treatment programmes. Davidson (1991) argues for an eclectic approach to treatment, in which all relevant professionals should intervene as necessary.

In carrying out his own work with the dependent individual, the nurse should be prepared:

- To identify the individual with a substance use problem
- To recognise the types of problems that are likely to be experienced by the individual
- To assist the individual in the process of acknowledging, exploring and understanding the substance use problem
- To appreciate the individual's own perception of the problem
- To consider with the individual the treatment options available
- To facilitate the individual's achievement of her chosen goal(s)
- To acquaint the individual with the services and facilities available to assist her
- To act in a non-judgemental way
- To provide nursing interventions in withdrawal
- To provide understanding and support should relapse occur.

Identifying substance use

Being aware of substance use and knowing when and how to seek advice can save valuable nursing time. Consider the example of a health visitor who is persistently requested to call on a mother and her crying baby. Each time, the mother is advised on feeding, comforting and how to rest while the baby sleeps. Despite these reassurances, the health visitor continues to receive requests to visit. Had the question of substance use been explored, it might have been realised that the woman's husband had a substance use problem. The couple was behind on rent, had insufficient money to buy food, and the husband was resorting to theft to fund his substance use. The mother's resultant anxiety was being sensed by the baby and expressed in the only way the child could, i.e. by crying. This example is not meant to imply that all parents with crying babies have substance use problems, but simply that substance use is a potential contributing factor in a wide range of problems and therefore should be considered and explored in initial and subsequent assessment.

Box 36.1 lists various signs that can indicate the existence of a substance use problem. The nurse should bear in mind, of course, that not every feature listed will apply to a given individual, nor does the existence of any one feature demonstrate conclusively that a substance use problem exists.

Box 36.1 Signs that may alert the professional to the existence of a substance-using client

- Physical health problem, e.g. vitamin deficiency, gastritis, infections, ulcers
- Mental health problem, e.g. anxiety, depression, suicide attempts
- Symptoms of substance use, e.g. tremor, shakes, sweating
- Problem at work, e.g. lateness, absenteeism, accidents
- Criminal offences
- Family problems, e.g. neglect, child disturbance, marital disharmony
- Requests for help, e.g. from the client, family or other professional
- Evidence of substance use, e.g. smell, used equipment
- Known history of substance use
- Family history of substance use
- Other, e.g. complaints of fatigue, lethargy, insomnia, restlessness

Nurses and substance use

It is equally important that nurses are aware of the high levels of stress that they experience in their professional lives, which can make them vulnerable to substance use problems (Coombs 1996). It is very hard for a nurse to broach this subject with a colleague whom he suspects of substance use. It is just as difficult for the nurse with a substance use problem to come forward and ask for help. The nurse who is beginning to face up to a substance use problem may find himself asking the following questions (Cooper & Faugier 1993):

- Will my colleagues find out details of my problem and treatment?
- If I cannot look after myself, how can others be entrusted to my care?
- Will treatment for a substance use problem be noted on my record and limit my professional development?
- How will I relate to the nurses who are caring for me?
- Will I be suspended, disciplined or asked to leave?
- Will I be considered responsible enough to continue in my profession if I accept help?
- How will I convince others that I can be trusted to hold drug cupboard keys?
- How can I impress on senior managers and nursing colleagues that any future time off from work is not due to the substance use?
- How will I arrange regular time off to keep my counselling appointments?

How nurses can get help

The nurse who has acknowledged to himself that he has a substance use problem should check to see if his health district has an 'alcohol (and drug) in the workplace' policy. If the problem has been brought into the open by a warning from an employer, then this policy will be invoked and the nurse referred to Occupational Health for further treatment. The nurse should make sure that the policy is duly followed. Although he will probably be under a contract by which improvement in work performance is required, the policy is usually in the nurse's favour, protecting his job security whilst he responds to agreed therapy and ensuring adequate time off to attend counselling and treatment sessions.

If the problem is one of alcohol use, the contract might not require the nurse to stop drinking altogether. However, if the problem is one of illegal substance use, total abstinence is the accepted outcome at the present time. The nurse will not, however, be rushed. It is normal procedure to refer an employee for professional help outside of the health district that employs him in order to ensure confidentiality.

The nurse does not have to be referred to Occupational Health by his employer. It is possible for him to approach Occupational

Health in confidence on his own. He will then be put in contact with a drug and/or alcohol advisory service. If the nurse has identified the problem himself, he may in fact wish to approach such an agency directly. Contact information can usually be found in the yellow pages or obtained from citizens' advice bureaux. Again, whether the agency is voluntary or statutory, it is bound by rules of confidentiality. It will, however, make contact with the nurse's Occupational Health department, if he so requires.

If a nurse feels that he has a substance use problem of any kind, which is affecting his work, it is best for him to seek help before formal measures by his employer become necessary. Following assessment, treatment goals can be set. The nurse should be free to progress at his own pace without the worry of being 'found out' and losing his job. He should not be considered weak at having to admit to a substance use problem or to feeling unable to cope with the stresses of his work. On the contrary — it takes courage and determination to come forward and make the first, and possibly most difficult, step towards change.

If the nurse's colleagues have already suspected the existence of a substance use problem, because of little errors (or larger ones) he has made at work, they may have already taken some responsibility away from him. As his improvement becomes apparent, their confidence will gradually be regained and responsibility will be handed back. It is important, however, that the nurse does not allow himself to be pushed into taking on more responsibility or a heavier workload than he feels ready for. Relapse is a real possibility and can be brought about by the nurse putting pressure on himself to make rapid change.

Approaching the patient with a suspected substance use problem

If the nurse suspects that a patient has a substance use problem, he should be careful to raise the question of the patient's substance use in a non-threatening manner. While the patient may be evasive or defensive at first, at least the nurse will have demonstrated his concern and made the first approach. The subject should not be belaboured at the initial stages, but the nurse should tactfully and sensitively try to progress at each contact. The nurse should remember that he is not a judge, but a facilitator, educator and carer.

Bedside conversations in large wards do not enhance confidentiality. Curtains round a bed do not block out sound. The nurse should consider where and how he would want to be approached if he were in the patient's situation and apply the same standards of confidentiality he would expect for himself in his interactions with others.

If the nurse feels unsure about how to proceed, he should seek advice and support and find out about local agencies that may be of benefit to his patient. The nurse should make contact with colleagues who have similar patients on their caseloads, as mutual support is essential in all areas of nursing.

Assessment

Any intervention can be undertaken only following a full and systematic assessment of the needs of the patient and her family. If treatment is to have a favourable outcome, a complete picture of the patient's substance use must be obtained. Moreover, a clear understanding of the patient's own treatment goals is essential. Does she want to achieve a reduction in use, a change to a less harmful substance, controlled use, withdrawal or total abstinence?

Many individuals with substance use problems 'sound out' a service before committing themselves to care. Therefore, any information given on treatment options should be clear and to the point, and should be communicated both verbally and in written form.

Assessment should include details of past and present substance use. In preparation, the patient could be asked to complete a diary similar to that shown in Figure 36.2. The following factors should always be considered in any assessment:

- psychological state
- work, social and cultural factors
- problematic effects of use
- motivation for treatment
- family psychodynamics
- relevant personal factors
- physical state and complications.

Prevention

Whether or not an individual develops a substance use problem often depends on the social resources available to her. It is vital that the problems and experiences that can set the stage for substance use problems are recognised by the caring professions and that the relevant agencies persevere in improving and developing preventive strategies at both local and national levels.

In recent years, campaigns such as 'No Smoking Day' and 'Drinkwise Day' have had some effect. Most health districts now have a drug and/or alcohol advisory service, as well as a health promotion officer dealing with HIV/AIDS-related issues (see Ch. 37). The introduction of such initiatives as outreach programmes and needle exchange schemes has also proved valuable in the early identification of substance users (see p. 1029).

Readers with a special interest in the area of prevention are referred to Keene (1997) and Watson (2000).

SUBSTANCE USE: SOME FACTS

LEGAL SUBSTANCES

Tea and coffee

> The sufferer is tremulous and loses his self-command; he is subject to fits of agitation and depression. He loses colour and has a haggard appearance. As with other agents, a renewed doses of the poison gives temporary relief, but at the cost of future misery (cited in Pickles 1991).

Coffee, tea, soft drinks such as Coca-Cola, and some analgesics contain caffeine, a substance that has a stimulating effect upon the central nervous system. Perhaps the reader will identify with some aspects of the above description of the effects of coffee drinking, written anonymously in 1909.

In the UK, 70% of the adult population drink coffee, whilst 86% drink tea. The daily caffeine consumption for this group has been estimated at 440 mg/person (Cosgrove 1992). The existence of a caffeine withdrawal syndrome is now accepted. Silverman et al (1992) stated that 'caffeine withdrawal can produce severe symptoms, and health care professionals should be aware of the problem'. Participants in their double-blind study underwent physical and psychological tests during a period of normal diet followed by a period of caffeine-free diet. Half the group, who received a caffeine supplement during the second period, reported

Day	Time drinking commenced and ended	Type and amount consumed	Mood prior	Mood after	Number of units consumed
Monday					
Tuesday					
Wednesday					
Thursday					
Friday					
Saturday					
Sunday					
Totals					

Fig. 36.2 Sample form for an alcohol use diary.

no significant change. The other half, who were given placebo drugs, recorded more headaches, increased use of analgesia and greater fatigue. Depression and anxiety scores were also abnormally high in this group.

Tobacco

It takes 7 seconds for the chemicals contained in tobacco smoke to produce an effect within the brain (Cosgrove 1992). These chemicals are stimulants and assist in the maintenance of performance in cases of fatigue and monotony. They alleviate stress and anxiety by producing relaxation and stimulation. The rapid decline of these effects, however, encourages further use, and dependence develops quickly. If tobacco use is stopped abruptly, depression, restlessness, irritability and craving may be experienced.

The United States Surgeon General's report for 1989 concludes that (US Department of Health and Human Services 1989):

- cigarettes and other forms of tobacco are addictive
- nicotine is the substance in tobacco that causes addiction
- the pharmacological and behavioural processes that determine tobacco addiction are similar to those that determine addiction to drugs such as heroin and cocaine.

The Health Education Authority (1996) reports that smoking is the largest single cause of preventable and premature deaths in the UK. In excess of 92 000 people die each year in England alone (HEA 1996). The estimated health cost of tobacco-related illnesses is between £1.4 and £1.7 billion a year (Centre for Health Economics and HEA 1997). It is estimated that 23% of 11-year-olds had at least tried smoking and by the age of 15 years old, 63% of girls and 59% of boys had done so (HEA 1996).

Consequences for health

The high cost of tobacco use to the nation's health is clearly demonstrated in Table 36.1. Tobacco use can also be a contributing factor in the development of pancreatic cancer, blood clots, lung infections, strokes, bronchitis, poor circulation, cancer of the mouth and throat, ischaemic heart disease, thrombosis and emphysema.

Women and smoking. A total of 28% of women smoke during pregnancy (HEA 1996), doubling the risk of underweight births, stillbirths and early infant deaths (HEA 1996). Krishna (1978) suggests that the health risks associated with tobacco use in women are increased in those 'who are poor, anaemic and have several children'. Fogelman & Manor (1988) also reported 'deficiencies in physical growth and intellectual development in children of women smokers'. It has been suggested that pregnant women who smoke run the risk of spontaneous abortion or of complications such as bleeding during pregnancy, premature detachment of the placenta and premature rupture of the membrane (Sidle 1982).

Reports have suggested a close link between smoking and sudden infant death syndrome (SIDS; Mitchell et al 1992, 1993). The incidence of cancer of the cervix is high among women who smoke heavily (HEA 1996), and women who smoke increase their risk of coronary heart disease, stroke, blood clots, pulmonary embolism, circulatory disease, and raised blood pressure and cholesterol levels (HEA 1996).

Table 36.1 Incidence of tobacco-related disease in the UK in 1988. (Adapted from HEA 1996)

Disease	*Number*
Lung cancer	32 300
Coronary heart disease	32 100
Chronic obstructive pulmonary disease (COPD)	22 000
Other cancers: buccal cavity, oesophagus, larynx, bladder, kidneys and cervix	11 300
Strokes	9000
Aortic aneurysm and atherosclerotic peripheral disease	2900
Peptic ulcers	1000

Passive smoking

Children and adolescents exposed to passive or second-hand smoking have been quoted as being at risk of the adverse effects of smoking. Impaired respiration, chest infections and asthma in children are more often associated with parental smoking than any other causative factor (Pagliaro & Pagliaro 1996).

The effect of this 'passive smoking' is receiving increased attention (Pagliaro & Pagliaro 1996). A report by the Independent Scientific Committee on Smoking and Health (Froggatt 1988) suggests that people who are subjected to the smoke of others have an increased risk (in the range of 10–30%) of developing lung cancer. The committee suggests that in view of the dangers of 'second-hand' smoke, 'non-smoking should be regarded as the norm in enclosed areas frequented by the public or employees, special provision being made for smokers, rather than vice versa'.

The effects of tobacco smoke on non-smokers can include nose, throat and chest irritations, breathing difficulties, coughing, red and runny eyes, headaches, dizziness, nausea, lack of concentration and decrease in lung function. Those with long-term health problems such as asthma, chronic bronchitis, allergies and heart problems are especially at risk. The WHO 'Charter against Tobacco' (see Box 36.2) is in part an attempt to assert the right of non-smokers to a healthy environment.

Box 36.2 WHO 'Charter against Tobacco'

- Fresh air, free from tobacco smoke, is an essential component of the right to a healthy and unpolluted environment
- Every child and adolescent has the right to be protected from all tobacco promotion and to receive all necessary educational and other help to resist the temptation to start using tobacco in any form
- All citizens have the right to smoke-free air in enclosed public places and transport
- Every worker has the right to breathe air in the workplace that is unpolluted by tobacco smoke
- Every smoker has the right to receive encouragement and help to overcome the habit
- Every citizen has the right to be informed of the unparalleled health risks of tobacco use

Cessation aids

It has been suggested that the majority of smokers would like to stop (Baldwin & Rogers 1996a). However, pharmacological and psychological dependence often prevents them from doing so. Some cessation aids contain nicotine, whilst others aim to reduce craving by producing an unpleasant taste when smoking takes place. It is not recommended that cigarette smokers switch to a pipe or cigars, as research has indicated that those who switch are more likely to inhale the smoke than those for whom these are the primary substance of use (Jarvis 1989). Baldwin & Rogers (1996a,b) produced a strong case for a controlled smoking programme involving gradual reduction in tobacco use.

Withdrawal symptoms experienced by smokers may last for a few weeks, although occasional cravings may occur for a few years after cessation.

The Health Education Authority produces two booklets which nurses may find useful for themselves or their patients: *How to Stop Smoking for You and Your Baby* and *A Smokers Guide to 'Giving Up'*.
Action on Smoking and Health (ASH) also produce a useful set of information sheets (see 'Useful addresses', p. 1032).

Alcohol

> 'I didn't really like the taste but the effect allowed me to be sophisticated and to feel good with others. I felt guilty at my unhappiness. I had a good husband, a nice house and healthy children. Everything I wanted really.
> 'I suppose I drank because I couldn't cope with the reality of life. As my drinking progressed I blamed others for any problems I had. If I couldn't cope with a problem, I would blot it out with alcohol.
> 'As my problems mounted I remembered as a teenager how alcohol took away my inhibitions, made me feel confident and able to converse. People liked me better then.' (A problem drinker.)

36.3 For a 1-week period, keep a daily diary of your alcohol consumption, using the format given in Figure 36.2. When you have read the following section, refer to your diary as you discuss with your colleagues your reactions to and reflections on your own alcohol use.

Alcohol is the most popular psychoactive substance used in modern society and is consumed by approximately 90% of the adult population in the UK. When used in moderation, it does little more than act as a social 'lubricant', lowering inhibitions and facilitating social interaction. Excessive, heavy and prolonged use, however, can have serious consequences for health.

Alcoholic drinks mainly comprise water and ethanol (alcohol) and are produced by the fermentation of fruits, vegetables or grain. Congeners are added to give the drink its distinctive flavour, taste and smell.

Units of alcohol

One unit of alcohol is that amount of a given drink which contains approximately 15 mg of pure ethanol. This is based on a standard measure purchased in a UK licensed premises of an average-strength drink, i.e. half a pint of beer, lager or cider, a single measure of spirits (e.g. whisky, gin, vodka), a standard glass of wine,

Table 36.2 Calculation of unit consumption for alcoholic drinks of various strengths. (Adapted from HEA 1989)

Type of drink	*Measure*	*Number of units*
Export beer	1 pint 1 can*	2.5 2
Strong beer or lager	1 pint 1 can*	4 3
Extra strong beer or lager	1 pint 1 can*	5 4
Strong cider	1 pint	4
Spirits	1 bottle	30
Table wine	1 bottle 1 L bottle	7 10
Sherry	1 bottle	13
Low-alcohol beers and lager	1 pint	0.66
Low-alcohol cider	1 pint	0.5

*1 can = $^{3}/_{4}$ pint.

a small glass of sherry or a measure of vermouth (or aperitif). Therefore, if a total of 2 pints of average-strength lager and a small sherry were consumed, the total number of units consumed would be 5.

However, since many varieties of alcoholic drinks of varying strengths are available, it can be very difficult to estimate how much alcohol one has consumed. Table 36.2 gives an approximate guide to the calculation of unit consumption for drinks of various strengths.

What is safe? It has been suggested that the following units represent maximum levels for 'safe' weekly consumption. Consumption above these levels can be expected to lead to health problems:

- *For men*: up to 21 units; not exceeding 4 units/day
- *For women*: up to 14 units; not exceeding 3 units/day.

Alcohol absorption and elimination

Alcohol is one of the quickest-acting orally administered substances. It is a toxic substance and the only organ capable of eliminating it from the body is the liver.

Alcohol passes chemically unchanged from the stomach into the blood supply within 5 minutes. Adding carbonated drinks, alternating alcohol with carbonated drinks, drinking on an empty stomach and drinking quickly may speed up absorption.

It takes approximately 30 minutes for alcohol levels to peak in the blood and 1 hour for the liver to eliminate 1 unit. Any other alcohol taken during this time will accumulate in the blood, awaiting processing. Therefore, if 8 units are consumed (e.g. 4 pints of lager or 4 double spirits) the liver will take approximately 8–9 hours to eliminate all the alcohol.

Health consequences of excessive alcohol use

Excessive, chronic or inappropriate alcohol use can lead to a wide range of health problems affecting virtually all parts of the body (see Fig. 36.3). In addition to the possible consequences of intoxication, excessive regular use and dependence (see Box 36.3), alcohol consumption (even at moderate levels) can interfere with the effects of many prescribed drugs such as oral contraceptives, antibiotics, anti-inflammatory agents, tranquillisers, antidepressants and diuretics. The habitual overuse of alcohol is associated with a number of psychosocial problems.

Long-term use and withdrawal. Tolerance develops quickly with the regular use of alcohol. Physical as well as psychological dependence can occur. Sudden withdrawal after excessive use can be accompanied by unpleasant symptoms such as sweating, increased anxiety, tremor, headache, thirst, nausea and occasional vomiting. Full delirium tremens and convulsions may also be experienced, but are rare.

Those who have suffered severe withdrawal symptoms in the past or who, following assessment, appear to be at risk will need a properly supervised withdrawal programme (Cooper 1994). Contrary to popular belief, it is possible for someone with an alcohol problem to return to 'normal' social drinking or controlled drinking.

Teenage drinking

The issue of teenage drinking in the UK has given rise to a certain degree of public alarm. Newspaper articles condemn the behaviour of young 'alcopop' drinkers and demand that underage drinking be stopped. Yet there is little evidence to suggest that the majority of teenagers do anything other than drink sensibly, or, indeed, that heavy consumption at an early age leads to excessive or chronic alcohol use in later life.

Box 36.3 Alcohol use: associated harm

Consequences of intoxication

- Accidents
- Acute poisoning
- Acute gastritis
- Drug overdose
- Epileptic-type seizures
- Head injury
- Suicidal behaviour

Consequences of excessive regular use

- Anxiety
- Cancer of the mouth/throat
- Depression
- Fatty liver
- Liver cancer
- Liver cirrhosis
- Pancreatitis
- Peripheral neuritis
- Phobic illness
- Sexual impotence
- Stomach haemorrhage

Consequences of dependence

- Alcoholic psychosis
- Anxiety
- Delirium tremens
- Depression
- Hallucination
- Paranoid states
- Polydrug abuse
- Withdrawal: epileptic seizures

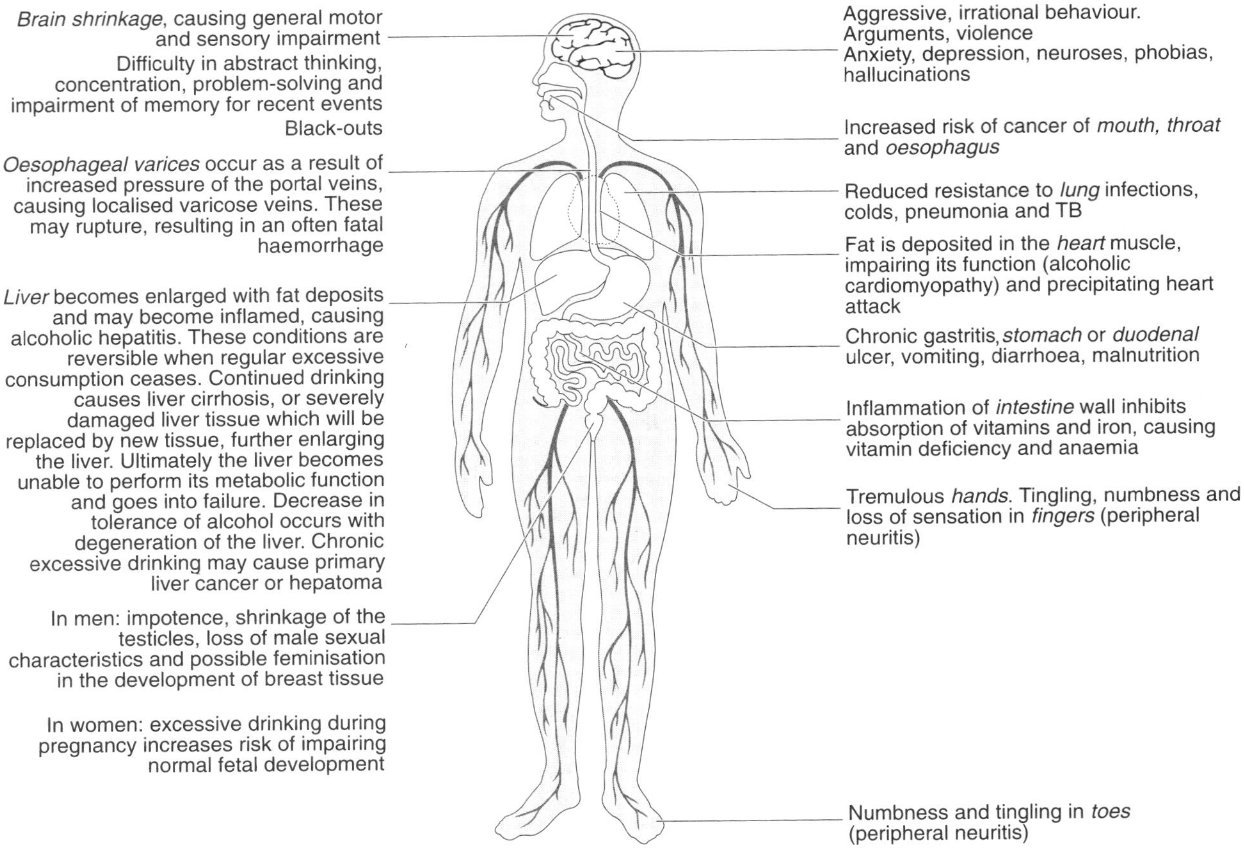
Brain shrinkage, causing general motor and sensory impairment
Difficulty in abstract thinking, concentration, problem-solving and impairment of memory for recent events
Black-outs
Oesophageal varices occur as a result of increased pressure of the portal veins, causing localised varicose veins. These may rupture, resulting in an often fatal haemorrhage
Liver becomes enlarged with fat deposits and may become inflamed, causing alcoholic hepatitis. These conditions are reversible when regular excessive consumption ceases. Continued drinking causes liver cirrhosis, or severely damaged liver tissue which will be replaced by new tissue, further enlarging the liver. Ultimately the liver becomes unable to perform its metabolic function and goes into failure. Decrease in tolerance of alcohol occurs with degeneration of the liver. Chronic excessive drinking may cause primary liver cancer or hepatoma
In men: impotence, shrinkage of the testicles, loss of male sexual characteristics and possible feminisation in the development of breast tissue
In women: excessive drinking during pregnancy increases risk of impairing normal fetal development
Aggressive, irrational behaviour. Arguments, violence
Anxiety, depression, neuroses, phobias, hallucinations
Increased risk of cancer of *mouth, throat* and *oesophagus*
Reduced resistance to *lung* infections, colds, pneumonia and TB
Fat is deposited in the *heart* muscle, impairing its function (alcoholic cardiomyopathy) and precipitating heart attack
Chronic gastritis, *stomach* or *duodenal* ulcer, vomiting, diarrhoea, malnutrition
Inflammation of *intestine* wall inhibits absorption of vitamins and iron, causing vitamin deficiency and anaemia
Tremulous *hands*. Tingling, numbness and loss of sensation in *fingers* (peripheral neuritis)
Numbness and tingling in *toes* (peripheral neuritis)

Fig. 36.3 Consequences of excessive consumption of alcohol. (Reproduced with kind permission from Alcohol Concern 1987.)

Children in our society do, however, encounter alcohol at an early age. Best & Barrie (1997) found that, in a sample of 147 young people aged 12–19 years, 91.9% drank alcoholic drinks. However, Coggans & McKellar (1995) suggest that 'despite the apparent high levels of alcohol-related disorders involving young people in recent years there is nothing new about the phenomenon'. The authors continue by suggesting that alcohol-related hooliganism has been with us for centuries!

Young people tend to be introduced to alcohol by their parents. Most are primed from an early age to accept alcohol as part of everyday life. While excessive alcohol use is a real problem for some teenagers, perhaps what is needed is not a demand for total abstinence among young people (since this would be unenforceable in practice anyway) but increased public education on the risks of inappropriate or excessive alcohol use, including the possible links with HIV/AIDS, promiscuous behaviour — including teenage pregnancy — and other substance use (Cooper 1998). Teenagers should be allowed to develop their own concepts about the appropriate use of alcohol in a straightforward and, most importantly, informed manner. A failure to be open in our approach to the subject of alcohol use may only serve to entice adolescents to explore this forbidden territory in a spirit of rebellion, without the benefit of adequate knowledge and experience.

Q **36.4** Do you think that there is a widespread teenage drinking problem in the UK? If so, how could you as a nurse help to prevent drinking problems among young people?

Women and alcohol use

It is generally acknowledged that alcohol-related problems amongst women are increasing (Plant 1997). However, this does not necessarily imply that women can consume the same quantities of alcohol as men before experiencing health consequences, since lower dose alcohol use can affects women's health. Women achieve a higher blood alcohol concentration than men. This occurs mainly because women have less body water than men, and therefore alcohol is less diluted within the body (Morgan 1992). There are key physical differences in the way a woman's body copes with alcohol. Factors concerning the female reproductive system can influence metabolism and play an integral part in alcohol-related problems (Plant 1997).

Women present to caring agencies with the same alcohol-related problems as men, e.g. gastritis, duodenal ulcers, peripheral neuritis, cancer of the mouth, throat or oesophagus, amnesic episodes and suicidal behaviour. However, women who drink excessively have a greater risk of acute inflammation of the liver than do men. Moreover, any damage to the liver in child-bearing years may increase in severity even after cessation (Plant 1997).

Stratton et al (1996) suggest that the heaviest drinking among women occurs in those aged under 30 years. Social factors such as marriage, a shortage of personal finance, responsibility for children and a lack of leisure time appear to moderate alcohol consumption (Plant 1997).

Societies still view women with substance use problems more critically than men and are quick to condemn women as weak, inadequate and as 'bad' mothers or wives when they have a substance use problem. When their partner develops a substance use problem, men appear to be generally less tolerant and supportive and more likely to leave a relationship than are women.

Women present to helping agencies with their own specific set of problems, which include guilt, low self-esteem and depression. This requires sensitive nursing skills. The individual needs to feel sufficiently at ease with a professional to disclose her substance problem. In order to gain the patient's confidence, the nurse must be non-judgemental, supportive and well informed about appropriate sources of help.

Alcohol in pregnancy. The Royal College of Psychiatrists (1987) suggested that whilst there is a link between excessive alcohol consumption and birth deformities, 'it is a misuse of that evidence to preach hellfire to every woman who takes a glass of wine during pregnancy'. The main problem is that, as yet, no one knows how much alcohol it is 'safe' to drink during pregnancy and few are willing to state a 'safe level'. The debate still continues, but there is a consensus that the greater the amount of alcohol consumed, especially during the early part of pregnancy (specifically pre- and post-conception in the phase when few would know of or have planned for conception), the greater is the risk to the future development of the fetus and child (Plant 1997).

There is, however, a recognised syndrome in babies of women who regularly consume large amounts of alcohol in pregnancy. Jones & Smith (1973) called this the 'fetal alcohol syndrome'. They recorded several features commonly found in babies of alcohol-dependent women, including growth deficiencies, delayed development, joint and heart abnormalities, microcephaly and fine motor dysfunction. Facial features included asymmetrical ears, receding chin, receding forehead, upturned nose and short palpebral fissure length.

Plant (1997) has attempted to put the problem into perspective by suggesting that there are several social factors which may influence birth defects, including tobacco and alcohol consumption and accommodation. Looking at specific levels of alcohol consumption during pregnancy, Plant found that 'women who consumed 10 units of alcohol on a single occasion during pregnancy were more likely than other women to have damaged offspring'. She suggested that low levels of alcohol consumption are not associated with birth defects.

Alcohol Concern's (1992) advice to women is as follows:

- drink in moderation
- avoid binge drinking
- cut down if you drink over 14 standard drinks per week; contact your GP, Alcohol Concern or your local alcohol advisory service
- take special care if you are pregnant.

36.5 Test your factual knowledge by answering the following questions.

(a) On average, how much (i) wine, (ii) spirits, (iii) beer, (iv) lager would you need to drink to be over the legal limit for driving?
(b) Which parts of the body are affected by alcohol, and what are the effects?
(c) What organ in the body breaks down alcohol?
(d) After drinking 1 pint of ordinary beer, how long will it take before the alcohol in it is completely burned up by the body?
(e) Which of these is an effective way of sobering up?
- Drinking a cup of strong black coffee
- Taking fresh air

36.5 *(cont'd)*
- Taking physical exercise
- Taking a cold shower
- Making yourself sick.

(f) What level of daily consumption is considered to lead to the possibility of alcohol dependence?
(i) 4 pints of beer
(ii) 8 glasses of wine
(iii) 2 single tots of whisky
(iv) 2 double tots of rum
(v) 6 glasses of fortified wine
(vi) 3 pints of lager.
(g) Is the recommended safe limit of drinking for women lower or higher than that for men?
(h) Equal amounts of alcohol have a greater effect on a young person than on the average adult male.
Why is this?
(i) What can speed up the effect of alcohol?

Alcohol and the older person

As the body ages, its ability to tolerate alcohol diminishes. The liver and kidneys become less efficient, and thus the elimination of alcohol from the body becomes slower. The effect of alcohol on reflexes, balance, self-control and judgement may compound existing health problems, increasing the risk of falls and other accidents. Equally, many older people take medication such as hypnotics, analgesics and anti-inflammatory drugs which, when mixed with alcohol, increase the risk of health problems.

Age can bring with it many difficulties such as financial hardship, loneliness, isolation, insomnia, pain and susceptibility to cold. (Note that a 'hot toddy' will not warm a person up. Alcohol dilates the blood vessels, allowing heat to escape and increasing the risk of hypothermia.) Many older people eat unbalanced diets and have a poor appetite; some may sacrifice food for alcohol.

Some older people may use alcohol to block out feelings of loneliness. Many of these individuals will find it hard to come forward for help, and it can sometimes be difficult for professionals to recognise alcohol and/or other substance use problems among this client group (Graham et al 1995, 1998, McKee 2000). The relatives of an elderly person may dismiss her drinking as a minor foible or take the view that alcohol helps her to cope. Nurses working in this field may hear relatives and carers expressing sentiments such as 'It will do her no harm' or 'What else has she got to live for?'. Even GPs have been known to suggest alcohol as a remedy for insomnia in older people. This can be unwise, as the physical, social and psychological effects of alcohol are often felt among this client group at a relatively low level of consumption.

Treatment. Older people who have come forward for help or who have been identified as having an alcohol-related problem often feel guilt and shame. In many cases, information on the sensible use of alcohol is all that is required to allay anxiety and enable the person to adopt healthier drinking habits. It is important to remember, however, that age does not make someone less able to make decisions about her own life. If the patient does not wish to reduce or modify her consumption, that is her choice. Professionals have a responsibility, nonetheless, to ensure that the individual has adequate information on which to base informed decisions (see Research Abstract 36.1).

See Graham et al (1995, 1998) and McKee (2000) for further reading on alcohol and the older person.

36.6 On the basis of the information given in this section, how would you define 'the sensible use of alcohol'? Can alcohol in any way be beneficial?

Tranquillisers

It is estimated that some 15% of the adult population of the UK have problems associated with prescribed medication (Cosgrove 1992). In 1995, nearly 13.9 million prescriptions for benzodiazepines were written in England alone (Government Statistical Service 1996). Among consumers of these drugs, women form the largest group, although there is a steady increase in prescriptions for men which appears to be associated with unemployment and poor employment prospects. The most commonly prescribed tranquillisers are benzodiazepines (diazepam, temazepam).

Seivewright (1998) suggested that tranquilliser withdrawal carries with it serious physical and psychological risks. Once dependent, it can be dangerous for the individual to cease abruptly. Therefore, it is essential that any withdrawal is gradual. Because the symptoms of withdrawal often mask the symptoms of the original complaint, dependence often goes unidentified until the substance is reduced or stopped or until tolerance develops. Symptoms are similar to phobic anxiety states and may include fear, agoraphobia, suicidal feelings and panic attacks.

Members of the caring professions have expressed concern over the lack of identification of those dependent on tranquillisers. Faugier (1992) claims that 'tranquilliser dependence has reached epidemic proportions, yet community nurses are not trained adequately to help those who are trying to cope with withdrawal'.

Many doctors have attempted to treat social problems with this group of drugs. Faugier (1992) remarks, however, that these drugs 'often produce quite disabling side effects which not only fail to solve the original problems, but, in fact, add to them significantly'.

Effects

The effects of tranquillisers commence within an hour of administration and last up to 12 hours. They include:

- relief from tension
- a sense of calm and relaxation
- decreased self-control, alertness, power of observation and level of dexterity
- control of anxiety
- short-term memory loss
- lowered inhibitions
- release of aggression
- the onset of sleep.

Research Abstract 36.1
A study of the effectiveness of brief interventions for problem drinkers in acute hospital settings

A consecutive series of 998 patients who were admitted to general medical, surgical, orthopaedic and short-stay wards of a large teaching hospital were screened to identify potential problem drinkers.

The screening procedure consisted of recording a retrospective diary of the previous week's level of alcohol consumption, a structured interview to assess the frequency of experience of alcohol-related problems and blood samples to estimate levels of gamma-glutamyl transferase (GGT), aspartate transferase (AST) and mean cell volume (MCV).

Of those screened, 24.5% reported levels of alcohol consumption during the previous week as being in excess of the recommended 'sensible limits' as suggested by the Health Education Authority (1989). On further investigation it was found that 153 patients were regular consumers of alcohol who had not previously received treatment for an alcohol problem. These were patients who were receiving treatment for a wide variety of health problems, which were not primarily alcohol-related.

The newly identified potential problem drinkers were assigned to one of four treatment groups as follows:

- *Group 1*. Patients in this group were given a copy of the Health Education Authority booklet entitled *That's the Limit: a Guide to Sensible Drinking*. This is a 14-page pamphlet, which contains advice about the effects of alcohol and how to reduce consumption to within recommended sensible limits.
- *Group 2*. Patients in this group were given brief advice in a one-to-one interpersonal interaction about the effects of alcohol consumption on health and about how to reduce consumption.
- *Group 3*. Patients were given both the booklet that was given to members of Group 1 and the advice as described for patients in Group 2.
- *Group 4* patients were given no intervention.

A nurse administered all the interventions.

One year later, 102 patients participated in follow-up interviews. It was found that the entire sample reported statistically highly significant reductions in the mean levels of alcohol consumption as recorded again by the diary method and also in the mean numbers of alcohol-related problems. These reductions were supported by statistically significant reductions in the mean levels of GGT and AST. Changes in MCV, however, did not reach the levels of statistical significance.

The patients in all groups, including the control group (who had received no treatment), demonstrated improvements in each of the self-report measures and also in liver function tests. The extent of the improvement reported by the control group was not significantly different from any of the three treatment groups.

It is possible that the nurse's detailed inquiry into the level of alcohol consumption at a time when people were unwell and therefore perhaps more receptive to advice relating to health was sufficient to cause them to consider their drinking habits and consequently reduce their consumption.

This does not require specialist experience of working with problem drinkers. The brief interventions described above are measures which can readily be carried out by nurses in a wide variety of health care settings. They are important because they have the potential to help nurses to recognise potential problem drinking at an early stage and, hopefully, to prevent the development of alcohol dependence.

Watson H E 1996 Minimal interventions for problem drinkers. Journal of Substance Misuse 1(2): 107–110

Box 36.4 Common tranquilliser withdrawal symptoms

- Convulsions
- Dry retching
- Hand tremor
- Headaches
- Increased tension/anxiety
- Irritability
- Loss of feeling/emotion
- Mental confusion
- Muscle pain/stiffness
- Nausea
- Nightmares
- Palpitations
- Panic attacks
- Personality change
- Profuse sweating
- Rebound insomnia
- Weight loss

With intoxication, the individual may experience dysarthria, ataxia, nystagmus and emotional lability.

It is not clear how long it will take an individual to become dependent, although an increase in anxiety has been noted after 4 weeks' use. By 6 months, the risk of dependency is greatly increased. Psychological dependence is common.

Tolerance can develop with both therapeutic and non-therapeutic use and withdrawal symptoms may occur even with therapeutic doses (see Box 36.4). Whilst these are not potentially fatal, they can be very unpleasant and have been described by some as worse than those experienced in heroin withdrawal.

Support during withdrawal

As withdrawal symptoms commence even after a small reduction in tranquilliser dosage, the withdrawal process needs to be undertaken in slow steps. It may take several months or even some years for the patient to be able to live comfortably without the substance.

Support, whether given individually or in a group, is essential. Nurses should be aware of the unpleasantness associated with tranquilliser withdrawal and the fear and emotional stress this process is likely to cause the individual and her family.

Useful information on the process of tranquilliser withdrawal can be found in Seivewright (1998).

Solvents

Many solvents, glues, gases and volatile substances are readily available in homes, shops, offices and factories. Under normal use, they are reasonably safe, but unfortunately they are sometimes inhaled specifically for their depressant effect on the central nervous system. Ives (1990) describes three kinds of solvent use among young people:

- experimental — by those who want to know what it is like
- recreational — by those who inhale solvents occasionally with friends
- dependent — regular, long-term use.

Seventy-five premature deaths per annum are associated with volatile substance use (Taylor et al 1998), with between 4 and 8% of secondary school youths claiming to have tried a volatile substance (Institute for the Study of Drug Dependence [ISDD] 1994).

The primary substances of use are adhesives, cleaning fluids, aerosols and fuels. The common street name for the use of these substances is 'huffing' or 'sniffing'. These substances are often inhaled in 'sniffing dens', which may be found by canals, in derelict buildings or on railway banks. These solvents are relatively easy to obtain and offer a cheap alternative to alcohol and other drugs.

Effects of solvent inhalation

Effects commence within 7 s of inhalation and last for approximately 30 min. Continual sniffing maintains the effect. As the level of intoxication is reduced, the user experiences nausea and headache. With the repetition and deep inhalation, overdose may result, causing loss of control, disorientation and unconsciousness. On cessation, recovery usually follows quickly. Concentration of the substance and intensification of effects can be achieved by placing a plastic bag over the head. This method brings with it the danger of asphyxiation.

It is not easy to identify use, as the presenting problems may appear to be similar to behaviour associated with 'normal' adolescent development, e.g. moodiness, aggression, loss of appetite, disinterest and aloofness. With regular use, tolerance may develop. Whilst physical dependence does not appear to occur, psychological dependence has been suggested as a problem in a small number of users.

Dangers of excessive and frequent use. It is important for the substance user to avoid exertion, as this may affect the function of the heart and increase sensitivity. Any exercise may lead to collapse and death. Other dangers include damage to the liver, lungs, kidneys, heart and central nervous system, as well as death by suffocation, accidents, direct toxic effect on the heart and inhalation of vomit. Gas squirted directly into the mouth can cause suffocation.

Ives (1990) itemises the range of approaches to prevention and intervention that are adopted in relation to solvent abuse:

- collecting information
- doing nothing
- using scare tactics
- policing
- providing information and education
- offering activity substitution: individual or group
- providing individual counselling or therapy
- encouraging parental education and involvement in treatment
- offering family counselling or therapy
- organising self-help groups for sniffers
- educating professionals
- organising community action.

36.7 As a nurse who may at some stage come into contact with solvent users, consider which method or combination of methods listed above would be most effective, and why? What other measures can you think of? How would you introduce them?

For practical advice on this area of care, the reader is referred to Ives (1990) and a report by the Advisory Council on the Misuse of Drugs (1995).

ILLEGAL SUBSTANCES

Rave or dance club culture

The 'rave' or dance club culture has become popular among some young people over recent years. It has been suggested that there is a strong link between the music played at events attended by young people and substance use. Case History 36.1 describes one teenager's brief flirtation with substance use, as recalled from diary entries.

Opiates and opioids

Opiates are derived from the sap of the opium poppy (*Papaver somniferum*). They are narcotic analgesics. Their synthetic equivalents are collectively known as opioids.

Heroin

Heroin ('H' or 'smack'), a narcotic made from morphine, can be sniffed, injected ('shooting' or 'mainlining') or smoked over tinfoil through a small tube ('chasing the dragon'). The purity of the drug is often unknown, and consequently accidental overdose can easily occur and may be lethal.

Heroin users who share needles and syringes ('works') are at risk of septicaemia, hepatitis and HIV/AIDS (see Ch. 37).

The effects of heroin include euphoria, drowsiness and a sense of well-being and raised self-esteem. Tolerance develops quickly, demanding increased intake to achieve the desired effect. Physical and psychological dependence may follow. Contamination of the substance often leads to severe allergic reactions, which may be exacerbated by poor diet and self-neglect. This degenerative process may lead to death if medical care is not available. Withdrawal is unpleasant and is often described as being 'like a severe dose of flu'. Other problems include constipation and vomiting. Complaints of diarrhoea, abdominal cramps and muscle spasm are common. Although it has been suggested that withdrawal from heroin is easier than withdrawal from nicotine or methadone, it should be attempted gradually, using reducing doses of methadone as a heroin substitute.

Case History 36.1 G

G is an 18-year-old art student. His illegal substance use commenced when he was 16 years old, when he first smoked 'grass' at a sixth form party. He is a smoker (10–20/day) and drinks alcohol, mainly for effect, i.e. to 'get merry'. His favoured drinks are 'Thunderbird' wine and 'Merrydown' cider, because they are cheap.

G's regular use of recreational 'ganja' (cannabis) began when he commenced college in October 1990. He took his first dose of 'speed' (5 g) in July 1991. On the second occasion, G also 'took a trip' (i.e. on 'half a paper' of LSD). He recalled:

> 'I felt very energetic and got the verbals. My arms and legs tingled and I kept getting head rushes when I stood up. These were very bad. I felt as if I had lost control. I knew where I was; it gave me a confidence boost. You can dance for ages at raves without feeling tired.
>
> 'In September 1991, I went to a college rave; I took half a gram of speed and half an E [ecstasy]. The effect depends on your mood. If you are in a thinking mood, it does your head in. I got very verbal that night.
>
> 'In November my parents found out and we had a row. I went out to an all-nighter. I took 1 g of speed and also used amyl nitrate. If you sniff this it gives you an amazing head rush, it distorts noises and you see spots in front of your eyes and feel really light.
>
> 'On Boxing day I took Triple X. It took 2 hours to work, then it started. I felt good and talked a lot. I had to keep on top of it, otherwise you get very confused, and you don't know what to do — dance, talk, stand up, sit down. Sometimes it's enjoyable, sometimes it isn't. The music really scared me. It was hard core and got really deep in my head. I just had to sit down. If you use Vicks inhaler on your eyelids or the back of the neck, or sniff it, it brings on a rush. Certain songs can also bring on a rush.'

Over the next 5 weeks G's drug intake increased. His diary extracts are as follows:

Jan 10th: Got 2 Es, white tablets, wasn't sure what they were. I did a lot of talking and got really worried. Real heavy head rushes; I started tripping badly. Curtains and carpets were moving in and out, a man was moving in and out of himself. I saw this picture, the eyes were moving, then a skeleton appeared and the hair grew. It was 26 hours before I could get to sleep. I was out of it, it got bad, and I just wanted it to stop. I felt paranoid, as if everyone was talking about me, they didn't like me. I smoked ganja to make me feel tired.

Jan 14th: Got 2 Es, £15 each, they must have been bad, I didn't get off.

Jan 11th: Took 1 1/3 trip and went off on a mission.

Jan 18th: 1 g of speed.

Jan 25th: Had 2 Es, started in 20 minutes.

Feb 3rd: 1 g speed. I got caught in disco toilets and was made to leave.

> 'I started to think what I was doing, making a mess of myself, getting in a mood with everyone. It seemed the night was all I was waiting for, I was getting off too often. When I first took them I swore it would be the only time, that I would never take E. Then only at raves. I realised I was getting in deep. Everyone had realised except me.
>
> 'If it were not for the drugs then there would be no raves. They are made for people on them, the music entices you. If I had carried on it would have turned nasty. I just felt very depressed all the time, except when I took drugs.
>
> 'I'm staying clear of the music. I think I'll be OK. Things actually got worse when my parents confronted me. I thought, mind your own business, you don't understand, it's my life, nothing to do with you.
>
> 'Dealers spot you; they just walk around and ask as soon as you walk in. I buy my drugs then supplement them with Pro-plus. I'd take 10 tablets [Pro-plus] and 1 g speed, it does give you a buzz but not like the hard stuff.
>
> 'I had offers to sell. It's OK taking them yourself, but not to give it to others. That's out of order. It's up to them.
>
> 'I don't think I'm the strongest person mentally, I get easily led. I suppose as a one-off it is worth it for the experience but it's not worth doing it. I've seen my mates mess themselves up, all they talk about is drugs and raves. It was a hard 5 weeks.'

Stimulants

Amphetamines

Amphetamines ('speed', 'amphs' and 'whizz') are currently very popular. These substances can be sniffed, injected or taken in tablet form. Initially introduced for the treatment of depression and as appetite suppressants, they are now rarely prescribed. Their main source of supply is therefore the illegal market.

The effects of these substances can last for up to 5 hours and include an increase in pulse and respiration, reduced fatigue and increased muscular activity. The individual becomes restless and over-talkative. Weight loss and excessive body fluid loss are potential complications.

The user may complain of headache, tiredness and lack of social interest. During intoxication, accidental injury and death may occur as a consequence of irrational behaviour. Amphetamine overdose may cause fever, paranoid psychosis, respiratory failure, hallucinations, seizures, coma, disorientation and cardiovascular collapse.

There are no specific withdrawal symptoms, although the user may complain of lethargy, prolonged sleep and excessive hunger. Psychological dependence is a major obstacle to successful withdrawal, and much individual support and counselling will be needed.

Cocaine

Cocaine ('coke', 'snow' or 'toot') is an alkaloid derived from the coca plant, a shrub native to South America. This white crystal-like powder is a powerful but short-acting stimulant. It can be sniffed ('snorted'), injected or smoked (in the form of 'crack'). Occasionally it is mixed with heroin to maximise the effect ('speedball'). When cocaine is treated with baking powder and water, it forms into tiny chalk-like lumps or 'rocks' and is referred to as 'crack'.

The effects of cocaine peak within 30 minutes and then gradually decrease. The user experiences a tremendous feeling of physical and mental power. This physiological arousal and euphoria lead to an indifference to pain and fatigue. Normal requirements for food are decreased. Large doses may lead to agitation, anxiety, hallucinations and erratic behaviour.

Dependence is usually psychological. The individual may complain of depression, fatigue and inability to cope. Chronic use may cause restlessness, nausea, sleeplessness, paranoid psychosis, hyperexcitability and severe depression. Repeated sniffing also leads to erosion of the nasal membrane.

Hallucinogens

Hallucinogens (psychedelics, psychotomimetics or psychotogens) include LSD (lysergic acid diethylamide), hallucinogenic mushrooms and cannabis. The prime effect of these substances is the alteration of perceptual functions of the brain.

Cannabis

It is generally believed that, when used occasionally, cannabis has no long-lasting effects and is safer than alcohol. Cannabis, a preparation of the hemp plant, is available in three forms:

- 'grass', a dried leaf (marijuana)
- resin, a compact block ('hash')
- oil, the most highly concentrated form.

It has been suggested that cannabis may play an important role in pain and symptom relief in multiple sclerosis sufferers and some cancers (Stimmel 1997). At present, such use is illegal according to UK law; however, the debate rightly continues around legalisation for specific medical use. One would eventually hope that common sense will prevail and legalisation will follow. Until then, a significant number of this client group is denied effective legal clinical intervention.

Cannabis is usually mixed with tobacco and smoked (as a 'joint'), although occasionally it is eaten or baked. The immediate effect is one of relaxation, talkativeness and hilarity. Intensification of sound and colour may also be experienced. There is a reduction in short-term memory function and in motor skill. Concentration is poor. These effects last up to 1 hour after social use.

High doses of cannabis can lead to confusion. However, the main health hazard appears to derive from the inhalation of tobacco smoke. The use of cannabis is often transient and it has been suggested that in order to experience the desired effects one has to be taught by a more competent user what to expect and how to inhale the smoke correctly to maximise effect and minimise the initial nausea (Emmet & Nice 1996).

Lysergic acid diethylamide (LSD)

LSD is a derivative of ergot, a fungus commonly found on rye and other grasses. An exceedingly potent substance, only minute doses of LSD are required to achieve a hallucinogenic effect.

The short-term user experiences a 'trip', in which hallucinations, disturbance of perception, increases in awareness, disorientation and disassociation from the body may occur. These experiences commence within 30 minutes following ingestion and peak 2–6 hours later, gradually fading after 10 hours.

Excessive and long-term use can cause prolonged psychological reactions and re-experiencing of past 'trips' ('flashbacks'). However, LSD is not known to cause physical dependence.

'Magic' mushrooms

There are approximately 12 varieties of mushrooms which contain hallucinogenic chemicals. The most common of these is *Psilocybe semilanceata* ('liberty cap').

'Magic' mushrooms contain two active ingredients, psilocybin and psilocin. The mushrooms may be crushed, eaten fresh, brewed in a tea or cooked in soup. The user experiences effects similar to those of LSD, along with euphoria, hilarity, increased heart rate and blood pressure, and dilated pupils. Commencing within 30 minutes, the effects peak at approximately 3 hours and last 4–10 hours.

Dependence, withdrawal and overdose are unlikely, the primary danger to health lying in the possibility that the individual may pick and consume a poisonous mushroom by mistake.

Ecstasy (E)

Ecstasy is, like heroin and cocaine, a class A substance. There is much debate about ecstasy's recreational drug use with much publicity following the death of an individual. It is acknowledged that the reader may have some preconceived views, experiences and attitudes about ecstasy use and it may be useful to provide some time for reflection.

36.8 Take 30 minutes to write down your feelings, attitudes and experiences relating to ecstasy. Once you have completed this task, read the following articles (cf. 'References', p. 1030): Pates (1998), Handy et al (1998), Fromberg (1998), Jones (1998) and Saunders (1998). These articles attempt to put the use of ecstasy into perspective. Once you have completed your reading, spend 30 minutes repeating the above essay and see how and/or if your opinions have changed and why you think this is.

36.9 Consider the evidence for and against the main aspects of substance legislation. Discuss the following quotations. How convincing are the arguments? Should illegal substances be legalised? Explain your reasoning.

(a) 'Legalising doesn't mean approval, it means control. It brings [the problem] into the open... [The legalisation of drugs would reduce drug-related problems by] saving money on law enforcement, unblocking courts and reducing prison overcrowding...[It would also] improve civil liberties and reduce the spread of HIV/AIDS.

[We should abolish] all offences related to cannabis. If this works it should be followed by other drugs...If consumption increases, [we should] stop and rethink the strategies. The sale of drugs to children should remain an offence, as it is with alcohol and tobacco...If someone becomes so addicted to a drug that he becomes a harm to others or his or her self, then the courts should be able to send him or her for treatment.' (Pickles 1991)

(b) 'Drug problems will not be beaten out of society by yet harsher laws, lectured out of society by yet more hours of "health education", or treated out of society by yet more drug experts. There is a place, however, for legislation and education and treatment.' (Royal College of Psychiatrists 1987).

SUPPORT AGENCIES

Outreach workers

There are three main kinds of outreach worker in the field of substance rehabilitation. Some, mainly nurses or health promotion officers, are employed professionals. Others are unpaid or paid scripted users or ex-users. Whatever their background, the aim of these workers is to facilitate access to caring services for individuals who want to deal with a substance use problem. An example of how outreach work might be carried out is given in Box 36.5.

Professional outreach workers

These workers are usually nurses or health promotion officers; some have dual qualifications. They work independently of the alcohol and/or drug advisory service and their main function is to provide health education and health delivery at the 'grass roots' level. Advice on general care issues, substance use and safe practices is given with the aim of increasing the number of substance users coming forward to seek professional help.

Existing scripted users: unpaid

These outreach workers already live, work and socialise with other users. Their aim is to deliver a health promotion message, e.g. harm minimisation and HIV/AIDS advice, and to promote the idea that local agencies are 'user friendly'.

Ex-users and existing users: paid

In most cases employed by alcohol and/or drug advisory services, these individuals are detached youth workers dealing with all welfare aspects of substance use. Their aim is to increase levels of understanding, to give information on safer substance-using practices and to encourage attendance at substance clinics for appropriate interventions.

Readers who would like to know more about this type of work are referred to Gilman (1992).

Box 36.5 Outreach work: an example

The outreach worker may go to a pub, dance club or 'rave'. During the evening, he may meet up with an existing contact, who during the course of a conversation may introduce the worker to an associate who would like to talk (this form of contacting is often referred to as 'snowballing'). This individual may be experiencing substance use problems or problems with her GP. In the case of a health care problem, the worker may be able to facilitate 'harm minimisation' (see below). For example, the user may be advised to go for a health check or for HIV/AIDS and hepatitis B and C testing, or she may be informed about how to obtain clean 'works'. In some cases, the worker undertakes these tasks, dealing with the problem on street level.

As the user's trust develops, the worker may bring a colleague along to a meeting or encourage attendance at a clinic. This process gradually leads to a deeper level of care and involvement with the community drug team.

Harm minimisation

Harm minimisation is a form of intervention which has given rise to much controversy. It is a process by which substance users are advised on safe methods of substance use rather than being urged to abstain. The user is offered blood tests and health checks, is given advice on safer using practices and is supplied with clean 'works' and condoms. The underlying philosophy is that while it may be impossible to eradicate altogether the illegal use of substances, it is nonetheless beneficial for individuals and society to make existing substance use as safe as possible (see Ch. 37).

Needle exchange schemes. Usually operated by drug and/or alcohol advisory services, these schemes aim to distribute clean needles, syringes and containers with a view to preventing the sharing of equipment and thus reducing the spread of infection. These schemes also allow for access to this equipment as well as health promotion materials and advice, e.g. on cleaning equipment and on safe sexual practices.

Some pharmacists, GPs and community psychiatric nurses offer this service. Needle exchange schemes also facilitate the safe disposal of used equipment and help in maintaining the link between the user and helping agencies.

Voluntary and professional agencies

Local services

Most health districts have a drug and/or alcohol advisory service, usually staffed by specialist nurses, social workers and administrators. Other professionals such as health promotion officers, occupational therapists, doctors/consultants and probation officers may also be attached to the team.

These teams offer help, advice, information, health education, treatment and counselling for the substance user and her family or close associates as well as for health care professionals. Some districts have a similar, voluntary service staffed by trained counsellors. Contact with these services can be made via the yellow pages, citizens' advice bureaux, community health councils or sector managers and nurse tutors. Some regional alcohol and/or drug treatment units still operate, offering outpatient and in-patient treatment, usually on a 6-week basis. However, access to these may be difficult to obtain and usually requires a doctor's recommendation.

National bodies

Technical information and advice relating to voluntary services may be obtained by making contact with the following organisations (relevant addresses are given on p. 1032):

- Alcohol Concern
- Standing Conference on Drug Abuse (SCODA)
- Re-Solv
- The Addictions Forum.

Support groups

Statutory and voluntary drug and/or alcohol advisory services may offer group therapy in a variety of formats. Membership of these groups may be open or closed, and may be for men only, women only or mixed. Some aim for total abstinence, others for controlled use. Some groups are set up to provide support for family members.

'Drinkwatchers' is organised on lines similar to 'Weight-watchers'. Total abstinence is not a requirement. Alcoholics Anonymous (AA) and Narcotics Anonymous (NA) are self-help organisations offering individual and group support. Total abstinence is required. Al-Anon, Al-Ateen and Families Anonymous are run on similar lines to AA and NA groups to provide self-help for the families and friends of substance users. Tranquilliser support groups have also been established to offer support and encouragement to individuals during the often long and difficult process of withdrawal.

Additional programmes undertaken by drug and/or alcohol advisory services may include group psychotherapy, social skills training, relaxation, family therapy, education and prevention, and telephone support. Most teams are able to access intensive residential courses, 'dry' hostels and other care facilities. Each of these offers a particular philosophy of care. The service provider usually agrees admission following assessment.

Q

36.10 *Tackling Drugs Together* (DoH 1995) suggests that all workers should have knowledge of the services and facilities available to them and how to access these. Produce your own 'resource catalogue' using the information and addresses contained within this chapter. In addition, to increase your familiarity with the services available in your own health district, carry out the following project:

(a) Research all local resources which may assist you in the care of your patient, whether this would be with advice, help, information or statistics. Don't forget self-help groups and counselling services such as the Samaritans, as well as mother-and-toddler groups, which may provide much-needed support for a mother under stress.
(b) Prepare a file card or computer database on each group, listing the contact name, address, phone number and type of help offered.

CONCLUSION

This chapter has attempted to provide an introduction for the nurse to the many issues surrounding the care of individuals who use substances and who may or may not have a problem with that use. While work with this client group can constitute a specialism within nursing, the need for nurses in every field to be aware of the signs and the consequences of substance use cannot be overemphasised (ENB 1995, 1996a,b).

Substance use problems occur in every age group and social class. Within the family, substance use problems may have serious implications not only for the individual directly affected, but also for her spouse or partner and children. Indeed, the nurse may first detect the existence of substance use not through his contact with the substance user, but through his interactions with family members. It is vital that nursing interventions undertaken in response to substance use are based on an assessment not only of the individual herself but also of her family circumstances.

As in many areas of nursing, prevention and education show the way forward (Watson 2000). When averting or changing from substance use, be that use problematic or otherwise, individuals must be given adequate information on which to base free and informed decisions. Nurses working with substance users may find that, in order to be more responsive to the needs of their clients, they must venture beyond traditional clinical settings into outreach work. In any event, rehabilitation will demand a holistic approach in which the unique identity of the individual is not lost sight of, and in which all aspects of her physical, mental and social well-being are addressed by the cooperative efforts of a multidisciplinary team.

One might add that nurses are in a privileged position by virtue of their close and frequent contact with patients. They are often seen as the 'human face' of community and hospital health services and are perceived to be 'on the patient's side' — practical, approachable and down-to-earth. Nurses are well placed to listen to, support, advise and inform their patients. Nursing the substance-using individual can offer a particularly challenging and rewarding context for the practice of these invaluable skills.

Q

36.11 Now that you have read through the chapter, repeat exercise 36.1, taking note of the following:

- Have your feelings changed? If so, in what way? What new information influenced this change?
- Are there any areas that you feel you need to investigate further? What are these and what sources could you use?

REFERENCES

Alcohol Concern 1987 Teaching about alcohol problems. Tutor and student manual. Woodhead & Faulkner, Cambridge

Alcohol Concern 1992 A woman's guide to alcohol. Alcohol Concern, London

Baldwin S, Rogers P 1996a Controlled smoking (part I): a last resort. Journal of Substance Misuse 1(2): 61–118

Baldwin S, Rogers P 1996b Controlled smoking (part II): a last resort. Journal of Substance Misuse 1(3): 119–178

Best D W, Barrie A 1997 Impact of illicit substance activity on young people. Journal of Substance Misuse 2(4): 181–224

Centre for Health Economics and the Health Education Authority 1997 Cost effectiveness of smoking cessation interventions. The University of York and the HEA, London

Coggans N, McKellar S 1995 The facts about alcohol, aggression and adolescence. Cassell, London

Coombs R H 1996 Addicted health professional. Journal of Substance Misuse, 1(4): 187–194
Cooper D B (ed) 2000 Alcohol use. Radcliffe Medical Press, Oxford
Cooper D B 1994 Alcohol home detoxification and assessment. Radcliffe Medical Press, Oxford
Cooper D B 1998 Editorial: If I pretend it does not exist will it go away? Journal of Substance Misuse 3: 4, 187–188
Cooper D B, Faugier J 1993 Substance misuse. In: Wright H, Giddey M (eds) Mental health nursing – from first principle to professional practice. Chapman and Hall, London
Cosgrove S 1992 Hooked: facts and myths surrounding drugs. Video (6 parts), Granada Television
Davidson R 1991 Facilitating change in problem drinkers. In: Davidson R, Rollnick S, MacEwan I (eds) Counselling problem drinkers. Tavistock, London, pp 3–20
Department of Health (DoH) 1995 Tackling drugs together: a strategy for England 1995–1998. HMSO, London
Emmett D, Nice G 1996 Understanding drugs: a handbook for parents, teachers and other professionals. Jessica Kingsley, London
English National Board for Nursing, Midwifery and Health Visiting (ENB) 1995 Training needs analysis. ENB, London
English National Board for Nursing, Midwifery and Health Visiting (ENB) 1996a Substance misuse – guidelines for good practice in education and training of nurses, midwives and health visitors. ENB, London
English National Board for Nursing, Midwifery and Health Visiting (ENB) 1996b Curriculum guidelines for education programmes for substance misuse. ENB, London
Faugier J 1992 What price tranquillity. Nursing Times 88(3): 22
Fogelman K R, Manor O 1988 Smoking in pregnancy and developing into adulthood. British Medical Journal 297: 1233–1236
Froggatt P 1988 Fourth report of the independent scientific committee on smoking and health. HMSO, London
Fromberg E 1998 Current opinion: ecstasy: the Dutch story. Journal of Substance Misuse 3(2): 89–94
Government Statistical Service 1996 Prescription cost analysis in England 1995. Department of Health. National Health Service Executive, London, pp 83–85
Graham K, Clarke D, Bois C, Carver V, Marsham J, Smythe C 1998 Depressant medication use by older persons in the broader social context relating to use of psychoactive substances. Journal of Substance Misuse 3(3): 161–169
Graham K, Saunders S J, Flowers M C, Birchmore Timney C, White-Campbell M, Ziedman Pietropalo A 1995 Addiction treatment of older adults: evaluation of an innovative client centred approach. Howarth Press, Canada
Handy C, Pates R, Barrowcliff 1998 Drug use in South Wales; who uses Ecstasy anyway? Journal of Substance Misuse 3(2): 82–88
Health Education Authority 1989 That's the limit: a guide to sensible drinking. HEA, London
Health Education Authority 1996 Health update: smoking. HEA, London
Institute for the Study of Drug Dependence 1994 Drug use in Britain. ISDD, London
Ives R 1990 Working with solvent sniffers. ISDD, London
Jarvis M 1989 Myths of cigar and pipes. Physician 8(2): 130
Jones C 1998 Why do people die from taking Ecstasy? Journal of Substance Misuse 3(2): 95–97
Jones K L, Smith D W 1973 Recognition of the foetal alcohol syndrome in early infancy. Lancet 2: 999–1001
Krishna K 1978 Tobacco chewing in pregnancy. British Journal of Obstetrics and Gynaecology 85(10): 726–728
McKee E 2000 Alcohol and the older person. In: Cooper D B (ed) Alcohol use. Radcliffe Medical Press, Oxford
Mitchell E A, Taylor B J, Ford R P K et al 1992 Four modifiable and other major risk factors for cot death: the New Zealand study. Journal of Paediatric Child Health 28(suppl 1): S3–8
Mitchell E A, Ford R P, Stewart A W et al 1993 Smoking and the sudden infant death syndrome. Paediatrics 91(5): 893–896
Morgan M 1992 Resume of paper 3: 'The medical background'. In: Royal College of General Practitioners (ed) Women and alcohol. HMSO, London
Pagliaro A M, Pagliaro L A 1996 Substance use among children and adolescents: its nature, extent and effects from conception to adulthood. John Wiley, New York
Parloff M 1980 Psychotherapy and research: an anaclitic depression. Psychiatry 43: 279–293
Pates R 1998 Guest editorial: the agony of ecstasy. Journal of Substance Misuse 3(2): 81
Pickles Judge J 1991 A futile war. 'Byline', BBC 1
Plant M L 1997 Women and alcohol: contemporary and historical perspectives. Free Association Books, London
Prochaska J O, Di Clemente C C 1983 Stages and process of self-change of smoking: towards an integrative model of change. Journal of Consulting and Clinical Psychology 51(3): 390–395
Prochaska J O, Di Clemente C C 1986 Towards a comprehensive model of change. In: Miller W R, Heather N (eds) Treating addictive behaviours: processes of change. Plenum, London
Royal College of Psychiatrists 1987 Drug scenes: a report on drugs and drug dependency. Gaskell, Oxford
Saunders B, Marsh A 1999 Harm reduction and the use of currently illegal drugs: some assumptions and dilemmas. Journal of Substance Use 4(1): 3–9
Saunders N 1998 Current opinion: how the media report ecstasy. Journal of Substance Misuse 3(2): 98–100
Schacter S 1982 Recidivism and self cure of smoking and obesity. American Psychologist 37: 436–444
Seivewright N 1998 Current opinion: theory and practice in managing benzodiazepine dependence and misuse. Journal of Substance Misuse 3(3): 170–177
Sidle N 1982 Smoking in pregnancy: a review. Spastic Society. Hera Unit, London
Silverman K, Evans S M, Stragin E C et al 1992 Withdrawal syndrome after the double-blind cessation of caffeine consumption. New England Journal of Medicine 327(16): 1109–1114
Stimmel B 1997 Pain and its relief without addiction. Haworth Medical Press, New York
Stratton K, Howe C, Battaglin F (eds) 1996 Foetal alcohol syndrome: diagnosis, epidemiology, prevention and treatment. Institute of Medicine and National Academy Press, Washington, DC
Taylor J C, Norman C L, Bland J M, Ramsey J D, Anderson H R 1998 Trends in death associated with abuse of volatile substances 1971–1996 (report no. 11). St George's Hospital Medical School, London
US Department of Health and Human Services 1989 Reducing the health consequences of smoking: 25 years progress. A report of the Surgeon General US Department of Health and Human Services, Public Health Services, Centre for Disease Control, Centre for Chronic Disease Prevention and Health Promotion, Office of Smoking and Health. DHHS Publication (CDC) 89: 8411
Watson H E 1996 Minimal interventions for problem drinkers. Journal of Substance Misuse 1(2): 107–110
Watson H E 2000 Alcohol: prevention, identification and health promotion. In: Cooper D B (ed) Alcohol use. Radcliffe Medical Press, Oxford
World Health Organization 1985 The use of essential drugs. Publication TRS722. WHO, Geneva

FURTHER READING

Advisory Council on the Misuse of Drugs 1995 Volatile substance abuse. HMSO, London
Cameron D 1995 Liberating solutions to alcohol problems: treating problem drinkers without saying no. Jason Aronson, Northvale, USA
Cameron D 2000 Alcohol use in perspective. In: Cooper D B (ed) Alcohol use. Radcliffe Medical Press, Oxford
Cooper D B 1994 Alcohol home detoxification and assessment. Radcliffe Medical Press, Oxford
Cooper D B 2000 Alcohol use. Radcliffe Medical Press, Oxford
Department Of Health 1991 Drug misuse and dependence: guidelines on clinical management. HMSO, London
Dorn N, Henderson S, South N (eds) 1991 AIDS: women, drugs and social care. Falmer Press, London
Fossey E 1994 Growing up with alcohol. Routledge, London
Gilman M 1992 Outreach. ISDD, London
Graham K, Saunders S J, Flowers M C, Birchmore Timney C, White-Campbell M, Ziedman Pietropalo A 1995 Addiction treatment of older adults: evaluation of an innovative client centred approach. Howarth Press, Canada

Graham K, Clarke D, Bois C, Carver V, Marsham J, Smythe C 1998 Depressant medication use by older persons in the broader social context relating to use of psychoactive substances. Journal of Substance Misuse 3(3): 161–169
Heather N, Robertson I 1981 Controlled drinking. Methuen, London
Institute for the Study of Drug Dependence 1989 The Misuse of Drugs Act explained. ISDD, London
Institute for the Study of Drug Dependence 1991 So you've chosen drugs for your project. ISDD, London
Ives R 1990 Parents: what you need to know about solvent sniffing. ISDD, London
Ives R 1990 Working with solvent sniffers. ISDD, London
Keene J 1997 Drug misuse: prevention, harm minimisation and treatment. Chapman and Hall, London
McKee E 2000 Alcohol and the older person. In: Cooper D B (ed) Alcohol use: the handbook. Radcliffe Medical Press, Oxford
Miller W R, Rollnick S 1991 Motivational interviewing — preparing people to change addictive behaviours. Guilford, New York
Pagliaro A M, Pagliaro L A 1996 Substance use among children and adolescents: its nature, extent and effects from conception to adulthood. John Wiley, New York
Preston A 1996 The methadone briefing. ISDD, London
Rassool G H, Gafoor M 1997 Addiction nursing: perspectives on professional and clinical practice. Stanley Thornes, London
Royal College of General Practitioners 1992 Women and alcohol. HMSO, London
Seivewright N 1998 Current opinion: theory and practice in managing benzodiazepine dependence and misuse. Journal of Substance Misuse 3(3): 170–177
Siney C 1995 The pregnant drug addict. Royal College of Midwives and Haigh and Hochland. Books for Midwives Press, Cheshire
Stimmel B 1997 Pain and its relief without addiction. Haworth Medical Press, New York
Strang J, Farrell M 1992 Hepatitis. ISDD, London
Stratton K, Howe C, Battaglin F (eds) 1996 Foetal alcohol syndrome: diagnosis, epidemiology, prevention and treatment. Institute of Medicine and National Academy Press, Washington, DC
Watson H E 2000 Alcohol: prevention, identification and health promotion. In: Cooper D B (ed) Alcohol use: the handbook. Radcliffe Medical Press, Oxford

USEFUL ADDRESSES

The Addictions Forum
Membership Secretary: Dr Moira Plant
Alcohol & Health Research Centre,
City Hospital,
Edinburgh EH1 5SB

AIDS Helpline: 0800 567123
Minority languages — phone AIDS Helpline for relevant language number
Hard of hearing — 0800 521361

Alcohol Concern
Waterbridge House
32–36 Loman Street
London SE1 0EE

ASH (Action on Smoking and Health)
16 Fitzhadinge Street
London W1H 9PL

Council for Involuntary Tranquilliser Addiction
Cavendish House
Brighton Road
Waterloo
Liverpool L22 5NG

Drinkline: 0345 320 202

GamCare
Suite 1, Catherine House
25–27 Catherine Place
London SW1E 6DU

ISDD (Institute for the Study of Drug Dependence)
Waterbridge House
32–36 Loman Street
London SE1 0EE

National Drug Helpline: 0800 77 66 00

Nursing Council on Alcohol and Drugs (NCAD)
Mr David B. Cooper
Development and Communications Contact
c/o Parkholme
Ashreigney
Chulmleigh
Devon EX18 7LY

QUIT
102 Gloucester Place
London W1H 3DA

Re-Solv (The Society for the Prevention of Solvent & Volatile Substance Abuse)
St Mary's Chambers
19 Station Road
Stone
Staffs ST15 8JP

SCODA (Standing Conference on Drug Abuse)
Waterbridge House
32–36 Loman Street
London SE1 0EE

Smokers' Quitline: 0800 00 22 00
Cantonese: 0800 18 11 53
Silhetti: 0800 18 13 48

Terrence Higgins Trust
52–54 Gray's Inn Road
London WC1X 8JU
Helpline: 0171 242 1010

Women's Alcohol Centre
66a Drayton Park
London N5 1ND

THE PERSON WITH HIV/AIDS

37

John Atkinson

INTRODUCTION

In June 1981, five young men in the USA were reported to have died of *Pneumocystis carinii* pneumonia (PCP), a rare infection. The only characteristics they had in common were their young age, their gender and the fact that they were homosexual. Later that year a patient with similar symptoms died in a London hospital (Pratt 1998). The condition we now call acquired immune deficiency syndrome (AIDS) had arrived. In 1983–84, in France and the USA, the causative agent, a virus from the family of retroviruses, (see p. 1035) was isolated. This virus was found to infiltrate and destroy human helper T lymphocytes, which promote both the ability of B-lymphocyte-derived plasma cells to produce antibodies and the activation of killer T lymphocytes (CD8+ cytotoxic cells), which are able to attack and kill those cells infected with viruses. The viruses which cause AIDS are known as the human immunodeficiency viruses.

This chapter will present the main historical features of the advent of HIV/AIDS along with a profile of the retrovirus. It will address the social and economic implications of HIV/AIDS and the effect of the disease on patients and their carers. Testing will be highlighted together with concomitant ethical and practical dilemmas. The final sections of the chapter will consider the clinical manifestations of HIV/AIDS, giving details of the treatments currently available. The contribution of nurses to the care of individuals with HIV/AIDS will be discussed. Whilst reading this chapter, the reader should remember that the person with HIV/AIDS will spend most of his time at home and not in hospital or other formal care settings.

By setting HIV/AIDS, at the outset, in a wide social context, this chapter is intended to emphasise that HIV/AIDS is both a clinical and a sociopolitical issue. It is hoped that nurses, armed with the information provided by this chapter, will be able to develop a knowledgeable and empathetic mode of practice with people who have HIV and related problems.

Definitions

In order for nurses to use the correct terminology relating to HIV/AIDS, they need to understand how this terminology developed.

The syndrome

The only clinical factor linking the original patients with AIDS was the fact that they were so profoundly immunodepressed that microorganisms which generally inhabit the body harmlessly took the opportunity to replicate wildly, disseminate and cause clinical illness, e.g. *Pneumocystis carinii* (PCP). Until that time, this infection was seen only occasionally, in patients who were immunodepressed with diseases such as leukaemia or whose immunity was suppressed as a side-effect of medication. These types of illness and neoplastic events, which only manifest themselves in persons who have a depressed immune system, are referred to as 'opportunistic diseases' and they are the hallmark of the syndrome now referred to as AIDS. As this immunodepressed state was not a primary (e.g. congenital) but a secondary immunodeficiency, it was called acquired immune deficiency (the main linking clinical factor) syndrome (a group of recognised clinical signs). In time it would be recognised that this particular immunodeficiency was secondary to specific viral infection.

HIV

The retroviruses, now called human immunodeficiency viruses (HIV), were isolated and designated the causative agents of AIDS. A blood test which could detect antibodies to HIV following infection was developed in 1985. An individual who becomes infected with HIV will respond by producing antibodies in a process known as seroconversion. When a person is found to have HIV antibodies, he is said to be HIV antibody-positive or, less correctly, HIV-positive (HIV+) and is considered to be infected with HIV.

Since the discovery of HIV, a major strain variation within the species human immunodeficiency viruses — HIV 2 — has been identified. It is most commonly found in certain countries on the west coast of Africa and in west India. HIV 2 is less able to be transmitted from an infected mother to her child (vertical transmission) and infection with HIV 2 is generally associated with a longer incubation period to an AIDS-defining illness.

AIDS diagnosis

A patient is diagnosed as having AIDS only if he is HIV antibody-positive and has one of the designated infections or diseases associated with AIDS. The classification of these diseases devised by the Centers for Disease Control (CDC 1987) in the USA is used globally and will be adopted in this chapter. Also current is the 'World Health Organization Clinical Staging System for HIV Infection and Disease'. This system attempts to address some of the anomalies which the CDC system presented. A helpful explanation of the staging system is given in Pratt (1998), Appendix 2.

The CDC classification also includes a description of the disease process from the time an individual contracts HIV until he becomes ill. Some people who have contracted HIV go through a short flu-like illness during which they develop antibodies; this is called acute seroconversion illness (CDC phase A; see Box 37.1). Many individuals will have the virus for some time without knowing it, and may be completely asymptomatic for several years (CDC phase B-1: the asymptomatic or dormant phase).

It is important to understand the following relationship between HIV antibodies and AIDS — everybody who has AIDS is HIV antibody-positive, but not everybody who is HIV antibody-positive has AIDS. It should also be pointed out that an individual who has a positive HIV antibody status may become ill without being diagnosed as having AIDS. This may be because he has not yet contracted one of the classified list of infections and diseases but is ill for some other reason, or because he is experiencing side-effects of, for instance, antiretroviral treatment.

Nurses will meet many people who have at some earlier time been diagnosed as having AIDS but who are presently well. This is increasingly common as people with the syndrome survive longer. When the author began working in the field, death 18 months to 2 years after diagnosis was the 'norm'. Now one may meet individuals who have survived 10–15 years. Thus the term AIDS can be unhelpful, and even misleading, because it does not necessarily reflect how the person is at a given moment. For nurses in particular, the term has little relevance. It is more helpful to consider the term 'persons living with HIV infection' rather than AIDS or HIV patients. The term conveys a continuum from the moment of infection to end-stage disease and death with early, middle and late events and issues affecting individuals.

Box 37.1 The phases of HIV/AIDS and associated infections and conditions

PHASE A: ACUTE SEROCONVERSION ILLNESS (CDC PHASE A, see p. 000)

PHASE B: ANTIBODY-POSITIVE PHASE

B-1: asymptomatic HIV infection

B-2: persistent generalised lymphadenopathy (PGL) or lymphadenopathy syndrome (LAS)

PHASE C: AIDS-RELATED COMPLEX (ARC)

PHASE D: AIDS — CONSTITUTIONAL DISEASE; HIV WASTING SYNDROME; OPPORTUNISTIC INFECTIONS

Protozoal infections
- *Pneumocystis carinii* pneumonia (PCP)
- Cryptosporidiosis
- Toxoplasmosis
- Isosporiasis

Viral infections
- Herpes simplex virus
- Cytomegalovirus (CMV)
- Progressive multifocal leucoencephalopathy (PML)

Bacterial infections
- *Mycobacterium tuberculosis* (TB)
- Salmonellosis
- *Mycobacterium avium* complex (MAC)

Fungal infections
- Candidiasis (thrush)
- Cryptococcus
- Histoplasmosis
- Coccidioidomycosis

Infestations

Secondary cancers (neoplasms)
- Kaposi's sarcoma (KS)
- Non-Hodgkin's lymphomas (B-cell lymphomas, undifferentiated lymphomas)

Neurological disease; HIV encephalopathy

Issues surrounding terminology

HIV/AIDS has become a deeply politicised disease phenomenon. The nurse as educator and advocate must be sensitive to the sociopolitical issues surrounding HIV/AIDS and its description. The patient has the right to expect that nurses will use terminology that is appropriate and technically correct, is not stigmatising, promotes well-being and does not give offence.

Although the term AIDS has limited clinical usefulness, it is the one most commonly used by the media and the public. Also common are the terms 'the AIDS virus' and 'the HIV virus'. Neither is strictly correct and nurses should try simply to use 'HIV' instead.

It is now generally accepted that 'person/s living with AIDS' (PLWA) or HIV is a more acceptable term than 'AIDS patient'.

The latter term is inappropriate as an individual may live a normal life for long periods without recourse to medical or nursing care. Calling an individual a 'victim' raises questions of guilt or innocence and, along with 'sufferer', implies that he is powerless to help himself.

VIRUSES AND NORMAL IMMUNOLOGY

The reader is referred to Chapter 16 for an outline of normal immunology.

Viruses

Viruses are not complete organisms. They can survive only as part of 'host' cells. Unlike bacteria, fungi, protozoans and other infective agents, all of which are complete and independently viable, viruses cannot replicate (multiply/reproduce) by themselves. They are also very small and cannot be seen by a light microscope. Viruses are made up of a core of nucleic acid (i.e. DNA or RNA, never both) and are enveloped in a protein shell.

Retroviruses

These viruses, to which HIV belongs, contain RNA. They have the ability to infiltrate the DNA of the host cell and implant their genetic material there, after which the host cell will have the capability to reproduce HIV.

DNA is present in almost all organisms. It plays a central part in heredity and, because of its structure (two interwoven strands of nucleotides connected by hydrogen bonds), can replicate, carrying the genetic blueprint to the next generation of cells. RNA is made up of a single strand of nucleotides and is involved in protein synthesis. It provides the genetic blueprint of some viruses, including HIV. HIV infects a variety of cells which contain CD4+ host cell receptors, including T lymphocytes of the helper subset. The presence of additional host cell receptors is known to be necessary in order for HIV to attach itself to a cell and infect it.

The importance of this disruption of the T lymphocytes must be understood within the context of the normal immune response (see Ch. 16). The various types of white blood cells have interlinking but quite distinct cell-mediated responses to seek and destroy invading microorganisms and malignant cells. For a stage-by-stage summary of this process, see Box 37.2. Given the essential role played by helper T cells in the immune system, it is clear that their invasion and destruction by HIV will have devastating results.

Box 37.2 The normal immune response

Warning
In response to the invading microorganism, helper T cells orchestrate defences by releasing chemicals which stimulate other cells of the immune system.

Preparation
Activated by these chemical signals, other kinds of T cells (cytotoxic cells and lymphokine producers) begin to proliferate, while B lymphocytes multiply and become plasma cells which start to manufacture antibodies.

Attack
Activated T cells and antibodies are released into the circulation, where they specifically target and destroy the invading organism.

Stand down
Once the foreign organism is routed and the infection is under control, the activity of the immune system is reduced, perhaps partly through the action of suppressor T lymphocytes.

THE TRANSMISSION OF HIV

Modes of transmission

The first stage of HIV infection occurs when the individual is infected with HIV through an exchange of body fluids and/or blood with an infected individual. Sexual contact and blood-to-blood contact are known as 'horizontal' methods of transmission, i.e. they move 'across' from one individual to another.

Transmission through sexual contact

Unprotected vaginal or anal intercourse is the most common means by which HIV can be transmitted from an infected to a non-infected person. It is difficult to determine absolutely whether other intimate sexual activities (e.g. oral sex) transmit the virus as they do not often occur in isolation, but some individual cases have been reported (Rothenberg et al 1998). There is much debate in the scientific and secular worlds about which sexual activities are the most 'dangerous'. Until recently anal sex was considered to be most risky. Also, women were thought to be more at risk from penis/vagina sex than men. More recent findings are leading to a re-examination of these assumptions, and the scientific debate still rages (O'Connell 1993).

It is important to inform patients that they may be at risk from any intimate sexual contact.

Transmission through blood and blood products

Blood transfusions. The spread of HIV in Western countries which have sophisticated blood transfusion services has been greatly reduced since the rigorous screening of donors was first instituted (1985 in most countries). In the UK it is now reckoned that there is a risk factor of less than one transmission in a million units of blood. This works out at fewer than three transmissions a year.

The best-known recipients of blood products are haemophiliacs and those with other blood-clotting disorders. Before 1985, many thousands of haemophiliacs and others became infected through blood products. Since 1985, these products have been heat-treated. The treatment is totally successful but reduces the efficacy of the products such that more of them are required.

Blood transmission through sharing of equipment. HIV transmission can occur through the sharing of syringes, needles and other blood-giving equipment. In Western countries this is commonly through the illicit, intravenous (i.v.) use of drugs. Here the probability of infection is often increased by the user 'flushing' the syringe with his blood before injection. In poorer countries it is also seen where there is re-use of medical equipment and insufficient sterilising facilities. The mode of transmission is the same in both cases.

Small amounts of infected blood remain in the equipment and are introduced straight into the bloodstream of the recipient. The recipient, in fact, receives a small and unintentional inoculation. So-called 'needlestick' injuries in which a used needle accidentally stabs an individual are also dangerous. However, there have been very few proven cases of infection by this mode (Hanrahan & Reutter 1997, Sistrom et al 1998).

Transmission through skin piercing procedures. Transmission is certainly a theoretical risk from procedures such as tattooing (Greif & Hewitt 1998), and cases have been reported of transmission by body piercing (Armstrong 1998) and skin grafting (Eastlund 1995).

Transmission through other bodily fluids. Infection with HIV takes place only when there is sufficient concentration of the virus. Infection through saliva, for instance, is therefore considered unlikely. Worldwide retrospective studies have shown that the number of workers contracting the virus through urine, faeces or saliva, for example, has been extremely small (WHO 1998).

Mother-to-child transmission

This form of transmission is known as 'vertical' transmission, i.e. down 'from' an infected mother to her child in the womb or during delivery, when the mother's blood and the child's blood become mixed. There is a possibility that transmission through amniotic fluid and ('horizontally') through breast milk can also take place (Mok 1993, Carlisle 1998).

From birth until 11–18 months, the baby will carry the mother's HIV and other antibodies. Therefore, all babies born to HIV-infected mothers are found to be HIV antibody-positive. At about 11–18 months, the baby will lose the mother's antibodies and go on either to being HIV antibody-negative (not carrying the virus) or to developing his own antibodies (being infected in his own right). A few go on to become HIV antibody-negative but positive to another test which isolates antigen (particles of the actual virus), so that they are carrying the virus but not the antibodies.

At the beginning of the HIV epidemic it appeared that about 50% of children born to HIV antibody-positive mothers became infected in their own right.

In countries where there are good antenatal facilities and the mother remains well throughout pregnancy, the rate of transmission from mother to child is dramatically lower. The babies still carry the mothers' antibodies, but only about 20% appear to go on to be infected in their own right.

Stages of HIV infection

The dormant or asymptomatic stage

In HIV-related illness, two main processes take place in the infected person's body:

- HIV destroys the helper T cells and replicates itself
- The body's immunity is inexorably weakened and is attacked by other infections. The body becomes increasingly unable to fight off these attacks.

Since viruses cannot multiply by themselves, they need to use the cell-building material of their host cells in order to reproduce themselves (see Fig. 37.1). When HIV enters the bloodstream, it attaches itself to the outer cell membrane of the helper T lymphocyte. Following this, it breaks into the cell and releases its genetic blueprint, which has the ability to replicate itself.

The disease process may then go no further for several months or even years. That is, the person is infected with HIV and may or may not have produced antibodies (this may take 3 months or more). If he has seroconverted (started to produce antibodies) he may or may not have become ill. If he did become ill with acute seroconversion illness (CDC phase A), the usually mild, flu-like symptoms were probably not recognised by the individual or his physician as a sign of HIV infection. The helper T lymphocyte blood count will still be normal and therefore the immune system will remain unaffected. The patient will continue to be well. This stage, often called the dormant stage, is referred to as 'Clinical stage one: 1. Asymptomatic' in the WHO staging system (Pratt 1998).

Some time in the future the infected T cells will start to replicate new HIV retroviruses. It is unclear what triggers this process. However, it seems that, if an individual keeps generally well and leads a healthy lifestyle, the stage at which HIV starts to replicate

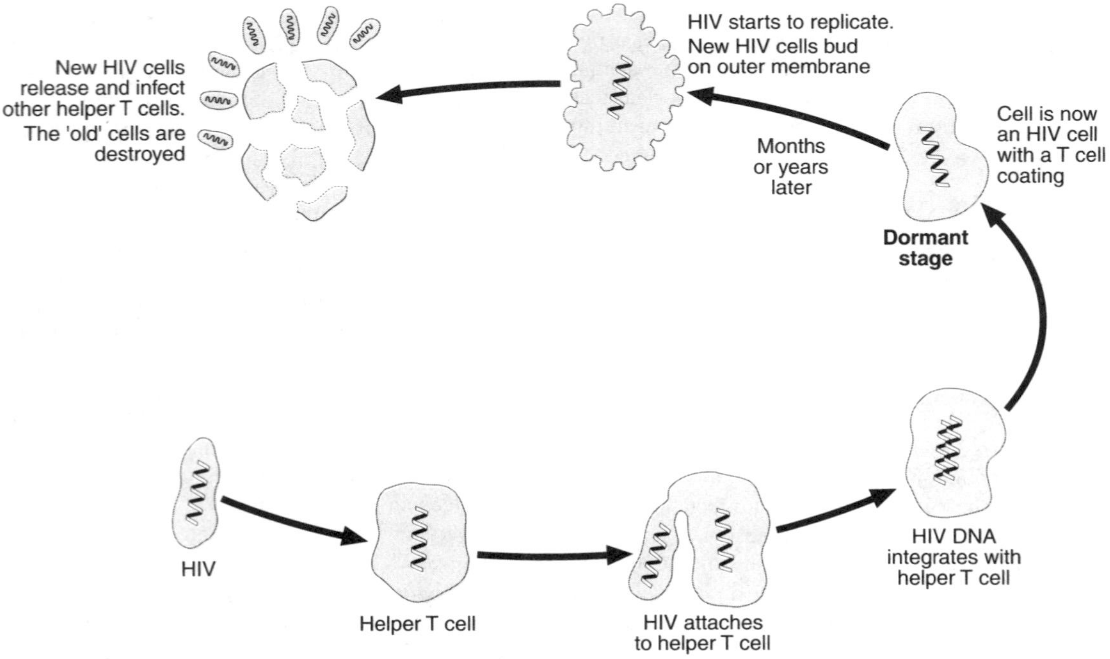

Fig. 37.1 The human immunodeficiency virus in action.

and destroy the T cells may be delayed. A clearer finding is that, in conditions of deprivation and poor health, the illness seems to progress faster.

The role of antibodies. Until quite recently, it was thought that HIV antibodies had no effect whatsoever. However, more recent research in various countries suggests that the maligned HIV antibody may have some effect in delaying the onset of replication and therefore the onset of HIV-related illness.

The replication stage

The first process. Some time (the timing is not precise) after HIV has been incorporated into the helper T lymphocyte, it begins to replicate itself within the cell walls using the cell's own material. The new viruses aggregate, start to destroy the outer cell membrane and break out of the helper T cell, encased in membrane stolen from the host cell and clinging onto the remnants of the cell. This is known as 'budding' (see Fig. 37.1). At this stage, the host cell dies. The new viruses then disperse throughout the bloodstream, infecting other helper T lymphocytes, and the process begins again.

The second process begins when other helper T cells have been infected and the level of normal, healthy helper T cells begins to fall. At this point the body's immunity to other infections will begin to be compromised. From the clinician's viewpoint this is a significant stage, as the depletion of normal helper T cells can be measured in a blood sample with the 'CD4 T cell subsets' procedure (see Appendix 1).

Also significant is the ratio between the helper T lymphocytes and the cytotoxic T lymphocytes, which are reckoned to assist in the 'stand down' phase of the normal immune response (see Box 37.2). Normally the ratio is 1.5 helpers to 1.0 cytotoxic (suppressors). As the number of healthy helper cells decreases, this ratio is changed. This may have a detrimental effect on the immune system. It is also one of the diagnostic signs used to confirm the presence of HIV-related illness. In other forms of immune deficiency illnesses, both helper and suppressor cell levels fall, and so the ratio between them remains roughly the same.

As the helper T cell level falls the body will become more susceptible to other infections. The individual may at first experience rather vague symptoms, progressing to debilitating but not life-threatening conditions and finally serious illness and death. (Information on the specific diseases which may appear is given later in the chapter.)

The illness profile represented in Figure 37.2 is a very general description. How HIV/AIDS actually manifests itself will vary dramatically from one person to another. Many people with extremely low helper T cell counts will seem healthy; others with what should be a 'good' count will be extremely ill. The nurse must rely on her own observations of and discussions with the patient in assessing his condition, rather than on abstract clinical indicators alone.

POLITICAL AND SOCIAL IMPLICATIONS OF HIV/AIDS

AIDS has been compared to the great plagues of the past in that it appears to be spreading unchecked and has, as yet, no cure. Like other infectious diseases which have reached epidemic or pandemic

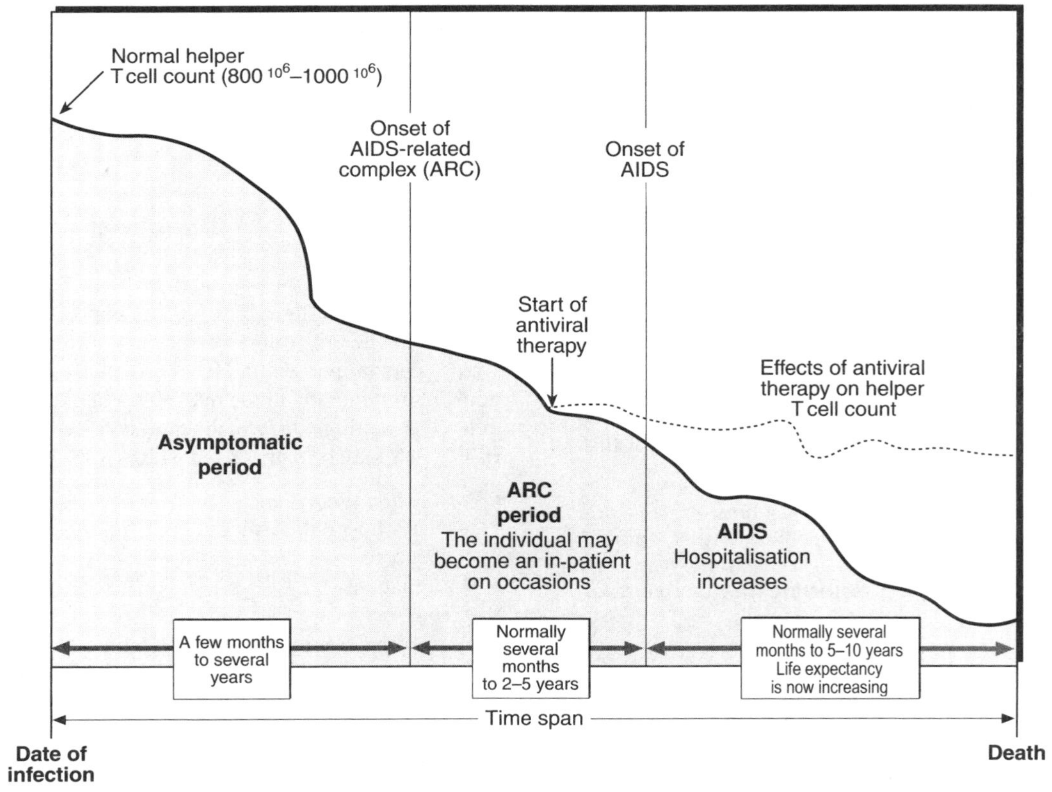

Fig. 37.2 Diagrammatic representation of the progress of HIV-related illness. Many people die when they get the first major opportunistic infection (onset of AIDS). It is very difficult to state when a person is going into the terminal stages of the disease. Many people make remarkable recoveries over a period of months or years.

proportions, HIV/AIDS has given rise to a great deal of fear and stigmatisation. In formulating health and social policies in response to AIDS, the government has a duty not only to safeguard the health and well-being of the population as a whole but also to protect the rights of those individuals affected by the disease.

The foundation for political and social responses to HIV/AIDS is provided by the work of epidemiologists, who define the disease, describe its typical progression and determine its national and international incidence. Also relevant is its prevalence, i.e. its incidence within particular groups. On the basis of these findings, predictions are made as to the future impact of the disease (Barker & Rose 1998). Armed with this knowledge, nursing, medical and scientific practitioners, along with the individuals and groups affected, endeavour to raise awareness of HIV/AIDS and to lobby the government to take appropriate action.

Although cases of HIV infection were known in 1981, it was not until 2 or 3 years later that HIV appeared officially to be recognised as a threat to the whole community. Various media campaigns were instigated from 1985 onwards and the first full debate was held in the House of Commons in November 1986 (Hansard 1986).

Some of the questions and issues raised by the epidemiology of HIV/AIDS are listed in Box 37.3.

Political challenges

The most intractable problem presented by HIV to policy makers is the length of time it takes for the disease to manifest itself after an individual becomes infected. This has the following profound epidemiological implications:

- Most people who are infected are not aware of it until they become ill.
- The government figures published regularly on people with AIDS do not reflect the prevalence of HIV at the present moment. They give, at best, an idea of the prevalence 5–10 years ago.
- It is more difficult to gauge specifically who is at risk, although some 'high-risk' activities can be identified (e.g. i.v. drug use, unprotected sexual intercourse).

It is therefore vital that data on AIDS are as specific as possible. In the UK, the following bodies collect, collate and distribute information on the incidence and prevalence of HIV and AIDS:

- Public Health Laboratory Service (PHLS), Colindale Avenue, London
- Communicable diseases surveillance units (CDSUs)
- Department of Health, AIDS Unit, Blackfriars Road, London
- Health boards and authorities under the direction of the AIDS (Control) Act 1987.

Until January 1991, the number of reported AIDS cases was published monthly. The main figure quoted was the cumulative total, i.e. the overall number known since reporting started. Since the implementation of the AIDS (Control) Act 1987 and other measures, it has been possible to gather more specific, local information from hospitals, clinics and health boards. There is now a yearly breakdown of HIV seropositive incidence, cases of AIDS, gender, high-risk activity (e.g. drug use) and age. The Department of Health also produces a quarterly press release (DoH 1998). Internationally, data collection has been improved by the coordination of research projects and the collation of information. There is an annual global AIDS medical conference and the European Association for Nurses in AIDS Care has established conferences in both Western and Eastern countries.

Box 37.3 Questions and issues raised by HIV/AIDS

- In the Third World, particularly Africa, HIV affects mainly heterosexual people. In the West, with some notable exceptions, the prevalence appears to be overwhelmingly among homosexual men and intravenous drug users. Why is the pattern so different, given that HIV is now present in all sections of the population in the West?
- In many cities in the USA and Africa, the prevalence of HIV among young heterosexuals is rising dramatically. It is now the most common cause of death in this group. Will this happen everywhere?
- Given that there is no cure for AIDS, just how effective are education and prevention policies? Some countries, notably the USA, have strict entry laws. What is the case for stringent political action, e.g. restricting the movements of known HIV-positive individuals?
- Is there a case for testing as many people as possible anonymously to get a more accurate profile of what is going on so that policymakers are better able to provide proper services?
- Is the nurse's primary responsibility to the individual patient and to his confidentiality and wishes? If so, what responsibility does the nurse have to protect the public at large? Can she meet both responsibilities at the same time?

Q **37.1** Obtain national and local AIDS/HIV-related statistics. Analyse trends over the last 5 years (PHLS & SCIEH 1999).

The impact of HIV/AIDS on health and social services

Although qualified nurses tend to work exclusively in either a hospital or a community setting, it is important to consider HIV in relation to the full range of services available to the (typically young) person living with HIV, particularly in the light of innovations in drug therapy in the mid-1990s and the longer life expectation. The settings in which care is given to individuals with HIV/AIDS may be categorised as follows:

- *Institutional/hospital*
  —ward: hospital/hospice
  —day care
  —outpatients
- *Community*
  —treatment room: health centre/clinic
  —home: with a district nurse, health visitor or other practitioner
  —home: self-care or with family/partner/friends
  —outreach: residential (hostels, prisons, caravans)
  —outreach: non-residential (drop-in centres, street work).

Hospital care. At first, HIV care was delivered almost exclusively in the ward setting. This was an expensive, labour-intensive and often 'patient-unfriendly' option. Individuals would spend many days or weeks in hospital per year, sometimes feeling relatively well but needing, say, i.v. therapy. The ward setting is now used for other purposes, including respite and day care. Day care units are now used extensively and often have flexible hours to facilitate patients' work commitments. Day care units and outpatient departments are used as places of treatment, monitoring, counselling and group work as well as traditional consultation.

Community care. Most procedures, including continuous i.v. therapy, can now be performed in the patient's home. The author looked after a young person who, having been in prison, was frightened of being in hospital. Even though the patient lived in a very poor area in a crowded home with young children, a high standard of nursing care was possible, including the successful care of a gangrenous ulcer. This patient very rarely went into hospital.

Outreach care is now a well developed area of health and nursing delivery, particularly in relation to HIV and drug misuse, providing drop-in centres where counselling, medical cover, family planning and antenatal care with direct access to the hospital services are available (GGHB 1998).

HIV has an enormous social impact on the individual and his carers. In order to provide the best possible care, it is essential to have an integrated, multidisciplinary service that addresses social as well as clinical concerns, particularly in discharge planning and follow-up (Pratt 1998). Creating an environment which enables an effective but confidential service is difficult, especially as more agencies become involved in care. The best principle to adopt is a 'need to know' policy of information disclosure involving the patient at every stage. This sometimes causes problems, as many professionals, quite wrongly, think they have a 'blanket' right to know a patient's details.

Manpower implications

The two main effects that HIV has had on health service manpower are:

- role change and extension of roles
- increased workloads and accompanying costs.

Role change has been seen both in hospital and in the community. By the 1970s it was felt that infectious disease nursing as a speciality was no longer needed and infectious diseases hospitals were increasingly used for other purposes. Now infectious disease hospitals and wards have once again become necessary. Special facilities for people with HIV/AIDS have been built, requiring a large number of new staff. To date there has been no audit of how many nurses in the UK have been deployed in this field. However, each authority has to publish a yearly report on activities and services under the 1987 AIDS (Control) Act.

Costs. Since 1995–96 (and the first edition of this book) these implications have changed again, particularly as individuals receive new therapies (see below) from an earlier stage in their illness with the result that many remain in better health for longer periods. This has a considerable impact on financial resources but has, at present, lessened the need for specialist in-patient facilities. Hospital admissions, mainly for the treatment of devastating opportunistic infections, increase costs considerably. Newer treatments, although expensive, are seen to be cost-effective as they delay the onset of advanced disease, AIDS, for which care is very expensive (Oddone et al 1993, Petrou et al 1996). More people are therefore able to stay well for longer, although the long-term influence of combination therapy (see p. 1048) on the infected population is unknown (King 1997, Howe 1998).

Increased workloads. In the community, HIV has had the effect of creating new fields of work for practitioners. District nurses, whose main workload lies in caring for elderly people, now have younger people on their caseloads with a variety of clinical needs.

Increased input by social services is needed by most affected people at one stage or another as their situation changes. Typically the individual is young, independent and employed; he may be living alone (paying a mortgage or rent) and may have no regular partner. As the disease progresses, these circumstances may change rapidly. In HIV units where there is no resident social worker, the nurse may need to act as advisor and advocate in helping the patient to obtain benefits, housing, domestic assistance, meal supplements and other services. For such nurses the key to success is to identify the appropriate services (without divulging the patient's personal details) and then, with the patient, to approach them for help. Without careful management, this extension of the nursing role can result in staff being 'spread too thinly'. Efficient and appropriate referral will be vital to the success of the shift towards community-based care (Faugier & Hicken 1996).

If one compares HIV therapy with another long-term disease and treatment — diabetes mellitus and insulin — where many individuals being treated from a young age may expect to live a fully functional life with normal longevity, the situation with HIV is still uncertain, especially as other factors, such as virus mutation with new disease patterns, manifest themselves (Josefson 1997). These patterns include drug resistance. A good description of the latest developments overcoming drug resistance is given by Clapham & Simmons (1997).

Statistics from the Public Health Laboratory Service show the cumulative totals of cases reported until January 1999 for HIV and AIDS. Although the largest proportion of people affected have been homosexual men, the most rapid increase is among heterosexuals. However, the reader should be cautioned that it is not good practice to multiply the figures ad infinitum to get projected numbers. At that rate, the whole world would eventually become infected. A more useful indicator is the number of new cases reported monthly and the increase (if any) in incidence that this represents.

37.2 What are the current statistics on *new* AIDS cases?

Social implications

The social impact of HIV/AIDS is felt in two ways: on society as a whole, and on the individual as a social being. Here we will consider the wider societal implications first.

Consider the following quotation (Connor & Kingman 1989):

> *At least one American senator was heard to say 'somewhere along the way we are going to have quarantine'.*

This typifies the way in which epidemics are often viewed by the makers of social policy. When the management of an epidemic is seen as being analogous to the management of acute illnesses in clinical practice (Barker & Rose 1998), the following equation is made:

The organism + the individual = the disease + the population = the epidemic

In this view an intervention must be made to prevent the transformation of 'organism' into 'epidemic'. Theoretically, the options are:

- to kill the organism
- to make the organism inoperative
- to ameliorate the effects of the organism on the individual
- to separate the individual from the organism
- to separate the individual from the population
- to separate affected groups from the rest of the population.

Looking at disease in this way, the reader may see the role of antibiotics and disinfectants (killing the organism), immunisation (making the organism inoperative), symptom control (ameliorating the effects), infection control and health education (separating the individual from the organism), quarantine (separating the individual from the population) and banishment/leper colonies (separating groups from the population).

It may also be seen that HIV does not present many options. There is no antibiotic and no vaccine. As HIV takes a long time to manifest itself and has no very clear presenting features, quarantine and isolation of potential and actual 'victims' are difficult. At present, only the amelioration of the effects, health education and infection control (including, in this case, the use of condoms) are available in the 'battle' against this epidemic.

These options may strike us as being very limited, and therein lies the key to public reaction to HIV and AIDS. In the eyes of society, those who have been appointed to protect the population from disease have not come up with a satisfactory solution for HIV/AIDS. This has led to a reaction of fear and to a willingness to stigmatise and even scapegoat those with HIV.

Fear. It is important for the nurse to appreciate the complex nature of fear. For example, the knowledge that one cannot catch HIV by shaking hands may not be enough to dispel someone's fear of such contact, for along with the fear of actual physical contamination may be the fear of the very idea of the disease. HIV is particularly frightening because there are very few factors which separate an individual from the virus. This in itself may lead people to distinguish their own behaviour from that of individuals affected by HIV in the hope of confirming their own 'immunity', as in: 'I can't get HIV because I'm not homosexual'. At the same time, this implies that individuals with HIV/AIDS are themselves to blame and that if everyone in society conformed to certain patterns of behaviour then everything would be all right.

Fear is also associated with lack of personal experience. Butterworth et al (1993), reporting on a sample of community nurses, observed different levels of concern depending on the actual experience of direct care of people with HIV.

Stigmatisation. Scapegoats are those chosen by society to take the blame for evil or misfortune. The selection of a scapegoat is either arbitrary or based in prejudice. This is clear in the case of HIV, which can infect anyone, particularly the sexually active. In the Western world, the virus happens to have affected large numbers of homosexual men first, followed by i.v. drug users. In other areas of the world, its epidemiology has followed other patterns. In any event, the appearance of the virus among one group or another has been a matter of historical accident only and has no inherent moral significance. Nonetheless, people with HIV have been stigmatised officially (e.g. by being refused insurance, employment or entry into certain countries) and unofficially (e.g. by physical and verbal abuse). Individuals affected often become isolated, and because they expect abuse they may start to avoid social interaction, thus compounding their isolation and stigmatisation.

Whether the person involved is a gay man, a drug user, a patient's mother or a child in the playground, fear and stigmatisation have devastating consequences. A thoughtful nurse often makes all the difference.

Effects on the individual. The psychological impact of HIV/AIDS is similar to that of other terminal illnesses. For a fuller discussion of the psychological implications of terminal illness the reader is referred to Chapter 33.

The sick role. Bond & Bond (1986) define 'the sick role' as 'the expectations of people in a society which define the rights and duties of its members who are sick'. Thus, individuals diagnosed as being ill are implicitly or otherwise 'given permission' to behave in certain ways.

Conditions which are seen as 'self-inflicted' tend to elicit less sympathy than others. The author has worked with a patient who, while receiving treatment for a malignant illness, became infected with HIV through a blood transfusion. The patient described to carers the shift in attitude which he then perceived. While the diagnosis was 'cancer', a great deal of sympathy was given. When the diagnosis became 'HIV', the sympathy was considerably less.

A patient who eventually becomes ill may think that he is to blame for not keeping fit enough and may feel guilty when he is forced to leave work or abandon his former social roles (Atkinson 1991).

The difficulties are compounded when the person, e.g. a young drug user who prostitutes, has a disordered or chaotic lifestyle. Combined with all of his other problems, a positive HIV diagnosis can be devastating.

It is often difficult for the patient to inform relatives of his diagnosis, thus cutting himself off from a potential source of support and practical help. The nurse can often help the patient and his family to achieve a mutually acceptable resolution. She must bear in mind that whereas a family caring for someone with, say, cancer may get support and practical help from neighbours and others, HIV often sets the scene for isolation, guilt, prejudice and despair. This can happen in any terminal illness, but is often a particularly acute problem in HIV.

Philosophical issues for nurses

The problems the patient experiences as a stigmatised member of society demand that nurses who seek to help are very clear about their own attitudes and professional philosophy. Central to any philosophy of nursing practice is the patient's right to 'quality health care in an atmosphere of human dignity without regard to age, ethnic or national origin, sex or sexual orientation, religion or presenting illness' (Pratt 1998). Coupled with this is the duty of nurses to look after all patients: unlike other professionals, nurses cannot choose whom they will look after.

Models of care

The so-called 'medical model' on which much of nursing practice is based tends not to provide a satisfactory approach to illnesses in which there is no cure. This model works best when the illness can be reduced to a few constituent parts which can then be treated, eliminated or made ineffective. HIV and AIDS offer little scope for such an approach, although the search for a 'cure' continues. The reductionist medical model tends to be less effective with multifaceted problems, especially those such as AIDS which are heavily influenced by sociopolitical factors.

Western care systems are based on humanist and utilitarian philosophies by which the individual is respected and recognised as being capable of independent moral judgement and action. This respect is the basis for the quotation from Pratt above. While most people accept this sentiment, there is always difficulty in its application, for it tends to be put into practice only when the individual asserts his rights (Downie & Telfer 1980). Those who have difficulty expressing their rights or who are considered as less worthy than others to do so are often treated as second-class citizens. Many people with HIV fall into these categories. Moreover, professionals and society at large may impose what may be called 'existential assumptions' upon a situation. One patient who is thought to be 'going somewhere' or to have 'been someone' may be considered to be more 'worthwhile' than another patient who is 'going nowhere'. So the death of a 'promising' young pianist, say, is considered sadder than the death of a young prostitute. This attitude pervades care delivery as professionals prioritise their care using these value judgements as well as formal clinical signs (Bishop & Scudder 1990).

Western models of care tend to hold that one person's rights and liberties must not impinge upon another's and that one may not interfere with a person, even for his own good, unless he is violating the rights of other people (Downie & Telfer 1980). In the case of people who are considered members of a 'minority', these principles often work against their right to high-quality care.

Another possible reaction is for the professional to look at a patient in difficulty and say, 'Who am I to interfere with this person's right to choose to live like this?', as if the young, homeless, ill, drug user has made the same kind of choices and been afforded the same opportunities as, for example, the nurse in training. This attitude is seen in specific cases where patients are 'left alone', and in general where whole groups of people are either ignored or given the minimum of care.

Finally, Western care models are structured on materialistic rationalism whereby only what is 'rational' is accepted as being 'real'. The reader is invited to consider how limiting this view is as an approach to someone whose mind, body and spirit are in turmoil. By being too rational the nurse may cut herself off from the patient's real lived experience.

Several research studies into nurses' knowledge and attitudes with regard to AIDS and related issues have been undertaken in the UK. These studies have shown that it is not enough for nurses to have information about AIDS. They must also have confidence in their knowledge and in their practice (Akinsanya 1991, Aggleton & AVERT 1993, Lewis & Bor 1994).

TESTING AND SCREENING

AIDS/HIV testing involves analysis for HIV antibodies. Testing for the actual virus, i.e. testing for HIV core antigen (particles of the virus), is used for clinical prognosis and management, not generally for diagnostic purposes. Blood samples are used at present for all forms of testing, although urine and saliva tests are being developed, especially for use in screening.

Screening. The term 'screening' is generally used to refer to the process by which blood samples undergo laboratory analysis by enzyme-linked immunosorbent assay (ELISA). This procedure is carried out on several samples at once and is used to find out the prevalence of HIV antibodies in a batch of samples. The process may stop here, as in the case of anonymous prevalence surveys. The screening assay has a 'built-in' false-positive rate which ensures that there are no false-negative readings. The analysts know the percentage false-positive rate of the assay and so when confronted with a batch of positive results can make a mathematical adjustment to get an accurate picture of the prevalence of HIV in the group.

Individual testing. While ELISA is an efficient method of mass screening, it is far from satisfactory for testing an individual, for whom a false-positive result would be devastating. Therefore in individual testing the sample first undergoes ELISA, and then immunoblotting or the Western blotting method (accurate to within thousandths of 1%) to confirm the diagnosis. This method is more complex and is available only in sophisticated laboratories. In poorer countries, samples may undergo repeated ELISA procedures instead of Western blotting to achieve maximum accuracy in difficult circumstances.

Timing

Generally, HIV antibodies are produced between 3 weeks and 3 months after the individual becomes infected with HIV. This period can, however, be much longer — lapses of 2 years and more have been known. The timing of a diagnostic test is therefore important. Individuals who have a test which proves negative are often advised to come back for repeat tests over a period of months. Because of this uncertainty and the personal impact of a positive result, HIV antibody testing should take place only with pre- and post-test counselling.

Forms of testing

There are various forms of HIV testing, some of which have become controversial. All types are defined here so that the reader can differentiate between them and enter into the continuing debate over their efficacy, need and ethics.

Named voluntary testing with pre- and post-test counselling. This form occurs when an individual seeks a test following a specific high-risk activity or contact or when the individual, for reasons of his own, wants to know his sero status. It is available at genitourinary clinics and HIV units, and from some GPs and other community practitioners. People found to be positive are automatically referred to medical/nursing services. Professionals and others agree that this form is the most acceptable, both practically and ethically.

Named voluntary testing with minimal or no counselling. Many people go for testing without being given the opportunity to discuss the implications of a positive or negative result. Many, on being found positive, are not referred to services. Others, on being found negative, think that they are 'safe' and need not worry or make behavioural changes.

Conditional named 'voluntary' testing. Increasingly, organisations, countries giving work permits, and insurance companies are asking applicants to have an HIV antibody test before gaining entry or obtaining services. The clinical value of these tests is doubtful as they are taken in isolation, often without counselling.

Patients on transplant and other medical waiting lists are often asked to be tested as a condition of entry onto the list. This is done mainly in a hospital setting.

Also increasing is the use of an HIV antibody test as part of a battery of tests seeking a diagnosis, especially for ill patients admitted with unusual or vague symptoms or for patients who appear to be from 'high-risk' groups. Nurses must be particularly careful in these cases. It is their legal duty, as well as the doctor's, to ensure that every patient gives his informed consent for the test. This may be difficult if the patient is very ill, but this does not change the nurse's legal and professional accountability.

Local anonymous HIV seroprevalence surveys. These surveys are carried out by hospital departments who use part of blood samples given for other purposes to screen for HIV seroprevalence in a given locality or patient group. This is perfectly legal as long as the patients are informed that this procedure may be carried out. The sample has to be made anonymous and the result is not given to the patient.

Controversy has arisen surrounding this form of testing, particularly when the results are published in medical journals and the media. This is because relatively small numbers of patients are highlighted. For example, 1000 or so pregnant women may be screened, of whom 15 are shown to be HIV antibody-positive. Some publications may break this down even further and state that, of this 15, eight came from a particular place. This narrows down the numbers so much that many people are of the opinion that it compromises anonymity. The Royal Colleges of Nursing and of Midwives have both strongly condemned the practice of publishing results in this manner (RCN Congress 1991).

National Anonymous Survey of the Seroprevalence of HIV. This is an ongoing survey directed by the Department of Health and organised by the Public Health Laboratory Service (PHLS). As in local surveys, surplus blood from patient samples is used. Again the patients do not have to give specific consent, but they must be informed that their blood may be used. This is done via a multilingual poster campaign and through the nursing and medical professions. The samples are made anonymous, but certain pieces of information, such as gender, age and geographical area, remain with the sample. The various governmental and professional organisations concerned, including nursing and midwifery, meet in a special forum to monitor and improve the project. The results are published nationally with a breakdown of regions and other groups.

Advantages and disadvantages of anonymous testing

Voluntary, informed testing with counselling allows the HIV seropositive individual to be referred to the appropriate services. Ethically and practically, this form is best for patient and professional carer alike. However, in the public perception, the risk of HIV appears to centre around minority groups. Most people do not feel they are at risk. Of those who do feel some risk, most do not think they need to be tested.

Anonymous testing is the compromise that has emerged to satisfy, on the one hand, the need of professionals to find out how many people are, or are likely to be, affected and, on the other, the personal and civil liberties of individuals. Some professionals argue that not enough political effort has been made to increase the uptake of voluntary named testing. As HIV care improves, it is becoming clearer that the earlier an individual knows the diagnosis and is referred into medical and nursing services, the better.

This presents one of the ethical dilemmas of anonymous testing. As the number of anonymous positive samples increases, it will become apparent that, for instance, X number of pregnant women and their babies are affected, but nothing can be done for them because they are unknown. Another objection made by some is that testing babies is an underhand way of testing mothers and that as the number of known but unnamed HIV-positive babies increases, the government will be forced to establish Draconian measures such as mandatory testing for all mothers. Many professionals would argue, however, that the more we know about national and local prevalence, the more we can target services.

In these matters, the rights of the individual must be balanced against the rights of the community. Nurses are bound to uphold the right of the individual, but they also have a duty towards the community. These obligations are not mutually exclusive, but require that the issues are considered from every viewpoint. The professional bodies provide guidelines on many of the more contentious issues. It may be fair to say, however, that the nurse should generally 'err' on the side of the individual patient, for she is often his only advocate (UKCC 1992).

Targeted screening. Until the National Survey, screening took place almost exclusively in specialist areas and among particular groups who were considered 'high risk'. Whereas the information gleaned from this work was useful, it was incomplete, yielding little knowledge about the population at large. Moreover, HIV would always seem to affect mainly homosexuals or drug users if most of the samples continued to be taken from those groups. In Glasgow, for example, one area which had a higher proportion of known HIV-positive drug users than other, similarly deprived areas received much research attention. Another similar area at the other side of the city had a 'lower' prevalence, but very few individuals had been tested. When looking at research, it is important to be aware of such factors which may distort results.

Counselling

While a comprehensive guide to counselling could hardly be presented here, the following offers a few pointers to assist the nurse to meet the challenge of HIV-related counselling:

- Counselling is a helpful tool, among other tools, which may be used to assist the patient. It is not an end in itself. One person with AIDS half-jokingly remarked: 'Nurses are so keen to counsel me, it seems they forget I have practical needs. Sometimes I feel I'm being counselled to death!'
- Counselling is not advice-giving. Patients often ask 'What would you do, nurse?', but the nurse must seriously consider the relevance of her reply. Advice of the 'If I were you…' type is rarely appropriate.
- Counselling is not about getting the patient to do the 'right' thing; for example, a young, pregnant, HIV-seropositive woman cannot be 'counselled' to have, or not to have, an abortion.
- Counselling is about helping someone come to his own decisions.
- Counselling is an exploration made by two people of issues and problems. The counsellor is an equal partner whose personal opinion is very often not relevant, although it may come up in the course of the conversation.
- It is difficult to counsel and do something else. On many occasions nurses gain the patient's confidence in the process of delivering clinical and personal services. This is a good entry into the counselling relationship, as is the provision of accurate information. To achieve the equality necessary, it is advisable to be in a neutral place on an eye-to-eye level. This is difficult if the patient is lying down with few clothes on with the nurse standing over him!
- Good counselling does not have to take a long time. Some practitioners think counselling is 'rather fancy' and too time-consuming for the busy clinical situation. This is not the case. Effective counselling can be achieved in half an hour or less, especially if the counsellor gives the individual her undivided attention.
- Know your limitations. During a session it may become apparent to the counsellor that she is getting into areas where one or both parties feel they cannot cope or are out of their depth. There is no shame in this. Seek appropriate help. No one is supposed to have all the answers.

Pre- and post-test counselling

Nurses are often asked to give pre- and post-test counselling. It is essential that the nurse is proficient before attempting this. Short courses are now available in many authorities. Counselling in other clinical areas, especially oncology, genetics and terminal care, can provide very good experience. The counsellor does not have to be an 'expert' on HIV, but she must have sound clinical knowledge, as she will often encounter unusual questions which are worrying the patient.

Pre-test counselling will involve the following:

- Establishing why the individual wants to be tested. Many people come armed with erroneous conceptions. Clinical factors must also be established. A patient of the author's came seeking the test and a termination of pregnancy. She thought her partner

was HIV-positive and that her baby would die of AIDS. When she was investigated it was found that she was, in fact, not pregnant. Her partner's HIV status was not known. Because she had been worrying, she had imagined the very worst.
- Exploring the pros and cons, for that individual, of having the test. Is it appropriate? Should he wait for 3–6 months? Has he been at risk?
- Considering the implications of a positive result. Most people come for a negative result, in order to be reassured.

Having decided to be tested the person usually has to wait about a week. Ideally the same counsellor should give the person the result, but in the hospital setting the result is often given by the doctor.

If the result is negative, it is important that the individual knows how to avoid risk in the future and whether it is advisable to come back for a repeat test in, say, 6 months' and 1 year's time. If the result is positive, the counsellor may want to be accompanied by a colleague who can be on hand to assist. There is no good way of divulging such devastating news. Experts in the field often say that every time they have to do it is different and that it does not get easier.

Q

37.3 When helping a person in distress with a condition such as HIV, black-and-white answers seldom fit. Here are some true situations. How can you help?

Remember: What you think is 'right' may not help you or the patient.

(a) A patient is found to be HIV-positive. He understands the 'duty' he has to tell his partner but does not know how to do it and 'cannot go through with it'. How do you help him?
(b) A patient who is demonstrating signs of serious illness has been advised to have the HIV test. She does not want to and asks you as the nurse to help her. What do you do?
(c) A colleague of yours receives a needlestick injury from a suspected drug user. There is pressure to test the drug user to see if he has HIV. What is your view of the matter?
(d) A patient with HIV tells you that he is scared of becoming ill and wants to die now. Is he depressed? Is there any hope? How do you cope when you can't say 'It'll be all right'?
(e) A patient tells you of a 'high-risk' activity he has engaged in. You want to help him. How do you reassure him without lying? On the other hand, how do you tell him the truth without panicking him or making him behave rashly?

In all of these situations where do your 'loyalties' lie? To whom are you accountable or responsible — the patient, the public, the government, yourself, your profession?

HEALTH EDUCATION AND PROMOTION IN HIV

Although treatment for AIDS is improving, it is still very limited. Health education must therefore take a central role in the fight against the disease. Caplan's (1961) classic model describes health education and promotion as having three parts:

- primary — preventing occurrence of the disease; providing education, raising awareness, giving information
- secondary — detecting disease early; screening, performing individual testing
- tertiary — preventing deterioration of individuals affected, giving support.

These general aims must be responsive to the physical, mental, emotional, spiritual and societal needs of the individual (Ewles & Simnett 1999).

Health promotion in HIV/AIDS entails more than raising general public awareness through mass media campaigns. It can also involve such activities as providing assertiveness training for individuals affected and helping them to learn self-care and nurturing skills. HIV awareness also has implications for the workplace, raising concerns about working practice and hiring policies. Legal and ethical issues must also be grappled with by nurses working with people who are involved in illicit drug use and prostitution and who consequently face particular difficulties (Faugier & Hicken 1996).

To become equipped to operate on so many levels, the reader is urged to read not only 'mainstream' publications on health promotion such as Ewles & Simnett (1999), but also books which take a particular perspective, such as Karpf's (1988) *Doctoring the Media*. These, while not specifically on HIV education, may help the reader to take a more analytical view of large-scale media campaigns. For regular updating of information, the reader may refer to the Department of Health AIDS Unit's press releases, issued quarterly. Several nursing journals publish HIV updates, which give recent research and articles on both clinical and educational issues; a good, comprehensive example is Howe (1998). In England and Wales, nurses may obtain information from the National Health Education Authority, and in Scotland from the Health Education Board. Help is also available locally from health promotion departments.

Elements of health promotion

Targeting the 'audience'

The way in which HIV educators convey their message sometimes seems to contradict the message itself. For example, the maxim that 'there are no high-risk groups, only high-risk activities' is generally 'targeted' at drug users, prostitutes, gay men, etc. Does this amount to ideological double talk?

The problem with labelling whole groups as being 'at risk' is that it is not precise. A gay man, for example, is not at risk if he refrains from unprotected sexual intercourse. An i.v. drug user who does not share injecting equipment is also not at risk. That is, these individuals are not at risk merely because they can be labelled 'gay' or 'drug user'. People are at risk if they undertake a high-risk activity.

Advertisers and health educators, however, record that certain groups have certain behaviour patterns in common. It makes sense, therefore, to target these groups with certain services and messages, always remembering that general patterns will not fully reflect the complexity of individuals.

Initiatives vary and take on cultural differences around the world, from the 'light touch' of fun days, health awareness messages on beer mats (seen from Hong Kong to London) to in-depth and detailed information to particular groups of individuals displaying high-risk behaviour, e.g. pregnant women who use illicit drugs intravenously. It should be remembered that individuals move through different groups. A good example in this context is the young, adult holidaymaker whose behaviour, during most of the year, would not be considered at risk but who may be considered high-risk when on holiday. Several initiatives around the world address this issue.

The right medium and the right message

Leaflets are frequently used in various kinds of information campaigns because they are very simple to distribute. Most people can read in the UK, and by means of leaflets, information can be placed unequivocally in the hands of the target audience. What could be better? Unfortunately, research over the years has shown that people tend not to read unsolicited leaflets. While they can be an excellent written adjunct to a spoken session, leaflets are of limited use 'cold' (AVERT 1992).

The first public message from the UK government came in the form of an open letter, warning of the risks of HIV, from the Chief Medical Officer at the Department of Health. This message was published in all the national papers. Following this there was a leaflet drop to every household in the UK and a poster and television campaign. The commercials and posters carried the slogan 'Don't die of ignorance' but did not go into clinical detail. They were designed to raise awareness. The National AIDS Helpline was set up where people could (and still can) phone free to speak to a trained telephone counsellor.

Research subsequently showed that general messages warning of danger and giving non-specific information were of limited efficacy. Over the years, mass media messages have therefore become much more specific, aiming at particular individuals and behaviour groups. Awareness and knowledge of HIV appear to be improving as a result (HEA 1998).

Although HIV education through the mass media has some degree of effectiveness, this kind of communication, no matter how expertly done, always has a high degree of 'wastage'. Even the most successful television advertising campaigns can only expect to 'reach', i.e. to elicit sales from, 2% of the adult population (Fletcher 1992a,b). But as long as this form of health promotion is successful in influencing the behaviour of some people for their own benefit and that of the larger community, mass media information campaigns must continue to constitute a vital part of the battle against HIV.

The nurse's role

Given the limitations of mass communications in influencing behaviour, the nurse must take every opportunity to make general messages relevant to the patients in her care. Nurses have always been involved in assisting patients to understand their treatment, and in answering their questions in terms that can be understood. In doing so they require sound clinical knowledge together with an understanding of the patient's needs, lifestyle and expectations, as obtained from the nursing assessment.

One of the nurse's greatest advantages as a health educator is that she is with the patient for long periods of time in a position of trust. Many other care professionals see the patient only during short visits and often have to work harder to establish a rapport (Bishop & Scudder 1990). Nevertheless, the nurse may still experience some difficulty in discussing sexual matters and sexuality with her patients. Public campaigns are restricted by legislation and 'public taste', and it may be left to the nurse to provide more explicit information. Personal value judgements, embarrassment and questions of status may present obstacles. Answering questions on, say, oral sex from a person of a different sexual persuasion to oneself may be difficult. Speaking to an underage person who is sexually active may be embarrassing and raise ethical questions. Many practitioners become expert at putting up verbal and non-verbal barriers so that such discussions are avoided.

Despite this potential for awkwardness or discomfort, it is clear, given the devastating effects of HIV, how important it is for nurses to fulfil their obligations as health educators. It is strongly suggested that the reader find an expert practitioner who can act as a role model and mentor. Attending an organised course may also help. It is not suggested that the nurse must necessarily change her mind about certain issues or that she must agree with what each patient has to say. However, her caring must be unconditional, answering to the patient's needs regardless of the nurse's personal judgement.

A mentor can also help the less experienced practitioner to deal with difficult ethical issues. Patients sometimes give the nurse information about past actions which places the nurse in a difficult position. In such cases, nurses at all levels should seek advice, whilst ensuring that patient confidentiality is maintained. Under the UKCC (1992) guidelines the nurse is judged both on confidentiality and on the accounts she gives of her actions in a difficult situation. To give an example, the author once looked after an HIV antibody-positive 15-year-old who was having penetrative sex with an underage partner who lived with her parents. The situation was discussed and acted upon, keeping the confidentiality of all parties. The 15-year-old was assisted to approach the partner and her parents accompanied by nursing staff. Although, in this case, the medical consultant had the power to make an approach without consent, sensitive work with the patient made this unnecessary and a good working relationship was maintained.

Health educators are sometimes faced with the dilemma that encouraging safe practice and encouraging someone to break the law seem to amount to the same thing. For example, nurses are now involved in giving drug users clean needles and syringes. This practice has government and professional support. Is it correct, however, for the nurse to tell the patient how to inject safely or to use one form of drug instead of another? (see Ch. 36). In the face of a bleak prognosis, the practitioner may see no option but to fall back on the pragmatic principle of 'harm reduction' rather than to insist upon an ideal. In such a situation the nurse should seek guidance and support from management.

Group work. Nurses are increasingly becoming involved in working with groups, particularly in the community. These may be self-help groups or people attending a clinic for a particular service. Whether the nurse sets the group up herself or 'piggy-backs' a service onto an existing group, the results can be dramatic. By speaking to a small number, answering questions they want to ask and offering individuals the opportunity to speak in private afterwards, the nurse can make health education messages personally relevant. Ewles & Simnett (1999) describe the formal and informal intricacies of setting up groups, agendas and action plans.

CLINICAL MANIFESTATIONS AND MANAGEMENT OF HIV/AIDS

People with HIV disease rarely get all of the diseases associated with AIDS (see Box 37.1), and often those that do occur manifest one at a time. The precise course of the illness is virtually impossible to predict. A patient of the author's seemed so close to death in late 1987 that it seemed cruel to persist with his medication. In 1995, he was still alive. Another patient was reasonably well but then developed a B-cell lymphoma and died within 2 months. Yet another, with the same diagnosis, became paralysed, recovered and lived for a further 2 years.

The treatment of AIDS is a rapidly developing field in which modifications are being made all the time. This section will therefore present a matrix of current approaches that can be used by the nurse as a conceptual and practical framework as the medical and nursing management of HIV/AIDS advances.

Approaches to nursing care

Pratt (1998) provides detailed strategies and philosophies for ward and service management and Faugier & Hicken (1996) exemplify a variety of nursing responses to people with HIV. The present author uses a process based on Roy's adaptation model (Roy & Andrews 1991) which takes into account the following aspects of the patient's illness experience:

- physiological adaptation — clinical signs, disease process
- self-concept adaptation — anxiety, aggression, grief, social belonging
- role function adaptation (e.g. as a father, a partner, a worker) — sense of failure, sense of conflict
- interdependency adaptation (loneliness, rejection, social interaction).

These four 'adaptive modes' are placed in the context of three 'stimuli':

- focal, e.g. the surrounding facilities, services available; other people
- contextual, e.g. space available, distance to toilet, room temperature
- residual, e.g. personal beliefs, prejudices, personal qualities.

The nurse applying this model, having identified a clinical problem (say, the patient's sudden inability to walk), will consider not only his medication and treatment but also his ability to function and adapt. This is then put alongside the practicalities of the stimuli. Are the facilities at home suitable? How far is it to the toilet? Can the patient put up with a commode in his front room? Will he let his wife or partner look after him?

Roy's model is also useful as it helps the nurse consider all the adaptations needed to make an individual service effective. Does the present service or nursing procedure need change? Does the environment suit the patient? Does the patient need to modify his lifestyle? How can the nurse help these factors come to fruition? The adaptation model encourages a flexible approach by nurse and patient using all the available hospital and community care settings.

People with HIV may present with seemingly minor problems which cannot always be diagnosed or predicted. For example, an individual may suffer weight loss, difficulty in swallowing, anorexia, night sweats, lethargy, mouth ulcers, diarrhoea, constipation and so on. In addition to this, he may become depressed and desperate, as such conditions, even if not in themselves life-threatening, can be very distressing. A patient of the author's had, over 2 years, contracted two serious bouts of *Pneumocystis carinii* pneumonia. He had borne these very well. However, he became severely depressed sometime later when he was back at work. Having contracted oral thrush, he could not swallow properly and was losing weight. This made him feel powerless and he said it was worse than the 'serious' illnesses. Such examples serve to remind the practitioner that the seriousness of a condition cannot be judged strictly by clinical criteria. Moreover, by taking notice of even the smallest signs and taking action, nurses can help many patients remain alive. Many HIV-related conditions, if diagnosed early, respond well to treatment.

Infection control

For general principles of infection control, the reader is referred to Chapter 16. The essence of infection control with HIV is to use universal precautions and to protect the patient (Howe 1998). Care should be taken with all body fluids, and gloves and aprons should be used for intimate procedures. Because of his damaged immune system, the patient may be more at risk from the nurse than the other way round. There is generally no need for reverse barrier nursing, however, as most individuals are not seriously at risk from their carers.

In the home, basic hygiene is to be encouraged and clothes and bedding should be washed in a washing machine. Disposal of medical waste should be carried out in accordance with local nursing procedures. Needles and syringes found in the street are the responsibility of the Environmental Health Department, although health care professionals finding them have a duty to minimise the risk of injury to themselves and others where possible.

CONDITIONS, TREATMENTS AND SPECIFIC NURSING INTERVENTIONS

What follows is a description of the main presenting infections, conditions and treatments associated with HIV and AIDS (see Box 37.1).

> For further information, the following are recommended: Pratt (1998) for discussion of nursing strategy; Flaskerud & Ungvarski (1994) for an American perspective; Adler (1991) for colour photographs and large illustrations; Sims & Moss (1994) from the Mildmay AIDS Hospice in London for palliative care; Butterworth et al (1993) for insight into community care discharge and referral patterns.

Articles relating to specific treatment and nursing care are referred to throughout the following sections.

At present there is no vaccine in general use against AIDS. Research is advancing and expectations of a vaccine to make people immune to HIV are still cited by various establishments as being from 5 to 10 years away. Although there are various treatments which ameliorate the effects of viruses, there has never been anything in the nature of a broad-spectrum antibiotic which actually kills viruses. Antiviral agents which suppress HIV will be discussed later.

Possibilities for fighting and killing the virus are therefore limited. The best successes so far have been in the area of symptomatic control, i.e. stopping or slowing the associated diseases and conditions which can kill the patient. The other main aim of care is to improve the patient's quality of life. There is thus a similarity between AIDS nursing and oncology and palliative care.

At the beginning of the epidemic, the life expectancy of someone diagnosed as having AIDS ranged from a few weeks to 2 years. Patients receiving care can now live for 5–10 years, sometimes more. As described earlier, when comparing HIV disease with other life-threatening conditions such as diabetes mellitus, which similarly depend on symptomatic control but for which there is a much longer life expectancy, it becomes apparent that the care of HIV-related illness continues to be in a developing stage.

The general progress of HIV-related illness is represented in Figure 37.2 (p. 1037).

Phases of HIV and AIDS

Phase A: acute seroconversion illness

In most individuals this illness is not recognised. It may be seen 2–6 weeks after exposure to HIV. Not everybody infected with HIV gets this flu- or glandular fever-like condition. It may be associated with joint pain and other non-specific signs. A skin rash is sometimes seen, as are swollen lymph glands (these usually reduce after some time). At this stage the body will be producing HIV antibodies (seroconversion). A few individuals may also show early signs of HIV affecting the central nervous system, particularly the layers of the brain (encephalopathy, meningitis; see Ch. 9).

Treatment of seroconversion illness is symptomatic and does not usually take place in hospital. For the alert doctor and nurse, the illness may be a useful diagnostic warning, rather as the presence of a thirst and boils suggest diabetes. However, the signs are very similar to those of many minor infections.

Phase B: antibody positive phase

B-1: asymptomatic HIV infection. As HIV has only been recognised for less than 20 years, one can only state that the period between infection and the onset of clinical signs may be anything from a few weeks to 18 or more years. From this fact, it may be seen that procedures such as contact tracing are not as simple or effective as in other sexually transmitted disease, as the asymptomatic period commonly covers much of an individual's sexually active life.

B-2: persistent generalised lymphadenopathy (PGL) or lymphadenopathy syndrome (LAS). This condition is sometimes the one which alerts medical services to investigate for HIV. The individual presents with swollen glands of more than 1 cm which persist for longer than 12 weeks. Although the individual may have swollen inguinal glands, he must also have other affected glands. Other reasons for swollen glands must be discounted before a diagnosis is given. As this is often the 'introductory' condition to HIV illness, monitoring of helper T cells and suppressor T cells (called the CD4 T-cell subsets procedure; see Appendix 1) and other investigations may begin. It is at this stage that the individual may be tested for HIV for the first time.

Phase C: AIDS-related complex (ARC)

This phase refers to a period in an individual's illness career where he may contract a variety of well-known conditions, but not major, life-threatening, opportunistic infections or cancers. Common bacterial, viral and fungal infections frequently occur and are often marked by their persistence and virulence. Oral and genital herpes or athlete's foot are good examples. In a normally healthy person, these conditions would resolve within a few days. When someone 'goes into' ARC, the duration of the infection is lengthened and the whole foot, for instance, may become affected. Other conditions such as oral hairy leukoplakia are sometimes seen.

Loss of weight (up to 10% body mass) may be seen at this stage. This may be due to a specific mechanical problem, such as mouth ulcers, or from persistent low-grade attacks from infections. At this stage a significant drop may be seen in the helper T cells. In day-to-day practice, nurses should bear in mind that young, healthy people should overcome common infections quickly without them becoming widespread. Any persistent condition (e.g. coughing, loss of weight) should be noted. While thrush (*Candida albicans*) is common in the vagina, it is very uncommon in the mouth of a young healthy person. Such an occurrence should immediately alert the practitioner to the fact that the individual may have an underlying condition such as HIV.

The nurse working with diagnosed patients should also be aware that, since the positive diagnosis, the individual will have been dreading the onset of illness. When weight loss, mouth ulcers or fungal infections occur, he may become acutely anxious, considering himself to be in imminent danger of death or pain. Other professionals, such as clinical psychologists, can assist the patient during these periods. Involvement of the patient in all stages of decision-making and treatment right from the start will assist him to take control of his condition and reduce his feeling of helplessness.

Box 37.4 summarises treatments and medications used in various conditions associated with ARC.

Box 37.4 Nursing care in AIDS-related complex (Flaskerud & Ungvarski 1994, Pratt 1998)

Diarrhoea
Immediate monitoring should start with the help of a dietician.

Weight loss
Measurements of muscle and fat loss should be included in the care programme. Eating patterns should be discussed along with ways of increasing intake, e.g. taking frequent, smaller meals and perhaps supplementary feeds such as Ensure (MacCallum 1991).

Fluid and electrolyte replacement is essential. Codeine phosphate, loperamide hydrochloride and diphenoxylate hydrochloride may be useful, but it is emphasised that medication should always be given in combination with dietary monitoring and therapy (see Chs 20 and 21).

Herpes simplex
Acyclovir is used. Prophylactic doses may also be given.

Herpes zoster
Mouth and lip care is important to prevent cracking and secondary infection. Soothing lotions and loose clothing may be appropriate for attacks of shingles. Sleep, fluid intake and diet should be monitored.

Seborrhoeic dermatitis/skin care
Salicylic acid and tar-based lotions are used. Low-dose steroids and steroid/antibiotic/antifungal combinations (e.g. Trimovate) are sometimes used for short periods. Responding to the individual patient's discomfort is important. Giving attention to small details in order to alleviate the irritation of skin conditions is one of the most appreciated nursing services (see Ch. 12).

Tinea pedis
Miconazole and clotrimazole creams are used topically. Systemic griseofulvin is used if the infection is persistent. Keeping the feet dry and comfortable can be helped by such measures as drying with a cool hair dryer and leaving the end of the bed covers loose.

Oral candidiasis
Nystatin antifungal topical drops may be used. However, oral thrush is often persistent in HIV illness, in which case systemic fluconazole is used (see Ch. 12). Mouth care is vital, as is a high fluid intake. Some patients find mouth rinsing with benzydamide hydrochloride, which has anaesthetic properties, helpful. Others rinse with fizzy water or diet cola to relieve discomfort, a valued practice that is not yet supported by research evidence.

Oral hairy leukoplakia
Acyclovir is used. Mouth care is again essential.

Phase D: AIDS — constitutional disease, opportunistic infections, secondary cancers

Constitutional disease: HIV wasting syndrome. The diagnosis of AIDS depends on an individual being diagnosed as HIV antibody-positive plus being diagnosed as having one of the life-threatening opportunistic infections or secondary cancers associated with HIV. Recently, a third criterion has come more to the fore, namely the constitutional or systemic condition known as HIV wasting syndrome. This has arisen from the experience in Africa, where AIDS is called 'slim disease'. In the West also it is increasingly recognised that some individuals become extremely ill, losing extreme amounts of weight (more than 10% body mass) and suffering from morbid weakness and loss of function with or without having the 'label' of one of the listed conditions. In the USA, 19% of adults with AIDS are diagnosed as having HIV wasting syndrome.

The causes of HIV wasting syndrome may be mechanical or systemic. As mentioned before, people lose weight if there are factors such as mouth ulcers and sickness which impede eating. Malabsorption may also be seen and may be due to the presence of a lesion such as Kaposi's sarcoma in the gut or to a more generalised dysfunction. In all these cases the patient is starved of nutrients.

Wasting may also occur as a result of metabolic changes. As in cancerous conditions, the body may go from its normal anabolic state into a catabolic crisis in which body mass is 'burnt up' at an increased and dangerous rate, often causing irreparable damage. These patients may recover some weight but they often do not recover muscle mass (Flaskerud & Ungvarski 1994).

Supervised nutritional rehabilitation is therefore necessary. This may include nutritional supplements and more invasive therapy such as continuous or intermittent parenteral feeding. However, it is as well to remember that the nurse can play a life-saving role in the attention she pays to the ordinary nutritional service to the patient. MacCallum's (1991) research found that nutritionally compromised patients were often losing weight in hospital because of the meal and nutrition service. He concluded that nursing care and nutrition are as much about 'knives and forks' as about sophisticated tube feeding.

Opportunistic infections: protozoal. Some of the protozoal infections which may occur in AIDS are as follows.

Pneumocystis carinii pneumonia (PCP; pneumocystosis). About 60% of individuals contract PCP as the first AIDS-related infection. Because the vast majority of people diagnosed as having AIDS have been unaware of their HIV status, many people who have contracted PCP for the first time present not to specialist units but to A&E departments, GPs' offices and other non-specialist areas.

Although PCP is the most common cause of death in AIDS, the organism responsible, *Pneumocystis carinii*, can be found, quite normally, in most human beings. Their immune system keeps the population of the organism at an acceptable level. When the immune system is compromised, the level rises and causes severe, life-threatening pneumonia. The individual usually presents with a 2–5 week history of increasing shortness of breath, weakness and dry cough; cyanosis is often seen.

Treatment is by i.v. pentamidine isethionate. Co-trimoxazole is also used, although some patients suffer from severe rashes caused by the high doses necessary. Pentamidine has side-effects, e.g. nephrotoxicity. Regular blood pressure observations and urinalysis are necessary. Diaminodiphenylsulfone is used as well as pyrimethamine. Aerosolised pentamidine is used as a treatment but is more commonly used as a prophylactic 2- to 4-weekly.

For more detail about PCP, see Flaskerud & Ungvarski (1994) and Pratt (1998).

Cryptosporidiosis. This condition has some notoriety because of the sometimes devastating diarrhoea it causes and because high levels of the organism in the general water supply are often reported in the news. It is caused by a protozoan which is normally present in small quantities in the water supply. In immunocompromised patients, it rises to high levels in the gastrointestinal tract and causes diarrhoea. The loss of fluid can be as much as 10–20 L/day, although less virulent attacks are also seen.

Cryptosporidiosis is generally seen only in patients who are already very ill and have suffered other infections. It is very difficult to manage this condition at home, as i.v. fluid replacement and constant bowel movements will need constant attention. For the patient, this condition may mean an extremely poor state of health and hospitalisation. In its worst form it is an extremely distressing condition for both the patient and his carers.

Treatments have varying success. Spiramycin and erythromycin are the main antibiotics used but combinations of others may also be tried. Diarrhoea may also be caused by isosporiasis and is usually treated by co-trimoxazole.

Toxoplasmosis. The causative protozoan is sometimes heard mentioned in association with cats and raw meat, although it does not generally manifest itself as a disease in healthy people. Its most common manifestation is cerebral toxoplasmosis. The organism causes space-occupying lesions in the brain. These create cerebral oedema and raised intracranial pressure. The patient suffers the usual signs of these conditions: paralysis and unconsciousness (see Ch. 9). Toxoplasmosis is often fatal and treatment must be prolonged as relapses are almost inevitable. The main medication is pyrimethamine given with sulphadiazine. Dexamethasone is also used to reduce cerebral oedema. In the most serious cases, constant nursing attention is needed as the patient's condition may deteriorate rapidly.

Opportunistic infections: viral. The most common of these are described below.

Herpes simplex virus. This condition has been mentioned in association with ARC, where it occurs in its less virulent forms. Serious and life-threatening forms (e.g. encephalitis) are sometimes seen, affecting the central nervous system (Pratt 1998). Acyclovir is used in treatment.

Cytomegalovirus (CMV). This virus is encountered in general practice and in midwifery, where it is known to cause spontaneous abortion. In HIV-related illness it is most commonly seen causing CMV retinitis. Small 'cotton buds' are seen on the retina on examination. The patient may then rapidly become blind. The author has cared for people to whom this has happened over a few days. Treatment with ganciclovir i.v. is given; trisodium phosphonoformate i.v. is also used. These may be given in the hospital setting, but increasingly (especially ganciclovir) are given at home. Improvement is seen with treatment but relapse occurs in almost all cases.

CMV retinitis can have a devastating affect on the patient's morale and state of mind. Two of the author's patients decided to stop all treatment once they became blind, whereupon other illness and death followed quite quickly. This demonstrated to the author the vital importance of the patient's will to live when combating HIV-related illness.

Progressive multifocal leucoencephalopathy (PML). This unusual disease is caused by a papovavirus and results in demyelination. Conditions most likely to be seen are blindness, hemiparesis, ataxia and aphasia (Adler 1991). No treatment is known for this crippling condition (Pratt 1998).

Opportunistic infections: bacterial. The following bacterial infections may be seen in people with AIDS (see also Ch. 16).

Mycobacterium tuberculosis (TB). Tuberculosis is now increasingly seen in patients with HIV and is often associated with poor social conditions. Work in prisons around the world has seen an increase in TB prevalence in some places where there is a high prevalence of HIV. Prisoners with HIV are affected, as are other vulnerable inmates (Drielsma 1994). Treatment is with rifampicin, ethambutol, isoniazid and pyrazinamide. TB in the general population, when treated, is not generally life-threatening. Patients with HIV infected with TB, however, are often made even weaker by the condition.

Salmonellosis. As with other compromised and vulnerable individuals this infection, generally associated with food poisoning, poses a particular danger to people with HIV. Scrupulous care should be taken in food preparation and delivery. Patients should avoid undercooking foods such as eggs and poultry. Hand hygiene is also important. Treatment is with chloramphenicol, ampicillin or amoxycillin.

Mycobacterium avium complex (MAC). People in advanced stages of HIV illness are sometimes found to have atypical mycobacteria in their lungs. The effect of this on prognosis is still unclear, although some minor clinical signs are associated with the condition. Treatment is not generally successful.

Opportunistic infections: fungal. Candidiasis is sometimes seen in virulent manifestations in people with advanced HIV illness. Infection may extend from the mouth to the alimentary tract. Vaginal candidiasis may be particularly persistent and distressing. Nystatin vaginal pessaries and other conventional treatments are used.

Cryptococcus is one of the systemic fungal conditions sometimes seen. Treatment is with amphotericin and fluconazole. Two others are histoplasmosis, which affects the lungs, liver and gastrointestinal tract, and coccidioidomycosis, which affects any organ, including the brain (Pratt 1998).

Infestation. Strictly speaking, infestation is not associated with HIV. However, it should be pointed out that if a patient with HIV happens to become infested with lice or scabies, particularly the variety known as Norwegian scabies, the infection may be particularly virulent, with several thousand times as many mites on the skin as in a patient who is not immunocompromised. Norwegian scabies occasionally strikes hospitals and institutions. Treatment is with gamma benzene hexachloride (Sims & Moss 1994).

Secondary cancers (neoplasms). The immune system has the function not only of fighting infection but also of fighting and inhibiting malignant cells. The following two forms of cancer are associated with HIV and an AIDS diagnosis.

Kaposi's sarcoma (KS). This purplish skin cancer was previously seen only in elderly men of certain races, e.g. Jewish men. With the advent of AIDS in the Western world, it was one of the first manifestations of the condition. As with the opportunistic infections, it is not seen in all patients. As a skin condition it is very disfiguring, particularly when on the face. If it remains in small patches, treatment is often confined to cosmetic camouflage, which the British Red Cross Society can provide. However, it sometimes forms into constricting bands on the skin (e.g. around the ankle). Internally it may also form gastrointestinal obstructions and it is sometimes found in the lungs and other internal organs. Irradiation treatment is sometimes used in these cases (Adler 1991).

Non-Hodgkin's lymphomas (B cell lymphomas, undifferentiated lymphomas). These cancers are seen in much higher numbers among people with AIDS than in the general population. They are found in the central nervous system, the bone marrow and the gastrointestinal tract. They are often rapidly fatal and treatment is often not successful. Various chemotherapies may be used (see Ch. 11).

Neurological disease; HIV encephalopathy. HIV neurological disease is not an opportunistic infection. It is the human immunodeficiency virus directly affecting the central nervous system, including the covering of the brain. It may manifest early on as peripheral neuropathy, in its many forms, and later progress to affect the individual's personality and lucidity. Eventually the person may become demented. One of the problems in diagnosing this condition is that changes in computed tomograms (CT scans) do not necessarily accompany changes in behaviour; it is possible for a patient with a normal CT to be demented.

Nursing care of the various conditions associated with neurological disease and encephalopathy is often challenging. Caring for an active young person who suffers from cerebral dysfunction demands a flexible approach. Remissions can be experienced and there can be periods of despair for the individual. One of the author's patients, who refused to be cared for in hospital (he had spent long periods in prison and was afraid of institutions), was cared for at home. He began to suffer from forgetfulness, personality changes and eventually showed signs of dementia. This was distressing for him, as he often had insight into his condition; in these lucid periods he would sometimes say he wanted to end his life.

On a more optimistic note, however, HIV neurological disease does appear to respond well to antiviral therapy. Many patients show a marked improvement as well as a slowing down of the advancement of the disease.

Antiviral treatment

Antiviral treatment of AIDS has, since the mid-1990s, developed considerably. Treatment is now based on 'combination' therapy. These treatments do not kill HIV, but interfere with the process of virus replication by inhibiting with the function of reverse transcriptase such as zidovudine (AZT) and didanosine (ddI). More recently, there is a new set of treatments known as protease inhibitors (Saquinavir, Ritonavir, Indinavir) and also non-nucleoside reverse transcriptase inhibitors (Lipsky 1996).

The main problems recognised with antiviral treatment are side-effects and, increasingly, resistance. Resistance following the treatment of individuals with only one antiviral drug (monotherapy) has led to the use of combination therapy, where two or three drugs are used. Serious side-effects are seen more commonly in the 'earlier' drugs such as AZT, which are toxic. The newer drugs are generally found to be less toxic with fewer side-effects. The Medical Control Agency (1997) provides a useful summary of reactions to the various HIV therapies.

Because virus replication is slowed down by antiviral treatment, the level of healthy helper T cells remains higher, giving the T cells a chance to recover and modestly increase.

When zidovudine first became available, it was used mainly for people who were already in advanced stages of illness. Side-effects were considerable, nausea and depletion of red blood cells being the most damaging. Following worldwide double-blind placebo-controlled trials, it was found that zidovudine was more effective if given to people earlier on, after some fall in helper T cell level had occurred. Side-effects were fewer and recovery better. This remains the clinical view today. Because zidovudine therapy is now given earlier with encouraging results, it has, some would say, strengthened the case for people to come forward, be tested and receive treatment. Didanosine (ddI) is a more recently developed antiviral agent which works in a similar way. Extensive clinical trials have been, and continue to be, undertaken with antiviral therapies (Lenderking et al 1994, Carpenter et al 1996).

One of the main problems with antiviral treatment is that it appears to have limited efficacy over long periods of time. Some patients find a loss of effect after 18 months to 2 years. Side-effects are still seen. The one which may affect the individual most is the loss of red blood cells, some patients requiring blood transfusions every 5–8 weeks. During the intervening period the patient may need help adapting to the varying levels of energy and lethargy he may experience. Headaches and insomnia are also experienced by some (Simberkoff et al 1996).

CONCLUSION

In the year 2000, HIV and its related diseases continue to challenge health services throughout the world. The irony, described earlier, of discontinuing the specialism of fever nurses, just when AIDS was first recognised, as though infectious disease were yesterday's problem, has been further compounded by the emergence of widespread resistant tuberculosis and hepatitis C. In future years, perhaps AIDS and other intractable infectious diseases will be considered together rather than as separate and distinct specialities.

Whatever the future of AIDS as a speciality it will remain important that nurses stay involved with their patients and not aloof. More than ever before, nurses appreciate that they are privileged to be admitted into the trust of their patients. In the field of HIV, as in other palliative care, nurses become very deeply involved in their patients' lives and in their experience of dying.

The nursing care of people with HIV has seen a real growth in innovative practice. Work with drug users, prisoners, prostitutes and other marginalised people has meant that nurses are increasingly working in non-traditional areas, using new procedures. Many myths have been shattered, particularly with regard to the amount of sophisticated equipment that was thought necessary to provide care. High-level nursing care is now given in the poorest areas and in the most difficult of circumstances (Faugier & Hicken 1996).

Family recognition. People with HIV and AIDS have, like the rest of the population, a variety of domestic arrangements and relationships, and the nurse would do well to take the widest view of the terms 'family' and 'next of kin'. It is distressing to watch courtesy and kindness being shown to the 'official' family and next of kin, who may be estranged, while the patient's lifelong partner and the people he chooses to spend every day with are pushed out of the picture. The author has seen this happen to both homosexual and heterosexual patients. In such matters, the nurse should take the lead from the patient, not from the admission form.

Spirituality does not always manifest itself as the embracing of a formal religion. When an individual is seriously ill, he may 'plug into the infinite' in many ways. One of my patients found solace in a trip to the opera (Atkinson 1989). Another, who had gone blind, particularly loved sweet-smelling flowers. As an aspiring professional, I used to be rather contemptuous of what I considered sentimental or superstitious behaviour. Experience, however, has taught me greater wisdom and humility.

Grieving and the nurse

Over 40 of the patients I have cared for have now died. The oldest was 70, the youngest 18. I remember them all, and they have enhanced my practice. As I wrote this chapter, their memory was close by, their faces very clear in my mind. I remember when each one died, and each time was an emotional experience. There is some debate as to whether it is a good thing to hang onto disturbing memories. My experience is that it is not a question of deliberately hanging on. When one becomes deeply involved in an individual's living and dying, his memory will live on. It is the nurse's role to bear witness to those memories and to the present experience of each patient alive today. This may be emotional sometimes, but it is not depressing. It is a positive attitude which improves care delivery.

One of my patients had a friend who, during their working life together, used to phone him in the morning: 'What news from the Rialto today, Bassanio?' he would quip. The two friends would then chat about their news, sometimes separated by the Atlantic, sometimes by a few streets. When my patient died, a dedication appeared in *Variety*. It sums up my feelings for all my patients: 'Farewell Bassanio, you are sadly missed'.

REFERENCES

Adler M (ed) 1991 ABC of AIDS, 2nd edn. BMJ Publications, London

Aggleton P, AVERT 1993 A study of the attitudes of student nurses to HIV/AIDS. AIDS Education and Research Trust, Goldsmith College, London

Akinsanya J A 1991 Who will care: a survey of the knowledge and attitudes of hospital nurses to people with HIV/AIDS. Department of Health, Anglia Polytechnic. HMSO, London

Armstrong M L 1998 Body piercing: a clinical look. Office Nurse 11(3): 26–29

Atkinson J 1989 A flexible friend. Community Outlook June: 4–6

Atkinson J 1991 Coping with the guilty ill. Nursing Standard 5(17): 42–44

AVERT 1992 HIV, AIDS and sex: information for young people. AIDS Education and Research Trust, Horsham, West Sussex

Barker D J P, Rose G 1998 Epidemiology in medical practice. Churchill Livingstone, Edinburgh

Bishop A H, Scudder J R 1990 The practical, moral and personal sense of nursing. State University of New York Press, NY, USA

Bond J, Bond S 1986 Sociology and health care. Churchill Livingstone, Edinburgh

Butterworth T, Faugier J, Brocklehurst N 1993 AIDS and community care discharge. Referral patterns and coordination. School of Nursing Studies, University of Manchester

Caplan G 1961 An approach to community mental health. Tavistock, London

Carlisle D 1998 HIV and breastfeeding: a global issue for midwives. RCM Midwives Journal 1(3): 78–80

Carpenter C C J, Fischi M A, Hammer S M 1996 Antiretroviral therapy for HIV infection in 1996. Recommendations of an International panel. Journal of the American Medical Association 276: 146–154

CDC 1987 A report by Council of State and Territorial Epidemiologists; AIDS Program, Centre for Infectious Diseases. Morbidity and Mortality Weekly Report (Suppl 36): 1S

Clapham P, Simmons G 1997 New targets for HIV therapy. MRC News. Medical Research Council Autumn (75): 40–43

Connor S, Kingman S 1989 The search for the virus. Penguin, Harmondsworth

Department of Health 1998 AIDS press release (January). HMSO, London

Downie R, Telfer E 1980 Caring and curing. Methuen, London

Drielsma P 1994 Tuberculosis and HIV: back to the bad old days? Venereology – The Interdisciplinary International Journal of Sexual Health 7(2): 77–79

Eastlund T 1995 Infectious disease transmission through cell, tissue, and organ transplantation: reducing the risk through donor selection. Cell Transplant 4(5): 455–477

Ewles L, Simnett I 1999 Promoting health: a practical guide to health education, 4th edn. Baillière Tindall, Edinburgh

Faugier J, Hicken I 1996 AIDS and HIV: the nursing response. Chapman and Hall, London
Flaskerud J H, Ungvarski P J (eds) 1994 HIV/AIDS: a guide to nursing care, 3rd edn. WB Saunders, Pennsylvania
Fletcher W 1992a Hit and miss of mass marketing. The Guardian (Media section), 23 March, p 29
Fletcher W 1992b A glittering haze. NTC Publications, London
GGHB 1998 Information from Greater Glasgow Health Board Department of Public Health Addictions, mental health and sexual health team. GGHB, Glasgow
Greif J, Hewitt W 1998 The living canvas. Advance for Nurse Practitioners. 6(6): 26-31, 82
Hanrahan A, Reutter L 1997 A critical review of the literature on sharps injuries: epidemiology, management of exposures and prevention. Journal of Advanced Nursing 25(1): 144–154
Hansard 1986 Parliamentary report on the debate on HIV and AIDS (November). House of Commons, London
HEA 1998 Information on the continuing mass media campaign. Health Education Authority, London
Howe J 1998 HIV clinical update. Primary Health Care 8(2): 17–22
Josefson D 1997 Antiretrovirals, combinations do not eliminate HIV entirely. British Medical Journal 315: 1488
Karpf A 1988 Doctoring the media: the reporting of health and medicine. Routledge, London
King E 1997 A cure for over optimism. Positive Nation 16(30): 11–12
Lemp G F, Hirozawa A M, Givertz D et al 1994 Seroprevalence of HIV and risk behaviours among young homosexual and bisexual men; the San Francisco/Berkeley Young Men's Survey. Journal of the American Medical Association 272(6): 449–454
Lenderking W R, Gelber R D, Cotton D J 1994 Evaluation of the quality of life associated with zidovudine treatment in asymptomatic human immunodeficiency infection. The AIDS Clinical Trials Group. New England Journal of Medicine 330: 738–743
Lewis S, Bor R 1994 Nurses' knowledge of and attitudes towards sexuality and the relationship of these with nursing practice. Journal of Advanced Nursing 20: 251–259
Lipsky J J 1996 Antiretroviral drugs for AIDS. The Lancet 348: 800–803
MacCallum A 1991 Nutrition and the patient with HIV. Report on Research Project for MSc. Royal Free Hospital/Department of Nursing, King's College, Waterloo
Medical Control Agency 1997 Summary of HIV therapies and their side effects. MCA, London
Mok J 1993 HIV-1 infection, breast milk and HIV-1 transmission. Lancet 341: 931
O'Connell C B 1993 Risk assessment interviewing for HIV. Physician Assistant 17(3): 35–36, 41–43, 122–124
Oddone E, Cowper P, Hamilton J 1993 Cost effectiveness analysis of early zidovudine treatment of HIV infected patients. British Medical Journal 307: 1322–1325
Petrou S, Dooley M, Whitaker L 1996 The economic costs of caring for people with HIV infection and AIDS in England and Wales. Pharmacoeconomics 9: 332–340
PHLS & SCIEH 1999 (and ongoing) AIDS/HIV quarterly surveillance tables. Public Health Laboratory Service, London, and the Scottish Centre for Infection and Environmental Health, Glasgow
Pratt R 1998 HIV & AIDS: a strategy for nursing care, 5th edn. Edward Arnold, London
RCN Congress 1991 Emergency Debate tabled by the Royal College of Nursing AIDS Nursing Forum on the practice of publishing results of local HIV prevalence screening. Harrogate
Rothenberg R B, Scarlett M, del Rio C, Reznik D, O'Daniels C 1998 Oral transmission of AIDS. AIDS 12: 2095-2105
Roy C, Andrews H A 1991 The Roy adaptation model – the definitive statement. Appleton and Lange, New York
Simberkoff M S, Hartigan P M, Hamilton J D 1996 Long-term follow-up of symptomatic HIV infected patients originally randomised to early versus later zidovudine treatment: report of a Veterans Affairs Cooperative study. Journal of Acquired Immune Deficiency Syndrome 11: 142–150
Sims R, Moss V 1994 Palliative care for people with AIDS. Edward Arnold, London
Sistrom M G, Coyner B J, Gwaltney J M Jr, Farr B M 1998 Concise communications. Frequency of percutaneous injuries requiring post exposure prophylaxis for occupational exposure to human immuno deficiency virus. Infection Control & Hospital Epidemiology 19(7): 504–506
UKCC 1992 Code of professional conduct, 3rd edn. United Kingdom Central Council of Nurses, Midwives and Health Visitors, London
WHO 1998 Information from the World Health Organization, Europe. WHO, Copenhagen.

FURTHER READING

Adler M (ed) 1991 ABC of AIDS, 2nd edn. BMJ Publications, London
Butterworth T, Faugier J, Brocklehurst N 1993 AIDS and community care discharge. Referral patterns and coordination. School of Nursing Studies, University of Manchester
Flaskerud J H, Ungvarski P J (eds) 1994 HIV/AIDS: a guide to nursing care, 3rd edn. WB Saunders, Pennsylvania
PHLS 1991 Proforma and guidance for the National Anonymous Survey of the Seroprevalence of HIV. Public Health Laboratory Service, London
Pratt R 1998 HIV & AIDS: a strategy for nursing care, 5th edn. Edward Arnold, London
Sims R, Moss V 1994 Palliative care for people with AIDS. Edward Arnold, London
UKCC 1990 Anonymous testing for HIV. Register Journal of the United Kingdom Central Council for Nurses, Midwives and Health Visitors, London

USEFUL ADDRESSES AND TELEPHONE HELPLINE

AVERT
AIDS Education and Research Trust
4 Brighton Road
Horsham
West Sussex RH3 5BA

Haemophilia Society
Chesterfield House
385 Euston Road
London NW1 3AV

National AIDS Helpline (24 hour)
Tel: 0800 567 123

Royal College of Nursing Sexual Health Forum
20 Cavendish Square
London W1M 0AB

Terrence Higgins Trust
52/54 Gray's Inn Road
London WC1X 8LT

ANSWERS

CHAPTER 8

8.15 The following arrangements and interventions can make life easier for patients on dialysis:

- Transport can be arranged by the hospital, if necessary.
- Little can be done to avoid the two or three sessions a week away from home, but by involving the social worker it may be possible to assess and solve some home problems.
- Try and work out the times that will best fit in with the patient's job. Try also to provide a quiet environment that will allow her to rest and sleep.
- Discuss with the patient her fluid intake and come to some compromise that will prevent overload of fluid.
- Seek help from the dietician. Involve the family in discussions about menus and permitted food.
- The social worker may be able to help with financial problems by informing the patient of help and benefits available, and also by assisting with any form-filling requirements.
- The patient should have regular access to medical staff to address problems and assess medication.
- Give psychological help by listening to the patient's expressions of fears and hopes. Above all, always leave the patient with hope.
- Counselling the family as well as the patient will help to keep stress to a minimum.

Patients can often gain a lot of support from other patients in a similar situation. They compare experiences and discuss their various problems and hopes between themselves. Do consider trying to treat patients who get on well together on the same shift.

CHAPTER 11

11.1 Liver, spinach, cauliflower, cabbage and peas.

11.2 In the small intestine, by commensal organisms.

11.3 Patients with:

- liver disease, because of reduced formation of clotting factors
- obstructive jaundice, because of reduced absorption due to lack of bile salts
- chronic diarrhoea.

11.4 (a) Any healthy person aged 18–64 years.

(b)
- Complete health questionnaire to exclude any person who might transmit an infection. This includes having, or contact with, syphilis, malaria, other tropical diseases, HIV, AIDS, hepatitis (type A, B or C), infectious diseases and skin infections. Other categories excluded are a person who has had tooth extractions or oral surgery within 72 h or who has been immunised with live attenuated vaccines (variable time limit).
  Other questions relate to the presence in the donor's blood of antigens (e.g. allergies or asthma), whether the patient has cancer, or the taking of any drugs. Other questions are to ensure the donor's health, e.g. recent donations, pregnancy and time of last meal.
- Health check, including height, weight, temperature, pulse, blood pressure and haemoglobin level.

(c) Important points include maintaining asepsis; the speed with which the unit of blood is withdrawn (450 mL over 15 min); the total amount of each donation (1 pint); labelling of the unit with the donor's name, blood group and rhesus factor immediately it is withdrawn; and screening each unit for hepatitis and HIV.

(d) Care of the donor includes explaining the procedure fully and taking the donation with the donor recumbent. After-care includes maintaining the donor in a recumbent position until she is able to sit up and get up without feeling dizzy or faint; recommending that she has a cup of tea and food and waits another 15 min before leaving the centre; and advising her to refrain from smoking (for 1 h) and drinking alcohol (3 h), and to increase fluid intake for 2 days and take a balanced diet for 2 weeks.

(e) Stored at 4°C for 35 days.

11.6 • Blood transfusion will increase blood volume and therefore stroke volume.
- There may be a degree of cardiac failure because of a lack of oxygen-carrying capacity to the tissues, with a resultant increase in heart rate to compensate. For this, the heart will also require adequate oxygen, and if this is lacking it will fail.

11.7 (a) Potential problems:
- Compliance with taking medication
- Balanced diet with adequate iron
- Financial problems
- Depression or loneliness
- Inability to buy or cook.

(b) Ways to resolve problems:
- Patient education about medication
- Advice from the dietician and nurses about a balanced diet. Use menu choice card as a teaching aid
- Advice from the social worker about social services benefits and budgeting
- Attendance at a day hospital or lunch club, or another social activity that appeals and is available in the patient's area
- Assessment of necessary skills in the OT department and a home visit for possible adaptations, e.g. to gas taps or plugs
- Someone to shop for him.

(c) Community services: health visitor, social services for home help, meals on wheels, lunch clubs, outings, attendance at day hospital, OT, physiotherapy, possible rehousing or sheltered housing, contact with self-help group for bereavement, e.g. Cruse, contact with local church.

11.8 The implications of this ongoing therapy might include:
- A need to understand the rationale for the treatment
- Recurring anxiety about health and about the injections themselves
- Disruption to social life. Where are the injections administered: GP surgery, health clinic or patient's home? Is transport available? Are there cost implications?
- A need to consider safety implications. How are needles and syringes stored and disposed of? Are there children in the home?

11.9 Green, leafy vegetables, liver, white fish, yeast extract (e.g. Marmite) and fortified cornflakes.

11.10 By not overcooking foods.

11.12 In sickle cell disease there is a structural abnormality of one of the globin chains of haemoglobin, causing erythrocytes to become sickle-shaped in certain circumstances (see text). In thalassaemia, there is reduced synthesis of one or more globin chains, resulting in chronic anaemia.

11.13 Blood transfusions every 4 weeks.

11.14 Iron overload and hepatitis C.

11.16 (a) Her fears and anxieties might relate to:
- losing the protection of a sheltered environment and immediate access to specialist nursing and medical advice
- her perceived inability to cope at home
- her future, e.g. her wedding, marriage and the possibility of having children
- the diagnosis, treatment and prognosis
- the prospect of meeting strangers, or friends who have not seen her since her admission.

(b) By giving her advice about wigs, turbans, hats or scarves to cover hair loss; make-up to disguise loss of eyebrows; jewellery and other fashionable accessories to distract attention from the alopecia.

(c) Community support available could include GP; clinical nurse specialist (if available); health visitor; self-help groups (e.g. Leukaemia Care Society, BACUP, Cancer Link); social worker; district nurse (if Hickman line catheter is in situ and the patient is unable to dress the exit site and heparinise the line herself); religious groups; DSS and/or citizens' advice bureau.

(d) How to take her own temperature and, if it is raised, who to contact; general advice on reducing the possibility of infections, e.g. avoiding crowded places; ongoing mouth care and personal hygiene; care of Hickman line; details about medication; dietary advice; return to normal activity and work; advice about going away on holiday.

CHAPTER 18

18.6 (a) Tachycardia is produced by an increase in sympathetic activity due to stressors such as fright, anxiety and pain. In the event of hypovolaemia, the heart is required to work much more quickly to maintain the same cardiac output. Infection is usually associated with a pyrexia and an increase in the metabolic demands of the body, and hence with a faster heart rate. Arrhythmias are frequently observed following a myocardial infarction and in the patient with cardiogenic shock.

(b) An increase of parasympathetic nervous activity produces a bradycardia. This finding is also associated with excessive vagal stimulation in the patient with spinal shock or myocardial infarction. A myocardial infarction may also cause an interruption in the heart's conducting mechanism and precipitate heart block and bradycardia. The traumatised and head-injured patient in shock frequently will have cerebral oedema, raised intracranial pressure and a reduced heart rate.

18.7 A low PAWP would indicate that the patient is depleted of fluid and needs rapid fluid replacement.

18.8 A high PAWP would indicate left ventricular failure, which if not corrected might lead to pulmonary oedema.

CHAPTER 20

20.1 The examples listed require different management to resolve the oedema, e.g. obstruction (deep venous thrombosis); inflammmation and/or cell damage (soft tissue injury); changes in blood flow and oxygenation (arterial insufficiency, cardiac failure) and osmotic effects (protein loss). Specific measures are required in each case.

20.2 Not only are the absorption and dissemination of the drug affected by the oedema, but the drug itself may damage the oedematous area, especially if there is cellular damage.

20.3 The shoe should be fitted to offer firm, uniform support to the entire foot and not constrict blood flow to or from the foot. High heels and loose thin straps are to be avoided with particular attention being focused upon the ankles.

20.4 Approximately 2.5 L/day, with an additional 500 mL to compensate for the pyrexia.

20.5 (a) Potenial causes of the reduced urinary output are: the opiate; pain and related stress factors; surgical losses and exposure in theatre; inadequate fluid replacement therapy; impaired renal function due to renal disease or diabetes; a blocked urinary catheter or urine retention.
(b) To establish the most likely cause, first assess the patient for signs of haemorrhage, shock or dehydration. Check the patency of the urinary catheter. Examine the urine for its concentration; analyse the fluid balance records to establish the likelihood of dehyrdration; check the patency of i.v. fluid lines; ensure the analgesia is effective and be knowledgeable concerning any existing medical problems or intraoperative problems that may affect the patient.

20.6 Dehydration, oxygen therapy, mouth breathing, electrolyte imbalance (hypernatraemia), diabetes insipidus.

20.10 There are numerous potential causes — typical examples include an inability to feed, drink or excrete; regulatory problems (hormonal, metabolic, electrolytic and temperature).

20.14 Some indicators of difficulties with i.v. therapies include difficulty in administration; changes in flow rate; pain or discomfort at the site; low-grade pyrexia; no indicator that the therapy is having an effect.

20.15 Anxiety and fear amongst carers; inadequate supervision of the site and equipment; poor maintenance; communication problems between carers and health care team; poor hygiene.

20.16 In both instances, it is important to be able to prevent or relieve and manage the vomiting episode, e.g. to be able to maintain a clear airway (i.e. suction, perhaps cut the jaw wires/bands), and quickly *but safely* to move the spinal-injured patient (i.e. have colleagues available).

20.17 This information may indicate the cause and severity of the vomiting (haemorrhage, obstruction, volume, nature), its likely triggers (smell, food, stress) and management (drugs, breathing exercises).

20.18 Glucose enhances the reabsorption of sodium and water from the intestines.

CHAPTER 24

24.13 (a) Four situations in which catheterisation would be justified are:
- during operations on the lower abdomen
- for precise measurement of urinary output
- where the bladder fails to empty, as in acute and chronic retention
- in cases of intractable incontinence.

It may also be used for irrigation purposes, cytotoxic therapy and urodynamic investigations.
(b) A Foley catheter is an indwelling flexible tube, retained in the bladder by a balloon, for the purpose of continuous drainage.
(c) To aid haemostasis following prostatectomy.
(d) For all catheterisation except that following prostatectomy, or where debris is a problem to drainage.
(e) Four other features which should be considered are:
- catheter material
- tips
- eyes
- balloon size.

Also: shaft size and length.
(f) PVC and plastic for in-and-out intermittent catheters and silicone, latex, Teflon and silicone elastomer or hydrogel materials for indwelling catheters.
(g) This type of catheter is called a Roberts catheter. It allows complete drainage of the bladder. It is not now available on prescription but may be available through the hospital service.
(h) No — only sterile water can be used. Air would make the balloon float. Other substances may cause the introduction of crystals or debris into the inflation channel and block it. Some degree of osmosis occurs between the balloon and the bladder, and harmful substances such as chlorhexidine are therefore not suitable. Prefilled balloons are available.
(i) 10 mL. If only 5 mL are used then only the shaft would be filled; the balloon requires a further 5 mL.
(j) Keep them on a shelf in strict date order in the boxes and packaging provided. Avoid sunlight and direct heat. Do not use rubber bands on the catheter or store in drawers. Avoid all contact with oil and spirit products such as petroleum jelly and paraffin-based items.

24.14 Potential entry points for infection.
Key to diagram:
A — urethral meatus and around catheter
B — junction between catheter and connection tube
C — sample port
D — drainage outlet.

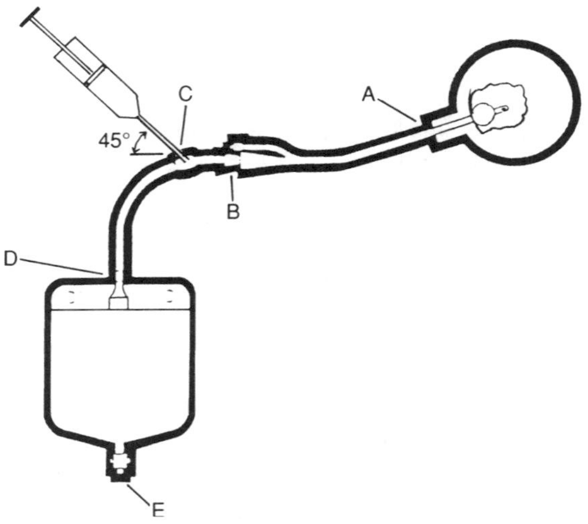

Fig. 24.7 Potential entry points for infection

Procedures to prevent infection:

A. Water should be used for washing the area of the vulva or penis and may be more suitable than antiseptics (Bard 1984). Female-length catheters should be used for women to avoid the 'piston' effect.
B. Catheters should not be disconnected, expect when the bag is being changed. Add-on bags should be attached to leg bags for extra drainage through the night.
C. Samples of urine should be taken only by using the special sleeve on the urine bag tubing, which may be clamped or folded back to allow urine to collect.
D. Urine bags should always be kept at a level below the bladder, and tubing should be occluded by being folded or clamped, if movement across the bed is required.
E. Each time the bags are emptied this should be viewed as a separate procedure for each individual; multipurpose jugs and containers should never be used. Hands should be washed before and after emptying and the bag should be kept on its stand with the tap clear of the floor. Care should be taken when emptying leg bags that the tap does not come into contact with the toilet. The tap should be dried or wiped with an alcohol swab after emptying.

CHAPTER 25

25.4 *Possible reasons:*

- Postoperative pain
  —at site of operation
  —backache
- Noise at night
  —telephone
  —bedpan macerator
  —noisy shoes (nurses and doctors)
  —nurses chatting or giggling
  —i.v. infusion pump alarms
  —other patients snoring/crying out
  —ambulances driving past
- Uncomfortable beds
  —hard mattresses
  —plastic covers on mattresses and pillows.

Nursing interventions:

- No unnecessary pain should be endured. Ensure that Mr B receives regular and careful assessment of pain, provision of analgesics and other comfort measures (positioning, support with pillows, etc.) and monitor the effect of these interventions.
- Positive efforts should be made to keep noise to a minimum during the night. Telephones should be kept off the main ward where possible. Used papier maché bedpans should be rinsed and left until the next morning to be macerated. All ward staff should wear quiet shoes. Nurses should try to keep as quiet as possible while in the main ward. Intravenous infusion pump alarms should be turned down (not off) where this is an option. Patients who snore should be positioned so that they are not on their backs (if appropriate to their care). Noisy patients and noise from outside the ward are more difficult to deal with. Mr B may find wax or silicone earplugs helpful, although not everyone finds these comfortable enough to use during sleep.
- The uncomfortable and unfamiliar beds found in hospital wards may take some adjusting to. A plastic drawsheet should not be left on Mr B's bed unless its presence is really necessary. Mr B is on an adjustable height bed which should be left low during the night, so that he can get out with a minimum of assistance.

Expected outcomes:

- Mr B's pain is well controlled throughout the night.
- The ward is as quiet as possible during the night.
- Mr B is as comfortable as possible in bed.
- Mr B is satisfied with his sleep.

CHAPTER 31

31.2 (a) False. Some forms of cancer, such as testicular teratoma and Hodgkin's disease, are now curable. Many people with cancer are elderly and die from other causes.
(b) False. Deaths due to cardiovascular disease are more prevalent than deaths due to cancer, although cancer is catching up!
(c) Partly true. The causes of cancer are not fully known. Epidemiological studies indicate that cancer may be a disease of lifestyle in the broadest sense. Social and environmental factors are as important as individual behaviour (see p. 915).

(d) Partly true. Some forms of cancer, particularly those of childhood, are hereditary. A small number of other cancers have a high incidence in certain families. Daughters or sisters of women with breast cancer are three times more likely to develop the disease than are others (Slattery & Kerber 1993).

(e) False. There is no evidence to substantiate this claim. However, personality may affect the way a person copes with cancer, and may even have an influence on prognosis (Greer et al 1979).

(f) False. Cancer cannot be 'caught' (see p. 915).

(g) False. Many forms of cancer cause little or no change in physical appearance. Modern surgical techniques tend to be far more conservative and to achieve better cosmetic results than those used in the past.

(h) True. Many tumours are curable, particularly if diagnosed in the early stages, e.g. cervical cancer, teratoma. Risk of recurrence reduces as time lengthens from the original diagnosis.

(i) False. Cancer cells are not alien or foreign to the body but derive from malignant changes in normal cells (see p. 910).

(j) False. The side-effects of intensive radiotherapy and chemotherapy may be severe, but the manifestation of side-effects varies greatly between individuals. Some treatments, such as tamoxifen therapy for breast cancer, have few side-effects.

(k) False. Approximately 60–80% of cancer patients develop moderate to severe pain (Fischer et al 1997). This is generally not until the later stages and is usually controllable (see Ch. 33).

CHAPTER 36

36.5 (a) (i) 5 glasses, (ii) 5 single measures, (iii) 2.5 pints, (iv) 2.5 pints.

(b) *Brain* — aggression, irrational behaviour, arguments, violence, depression, nervousness, chronic anxiety, unknown fears, hallucination, serious mental health problems, epilepsy, dementia, memory loss, blackouts, damage to nerves, impaired balance and slurred speech.
Liver — damage to cells, leading to cirrhosis and liver cancer.
Heart — weakness of heart muscle and heart failure.
Stomach — inflammation of stomach, vomiting, diarrhoea and malnutrition.
Oesophagus — haemorrhage and cancer.
Lungs — increased risk of pneumonia and tuberculosis.
Large intestine — duodenal ulcers.
Nerves — numbness, tingling of extremities, peripheral neuritis, impairment of sensory organs and motor control.
Blood — anaemia and impaired blood clotting.
Reproductive system — impotence in male and increased risk of fetal damage in pregnant females.

(c) The liver.

(d) 2–3 hours.

(e) None.

(f) (i) and (ii).

(g) It is lower in women.

(h) Lower body weight, lower tolerance level and the tendency to add carbonised mixers to alcohol.

(i) An empty stomach, low body weight, adding carbonised drinks to alcoholic drinks, alternating carbonised and alcoholic drinks, drinking rapidly and low tolerance.

GLOSSARY

Achalasia. A failure of the smooth muscle of the GI tract to relax. The cause is unknown, but it occurs due to degeneration of the ganglionic cells. The failure is most notable in the lower oesophagus which fails to relax with swallowing.

Adjuvant therapy. Any therapy which is deliberately planned in conjunction with another form of therapy, e.g. adjuvant chemotherapy following surgery for breast cancer.

Advocate. An aspect of the nursing role essential to humanistic care whereby the nurse assists the patient to make decisions in a self-determined manner.

Affective. Refers to affect, an outward manifestation of a person's feelings or emotions.

Afferent nerve fibre. This is the sensory nerve fibre which runs from the tissues to the central nervous system.

Allodynia. 'Pain due to a stimulus which does not normally provoke pain' (IASP 1986, p. S217).

Anticholinergic. Inhibitory to the action of a cholinergic nerve by interfering with the action of acetylcholine.

Antihistamine labyrinthine sedatives. Sedatives that have an anti-inflammatory action and also reduce the levels of dizziness and nausea.

Antinociceptive. This describes something that helps to reduce or stop the response to noxious stimulation.

Antroscopy. Endoscopic examination of the maxillary sinuses.

Appraisal. The individual's assessment of a stressful situation and how it will affect him.

Arteriogram. A radio-opaque dye is injected into an artery and a series of X-rays taken to show the path of the dye in the arteries and to pinpoint any obstruction to blood flow.

Ascites. An abnormal collection of fluid in the peritoneal cavity.

Atopy. Hereditary tendency to a clinical hypersensitivity state.

Attico-antral disease. Bone erosion of the middle ear, caused by chronic infection.

Auriscope. An instrument which incorporates magnification and illumination, and can be used for examining the ear.

Autonomy. To act with self-determination.

Biofeedback. Presentation of immediate visual or auditory information about usually unconscious body functions.

Buchanan laryngectomy bib protector. A humidifying covering for the stoma of a laryngectomy.

Bulbospongiosum. Muscle that evacuates the bulb of the urethra. Responds to manual compression of the urethral bulb to prevent postmicturition dribbling in men.

Bulla. Large visible collection of fluid more than 1 cm in diameter.

Burrow. Tunnel in the skin caused by a parasite (scabies).

Causalgias. 'A syndrome of sustained burning pain, allodynia and hyperpathios after a traumatic nerve lesion' (IASP 1986, p. S218).

Cell architecture. The distinct cell pattern or structure that means the pathologist can identify the pathological disorder, in this case Hodgkin's lymphoma or any of the non-Hodgkin lymphomas.

Cholangiocarcinoma. Cancer of the bile ducts.

Choledocholithiasis. Stones in the bile ducts.

Cisplatin-based. Chemotherapeutic agents of similar chemical structure and use as cisplatinum, e.g. carboplatin.

Cognitive. Refers to cognition, the mental process characterised by knowing, thinking, learning and judging.

Collaborative relationships. Relationships within which the nurse, the patient and the patient's significant others work together as a cohesive team with shared responsibilities.

Comedone. Plug of sebum and keratin in the pilosebaceous gland.

Complementary therapies. Those methods of diagnosis and therapeutic practice which do not necessarily adhere to the principles which guide conventional scientific medicine, e.g. acupuncture, aromatherapy and homeopathy.

Coping. The various strategies individuals utilise to deal with the effects of stress in their lives.

Crust. Dried exudate on skin (serum, blood, pus).

Curettage. The scraping of tissue from a cavity using an instrument known as a 'curette'. Scrapings of the endometrium of the uterus are analysed in a pathology laboratory to aid diagnosis.

Decerebration. Characterised by extension and pronation of the arms, extension of the legs and plantarflexion (i.e. hyperextension of all limbs). The condition may progress to opisthotonus.

Decortication. Characterised by hyperflexion and adduction of the upper limbs, and hyperextension, internal rotation and plantarflexion of the lower limbs. It occurs when there is severe damage to the cerebral hemispheres or the internal capsule.

Demography. The study of statistics relating to population variables such as age gender, income and dependency.

Dermatitis artefacta. Psychological problem where patient presents with self-induced skin lesions.

Dermatome. An area of skin mainly innervated by a particular spinal cord segment.

Desmopressin. Artificial antidiuretic hormone. In spray form, used intranasally for short relief of symptoms of nocturnal enuresis.

Differentiation. The development process during which immature cells and tissues become more complex and specialised.

Disability. An enduring incapacity arising from congenital defect, disease, injury or old age.

Disseminated disease. Disease which is distributed over a considerable area of the body, e.g. metastatic cancer.

Dysmorphobia. Patient complains of severe skin problems but investigations are normal. Often associated with clinical depression and delusions of body image.

Dyspareunia. Difficult and/or painful sexual intercourse experienced by the woman. The discomfort may be described as superficial or deep.

Echocardiogram. A non-invasive technique which uses pulses of high-frequency sounds (ultrasound) emitted from a transducer to evaluate cardiac anatomy, pathology and function. The procedure involves an operator applying a lubricant to the skin surface of the chest wall and moving the transducer or probe back and forth by hand across the surface.

Embolism. The plugging of a blood vessel by material which has been carried through the larger vessels by the bloodstream. Usually due to fragments of a clot, but can be due to other factors such as a mass of air bubbles or bacteria.

Emollients. Agents that soften and soothe skin.

Empowering. Action which enables individuals to mobilise their personal resources and exercise control in everyday life.

Equianalgesic. A specified drug dose or route of administration that will give about the same analgesic effect as another specified drug dose or route. The term is often applied to an equianalgesic chart. This chart is useful to help maintain the same level of analgesia when changing the type of drug and/or the route of administration. Morphine is usually used as a standard for comparison. This chart can be used, for example, to see how much pethidine would have the same effect as 10 mg morphine. It also shows how much of an oral dose would be needed to equate in analgesic effect to a previous i.m. or i.v. dose, or vice versa.

Erythema. Redness of skin caused by vascular dilatation.

Excoriation. Superficial abrasion caused by scratching.

Exfoliation. Shedding of tissue in layers.

Extravasation. Accidental infiltration of vesicant/irritant fluids/drugs into subcutaneous tissues surrounding the site of administration.

Fine-needle aspiration (FNA). A means of tissue diagnosis by withdrawing fluid or tissue from a swelling, e.g. in the neck.

Fissure. Linear split in the epidermis.

Gastrocolic reflex. Sensory stimulation arising on entry of food into the stomach, resulting in strong peristaltic waves in the colon.

Haemolysis. The breakdown of red blood cells with the liberation of haemoglobin.

Haemorrhagic telangiectasia. A group of leaking dilated capillaries, often obvious on the surface of the skin.

Haemostasis. The homeostatic process which prevents the loss of blood from the vascular system and ensures the patency of the blood vessels.

Hepatic encephalopathy. A neuropsychiatric syndrome present only in significant liver disease. Features can range from barely detectable changes in ability to concentrate through to violent behaviour and eventually coma.

Hydrocephalus. An excess of cerebrospinal fluid inside the skull due to an obstruction to normal cerebrospinal fluid absorption.

Hyperpathia. 'A painful syndrome, characterised by increased reaction to a stimulus, especially a repetitive stimulus, as well as an increased threshold' (IASP 1986, p. S219).

Hypertrophy. Increase in size which takes place in an organ as a result of an increased amount of work demanded of it.

Impairment. Physiological or anatomical abnormalities caused by disease processes.

Infestation. Presence of animal parasites in or on the human body.

Interferential. Electrically induced impulses that can be used to strengthen the muscles of the pelvic floor, e.g. in the management of incontinence.

Intra-aortic balloon pump. Intra-aortic balloon counterpulsation is a mechanical means of supporting the acutely failing left ventricle. The balloon is introduced under local anaesthetic, usually via the femoral artery, into the descending thoracic aorta. During diastole the balloon is inflated with helium and blood is driven out of the aorta into the distributing arteries. The balloon is deflated at the end of diastole just prior to the opening of the aortic valve, reducing afterload and left ventricular work.

Irritant. Drug/solution which has the potential to cause pain or irritation at the site of administration.

Isometric exercises. Exercises that increase muscle tension by applying pressure against stable resistance, e.g. making a limb push against an immovable object.

Laparoscopy. The surgical procedure of insertion of a fibreoptic endoscope, known as a 'laparoscope', into the abdominal cavity for the purpose of examination of the pelvic organs and carrying out surgical procedures such as biopsies, aspiration of cysts, collection of ova from ripened follicles, division of adhesions or ligation of the uterine tubes for sterilisation.

Lemniscal tract. Transmits impulses for more discriminating touch and pressure sensations.

Macule. Non-palpable localised area of change in skin colour.

Marsupial pants. Incontinence aids having an external pouch, with a pocket to contain a pad.

Melaena. Black tarry stools due to the presence of partly digested blood from further up in the digestive tract. Melaena is not apparent in an adult unless 500 mL of blood has entered the gut.

Meridians. In Eastern medicine these are believed to be connected channels through which energy (or *ki*) flows throughout the body. Each meridian is linked to an organ or psychophysical function, and its *ki* can be contacted at certain points along its path. For example, in acupuncture these are the places where needles would be placed.

Mesencephalon. The midbrain (which is one of three parts of the brain stem), lying just below the cerebrum and just above the pons.

Mesenteric adenitis. Inflammation of the lymph glands in the membranous support of the intestines: the mesentery. This condition must be ruled out when diagnosing appendicitis.

Metastases. The transfer of disease from one organ or part of the body to another not directly connected with it. Most commonly used to describe secondary growth of malignant tumours.

MMR vaccination. Measles, mumps and rubella vaccination.

Mortality. A measure of causes of and age at death for a given population which can provide information on changes in life expectancy but may not indicate quality of life experienced.

Neoplasm. Any new and abnormal growth, a tumour. Neoplasms may be benign or malignant.

Nephrotoxicity. The degree to which a substance may impair kidney function.

Neuralgias. 'Pain in the distribution of a nerve or nerves' (IASP 1986, p. S220).

Neutropenia. Reduction in number of neutrophils, usually less than 1000×10^9 cells/L, resulting in the neutropenic patient being highly susceptible to infection.

Nociceptor. This is a receptor which responds to noxious stimuli or injury.

Nodule. Small node or swelling.

Nulliparous. A woman who has not borne a child.

Nystagmus. Rapid and involuntary movements of the eyes which may be vertical, horizontal or rotatory. The condition may be congenital and associated with poor sight or may occur due to disorders in the part of the brain responsible for movements and coordination. Vestibular nystagmus results when there is labyrinthine damage in the ear.

Opisthotonus. Arching of the back with backward flexion of the head and feet. This posture occurs when there is damage to the midbrain and pons. Opisthotonus can also occur in meningitis, due to severe inflammation of the meninges.

Orthopantomogram (OPT). Panoramic radiograph giving consistent image quality, usually of mandible or maxilla, for suspected neoplasia. Also in maxillofacial surgery for middle third fracture of facial bones.

Ototoxicity. The degree to which a substance may cause damage to the ear.

Palliative therapy. Therapy used to treat distressing symptoms and improve quality of life where no cure is thought possible, e.g. radiotherapy to painful bone metastases.

Pancytopenia. Reduction in the number of red blood cells, neutrophils and platelets, i.e. there is an anaemia, neutropenia and thrombocytopenia.

Papule. Circumscribed disc-shaped elevated area of skin less than 1 cm in diameter.

Parous. Having given birth to a child.

Passive exercise. The moving of parts of the body, e.g. a limb, by an outside force, with no voluntary contribution by the individual.

Paterson–Kelly/Plummer–Vinson syndrome. A combination of dysphagia, glossitis and nutritional iron deficiency anaemia. Dysphagia is caused by a fibrous web in the post-cricoid region of the oesophagus. Oral iron therapy usually leads to complete recovery.

Patulent. The external sphincter lacks tone and is open, due to a grossly overloaded rectum.

Perineometer. Pressure gauge inserted into the vagina or rectum to register the strength of contraction of the pelvic floor.

Phenomenological. Offering an account of the person's own experience as a unique event or phenomenon.

Photophobia. Inability to expose the eyes to light.

Piston effect. Movement of catheter up and down within the urethra.

Plaque. Palpable elevation of the skin more than 2 cm in diameter.

Pluripotent or stem cell. A blood stem cell is the original blood cell from which all other blood cells are derived.

Portage. Pre-school training programme, which takes place in the home, aimed at improving the child's continence abilities. Often used in the context of learning disability.

Prognosis. A forecast of the probable course and outcome of a condition and the prospects of a recovery.

Proprioceptors. Any sensory nerve ending, such as those located in muscles, tendons, joints and the vestibular apparatus, that respond to stimuli regarding movement and spatial positions.

pruritus. Itching that may result from many skin and systemic disorders. In liver disease, the cause of the itching is unclear, although the deposition of bile salts is implicated.

Pseudocyst. An abnormal dilated space which resembles a cyst but has no epithelial lining, e.g. pancreatic pseudocyst where the sac contains pancreatic enzymes, debris and blood within a lining of inflammatory tissue.

Purpura. Extravasation of blood from the capillaries into the skin or onto or into the mucous membranes. Appears as small red dots (petechiae) or large bruises.

Pustule. Visible collection of pus.

Quality assurance. An ongoing process of assuring the client of a specific standard of excellence through measurement and evaluation of a product or service.

Quality audit. A systematic and independent examination of the effectiveness of the quality system or its parts.

Response. A psychological or physiological reaction to stimulation.

Reticular. From the Latin word *reticulus* (net-like), meaning a Roman gladiator who fought with a net.

Roger's crystal spray. A glass atomiser with saline to spray at the tracheostomy stoma or bib protector, in order to moisten it.

Salpingolysis. The breaking down of adhesions in a uterine tube.

Salpingostomy. The surgical opening of the uterine tubes for reparative procedures following inflammatory disease or sterilisation. The aim is to restore patency to the tubes by anastomoses of the cut ends from either side of the blockage.

Saltatory conduction. A means of increasing the speed of nerve conduction, whereby the impulse 'jumps' from one node of Ranvier to the next.

Sclerotherapy. The injection of an irritant substance into varicose veins, which causes thrombophlebitis and encourages obliteration and subsequent scarring of the tissue.

Sialogram. Radiograph following injection of contrast medium into salivary duct and gland.

Slit lamp. An instrument used in opthalmology for the examination of the conjunctiva, the lens, the vitreous humor, the iris and the cornea. A high-intensity beam of light is projected through a narrow slit and a cross-section of the illuminated part of the eye is examined through a magnifying lens.

'Sounds'. Medical probes of different sizes used to explore or expand a cavity, e.g. dilatation of the urethra.

Spider telangiectasis. A localised collection of distended blood capillaries arising from a central point, thereby resembling a spider's web (also known as 'spider naevi').

Spinothalamic tract. Transmits impulses for crude touch, pain and temperature sensations.

Staging. A process of identifying the stage of progression of a disease, e.g. the size of a tumour and the extent of any spread.

Sterilisation. The process of rendering an individual incapable of reproduction. Female sterilisation is most commonly carried out via a laparoscopic procedure. The uterine tubes are occluded by the application of clips, cautery, thermal coagulation or laser vaporisation with photocoagulation.

Stimulus. Any factor such as heat, light, cold or drugs that will cause a response in a person or an organism. The term can also apply to any event causing emotional distress.

Stoma button. A stoma button is a small Silastic appliance approximately 2.5 cm in length. It has an external flange and is designed to sit firmly in a laryngectomy stoma in the same way as would a laryngectomy tube.

Stomatitis. Inflammation of the oral mucosa.

Support and supervision. Regular contact with another person undertaking similar clinical work with the purpose of sharing and learning from difficult or painful situations.

Synapse. The point of communication between two adjacent neurones.

Thalamus. A collection of grey matter located within the forebrain or prosencephalon.

Thrombocytopenia. Reduced number of platelets, usually less than 100×10^9 cells/L, which can result in the occurrence of purpura and spontaneous bleeding.

Thrombosis. Formation of a blood clot within the blood vessels or the heart. The indirect cause is usually some damage to the smooth lining of the blood vessels brought about by inflammation or the result of atheroma.

Titration. A method whereby the amount of solute in a solution can be measured. The solution is added in small measured quantities to a known volume of a standard solution until the required reaction occurs.

Transactional. Representing an interaction between the perception of the person and the object of the person's stress.

Trichotillomania. Compulsive plucking of hair — often a transient compulsive habit, but can be a sign of disturbed behaviour.

Ventricular assist device. This is a device that provides temporary circulatory support in heart failure in order to promote optimum myocardial tissue recovery. Ventricular assist devices partially bypass either the left or right ventricle using an artificial pump that maintains systemic circulation. A median sternotomy is made, blood is diverted away from the heart, bypasses the ventricle and is returned to the patient.

Ventrosuspension. The round ligaments of the pelvis may be folded, ligated, plicated or transplanted at operation with the aim of pulling the retroverted uterus forward.

Vesicant. Drug or solution which has corrosive properties and therefore the potential to cause tissue destruction in the event of extravasation.

Vesicle. Small visible collection of fluid less than 1 cm in diameter.

Viability. The capacity of a fetus for living a separate existence from its mother. A fetus is considered viable or capable of survival from the 24th week of pregnancy. This viability is recognised and safeguarded in the Human Fertilisation and Embryology Act 1990.

Videofluoroscopy. Video recording of swallowing mechanism, using fluorescent fluid, an 'action X-ray'.

Weal. Circumscribed, elevated area of cutaneous oedema.

Wilson's disease. An inborn defect of copper metabolism that results in free copper being deposited in the liver, causing jaundice and cirrhosis. Deposits can also occur in the brain, resulting in intellectual impairment. The condition is treated with penicillamine, a derivative of penicillin, which chelates (binds) the copper in order to remove excess from the body.

REFERENCE

International Association for the Study of Pain (IASP) 1986 Pain terms: a current list with definitions and notes on usage. Pain 27: S215–S221

APPENDICES

APPENDIX 1

TESTS AND INVESTIGATIONS

The following tests and investigations should be seen as terms defined rather than processes described and are used to supplement and clarify reference made to them in the text.

Angiography

This involves the injection of contrast medium to outline blood vessels. The contrast is injected and rapid serial X-ray films are taken. The presence and location of aneurysms and other blood vessel anomalies such as stenosis are demonstrated. Angiography is not without risk and its performance may be delayed in the patient who is in a poor clinical condition.

Arteriography

A radio-opaque dye is injected into an artery and a series of X-rays are taken to show the path of the dye in the arteries and pinpoint any obstruction to blood flow.

Arthroscopy

The direct examination of a joint by the surgical insertion of an arthroscope. The procedure can be performed on an outpatient basis and is used in the diagnosis of injuries. Although it is most commonly used for the knee joint, arthroscopic techniques can also be used for the hip, shoulder, wrist and ankle.

Barium studies

When plain radiography is inadequate to study an area of interest, contrast media can be used. Barium sulphate is an aqueous suspension, which is non-irritant and radiodense. Administered orally or rectally, it allows the gastrointestinal tract to stand out when viewed through a fluoroscope or on a radiograph. Barium studies of the gastrointestinal tract can help in the diagnosis of disorders such as peptic ulceration, malignant tumours, diverticulitis and colitis.

Blood count

Calculation of the number of red blood cells, white blood cells and platelets in a litre of blood. A differential blood count is the estimation of the relative proportion of the different white blood cells in the blood.

Blood film

Microscopic examination of the cellular components of the blood (i.e. red and white blood cells and platelets).

Red cells

Size:

- Microcytic — smaller than normal
- Normocytic — normal size
- Macrocytic — larger than normal
- Anisocytic — inequality in size.

Shape. Poikilocytic — marked irregularity in shape.

Colour:

- Hypochromic — red cells contain less haemoglobin than normal, resulting in a pale colour
- Normochromic — normal amount of haemoglobin in red blood cells and therefore normal colour.

White cells

Size. Usually 10–15 μm in diameter.

Structure:

- Staining characteristics of granules are different for neutrophils, eosinophils and basophils
- Excessive nuclear lobulation in neutrophils (indication of megaloblastic anaemia, iron deficiency, renal failure).

Cell differentiation between different granulocytes, lymphocytes and monocytes can be performed and commented on in the blood film report.

Platelets

Size. 2–4 μm in diameter.

Structure. Smaller or larger than average occur in certain haematological conditions, e.g. large platelets occur in thrombocytopenia due to platelet loss or destruction or postsplenectomy.

Cardiotocography

The simultaneous monitoring of the fetal heart rate and maternal uterine contractions as a means of monitoring fetal well-being.

Cholecystography

Radiological examination of the gall bladder using a radio-opaque contrast medium taken orally. A normal liver will normally remove the radio-opaque drugs from the bloodstream and store and concentrate them in the gall bladder. Radiographs taken will show the dye-filled gall bladder as a dense shadow. Gallstones may be seen as filling defects. This technique will not outline the gall bladder when the serum bilirubin concentration is elevated

(> 34 mmol/L), as insufficient contrast medium is excreted. Although oral cystography is a reliable means of detecting gallstones in non-jaundiced patients, it has been largely superseded by ultrasonography.

Computerised (axial) tomography (CT scan)

The patient lies on a couch and the head is placed in an opening in the front of the scanner. A series of X-rays are beamed through the patient's head in transaxial slices of various sizes and, depending upon the density of the tissue, are either transmitted or absorbed. Those that are transmitted are detected by a battery of sensitive crystals and this information is then fed to a computer, which creates an image of the scanned structures, e.g. brain tissue. Once one 'sweep' is complete, the machine moves through 1° until an 180° arc has been completed. CT scanning may reveal alterations in tissue density, displacement of structures and abnormalities. Certain types of lesion are better demonstrated with the use of contrast enhancement; this involves the injection of an intravenous contrast and then scanning the patient as already described.

Coombs' test

Test to detect antibodies to red blood cells.
Direct Coombs' test detects those bound to the red blood cells.
Indirect Coombs' test detects those not bound to the red blood cells but circulating in the serum.

Countercurrent immunoelectrophoresis (CCIE)

A laboratory method for the detection of specific antibodies or antigens.

Culture (bacterial)

The specimen material is smeared onto a culture medium plate (containing nutrients and moisture), and then incubated at 37°C to allow any bacteria present to grow and multiply. After 18–24 h, the culture plate is examined and bacteria can be identified.

Cystography/cystourography

Via a urinary catheter, the bladder is filled to capacity with a contrast medium and X-rayed. By so doing, bladder abnormalities may be revealed. The catheter is then removed to observe the function of the bladder and upper urethra during micturition — a cystourogram.

Cystometry

This investigation measures changes in the pressure in the bladder. A urinary catheter is inserted and the bladder drained. Water at body temperature is then introduced into the bladder at a slow and constant rate and, in response to the increasing volume, the bladder pressure is recorded using a pressure-measuring device, which produces a cystometrogram.

Cytology

Cytology is the study of the structure and function of cells, both normal and abnormal. Body cells may be collected by a variety of methods, e.g. from a specimen of urine or sputum, scraped from a skin lesion or from the cervix during a Papanicolaou smear test, or from aspirate of a lump or bone marrow. The cells are then examined microscopically for abnormalities.

Echocardiography

A non-invasive technique which uses pulses of high-frequency sound (ultrasound) emitted from a transducer to evaluate cardiac anatomy, pathology and function. The procedure involves an operator applying a lubricant to the skin surface of the chest wall and moving the transducer or probe back and forth by hand across the surface.

Electroencephalography (EEG)

A graphic recording of the electrical activity of the brain. Electrodes are attached to the scalp and the electrical activity is noted with a sensitive recorder. Some patients who are prone to seizures will demonstrate an abnormal waveform even while seizure-free.

Enzyme-linked immunosorbent assay (ELISA)

A laboratory method for the detection of specific antibodies or antigens.

Erythrocyte sedimentation rate (ESR)

Measurement of the height of red blood cells at the foot of a column of blood after the blood has been left standing in the narrow tube for 1 h (normal value < 10 mm).

Evoked responses

In this test, one of the sensory systems is artificially stimulated and the response noted with the use of appropriately placed electrodes, which detect disturbances of conduction. Visual evoked responses involve stimulating the patient by getting him to look at a reversing checkboard pattern or flashing lights. Electrodes placed on the scalp over the occipital lobes will detect if there is any delay in conduction along the optic pathway, such as may occur in the patient with multiple sclerosis.

Gonioscopy

Gonioscopy is performed to assess the angle of the eye, between the cornea and iris. A narrowed angle is indicative of closed-angled glaucoma.

The eye is anaesthetised with short-acting eye drops. A contact lens in which an angled mirror has been incorporated (gonioscope) is lubricated with methylcellulose eye drops and applied to the cornea. The eye is then examined through a slit lamp.

Haemoglobin estimation

Estimation of the amount of haemoglobin present in 100 mL of blood (normal values: men, 130–180 g/L; women, 115–165 g/ L).

Haemostasis (clotting) tests

Kaolin cephalin clotting time (KCTT) or partial thromboplastin time (PTT). A coagulation test of the intrinsic clotting pathway. Kaolin is added to plasma and activation of factors XI and XII. Cephalin reagent is added and the mixture recalcifies at 37°C. The clotting time depends on the presence of the components of the intrinsic pathway. Abnormalities in the test result from deficiencies of intrinsic pathway factors and final pathway factors (normal result: 40 s).
Prothrombin clotting time (PCT). Tests the extrinsic pathway of blood coagulation. The test requires the presence of functional quantities of factor VII and vitamin K-dependent factor X. The result is expressed as the ratio of patient:control. (Normal result: clot forms in 13 s; normal ratio: 1.0–1.3.)
Thrombin clotting time (TT) tests the final reaction in the final pathway, i.e. fibrinogen converted to fibrin (normal value: about 10 s).
Bleeding time. Time taken to stop bleeding after making a standardised superficial skin incision, e.g. with a lancet (normal value: up to 9 min).

Immunocoagglutination
A laboratory method for the detection of specific antibodies or antigens.

Immunodiffusion
A laboratory method for the detection of specific antibodies or antigens.

Immunoelectrophoresis
A laboratory method for the detection of specific antibodies or antigens.

Intravenous cholangiography
Contrast medium, given intravenously, is excreted into the biliary system. Serial radiographs are taken. However, this technique is not commonly used as results are often of poor quality, are of no value in jaundiced patients and also carry a small but significant risk of an anaphylactic reaction to the contrast medium. As a result, methods that allow direct injection of the contrast into the biliary tree are preferred, e.g. percutaneous transhepatic cholangiography (PTC), endoscopic retrograde cholangiopancreatography (ERCP), operative cholangiography and T-tube cholangiography.

Intravenous fluorescein angiography
This technique is used as an aid in the diagnosis and treatment of many of the vascular disorders of the retina. A 5 mL i.v. injection of 10% fluorescein sodium is given into a vein in the arm. A series of photographs are taken through a dilated pupil at timed intervals, using a fundal camera. Any defect in the retinal vessels will show up as a leakage of dye or occlusion of the vessel.

The patient may feel nauseated after the procedure. He should be informed that his sclera and skin will take on a yellow colour for about 24 h and that his urine will be greenish for 24–48 h as the dye is excreted through the kidneys. Diabetic patients who carry out urine testing should be advised to test their blood sugar instead, as the dye can affect the results obtained by urine test strips.

Lymphangiogram
An X-ray of the lymphatic channels and lymph nodes, often used to diagnose lymphatic cancers or metastases. An oily radio-opaque medium is injected into a small lymph channel in the patient's foot. As this medium travels slowly upwards through the body, X-rays are taken at various stages. This involves the patient waiting in the X-ray department for several hours one day and returning the following day. The small incision in the foot is sutured. The medium may cause temporary blue discoloration of the urine and of the skin over the incision.

Lumbar puncture
This is the most common neurological investigation. It involves the insertion of a sterile needle and trocar between lumbar vertebrae 3 and 4, or 4 and 5, and the withdrawal of a quantity of CSF for analysis. The procedure is usually performed in the ward under local anaesthetic. The lumbar CSF pressure may also be measured prior to the removal of CSF. The normal constituents and their values of CSF may be altered in the presence of a disorder, e.g. the number of red blood cells in the CSF following subarachnoid haemorrhage will be markedly elevated.

Magnetic resonance imaging (MRI)
This investigation is based on the use of a magnetic field and radio pulse waves, instead of traditional irradiation. The patient lies on a couch and is then completely enclosed in a tunnel within the scanner. A strong magnetic field is applied and the nuclei within the tissues, which were previously spinning in a random fashion, line up in a north–south magnetic field orientation. A radio pulse wave is introduced at a right angle to the magnetic field and the nuclei are tipped out of alignment, causing uniform resonance. The pulse waves are stopped and the resonating nuclei will return to their previous state. Minute radiofrequency signals are given off as the nuclei enter this relaxed state and these are monitored by the scanner. By pre-programming the computer to simulate a non-uniform magnetic field, the positively charged particles in different parts of the magnetic field will resonate at different speeds. Variable radio pulse waves result in differences in the emission of radiofrequency data. The computer assimilates this data and constructs a tissue image.

This type of scanning has a particular use in detecting cerebral and spinal oedema, and cerebral and spinal blood flow-related disorders, such as infarction, haemorrhage and arteriovenous malformation.

Mantoux test
An intradermal injection of tuberculin purified protein derivative (PPD), which is a sterile preparation 'made from the heat-treated products of growth and lysis of the mycobacterium' (DOH 1996). The result is read after 48-72 hours. A positive result is described as induration of at least 5 mm diameter at the injection site. This indicates that the individual has sensitivity to the tuberculin protein, and a strong reaction may indicate active disease.

Mean corpuscular haemoglobin concentrate (MCHC)
This is the average concentration of haemoglobin in a red blood cell and is calculated as follows:

haemoglobin level/PCV (see below)

(Normal range: 30–35 g/100 mL.)

Mean corpuscular or cell volume (MCV)
The average red cell volume (normal: 85 fl [75–95 fl]).

Microscopy
Direct visualisation of microorganisms using a light microscope or an electron microscope (uses a beam of electrons rather than light rays).

Myelography
This involves the injection of a water-soluble contrast into the subarachnoid space, usually via lumbar puncture. Cervical myelogram would require a cervical puncture. The patient is placed on a tilting table to encourage the contrast to flow up and down, thus highlighting the spinal cord and roots. X-ray pictures can then be taken at appropriate levels to detect blockage of, or interruption to, the flow of contrast, indicative of intraspinal pathology.

Magnetic resonance imaging of the spinal cord (magnetic myelography) has recently evolved and now provides greater detail of spinal pathology at less risk to the patient. Spinal CT scan may also be of some benefit.

Orthopantomogram (OPT)
Panoramic radiograph giving consistent image quality, usually of mandible or maxilla, for suspected neoplasia. Also in maxillofacial surgery for middle third fracture.

Packed cell volume (PCV) or haematocrit

This list measures the relative red cell mass to plasma, i.e. the proportion of the blood sample composed of packed red blood cells to plasma (normal values: men, 0.47; women, 0.42).

Paul–Bunnell (monospot) test

A method of determining the diagnosis of infectious mononucleosis (glandular fever), which may result from the Epstein–Barr virus (EBV). During the second week of the infection, specific EBV IgM antibodies indicate recent infection by the virus.

Positron emission tomography (PET) scans

A computerised radiographic technique that employs radioactive substances to examine the metabolic activities of various body structures. It involves the injection into the bloodstream of a solution containing a very short-lived radioactive agent which then emits positively charged particles — positrons. These combine with negatively charged electrons normally found in body cells and emit gamma rays. It is these rays that are picked up by the PET computer and converted to colour-coded images that indicate the intensity of metabolic activity of the organ involved.

PET scans have proved useful in studying the blood flow and metabolism in the heart and blood vessels, in diagnosing and studying cancer, in understanding the biochemical activity in the brain in such disorders as multiple sclerosis and Parkinson's disease, and even, more recently, in demonstrating which parts of the brain are active when people are in pain.

Precipitin test

A laboratory method for the detection of specific antibodies or antigens.

Radioisotope scanning

Radioisotope scans involve the use of small amounts of various radioactive substances, which are differentially taken up by normal and abnormal (malignant) tissue. The most common radioisotope scans are those of the liver, brain and bones. The radioisotope is injected intravenously, and the scan occurs several hours later. Patients should be reassured that the radioactivity of their bodies during this waiting time is minimal and that they are not a danger to others.

Radioallergosorbent test (RAST)

A laboratory method for the detection of specific antibodies or antigens.

Red cell mass

Estimation of the total volume of circulating red cells performed by labelling a sample of the patient's own red blood cells with isotope ^{51}Cr or ^{99m}Tc. A measured amount is reinjected and a sample is taken after a specific period of time when the dilution can be calculated (normal value: men, 25–35 mL/kg; women, 20–30 mL/kg).

Radioimmunoassay (RIA)

A laboratory method for the detection of specific antibodies or antigens.

Renography

This is a radiological study to assess renal function. Some elements that the kidneys normally concentrate and excrete can be labelled with radioactive isotopes. These are administered intravenously and, by so doing, the function of the kidneys can be traced by recording the rate at which the isotopes are removed from the blood and passed into the urinary collecting system.

Reticulocyte count

The number of reticulocytes in the peripheral blood (normal range: 0.2–2.0% of red blood cells).

Schilling test

Estimation of the gastrointestinal absorption of radioactive vitamin B_{12} (normal range > 10% of administered oral dose in 24-h urine sample).

Sensitivity

A test used to determine which antibiotics will kill the bacteria in the specimen. It is done by placing antibiotic-impregnated discs over a film of cultured bacteria on a culture plate and then reading the plate some hours later. A zone of inhibition around the disc indicates that the organism is sensitive to that antibiotic. If an organism is resistant, there will be growth right up to the disc.

Serology

The examination of blood serum, often to ascertain if infection is present by identifying antigen/antibody.

Sialogram

Radiograph following injection of contrast medium into a salivary duct and gland.

Skeletal survey X-rays

A skeletal survey involves X-rays of the skull, spine, ribs, pelvis and the femoral and humeral heads. Primary bone tumours and bone metastases from other tumours may be detected in this way.

T-cell immunophenotyping (CD4 T-cell subsets)

This procedure, used particularly for patients with HIV disease, shows the level of healthy T-helper cells the patient has. This is a vital prognostic tool. The test uses a monoclonal antibody, which binds to a specific antigen on the T4 helper cells. The test counts these and presents them as a ratio of the total T cells.

Tonometry

Tonometric tests measure intraocular pressure (IOP). The normal range is 12–20 mmHg.

Applanation tonometry. Fluorescein and anaesthetic drops are instilled prior to this procedure. A prism attached to a slit lamp (or a portable Perkins' tonometer) is used to flatten a defined area of the cornea. The greater the force required to flatten the area, the higher the IOP.

Non-contact (air puff) tonometry uses a computerised instrument to direct a fine, high-pressure jet of air onto the cornea. The increase in force progresses linearly until the cornea becomes flat. At this point the cornea acts like a mirror and reflects light to a photoelectric sensor, which immediately shuts off the puff of air. The force required to flatten the cornea is recorded and converted into an IOP reading.

Tumour markers

Some malignant tumours produce substances that can be detected in the blood. These may serve as 'markers' of the presence or recurrence of the tumour, and sometimes as an indicator of its size and, therefore, response to treatment. For example, alpha-fetoprotein (AFP) and beta-human chorionic gonadotrophin (BHCG) are produced by testicular tumours, and acid phosphatase by prostatic tumours.

Urinary flow rate
The voiding flow rate is measured using specially equipped facilities which allow the patient to void in privacy but where a machine can record the characteristics of the flow. The test will identify such things as peak flow, average flow and total flow time.

Urethroscopy
This is the endoscopic examination of the male urethra and prostate gland.

Videofluoroscopy
Video recording of the swallowing mechanism, using fluorescent fluid.

Water depletion test (diabetes insipidus)
Fluids are withheld for 8–12 h or until 3% of the body weight has been lost. Regular measurements of plasma and urine are taken. The inability to increase urinary specific gravity and osmolality in response to water depletion is indicative of diabetes insipidus. The test must be closely supervised as the patient will experience excessive thirst. The test is terminated if signs of tachycardia, hypotension or obvious dehydration occur.

REFERENCE

Department of Health 1996 Immunisation against infectious disease. HMSO, London

APPENDIX 2

NORMAL VALUES

NOTES ON INTERNATIONAL SYSTEM OF UNITS (SI UNITS)

Examples of basic SI units

Length	metre (m)
Mass	kilogram (kg)
Amount of substance	mole (mol)
Energy	joule (J)
Pressure	pascal (Pa)

Examples of decimal multiples and submultiples of SI units

Factor	Name	Symbol
10^{6}	mega-	M
10^{3}	kilo-	k
10^{-1}	deci-	d
10^{-2}	centi-	c
10^{-3}	milli-	m
10^{-6}	micro-	μ
10^{-9}	nano-	n
10^{-12}	pico-	p
10^{-15}	femto-	f

Volume. The basic SI unit of volume is the cubic metre (1000 litres). Because of its convenience the litre is used as the unit of volume in laboratory work.

Mass concentration (e.g. g/l, μg/L) is used for all protein measurements, for substances which do not have a sufficiently well defined composition and for serum vitamin B_{12} and folate measurements.

SI units are not employed for enzymes, nor usually for immunoglobulins.

BIOCHEMICAL VALUES

Reference ranges are largely those used in the Department of Clinical Biochemistry, the Lothian University NHS Trust. These can vary from laboratory to laboratory, depending on the assay method used and other factors; this is especially the case for the enzyme assays. Although the SI system of units is widely used in the UK, *units* of measurement can vary and lead to laboratory differences.

No details are given of the collection requirements which may be critical to obtaining a meaningful result.

Unless otherwise stated, reference ranges apply to adults; *values in children may be different.*

The values quoted for blood, except for Table A2.1, refer to plasma or serum. Serum is preferred for some analyses, especially certain hormones and electrophoretic studies.

Table A2.1 Arterial blood analysis

Analysis	*Reference range*	*Units*
Bicarbonate	21–27.5	mmol/L
Hydrogen ion	36–44	mmol/L
P_aCO_2	4.4–6.1	kPa
P_aO_2	12–15	kPa
Oxygen saturation	Normally >97	%

Table A2.2 Cerebrospinal fluid

Analysis	*Reference range*	*Units*
Cells	Up to 5 (all mononuclear)	cells/mm^3
Chloride	120–170	mmol/L
Glucose	2.5–4.0	mmol/L
IgG index*	<0.65	
Total protein	100–400	mg/L

* A crude index of increase in IgG attributable to intrathecal synthesis.
Pressure (adult) 0–15 mmHg.

Table A2.3 Reference values in venous plasma for the more common analytes in adults

Analysis	*Reference range*	*Units*
α_1-Antitrypsin	1.7–3.2	g/L
Alanine	10–40	U/L
aminotransferase (ALT)		
Albumin	36–47	g/L
Alkaline phosphatase	40–125	U/L
Amylase	50–300	U/L
Aspartate	10–35	U/L
aminotransferase (AST)		
Bilirubin (total)	2–17	μmol/L
Calcium	2.12–2.62	mmol/L
Carboxyhaemoglobin	Not normally detectable Up to 1.5% in non-smokers	%
Caeruloplasmin	150–600	mg/L
Chloride	95–107	mmol/L
Cholesterol (total)	[See note 1]	
HDL cholesterol	0.5–1.6 (M) 0.6–1.9 (F)	mmol/L
Copper	13–24	μmol/L
Creatine kinase (MB isoenzyme)	Normally <6% of total CK	
Creatine kinase (total)	30–200 (M) 30–150 (F)	U/L
Ethanol	Not normally detectable 65–87 (marked intoxication) 87–109 (stupor) >109 (coma)	mmol/L

Table A2.3 *(cont'd)*

Analysis	*Reference range*	*Units*
Creatinine	55–150	μmol/L
Ferritin	15–350 (M) 8–300 (F)	μg/L
Gamma-glutamyl transferase (GGT)	10–55 (M) 5–35 (F)	U/L
Glucose (fasting)[2]	3.6–5.8	mmol/L
Glycated haemoglobin (HbA_1)	4.5–8	%
Immunoglobulin A	0.5–4.0	g/L
Immunoglobulin G	5.0–13.0	g/L
Immunoglobulin M	0.3–2.2 (M) 0.4–2.5 (F)	g/L
Iron	14–32 (M) 10–28 (F)	μmol/L
Iron binding capacity	45–72	μmol/L
Lactate	0.4–1.4	mmol/L
Lactate dehydrogenase (total)	230–460	U/L
Lead[3]	<1.7	μmol/L
Magnesium	0.75–1.0	mmol/L
Osmolality	280–290	mmol/kg
Phosphate (fasting)	0.8–1.4	mmol/L
Potassium (plasma)	3.3–4.7	mmol/L
Potassium (serum)	3.6–5.1	mmol/L
Protein (total)	60–80	g/L
Sodium	132–144	mmol/L
Total CO_2	24–30	mmol/L
Transferrin	2.0–4.0	g/L
Triglycerides (fasting)	0.6–1.7	mmol/L
Urate	0.12–0.42 (M) 0.12–0.36 (F)	mmol/L
Urea	2.5–6.6	mmol/L
Zinc	11–22	μmol/L

Notes

1. Cholesterol (total)
   - ideally <5.2 mmol/L
   - mild increase 5.2–6.5 mmol/L
   - moderate increase 6.5–7.8 mmol/L
   - severe increase >7.8 mmol/L

(as defined by the European Atherosclerosis Society).

2. Values quoted for venous plasma or serum.
3. Up to 1.2 μmol/L in children.

Table A2.4 Reference values for the more common analytes in urine

Analysis	*Reference range*	*Units*
Albumin	[See note 1]	
Calcium	1.2–3.7 (low calcium diet) Up to 12 (normal diet)	mmol/24 h
Copper	Up to 0.6	μmol/24 h
Cortisol	9–50	μmol/mol creatinine
Creatinine	10–20	mmol/24 h
5-Hydroxyindole-3-acetic acid (5-HIAA)	< 60	μmol/24 h
Metanadrenalines Normetadrenaline Metadrenaline	 0.4–3.4 0.3–1.7	 μmol/24 h μmol/24 h
Oxalate	80–490 (M) 40–320 (F)	mmol/24 h mmol/24 h
Phosphate	15–50	mmol/24 h
Potassium[2]	25–100	mmol/24 h
Protein	Up to 0.3	g/L
Sodium	100–200	mmol/24 h
Urate	1.2–3.0	mmol/24 h
Urea	170–600	mmol/24 h

Notes

1. Albumin/creatinine ratio (ACR) and urinary albumin excretion rate (AER) are used to detect microalbuminuria, i.e. excessive albumin excretion in patients with diabetes mellitus, which is of predictive value in identifying patients at risk of progression to diabetic nephropathy. The test should only be carried out in the absence of overt proteinuria (Dipstix negative).

ACR

Reference range:	<3.5 mg albumin/mmol creatinine
'Borderline':	3.5–10 mg albumin/mmol creatinine
Positive test:	>10 mg albumin/mmol creatinine

AER

Reference range:	<20 μg albumin/min
Microalbuminuria:	20–200 μg albumin/min

2. The urinary output of electrolytes such as sodium and potassium is normally a reflection of intake. This can vary widely, especially on a cultural, worldwide basis. The values quoted are more appropriate to a 'Western' diet.

Table A2.5 Hormones

Hormone	*Reference range*	*Units*
Adrenocorticotrophic hormone (ACTH)	7–51 (07.00–09.00 h)	mg/L
Cortisol	150–550 (at 08.00 h) <200 (at 22.00 h)	nmol/L
Follicle-stimulating hormone (FSH) (male)	1.5–9.0	U/L
Follicle-stimulating hormone (FSH) (female)*	3.0–1.5 (early follicular) Up to 20 (mid-cycle) >30 (postmenopausal)	U/L
Gastrin	Up to 120	ng/L
Growth hormone (GH)	Very variable, usually less than 2, but may be up to 50 with stress	mU/L
Insulin	Highly variable and interpretable only in relation to plasma glucose and body habitus	mU/L
Luteinising hormone (LH) (female)*	2.5–9.0 (early follicular) Up to 90 (mid-cycle) >20 (postmenopausal)	U/L
Luteinising hormone (LH) (male)	1.5–9.0	U/L
Oestradiol-17β (female)	110–180 (early follicular) 550–1650 (mid-cycle) 370–770 (luteal) <150 (postmenopausal)	pmol/L
Oestradiol-17β (male)	<200	pmol/L
Parathyroid hormone (PTH)	10–65	ng/L
Progesterone (male)	<2.0	nmol/L
Progesterone (female)	<2.0 (follicular) >15 (mid-luteal) <2.0 (postmenopausal)	nmol/L
Prolactin (PRL)	60–390	mU/L
Testosterone (male)	10–30	nmol/L
Testosterone (female)	0.4–2.8	nmol/L
Thyroid-stimulating hormone (TSH)	0.15–3.15	mU/L
Thyroxine (free) (free T_4)	10–27	pmol/L
Tri-iodothyronine (T_3)	1.0–2.6	nmol/L
TSH receptor antibodies (TRAb)	<7	U/L

* Luteal phase values similar to follicular phase.

Notes
1. A number of hormones are unstable, and collection details are critical to obtaining a meaningful result. Refer to local hospital handbook.
2. Values in the table are only a guideline; hormone levels can often only be meaningfully understood in relation to factors such as sex (e.g. testosterone), age (e.g. FSH in women), time of day (e.g. cortisol) or regulatory factors (e.g. insulin and glucose, PTH and [Ca^{2+}]). Also, reference ranges may be critically method-dependent.

HAEMATOLOGICAL VALUES

Table A2.6 Haematological values

	SI units	*Other units*
Bleeding time (Ivy)	< 8 min	
Body fluid (total)		50% (obese)–70% (lean) of body weight
Intracellular		30–40% of body weight
Extracellular		20–30% of body weight
Blood volume		
Men	75 ± 10 mL/kg	
Women	70 ± 10 mL/kg	
Erythrocyte sedimentation rate*		
Adult male	0–5 mm/h	
Adult female	0–7 mm/h	
Fibrinogen	1.5–4.0 g/L	
Folate		
Serum	1.9–9.0 μg/L	
Red cell	150–500 μg/L	
Haemoglobin		
Men	130–180 g/L	
Women	115–165 g/L	
Haptoglobin	0.3–2.0 g/L	
Leucocytes — adults	$4.0–11.0 \times 10^9/L$	
Differential white cell count		
Neutrophil granulocytes	$2.0–7.5 \times 10^9/L$	40–75%
Lymphocytes	$1.5–4.0 \times 10^9/L$	20–45%
Monocytes	$0.2–0.8 \times 10^9/L$	2–10%
Eosinophil granulocytes	$0.04–0.4 \times 10^9/L$	1–6%
Basophil granulocytes	$0.01–0.1 \times 10^9/L$	0–1%
Mean corpuscular haemoglobin (MCH)	27–35 pg	
Mean corpuscular haemoglobin concentration (MCHC)	31–35 g/dL	30–35%
Mean corpuscular volume (MCV)	76–98 fL	
Packed cell volume (PCV) or haematocrit		
Men	0.40–0.54	
Women	0.35–0.47	
Platelets	$150–400 \times 10^9/L$	
Prothrombin time	10.5–14.5 s	
Prothrombin ratio	2.0–4.5	
APTT (heparin control)	1.5–2.5	
Red cell count		
Men	$4.5–6.5 \times 10^{12}/L$	
Women	$3.8–5.8 \times 10^{12}/L$	
Red cell life span (mean)	120 days	
Red cell life span $t_{1/2}$(^{51}Cr)	25–35 days	
Reticulocytes (adults)	$10–100 \times 10^9/L$	0.2–2%
Vitamin B_{12}	280–900 ng/L	

*Higher values in older patients not necessarily abnormal.

INDEX

Page numbers in colour indicate main discussions;
those in *italics* refer to figures, tables or boxes.
The alphabetical arrangement is letter-by-letter.

INDEX

A

B

C

colour = **main discussion;** *italics* **= Figures, Tables, Boxes, etc.**

colour = **main discussion;** *italics* = **Figures, Tables, Boxes, etc.**

colour = **main discussion;** *italics* = **Figures, Tables, Boxes, etc.**

E

F

G

H

I

J

K

L

colour = **main discussion;** *italics* = **Figures, Tables, Boxes, etc.**

M

N

O

P

colour = **main discussion;** *italics* = **Figures, Tables, Boxes, etc.**

Q

R

S

colour = **main discussion;** *italics* = **Figures, Tables, Boxes, etc.**

T

colour = **main discussion;** *italics* = **Figures, Tables, Boxes, etc.**

U

V

W

X

Y

Z